Mosby's Comprehensive Dental Assisting

A CLINICAL APPROACH

Mosby's
Comprehensive
Dental Assisting

A CLINICAL APPROACH

BETTY LADLEY FINKBEINER, CDA, RDA, BS, MS

Chairperson, Dental Assisting Program,
Washtenaw Community College,
Ann Arbor, Michigan

CLAUDIA SULLENS JOHNSON, RDA, BS

Clinical Instructor, Dental Assisting Program,
Washtenaw Community College,
Ann Arbor, Michigan

with 11 contributors
and 1000 illustrations

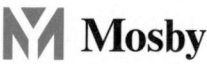 **Mosby**

St. Louis Baltimore Boston Carlsbad Chicago Naples New York Philadelphia Portland
London Madrid Mexico City Singapore Sydney Tokyo Toronto Wiesbaden

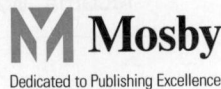

Mosby
Dedicated to Publishing Excellence

A Times Mirror
Company

Executive Editor: Linda L. Duncan
Developmental Editor: Penny Rudolph
Project Manager: Patricia Tannian
Senior Production Editor: Barbara Jeanne Wilson
Senior Book Designer: Gail Morey Hudson
Manufacturing Supervisor: Karen Lewis

Printed in the United States of America
Composition by Graphic World, Inc.
Printing/binding by Von Hoffmann Press, Inc.

Mosby-Year Book, Inc.
11830 Westline Industrial Drive
St. Louis, Missouri 63146

Library of Congress Cataloging in Publication Data

Mosby's comprehensive dental assisting: a clinical approach / [edited by] Betty Ladley
  Finkbeiner, Claudia Sullens Johnson with 11 contributors.
        p.   cm.
    Includes bibliographical references and index.
    ISBN 0-8151-3239-5
    1. Dental assistants.   I. Finkbeiner Betty Ladley, 1939-   .
II. Johnson, Claudia Sullens.
    [DNLM: 1. Dental Assistants.   WU 90 M894 1995]
    RK60.5.M63   1995
    617.6—dc20
    DNLM/DLC
    for Library of Congress   94-31991
                                                              CIP

94 95 96 97 98 / 9 8 7 6 5 4 3 2 1

Contributors

JOHN G. CLINTHORNE, DDS, MS

Orthodontist,
Private Practice,
Ann Arbor, Michigan

VIRGINIA A. MERCHANT, MS, DMD

Professor, Department of Biomedical Sciences,
University of Detroit Mercy,
School of Dentistry;
Antemortem Section Leader,
Michigan Dental Association's
   Forensic Dental Identification *Go Team,*
Detroit, Michigan

JOHN A. MOLINARI, PhD

Department of Biomedical Sciences,
University of Detroit Mercy,
School of Dentistry,
Detroit, Michigan

LINDA L. OTIS, MS, DDS

Assistant Professor,
Department of Oral Diagnosis,
Division of Maxillofacial Radiology,
University of Connecticut Health Center,
Farmington, Connecticut

JERRY C. PATT, BS

Instructor Emeritus,
Washtenaw Community College,
Ann Arbor, Michigan

FRIEDA A. PICKETT, RDH, MSDHEd

Former Associate Professor,
Caruth School of Dental Hygiene,
Baylor College of Dentistry,
Dallas, Texas

SUSAN A. ROYAL, RDA, RDH

Department of Dental Assisting,
Washtenaw Community College,
Ann Arbor, Michigan

JEANNE C. SCHERER, RN, BSN, MS

Formerly Assistant Director and Medical-Surgical Coordinator,
Sisters Hospital,
School of Nursing,
Buffalo, New York

ELEANOR D. VANABLE, CDA, RDH, MA, EdD

Professor, Department of Dental Health,
Community College of Rhode Island,
Lincoln, Rhode Island

ALLEN J. WARNICK, DDS

Chief Forensic Dental Consultant,
Wayne County Medical Examiner's Office,
Livonia Michigan;
Clinical Assistant Professor,
Forensic Dentistry,
University of Detroit Mercy School of Dentistry;
Team Leader,
Michigan Dental Association's
   Forensic Dental Identification *Go Team;*
Private Practice,
Detroit, Michigan

HELEN M. ZYLMAN, DDS

Maxillofacial Oral Surgeon,
Private Practice,
Ann Arbor, Michigan

To the memory of

Harry Arthur Sullens

who provided love, support, and encouragement
throughout all his years

and to

The Dental Assistant Advisory Committee
of Washtenaw Community College's Dental Assistant Program

for their support of educated dental assistants

Preface

The dental assistant faces several challenges in education today. Complex procedural steps need to be learned quickly to maximize production. Yet, the dental assistant must gain a comprehensive knowledge of procedures and concepts to procure the necessary credentials to ensure a credible position on the dental health team. The authors of this textbook have provided the basic concepts of dental assisting in two forms: easy-to-read tables are provided for learning basic procedures, and detailed descriptions offer the cognitive knowledge for the concepts or procedures.

Further, this textbook provides the dental assistant student with practical applications of these concepts by illustrating many of the daily activities that the employed assistant encounters in scenario or case study format. Information concerning drugs that are used in dentistry is covered extensively to provide the assistant with a thorough understanding of drug interaction and the consequence of drug use in dentistry.

The workbook that is designed for this text provides an opportunity for the reader to validate learning. It is designed not only with a traditional format that seeks objective feedback, but also presents the reader with the opportunity to enjoy learning through the use of puzzles and critical thinking activities.

The authors recognize the role of the dental assistant in the twenty-first century. The dental assistant today must be aware of new technology, practice safely, think critically, promote quality care standards, practice quality assurance, respond to patient needs, and realize that the product of the modern dental office in the twenty-first century is service—perhaps the most valuable product in dentistry today. For this reason the authors have alerted the dental assistant reader to the need for safe practice by the use of periodic symbols throughout the book and offer suggestions for daily interactions with patients. Further, the authors realize the emphasis in a dental assistant textbook should be on the history of dental assisting. Thus, a complete chapter on the evolution of the dental assistant is presented. For creative learning, historical periods in dentistry have been placed in appropriate chapters to indicate a significant moment in history that reflects on the chapter's content.

In today's modern world it is difficult to write a single textbook that covers each discipline of dental assisting that is all inclusive. This textbook is designed to provide a comprehensive overview of each of the topics, with emphasis on the clinical approach to dental assisting. Consequently, the reader whose primary responsibility is dental practice management, dental radiography, or dental laboratory procedures will likely use this text as an introduction to these topics. From this text the assistant can gain an understanding of how these areas of dental assisting interrelate with clinical dental assisting and will likely seek specialty texts in each of these areas for advanced study.

This textbook is unique in the combination of its authors. It brings about an oft-dreamed-for opportunity of many teachers, the chance to work with a former student to create a masterpiece. In this situation the former student, who now is a teaching colleague, offers new technology and challenges for the future, while the experienced teacher offers levity and wisdom of experience. Most importantly this experience to work together as a team has documented the passage of standards of quality, ethics, and knowledge from one generation to the other.

No book is written by the authors alone. It is from the help and encouragement of many supportive people that such a project comes to fruition. Our first appreciation must be extended to our spouses, Charles Finkbeiner and David Johnson, who survived this project. Their willingness to endure neglect, assume additional responsibilities, and survive our deadlines is evidence of their support and good humor. Without Charles' final rush of computer expertise our deadlines could never have been met. We give special thanks to Kathy Weber, Carl Read, Suzan Harden, Charlotte Hanson, Debbie Shillington, and Linda Stakley for the time they gave to photography and manuscript development. To Jaye Scheslinger, a special acknowledgement, not only for her technical art skills, but also for her friendship, which made a difficult task so enjoyable. To Carolyn Jaissle, Debra Griffin, Dr. Richard Zillich, Dr. Jeffrey Shotwell, Dr. Don Wurtzel, Dr. William Sorenson, Dr. Kimberly Rice, Joseph L. Flack, Jr., Avraam Piniatoglou of Sharp Dental Laboratory, Jane McCaw at Sycom, Jim Wells of Health Science Products, Diane Ohlmacher Hough and staff at Ivory Photo, and the many representatives of dental manufacturing companies who contributed illustrations, we owe thanks for their technical expertise. For their continued support and encouragement we offer our thanks to Shirley Wilson, Jean Sullens, Karen Hart, Dr. John Fleszar, and Phyllis Grzegorczyk. Finally, a very special thanks to Linda Duncan, Executive Editor, Barbara Wilson, Senior Production Editor, and Gail Morey Hudson, Senior Book Designer, for the tremendous support and creativity they brought to this project.

Betty Ladley Finkbeiner
Claudia Sullens Johnson

STEPS TO SUCCESS: A MESSAGE TO THE READER

Since this textbook is intended for a student in a dental assisting program or a new employee in a dental practice, it seems appropriate that the authors make suggestions for its use. The perceived difficulty of this text will depend on the background of the individual reader. The following suggestions are intended to guide a person through basic to complex concepts and should benefit each reader.

Skim over the chapter in a cursory review. Before reading an entire chapter, a brief glance through the chapter will identify the basic concepts that are being presented. Look at the illustrations and tables to discern familiar and new ideas.

Decide where there are natural breaks in the subject material; then determine how long it will take to read the chapter and to set a deadline for completing the material.

Read the text material. Divide the chapter into segments if it appears too difficult to read in one sitting. Each time you return to the material, review the previous material. For positive reinforcement you may wish to reward yourself for completing the task.

Outline or underline key concepts. On separate paper outline the key concepts or list steps to a procedure in an abbreviated form. Don't hesitate to use markers or pencils to highlight important information in the textbook that may be needed for later reference. Choose only key words to underline rather than an entire paragraph or section.

List unfamiliar words in a notebook. When new words are encountered, write them down in a reference notebook. If the term is not clearly defined, refer to the glossary or to a technical dictionary. Break words down into root, prefix, and suffix for easier identification.

Discuss the material with another student or dental professional. Explaining what you have read with another person often aids in understanding a concept or procedure. Discussing a specific reading assignment with another person can create a dialogue that may clear up some misunderstanding or may create a critical discussion about a concept. It may even challenge the reader to go back to the text material to determine whether he or she has read and understood the material accurately.

Identify concepts or terms that are not clearly understood. If some part of the material is unclear, write out questions to ask in a structured class setting or to clarify in other text references or with a dental professional. Compare questions and notes with others who have read the material to determine if they have similar questions.

Ask questions. When you do not understand something, be certain to seek out help and to ask questions. Be specific about what it is that you do not understand. Refer to a special sentence or paragraph. It is often wise to write out the question to be certain that it is not forgotten.

Be a good listener. When you ask a question, listen to the answer and carry on a dialogue with the respondent, until you understand the material thoroughly. Repeat what you think you understood the respondent to say to determine if what you understood is correct.

When other people ask questions, listen to the questions and to the responses. Many times, others have the same question, or your question may be answered during the discussion.

Express appreciation to the resource person for his or her efforts in helping you understand a concept.

Continue studying. If something is unclear, don't give up; continue to read, study, and be inquisitive. Often times, if one concept is not understood it may later be clarified if you continue to read and study. Also, accept responsibility for your own learning.

Betty Ladley Finkbeiner
Claudia Sullens Johnson

Contents

Mosby's Comprehensive Dental Assisting

A CLINICAL APPROACH

UNIT 1 THE MODERN DENTAL HEALTH TEAM

1 The Modern Dental Health Team

LEARNING OBJECTIVES

You will have mastered the material in this chapter when you can:
- Define the key terms
- Describe the role of each member of the dental health team
- Identify the members of the dental health team
- Describe the background of the dentist and the dental auxiliaries
- Identify and describe each of the dental specialties
- Describe the advanced functions
- Identify acronyms common to the dental profession
- Identify the factors or programs that have influenced changes in dentistry
- Explain the concept of team dentistry
- Identify the objectives of dentistry

KEY TERMS

Advanced functions
American Dental Association (ADA)
Certified Dental Assistant (CDA)
Certified Dental Technician (CDT)
Certified Orthodontic Assistant (COA)
Certified Dental Practice Management Assistant (CDPMA)
Certified Oral and Maxillofacial Surgery Assistant (COMSA)
Chairside assistant
Doctor of Dental Surgery (DDS)
Dental assistant
Dental Assistant National Board (DANB)
Dental health team
Dental laboratory technician
Dental practice act
Dental public health

Dentist
Dentistry
Doctor of Dental Medicine (DMD)
Endodontics
Etiology
General practitioner
Oral maxillofacial surgery
Oral pathology
Orthodontics
Pediatric dentistry
Periodontics
Prosthodontics
Registered Dental Assistant (RDA)
Registered Dental Assistant Expanded Functions (RDAEF)
Registered Dental Hygienist (RDH)
Specialty
State Board of Dentistry

The dental health team is the primary care unit within the profession of dentistry. The team consists of the dentist, the dental assistant, the dental hygienist, and the dental laboratory technician. This chapter will provide an overview of each member of the dental health team and will discuss the role that each plays in the total care of the dental patient.

Dentistry as Health Care System

Dentistry is a healing art and science that is concerned with the teeth, oral cavity, and associated structures. Dentistry encompasses several major areas including the following:

1. Maintaining dental health
2. Diagnosing and treating oral diseases
3. Preventing dental diseases
4. Restoring defective teeth
5. Replacing missing teeth and oral tissues
6. Preventing, intercepting, and maintaining proper occlusion
7. Providing function in mastication and speech
8. Providing esthetics

Dentistry, as a health care system, is a dynamic profession, and dental assisting is a vital professional component. As the number and complexity of jobs within the field have expanded, the dental assistant has become more valuable.

 Robert Tanner Freeman (first an apprentice to Dr. Noble of Washington, D.C.) became the first black man to graduate from an American Dental School: Harvard School of Dental Medicine, in 1869.

State Board of Dentistry

State government has a direct control over the practice of dentistry and over the function and status of the dentist and the dental auxiliaries. The state is responsible to enact laws that protect the public from harm. As a result, states have written **dental practice acts** to protect the health of the public by providing standardized safe dental care. On February 6, 1868, Kentucky became the first state to create a dental practice act. Later that same year New York and Ohio followed suit. In 1915 Connecticut became the first state to include dental hygiene in its dental practice act. Since that time the practice of dental hygiene has been written into every dental practice act in the United States. The practice of dental assisting varies in each state, and licensure is not mandatory in every state.

Each state's practice act defines the **State Board of Dentistry**—the body that supervises the practice of dentistry. The composition of the State Board of Dentistry varies from state to state, but generally it includes several dentists, who have varying dental and geographic backgrounds; hygienists; assistants (if they are included in the state practice act); and public members. Appointments to a dental board are commonly made by the governor of a state, with recommendations from dental organizations.

The Dental Health Team

To understand how staff members interact in the delivery of dental services, the dental assistant must be familiar with common procedures, as well as with the duties of each auxiliary. The members of the dental health team include the dentist, the dental assistant, the dental hygienist, and the dental laboratory technician (Fig. 1-1). The **dental health team** is a group of qualified individuals who work together efficiently to provide quality dental health care. The dentist acts as the leader of the team; however, the most important person in the office is the **patient.** It is the patient around whom all activities take place, and each member of the team must understand that without the patient, the services of the dental staff would not be needed. An attitude of cooperative teamwork should exist among staff members as they interrelate while treating the patient. The following

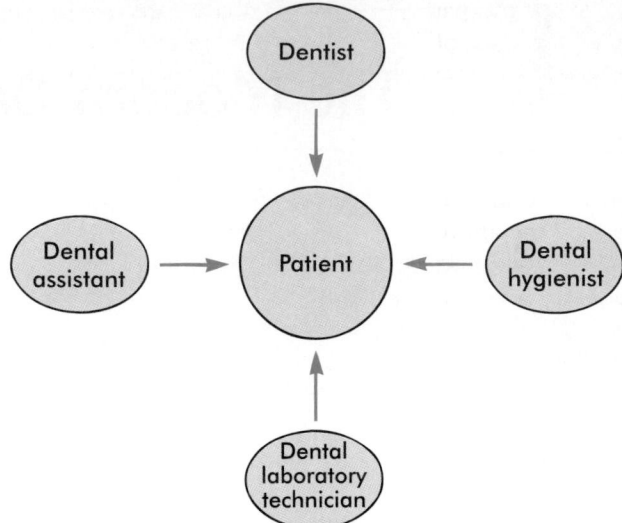

FIG. 1-1   The dental health team: the patient is the center of all activity.

descriptions will aid in understanding the background and role of each member of the dental health team.

▶ The Dentist

The **dentist,** as a professional, has the privilege of self-government; however, he or she also has an obligation to the public to maintain a standard of quality care and ethical conduct. The mission of the profession is to encourage the improvement of the public's health, to promote the art and science of dentistry, and to represent the interests of the dental profession, as well as the public it serves.

The typical dentist of past decades operated from a modest office, often as a solo practitioner, with an assistant or a receptionist serving as the only dental auxiliary. Approximately 60% of the dentists in the United States still practice autonomously; however, they have increased productivity and efficiency by employing a number of dental auxiliaries to assist in a variety of procedures. These auxiliaries include one or more chairside assistants and dental hygienists, an office manager, clerical assistants, and possibly a laboratory technician.

 Paul Revere, in addition to earning a living as a silversmith and a copper plate engraver, also worked as a dentist.

With the many state and federal regulations placed on the profession today, a dentist can ill afford to hire inexperienced and noncredentialed personnel. Concerns for the patient's safety in dental radiography and infection control alone warrant hiring the most skilled auxiliaries. A team of highly trained auxiliaries is needed to maximize efficiency and production and to maintain safe practice in the dental office.

The team's leader, the dentist, will have completed an extensive and formal education and will have successfully passed the appropriate examinations, thereby earning a license to practice within a specific state. Formal education begins with predental studies for 2 or more years in liberal arts and science courses, ultimately leading to a Bachelor of Science (B.S.) degree. Graduation from a dental school accredited by the American Dental Association's Commission on Dental Accreditation requires 3 to 4 years of additional study. The dental school will award the dentist either a **D.D.S.** (Doctor of Dental Surgery) or a **D.M.D.** (Doctor of Dental Medicine) degree. After graduating from dental school, the dentist must meet the requirements for licensure as specified by the board of dentistry of the state in which the dentist plans to practice.

A dentist may be in a partnership or a group practice or may be in a clinic or a diversified unit. A dentist may provide a variety of treatments, limit the practice to a specialty, or become involved in hospital dentistry or dental public health.

Each state, except Delaware, requires that a dentist pass a written national board examination administered by the Joint Commission on National Dental Examinations. The dentist must also pass a clinical examination. In most states a regional examination serves as a qualification for licensure. However, some states, such as California, Florida, Texas, and Washington, require state clinical examinations rather than regional examinations. Once the dentist has been licensed by the state, he or she must adhere to the dental practice act or to other laws that are implemented by the state or federal government to govern dental practices. Failure to abide by these laws can result in a fine or a license revocation.

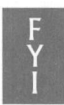 On March 6, 1840, the first dental college in the country, the Baltimore College of Dental Surgery, was founded in the state of Maryland through the efforts of Horace Hayden and Chapin Harris.

▶ Dental Specialties

A dentist who practices all phases of dentistry, including restorative, surgical, prosthetic, and preventive procedures, is referred to as a **general practitioner.** In some cases the required treatment for a patient may extend beyond the general practitioner's scope of knowledge, skill, or desire to perform. The general practitioner then should refer the patient to a dental specialist: a person

who is licensed by the state to practice a **specialty** or a specific category of treatment. The specialist has received additional education designed to comply with the state dental practice act.

Responsibilities may overlap among the recognized areas of dental practice. The specialist and the general practitioner work together as a team to provide total patient care. As the primary care giver the general practitioner may refer a patient to a specialist to obtain a second opinion, to confirm a diagnosis, or to receive treatment that is beyond the scope or the desire to perform of the general practitioner; or the patient may be referred by the general practitioner to ensure that the patient will receive treatment by someone who is knowledgeable in current concepts and who is skilled in using the most recently developed equipment in a particular specialty. A good example of such team interaction is when a general practitioner has observed that a child's tooth development does not appear normal and that the dental arch appears too small for the size of the erupting permanent teeth. The dentist may refer the child to an orthodontist for a consultation. The orthodontist informs the dentist of the diagnosis and may request that some teeth be removed. The dentist may then refer the child to an oral surgeon who will remove the teeth. During this time the patient is still under the care of the family dentist for routine preventive and restorative treatment. The specialists perform only the duties for which they have been trained. It should be noted that some general practitioners may limit their practice to specific types of treatment. This circumstance is not to be confused with a *specialty*. To practice as a licensed specialist, a dentist must have met the requirements of the state's dental practice act for a particular specialty.

The **American Dental Association (ADA)** is the national professional organization for dentists. The ADA recognizes eight specialties of dentistry. In most instances a dental specialty is referred to by the suffix *ics* or *ia* (e.g., orthodont*ics* or orthodont*ia*). The person practicing the specialty is designated with the suffix *ist*, (e.g., orthodont*ist*).

DENTAL PUBLIC HEALTH. The science and art of preventing and controlling diseases and promoting health through organized community efforts is referred to as public health. **Dental public health** is a form of dental practice that considers the community as the patient rather than the individual, controlling dental disease and promoting dental health. This specialty is concerned with public education, applied dental research, and the administration of group dental care programs, as well as the prevention and control of dental diseases on a community-wide basis. Commonly the public health dentist is involved with the implementation of public health programs, such as Head Start, fluoridation, or similar types of programs that provide treatment to a designated group.

ENDODONTICS. This specialty of **endodontics** is concerned with the morphology, physiology, and pathology of the dental pulp and associated tissues. A specialist in this area, an endodontist, must have a broad understanding of the biology of the normal pulp; common diseases and their **etiologies** or causative factors; diagnosis, prevention, and treatment of these diseases; and common injuries of the pulp and associated tissues.

ORAL PATHOLOGY. The specialty that deals with the nature of the diseases that affect the oral cavity and the adjacent structures is referred to as **oral pathology.** The specialist, the oral pathologist, works *behind the scenes* to aid the dentist in making a diagnosis. One of the common functions of this specialist is to analyze tissues and to identify structural changes caused by disease. An oral surgeon works closely with the oral pathologist when a biopsy is to be done to determine the disease and its causes. The oral pathologist not only can help make the diagnosis, but also he or she can aid the oral surgeon in determining the prognosis for future structural changes and thus can aid in maintaining the health of the patient. An oral pathologist must have an extensive knowledge of clinical, microscopic, radiographic, biochemical and other laboratory examinations or procedures that may be required to establish a diagnosis for a patient.

ORAL MAXILLOFACIAL SURGERY. Formerly known as oral surgery, the specialty of **oral maxillofacial surgery** is responsible for the diagnosis and surgical treatment of diseases, injuries, and defects of the oral and maxillofacial region. This specialist works with many other dentists, general practitioners and other specialists, in the total treatment of a patient. Patients commonly associate an oral surgeon with the practice of extracting teeth in preparation for dentures or with the removal of third molars. Such procedures are only a small phase of the total responsibility of this specialty. For instance, an oral maxillofacial surgeon may see a patient who has been severely injured in an accident to reset the mandibular jaw and to work closely with the orthodontist and perhaps even a plastic surgeon to restore the patient to normal appearance, as well as to normal oral function. Another aspect of oral maxillofacial surgery involves implantology and facial cosmetic surgery.

ORTHODONTICS. Most people associate this specialty with braces or appliances; however, **orthodontics** more specifically is concerned with the supervision, guidance, and correction of the growing or mature dentofacial structures, including those conditions that require moving the teeth to correct a malocclusion or to correct a malformation of the jaw. Major responsibilities of an orthodontist include the diagnosis, prevention, interception, and treatment of all forms of malocclusion of the teeth and associated structures; the design, application, and control of functional and corrective appliances; and the movement of the dentition and supporting structures

into optimal occlusal relationship to provide improved function and esthetics (good appearance).

PEDIATRIC DENTISTRY. The specialty of **pediatric dentistry** is defined as the practice and teaching of comprehensive preventive and therapeutic oral health care of children from birth through adolescence, including care for special patients beyond the age of adolescence who demonstrate mental, physical, and/or emotional problems and who require specialized care. Often a pediatric dentist will receive patients with behavior problems who have been referred by a general practitioner.

PERIODONTICS. The diagnosis and treatment of diseases of the supporting and surrounding tissues of the teeth are the focus in the specialty of **periodontics**. The periodontist also is concerned with the maintenance of the health of these structures and tissues, which can be achieved through periodontal treatment procedures. A periodontist must work closely with the patient's general practitioner. The success of restorative dentistry is dependent on good periodontal health; to achieve this goal the periodontist must rely on the general practitioner to place restorations or appliances in the patient's mouth that will enhance periodontal health, not impede it. A periodontist may recommend that the general practitioner replace faulty restorations or missing teeth. In this situation the patient would continue to see the general practitioner for routine care and restorative treatment and would maintain regular visits for periodontal treatment with the specialist.

PROSTHODONTICS. This branch of dentistry, called **prosthodontics,** pertains to the restoration and maintenance of oral functions, comfort, appearance, and health of the patient by the restoration of natural teeth or by the replacement of missing teeth or oral structures with artificial devices: dental prostheses. Two basic types of dental prostheses are fixed and removable. Examples of fixed prostheses include full gold crowns, bridges, and porcelain veneer crowns. A removable prosthesis is a full denture, a partial denture, or a precision partial denture.

▶ The Dental Assistant

The educated **dental assistant** has become a vital member of the dental health team in the modern dental practice. Studies have proven that a highly skilled assistant at chairside can reduce stress on the patient, the dentist, and the assistant; can increase productivity; and can improve the quality of care. As dentists delegate more **advanced functions,** such as specific intraoral clinical functions that go beyond basic chairside skills, to chairside dental assistants and as they continue to place more management responsibilities on assistants in the business office, the dental assisting profession will become even more vital to dentistry. Keep in mind two important factors about the dental assistant's job: (1) the dental assistant should perform only duties that do not require the dentist's professional skill and judgment; and (2) the dental assistant should perform only those duties that are delegatable by the state dental practice act in the state in which the dentist practices.

The dental assistant's role is multifaceted, providing an opportunity for both variety and specialization. Primary roles might include any of the following:

▶ *Chairside assistant* assists in specialized duties during operative, preventive, or surgical procedures. A person having a credential as a **Certified Dental Assistant (CDA)** (see Chapter 2) will have a broad background in chairside procedures, dental radiography, laboratory and business procedures, infection control, and patient education and will have passed an examination administered by the **Dental Assisting National Board (DANB)**—a national agency granting certification to dental assistants. Examinations are offered by this organization for assistants in two specialties: orthodontics and maxillofacial oral surgery. Credentials for these individuals are the **Certified Orthodontic Assistant (COA)** and the **Certified Oral and Maxillofacial Surgery Assistant (COMSA)**.

▶ *Office manager* is responsible for all aspects of the business office, including telephone and appointment management, accounts receivable, banking, and insurance. An ideal combination for an office manager is a person with chairside experience, who has a background in business office systems, bookkeeping, insurance management, and computer systems. A person skilled in business management with a broad knowledge of dentistry is eligible to take a specialty examination offered by DANB and become a **Certified Dental Practice Management Assistant (CDPMA)**. Several staff levels may exist in the business office including a receptionist, records or insurance clerk, and the office manager. The size of the business staff will vary with the size of the practice; however, with increased record keeping it is likely that the qualifications for the staff in this area will be increased.

▶ *Generalist* performs duties in all areas of the dental office.

▶ *Advanced (expanded) functions assistant* is able to perform specific advanced clinical functions that, by the dental practice act within the state, are delegatable to this person, providing that she or he meets the state's requirements for these duties. Many states require evidence of additional education for advanced functions and require the person to take a written or clinical examination given by the state licensing agency.

The credential granted as evidence of successful performance in some states is the **Registered Dental Assistant (RDA)** or **Registered Dental Assistant in Extended Functions (RDAEF)**. Other acronyms synonymous with this type of auxiliary are EFDA (Expanded Functions Dental Assistant) or EDDA (Extended Duties Dental Assistant). EFDA and EDDA are not licensed credentials but are merely accepted abbreviations that can be used when referring to a person who performs advanced functions.

Today the use of acronyms for dental assistants can pose a challenge to the dental assistant student. Since each state establishes credentialing requirements and not all states include the dental assistant in the practice act, many variables exist in definitions of the credentials of an assistant (Box 1-1).

BOX 1-1

ACRONYMS FOR IDENTIFICATION OF DENTAL ASSISTANTS

CDA

Certified Dental Assistant

    National credential granted by the DANB to recognize successful completion of the national certification examination. This credential may be recognized as a licensure requirement for dental assistants in some state practice acts.

CDPMA

Certified Dental Practice Management Assistant

    National credential granted by the DANB to recognize successful completion of the specialty examination in Dental Practice Management.

COA

Certified Orthodontic Assistant

    National credential granted by the DANB to recognize successful completion of the specialty examination in Orthodontics.

COMSA

Certified Oral and Maxillofacial Surgery Assistant

    National credential granted by the DANB to recognize successful completion of the Oral and Maxillofacial Surgery specialty examination.

RDA

Registered Dental Assistant

    A credential given by some states to indicate that specific requirements have been met to practice expanded and advanced functions for that state.

RDAEF

Registered Dental Assistant in Expanded Functions

    A credential given by some states to indicate specific requirements have been met to practice expanded and advanced functions in that state.

OJT

On-the-job trained assistant

    This is *not* a credential but a status of level of knowledge, learned *on–the–job*.

BOX 1-2

ADVANCED FUNCTIONS

The following list of duties include some of the advanced functions (additional intraoral tasks that can be performed independent of the dentist) delegated to dental assistants in several states:

- Inspecting the oral cavity
- Applying topical anesthetics
- Assisting in the administration of nitrous oxide analgesia or sedations
- Applying anticariogenic agents topically
- Polishing coronal surfaces of the teeth
- Determining root length and endodontic file length
- Fitting trial endodontic file points
- Exposing radiographs
- Making impressions for intraoral appliances
- Making impressions for study casts
- Removing sutures
- Performing preliminary oral examinations
- Replacing and removing wedges and matrices
- Placing and removing sedative or temporary restorations or crowns
- Removing excess cement from the coronal surfaces of teeth
- Preparing the teeth for bonding by etching
- Placing and removing the rubber dam
- Placing and removing periodontal dressings
- Placing, condensing, and carving amalgam restorations
- Placing and finishing composite resin restorations
- Applying cavity liners and bases

SOURCES OF INFORMATION

American Dental Association
Commission on Dental Accreditation
211 East Chicago Avenue
Chicago, IL 60611

Dental Assistant National Board
216 East Ontario
Chicago, IL 60611

Appendix A lists specific duties that are delegated to either the dental assistant or to the dental hygienist in those states that allow delegation of advanced functions. Before any duties are performed, an assistant or a hygienist should acquire the necessary education and credentials that are needed and that are legally delegatable (Box 1-2).

The education of the dental assistant varies according to state requirements. The OJT (on-the-job trained) assistant has no credentials and is limited in performing many intraoral duties. Educational programs (discussed more completely in Chapter 2, *Evolution of the Dental Assistant*) vary in length; the maximum time requirement is generally 2 years in a postsecondary educational institution. A graduate of an ADA accredited program is eligible to become a Certified Dental Assistant through the Dental Assistant National Board (DANB). Each state establishes specific criteria and educational requirements for licensure. You can obtain information regarding legal duties for any dental auxiliary by contacting the State Board of Dentistry in your state. For specific information about accredited programs or credentials in your area contact the ADA or DANB.

▶ The Dental Hygienist

The primary role of the **dental hygienist** is preventive care. Traditionally, this important role includes such duties as the oral prophylaxis (scaling and polishing the teeth); charting oral conditions; polishing restorations; applying anticariogenic agents; providing patient education in oral hygiene and nutrition; and exposing, processing, and evaluating dental radiographs. The individual state dental practice act determines if the dental hygienist may perform additional intraoral duties that are recognized as advanced functions (see Appendix A). The education of a dental hygienist requires at least 2 years of postsecondary education, resulting in a certificate or associate degree. Advanced education of 2 or more years will lead to a Baccalaureate (B.S. or B.A.) or Master's (M.S.) degree. The dental hygienist must pass a written and clinical examination in accordance with criteria determined by the state in which the person plans to practice dental hygiene. The hygienist licensed by the state is called a **Registered** or **Licensed Dental Hygienist (RDH** or **LDH)**.

▶ Dental Laboratory Technician

A **dental laboratory technician** performs extraoral functions in a private dental office, a commercial laboratory, or a dental school. This dental team member's primary duty is the construction of prosthetic devices and restorations (i.e., crowns, bridges, or dentures). The dental laboratory technician works according to the written prescription of a licensed dentist.

The duties of the laboratory technician require extensive mechanical and technical skills and a thorough knowledge of dental anatomy. This education is attained through ADA-accredited programs, apprenticeships, postsecondary schools, the armed forces, or proprietary schools. A person may receive a credential as a **Certified Dental Technician (CDT)** by taking the examination. No state licensure is available for this dental auxiliary. Today the military service is a major source of skilled technicians.

PROFESSIONAL ORGANIZATIONS FOR THE DENTAL HEALTH TEAM

DENTIST

American Dental Association (ADA)
Michigan Dental Association (MDA)
Central District Dental Society (CDDS)*

DENTAL ASSISTANT

American Dental Assistants' Association (ADAA)
Michigan Dental Assistants' Association (MDAA)
Central District Dental Assistants' Society (CDDAS)*

DENTAL HYGIENIST

American Dental Hygienists' Association (ADHA)
Michigan Dental Hygienists' Association (MDHA)
Central District Dental Hygienists' Society (CDDHS)*

DENTAL LABORATORY TECHNICIAN

National Association of Dental Laboratories (NADL)+

* These acronyms are based on cities, counties, or districts.
+ Membership is based on laboratory membership rather than individual membership.

Professional Organizations

Voluntary educational organizations are available for each member of the dental health team at the national, state, and local levels. Each of these organizations provides educational publications, legislation, and other activities for its members. Each national organization is composed of members who have memberships in constituent (state and dependency) societies. The constituent societies in turn are composed of component (local) societies. The acronyms for each of the organizations are derived from the state and local districts of residence or practice. Box 1-3 lists some organizations to which a dental team member living in Lansing, Michigan, might belong.

The American Board of Dental Public Health was established in 1950 to promote dental health throughout the world.

Societal Impact on Dentistry

Several factors have influenced the practice of dentistry in the past 50 years. From 1950 through the 1960s the federal government played a major role in legislation to alleviate the dental labor shortages. The government enacted programs for Dental Auxiliary Utilization (DAU), Training in Expanded Auxiliary Management (TEAM), and Expanded Functions Dental Auxiliary (EFDA). These programs all placed emphasis on increasing the produc-

tion of the dental profession, maintaining quality of care, and providing cost containment for the consumer.

In 1965 the Office of Economic Opportunity (OEO) enacted the Head Start Program to provide educational health and social services to preschool children of the needy. The Head Start program assures that each child enrolled will receive total basic dental services. Evidence shows that these programs have been effective and follow up on children from the early programs who have performed better in school, had a higher employment rate, and increased self-esteem. With government cost containments these programs could face difficult times in the future.

The 1970s was the decade of dental insurance. Though insurance emerged as early as 1950, its impact was not felt on the profession until the 1970s. Dental insurance today is considered one of the most desirable benefits for an employee. Early growth of dental insurance came from organized labor; however, today employees with small businesses are purchasing dental plans for employee benefits.

The 1970s brought consumerism to state dental boards. During these years many states changed the composition of the dental boards to include laypersons. This impetus continues as the profession seeks to be more progressive and to satisfy the needs of the consumer.

The 1980s and the 1990s have been known for the impact of renewed safety: infection control and radiography regulations. The federal regulations of Occupational Safety and Health Administration (OSHA) on infection control and management of medical and dental wastes and state regulations on dental radiography have resulted in a need to alter methods of delivering dental care. Today the dental staff uses universal barrier techniques, including gloves, masks, and eye protection; is responsible for waste management; and regulates the exposure of dental radiographs in many states to educated or credentialed dental personnel.

Dentistry's Changing Profile

Figures today tell us that many changes have taken place in dentistry. In 1987 data indicated that there were just over 126,000 practicing dentists of whom approximately 7400 were female. The male-female ratio is rapidly changing. In a 1980-1981 survey of dental school enrollments, just under 17% of the dental students were female, and in the 1990-1991 survey of dental schools the percentage of females was 34.4% with an increase of women expected to continue. Though it is more difficult to determine the exact number of dental assistants in the United States, it is estimated that in 1990 there were approximately 225,000 assistants, with approximately 1% being male. In 1988 dental hygienists numbered about 98,000; less than 1% of these hygienists were male. The male ratio in both of these auxiliary programs appears to be increasing. It is interesting to note that the age of the auxiliaries is changing since the demographics of the population is changing. There is less population in the 18-year to 25-year age group, and thus many students enrolled in auxiliary programs may be returning to school for a career change or may be attending school for the first time after raising a family.

 Lucy Beaman Hobbs graduated from the Ohio College of Dental Surgery in 1866, thereby becoming the first woman in the world to receive a dental degree.

The Team Approach to Dentistry

Whenever a group of people work together to achieve a common objective, they form an organization: a team. In dentistry this team forms the dental practice, and the common objective is treatment for the patients. Within the dental practice other objectives must be met: employment and satisfaction for the staff, service to the patients, and profit for the owner and the dentist. It is at this point that one must realize that although dentistry is a health care profession, it is also a business, and its major product is service. The ADA has identified the following basic objectives of the profession that can become the objectives for each practice:

- Provide relief of pain from dental origin
- Help prevent pain by practicing preventive dentistry
- Help maintain personal appearance
- Help masticate food throughout a lifetime
- Maintain good oral health

As discussed in this chapter, each member of the dental health team must assume specific legal and professional responsibilities. In addition, each member has a responsibility to the dental team to maintain maximum productivity and a responsibility to the patient to provide quality care. To ensure that productivity is met with quality assurance each member should adhere to the following:

- Perform only those duties that are legally delegable to them
- Obtain skills and credentials for all legally delegatable duties in the state
- Participate in professional activities
- Be willing to assist other staff members in performing their duties: the hygienist, the assistant, and the office manager help one another to get the job done
- Participate in staff meetings for the purpose of improving the overall dental practice
- Be a team player who gives others credit and respect for their various roles on the team
- Promote the dental practice, and be committed to its objectives

KEY POINTS

- Dentistry is a healing art and science that is concerned with maintaining dental health, treating and preventing oral disease, restoring defective teeth, replacing oral structures and restoring function and esthetics to the oral cavity.
- A state board of dentistry controls the practice of the profession, the function, the dentists, and the auxiliaries.
- A state dental practice act protects the health of the public by providing them with standardized, safe dental care.
- The dental health team includes the dentist, the dental assistant, the dental hygienist, and the laboratory technicians, who work together to provide quality dental care in an efficient manner.
- The ADA recognizes the following eight specialties: dental public health, endodontics, oral pathology, oral maxillofacial surgery, orthodontics, pediatric dentistry, periodontics, and prosthodontics.
- The dental assistant is a vital member of the dental health team and may assume roles such as chairside assistant, office manager, generalist, and advanced functions assistant.
- The primary role of the dental hygienist is preventive care.
- The primary duty of the dental laboratory technician is the construction of prosthetic devices and restorations.
- Voluntary professional organizations are available to all members of the dental health team at national, state, and local levels.
- Several societal factors have influenced the practice of dentistry, including government programs, such as DAU, TEAM, Headstart, as well as dental insurance, consumerism, and OSHA requirements.
- The profile of dentistry is changing. The number of females entering dentistry is increasing, the demographics of the population is changing, and the male ratio in auxiliary programs is increasing.
- Dentistry is a health care profession, as well as a business, and its major production is service. To provide the service each member of the dental staff works together as a team.

BIBLIOGRAPHY

American Dental Association, Department of Educational Surveys: *Annual Report, 1992-93, Allied Dental Education,* Chicago, Il, 1993, The Association.

American Dental Hygiene Association: *Membership Department Survey,* 1988, The Association.

Commission on Dental Accreditation, Council on Dental Education of the American Dental Association: *New faces for allied dental education,* Chicago, 1993, The Association.

Hengl R: *Dental Assistant National Board Research,* 1990, The Board.

Miller CH, Palenik CJ: *Infection control and management of hazardous material for the dental team,* St Louis, 1993, Mosby.

U.S. Bureau of Economics and Behavioral Research, *ADA Distribution of Dentists 1987,* The Bureau.

2 Evolution of the Dental Assistant

LEARNING OBJECTIVES

You will have mastered the material in this chapter when you can:

▶ Define the key terms
▶ Describe the role of the modern dental assistant
▶ Explain the origin of dental assisting
▶ Describe a brief history of dental assisting
▶ Define the purpose of the American Dental Assistants' Association
▶ Describe the evolution of education for the dental assistant
▶ Identify credentialing processes for dental assistants
▶ Identify individuals who have made significant contributions to the history of dental assisting
▶ Explain the impact of DAU on the profession of dental assisting
▶ Discuss changes that have impacted the dental profession in recent decades
▶ Explain potential job sources for dental assistants

KEY TERMS

American Association of Dental Schools (AADS)
American Dental Assistants' Association (ADAA)
Commission on Dental Accreditation (CDA)
Council on Dental Education (CDE)
Dental Auxiliary Teacher Education (DATE)
Dental Auxiliary Utilization (DAU)
Four-handed dentistry

Dental assisting is a diverse allied health profession. It offers many exciting opportunities in various settings. The profession has grown from the early days when an assistant merely prepared instruments and materials for a dentist or provided housekeeping and secretarial duties to the exciting and challenging profession it is today.

This chapter will track the dental assistant profession as it has evolved from *lady in attendance* to *valued member* of the modern dental health team. The development of the educational programs and the advancement of auxiliary utilization are explored in this chapter, as are the roles of pioneers who have reached beyond the private dental office to promote the profession. A dental assistant has much to look forward to as the profession advances into the twenty-first century, and many states continue to expand the assistant's duties. This profession is young and strong. The 1991-1992 edition of the *Occupational Outlook Handbook,* published by the U.S. Department of Labor's Bureau of Labor Statistics, states that employment of dental assistants is expected to grow as fast as most other allied health occupations through the year 2000.

Dental Assisting Today

On an average, dentists today employ about four staff members, including assistants, hygienists, and dental

Career Opportunities in Dental Assisting

A career in dental assisting includes the following opportunities:
▶ Assist a dentist in general restorative dentistry
▶ Assist in various specialty practices
▶ Assist in a hospital operating room
▶ Provide patient education
▶ Care for a geriatric patient
▶ Comfort a young child
▶ Place and carve amalgam restorations
▶ Manage a dental business office
▶ Expose and process dental radiographs
▶ Teach in a college or vocational program
▶ Work in a major dental manufacturing or insurance company
▶ Work in a state or federal government dental clinic
▶ Work as a sales representative for dental equipment or supply company
▶ Serve in the armed forces
▶ Work in research and development in a dental school or other agency
  Some duties require appropriate education and credentials and may be regulated in certain states.

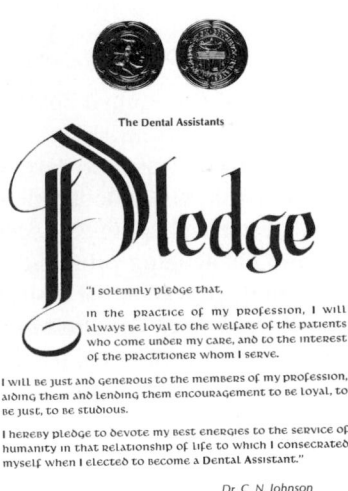

The Dental Assistants

Pledge

"I solemnly pledge that,

in the practice of my profession, I will always be loyal to the welfare of the patients who come under my care, and to the interest of the practitioner whom I serve.

I will be just and generous to the members of my profession, aiding them and lending them encouragement to be loyal, to be just, to be studious.

I hereby pledge to devote my best energies to the service of humanity in that relationship of life to which I consecrated myself when I elected to become a Dental Assistant."

Dr. C. N. Johnson

Printed and distributed through the American Dental Assistants Association by courtesy of Dentsply International Inc.

laboratory technicians. The number of these auxiliaries increased from an average of 3.0 in 1983 to 3.5 in 1990, to the current 4.0. Many dentists employ two or more dental assistants; therefore the employment opportunities are excellent. The economics of dental assisting vary widely across the country, depending on the specific position, responsibilities, and geographic location of the practice. The average national wage of a dental assistant in 1992-1993 was approximately $10.00 per hour. These data were reported in the *Select* career guidance program

that was sponsored by the ADA and the **American Association of Dental Schools (AADS),** a professional organization for educators and schools of dentistry or dental auxiliaries. Dental assistants possessing formal education and certification or registration may receive significantly higher salaries.

Dental assistants can receive varied benefit packages, including one or several of the following options: health (medical and dental) and disability insurance, membership in professional organizations, uniform or clothing stipends, hepatitis vaccine, paid vacations, wellness days, day care allotments, educational stipends, retirement plans, and profit sharing. Dental assisting provides an opportunity for full- or part-time employment. In private practice the dental assistant rarely works on holidays and works on weekends only on an optional basis. Many assistants find this profession satisfies an interest in working in the health care field without having to work in a hospital or with critically ill patients.

Early Times

Dr. C. Edmund Kells, who is remembered in dental history for his early contributions in the use of radiation for diagnostic purposes, is credited with hiring the first dental assistant. Kells was an innovator and writer, and in 1887 in the *Ohio Journal of Dental Science* first mentioned *the lady in attendance.* In 1893 Kells expressed his views on auxiliary utilization when he stated that someday *the lady assistant* would be found in every dental office in the land. He further enumerated the functions of an assistant: "To be a successful assistant, a young lady must be quick, quiet, gentle, attentive without being obtrusive and intelligent." He went on to explain that the dental assistant would be responsible for cleaning the handpieces once a week, and at chairside

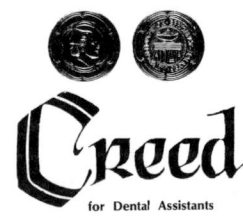

Creed

for Dental Assistants

To be loyal to my employer, my calling and myself.
To develop initiative—having the courage to assume responsibility and the imagination to create ideas and develop them.
To be prepared to visualize, take advantage of, and fulfill the opportunities of my calling.
To be a co-worker—creating a spirit of co-operation and friendliness rather than one of fault-finding and criticism.
To be enthusiastic—for therein lies the easiest way to accomplishment.
To be generous, not alone of my name but of my praise and my time.
To be tolerant with my associates, for at times I too make mistakes.
To be friendly, realizing that friendship bestows and receives happiness.
To be respectful of the other person's viewpoint and condition.
To be systematic, believing that system makes for efficiency.
To know the value of time for both my employer and myself.
To safeguard my health, for good health is necessary for the achievement of a successful career.
To be tactful—always doing the right thing at the right time.
To be courteous—for this is the badge of good breeding.
To walk on the sunny side of the street, seeing the beautiful things in life rather than fearing the shadows.
To keep smiling always."

— Juliette A. Southard

Printed and distributed through the American Dental Assistants Association by courtesy of Dentsply International Inc

she would keep the cavity free from chips with the chip blower; prepare the filling material, whether it be gold, amalgam, or cement; and ensure that supplies of all kinds were always on hand. Kells also stated, "It should be her duty to receive all patients, make appointments, attend to correspondence, look after the linens, and take a general interest in the welfare of the office." For the late 1800s Dr. Kell's approach to dental practice appeared to be advanced. Although several of his statements seem archaic by today's standards, they depict the philosophy of the times, and his general concepts reflect a growing trend to use dental assistants.

One of Dr. Kells' assistants, Malvina Cueria, became a pioneer in the profession of dental assisting. Cueria was employed by Dr. Kells in 1920. In 1935 she attended the ADA annual session in New Orleans and became involved in organizing the New Orleans Dental Assistants' Society; later she became one of its charter members. In 1948 she was granted certification under the *grandmother* clause provided by the Certifying Board of the ADAA. Such a clause enabled experienced assistants to obtain certification, for a specific period of time, based on their employment and specific requirements identified by the ADAA's Certifying Board. During World War II, Cueria helped start one of the original 104-hour study courses for dental assistants, and from 1953 to 1956 she served as an ADAA Trustee. At the urging of the Dean of Loyola University's Dental School in Louisiana, Malvina Cueria came out of retirement to recruit certified dental assistants for the **dental auxiliary utilization** (DAU) program—a federal program designed to teach dental students how to work and how to use dental auxiliaries most effectively. Later, she served as supervisor of the program until the dental school closed. Based on these achievements it would appear that the dentist who originated the idea of a *lady in attendance* certainly had an impact on the profession of dental assisting.

 World War II had an impact on dental assisting when in 1942 the annual session of the ADAA in Boston was cancelled by government order because of the war and traveling conditions. Later in 1945 the House of Delegates Meeting was cancelled for similar reasons. Both times special meetings of the Board of Trustees substituted for annual meetings. A special committee entitled War Service was created during this time for the purpose of coordinating the war efforts of dental assistants throughout the country.

The American Dental Assistants' Association

In 1921 Juliette Southard organized dental assistants into the Education and Efficiency Society, which later became the American Dental Assistants' Association (ADAA), a national organization that represents the interests of dental assistants. Her goal was "an educated, efficient dental assistant with her own place in the profession of dentistry." Juliette Southard was able to see her dream become reality.

Southard's interest in the profession began in 1911 when she was a patient for Dr. Henry Fowler, a noted gold specialist in New York City. She was fascinated by the work being done for her and asked if she could observe the laboratory procedures. It was the beginning of a long career. She worked for Dr. Fowler for 23 years until his death in 1934.

In 1921 there was a move to organize dental assistants throughout the nation. Southard, who had initiated the Education and Efficiency Society of New York, was to see the creation of groups throughout the country. A born organizer, she began to mobilize these local groups into a national organization. She petitioned the ADA for permission to register women attending the 1923 ADA convention in Cleveland and initiated a letter-writing campaign inviting all dental assistants' groups to send representatives to Cleveland. From this activity evolved a national organization to represent the interests of dental assistants—the American Dental Assistants' Association.

▶ The ADAA Journal

In 1933, under the presidency of Ruth Rodgers, the official publication of the ADAA, *The Dental Assistant*, was adopted (Fig. 2-1). In 1934 *The Dental Assistant* became accepted as a member publication of the American Association of Dental Editors. Over the years this journal has continued efforts to promote dental education and to address comprehensive, controversial, and societal issues that affect the profession of dental assisting. The efforts of its many editors have not gone unnoticed. Violet Crowley, editor for 10 years, received the American Association of Dental Editors Distinguished Service Award in 1971 and was honored in 1973 with an Award of Merit for her outstanding contributions in the advancement of the dental profession. Later Joan Keisel, editor from 1962 to 1973, received the 1973 International College of Dentists' Golden Pen Award for the most outstanding article published in a dental journal.

▶ ADAA Insignia

At the time the *ADAA Journal* was adopted, the association also adopted an official cap (Fig. 2-2). The emblem worn on this cap indicated that the assistant was certified. Today the cap is no longer worn. An official pin representing membership in the ADAA contains the organization's motto, "Education, Efficiency, Loyalty, and Service" (Fig. 2-3).

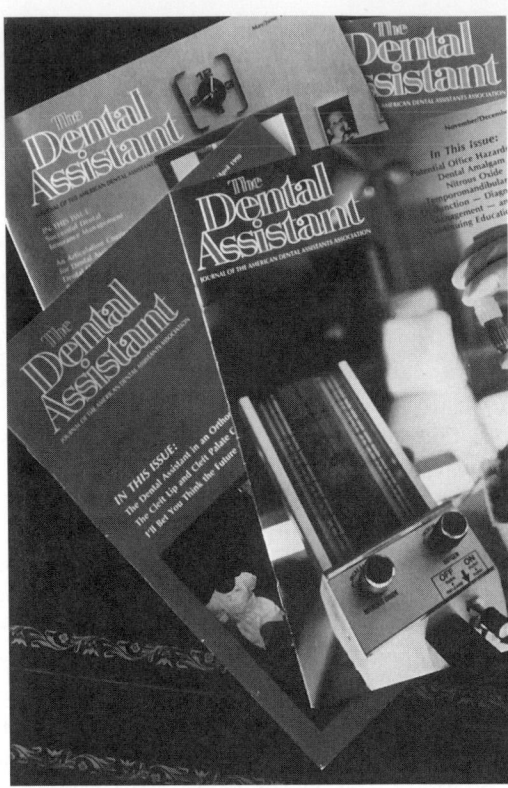

FIG. 2-1   Dental Assistant Journal.

(Courtesy of the American Dental Assistants Association.)

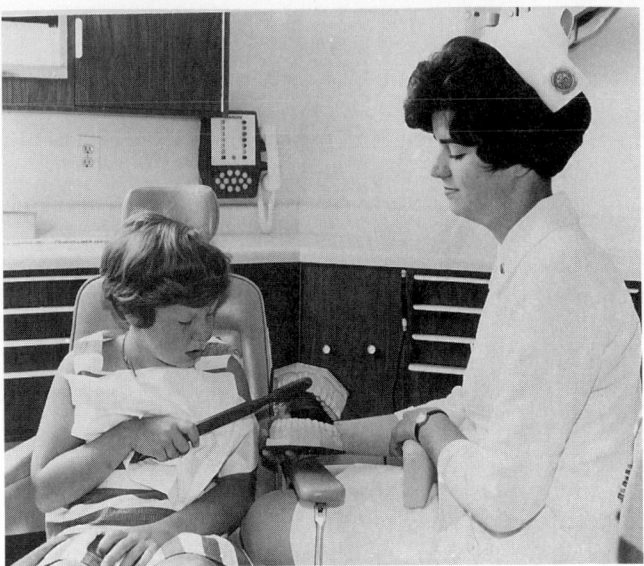

FIG. 2-2   Official cap previously worn by dental assistants. The emblem indicates that the assistant is certified.

(Courtesy of the American Dental Assistants' Association.)

Formal Education for Dental Assistants

Efforts to provide formal education for the dental assistant began as early as the Southard era, but these efforts were not recognized until 1947, when the Certifying Board of the ADAA was established to administer examinations and to certify dental assistants. In 1948 programs known as the *104-hour study courses* were designed by the ADAA to be offered by local ADAA chapters throughout the country; their aim was to prepare an employed dental assistant for certification. These courses provided the dental assistant with basic skills and cognitive knowledge about dentistry and required a minimal employment time before taking the certification examination, which included written and clinical elements.

While many dental schools around the country made significant contributions to the advancement of four-handed dentistry, the University of North Carolina (UNC) can be credited with some of the greatest contributions in promoting education for the dental assistant. **Four-handed dentistry** is the concept of four hands working together to perform treatment in the oral cavity. For many

years, dentistry was faced with a twofold problem: the lack of training facilities for dental assistants and the lack of training of dental students in the use of dental assistants. By 1954 the UNC had made efforts to correct both of these problems. Dr. John Brauer, Dean of the University of North Carolina, headed a program that designed a correspondence course for dental assistants. The total program included seven courses; five were correspondence courses, and two courses retained the option of residence or correspondence. These courses were not for college credit but were intended to provide working dental assistants with practical and theoretical knowledge that would enable them to successfully complete the national certification examination.

In 1957 the University of North Carolina School of Dentistry, in conjunction with the Division of Dental Resources, Public Health Service of the U.S. Department of Health, Education, and Welfare, inaugurated an educational program for training dental assistants in the School of Dentistry. UNC was one of five pilot programs (each designed differently) that operated in the United States. The UNC placed its emphasis on education for dental assistants, while teaching dental students how to utilize dental assistants in the practice of four- or six-handed dentistry. This pilot program was highly successful and resulted in the establishment of similar courses, not only in dental schools, but also in community colleges. Dr. Roger Barton continued to be director of this program until 1966 when Ethel Earl, a Certified Dental Assistant, became the director and the program became accredited by the ADA. Earl participated in the

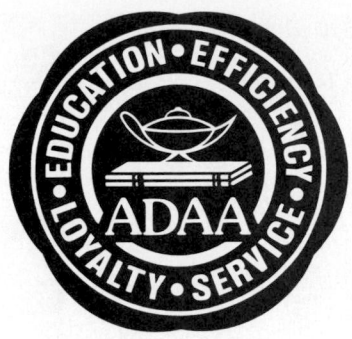

FIG. 2-3   Official pin of the ADAA.
(Courtesy of the American Dental Assistants' Association.)

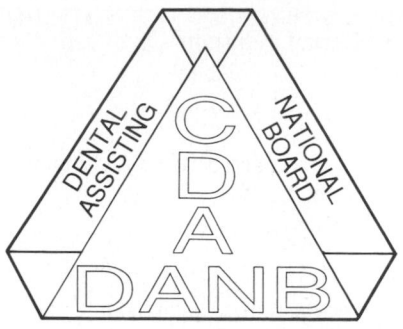

FIG. 2-4   Artist's sketch of DANB certification pin.

UNC teacher workshop sponsored by the W.K. Kellogg Foundation and has made significant contributions to dental assisting as an author and consultant to the DANB test construction committee and the ADA Commission on Dental Accreditation, and as an officer on the local, state, and national levels of the ADAA.

In 1967 a model curriculum leading to a Bachelor of Science Degree in **Dental Auxiliary Teacher Education (DATE)** was developed by the University of North Carolina School of Dentistry. This program offered an opportunity for dental assistants, hygienists, and laboratory technicians to enroll in a teacher-preparation program. By 1979 a Master of Science Degree was implemented in the DATE program, adding another step on the ladder of education for the dental assistant.

The Commission on Dental Accreditation

The ADA's **Council on Dental Education (CDE)** was the agency responsible for accrediting dental schools and related dental programs from the early 1940s until 1975. In January 1975 the Council's authority was transferred to the **Commission on Dental Accreditation (CDA)** and Dental Auxiliary Educational Programs, an organization that would be representative of accreditation for all dental education groups. In 1979 the name of the Commission was changed to the Commission on Dental Accreditation. Each auxiliary was represented on this commission.

The task of accreditation is still the primary responsibility of this commission as it accredits dental schools and educational programs in dental assisting, dental hygiene, and dental laboratory technology. Its mission is to maintain and improve the quality of dental education, to evaluate the program to ensure that approved accreditation standards are met, to encourage innovative educational programs based on sound educational principles,

and to provide consultation for continuing program development.

The 1950s were a busy time for the advancement of dental assistant education. In 1957 the ADA's CDE conducted a workshop on dental assisting and invited practicing dentists, dental educators, and dental assistants to participate. Out of this workshop came recommendations for education and certification of dental assistants, laying the groundwork for the development of the "Requirements for an Accredited Program in Dental Assisting Education." These standards were revised to meet the needs and changes of the profession; they continue to be the accreditation standards for dental assistant education programs today. During this time the ADA officially recognized the Certifying Board of the ADAA. Until these standards were adopted, programs varied from the 104-hour program to programs lasting 2 academic years. The CDE granted *provisional approval* initially to programs approved by the ADAA that were for at least 1 academic year, until site visits could be arranged to accredit the programs. Twenty-six programs appeared on the initial list of accredited dental assisting programs in 1961. This list grew to 294 in 1979; however, by 1991 the list had decreased to 248. Cost containment in schools; the demographics of prospective students; changing roles of women, who made up the major work force of dental assistants; and a lack of recruitment activities may all be contributing factors to this decline. Data in 1992 indicate that the number of programs is being maintained and enrollment in many of the dental assisting programs is increasing.

Dental Assistants' National Board

The Dental Assistants' National Board (DANB) assumes the responsibility for dental assistant certification and is independent of the ADAA. Successful completion of the DANB examination enables an assistant to use the credential of Certified Dental Assistant (CDA), wear the official certification pin (Fig. 2-4), and display the

Pathways to Dental Assistant Certification through the DANB

PATHWAY I

▶ Graduate of an accredited Dental Assistant or Dental Hygiene program
▶ Current CPR card

PATHWAY II

▶ High school graduation or equivalent
▶ Current CPR card
▶ Two years of full-time employment or 3500 hours
▶ Recommendation of dentist employer

PATHWAY III

▶ Previous certification with a lapsed status of 18 months
▶ Current CPR card

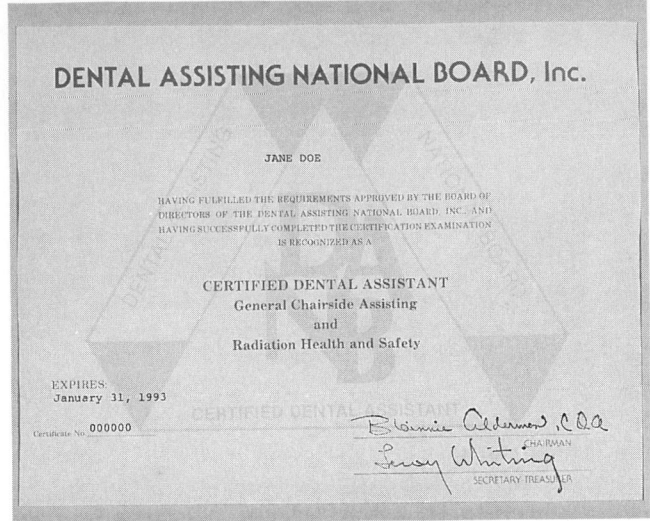

FIG. 2-5   An example of the DANB certificate awarded for successful completion of the DANB examination.

(Courtesy of the Dental Assistants' National Board.)

certificate (Fig. 2-5). Three pathways lead to this national credential.

Credentialling examinations provided by DANB include the general chairside, radiographic hygiene, and infection control tests, as well as specialty examinations in dental office management, oral maxillofacial surgery, and orthodontics. More information on this credential is available by writing to the Dental Assistants' National Board, 216 East Ontario St., Chicago, IL, 60611.

State Credentialing

Minnesota was the first state to license dental assistants. Helen Tuchner, CDA, RDA, educator, and the first dental assistant commissioner on the Commission on Dental Accreditation of the ADA, was a leader in the movement to license dental assistants. Minnesota was the first to include a dental assistant on the State Board of Dentistry and has enjoyed a close working relationship with the Minnesota Dental Assistants' Association (MDAA) and the Minnesota Educators Association of Dental Assistants (MEADA). Tuchner's strong commitment to education and the credentialing process in Minnesota brought her national recognition as she worked to achieve this credential for assistants in her state. Today assistants in other states benefit from the foresight of Helen Tuchner.

Credentials for dental assistants vary from state to state. In some states, certification from DANB is a prerequisite to eligibility for a state examination, while in other states specific course work or employment may be the criterion. For specific information about legal duties, educational requirements, and credentialing, an assistant can write to the State Board of Dentistry in the state for which this information is desired.

Each credential verifies to both patients and employer a person's professional credibility in a specific area. A credential builds self-esteem and provides an assistant with bargaining power during salary negotiations. It is important that an assistant seek to obtain as many credentials as possible.

Beyond the Dental Office

Many individuals, including dentists, assistants, and hygienists, have made significant contributions to the profession of dental assisting. In a text such as this it is impossible to identify all contributors to the profession; however, it seems appropriate to recognize a group of pioneers who can serve as role models for dental assistants today. The authors have chosen a handful of individuals who dared to accept a challenge and go beyond the dental office to use their skills for the advancement of the profession.

▶ The ADA

The Commission on Dental Accreditation of the ADA has sought out leaders in education to represent the profession. Joyce Sigmon became the first Director of Dental Assisting Education for the ADA's CDE and CDA in 1971. Her career has ranged from dental assisting in a general practice, to being an educator in the North Carolina Community College System, to serving in association management with several agencies within the ADA. In addition to her dental assisting credentials, she obtained a baccalaureate degree from UNC at Chapel Hill as one of the original graduates of the DATE program along with Ethel Earl and Chris Lemoine. Sigmon later obtained a master's degree from Loyola University of Chicago.

Like Joyce Sigmon, Judy Nix's advancement in the field exemplifies a potential career ladder for a dental assistant today. Her present role as Assistant Director, Advanced Dental Education on the ADA's CDA/CDE was attained after her experience as a chairside assistant in private practice and later as an assistant in the Dental Auxiliary Utilization Program at Loyola University School of Dentistry in Chicago. The latter experience inspired her to obtain a degree from the State University of New York at Buffalo in the Allied Health Teacher Training Program. Later, she taught at Morton College in Cicero, Illinois, which led to an appointment as an accreditation consultant to the ADA's CDA program of the American Dental Association. Before working with the ADA, she was the Director of Education for the ADAA.

▶ Federal Government

In 1963 Lois Kryger was employed by the Education Development Branch of the Division of Dentistry and became a consultant for the Public Health Service Health Resources Administration of the Department of Health, Education, and Welfare (HEW) of the federal government. Until her retirement from this position, she assumed the primary responsibility for independently planning, conducting, and evaluating national programs for studying, implementing, and improving dental assisting education activities; for providing consultation to state and local health educational agencies regarding dental assisting programs; for advising program staff in developing programs for utilizing dental assistants; and for consulting with national professional groups and other federal agencies about programs in this field. Before her employment with the federal government, she was a chairside assistant in Seattle and completed teacher education at the Washington State Department of Vocational Education. An avid student, Kryger attended many seminars, taught dental assisting at Seattle Central Community College, became president of the ADAA in 1960, developed continuing education courses for the ADAA Education Committee, and was a consultant to the ADA's CDE program.

▶ Dental Assistant Literature

Today many textbooks are written for the dental assistant, but in the early days few resources existed. In 1948 G. Archanna Morrison wrote *In the Dentist's Office.* Morrison was a business assistant in Boston where she gained experience in a wide range of offices. She realized that not all dentists were able to spend time and effort in training an assistant; she wrote a book to address the

situation. An enthusiastic lecturer, Morrison toured the country in the late 1950s and promoted greater utilization of dental auxiliaries. She challenged dental assistants to ask themselves "How can I advance myself to become more valuable to my employer?" She challenged the dentist to ask "How can I train my assistants so that they can assume executive responsibilities, thereby enabling me to concentrate on scientific services?" Morrison was an inspiration to dental assistants who were eager to advance their careers and to expand their responsibilities. Throughout her lectures Morrison maintained that the duties of the dentist and the dental assistant are interdependent. A deficiency in one automatically reflects in the other.

The Dental Assistant by Drs. John C. Brauer and Richard E. Richardson, written in 1955, provided the dental assistant with one of the first comprehensive textbooks in dental assisting. This text was the primary reference used in many of the 104-hour study courses offered around the country.

Ann Ehrlich was a coauthor of *Dental Practice Management—The Teamwork Approach,* written in 1969, which was the first reference to place emphasis on the dental assistant in the business office. Ehrlich, a Certified Dental Assistant, has been a dental assistant in private practice, an educator, an author, and a consultant to the Dental Assistant National Board; however, she is best known for her extensive work in the application of work simplification in the dental business office.

One of the major textbooks from 1976 to today has been *Modern Dental Assisting,* written by Hazel Torres and Ann Ehrlich. Although other textbooks were on the market earlier, this text was the first major work written *by* dental assistants *for* dental assistants. Torres, like Ehrlich, has been a dental assistant in private practice, an educator, an author, and a consultant and has also served as president of the ADAA.

The collage in Fig. 2-6 identifies many of the pioneers who have contributed to the dental assisting profession. Chance may have been the reason each of these individuals entered dental assisting; however, it was not chance that made them successful. Hard work, determination, and strong motivation led them to shape a career that would serve as an example for future generations.

Dental Auxiliary Utilization Movement

The middle of the twentieth century saw the greatest advances in the utilization of dental assistants. These advances were realized with the increase in formal educational programs for dental assistants in postsecondary schools, accreditation of these programs by the ADA, federal funding of auxiliary utilization programs in dental

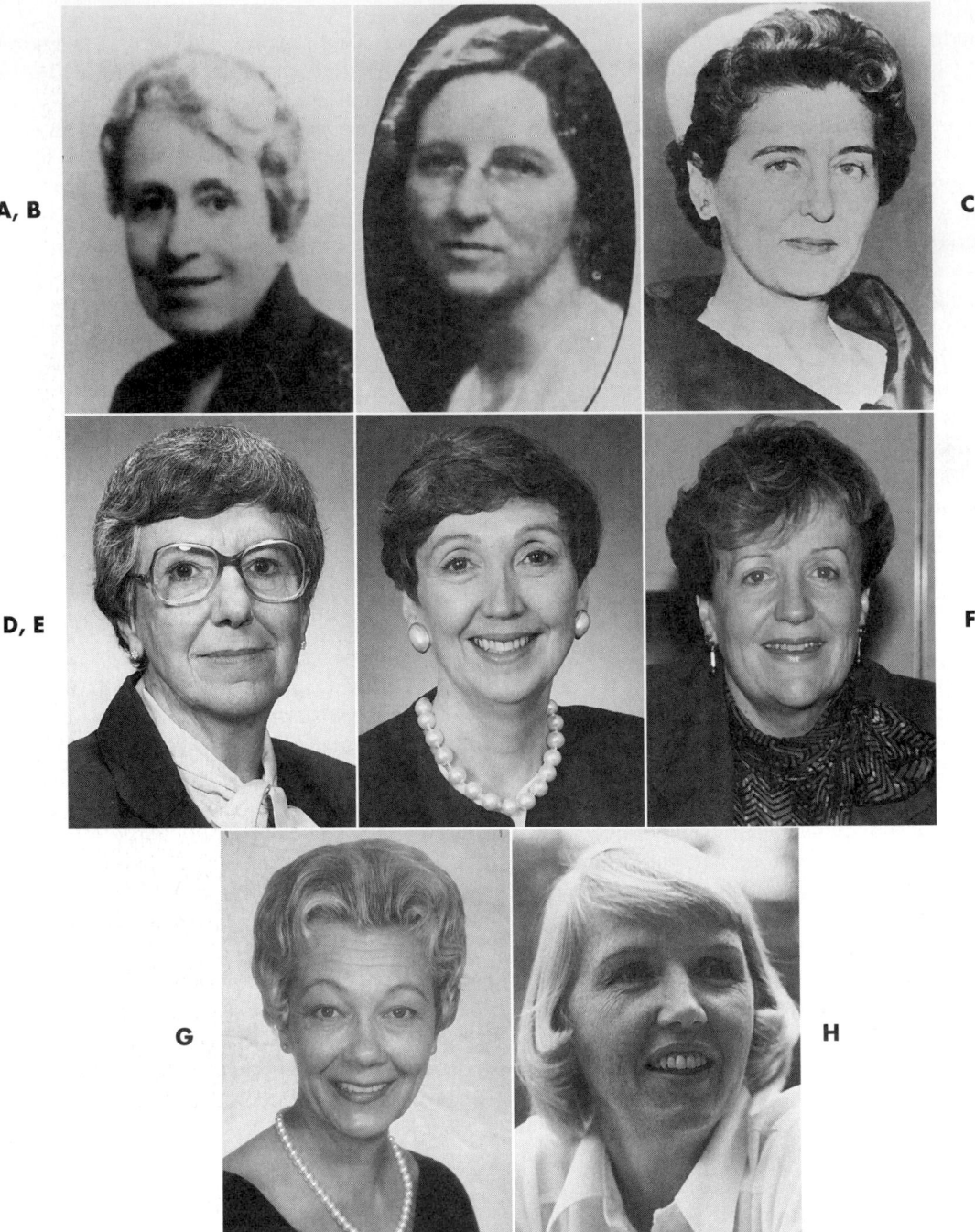

FIG. 2-6 *A,* Juliette Southard was founder of the ADAA. *B,* Under the presidency of Ruth Rodgers in 1933 the *Dental Assistant,* the official publication of the ADAA, was adopted. *C,* Violet Crowley made significant contributions to the advancement of dental assisting through her contribution to dental literature. *D,* Ethel Earl participated in the original University of North Carolina (UNC) teacher workshop and became director of the UNC dental auxiliary utilization program—one of the original in the country. *E,* Joyce Sigmon became the first director of dental assisting education for the ADA Council on Dental Education. *F,* Judy Nix has demonstrated the potential career ladder for a dental assistant today, from private practice to the role as assistant director on the ADA's Council on Dental Education. *G,* Lois Kryger Miller was the first dental assistant to be employed by the education development branch of the division of dentistry and became a consultant to the Health, Education, and Welfare (HEW) agency. *H,* Ann Ehrlich coauthored the first practice management textbook for dental assistants, *Dental practice management: the teamwork approach.*

(*A* and *C* courtesy of the American Dental Assistants' Association.)

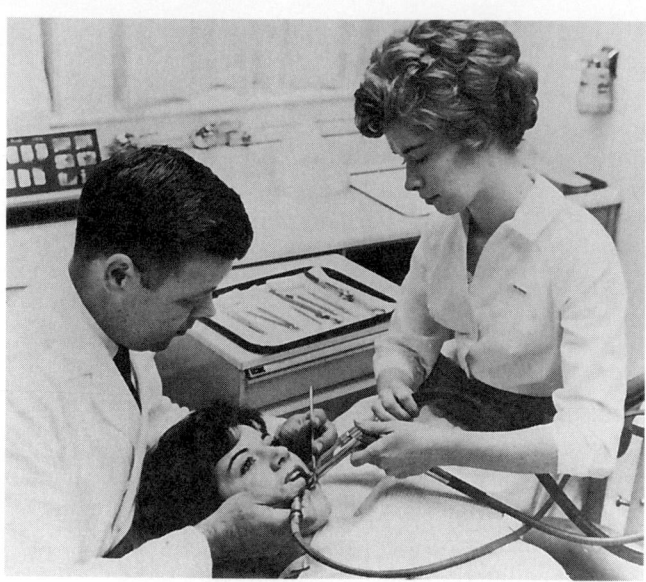

FIG. 2-7   DAU program at the University of Alabama, circa 1950s.

(Courtesy of the University of Alabama—School of Dentistry.)

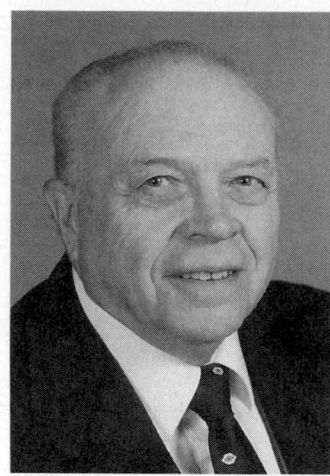

FIG. 2-8   Dr. Richard Barton, author and pioneer in four-handed dentistry.

(Courtesy of the University of North Carolina—School of Dentistry.)

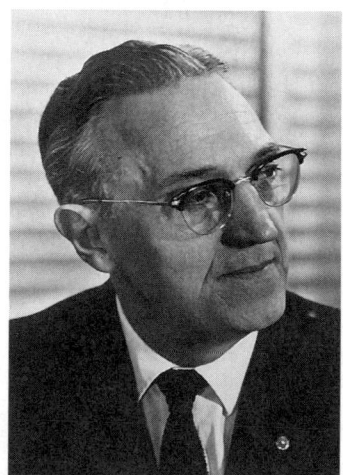

FIG. 2-9   Dr. Richard Brauer, innovator of four-handed dentistry.

(Courtesy of the University of North Carolina—School of Dentistry.)

schools, and the increase in seminars on four-handed dentistry throughout the country by noted dentists and assistants. The major change came in 1956 when the federal government provided funds for a few dental schools to expand the use of chairside assistants. By 1960 the project was so successful and the desire to increase the productivity of dentists was so evident that the federal government made funds available to all dental schools in the United States. The dental auxiliary utilization (DAU) grants were used by dental schools to teach their students to work efficiently with chairside assistants (Fig. 2-7). This milestone for dental assistants opened the door to more effective utilization of their skills. Likewise, it created a need for the dental assistant to obtain a basic theoretical and clinical knowledge of dental assisting. Programs began to develop at a greater rate within dental schools, as well as within postsecondary and technical institutions. Today, these programs, like those for dental hygienists and dental laboratory technicians, are eligible for accreditation by the ADA's CDA.

As a result of this increased interest in DAU, staff members in dental schools and private practitioners became deeply involved in four-handed dentistry. Great emphasis was placed on increased chairside production and reduced stress for practitioners and their staffs. Private practitioners were eager to attend seminars to learn about new concepts in instrument transfer, high-velocity evacuation, preset trays, and developments in major equipment that would impact both their practices and the delivery of dental treatment in the 1960s.

To satisfy the needs of the staff in dental schools and those in private practitioners, leaders around the country created practical applications for the new four-handed dentistry concepts. Dr. Richard Barton (University of North Carolina) (Fig. 2-8), Dr. John Brauer (University of North Carolina) (Fig. 2-9), Dr. James Bush (University of Michigan) (Fig. 2-10), Dr. Shailer Peterson (University of Tennessee) (not pictured), and Dr. Harold Kilpatrick (not pictured) were only a few of the innovators who lectured on new concepts in dental auxiliary utilization. The central theme in all of their messages was increased production and reduced stress

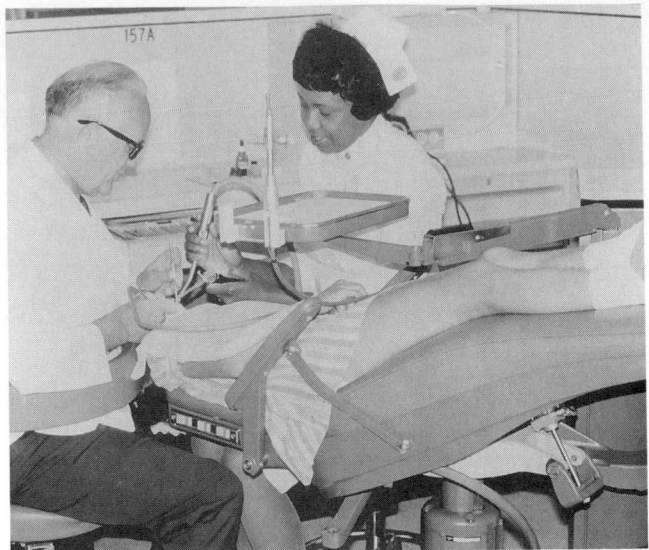

FIG. 2-10   Dr. James Bush and Mamie Crawford, RDA, using four-handed dentistry techniques in the 1960s at the University of Michigan.

(Courtesy of the University of Michigan—School of Dentistry.)

through the use of sit-down, four-handed dentistry, employing the results of time and motion studies.

Extensive DAU studies were also conducted at the University of Alabama. The team of Drs. G.E. Wuerhmann and Glen Robinson, the team assistant Gertrude (Trudy) Sinnet, and equipment designer Ed McDivitt (Fig. 2-11, *A* through *E*) committed tireless energies to the promotion of four-handed dentistry for dental students and practicing dentists—a program that still affects dentistry today. The University of Alabama team was integral in designing equipment (see Fig. 2-7) that was customized primarily for use with four-handed dentistry concepts. Many of those equipment styles are still produced today. Courses were conducted in the 1960s at the University of Alabama to train dental teams, practicing dentists, and their assistants concerning the concepts of four-handed dentistry and to adapt their offices to this new work style.

By the early 1970s DAU was phased out and the inception of training in expanded auxiliary management (TEAM) grants were made available on a limited basis. Although no dramatic effect was felt from the TEAM grants, the concept that a dentist needs to be taught how to manage a staff of auxiliaries trained in advanced techniques was accepted.

Changes Impacting The Role Of Dental Auxiliaries

Significant changes have taken place concerning female representation in the dental profession. As noted in

Chapter 1, the number of women in dental schools has increased significantly in the last 2 decades.

Another impact on dental care occurred in the 1950s when third-party payments became more evident. Major industries began to provide dental insurance as a benefit for their employees. In 1965 about 1.9 million Americans were covered by some form of dental insurance, and by 1990 over 100 million Americans received this benefit.

One of the most important changes in dentistry has been the recognition of dental auxiliaries in state dental practice acts. Many states realized by the 1950s that expanded use of dental auxiliaries would require changes in existing state dental practice acts. The need to increase production resulted in a need to delegate more duties to dental assistants and hygienists. Thus, today, state dental boards and legislators continue this extensive process of changing the existing dental laws. Both the dental assistant and the hygienist are affected by these changes. In most cases, additional duties are being delegated, and the education that is needed to perform these duties has been upgraded.

Job Sources

As a dental assistant enters the profession, thoughts generally turn to potential employment possibilities. Today the job market that awaits a highly skilled, well-educated dental assistant is limitless. In the past the primary source of employment may have been private dental practice, but now the field offers employment in many settings.

Private Dental Offices. An assistant may choose to work in a general or a specialty practice in a small office or a large multidentist practice. The number of employees may vary from 2 to 20 or more. These types of practices provide the opportunity for varied experiences at chairside, in a business office, or in the laboratory and in most settings will allow the novice to develop a close rapport with patients who are seen regularly and to develop the skills that are needed to become a valuable asset in the dental practice.

Dental Schools. A dental school offers various opportunities that range from working with dental students in four-handed dentistry procedures, clinical supervision, sterilization, or business office/records management; to working on research projects, or assisting professors in a clinical setting.

Public/State or Federal Clinics. A dental assistant may opt for employment in a federal dental clinic at a Veterans Administration Hospital, in a prison, or in a public clinic set up by some form of state or federal agency. Benefits and regulations are generally standardized within the realm of government. The environment obviously varies

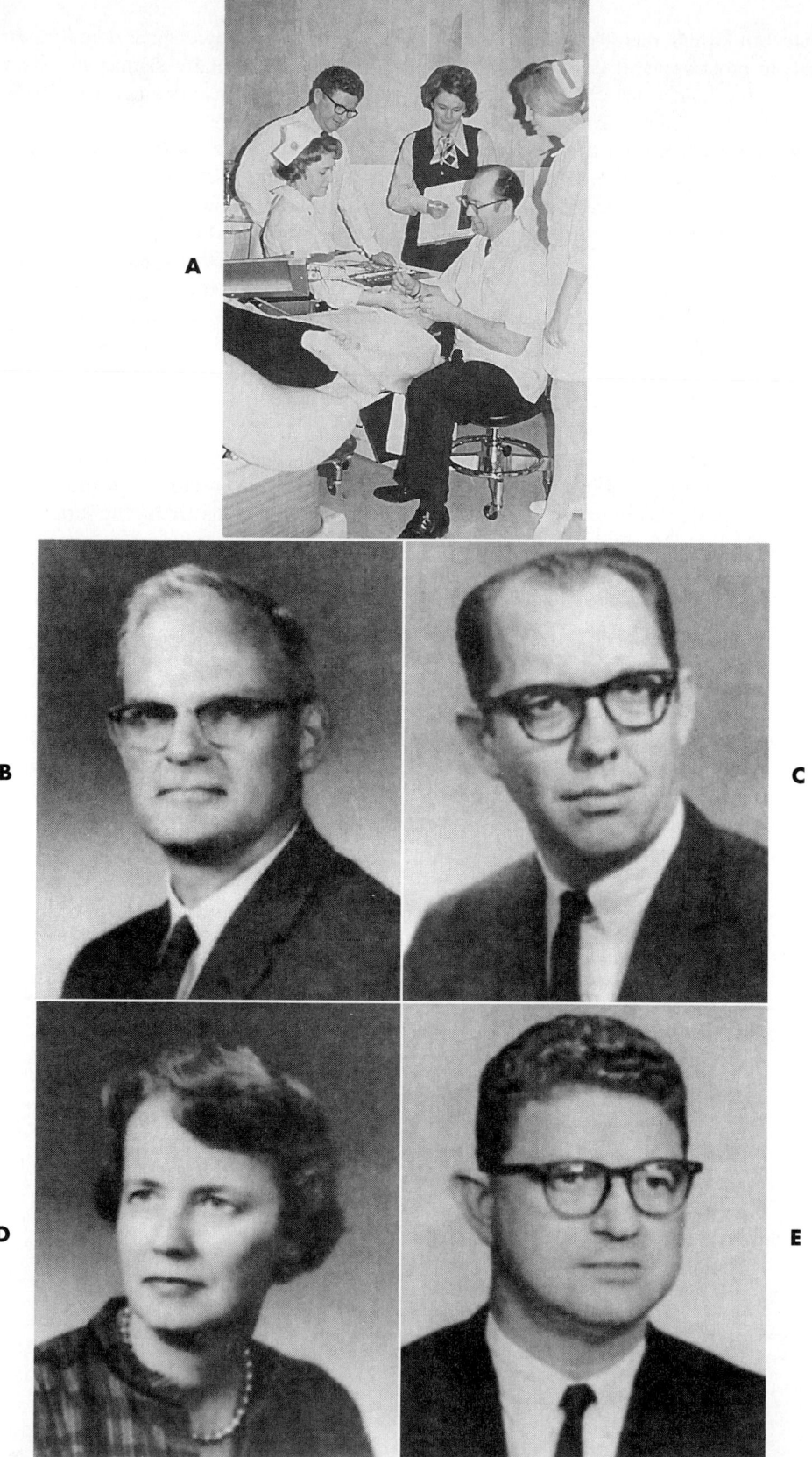

FIG. 2-11   *A,* University of Alabama team who promoted four-handed dentistry for dental students and practicing dentists. *B,* Dr. G. E. Wuerhmann; *C,* Dr. Glen Robinson; *D,* Gertrude (Trudy) Sinnet; and *E,* Ed McDivitt.

(Courtesy of the University of Alabama—School of Dentistry.)

from clinic to clinic but offers many opportunities to practice varied skills in most areas of dentistry.

Corporate/Department Store Clinics. Today, many large corporations are providing clinics for their employees. Department stores also have opened dental clinics for the public. Depending on the size of the organization, these clinics are generally operated in the same manner as a private dental practice.

Hospitals. Many large university hospitals and some general hospitals have dental clinics within their facilities. The patients often have special needs and require a hospital setting; some patients are terminally ill, or are physically or mentally disabled. The treatment is the same as in routine restorative or preventive dentistry; however, the environment is a hospital operating room, and in most situations the patients are treated while they are under general anesthesia. The patient/staff relationships may vary in these settings; however, the hospital clinic presents a great opportunity to work with patients who have special needs (Fig. 2-12).

Armed Forces. An advanced standing in the various branches of the armed forces often awaits dental assistants with education and skills in the field of dentistry. It is possible to receive training in the armed forces and then continue this career after leaving the service. Alternatively, a person may enter the armed forces with previously learned skills that can affect the entry-level rank.

To this point, job opportunities have included gener-

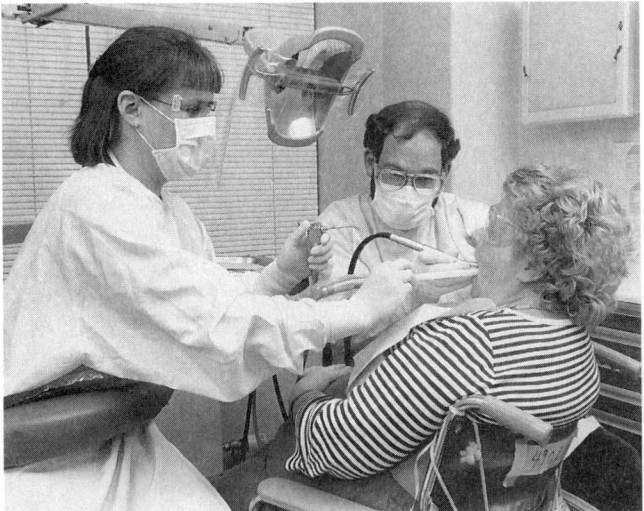

FIG. 2-12   Hospital dentistry employment.

(Courtesy of the Veterans Administration Hospital, Ann Arbor, Michigan.)

alized skills. However, a dental assistant who possesses interests in dental assisting and who has skills in other areas might consider one of the following careers.

Teaching. After a dental assistant completes a basic program and has worked for a period of time, teaching often becomes an attractive career goal. Colleges and universities around the country offer programs in occupational or health education. In many instances course credits can be transferred into a baccalaureate degree program and the dental assistant is then qualified to teach in a postsecondary program in dental assisting. Career-ladder mobility can also lead to a master's or a doctoral degree.

Publishing/Public Relations. Dental assistants with artistic talent may secure a position as a dental illustrator. These individuals are highly sought by dental schools and authors of dental texts. Having the credentials of a dental assistant and the skills of an artist opens the door to vast opportunities through publishers and hospital medical media departments.

Medical/dental publishers are always looking for ambitious people who are interested in dental literature, who have backgrounds in dentistry, and who have an ability to write. Such skills and talents can lead to employment as a textbook reviewer or an editor.

Insurance Companies. Insurance companies seek educated assistants with some dental office experience to process claim forms and work in the customer relations department. This offers an excellent opportunity for the dental assistant who has a good dental background and has an interest in business and computers. Advanced positions that involve supervision and education are also available in large insurance companies.

Dental Manufacturers and Suppliers. An enthusiastic dental assistant with an eagerness for sales may find fulfilling employment in a manufacturing or supply company. Large companies often provide travel opportunities, and dental representatives frequently present educational seminars. In other instances, companies may seek such an employee for research and development.

KEY POINTS

▷ Career opportunities for dental assistants today are available throughout various industries and can range from general to specialty practices.

▷ The ADAA was founded by Juliette Southard and today is the professional organization for dental assistants.

▷ Formal education programs for dental assistants began in 1948 with a *104-hour study courses* and have evolved into accreditation programs in postsecondary institutions.

◗ The Commission on Dental Accreditation is responsible for maintaining program standards in dentistry and dental auxiliary programs.

◗ The Dental Assistants' National Board is responsible for administering the Dental Assistant Certification Examination and offers three pathways to the credential.

◗ Credentials for dental assistants vary from state to state and are defined in the state's Dental Practice Act.

◗ Significant contributions have been made to the profession of dental assisting, including pioneers with backgrounds in teaching, federal service, national professional organizations, and writing.

◗ Dental auxiliary utilization grants were the impetus for four-handed dentistry. These grants were used by dental schools to teach dental students to work efficiently with dental assistants.

◗ The implementation of dental insurance, changes in state dental practice acts, and changing demographics of the population have had an impact on the roles of dental auxiliaries by requiring them to assume additional duties.

◗ Job opportunities for dental assistants include employment in the private and public sectors, educational institutions, health care, and health-related agencies.

BIBLIOGRAPHY

ADAA golden anniversary, *Dent Assist J,* 1974.

American Dental Assistants' Association: *Highlights of the 50 years history of the American Dental Assistants' Association,* Chicago, 1974, The Association.

American Dental Association, Council on Dental Education: *1992 annual surveys of allied dental education programs,* U.S. Department of Health and Human Services, U.S. Department of Labor (revised August 1993).

American Dental Association, Department of Educational Surveys: *Number of accredited dental hygiene programs,* Chicago, 1993, The Association.

American Dental Association, Department of Educational Surveys: *Number of C.D.A. accredited programs in dental assisting,* Chicago 1993, The Association.

Dental Assistant 1887, *Dent Assist J,* August 1971.

Helgeson B: American dental assistants commemorate 50th anniversary, *JADA* 89: 1924-1974, Sept 1974.

Johnson E: *Stepping forward: a history of the American Dental Assistants,* LaPort, Ind, 1962, ADAA Certification Board.

U.S. Bureau of Economics and Behavioral Research: *Distribution of dentists 1987,* Chicago, 1987, ADA.

UNIT II BASIC SCIENCES IN DENTISTRY

3

Basic Anatomy and Physiology

LEARNING OBJECTIVES

You will have mastered the material in this chapter when you can:

▶ Define the key terms
▶ List common prefixes and suffixes relative to dentistry
▶ Describe anatomic position
▶ Describe anatomic body locations
▶ Explain the different body planes
▶ Explain the human organism and cell components
▶ Identify the basic systems of the body as they relate to dentistry
▶ Identify and locate the bones and other important landmarks of the skull
▶ Identify and locate muscles of mastication and facial expression and the origin and insertion of each
▶ Identify the oral cavity and facial landmarks
▶ Identify and list the parts and name the purpose of the temporomandibular joint
▶ Identify the location and the purpose of the salivary glands and the surrounding structures
▶ Identify and describe the paranasal sinuses and the functions of each

KEY TERMS

Alveolar process	Anomalies
Anatomic position	Anterior
Anatomy	Artery
Atria	Orbit
Blood	Organ
Body planes	Origin
Bone	Osteoblast
Canal	Osteoclast
Cells	Papilla
Condyle	Periosteum
Cranial bones	Physiology
Deglutition	Posterior
Distal	Process
Dorsal	Protuberance
Extrinsic	Proximal
Facial bones	Ramus
Foramen	Sagittal
Fossa	Salivary glands
Frenum	Septum
Frontal	Sinus
Gingiva	Superior
Inferior	Suture
Insertion	Symphysis
Intrinsic	Synovial
Lateral	System
Longitudinal	Temporomandibular joint
Mandible	Tissue
Maxilla	Transverse
Meatus	Tubercle
Medial	Vein
Mesial	Ventral
Muscles of facial expression	Ventricle
Muscles of mastication	Vestibule
Neuron	

Before a dental assistant can develop a thorough understanding of oral and dental anatomy, it is necessary to develop an understanding of basic human anatomy. This chapter will not present an in-depth study of human anatomy and physiology, but rather it will provide an overview of basic anatomic terms and the systems of the body as they relate to dentistry. In addition, a thorough review of head and neck anatomy will be presented as it relates to the role of the dental assistant.

To communicate effectively in the dental profession

BOX 3-1

COMMON PREFIXES AND SUFFIXES

COMMON PREFIXES

a or ab - away from
a or an - without
adeno - gland
album - white
ante - before or preceding
ant or anti—against
bi, bin, bis—two or twice
bio - relating to living organism
blast - formative cell
cardio - heart
cephal - head
cheil - lip
chemo - relating to chemistry
contra - against
crani - skull
cyano - blue
cyst - sac, bladder, bag
cyt - cell
de - away
deci, deca - ten
dento, denti - tooth or dental
dermato, dermo - skin
di - two
dis - free of, separation, reversal
dys - difficult, painful, faulty
e, ex - out, away from, without
ecto, exo, extra - without, on the outside
encephal - brain
erythro - red
galact - milk
gastro - stomach
glosso - tongue
hemato, hemo, hema - blood
hepato, hepatico - liver
histo - tissue, web-like
homo - alike, same
hydro - water
hypo - below
infra - under
inter - between
intro - into
kerato - horn or corn
kin - movement
labia - lip
latero - to the side of
lith - stone
macro - great
mast - breast
media, medial - middle
meta - change
micro - small
milli - thousand
mono - one

morpho - form
myo - muscle
narco - numbness
naso - nose
necro - dead
neo - new
neuro - nerve
nona - ten
octo - eight
odonto - tooth or teeth
ortho - straight, correct
osteo - bone
oti - ear
para - beside, alongside of
path - disease
penta - five
pedo - child
per - between, through, across
peri - around
pharm - drugs
phlebo - vein
pneum - air
poly - many
post - behind or after
pre - before
pro - in front
pros - toward
pseudo - false
psycho - soul or mind
pyo - pus
re, retro - behind, backward, again
rhino - nose
rube - red
semi - half
septa - seven
septic - poison
sial - saliva
sphygmo - pulse
sub - less, deficient
super, supra - above, over, excess
thermo - heat
tachy - fast or swift
ter, tri - three
tetra - four
thermo - heat
thrombo - clot
toxi, toxo - poison
tracheo - windpipe or air passageway
trans - across or through
uni - mono or one
ultra - beyond or excess
vaso - vessel
xero - dry

COMMON SUFFIXES

-al - act or process
-algia, -algesia - pain
-agra - seizure or acute pain
-ago, igo - disease
-cide - destroyer, killer
-eal, -eous - of the nature of
-ectomy - to excise or remove
-emesis - vomiting
-emia - condition of the blood
-gnosis - knowledge
-ia, -iasis, -id, -ism - abnormal, diseased
-iasis - a condition
-ics - science or art of
-ist - person who does
-itis - inflammation
-ize - action or treatment
-less - without
-lith - stone
-logy - study of
-oid, -oides - like or resembling
-oma - tumor
-osis - condition or state
-oscopy - inspection of
-ostomy - an opening
-otomy - incision or cut
-pathy - disease
-phagy or -phage - swallowing
-phonia - voice or sound
-phylaxis - protection
-plasty - repair, reconstruction by surgery
-pnea - breathing
-rrhage - excessive flow
-rrhaphy - suture
-stasis - stopping the flow
-staxis - dripping, oozing
-therapy - treatment, healing
-uria - condition of the urine

the dental assistant must have a general understanding of terminology that relates to the anatomy and physiology of the human body and specifically of the head and neck regions. An understanding of anatomic terminology enables a dental assistant to communicate with other professionals and to identify specific locations of anatomic structures in a universal professional language. This section will present various body systems, the body planes, anatomic structures, and key terminology.

Prefixes and Suffixes

Dental terminology is easier to comprehend when prefixes and suffixes are understood. A prefix is a single letter or group of letters placed at the beginning of a word. For instance, the prefix *uni* means one and the prefix *bi* means two. When these prefixes are added to the root word *lateral,* which means side, the following meanings are derived:

uni + lateral = unilateral = one side
bi + lateral = bilateral = two sides

The applications of these words to dentistry are common. If a patient is to have a unilateral partial denture made, it simply means that a partial denture will be placed on one side of the patient's arch. If the patient requires a bilateral partial denture, it will be placed on two sides or both sides of the dental arch.

Whereas a prefix is added before the root word, a suffix is a single letter or group of letters placed at the end of a word. A suffix can describe either the prefix or the root word. A common example of a suffix is *itis,* meaning inflammation. Since the term *glosso* refers to tongue, glossitis, then, is an inflammation of the tongue.

It is also common in dentistry to add both a prefix and a suffix to a root word. From a combination of prefix + root word + suffix can come a term such as *periodontics.* Note that when two vowels are joined together, as in the root word and the suffix, the O is dropped before the suffix is added. Thus, *peri + odonto + ics = periodontics* (around + tooth + science or study of), which refers to the specialty involved with treatment of the tissues around the tooth. If the suffix *ist* (which refers to the person who studies) were substituted for *ics,* the term would be *periodontist* and would refer to the person who practices the specialty of periodontics. Box 3-1 displays the common prefixes and suffixes that a dental assistant will use in daily professional communication. Review of this list is recommended to become familiar with the meanings of each term.

Descriptive Terms Identifying Areas of the Body

To communicate effectively about specific areas of the body, all health professionals need to use standardized language. When regions of the body are discussed, the terms that are used refer to the body when it is in an anatomic position. **Anatomic position** refers to the body when it is in a vertical position, with the face and the palms of the hands facing forward. When the body is in the anatomic position, specific descriptive terms can be used to locate areas on the body. Box 3-2 contains a list of common terms. Their relationship to the human form is illustrated in Fig. 3-1.

Body Planes

A **body plane** is an imaginary line that divides the body into segments or sections. This division provides for ease in locating specific body areas. The planes are referenced relative to the body in the anatomic position. Box 3-3 defines these planes, and Fig. 3-2 indicates their location on the human body.

Knowledge of the body planes should provide the dental assistant with a basic understanding that allows easy identification of anatomic structures. For instance, as the dental assistant becomes responsible for records management, it may be necessary to describe a section of tissue that has been removed for pathologic study. To define the location and type of tissue sample used for a biopsy, it will be necessary to describe it using anatomic terminology, such as:

The tissue is a longitudinal section of the alveolar process superior to the maxillary right cuspid.

BOX 3-2

COMMON ANATOMIC TERMS USED IN DESCRIBING BODY LOCATIONS

Anterior - situated in front, toward the front of the body

Distal - away from the midline of the body, structure, or organ, or the median sagittal plane

Dorsal - toward the back surface or posterior of an organ

Inferior - below or lower part, farthest from the head on the body

Lateral - toward the outside of the body or to the left or right of the midsagittal plane

Medial - toward the midline or middle line of the body

Mesial - toward the midline or middle line of the body

Posterior - toward the back of the body, structure, or organ

Proximal - part closest to the source, part of limb closest to the trunk

Superior - area or part closest or nearest to the head

Ventral - front or abdominal area of the body

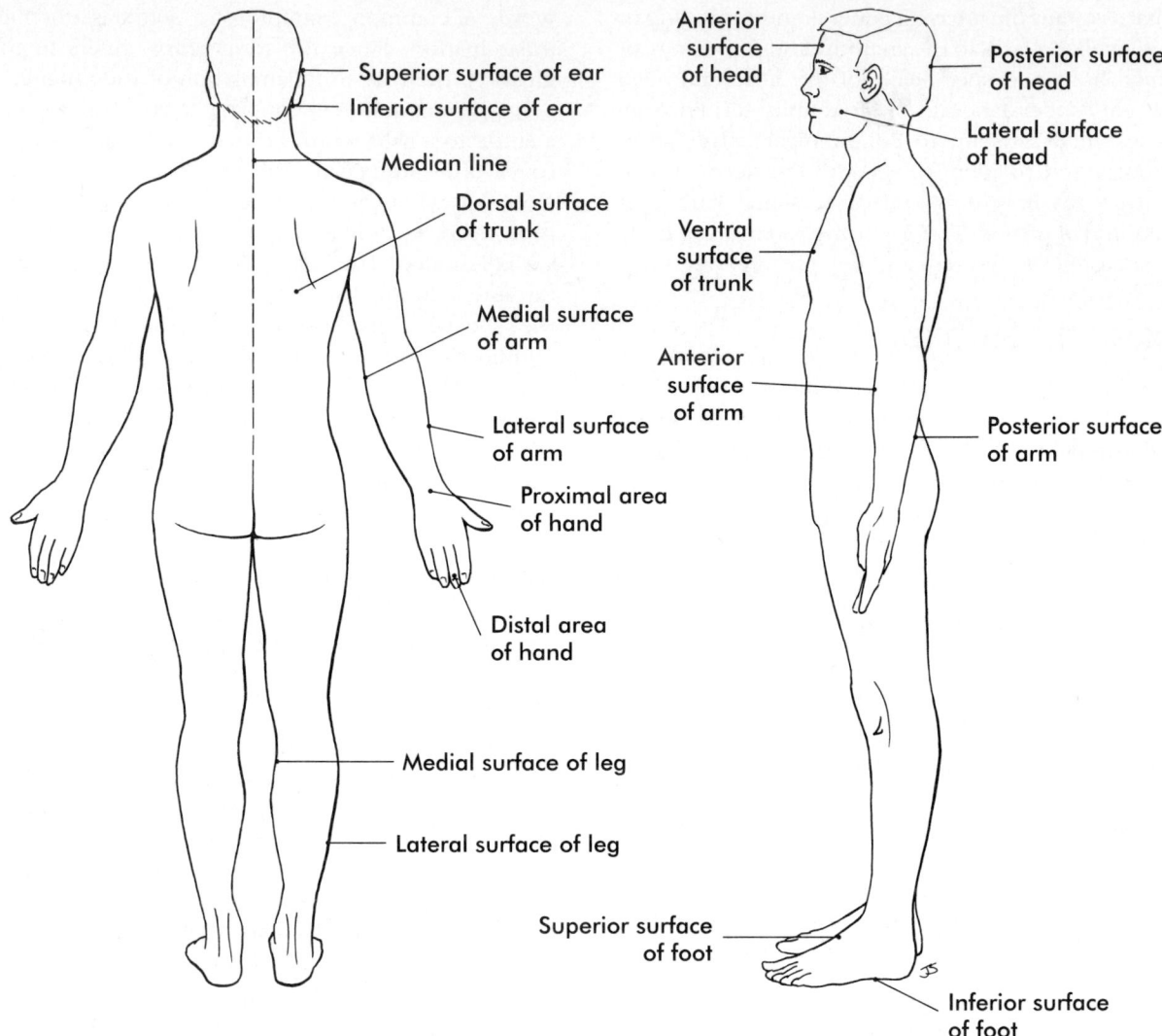

Superior surface of ear
Inferior surface of ear
Median line
Dorsal surface of trunk
Medial surface of arm
Lateral surface of arm
Proximal area of hand
Distal area of hand
Medial surface of leg
Lateral surface of leg
Superior surface of foot

Anterior surface of head
Posterior surface of head
Lateral surface of head
Ventral surface of trunk
Anterior surface of arm
Posterior surface of arm
Inferior surface of foot

FIG. 3-1   Common terms used in describing locations on the human body.

Such a description indicates that the tissue was cut in a plane running the length of the long axis of the body and was taken from the alveolar process above the upper right cuspid.

Learning some of the basic terminology should aid in understanding each of the body systems that are presented in this chapter. Simple variations in the position of anatomic structures may occur with each individual, but this background knowledge will simplify the location and identification of anatomic structures.

The Body Systems and Tissues

According to *Webster's Dictionary,* **anatomy** is the study of "the structures of a body," and **physiology** is "the function and vital process of an organism." The following discussion presents an overview of anatomy and physi-

ology as it relates to dentistry. Eleven systems of the human body are listed in Box 3-4.

All human bodies are made up of **cells**, which are the basic unit of structure and function. Different cells have different functions. For instance, muscle cells contract, and red blood cells carry oxygen, whereas skin cells protect the body from disease. Cells that are alike are grouped into tissues.

The Human Organism

Since human beings belong to a multicellular living species, it is at the cellular level that health can be affected positively or negatively. Human oral health is also affected by cellular changes; therefore, it is important for the dental health care worker to understand

IMAGINARY BODY PLANES

Transverse or Horizontal - A plane dividing the body into two portions, superior and inferior, by cutting across the long axis of the body, thereby creating a cross-section; the superior portion of the body is above the horizontal plane and the inferior beneath it

Sagittal Plane - A vertical plane from the top of the body down, leaving right and left segments

Midsagittal Plane - A sagittal plane dividing the body into equal segments, running from the front to the back through the sagittal suture of the skull down through the body

Longitudinal Plane - The plane that runs the length of the long axis of the body with the body in the anatomic position

Frontal or Coronal Plane - A vertical plane at a right angle to the sagittal plane, dividing the body into anterior and posterior segments

ELEVEN SYSTEMS OF THE HUMAN BODY

Skeletal	Urinary
Muscular	Reproductive
Nervous	Endocrine
Circulatory	Sensory
Respiratory	Lymphatic
Digestive	

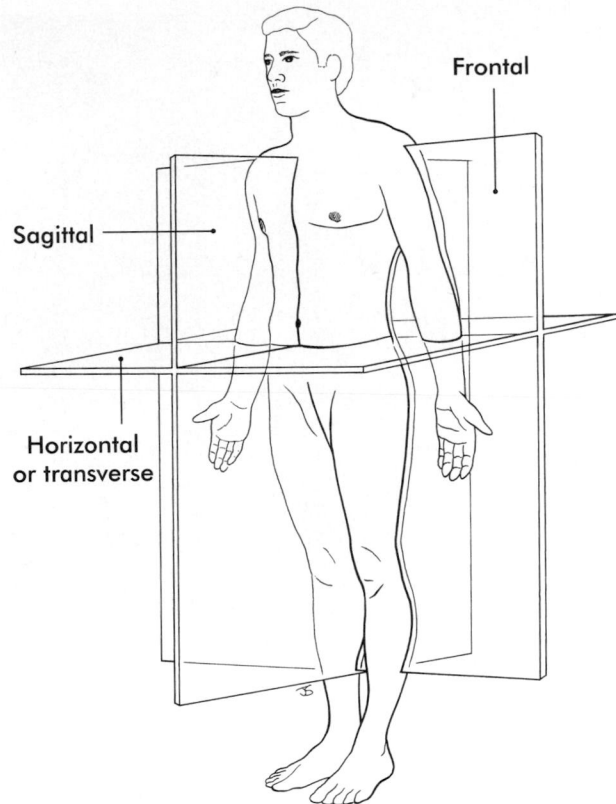

FIG. 3-2   Planes of the body.

the functions of the body from the level of cell structure to that of an organ system.

▶ Cells

Cells, the smallest structures of life, work together to comprise the human body. Each human cell is surrounded by a membrane consisting of organelles, which are specialized structures with specific functions. The membrane allows passage of molecules and provides direction for the organelles' functions.

Within the cell membrane exists the **cytoplasm** (ground substances of colloidal solution), which surrounds the **nucleus**: the control center for cell activity (Fig. 3-3). The nucleus is encapsulated by a nuclear membrane that provides a barrier for the nucleus from other materials in the cell structure. Organelles, or little organs, are also found in the cytoplasm. Types of organelles include the endoplasmic reticulum, which

assists in allowing passage through the membrane; ribosomes, which are attached to the endoplasmic reticulum and function as enzymes responsible for the control of protein synthesis; mitochondria, the center of respiration for the cell; lysosomes, the enzymes that assist in digestion; Golgi apparatus, which receives molecules of protein from the endoplasmic reticulum; plastids, which are responsible for forming carbohydrates; and vacuoles, fluid-filled cavities that control molecular movement from the vacuole to the remaining cell.

Cell Membrane

The cell membrane, also known as the plasma membrane, provides a barrier between the inside and the outside of the cell. The membrane allows passage of certain molecules to and from the cytoplasm; thus, the membrane is considered selectively permeable. Passage through the membrane of lipid-soluble molecules, including gases and water, occurs by diffusion. Diffusion is the movement from an area of greater concentration to one of lesser concentration to attain equilibrium (Fig. 3-4).

Osmosis is another form of molecular movement. When a greater concentration of water exists on one side of a permeable membrane, water crosses (osmosis) to

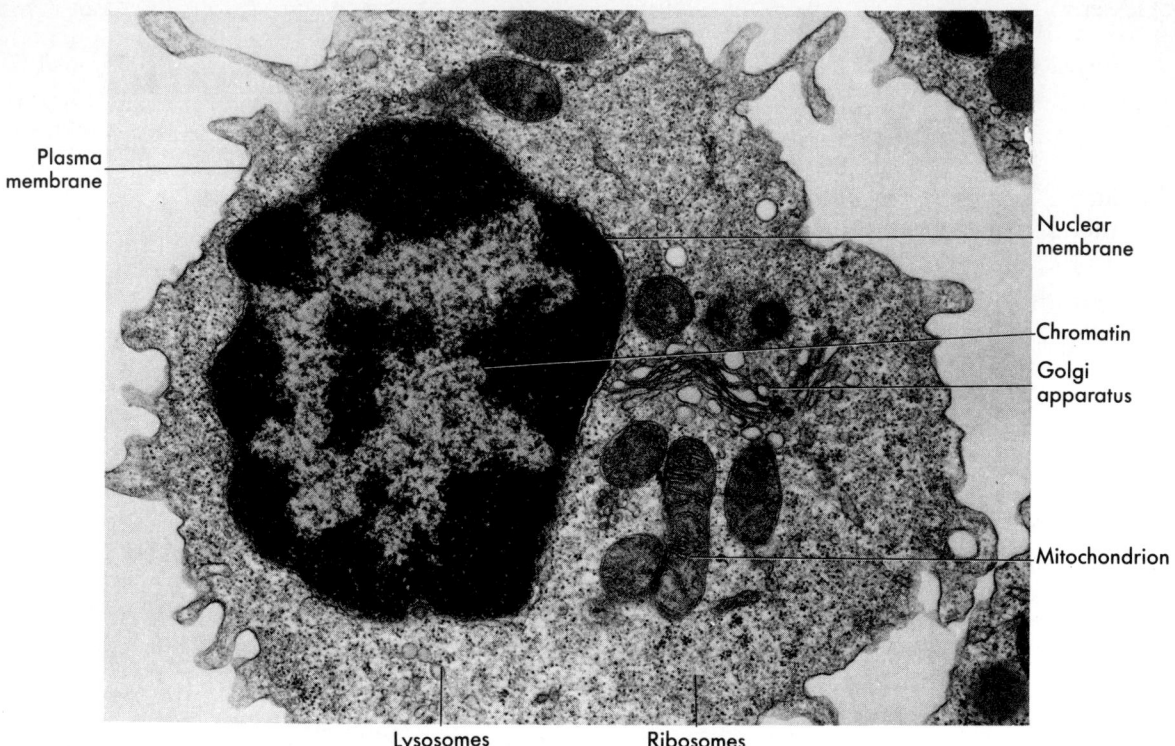

Plasma membrane

Nuclear membrane

Chromatin

Golgi apparatus

Mitochondrion

Lysosomes   Ribosomes

FIG. 3-3   Color-enhanced electron micrograph of a cell.

(From Thibodeau GA, Patton KT: *Anatomy and physiology*, ed 2, St Louis, 1992, Mosby.)

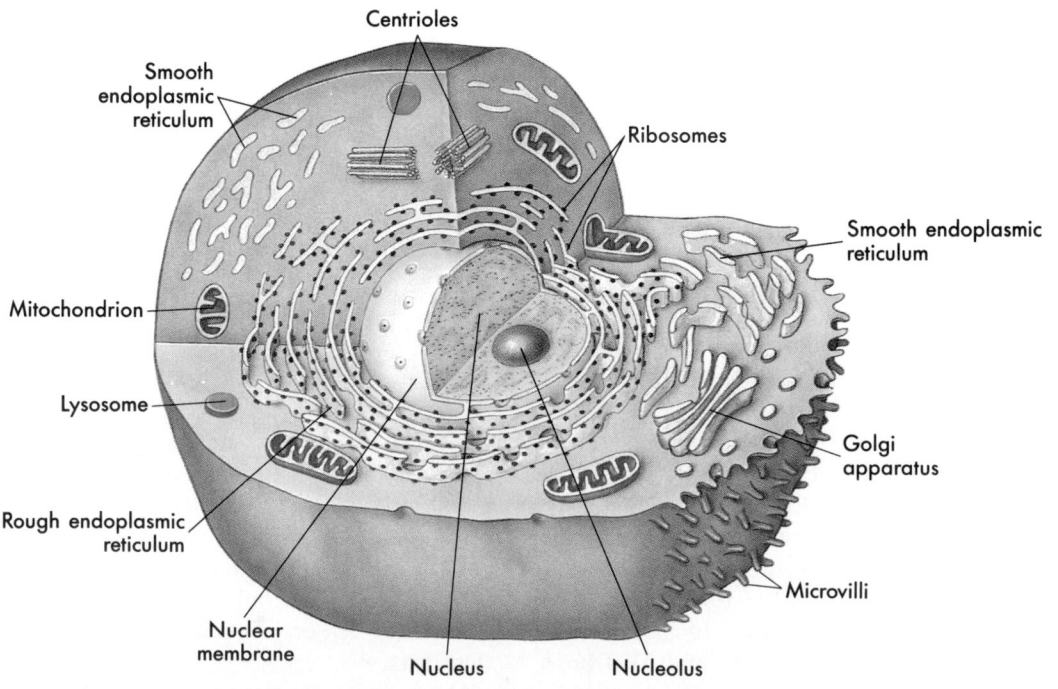

Centrioles

Smooth endoplasmic reticulum

Ribosomes

Smooth endoplasmic reticulum

Mitochondrion

Lysosome

Golgi apparatus

Rough endoplasmic reticulum

Microvilli

Nuclear membrane

Nucleus   Nucleolus

FIG. 3-4   Cell structure.

(From Thibodeau GA, Patton KT: *Anatomy and physiology*, ed 2, St Louis, 1992, Mosby.)

the side of lesser water concentration until equilibrium is reached.

To achieve homeostasis, or an internal stability within a living structure, an organism of any form must undergo change. The change of conditions may be from within or from an external environment to maintain balance and continue to survive. A living cell has this capability, as shown with the mechanisms of diffusion and osmosis.

▶ Tissues and Organs

Each system is composed of different and specialized cells, including the following basic tissues: **connective**, **epithelial**, **muscle**, **blood**, and **nervous tissue**. A **tissue** is a combination of cells, crystals, fibers, and fluids that have similar shape and function. For instance, the cells that make up the tissue that lines the digestive tract can make chemicals that digest and absorb the food a person eats.

An **organ** is made of a group of tissues that work together to carry out a specific function. Different tissues, such as blood and nerve tissue, are found together in organs. For example, the tooth is an organ made of connective, blood, and nerve tissues. The following list of body tissues describes the various functions:

Connective tissue—provides support to body structures

Epithelial tissue—covers the outer body and inner structures to provide protection

Muscle tissue—provides motion through contraction and stretching

Blood—type of connective tissue that supplies food and oxygen throughout the body while fighting infection

Nerve tissue—provides stimulation to and from parts of the body

TABLE 3-1   ORGAN SYSTEMS

Organ system	Function/responsibility	Relationship to dentistry
Muscular	Responsible for body movement and heat.	Assists in deglutination, phonetics.
Nervous	Regulates all body activity learning and memory.	Major nerve affecting the area of head and neck; includes the trigeminal nerve.
Respiratory	Exchanges gaseous substances between the environment and the blood.	The head is the first source of breathing for both internal and external respiration; mouth breathing as a source of respiration causes complications in the oral cavity.
Circulatory	Transports life-necessary substance to cells and removes metabolic waste from cells.	Use of a vasoconstrictor to obtain anesthesia in the oral cavity may have an effect when the patient has contraindications to this therapy. Hematologic studies would verify systemic disease.
Skeletal	Provides framework and supports structures and flexibility for movement of the body; produces blood cells.	The skull as part of the skeletal system includes the only movable part, which is the mandible working on a hinge. Anomalies in skeletal development relate to malocclusion and facial development.
Lymphatic	Provides body immunity, drains body fluids, and absorbs fats.	It is important to protect the lymphatic system, particularly the area of head and neck, from radiation exposure. This system produces fluids at the site of infection.
Urinary	Filters blood and maintains the volume as well as chemical composition of blood.	Secretions from this system are used to test for systemic diseases.
Endocrine	Secretes hormones for regulation with chemicals in the body.	Radiation to the thyroid during diagnostic radiography can cause abnormal behavior in the gland.
Digestive	Continues the function of breaking down and absorbing food.	Digestion begins in the oral cavity through mastication. A patient with dental pain may not be able to masticate easily.
Male reproductive	Produces sperm and transfers the sperm to the female reproductive system.	Radiation used in the diagnosis of oral anomalies can cause damage to male reproductive ability.
Female reproductive	Produces ova and receives sperm from the male; area where fertilization of ovum, implantation, and development of embryo to fetus and delivery of the fetus take place.	Radiation used in the diagnosis of oral anomalies can cause damage to female reproductive ability. Diet during pregnancy may affect the development of the fetus.

▶ Body Systems

A body **system** is a similar group of tissues or organs that perform like functions. Many of the systems are directly related to dentistry, while others are more abstract in their relationship (Table 3-1).

Skeletal System

This system is a combination of bones that provides the underlying structure or frame for the body. The skeleton shapes and supports the body and provides protection for internal organs. The skeleton is the framework to which muscles are attached, and it also stores certain chemicals for use by the body (Fig. 3-5, *A*).

Relationship of Skeletal System to Dentistry. This system provides the maxilla (upper jaw) and the mandible (lower jaw), which support the teeth. The cranium and facial structure are formed by the skeletal system; thus this system is one of the primary systems to be studied in dentistry.

Muscular System

The muscular system provides the tissue that allows for movement of all the parts of the body. Muscles are used when a person walks, talks, blinks, chews, breathes, and listens. The human body contains three kinds of muscle fibers: smooth, striated, and heart or cardiac (Fig. 3-5, *B*).

Relationship of Muscular System to Dentistry. Muscles are important to dentistry. They aid in talking, chewing, swallowing, eating, and smiling. In addition, muscles provide a person the ability to change facial expressions. There are more than 300 muscles in the human body, with various muscles involved with the head and neck area. Muscles make up to 30% to 40% of a person's weight. Muscles that are not exercised regularly can become weak, soft, and flabby. This is evidenced in dentistry when individuals lose their teeth and become edentulous. The muscles of the face begin to sag from loss of support and normal use, often causing these people to look older than their chronologic age.

Nervous System

The nervous system is a combination of the brain, spinal cord, and nerve cells, or neurons, that run throughout the body. A **neuron** is the structural and functional unit of nervous tissue. Nerves carry messages back and forth between the brain and the rest of the body. The muscles of the body are controlled by the nervous system. For instance, the following sequence occurs when a dental assistant passes dental instruments: (1) the nervous system sends messages to contract the voluntary, striated muscles in the person's arms and hands; (2) messages are then sent through nerves to the brain and to the eyes, causing the eyes to focus on an instrument; and (3) then other messages are sent, causing the hands to pick up an instrument, grasp it, and transfer it to the dentist (Fig. 3-5, *C*).

Relationship of the Nervous System to Dentistry. The nervous system is important to dentistry because nerves innervate and control the senses emanating from the area of the head and neck. The dental assistant will need to understand the function and location of nerves in the head and neck area, which will be discussed later in this and in the chapter on anesthesia. As the assistant prepares anesthesia for treatment procedures, it will be necessary to know which nerves are to be anesthetized or numbed.

Each tooth is supplied with one or more nerves, depending on its anatomic structure. Also, when a patient complains of certain types of pain, the dentist will seek to determine if there has been trauma, disease, or degeneration of the nerve. Thus the nervous system is directly related to dental treatment.

Circulatory System

The major parts of the human circulatory, or cardiovascular, system are the blood, blood vessels, heart, and lymph. This system is responsible for moving food, water, and oxygen throughout the body to sustain life and growth (Fig. 3-5, *D*).

The heart is a pump that forces blood out to the tissues of the body through blood vessels. Blood vessels include arteries, veins, and capillaries. An artery carries blood away from the heart; a vein carries blood to the heart; and capillaries are small vessels that connect arteries to veins. Arteries have thick, elastic walls, whereas veins have thin walls with valves to prevent the backflow of blood. Capillaries have walls that are only one cell thick.

Blood is the fluid that transports all of the body substances. It is a special type of connective tissue that consists of a solid part, called blood cells, and a nonliving substance called plasma. Three types of blood cells exist: white cells or leukocytes, red cells or erythrocytes, and platelets or thrombocytes. These cells are scattered throughout the plasma. Plasma is composed of water, proteins, digested food, mineral salts, organic nutrients, and cell wastes.

Red cells are shaped like discs and do not have a nucleus. These cells contain a red pigment called hemoglobin, a protein substance that is essential to life. White blood cells are larger than red ones, have a nucleus, contain no hemoglobin, are colorless, and are capable of ameboid movement. There are fewer white cells than red cells in the body, with approximately one white cell for every 600 red cells. White blood cells are an important defense for the body against infection. In fact, whenever a person develops an infection, the white blood cell count rises as white cells collect in the infected area, ingest, and destroy bacteria. The remains of dead bacteria, white blood cells, and tissue fluid are referred to as *pus*.

Platelets are much smaller than red blood cells, are shaped irregularly, and are colorless; they are formed in the red marrow. These cells are incapable of moving on their own and simply float along in the bloodstream. Platelets are important in forming blood clots. Clotting occurs when chemical and physical changes take place in the blood. If an area of the body is wounded and bleeds, platelets disintegrate as the blood leaves a vessel. As the platelets disintegrate, thromboplastin, an agent in clotting, is released. Thromboplastin reacts with prothrombin, which is produced by the liver, in the presence of calcium, which allows the formation of thrombin. Thrombin changes the soluble blood protein of the fibrinogen to fibrin in the injured area. Fibrin is a network of tiny threads that traps blood cells, forming a clot in the area of tissue damage and stopping additional blood from leaving the area.

Relationship of the Circulatory System to Dentistry. Circulation is vital to dentistry. The alteration of blood pressure, which is the measure of the pressure of blood in arteries, from normal can be a contraindication or negative factor in the treatment of a patient. Other factors, such as poor circulation, coronary disease, clotting anomalies, or other blood diseases can be reasons to carefully examine the patient before beginning treatment.

A patient's blood count can be important when a surgical procedure is undertaken. A person who is taking blood-thinning medication may have an inadequate amount of platelets to promote clotting; surgery may be postponed or consultation with the physician may be necessary to alter the dosage of medication.

Just as nerves supply the teeth, blood is supplied to each tooth and provides nourishment. When trauma occurs to a tooth, the blood supply may be reduced or lost, possibly causing the loss of tooth vitality.

Respiratory System

The respiratory system includes the nose, pharynx, larynx, trachea, bronchi, sinuses, and lungs. The body cells need a continuous supply of oxygen. The oxygen that is carried to the cells by the circulatory system comes from the air a person breathes. Breathing and supplying the blood with oxygen are two functions of the respiratory system. This system also removes carbon dioxide from the blood (Fig. 3-5, *E*).

As air passes through the nose, it is warmed. Moisture is added to the air, and it then passes toward the trachea. The trachea is the tube that transports air into the lungs. At the top of the trachea is a structure called the larynx, which is composed of cartilage and contains the vocal cords. When air passes over these vocal cords during movements of the mouth and tongue, sounds are produced, creating speech. The trachea and larynx are protected by the epiglottis, a flap of cartilage. Most of the time the trachea is open. However, when a person swallows, the epiglottis covers the top of the trachea, preventing food from entering it.

As the air continues to pass into the chest cavity, the trachea divides into slightly smaller tubes called *bronchi,* then into bronchioles, which terminate as alveoli, small, thin-walled air-filled sacs. Each alveolus is surrounded by capillaries. When a person inhales, the alveoli fill with air. Oxygen from the air diffuses through the alveolar walls and then through the capillary walls into the blood. The blood carries the oxygen to body cells. At the same time, carbon dioxide, a waste product of the body cells, diffuses into the blood and is carried back to the alveoli. The carbon dioxide is pushed out of the lungs as the person exhales.

Relationship of the Respiratory System to Dentistry. The respiratory system plays a significant role in dentistry. Blockage of the nose and sinuses can force a person to become a mouth breather, possibly damaging the oral tissues over a long period of time. Sinus pain can also be confused with dental pain because of the location of the sinuses. The use of nitrous oxide analgesia must be followed up with an appropriate inhalation of oxygen to prevent damage to the lungs.

Digestive System

The mouth, teeth, salivary glands, pharynx, esophagus, stomach, intestines, liver, gallbladder, and pancreas are organs of the digestive system that work together to process food for use by the body. Digestion begins in the mouth. The teeth break off and grind the food as the **salivary glands** secrete enzymes that begin the digestive process. As foods move throughout the digestive tract, they undergo a series of chemical changes. During each step, a specific enzyme is secreted (Fig. 3-5, *F*).

Relationship of the Digestive System to Dentistry. Without teeth and salivary glands to aid in mastication, the digestive process is inhibited.

Excretory System

The kidneys, ureters, urinary bladder, urethra, and skin are the organs of the excretory system, which is also

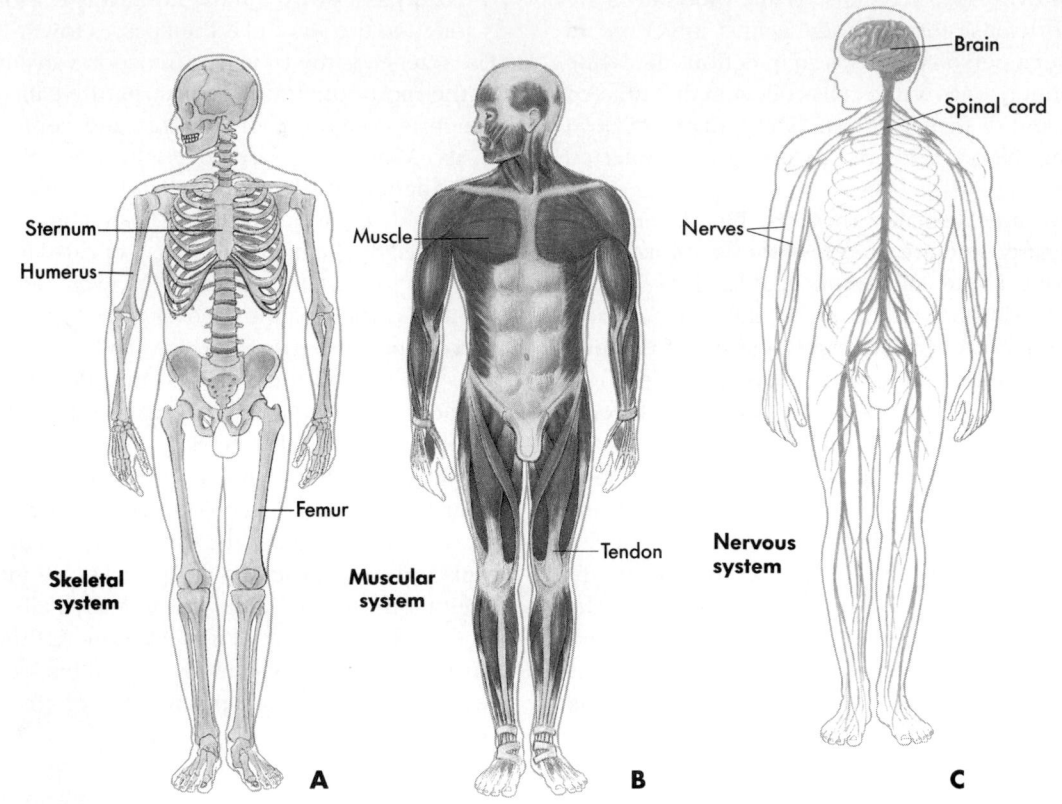

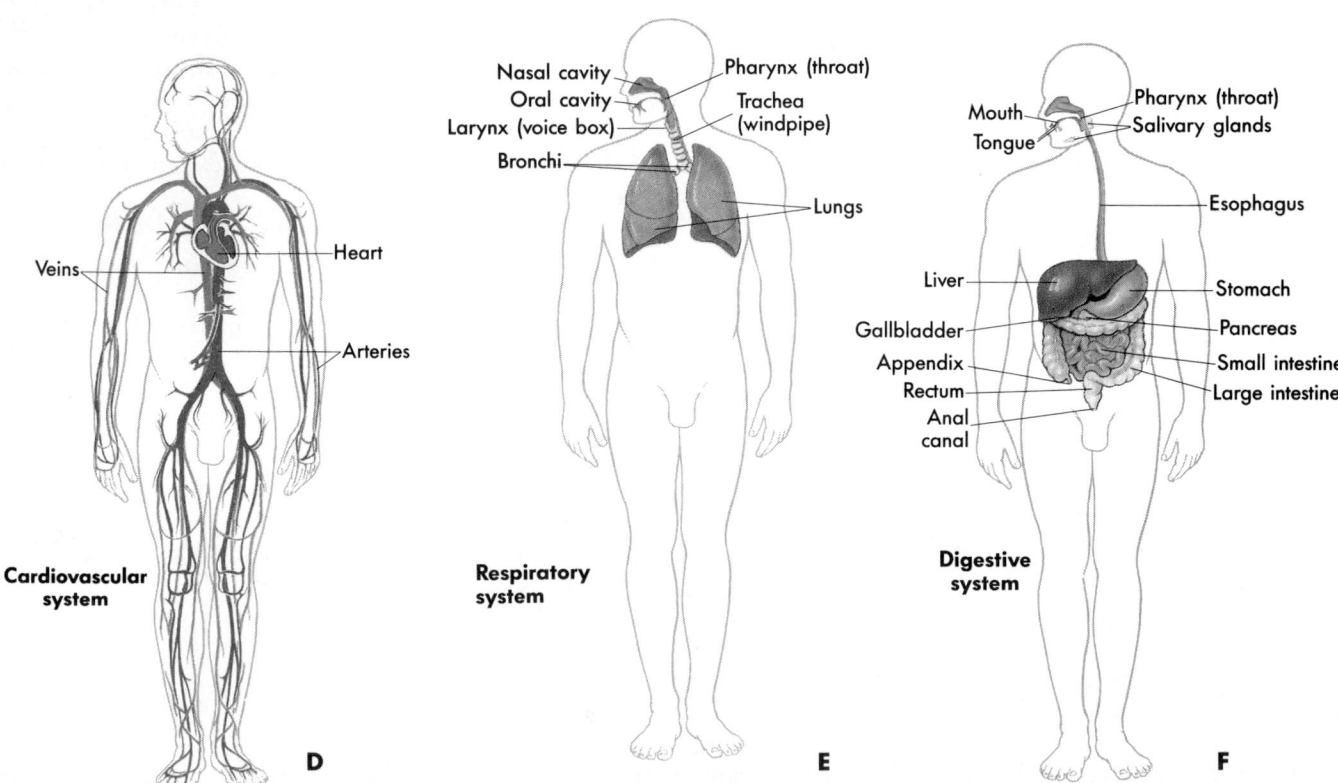

FIG. 3-5   The eleven systems of the body.

(From Thibodeau GA, Patton KT: *Anatomy and physiology*, ed 2, St Louis, 1992, Mosby.)

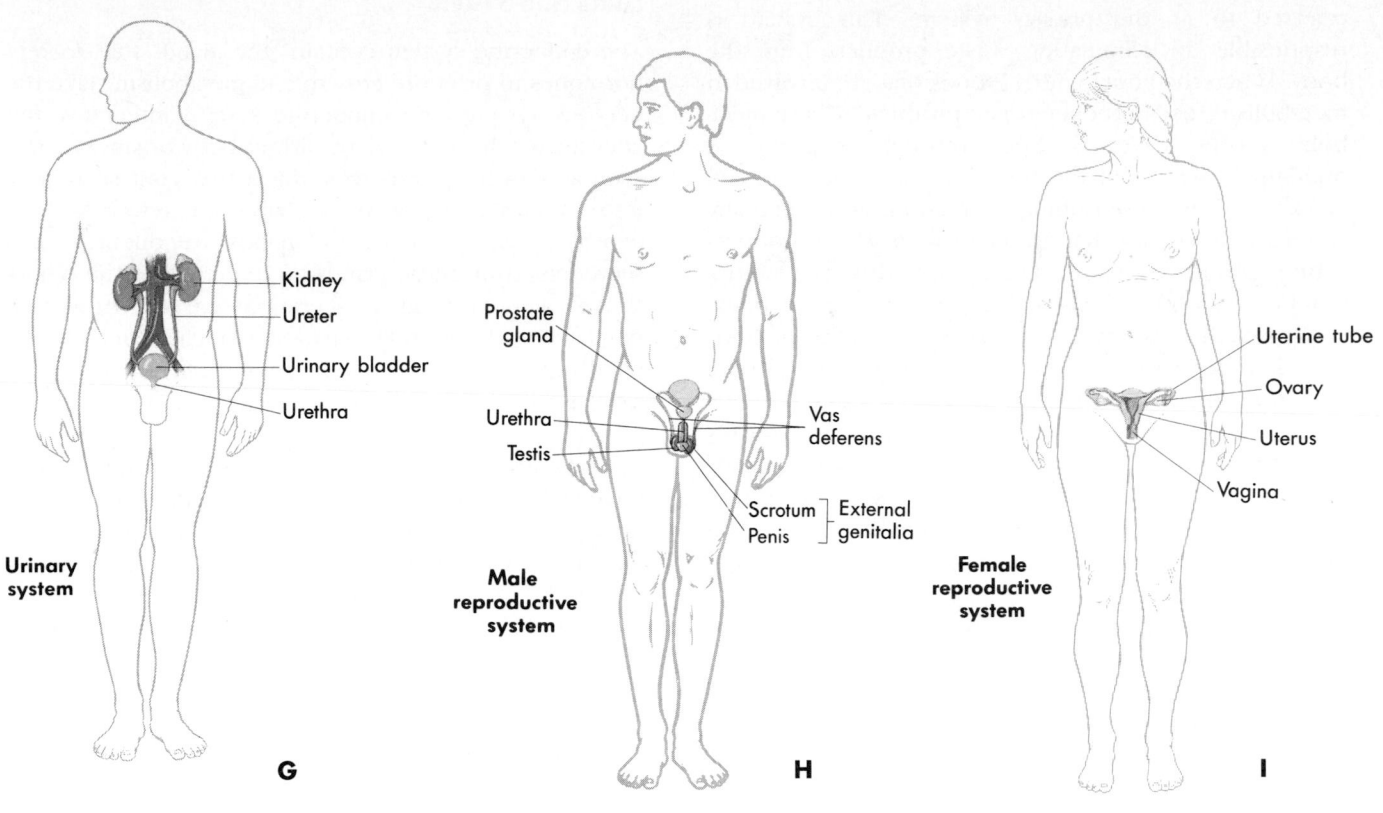

Kidney
Ureter
Urinary bladder
Urethra

Urinary system

G

Prostate gland
Urethra
Testis
Vas deferens
Scrotum
Penis
External genitalia

Male reproductive system

H

Uterine tube
Ovary
Uterus
Vagina

Female reproductive system

I

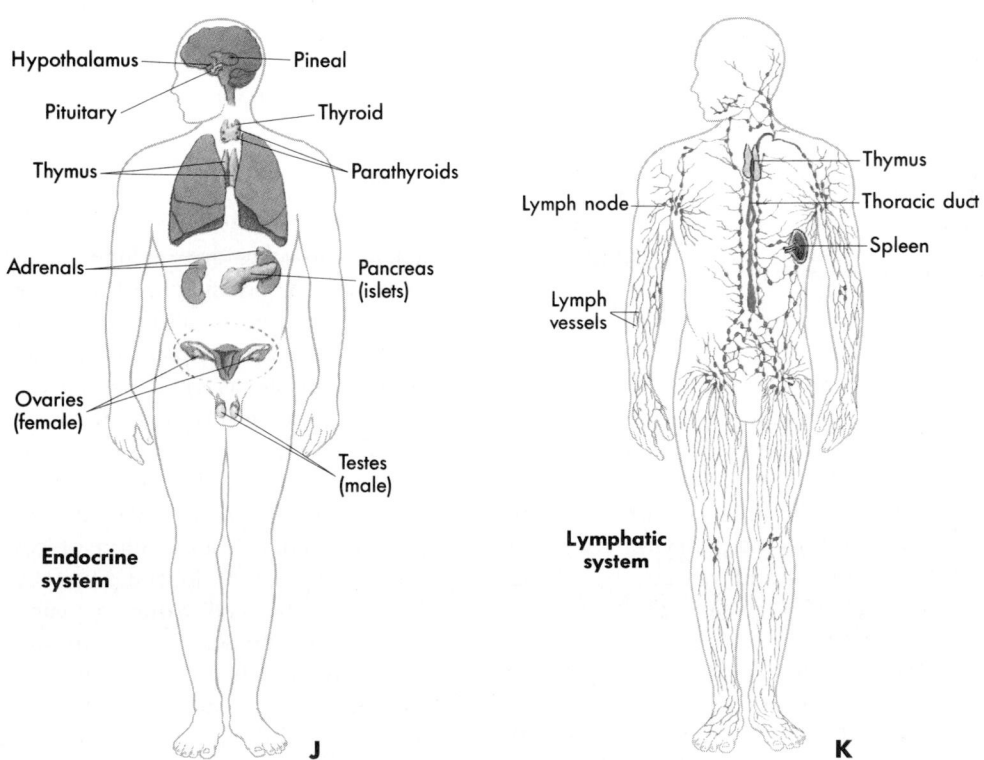

Hypothalamus
Pineal
Pituitary
Thyroid
Thymus
Parathyroids
Adrenals
Pancreas (islets)
Ovaries (female)
Testes (male)

Endocrine system

J

Thymus
Lymph node
Thoracic duct
Spleen
Lymph vessels

Lymphatic system

K

FIG. 3-5, cont'd.   The eleven systems of the body.

referred to as the urinary system. This system is responsible for eliminating waste products from the body. When the body oxidizes foods that are involved in metabolism, cells produce waste products. These metabolic wastes leave the body through excretion. A build-up of wastes in the tissues is dangerous and can cause rapid tissue poisoning, starvation, and eventually suffocation. Tissues that are filled with waste products cannot absorb food or oxygen, and thus the body's functioning cannot be sustained. In the human body, cells discharge their waste materials into the tissue fluid. This fluid flows to the bloodstream and is carried to the excretory organs for elimination (Fig. 3-5, *G*).

The kidneys are the primary excretory organs. Wastes are brought to the kidneys through the bloodstream, and, after an elaborate filtering process, the waste, or urine, passes to the ureters. The ureters carry the urine to the urinary bladder, and the urine is then excreted through the urethra.

The skin is also an excretory organ. It is made of the epidermis (outer layer) and the dermis (the layer beneath the epidermis). Excretion through the skin is in the form of perspiration, which helps to regulate body temperature.

Relationship of the Excretory System to Dentistry. The excretory system does not have a primary relationship to dentistry. However, the oral cavity aids in the beginning of the digestive processes that ultimately produce the wastes excreted from the body. A patient with systemic diseases of the organs of this system may be taking medication that could potentially contraindicate dental treatment. Symptoms of disease are often indicated by this system; for example, when infection is evident, the skin may be warm or it may be red and clammy.

Reproductive System

The reproductive system provides new life through the combination of ovaries, fallopian tubes, uterus, vagina, mammary glands, testes, and penis. The primitive germ layers—the ectoderm, mesoderm, and endoderm—actively form structures of skin, cartilage, nervous system, lining of the mouth to the pharynx, connective tissue, bone, muscles, blood and vessels, lymphatics, trachea, and other structures (Fig. 3-5, *H* and *I*).

Relationship of the Reproductive System to Dentistry. Genetic **anomalies** (abnormalities) that develop from this system may be identified in the dental arches of the child. Toxins from dental infections of the mother can be dangerous to a fetus. Care should be taken to protect pregnant patients from exposure to dental radiography during the second week through the sixth week of gestation to safeguard the development of the fetus.

Endocrine System

The endocrine system contains the glands that secrete hormones to promote growth and metabolism. Like the nervous system, the endocrine system integrates and coordinates the activities of various body organs. Glands such as salivary glands have ducts that emit secretions into an organ. These duct glands are referred to as exocrine glands. Endocrine glands are ductless, and secretions from these glands go directly into the bloodstream. Endocrine gland secretions are known as hormones. Glands that are in this system include the thyroid, parathyroid, pituitary, adrenal, pancreas, thymus, ovaries, testes, and hypothalamus (Fig. 3-5, *J*).

Relationship of the Endocrine System to Dentistry. The relationship of the endocrine system to dentistry is both direct and indirect. Directly, this system is responsible for the metabolism of sugars and starches that takes place during the digestive process, which of course begins in the oral cavity.

Indirectly, this system affects the practice of dentistry when a patient presents for treatment and has a disease in any of the organs of this system. For instance, a patient with diabetes mellitus is unable to store or oxidize sugar properly—the result of a poorly functioning pancreas. Healing is affected in this patient, and treatment may need to be altered to compensate for any medications that the patient may be taking for the disease. Similar situations can develop if a patient has a history of disease in any other endocrine organ.

Sensory System

Organs that provide the sense of vision, hearing, touch, smell, and taste are included in the sensory system. Special sense organs called receptors are located in the skin. There are five different kinds of receptors, including touch, pressure, pain, heat, and cold. Obviously the sense of taste is in a person's mouth, specifically involving the taste buds on the tongue. The four flavors that can be recognized—sweet, sour, salty, and bitter—originate from papillae on the tongue.

The sense of smell, like the sense of taste, results from a chemical stimulation of certain nerve endings; these are located in the nose. A person's sense of hearing is derived from the ear—a complex organ. Vision, of course, comes from the eye. Later, in discussing the anatomic structure of the head and neck, each of these organs will be involved, since they are all close to the mouth and often have nerves and blood vessels that supply the same areas.

Relationship of the Sensory System to Dentistry. The sensory system is closely related to dentistry, since many of the organs responsible for these senses are located within close proximity to the oral cavity. When a patient has lost complete use of any of these senses, the dental assistant must provide special attention. For instance, special efforts to communicate with the patient whose vision or hearing is impaired will need to be made.

Lymphatic System

Lymph fluid, a tissue fluid, carries nutrients and oxygen to the cells, as well as removes wastes and other products from the cells. Tiny lymph vessels group together, forming larger vessels that enlarge to create lymph nodes or glands.

The function of lymph nodes is to cleanse lymph fluid before it returns to the blood. The area of the head and neck contains many lymph nodes, such as the tonsils and adenoids (Fig. 3-5, *K*).

Relationship of the Lymphatic System to Dentistry. The lymphatic system has both a direct and an indirect relationship to dentistry. The tonsils, which are found in the oral cavity, may become inflamed and swollen with infection, making dental treatment uncomfortable, if not difficult, for the patient. Lymph nodes that are found to be enlarged during an extraoral examination may prompt the dentist to refer the patient to a physician for further examination.

▶ The Skeletal System

The skeletal system consists primarily of a hard connective tissue called **bone** that forms the framework of the body. Periosteum is a form of connective tissue that covers bones throughout the body.

There are two types of bone: *compact* and *cancellous.* Compact or cortical bone is strong, hard, and dense. Cancellous or spongy bone is not as strong and weighs less than compact bone. Both of these bone types are formed by cells called **osteoblasts**. Osteo means *bone* and blast refers to *former.* Bone may be destroyed by cells called **osteoclasts**—*clasts* meaning something that destroys. Under certain conditions, particularly under orthodontic treatment, the two cells may work together in response to stress placed during the treatment. Bone may be disturbed during the movement of teeth through osteoclast activity, while osteoblasts assist in forming new bone growth around the new position of the teeth.

Bones of the Skull

The bones of the skull consist of cranial and facial bones, for a total of 22; they are found in pairs or as single bones. Table 3-2 lists the name of the bones found in both categories. Fig. 3-6, *A* through *D,* illustrates the location of the bones of the skull.

TABLE 3-2   CRANIAL BONES

Name of bone	Number of bones
Ethmoid	1
Frontal	1
Occipital	1
Parietal	2
Sphenoid	1
Temporal	2
Total	8

FACIAL BONES

Name of bone	Number of bones
Inferior nasal conchae	2
Lacrimal	2
Mandible	1
Maxilla	2
Nasal	2
Palatine	2
Vomer	1
Zygomatic	2
Total	14

The following are important terms that pertain to the location of the bones of the skull:

Canal - a long tube opening through bone

Condyle - a rounded surface at the articular end of a bone

Foramen - a short opening in a bone or other structure

Fossa - a pit, hollow, or depression in bone

Meatus - an opening or tunnel through the body

Process - a distinct projection of bone

Septum - a thin bony layer separating two areas, such as the nasal cavities

Sinus - a hollow space or opening, a cavity

Suture - a rigid joint formed between two bones by cartilage, connective tissue, or bone

Tubercle - a rounded elevation on the surface of tissue

By viewing the various aspects of the skull found in Fig. 3-6, *A* through *D.* Most of these structures can be located.

F
Y
I

Leonardo da Vinci (1452-1519) completed some of the original studies of the skull. His drawings of the skull and teeth illustrate a distinction between molars and premolars, which had not previously been distinguished.

Cranial Bones

The ethmoid bone is a single cranial bone that houses the paranasal sinuses. Combined with the vomer and cartilage, it forms the *nasal septum.* The *cribriform plate,* which is the horizontal portion of the ethmoid, is a

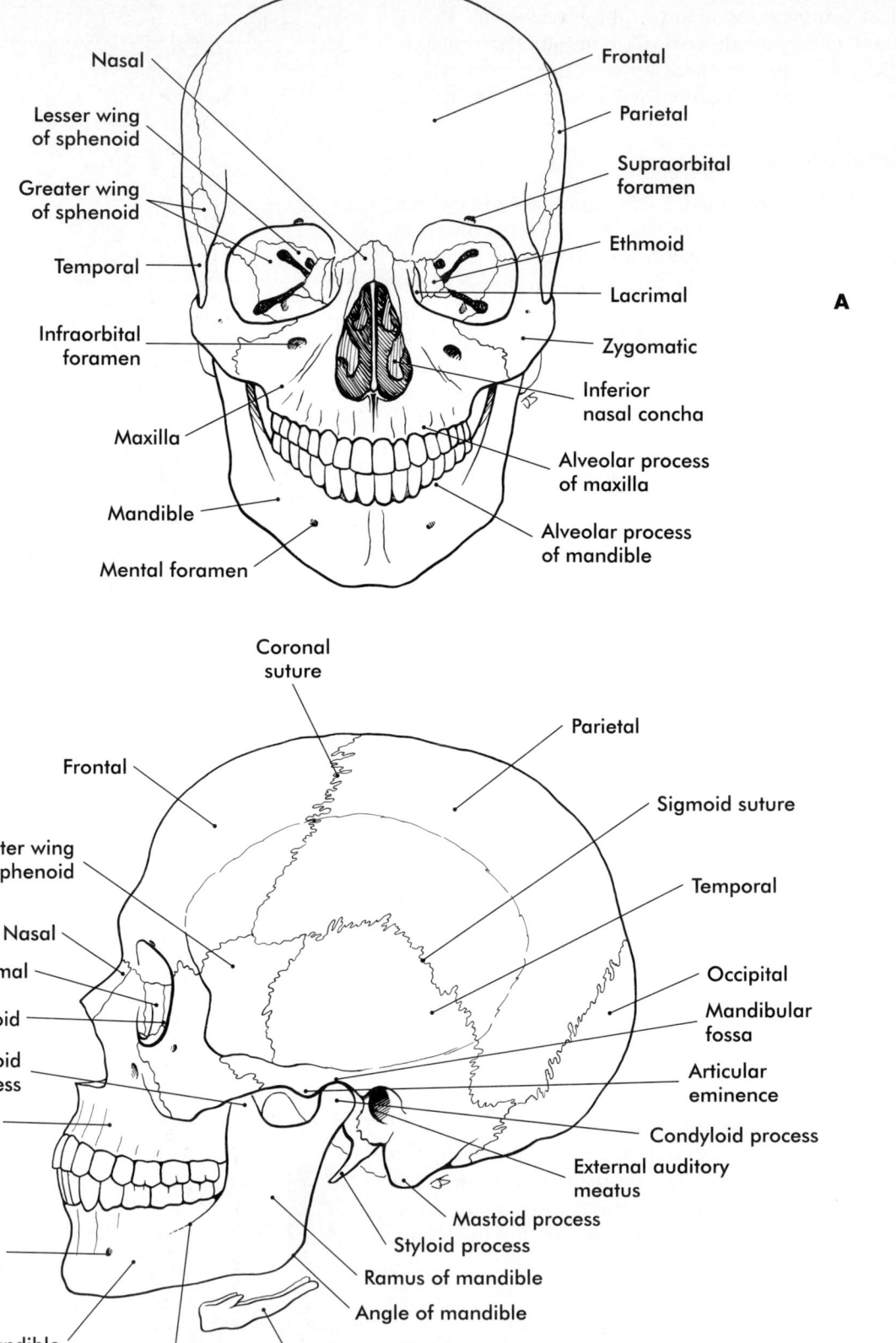

FIG. 3-6 *A,* Frontal view of the skull. *B,* Lateral view of the skull.

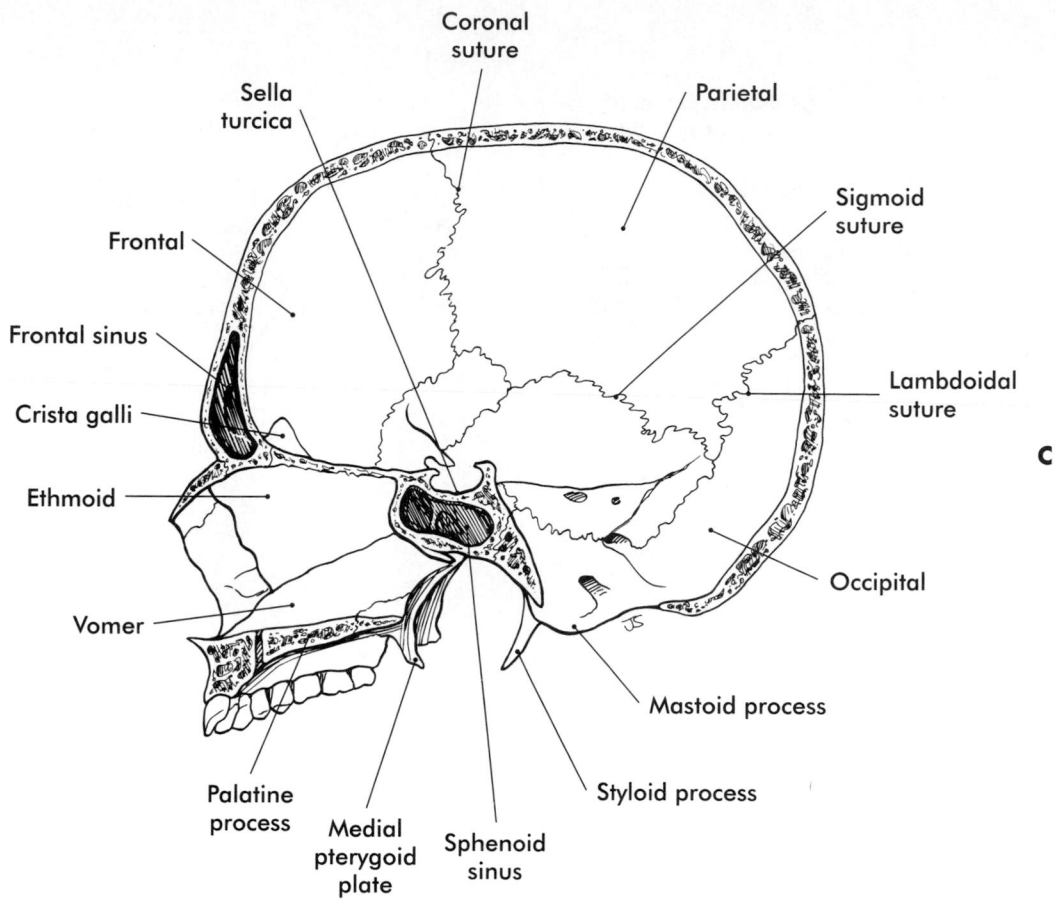

FIG. 3-6, cont'd.   *C,* Cross-section of the skull.

passageway for the olfactory nerves to the brain. The superior portion, called the *crista galli,* also projects through the frontal bone and attaches to the layers of the brain tissue.

The frontal bone, a single bone, forms the anterior portion of the skull, the forehead, the orbits of the eye, and the nasal cavity. As the frontal bone extends laterally, it contacts the *zygomatic arch.*

The occipital bone, another single bone, forms the inferior and posterior portion of the skull. It contains the *foramen magnum*—the passageway for the spinal cord. It also joins with the parietal bones to form the *lambdoid suture.*

The parietal bones form a contact with the frontal, sphenoid, and occipital bones. The two parietal bones meet at the top of the head, at the site of the *coronal suture,* and at the lambdoid suture.

The sphenoid bone is divided into two segments: the greater wing and the lesser wing. The greater wing contacts the temporal bone on both sides of the skull and contacts the frontal bone and zygomatic arch anteriorly, forming part of the orbit. The lesser wing also forms part

of the orbit by articulating with the ethmoid and frontal bones. The sphenoid also contains the sphenoid sinuses.

The temporal bones form the sides of the skull and the base of the cranium. The bone radiates anteriorly to the zygomatic process. The area inferior to the zygomatic arch is where the temporal bone encompasses the *glenoid fossa.* Here the *mandibular condyle* articulates with the glenoid fossa and forms the temporomandibular joint. The mastoid and styloid processes are also projections of the temporal bone (Fig. 3-6, *A* through *D*).

Facial Bones

The inferior nasal conchae are small bones in the floor of the nasal cavity that attach to its lateral walls. The lacrimal bones are also small bones that are a part of the orbit of the eye. These bones form the medial surface of the orbit and articulate with the **maxillae**, or the upper jaw. The *lacrimal fossa,* which is located in the lacrimal bones, houses the *lacrimal sac*—the collection site of tears that are secreted through the *lacrimal gland.*

The **mandible** is the lower jaw and the only movable

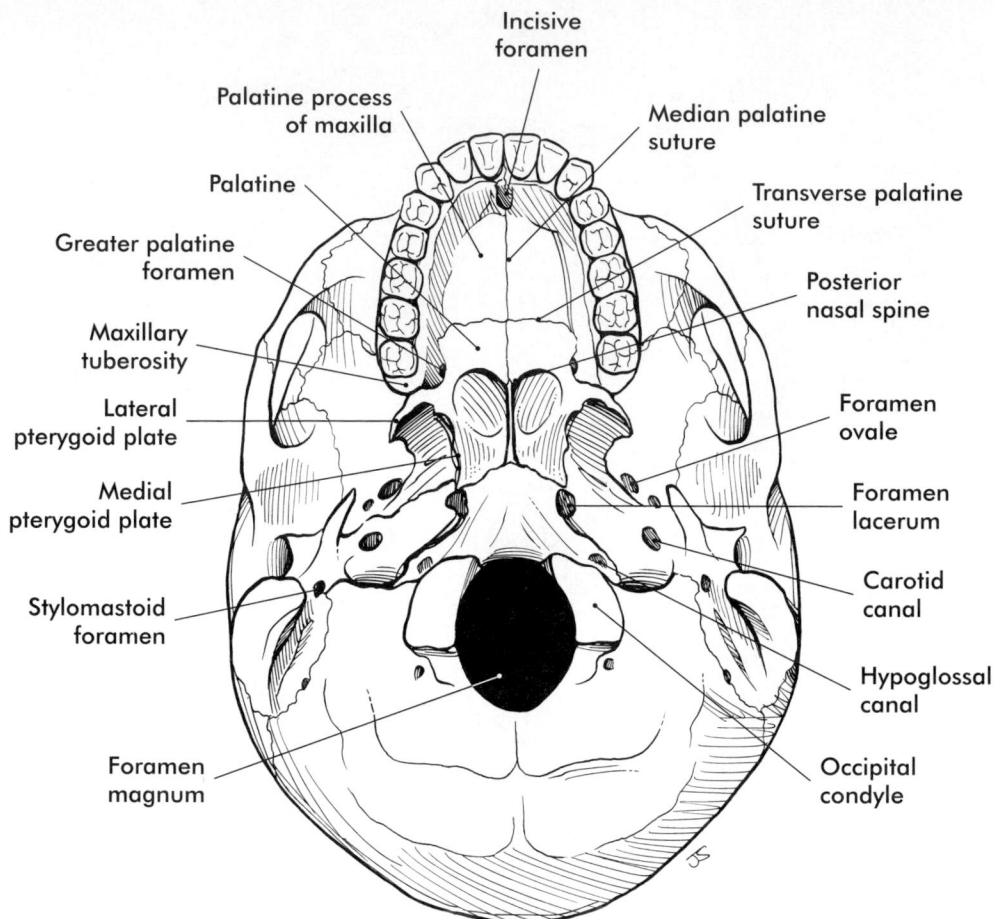

FIG. 3-6, cont'd.   *D,* Inferior view of the skull (minus the mandible).

bone in the skull. The mandible consists of the body, the horizontal portion or **alveolar process,** the portions that surround the teeth, and the **ramus** or vertical segment. The mandible supports the teeth and forms the shape of the lower face. It also provides a framework for the floor of the mouth and is the area of attachments for muscles involved in mastication and facial expression (Fig. 3-7).

The **symphysis,** the chin, is where the two halves of the mandible meet. The exact point of the junction is called the *mental protuberance.* The *mental foramina,* which contain the pathways for blood and nerve vessels in the mandible, are just posterior to the protuberance. The *genial tubercles* are also located near the mental protuberance on the medial surface. The body of the mandible extends and meets the *angle of the mandible,* which is the division between the ramus and the body of the mandible. The most anterior portion of the vertical segment of the ramus is the *coronoid process.* The coronoid process is positioned anterior to the *coronoid notch,* which is anterior to the condyle and posterior to the ramus. Contained within the structure of the ramus are the *mandibular foramina,* located on the medial

surface. Two additional fossae are found in the mandible: the *sublingual fossa* and the *submandibular fossa,* which contain the salivary glands.

Two ridges also exist on the mandible: on the lingual surface, the *mylohyoid ridge* or *groove,* and on the external surface near the ramus, the *oblique ridge* or *line.* Superior to the mylohyoid ridge is the *internal oblique line.*

The *mandibular notch* is positioned below the mandibular foramen and anterior of the angle of the mandible.

The maxillary bones combine to form the upper jaw, or maxilla, providing shape to the upper part of the face. The maxilla also provides the *hard palate,* the maxillary alveolar process, the floor of the orbit, and the lateral wall of the nose. Within the maxilla is the *maxillary sinus; the palatine process,* where the *palatine suture* is located; the *anterior nasal spine;* the *canine eminence;* and the *canine fossa.* A bony extension posterior to the maxillary teeth is called the *maxillary tuberosity;* it is similar to the retromolar pad found in the mandible.

Nasal bones combine to create the bones for the bridge

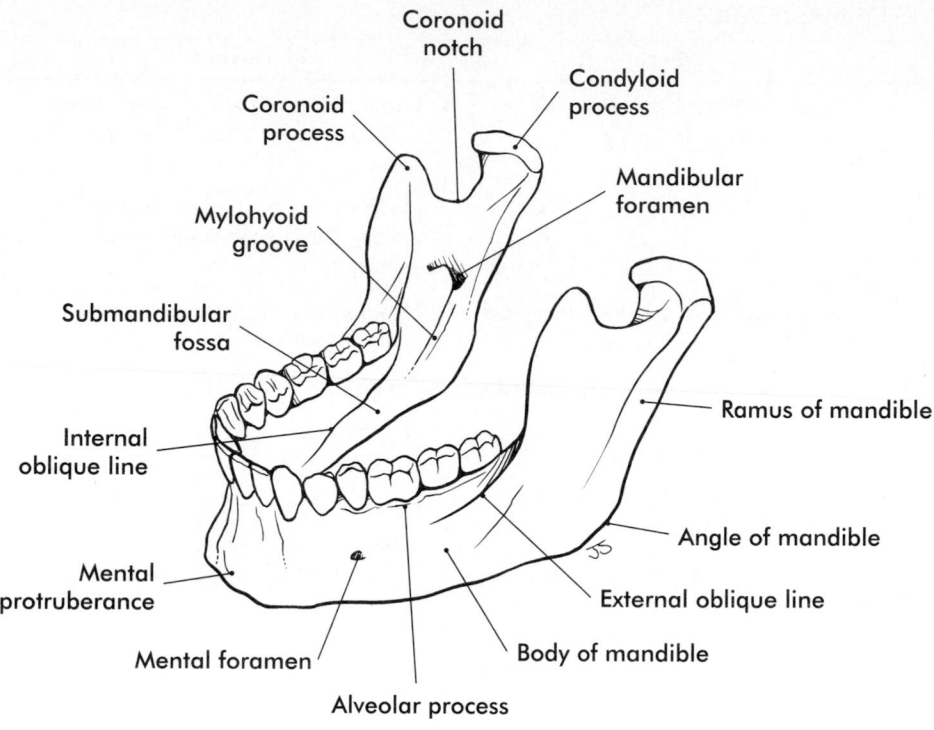

Coronoid notch

Condyloid process

Coronoid process

Mandibular foramen

Mylohyoid groove

Submandibular fossa

Ramus of mandible

Internal oblique line

Angle of mandible

Mental protruberance

External oblique line

Mental foramen

Body of mandible

Alveolar process

FIG. 3-7 The mandible.

of the nose. The nasal bones articulate with the frontal bone and the maxilla. The vomer, a single bone, forms the base of the nasal septum.

The palatine bones contact both the maxilla and the sphenoid bones. Within the palatine bones are found the palatine foramen and the *median* and *transverse palatine sutures.*

The zygomatic bones form the cheeks of the facial structure. It connects with the zygomatic process and the temporal and frontal bones. The prominence of the cheek is created by the combined zygomatic process and temporal bone forming the zygomatic arch.

The hyoid bone is an integral aspect of the skull. It is suspended between the mandible and the larynx; it provides support for the tongue and other muscles. It is not always considered a portion of the skull but is a necessary bone to several functions (see Fig. 3-6, *B*).

▶ The Muscular System

The muscles of mastication and those muscles that are responsible for facial expression allow for movement in the skull, as do muscles in the rest of the human body. All muscles have an **origin**: the end of the muscle that is attached to a nonmovable structure; and an **insertion**: the end of the muscle that is attached to a movable structure. The body of the muscle is the area between the origin and the insertion. The origin and insertion of the muscles

normally attach to bone, but in some circumstances the attachments may be to soft tissue.

The Muscles of Mastication

Four pairs of muscles are grouped as the **muscles of mastication** and are the muscles that are responsible for chewing, tearing, and grinding food. These muscles are attached to the mandible (insertion) and the upper two thirds of the skull (origin). They provide the following movements of the mandible: protrusion, retrusion, elevation, and lateral movement. The four sets of muscles are paired and work in conjunction to contract, allowing the mandible to open and close. Box 3-5 defines the functions of the muscles of mastication.

The muscles are innervated by an area of the third

BOX 3-5

FUNCTIONS OF MUSCLES OF MASTICATION

Elevation	Moves the mandible up or in closing
Protrusion	Moves the mandible forward
Retrusion	Moves the mandible back
Depression	Lowers or opens the mouth
Lateral excursion	Moves the mandible sideways

TABLE 3-3   MUSCLES OF MASTICATION

Name	Origin	Insertion	Function
MASSETER	Lower, border, and medial surface of zygomatic arch	Lateral surface of coronoid process and along the anterior border of the ramus	Closes jaw
TEMPORALIS	Temporal bone	Medial surface of coronoid process and along the anterior border of the ramus	Closes jaw, retracts, or pulls back
MEDIAL PTERYGOID	Medial surface of the lateral pterygoid plate	Medial surface of the angle and ramus of mandible	Closes jaw and aids in protrusion
LATERAL PTERYGOID	Lateral surface of the lateral pterygoid plate	Condyle and disc of TMJ	Opens jaw and aids in protrusion

ACCESSORY MUSCLES			
Name	Origin	Insertion	Function
BUCCINATOR	Alveolar portion of maxilla and anterior portion of ramus	Corner of mouth and lips	Keeps lips against teeth
SUPRAHYOID	From hyoid	To mandible	When contracted, opens jaw
INFRAHYOID	From hyoid	To sternum	Aids in swallowing
ORBICULARIS ORIS	Encircles mouth		Draws lips together

division of the trigeminal nerve, which is discussed in greater detail later in this chapter. The blood supply for these muscles is derived from the external carotid artery via the maxillary artery.

The Masseter Muscle

The *masseter muscle* is usually considered the most powerful of the muscles of mastication. This muscle's origin is on the zygomatic arch in two areas—the inferior border of the arch, and the medial surface of the zygoma. The insertion is at the lateral surface of the mandible, as the fibers of the muscle run downward and posteriorly from the origin. The function of this muscle is to close the mouth. This occurs when the muscle contracts, elevating the mandible.

The Temporal Muscle

The *temporal muscle* is a large muscle whose origin spans the temporal fossa on the lateral surface of the skull. The fibers of the muscle run vertically in the anterior, but as they move to the posterior, they run almost in a horizontal plane over the ear. The fibers insert into the coronoid process of the mandible and may extend to the anterior border of the ramus of the mandible. The function of this muscle is to elevate the

mandible, thereby closing the mouth. This function occurs when the muscle contracts and the mandible retrudes as it is pulled posteriorly.

The Medial Pterygoid Muscle

The *medial pterygoid* muscle has two origins, the larger being the medial surface of the lateral pterygoid plate and the pterygoid fossa. The smaller origin is anterior to these, from the maxillary tuberosity. The insertion is the medial surface of the angle of the mandible. The fibers of the muscles run downward from the origin to aid in its function, to elevate or close the mandible, while working with the masseter muscle.

The Lateral Pterygoid Muscle

The *lateral pterygoid* muscle also has two origins, and it is the shortest of the masticatory muscles. The smaller or superior origin is at the greater wing of the sphenoid, at an area called the infratemporal crest. The larger or inferior origin attaches at the lateral surface of the lateral pterygoid plate. Note that the lateral pterygoid origins are just the opposite of the medial pterygoid muscle. The fibers of this muscle are running in a mostly horizontal direction from anterior to posterior. The insertion of the superior origin is at the capsule of the temporomandibular joint and into the joint disc. The insertion of the inferior origin is at the neck of the condyle.

The function of the inferior segment of the lateral pterygoid muscle is seen as the muscle contracts and pulls the disc and condyle forward, protruding the mandible and opening the mouth. It does have a secondary function, allowing the mandible to move laterally. This occurs when one lateral pterygoid muscle contracts on a single side, allowing lateral excursion to the opposite side of the mouth. The function of the superior insertion of this muscle is in the biting action. It guides the posterior movement of the condyle and disc back into a normal or centric position (Fig. 3-8). Fig. 3-9 illustrates the position of the muscles in another view.

The four sets of muscles, as discussed, are the major muscles of mastication. With the exception of the lateral pterygoid muscle, they are all responsible for closing the mouth. The mandible must be depressed or pulled toward the chest, opening the mouth, and this is accomplished by a group of muscles called the *hyoid muscles*. This group is sometimes referred to as the accessory muscles of mastication. They all have contact with the hyoid bone, which is a horseshoe-shaped bone that is found inferior to the mandible.

The hyoid muscles are divided into two groups, the *suprahyoid muscles*, found superior to the hyoid bone, and the *infrahyoid muscles*, found inferior to the hyoid bone. The suprahyoid muscles are the *digastric, mylohyoid, geniohyoid*, and *stylohyoid muscles*. The infrahyoid muscles are the *omohyoid, sternohyoid, sternothyroid*, and *thyrohyoid muscles*.

The Suprahyoid Muscles

The *digastric muscle* is unusual in that it is considered to have two origins. The posterior origin is at the digastric notch, medial to the mastoid process, and runs anterior and down toward the tendon loop that attaches to the hyoid bone. The anterior origin has muscle fibers attached to the digastric fossa, near the inferior surface of the symphysis, and inserts into the same tendon loop.

The anterior fibers of the muscle pull the hyoid bone anteriorly, while the posterior fibers pull it posteriorly. When the two sets of fibers of the muscle work in unison, they elevate the hyoid muscle from its normal position. The function of the digastric muscle then becomes retruding and depressing the mandible and elevating the hyoid bone.

The origin of the *geniohyoid muscle* is found on the mandible at the inferior genial tubercles. The insertion is found at the hyoid bone as the muscle runs posteriorly and down. The function of the muscle is to elevate the hyoid bone and depress the mandible to open the mouth.

The *mylohyoid muscle* creates the floor of the mouth, with the origin on the medial surface of the mandible at the mylohyoid or oblique line. The pair of muscles on either side of the mandible run toward the midline and meet at the mylohyoid raphe. The muscle inserts at the hyoid bone and allows it to depress the mandible as its function.

The *stylohyoid muscle* originates at the styloid process of the temporal bone. The stylohyoid muscle then runs anteriorly and downward to insert on the posterior part of the hyoid bone. The function of this muscle is to pull the hyoid bone posteriorly and upward, aiding in the **deglutition** (swallowing) process.

The Infrahyoid Muscles

The *omohyoid muscle* is separated by the intermediate tendon into two segments, with the origins at the upper border of the scapula. The muscle inserts at the hyoid bone, allowing it to depress and fix the hyoid bone.

The origin of the *sternohyoid muscle* is at the upper border of the sternum, running vertically to the insertion, which is the anterior segment of the hyoid bone. The function of this muscle is also to depress and fix the hyoid bone.

The *thyrohyoid muscle* has its origin at the oblique line on the lateral surface of the thyroid cartilage, which is also the insertion of the sternothyroid muscle. The muscle runs vertically and inserts at the hyoid bone. The function of this muscle is to depress the larynx.

The Muscles of Facial Expression

The **muscles of facial expression** are responsible for movement of the cheeks and lips to reveal emotions, as well as motion during mastication and speech. The muscles work together to be able to provide these movements. Other muscles are responsible for movement in areas of the head, but we will deal specifically with those pertaining to the area of the mouth.

The *orbicularis oris* is the muscle that surrounds the mouth, specifically, the lips. This muscle allows a person to purse and to close the lips.

The *depressors* of the lip are a combination of muscles: the *mentalis, depressor labii inferiorus, depressor anguli oris*, and *platysma* muscles. The first two muscles either protrude or depress the lower lip. The third, the depressor anguli oris, depresses the corners of the mouth. The fourth muscle, the platysma, draws the outer area of the lower lip down and back and raises the skin of the neck.

The *elevators of the lip* consist of the *levator labii superioris, levator labii superioris alaeque nasi, levator anguli oris, zygomaticus minor*, and *zygomaticus major* muscles. The first muscle elevates the upper lip, as does the second muscle, but it also dilates the nostril. The third muscle, the levator anguli oris, pulls the

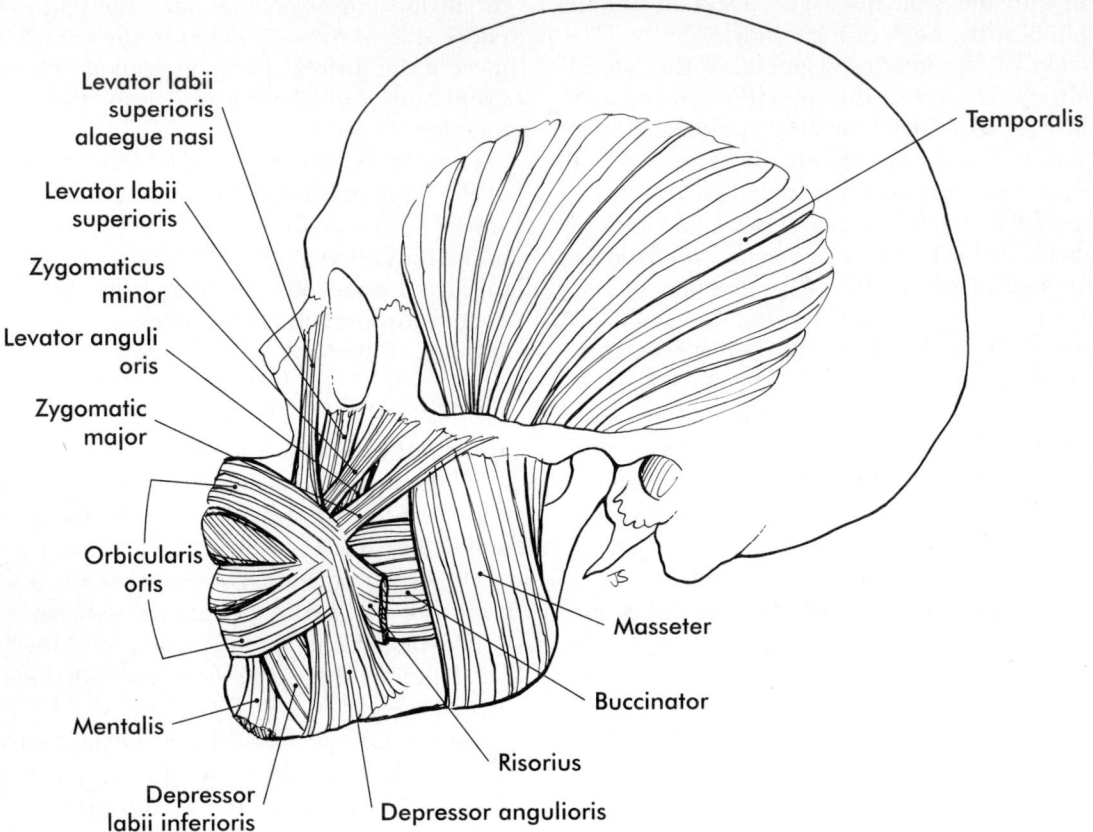

Levator labii superioris alaegue nasi

Levator labii superioris

Zygomaticus minor

Levator anguli oris

Zygomatic major

Orbicularis oris

Mentalis

Depressor labii inferioris

Depressor angulioris

Risorius

Buccinator

Masseter

Temporalis

FIG. 3-8   The muscles of mastication and facial expression.

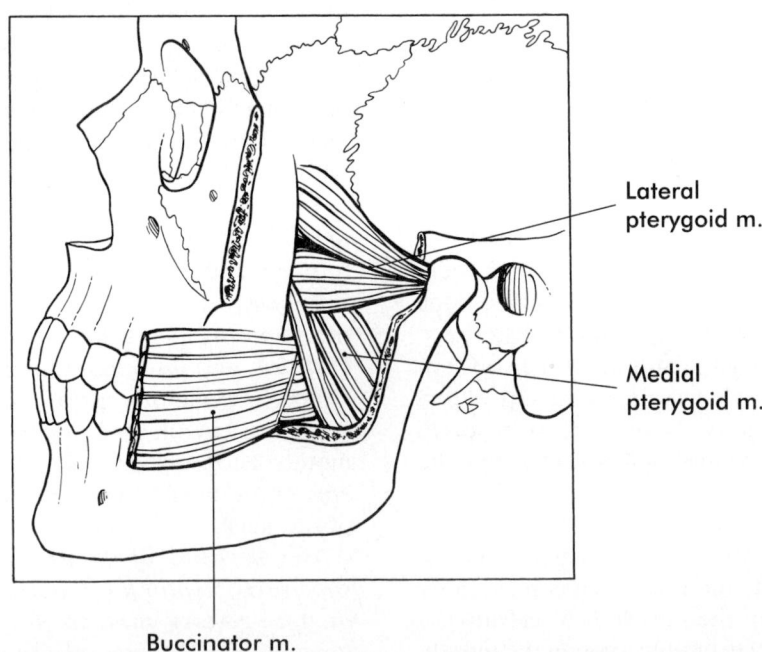

Lateral pterygoid m.

Medial pterygoid m.

Buccinator m.

FIG. 3-9   Resected portion of the ramus provides additional visualization of the lateral and medial pterygoid muscles and the buccinator muscle.

corners of the mouth upward. The fourth muscle, the zygomaticus minor, raises the upper lip, and the zygomaticus major pulls the corners of the mouth upward and laterally, aiding in the formation of a smile.

The *risorius muscle* is responsible for pulling the corners of the mouth laterally. This motion creates movement of the mouth, forming a smile.

The *buccinator muscle* is considered a muscle of mastication by some, since it has an active role in the mastication of food. It lies within the tissues of the cheek between the maxilla and the mandible (see Fig. 3-10). The muscle draws the corner of the mouth toward the midline, pressing the mucosa of the cheek against the teeth. The buccinator muscle aids in a blowing action of the mouth and controls the tautness of the cheeks when the mouth is opened and closed.

▶ Temporomandibular Joint

The **temporomandibular joint** or TMJ, as it is sometimes called, is the joint responsible for movement of the mandible. It is the only movable joint that exists in the skull, with the hinging of the mandible to both temporal bones. The hinged joint allows for a gliding motion, as well as for the hinge action. The temporomandibular joint is composed of a combination of structures. The coordination of these structures, some of which have previously been discussed, creates an articulation of both the joints on the opposing sides of the skull.

The mandible, particularly the **condyle** and the neck, make up the mandibular segment of the temporomandibular joint. Between the mandibular condyle and the *temporal bone* (the *articular eminence*) and in the glenoid or mandibular fossa lies the *articular disc* or *meniscus.* The superior surface of the articular disc is concavo-convex in shape to complement the shape of the mandibular fossa and the articular eminence. The inferior surface of the disc is concave to complement the shape of the condyle. The disc consists of a thick collagen tissue that protects the joint during stress-bearing action.

Found on both surfaces of the meniscus are saclike areas that are called **synovial cavities**. The cavities are lined with epithelial tissue that is responsible for secreting lubricating liquid, *synovial fluid,* onto surfaces. This fluid aids in the avoidance of friction and irritation to the structures of the temporomandibular joint.

Both joints are surrounded by a fibrous capsule or sac, called the *articular capsule.* The temporomandibular

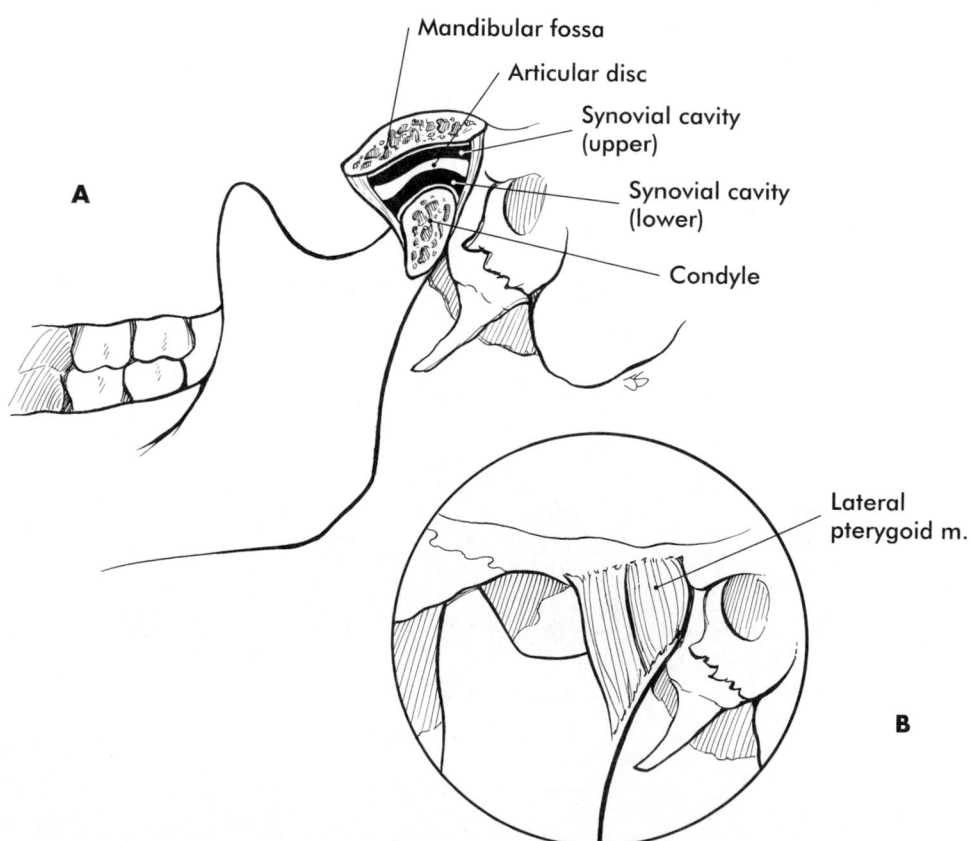

FIG. 3-10 *A,* Cross-section of the temporomandibular joint. *B,* Insert shows the temporomandibular joint with the lateral pterygoid muscle over the lateral surface.

ligament is a thickening of the capsule on the lateral surface that prevents displacement of the capsule. The fibers of the articular capsule are attached to all the bony structures of the skull components and extend to encompass the neck of the condyle.

The muscles of mastication play an active role in the movement of the joint. As the muscles attain a relaxed position, the maxilla and the mandible are not touching or articulating. The temporomandibular joint provides movement of the mandible to open, close, protrude, and perform lateral displacement. As the mandible opens and closes the articular disc glides across the articular tubercle, and the condyle then rotates on the disc. When a person is eating and using the power stroke, other action may take place. The mandible is in the open position and is forced down on a piece of food to chew on the right side. On the opposite side, correct positioning occurs between the condyle, disc, and temporal bone, but on the right side, the condyle, disc, and temporal bone will still be apart. With this difference between the joints, the mandible is not centered properly and injury may occur as the structures bounce off one another. Without the joint movement, use of the mandible would be impossible (Fig. 3-10, *A* and *B*).

▶ Paranasal Sinuses, Nasal Cavity, and the Orbits of the Eyes

The paranasal sinuses are located in the areas surrounding the *nasal cavity*. The nasal cavity is divided in half by the *nasal septum*. Each half is the opening of the nasal cavity into the skull and is referred to as the *nasal aperture*. The nasal septum's most posterior section reaches the posterior nasal aperture.

The nasal cavity is surrounded by numerous bones of the skull to provide its shape. The superior portion of the cavity is bounded by the nasal bones, while the inferior portion extends to the maxillae and the palatal bones. The lateral portion of the nasal cavity combines with the maxilla, ethmoid, and inferior nasal concha. The medial portion of the nasal cavity, the area of the nasal septum, is formed by the vomer and the ethmoid.

Superior to the nasal cavity toward the lateral area are the **orbits**, the bony openings of the eyes. Some of the same bones that make up segments of the nasal cavity are also included in the orbit. The superior bones of the orbit are the frontal and sphenoid. Inferior to these are the zygoma, maxilla, and palatal bones. The posterior portion of the orbit is composed of the greater and lesser wings of the sphenoid bones, while the lateral surface is a combination of the zygoma and the sphenoid. The medial area combines the lacrimal, ethmoid, maxilla, and sphenoid to form the surface.

The paranasal sinuses are paired and are found within many of the previously mentioned structures. The main functions of the sinuses are to (1) lighten the skull; (2) provide resonance chambers for the voice; and (3) warm inspired air for the respiratory system.

The sinuses are covered with an epithelial lining called the *respiratory epithelium*. The *olfactory epithelium* is also found in the superior nasal cavity and provides the perception of taste via the nerve fibers.

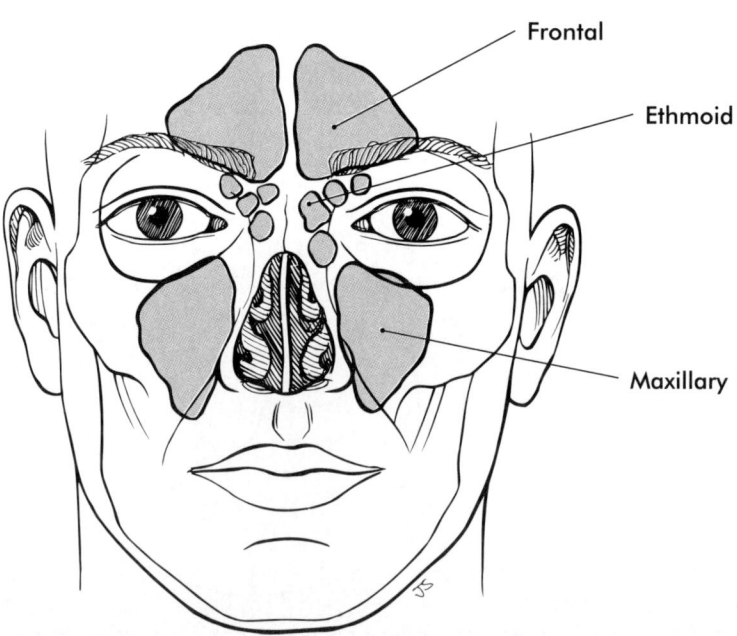

FIG. 3-11   Frontal view of the sinuses of the skull.

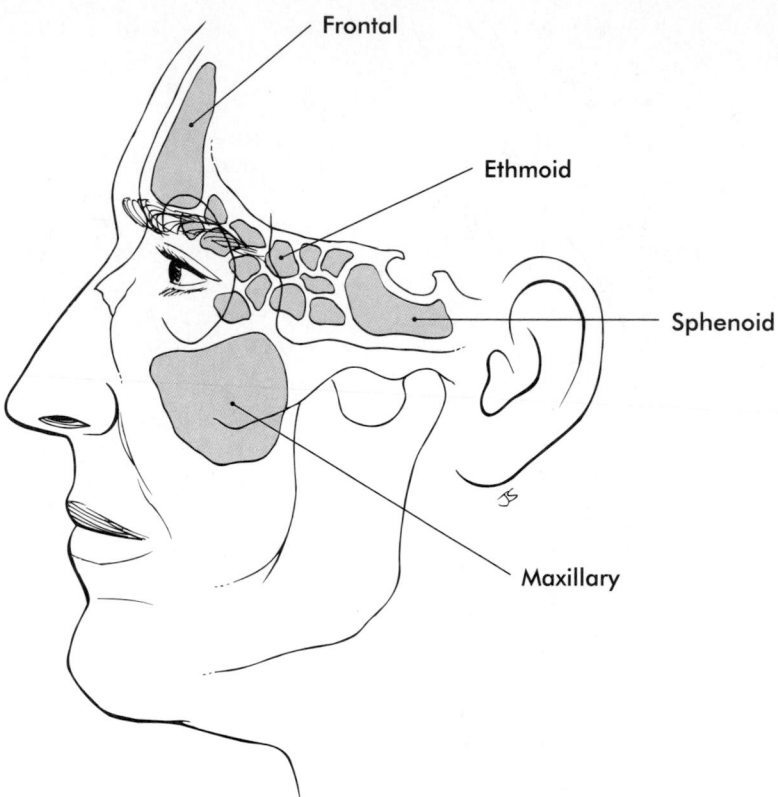

FIG. 3-12   Lateral view of the sinuses of the skull.

The size of the sinus varies with the location of each pair. The *maxillary sinuses* are the largest and are found in the body of the maxilla. The *frontal sinuses* are located superior to the orbit of the eye within the frontal bones. The *sphenoid sinuses* are found in the area of the *pituitary fossa* in the sphenoid bone. The *ethmoid sinuses* are not paired but are divided into the *anterior, middle,* and *posterior ethmoids* and are referred to as *ethmoid air cells* (Fig. 3-11).

Often the floor of the maxillary sinus extends down further into the area of the maxilla, and the roots of the posterior teeth may be close to or inside the sinus opening. This may result in more tooth discomfort during infections of the mucosal linings or during the process of tooth extraction (Fig. 3-12).

▶ Salivary Glands

Saliva, the fluid of the oral cavity, is secreted from *salivary glands.* Its purpose is to cleanse the oral cavity and to moisten food during mastication so that it will pass easily through the esophagus, which is the initial stage of digestion. It also protects the mucosal lining from dryness and moistens tissues for ease in speech. The consistency of saliva may vary from serous, or watery, to mucous, which is thick and may be ropelike. Three major glands secrete the majority of fluid into the oral cavity, but smaller additional glands also exist.

The *parotid gland* is a major salivary gland that can be found on both sides of the face within the confines of the cheek. It is specifically located anterior and inferior to the ears, close to the maxillary first molars. These glands are responsible for the secretion of approximately 25% of the total salivary production. The saliva exits into the oral cavity through the parotid duct, or *Stenson's duct,* and is considered to be of serous consistency. The specific exit site can be observed on the buccal mucosa by locating the parotid papilla, which is a raised area.

The *submandibular* or *submaxillary gland* is the second largest of the salivary glands and is responsible for the secretion of approximately 60% to 65% of serous and mucous saliva into the oral cavity. The gland is located in the submandibular fossa on the medial surface of the mandible and extends to the hyoid bone. The secretions enter the oral cavity by way of the submandibular or *Wharton's duct.* As the parotid duct exits can be located by the parotid papilla, near the maxillary first molars, the opening for the submandibular gland is located by the **sublingual caruncle,** or the small raised area on both sides of the lingual frenum.

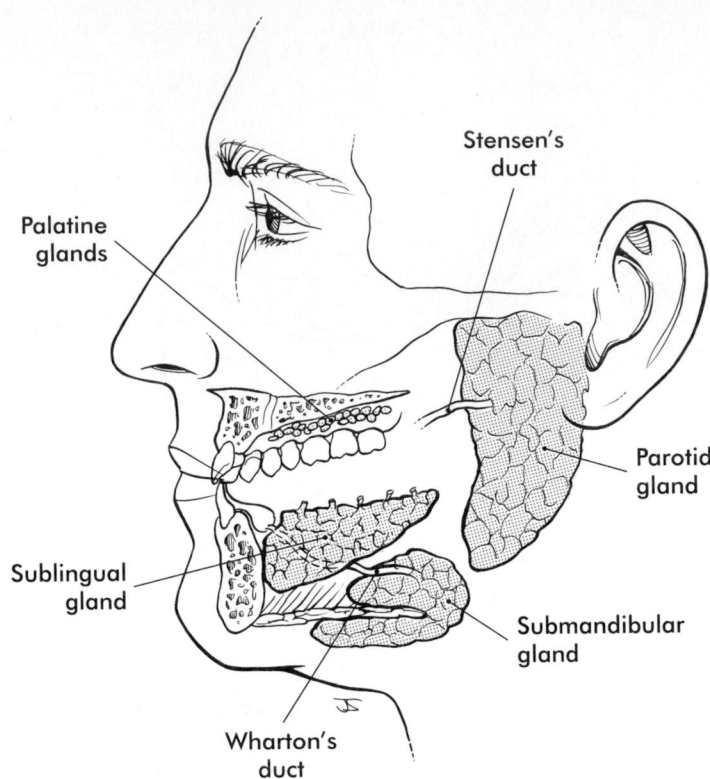

FIG. 3-13   Positions of the major salivary glands.

The *sublingual gland* is the smallest of the major salivary glands and is responsible for only 10% of the salivary fluids in the oral cavity. It is located near the mandibular canines but inferior to the floor of the mouth. The secretion consists predominantly of a mucous fluid, with a small amount that is of serous consistency. The sublingual gland exits into the oral cavity by way of *Bartholin's duct* into the submandibular duct and other openings along the lingual surface of the tongue (Fig. 3-13).

The minor salivary glands are located throughout the rest of the oral cavity, labially, buccally, palatally, lingually, and glossopalatally. They are primarily responsible for secreting small amounts of saliva to maintain moisture on the mucosal surfaces. The minor salivary glands are basically found in clusters rather than in a duct pattern as are the major salivary glands. The glands are the *labial, buccal, palatine, glossopalatine,* and *lingual glands.* The lingual glands are divided into groups: the *anterior lingual glands, the lingual glands of von Ebner,* and the *posterior lingual glands.* These glands may be purely serous, purely mucous, or a combination of both.

The amount of saliva that exists in any mouth varies from person to person. One factor that may have some bearing on the amount of saliva may be medications that are being ingested by the individual.

▶ Circulatory and Nervous System
Circulatory System

The circulatory system is a network of channels through which blood flows throughout the body. As with other areas of the body, it is necessary to know about blood and the circulatory system of the head and neck. The three parts of the circulatory system are the heart, the blood, and the blood vessels. The heart is divided into chambers: two **atria**, or upper chambers; and two **ventricles**, or lower chambers. The atria and ventricles are further divided into the right and left, with the right receiving and the left carrying blood (Fig. 3-14).

Blood is moved from the atria and ventricles via blood vessels called arteries, veins, and capillaries. A **vein** carries blood to the heart from all areas of the body, whereas an **artery** carries it away from the heart. A **capillary** connects the venous and arterial systems and slows the movement of blood by dispersing it into smaller vessels over a greater area.

Major arteries in the head and neck area must be familiar to the health care provider in dentistry. The *aorta* extends from the left ventricle of the heart and provides for the *common carotid artery,* which is divided into the *internal* and *external carotid* vessels. The internal carotid artery does not supply blood to the

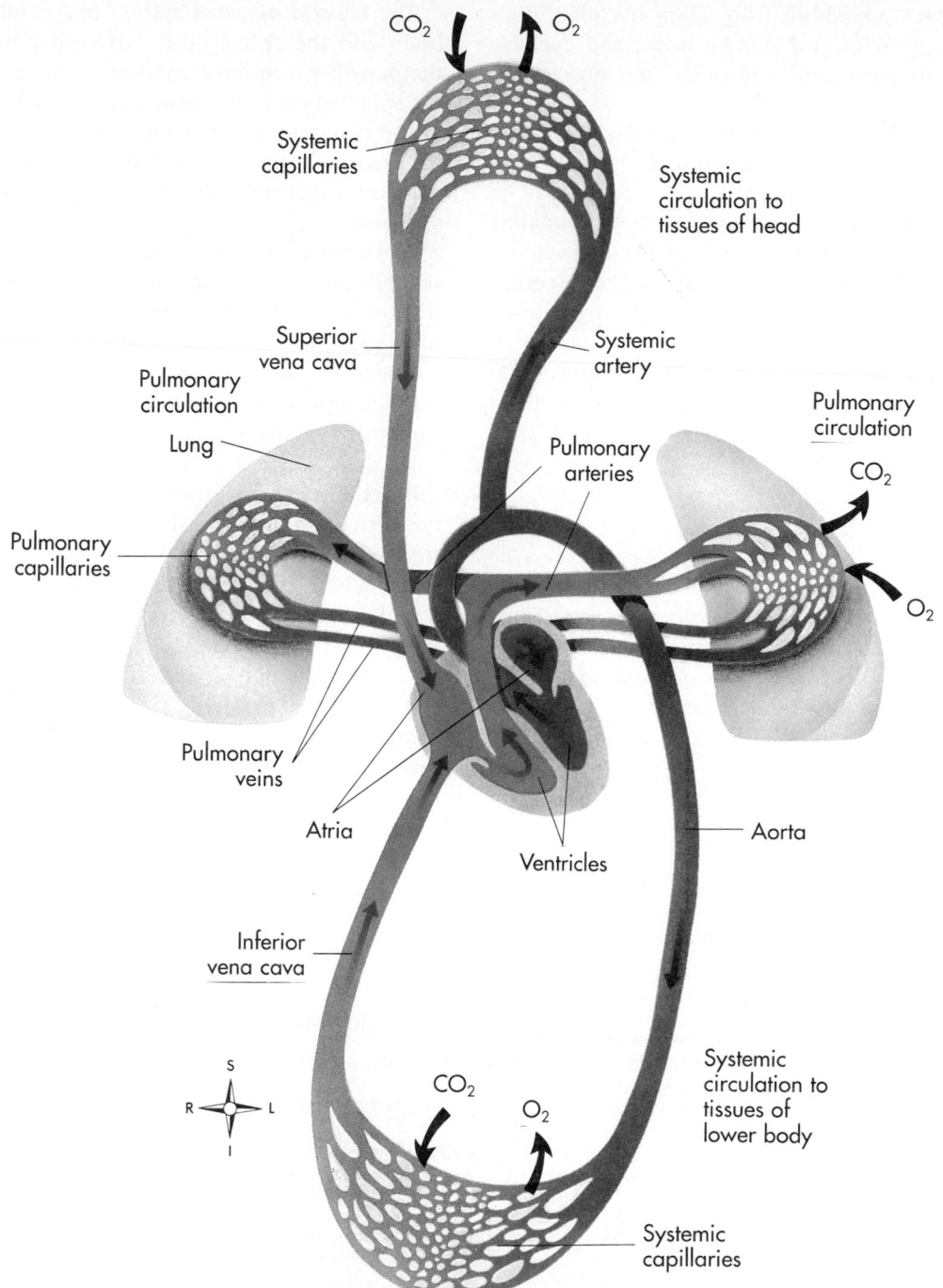

FIG. 3-14   Blood flow through the circulatory system.

(From Thibodeau GA, Patton KT: *Anatomy and physiology,* ed 2, St Louis, 1992, Mosby.)

mouth but branches off to supply the brain and the eyes. The external carotid artery extends throughout the head and neck, providing the blood supply to eight branches serving various anatomic structures (see Fig. 3-14). The external carotid artery rises from the heart to the mandible, crossing the face and scalp. The eight branches of the artery and the areas supplied are as follows:

Ascending pharyngeal - pharynx and surrounding muscles

Superior thyroid - thyroid gland and surrounding muscles

Lingual - floor of mouth, sublingual gland, mylohyoid muscles, tonsils, soft palate, epiglottis

Facial - soft palate, pharynx, pharyngeal muscles, tonsils, sublingual and submandibular glands, mylohyoid muscles, mandibular lip, chin, maxillary lip, facial skin, muscles and skin of nose, and eyelids

Occipital - scalp, surrounding muscles, and muscles of the neck

Posterior auricular - outer ear and surrounding scalp

Superficial temporal - temporalis muscle

Maxillary - facial structures

One of the most important arteries arising from the external carotid artery is the *maxillary artery.* It provides the blood supply to the mandibular and maxillary teeth, the palate, the masticatory muscles, and the nasal and oral cavities.

The veins of the head and neck basically correspond with the arteries and have similar names. One such vein is the *maxillary vein,* which drains blood into the *internal jugular vein.*

Nervous System

The nervous system communicates with the body by carrying messages to and from the brain. Messages from the brain to a body structure to perform an action or function are referred to as *motor* or *efferent messages.* Messages that originate in a body structure and are then transferred to the brain are referred to as *sensory* or *afferent messages.*

The *central nervous system* is a combination of the brain and the spinal cord. The other nervous system, the *peripheral nervous system,* includes the cranial and the spinal nerves. The **neuron** is the cell working in each of these systems to transmit messages via a small electrical current into information, depending on the type of neuron that delivers the message, whether motor or sensory.

The cranial nerves are 12 pairs of nerves that act as sensory or motor nerves. They are named according to the area or type of function they assist and are referred to by name and/or Roman numeral. Table 3-4 reflects the 12 pairs of cranial nerves and the function of each; Fig. 3-15 illustrates the location of each nerve and the areas of the body that are served.

Because of the practice of administering anesthesia in the oral cavity, the trigeminal and facial nerves are of concern to the dental team. The terminal branches of the trigeminal and facial nerves communicate, explaining why, when the division of the trigeminal nerve is anesthetized, motor capabilities may be reduced on the patient's face. The patient may experience displeasure with the reduction of facial motor skills.

The trigeminal nerve divides into three branches: the *mandibular,* the *maxillary,* and the *ophthalmic.* The mandibular division is separated into the buccal nerve,

TABLE 3-4   CRANIAL NERVES

Nerve	Type	Function
OLFACTORY NERVE	Sensory	Provides sense of smell
OPTIC NERVE	Sensory	Provides sense of sight
OCULOMOTOR NERVE	Motor	Provides movement of the muscles of the eye
TROCHLEAR NERVE	Motor	Provides movement for a single muscle of the eye
TRIGEMINAL NERVE	Motor and sensory	Divided into three parts; largest and most important nerve to dentistry
OPHTHALMIC DIVISION	Sensory	Supplies the eyes and forehead
MAXILLARY DIVISION	Sensory	Supplies the maxillary arch and related structures and innervates the maxillary teeth
MANDIBULAR DIVISION	Motor and sensory	Supplies the mandibular arch and sensory-related structures and innervates the mandibular teeth
ABDUCENS NERVE	Motor	Provides movement for one muscle of the eye
FACIAL NERVE	Motor and sensory	Provides movement to facial muscles and salivary glands; supplies sense of taste
ACOUSTIC NERVE	Sensory	Provides hearing and sense of balance
GLOSSOPHARYNGEAL NERVE	Motor and sensory	Provides movement for muscles of soft palate, throat, and salivary glands; provides sense of taste, pain, temperature, and pressure
VAGUS NERVE	Motor and sensory	Provides movement for larynx and pharynx, muscles of the soft palate, and smooth and cardiac muscles; provides sense of taste from the root of the tongue and sensory information from the skin around the ear
ACCESSORY (SPINAL) NERVE	Motor	Provides movement for muscles of the shoulder
HYPOGLOSSAL NERVE	Motor	Provides movement for muscles of the tongue

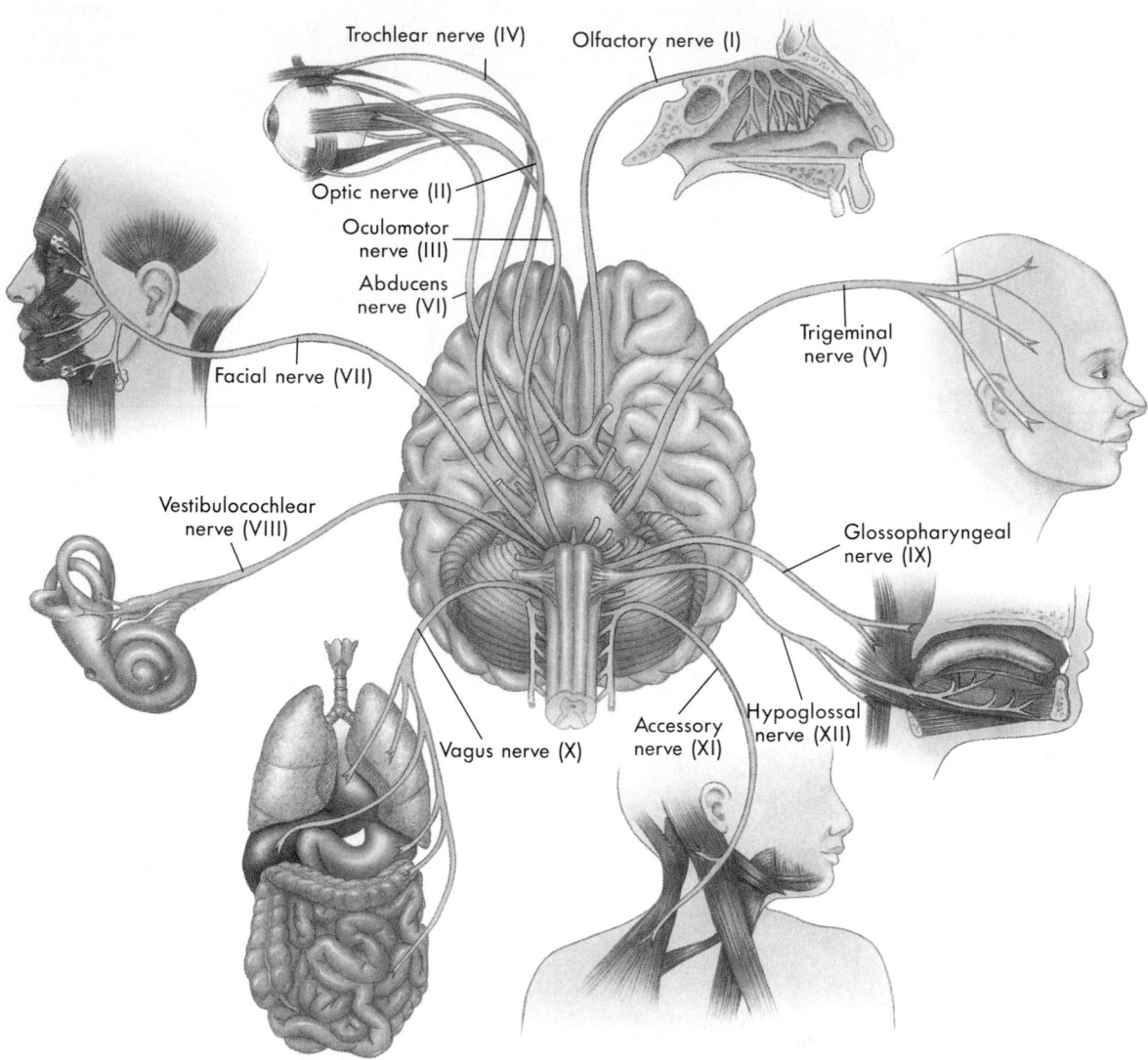

FIG. 3-15   Ventral surface of the brain showing attachments of the cranial nerves.

(From Thibodeau G, Patton K: *Anatomy and physiology,* ed 2, St Louis, 1992, Mosby.)

which supplies the buccal mucous membrane and the mucoperiosteum of the molars, and the lingual nerve, which supplies the anterior two thirds of the tongue, the lingual mucosa, and the mucoperiosteum. The third branch of the mandibular division of the trigeminal nerve is the inferior alveolar nerve, which branches into four subdivisions. The mylohyoid nerve supplies the mylohyoid and digastric muscles. The incisive nerve breaks into small branches that supply the central and lateral incisors and the cuspids. The mental nerve supplies the mucosa of the mandibular lip and the chin. Finally, the small dental nerves supply the periosteum, alveolar process, molars, and premolars.

The maxillary division of the trigeminal nerve branches into the anterior palatine nerve, which supplies the mucoperiosteum, while combining with the nasopalatine nerve, which supplies the mucoperiosteum of the

palate to the anterior teeth. The maxillary division also branches to include the anterior, middle, and posterosuperior alveolar nerves. These three nerves supply the following structures: anterior alveolar—central and lateral cuspids, periodontal membranes, and gingiva; middle alveolar—first and second premolars, mesiobuccal root of the first molar, and maxillary sinus; and posterosuperior alveolar—the rest of the first molar roots, second and third molars, and lateral wall of the maxillary sinus (Fig. 3-16, *A* through *C*).

▶ Oral Facial Structures and the Oral Cavity

The oral cavity is where the first step in the digestive process takes place. The oral cavity also actively participates in the respiratory system and contains the taste

FIG. 3-16 *A,* Areas of distribution on facial skin of three divisions of the trigeminal nerve. *B,* The general distribution of the maxillary division of the trigeminal nerve. *C,* A partial diagram of the maxillary (V_2) and the mandibular (V_3) nerves.

(From Brand RW, Isselhardt DE: *Anatomy of Orofacial Structures,* ed 4, St Louis, 1990, Mosby.)

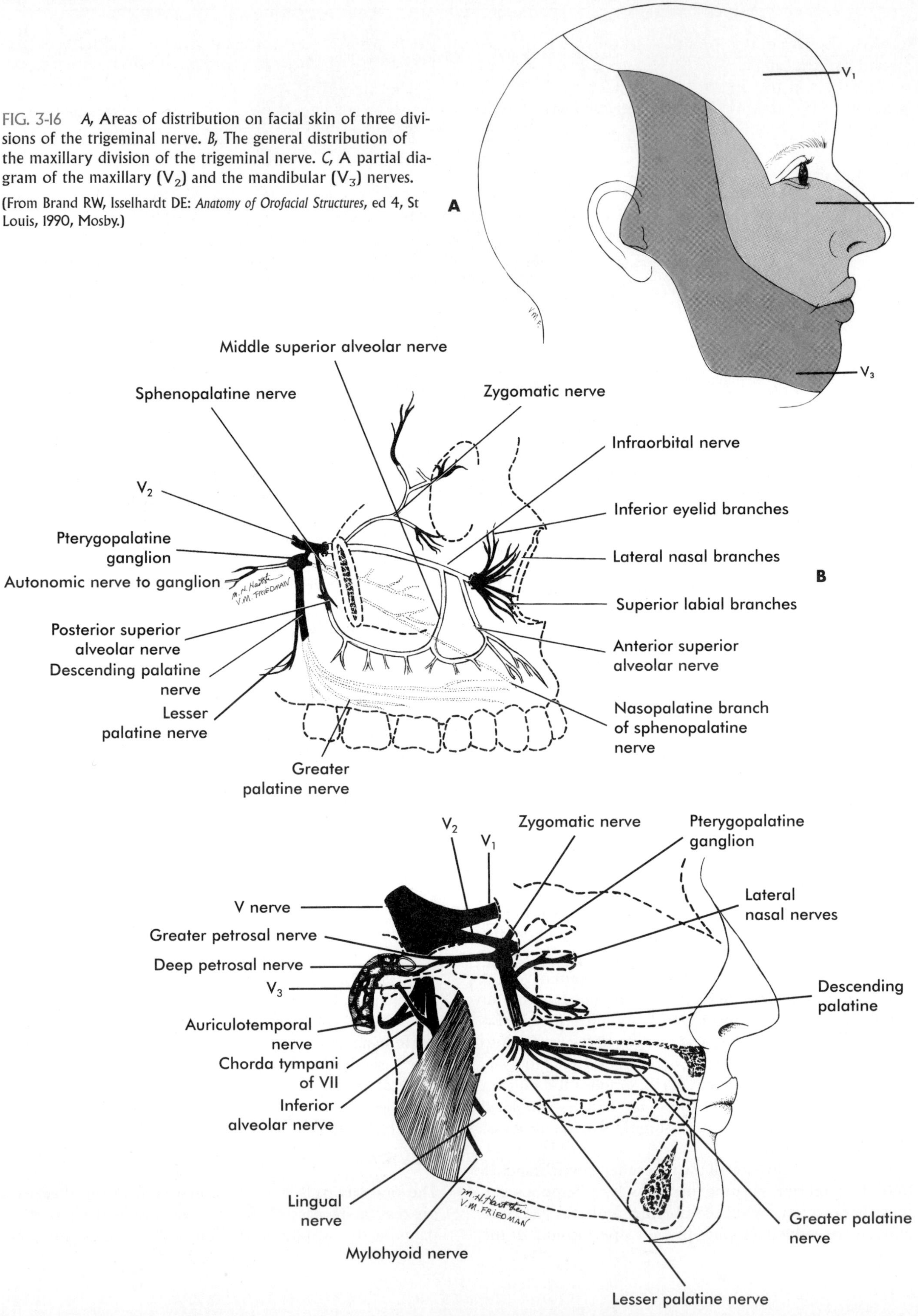

organs. The area of the oral cavity is bordered by the lips anteriorly, the anterior pillars posteriorly, the palate superiorly, and the muscles of the floor of the mouth inferiorly. The oral cavity is commonly divided into two segments: the **vestibule** and the **oral cavity proper**.

VESTIBULE

The vestibule is the space or cavity that serves as the entrance to the oral cavity. The outer borders of the vestibule are the lips and cheek, and the inner borders are the facial surfaces of the teeth and the alveolar processes, which create a trough-like space. The skin that covers the face and stops at the edge of the lips is called keratinized stratified squamous epithelium. This type of epithelium is found throughout the body. The *mucosa* is the tissue that covers the oral cavity, and it is termed *parakeratinized stratified squamous epithelium*. The area of the lips that appears redder, where the two kinds of epithelium join, is highly vascular and is called the *vermilion border*. The contact point for the upper and lower lip in the corner of the mouth is referred to as the *labial commissure*.

Various landmarks should be learned concerning the lips and cheeks. The *nasolabial groove* is found unilaterally on the upper lip and separates the lip from the cheek. The nasolabial groove runs from the *alae of the nose,* which are its flared outer surfaces, to the labial commissure. Lying between the nasolabial grooves, inferior to the nose but superior to the upper lip, is a depressed area known as the *philtrum*. The *labial tubercle* is just inferior to the philtrum and is a raised tissue area that varies in size.

In the same way that the maxillary lip is divided by landmarks, so is the mandibular lip. The *labiomental groove* separates the lower lip from the chin or *symphysis* (Fig. 3-17). Between the internal and external segments of the vestibule the buccinator muscle runs horizontally. As the mouth opens, the posterior border of the buccinator muscle, the *pterygomandibular raphe,* can be seen. It appears to be a taut fold of tissue from the maxillary to the mandibular arches near the maxillary second molars and the parotid papilla.

Muscle and fiber attachments are found within the vestibule and oral cavity. They are named according to location. The attachments are composed of connective tissue and are known as frenum (plural, frena). The frena are responsible for connecting the lips, cheeks, and tongue to the alveolar processes. They are as follows:

Maxillary labial frenum attaches the upper lip and the alveolar process and may create a diastema (space) if it extends too far to the central incisors

Maxillary buccal frena attach to the maxillary alveolar process and to the upper lip on both the right and left sides of the mouth to the area of the maxillary premolars

Mandibular labial frenum connects the lower lip and the mandibular alveolar process between the mandibular central incisors

Mandibular buccal frena attach to the mandibular alveolar process and the lower lip on both the right and left sides of the mouth in the area of the mandibular premolars

Lingual frenum attaches the dorsal surface of the tongue to the floor of the mouth; if it extends too far to the anterior segment of the tongue, this may result in tongue tying (Fig. 3-18)

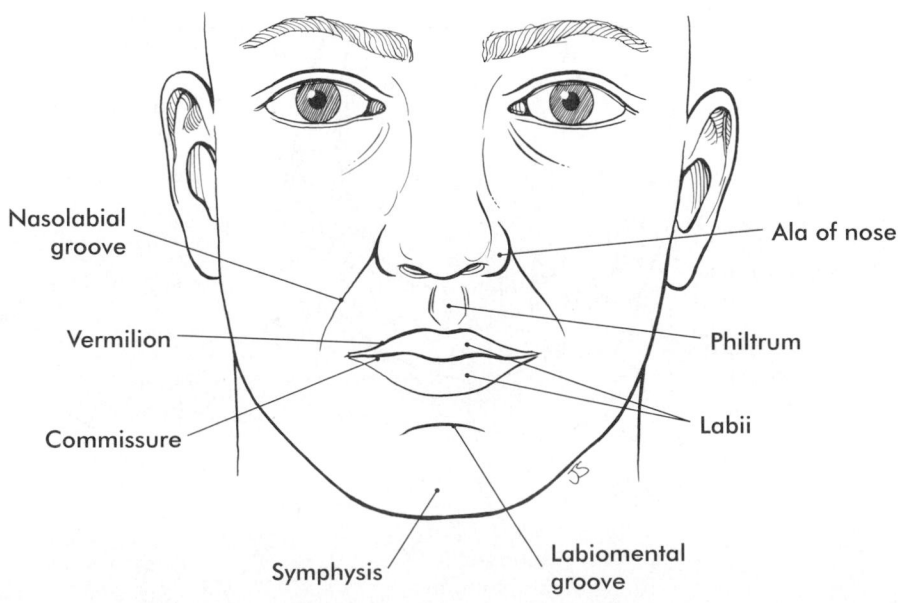

FIG. 3-17 Oral facial structures of a frontal view of the face.

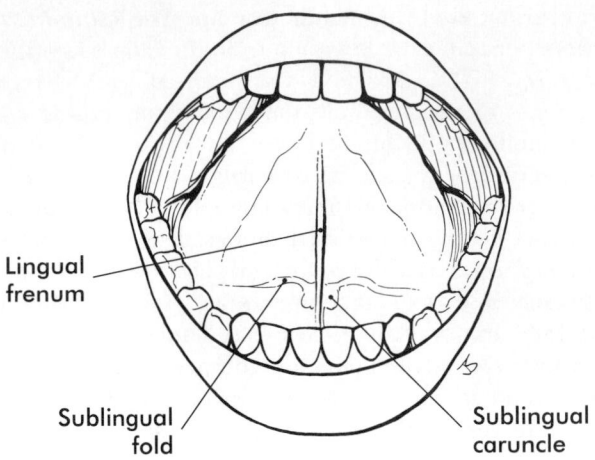

Lingual frenum

Sublingual fold

Sublingual caruncle

FIG. 3-18   Opened oral cavity with tip of tongue elevated.

The *mucobuccal fold or fornix* is where the alveolar buccal mucosa joins with the cheek mucosa. The mucolabial fold or fornix is found in the anterior segment of the maxillary and mandibular arches where the labial mucosa joins with the alveolar mucosa.

The oral mucosa that surrounds all the teeth is designated as **gingiva** (Fig. 3-19). The gingiva appears to differ in color from the *lining mucosa* of the lips and cheeks and from the *alveolar mucosa* that lies between the lining mucosa and the gingiva. This difference in color is due to the increased vascular supply, with the alveolar mucosa appearing redder than the gingiva, which is pink to brown, depending on the genetic background.

The gingiva is divided into *free gingiva* or *marginal gingiva* and *attached gingiva.* The free gingiva covers the neck of the teeth and extends to a depth of 1 to 3 mm before it reaches the attached gingiva. The attached gingiva covers the alveolar bone and a portion of the

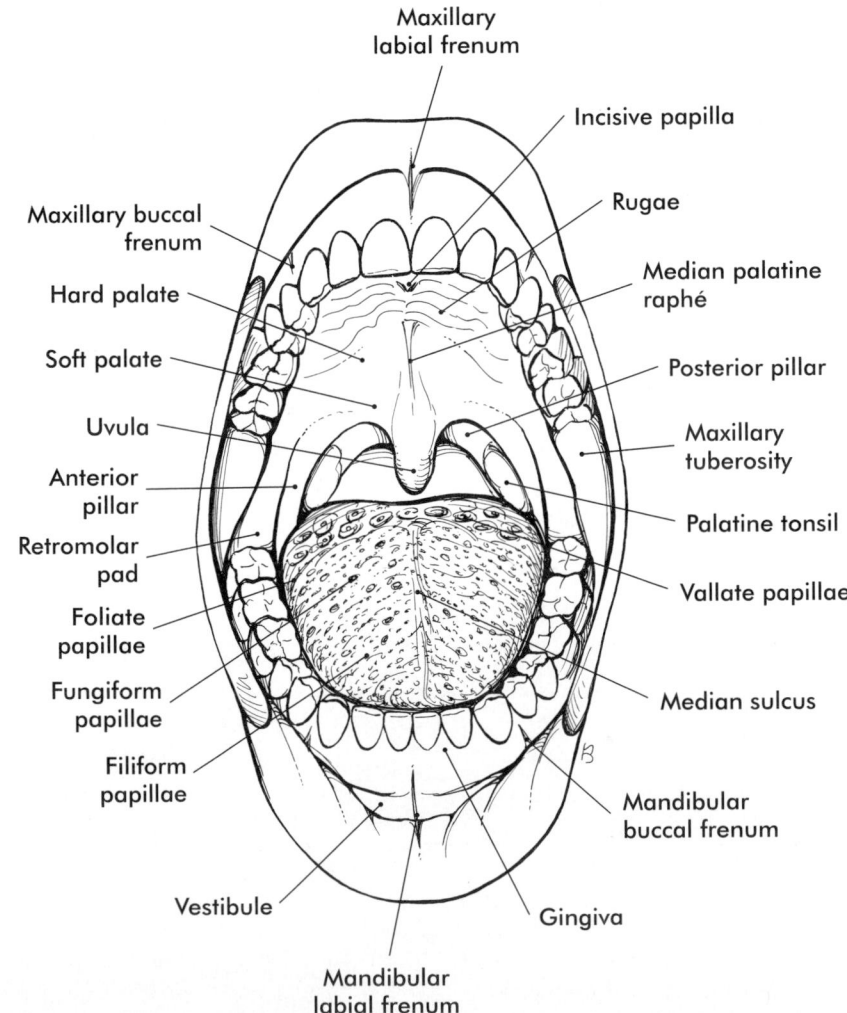

Maxillary labial frenum

Incisive papilla

Maxillary buccal frenum

Rugae

Hard palate

Median palatine raphé

Soft palate

Posterior pillar

Uvula

Maxillary tuberosity

Anterior pillar

Palatine tonsil

Retromolar pad

Vallate papillae

Foliate papillae

Fungiform papillae

Median sulcus

Filiform papillae

Mandibular buccal frenum

Vestibule

Gingiva

Mandibular labial frenum

FIG. 3-19   Opened mouth showing numerous intraoral structures.

cementum of the teeth. A detailed drawing of this area is found in Chapter 6.

ORAL CAVITY PROPER

As mentioned earlier, the oral cavity proper (see Fig. 3-19) is bounded by the internal surface of the alveolar process and the teeth; it therefore lies between the dental arches and includes the tongue. The bony roof of the mouth—the maxilla—includes the *palate,* which can be divided into the *hard* and the *soft palates.* Both are covered by palatal mucosa, with the hard palate having the mucosa attached to it. The hard palate is so named because the bone of the maxilla is superior to it, while the soft palate has no bone-based support.

Located on the hard palate, posterior to the maxillary central incisors, is a V-shaped tissue elevation, the *incisive papilla* or *palatine papilla,* which covers the maxillary incisive foramen. Extending from the anterior portion of the maxilla down the palate's midline is a ridge called the *palatine raphe.* This is the palatal mucosa covering the palatine suture line. The irregular folds or ridges of connective tissue extending from the anterior of the maxilla to the area of the maxillary first molars from the palatal raphe are the *palatine rugae.* These structures aid in speech and mastication.

The soft palate is posterior to the hard palate and is referred to as soft because, as mentioned earlier, there is no bony support. An extension of the soft palate is the *uvula,* a vertical segment of muscle, connective tissue, and glands that hang in the back of the throat. The uvula closes the nasopharynx and prevents the entry of objects into the nasal cavity.

Where the soft and hard palates meet, small pits in the mucosa may be visible. These are the *palatine foveae,* where some of the palatine saliva glands empty.

The posterolateral areas of the mouth house the posterior folds, which are two folds of muscles and tissues. The larger of the folds is referred to as the *posterior pillar,* or *palatopharyngeal pillar or fold.* The folds are located behind the palatine tonsil. Anterior to the palatine tonsil are the *anterior pillars* or *palatoglossal pillar or fold.* The open area between the sets of pillars on either side of the mouth is referred to as the *fauces.* This is where the oral cavity opens into the pharynx.

Three sets of tonsils are located in the posterior segment of the oral cavity. The *pharyngeal adenoid tonsils* are superior and near the soft palate; the *palatine tonsils* are directly inferior to this area; and the *lingual tonsils* are on the inferior lateral surface at the base of the tongue.

Anterior to the tonsils on the maxilla, and posterior to the third molars, is a mass of bone called the *maxillary tuberosity.* Usually inferior to the maxillary tuberosity and posterior to the mandibular third molars is the

retromolar pad. This forms the inferior portion of the anterior border of the ramus and is a raised area of tissue.

TONGUE AND FLOOR OF THE MOUTH

The tongue is a highly muscular and vascular structure covered by epithelium. It is extremely well coordinated and has acute tactile sense. Its functions include forming words for speech, assisting in mastication and swallowing, and providing taste sensation from the taste buds located on its surface.

The tongue is divided into two portions: the posterior or base and the anterior or body of the tongue. On the dorsal surface of the body, a line can be seen dividing the tongue into a right and a left segment. This line separates approximately two thirds of the body of the tongue and is called the *median sulcus* or *fissure.* The median sulcus extends to the posterior of the tongue and then to the *circumvallate papillae.* Posterior to the circumvallate papillae is a developmental line called the *terminalis sulcus,* which divides the anterior from the posterior portion of the tongue (see Fig. 3-19).

Besides the circumvallate papillae, three other papillae are of importance: the *fungiform, filiform,* and *foliate* (see Fig. 3-19). The papillae are elevated structures on epithelial tissues of the tongue, and they are responsible for the sensation of taste. As mentioned previously, the circumvallate papillae are on the posterior segment of the tongue and form a V anterior to the terminalis sulcus. The taste buds are rounded with deep grooves surrounding them. Beneath and surrounding the taste buds are many small salivary glands that wash the papillae constantly to accommodate new taste sensations. The circumvallate papillae receive the bitter tastes. A large salivary gland, the *Von Eber gland,* also exits at this site.

The other three types of papillae are located on the body of the tongue. The fungiform papillae cover the anterior two thirds of the tongue and appear as small raised areas of tissue. The buds on the dorsal surface of the tongue are responsible for sensing sweet sensations; those toward the lateral surface sense salty tastes.

The foliate papillae are found on the posterior third and on the lateral surfaces of the tongue in the folds. Often the tongue must be extended to easily see the area where the foliate papillae are positioned. These papillae are responsible for sensing sour taste sensations.

The filiform papillae are somewhat hairlike in appearance and are located completely over the dorsal surface of the tongue in large quantities. They detect no taste sensations, but are sensitive to tactile sensations on the surface. In certain circumstances, pathologic conditions may develop in the area of the filiform papillae, such as hairy tongue and glossitis. The epithelium grows longer on the tongue and, as the name suggests, seems hairy, which can be the source of oral bacteria. Glossitis results when the epithelium becomes smooth as a result of various diseases.

The muscles of the tongue are divided into two groups: the **extrinsic** (outside the muscle) and the **intrinsic** (inside the muscle). The intrinsic muscles consist of four groups and are found within the tongue itself. The muscles are the superior longitudinal, transverse, vertical, and inferior longitudinal. The muscles function during mastication, speech, and deglutition.

The extrinsic muscles also consist of four groupings: the genioglossus, hyoglossus, palatoglossus, and styloglossus. These muscles suspend and anchor the tongue, as well as allow the tongue to move in a protruding or depressing movement.

KEY POINTS

▸ Prefixes and suffixes are single letters or groups of letters before or after the root word. Dental terminology often has a prefix and a suffix surrounding the root word.

▸ Commonly used descriptive terminology allows a dental professional to communicate the correct location and description of an area.

▸ Identification of body planes provides for specific descriptions of the surface/anatomic segment of the body in records management.

▸ Complete understanding of anatomy and physiology and the relationship of the systems in the human body to dentistry is necessary to provide complete care to the dental patient.

▸ The human organism, the relationship of the cells to the systems, and the function of each system all impact the type of care provided during dental treatment.

▸ The dental assistant should develop a thorough knowledge of head and neck anatomy, including cranial and facial bones, muscles of mastication and facial expression, trigeminal nerve, and oral/facial landmarks.

▸ Salivary glands and sinuses are directly related to dental care. The location and function of each of these should be understood by the dental assistant.

BIBLIOGRAPHY

Brand RW, Isselhard DE: *Anatomy of orofacial structures,* ed 5, St Louis, 1994, Mosby.

Moffett D, Moffett S, Schauf D: *Human physiology, foundations and frontiers,* ed 2, St Louis, 1993, Mosby.

Reed GM, Sheppard VF: *Basic structures of the head and neck,* Philadelphia, 1976, WB Saunders.

Thibodeau GA, Patton KT: *Anatomy and physiology,* ed 2, St Louis, 1993, Mosby.

4 Intraoral Structures

LEARNING OBJECTIVES

You will have mastered the material in this chapter when you can:

▶ Define the key terms
▶ Identify each dentition
▶ List the teeth and the characteristics of each dentition
▶ Locate the dentition, arch, and quadrant of each
▶ Describe common tooth numbering systems as they correlate to specific teeth
▶ Describe oral histology and embryology and their relationship to the oral cavity
▶ Describe the functions of the teeth and surrounding tissues
▶ Explain the difference between the anatomic and clinical crown
▶ List and identify the parts of the tooth
▶ Describe the development of the tooth from bud stage through eruption
▶ List the sequence of eruption of both dentitions

KEY TERMS

Ameloblast	Attrition	Buccal
Angle	Axial	Bud
Apical foramen	Bell stage	Canine
Cap stage	Endoderm	Occlusal
Cementoblast	Facial	Occlusion
Cementum	Fibroblast	Odontoblasts
Cingulum	Fossa	Overbite
Concave	Furcation	Overjet
Contact	Gingiva	Papilla
Convex	Groove	Periodontium
Crown	Incisal	Permanent
Curve of Spee	Incisor	Premolar
Cusp	Histology	Primary
Cuspid	Labial	Primordium
Deciduous	Lamina dura	Proximal
Dentin	Lingual	Pulp
Dentinal tubule	Lobe	Quadrant
Dentition	Mamelon	Ridge
Diastema	Mandible	Secondary
Ectoderm	Maxilla	Segment
Embrasure	Mesoderm	Succedaneous
Embryology	Molar	Sulcus
Enamel	Mucosa	Supernumerary
Enamel cuticle	Oblique	Tubercle

The Dental Arches

When the structures of the oral cavity are observed, the dental arches are the first to be examined. In a human mouth there are two dental arches, the **maxilla** and the **mandible**. The lay person may refer to the maxillary arch as the upper jaw and the mandibular arch as the lower jaw.

▶ Dentition

The arches support a combination of teeth that are referred to as **dentition**. In a lifetime it is normal to have two sets of dentition. The **primary or deciduous** dentition (sometimes referred to as the baby teeth by the lay person), is the first to develop in an infant's mouth; it begins to erupt at approximately 6 months and consists of 20 teeth. The primary or deciduous dentition is replaced by the **secondary or permanent** dentition, which include a maximum of 32 teeth. The secondary

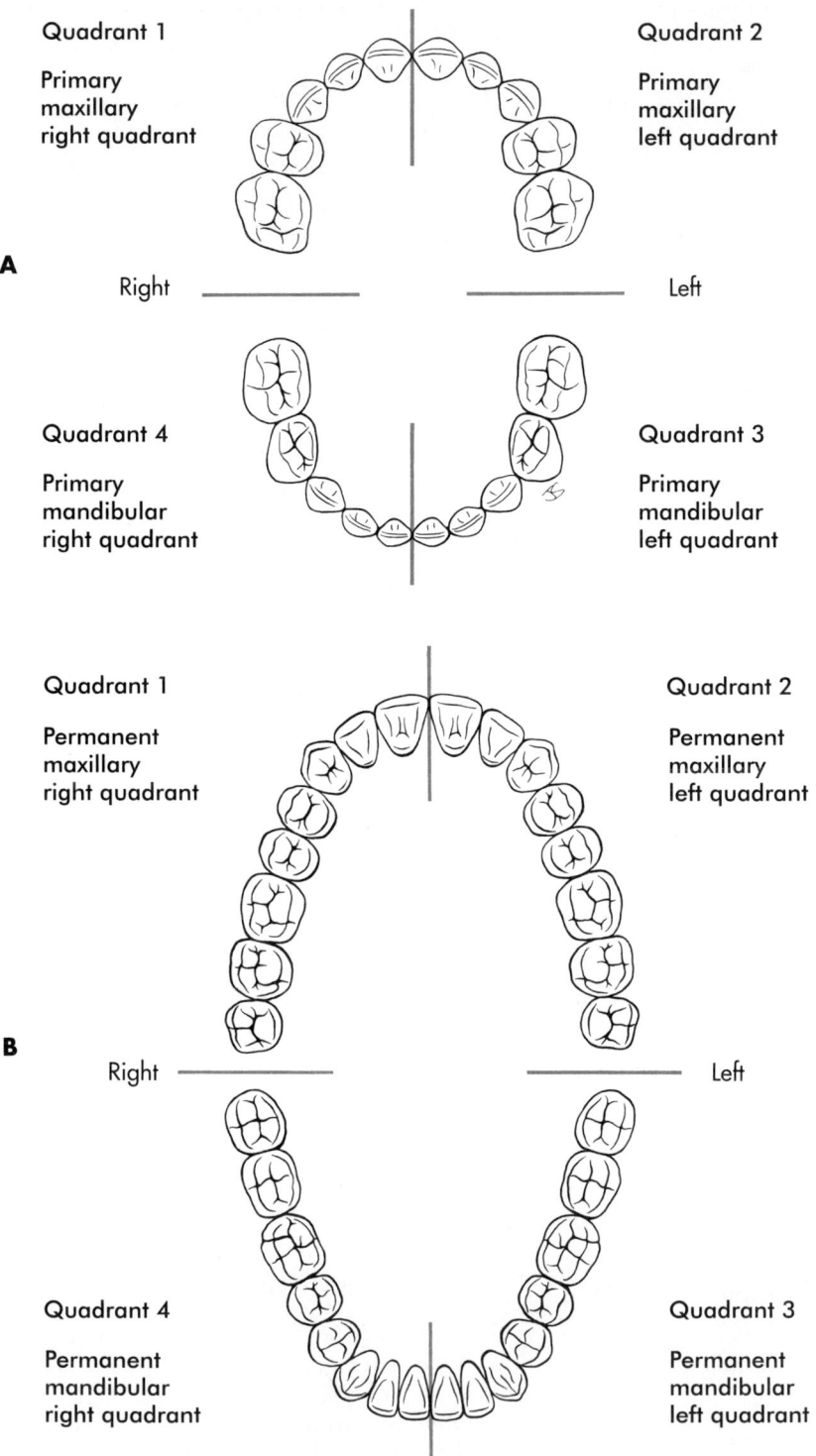

FIG. 4-1   *A,* Primary and, *B,* permanent dentition separated into quadrants.

teeth begin to erupt at approximately 6 years of age. The number of permanent teeth varies, depending on whether the third molars or wisdom teeth erupt.

Since the maxillary and mandibular arches each represent one half of the mouth, each arch accommodates the same number of teeth. In the primary dentition an arch contains 10 teeth, while in the permanent dentition the arch comprises 16 teeth, giving a total of 20 teeth in the primary and 32 teeth in the permanent dentition.

 Aristotle recorded in his early writings the belief that men have more teeth than women and that teeth continue to grow throughout a person's lifetime.

The arches can be divided in half. Each half of the arch is referred to as a **quadrant** or one quarter of the mouth. Each arch has two quadrants, totaling four quadrants in a full dentition. Each quadrant extends from the midline of the arch to the most posterior area of the arch.

Ideally each quadrant in a person's arch will be symmetric: the same number, type, and alignment of teeth are in each quadrant. A quadrant in the primary dentition will consist of five teeth, with eight teeth in each quadrant of the permanent dentition (Fig. 4-1, *A* and *B*). Each arch also can be divided into **segments** rather than quadrants. A segment is a section of the arch. Three segments are in each arch, totaling six segments in the dentition. A dental arch is divided into an anterior segment and two posterior segments, right and left. The anterior and posterior segments are found on both the maxillary and mandibular arches. The anterior segment consists of the anterior teeth, the four incisors and the cuspids or canines. The posterior segments consist of the remaining teeth of the arch: the premolars and molars (Fig. 4-2).

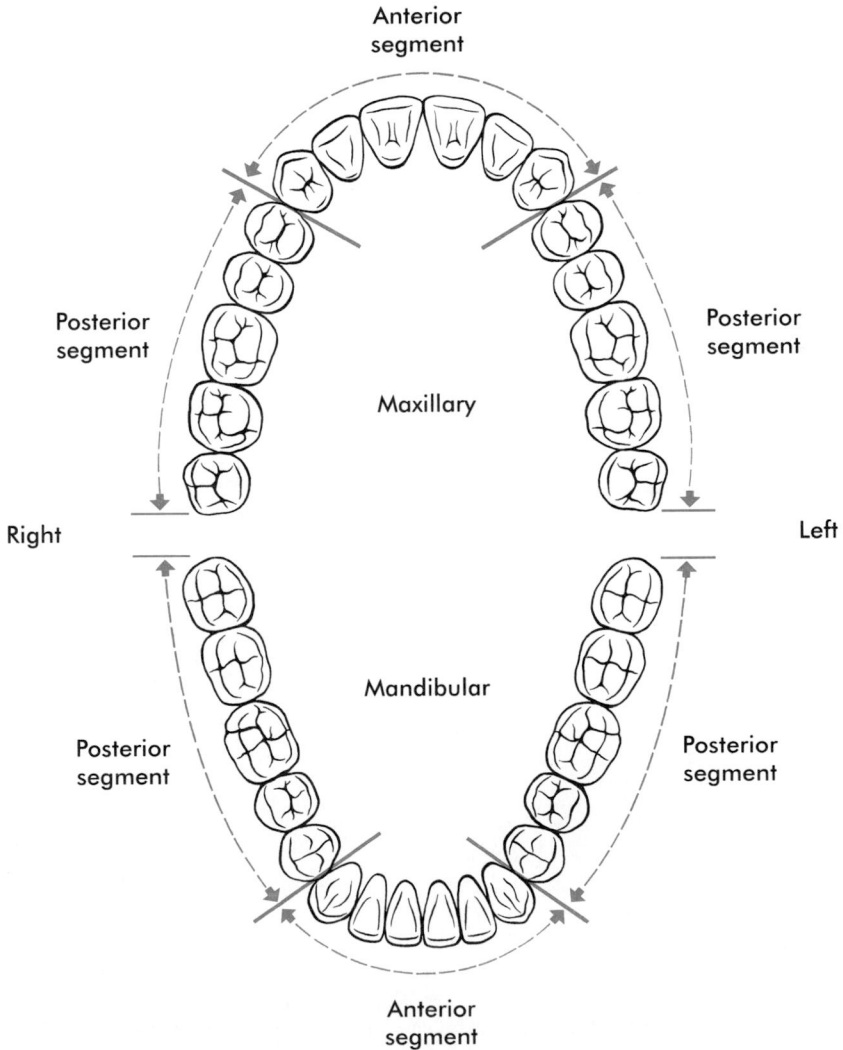

FIG. 4-2   Permanent dentition separated into segments.

▶ The Primary Dentition

PRIMARY DENTITION

The primary dentition consists of 20 teeth. Each arch includes the following:
two central incisors
two lateral incisors
two cuspids
two first molars
two second molars
Total: ten in each arch

The function of the primary dentition is similar to that of the permanent dentition, which will be discussed later in this chapter. One additional purpose of the primary dentition is to provide a guide for the permanent teeth as they develop and erupt into the oral cavity. The position of the primary teeth in the dental arches is completed at approximately 2 to 3 years of age. As the dental arches grow, the position of the primary teeth changes slightly to allow for the permanent dentition to assume its place in the arches. The change in position creates spaces between the teeth, known as a **diastema**. Many parents become concerned when they see the diastemas in a child's mouth and the dental professional must assure the parent that this is a desirable characteristic in development and that diastemas may ensure adequate space for the permanent tooth eruption.

▶ The Permanent Dentition

PERMANENT DENTITION

A full complement of permanent dentition includes 32 teeth. Each arch includes the following:
two central incisors
two lateral incisors
two cuspids
two first premolars
two second premolars
two first molars
two second molars
two third molars (may not develop)
Total: 16 in each arch (including the third molars)

Teeth provide esthetics or good appearance; support for other structures; aid in swallowing, mastication, and digestion; and aid in producing speech and phonetics. During mastication, eating, and chewing, each tooth type has a specific purpose as the dentition works to prepare food for swallowing and digestion. **Incisors** have sharp biting edges that aid in cutting and incising food; **cuspids or canines** have pointed cusps, which aid in holding and tearing food; **premolars** are used to crush and tear food, and the **molars** with their broad biting surfaces aid in chewing and grinding food. Box 4-3 provides a diagram of each of these teeth, including the identifying characteristics of each type of tooth.

Box 4-3

Left

MAXILLA

Third molar · Third molar

Second molar · Second molar

First molar · First molar

Second premolar · Second premolar

First premolar · First premolar

Canine (cuspid) · Canine (cuspid)

Lateral incisor · Lateral incisor

Central incisor · Central incisor

Central incisor · Central incisor

Lateral incisor · Lateral incisor

Canine (cuspid) · Canine (cuspid)

First premolar · First premolar

Second premolar · Second premolar

First molar · First molar

Second molar · Second molar

Third molar · Third molar

MANDIBLE

Right

BOX 4-3

CHARACTERISTICS AND DIAGRAM OF EACH TYPE OF TOOTH

MAXILLARY RIGHT AND LEFT CENTRAL INCISORS

Universal numbering system - #8 and #9
Palmer numbering system - 1| and |1
FDI numbering system - #11 and #21
Identifying characteristics:

Largest and widest of the incisor teeth in the mouth
Well-developed cingulum on lingual surface
The mesioincisal point is more acute, while the distoincisal is more blunted in shape
Has triangular-shaped root tipped toward the distal
The mesial contact with the abutment tooth is near the mesioincisal angle
Single root

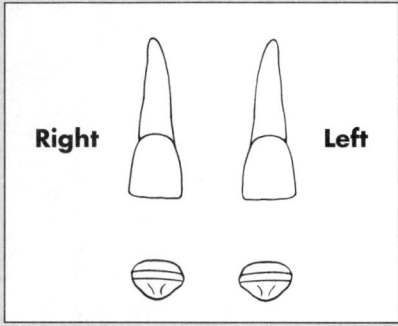

MAXILLARY RIGHT AND LEFT LATERAL INCISORS

Universal numbering system - #7 and #10
Palmer numbering system - 2| and |2
FDI numbering system - #12 and #22
Identifying characteristics:

Crown is smaller in size than the maxillary central incisor, but root length is similar
Smaller cingulum than maxillary central incisor and has distinct lingual pit and fossa
Mesioincisal point is more rounded than the maxillary central incisor
Mesial contact with abutment tooth is near the incisal and middle third of tooth
Distal contact with abutment tooth is near middle third of tooth
Single root

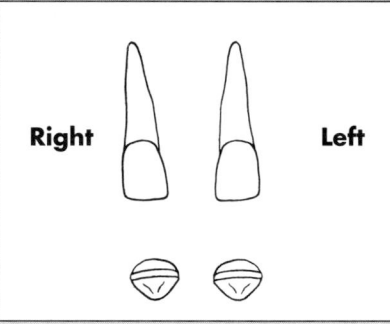

MANDIBULAR CENTRAL INCISORS

Universal numbering system - #24 and #25
Palmer numbering system - 1| and |1
FDI numbering system - #31 and #41
Identifying characteristics:

Usually is the smallest incisor in the mouth
Usually smaller than the mandibular lateral incisors
The mesial-distal crown width is small
Has a flat cingulum
The root is oval in shape in a cross-section
Single root that may curve slightly towards the distal

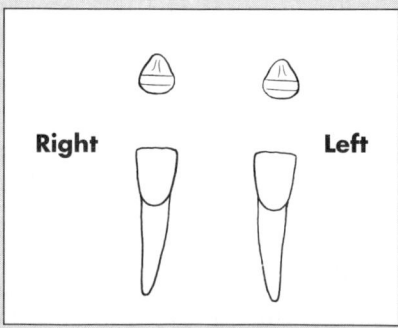

MANDIBULAR LATERAL INCISORS

Universal numbering system - #23 and #26
Palmer numbering system - 2| and |2
FDI numbering system - #32 and #42
Identifying characteristics:

The mesial contact is near the incisal third, and the distal contact is near the middle third
The distal incisal edge slopes apically
The mesial-facial line angle is longer than the distal-facial line angle
The cingulum is positioned slightly towards the distal
The incisal edge wears more towards the distal surface
Single root

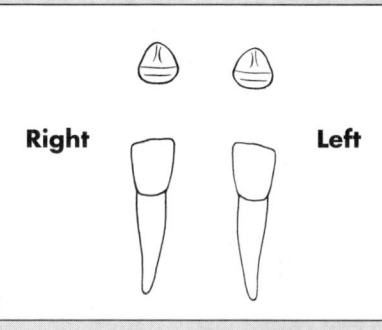

BOX 4-3

CHARACTERISTICS AND DIAGRAM OF EACH TYPE OF TOOTH

MAXILLARY RIGHT AND LEFT CUSPIDS (CANINES, SINGLE CUSP)

Universal numbering system - #6 and #11
Palmer numbering system - 3| and |3
FDI numbering system - #13 and #23
Identifying characteristics:
  Has no incisal edge, has a cusp instead
  Length of distal cusp ridge is longer than mesial cusp ridge
  Mesial contact with abutment tooth is near cusp apex
  Distal contact with abutment tooth is near cervical area
  Prominent cingulum in cervical half of clinical crown
  Longest single-rooted tooth in mouth

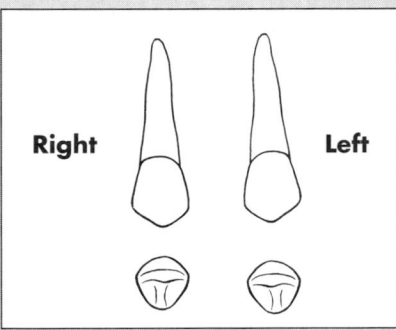

MANDIBULAR CUSPIDS (CANINES, ONE CUSP)

Universal numbering system - #22 and #27
Palmer numbering system - 3| and |3
FDI numbering system - #33 and #43
Identifying characteristics:
  Has smooth lingual anatomy with a cingulum in the cervical third
  Has cusp, no incisal edge
  The distal cusp ridge is longer than the mesial cusp ridge
  Has smaller mesiodistal width than the maxillary cuspids
  Receives much wear on facial surface
  Single root that curves toward the distal

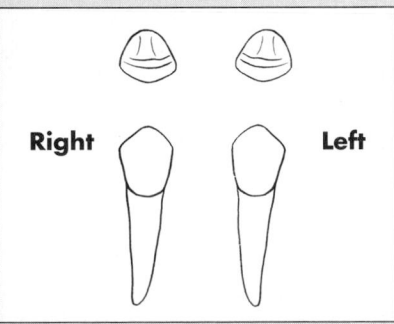

MAXILLARY RIGHT AND LEFT FIRST PREMOLARS (BICUSPIDS, TWO CUSPS)

Universal numbering system - #5 and #12
Palmer numbering system - 4| and |4
FDI numbering system - #14 and #24
Identifying characteristics:
  Crown of tooth has a hexagonal shape
  Has both a buccal and lingual cusp, with buccal cusp usually being longer
  Buccal cusp is wider from the mesial to distal than the lingual cusp
  Central occlusal groove crosses the mesial marginal ridge
  Buccal cusp ridge slopes towards the mesial of the tooth
  Usually double rooted with one buccal and lingual root, but may be single rooted

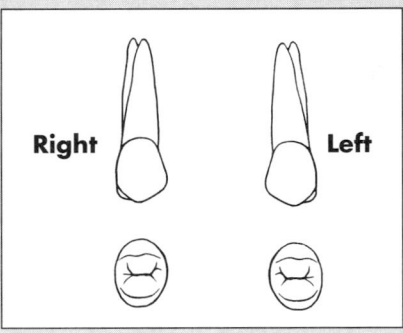

MANDIBULAR RIGHT AND LEFT FIRST PREMOLARS (BICUSPIDS, TWO CUSPS)

Universal numbering system - #21 and #28
Palmer numbering system - 4| and |4
FDI numbering system - #34 and #44
Identifying characteristics:
  Smaller in size compared to the mandibular second premolar
  Lingual cusp(s) are nonfunctional
  Has large cusp with one or two smaller and shorter lingual cusps
  Has transverse ridge across the occlusal surface
  Single root is smaller than the mandibular second premolar

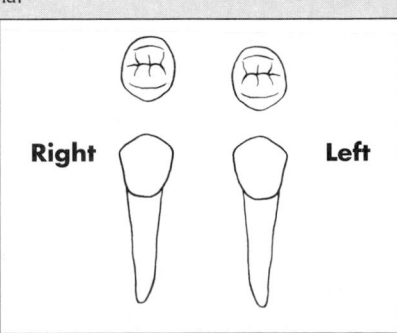

Continued.

BOX 4-3

CHARACTERISTICS AND DIAGRAM OF EACH TYPE OF TOOTH

MAXILLARY RIGHT AND LEFT SECOND PREMOLARS (BICUSPIDS, TWO CUSPS)

Universal numbering system - #4 and #13
Palmer numbering system - 5⌋ and ⌊5
FDI numbering system - #15 and #25
Identifying characteristics:

Has buccal and lingual cusp that are similar in length
No depression on the mesial or distal crown surfaces
Size of crown wider from buccal to lingual than from mesial to distal
Tooth has central groove that doesn't cross the marginal ridge
Buccal cusp ridge is parallel to the central groove
Single root

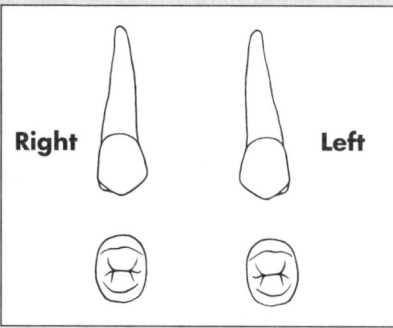

MANDIBULAR RIGHT AND LEFT SECOND PREMOLARS (BICUSPIDS, THREE CUSPS)

Universal numbering system - #20 and #29
Palmer numbering system - 5⌋ and ⌊5
FDI numbering system - #35 and #45
Identifying characteristics:

Has single buccal cusp with one or two lingual cusps
Lingual cusps are more functional than mandibular first premolar
If the tooth has single lingual cusp, occlusal pattern is usually U or H shaped
If the tooth has two lingual cusps, occlusal pattern is usually Y shaped
Larger and longer root than the mandibular first premolar
Has single root

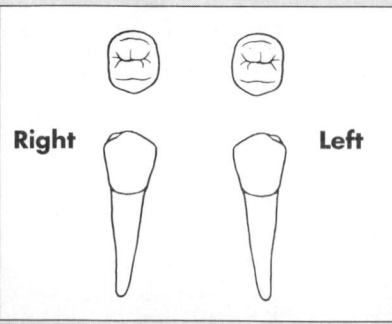

MAXILLARY RIGHT AND LEFT FIRST MOLARS

Universal numbering system - #3 and #14
Palmer numbering system - 6⌋ and ⌊6
FDI numbering system - #16 and #26
Identifying characteristics:

Usually the largest maxillary tooth
Has four defined cusps: mesiolingual, mesiobuccal, distobuccal, and distolingual, with the mesiolingual being the largest and the distolingual the smallest
Has a supplemental cusp called cusp of Carabelli that is lingual to the mesiolingual cusp
The crown shape is rhomboidal
Has a strong and defined oblique ridge
Has three roots being trifurcated—mesiobuccal, distobuccal, and lingual

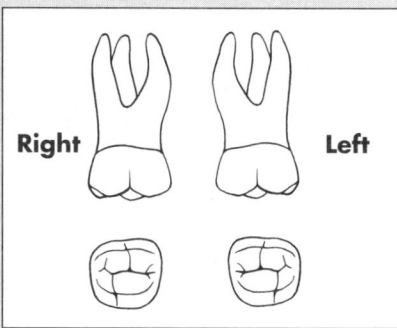

MANDIBULAR RIGHT AND LEFT FIRST MOLARS

Universal numbering system - #19 and #30
Palmer numbering system - 6⌋ and ⌊6
FDI numbering system - #36 and #46
Identifying characteristics:

Usually the largest mandibular tooth
Has five well-developed cusps: mesiobuccal, mesiolingual, distolingual, distobuccal, and distal
Has two buccal grooves with three cusps
Has one lingual groove and two cusps
Crown shape is somewhat rectangular
Has two roots, one mesial, and one distal; they are spaced wide apart

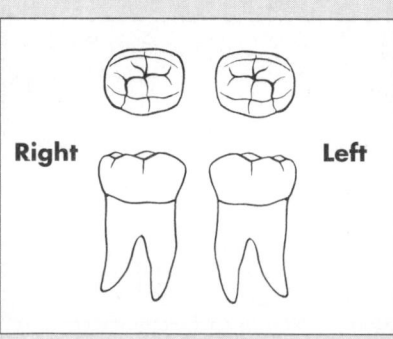

BOX 4-3

CHARACTERISTICS AND DIAGRAM OF EACH TYPE OF TOOTH

MAXILLARY RIGHT AND LEFT SECOND MOLARS

Universal numbering system - #2 and #15
Palmer numbering system - 7⌋ and ⌊7
FDI numbering system - #17 and #27
Identifying characteristics:

Has four defined cusps: mesiolingual, mesiobuccal, distobuccal, and distolingual

Also has oblique ridge, but it is crossed by the central groove

Crown of tooth is usually shorter in length than the maxillary first molar

The distolingual cusp usually is smaller than that of the maxillary first molar

The roots tend to be closer together than the maxillary first molar

Has three roots being trifurcated: mesiobuccal, distobuccal, and lingual; the roots usually are longer than the maxillary first molar roots

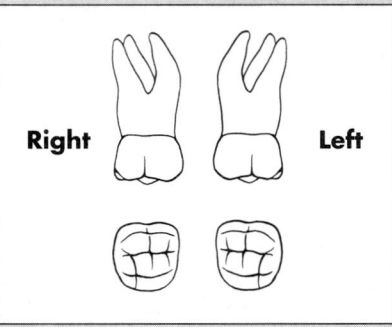

MANDIBULAR SECOND MOLARS

Universal numbering system - #18 and #31
Palmer numbering system - 7̅⌋ and ⌊7̅
FDI numbering system - #37 and #47
Identifying characteristics:

Has four cusps: mesiobuccal, mesiolingual, distobuccal, and distolingual

Has two buccal cusps, and one groove

Lingual cusps are more pointed and longer than the buccal cusps

Has three occlusal pits

Buccal cusps tip toward the lingual

Has two roots, mesial and distal, that are not spread as far apart as the mandibular first molars

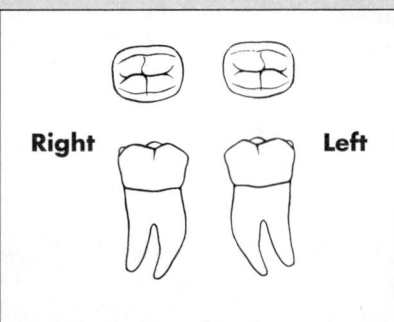

MAXILLARY RIGHT AND LEFT THIRD MOLARS

Universal numbering system - #1 and #16
Palmer numbering system - 8⌋ and ⌊8
FDI numbering system - #18 and #28
Identifying characteristics:

Usually no oblique ridge

Size, shape, and contour may differ greatly because the teeth are developmental anomalies

Roots curve toward the distal

Roots are often fused together

The number of roots may vary: one, two, or three

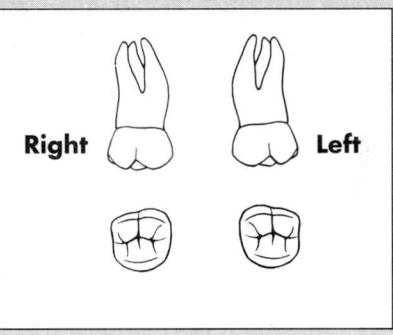

MANDIBULAR THIRD MOLARS

Universal numbering system - #17 and #32
Palmer numbering system - 8̅⌋ and ⌊8̅
FDI numbering system - #38 and #48
Identifying characteristics:

Size, shape, and contour may differ greatly because these are developmental anomalies

Roots are usually fused together

Roots are usually curved distally

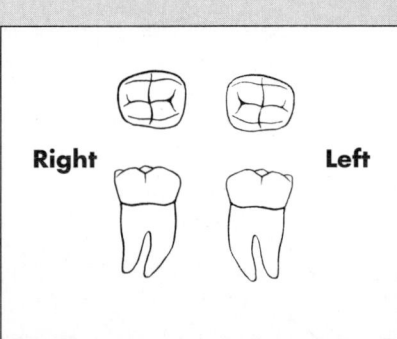

▶ Mixed Dentition

Mixed dentition usually exists in a person's oral cavity from approximately 6 to 12 years of age. This mixed dentition is a combination of primary and permanent dentition. Mixed dentition occurs as the permanent teeth begin to erupt within the oral cavity, while some of the primary teeth are still present. This is common, for instance, in a child who is about 7 years old. He or she may have lost the primary central incisors and the first permanent molars may have erupted. Occasionally, this occurs in an adult when a primary tooth is retained and not replaced by a permanent tooth.

 Hippocrates wrote that the first teeth are formed by the nourishment the fetus receives in the womb, and then after birth, by the mother's milk. After these first teeth are lost the replacement teeth are formed by food and drink. These first teeth are shed generally at about 7 years of age. Those that come after this "grow old with the man," unless some illness destroys them.

As the teeth of the primary dentition are naturally lost, they are replaced by the permanent teeth, which are called **succedaneous** teeth: a group of teeth that follow the first set. Any teeth of the permanent dentition that do not replace primary teeth are referred to as nonsuccedaneous teeth. Normally the teeth considered nonsuccedaneous are the permanent molars, since they erupt distal to the primary teeth and do not replace any primary teeth.

Teeth can also be **congenitally missing**, or the tooth bud is not present at birth; this could occur with a primary or permanent tooth. If a primary tooth is congenitally missing, if the tooth never developed, a space maintainer may be placed in the arch to allow for the correct positioning of the permanent tooth as it erupts. If the permanent tooth is congenitally missing, the primary tooth can be maintained in the arch or if it is lost, a prosthesis can be used to replace the missing tooth. Another abnormality that is observed in dentistry is the existence of **supernumerary teeth**. This is the existence of additional tooth bud(s) that erupt as a third tooth or teeth on the dental arch(es). It is common practice to remove the additional tooth or teeth to maintain good oral hygiene conditions and to avoid decay.

Tooth Morphology

It is important to understand the correct identification of a tooth within the oral cavity and the sequence of the terms for its identification. When the order of identification of a tooth is confused it can result in many communication problems. The correct sequence of identification should first be the dentition, then the arch, then the quadrant, and finally the specific tooth about which you are talking (Box 4-4).

BOX 4-4

SEQUENCE FOR TOOTH IDENTIFICATION

DENTITION	SIDE
Permanent	Right
Primary	Left

ARCH	TOOTH NAME
Maxillary	First Premolar
Mandibular	Central Incisor

Thus, when describing a specific tooth about which a patient is having discomfort, you would define the condition as being on the permanent maxillary right first molar. This sequence of order is a commonly accepted method used in dental offices.

The permanent dentition has the same teeth in each quadrant from the most posterior area of the mouth to the midline of the mouth. The teeth are as follows:

Third molar
Second molar
First molar
Second premolar (second bicuspid)
First premolar (first bicuspid)
Cuspid (canine)
Lateral incisor
Central incisor

The primary dentition has the same teeth in each quadrant from the most posterior area of the mouth to the midline of the mouth. The teeth are as follows:

Second molar
First molar
Cuspid (canine)
Lateral incisor
Central incisor

▶ Tooth Numbering Systems

Every dental office has a specific numbering system that is used when charting a patient's oral cavity or when referring to dental treatment that is to be performed. Several numbering systems exist, and the doctor and staff choose which system will be used. The objective of a numbering system is to name and code each tooth in the oral cavity, either numerically or alphabetically. This number or letter provides an abbreviated form of tooth reference and aids in consistency in records management. The most common types of numbering systems include the Universal Numbering System, Palmer Notation System and Federal Dentaire Internationale System. Each of these is described in detail in the following narrative.

UNIVERSAL NUMBERING SYSTEM

The most popular of these systems is the *Universal numbering system*. It uses the Arabic numbering system from *1* through *32* for the permanent dentition and uses letters for the primary dentition from *A* through *T*. Mixed dentition may include permanent and primary teeth, so there may be numbers as well as letters in a charting sequence for a particular patient using this system.

The universal system begins numbering the teeth with the most posterior tooth on the patient's maxillary right quadrant, the third molar, being tooth #1 or the permanent maxillary right third molar. If the numbering is for the primary dentition, the tooth would be A for the primary maxillary right second molar. The numbering continues toward the anterior midline to the central incisor or tooth #8 of the permanent or tooth #E for the primary tooth.

The numbering continues to the maxillary left quadrant, from the midline to the most posterior tooth either #16 of the permanent or #J of the primary dentition. The numbering then drops to the mandibular left quadrant to permanent tooth #17 and the primary to tooth #K across the arch to the mandibular right most posterior tooth or #32 or #T (Fig. 4-3, *A* and *B*).

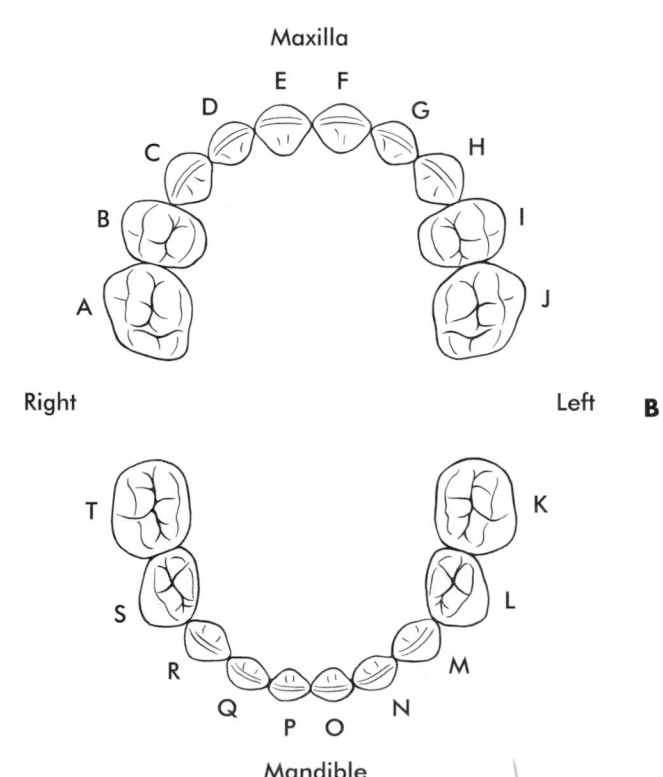

FIG. 4-3 Universal numbering system for the, *A*, permanent and, *B*, primary dentition.

PALMER NOTATION SYSTEM

The *Palmer notation system* assigns each of the four quadrants a bracket to designate the area of the mouth in which the tooth exists. As you look at a chart shown in either Fig. 4-4, *A*, or Fig. 4-4, *B*, the left side of the chart represents the patient's right side and the right side of the chart is the patient's left side.

Example: Maxillary right   Maxillary left
            Mandibular right   Mandibular left

Each particular permanent tooth in any quadrant is assigned the same number with #1 beginning at the midline and increasing to #8 distally. For instance:

Maxillary right central incisor = 1⌋
Maxillary left central incisor =⌊1
Mandibular left central incisor =⌈1

Mandibular right central incisor = 1⌉
The direction of the bracket determines the arch and the number within the bracket determines the tooth.
Maxillary right third molar is 8⌋
Maxillary left second molar is⌊7
Mandibular right first premolar is 4⌉
Mandibular left lateral incisor is⌊2

In this system, the primary dentition uses the bracket system to assign a quadrant, but the teeth are designated by letters, *A* through *E*, instead of numbers. The *A* specifies the central incisors and the *E* the second molars.

Examples of each dentition are as follows:
⌊5 is the permanent maxillary left second premolar
D⌉ is the primary mandibular right first molar

FIG. 4-4   Palmer notation system assigned to, *A*, primary and, *B*, permanent dentition.

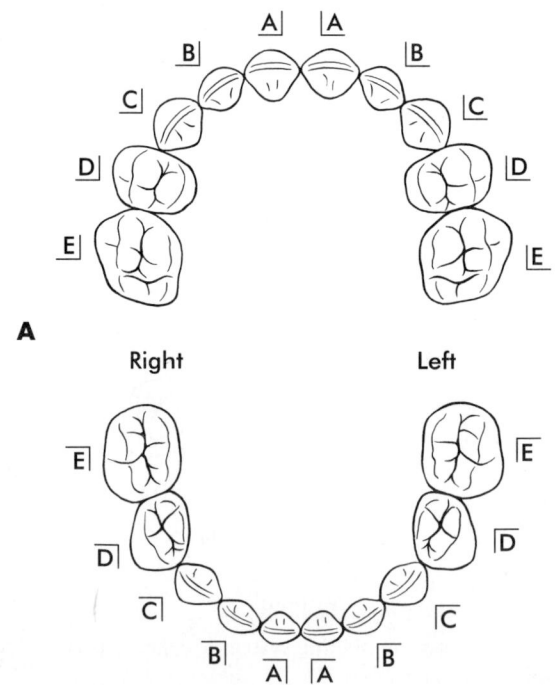

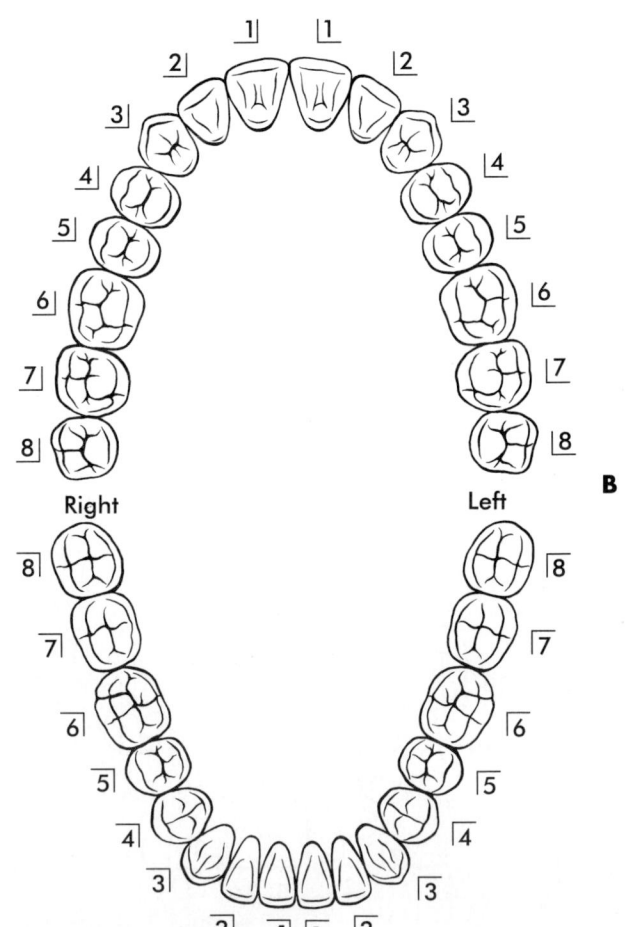

THE FEDERAL DENTAIRE INTERNATIONALE

The *Federal Dentaire Internationale (FDI)* system assigns a two-digit number to each tooth in any quadrant. The first number indicates the quadrant in which the tooth is positioned and the second number identifies the specific tooth. The first digit numbers 1 through 4 are assigned to the permanent dentition and 5 through 8 are assigned to the quadrants of the primary dentition.

Quadrant Number	Identification of Quadrant
1	Permanent maxillary right
2	Permanent maxillary left
3	Permanent mandibular left
4	Permanent mandibular right
5	Primary maxillary right
6	Primary maxillary left
7	Primary mandibular left
8	Primary mandibular right

The second number identifies the specific tooth in the arch. The numbers 1 through 8 are the second digit assigned to the permanent dentition and numbers 1 through 5 are for the primary dentition. The #1 in both instances begins with the central incisors and the numbering of the teeth proceeds posteriorly so that the last tooth in the quadrant is the highest number in the sequence. Using this two-digit system the following are true:

Permanent maxillary right central incisor is #11 or #one one

Permanent maxillary left central incisor is #21 or #two one

Permanent mandibular left central incisor is #31 or #three one

Permanent mandibular right central incisor is #41 or #four one

The primary dentition is handled in the same manner, but since there are only five teeth per quadrant, the numbers would range from 1 through 5 for each tooth and from 5 through 8 for the quadrants (Fig. 4-5, *A* and *B*). The following are examples:

Primary maxillary right first molar is #54

Primary mandibular left lateral incisor is #72

FIG. 4-5   Federal Dentaire Internationale system assigned to, *A*, primary and, *B*, permanent dentition.

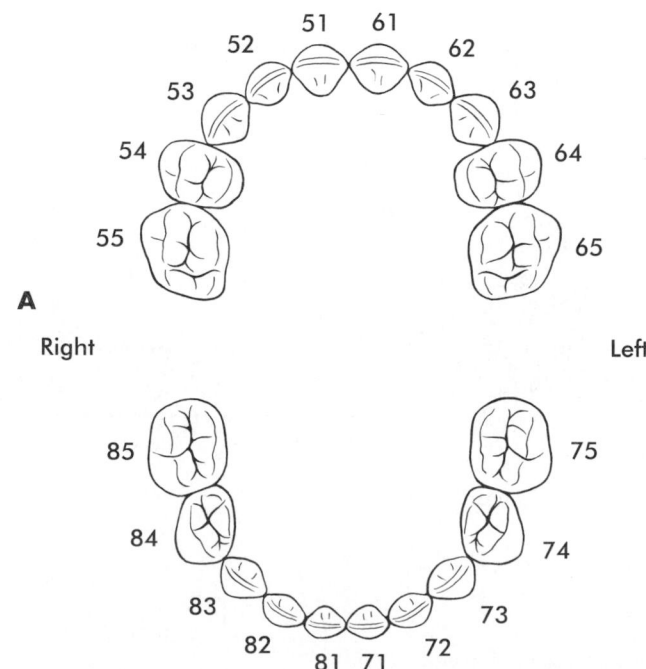

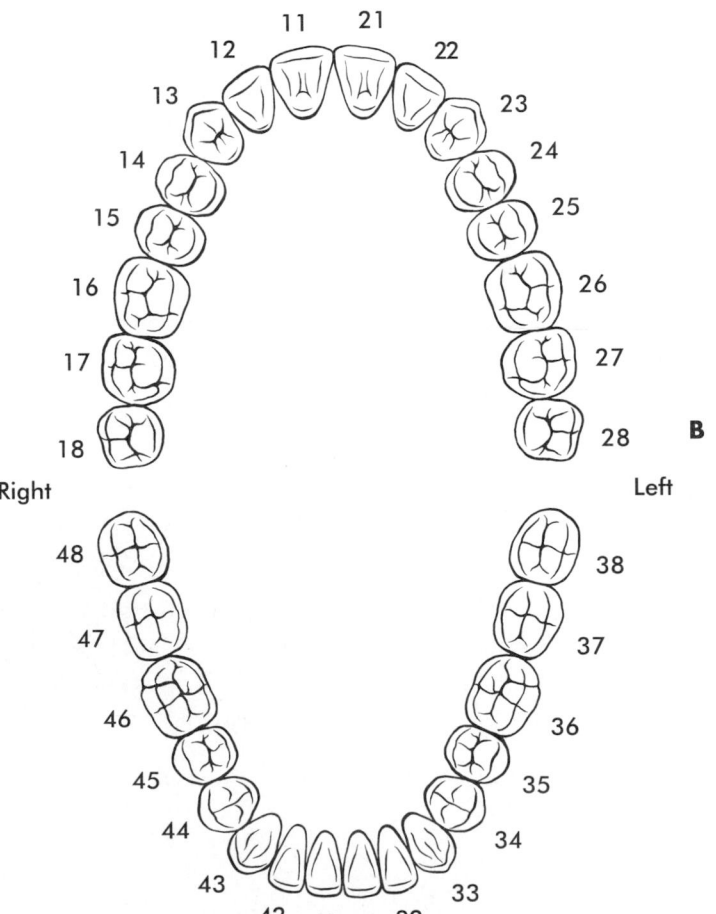

▶ Tooth Surfaces

As the dental team performs a complete oral examination on a patient, it is necessary to use a standardized system, not only for tooth numbering, but also for tooth surface annotation. By combining both of these forms of communication, it becomes easy to identify a specific location on a tooth with dental decay, a fracture, or a restoration. All crowns of the teeth are divided into surfaces. These surfaces are identified by the position they take in relation to the oral cavity. For instance, those surfaces which are nearest the lips are referred to as the labial or facial surfaces.

The posterior teeth, premolars, and molars have five surfaces. The anterior teeth, incisors, and canines have four surfaces with a ridge. Of these surfaces, both anterior and posterior teeth have four **axial** surfaces. Axial surfaces are those surfaces that run vertically from the biting surface to the apex of a tooth. The posterior teeth have one additional surface, the **occlusal** surface, which is a horizontal surface running perpendicular to the other axial surfaces.

The surfaces of the teeth are not only named but are also identified by letters or numbers. This surface annotation is used to chart notations and is used in all insurance claim reporting. This letter or number is commonly placed as a superscript (above the print line) next to the tooth number. An example of this is the permanent maxillary left first molar involving the mesial surface using the Universal Numbering System; #14^m or #14^1.

Surfaces of the Teeth

Mesial surface (M or 1) is the axial surface of teeth that is closest to the midline of the mouth. It is directly opposite on the tooth from the distal surface.

Distal surface (D or 2) lies directly opposite the mesial surface on all teeth and is the axial surface furthest from the midline.

Facial surface (F or 3) is the surface of a tooth that faces the cheek and lips, or the exterior of the mouth.

Labial surface (LA or 3) is the same as the facial surface but is found facing only the lips on the anterior teeth.

Buccal surface (B or 3) is the same as the facial surface but is found on posterior teeth only facing the cheeks.

Lingual surface (L or 4) is the surface closest to the tongue on all teeth, anterior or posterior.

Occlusal surface (O or 5) is found only on posterior teeth on a vertical plane on the biting surface of the teeth.

Occlusal surface (O or 6) is found only on posterior teeth where a ridge divides the surface into two parts. The portion designated as surface 6 is the distal segment.

Incisal ridge/edge/surface (I or 5) is found only on anterior teeth where there is a biting edge.

The **proximal area or surface** are the surfaces of two teeth that abut or face each other. On any given two, there are two proximal surfaces: the mesial and the distal. In the situation of the third molars though, only the mesial surface may be considered a proximal surface (Fig. 4-6).

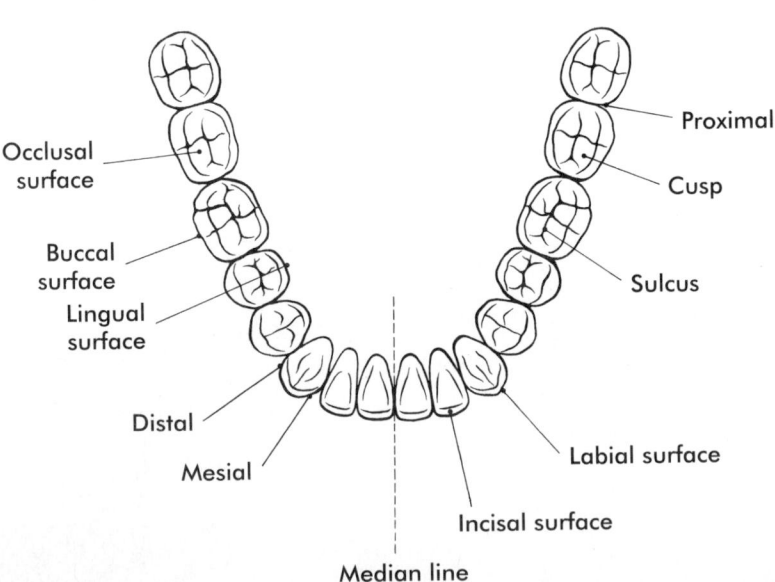

FIG. 4-6   Surfaces of the anterior and posterior teeth.

When more than one surface is involved, such as the mesial, occlusal, and distal surfaces, the surface annotations are placed in order from mesial to distal. For instance, #19^{MOD}, instead of 19^{DOM}, or 19^{ODM}. Again this standardization provides for uniform communication between dental professionals.

The area where two surfaces on a tooth meet is a **line angle**. The angles on teeth are named by the two surfaces that meet (Fig. 4-7). Examples of line angles for anterior and posterior teeth are seen in Box 4-5 and illustrated in Fig. 4-7, *A* and *B*.

Since a line angle is where two surfaces meet, a point angle is the area where three surfaces meet at a point. Examples of point angles for anterior and posterior teeth are found in Box 4-6 and illustrated in Fig. 4-8, *A* and *B*.

The names formed to describe either line or point angles are developed from the surfaces that are joined together. In each case when the multiple surfaces are joined together to form one term the *al* suffix is dropped and replaced with the letter *o*.

BOX 4-5

LINE ANGLES OF ANTERIOR AND POSTERIOR TEETH

ANTERIOR TEETH

DISTOLABIAL	DISTOLINGUAL
MESIOLABIAL	MESIOLINGUAL
LABIOINCISAL	LINGUOINCISAL

POSTERIOR TEETH

DISTOBUCCAL	BUCCO-OCCLUSAL
MESIOBUCCAL	LINGUO-OCCLUSAL
DISTOLINGUAL	DISTO-OCCLUSAL
MESIOLINGUAL	MESIO-OCCLUSAL

BOX 4-6

POINT ANGLES OF ANTERIOR AND POSTERIOR TEETH

ANTERIOR TEETH	POSTERIOR TEETH
MESIOLABIOINCISAL	MESIOBUCCO-OCCLUSAL
DISTOLABIOINCISAL	DISTOBUCCO-OCCLUSAL
MESIOLINGUOINCISAL	MESIOLINGUO-OCCLUSAL
DISTOLINGUOINCISAL	DISTOLINGUO-OCCLUSAL

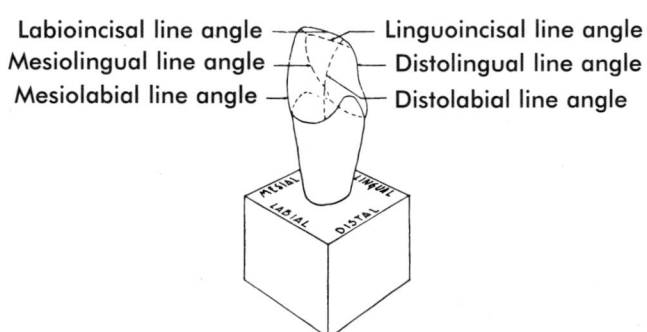

Labioincisal line angle — Linguoincisal line angle
Mesiolingual line angle — Distolingual line angle
Mesiolabial line angle — Distolabial line angle

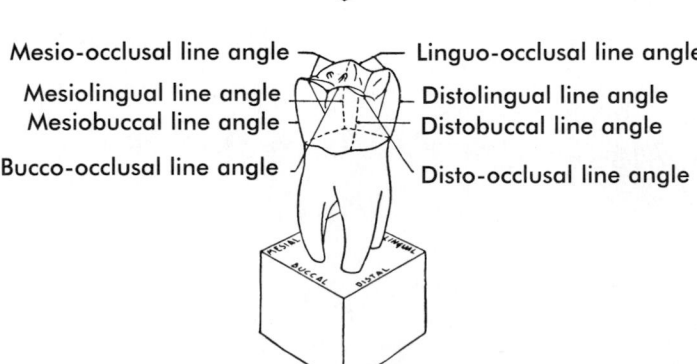

Mesio-occlusal line angle — Linguo-occlusal line angle
Mesiolingual line angle — Distolingual line angle
Mesiobuccal line angle — Distobuccal line angle
Bucco-occlusal line angle — Disto-occlusal line angle

FIG. 4-7   Relationship of line angle to surfaces on a tooth.

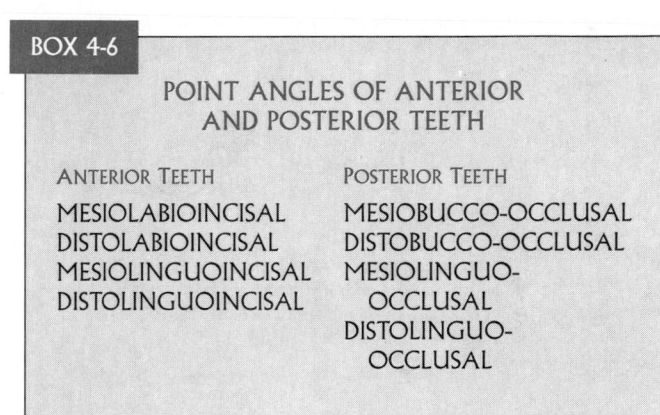

Mesiolabioincisal point angle — Distolabioincisal point angle
Mesiolinguoincisal point angle — Distolinguoincisal point angle

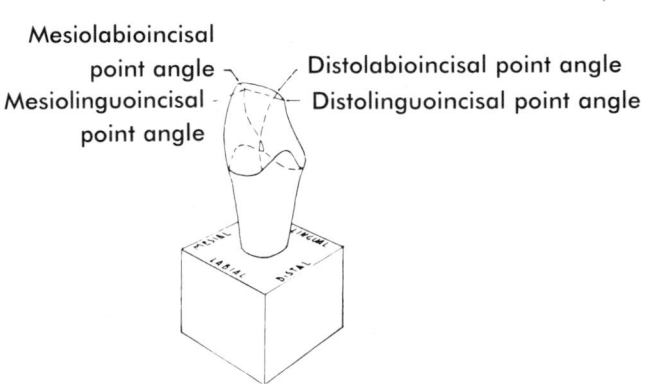

Mesiolinguo-occlusal point angle — Distolinguo-occlusal point angle
Mesiobucco-occlusal point angle — Distobucco-occlusal point angle

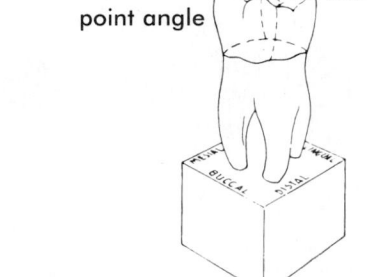

FIG. 4-8   Relationship of point angle to surfaces on a tooth.

▌Dental Anatomy

Before studying the anatomy of individual teeth, the dental assistant should become familiar with several anatomic terms in relation to tooth anatomy (Box 4-7).

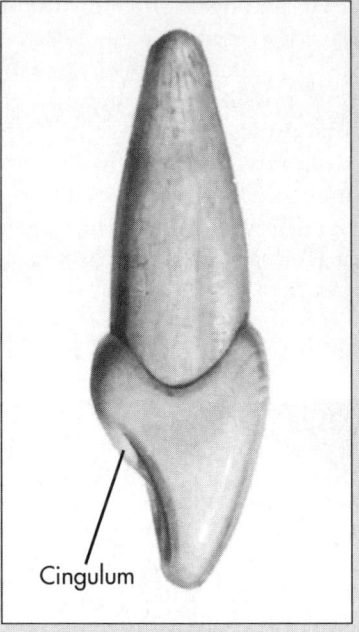

Cingulum

ANATOMIC TERMS

Cingulum - a prominence of enamel on the lingual surface of anterior teeth and referred to as a lobe

Concave - a curvature that leans inward, opposite of convex

Contact area - the area of a tooth that physically touches the abutment tooth; the contact areas occur on the proximal surfaces of teeth

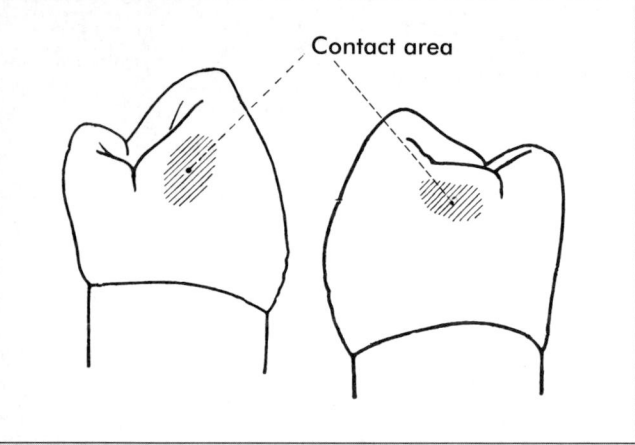

Contact area

Convex - a curvature that extends outward, opposite of concave

Curve of Spee - the curve upward that the maxillary and mandibular arches form when the two are in occlusion

Cusp - a prominence of large tooth structure found on canines, premolars, and molars

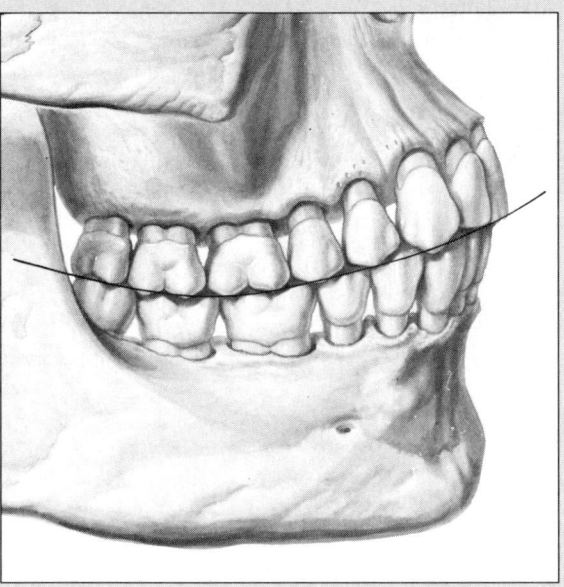

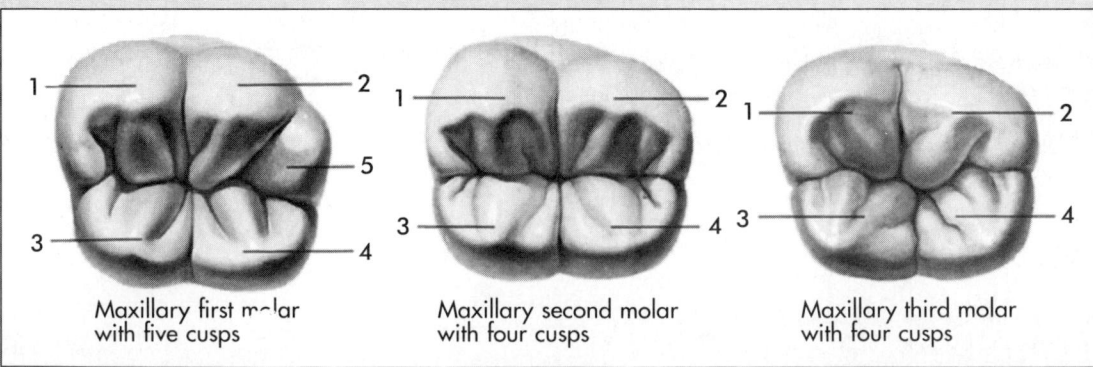

Maxillary first molar with five cusps

Maxillary second molar with four cusps

Maxillary third molar with four cusps

BOX 4-7

ANATOMIC TERMS—cont'd

Developmental groove - a line on the surfaces of the tooth that separate distinct portions of the tooth from each other

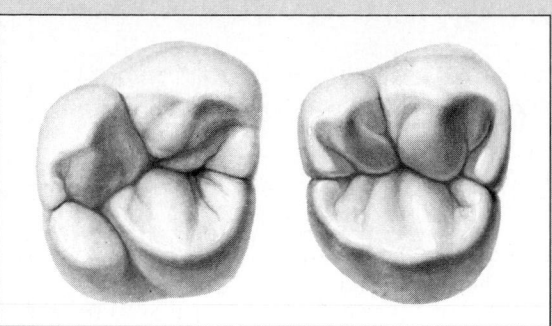

Diastema - a spacing between two adjacent teeth

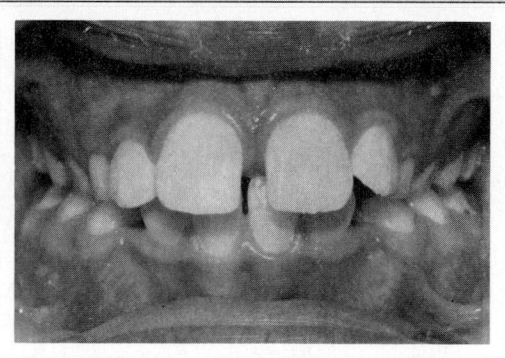

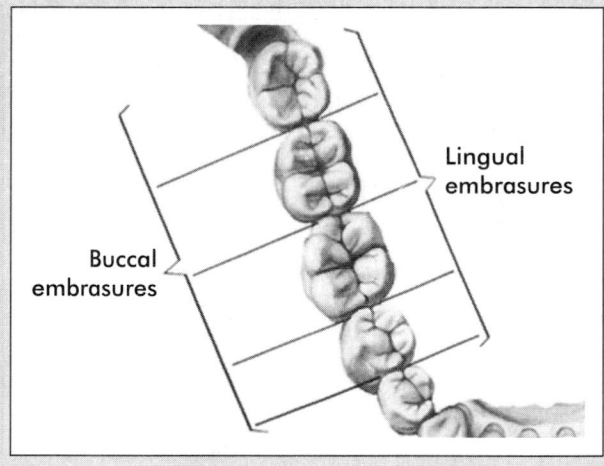

Fossa - an area on a tooth that has a concave surface and is usually named for the area that it is found

Embrasure - a V-shaped space that exists between proximal surfaces of abutment teeth; the different embrasures are: gingival, incisal, facial, lingual, and occlusal

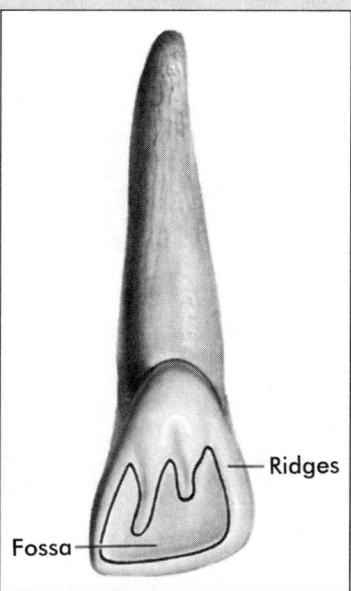

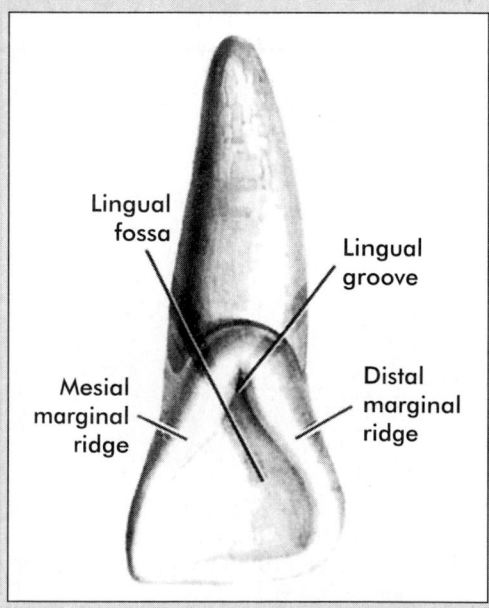

Lingual groove - a line that separates the cingulum from the other lobes that exist on the tooth

Continued.

BOX 4-7

ANATOMIC TERMS—cont'd

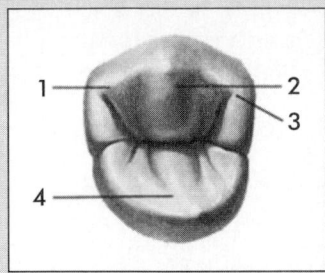

Lobes - a growth center that forms together with other developmental structures to combine as the crowns of teeth

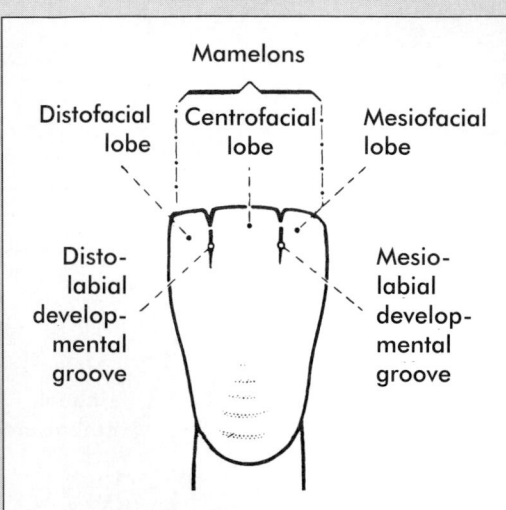

Mamelon - a rounded prominence at the incisal edge of newly erupted teeth that wears away with use

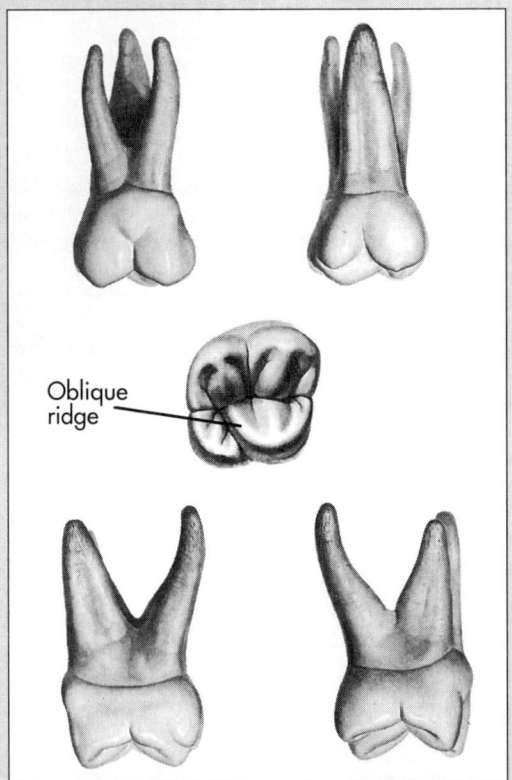

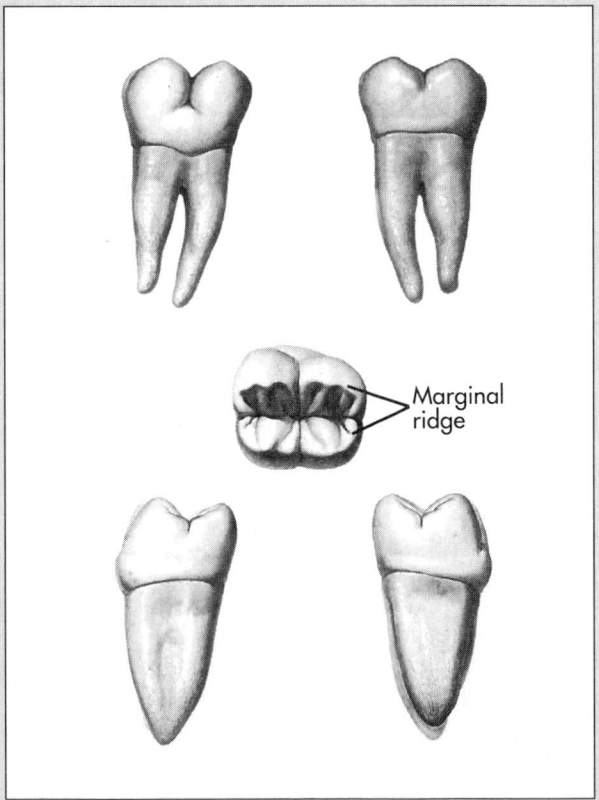

Marginal ridge - rounded areas on the proximal surfaces of teeth where contact may exist with the abutment teeth, creating embrasures

(Courtesy of Zeisz and Nuckolls.)

Oblique ridge - an elevated line on the occlusal surface crossing from mesiolingual cusp to the distobuccal cusp of maxillary molars

(Courtesy of Zeisz and Nuckolls.)

BOX 4-7

ANATOMIC TERMS—cont'd

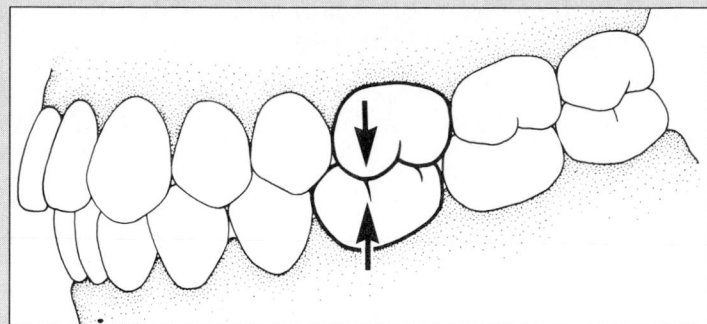

Occlusion - the contact that is made between the maxillary and mandibular teeth when the mandible is in a closed position

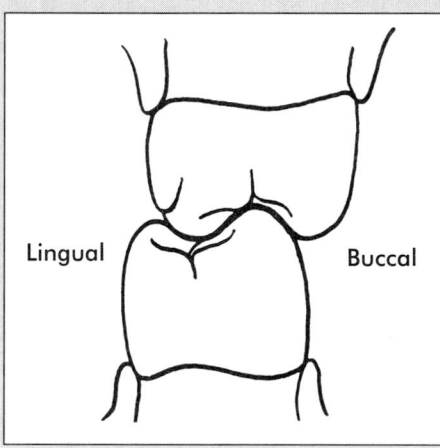

Lingual Buccal

Centric occlusion - contact that is made when the maxillary and mandibular jaws are closed in the most stable position

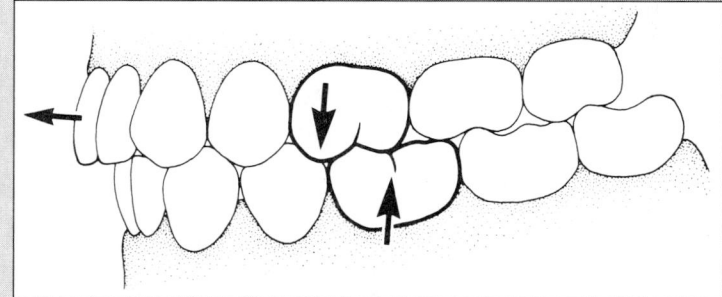

Malocclusion - a position of the maxillary and mandibular jaws to each other that is abnormal or out of position: P-2 and Q-2

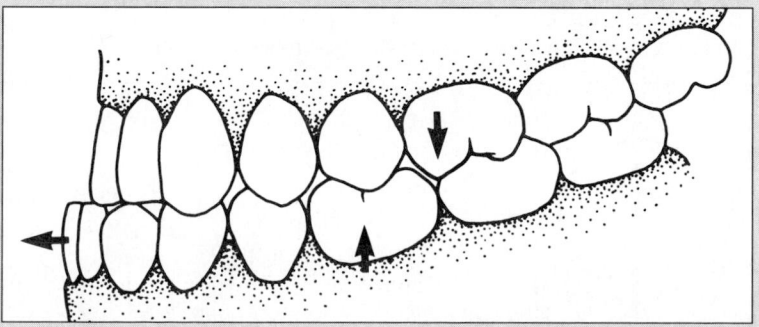

Functional occlusion - the contact that is made between the maxillary and mandibular jaws when chewing takes place

Continued.

BOX 4-7

ANATOMIC TERMS—cont'd

Overbite - the overlap of the maxillary teeth over the mandibular teeth when the mouth is closed

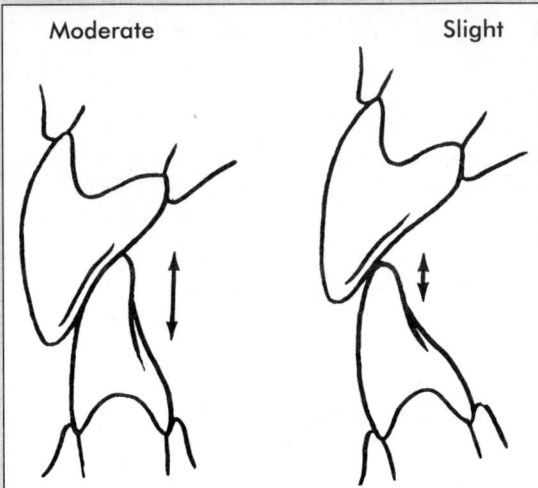

Moderate   Slight

Overjet - the horizontal projection of the maxillary teeth when they are occluded with the mandibular teeth

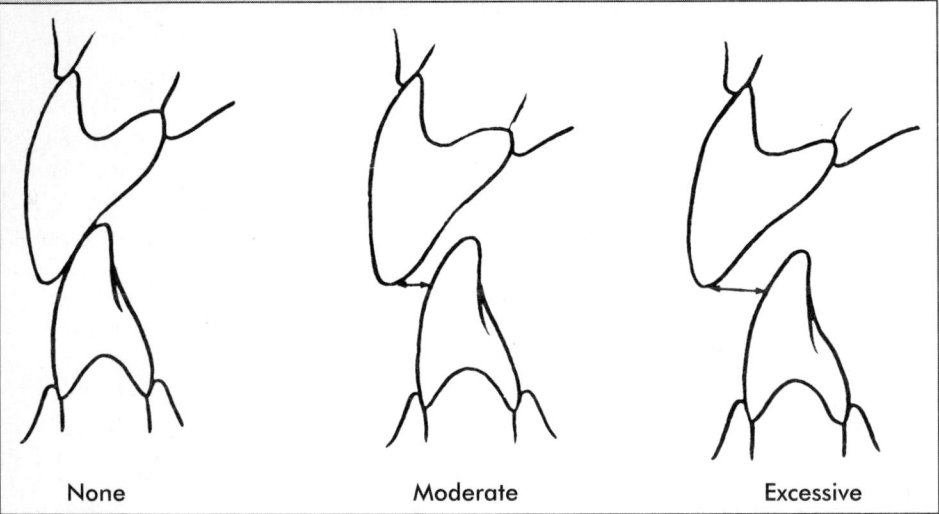

None   Moderate   Excessive

Transverse ridge - the combination of the buccal and lingual triangular ridge; this crosses the occlusal surface of posterior teeth, dividing it into two segments

Triangular ridge - a line that runs from the tip of a cusp to the occlusal surface

Tubercle - a small layer of enamel on the crown of a tooth

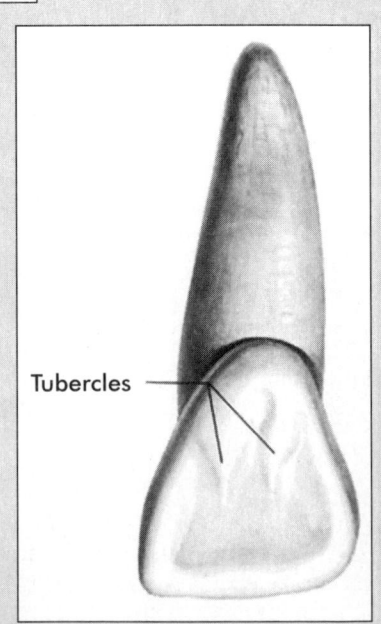

Tubercles

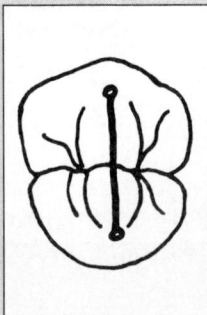

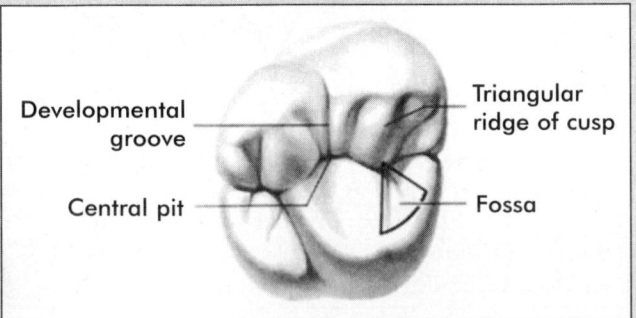

Developmental groove

Central pit

Triangular ridge of cusp

Fossa

Tooth Identification

In a dental office the correct identification of teeth is important for treatment and record keeping. Correct identification of teeth relates directly to patient treatment planning, treatment, insurance claim forms, malpractice suits, and forensic identification purposes. The anatomy of any individual tooth may vary among patients. Standard characteristics are common to most teeth. A complete understanding of the anatomy of a specific tooth is necessary to ensure correct identification of the tooth. For example, a second molar may be found where a first molar is expected to be positioned. It is possible that the patient may have lost a first molar or that the first molar may not have erupted and the second molar may have drifted into its space. It is important to have a complete understanding of the criteria that determine whether a first molar is a first molar or a second molar is a second molar. The specific characteristics that aid in the identification of teeth are located in Box 4-3.

Oral Embryology and Histology

Embryology is the science that deals with the origin and development of an individual organism. Oral embryology specifically examines the development of the tissues in the oral cavity. The study of living tissues, their composition, and their function is referred to as **histology**. The study of the tissues of the teeth and the surrounding structures is called **oral histology**.

Although the dental assistant does not study either of these sciences in depth, it is wise to have an understanding of the basic concepts in each of these areas.

Long before the primary teeth of an infant have erupted into the oral cavity, development and growth have occurred in the body that allow tooth eruption to evolve. When a fetus is examined, cells are discovered to be proliferating, differentiating, and integrating to form the primary embryonic cell layers that eventually become the human body. The embryonic layers of the fetus are as follows:

ECTODERM

Forms the epithelium, nervous system, organs of special sense, mucosal tissues, tooth enamel, and hair and nails on the body

ENDODERM

Produces lining for the cavities and passages of the body and internal organs

MESODERM

Forms the dentin, cementum, and pulp of the teeth, as well as circulatory and reproductive systems, kidneys, bones, connective tissue, muscles, blood, and abdominal lining

The **branchial arches**, apparent during the fourth week of fetal development, are five defined areas that develop into structures of the head and neck. The branchial arches produce the human face at approximately 5 to 8 weeks, with increased development of the dental arches and face. During the fourth month the hard and soft palates of the fetus and the primary dentition have begun to form. The increased growth activity and development of the fetus produce a head and face that will continue to grow after birth. The oral cavity of the infant continues to change during the modeling or alteration that occurs during growth.

When one studies the oral cavity, emphasis is placed on the teeth. A tooth has a crown and one or more roots made up of many tissues. But the oral cavity contains more than just teeth. The oral cavity consists of hard and soft tissues that contribute to many functions. The teeth and surrounding tissues provide for the following functions:

Esthetics

Swallowing

Mastication and digestion

Support for structures

Proper speech or phonetics

Each tooth has a crown and a root. The crown is covered with **enamel**, and the root, with **cementum**. The area where the enamel and cementum meet is the **cementoenamel junction (CEJ)** or cervical line. The portion of the crown that is visibly seen above the gingival or tissue line is the **clinical crown**. A portion of the crown that extends below the gingival line and includes the clinical crown is referred to as the **anatomical crown** (Fig. 4-9). Throughout the life cycle of the tooth, the anatomical crown remains the same as it extends from the occlusal/incisal edge of the tooth to the CEJ. The clinical crown may vary with age as soft tissue recedes. During the early eruption period of the tooth the clinical crown has a minimal amount of exposed crown structure. With final eruption levels and possible gingival resorption, a greater tooth structure may be exposed orally, beyond the anatomic crown.

The tooth must erupt through bone and gingival tissue for the crown to be visible, but the root remains within the alveolar process, specifically in the alveolus. The root may be single or multiple. The anatomic junction of the roots and crown is referred to as the **furcation**. If the tooth has multiple roots, this area is either a *bifurcation*, a division into two roots, or a *trifurcation*, a division into three roots (Fig. 4-10, *A* and *B*). Whether there are one, two, or three roots, each root has an **apex** or end that is set in the dental arch.

The tissues of the tooth are either hard or soft. The hard tissues include the **enamel**, the **dentin**, and the **cementum**. The soft tissue is the **pulp** (Fig. 4-11). The enamel is the outer layer of the anatomic crown that ends at the cervical line and that is formed from **ameloblasts**—enamel producing cells.

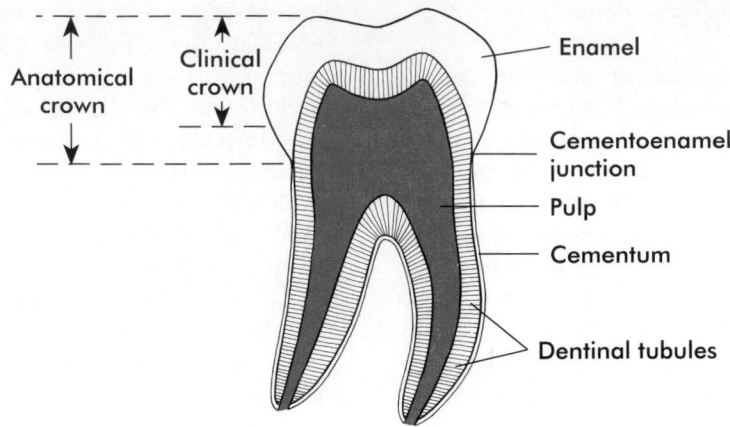

FIG. 4-9   Tooth diagram denoting enamel, cementum, cementoenamel junction (CEJ), and clinical and anatomical crown.

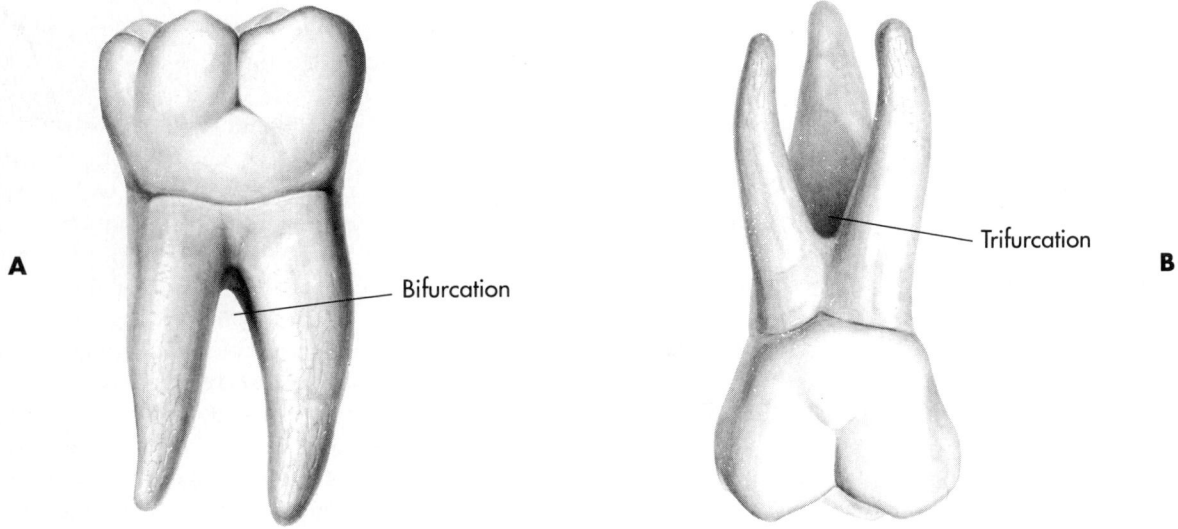

FIG. 4-10   *A,* Bifurcation, *B,* trifurcation, and apex identified.

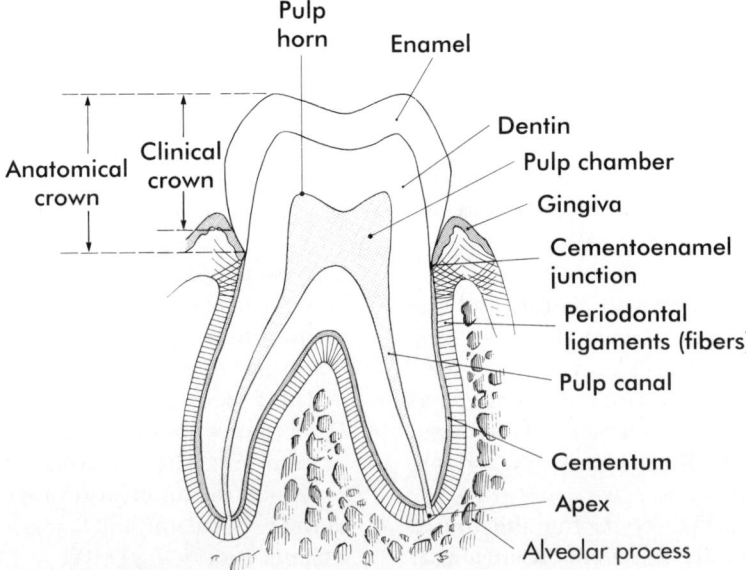

FIG. 4-II   Various parts of the tooth with surrounding periodontium and gingival tissues.

Enamel is a hard calcified tissue composed of 96% inorganic and 4% organic material and water. The hardness is attributed to hydroxyapatite, or calcium, which provides protection to the other softer tooth tissues. This hardness can withstand excessive pounds of pressure during mastication and consequently provides resistance to wear of the tooth surface. The color of enamel varies from tooth to tooth, depending on the thickness and mineralization of the tissue. At a thick point of enamel, such as the middle of the crown, the enamel appears whiter. As the enamel becomes thinner, the color and translucency vary, possibly showing the yellow of the underlying dentin. This is common at the cervical line.

The **dentin** lies under the surrounding enamel and cementum that cover the crown and the root, contributing to the largest portion of tooth tissue. Dentin is also a calcified tissue, but is not as hard as enamel. It is yellow in color and contributes to the difference in tooth coloring because of the varying degrees of enamel translucency. The dentin consists of approximately 70% inorganic and 30% organic material and water.

Dentin is formed from **odontoblasts**—dentin-producing cells—just as enamel is formed from ameloblasts. However, unlike enamel, dentin is able to repair itself from trauma; this occurs as the odontoblasts form **secondary dentin** or **reparative dentin** to protect the pulpal tissues in the area disturbed by the trauma. The formation of this reparative tissue is unique in that dentin is the only tooth tissue that can be formed after the eruption process has been completed. Dentin is also a porous tissue that forms as microscopic tubes (known as **dentinal tubules**) that run throughout. Dentinal tubules begin at the pulpal tissues and extend to the enamel or cementum junctions. As decay penetrates the enamel tissues to the dentin, the carious bacteria may travel quickly through the dentinal tubules to the pulp.

Cementum is the tooth tissue that covers the root of the tooth and the dentin of this area. Cementum consists of approximately 50% organic and 50% inorganic material, resulting in a softer tissue than enamel and dentin. The function of cementum is to provide an attachment for the periodontal fibers to the alveolar bone where the tooth rests in the alveolar socket.

Cementum is similar to bone in its consistency; however, it does not have the same resorption ability as bone. Cementum is thinner at the cervical line, the point where the **dentin** and **cementum** meet, the dentinocemental junction, than it is at the apex of the root. Cementum is formed by **cementoblasts**, cementum-producing cells, which are acellular and cellular cementum. The acellular cementum forms and covers the complete root as it develops. The cellular cementum is found only in the apical third of the root and is able to regenerate, as does dentin. During a patient's life,

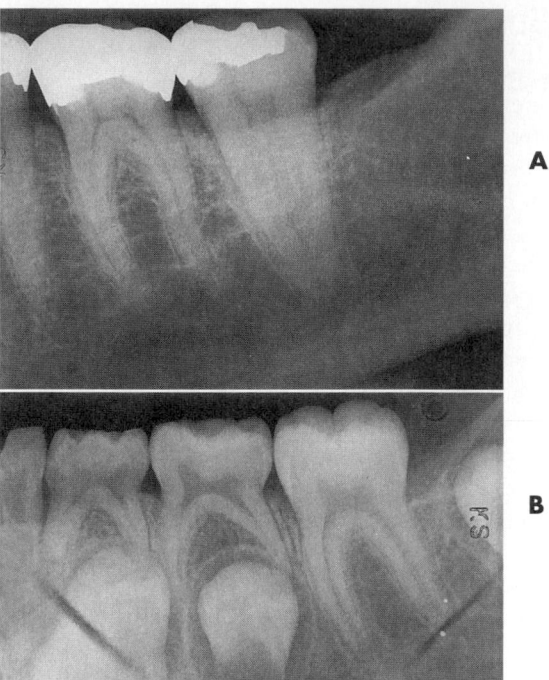

FIG. 4-12   Radiographs showing the difference of pulp chamber sizes. *A,* Large pulp of a young person. *B,* Smaller pulp of an older person.

attrition, or wearing of the crown surface occurs. Cellular cementum can lay down additional cell layers in the apical area, aiding in additional occlusal eruption and maintaining occlusal balance.

Blood and lymphatic vessels, nerve and connective tissues, and odontoblasts all combine to form the **pulpal tissues** or **pulp chamber**. In a young person the pulp chamber (found in the coronal portion of the tooth) is larger than it is in that of an older individual (Fig. 4-12, *A* and *B*). The odontoblasts (found immediately surrounding the pulpal tissues) continue to form layers of secondary dentin as trauma occurs, decreasing the size of the pulp.

The **coronal pulp** or pulp chamber (found in the crown of the tooth) has peaks that extend toward the cusps and are referred to as **pulp horns**. The **pulp canal** or **root canal** extends the length of the root carrying the blood and nerve vessels to the **apical foramen**. The apical foramen is a channel connecting the blood, nerve, lymph, and connective tissues to the interior of the tooth to provide necessary nourishment. When the pulpal tissues are invaded by bacteria or when damage occurs by other means, the reparative dentin is formed for protection. If the trauma is too severe, the vascular supply may diminish or disappear, causing subsequent death of the tooth.

▶ Supporting Tissues of the Oral Cavity

The emphasis to this point has been on the tooth and the tissues of the tooth. It is also necessary to discuss other tissues that contribute to the function of the tooth within the oral cavity, such as the **periodontium**. The periodontium is the connective tissue found between the cementum of the root and the bony alveolar process. It is formed by cells called **fibroblasts**. The periodontium supports and suspends the tooth in the alveolus. It also protects the tooth and provides nourishment and sensory reception. Protection is provided during mastication, acting as a cushion surrounding the root as biting force is applied. This cushion prevents forces from crushing the root into the socket of the alveolar process. The periodontium is also vascular with the supply arriving from the bone, proceeding through the alveolus and into the periodontal ligament. The parts of the periodontium are listed in Box 4-8.

The bone of the alveolar process to which the periodontal ligament attaches is referred to as the **lamina dura**. The lamina dura can be seen as a radiopaque or dark line on a radiograph because of the dense nature of the bone (Fig. 4-13). The blood and lymph vessels and the nerve supply of the tooth travel through openings in the lamina dura at the apex of the tooth. As the periodontal ligament attaches to the lamina dura of the alveolar process, the fibers that attach to the cementum are called *Sharpey's fibers*.

The oral mucosa consists of the **lining mucosa** and the **masticatory mucosa**. The lining mucosa is found on the cheeks, lips, vestibule, and floor of the mouth, as well as on the soft palate and underside of the tongue. These tissues are highly vascular and flexible, allowing for ease in movement during speech and mastication. Some of the tissues in the cheeks, lips, vestibule, and palate are smooth in appearance and are less susceptible to injury compared to the floor of the mouth and the underside of the tongue.

The masticatory mucosa is stronger than the lining mucosa to withstand trauma during the act of mastication. This tissue is not as flexible; it covers the free and attached gingiva, hard palate, and dorsal surface of the tongue.

BOX 4-8

THE PERIODONTIUM

Periodontal ligament - Supports and suspends the tooth in position with fibers that attach to the alveolar process or the cementum

Cementum - Has fibers that attach to it from the periodontal ligament

Alveolar process - Provides support and stabilization to the tooth

Attached and free gingiva - The visible portions of the periodontium

The *free gingiva*, by covering structures, fills the interdental spaces, is the interdental papilla, and creates the gingival sulcus.

The *attached gingiva* is the keratinized (leathery) tissue that is firmly attached to bone and cementum; it connects to the free gingiva at the free gingival junction and extends apically until it meets the alveolar mucosa

---

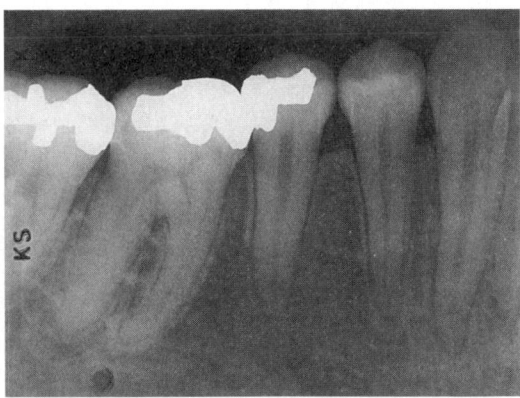

FIG. 4-13   Radiograph showing lamina dura.

▶ Tooth Development and Eruption

The tooth, as a vital structure in the oral cavity, is a living functional organ. The development of a tooth is seen in stages that begin during the fifth or sixth week *in utero,* with small **tooth buds** forming. The tooth buds will eventually grow and become known as **developmental lobes**, that will evolve into one object, the tooth. During this time there is a thickening of the oral epithelium, which is the **dental lamina**. The dental lamina is a U-shaped band of tissue on the future developing alveolar arches. The thickening develops throughout the arches in different areas, 10 in the maxillary and 10 in the mandibular. This thickening eventually evolves into the enamel of the primary dentition. The enamel forms from the ectoderm, which is the outer embryonic germ layer.

Eventually the thickening and the downward development of the dental lamina become the **bud stage**. As the bud or **enamel organ** extends downward into the tissue, the oral epithelium is segregated. The cells from the deepest extension of the bud are from the basal or deep layer of the oral epithelium, and the cells from the middle of the bud are from superficial or outer layers (Fig. 4-14). As the downgrowth continues, the bud becomes concave at the deepest extension. At this point, the enamel organ is developing into the **cap stage** (Fig. 4-15).

The enamel organ consists of the **outer enamel (dental) epithelium**, **inner enamel (dental) epithelium**, and the **stellate reticulum**. The concave area of the enamel organ deepens, and the **bell stage** begins (Fig. 4-16). The primitive cells of the cap stage histodifferentiate or change, and their function becomes specialized. They then form three main parts of the bud: the **dental organ**, the **dental papilla**, and the **dental sac** during the eighth week *in utero* (Fig. 4-17).

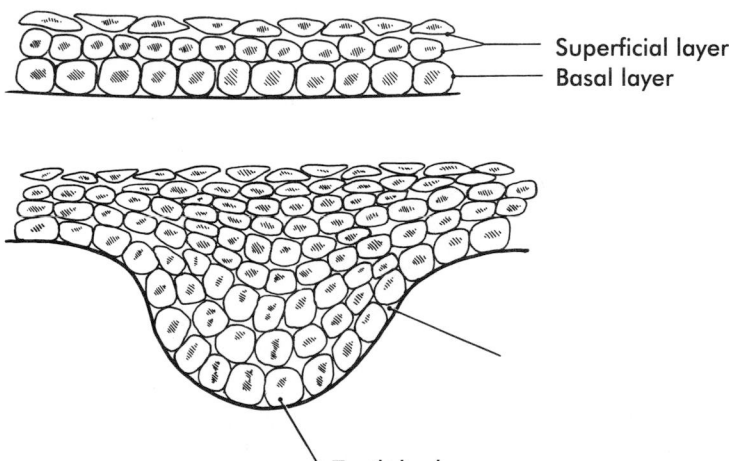

FIG. 4-14   The dental lamina thickens and extends downward.

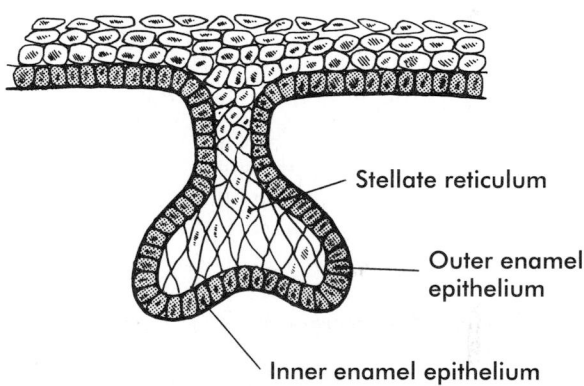

FIG. 4-15   The continued downgrowth, with the bud becoming concave in shape.

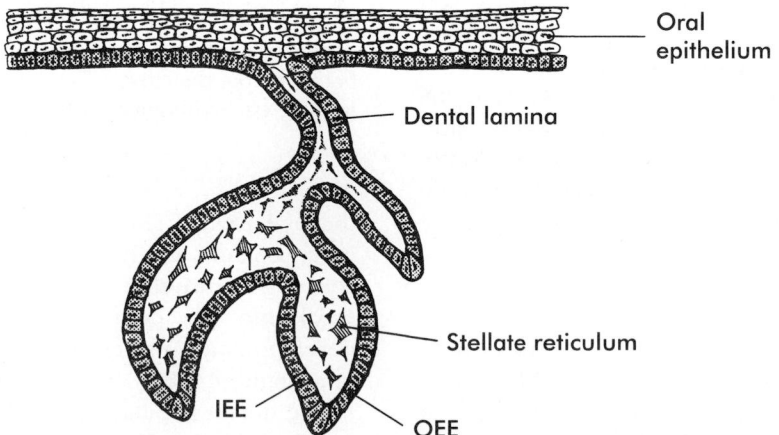

FIG. 4-16   The deepening concave area of the enamel organ and the bell stage begins.

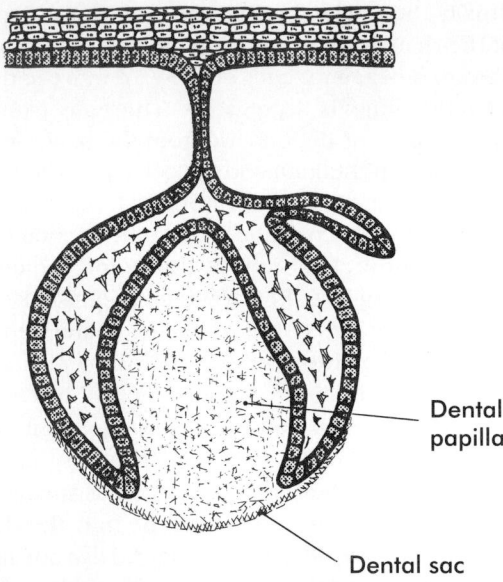

FIG. 4-17   During histodifferentiation the cells of cap stage change, becoming the dental organ, papilla, and dental sac.

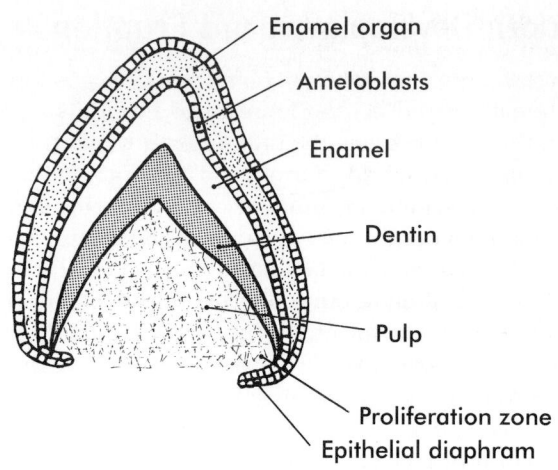

FIG. 4-18   The fourth part of the bell stage, the stratum intermedium, develops. The parts of the bell stage begin to create enamel, dentin, cementum, and the periodontal ligament.

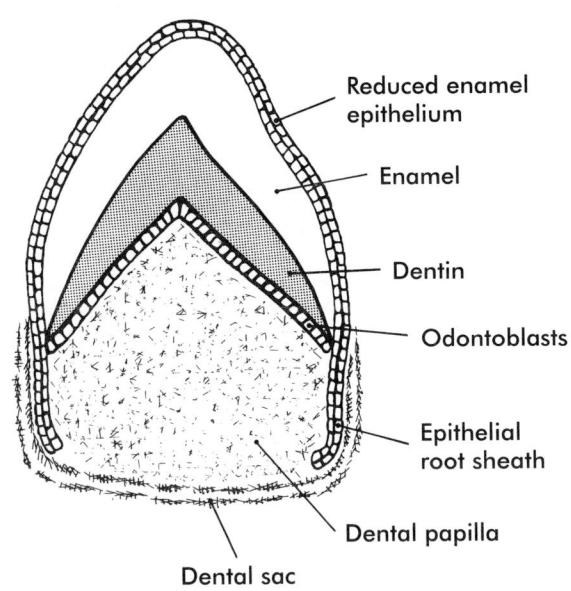

FIG. 4-19   Root formation, the first step of eruption, begins as the enamel and dentin form an outline of the crown. The organ collapses; and a thin layer of cells, the Nasmyth's membrane, overlie the crown. The dentin and cementum continue forming establishing root shape and length.

A fourth layer develops in the bell stage near the fourteenth week In Utero. This layer is called the **stratum intermedium** and is located between the inner enamel epithelium and the stellate reticulum. During the bell stage the inner enamel epithelium is producing cells: **ameloblasts** or enamel-producing cells. The dental papilla converts some cells to **odontoblasts** or dentin-producing cells (Fig. 4-18). The dental lamina produces the **primordium**, superior to the primary tooth bud, which is the area responsible for the formation of the permanent tooth bud. This area is also referred to as the **successional lamina**. The dental sac cells differentiate into **cementoblasts**, cementum-producing cells, or **fibroblasts**, periodontal-ligament–producing cells. The alveolar bone is also developing around the tooth bud.

The **advanced bell stage** begins during the eighteenth week in utero. The ameloblasts and odontoblasts begin to produce enamel and dentin, which means that **amelogenesis** and **odontogenesis** are occurring, forming the crown of the tooth. The dental papilla develops into the pulp, which consists of blood vessels and lymphatic, nerve and fibrous tissues, as well as odontoblasts. The dental lamina disappears at this time, and the primordium migrates to the lingual side of the continually developing bud.

The formation of the root of the tooth is the first stage of the eruption cycle and begins after the enamel and dentin have completely formed an outline of the crown. The dental organ has collapsed and the ameloblasts have reduced function to only the **enamel cuticle** or **Nasmyth's membrane**. This is a thin coating on the surface of the tooth that abrades away as the tooth enters the oral cavity. The outer enamel epithelium and the inner enamel epithelium form layers referred to as **Hertwig's epithelial root sheath**. The cells grow downward into the connective tissue, forming the root development. This development may take on the growth of a single, double- or triple-rooted tooth.

The dental papilla lies within the forming root structure and the dental sac outside, aiding in the formation and shaping of the root and allowing odontoblasts and cementoblasts to continue their functions. The root sheath grows inward forming the epithelial diaphragm that develops the shape and the number of roots for each tooth. With the continued formation of dentin and cementum, the growth of the tooth or apposition is occurring (Fig. 4-19).

As the development of the tooth occurs, so does the development of the alveolar process. The combination of both these actions forces the tooth into the proper position in the oral cavity. As the tooth begins to erupt through the oral mucosa into the oral cavity, only a fragment of the root has actually formed. It will involve 1 to 3 years for a deciduous tooth and nearly 3 years for a permanent tooth to completely erupt, with the deposition of the hard tissues of the root.

▶ Eruption Sequence for Primary and Permanent Dentition

The primary and permanent dentition erupt at different times in the life of a human, even though the teeth are forming in utero. The first eruption of the primary teeth usually transpires around 6 to 8 months of age. The succeeding teeth erupt at different times dependent upon the individual. The permanent teeth normally begin to erupt near age 6. Table 4-1 lists the common eruption sequence for both primary and permanent dentition as provided by the American Dental Association.

The eruption periods that have just been listed are part of the **active eruption** process, as the teeth/crowns become properly positioned in the dental arch. A second phase of eruption may occur: **passive eruption**, which arises when additional tooth structure is exposed supragingivally. **Attrition** may also occur: the wearing away of the tooth structure caused by contact with other surfaces, thereby causing passive eruption.

KEY POINTS

▶ Two arches, the maxilla and the mandible, will support, in a person's lifetime, the primary dentition of 20 teeth and the permanent dentition of possibly 32 teeth.

▶ Each arch can be divided into two quadrants or three segments: one anterior and two posterior.

▶ Correct identification of a tooth includes naming in sequence the dentition, the arch, the side of the mouth, and the name of the tooth.

▶ Several tooth-numbering systems, using numbers and/or letters, are used to consistently identify specific teeth.

▶ Each tooth has either four or five surfaces that are identified by the relation of the position in the oral cavity.

▶ The relationship of oral embryology and histology in understanding basic concepts of dentistry is necessary to develop an awareness of oral structures.

▶ Embryonic layers, ectoderm, endoderm and mesoderm, which produce structure/organs are significant to dentistry.

▶ The teeth and surrounding tissues provide several functions.

▶ Specific cell types: *blasts* produce enamel, dentin, cementum, and fiber, while other specific cells, *clasts,* destroy cells.

▶ The tooth develops in utero from a thickening and downgrowth of the lamina dura, to the bud stage, the bell stage, the advanced bell stage, and then root development through eruption.

TABLE 4-1   TOOTH ERUPTION SEQUENCE

Primary teeth	Normal eruption time in months
Mandibular central incisors	6
Mandibular lateral incisors	7
Maxillary central incisors	7½
Maxillary lateral incisors	8
Mandibular first molars	12 to 16
Maxillary first molars	14
Mandibular canines	16
Maxillary canines	18
Mandibular second molars	20
Maxillary second molars	24

Permanent teeth	Normal eruption time in years
Mandibular first molars	6 to 7
Maxillary first molars	6 to 7
Mandibular central incisors	6 to 7
Mandibular lateral incisors	7 to 8
Maxillary central incisors	7 to 8
Maxillary lateral incisors	8 to 9
Mandibular canines	9 to 10
Maxillary first premolars	10 to 11
Mandibular first premolars	10 to 12
Maxillary second premolars	11 to 12
Mandibular second premolars	11 to 12
Maxillary canines	11 to 12
Mandibular second molars	11 to 13
Maxillary second molars	12 to 13
Third molars	17 to 21

BIBLIOGRAPHY

Berkovitz BKB, Holland GR, Moxham BJ: *A color atlas and text of oral anatomy, histology, and embryology,* ed 2, St Louis, 1992, Mosby.

Bhaskar SN: *Orban's oral histology and embryology,* ed 11, St Louis, 1991, Mosby.

Brand RW, Isselhard DE: *Anatomy of orofacial structure,* ed 5, St Louis, 1994, Mosby.

Massler M, Schour I: *Atlas of the mouth,* ed 2, Chicago, 1982, American Dental Association.

Ring ME: *Dentistry: an illustrated history,* St Louis, 1985, Mosby.

5 Nutrition and Dental Health

LEARNING OBJECTIVES

You will have mastered the material in this chapter when you can:

▶ Define the key terms

▶ Explain the difference between the USRDA and RDA

▶ Explain the food guide pyramid

▶ Explain energy balance and how it relates to weight gain and loss

▶ List the major function, food sources, and calories provided per gram for carbohydrates, fats, and proteins

▶ List water-soluble vitamins, their function, and food sources

▶ List fat-soluble vitamins, their function, and food sources

▶ Distinguish between major and trace minerals, and identify their function and food sources

▶ Explain how to read a food label

▶ Describe the food exchange system

▶ Discuss the positive and negative aspects of *fast food* consumption

▶ Discuss the relationship of monosaccharides, disaccharides, and polysaccharides in caries production

▶ Identify health risks related to diet

▶ Explain the effect of medicine and drugs on nutrition

▶ Discuss dietary management of patients with special needs

KEY TERMS

Calorie	Glucose	Protein
Carbohydrate	kcalorie	Saccharin
Disaccharide	Metabolize	Sucrose
Fat	Mineral	Vitamin
Fat soluble	Monosaccharide	Water soluble
Fructose	Nutrient	
Galactose	Polysaccharide	

The human body is a miraculous machine. As with all machinery, routine care and periodic maintenance are needed to ensure that it continues to function. The body needs to be exercised and rested if it is to function, grow, heal, and reproduce normally. Without the proper amount and type of *fuel*, the body is unable to perform to its maximum (Fig. 5-1). As a health care provider the dental assistant has a dual responsibility in the study of nutrition. First, it is necessary to understand how proper nutrition nourishes the body and maintains it in optimum condition. Second, as a health care professional, the dental assistant is a resource person for the patient who seeks answers to nutritional questions. The study of nutrition changes rapidly as research continues to unfold new discoveries. Consequently, frequent reviews of nutritional literature and updates are necessary to remain current with trends. This chapter will provide a basic knowledge of nutrition, as it pertains to you, to the patient, and to good oral health.

In this chapter the basic nutrients, that is, vitamins, minerals, fats, carbohydrates, water, and proteins, will be discussed. In addition, the nutritional labeling of processed foods will be interpreted to enable the dental assistant to not only make wise choices regarding personal diet, but also to make appropriate suggestions to patients. The effect of nutrition on a patient's general health often relates to dental health. Therefore in this chapter the effect of each nutrient is related to dental health, when applicable, as well as to a patient's general health.

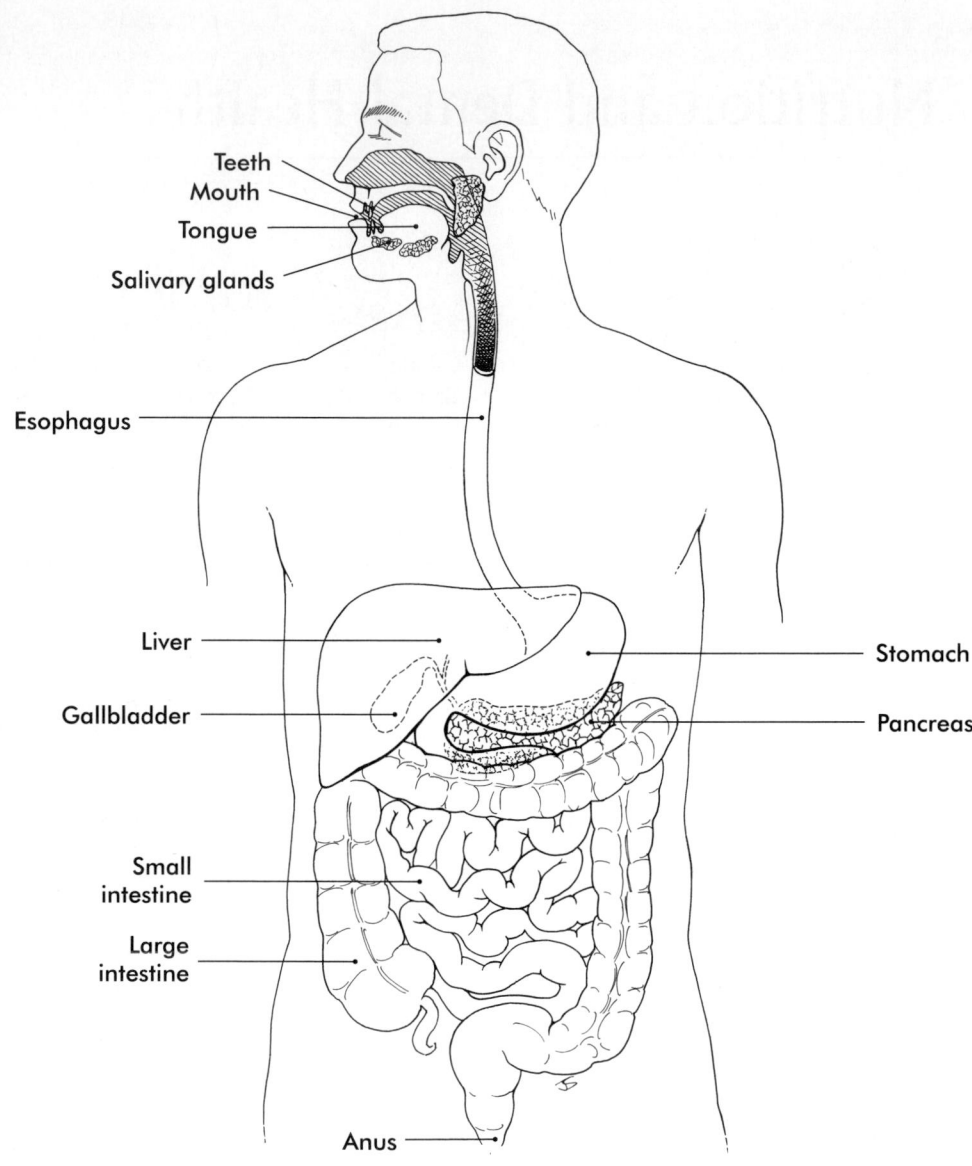

Teeth
Mouth
Tongue
Salivary glands
Esophagus
Liver
Gallbladder
Small intestine
Large intestine
Anus
Stomach
Pancreas

FIG. 5-1   The digestive system.

Digestion

For the body to use the food it receives, the food must first be broken down, digested, and absorbed. Only after these processes occur can nutrients be metabolized by the individual cells and used for energy, tissue growth and maintenance. Digestion takes place in two forms: mechanical and chemical. The digestive process is described in Chapter 3, Anatomy and Physiology.

▶ Mechanical Digestion

Mechanical digestion occurs in both the oral cavity and the stomach. The teeth and tongue break down the larger mass of food into smaller, easier-to-digest pieces. As the food reaches the stomach, it is further broken down mechanically for easier absorption into the system.

▶ Chemical Digestion

Chemical digestion involves enzymes and other body chemicals. It begins in the mouth as the enzyme ptyalin, or salivary amylase, is combined with the food. The primary function of this enzyme is to chemically digest carbohydrates. The partially digested food is then passed to the stomach through the pharynx and esophagus. Once in the stomach, mechanical mixing takes place with the gastric juice, which contains hydrochloric acid and enzymes, such as protease (pepsin), which acts on proteins; rennin, which breaks down dairy products; and lipase, which helps digest emulsified fats.

The small intestine is the next organ in the process of digestion. Here bile, which is produced by the liver and stored in the gallbladder, is used to further chemically reduce the fat molecules. The pancreas also produces enzymes, called pancreatic juices, that are released into the small intestine during the digestion process. These include protease, lipase, and amylase and are used to break down proteins, fats, and carbohydrates, respectively. Additional enzymes are created by the small intestine itself. Intestinal juices are a blend of lactase, maltase, and sucrase, all of which act on carbohydrates, and peptidases, which aid in the digestion of proteins.

The food products then progress to the large intestine, where bacterial enzymes break down dietary fiber. The large intestine also absorbs water and minerals and synthesizes some of the B complex vitamins and vitamin K. Digestion is thereby completed in the large intestine. Any undigested products and waste materials are excreted from the body.

After a food product has been sufficiently digested into usable molecules, it can be absorbed into the fluids of the body, primarily blood and lymph. The small intestine is the primary site for this absorption and its inside walls are specifically designed to absorb these nutrients into the blood and lymph fluids. Once absorbed, the nutrients are available to be metabolized or used by the body tissues to perform specific body functions.

Nutrition and Nutrients

Nutrition is a science that relates diet to health. It is concerned with how the body uses food for the growth, development, and maintenance of tissues and structures.

Nutrients are the chemical parts of a food that are needed by the body to carry on its activities. A nutrient can be as simple as a molecule of water, which although it furnishes no energy, is essential to life itself. A nutrient can be as complex as a protein molecule in hemoglobin. The nutrient protein, as with carbohydrate and fat nutrients, releases energy.

After a food is eaten, the body metabolizes or *burns* the food (or fuel). As it burns, heat is produced and energy is released, allowing the body to carry on its many functions. The heat produced is measured in units called *calories,* also known as *kilocalories* (kcalories), which are units of 1000 calories. Some nutrients do not release energy or heat and therefore do not contain kcalories. These nutrients include vitamins, minerals, and water. Fat, the most concentrated form of energy, contains 9 kcalories per gram (1 ounce equals approximately 30 grams). Carbohydrates and protein each contain 4

kcalories per gram. Although the other nutrients do not release any energy, they are essential to complete body health and aid in the overall metabolism of food and many other body functions.

▶ Diet and Nutrition

The word *diet* often conjures up negative feelings of giving up favorite foods in hopes of losing a few pounds of excess body weight. In this chapter, the term *diet* refers to the total food (or nutrient) intake, and the consumption pattern of these foods. A person will always have favorite foods that he or she enjoys, but other factors, such as family tradition, religious beliefs, aging, socioeconomic factors, food sensitivities, or a preference for vegetables, may dictate the components of a person's diet. Availability and convenience of certain foods, as well as a person's interest in food, may also play a role in food selection. Because of these reasons and others, dietary counseling and the altering of food habits can often be challenging.

▶ Recommended Dietary Allowances (RDA)

The development of the RDA goes back to 1941 when the National Nutritional Conference for Defense was held. The findings of this group were published by the U.S. government in 1943 as a guide for nutritional workers in national defense and for the nutritional needs of the general population. Since that time, a new edition of the RDA has been published approximately every 5 years. The current, 1989 revision of the RDA is contained in Table 5-1. The publication is a joint effort of scientists from the Food and Nutrition Board affiliated with a division of the National Academy of Sciences in Washington, D.C., and the Committee on Dietary Allowances.

The RDA offers guidelines for daily nutrient consumption for healthy individuals in the U.S. population. It is not a requirement for each specific person. The amounts stated in the RDA include a margin of safety to cover most healthy people. The needs of persons with medical problems are not contained in this listing. The acronym USRDA represents the United States Recommended Daily Allowances, which are based on the RDA. The USRDA are used on food labels to help the consumer understand the content of the package and the nutritional value obtained when the food is ingested. There are currently four different USRDA listings:

▶ Infants up to age 1 year
▶ Children from age 1 to 4 years
▶ Pregnant and lactating women
▶ Healthy individuals age 4 years and older

TABLE 5-1   FOOD AND NUTRITION BOARD, NATIONAL ACADEMY OF SCIENCES NATIONAL RESEARCH COUNCIL RECOMMENDED DIETARY ALLOWANCES[a]; REVISED 1989

Category	Age (years) or condition	Weight[b] (kg)	Weight[b] (lb)	Height[b] (cm)	Height[b] (in)	Protein (g)	Fat-soluble vitamins Vitamin A (µg RE)[c]	Vitamin D (µg)[d]	Vitamin E (mg α-TE)[e]	Vitamin K (µg)
Infants	0.0-0.5	6	13	60	24	13	375	7.5	3	5
	0.5-1.0	9	20	71	28	14	375	10	4	10
Children	1-3	13	29	90	35	16	400	10	6	15
	4-6	20	44	112	44	24	500	10	7	20
	7-10	28	62	132	52	28	700	10	7	30
Males	11-14	45	99	157	62	45	1000	10	10	45
	15-18	66	145	176	69	59	1000	10	10	65
	19-24	72	160	177	70	58	1000	10	10	70
	25-50	79	174	176	70	63	1000	5	10	80
	51+	77	170	173	68	63	1000	5	10	80
Females	11-14	46	101	157	62	46	800	10	8	45
	15-18	55	120	163	64	44	800	10	8	55
	19-24	58	128	164	65	46	800	10	8	60
	25-50	63	138	163	64	50	800	5	8	65
	51+	65	143	160	63	50	800	5	8	65
Pregnant						60	800	10	10	65
Lactating	1st 6 months					65	1300	10	12	65
	2nd 6 months					62	1200	10	11	65

[a]The allowances, expressed as average daily intakes over time, are intended to provide for individual variations among most normal persons as they live in the United States under usual environmental stresses. Diets should be based on a variety of common foods in order to provide other nutrients for which human requirements have been less well defined. See text for detailed discussion of allowances and of nutrients not tabulated.
[b]Weights and heights of Reference Adults are actual medians for the U.S. population of the designated age, as reported by NHANES II. The use of these figures does not imply that the height-to-weight ratios are ideal.

Food Pyramid

The *basic four* food groups—dairy, meat, fruit/vegetable, and bread/grain—issued by the U.S. Department of Agriculture (USDA) have been used for menu planning since 1958. They offered guidelines as to the types and amounts of food deemed necessary in the daily diet of a healthy individual. The *basic four* food groups identified those foods and recommended amounts that would best provide the nutrients suggested in the RDA.

To improve the way Americans are eating, the USDA introduced in 1992 a new guide to good nutrition titled *The Food Guide Pyramid* (Fig. 5-2). The new pyramid has five food groups: grains, fruits, vegetables, dairy products, and meats. By increasing the number of servings in the grain, fruit, and vegetable groups (which are naturally lower in fat and kcalories) and including a notation at the *peak* of the pyramid to use fats, oils, and sweets sparingly, the public is encouraged to develop healthier eating habits. The concept in the pyramid suggests that the base of the pyramid is the foundation of the diet from which the greatest daily consumption should be derived. As the pyramid decreases to the top, so the amounts from each of these groups should decrease to provide a healthier diet. The four basic food groups did not provide guidance in the areas of fat and kcalorie intake nor did they emphasize the importance of grains, vegetables, or fruit. The latest development in nutritional guidance by the USDA illustrates a positive addition to the health of the general public (Fig. 5-3).

▶ Energy-Releasing Nutrients

Energy-releasing nutrients are so named because they contain *fuel* or kcalories that the body can use for energy. These nutrients provide the energy needed to get up in the morning and to go about a busy day, energy to build and repair body cells, and energy to simply digest the food eaten. With little or no fuel provided in food eaten, the body will be unable to carry on necessary activities, and it will cease to function. Table 5-2 summarizes each of these energy-releasing nutrients as they apply to dentistry.

CARBOHYDRATES

Of the three energy-releasing nutrients, carbohydrates are the body's main source of energy. The brain and the

Designed for the Maintenance of Good Nutrition of Practically All Healthy People in the United States

Water-soluble vitamins							Minerals						
Vitamin C (mg)	Thiamin (mg)	Riboflavin (mg)	Niacin (mg NE)^f	Vitamin B$_6$ (mg)	Folate (μg)	Vitamin B$_{12}$ (μg)	Calcium (mg)	Phophorus (mg)	Magnesium (mg)	Iron (mg)	Zinc (mg)	Iodine (μg)	Selenium (μg)
30	0.3	0.4	5	0.3	25	0.3	400	300	40	6	5	40	10
35	0.4	0.5	6	0.6	35	0.5	600	500	60	10	5	50	15
40	0.7	0.8	9	1.0	50	0.7	800	800	80	10	10	70	20
45	0.9	1.1	12	1.1	75	1.0	800	800	120	10	10	90	20
45	1.0	1.2	13	1.4	100	1.4	800	800	170	10	10	120	30
50	1.3	1.5	17	1.7	150	2.0	1200	1200	270	12	15	150	40
60	1.5	1.8	20	2.0	200	2.0	1200	1200	400	12	15	150	50
60	1.5	1.7	19	2.0	200	2.0	1200	1200	350	10	15	150	70
60	1.5	1.7	19	2.0	200	2.0	800	800	350	10	15	150	70
60	1.2	1.4	15	2.0	200	2.0	800	800	350	10	15	150	70
50	1.1	1.3	15	1.4	150	2.0	1200	1200	280	15	12	150	45
60	1.1	1.3	15	1.5	180	2.0	1200	1200	300	15	12	150	50
60	1.1	1.3	15	1.6	180	2.0	1200	1200	280	15	12	150	55
60	1.1	1.3	15	1.6	180	2.0	800	800	280	15	12	150	55
60	1.0	1.2	13	1.6	180	2.0	800	800	280	10	12	150	55
70	1.5	1.6	17	2.2	400	2.2	1200	1200	300	30	15	175	65
95	1.6	1.8	20	2.1	280	2.6	1200	1200	355	15	19	200	75
90	1.6	1.7	20	2.1	260	2.6	1200	1200	340	15	16	200	75

^{c}Retinol equivalents. 1 retinol equivalent = 1 μg retinol or 6 μg β-carotene.
^{d}As cholecalciferol. 10 μg cholecalciferol = 400 IU of vitamin D.
^{e}α-Tocopherol equivalents. 1 mg d-α tocopherol = 1 α-TE.
^{f}1 NE (niacin equivalent) is equal to 1 mg of niacin or 60 mg of dietary trytophan.

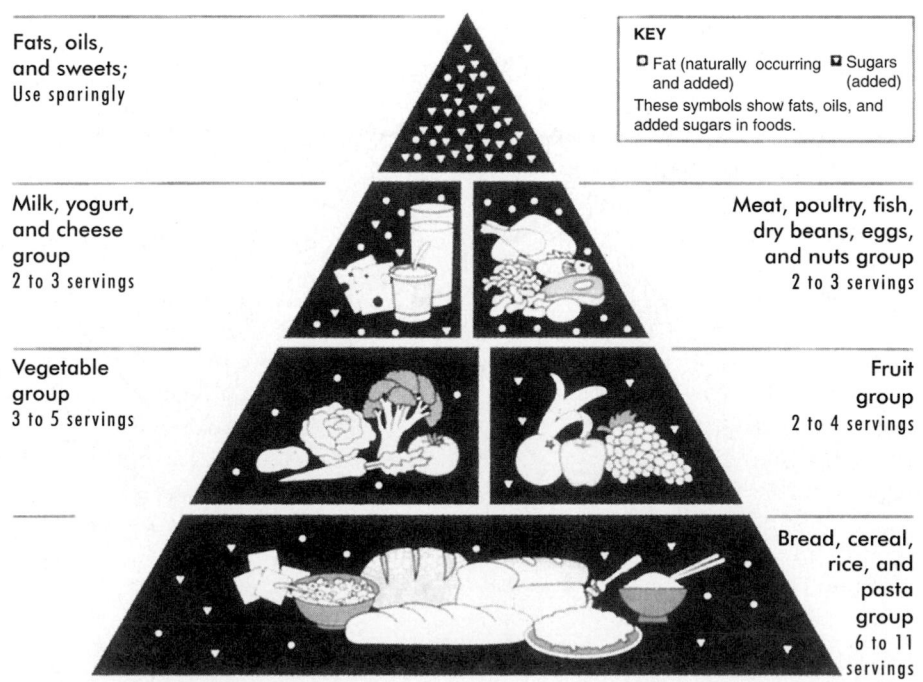

FIG. 5-2   *Food Guide Pyramid:* a guide to daily food choices.

(Adapted from the U.S. Department of Agriculture, 1992).

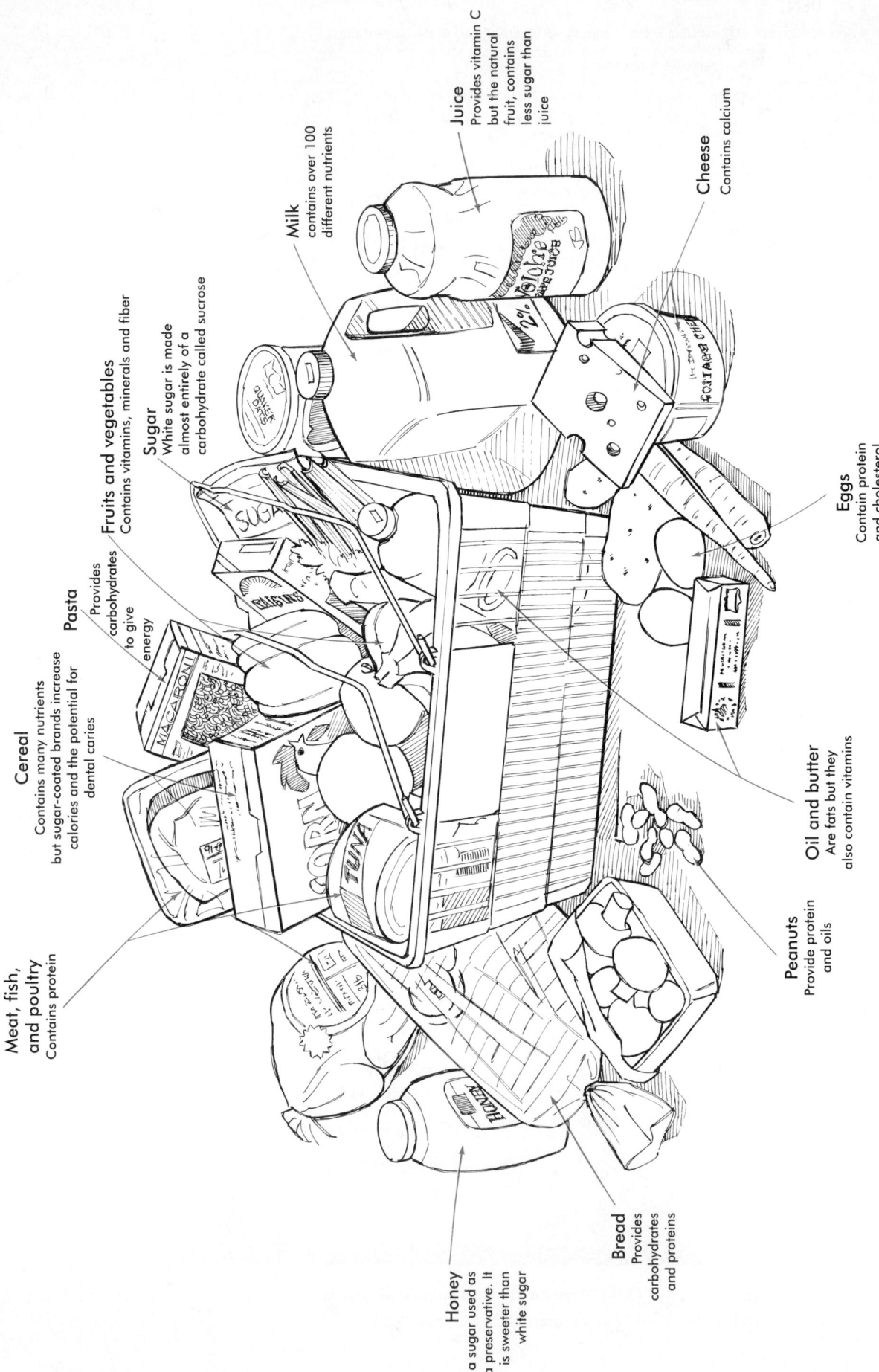

Milk contains over 100 different nutrients

Juice Provides vitamin C but the natural fruit, contains less sugar than juice

Cheese Contains calcium

Fruits and vegetables Contains vitamins, minerals and fiber

Sugar White sugar is made almost entirely of a carbohydrate called sucrose

Eggs Contain protein and cholesterol

Pasta Provides carbohydrates to give energy

Cereal Contains many nutrients but sugar-coated brands increase calories and the potential for dental caries

Oil and butter Are fats but they also contain vitamins

Meat, fish, and poultry Contains protein

Peanuts Provide protein and oils

Honey Is a sugar used as a preservative. It is sweeter than white sugar

Bread Provides carbohydrates and proteins

FIG. 5-3 Sources of nutrition.

TABLE 5-2 DENTAL NUTRIENT FUNCTION/EFFECT CHART

Nutrient	Source	Function	Effect on dental health
Carbohydrates	Grains, fruits, vegetables, legumes, tubers	Primary energy source for the body Contributes 4 kcalories of energy per gram	Refined carbohydrates *(simple sugars)* are a main component in production of dental caries
Protein	Meats, poultry, fish, eggs, legumes, nuts	Building and maintenance of body tissues Components of hormones, enzymes, and antibodies Contributes 4 kcalories of energy per gram	Noncariogenic Necessary for growth and proper development of teeth and oral structures Component of collagen, the protein glue that holds cells together and aids in healing Deficiency can result in slow healing, for example, gingival treatment or periodontal and oral surgery
Fat	Red meat, butter, margarine, eggs, salad oils and dressings, nuts	Cushion for vital body organs Insulation to prevent body heat loss Transport of fat-soluble vitamins Contributes 9 kcalories of energy per gram	Noncariogenic May buffer effects of acidic saliva on tooth structure
Water	Drinking water, beverages	Transport of water-soluble vitamins Solvent and lubricant in numerous body functions Contributes no kcalories of energy	Can buffer acidic saliva Deficiency can cause decreased flow of saliva, less tissue lubrication, and greater caries potential
Sodium	Table salt, processed foods	An electrolyte that helps maintain body fluid balance	Increase can cause decreased saliva flow, greater caries potential, less tissue lubrication, and increased tissue irritation
Potassium	Widely distributed in foods: legumes, grains, potatoes, green leafy vegetables, oranges, bananas	An electrolyte that helps maintain body fluid balance	Necessary for proper amount and quality of saliva
Chloride	Table salt, processed foods	An electrolyte that helps maintain body fluid balance	Necessary for proper amount and quality of saliva
Calcium	Milk, cheese, yogurt, dark green leafy vegetables	An aid in blood coagulation and muscle contraction Strength and stability for bones and teeth	Major component of teeth and bones
Phosphorus	Widely distributed in foods: lean meat, milk	Mineralization and maintenance of bones Necessary for proper energy metabolism	Mineralization of teeth Second most abundant mineral in tooth structure
Magnesium	Dark green leafy vegetables, nuts, legumes, whole grains	Cell respiration Stabilization of bones	Stabilizes components of teeth once formed Third most abundant mineral in tooth structure Deficiency can cause hypoplasia during tooth development and compromised formation of periodontium
Fluoride	Drinking water, tea, seafood	Source of strength to bone structure, reducing susceptibility to osteoporosis	Adds strength and caries resistance to developing teeth Excessive amounts can cause endemic fluorosis (mottled enamel)
Iron	Meat, eggs, enriched/fortified grains	Required for manufacture of protein hemoglobin Cell respiration and oxygen transport	Deficiency can cause glossitis, angular cheilosis, atrophy of oral tissues
Zinc	Meat, eggs, fish, legumes, whole grains	Component of numerous body enzymes, including insulin Essential for tissue growth and wound healing	Necessary for healing of oral tissues, for example, in gingivitis, periodontal surgery, or oral surgery Deficiency can result in slow/difficult healing of tissues

Continued.

TABLE 5-2   DENTAL NUTRIENT FUNCTION/EFFECT CHART—cont'd

Nutrient	Source	Function	Effect on dental health
Iodine	Iodized table salt, seafood	Required for manufacture of thyroid hormone thyroxine	Deficiency can cause late tooth eruption, small jaw size
Copper	Organ meats, shellfish, legumes	Component in manufacture of proteins hemoglobin and collagen	Collagen needed for growth and healing of epithelial cells in the oral tissues
Selenium	Seafood, meat, organ meats, legumes, milk products	Antioxidant	Found in the protein component of the teeth
Vitamin A	Dark green leafy vegetables, bright orange/yellow fruits and vegetables, liver, egg yolks	Antioxidant Necessary for bone remodeling, proper vision, health of the mucous membranes	Maintenance of health and secretions of mucous membranes Needed for development of ameloblasts during tooth formation
Vitamin D	Sunshine, liver oils, fortified milk	Absorption of calcium and phophorus in bone mineralization	Needed for proper tooth calcification and *on–time* eruption Deficiency can cause hypoplasia
Vitamin E	Eggs, liver, vegetable oils, dark green leafy vegetables	Antioxidant Stabilization of red blood cell walls	Unknown
Vitamin K	Dark green leafy vegetables, liver, egg yolks, bacteria in gastrointestinal tract can synthesize vitamin K	Essential in blood clotting Component in manufacture of protein prothrombin	Deficiency can cause increased gingival bleeding
Vitamin B_1	Pork, legumes, whole/enriched grains	Coenzyme in nutrient metabolism, especially carbohydrates	Deficiency can cause a *burning* tongue, sensitive oral tissues
Vitamin B_2—riboflavin	Meat, fish, poultry, whole grains	Coenzyme in nutrient metabolism	Deficiency can cause glossitis, angular cheilosis, swollen lips
Niacin	Dairy products, whole grains, meat	Coenzyme in nutrient metabolism	Deficiency can cause angular cheilosis, glossitis
Vitamin B_6—pyridoxine	Chicken, pork, fish, organ meats, whole grains	Coenzyme in nutrient metabolism, especially proteins	Deficiency can cause glossitis, angular cheilosis
Folacin	Dark green leafy vegetables, legumes, liver	Necessary in manufacture of red blood cells	Deficiency can cause *burning* of tongue and oral tissues, angular cheilosis, gingivitis
Pantothenic acid	Legumes, liver, eggs, whole grains	Coenzyme in nutrient metabolism	Unknown
Biotin	Organ meats, milk, egg yolks, intestinal bacteria able to synthesize biotin	Coenzyme in nutrient metabolism	Glossitis
Vitamin B_{12}—cobalamin	Liver, milk, eggs, cheese, fish	Coenzyme in nutrient metabolism An aid in blood cell formation	Glossitis (atrophic)
Vitamin C—ascorbic acid	Citrus fruits, green and red peppers, broccoli, cabbage, spinach	Essential in synthesis of protein collagen	Necessary for proper tooth and bone formation/maintenance Deficiency can cause enlarged gingiva that bleeds easily, slow/difficult healing of oral tissues

central nervous system depend on a constant supply of carbohydrates, in the form of glucose, to function. Without sufficient carbohydrates the body may use protein as an alternative energy source. The use of protein in this way interferes with its function to build and repair body cells.

This nutrient group includes sugars, starches, and fiber. Carbohydrates provide 4 kcalories per gram and usually make up approximately 50% of daily kcalorie intake. Carbohydrates by themselves are not fattening.

When eaten in excess, or when added to other high-fat ingredients, they tend to cause weight increase. For example, a baked potato by itself is an excellent nonfat carbohydrate source, supplying simple energy. But add a pat or two of butter and/or a spoonful of sour cream, and you have added a substantial amount of fat and kcalories.

Carbohydrates consist of saccharide or sugar units. Saccharides can be categorized as monosaccharides, single sugars; disaccharides, double sugars; and polysaccharides, which are multiple units of sugar.

MONOSACCHARIDES

The single sugars, *monosaccharides,* are glucose, fructose, and galactose. These are the simplest units, which need no further digestion. Glucose, also called *dextrose,* is the *blood sugar* required by the brain and nervous system. It is found in almost all plant foods in the form of starch. The body converts this starch to glucose to supply needed energy.

Found often in fruits and honey, fructose is the sweetest of all monosaccharides. This single sugar is also converted to glucose by the body. Galactose is not found as a single sugar unit in foods. Instead it is a component of the disaccharide lactose. Similar to fructose, galactose can be converted by the body to glucose.

DISACCHARIDES

Disaccharides, or *double sugars,* are combinations of two monosaccharides. These must be metabolized by the body to single sugar units in order to provide energy. White table sugar is actually disaccharide sucrose. One unit of glucose and one of fructose join together to form one molecule of sucrose. Along with table sugar, sources of sucrose are powdered and brown sugar, molasses, and some fruits and vegetables.

Lactose or *milk sugar* is another type of disaccharide. It is the main carbohydrate in milk and can be the primary source for *milk bottle caries.* A single unit each of glucose and galactose combine to form this sugar. The disaccharide maltose is composed of two glucose units. Also called *malt sugar,* it is found in germinating seeds, although it is not commonly found in the daily diet. Maltose is obtained by the body through starch metabolism.

POLYSACCHARIDES

Polysaccharides are the third classification of carbohydrates. Sometimes called *complex carbohydrates,* these include starch, glycogen, and cellulose. The prefix *poly* indicates that there are many single units of sugar joined together to form these large molecules. For example, one molecule of starch may contain 3000 single glucose units. The starches are an important part of the diet and are found in plant sources—especially grain products, such as rice, wheat, corn, barley, and oats. Peas and beans, known as *legumes,* and tubers, such as potatoes and yams, are also significant sources of this nutrient.

Processed foods contain surprisingly large amounts of sugar. For the dental assistant and patient who are discussing the amount of sugar in common foods, Table 5-3 may be of assistance.

GLYCOGEN

Glycogen is not found by itself in plant sources. It is actually a storage product, made by the body from glucose and reserved in the liver and muscle tissue. The body can *draw* on these glycogen reserves whenever additional or emergency energy is required.

FIBER

Dietary fiber, or cellulose, has been receiving much attention in the United States recently. The public has been encouraged to increase their consumption of fiber. Although our diets contain approximately 50% carbohydrates, a large percentage of those come from refined carbohydrates (monosaccharides and disaccharides). Increasing the cellulose in the diet from an average 10 to 15 grams daily to 20 to 30 grams is recommended for a healthier diet and for better digestion and elimination. Cellulose is found in plant sources, particularly grains, legumes, fruits, and vegetables. These contain little or no fat but provide plenty of energy. Because of the large size of the cellulose molecules, the body takes more time to metabolize them. Thus, the feeling of fullness lasts for a long period of time after eating cellulose.

FATS

Fats or lipids are the most concentrated form of the energy-releasing nutrients, providing 9 kcalories per gram. Fat is necessary in the diet for various reasons. Fats are an alternative source of energy when carbohydrates are not available. Fat also provides a cushion for vital organs; for example, a layer of fat padding around the kidneys protects them from mechanical shock. Fat also acts as insulation under the skin to prevent body heat loss and aids the transport and absorption of vitamins A, D, E, and K: the fat-soluble vitamins.

Essential Fatty Acids

Fats can be further divided into smaller components called essential fatty acids. The essential fatty acids

TABLE 5-3   SUGAR IN PROCESSED FOODS

Food	Sugar content (tsp)
1.6 oz bran muffin	1.2
5 oz canned corn	3
½ c canned fruit	4
1 T ketchup	1
12 oz soft drink	8
¾ c beans and franks	3.3
8 oz yogurt (frost on the bottom)	7
1 T creamer	2
2 oz chocolate	8

linolenic and arachidonic acid cannot be produced by the body itself in sufficient amounts for proper body function. These must be acquired from dietary sources. Technically, linolenic acid is the only true essential dietary fatty acid. When sufficient amounts are present, the body itself can synthesize the other two. Metabolism of other fats and cholesterol and cell membrane strength are associated with an adequate intake of these nutrients. Deficiency symptoms include dermatitis and compromised wound healing. Important sources of these nutrients include the oils: corn, cottonseed, peanut, soybean, and safflower.

Foods that provide fat include meats, nuts, salad oils and dressings, olives, avocados, eggs, milk, butter, and margarine. The American diet contains an average of 40% to 45% fat. The American Heart Association has suggested lowering that amount to a healthier 30% to reduce the risks of some forms of cancer and heart disease.

PROTEIN

The major function of protein is the building and maintenance of body tissue, as well as aiding in nutrient metabolism. Proteins are necessary components of the body hormones, enzymes, and antibodies. Similar to carbohydrates, protein provides 4 kcalories per gram.

Protein can be used by the body as an optional energy source, but only when carbohydrates and fats are not in ample supply. To use protein in this manner diminishes the body's ability to manufacture and repair cells.

Amino acids are the building blocks of the protein molecule. They link together in the body to form individual tissue proteins. There are 20 to 22 amino acids, 8 to 10 of which are classified as *essential*. Unlike the other amino acids, essential amino acids cannot be made or synthesized by the body and must be obtained from food. In addition, proteins are also classified as *complete* or *incomplete*. An egg is an example of a complete protein because it possesses all of the essential amino acids. It is likewise a *high-quality* protein because it contains all of the essential amino acids in the exact amounts needed by the body.

Complete and high-quality proteins are usually derived from animal sources, such as meat, fish, poultry, eggs, milk, and cheese. Plant sources, such as legumes, grains, seeds, and nuts, also provide essential amino acids but often not in the amounts needed. Thus, they are referred to as incomplete proteins. By eating a combination of these foods, the body will acquire the necessary components to *build* a complete protein. A diet containing a variety of these lower quality proteins is known as *protein complementation*. Examples would be peanut butter and bread, or macaroni and cheese. In summary, eating a variety of proteins daily ensures that the body is receiving essential amino acids in the correct quantities.

▶ Non–energy-releasing Nutrients

Nonenergy-releasing nutrients (as their name implies) contain no kcalories for use by the body. They are, however, essential to many important body functions, including nutrient metabolism and formation of blood cells, enzymes, and healthy bones and teeth. If these nutrients are not obtained through the diet, numerous body functions will be impaired and deficiency symptoms will become evident. Table 5-2 also summarizes how each of these nonenergy-releasing nutrients applies to dentistry.

VITAMINS

In 1912 the word *vitamine* was introduced, meaning an organic compound vital to life. Since then, the *e* has been dropped and 13 vitamins have been discovered and named. Vitamins are essential nutrients that provide no energy, contain no kcalories, and are needed in only small amounts. The body is unable to synthesize most of these nutrients, so vitamins must be obtained from food. In a general sense, the major function of vitamins is to assist in the metabolism of other nutrients to release energy for the body's use. Vitamins also aid in the prevention of certain dental anomalies, such as glossitis; help prevent periodontal disease; and promote healing of oral tissues.

Water-Soluble Vitamins

Water-soluble vitamins include vitamins B_1 or thiamin, B_2 or riboflavin, niacin, B_6 or pyridoxine, B_{12} or cobalamin; B complex (folacin, pantothenic acid, biotin), and C. All nine water-soluble vitamins share the following characteristics:
  ▶ Needed every day
  ▶ Not stored in the body
  ▶ Deficiencies show up quickly
  ▶ Organic, contains nitrogen
  ▶ Easily destroyed in cooking and processing
  ▶ Not usually toxic unless taken in large doses
  ▶ Excess amounts excreted in the urine

Vitamin B_1, also known as thiamin, is important as a coenzyme in the metabolism of food, especially carbohydrates. The disease beriberi results from a thiamin deficiency. Symptoms of beriberi include muscle weakness, nerve damage, and possible heart failure. This deficiency disease is not seen often in the United States except in habitual alcoholics. Good sources of thiamin include lean pork, legumes, and whole and enriched grains.

Vitamin B_2, or riboflavin, functions in nutrient metabolism as a coenzyme. Riboflavin deficiency can cause angular cheilosis or cracks at the corners of the mouth;

glossitis, involving swollen lips and an enlarged, reddened tongue; and generalized dermatitis.

Important food sources of riboflavin include milk, meat, fish, poultry, and grain products. Riboflavin is sensitive to and easily destroyed by light; so proper storage of these foods is necessary to preserve their nutritive value. For this reason, milk is frequently packaged in tinted containers or paper cartons to protect against exposure to light.

Niacin is another of the B complex vitamins. It serves as a coenzyme in nutrient digestion. Pellagra marked by severe dermatitis, gastrointestinal complications, and glossitis is characteristic of a niacin deficiency. Niacin is found in meats, whole grains, and dairy products. The body can make its own niacin in the event of a dietary deficiency if enough of the essential amino acid tryptophan is present. Dairy products contain large amounts of tryptophan.

Vitamin B$_6$, or pyridoxine, is important in nutrient metabolism, especially that of protein. Deficiencies in this vitamin are rarely seen, since pyridoxine is found in so many food items. If a deficiency does occur, anemia and convulsions can result. Foods containing substantial amounts of pyridoxine include chicken, pork, fish, liver, kidney, and whole grains.

The B complex vitamin *folacin (folic acid)* acquired its name from a Latin term for *leaf.* It was found that an important source of this nutrient is leafy dark green vegetables, such as romaine lettuce or spinach. Other sources of folacin include brewer's yeast, legumes, asparagus, and liver. This B-complex vitamin acts as a coenzyme in nutrient metabolism and in red blood cell formation. In a deficiency, symptoms include a form of anemia, gastrointestinal complications, and compromised cell growth and division.

Vitamin B$_{12}$, cobalamin, is an important coenzyme aiding in the metabolism of proteins and in red blood cell formation. Sources include primarily animal products, such as meats, liver, kidney, milk products, and eggs. For this reason, some groups of vegetarians may have difficulty getting enough of this vitamin in their chosen diet. Pernicious anemia is the deficiency disease associated with cobalamin. In this disease, the person may be unable to acquire the nutrient from food because of the lack of a specific *intrinsic factor* that is secreted in the gastric tissues and that is necessary for the absorption of cobalamin. Periodic injections of this vitamin are used to correct the problem.

The B-complex vitamin *pantothenic acid* is essential in nutrient metabolism, especially fats, and in the formation of hormones. Good sources of this vitamin are found in liver, whole grains, and legumes. A deficiency of this vitamin is not often seen, but if it does occur, gastrointestinal malfunctions, sleep disorders, and headaches are some of the symptoms.

Biotin is a B-complex vitamin similar to pantothenic acid in its food sources: legumes, whole grains, and liver. However, the body can also synthesize biotin via microorganisms in the intestinal tract. Biotin is needed daily for general nutrient metabolism. A deficiency can be produced by the ingestion of large amounts of egg whites. Avidin, a glycoprotein in egg whites, binds with the biotin, making it unavailable for use by the body. Various antibiotics can also destroy the bacteria necessary for intestinal biotin synthesis, which causes deficiency symptoms such as dermatitis, digestive disorders, glossitis, and depression.

Vitamin C. In 1747, in the first documented human nutrition experiment, British doctor James Lind was searching for a cure for the serious and often fatal disease *scurvy.* This illness often struck British sailors who were on long voyages with no ample supply of fresh fruits and vegetables. Their symptoms included bleeding gums, tooth loss, hemorrhages under the skin, and injuries that would not heal. Through this experiment, Dr. Lind found that administering citrus fruits to sailors with scurvy quickly cured their symptoms. Sometime after this discovery, all ships were required to stock an adequate supply of limes to prevent this disease; hence the British sailor's nickname—*limey.*

Vitamin C or ascorbic acid is a water-soluble vitamin that is needed every day. It is easily lost from foods, so care should be taken in processing and cooking. Vitamin C is vital to the body for the production of the protein *collagen.* Collagen is the *glue* that holds tissue cells together. Without it, the body is easily bruised, capillaries readily rupture, and wound healing is greatly compromised. This vitamin is also an important *antioxidant:* it protects other body substances from being destroyed or *oxidized.* In a dental sense, vitamin C is essential for proper healing of gingivitis and for complete repair of tissues after periodontal or other oral surgery.

Vitamin C is found in many fruits and vegetables, especially in citrus fruits, such as grapefruit, oranges, lemons, and limes. Other sources include tomatoes, green peppers, strawberries, broccoli, and brussels sprouts.

Fat-Soluble Vitamins

Vitamins A, D, E, and K fall into the category of *fat-soluble vitamins.* These four all possess the following characteristics:

- Not excreted
- Not needed every day
- Excess amounts can be toxic
- Organic
- Stored in the body in liver and fatty tissue until used

Vitamin A. One of the important roles that vitamin A or retinol plays in the body is in the health of the eyes. The ability of the eye to adjust to changes in light and dark depends on the pigment rhodopsin. Rhodopsin is found in the rod cells of the eye and is composed of vitamin A. A lack of this vitamin can cause *night blindness,* where the eye cannot recover from a sudden burst of bright light. Vitamin A is also necessary to keep the eye moist and healthy. The mucous membranes need vitamin A to keep them smooth and to ensure adequate mucous secretions. In bone growth this nutrient helps *remodel* small bones so that they grow into larger bones. Deficiencies in vitamin A produce eye and vision problems, retarded bone development, and impaired tooth formation. Decreased mucus production along with a hardening or *keratinization* of the mucous membranes may also be present with this deficiency.

Sources of vitamin A include liver, egg yolk, milk, dark green leafy vegetables, sweet potatoes, squash, apricots, and cantaloupe.

Vitamin D. Another vitamin that is in the fat-soluble group, vitamin D, is essential for adequate bone mineralization. Vitamin D enhances the body's absorption of the major minerals calcium and phosphorus. This in turn provides the proper amounts of these minerals for use in bone construction. Without enough vitamin D, the body cannot build healthy, strong bones. The result can be the vitamin D deficiency disease known as *rickets.* Persons with rickets may exhibit bowed legs or other malformed bones and stunted growth. Dentally speaking, insufficient vitamin D can cause teeth that are not well formed and late eruption of the permanent dentition. Vitamin D is found naturally in few sources, mostly fish and liver oils.

The most common food source that people probably enjoy is fortified milk. Since milk naturally contains calcium and phosphorus, fortifying it with vitamin D to increase the body's absorption of these minerals, was a good choice. Vitamin D is also referred to as the *sunshine vitamin.* As the skin is exposed to sunlight, the body is able to make its own vitamin D. Fortified milk, however, is still the most dependable source of this nutrient.

Vitamin E. Discovered in 1922, vitamin E, like vitamin C, is an antioxidant, protecting other body substances, especially vitamin A, from being oxidized or destroyed. Unlike vitamin C, vitamin E is fat soluble and is not needed every day. Red blood cells also depend on vitamin E to keep their cell walls stable so that they are less susceptible to destruction. Deficiencies in this nutrient are rare, since it is found naturally in many foods, including vegetable oils, eggs, liver, nuts, and green leafy vegetables.

Vitamin K. Vitamin K is essential in proper blood clotting and coagulation. Without this vitamin the body is unable to manufacture prothrombin, which is one of the main blood clotting proteins. A deficiency, therefore, results in bleeding disorders. Food sources for vitamin K include green leafy vegetables, egg yolks, and liver; however, a major source of vitamin K is the body's ability to synthesize it. Specialized bacteria in the intestines are able to produce adequate amounts of vitamin K for the body to use. These bacteria are not found in the newborn infant because the intestinal tract is sterile at birth. An initial injection of vitamin K is often given shortly after birth for protection until the infant's body can manufacture its own supply. Some antibiotics, including sulfa drugs, can destroy essential intestinal bacteria and thereby cause a deficiency of vitamin K.

Minerals. Minerals are similar to vitamins in that they provide no energy. Minerals, however, are *inorganic,* and they contain no nitrogen. Minerals are needed in various amounts, depending on their function. These nutrients are divided into two groups: the major minerals, or macrominerals, and the trace minerals, or microminerals. This division is based on how much of each mineral is required daily.

MAJOR MINERALS

Minerals are categorized based on two factors: how much of the mineral is present in the body and how much of the mineral is needed in the daily diet. Seven minerals are included in the major mineral classification: calcium, phosphorus, magnesium, sulfur, potassium, chloride, and sodium. To be named a major mineral it must be present in the body in amounts larger that 5 grams, and the daily dietary requirement must be at least 100 mg per day.

Calcium. Calcium is the most abundant mineral in the body, found mostly in the skeleton and teeth. Obviously, calcium is needed for bone and tooth construction, but it is also required daily for their maintenance. Bones, as well as the cementum and dentin of the tooth, need a supply of calcium nutrient to remodel and repair themselves as necessary. Calcium is also important in blood clotting, normal muscle movements, and the transmission of nerve impulses.

The best sources of calcium are dairy foods, including milk, cheese, and yogurt. A deficiency in calcium can result in poor tooth and bone formation. Osteoporosis may occur when a person ages and this happens when sufficient calcium is not ingested daily so that the calcium that is stored in the bone is depleted. This leaves the bones porous and vulnerable to fracture.

Phosphorus. The major mineral phosphorus is important in bone and tooth formation and daily maintenance. Similar to calcium, the majority of this mineral, approximately 85%, is located in the skeleton and teeth. Phosphorus also plays an important role in energy metabolism, where it is often associated with the B-complex vitamins. Since numerous foods containing phosphorus exist, a deficiency is rarely seen. Protein foods, such as those from the meat and dairy groups, offer good sources of the nutrient. In the presence of vitamin D, phosphorus and calcium are more readily absorbed by the body.

Magnesium. Magnesium is needed by the bones and teeth, especially in stabilizing their components once they are formed. Magnesium also aids in protein manufacture and energy metabolism. Food sources of magnesium are widespread, including milk, legumes, grains, green leafy vegetables, nuts, and cocoa. A deficiency in magnesium does not usually occur. If it does, it is often due to another illness.

Sulfur. Sulfur is needed by the body as part of the protein molecule. It helps stabilize some of the more *rigid* proteins, such as hair and nails. Sulfur can be found in meat, eggs, milk, and legumes. There is no RDA for this mineral, nor are there any documented deficiencies.

Water, Potassium, Chloride, and Sodium. These four elements will be discussed together because they all play a role in the fluid balance of the body. Water has been referred to as the *universal solvent*. In the human body, water is indeed a solvent and *carrier* for numerous substances, including the B-complex vitamins, vitamin C, and many of the minerals such as potassium, chloride, and sodium, also known as electrolytes. In addition, water:

- Is found in all body cells
- Lubricates various body joints
- Composes 50% to 60% of body weight
- Helps regulate the temperature of the body
- Is a necessary *agent* for many chemical reactions in the body

Aside from the ordinary drinking supply, the body acquires water from other beverages: milk, tea, coffee, and soda. There is also a high percentage of water in fruits and vegetables. Since the body weight is composed of approximately half water and is involved in so many activities, a deficiency (dehydration) is very serious.

The major minerals sodium and chloride work together mainly outside of the body cells. Potassium, on the other hand, is used within the cell walls. These minerals protect and equalize the fluids in and around all body cells. Each cell can pump these minerals back and forth through the cell wall to carry on various body functions. The transmission of nerve messages and muscle movements necessitates this cell *pump*. Upsetting the amounts of these nutrients in the body, as in excessive salt (sodium chloride) intake or depletion of potassium caused by diuretics or illness, will cause certain body systems to malfunction. Blood pressure and the action of the heart muscle itself are directly related to body fluid balance. Although an increased amount of salt may appear to be deleterious, salt can be a source of healing when used as an oral rinse after an invasive dental procedure.

Sodium and chloride are commonly found in table salt. Processed foods are yet another source of sodium, as either a seasoning or a preservative. Check product labels and you will be surprised. Suggested sodium intake ranges from 1100 mg to 3000 mg daily. (NOTE: 1 teaspoon of salt equals approximately 2000 mg of sodium!) Potassium is distributed in many natural foods. Among the best sources are bananas, oranges, leafy green vegetables, potatoes, and milk.

Trace Minerals. Trace minerals, or microminerals, are so named because of the small amounts (less than 100 mg) needed daily by the body for proper function. Many necessary trace minerals exist, but only a few have an actual RDA or an established safe and adequate dose. Trace minerals include iron, zinc, iodine, selenium, copper, and fluorine.

Iron. Iron is a well-known necessary body nutrient. Approximately 70% to 80% of the body's iron is found in the blood. Consequently, a loss of blood for any reason can quickly deplete the body of this essential nutrient. Iron is required for the manufacture of hemoglobin, a protein in the red blood cells that carries oxygen through the body. The B-complex vitamins cobalamin and folacin join with iron in the manufacture of this protein. Iron is found in liver, meats, eggs, enriched/fortified and whole grains, and of course spinach. The absorption of iron can be inhibited in the presence of the minerals calcium and magnesium. Coffee and tea consumption can also reduce the amount of iron available for use by the body. Conversely, absorption is increased in an acidic environment or when eaten with foods containing ascorbic acid (vitamin C) or amino acids (protein). A deficiency in iron may cause anemia, with symptoms that include fatigue, pallor, headaches, and a low level of energy. Anemia causes hypoplasia of the bone marrow because of a shortened life span of the erythrocytes. This creates distortion of the alveolar process, resulting in malposition of the teeth. Deficiency also may be indicated by glossitis, angular cheilosis, and gray mucous membranes.

Zinc. As a component of many enzymes, including

insulin, zinc is a notable trace mineral. It is important in nutrient metabolism, especially that of proteins. Best sources of this mineral are animal in nature: meat, eggs, and seafood. Lesser amounts can be found in legumes and whole grains. Zinc is also necessary in wound healing, together with the water-soluble vitamin C. In gingivitis or periodontal or oral surgery, a deficiency of this nutrient may result in slow healing, but deficiency symptoms can also include retarded growth, poor appetite, and decreased absorption of other essential nutrients.

Iodine. Goiter, an enlargement of the thyroid gland cells, is a visible sign of iodine deficiency. In years past, goiter could be seen frequently, particularly in areas where the soil contained no iodine. In 1924 iodized salt was introduced to the American public. Since that time, goiter has not been a major problem. The body uses iodine to manufacture the thyroid hormone thyroxine. This hormone plays an important role in regulating the body's entire metabolism. Therefore, a deficiency in iodine can slow the metabolic rate, thereby causing weight gain and decreased energy. In addition to iodized table salt, seafood provides a good source of iodine.

Selenium. Selenium is a trace mineral important in proper heart function. In addition, it is a notable antioxidant, similar to vitamin E, and aids in the protection of other body substances from possible destruction. Specific to dentistry, selenium is found in the protein component of the teeth. Deficiency symptoms include enlargement of the heart muscle, compromised function, and possible heart failure. Food sources are meats, seafood, kidney, liver, legumes, and milk products.

Copper. Even though copper has not received an official RDA rating, a *safe and adequate* dose has been assigned. Copper is used by the body in conjunction with the trace mineral iron. These two are required in the formation of the protein hemoglobin. Copper is also necessary in the synthesis of collagen and so plays a part in wound healing. Sources of this nutrient include organ meats, shellfish, legumes, and grain products.

Fluorine. From a dental perspective, fluorine or fluoride plays an important role in the formation of teeth and the reduction of dental caries. Fluorine is also a notable component of strong bone structure. Some studies have indicated that fluorine that is deposited in bones makes them more resistant to the degenerative disease osteoporosis. Fluorine is a naturally occurring element in many water supplies, in soil, and in the beverage tea. An RDA has not yet been established for fluorine, but a safe and adequate dose has been documented. The addition of 1 part per million (ppm) of fluorine has been recommended for use in public water supplies. The use

of fluoride in dentistry is discussed in Chapter 26.

Some individuals believe that supplementing communal drinking water is unsafe and that it may cause some forms of cancer. At this time the American Dental Association continues to support the use of fluoride in public water supplies, since evidence is insufficient to suggest the correlation between cancer and fluoride.

Nutritional Information

To ensure that individuals are making proper food selections based on needed nutrients, many agencies, such as the American Diabetes Association, American Heart Association, and American Dietetic Association, have provided specialized diet exchange menus. Cookbook publishers, the press, and the RDA have expended much expertise in providing nutritional information to the public concerning food labels and recipes, as shown in Box 5-1.

▶ Using Food Exchange Diets

Food exchange is a common phrase in diet management. Many patients who are on specialized diets, such as diabetics, cardiovascular patients, or individuals on a weight reduction diet, use this concept in managing the daily intake of food. The concept refers to the exchange of various foods within one of the basic groups: milk or dairy, meat, bread or starch, vegetables, fruit, or fat. For instance, a diabetic patient may work with a nutritionist to determine the needed daily caloric intake. From that total intake it can be determined that the patient may select a specified number of exchanges in each of the food groups from the chart shown in Table 5-4. For instance, if it was recommended to the patient that he or she should be on a 1200-calorie diet based on diabetic status, weight, and energy needs, the following exchanges could be selected:

5 breads	=	400 calories
4 meats	=	220 calories
2 milks	=	180 calories
3 vegetables	=	75 calories
3 fruits	=	180 calories
3 fats	=	125 calories
TOTAL		1180 calories

Then from a prepared list, such as that provided by the American Diabetic Association, foods can be selected that have been determined to be equal to a single exchange of each of the food groups. For instance, a patient could choose from the starch or bread exchange four exchanges that might include any one of the following:

½ bagel; ½ C cooked brown or white rice; ⅓ C cooked dried peas; ½ C corn; 1 C of winter squash; or one small baked potato. (NOTE: This is only a small selection from the suggested group.)

BOX 5-1

RECIPE
Three-Bean Baked Beans

½ lb bacon, diced
½ lb ground beef
1 large onion, peeled ends removed, chopped
½ c brown sugar
½ c granulated sugar
¼ c ketchup
¼ c barbecue sauce
2 tsp prepared mustard
2 tsp molasses

½ tsp chili powder
1 tsp black pepper
½ tsp salt
1 16 oz can butter beans, drained
1 16 oz can kidney beans, drained
1 31 oz can pork and beans, drained

Preheat oven to 350° F. In a large skillet, brown bacon, beef, and onion over medium heat; drain. Transfer to a 3- to 4-quart baking dish, and mix in brown sugar, granulated sugar, ketchup, barbecue sauce, mustard, molasses, chili powder, pepper, salt, butter beans, kidney beans, and pork and beans.

Bake 1 hour. Remove from oven and serve. Serves 8 to 10 people. **Cook's Note:** To reduce the calories, fat, and sodium, make these changes: Use ¼ lb diced bacon, ¼ lb ground beef, ¼ c granulated sugar, and ¼ c low-sodium ketchup; omit the salt; drain and rinse the beans. Note the difference in the following nutritional information.

Nutritional details per serving

Original Recipe			Healthier Version		
Calories................449			Calories................340		
% of calories from fat.....36%			% of calories from fat.....27%		
Fat	Protein	Carbohydrates	Fat	Protein	Carbohydrates
18 gm	16 gm	56 gm	10 gm	13 gm	51 gm
	Cholesterol	Sodium		Cholesterol	Sodium
	40 mg	1,070 mg		23 mg	590 mg
Diabetic Exchanges			Diabetic Exchanges		
2¼ starch, 1 lean meat			2¼ starch, ½ lean meat		
¼ vegetable, 1½ fruit, 3 fat			¼ vegetable, 1 fruit, 1½ fat		

The individual could select four different exchanges or could use all four of the exchanges for one food item.

The exchange concept provides patients with options. They are able to exchange one food for another as long as they adhere to the specified quantities. This concept could also work for dental patients. The aim would be to provide an adequate caloric intake for energy and normal growth and would reduce starches and sugars, which could contribute to the creation of dental caries.

To apply this to dentistry, consider the same diabetic patient with a high caries rate. It would be necessary to examine his or her food intake and perhaps alter the number of breads and fruits by increasing exchanges in other food groups, since high carbohydrate intake relates to caries development.

TABLE 5-4   FOOD EXCHANGE LISTS

Exchange list	Carbohydrate (gm)	Protein (gm)	Fat (gm)	Calories
Starch/bread	15	3	Trace	80
Meat				
Lean	—	7	3	55
Medium-fat	—	7	5	75
High-fat	—	7	8	100
Vegetable	5	2	—	25
Fruit	15	—	—	60
Milk				
Skim	12	8	Trace	90
Low-fat	12	8	5	120
Whole	12	8	8	150
Fat	—	—	5	45

▶ Reading Food Labels

Walk down the cereal aisle of the grocery store and note the product advertising on the boxes. Low fat! No sugar added! High fiber! No cholesterol! It is difficult to comprehend all of these product claims. When you learn how to read and interpret food labels, you will no longer have to rely on the advertising and you will be properly prepared to make your own choices based on sound knowledge.

In 1990 Congress passed the Nutritional Labeling and Education Act. This act made the Food and Drug Administration (FDA) and the USDA accountable for updating the previous labeling laws. The law went into effect in May 1994, and requires manufacturers to list all ingredients in the product. This means that standards of identity that were formerly allowed (white bread, soup, condiments, etc.) must now include a list of all ingredients. Prepackaged products are required to use metric, as well as standard, units of measurement. Fig. 5-4 is an example of a food label.

Various nutrients are listed on the labels, including total calories, calories from fat, total fat, saturated fat, cholesterol, sodium, total carbohydrates, dietary fiber, sugars, protein, vitamin A, vitamin C, calcium, and iron.

Nutritional labeling will attempt to control manufacturers' specific health and food claims. This labeling should also aid individuals with special dietary needs and make it easier to plan meals and snacks.

INGREDIENTS

With a few exceptions almost any packaged food item purchased today contains a list of ingredients and USRDA labeling (explained earlier in this chapter). The ingredients are listed by their weight or predominance in the food product, with the most prevalent ingredient listed

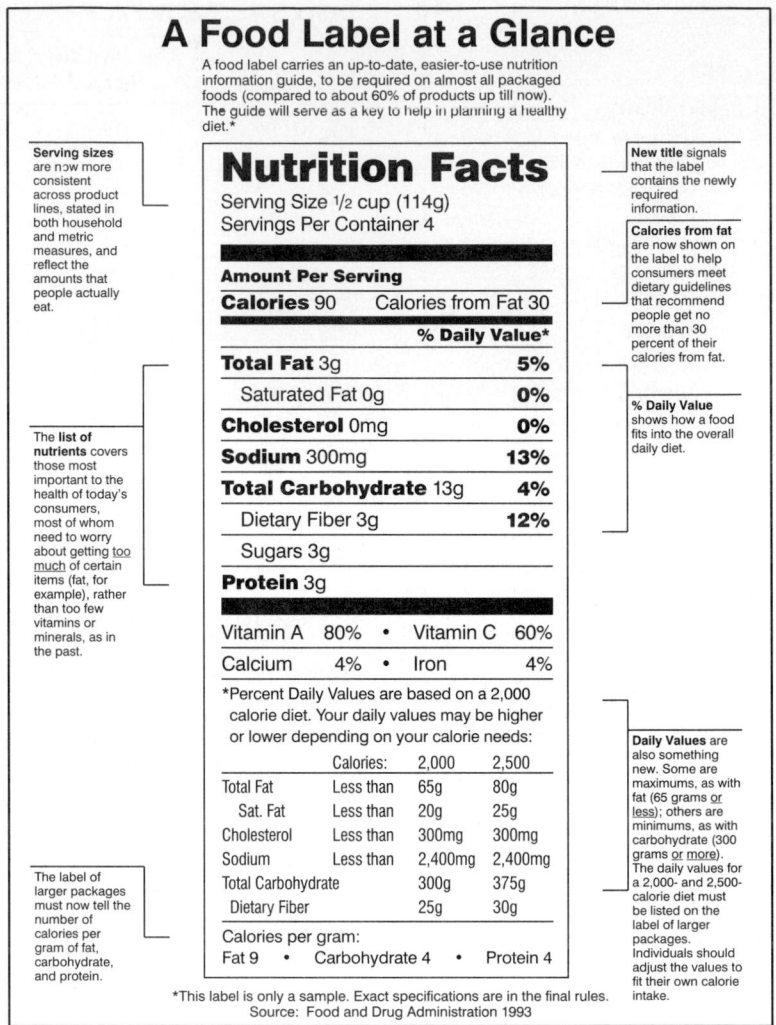

A Food Label at a Glance

A food label carries an up-to-date, easier-to-use nutrition information guide, to be required on almost all packaged foods (compared to about 60% of products up till now). The guide will serve as a key to help in planning a healthy diet.*

Serving sizes are now more consistent across product lines, stated in both household and metric measures, and reflect the amounts that people actually eat.

New title signals that the label contains the newly required information.

Calories from fat are now shown on the label to help consumers meet dietary guidelines that recommend people get no more than 30 percent of their calories from fat.

The **list of nutrients** covers those most important to the health of today's consumers, most of whom need to worry about getting <u>too much</u> of certain items (fat, for example), rather than too few vitamins or minerals, as in the past.

% Daily Value shows how a food fits into the overall daily diet.

The label of larger packages must now tell the number of calories per gram of fat, carbohydrate, and protein.

Daily Values are also something new. Some are maximums, as with fat (65 grams <u>or less</u>); others are minimums, as with carbohydrate (300 grams <u>or more</u>). The daily values for a 2,000- and 2,500-calorie diet must be listed on the label of larger packages. Individuals should adjust the values to fit their own calorie intake.

Nutrition Facts

Serving Size 1/2 cup (114g)
Servings Per Container 4

Amount Per Serving

Calories 90   Calories from Fat 30

	% Daily Value*
Total Fat 3g	**5%**
Saturated Fat 0g	**0%**
Cholesterol 0mg	**0%**
Sodium 300mg	**13%**
Total Carbohydrate 13g	**4%**
Dietary Fiber 3g	**12%**
Sugars 3g	
Protein 3g	

Vitamin A	80%	•	Vitamin C	60%
Calcium	4%	•	Iron	4%

*Percent Daily Values are based on a 2,000 calorie diet. Your daily values may be higher or lower depending on your calorie needs:

		Calories:	2,000	2,500
Total Fat	Less than		65g	80g
Sat. Fat	Less than		20g	25g
Cholesterol	Less than		300mg	300mg
Sodium	Less than		2,400mg	2,400mg
Total Carbohydrate			300g	375g
Dietary Fiber			25g	30g

Calories per gram:
Fat 9   •   Carbohydrate 4   •   Protein 4

*This label is only a sample. Exact specifications are in the final rules.
Source: Food and Drug Administration 1993

FIG. 5-4   The nutrition label required by the Nutritional Labeling and Education Act of 1990.

first and the other ingredients following according to their decreasing weight. Using the label in Fig. 5-5, it is evident that the predominant ingredient in this product is water. This label lists additives that include modified food starch, assorted seasonings, salt, flavorings, spices, soybean oil, and beta carotene. Salt has other names that may not be recognizable at first but that include terms that are related to sodium. The two words on some labels that indicate that salt is in the product are *monosodium glutamate* (MSG).

ADDITIVES

Sugar is another ingredient that goes by many names: sucrose, dextrose, fructose, corn syrup, and honey. When you begin to conscientiously read labels, you will be surprised to see how many different processed foods contain a form of sugar.

USING NUTRITIONAL INFORMATION

Next, look at the *nutrition information per serving.* Check first how many servings are in this item and the size of the serving. The label in Fig. 5-5 indicates that there are two servings in this container, each being 8.0 ounces. If a person were to eat the entire package (two servings), it would be necessary to double all of the other numbers and percentages. For example, 200 kcalories would be consumed, instead of 100, but 25% of the USRDA for vitamin A would also be consumed.

With the new labeling a person is able to look at a label and quickly determine the percentage of calories, saturated fat, maximum daily cholesterol, and sodium, as well as diet exchange information.

Applying nutritional labeling to dentistry, a patient concerned about good dental health must be aware of the sugar content in foods. A patient with a high caries rate would need to be concerned when eating cereal, as

Nutrition Facts

Serv. Size: 8 oz.
Serv./Container: 2

Calories 100
Fat Cal.

*Percent Daily Values (DV) are based on a 2,000 calorie diet
**Less than 1 g

Amount/serving	% DV*	Amount/serving	% DV*
Total Fat 1 g	9%	**Total Carb.** 23 g	0%
Sat. Fat **	0%	Fiber 1 g	0%
Cholest. 0 mg	0%	Sugars 1 g	0%
Sodium 540 mg	0%	**Protein** 3 g	5%

PERCENTAGE OF U.S. RECOMMENDED DAILY ALLOWANCES (U.S. RDA)

Protein 5	Thiamine 3	Calcium 2
Vitamin A 25	Riboflavin 3	Iron 1
Vitamin C 5	Niacin 6	

INGREDIENTS: WATER • VEGETABLES (CARROTS • POTATOES • CELERY • ONIONS • CORN) • LEGUMES (PEAS • GREEN BEANS • LIMA BEANS) • FLAVORINGS • TOMATOES IN JUICE (CONTAINS SALT • CITRIC ACID • AND CALCIUM SALT) • TOMATOES (CONTAINS ADDED CITRIC ACID) • MODIFIED FOOD STARCH • SEASONINGS (SALT • SPICES • SOYBEAN OIL • BETA CAROTENE).

FIG. 5-5   Nutrition facts on a soup can label.

noted in Fig. 5-6. This cereal label indicates a major content of complex carbohydrates and sugars. The patient with a high caries rate should be encouraged to purchase and consume a cereal with lower carbohydrate and sugar content. The patient should also be reminded that sugar added to cereal will result in increased caries and should be replaced with a sugar substitute. Knowing how to read package labels and nutrition information will allow the dental professional and the patient to be wise consumers.

▶ Fast Food

As patients are counseled in the dental office to change their diets, the dental care professional must be aware of the patient's lifestyle. It may not be possible to discour-

Nutrition Facts

Serving Size   1 Cup (28g/1.0 oz.)
Servings per Container   12

Amount Per Serving	Cereal	Cereal with ½ Cup Vitamins A & D Skim Milk
Calories	100	140
Fat Calories	0	0

	% Daily Value**	
Total Fat 0g*	0%	0%
Saturated Fat 0g	0%	0%
Polyunsaturated Fat 0g		
Monounsaturated Fat 0g		
Cholesterol 0mg	0%	0%
Sodium 290mg	12%	15%
Potassium 35mg	1%	7%
Total Carbohydrate 24g	8%	10%
Dietary Fiber 1g	3%	3%
Sugars 2g		
Other Carbohydrate 25g		
Protein 2g		
Vitamin A	12%	16%
Vitamin C	21%	21%
Calcium	0%	10%
Iron	5%	5%
Vitamin D	4%	8%
Thiamin	19%	24%
Riboflavin	15%	30%
Niacin	15%	30%
Vitamin B$_6$	15%	30%
Folate	15%	30%

*Amount in cereal. One half cup skim milk contributes an additional 40 calories, 65mg sodium, 6g total carbohydrate (6g sugars), and 4g protein.

**Percent Daily Values are based on a 2,000 calorie diet. Your daily values may be higher or lower depending on your calorie needs.

		Calories	2,000	2,500
Total Fat	Less than		65g	80g
Sat. Fat	Less than		20g	25g
Cholesterol	Less than		300mg	300mg
Sodium	Less than		2,400mg	2,400mg
Potassium			3,500mg	3,500mg
Total Carbohydrate			300g	375g
Dietary Fiber			25g	30g

Calories per gram:
Fat 9 • Carbohydrate 4 • Protein 4

Ingredients: Wheat, sugar, salt, malt flavoring, corn syrup.
Vitamins and Iron: ascorbic acid (vitamin C), niacinamide, iron, pyridoxine hydrochloride (vitamin B$_6$), riboflavin (vitamin B$_2$), vitamin A palmitate, thiamin hydrochloride (vitamin B$_1$), folic acid, and vitamin D. To maintain quality, BHT has been added to the packaging.

FIG. 5-6   Nutrition facts from the label found on a cereal box.

age patients from using fast food restaurants, but suggestions can be made to alter the food intake and to raise each patient's consciousness level. These suggestions include the following:

- Suggest the patient consider other options when eating in restaurants. Instead of a burger, fries, and a regular cola, suggest a broiled chicken or fish sandwich, salad with light dressing, and a diet drink or water. Use mustard, low-sugar barbecue sauce, or ketchup as alternative condiments to mayonnaise.
- Encourage the patient to ask about the nutritional value of foods served in the restaurant. Suggest that he or she look for charts posted in the restaurant or obtain nutritional pamphlets from the restaurant to discuss later.
- Suggest the use of sugar-free syrups in place of honey or regular syrup when eating pancakes or similar types of foods.
- Encourage the patient to look for alternative snacks. Instead of a chocolate frosted donut with coffee and sugar, suggest a bagel with light cream cheese or low-sugar fruit spreads or a low-fat/low-sugar muffin. Sugar substitutes can be added to coffee to eliminate regular sugar.
- Look for sugar-free candies and treats. Choose sugar-free and fat-free frozen yogurt and ice creams.
- Follow meals with tooth cleansing from vegetables or fresh fruits. Carrots, cabbage, or other rough, coarse vegetables cleanse by scrubbing the tooth surfaces and stimulating soft tissues.

Energy Balance

Energy balance refers to the number of kcalories a person consumes in relation to how many kcalories the body uses. If weight loss or weight gain occurs, the energy input versus output is no longer balanced. Three factors influence the amount of energy needed for this balance:

- **Basal metabolic rate (BMR).** This is controlled largely by the hormones produced in the thyroid gland. It can be defined as the amount of energy (kcalories) required by the body to maintain life-supporting functions while the body is at rest. The BMR is also called *resting energy expenditure* (REE).
- **Specific dynamic action (SDA).** The energy needed for the digestion and absorption of food accounts for the SDA. Also included is how the body metabolism is stimulated by various nutrients.
- **Activity level.** The energy that the body expends during various levels of activity, such as typing, walking, or running, influences this factor.

Take, for example, a body that requires 2000 kcalories daily to maintain a certain weight and activity level. If the energy intake increases by 500 kcalories per day, and the activity level stays the same, a body weight gain of approximately 1 pound per week will occur, since 3500 kcalories equals 1 pound. The body's energy balance has been disrupted. The opposite happens when too few kcalories are ingested over a period of time and the level of activity remains the same. A weight loss will occur.

Carbohydrates and Dental Caries

Numerous carbohydrates can be a factor in the onset of dental caries. Each one has its own rate of caries production, that is to say, its level of cariogenicity. This level is based on its texture, how sticky the food is, and what type of carbohydrate it is: a polysaccharide, disaccharide, or monosaccharide. A simplified formula for the formation of dental decay is as follows:

$$Sugar + Plaque = Acid;$$
$$Acid + Tooth = Decay$$

Based on this formula, plaque, or more specifically *Streptococcus mutans* (a bacterial component of plaque), is a necessary ingredient in caries formation. This type of bacteria requires a carbohydrate energy source to produce the acid that leads to decay. Fats and proteins do not provide a suitable alternative and are not considered to be cariogenic substances. Acid formation takes place within 20 seconds after a carbohydrate has been broken down to sucrose in the mouth. The normal pH of saliva ranges from 6.2 to 7.0. During an acid *attack*, the saliva pH falls. Enamel decalcification and dental decay occur in the critical pH level of 5.0 to 5.5. Each repeated introduction of a suitable carbohydrate into the mouth causes the pH level to remain at this detrimental number for 20 to 30 minutes. Meanwhile, the teeth are being bathed in an acid solution. This is why frequent eating or snacking is so damaging to the teeth. Further exposures to sucrose add up to more acid production, longer subjection to acidic saliva, and increased tooth decay.

EVALUATING CARBOHYDRATE INTAKE

A diet history, whether documented over a 3- or 5-day period, is a useful tool in detecting cariogenic carbohydrates and hidden sugars in the patient's diet. Ask the patient who is experiencing a high rate of decay to record food intake, including the amounts of food, the time of day that food is eaten, and the condiments that are used, for a specific number of days. When the diary is complete, review it with the patient. It may be advantageous to circle or highlight those carbohydrates that can easily promote acid production. Note the following:

- What carbohydrate is eaten? What is the texture of this food? Is it sticky, and does it remain on the teeth for a long period of time, like a caramel or raisins? Or does it have a high water content, such as fruit, and leave the mouth quickly?

- When the carbohydrate is eaten. Is the carbohydrate eaten during a meal when the saliva is flowing freely? Or at bedtime when the saliva flow tends to slow down and less acid-buffering action is available?
- What is eaten with the carbohydrate. Is the carbohydrate eaten alone or with other fats and proteins that offer some degree of acid neutralization? Certain cheeses are currently being studied and show some acid-buffering ability when eaten after a cariogenic food item.
- How often are carbohydrates eaten. Does the patient eat three distinct meals, or is there a pattern of frequent snacking during the day? With each additional incidence of carbohydrate intake comes the probability of subsequent acid production and tooth demineralization.

PROMOTING SUGAR ALTERNATIVES

Sugar alternatives have their place for those persons who wish to decrease or to totally avoid the use of sugar. Caution should be used when reading food labels that advertise *sugar free* or *no sugar added*. This simply indicates that sucrose or table sugar was not used as an ingredient in this product. It also may mean that the food contains other forms of sugar, such as fructose or honey. These items could contain as many kcalories as those sweetened with table sugar.

Sugar alcohols are one classification of alternative sweeteners and include sorbitol, mannitol, and xylitol. These are carbohydrates but are metabolized much more slowly in the mouth than sucrose. Therefore sugar alcohols do not possess a high rate of cariogenicity. An exception to this occurs when the patient is experiencing xerostomia, wherein there is no salivary buffering action. Studies have shown that xylitol, in particular, may actually help prevent dental caries and even inhibit the growth of cariogenic bacteria.

Aspartame or NutraSweet is a relatively new alternative sweetener derived from the essential amino acid phenylalanine. Accepted for use in 1981, aspartame does not promote dental decay because of its amino acid composition. It contains 4 kcalories per gram, but since it is used in such small amount because of its sweet taste, it can be considered practically kcalorie free. You can find aspartame in numerous products, from tabletop sweeteners, to soda, to pudding. Read the labels.

Saccharin, used today as a table sweetener or as an additive in some sodas, came into existence around 1900. Some have debated its safety for human consumption. Even though it has not been proven to cause cancer in humans, bladder tumors have been seen in test animals. Saccharin is labeled a nonnutritive sweetener because it contains no kcalories. Oral bacteria are unable to use saccharin as an energy source to produce acid, so it is considered noncariogenic.

▶ Health Risks Related to Diet

The health risks related to diet, in contrast to those of infectious diseases, such as tuberculosis, HIV, or HBV, can be attributed to environmental, behavioral, social, or genetic factors. A person's lifestyle presents many risk factors.

A person's behaviors, including food behaviors, are interwoven with many conditions. The choice to eat high-fat foods, for example, increases the probability of obesity and thereby contraction of several diseases: cancer, hypertension, diabetes, atherosclerosis, or other diseases. Table 5-5 summarizes the signs to watch for in nutrition.

Assessment and counseling for dental patients are a vital part of nutrition related to the prevention of oral disease. For this reason the process of diet analysis is addressed in Chapter 26.

▶ Diet Suggestions for Patients With Special Needs

At different stages of life or during dental treatment, patients may require a specialized diet plan. The following section includes suggestions for meeting those dietary concerns, based on patient need.

THE PREGNANT PATIENT

The pregnant female should be attuned to how much weight she gains during her pregnancy. But she must also be sure to take in an ample amount of kcalories and nutrients to supply her body, as well as that of the fetus. The foods and other substances eaten and used during this time all have an effect on the developing child. Care should be taken to make wise choices. During this period of rapid fetal growth, there is an increased need for many nutrients. Protein, the minerals calcium and iron, and vitamins A, C, D and B complex are examples of these. The patient's dentist and physician can both provide appropriate counseling and literature on the effect of nutrition on the mother and fetus during pregnancy. Further information should also be provided to the pregnant patient concerning the dental development of the fetus and the steps that will be needed to maintain good oral health and to avoid early dental problems in the newborn. One such concern is nursing bottle syndrome, which is addressed in Chapter 36.

It is also important to stress to the pregnant patient that continued good oral hygiene must be maintained to avoid infections in the oral cavity. This can be followed up by suggesting that the expectant mother monitor her food intake to avoid an increase in food items that are not nutritional and may be high in sugar content.

TABLE 5-5   CLASSIC SYMPTOMS OF POOR NUTRITIONAL STATUS

Area examined	Symptom	Possible nutrient imbalance
Skin	Follicular hyperkeratosis *(calloused dry, thickened)*	↓ Vitamin A
	Petechiae *(tiny, purple–red spots)*	↓ Vitamin C
	Dark dermatitis in areas exposed to sunlight	↓ Niacin
	Flaky dermatitis	↓ Protein—energy
	Pallor	↓ Iron, folate, vitamin B_{12}, copper
Eyes	Xerosis *(dry tissue)*	↓ Vitamin A
	Keratomalacia *(ulcerated cornea)*	
	Bitot's spot *(thick white deposits)*	
	Inflamed conjunctiva	
Mouth and tongue	Cheilosis *(scales and fissure on lips)*	↓ Riboflavin
	Glossitis *(magenta tongue)*	↓ Niacin, folacin, iron
	Gingivitis *(bleeding, spongy gingiva)*	↓ Vitamin C
	Carious teeth	↓ Fluoride
		↑ Sugar
	Mottled enamel	↑ Fluoride
Glands	Thyroid, parotid enlargement	↓ Iodine
		↓ Protein
Hair	Depigmentation	↓ Protein—energy
	Thin, sparse, poor texture	↓ Protein—energy
Nails	Koilonychia *(spoon nails)*	↓ Iron
Subcutaneous fat	Little fat	↓ Protein—energy
	Excessive fat	↑ Energy nutrients
	Edema	↓ Protein—energy
Musculature	Wasted muscles	↓ Protein—energy, thiamin
	Paralysis at extremities	↓ Thiamin, vitamin B_{12}
Skeletal structure	Bowed legs, knock-knees	↓ Vitamin D
	Rosary beading of ribs	↓ Vitamin C

THE OLDER ADULT PATIENT

As a person ages the basal metabolic rate tends to slow down. This calls for a modification in kcalorie intake to maintain an appropriate energy and weight level. The nutrient needs, however, remain the same. Some studies indicate that increased calcium consumption at this time in life gives added protection against osteoporosis. Many elderly people live alone and may not prepare balanced meals for themselves. However, nutrition is still important to maintain bodily functions. The dental professional must stress the importance of consuming nutritious meals to prevent oral diseases and to maintain function.

The older adult patient's diet must be examined to determine if he or she is eating balanced meals or is simply snacking on nonnutritional foods throughout the day. The patient may feel lonely or bored or may not have the emotional or physical ability to prepare nutritious meals. Therefore the following alternative suggestions might be made:

▶ Contact a local agency to deliver a nutritious meal to the home of the patient. This experience not only offers food but provides social contact for the elderly person.

▶ Suggest that perhaps an outside person purchase prepared meals to be delivered and easily heated at the patient's home.

▶ Suggest to the patient who has been used to cooking for a family that he or she continue to do so, but freeze the excess food in appropriate-sized portions for later meals.

▶ Suggest to the lonely patient that he or she prepare an attractive eating area, structure eating around a regular activity, or even invite another person to share meals.

▶ Inform the patient who is unable to eat solid foods that liquid supplements are available that contain adequate nutritional value.

PATIENTS WITH FOOD ALLERGIES

A true food allergy differs from a food intolerance in that it involves the body's immune system. An intolerance or *food sensitivity* may involve the body's inability to digest the nutrient, perhaps because of the lack of a necessary enzyme, thereby causing numerous problems. Protein foods head the list of common food allergies, including milk products, eggs, nuts, shellfish, and wheat. Food allergies are difficult to diagnose. Symptoms may include nausea, vomiting, skin rash, and asthma. These allergies are often discovered by removing certain foods from the diet, thereby eliminating the body's *allergic reaction.* Skin tests and blood tests are also used in food allergy detection. In a situation of food intolerance, abdominal bloating, cramps, nausea, and diarrhea may be present. For example, a lactose-intolerant person does not possess enough of the enzyme *lactase,* which breaks down the milk sugar known as *lactose.* Considerable physical discomfort can occur as a result of consuming a lactose-containing food item, such as milk, ice cream, or cottage cheese. Available on the market currently are numerous dairy products that have added the enzyme lactase, enabling the lactose-intolerant person to enjoy them.

VEGETARIAN PATIENTS

The person who chooses to eat a vegetarian diet must be especially well informed nutritionally. The trend toward this type of diet has steadily increased since 1970, along with vegetarian restaurants, markets, and cookbooks. Various reasons underlie this pattern of eating, including religious beliefs, health and economic concerns, and regard for the environment. Vegetarians or vegans who remove all animal products or the majority of animal products from their diet may have difficulty obtaining adequate amounts of vitamin B_{12} (cobalamin), iron, and zinc. However, those choosing to eliminate meats simultaneously lower fat consumption, which may prevent heart disease and some forms of cancer. Most vegetarian diets also provide plenty of complex carbohydrates, B-complex vitamins (except B_{12}), vitamins A and C, and numerous minerals. Consuming enough protein and iron may be a concern. Protein complementation, discussed earlier in this chapter, is one solution. Foods from the legume group can offer good sources of protein and iron. When eaten along with items containing vitamin C, the iron absorption is greatly enhanced. To reinforce an earlier statement, those persons electing this diet regimen should plan their food choices wisely in order to ensure adequate nutrient intake and proper body function.

PATIENTS WITH HEART DISEASE

Coronary heart disease is the number one cause of death in this country. Those persons fortunate enough to be only *warned* of an impending problem are well advised to carefully monitor their diet. It is generally accepted that fatty *plaque* accumulations (artherosclerosis) on the walls of arteries lead to *hardening of the arteries* (arteriosclerosis). Over a period of time, this can create

---

BOX 5-2

THE AMERICAN HEART ASSOCIATION DIETARY GUIDELINES FOR REDUCING THE RISK OF HEART DISEASE

- Drink skim milk and eat low-fat dairy foods
- Reduce total fat intake to about 30% of the day's kcalories
- Reduce sodium (*salt*) intake, using spices and herbs instead
- Increase consumption of fresh fruits, vegetables, breads, cereals, and pasta
- Avoid eating too many foods that contain saturated fat and/or cholesterol; eat less than 300 mg of cholesterol and 10% or less saturated fat in the daily diet

---

a blockage causing a *heart attack* if the coronary arteries are involved, or a *stroke* if the blockage occurs in a vessel leading to the brain. In either situation, the person should adjust the diet accordingly and learn to read and understand product labels.

Patients with heart disease should substitute lean meats for well-marbled varieties, lunch meats, and organ meats. To figure the percentage of fat content, they can use the formula presented earlier in this chapter. Caution should be taken when using food products labeled *no cholesterol* or *cholesterol free,* since they do not necessarily mean that these foods contain no fat. In addition, watch for the *tropical oils:* those foods with the names cocoa, coconut, palm, and palm kernel oil. Although these contain no cholesterol, they are high in saturated fats and should be avoided when following the American Heart Association recommendations. Vegetable oils containing monounsaturated and polyunsaturated fats, such as corn, safflower, sunflower, and canola, are a better choice in the diet of the heart patient.

Reading the nutritional information on the product labels will also assist in figuring the sodium content. Convenience and processed foods, such as microwave meals, often contain high levels of added salt. Some canned soups and products containing monosodium glutamate (MSG) also contribute large and unneeded amounts of sodium to the diet.

DIABETIC PATIENTS

Those individuals diagnosed with the disease *diabetes mellitus* are either not able to produce enough of the hormone *insulin* or else their body cannot use the insulin it produces effectively. In both instances, the blood glucose or sugar level remains too high because the insulin is not available to allow the body to metabolize it. With this condition, patients must monitor their food intake carefully to keep the blood glucose level stable. Precise diet *plans* are recommended, including specific foods, eating times, and serving sizes. Working regularly with a dietician will provide an individualized program for this purpose. The food *exchange* program discussed earlier in this chapter was first introduced in 1950 by the American Dietetic Association and the American Diabetes Association. It since has been revised and is currently used today not only for diabetic patients, but also for other special needs patients and those that are concerned for good basic nutrition. One of the primary concerns of the diabetic patient is to eliminate foods containing *simple* sugars and focus on consuming more complex carbohydrates. Emphasis is placed on breads, cereals, starches, and high-fiber foods, such as pasta, rice, potatoes, and legumes, while avoiding processed sweets, such as cookies, cakes, and candies. When making dietary suggestions for the diabetic patient, be certain that recommendations do not conflict with dietary needs.

SURGERY PATIENTS

Whether the patient has had periodontal or maxillofacial oral surgery, special dietary suggestions may be necessary. Although periodontal disease is not caused by a lack of specific nutrients, the healing process can be affected by diet. When present in adequate amounts, vitamins A and C will encourage desired tissue repair. Foods containing sufficient levels of protein, calcium, iron, zinc, and folic acid are also important. The restoration of oral tissues to normal health can be impaired when these nutrients do not exist in adequate amounts. The dental professional can suggest to the surgical patient that he or she consume a bland, soft diet. Furthermore, spicy foods should be avoided, since they may irritate sensitive oral tissues, and foods that are difficult to chew may disrupt tissue healing.

ORTHODONTIC PATIENT

Two factors are an issue in diet for the orthodontic patient: texture of food and sugar content. For the patient with orthodontic devices or appliances, special cautions should be followed:

 ▶ Avoid sticky foods, such as taffy, caramels, or gum
 ▶ Take care when eating hard foods to avoid displacement of orthodontic devices
 ▶ Since flossing may not be possible, reduce sugar intake or avoid stringy foods that would be difficult to remove from interproximal spaces

▶ Medicine, Drugs, and Nutrition

Patients often think that a medicine is unlike other drugs and provides a benefit and no harm. Not only do drugs

TABLE 5-6 FOOD EFFECT ON DRUG ABSORPTION

Absorption reduced by food	Absorption delayed by food
Amoxicillin	Acetaminophen
Ampicillin	Amoxicillin
Aspirin	Aspirin
Demethylchlortetracycline	Cephalexin
Doxycycline	Cephradine
Isoniazid	Digoxin
Levodopa	Furosemide
Methacycline	Sulfadiazine
Oxytetracycline	Sulfamethoxazole
Penicillin G, V(K)	Sulfamethoxypyridazine
Phenethicillin	Sulfanilamide
Phenobarbital	Sulfisoxazole
Propantheline	
Rifampin	
Tetracycline	

Adapted from Roe DA: Interactions between drugs and nutrients, *Med Clin North Am* 63:985, 1979; and Roe DA: *Diet and drug interactions*, ed 2, New York, 1989, AVI Books.

interact with each other, as discussed in Chapter 10, but drugs also interact with nutrition. This relates to prescription drugs, as well as over-the-counter (OTC) drugs. For the dental patient who is given a prescription or who uses an OTC drug, the following information is important:

 ▶ Foods can slow down the absorption of drugs in the digestive system
 ▶ Drugs can make nutrients unavailable for absorption
 ▶ Drugs can modify taste or alter appetite
 ▶ Nutrients can interfere with the action or excretion of drugs
 ▶ Drugs can also interfere with the action or excretion of nutrients
 ▶ Examples of how food can affect the absorption of certain drugs are shown in Table 5-6.

KEY POINTS

 ▶ Nutrition is a science that relates diet to health. It is concerned with how the body uses food for the growth, development, and maintenance of tissues and structures. For the dental assistant, it is necessary to understand how nutrition relates to dental health, evaluate a patient's diet, and make suggestions for change that can affect dental disease.
 ▶ *The Food Guide Pyramid* has five food groups: grains, fruits, vegetables, dairy products, and meats. The concept in the pyramid suggests that the base of the pyramid illustrates the foundation of the diet (grains), from which the greatest daily consumption should be derived. As the pyramid decreases to the top (fats and oils), so the amounts from each of these groups should decrease to provide a healthier diet.
 ▶ Food exchange is a common phrase in diet management. Many

patients who are on specialized diets, such as diabetics, cardiovascular patients, or individuals on a weight reduction diet, use this concept in managing daily intake of food. The concept refers to the exchange of various foods within one of the basic groups: milk or dairy, meat, bread or starch, vegetables, fruit, and fat. Food exchange diets are available from many organizations, such as the American Heart Association and the American Diabetes Association.

▶ The Nutritional Labeling and Education Act has impacted the manufacturers' method of labeling foods. This law requires manufacturers to list all ingredients in the product. This means that standards of identity that were formerly allowed (white bread, soup, condiments, etc.) must now include a list of all ingredients. The nutritional labeling will attempt to control manufacturers' specific health and food claims. This labeling should also aid individuals with specific diet needs and make it easier to plan meals and snacks.

▶ The dental professional must spend time in the market to become acquainted with the products with which patients are frequently confronted to aid them in making wise choices that can affect their diet and alter their dental health.

BIBLIOGRAPHY

American Diabetes Association, American Dietetic Association: *Exchange lists for meal planning,* 1989, The Associations.

American Heart Association: *Recipes for low-fat low-cholesterol meals,* Dallas, 1992, The Association.

American Heart Association: *The American Heart Association diet: an eating plan for healthy Americans,* Dallas, 1991, The Association.

Ehrlich A: *Nutrition and dental health,* Albany, NY 1987, Delmar Publishers.

Gershoff S: *The Tufts University guide to total nutrition,* New York, 1990, Harper & Row.

Hamilton EMN, Whitney EN, Sizer FS: *Nutrition, concepts and controversies,* St Paul, Minn, 1991, West Publishing.

Nizel AE, Papas AS: *Nutrition in clinical dentistry,* ed 3, Philadelphia, 1989, WB Saunders.

Subcommittee on the 10th edition of the RDAs, Food and Nutrition Board, Commission on Life Sciences, National Research Council: *Recommended dietary allowances,* ed 10, Washington, DC, 1989, National Academy Press.

Williams SR: *Nutrition and diet therapy,* ed 6, St Louis, 1994, Mosby.

6 Diseases of the Teeth and Supporting Tissues

LEARNING OBJECTIVES

You will have mastered the material in this chapter when you can:

▶ Define the key terms
▶ Recognize normal periodontal tissues
▶ Recognize the basic signs of periodontal disease status
▶ Differentiate between healthy and unhealthy gingival tissue
▶ Describe the progression of periodontal disease, its etiology, and its treatment
▶ Classify the diseases and conditions affecting the calcified portions of the teeth
▶ Explain the developmental processes of diseases and conditions affecting the calcified portions of the teeth
▶ Explain the G.V. Black cavity classification
▶ Describe the classification of cavity forms
▶ Distinguish between cavity walls, floors, and angles used in cavity preparation

KEY TERMS

Abrasion
Acute herpetic gingivostomatitis
Acute necrotizing ulcerative gingivitis (ANUG)

Acute periodontal abscess
Acquired pellicle
Adenopathy
Attrition
Calculus
Caries
Cavity preparation
Cavity wall
Convenience form
Erosion
Extrinsic stain
Floor
Gingivitis
Inflammation

Intrinsic stain
Line angle
Materia alba
Nursing bottle mouth
Outline form
Periocoronitis
Periodontitis
Point angle
Recurrent decay
Reparative dentin
Resistance form
Resorption
Retention form

Diseases of the teeth and supporting tissues can be classified into diseases of the calcified portions of the teeth, periodontium, and pulp. Since the majority of a general dental practice is dedicated to treating diseases of the calcified portions of the teeth and the periodontium, this chapter will be devoted to these two categories of diseases. In Chapter 7 a thorough discussion of oral pathology will be presented, and the diseases of the pulp will be discussed in detail in Chapter 33, *Endodontics.*

Normal Periodontium

To understand the diseases of the periodontium, it is necessary to recognize the constituents of a healthy periodontium. In Chapter 4, *Intraoral Structures,* a description of the periodontium consisting of the gingivae, periodontal ligament, alveolar process, and cementum was provided. The periodontium develops during the eruption of the teeth, and through the forces of normal mastication its integrity is maintained. The loss of the alveolar process can occur gradually if the supporting tissues of the teeth become diseased and teeth are lost.

A diagram of a healthy periodontium is illustrated in Fig. 6-1, and the physical characteristics are described in Box 6-1. Clinically, the gingiva is uniformly coral pink in color, but no single color can be considered normal. The exact color of a healthy gingiva depends on the

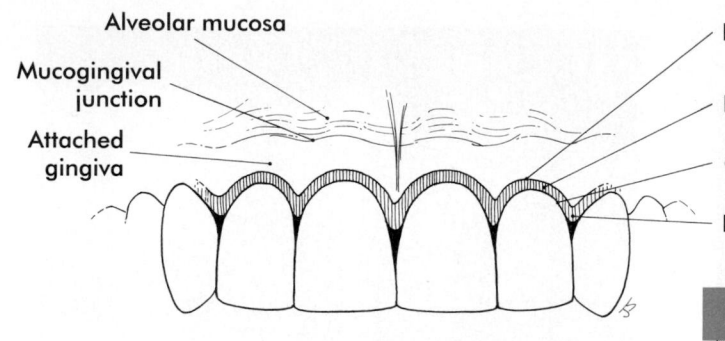

FIG. 6-1 Diagram of healthy periodontium.

Labels: Alveolar mucosa, Mucogingival junction, Attached gingiva, Free gingival groove, Free marginal gingiva, Gingival margin, Interdental papilla

pigmentation of the individual. A sharp distinction in color can be made between the gingiva from the alveolar mucosa at the mucogingival junction. The gingival surface is fully keratinized, and the margin of the tissue is knife edged and circumscribes the teeth in a collarlike fashion (Fig. 6-2). The depth of the healthy gingival sulcus is 0.5 to 1 mm. When it is probed, the tissue does not bleed and there is an absence of exudate. Radiographs of a healthy periodontium (Fig. 6-3) indicate an unerupted lamina dura (*darkened line*) surrounding the roots of the teeth. The alveolar crest bone is located slightly apical to the cementoenamel junction (CEJ) and appears pointed as the lamina dura approaches the crest of the alveolar bone.

Etiology of Periodontal Disease

The etiology or causative factors contributing to the development of periodontal disease can be classified into local and systemic factors. Local factors include inflammation and anomalies that contribute to the accumulation of plaque and trauma. Systemic factors are influenced by nutritional and hormonal deficiencies, metabolic disturbances, or the use of various medications or other substances.

Each of these factors can be described with various terms when the patient's gingival tissues are examined. The severity of the disease will be described as slight, moderate, or severe. The distribution of the disease can be any of the following:

Localized: Involves a small region, either a single tooth or a segment of teeth

Generalized: Exists throughout the mouth or is generalized to a specific arch or quadrant

Marginal: Confined to the free or marginal gingiva

Papillary: Involves a papilla but not the rest of the free gingiva around a tooth

Diffuse: Occurs when both the attached and free gingiva are involved; commonly, a diffuse change is localized rather than generalized

---

BOX 6-1

CLINICAL APPEARANCE OF GINGIVAL TISSUES IN HEALTHY AND DISEASED STATES

COLOR

Normal
Uniform in color; variations in pigmentation may occur in different races and complexions; darker pigment evident in people with darker complexions

Diseased tissue
Subtle change occurs in interdental papilla from light pink to red
Acute inflammation: bright red
Chronic condition: bluish pink to bluish red; magenta or deep blue

SHAPE

Normal
Knife-edged marginal gingiva; follows contour of the tooth; papillae are pointed and fill the interproximal space

Diseased tissue
Swollen; edematous interdental papilla; marginal gingiva is rolled or rounded; papillae may be bulbous, blunted, or cratered

SIZE

Normal
Free gingiva flat, not enlarged; fits securely around the tooth

Diseased tissue
Enlarged; edematous

TEXTURE

Normal
Free gingiva is smooth; attached gingiva is stippled

Diseased tissue
Acute condition: smooth, shiny gingiva
Chronic condition: firm stippling may be more pronounced

CONSISTENCY

Normal
Firm; attached gingiva securely adherent to underlying bone

Diseased tissue
Acute stage: soft and spongy; bleeds easily on probing
Chronic inflammation: firm gingiva; resists probing; bleeding in deeper part of a pocket, not near margin

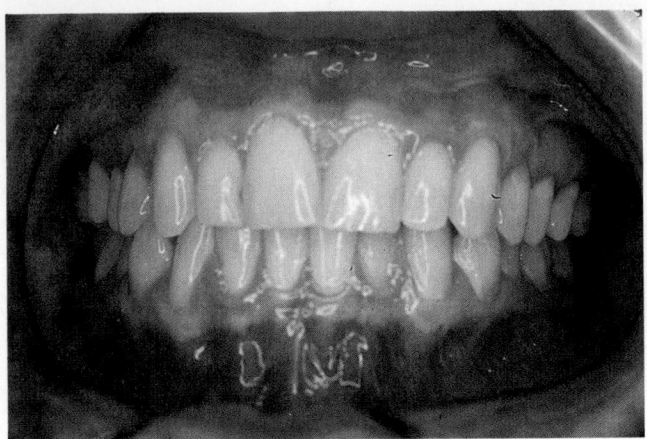

FIG. 6-2   Healthy gingival tissue is characterized by a knife-edge margin of tissue that surrounds the tooth in a collarlike action. The depth of the gingival sulcus is 0.5-1 mm.

(Courtesy of William Sorenson, D.D.S., M.S., Ann Arbor, Mich.)

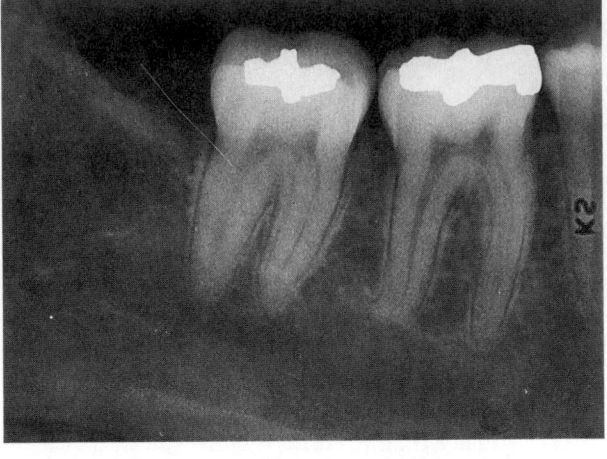

FIG. 6-3   Radiograph of the mandibular right molar region, indicating a healthy periodontium. The lamina dura *(white line)* is well defined as it surrounds the roots of the teeth.

(Courtesy of William Sorenson, D.D.S., M.S., Ann Arbor, Mich.)

▶ Inflammation

Inflammation is the response of tissue to an irritant. Signs of inflammation include redness, heat, swelling, and pain. Inflammation of the gingival tissues can be attributed to the presence of plaque, calculus, stain, food impaction, and mouth breathing.

Through the media today the terms *plaque* and *tartar* have become familiar to the general public. Much of this can be attributed to the impact that manufacturers have made through the development of products that claim to fight plaque and calculus (tartar), and yet current clinical research does not support all of the manufacturers' claims. Consequently, these two deposits still plague patients and continue to be major contributors to periodontal disease.

To understand the effects of plaque and calculus, you must have an understanding of these deposits. The following discussion describes the composition and appearance of common dental deposits and the consequences of these accretions.

ACQUIRED PELLICLE OR CUTICLE

Acquired pellicle is composed primarily of nonbacterial acellular salivary glycoproteins. This deposit forms within minutes after a professional prophylaxis; it is a thin coating covering the teeth, restorations, calculus, and even the fixed and removable prostheses. When a disclosing agent is applied, the pellicle takes on a light color and a *filmlike* appearance. Acquired pellicle provides a primary attachment where the plaque bacteria form and colonize. A professional prophylaxis is necessary for removal of this deposit.

PLAQUE

Plaque is a structured yellow-gray, transparent or near-transparent mass of colonizing bacteria that adheres to the acquired pellicle and supporting tissues. This thin layer of plaque is not visible to the patient. Plaque that is coronally at or above the gingival margin is referred to as supragingival plaque. Plaque that forms apically beneath the gingival margin within the sulcus is subgingival plaque. After 1 or 2 days the main constituents of supragingival plaque are *Streptococcus mutans,* the acidogenic microorganisms responsible for enamel caries. As the plaque remains for longer periods of time, changes take place in the bacterial structure that later can develop into dense pockets of spirochetes and vibrios, which can create a gingival inflammation. Subgingival plaque, on the other hand, creates a different environment for microorganisms. The plaque may be either adherent or nonadherent, depending on the bacterial composition. Adherent plaque develops within the sulcus on the root surface of the tooth and can contribute to gingival irritation. Nonadherent plaque consists of anaerobic bacteria that are motile and move about freely on soft tissues, causing inflammatory lesions.

In addition to being unsightly and a factor that contributes to halitosis, plaque can also be the beginning state for caries development, calculus formation, gingival inflammation, and periodontal disease (Fig. 6-4). Plaque commonly occurs in the following areas:

- ▶ Cervical one third of the tooth
- ▶ Proximal areas
- ▶ Lingual aspect of mandibular molars
- ▶ Pit and fissure areas
- ▶ Areas where it is difficult to maintain hygiene

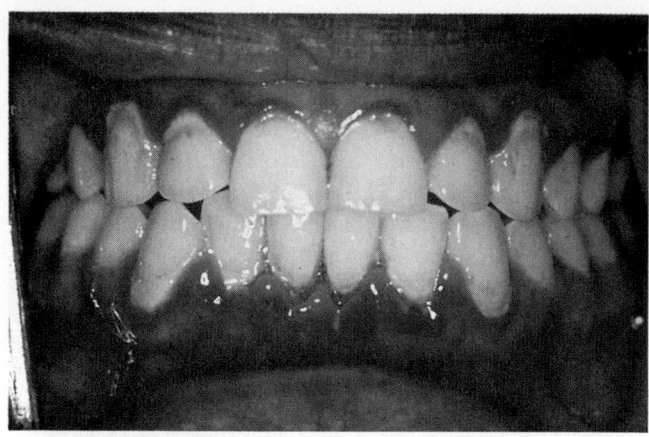

FIG. 6-4   Plaque left on the teeth appears as a white chalky substance causing gingival irritation.

(Courtesy of Hoyt Laboratories: *Oral Lesions*, ed 3, Colgate-Hoyt/Gel Kam, Director of Colgate Palmolive, Canton, Mass., 02021.)

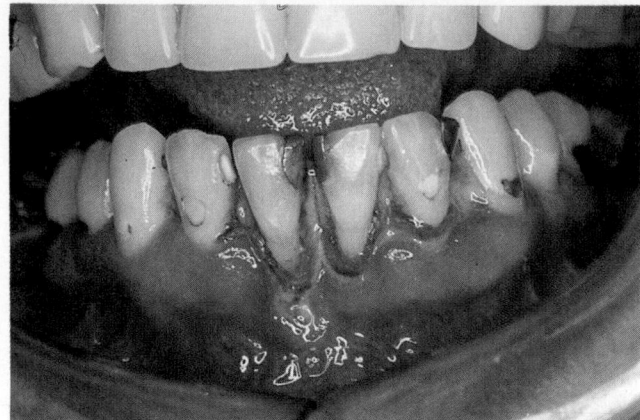

A

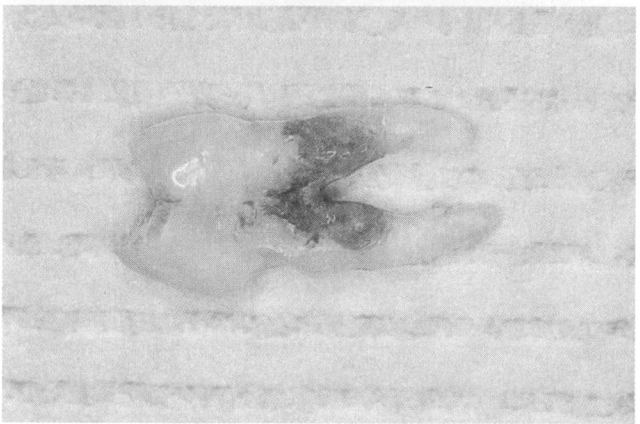

B

FIG. 6-5   *A* and *B,* Supragingival calculus.

(Courtesy of William Sorenson, D.D.S., M.S., Ann Arbor, Mich.)

MATERIA ALBA

Materia alba is a soft deposit whose composition differs from that of plaque. It is a loosely adherent mass of bacteria and cellular debris that covers plaque deposits. Materia alba is white or gray in color, with no uniform structure, and it can be removed by vigorous water irrigation and brushing. Components also include salivary proteins and food particles. Materia alba has a thick appearance that can feel fuzzy to the patient and is commonly found at the cervical one third of the tooth and in the interproximal areas. When a disclosing agent is used on materia alba, it acquires a dark hue. This soft deposit may contribute to gingival irritation.

CALCULUS

Calculus denotes the commonly chalky yellow or white crustaceous deposits found on the lingual aspect of mandibular anterior teeth and on the buccal surface of the maxillary molars. Both of these areas are related to the openings of salivary ducts. Calculus may also be found in the interproximal areas of the individual who has inadequate flossing habits.

Calculus formation begins with the attachment of bacterial plaque to the acquired pellicle. Minerals from the saliva, most commonly calcium and phosphate, are deposited into the plaque matrix. The once-soft deposit then becomes mineralized. The calcification process can take 10 to 20 days to form the mature calculus. This time varies, based on the patient's saliva composition and oral hygiene skills. Calculus deposits can form both above the gingiva (supragingival calculus) (Fig. 6-5, *A*) and below

the gingiva (subgingival calculus). In either case, calculus is irritating to the soft tissue and supporting periodontium because of its bacterial content and rough surface texture. Subgingival calculus differs from the chalky yellow-white supragingival calculus in that it will usually be darker because of blood pigments in the sulcus. Because of the tenacious nature of calculus, its removal cannot be accomplished with simple brushing and flossing. A professional prophylaxis is needed to remove calculus and restore the teeth and gingiva to a healthy state.

FOOD IMPACTION

Food impaction can also be a contributing factor in periodontal disease. When food is forced into the interdental space by the masticatory process, it acts as an irritant and can cause inflammation of the tissues. Other factors that lead to food impaction include open contacts, fractured teeth, or defective restorations. Partially erupted teeth can also create an environment for food impaction.

MOUTH BREATHING

In patients who are unable to breathe through the nasal opening effectively, mouth breathing can contribute to potential gingival inflammation. These patients may experience dehydration and chafing, as well as an enlargement of the lips.

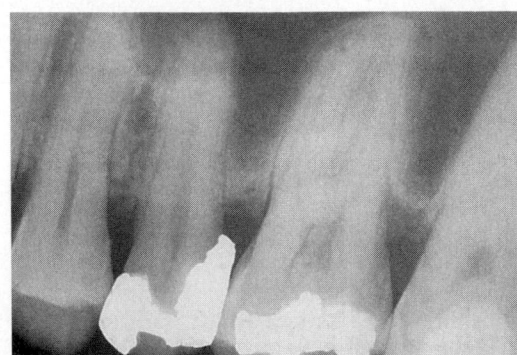

FIG. 6-6   A radiograph denoting an overhang on the distal of the amalgam restoration on the permanent maxillary left premolar.

(Courtesy of William Sorenson, D.D.S., M.S., Ann Arbor, Mich.)

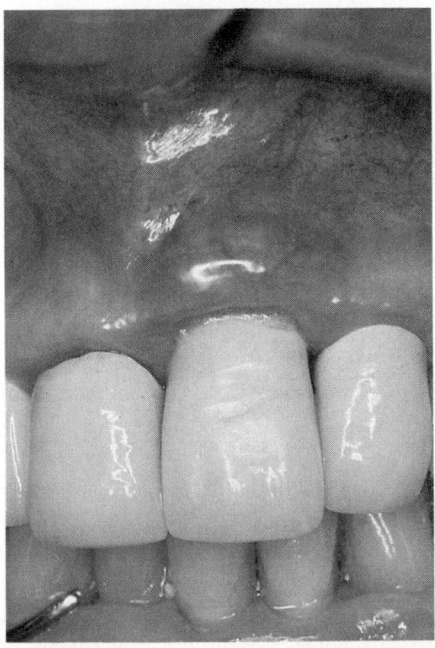

FIG. 6-7   An incorrectly contoured restoration on the permanent maxillary left central incisor has caused a reaction of the gingival tissues.

(Courtesy of William Sorenson, D.D.S., M.S., Ann Arbor, Mich.)

DEFECTIVE RESTORATIONS

Defective restorations can contribute to the accumulation of plaque. An overhanging restoration, such as the one shown in Fig. 6-6, creates an environment for the accumulation of plaque and food and ultimately for the formation of calculus. Fig. 6-7 illustrates the reaction of the gingival tissue to the incorrect contour of the gingival margins of a restoration. It is obvious that the gingivitis results from the defective restoration, since the inflammation is localized.

MISCELLANEOUS LOCAL CONTRIBUTING FACTORS

Additional contributing factors that result in localized gingival inflammation could include an abnormally attached frenum or gingiva (Fig. 6-8) or a malalignment of teeth (Fig. 6-9, *A* and *B*.). Trauma to the gingival tissues can occur through finger or nail biting, tongue thrusting, finger sucking, bruxism, or traumatic occlusion (Fig. 6-10).

SYSTEMIC DEFICIENCY

The lack of proper nutrition and metabolic and hormonal changes can contribute significantly to periodontal health. Two obvious examples of hormonal changes that have an effect on oral tissues are puberty and pregnancy. Either of these hormonal changes may cause enlargement and inflammation of the gingival tissues. In pubertal enlargement the tissues are soft and bleed readily, but after the removal of local irritants and a reestablishment

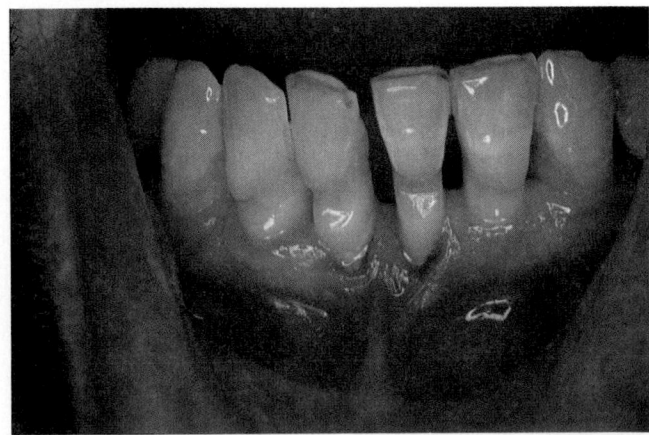

FIG. 6-8   The abnormally attached mandibular frenum has caused gingival disturbance.

(Courtesy of William Sorenson, D.D.S., M.S., Ann Arbor, Mich.)

of hormonal balance, the tissues will likely return to a healthy state. Similarly, gingival irritation may occur during pregnancy, but once the irritants are removed and parturition occurs, the enlargement usually subsides. The pubescent child and the pregnant woman are susceptible to changes in eating habits that may lead to nutritional deficiencies. These same nutritional deficiencies are evident in other patients, including older adult patients and anorexic, handicapped, or depressed patients.

The results of metabolic and chemical disturbances are often seen concurrently in the oral cavity. For instance, metabolic disturbances, such as epilepsy, may require drug therapy to control the disease (Fig. 6-11). Such therapy may result in gingival enlargement that could eventually cover the teeth completely. Contributing factors to the progression of the enlargement can be local irritations. Plaque control and regular prophylaxis can minimize this disturbance of the gingival tissues.

Periodontal Disease

Periodontal disease refers to diseases of the periodontium, which include the gingiva, the connective tissues, and the alveolar process. However, recent reports have shown that periodontal disease in the United States is lower than was previously reported. The reduction perhaps can be attributed to an increase in dental care, the use of antibiotics, and a higher degree of education among the public about dental care. Periodontal diseases are classified as those that involve the gingiva alone and those that involve the gingival tissue and the periodontium. Table 6-1 describes changes in the tissue from a normal to an abnormal state.

A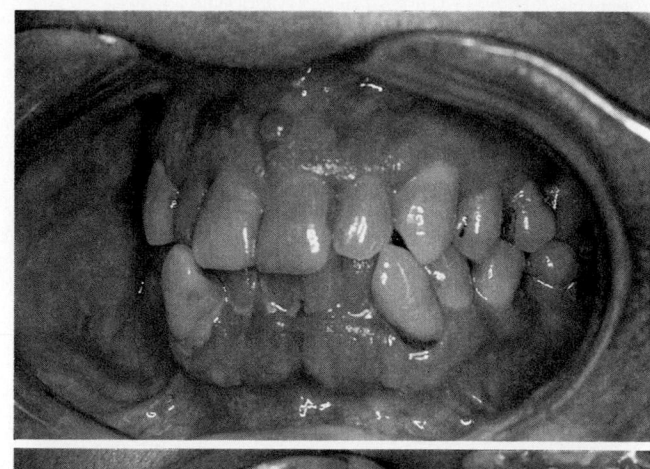

B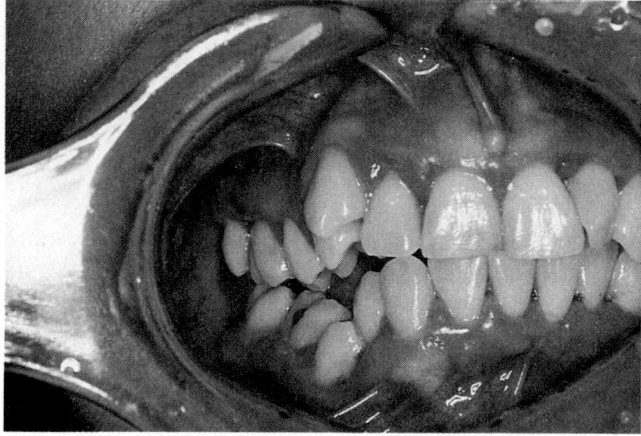

FIG. 6-9   *A* and *B,* Malalignment of teeth causing gingival disturbance.

(Courtesy of William Sorenson, D.D.S., M.S., Ann Arbor, Mich.)

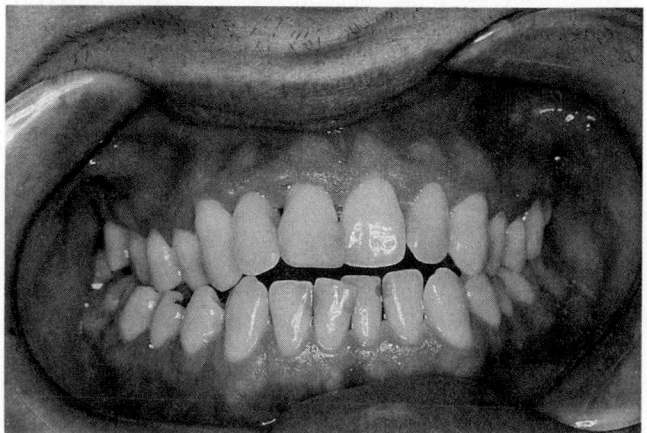

FIG. 6-10   Finger sucking or tongue thrusting may result in gingival trauma.

(Courtesy of William Sorenson, D.D.S., M.S., Ann Arbor, Mich.)

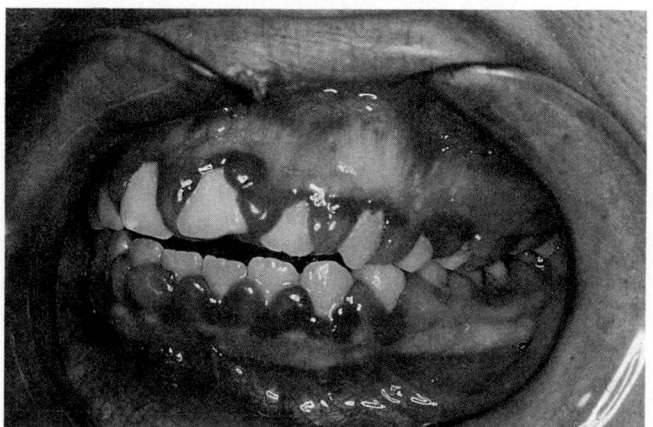

FIG. 6-11   Gingival enlargement as a result of Dilantin therapy.

(Courtesy of William Sorenson, D.D.S., M.S., Ann Arbor, Mich.)

TABLE 6-1   GINGIVAL ASSESSMENT: CLINICAL CHARACTERISTICS

Clinical characteristic	Ideal / Normal	Abnormal
Color	Uniformly coral pink Variations may occur depending on patient's complexion and race	Acute—bright red Chronic—red, bluish red, dark pink Color changes may be restricted to papilla or extend to marginal and attached gingiva
Contour	Margins are knifelike Contour of free margin forms regular parabolic curve as it goes around teeth Papillae are pointed and fill embrasure space	Margins become rolled, bulbous, enlarged; irregular contour may be noted; clefting or festooning Papillae may be flattened, bulbous, blunted, or cratered
Size	Free margin is near cementoenamel junction (CEJ) Margin adheres closely to tooth	Enlarged because of excess fluid in tissues (edematous) or buildup of collagen fibers (fibrotic) Margin may be retracted away from tooth with air or instrument
Consistency	Firm	Edematous, soft, spongy; pressure on tissues with an instrument will leave a dent Fibrotic, firm, hard tissue
Surface texture	Smooth free gingiva Stippled attached gingiva	Acute—loss of stippling; smooth and shiny Chronic—stippling present; may increase in occurrence
Position of gingival margin	1 to 2 mm above CEJ in fully erupted teeth	May be enlarged so that margin is more coronal than CEJ May show apical recession so that root surface is exposed
Position of junctional epithelium	At CEJ in fully erupted teeth	Apical migration onto root surface
Mucogingival junction	Clear distinction between appearance of attached gingiva (pink, stippled, immobile, firm) and alveolar mucosa (red, shiny, smooth, mobile)	Lack of attached gingiva determined by 1. Loss of junctional line 2. Mobility of all existing tissues 3. Probing extends beyond mucogingival junction
Bleeding	No bleeding detectable with palpation or probing	Spontaneous bleeding Bleeding resulting from probing
Exudate	No exudate with palpation or probing	Increase in amount of clear crevicular fluid Presence of white fluid (pus) with palpation

From Woodall IR: *Comprehensive dental hygiene care,* ed 4, St Louis, 1993, Mosby. Compiled from Goldman HM, Chohen DW: *Periodontal therapy,* ed 6, St Louis, 1980, Mosby; and Wilkens E: *Clinical practice of the dental hygienist,* ed 5, Philadelphia, 1989, Lea & Febiger.

▶ Gingivitis

When the gingiva alone is inflamed, the disease is known as **gingivitis.** If the inflammation is left untreated, it may progress to a subsequent form of disease referred to as acute necrotizing ulcerative gingivitis (ANUG). If neglected, gingivitis can progress into periodontal disease—a more serious disease that may result in the loss of bone support and ultimately the loss of teeth. Periodontitis is a chronic disease that results from gingival inflammation, periodontal pocket formation, bleeding and exudate from the pocket, tooth mobility, resorption of the alveolar process, and finally tooth loss if the disease is not treated.

ACUTE NECROTIZING ULCERATIVE GINGIVITIS (ANUG)

Trench mouth, Vincent's gingivitis or inflammation, Vincent's gingivostomatitis, and necrotizing gingivitis are

also known as acute necrotizing ulcerative gingivitis (ANUG). It is most common in patients between the ages of 18 and 30 and is associated with poor oral hygiene, smoking, and emotional stress. Clinical signs indicating ANUG include ulceration of the marginal gingiva and interdental papilla (Fig. 6-12). The inflammation begins with a necrotic ulcer on the papilla and rapidly progresses to destroy the papilla. Then it spreads to adjacent marginal gingiva and continues to destroy other papillae. As the ANUG spreads, the tissues become red, raw, and exposed, causing severe discomfort, spontaneous bleeding, and a foul odor.

Initial treatment of ANUG includes the removal of local irritants, often with an ultrasonic scaler, since manual scaling can cause more discomfort. When the pain and discomfort subside, the patient can be seen for further scaling and curettage. In the meantime the patient should be instructed to improve home care and perform thorough plaque control through gentle brushing, flossing, and rinsing the mouth often with warm water and hydrogen peroxide or other recommended oral rinses.

ACUTE HERPETIC GINGIVOSTOMATITIS

Acute herpetic gingivostomatitis is an infection caused by the herpes simplex virus and is noted clinically by edema, pain, and redness of the mucosa (Fig. 6-13). The discomfort is created by small painful ulcers resulting from the rupture of vesicles; chewing, eating, drinking, and talking are uncomfortable for the patient. Typically the disease lasts 2 to 3 days in its acute stage and will resolve in approximately 7 to 10 days. Although this disease is more common in young children, it may occur in adolescents and adults.

PERICORONITIS

Pericoronitis is a localized gingivitis that occurs around a partially erupted tooth (Fig. 6-14). When the gingival tissue lays over the partially erupted crown, it creates an environment in which food and plaque can become impacted. Severity of the inflammation may range from acute to chronic. Often this condition is characterized by edema, redness, exudate, foul odor, and pain that may radiate from the point of origin to the ear, throat, or floor of the mouth. Patients may indicate a tenderness of the lymph nodes, facial edema, difficulty in closing the mouth, and a possible increase in body temperature.

Treatment typically involves the removal of the bacteria and local irritants. This can be accomplished with antibacterial or antiseptic oral rinses and may require a drug therapy regimen.

More extensive treatment may result in surgical removal of the gingival tissue or the involved tooth, especially in the case of third molars.

ACUTE PERIODONTAL ABSCESS

An **acute periodontal abscess** is an acute purulent infection of the soft tissues of the periodontium and is typically treated as an emergency procedure in a dental office. The area involved becomes swollen and painful, and exudate may distend the gingival tissues. Other common symptoms of the abscess are **adenopathy**, extrusion of the tooth involved, and loosening and tenderness to slight percussion. Often the diagnosis of a periodontal abscess can be confused with a periapical lesion. A periodontal abscess may be an extension of chronic periodontal disease.

The primary objective in treating the periodontal abscess is to relieve pain by establishing a route of drainage for the site. As with other types of infections, the release of pressure through the evacuation of the exudate often provides immediate relief. Drainage may be established by locating the opening of the periodontal

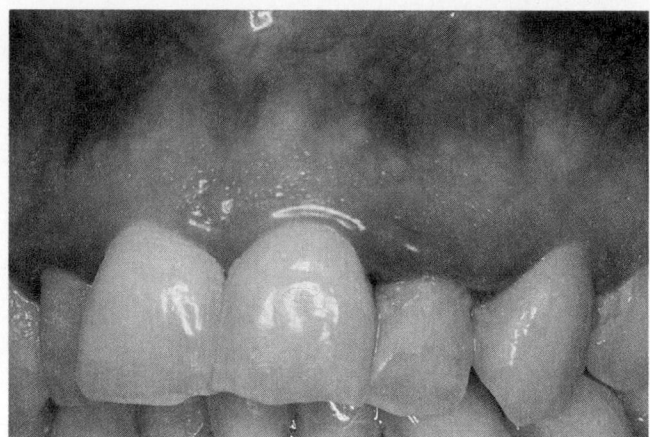

FIG. 6-12   Ulceration of the marginal gingiva and interdental papilla as a result of ANUG.

(Courtesy of William Sorenson, D.D.S., M.S., Ann Arbor, Mich.)

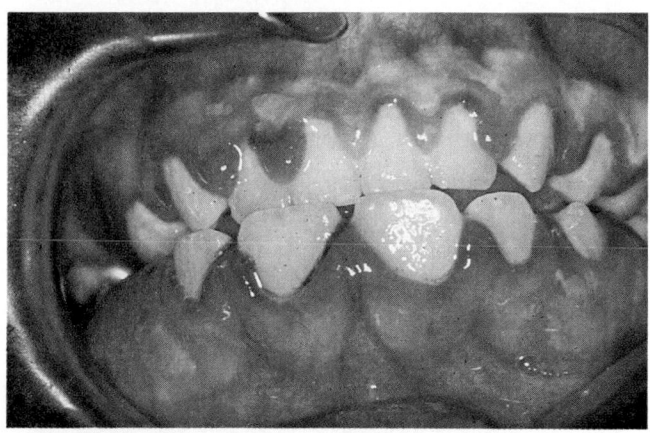

FIG. 6-13   Herpetic gingivostomatitis.

(Courtesy of Hoyt Laboratories: *Oral Legions,* ed 3, Colgate-Hoyt/Gel Kam, Director of Colgate Palmolive, Canton, Mass, 02021.)

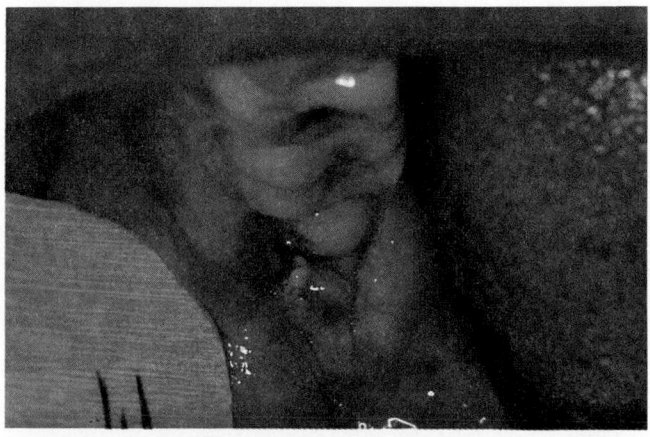

FIG. 6-14   Pericoronitis, an inflammation of gingival tissues surrounding a partially erupted tooth.

(Courtesy of Hoyt Laboratories: *Oral Legions,* ed 3, Colgate-Hoyt/Gel Kam, Director of Colgate Palmolive, Canton, Mass, 02021.)

pocket and gently forcing the release of the exudate or by making an incision to provide drainage.

▶ Periodontitis

Once the gingival disease has progressed to the deeper structures of the periodontium, the result is periodontitis. The progression of this disease includes resorption of the alveolar bone and loss of gingival attachment followed by the formation of periodontal pockets. A healthy periodontium is illustrated in the radiograph in Fig. 6-15. A normal periodontal depth measured in the gingival sulcus is expected to be 1 to 3 mm (Fig. 6-16). The space between the detached gingiva and the tooth is called a pocket. As periodontal disease advances, the pocket depth increases and the alveolar bone resorbs.

In mild periodontitis the gingival tissues are red and swollen, with bleeding evident and periodontal pockets measuring 3 to 5 mm. As the disease progresses into a chronic moderate periodontitis, a more definitive loss of the attached gingiva is evident and pocket depths progress to 6 to 7 mm (Fig. 6-17). In advanced periodontitis there is severe bleeding, exudate, and tooth mobility. In a radiograph of the advanced condition the loss of the alveolar process is evident (Fig. 6-18). Fig. 6-19 illustrates the progression of periodontal disease from the normal periodontium through advanced periodontitis. Often an illustration will be useful in patient education.

Treatment of periodontal disease may require several different approaches, but the initial treatment is the thorough removal of all local irritants from the gingival sulcus and around the teeth. Once this periodontal scaling has been completed and appropriate home care instructions have been given to the patient, careful follow-up of the patient is necessary. If improved results are not noted quickly, it may be necessary to proceed with additional treatment, including root planing to smooth rough root surfaces; gingival surgery to remove

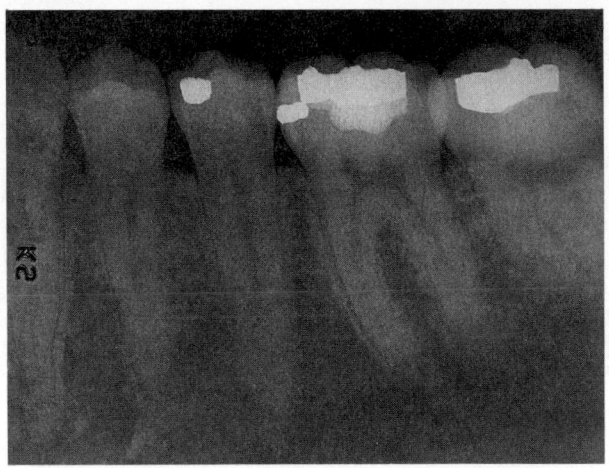

FIG. 6-15   Radiograph of healthy periodontium.

(Courtesy of William Sorenson, D.D.S., M.S., Ann Arbor, Mich.)

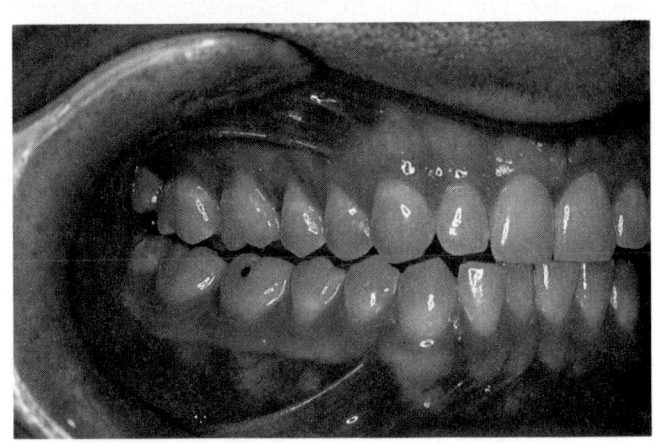

FIG. 6-16   Normal healthy gingival tissues.

(Courtesy of William Sorenson, D.D.S., M.S., Ann Arbor, Mich.)

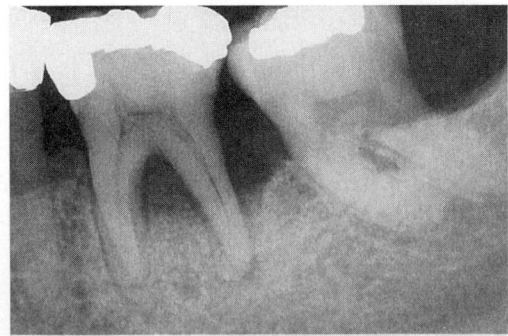

FIG. 6-17   Radiograph depicting extensive pocket depth progression. Note the significant bone loss around the molars.

(Courtesy of William Sorenson, D.D.S., M.S., Ann Arbor, Mich.)

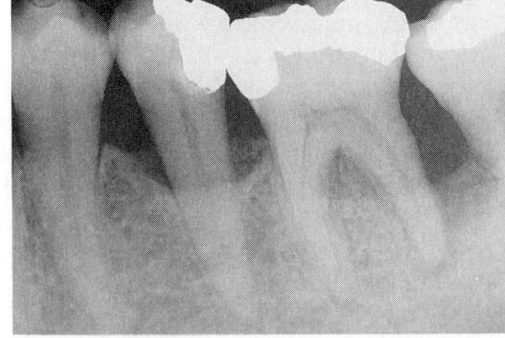

FIG. 6-18   Radiograph illustrating a continuation of pocket depth progression.

(Courtesy of William Sorenson, D.D.S., M.S., Ann Arbor, Mich.)

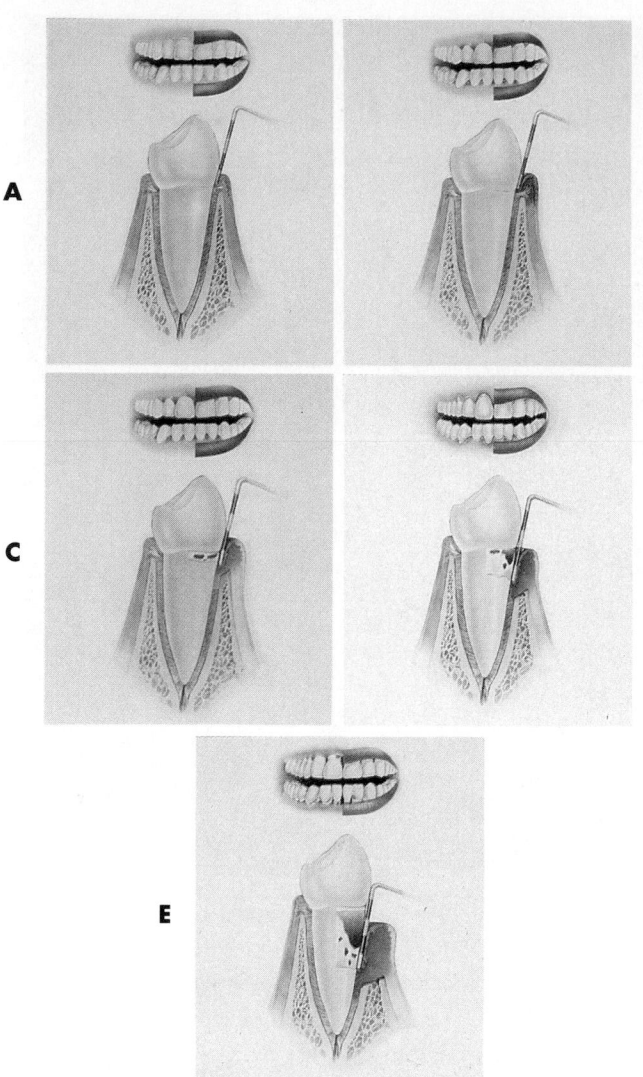

FIG. 6-19 Progression of periodontal disease from normal periodontium to advanced periodontitis.

(Courtesy of William Sorenson, D.D.S., M.S., Ann Arbor, Mich.)

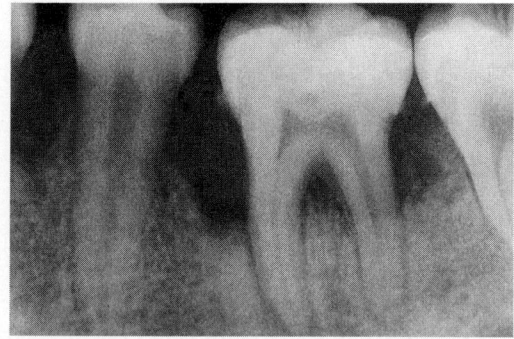

FIG. 6-20 Radiograph of juvenile periodontitis.

(Courtesy of William Sorenson, D.D.S., M.S., Ann Arbor, Mich.)

and eliminate periodontal pockets; occlusal adjustment to eliminate excessive trauma; orthodontic treatment to improve occlusal alignment; and restorative procedures to remove faulty restorations and to establish proper contacts and contours of the teeth. In Chapter 34, *Periodontics,* a review of several of these surgical procedures is offered.

JUVENILE PERIODONTITIS

Juvenile periodontitis is a disease of the periodontium that occurs in relatively healthy juveniles. The disease has often been associated with a genetic etiologic pattern. This condition is best identified by its rapid loss of alveolar bone around one or more teeth. Although the condition appears to be generalized, the most common areas of the mouth to experience the bone loss are the incisors and first molar regions (Fig. 6-20).

Diseases Affecting the Teeth

The diseases of the teeth and supporting tissues involve three groups of tissues: the calcified portion of the teeth, the periodontium, and the pulpal tissues. The calcified portions of the teeth are affected by several conditions and external factors. These factors or conditions include attrition, abrasion, erosion, stains, fractures, resorption, and carious activity. All of these cause a condition that is abnormal to the mouth. The condition may result in the loss of teeth, particularly without the intervention of dental treatment.

▶ Attrition

A building that has been built near the open sea, with no vegetation nearby, will eventually show wear from the sand and salt water plummeting against the side of the structure. Given normal environmental conditions, it can be anticipated that such a building will show wear and destruction over a period of time.

Similarly, the oral cavity undergoes changes during normal wear. The physiologic loss of the surfaces of the teeth through mastication is called **attrition**. Factors that facilitate attrition include bruxism and premature centric or eccentric contacts. Teeth that are abnormal in shape, size, and position can also contribute to attrition. Fig. 6-21, *A* and *B,* illustrates the appearance of attrition in the oral cavity. Wear facets found in areas of occlusal contact, particularly evident on the canine teeth, are caused by malocclusion and the wearing away of the tooth surface.

▶ Abrasion

Besides the normal loss of tooth structure attributed to attrition, **abrasion** can be caused by external sources.

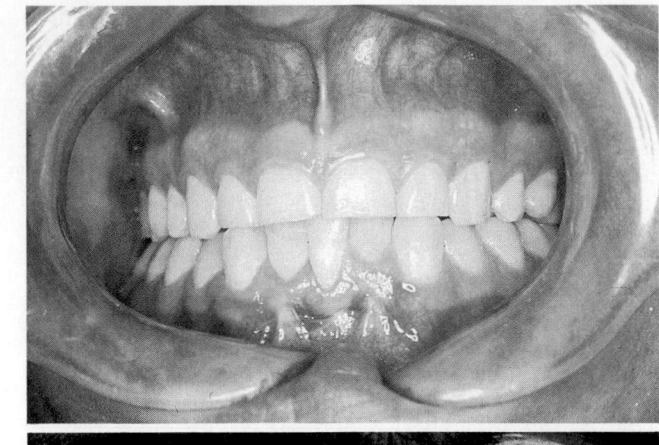

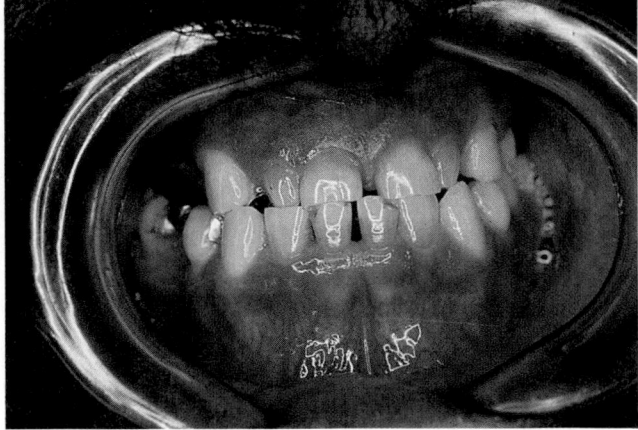

FIG. 6-21   *A* and *B,* Dental attrition.

(Courtesy of William Sorenson, D.D.S., M.S., Ann Arbor, Mich.)

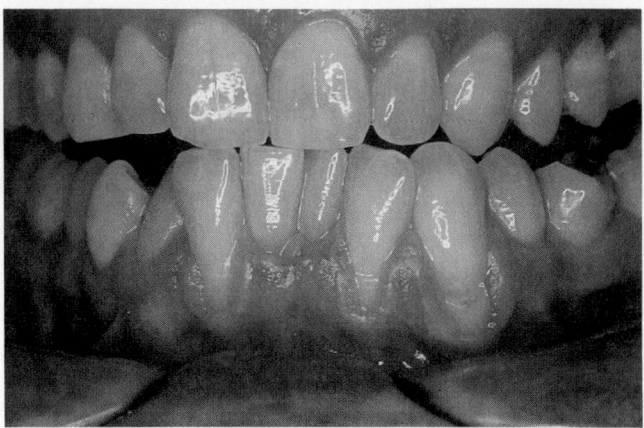

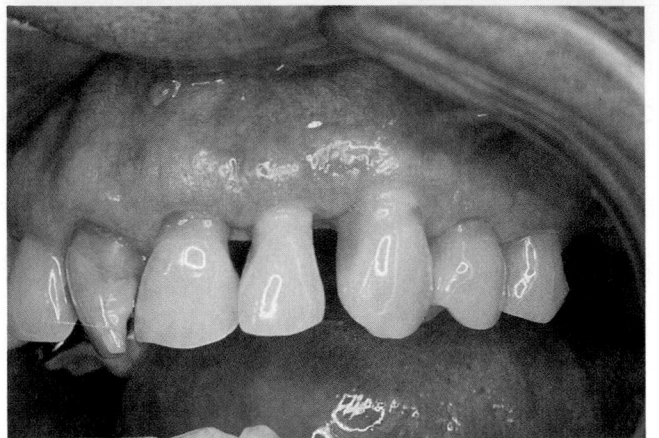

FIG. 6-22   *A* and *B,* Abrasion with marked clefting at the cervical line of the teeth.

(Courtesy of William Sorenson, D.D.S., M.S., Ann Arbor, Mich.)

Clinically it is difficult to distinguish abrasion from attrition. If wear can be attributed to an external source, the condition can be considered abrasion.

Abrasion may be caused by the vigorous use of a toothbrush and dentifrice on tooth surfaces. This action creates a marked clefting on the tooth, usually around the cervical margin, as noted in Fig. 6-22, *A* and *B.* The canine tooth is commonly affected by abrasion because of its prominence, but lateral incisors and premolars are also often involved. Toothbrush abrasion can be found on root surfaces of teeth with gingival recession. An interesting phenomenon can be found intraorally when abrasion is determined to be on the side of the mouth opposite the hand orientation of the patient. For instance, if the patient is right-handed, abrasion may occur on the buccal surface of the left side of the mouth, and vice versa. This phenomenon is the result of excessive force applied with the dominant hand.

Tobacco chewing is an external force that is routinely introduced to the oral cavity by some patients, causing abrasion of the teeth. The abrasion is more commonly found on the lingual surfaces of the maxillary teeth and

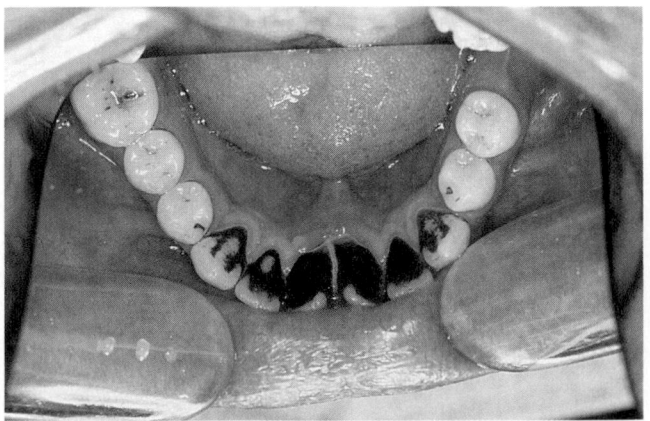

FIG. 6-23   Heavy staining as a result of the use of tobacco products.

(Courtesy of William Sorenson, D.D.S., M.S., Ann Arbor, Mich.)

the buccal cusps of the mandibular teeth. The habitual use of tobacco creates wear patterns, as well as heavy staining on the teeth (Fig. 6-23).

A seamstress who holds a needle in the mouth between the same teeth over an extended period of time can eventually create a wear groove on the incisal edges of the teeth. Other objects held between the teeth regularly, such as toothpicks, bobby-pins, or a pipe, may cause the same condition.

▶ Erosion

The loss of calcified tooth surface can also result from **erosion** caused by an abnormal substance in the mouth. Usually erosion is caused by the wearing away of a tooth or surface by acid and may be found in the mouth of individuals who regularly eat lemons. More commonly, erosion is caused by the repeated introduction of gastric acids to the mouth, as evidenced in the case of a bulimic patient. The bathing of the teeth in gastric acid after a period of time causes enamel erosion and the eventual exposure of dentin. Increased carious activity often results from the loss of tooth structure.

▶ Stains

Stains of the teeth emanate from two origins: **intrinsic**, from within the tooth, or **extrinsic**, from outside the tooth and usually through an accumulation of debris on the tooth surface. Tetracycline stain, discussed in Chapter 36, is an example of intrinsic stain. The stain is usually the result of a medical condition or of the medication given to treat a medical condition or disease. Stain may cause discoloration of the dentin during the developmental period of the dentition it affects, either primary or permanent.

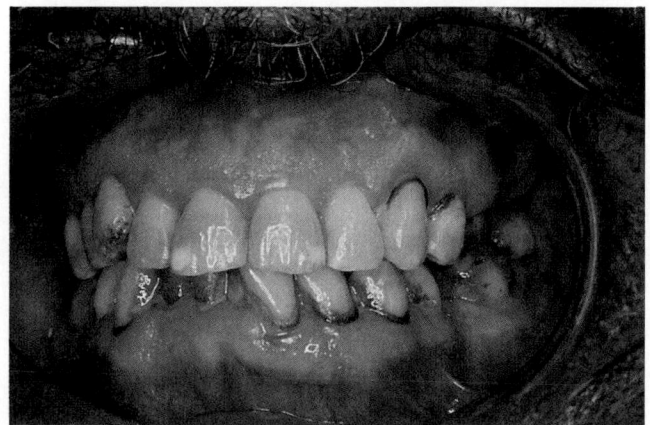

FIG. 6-24 **Extrinsic stain.**
(Courtesy of William Sorenson, D.D.S., M.S., Ann Arbor, Mich.)

Extrinsic stain is most often seen when oral hygiene is not maintained properly. The accumulation of soft deposits or calculus on the teeth coupled with poor oral hygiene may result in a green stain, often seen on the teeth of children, or in a brown pellicle. The use of a dentifrice with an abrasive ability will remove the soft deposits. However, the stain that is contained in calculus will need to be removed through a professional prophylaxis. Extrinsic stain may also originate from the use of drugs, certain types of foods, microorganisms, and tobacco (Fig. 6-24). The stain need not return if proper hygiene habits are continued.

▶ Root Fractures

Fractures of the root are usually the result of trauma. The treatment for root fractures is discussed in Chapter 33. Since fractures may not be obvious, they are often difficult to diagnose. The most common means of identifying a root fracture is through the use of a periapical radiograph. Even then the fracture may not be visible on the radiograph, but if the patient continues to complain of symptoms, the possibility of a fracture must be considered. A root that is fractured below the dentogingival attachment may heal without additional treatment, although immobilization of the crown may be necessary.

▶ Resorption

Two forms of resorption exist: internal and external. Either form results from a pathologic process that causes loss of some structure. Internal resorption involves a change in tooth structure within the tooth, enamel, dentin, or pulp. This change may result in an appearance of transparency. External resorption other than that seen in primary teeth causes changes in the root structure.

▶ Dental Caries

Dental caries, an abnormal condition of the tooth characterized by decay, if left unchecked, leads to the loss of tooth structure, mouth odors, poor aesthetic appearance, lowered self-esteem, and other dental problems. Dental caries is also known as tooth decay. Caries is caused by various microorganisms, such as *Streptococcus mutans* or *S. sobrinus* and lactobacilli, that cause a breakdown in the integrity of enamel, dentin, or cementum surfaces. This breakdown results in cavities or lesions on a tooth.

Areas of the teeth that are normally susceptible to dental caries are usually deep occlusal pits and fissures, interproximal surfaces, areas surrounding gingival margins that are exposed because of recession, and defective surfaces. It is possible that some of these sites are more

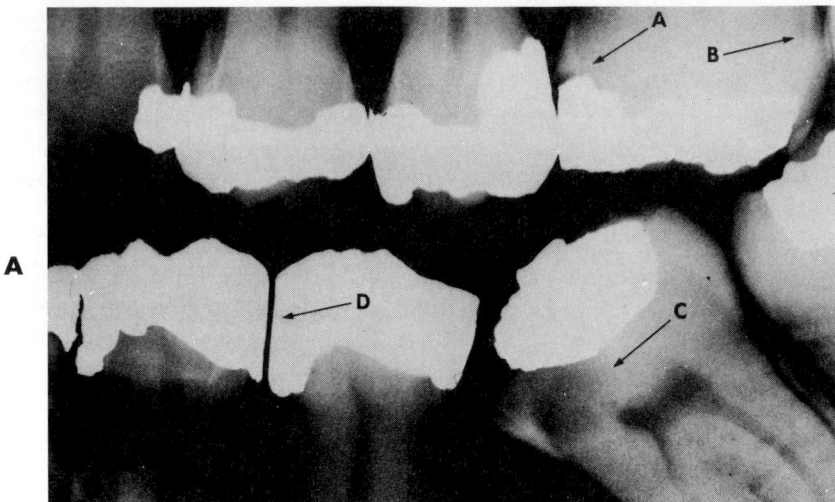

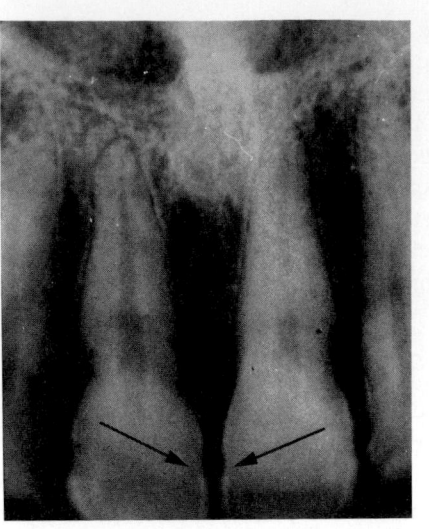

FIG. 6-25   *A,* Interproximal caries on bite-wing radiograph; *a,* recurrent; *b,* incipient; *c,* advanced at open contact. *B,* Caries seen on periapical film of maxillary incisors.

(Courtesy of William Sorenson, D.D.S., M.S., Ann Arbor, Mich.)

difficult to reach during normal oral hygiene. Consequently, dentobacterial plaque and debris are not removed, thus making the teeth more susceptible to the decay process.

Plaque forms enzymes that produce carbohydrates from food substances, which are then transformed to acid. The acid in the matrix of plaque is held in place on the tooth, attacking the surface by demineralization of the enamel, dentin, or cementum. The demineralization begins with the process of decalcification, the loss of calcium salts from tissues, which appears as a white spot on the tooth. Decalcification eventually leads to the beginning of the breakdown of the enamel surface known as incipient decay. In Chapter 5, a formula for caries development was presented in relationship to diet and nutrition; it is worthwhile to review it at this time. This process of change in the tooth surface through caries development can never be reversed, but the decay process can be stopped or arrested through proper hygiene habits and a reduction in the frequency of intake of refined carbohydrates.

If decay reaches the dentin layer of the tooth, it will progress into the internal tissues at a much quicker pace, sometimes leading to pulpal involvement. The involvement of the pulpal tissues during the decay process may require extensive dental treatment. If the pulpal tissue is offended by a carious lesion, pulp capping or a pulpectomy procedure may be needed, as discussed in Chapter 33, *Endodontics.* Fig. 6-25, *A* through *C,* illustrates dental caries at successive stages.

REPARATIVE DENTIN

As decay invades the tooth beyond the enamel, dentinal calcification, sclerosis, or **reparative dentin** begins to provide protection from the invasion of decay. Reparative dentin may develop at this stage or as a result of cavity preparation, abrasion, attrition, or erosion of the teeth. Odontoblasts react from any of these stimuli; the odontoblastic activity results in an increase in dentin formation in the traumatized area. As a person ages, odontoblastic activity continues in the pulp chamber through the protective layering of dentin on the pulpal surfaces, referred to as secondary dentin.

RECURRENT DECAY

Another form of decay found in the oral cavity is **recurrent decay.** Recurrent decay may be observed under existing dental restorations, often caused by incorrectly designed cavity preparations, improperly placed restorations, and/or poor oral hygiene with subsequent bacterial invasion. Although there may be other contributing factors, these situations can lead to loss of integrity of the cavosurface margins, the beginning of the carious process.

NURSING BOTTLE MOUTH

Nursing bottle mouth, discussed in more detail in Chapter 36, is extensive decay found in the mouth of an infant. This decay is caused by the constant bathing of the mouth with sweetened liquid throughout the day, but particularly during sleep. The liquid containing sugar combines with the bacteria in the oral cavity, forming acid. This acid barrages the teeth, causing a breakdown in the enamel and the beginning of the decay process.

ARRESTING DENTAL CARIES

Three important factors must be considered when attempting to reduce and eliminate the decay process. Each of these is discussed extensively in Chapter 5, *Nutrition and Dental Health*. The first is the decrease in total intake of carbohydrates, and the second is a reduction of the frequency of intake. The third factor is to change the consistency of the sugar-containing foods that are ingested. Today's lifestyle may create situations that necessitate eating prepared meals or snacks that are not as healthy as other choices. The repeated exposure of the teeth to carbohydrates and sugar results in increased carious activity. Efforts must be made to inform the patient about the need to change diets regardless of lifestyle. Suggestions for patient education are made in Chapter 5.

Cavity Forms and Classification

When carious activity invades the structure of a tooth, definitive action must be taken to avoid further involvement of the remaining areas. This action usually involves the removal of the carious tissue and the preparation of the tooth into a specific shape to accept some type of dental material as a restoration.

G.V. Black, sometimes referred to as the father of scientific dentistry, developed standardized classifications of cavities and rules for cavity preparations of all teeth that are to receive different restorative materials. As this text progresses into procedural techniques and as you gain experience in operative dentistry, you will need a thorough understanding of cavity nomenclature and preparation. A standardized method of classifying cavities enables the members of the dental team to communicate more effectively with each other about the patient, make accurate entries on patient records, and complete standardized forms used in third-party payments.

▶ Cavity Classifications

G.V. Black categorized dental lesions to provide a standard for dentistry. This classification is based on the clinical location of the carious lesions and is described in Box 6-2.

Since Black's original description of this classification, minor changes have taken place in its format. Originally Black had devised the system using Roman numerals; later

W.C. Davis used Arabic numerals. Today both systems appear to be interchanged. In the original classification, Black provided five categories. In some areas of the United States a modification has been made in complex cavity descriptions, with a sixth category being added. The first classification, Class I, identifies pit-and-fissure cavities, and the other classes refer to smooth-surface lesions.

Once you are able to identify the cavity classification, it is necessary to transpose this into surface annotations. It is not enough to simply state that you are going to treat a Class II cavity on #18. Since there are two proximal walls on this tooth, you must identify which surfaces are involved. Thus, it is necessary to use surface letters or numbers in such identification. Cavities involving a single surface, such as the buccal, lingual, or occlusal, are referred to as a single surface. When two or more surfaces of a tooth are involved, such as the mesial and occlusal (MO), the cavity becomes complex. To note such information on a patient's clinical record, a superscript number or letter is used. For instance, a Class I cavity on the occlusal surface of #18 would be written as 18° or 18^5. A Class II cavity, involving the distal occlusal surfaces of tooth, #30 would be written 30DO or 30^{25}. A complex cavity classification, such as the mesial occlusal and distal surfaces of #30, might be considered as two Class II restorations or a Class VI. Regardless of the cavity classification, the annotation is written as 30^{MOD} or 30^{152}. The G.V. Black system of cavity classification can be transposed to either alpha or numeric nomenclature, as seen in Box 6-3.

▶ Cavity Preparation

Although actual cavity preparation, by law, is the sole responsibility of the dentist, the practice of four-handed dentistry at chairside can only be enhanced by a dental assistant who has a thorough understanding of the restorative procedure. For an assistant to simply sit at chairside and wait to be asked for the next instrument in a procedure may increase production somewhat, but to observe the procedure, have an understanding of the process, and be prepared to offer the next instrument or material to be used in advance of the operator's need can be the difference between mediocrity and efficiency.

Cavity preparation is the process of mechanically removing tooth tissue to expose the carious lesion, remove the diseased tissue, and shape the remaining dentin and enamel so that the tooth can mechanically and biologically retain a restoration. The objectives of the dentist during cavity preparation of the tooth are as follows:

▶ Provide margin placement in accessible areas
▶ Provide adequate resistance in the tooth and resto-

BOX 6-2

G.V. BLACK CAVITY CLASSIFICATION

Class I
- Caries on occlusal surfaces of premolars (bicuspids) and molars
- Caries on buccal and lingual pits of molars and the lingual surface of anterior teeth

Class II
- Caries on proximal surfaces of premolars and molars

Class III
- Caries on the proximal surface of canines (cuspids) and incisors that do not involve the incisal edge

Class IV
- Caries on the proximal surface, including the incisal angle or edge of canines (cuspids) and incisors

Class V
- Caries on the facial and lingual gingival third of any tooth

Class VI
- Abraded incisal edges and occlusal tooth surface

Modification
- Caries on both mesial and distal proximal surfaces of premolars and molars that will be connected as one restoration

BOX 6-3

TRANSPOSITION OF CAVITIES FROM CAVITY CLASSIFICATIONS TO SURFACE ANNOTATIONS

Class I	Alpha 18^L, 30°, 7^L, or 12°
	Numeric 18^4, 30^5, 7^4, or 12^5
Class II	Alpha 18MO, 30DO, 14DO, 14MO
	Numeric 18^{15}, 30^{25}, 14^{26}, 14^{25}
Class III	Alpha 7^M, 24^D
	Numeric 7^1, 24^2
Class IV	Alpha 7^{MI}, 24^{DI}
	Numeric 7^{15}, 24^{25}
Class V	Alpha 18^B, 7^L, 30^L
	Numeric 18^3, 7^4, 30^4
Class VI (modification)	Alpha 18^{MOD}, 30^{MOD}
	Numeric 18^{152}, 30^{152}

ration to withstand the future stresses of normal mastication
- Provide adequate retention of the restoration
- Protect the vital pulp

The system of cavity preparation identified by G.V. Black provides a sequential pattern for cavity design and leads to achieving the goals of the dentist during the cavity preparation. Once the tooth is opened, the dentist will provide outline form, obtain retention and resistance form, establish convenience form, remove any remaining carious dentin, finish the enamel walls, and provide extension for prevention. Once this is completed, the cavity preparation is cleansed and medicated according to its depth. Each of the phases shown in Box 6-4 can be related to the need for specific instruments to be used in future restorative procedures. Thus, it is important for the assistant to understand the various phases of cavity preparation in order to prepare the appropriate instrument or material as the dentist progresses from one phase

G.V. BLACK ORDER OF PROCEDURE IN CAVITY PREPARATION

OUTLINE FORM

The form of the cavity preparation as it meets the tooth surface when it has been expanded to include all carious areas

RESISTANCE FORM

A shape that is given to a cavity to provide a filling that has the ability to withstand the stress brought on it in mastication

RETENTION FORM

The shaping of the cavity preparation to prevent the filling from being displaced; a large part of this is provided by the resistance form; in most cavities the retention form is made by shaping certain of the opposing walls so that they will be parallel or slightly undercut

CONVENIENCE FORM

The changes that are made in the basic outline form to facilitate visibility and placement of the restorative material

REMOVAL OF CARIES

The actual removal of carious or decalcified tissue from the tooth

FINISHING OF ENAMEL WALLS AND MARGINS

The placement of angles and bevels in the cavity preparation and the final smoothing of the cavity walls

EXTENSION FOR PREVENTION

The extension of the original cavity preparation to include pits and fissures that could become carious at a later time; to apply this principle to a carious lesion on the proximal surface will generally require the inclusion of the occlusal surface; even though the occlusal surface is not carious, it is the only feasible access to the proximal surface

to the next. All restorative procedures, such as amalgam, composite, and cast gold, progress through this systematic process of cavity preparation with variations in instruments and technique.

Nomenclature of Cavity Walls, Floors, and Angles

As a dental assistant develops a sophisticated understanding of the clinical preparation of a cavity design, a complete working knowledge of terms associated with basic cavity preparations will become more valuable. A dentist may indicate the need to place a medication or dental material in a specific area of the preparation or may indicate a need to sharpen a line angle in the proximal box of the preparation. Consequently, the dental assistant who has a clear understanding of the cavity design will more readily anticipate needs during the procedure. The following descriptions will help you become familiar with the nomenclature used in designing a cavity preparation.

Terms basic to most cavity designs include walls, floors, line angles, and point angles. **Cavity walls** are generally vertical and superior to the pulp, while a floor is horizontal to the pulp. The meeting of two walls of a cavity preparation is referred to as a **line angle**. Where three walls unite, a **point angle** is created. The walls, floors, and angles take their names from the names of the surfaces they approximate. To understand this nomenclature is not unlike standing in a room in a house where the vertical structures around and above you are the cavity walls and the place where your feet rest is the cavity floor. In the Class I restoration of #18° there are four walls and one floor: distal, buccal, mesial, and lingual walls and a pulpal floor, as shown in Fig. 6-26. In a Class III preparation on #9^D there would be axial, labial, incisal, and gingival walls, as shown in Fig. 6-27.

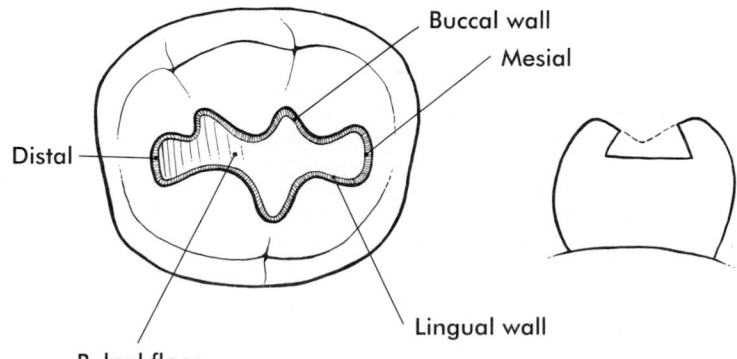

FIG. 6-26   Class I preparation illustrating various cavity walls.

(Courtesy of William Sorenson, D.D.S., M.S., Ann Arbor, Mich.)

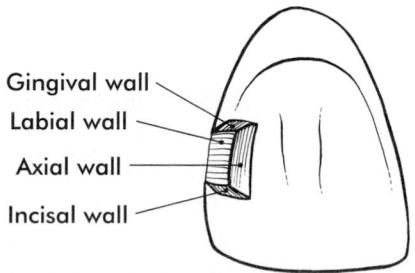

FIG. 6-27   Class III preparation illustrating various cavity walls.

(Courtesy of William Sorenson, D.D.S., M.S., Ann Arbor, Mich.)

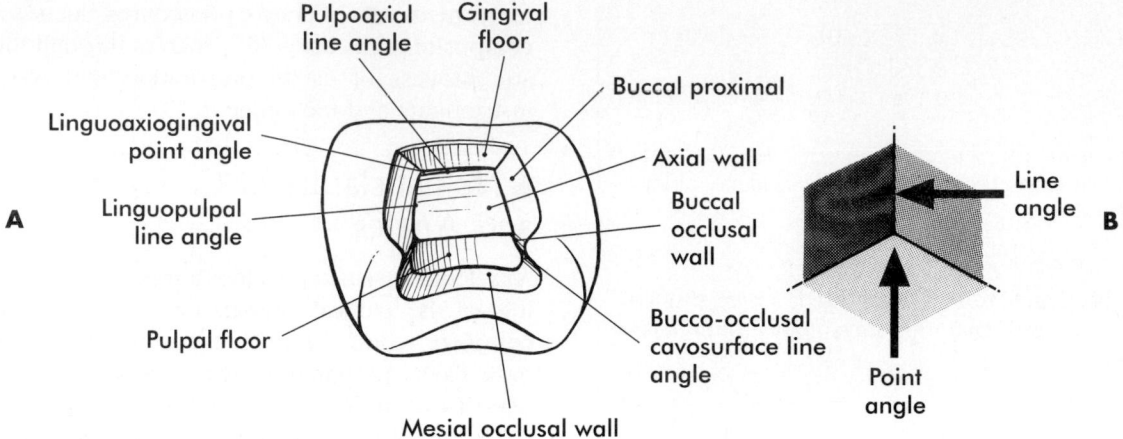

FIG. 6-28   *A* and *B,* Class II preparation illustrating various line and point angles, cavity floors, and walls.

(Courtesy of William Sorenson, D.D.S., M.S., Ann Arbor, Mich.)

In a complex preparation, such as a Class II on #30MO, there would be two sets of walls: a proximal set and an occlusal set. The differentiation is obvious once you try to name them, since there will be two buccal and lingual walls, one in the occlusal segment and one in the proximal segment. Fig. 6-28, *A* and *B,* illustrates the naming of these walls and various line and point angles in the preparation.

KEY POINTS

▶ Diseases of the teeth and supporting tissues can be classified into diseases of the teeth, periodontium, and pulp.

▶ Normal periodontium includes uniform color of the gingiva, varying with pigmentation of the patient, and sharp distinction between gingival and alvolar mucosa, with knife-edged margins circumscribing the teeth in a collarlike fashion.

▶ Periodontal disease can result from local or systemic factors. Local factors include inflammation and anomalies that contribute to the accumulation of plaque and trauma; systemic factors are influenced by nutrition or hormone deficiencies, metabolic disturbances, or various medications. Periodontal disease may be localized, generalized, or marginal and may involve papillary or diffuse change.

▶ Unhealthy gingival tissue is marked by inflammation, redness, and blunting of the interdental papilla.

▶ Periodontal disease progresses from gingivitis to ANUG and then to acute, mild, and eventually advanced periodontitis.

▶ Diseases or conditions that include the calcified tissue include attrition, abrasion, erosion, staining, root fractures, resorption, and dental caries.

▶ The process of disease in the calcified portion of the teeth begins with the decalcification of the enamel. The first stage is incipient

decay. As the decay progresses into the dentin, it advances at a more rapid pace, sometimes invading the pulpal tissues. The decay process cannot be reversed, although a change in diet and proper oral hygiene may arrest the progression.

▶ The G.V. Black system of cavity classification identifies dental lesions according to their clinical location into five categories with an optional sixth category.

▶ Cavity preparation is the process of mechanically removing tooth tissue to eliminate diseased tissue and shape the tooth to receive a restoration. Basic steps in cavity preparation include opening, outline, retention, and resistance forms.

▶ Cavity walls, floors, and angles refer to the surface interior landmarks of a cavity preparation and take their name from the corresponding anatomic positions.

BIBLIOGRAPHY

Charbeneau GT: *Principles and practice of operative dentistry,* ed 3, Philadelphia, 1988, Lea & Febiger.

Genco RJ, Goldman HM, Cohen DW: *Contemporary periodontics,* St Louis, 1990, Mosby.

Grant DA, Stern IB, Listgarten MA: *Periodontics,* ed 6, St Louis, 1988, Mosby.

Hoag PM, Pawlak EA: *Essentials of clinical periodontology,* St Louis, 1990, Mosby.

Incorporating new technologies in periodontal diagnosis into training programs and patient care: a critical assessment and a plan for the future, *J Periodont* 63(4):383-393, 1992.

Periodontal disease, *N Engl J Med* 332(6):373, 1990.

Ring ME: *Dentistry: an illustrated history,* St Louis, 1985, Mosby.

Schluger S, Yuodel R, Page R, Johnson RH: *Periodontal diseases,* ed 2, Philadelphia, 1990, Lea & Febiger.

Waite I, Strahan JD: *Color atlas of periodontology,* ed 2, St Louis, 1990, Mosby.

Woodall IR et al: *Comprehensive dental hygiene care,* ed 3, St Louis, 1989, Mosby.

7

Oral Pathology

LEARNING OBJECTIVES

You will have mastered the material in this chapter when you can:
- Define the key terms
- Identify clinical features, etiology, and treatment information for all conditions
- List the four signs of inflammation
- Identify historical information that should be gathered when suspicious lesions are found
- Identify the relationship between foliate papillae and the lingual tonsil
- List a differentiating feature between torus mandibularis and exostoses
- Identify oral hygiene information that is appropriate for the patient with a fissured tongue and a hairy tongue
- Identify the time schedule to repair the cleft lip and cleft palate
- Identify the area of the mouth where filiform papillae would be located and the conditions with which they are associated
- Differentiate between characteristics of herpes simplex ulcers and aphthous ulcers
- List features of the four forms of herpetic ulcerations
- Identify precipitating factors for recurrent aphthous ulcers and herpetic ulcers
- Identify the relationship between desquamative gingivitis and lichen planus
- Discuss the rationale for biopsy of leukoplakia and erythroplakia and identify the more dangerous of the two lesions
- Identify the role of early detection when squamous cell carcinoma is present in the mouth
- Compare the similarities and differences between basal cell and squamous cell carcinoma and between carcinoma-in-situ and squamous cell carcinoma
- List conditions that form as a result of frequent irritation
- Describe the differences between hyperplasia and hypertrophy
- Identify the conditions associated with *Candida albicans*
- List drugs reported on the medical history that may manifest orally as gingival hyperplasia
- Discuss the role of opportunistic infection in AIDS
- Identify infection control procedures that prevent the transmission of infectious diseases to dental personnel
- List conditions that can only be identified by radiographs

KEY TERMS

Atrophy	Genetic	Metastasis
Benign	Hyperkeratinization	Neoplasm
Bilateral	Hyperplasia	Nodule
Biopsy	Hypertrophy	Obturator
Carcinoma-in-situ	Idiopathic	Odontogenic
Clinical description	Inflammation	Opportunistic
Congenital	Innocuous	Oral pathology
Dysplasia	Lesion	Palpation
Erythematous	Leukoplakia	Tumor
Etiology	Localized	Unilateral
Exophytic	Malignant	

Oral pathology is defined as the study of disease that occurs in the mouth. A basic knowledge of oral pathology is necessary to differentiate between normal oral structures and abnormal findings in the oral cavity. Common pathologic conditions likely to be found in the head and neck region, as well as in the oral cavity, are discussed in this chapter.

The study of oral pathology includes discussion of diseases from common canker sores or aphthous ulcers, herpes virus, and candidasis to oral cancer. Oral pathology includes descriptions of disturbances in the soft and hard tissues of the mouth, as well as diseases of the oral cavity. The discussion of dental caries as a disease is reviewed in Chapter 6.

Diseases, including oral disease, may be caused through genetic changes or from external sources, such as microorganisms, drugs, chemicals, trauma, temperature change, radiation, inadequate nutrition, and immunologic causes.

Systemic diseases, such as mumps, tetanus, and measles, may involve the oral cavity, and the symptoms may become troublesome to a patient. Mumps and measles are often considered childhood diseases, but each can occur in the adult patient.

Mumps is an acute, contagious disease that is characterized by inflammation of the parotid glands and other salivary glands. Swelling of the glands is usually inferior and anterior to the ear. Movement of the jaw may be painful and restricted.

Tetanus is an acute infectious disease resulting from the toxin of tetanus bacillus. Tetanus may be localized at a wound site or manifest in muscle or joints, e.g., TMJ. The first symptom of tetanus in the head and neck is stiffness of the jaw, of the esophageal muscles, and of some muscles in the neck.

Measles is a highly communicable disease that is characterized by various symptoms, such as fever, general malaise, and skin rash eruptions. Orally, bluish white spots on the buccal mucosa, known as Koplik's spots, may occur.

An additional disease, tic douloureux, is a degeneration of, or a pressure on, the trigeminal nerve, which results in neuralgia of the nerve. Acute and severe pain radiates from the angle of the jaw along one of the involved nerve branches.

Most pathologic conditions in the oral cavity result from **inflammation**—a normal immune response of the body. The four signs of inflammation are *heat, redness, pain,* and *swelling.*

The immunologic system of the body responds immediately to protect the body when disease attacks. As discussed in Chapter 8, the immunologic system protects the body against pathogenic organisms and other foreign bodies. When a site becomes inflamed, the connective tissue cells encapsulate the inflamed site, forming a barrier of fibrin and fibrous tissue and localizing the inflammation. The healing process begins with the development of granulation tissue: soft fleshy projections of cells that form around the wound. If the body is unable to protect itself, it is because the immune system is not functioning properly; the body is then susceptible to the invasion of other pathogens and disease.

The dental assistant can be a keen observer of skin and oral mucosal irregularities and assist the dentist in identifying abnormal tissue conditions, called **lesions**, for the dentist's preliminary diagnosis. Lesions are usually found below the surface, above the surface, flat, or raised. Box 7-1 lists the categories of lesions and the characteristics of each.

Often the specific cause of the lesion, or **etiology**, can only be identified after tissue is surgically removed and examined under the microscope; such a procedure is called **biopsy**. The **clinical description** (features of the lesion that can be seen by the clinician) must always be recorded and submitted to the pathologist with the biopsy specimen to assist in the final diagnosis. Clinical features usually include the lesion's color, its surface texture, its location, and the tissue consistency.

When the lesions are examined, the general rules to follow are these:

1. The affected side is compared with the opposite side for similarities or differences.
2. Conditions that appear to be abnormal but that look the same on both sides of the oral cavity are considered normal for that particular patient and are usually not pathologic.
3. A history of the lesion is gained from the patient.

The dental assistant may be assigned the task of recording the clinical description and history of the lesion in the treatment record. Historic information may include (1) the patient's perception of what caused the lesion; (2) how long the lesion has existed; (3) whether the lesion is painful; and (4) the treatment the patient has been using.

CATEGORIES OF ORAL LESIONS

Lesions that are found below the mucosal surface include the following:

Cysts—Closed sac that is lined with epithelium containing fluid or semisolid material

Ulcers—Craterlike lesion that may also involve inflammation and infectious or malignant activity

Abscess—A cavity or area containing pus with inflamed tissue

Erosion—Mucosal defects that result from inflammation or injury

Lesions that are found above the mucosal surface include the following:

Vesicles—Small blister that is thin walled and contains clear serous fluid

Plaques—Flat or raised patch

Bullae—Thin-walled blister that is greater than 1 cm in diameter, containing clear serous fluid

Pustules—Small, circumscribed elevation of the skin that usually contains fluid

Hematoma—Collection of blood trapped in tissues that usually results from trauma

Papules—Small, solid, raised lesion that is less than 1 cm in diameter

Lesions that are considered flat surface include the following:

Patch—Small spot of surface tissue that differs from surrounding tissue in color, texture, or both

Petechiae—Tiny purple or red spots that appear as a result of minute hemorrhages

Purpura—Bleeding disorder that results in hemorrhage in tissues

Macules—Small blemish or discoloration

Lesions that are considered flat or with a raised surface include the following:

Granuloma—Chronic inflammation lesion with a tumor-like mass or nodule of granulation tissue

Nodules—Small node or rounded mass

Tumors—Swelling or enlargement that occurs in inflammatory conditions, which may be categorized as benign or malignant

WHITE LESIONS

Genokeratoses
Leukoedema
White sponge nevus
Hereditary benign intraepithelial dyskeratosis
Leukoplakia
Focal hyperkeratosis
Snuff dipper pouch
Nicotine stomatitis
Idiopathic leukoplakia
Hairy leukoplakia
Candidiasis
Mucosal burns
Lichen planus
Geographic tongue

something that occurred during pregnancy and disrupted the development of the fetus. Acquired malformations can occur in the fetus if the mother ingested any of a variety of drugs; they can occur if diseases (such as German measles) are contracted; or they can occur from **idiopathic** (unknown) reasons. **Congenital** conditions are present at birth; they can be either inherited or acquired. Most of the conditions included in this discussion are **innocuous**, or harmless, and require no treatment. Some conditions are simply variants of normal structures in that they look different from the usual anatomic structure. Although the dental assistant doesn't diagnose oral pathology, he or she may be asked to record a clinical description, and, at a later date, to record changes in lesions as part of the monitoring process.

Lesions may be characterized as white lesions, ulcerative lesions, or pigmented lesions. The white lesion is usually found intraorally as a thickened surface layer or keratin, as a thickened layer of epithelium, or as edematous epithelial cells. White lesions are listed in Box 7-2.

Lesions, abnormal in color, are divided into two primary groups: pigmented lesions and vascular lesions, with a smaller third group: yellow lesions. Pigmented lesions usually appear dark (brown to black) because of the production of melanin (Box 7-3). Lesions that are yellow contain lymphoid material, lipid, pus, or exudate.

The following includes descriptions, etiology, and treatment for a variety of pathologic conditions that are found in the oral cavity.

This chapter will include common conditions that affect oral structures: conditions that are precancerous and those that have developed into a true malignancy, lesions that are associated with the AIDS patient, as well as several common miscellaneous lesions.

Developmental Conditions

Abnormal conditions can include those that are formed during development of the fetus or those that develop after birth. **Genetic** (inherited) disorders are passed on through the genes. Acquired malformations result from

▶ Foliate Papillae

Foliate papillae are part of the collection of normally occurring papillae on the tongue.

PIGMENTED LESIONS

Pigmentations—Brown, blue, black
  Melanin
    Physiologic pigmentation
    Ephelis (freckle)
      Peutz-Jegher's syndrome
      Addison's disease
    Cafe-au-lait spots
      Neurofibromatosis
      Fibrous dysplasia
    Lentigo (age spot, liver spot)
    Nevus (mole)
      Intradermal
      Junctional
      Compound
      Blue
    Melanotic macule
    Melanoma
      Superficial
      Nodular
    Neuroectodermal tumor of infancy
  Silver—Amalgam tatoo
Yellow Lesions
  Fordyce granules
  Ectopic lymphoid tissue (oral tonsils, lymphoepithelial cyst)
  Lipoma
  Xanthoma
  Gingival cyst
  Parulis

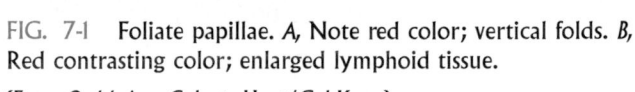

FIG. 7-1   Foliate papillae. *A,* Note red color; vertical folds. *B,* Red contrasting color; enlarged lymphoid tissue.

(From *Oral lesions,* Colgate-Hoyt / Gel-Kam.)

Clinical appearance: They appear as vertical folds of **erythematous**, or reddish colored tissue, on both sides of the posterolateral aspect of the tongue; they are positioned perpendicular to the dorsal surface and at a right angle. Foliate papillae are best seen when the tongue is extended and turned and the extreme posterior area of the side of the tongue is in view. In most people these structures are small and inconspicuous, but occasionally, they are enlarged, have a prominent red color, and appear to be inflamed and swollen (Fig. 7-1, *A* and *B*).

Etiology: Lymphoid tissue is found in the soft palate, pharynx, and posterior area of the tongue and is often reddish. When lymphoid tissue is found in the area of the foliate papillae, it appears as an enlarged, red lesion. Some texts call this condition *lingual tonsil* to denote the lymphoid tissue that is combined with the foliate papillae structure.

Treatment: Foliate papillae require no treatment; but they can be mistaken for **malignant** or cancerous tissue because of the common occurrence of malignant lesions on the posterolateral area of the tongue. Comparison of one side of the tongue to the opposite side helps to determine if the red enlargement is normal for the patient, or if it is potentially pathologic. Dentists may observe the lesion for a short period of time to determine if it enlarges or changes in any way before they consider performing a biopsy procedure.

▶ Varix

A varix is a dilated blood vessel that is associated with the aging process (plural: varices).

Clinical appearance: Varices appear as dark blue, purple, or black elevated lesions. They can occur in any mucosal location; however, they are more likely to be found under the tongue or on the buccal mucosa (Fig. 7-2).

Etiology: The lesion probably represents a distended vein weakened by the aging process. It is the oral counterpart of a *varicose vein.*

Treatment: No treatment is required; however, the lesion

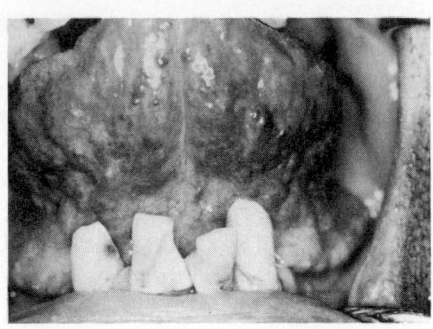

FIG. 7-2   Varix; note multiple lingual varicosities.

(From Wood NK, Goaz PM: *Differential diagnosis of oral lesions,* ed 3, St Louis, 1985, Mosby.)

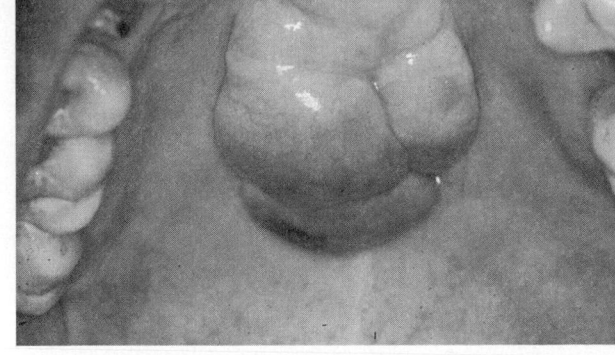

A

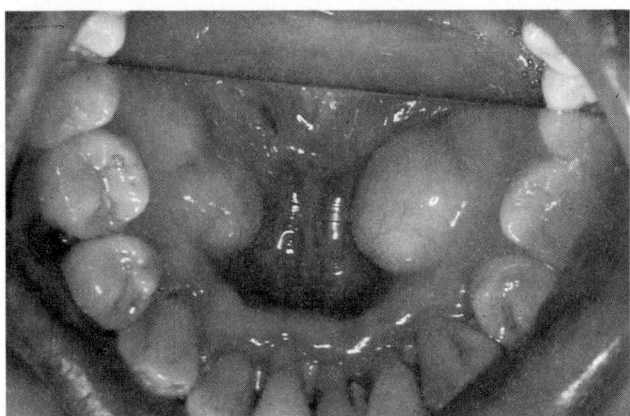

B

should be described, and the location should be noted in the treatment record.

▶ Tori

Tori are **benign tumors** of bone. *Benign* denotes normal, nonmalignant tissue. When tori are found in the palate, they are called *torus palatinus;* when tori are located in the lingual aspect of the mandible apical to the canine-premolar region, they are called *torus mandibularis.* Excess bony growths can also occur on the labial aspect of both the maxilla and the mandible. When they occur in that area, they are referred to as *exostoses.*

Clinical appearance: Tori appear as single or multiple **nodules,** or lumps, extending from the surface and covered by normal epithelium (Fig. 7-3, *A* and *B*). **Palpation** (feeling the tumor with the fingers) reveals a hard consistency. Mandibular tori are usually **bilateral** and occur on both sides of the mandible.

Etiology: The cause is unknown, but tori are probably hereditary.

Treatment: No treatment is indicated for tori unless the patient needs a removable prosthetic appliance, such as a denture. The tori must then be surgically removed to accommodate the appliance. Radiographs may be painful for the patient who has tori and require alterations in technique.

FIG. 7-3   Tori. *A,* Palatine torus. *B,* Bilateral torus mandibularis.

(From *Oral lesions,* Colgate-Hoyt/Gel-Kam.)

▶ Fissured Tongue

Fissured tongue is a common condition found on the dorsal surface of the tongue.

Clinical appearance: Furrows or cracks can be seen on the dorsal surface of the tongue (Fig. 7-4). It may be painful if a fissured tongue is secondarily infected by bacteria. Retained food can be caught in the fissures and promote the growth of microorganisms.

Etiology: The cause is probably hereditary; Kullaa-Mikkonen reports finding a gene for fissured tongue.

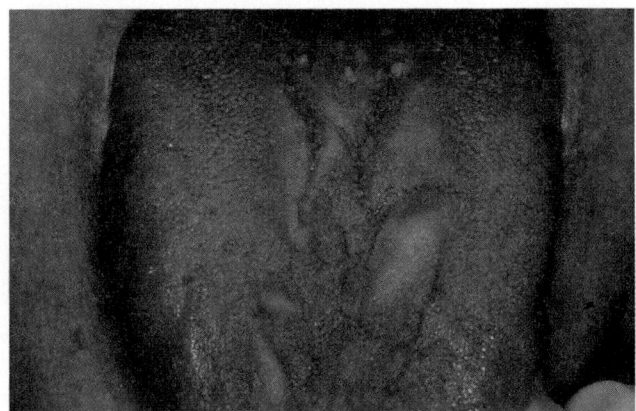

FIG. 7-4   Fissured tongue. Fissures are opened to view deep craters.

(*A* from Huffines R: VA Dental Center, Johnson City, Tennessee. *B* from Pickett F: *Files of Baylor College of Dentistry.*)

Some cases may be associated with irritation. Fissured tongue is more common in older individuals; however, it is not known why the condition appears late in life.

Treatment: When pain is associated with a fissured tongue, the patient should be instructed to clean retained food debris from the furrows.

Fordyce's Granules

Fordyce's granules represent a common deviation from normal found in some individuals, usually occurring at puberty.

Clinical appearance: Fordyce's granules are multiple, yellow round structures found in oral mucosa. They appear just below the surface most often on the buccal mucosa, but they can be found on any mucosal area (Fig. 7-5).

Etiology: These structures are sebaceous glands on the surface of the epithelium. Sebaceous glands usually surround hair follicles, but they are not associated with hair follicles in the mouth. It is not known why Fordyce's granules appear on oral mucosa—a location where hair is never found.

Treatment: No treatment is required. These are innocuous structures considered normal for the person who has them.

Cleft Lip and Cleft Palate

The most common clefting disorders of the head and neck region are cleft lip and cleft palate. These conditions can occur separately (cleft lip only, cleft palate only) or can be combined. Combined cleft lip and cleft palate occur more frequently than either condition occurs separately, with an incidence of 1 in every 800 births.

Clinical appearance: Cleft lip appears as an absence of tissue between the center of the lip and the adjacent lip area. It is usually a **unilateral** defect that occurs on one side only, but the defect can affect both sides of the lip (Fig. 7-6, *A* and *B*). The nose is often misshapen on the affected side. Cleft palate displays an open space anywhere from the uvula up through the median palatine raphe, depending on the severity of the cleft. A bifid uvula has been called the mildest form of cleft palate.

Etiology: Heredity is considered the single most likely cause of clefting disorders, although not all cases are inherited. Cleft lip results from a failure of embryonic mesodermal cells to penetrate the epithelial groove between the medial and lateral nasal processes. Cleft palate occurs when the palatal processes fail to fuse at the median line.

Treatment: Cleft lip is surgically repaired by 1 month of age and cleft palate, by 18 months of age. If the palatal cleft is large, a prosthetic appliance called an **obturator** is prepared to fill in the open defect. It looks much like a maxillary denture without teeth (see Chapter 31, *Prosthodontics*).

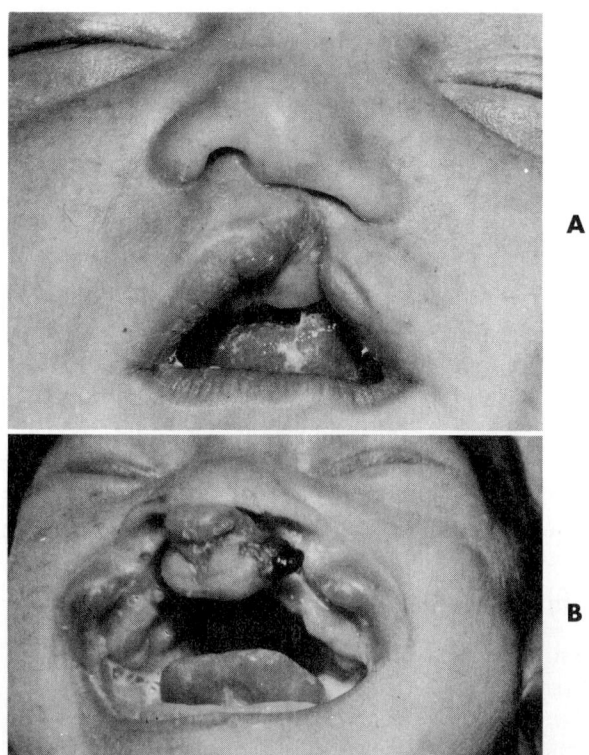

FIG. 7-6   Cleft lip and cleft palate. *A,* Unilateral cleft lip. *B,* Bilateral cleft lip and cleft palate.

(From Wood NK, Goaz PM: *Differential diagnosis of oral lesions,* ed 3, St. Louis, 1985, Mosby.)

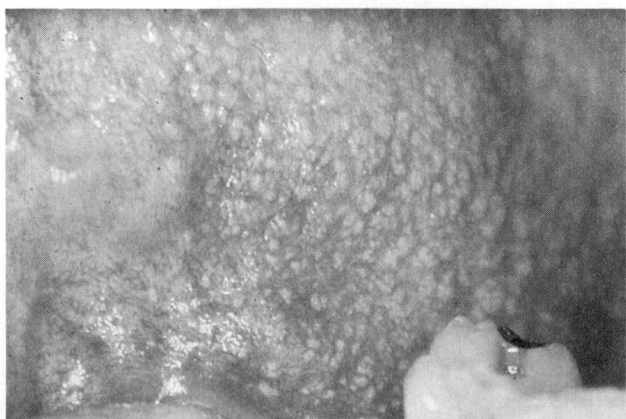

FIG. 7-5   Fordyce's granules.

(From *Oral lesions,* Colgate-Hoyt/Gel-Kam.)

Diseases of Mucous Membranes

Abnormal conditions that the dental assistant will likely observe are included in this section. Most are innocuous; however, lesions can be contagious, so appropriate infection control and patient-management procedures must be followed. Patients who have lesions often ask the dental assistant to explain the cause and the management of the condition.

▶ Geographic Tongue

Geographic tongue is a condition where filiform papillae atrophy in patches. Another name for geographic tongue is *benign migratory glossitis,* which describes the course of the disease in that lesions appear, heal, then seem to *migrate* to another area of the tongue.

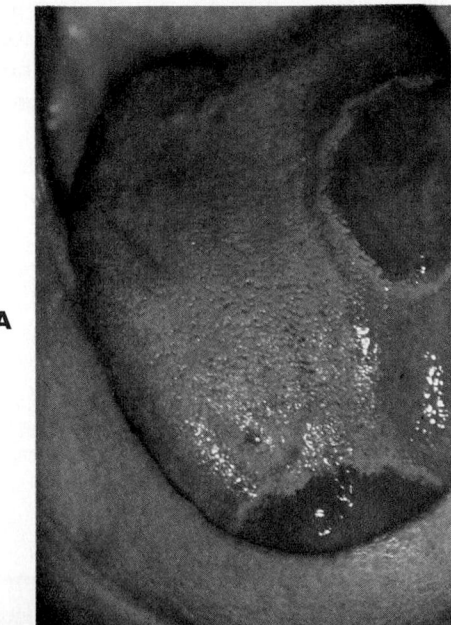

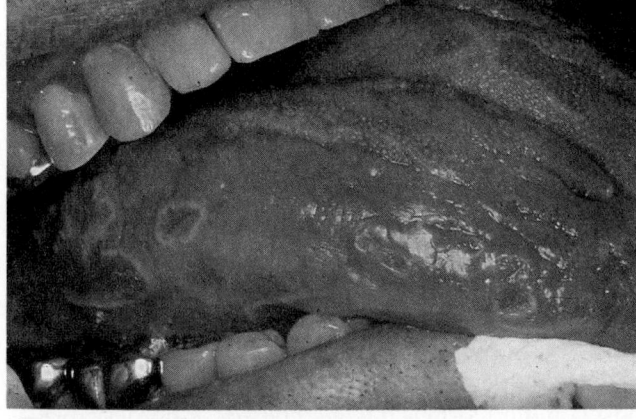

FIG. 7-7   Geographic tongue. *A,* Dorsal lesions. *B,* Lesions on lateral border.

(From *Oral lesions,* Colgate-Hoyt / Gel-Kam.)

Clinical appearance: The condition is characterized by circular pink-to-red areas on the dorsal surface of the tongue that are surrounded by yellow borders of necrotic filiform papillae (Fig. 7-7, *A* and *B*). It is most common on the tongue, but it can occur on other mucosal areas of the mouth. All ages are affected, and multiple or single lesions can occur at the same time. Symptoms range from a mild stinging sensation with tenderness to none at all. Occasionally the patient is not aware of having the condition until it is identified in an oral examination.

Etiology: The cause is unclear; however, there are several reports in the literature that support an hereditary etiology.

Treatment: No treatment is required. The patient should be informed of the innocuous nature of the condition to relieve any anxiety.

▶ Hairy Tongue

A tongue where filiform papillae are elongated making it appear *coated* and discolored, is called a *hairy tongue.* Tobacco products can stain it a dark color, giving it the name *black hairy tongue.*

Clinical Appearance: The filiform papillae become elongated and are light colored unless they are stained by substances that are taken into the mouth (Fig. 7-8). The tongue is not painful, but the papillae can become so long that they are reported to cause a gagging reflex.

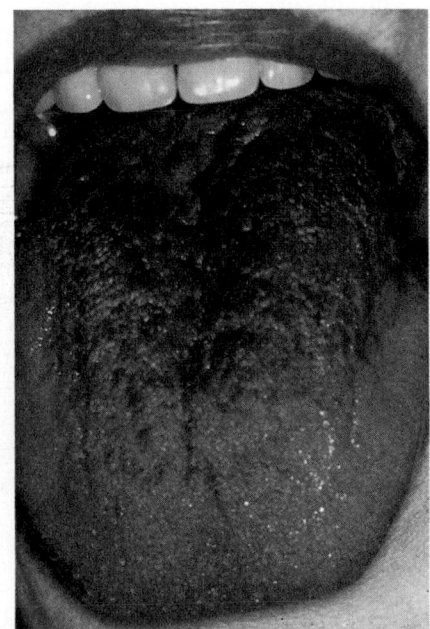

FIG. 7-8   Black hairy tongue in heavy smoker.

(From *Oral lesions,* Colgate-Hoyt / Gel-Kam.)

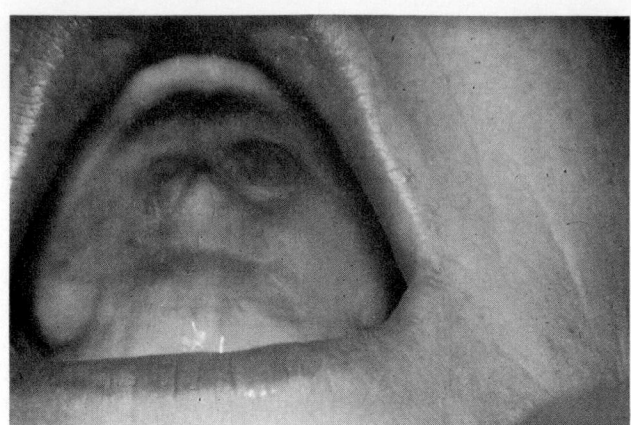

FIG. 7-9   Denture-related traumatic ulcer.

(From *Oral lesions*, Colgate-Hoyt/Gel-Kam.)

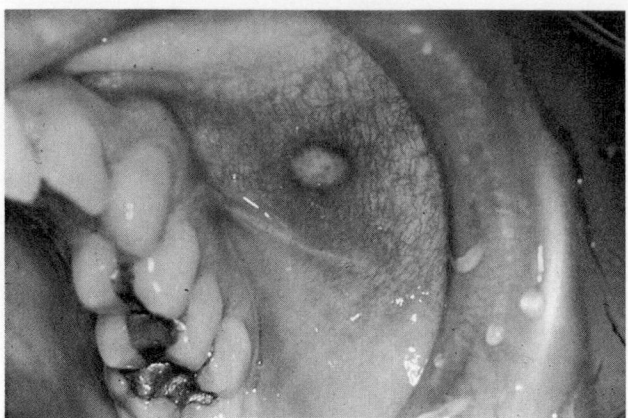

FIG. 7-10   Aphthous ulcer on movable mucosa.

(From *Oral lesions*, Colgate-Hoyt/Gel-Kam.)

Etiology: The cause is related to irritation from several factors, such as inadequate tongue cleaning, frequent use of a hydrogen peroxide mouthrinse, tobacco, *Candida albicans* yeast infection, and antibiotics. Other cases are **idiopathic:** they have no known cause.

Treatment: Patients are advised to improve tongue brushing techniques, and this eventually causes the condition to resolve. If the cause is apparent, it should be discontinued. Papillae that have reached an extreme length can be clipped off to reduce gagging.

Traumatic (Decubitus) Ulcer

The traumatic ulcer is the most common ulceration found on oral mucosa. It results from an injury that cuts or abrades the epithelium.

Clinical Appearance: The ulcer resembles most oral ulcerations; it is a shallow, depressed circular lesion that is usually covered by a yellow or white necrotic membrane (Fig. 7-9), and may have a red border. Lesions are usually painful and last from a few days to several weeks. Tongue-related ulcers often persist for a longer time.

Etiology: Injury can be caused by a variety of sources, such as cheek biting, sharp teeth or restorations, denture irritation, removal of dry cotton rolls from the vestibule after dental treatment, or burns from hot food.

Treatment: Removal of the cause to prevent further injury and to allow healing of the ulcer is important. Use of topical anesthetic agents and corticosteroids to relieve pain is recommended. Ulcers that do not heal in 3 weeks should be biopsied to rule out malignancy.

Recurrent Aphthous Ulcers (RAU)

Aphthous ulcers are common oral ulcerations that tend to recur throughout the patient's lifetime. They affect both sexes and all ages but are more common in women. The layman's term is *canker sore.*

Clinical Appearance: Lesions appear as shallow, circular ulcers with a yellow **necrotic** center where the epithelium has died. An erythematous halo often surrounds the ulcer (Fig. 7-10, *A* and *C*). They range in size from 1 mm to 2 cm, with the smaller lesions (2 to 5 mm) appearing more commonly. They appear on mucosa that is movable, such as the lips, cheeks, floor of the mouth, vestibule, or soft palate. RAU are *not* thought to be preceded by blisters. They can be painful and last from 10 to 14 days.

Etiology: The cause is unknown, but it is thought to involve a disorder of the immune response. Recurrences are associated with hormonal changes, emotional stress, food or drug allergies, and hereditary predisposition.

Treatment: Treatment is mostly aimed at reducing pain. Topical anesthetics are used to allay pain, and topical steroid preparations are used to reduce inflammation. Tetracycline rinses are reported to resolve the lesion in a few days. RAU are not contagious, but care should be taken not to cause discomfort during dental treatment. Some ulcers may be so painful that dental treatment will need to be postponed until the area has healed.

Herpetic Ulcers

The *herpes simplex I* virus causes oral ulcerations that look similar to small aphthous ulcerations; however, herpetic ulcers are usually differentiated from aphthous ulcers in that they are found on mucosa bound to bone, such as gingiva or palatal attached mucosa. The viral infection is contagious and occurs in four forms. The most common form is the *fever blister,* or herpes labialis, on the lips. The intraoral counterpart most often occurs on the palate and is called intraoral recurrent herpetic ulceration. Both of these are secondary infections that

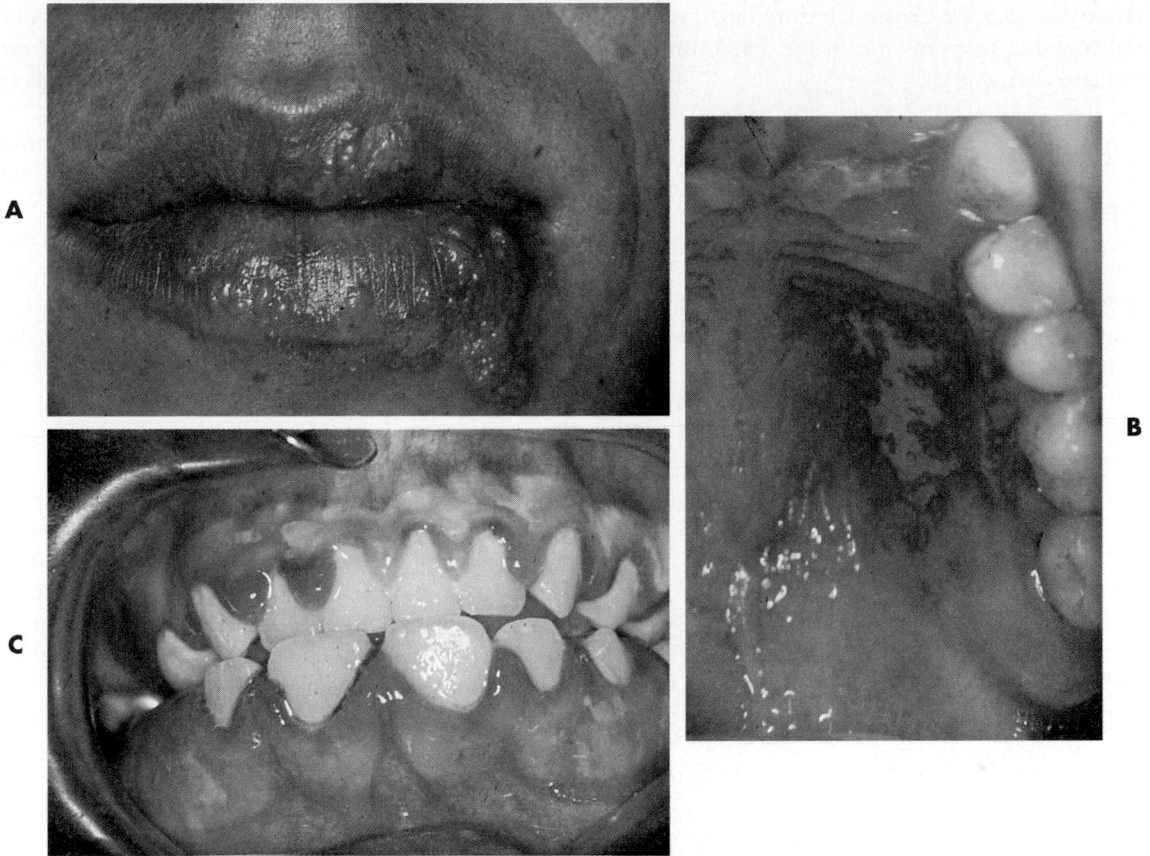

FIG. 7-11 Herpetic ulcers. *A,* Herpes labialis. *B,* Palatal herpetic lesion; recurrent. *C,* Primary herpetic gingivostomatitis.

(From *Oral lesions,* Colgate-Hoyt/Gel-Kam.)

occur after the initial (primary) herpetic infection. The third form is the initial infection called primary herpetic gingivostomatitis. This form usually occurs in children and is characterized by oral ulceration of all mucosal areas, both movable and attached, high fever, enlarged and tender lymph nodes and an individual who is ill. Most primary infections are subclinical—meaning that no lesion develops or that the lesion is so mild that the patient is unaware of it. Infection of the finger, or herpetic whitlow, is the fourth form. Wearing gloves will prevent the occurrence of this lesion on the fingers of dental personnel.

Clinical appearance: The lesion on the lips appears as a painful solitary blister or collection of blisters. The intraoral recurrent lesion appears as small pinpoint ulcers in a cluster (Fig. 7-11, *A* through *C*). The ulcers may or may not be covered with a necrotic membrane. An area of redness and inflammation often surrounds the ulcers. The ulcers in the primary infection are severe, covering intraoral mucosa, gingiva, and lips. Pain can be significant, causing the patient to be unable to eat. Herpetic whitlow appears as a swelling close to the nailbed with vesicles that break and form crusted, painful sores. These lesions can recur throughout life.

Etiology: The *herpes simplex I* virus causes these lesions. It is prevalent among the population, and children can contract the virus at a young age via kisses from family members who have fever blisters. Lesions are infectious in both the vesicular stage and the crusted stage. Fortunately, most primary infections are subclinical infections and no oral ulceration occurs, or the ulceration is mild. Precipitating factors that provoke a recurrent attack include sun exposure, stress, trauma, fever, and menstruation. It is interesting to note that the same precipitating factors can cause recurrence of the aphthous ulcer.

Treatment: Topical application of the drug acyclovir during the early stage of the lesion may reduce the severity of the episode and shorten the duration of the lesion. Other remedies have been tried with little success. Patients with multiple lesions and fever should drink plenty of liquids to prevent dehydration. Pulling or stretching the lips while a lesion is present can cause the virus to spread and may be painful to the patient. Most authorities advise against working in the mouth when vesicles or crusted lesions are present because of possible transmission of the virus through aerosols to the dental staff.

▶ Lichen Planus

Lichen planus is a skin disease with oral manifestations. Skin lesions appear as brown, crusted lesions on legs, wrists, and ankles. Oral lesions of lichen planus appear in two main forms. The reticular form is the mildest and is often asymptomatic, with the patient unaware that it exists. The erosive form results in loss of oral epithelium in affected areas and is painful.

Clinical appearance: The reticular form is characterized by white lines that intersect in a *lacy fashion* and a circular pattern (Fig. 7-12, *A* and *B*). The buccal mucosa is a common location for oral lesions. In the

erosive form the reticular pattern is found along with ulcerated areas. Lesions can occur on the gingiva or mucous membranes. When they affect the gingiva, the lesions are called *desquamative gingivitis.*

Etiology: The cause is related to an immunologic disorder. Erosive lesions tend to worsen when the patient is under emotional stress.

Treatment: No treatment is needed for asymptomatic lesions. Painful erosive lesions are treated with topical application of antiinflammatory drugs, such as Lidex, to relieve symptoms and severity. Patients should be reexamined twice a year because a small percentage of cases have transformed into malignancy.

▶ Angular Cheilosis

Cracking at the corners of the mouth has been called angular cheilosis, angular cheilitis, and perleche. Angular cheilitis is associated with a fungal infection or with the loss of vertical dimension in a denture patient when the occlusal plane is worn down and the nose and chin become closer together.

Clinical appearance: Crusted and fissured areas at the corners of the mouth occur, usually bilaterally (Fig. 7-13). Retained saliva in the corners of the mouth promotes colonization by microorganisms because of the warm, moist environment. Pain is minimal.

Etiology: Loss of vertical dimension is a major predisposing factor. This occurs in patients who wear worn dentures or wear no dentures at all. Vitamin B deficiency is also listed as a cause in malnourished individuals. The fungal organism *Candida albicans* has been found in a high number of lesions, supporting the theory of a fungal infection.

Treatment: Elimination of the causative factor will allow the area to heal. Candidal infections are treated with antifungal drugs.

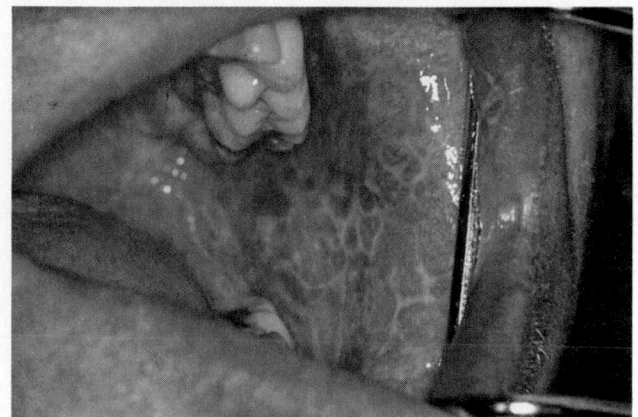

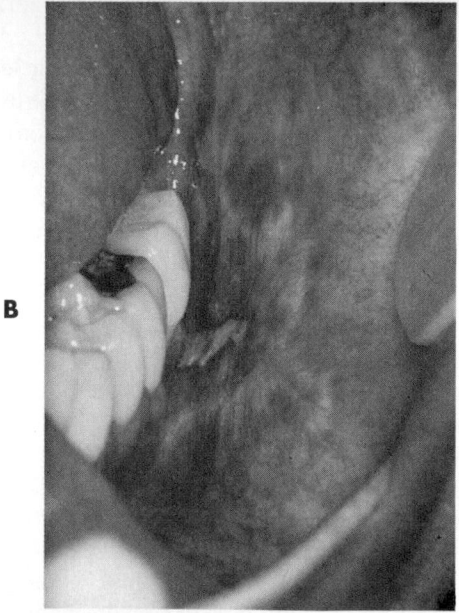

FIG. 7-12   Lichen planus. *A,* Reticular form of lichen planus. *B,* Erosive form.

(From *Oral lesions,* Colgate-Hoyt/Gel-Kam.)

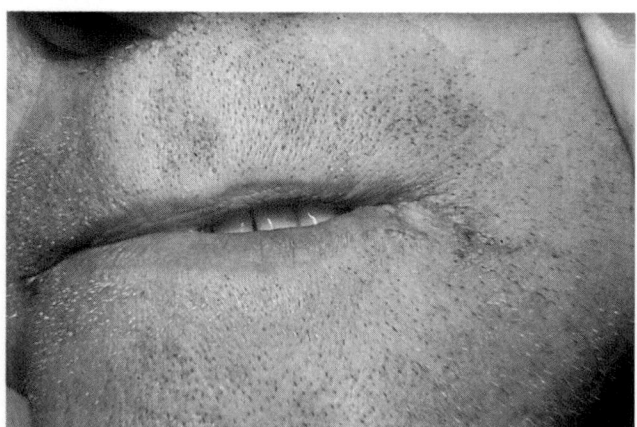

FIG. 7-13   Angular cheilosis.

(From *Oral lesions,* Colgate-Hoyt/Gel-Kam.)

Thrush

Thrush is another form of fungal infection that is found within the oral cavity of the newborn or of the older adult patient. When it occurs in the adult, it is called candidosis.

Clinical appearance: Mucous membranes develop a white, curdlike covering that represents colonies of yeast overgrowth that is mixed with necrotic epithelium (Fig. 7-14). The white membrane can be removed by wiping with a gauze pad. Thrush can occur on any mucous membrane.

Etiology: Candida albicans can be introduced into the newborn's mouth during birth as the baby moves through the birth canal. The warm moist environment of the oral cavity and the underdeveloped immune system cooperate to allow overgrowth of this fungal microorganism.

Treatment: Topical antifungal drugs are applied after wiping white colonies from the mouth.

Amalgam Tatoo

Occasionally, during placement of dental restorations or during oral surgery pieces of amalgam are embedded into adjacent soft tissue and the wound heals, entrapping the metals.

Clinical appearance: The condition appears as a **localized** (in one area) blue-to-gray color of the soft tissue. It is found adjacent to an area where amalgam has been placed or removed, as in a tooth restoration or a crown preparation (Fig. 7-15). It is asymptomatic and innocuous.

Etiology: When amalgam particles accidentally become embedded in a wound, an amalgam tatoo can form.

Treatment: No treatment is required. To prevent an amalgam tatoo, the dental assistant should cover any cut places that surround the restoration site and then flush the area at the end of treatment to remove metal particles. Use of a rubber dam helps to prevent this condition.

Nicotine Stomatitis

Tobacco-related injuries are fairly common in the mouth and are associated with premalignant conditions. Nicotine stomatitis is one tobacco-related injury that is not considered to be premalignant. It occurs frequently enough that the dental assistant is likely to see it.

Clinical appearance: The palatal mucosa may be fissured with a light-colored hyperkeratinized appearance (Fig. 7-16). **Hyperkeratinization** is the buildup of surface keratin on epithelium as a protective measure after frequent irritation. The minor salivary glands are affected and the **orifice**, or opening, of the ducts is red and inflamed. Sometimes the gland is enlarged, giving a rolled appearance around the opening.

Etiology: Pipe smoking is a frequent cause of stomatitis, but it can occur with heavy use of all forms of smoking tobacco.

Treatment: No treatment is recommended except to inform the patient of the cellular damage that has occurred and to suggest that smoking be discontinued. The condition usually disappears after the patient stops smoking.

Studies done by the Kaiser Permanente Center for Health Research in Portland, Oregon, show that 78.6% of smokeless tobacco users had observable oral lesions; 23.6% of them were in the most clinically advanced category. By comparison, only 6.3% of the 223 non-smokeless tobacco users studied had observable lesions.

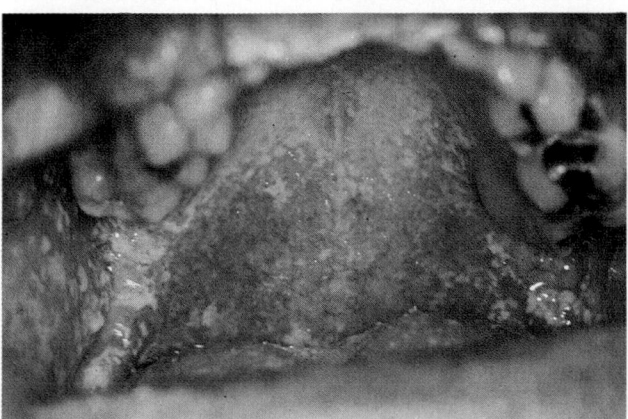

FIG. 7-14   **Thrush.**
(From *Oral lesions,* Colgate-Hoyt/Gel-Kam.)

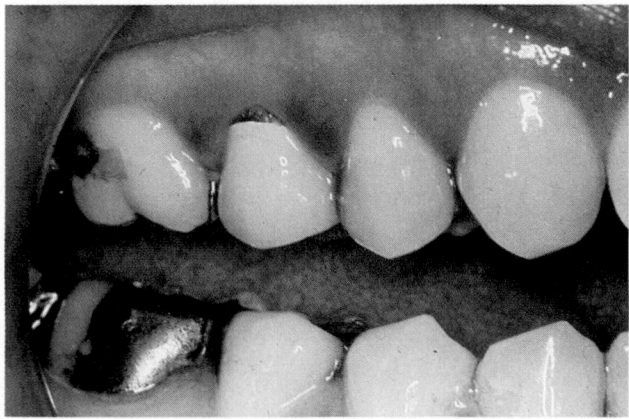

FIG. 7-15   **Amalgam tattoo.**
(From *Oral lesions,* Colgate-Hoyt/Gel-Kam.)

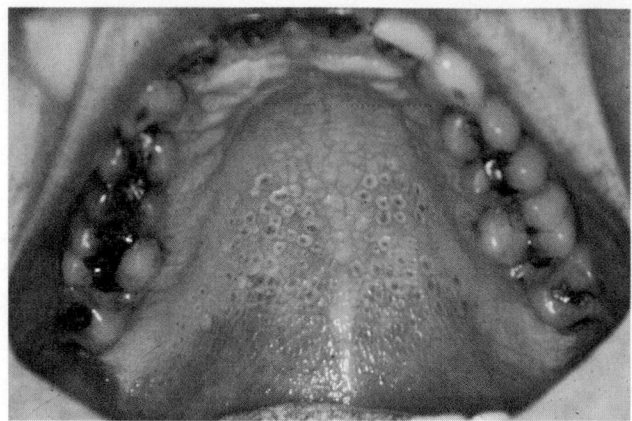

FIG. 7-16   Nicotine stomatitis.

(From *Oral lesions,* Colgate-Hoyt / Gel-Kam.)

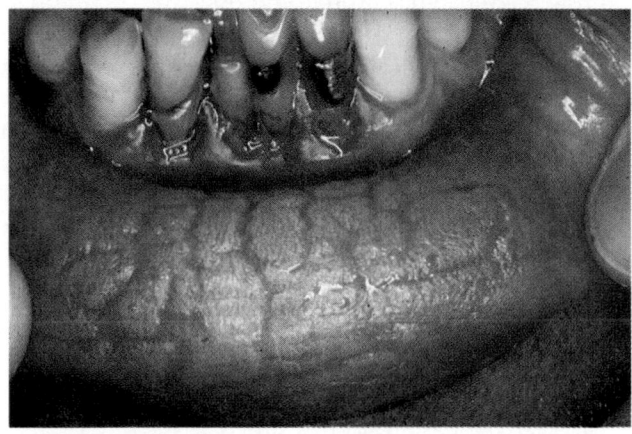

FIG. 7-17   Snuff lesion.

(From *Oral lesions,* Colgate-Hoyt / Gel-Kam.)

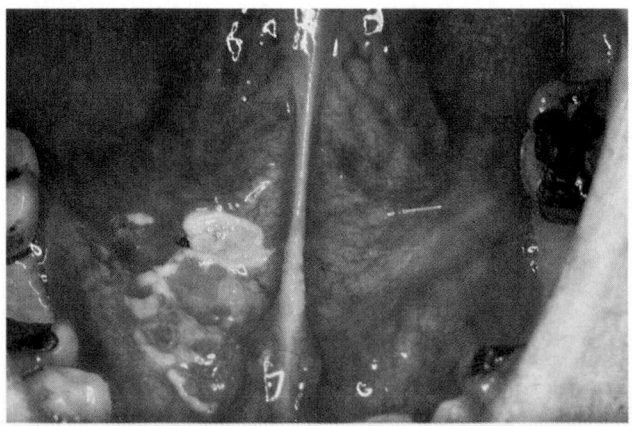

FIG. 7-18   Leukoplakia.

(From *Oral lesions,* Colgate-Hoyt / Gel-Kam.)

▶ Snuff Lesion

Snuff lesion is a fairly common tobacco-related injury that is caused by smokeless tobacco. It is increasing in incidence and is being seen in younger individuals than in the past because of the marketing of smokeless tobacco products. Snuff is frequently held in the oral vestibule, causing the lesion to form.

Clinical appearance: The mucosa under the smokeless tobacco product is wrinkled and has an opaque-to-white color caused by hyperkeratinization from frequent irritation (Fig. 7-17).

Etiology: Irritation from tobacco components that are applied on a frequent basis causes the soft tissue changes.

Treatment: No treatment is recommended except that the soft tissue changes should be shown to the patient, along with advice to stop the behavior. The lesion will disappear if the habit is discontinued. The lesion can transform into malignancy.

Malignant and Premalignant Lesions

Some intraoral lesions, as well as some head and neck lesions, may be observed during patient examination. Because of the potentially dangerous nature of these lesions the dental assistant should be familiar with the clinical appearance of, and the risk factors for, developing these conditions. The excessive growth of tissue in some of these lesions is called a **neoplasm**. Neoplasms don't return to normal size after the stimulus for overgrowth has been removed. They can be benign or malignant growths of tissue.

▶ Leukoplakia

Leukoplakia is defined as a white patch. Other white lesions already discussed could technically be called areas of *leukoplakia;* however, this discussion will involve white lesions of the mucosa that are unassociated with lichen planus or candidiasis. Biopsy is required to identify the cause of most areas of leukoplakia. This condition is called premalignant in that a small percentage will undergo malignant transformation.

Clinical appearance: The white patch of leukoplakia can be found on any mucous membrane, will not wipe away with gauze, and is often leathery in surface texture (Fig. 7-18). It can be in a small, localized area or can cover a large surface area.

Etiology: Smoking is considered a major causative factor. Other factors include excessive alcohol intake, trauma, and vitamin A deficiency. Biopsy of most white patches reveals hyperkeratinization. A small percentage of biopsies reveal either **dysplasic** (abnormal) cells or malignant cells.

Treatment: Treatment depends on biopsy results. Hyperkeratinized tissue is treated by advising the patient to discontinue the causative behavior, whereas dysplasia or malignant cells are surgically removed followed by chemotherapy or radiation in some instances.

▶ Erythroplakia

Erythroplakia presents as a velvety red lesion of oral mucosa. It is likely to be malignant at the time of biopsy, and for that reason it is considered to be a dangerous lesion.

Clinical appearance: The velvety red surface may be roughened or may have a smooth surface texture (Fig. 7-19). It may be in a small area, or it may cover a large area. Erythroplakia sometimes is *speckled* or contains white areas. Usually the patient is unaware that it exists, and no symptoms are reported. It is often found on the floor of the mouth or on the lateral borders of the tongue, areas that are considered at high risk for malignancy. Erythroplakia has also been found on other mucosal areas.

Etiology: These lesions have numerous causes, but alcohol and tobacco are highly rated as causative factors.

Treatment: Treatment includes eliminating the cause of the lesion, surgical excision, and, for those lesions where **metastasis** or the spreading of malignant cells into the body has occurred, appropriate chemotherapy and radiation.

▶ Squamous Cell Carcinoma

The oral cavity is lined by stratified squamous epithelium; therefore malignancy in this tissue is called squamous cell carcinoma. When lesions have malignant cells which have remained within the epithelial layer and have not metastasized past the basement membrane of epithelium, this is called **carcinoma-in-situ.** Cancer at this stage is easily removed with no chance of recurrence. It is not known how long a malignancy can exist before cells metastasize and infiltrate deeper tissues. Carcinoma travels throughout the body through the lymphatic system, which is why some surgeons remove regional lymph nodes along with the malignant tumor. Once malignant cells have metastasized, the prognosis for cure is reduced, which explains why early detection and removal are important for a favorable prognosis for cure.

Clinical appearance: The typical lesion is a white, red, or speckled ulcerated area that fails to heal (Fig. 7-20, *A* and *B*). The lesion is painless unless secondarily infected. The lateral borders of the tongue and floor of the mouth are the most common locations of squamous cell carcinoma. When the tongue is examined, it should be extended and the sides observed for lesions. The tongue should be lifted and the floor of the mouth should be examined for changes in color, texture, and consistency. This malignancy is more common in men

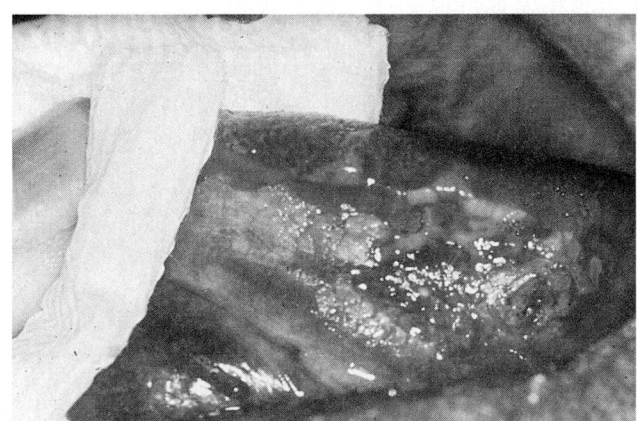

A

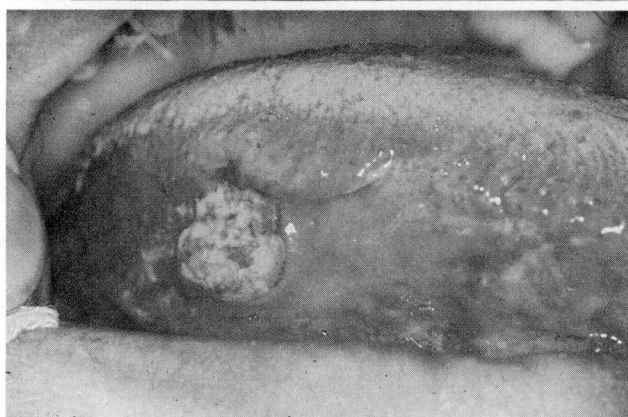

B

FIG. 7-20   Squamous cell carcinoma. *A,* Speckled lesion. *B,* Nonhealing ulcer of squamous cell carcinoma.

(From *Oral lesions,* Colgate-Hoyt / Gel-Kam.)

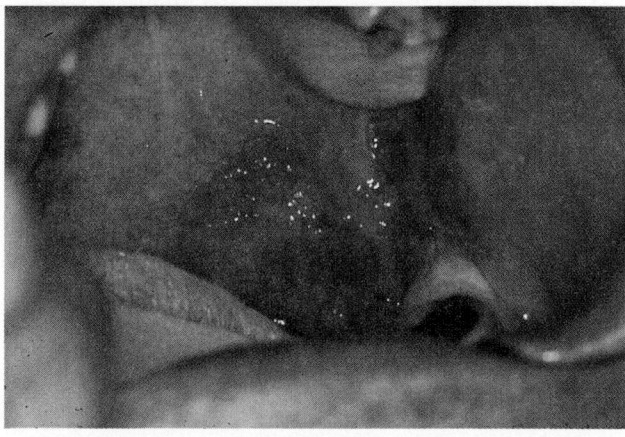

FIG. 7-19   Erythroplakia.

(From *Oral lesions,* Colgate-Hoyt / Gel-Kam.)

over the age of 40 years. It ranks as the ninth most common cancer in the United States.

Etiology: Several factors evidently cause oral malignancy; however, tobacco and alcohol are the prime suspicious factors. Viruses, such as the herpes and papillomavirus, are possible causes of some cases.

Treatment: Treatment involves the surgical removal of malignant tissue and regional lymph nodes, if metastasis is suspected, combined with radiation and chemotherapy. Early detection and removal greatly enhance the survival rate.

▌ Basal Cell Carcinoma

The most common carcinoma is a malignancy of the skin called basal cell carcinoma. It is found most often in skin that has been exposed to sunlight. In the head and neck region these lesions are usually found on the face, nose, and lips. Unlike squamous cell carcinoma, malignant cells are not likely to metastasize. They invade local areas by growing laterally and vertically: by direct invasion. An untreated basal cell carcinoma on the scalp could ultimately grow through the skull and invade the brain, causing death. Like squamous cell carcinoma, this malignancy is most common in men over the age of 40 years.

Clinical appearance: The lesion most often appears as a painless crusted lesion with rolled borders (Fig. 7-21). The rolled borders represent tumor cells that are growing laterally.

Etiology: Fair-complexioned people who have been frequently exposed to sunlight are those who are most likely to develop basal cell carcinoma.

Treatment: The tumor is surgically removed, and care is taken to excise all malignant cells. The area is checked at recall appointments to ensure that no recurrence has developed. It is not uncommon for people who have had one basal cell lesion to develop other, separate lesions.

Hyperplastic Lesions

Hyperplasia is defined as an increase in the number of cells. It is through this process that tumors are formed. Most hyperplastic overgrowths of tissue are benign and are commonly found in the mouth. They form as a result of chronic irritation. Some authors refer to this group as *reactive lesions,* since the cells *react* to irritation by forming more cells. Hyperplasia is sometimes confused with **hypertrophy,** which is defined as an increase in the size of a cell; it occurs as part of the inflammatory response. Hypertrophy causes a temporary increase in size, which will return to normal when the inflammation is resolved. However, hyperplastic tissue usually will not resolve by itself; it must be surgically removed.

▌ Irritation Fibroma (Fibroma)

The most common benign oral soft tissue growth is a fibroma. This lesion is found frequently on the buccal mucosa where the teeth occlude—a location that is commonly exposed to irritation.

Clinical appearance: The fibroma is hyperplasia of connective tissue covered by normal epithelium (Fig. 7-22). It is most often found on the buccal mucosa; however, it can occur in other oral locations. Fibroma is dome shaped, is pink in color, is usually less than 1 cm across, and is painless.

Etiology: Connective tissue growth is stimulated in the presence of repeated trauma. Fibroma is often seen in the patient who has a habit of cheek biting.

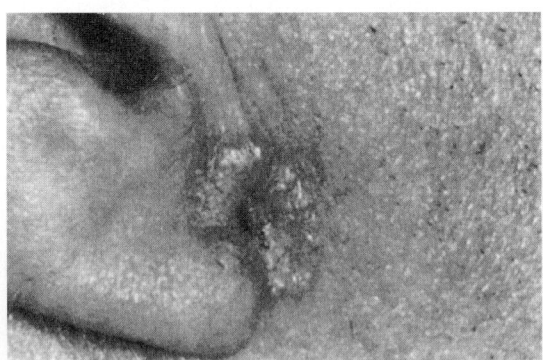

FIG. 7-21   Basal cell carcinoma.

(From Coleman GC, Nelson JF: *Principles of oral diagnosis,* St Louis, 1992, Mosby.)

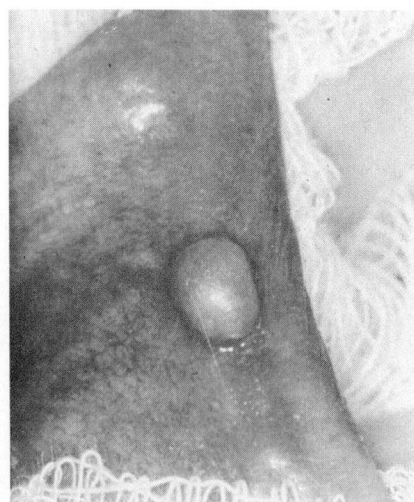

FIG. 7-22   **Fibroma.**

(From *Oral lesions,* Colgate-Hoyt/Gel-Kam.)

Treatment: Surgical removal is the recommended treatment. Since it is a benign growth, it is often left untreated.

Epulis Fissuratum (Redundant Tissue)

Epulis fissuratum is a hyperplastic lesion that is found in the oral vestibule of a denture patient.

Clinical appearance: The excess mass of hyperplastic tissue is covered by normal epithelium and is the same reddish color as vestibular mucosa. It grows over the flange of the ill-fitting denture (Fig. 7-23).

Etiology: Chronic irritation from the flange of a denture that extends too far into the vestibule causes the lesion.

Treatment: The excess tissue is surgically removed, the denture is recast, and the tissue overgrowth does not recur.

Papillary Hyperplasia

Irritation to palatal mucosa under a maxillary denture can result in a unique hyperplastic lesion of numerous polyps of tissue. Malignant transformation does not occur in this tissue.

Clinical appearance: In the early stage of the disease the palate is red and inflamed. A pebbly texture appears in the central area of the palate as the condition progresses (Fig. 7-24, *A* and *B*). In the late stage, numerous round red-to-pink papillary nodules fill the vault of the hard palate.

Etiology: A combination of factors is responsible for this lesion. *Candida albicans* is usually cultured from the overgrowth of tissue and from the maxillary denture. Chronic irritation from the untreated infection causes the lesion to form under an appliance that fits poorly.

Often, the denture is worn throughout the night, rather than taking it out.

Treatment: Lesions are treated with topical antifungal drugs, such as nystatin or clotrimazole. Patients are instructed about proper denture hygiene and are warned against wearing dentures during the night. Ill-fitting appliances are relined, or a new denture is constructed. If the hyperplastic tissue is excessive, surgical removal may be necessary before remaking the denture.

Pyogenic Granuloma

Pyogenic granuloma is a hyperplastic reactive lesion that was once called a *pregnancy tumor;* however, it also occurs in males and in nonpregnant females, so this terminology has been discontinued. It is more common in females, however, and it frequently develops during pregnancy. The *pyogenic* part of the name is a misnomer, since no pus is associated with this hyperplasia.

Clinical appearance: The lesion appears as a red, rounded, painless growth of tissue that extends from the surface of the mucosa (Fig. 7-25). The gingival

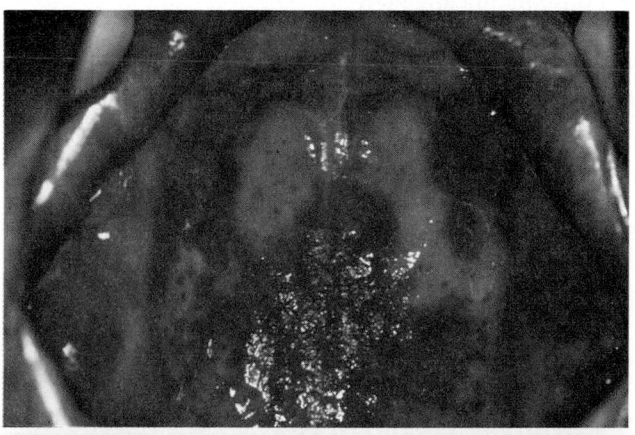
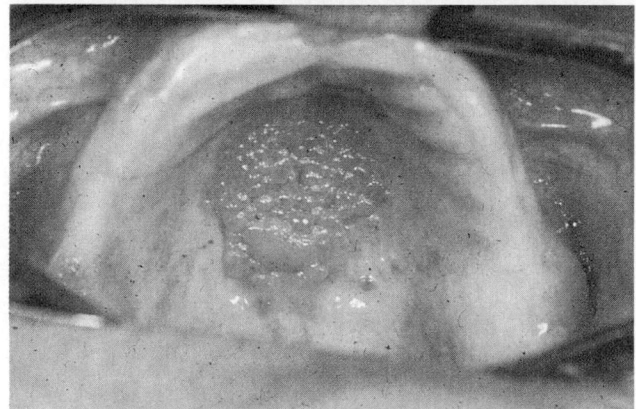

FIG. 7-24 Papillary hyperplasia. *A,* Early lesion. *B,* Typical lesion.

(From *Oral lesions,* Colgate-Hoyt/Gel-Kam.)

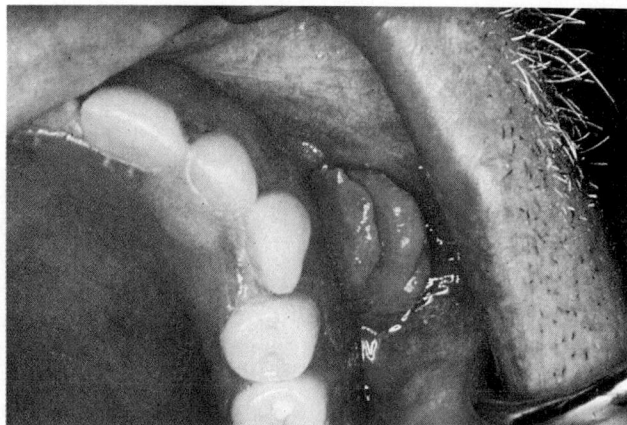

FIG. 7-23 Epulis fissuratum.

(From *Oral lesions,* Colgate-Hoyt/Gel-Kam.)

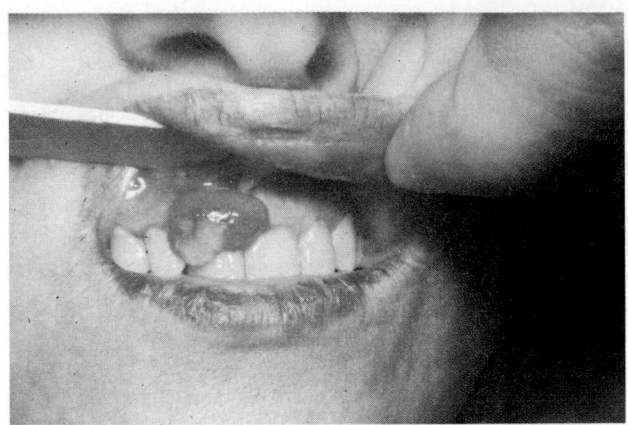

FIG. 7-25   Pyogenic granuloma.

(From *Oral lesions,* Colgate-Hoyt / Gel-Kam.)

FIG. 7-26   Gingival hyperplasia.

(From *Oral lesions,* Colgate-Hoyt / Gel-Kam.)

papilla is a common site followed by the lips, tongue, and lining mucosa of the mouth. The tumor is filled with capillaries and bleeds easily. Sizes range from 1 to 4 cm, making this growth fairly large. If the pyogenic granuloma is not surgically removed, the inflammatory component can resolve or *scar down* and form a lesion that looks like a fibroma.

Etiology: Chronic inflammation from bacterial plaque and local irritation from subgingival calculus may play a primary role in forming gingival lesions. Hormonal changes may cause an exaggeration of the inflammatory response. Lesions on the tongue, lips, and other mucosal areas may form as a result of chronic, mild trauma to the area.

Treatment: Lesions are surgically removed. A biopsy can provide a definite diagnosis, since the pyogenic granuloma can resemble other soft tissue tumors.

▶ Gingival Hyperplasia

Overgrowth of the connective tissue component in gingivae is commonly seen in dental patients. It is a reactive overgrowth of various causes. When it is seen, the area is examined for evidence of chronic irritation and a history of the condition is obtained from the patient.

Clinical appearance: The overgrown gingivae cover a good portion of the adjacent teeth (Fig. 7-26). The color is pale pink, and unless the marginal area is secondarily infected from retained bacterial plaque, the tissue does not bleed. Most cases are painless.

Etiology: There are various causes for this condition. Chronic irritation can occur from retained plaque because of orthodontic appliances, malaligned teeth, etc. Other cases result from the side effects of some drugs, such as sodium dilantin, which is taken for

epilepsy; nifedipine or diltiazem, which is taken for cardiovascular disease; or cyclosporine, which is taken by organ transplant patients to keep the body from rejecting the organ. Still other cases result from an hereditary etiology. The problem arises for patients who have hereditary gingival hyperplasia in that the tissue regrows after surgical removal, and it must be removed again and again. The clinical appearance of the tissue is the same no matter what has caused the overgrowth.

Treatment: Removal of bacterial plaque on a regular basis results in reduced inflammation; however, the hyperplastic tissue must be removed surgically. Drug-induced hyperplasia will resolve if the drug is discontinued. Removal of teeth has resulted in reduction of tissue size, called **atrophy,** although this is a drastic measure.

▶ Papilloma

Another name for papilloma is *squamous papilloma,* identifying the type of epithelium from which the tissue grows. This lesion is not hyperplastic because it does not occur from chronic irritation; it is classified as a reactive lesion that occurs after infection by a virus.

Clinical appearance: Papilloma is unique in appearance and extends from the surface as a cluster of papillary projections that resemble a mulberry (Fig. 7-27). It is found on any mucosal area but more frequently on the palate and uvula. Generally, the color is white because the blood supply is minimal. Pink lesions have a greater blood supply.

Etiology: The human papilloma virus (HPV) may be responsible for this condition. Over 60 subtypes of this virus exist; several different subtypes have been discovered in growths that resemble the papilloma.

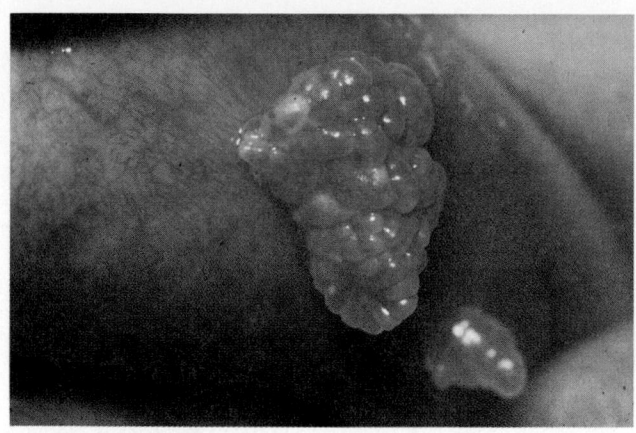

FIG. 7-27 **Papilloma.**

(From *Oral lesions,* Colgate-Hoyt / Gel-Kam.)

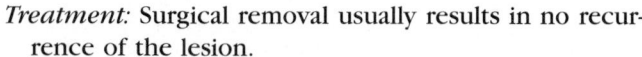

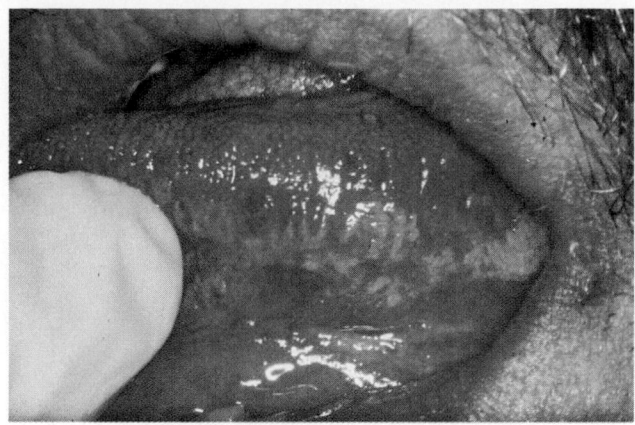

FIG. 7-28 **Candidosis.**

(From *Oral lesions,* Colgate-Hoyt / Gel-Kam.)

Treatment: Surgical removal usually results in no recurrence of the lesion.

AIDS-Associated Lesions

The disease called acquired immunodeficiency syndrome (AIDS) results in destruction of T lymphocytes; which are immune cells that protect us from many infections. People who suffer from AIDS have numerous **opportunistic infections,** which are caused by microorganisms that cannot cause diseases in individuals who have healthy immune systems. Infections that are potentially transmissible to health care workers include candidosis, tuberculosis, herpes virus infections, and hepatitis B (HBV). It is impossible to identify infected people by reviewing their medical histories; therefore all patients must be considered potentially infected. Use of barriers, such as masks, gloves, and glasses, is required, and an HBV vaccination reduces the risk of becoming infected. The Centers for Disease Control and Prevention (CDC) have stated that health care workers who use barrier protection when engaged in dental treatment should not be at risk for HIV infection. If barriers are broken—a puncture wound from an unprotected needle or a blood-contaminated instrument—the health care worker should see a physician immediately and receive an immune vaccine to boost the immune system and prevent infection. HIV is most often spread through sexual contact and through the use of an HIV-infected needle to inject drugs.

Since the identification of the AIDS in the late 1970s, oral manifestations that are unique to this disorder have been noted. Those conditions that are generally seen in patients who are infected with the causative virus, the human immunodeficiency virus (HIV), will be discussed here.

▌ Pseudomembranous Candidosis

Pseudomembranous candidosis (sometimes called candidiasis) is the most common and earliest oral manifestation of HIV infection. Infection from *Candida albicans* occurs in patients who are immunocompromised from various other reasons, such as after cancer chemotherapy and head and neck radiation, and in uncontrolled diabetes mellitus. It also can occur after long-term antibiotic therapy.

Clinical appearance: The lesion usually appears as a white membrane in a round or linear pattern on oral mucosa (Fig. 7-28). Wiping with gauze will remove the membrane, leaving a red, irritated surface. Patients may complain of a burning sensation. The infection can occur on any oral mucous membrane and extend into the pharynx and esophagus.

Etiology: Lesions described as thrush are caused by the same fungal organism that causes candidosis: *Candida albicans.*

Treatment: Antifungal drug therapy, both topical and systemic, is used.

▌ Hairy Leukoplakia

Hairy leukoplakia is a unique lesion that was discovered in the 1980s. It is associated with opportunistic infection in AIDS patients, but it can occur in immunocompromised patients who are not infected with HIV.

Clinical appearance: A corrugated pattern of white lines on the lateral borders of the tongue is the usual appearance of the lesion (Fig. 7-29). It looks similar to candidosis; however, it cannot be removed by wiping with gauze.

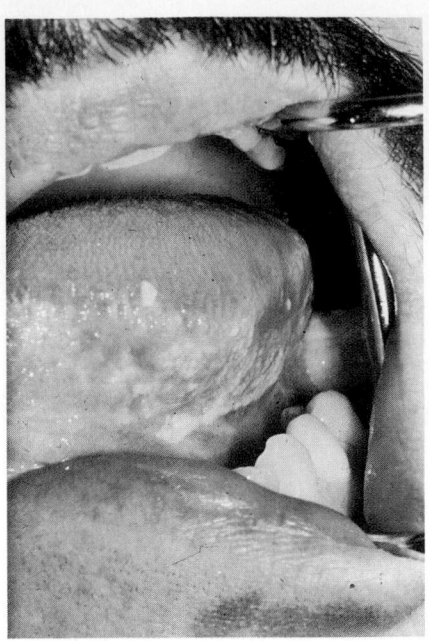

FIG. 7-29   **Hairy leukoplakia.**
(From *Oral lesions,* Colgate-Hoyt/Gel-Kam.)

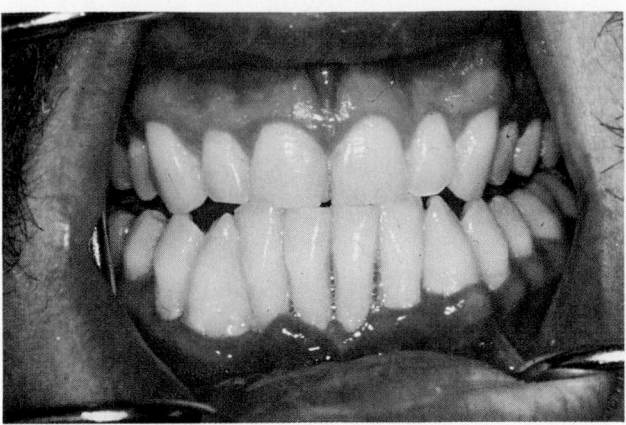

FIG. 7-31   **Gingival lesion in AIDS.**
(From *Oral lesions,* Colgate-Hoyt/Gel-Kam.)

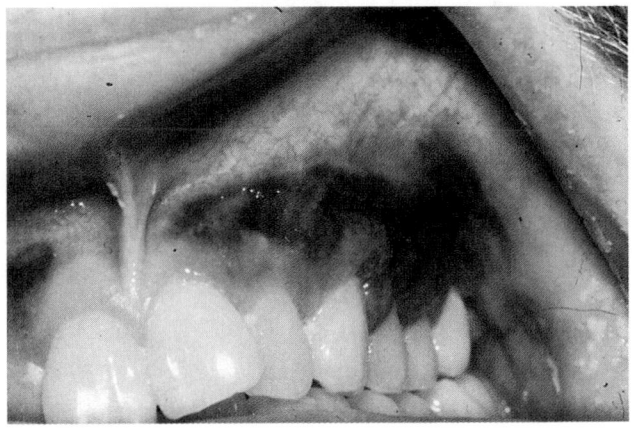

FIG. 7-30   Kaposi's sarcoma.
(From *Oral lesions,* Colgate-Hoyt/Gel-Kam.)

Etiology: The Epstein-Barr virus is considered the causative organism in hairy leukoplakia.

Treatment: No treatment is available for hairy leukoplakia; the clinician usually refers the patient for a blood test to evaluate for possible HIV infection.

▶ Kaposi's Sarcoma

AIDS patients are vulnerable to various malignant conditions, such as malignant lymphoma and squamous cell carcinoma. A unique cancer that is seen more often in AIDS patients is a malignancy of blood vessels called Kaposi's sarcoma. It affects about a third of AIDS patients.

Clinical appearance: This malignancy occurs on the skin and in the oral cavity, usually on the palate. The lesion is purple, blue, or red; it may be flat or nodular. As the tumor grows, it forms a hemorrhagic mass (Fig. 7-30). The cancer invades the tissue and causes bleeding and pain.

Etiology: It is not known what occurs in the AIDS patient to cause malignant transformation of the endothelial cells that form the blood vessels.

Treatment: Chemotherapeutic drugs and low-dose radiation have been used. No single treatment is successful for all patients.

▶ Gingival and Periodontal Lesions

Gingival lesions in HIV-infected patients can be severe and progress to a stage of rapid bone loss within a short time. They usually do not respond well to conventional scaling, root planing, and plaque control treatment regimens.

Clinical appearance: Gingivae may be red, inflamed, and bulbous (Fig. 7-31). Some patients have necrotic areas on the marginal and papillary areas, representing dead tissue. The area is painful and bleeds easily.

Etiology: Gram-negative bacteria and spirochetes are found in large numbers in subgingival plaque, along with large numbers of yeast organisms.

Treatment: Scaling and root planing, rinsing with chlorhexidine mouthwash to facilitate oral hygiene measures, and use of the antibiotic metronidazole have been employed with varying degrees of success.

Miscellaneous Conditions

Several common oral pathologic conditions that are seen by the dental assistant fall outside the categories already identified. These will be discussed here. The first two, mucocele and pleomorphic adenoma, involve problems of the salivary glands. The rest of the conditions are not seen clinically because they are found within the alveolar bone; however, these conditions can be identified in a radiograph.

❯ Mucocele

Mucocele occurs as a result of trauma to a minor salivary gland. The patient may report a history of the lesion filling with fluid and enlarging and then shrinking when the fluid is expressed from the swelling.

Clinical appearance: The mucocele is a blue elevation of the mucosa (Fig. 7-32). The lesion is caused by fluid collection within the soft tissue when the duct has been severed from the minor salivary gland. It can occur anywhere that minor salivary glands are located, but the lower lip is often affected.

Etiology: Usually, trauma to the area causes the duct to be severed from the minor salivary gland, resulting in the mucocele. Less frequently a stone may form in a duct, resulting in a fluid backup in the gland and causing an elevation of tissue.

Treatment: Removal of the affected gland and duct resolves the condition.

❯ Pleomorphic Adenoma

The most common benign tumor of the salivary glands is the pleomorphic adenoma. It can occur in both minor salivary glands and major salivary glands. The tumor is most commonly found in the parotid salivary gland; however, when it is found in minor salivary glands, the most common location is the palate.

Clinical appearance: The slowly growing tumor produces an enlargement within the affected gland. When it occurs in the parotid, the enlargement occurs inferior and anterior to the ear. The skin overlying the gland is normal. When the tumor affects the intraoral minor salivary gland, it produces a painless, firm, dome-shaped enlargement that is covered by normal epithelium (Fig. 7-33). Questioning the patient may reveal that the enlargement has been present for a year or more.

Etiology: The cause is unknown.

Treatment: The mass should be surgically removed and submitted for biopsy, since a small percentage of these lesions will undergo malignant transformation. It is impossible to differentiate between benign and malignant salivary gland tumors in their early stages.

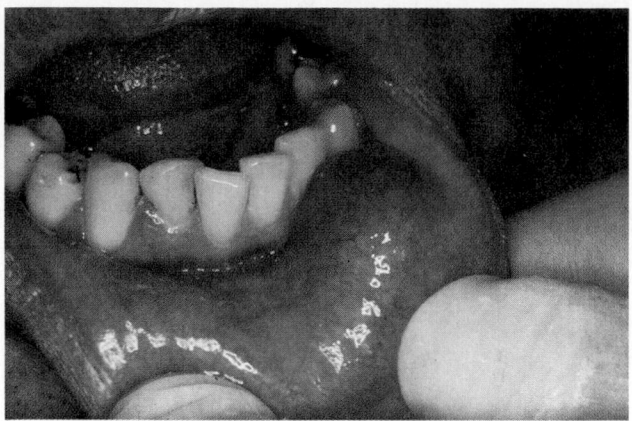

FIG. 7-32 **Mucocele.**
(From *Oral lesions,* Colgate-Hoyt/Gel-Kam.)

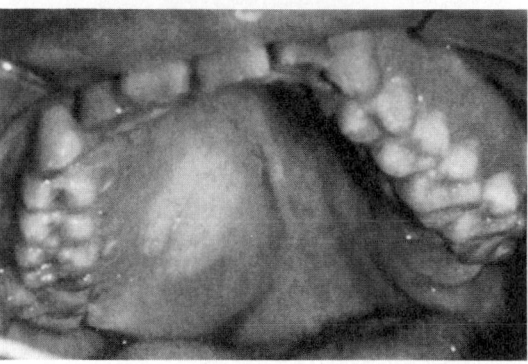

FIG. 7-33 **Pleomorphic adenoma.**
(From Coleman GC, Nelson JF: *Principles of oral diagnosis,* St Louis, 1992, Mosby.)

❯ Nasopalatine Canal Cyst

The nasopalatine canal cyst has been called incisive canal cyst and nasopalatine duct cyst. It formerly was classified as a different cyst from the median palatine cyst, which lies behind the incisive canal in the midline of the palate. It is now believed that both are the same cyst types, occurring in the anterior or posterior section of the canal.

Clinical appearance: This cyst usually is not seen clinically but is identified in a radiograph as a round radiolucency that is apical to the maxillary central incisor roots (Fig. 7-34). It is frequently found in edentulous patients. Occasionally the cyst becomes large enough to cause a swelling of tissue in the palate under the cyst; however, it is usually found as part of a routine radiographic survey and the patient is unaware that it exists. Cysts in the posterior portion of the canal occur in the midline of the palatal area.

Etiology: The cyst forms from remnants of epithelium left by embryonic fusion of the premaxilla and lateral palatine processes. The stimulus for cyst formation from this tissue is not known.

Treatment: The cyst is removed surgically. Recurrence is rare.

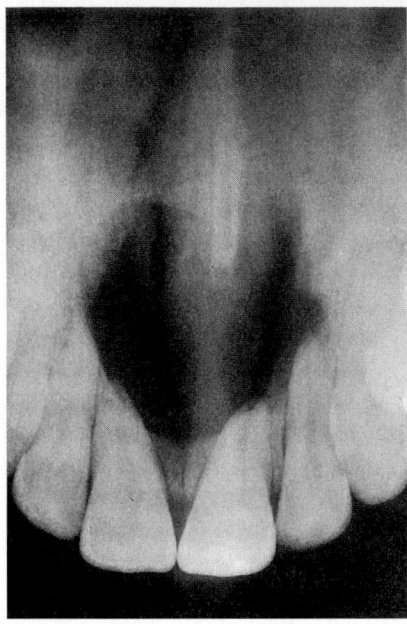

FIG. 7-34   Nasopalatine canal cyst; radiographic appearance.

(From *Oral lesions,* Colgate-Hoyt / Gel-Kam.)

▶ Periapical Cemental Dysplasia

Periapical cemental dysplasia is not a tumor, but rather an unusual reaction of normal bone for unknown reasons. It was formerly called a *cementoma.*

Clinical appearance: Since this condition occurs within apical bone, the only means to identify it is through dental radiographs. It has no symptoms, pulp tissue is vital, and the condition is usually discovered on a routine radiographic survey. There are three stages of the lesion. Initially, bone resorption occurs below the apices of roots, causing multiple radiolucencies that resemble periapical pathology. In the next stage, new resorptive areas occur and older areas begin to calcify, leaving areas of radiolucency and radiopacity within the apical bone. In the last stage, bone calcifies, leaving radiopaque areas (Fig. 7-35, *A* and *B*). The entire process usually takes years to complete. The condition is most common in the lower anterior area but can occur in other locations. It is seen predominantly in African American females.

Etiology: The cause is unknown.

Treatment: There is no treatment. The teeth are vital, and the condition is innocuous.

KEY POINTS

▶ A basic knowledge of oral pathology, the study of disease in the oral cavity, is needed for the dental assistant to be able to observe and identify irregularities of the skin and oral mucosa.

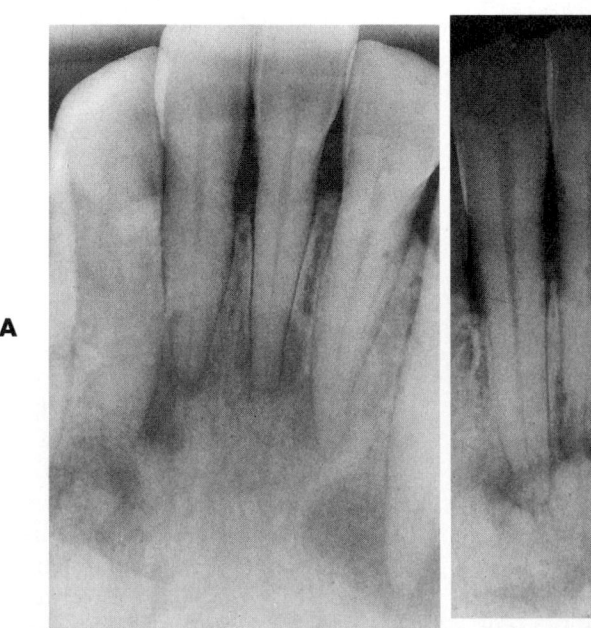
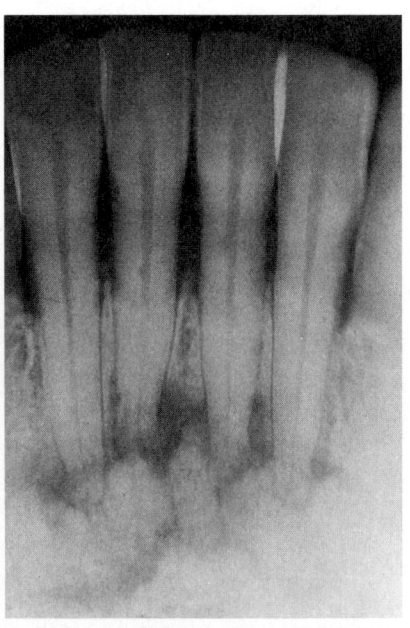

FIG. 7-35   Periapical cemental dysplasia. *A,* Initial stage. *B,* Mature stage of same lesion.

(From *Oral lesions,* Colgate-Hoyt / Gel-Kam.)

▶ Identification of lesions, their etiology, and their clinical descriptions becomes working knowledge for the dental assistant responsible for charting clinical features.

▶ When lesions are examined, the operator compares normal to nonnormal tissue and determines whether a condition may be normal for the patient, particularly if the *abnormality* is bilateral and may not be pathologic in origin.

▶ Abnormal conditions may be genetic, idiopathic, congenital, or innocuous in nature and origin. Conditions may require further observation, removal, follow-up examination, and treatment.

BIBLIOGRAPHY

Crawford JM: Human immunodeficiency virus-associated periodontal diseases: a review, *J Dent Hyg* 67(4):198-207, 1993.

Eisenberg E et al: Incidental oral hairy leukoplakia in immunocompetent persons: report of two cases, *Oral Surg Oral Med Oral Pathol* 74(3):332-333, 1992.

Eisenberg E et al: Lichenoid lesions of oral mucosa: diagnostic criteria and their importance in the alleged relationship to oral cancer, *Oral Surg Oral Med Oral Pathol* 73(6):699-704, 1991.

Fotos PG et al: Candida and candidosis: epidemiology, diagnosis and therapeutic management, *Dent Clin North Am* 36(4):857-878, 1992.

Garlick JA et al: Detection of human papillomavirus DNA in focal epithelial hyperplasia, *J Oral Pathol Med* 17:273-278, 1989.

Haring JI: Case #6 Mucocele, *RDH* 10(6):12, 16, 1990.

Haring JI: Case #1 Pyogenic granuloma, *RDH* 11(1):14-15, 1991.

Haring JI: Case #4 Irritation fibroma, *RDH* 11(4):10, 12, 1991.

Haring JI: Case #6 Squamous papilloma, *RDH* 11(6):12, 36, 1991.

Haring JI: Case #2 Pleomorphic adenoma, *RDH* 14(2):10, 36, 1994.

Jasmin JR et al: Local treatment of minor aphthous ulceration in children, *ASDCJ Dent Child* 60(1):26-28, 1993.

Kaugars GE et al: The prevalence of oral lesions in smokeless tobacco users and an evaluation of risk factors, *Cancer* 70(11):2579-2585, 1992.

Kullaa-Mikkonen A: Familial study of fissured tongue, *Scand J Dent Res* 96(4):366-375, 1988.

Miller CS et al: Diagnosis and management of orofacial herpes simplex virus infection, *Dent Clin North Am* 36(4):879-895, 1992.

Pindborg JJ et al: Classification of oral lesions associated with HIV infection, *Oral Surg* 67:292, 1989.

Rodu B et al: Oral mucosal ulcers: diagnosis and management, *JADA* 123(10):83-86, 1992.

Yetter JF: Cleft lip and cleft palate, *Am Fam Physician* 46(4):1211-1221, 1992.

BOOKS

Coleman GC: *Principles of oral diagnosis,* St Louis, 1993, Mosby.

Dunlap C, Barker BF: *Oral lesions,* ed 3, Kansas City, Mo, 1991, Colgate-Hoyt.

Public Health Department, Fall, 1992.

Wood NK, Goaz PW: *Differential diagnosis of oral lesions,* ed 4, St Louis, 1993, Mosby.

8 Infection Control

LEARNING OBJECTIVES

You will have mastered the material in this chapter when you can:

- Define the key terms
- Describe the methods of infection transmission
- Describe HIV, AIDS, HBV, and other infectious diseases
- Explain infection control
- Explain cross-contamination
- Identify the agencies regulating the dental profession
- Explain the techniques employed to eliminate transmission of infectious diseases
- Describe task categorization
- Describe universal precautions
- Explain the OSHA hazard communication program
- Explain common disinfection and sterilization procedures

KEY TERMS

Acquired immunodeficiency syndrome (AIDS)
Antimicrobial
Antiseptic
Autogenous
Asepsis
Aseptic technique
Bioburden
Blood-borne pathogens
Centers for Disease Control and Prevention (CDC)
Cold disinfection
Contamination
Cross-infections
Direct contact
Disinfection
Environmental Protection Agency (EPA)
Hepatitis B virus (HBV)
Human immunodeficiency virus (HIV)
Immunizations
Indirect contact
Infection control
Inhalation
Material Safety Data Sheet (MSDS)
Occupational Safety and Health Agency/Act (OSHA)
Polynitral gloves
Sanitization
Sterilization
Tuberculosis
Universal precautions

Research leading toward the control of infectious diseases has historically been marked by steady progress punctuated with extraordinary individual achievements. One of the earliest infection control milestones is exemplified by the successful development and introduction of a smallpox vaccine by Dr. Edward Jenner in the 1790s. Numerous developments have occurred since then in the culture and isolation of microbial forms, serologic techniques, and diagnosis and management of infections.

Principles of Infection Transmission

The realism of infection transmission is an important factor in providing dental care. Several sources of infectious diseases are present during dental treatment, including blood, saliva, nasal discharge, dust, hands, clothing, and hair. Any of these sources can potentially transfer microbial and viral infections.

When defining infections common to dental treatment, two categories must be considered—**autogenous infections and cross-infections**. In autogenous infections the patient is the source of the infection; an example is a patient who receives dental treatment, specifically an extensive scaling and polishing of the teeth. Subsequently, the patient develops endocarditis, which can result from the introduction of virulent organisms, such as staphylococci or pneumococci, that reside in the mouth and can be introduced into the bloodstream during the prophylaxis. The patient is the source of the endocarditis. Cross-infections are transferred from one patient or person to another.

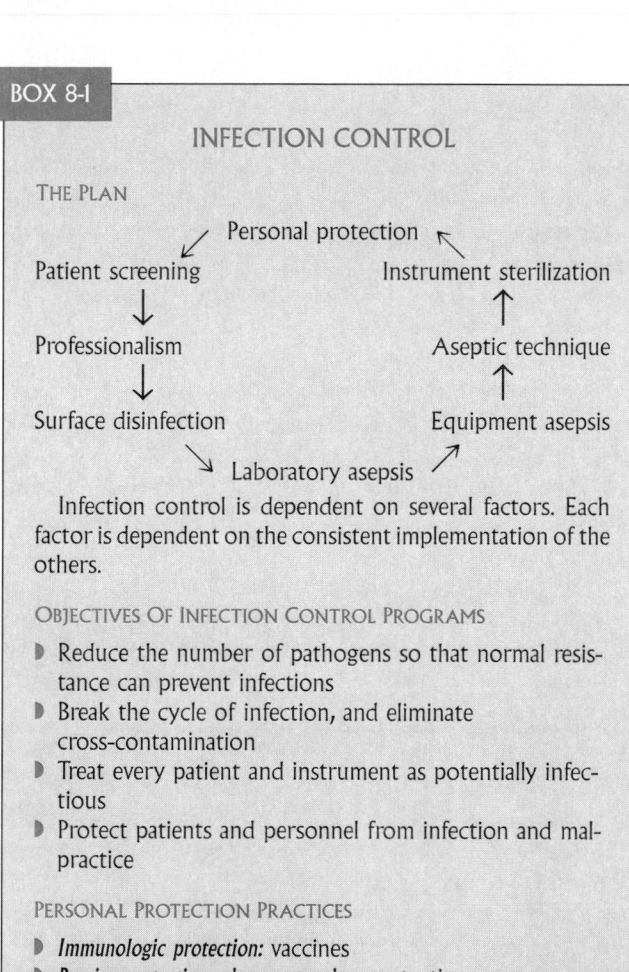

BOX 8-1

INFECTION CONTROL

THE PLAN

```
              Personal protection
            ↗                    ↖
Patient screening         Instrument sterilization
     ↓                              ↑
Professionalism              Aseptic technique
     ↓                              ↑
Surface disinfection         Equipment asepsis
            ↘                    ↗
              Laboratory asepsis
```

Infection control is dependent on several factors. Each factor is dependent on the consistent implementation of the others.

OBJECTIVES OF INFECTION CONTROL PROGRAMS

▸ Reduce the number of pathogens so that normal resistance can prevent infections
▸ Break the cycle of infection, and eliminate cross-contamination
▸ Treat every patient and instrument as potentially infectious
▸ Protect patients and personnel from infection and malpractice

PERSONAL PROTECTION PRACTICES

▸ *Immunologic protection:* vaccines
▸ *Barrier protection:* gloves, masks, protective eyewear, dams, uniforms

ROUTES OF TRANSMISSION OF POTENTIAL MICROBIAL PATHOGENS IN A DENTAL OFFICE

▸ *Direct transmission:* direct physical contact with infectious lesions or infected saliva and/or blood
▸ *Indirect transmission:* transfer of microorganisms from an intermediate contaminated object to another person
▸ *Aerosolization (spatter):* airborne transfer of infected blood, saliva, and/or nasopharyngeal secretions

▸ Routes of Transmission

Microbial transmission by dentistry-related secretions and exudates occurs by three general routes:

1. **Direct contact** with a lesion, organisms, or debris when performing intraoral procedures
2. **Indirect contact** via contaminated dental instruments, equipment, or supplies
3. **Inhalation** of microorganisms aerosolized from a patient's blood or saliva while using high-speed or ultrasonic equipment

In many dental practices, treatment providers may not comprehend or appreciate the dissemination potential of saliva and/or blood by these routes. Potential dangers are often missed, since much of the spatter coming from the patient's mouth is not readily noted. This may occur because the bioburden (blood, saliva, exudate) may be transparent or translucent, drying as a clear film and contaminating surfaces.

A demonstration was first developed in the 1970s using the premise: *if saliva were red.* This was later expanded to include restorative dentistry and dental prophylaxis techniques. The resultant salivary spatter was visible as red droplets on multiple tissue, instrument, and operatory surfaces (Fig. 8-1, *A* through *F*) during the procedures.

These guidelines apply to all dental professionals, but in most practices, dental assistants are responsible for much of their actual implementation. By routinely adhering to an infection control program the dental team can work to minimize infectious disease risk between patients and attending personnel. An effective program includes proper **sterilization**, the **destruction of all microbial life**, and **disinfection**, the killing of pathogenic organisms and clinical aseptic procedures (Box 8-1).

COMMON BLOOD-BORNE PATHOGEN DISEASES

Blood-borne pathogens are microorganisms that are found in human blood and that can cause disease. A brief section on blood-borne pathogens is being included here to elaborate on recognized health care worker occupational considerations. Several infectious diseases are of concern to health care workers, including **viral hepatitis** (HBV); human immunodeficiency virus (HIV), a retrovirus that causes a disease which alters the function of the immune system; and tuberculosis, a chronic bacterial infection of the lungs. Recognized infectious risks for health professionals have been documented for many years; however, HBV and HIV have had the greatest impact on the practice of dentistry regarding **infection control**. Infection control refers to all the processes used to eliminate the transmission of disease.

FIG. 8-1   A dental operatory following an oral prophylaxis procedure when using a red dye to trace saliva throughout the procedure. The saliva of a patient can contaminate the operating site as it is transferred (1) from the mouth; (2) to the operator or assistant's hand; (3) to the operating light; (4) to the preset tray; (5) to the A/W syringe; and(6) to other armamentarium.

(Courtesy of John Molinari.)

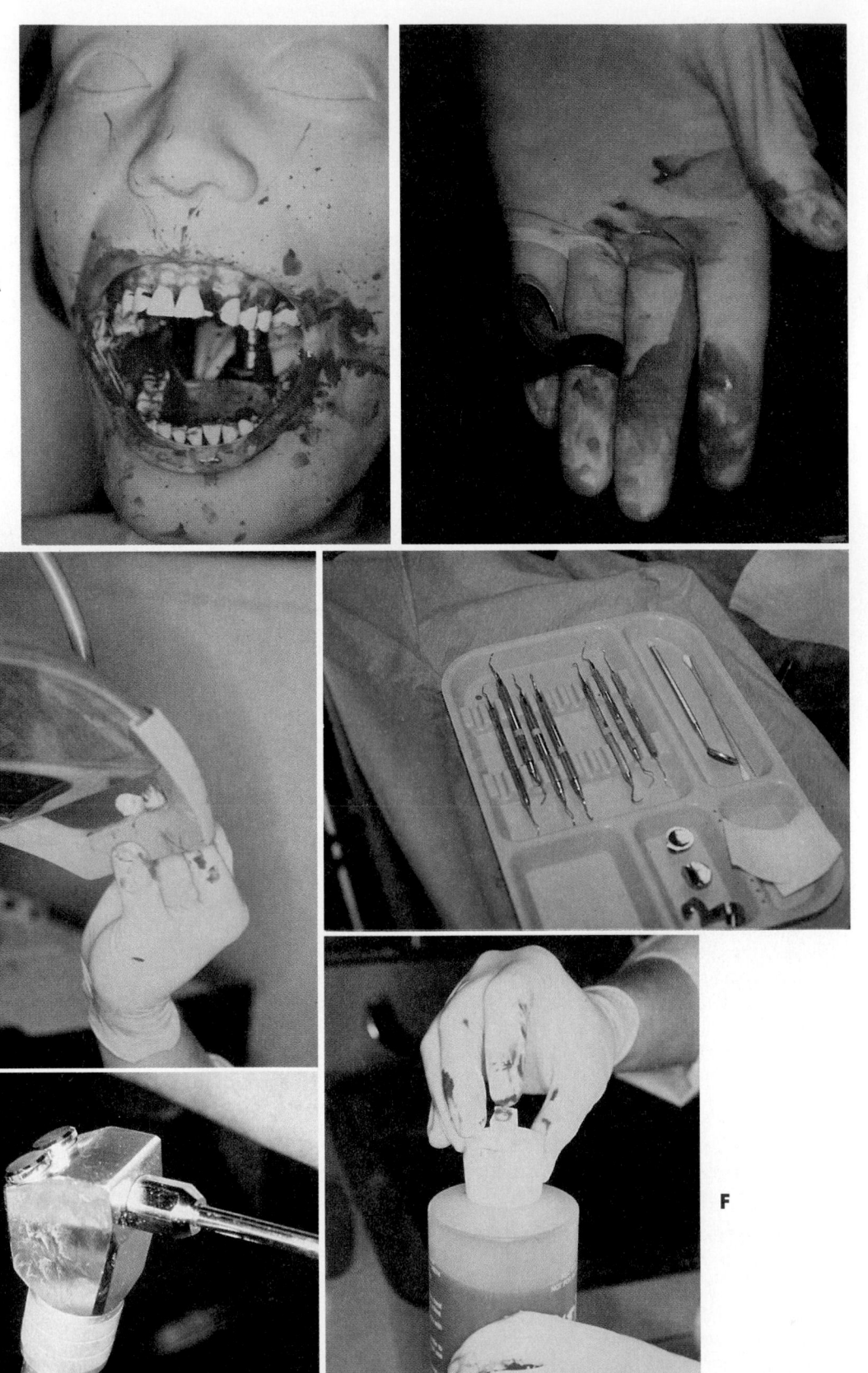

TABLE 8-I COMPARISON OF HBV AND HIV INFECTION

Feature	HBV	HIV
Can prevent exposure/infection	Yes	Yes
Patient prevalence	Increased	Increased
Virus titer/ml	>1 million	100 to 1000
Infection risk (%)	10 to 35	<1
HCW prevalence (%)	10 to 50	<<0.01
Annual HCW deaths	200 to 300	0 to 5(?)
Infectivity markers	Yes (HB$_e$)	Yes
Infection outcome:		
Resolved	90% to 95%	0%
Death	2%	100%
Incubation period	2 to 6 months	>2 years
Postexposure prophylaxis	Yes	No
Infectivity	Variable	Life
Treatment	Interferon	No

Adapted from Hadley WK: Infection of a health care worker by HIV and other bloodborne viruses: risks, protection and education, *Am J Hosp Pharm* 46:54-57, 1989.

BOX 8-2

FEATURES ASSOCIATED WITH HIV

Pneumocystis carinii (Pneumonia and respiratory failure) Fungal infections candidiasis
  Angular cheilitis
  Hyperplastic candidiasis
  Pseudomembranous form
  Florid form
  Atrophic form
  Lingual candidiasis
  Candidal lesions
  Gingival and mucosal candidiasis
Viral infections
  Herpes simplex virus
  Epstein-Barr virus
  Leukoplakia
  Varicella virus (zoster, shingles)
  Cytomegalovirus
  Human papillomavirus
Bacterial infections
  Gingivitis
  Periodontosis
  Nonoral flora opportunists
HIV-associated malignancies
  Kaposi's sarcoma
  Lymphomas
  Carcinoma
Other HIV-associated manifestations
  Recurrent aphthous stomatitis
  Hypersensitivity, lichenoid reactions
  Thrombocytopenia
  Sialadenitis
  Xerostomia

Certainly HIV infection and acquired immunodeficiency syndrome (AIDS) have received wide publicity because of fear, ignorance, and emotionalism. Yet when all of the scientific data are examined and the transmission risks delineated, it is evident that viral hepatitis, hepatitis B in particular, presents a greater challenge to infection control.

It is well established that HBV remains the major occupational infection for health care professionals. This information becomes more clinically relevant in the arena of infection control when it is compared with features that are associated with HIV infection (Box 8-2 and Table 8-1). The concentration of HBV in the blood of an infected individual can range from 1 to 100 million virus particles per milliliter, as compared with approximately 100 to 1000 HIV particles per milliliter in HIV-infected persons. The documented occupational risks to health care professionals for a multitude of bacterial, viral, and other microbial pathogens led to the development of recommended infection control precautions initially directed at preventing HBV transmission. The same basic protocol was later recommended for the treatment of HIV-positive patients in dental clinics and offices. Statements in subsequent published guidelines reinforced the position that infection control procedures must be used routinely to minimize the transmission of all occupational infectious diseases. Representative infections are presented in Table 8-2.

 If 1 ml of blood is taken from an HBV carrier and is placed into 24,000 gallons of water and if 1 ml of this dilution is injected into a susceptible person, the person will contract hepatitis B.
  When 1 ml of blood is taken from a person with AIDS and is placed in a quart of water and 1 ml of this dilution is injected into a susceptible person, there is a 1:10 chance the person will acquire an HIV infection.

Infection Control in Dentistry

Recognition of the potential for cross-contamination should lead to the application of a few general guidelines regarding universal precautions. Universal precautions include the following:

1. Reducing the concentration of pathogens so that normal host resistance mechanisms (those immune systems in a person) can prevent infections
2. Breaking the cycle of infection and eliminating cross-infection
3. Treating every patient and instrument as potentially infectious
4. Protecting patients and personnel from occupational infections (Fig. 8-2)

TABLE 8-2   REPRESENTATIVE INFECTIOUS DISEASE RISKS IN DENTISTRY

Disease	Etiologic agent	Incubation period
BACTERIAL		
Staphylococcal infections	*Staphylococcus aureus*	4 to 10 days
Tuberculosis	*Mycobacterium tuberculosis*	Up to 6 months
Streptococcal infections	*Streptococcus pyogenes*	1 to 3 days
Gonorrhea	*Neisseria gonorrhoeae*	1 to 7 days
Syphilis	*Treponema pallidum*	2 to 12 weeks
Tetanus	*Clostridium tetani*	7 to 10 days
VIRAL		
Recurrent herpetic lesion	Herpes simplex, types 1 and 2	Up to 2 weeks
Rubella	Rubella virus	9 to 11 days
Hepatitis A	Hepatitis A virus	2 to 7 weeks
Hepatitis B	Hepatitis B virus	6 weeks to 6 months
Delta hepatitis (hepatitis D)	Hepatitis D virus	Weeks to months
Infectious mononucleosis	Epstein-Barr virus	4 to 7 weeks
Hand-foot-mouth disease	Primarily Coxsackievirus A16	–2 days to >3 weeks
Herpangina	Coxsackievirus group A	5 days
AIDS	HIV	Months to years
FUNGAL		
Dermatomycoses (superficial skin infections)	*Trichophyton, Microsporum, Epidermophyton,* and *Candida* genera	Days to weeks
Candidiasis	*Candida albicans*	Days to weeks
MISCELLANEOUS		
Infections of fingers, hands, and eyes from dental plaque and calculus	Variety of microorganisms	1 to 8 days

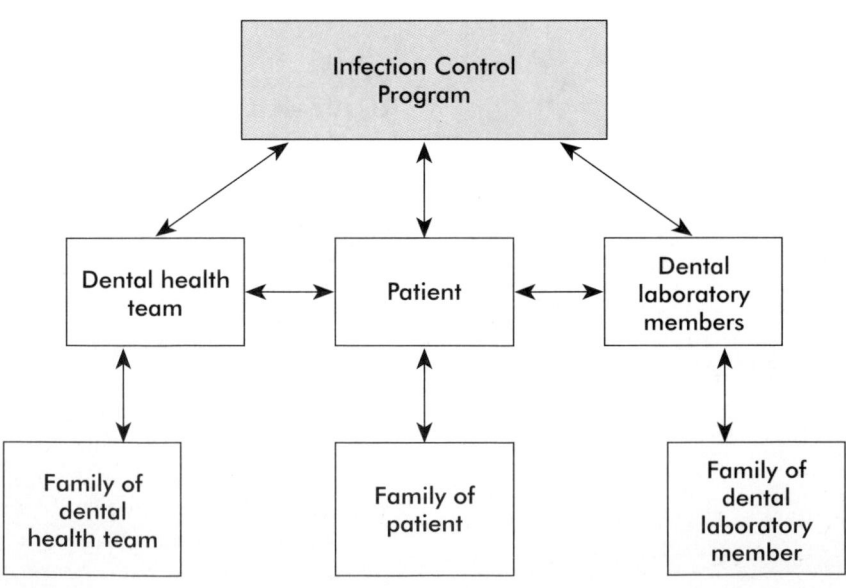

FIG. 8-2   Breaking the cycle of cross contamination.

▶ Basic Principles

Basic principles of infection control, such as using proper sterilization, disinfection, and clinical aseptic procedures, minimize the infectious risk that certain patients present to attending personnel. In this chapter the major areas considered include the following:

1. Patient screening
2. Aseptic technique
3. Personal protection
4. Instrument sterilization
5. Disinfection procedures
6. Equipment asepsis
7. Dental laboratory asepsis

The goal of antimicrobial sterilization, the process of completely removing or destroying all microorganisms, and disinfection, killing some microorganisms, is to reduce the spread of infectious agents. This necessitates an understanding of *cross-infections:* the passage of microorganisms from one person to another. The potential for cross-infection in the dental office exists for direct or indirect transmission, as well as via aerosols routinely created during clinical procedures.

▶ Governmental Regulations

Compliance with current guidelines and regulations for the implementation of policies regarding infection control, hazard communications, and medical waste disposal is expected from all dental professionals. Several agencies are responsible for providing the dental professional with current information regarding the regulations governing these areas. Current regulations will be discussed in this chapter.

In 1986 the **Occupational Safety and Health Agency (OSHA)**, a federal regulatory agency, reacted to requests from health care employees to establish guidelines to protect workers from occupational exposure to blood-borne diseases. OSHA's action resulted in Instruction CPL2-244A of August 1988, which provides regulations that require compliance through the use of **universal precautions** for employees who are in direct contact with blood that contains infectious materials and substances. On December 6, 1991, OSHA released a final rule with an effective date of March 6, 1992 (Boxes 8-3 and 8-4).

BOX 8-3

UNIVERSAL PRECAUTIONS

▶ Each work place must be safe or free from hazards that could cause harm or death.
▶ Provide personal protective clothing and equipment.
▶ Place poster 2203 in a prominent location.

BOX 8-4

1992 OVERVIEW OF REQUIRED FEDERAL OSHA STANDARDS

▶ Employers must identify and train workers who are *reasonably anticipated* to be at risk of exposure; reduce or eliminate exposure; and offer medical care and counseling.
▶ Employers must have written exposure control plans that will identify workers with occupational exposure to blood and other infectious materials and will identify the means to protect and train those workers.
▶ Employers must have a plan that includes a protocol for barrier techniques; sterilization; disinfection; hepatitis B vaccination; handling of office accidents, including postexposure to infectious materials; and plans to protect and train employers, with annual reviews and updates of the plan that are readily available to employees.
▶ Puncture-resistant containers must be used, hands must be washed as gloves are changed, and proper personal protective equipment is required to be worn.
▶ To launder protective clothing at home is prohibited.
▶ Recapping of sharps must be accomplished with a one-handed technique or by using a mechanical recapping device.
▶ Employees are required to wear gowns and gloves when there is risk of exposure of skin to blood, body fluids, or saliva.
▶ General work clothes are not considered protection against exposure to blood, body fluids, or saliva.
▶ Employees must wear masks, eyewear, or a face shield during exposure to splashes, spray, spatter, droplets of blood, body tissue, or saliva.
▶ Solid eyewear must have sideshields.
▶ Employers must provide personal protective equipment to be worn by all employees, including gowns, gloves, masks, and eyewear, at no expense to employees.
▶ Sharps containers must be labeled and easily accessible to the area of sharps use.
▶ Hepatitis B vaccinations must be offered to employees at no cost after training is completed but within 10 days of placement in a position that involves occupational exposure. If a worker declines the hepatitis B vaccination, access is still required if the employee has a change of mind.
▶ Employers must provide a training program during working hours to all employees in occupational exposure positions by June 4, 1992 and annually in subsequent years.
▶ Training records must be kept for 3 years following the training sessions.
▶ The standard requires that the following be handled as infectious waste by placement in special, labeled containers: Pathological waste; sharps; blood and body fluids; items that release blood, body fluid, or saliva when compressed; items caked with dried blood, body fluid, or saliva if they can release these materials during handling

There are several other specific regulations that commonly apply to the practice of dentistry. As a health care provider it is your responsibility to maintain current knowledge of the regulations that apply to dentistry. OSHA continuously reviews regulations and periodically makes changes that affect dentistry.

The **Environmental Protection Agency (EPA)**, a federal regulatory agency, in response to the Medical Waste Tracking Act (MWTA) of 1988, developed a program overseeing the handling, tracking, transportation, and disposal of medical waste once it has left the dental office.

The **Centers for Disease Control and Prevention (CDC)**, a division of the U.S. Public Health Service, comprise another regulating entity involved in providing recommendations to health care workers. This agency is responsible for the investigation and control of various diseases, an example of which is tuberculosis (a disease in which the instances are on the rise).

Task Categorization

All individuals working in a health care provider environment face the potential exposure to health risks. All infection control programs implemented into a health care provider setting should include a designation for task categorization. These tasks should be designated in accordance with OSHA guidelines (Box 8-5).

▶ Category I

Tasks that involve exposure to blood, body fluids, or tissues.

All procedures or other job-related tasks that involve an inherent potential for mucous membrane of skin contact with blood, body fluids or tissue, or a potential for spills or splashes of them are in Category I tasks. Use of appropriate protective measures should be required for every employee engaged in Category I tasks.

Most, although not necessarily all, tasks performed by the dentist, dental hygienist, dental assistant, and laboratory technician would fall into this category. The American Dental Association (ADA) recommends that these office personnel and the tasks that they perform be classified as Category I.

▶ Category II

Tasks that involve no exposure to blood, body fluids, or tissues, but employment may require performing unplanned Category I tasks.

The normal work routine involves no exposure to blood, body fluids or tissues, but exposure or potential exposure may be required as a condition of employment. Appropriate protective measures should be readily available to every employee engaged in Category II tasks.

Clerical or nonprofessional workers who may, as part of their duties, help clean up the office or handle instruments or impression materials, as well as those who send out dental materials to laboratories would be classified as Category II.

▶ Category III

Tasks that involve no exposure to blood, body fluids, or tissue.

The normal work routine involves no exposure to blood, body fluids or tissue. Persons who perform these duties are not called upon as part of their employment to perform or assist in emergency medical care or first aid or to be potentially exposed in some other way.

A front office receptionist, bookkeeper, or insurance clerk who does not handle dental instruments or materials would be a Category III worker.
NOTE: These classifications are not rigid, and there may be crossovers, depending on the jobs performed.

When working with employees who fall within these categories, it is necessary, because of OSHA requirements, to implement standardized record keeping. These records should include the following forms and dates of occurrence:

Exposure determination forms
Infection control program
HBV vaccination availability/requirement/
  implementation
Postexposure evaluation and follow-up
Training
Record keeping

BOX 8-5

TASK CATEGORIZATION

Category I
  ▶ Tasks that have exposure to blood, body fluids, or tissues.
  ▶ Individuals usually classified in this category are dentists, hygienists, assistants, and laboratory technicians.
Category II
  ▶ Tasks that involve no exposure to blood, body fluids, or tissues, but may have unplanned exposure to Category I tasks.
  ▶ Individuals classified in this category may include clerical or nonprofessional workers.
Category III
  ▶ Tasks that involve no exposure to blood, body fluids, or tissues.
  ▶ Individuals classified in this category may include receptionists, bookkeepers, and insurance clerks.

Hazard Communication Program

OSHA's Hazard Communication Standards require that all dental professionals take steps to come into or to maintain compliance with the existing standard. Specifically, a program must be developed and implemented that instructs all individuals, compiles a list of hazardous chemicals, obtains and files Material Safety Data Sheets, and labels all chemicals properly. This program must apply to all activities where an individual may be exposed to hazardous chemicals under normal working conditions or during an emergency situation.

One individual should be designated as the hazard communication program coordinator and is thus responsible for the following:

- Disseminating information regarding the contents of the program
- Recognizing the hazardous properties of the chemicals found within the work place
- Knowing safe handling procedures of chemicals
- Implementing measures to protect oneself from hazardous chemicals

This is accomplished by making and maintaining a list of all products in the facility that contain hazardous chemicals. A **Material Safety Data Sheet (MSDS)** is a government-approved form or an equivalent form that provides specific information on the chemicals purchased for use in a work place. Sheets for all products with hazardous potential are compiled, filed, and updated in a master list available to all individuals. Included on an MSDS for a hazardous chemical should be the manufacturer's name and address, product name, generic name if applicable, potential routes of entry, organs affected by the chemical, and means of protecting or reducing the effects of chemical exposure, e.g., eyewash.

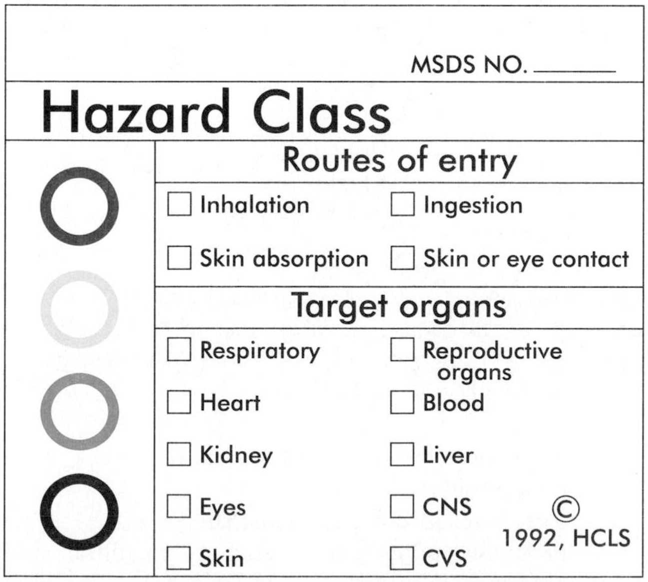
MSDS NO. ______
Hazard Class
Routes of entry
☐ Inhalation ☐ Ingestion
☐ Skin absorption ☐ Skin or eye contact
Target organs
☐ Respiratory ☐ Reproductive organs
☐ Heart ☐ Blood
☐ Kidney ☐ Liver
☐ Eyes ☐ CNS
☐ Skin ☐ CVS
© 1992, HCLS

FIG. 8-3 Hazard label required by OSHA regulations. (Courtesy of Health Career Learning Systems, Inc.)

Labels

The hazard communication program coordinator is also responsible for properly affixing labels to hazardous chemicals or substances. Many products purchased from dental supply companies arrive with permanently affixed information regarding hazardous chemicals. When purchasing items in bulk and placing the materials in smaller containers, it is necessary to complete hazard communication labels for these containers. An example would be the bulk purchase of antimicrobial soaps and the resulting placement into smaller, less obtrusive containers in the treatment room. These containers must include labels that (1) indicate that MSDS sheet information was obtained; (2) designate the hazard class of the chemical included; (3) outline routes of entry into the body; and (4) list the organs that are affected after entry has occurred (Fig. 8-3).

Several chemicals not considered of potential concern contain hazardous materials (Box 8-6). Table 8-3 lists various hazardous chemicals and where they may be found. Whenever there is specific information needed on a product, always refer to the MSDS.

Equipment to Meet Hazardous Situations

Certain equipment and devices should be present in a dental office to assist when a situation arises with hazardous chemicals. Spills of chemicals, gypsum products, and flammables require different reactions depending on the hazardous chemical. The following equipment

BOX 8-6

GENERAL PRECAUTIONS WHEN HANDLING HAZARDOUS CHEMICALS

The following are recommended general precautions to observe whenever working with hazardous chemicals:
Handle chemicals properly in accordance with manufacturer's or supplier's instructions.
Avoid skin contact with chemicals.
Minimize chemical vapor in the air.
Do not leave chemical bottles open.
Do not use a flame near flammable chemicals.
Do not eat or smoke in areas where chemicals are used.
When appropriate, wear protective eyewear and masks.
Dispose of all hazardous chemicals in accordance with MSDS instructions and applicable local, state, and federal regulations.

TABLE 8-3 HAZARDOUS CHEMICALS AND THE DENTAL PRODUCTS IN WHICH THEY ARE FOUND

Chemical name	May be found in	Chemical name	May be found in
Acetic acid	Photographic solutions	Methyl alcohol	Denatured alcohol
Acetone	Solvents	Methylene chloride	Solvents
Aluminum oxide	Polishing disks	Methylene methacrylate	Denature base resins
Aluminum soluble salts	Astringent agents	Methyl acetate	Solvents
Asbestos	Some cast ring liners	Molybdenum, insoluble	Casting alloys, chromium-cobalt alloys, stainless steel
Benzoyl peroxide	Resin systems, denture resins	Nickel, metal and soluble	Nickel-based casting alloys, stainless steel orthodontic appliances
Beryllium	Nickel-based casting alloys	Nitric acid	Pickling solutions, some bleaching solutions
Calcium carbonate	Polishing agents	Nitrous oxide	Nitrous oxide
Carbon tetrachloride	Solvents	Oil mist, mineral	Handpiece lubricants
Chloroform	Solvents	Petroleum distillates	Solvents, waxes, jellies
Chromium	Casting alloys	Phenol	Disinfectants
Cobalt	Casting alloys	Phosphoric acid	Etching agents, phosphate cements
Copper	Amalgam, casting alloys	Phthalic anhydride	Resins
Cresol, all isomers	Endodontic materials	Picric acid	Pickling solutions
Cyanide as CN	Plating solutions	Platinum	Casting alloys
Dibutylphthalate	Impression materials	Platinum soluble salts	Impression materials (addition silicones)
Ethyl acetate	Solvents	Propane	Burners
Ethyl acrylate	Resins	Rouge	Polishing agents
Ethyl alcohol	Solvents, sterilizing agents	Silica, amorphous including natural diatomaceous earth	Composite resins
Ethyl chloride	Solvents, topical refrigerants	Silica, crystalline	Composite resins, porcelain investments
Ethyl silicate	Silicate investments, impression materials (condensation silicones)	Silicon carbide	Polishing disks, cutting wheels
Ethylene oxide	Sterilizing agents	Silver, metal and soluble	Amalgam, endodontic points, casting alloys, photographic solutions
Fluoride dust	Fluoride-containing composites	Sulfuric acid	Etching agents for alloys, copper plating solutions
Formaldehyde	Sterilizing agents	Talc, nonasbestos form	Gloves
Glutaraldehyde	Sterilizing agents	Tantalum	Nickel-chromium-cobalt alloys
Hydrochloric acid	Pickling solutions, bleaching agents	Tin, inorganic compounds	Amalgam, polishing pastes
Hydrogen fluoride	Etching agents for porcelain	Tin, organic compounds	Impression materials (condensation silicones)
Hydroquinone	Methacrylate and denture base resins, photographic solutions	Titanium dioxide	Porcelain, impression materials
Iodine	Iodophor disinfectants and antimicrobial hand cleansers	Toluene	Solvents
Isopropyl alcohol	Solvents, wiping agents	Trichloromethane	Solvents
Lead, inorganic lead	Impression materials (some polysulfides)	Uranium, insoluble	Porcelain
Liquid petroleum gas (LPG)	Burners	Vinyl chloride	Maxillofacial plastics, mouth guard trays
Mercury	Amalgam	Xylene	Solvents
Mercury, organic	Topical antiseptics	Zirconium compounds	Porcelain, polishing agents

and recommendations will assist in the event of a hazardous spill:

1. Fire extinguisher
2. Eyewash stations
3. Amalgam spill kit
4. National Institute of Occupational Safety and Health (NIOSH) approved masks
5. Protective clothing (long sleeves, high neck, fluid impervious)
6. Kitty litter, broom, and dustpan
7. Protective utility gloves, such as polynitral, and glasses
8. Bags to seal spilled materials and contaminated objects

9. Well-ventilated areas for work where ventilation can be turned off in the event of an accident
10. Scavenging system when nitrous oxide is utilized

Infection Control Techniques

Throughout the course of providing dental treatment to patients, equipment, surfaces, instruments, and other devices become contaminated with bioburden or are simply not clean. The goal of any infection control program must be to maintain sterile techniques and to avoid the potential of cross-infection through aseptic technique.

▶ Aseptic Technique

Aseptic technique, or asepsis, refers to the use of procedures that break the circle of infection and, ideally, eliminate cross-contamination. Cross-contamination is a condition of a previously sterile environment being exposed to harmful agents. Implementation of effective, logical aseptic techniques also provides a thread that binds the other areas of infection control into an effective preventive program. This includes minimizing surface exposure and contact during treatment, minimizing the number of items that are contaminated during treatment procedures, and preventing interruptions in patient treatment.

The use of coverings on surfaces, treatment of exposed surfaces, and care of contaminated items are all important to aseptic technique, but each team member must also be keenly aware of his or her own actions. Movements of contaminated gloved hands to protective eyewear, masks, and hair all increase the potential for cross-infections. All of these movements should be eliminated during and after treatment.

The following techniques are examples of steps that can be taken to minimize contamination and cross-contamination during treatment procedures.

ANTISEPTIC MOUTH RINSES

The routine use of a pretreatment antiseptic mouth rinse that contains a substance to inhibit the growth of some microorganisms can lower the microbial load at a primary source for infection in the patient's mouth. Initial studies on the use of mouth rinses as part of an infection control regimen were performed in the early 1970s and demonstrated the efficacy of mouth rinsing to reduce the total number of microbes in the mouth. Relatively few advances were made in this area regarding infection control until a mouth rinse with documented residual antimicrobial activity (0.12% chlorhexidine gluconate) was formulated and made available. Such a mouth rinse can reduce the number of oral microbes while dental procedures are being performed.

Using an antiseptic mouth rinse as an infection control measure is not included in the 1988 ADA recommendations, nor is it in the 1993 CDC Guidelines for Infection Control in Dentistry; however, it is included in the American Heart Association's (AHA) recommended prophylaxis for patients who are at risk of infective endocarditis, an infection of the endocardium caused by bacteria that can destroy the valves of the heart and cause cardiac failure. For many of the same reasons as listed in the AHA recommendation, the state-of-the-art procedure in this area uses mouth rinses, with residual activity as an infection control procedure.

ANTISEPTIC HAND WASHING

All infection control recommendations and guidelines for dentistry stress hand washing. The rationale for using a hand washing agent with residual action is similar to the rationale for mouth rinses with the same property. The residual action in a hand wash combats the tendency for increased skin microbe replication while gloves are worn. Residual activity becomes evident after the eighth hand wash of the day and builds through the day's fifteenth hand wash (particularly with those containing 4% chlorhexidine gluconate as the active ingredient). Therefore antimicrobial hand washing agents should be used regularly throughout the day, not only a few times, such as before and after lunch.

Hands must be washed thoroughly just before and immediately after the treatment of each patient. The use of gloves does not serve as a substitute for routine hand washing with an effective liquid antiseptic. The rationale here includes the recognition that (1) gloves may tear or perforate during patient treatment; and (2) bacteria either remaining on the skin after washing or entering through a compromised glove can multiply rapidly under the glove.

Substituted phenol preparations, such as chlorhexidine gluconate (a bis-phenol) and parachlorometaxylenol (PCMX), are the best hand washing agents currently available. Both agents require repeated washings throughout the day to attain maximal effectiveness. Hands should be dried with air or disposable paper towels, not with reusable cloth towels.

An **antimicrobial hand wash** (using a substance that inhibits growth of microorganisms) involves wetting the hands with cold water to close the pores of the skin. The wash should take at least 10 seconds, working the lathered soap completely over the hands and up onto the forearms. The areas between the fingers should be cleaned thoroughly, as well as cleaning the nail area. Nails should be maintained short and without polish.

MEDICAL EVALUATION AND PATIENT SCREENING

In dentistry, it has been recommended routinely that a comprehensive medical history be taken for each patient

> **BOX 8-7**
>
> ### INFECTIOUS DISEASES THE HEALTH PROFESSIONAL ENCOUNTERS
>
> Common cold
> Acute pharyngitis
> Tuberculosis
> Chickenpox
> Hand-foot-mouth disease
> Rubeola
> Cytomegalovirus (CMV)
> Herpes labialis
> Recurrent intraoral infections
> Gonococcal infections
> Trichomonal infections
> Hepatitis
> Acute and chronic sinusitis
>
> Pneumonia
> Tuberculous infection
> Herpangina
> Rubella
> Mumps
> Herpetic infections
> Acute herpetic gingivo-stomatitis
> Herpetic whitlow
> Chlamydia infections
> Syphilis
> Acquired immuno-deficiency syndrome (AIDS)

and that this medical history be reviewed and updated at subsequent appointments. Although the medical history is usually obtained and reviewed, it appears not to be updated as often as desirable. One purpose of the medical history is to alert the dental team to medical problems that could, in conjunction with dental treatment, adversely affect the patient. However, not all patients with infectious diseases can be identified by medical history, physical examination, or laboratory tests; therefore the medical history should not be used to identify the *infectious disease risk* of a patient. Box 8-7 lists many of the infectious diseases the health professional faces during contact with the dental patient. Because the medical history is a poor indicator of prior infectious diseases, every patient must be considered infectious and subject to the same infection control procedures.

The basis of *universal precautions* (that is, treating all patients as though they are potentially infectious with HIV/HBV or other infectious diseases) was first recommended by the Centers for Disease Control in 1987. This concept of universal precautions is difficult for some dental offices to put into practice. Intellectually it is accepted; when providing treatment for a patient who is HIV seropositive, however, many practitioners continue to use extra infection control barriers. When universal precautions are used, additional procedures are not necessary when treating a patient who is known to have an infectious disease.

The medical history also can alert dental professionals to patient problems and discomforts resulting from previous dental office visits. For example, an inquiry about the posttreatment appearance of raised red hives or small ulcerations may suggest a patient's allergic reaction to latex. Just as we are observing an increasing incidence of latex allergies in health professionals, more health care facilities are finding that certain patients are developing either localized immediate or delayed hypersensitivity reactions to the individual components of latex gloves.

Under OSHA standards, employees are entitled to have access to patient health history information; this is especially important after an employee is exposed to blood-borne pathogens in the occupational setting of the dental office. This information is maintained as part of a confidential medical record for employees. OSHA requires that such records be kept for all employees at risk of blood-borne pathogen transmission in an occupational setting such as the dental office.

As already noted, all patients should be treated the same—that is, as potentially infectious for HBV, HIV, or other blood-borne pathogens. Consistent adherence to universal precautions is therefore a major professional standard of care and reduces the guesswork used to determine a patient's infection status.

Personal Protection

Repeated exposure to saliva and blood during intraoral, often invasive procedures can challenge the health professional's immune defenses with a wide range of microbial agents. Personal protection in this context thus involves two basic considerations: immunologic protection and barrier protection. Dental treatment providers should receive appropriate vaccines to prevent the onset of clinical or subclinical infection when the symptoms of the disease are not apparent. The occupational risks for HBV, measles, rubella, influenza, and certain other microbial infections can be minimized considerably by the stimulation of artificial active immunity. Approved vaccines are available for each of these and should be utilized by individuals providing patient care.

▶ Immunization

Immunization is the process by which resistance to an infectious disease is induced or augmented. The human body can produce immunity to particular diseases or conditions. When no immunity exists for a disease, immunization is provided through vaccinations.

Immunization to prevent and control cross-infection is an important aspect for dental health care providers. The availability and effectiveness of the HBV vaccination is widespread, but several other diseases may also pose threats to the health and well-being of dental personnel and potentially to patients.

Initially the transient immunity received from immunoglobulins from the mother's placenta provides the child with some protection against disease. But eventually the child's system increases in its ability to protect against other infections. To assist our systems in the fight against communicable diseases, immunizations are available. Common childhood immunizations may be received for several diseases, including diphtheria, tetanus, pertussis, polio, and rubella. Other vaccinations assist in avoiding rubeola, mumps, and influenza. Tuberculosis (TB) tine tests are available to determine whether an individual has or has been exposed to tuberculosis. These tests have become extremely important because TB, once thought to be almost nonexistent in North America, is increasing.

 Recent studies report that when children are given the choice, they prefer dental practitioners who wear personal protective equipment versus those who dress in street attire. When children were shown pictures of dentists in street attire and in personal protective equipment, including mask, eyewear, gloves, and gown; some school-aged children found the photos of the dentists in street attire frightening because they didn't appear safe or professional.

▶ Barriers

While vaccines are effective in minimizing the transmission of certain infections, they are not sufficient for protection against the wide variety of potential pathogens encountered during patient treatment. As a consequence, physical barriers are a fundamental component of the infection control program. The routine use of disposable gloves, face masks, and protective eyewear during treatment procedures minimizes exposure to infection.

GLOVES

Properly fitting gloves protect the dental care provider from exposure through cuts and abrasions often found on the hands. Even scrupulous hand washing cannot replace the use of gloves. Glove reuse is not recommended, since washing of gloves with hand washing antiseptics increases both the size and number of pinholes in the gloves and basically compromises commercial glove integrity. The latex examination gloves employed during routine nonsurgical treatment were not formulated to withstand prolonged exposure to secretions or chemical agents. Glove integrity may also be compromised during extensive procedures that require long treatment periods. Because of these factors, gloves may need to be changed while treating a single patient. Continued advances in the quality and manufacture of gloves can only expand the protection afforded by this important barrier.

A current alternative for latex gloves is to use medical-grade vinyl gloves. This may be necessitated when a treatment provider develops a documented allergy to latex or to glove powder. Individuals who wear vinyl gloves often immediately note the difference between vinyl and latex gloves. Tactile sensation with vinyl gloves may be altered, and the gloves may also tear more easily because they are more rigid. Newer generations of gloves of this type have attempted to correct these inherent differences in the original polyvinyl products.

Gloves may also be manufactured with talc or cornstarch on the inside surfaces. Either of these substances coats the gloves to assist in placement over hands, but may cause allergic reactions or hypersensitivities. An alternative to the gloves touching the health care worker's skin is to place a sealer over the skin to provide a barrier between the skin and the gloves. Many different products are available for this purpose. Wearing cloth gloves under the examination gloves provides an alternative barrier as well.

Additional types of gloves are used in situations that require patient contact or exposure. Overgloves, which are thin, oversized, clear plastic gloves, offer an alternative in maintaining cross-contamination control in a treatment room. Overgloves should be worn when retrieving devices from the mobile cabinet, mixing dental materials, leaving the treatment room for a short time, and touching patient records. The use of overgloves reduces the need for disinfection of devices and surfaces when used effectively.

Polynitrile gloves, heavy-duty utility gloves, are recommended for use when tearing a room down after treatment, when cleaning high velocity evacuation (HVE) (suction) systems, and during the processing of instruments. This type of glove provides greater protection against instrument punctures and tears as a result of excess stress during activities. Polynitrile gloves can be sterilized because they are resistant to the heat and chemicals found in sterilizing units. Eventually the gloves deteriorate, and when visible breaks or cracks are evident, they should be discarded.

Clinical Application. As gloves are removed, the clinician grasps the end of the cuff and turns the glove inside out. The second glove is grasped by the cuff and turned inside out over the first glove (Fig. 8-4, *A* through *E*). The glove surfaces exposed are those that have contacted the clinician's hands. Then the gloves can be discarded.

PROTECTIVE EYEWEAR

The eyes are particularly susceptible to physical and microbial injury by virtue of their limited vascularity and diminished immune capacities. Aerosolized droplets containing microbial contaminants can lead to the development of conjunctivitis, an eye infection also known as pink eye, in dental personnel. This may keep the individual away from work for a minimum of 1 to 2 weeks. Protective eyewear or an appropriate face shield should therefore be worn during treatment procedures,

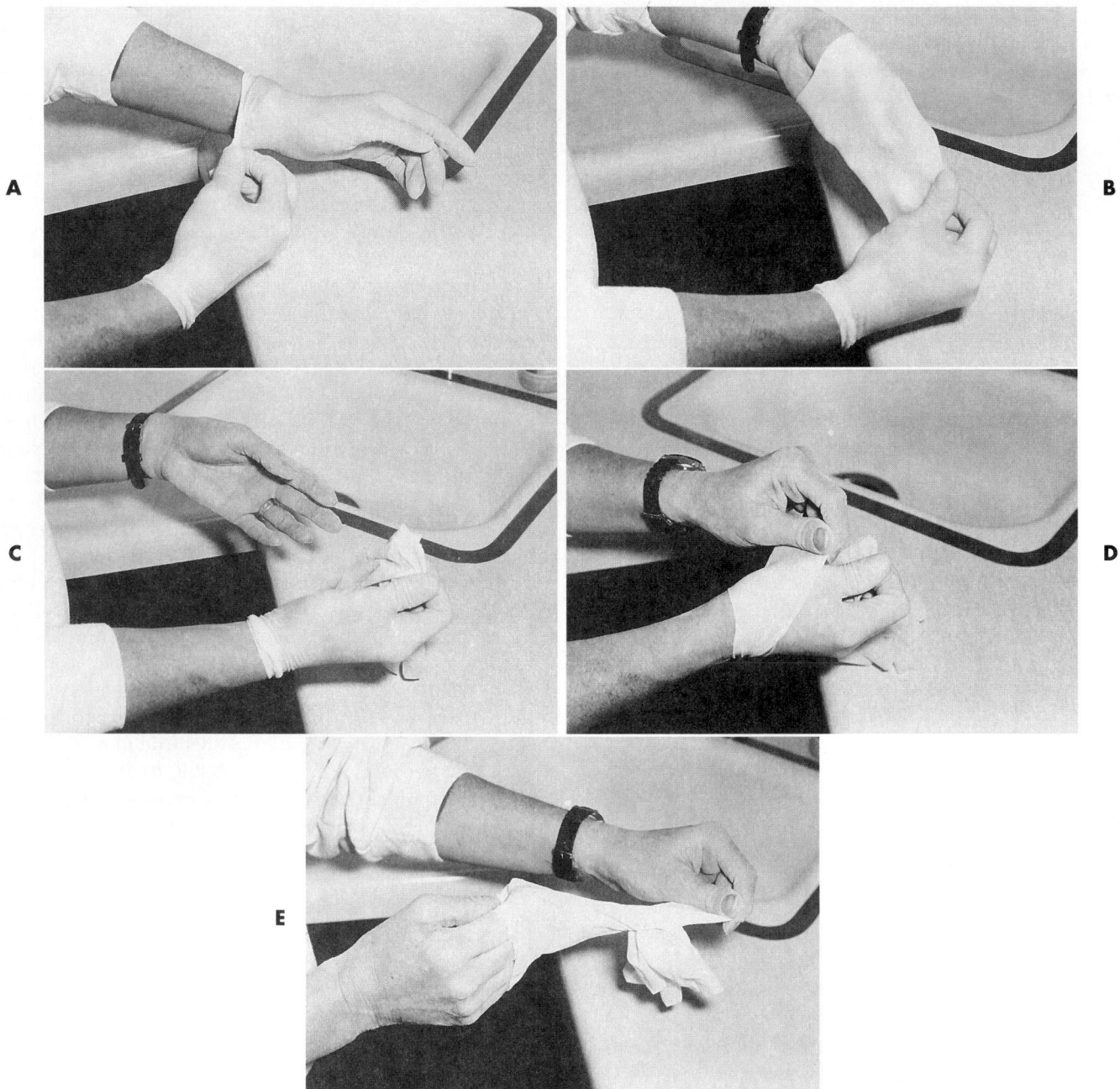

FIG. 8-4   Contaminated gloves are removed by grasping the cuff, *A*, and pulling the first glove off the hand inside out, *B*. The contaminated glove is completely removed and held in the hand of the remaining glove, *C*. The cuff of the second glove is pulled inside out over the first contaminated glove, *D* and *E*.

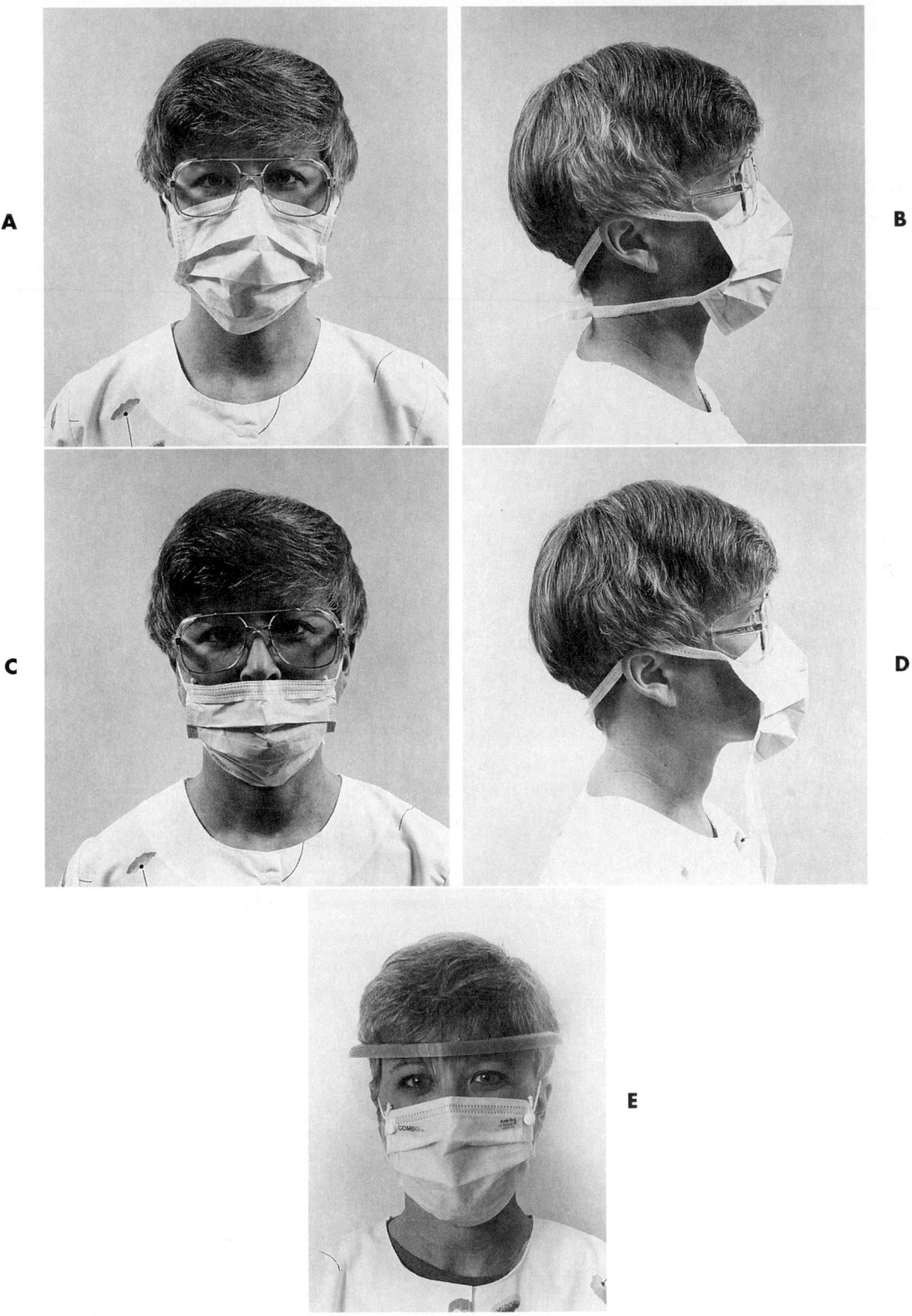

FIG. 8-5   *A,* Properly placed mask and glasses. *B,* Lateral view of properly positioned mask and glasses. *C,* Improperly placed mask. *D,* Lateral view of improperly positioned mask. *E,* Another example of protective face and eyewear.

in the dental laboratory, and in the sterilization/disinfection area when chemicals are mixed and poured.

If the dental employee wears prescription eyeglasses, side shields can be affixed to provide protection. If side shields are not used, face shields are recommended.

Clinical Application. Protective eyewear with side shields is placed before patient treatment and removed with gloves in place after treatment is completed. The eyewear can remain in place but should not be touched with ungloved hands. Protective eyewear should be disinfected after use (Fig. 8-5, *A* to *E*). Protective eyewear should also be provided for each patient and disinfected after use.

MASKS

The use of an approved face mask will protect the dentist, hygienist, assistant, and laboratory technician from microbe-laden aerosolized droplets. According to current technology and recommendations, the best masks are those which can filter at least 95% of droplet particles 3.0 to 3.2 μ in diameter.

In addition, a proper fit is required for both wearer comfort and barrier efficiency. As in the case of gloves, masks should be changed for each patient, since a mask's efficiency decreases as it traps moisture during dental procedures. The wet fabric serves as a vehicle for microbial transfer through the mask. Further protection needed in laboratory situations while using silicates or other potentially harmful products can be obtained through the use of NIOSH-approved filtering respirator masks.

If plastic face shields are worn, they efficiently protect only the eyes and not the mouth and nose. It is recommended that face masks be worn in conjunction with this type of shield.

Clinical Application. Masks are donned before gloves for ease of placement. Each mask is adjusted to facial configurations for proper adaptation and is changed before working with each patient or as moisture is absorbed into the mask during a procedure. A mask should not be allowed to hang below the clinician's chin after use; complete removal of the mask is recommended.

OPERATORY ATTIRE

Appropriate uniforms or gowns must be worn for all dental treatment. Debate regarding the appropriateness of either long-sleeved or short-sleeved uniforms or clinic jackets continues, with positive and negative features inherent with each type. Changing the gown or uniform or wearing a protective cover over the uniform when an aerosol spray is being generated is recommended. All clinical attire should be of synthetic material so that contaminants are not easily absorbed into the material. Seams, buttons, and buckles should be kept to a minimum for the same reason.

In some treatment situations, such as oral or periodontal surgery and hospital dentistry, additional coverings may be considered. Hair and shoe coverings offer greater protection to the health care provider.

Clinical Application. Clinical attire should be removed at the end of the day when all clinical activities are completed. The ability to shower and change all clinical attire before leaving the facility is recommended. This action breaks the cross-contamination cycle that may be extended to include family and friends. Clinical attire should not be worn during food breaks or taken home to be laundered. As indicated earlier, clinical attire is not considered general clothing that is worn on a daily basis.

The wearing of all jewelry, necklaces, bracelets, earrings, and rings should be eliminated or at least reduced. It is a common practice for health care workers to continue to wear wedding and engagement rings. Care must always be taken not to puncture protective gloves with the rings.

OTHER BARRIERS

Most students in dental schools learn to use a rubber dam when performing restorative or endodontic procedures. A rubber dam is helpful when water-spray handpieces are used. A combination of the high-speed evacuation device and rubber dam can sharply reduce the microbial load in

---

BOX 8-8

CDC CATEGORIES

Critical: Surgical and other instruments used to penetrate soft tissue or bone are classified as critical and should be sterilized after each use. These devices include forceps, scalpels, bone chisels, scalers, and burs.

Semicritical: Instruments, such as mirrors and amalgam condensers, that do not penetrate soft tissues or bone but contact oral tissues are classified as semicritical. These devices should be sterilized after each use. If, however, sterilization is not feasible because the instrument will be damaged by heat, the instrument should receive, at a minimum, high-level disinfection.

Noncritical: Instruments or medical devices such as external components of x-ray heads that come into contact only with intact skin are classified as noncritical. Because these noncritical surfaces have a relatively low risk of transmitting infection, they may be reprocessed between patients with intermediate-level or low-level disinfection or detergent and water washing, depending on the nature of the surface and the degree and nature of the contamination.

the aerosols produced. The use of disposable covers or drapes on operatory surfaces also diminishes the collection of spatter on equipment that can only be disinfected.

▶ Sterilization

A complete understanding of the concepts of disinfection and sterilization is mandatory for an effective infection control program. **Disinfection** is the inhibition or destruction of most pathogens—but not spores on a given surface, whereas sterilization is the destruction or removal of all forms of life, with particular reference to microorganisms. The ultimate requirement for sterilization is the destruction of bacterial and fungal spores. Sterilization methodologies applicable to dentistry include prolonged dry heat, unsaturated chemical vapor, steam under pressure, ethylene oxide, and certain chemical sterilants.

The CDC have three classification categories for instruments and devices, depending on the risk of transmitting infection and the need to sterilize. The three categories are **critical**, **semicritical**, and **noncritical** (Box 8-8).

Cold disinfection refers to disinfection of instruments at room temperature by immersion in a chemical solution. Often referred to as immersion disinfection, this process represents an often abused aspect of office asepsis. Since the solutions are often misused and thus cannot guarantee destruction of all microbial forms, cold disinfection should not be confused with acceptable methods of sterilization.

Sanitization is a frequently used process involving the use of agents to maintain the microbial flora at safe public health levels. This particular process is not considered part of an effective aseptic program.

Although complete sterilization is the ideal for surfaces that are contaminated during dental treatment, it is not always practical. Mobile and fixed cabinets, dental units, and chairs do not lend themselves to sterilization procedures. However, disinfecting the surfaces provides the next best alternative.

Certain routine steps must be employed to sterilize all instruments, mirrors, burs, metal bands, and other intraoral materials that can withstand effective techniques. The following section will consider the most appropriate physical methods of sterilization; steam under pressure, autoclaving, dry heat, and chemical vapor, as well as other physical modes are useful in microbiology as sterilizing systems. Each method of sterilization has certain advantages and disadvantages, as seen in Table 8-4.

Whenever a sterilization processing area is designed, certain factors should be considered that would reduce confusion and the possibility of error in processing. The sterilization area ideally has two places for entry and exit, reducing congestion. Areas that are designated for contaminated and sterile instruments avoid the accidental contamination of sterile instruments. A sterilization area that has one work area that is used for processing contaminated and sterile instruments increases the potential for sterile items to become contaminated. This is especially important when more than one person is responsible for processing instruments.

TABLE 8-4 FEATURES OF STERILIZATION METHODS

Method	Advantages	Disadvantages
Steam under pressure	Short cycle time Good penetration Wide range of materials can be processed without destruction	Corrosion of unprotected carbon steel instruments Dulling of unprotected cutting edges Packages may remain wet at end of cycle May destroy heat-sensitive materials
Dry heat	Effective and safe for sterilization of metal instruments and mirrors Does not dull cutting edges Does not rust or corrode	Long cycle required for sterilization Poor penetration May discolor and char fabric Destroys heat-labile items
Unsaturated chemical vapor	Short cycle time Does not rust or corrode metal instruments, including carbon steel Does not dull cutting edges Suitable for orthodontic stainless wires	Instruments must be completely dried before processing Will destroy heat-sensitive plastics Chemical odor in poorly ventilated areas
Ethylene oxide	High capacity for penetration Does not damage heat-labile materials (including rubber and handpieces) Evaporates without leaving a residue Suitable for materials that cannot be exposed to moisture	Slow—requires extended cycle times Retained in liquids and rubber materials for prolonged intervals Causes tissue irritation if not well aerated Requires special *spark–shield*—explosive in the presence of flame or sparks

PROCESSING INSTRUMENTS

The processing of dental instruments and armamentarium requires the use of utility gloves for protection. Instruments removed from a treatment room are often covered with debris from the procedure. Before sterilization the instruments must be cared for properly. They can be placed in a holding or soaking tank to loosen hardened debris and then moved to an ultrasonic cleaner (Fig. 8-6, *A* and *B*). To reduce multiple handling of the instruments, before placement in the holding tank or ultrasonic unit, they can be put in metal baskets for transfer. The instruments can also be placed directly into the ultrasonic cleaner to be cleansed of any debris. The ultrasonic cleaner uses sound waves in a specialized solution to remove any debris, thus avoiding hand scrubbing of instruments, which can lead to puncture wounds during handling.

Ultrasonic cleaning *does not sterilize* instruments, but simply removes any debris that could compromise the sterilization process. After the instruments are removed from the ultrasonic cleaner, they must be rinsed thoroughly and tapped or blotted dry of excess water.

The sterilization process will vary with the machine

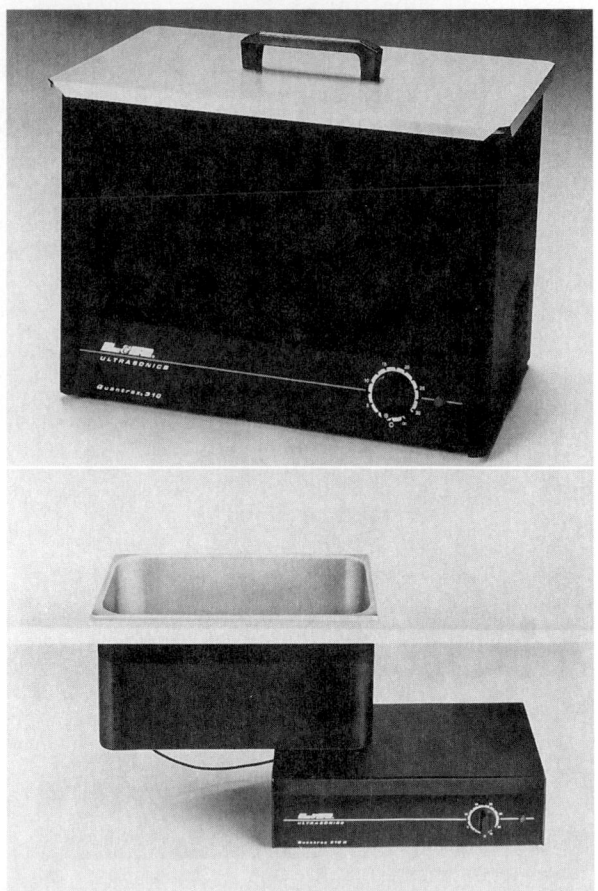

FIG. 8-6 An example of an ultrasonic instrument cleaning device.

(Courtesy of L & R Company, Kearney, New Jersey.)

that is used, but the end result is the same: sterilization of the instruments. If the instruments are to be placed in cold disinfection because of their melting point, this is done immediately after rinsing under water. If the instruments are to be placed in dry heat or chemical sterilization, the instruments must be dried completely. If they are not dried thoroughly, corrosion of the metal may occur, resulting in dulled cutting edges and rusted joints.

Instruments that are to be sterilized in steam under pressure must be handled differently than with the sterilization procedures previously outlined. Steam under pressure, as the name implies uses moisture at a high temperature to sterilize instruments. Moisture is corrosive to metal, so metal instruments, particularly those with sharp cutting edges or hinged parts, must be placed in a surgical milk or liquid emulsion. This oil emulsion coats the metal and protects it from corrosion. Certain instruments are not recommended to be placed in the oil emulsion, such as the mirror, amalgam carriers, anesthetic syringes, and endodontic instruments.

To maintain the sterile process, many dental professionals will bag instruments before the sterilization process. Bagging instruments aids in verifying their sterility. Color-coded indicators signify whether an instrument bag has reached sterilizing temperatures. Instruments are also bagged as tray set-ups to aid in the efficiency of the dental professional. If all instruments used in a treatment procedure are sterilized in a group, the ease in preparing the tray set-up is increased dramatically. When instruments are placed in bags or metal containers for sterilization, care must be taken not to overload the bag or basket, which would reduce the effectiveness of the sterilant to reach all the instruments. A container may be wrapped, sealed, and sterilized as a unit. A guide to use to determine whether a metal container is overloaded is not to stack more than 2 or 3 instruments. When metal containers are placed in sterilization unit trays that are designed by the manufacturer to fit in an individual unit, the trays should not be stacked on top of each other. Individual bags of instruments should lie flat on the trays or be loosely packed on the side to allow penetration of the sterilant.

Instruments used on a highly infectious patient, such as one with HBV should be processed differently. The used instrument tray should be tagged with a signal that is recognized by all personnel to indicate that the instruments were used on an infectious patient. Then instead of processing these instruments through the normal routine, the instruments are all sterilized first and then separated and run through the normal steps. Articles on the tray set-up or from the treatment room that cannot be sterilized because they may melt or become flammable should be placed in a red or bright fluorescent orange *biohazard*-labelled bag and disposed of after one use (Fig. 8-7).

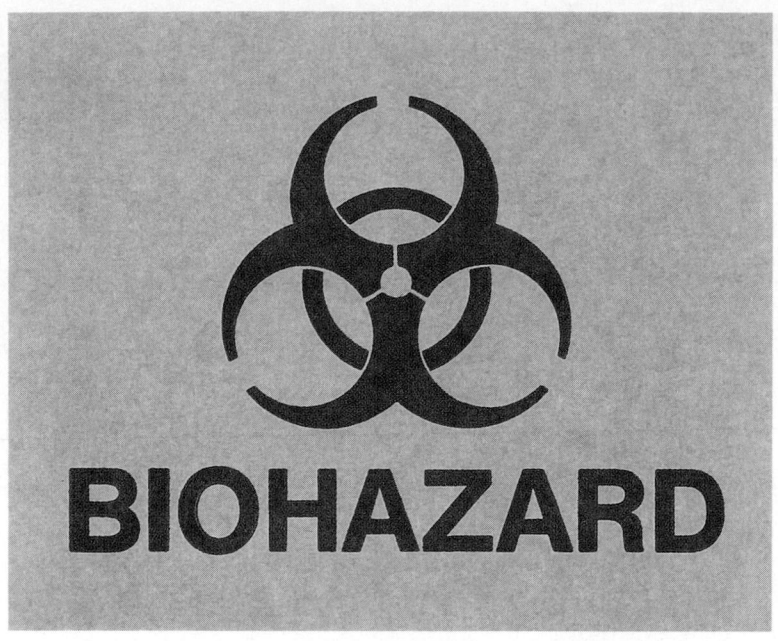

FIG. 8-7   Biohazard label as required by OSHA regulations for placement on designated bioburden container.

STEAM STERILIZATION

Complete sterilization is achieved by the use of moist heat at higher temperatures in the form of saturated steam under pressure in airtight vessels, such as an autoclave or omniclave. Under the appropriate conditions, autoclaving represents an efficient sterilization process. Steam may also be employed as free-flowing at atmospheric conditions, although at 1 atmosphere pressure its effectiveness equals that of boiling water.

Most commonly, a temperature of 121° C (250° F) is applied for 15 to 20 minutes. These conditions yield 15 pounds pressure of steam at sea level. Direct exposure to saturated steam at 121° C for 10 minutes normally destroys all forms of life. In practice, an additional *safety factor* interval must be allowed for the temperature to reach this point in the center of thick packages of dressings or large containers of liquids. In most instances, a sterilization period of 30 minutes suffices. Alternative methods using higher temperatures and pressures for shorter periods of time are employed with the newer equipment used in many dental facilities (Fig. 8-8, *A* and *B*).

As efficient as steam under pressure can be in instrument sterilization, this procedure is effective only when suitable conditions are present in the pressurized chamber. Inadequate sterilization of instruments may be caused by the following (Box 8-9):

▸ Faulty preparation of materials for sterilization (packaging that does not allow for penetration of the sterilant)

BOX 8-9

POTENTIAL STERILIZER PROBLEMS

STEAM UNDER PRESSURE

Faulty preparation of materials
Improper loading
Faulty seals, heating coils, traps, exhaust lines
Air in the chamber
Wet steam

DRY HEAT

Excessive temperature
Mistimed cycle
Interrupted cycle
Heat-sensitive materials
Packages not correctly spaced
Longer sterilization interval
Charred wrapping materials
Use of inappropriate equipment, e.g., toaster and conventional oven

UNSATURATED CHEMICAL VAPOR

Wraps not designed or intended for chemical vapor units
Improper instrument wraps, such as sealed containers, foil, or cloth
Wraps not loose enough to allow vapor penetration
Inadequate spacing of packs
Faulty door gasket or seals, e.g., worn from exposure to chemical vapor
Unit not located in a well-ventilated area of prep room
Instruments not dry before being placed in the sterilizer

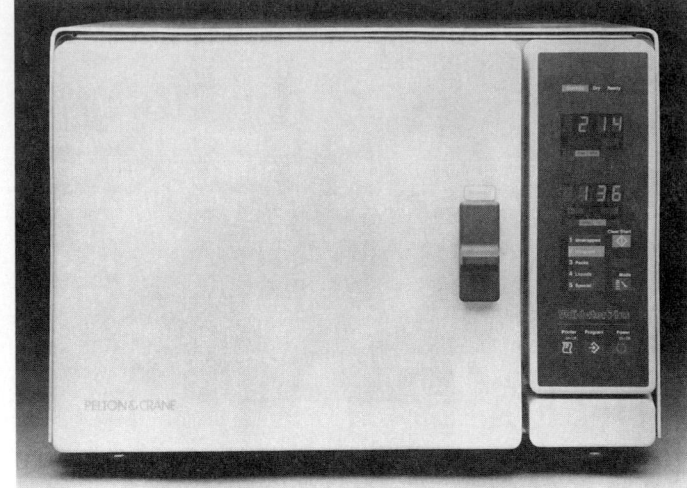

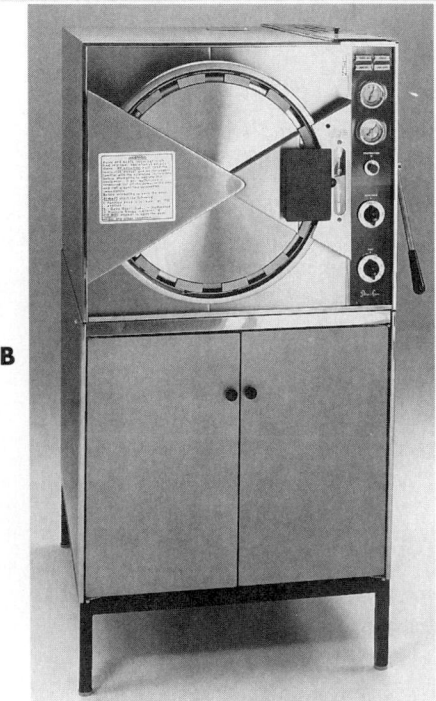

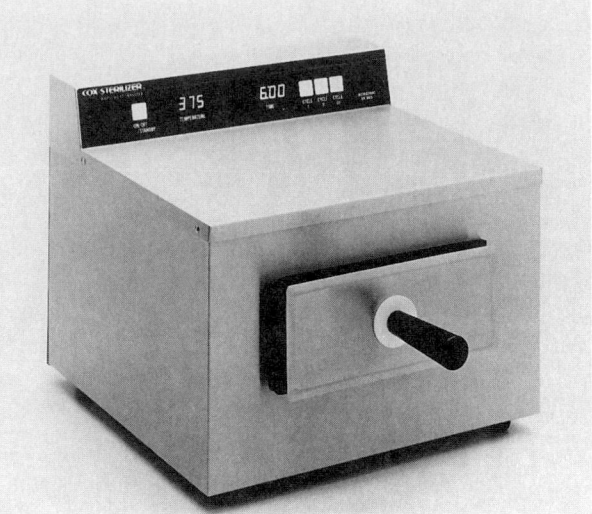

FIG. 8-9   Flash point sterilizer that is often used for hand-piece sterilization.

FIG. 8-8   Steam/dry heat sterilizer. *A,* Validator plus. *B,* Magnaclave.

(Courtesy of Pelton and Crane Company.)

▶ Improper loading of the instrument chamber
▶ Improper functioning of the sterilizer (failure to reach temperature and/or pressure)
▶ Presence of air in the chamber (may delay microbial destruction up to 10 times longer)
▶ Excess water in the steam (can serve as passageway for microorganisms to get through wet instrument packages)

Operator failure may also be a contributing factor to inadequate sterilization. If the operator of the sterilization unit does not allow it to reach sterilizing levels before timing the sterilization process or if the sterilizing temperature is not reached, the process is incomplete. It is always extremely important for the operator of sterilizing equipment to follow manufacturer's directions carefully.

Newer and quicker sterilization units, such as flash sterilizers, are available today and are used primarily to sterilize dental handpieces and other instruments. The 8- to 10-minute processing time available with these units makes them more attractive for use when the purchase of multiple numbers of costly instruments is impractical (Fig. 8-9).

Several sterilizing units are equipped with drying cycles to ensure that paper instrument bags are thoroughly dried in order to prevent punctures or rips during the handling of moist bags. The efficient use of units without drying cycles and allowing instruments to dry thoroughly before handling will also reduce the possibility of tears.

UNSATURATED CHEMICAL VAPOR

Chemical vapor sterilization in dental practices and clinics is considered an acceptable method of sterilization by the Council on Dental Therapeutics, and its use has increased substantially in recent years. This system depends on a combination of heat, water, and chemicals in a pressurized system to be effective (Fig. 8-10). The chemicals include mixtures of alcohols, formaldehyde, ketone, acetone, and water. As shown in Table 8-5, the temperature and pressure required with chemical vapor sterilizers vary from other methods of sterilization. The principle of operation has similarities with steam sterilizers, as well as some important distinctions. The solution of premixed chemicals added to the jacket

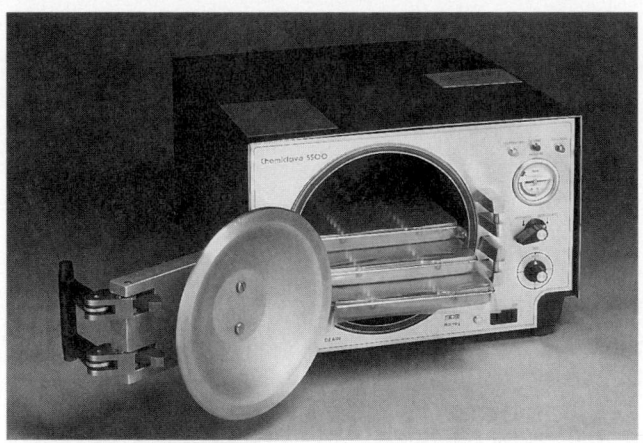

FIG. 8-10 **Chemical vapor sterilizer.**
(Courtesy of MDT Company, North Charleston, South Carolina.)

reservoir in the sterilizer must be purchased from the manufacturer, since the ratio of each chemical in the preparation is critical. After the apparatus is preheated, clean, dry, loosely wrapped instruments are placed in the chamber. The package wraps must be loose to allow the chemical vapors to condense on the instrument surfaces during the cycle. Thick, tightly wrapped items require longer exposure because the unsaturated chemical vapors cannot penetrate under pressure as well as can saturated steam. Metal instruments must be dry before sterilization or chemicals will accumulate in the wetted surfaces and corrosion will occur.

The major advantages of chemical vapor sterilization are as follows: (1) a short cycle time when compared with that of steam under pressure; (2) no rusting of instruments and burs in contrast to steam sterilization; (3) instruments are dry when the cycle is complete; and (4) the cycle timing is automatic. The presence of only about 8% to 9% water vapor in the chemical solution is significantly below the 15% minimum for rusting and dulling, and this property prevents destruction of dental items, such as endodontic files, orthodontic pliers, wires and bands, burs, and carbon steel instruments caused by rusting and corrosion. Thus, a wide range of items can be routinely sterilized. However, a requirement for adequate ventilation can constitute a problem for practitioners who use this type of apparatus. Chemical vapors, particularly formaldehyde, can be released when the

chamber door is opened at the end of the cycle, and these leave a temporary unpleasant odor in the area. Although numerous toxicity studies by the manufacturer indicate little chance of eye irritation from these residual vapors, dental personnel occasionally report some discomfort if the sterilizer is in an area with poor air circulation. To counteract this detrimental aspect, later models are equipped with a special filtration device that further reduces the amount of vapor left in the chamber at the end of the cycle.

Formaldehyde, sometimes used in chemical vapor sterilization units, is a known carcinogenic chemical. Exposure to vapors is dangerous to dental personnel. After degassing the chamber, a minimum of 3 minutes should elapse before the chamber door is opened to remove the sterilized instruments. Protective eye, hand, and face wear should be worn while depressurizing a chamber or when handling the sterilant chemicals.

DRY HEAT

The destruction of all forms of microbial life in the absence of moisture requires different conditions than those discussed previously. As proteins dry, their resistance to denaturation increases. Thus, at a given temperature, dry heat sterilizes much less efficiently than moist heat, and, as shown in Table 8-5, higher temperatures are required for a properly functioning hot air oven.

Destruction of microorganisms by dry heat is accomplished either by incineration or placement of items in a hot air oven. Obviously, direct flaming constitutes the most drastic application of dry heat, yet it is also one of the simplest procedures. No special apparatus is necessary, and 100% effectiveness is guaranteed. Disposal of infectious materials and organic wastes is safely accomplished using large incinerators; however, the practical application of this method in clinical areas is limited at best. Flaming is done during endodontic treatment and in gold foil procedures to sterilize the tips of instruments for immediate use. But aside from the flaming of wire loops in the microbiology laboratory before the sterile inoculation of cultures, other metallic items are unable to maintain their integrity with repeated flaming.

The proper use of a dry heat oven is recognized as an effective means of sterilization in dental practices. Since dry air is not as efficient a heat conductor as moist heat

TABLE 8-5 STERILIZATION TIME / TEMPERATURE / PRESSURE CHART

Type of sterilization	Time	Temperature (° F)	Pressure
Steam under pressure	15 to 20 minutes	250 to 270	15 to 20 pounds
Unsaturated chemical vapor	20 to 30 minutes*	270	Automatic
Dry heat	1 hour	320 to 350	0 pounds

*The cycle length or time is reduced in some machines.

at the same temperature, a much higher temperature is required for sterilization. The usual recommended practice is to hold the temperature at 160° C for 2 hours. A 1-hour exposure at 170° C or 238° F is also effective. These conditions are suitable for sterilizing glassware and metal instruments that rust or dull in the presence of water vapor. Many dental practitioners prefer the use of dry heat sterilizers in their offices because of the preservation of sharp cutting edges on their surgical instruments. In addition, many types of oils and powders with high heat resistance can be sterilized at 160° C to 170° C. However, these high temperatures will destroy many rubber- and plastic-based materials, melt the solder of most impression trays, and weaken some fabrics, as well as discolor other fabrics and paper materials. As with the design of newer generations of autoclaves, advances in the technology for dry heat sterilization continue. Dry heat convection units are currently available that use higher temperatures and require substantially shorter sterilization intervals.

One of the most common problems with using a dry heat sterilizer is the failure of clinical personnel to properly time the sterilization interval. Since the penetration of dry heat into the center of the pack is slow and dependent on both the size of packages and the type of wrapping material, a proper temperature must be attained in the chamber (preheating) before setting the timer. Thick wraps and larger-than-normal packages can significantly increase the interval required for assured sterility. Some individuals also view the prolonged exposure times for dry heat as a disadvantage. Some argue that if only one sterilizer is available, the 1- to 2-hour period plus cooling time disrupts a smooth flow of instrument recirculation. These aspects may be compared with those inherent for autoclaving and chemical vapor that are shown in Table 8-5.

MONITORING OF STERILIZATION

An integral component of office sterilization procedures is monitoring the efficiency of the system. A multitude of factors may diminish the effectiveness of an autoclave, dry heat sterilizer, or unsaturated chemical vapor apparatus. Frequent problems that are encountered include improper wrapping of instruments, which prevents adequate penetration to the instrument surface; human error in timing the cycle; defective control gauges that do not reflect actual conditions inside the sterilizer; and sterilizer malfunction.

Chemically treated tapes that change color or biologic controls to check for the proper functioning of an office sterilizer can be used. Materials that change color generally inform the practitioner that sterilized conditions have been reached but do not necessarily indicate that sterilization of the chamber contents has been

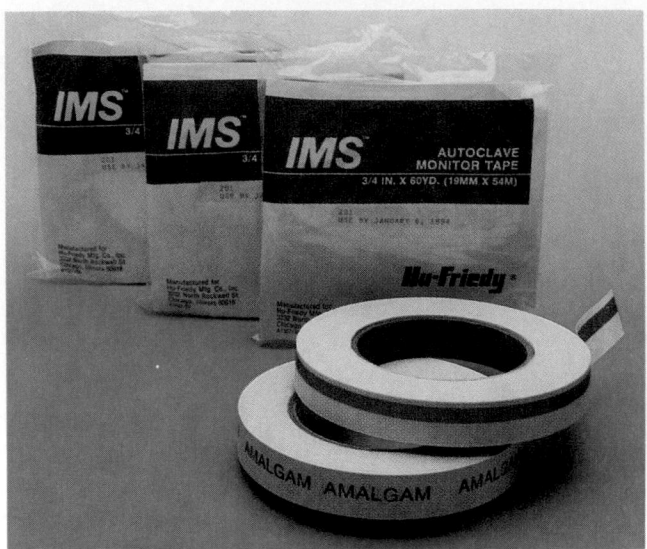

FIG. 8-11 In-office, biologic monitoring and testing system. (Courtesy of IMS Company.)

achieved. In addition, certain indicators change color long before sterilization occurs and before appropriate conditions are met. Autoclave tape is probably the worst offender in this regard, as it will change to show the striped markings following brief exposure to steam, which does not necessarily mean sterilization has occurred. It appears that the major use of specific chemical indicators to monitor sterilization is a routine check for each load of items processed through the sterilizer. Gross malfunctions can usually be detected quickly by using indicator labels, strips, and steam pattern cards (Fig. 8-11).

The use of calibrated biologic controls remains the main guarantee of sterilization. A test strip with harmless active spores is placed in the sterilization chamber with a normal load of instruments. The test strip is returned to the manufacturer or monitoring agency to verify that sterilization has occurred. The office is provided with written documentation that is maintained as a record. These preparations of bacterial spores are more resistant to heat than viruses and vegetative bacteria. Since a spore vehicle designed for one sterilization method is not necessarily the proper mode to use for other procedures, manufacturers produce both glass vials containing spores and biological test strips. The organisms most used are calibrated concentrations of either *Bacillus stearothermophilus* or *Bacillus subtilis* spores. These are either suspended in a nutrient medium (ampule form) or impregnated onto a test strip with the broth in an adjacent capsule. A pH indicator in the medium is also present; this changes color when spores germinate, thereby visually demonstrating a failure to sterilize. Since the spore preparations are relatively heat resistant, the proof of their destruction after exposure to the sterilization cycle is used to infer that all microorganisms exposed to the same conditions have been destroyed. The demonstration of sporicidal activity by an office sterilizer thus represents the most sensitive check for efficiency.

CHEMICAL AGENTS

Antiseptics and disinfectants are the most widely used of all drugs in public health practice, hospital practice, sanitation, and the household. These agents are used extensively in dental practices and hospitals despite the demonstrated limited effectiveness of certain substances. Many are applied to the skin of the patient or to the hands of the health professional (both, animate objects) and to environmental surfaces for disinfection of inanimate objects for use in controlling microbial contamination.

IDEAL PROPERTIES

Various chemical disinfectants and antiseptics may be employed. The antimicrobial spectra of these agents range from limited to broad. The most appropriate agent may be difficult to determine, since exaggerated claims may cloud actual performance capabilities. It is therefore advisable to compare the qualities of any product with the desirable properties for an *ideal* agent. It is always recommended to follow the manufacturer's directions regarding dilution rates, shelf life, reuse life, and effective usage time.

INSTRUMENT RECIRCULATION

Processing reusable items includes cleaning, packaging, sterilizing, monitoring, and storing packaged instruments. Accumulated debris, such as blood and saliva, can lengthen the interval required for sterilization or even prevent sterilization under certain conditions. Effectively, sterilization will not occur if debris is still present.

The initial requirement for instrument recirculation is to remove any collected organic matter. Hand scrubbing can accomplish this cleaning, although caution must always be exercised to prevent punctures. Puncture-resistant utility gloves should be worn to prevent this type of accident. An alternative or additional method of cleaning instruments uses an ultrasonic bath. This apparatus must be operated with a cover to prevent aerosolization of contaminants. Cleaning solutions are manufactured that are compatible with this type of unit and are changed regularly, depending on the rate of use. The metal container within the ultrasonic unit should be emptied and wiped with a suitable cleanser and/or disinfectant at frequent intervals (i.e., periodically during the day or after each use, depending on instrument load size).

The packaging of recirculated items for heat sterilization depends on the type of sterilizer used and the characteristics of the instruments. Cleaned instruments should be placed in heat-stable wraps, sealed, and dated. Sterilized instruments should remain wrapped until use. Many commercial wraps and sealed plastic pouches are able to maintain sterility for months if they remain unopened. Taking sterilized instruments out of a package and placing them in cabinet drawers for later use is *not* recommended. An updated list formulated by the ADA, regarding the application of various sterilization modalities for instruments and other intraoral items, is available for dental professionals. Corrosion or rusting of metallic instruments is a major fault of using steam under pressure for sterilization. Even the best autoclaves contain sufficient oxygen to cause corrosion of carbon steel during sterilization. An approach has been made using chemicals that vaporize in the autoclave and protect iron or steel from oxidation by hydrolysis. The use of a dry heat oven, chemical vapor sterilizer, or ethylene oxide unit prevents this adverse effect (Fig. 8-12, *A* and *B*). Table 8-6 contains a list of instruments and devices with suggested methods of processing.

The processing of dental instruments is a primary responsibility of the dental assistant, who must make decisions during instrument processing about whether an item should be discarded or sterilized. If the item is to be discarded, where should it be placed? Also the

---

BOX 8-10

STAGES OF CONTAMINATED TRAY PROCESSING

▶ Determine if the patient was a high-risk patient, and handle appropriately.
▶ Discard disposables.
▶ Place instruments in a holding tank for the prescribed time.
▶ Clean instruments in an ultrasonic cleaner.
▶ Rinse instruments thoroughly, and tap or blot dry.
▶ Determine method of sterilization or disinfection if appropriate.
▶ If steam under pressure is used, dip sharp and hinged instruments in protective emulsion.
▶ If chemical vapor is used, dry instruments completely before processing.
▶ If cold chemical is used, place instruments into the container, and cover with solution. If instruments are added after cycle timing has begun, the cycle must be restarted.
▶ Before the sterilization process begins, instruments can be packaged for the appropriate sterilization method.
▶ Remove the instruments from the sterilizer or disinfection solution.
▶ Return the instruments to storage area.

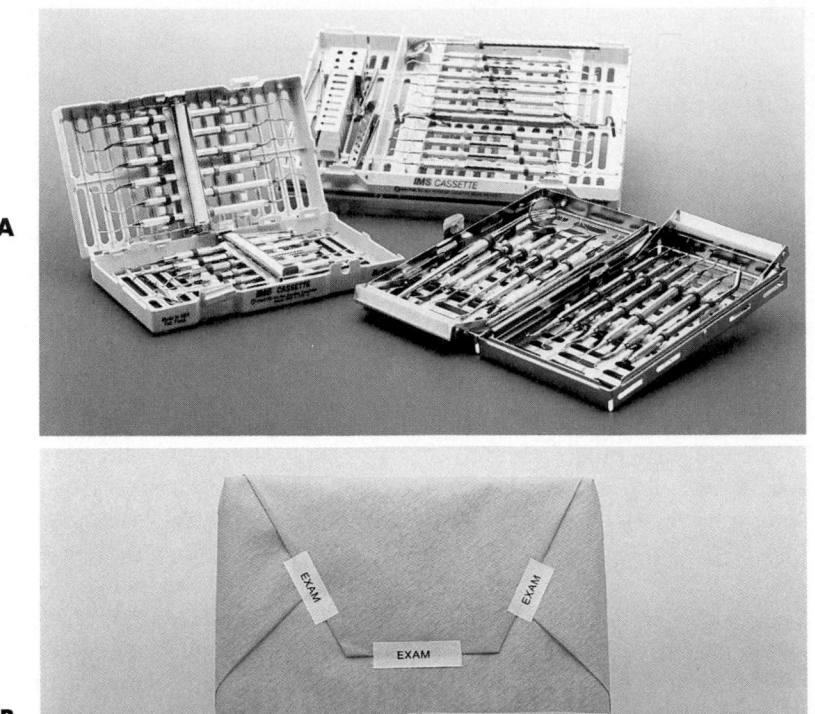

FIG. 8-12   **Cassette instrument sterilizing system.**
(Courtesy of Hu-Friedy.)

assistant must be aware of the types of instruments that need to be placed in an emulsion solution to protect sharp edges and hinged parts. The following steps are a synopsis of the processing stages of a contaminated tray (Box 8-10). Table 8-6 also provides methods for care of a selection of items with which the dental professional has daily contact.

HANDPIECE ASEPSIS

The issue of handpiece sterilization has been actively addressed recently. Previously, heat sterilization was not feasible for this equipment because handpieces were unable to withstand elevated temperatures. As a result, practitioners became used to disinfecting the outer surfaces of the handpiece. Asepsis of internal components, which are also exposed to saliva and blood, was not accomplished. Advances in technology are resolving many of these problems, with the result being that there is now routine manufacture and sale of heat-sterilizable

handpieces for dental practice. As a result, current infection control guidelines include a statement for the sterilization of dental handpieces each time they are used.

The current recommended methods for heat sterilization of handpieces are use of an autoclave or an unsaturated chemical vapor sterilizer, although newer generation, shorter cycle dry heat units also appear to be feasible. For handpieces that cannot withstand heat, the CDC has outlined a compromise precleaning and disinfection protocol. It should be noted here that handpieces should never be immersed in a disinfectant solution or treated with 2.0% to 3.0% glutaraldehyde preparations. Such misuse of these chemicals will shorten handpiece life dramatically, as well as increase the chances for glutaraldehyde toxicity reactions during operator handling.

Handpieces should also be properly lubricated before they are wrapped for sterilization. Failure to maintain the handpiece properly in this manner can also diminish its

TABLE 8-6 PREPARATION AND STERILIZATION PROCESS

List of instruments*	Sterilize before processing	Place in holding tank	Discard in biohazard bag	Discard in sharps container	Discard in trash receptacle	Discard in glycerine	Ultrasonic cleaning	Rinse in water and drain	Dip in emulsion and drain †	Dry instruments thoroughly ‡	Immerse in disinfectant	Sterilize in steam under pressure†	Sterilize in dry heat
Mirrors		X					X	X				X	
Explorer		X					X	X	X			X	
Cotton pliers		X					X	X	X			X	
Spoon excavator		X					X	X	X			X	
Articulating paper					X								
Cotton pellets					X								
2×2 cotton gauze					X								
Glass dappen dish		X										X	
Prophylaxis polishing cup					X								
Prophylaxis polishing brush					X								
Patient napkin, HBV patient	X												
Operator's protective glasses		X					X	X			X		
Amalgam carrier		X					X	X				X	
Leftover amalgam						X							
Plastic saliva ejector					X								
Endodontic file		X					X	X		X			X
Anesthetic syringe		X					X	X				X	
Anesthetic needle				X									
Anesthetic syringe, HBV patient	X		X										
Extracted tooth with granuloma			X	X									
Burs		X					X	X	X			X	
Unused activated amalgam capsule						X							
Contra angle							X	X	X			X	
Diamond stone		X					X	X	X			X	
Composite finishing disk					X								
Scissors		X					X	X	X			X	
Rubber dam					X								
Rubber dam frame		X					X	X				X	
Metal air/water syringe tip		X					X	X				X	
Nu-tip a/w sheath					X								
Plastic impression tray		X					X	X			X		

*Contaminated instruments, not otherwise noted, have been used on patients where there is no indication of HIV or HBV noted in patient record.

†This step is used only with steam under pressure method of sterilization.

‡This step is used when dry heat or unsaturated chemical vapor sterilization is used.

§An alternative to steam under pressure is unsaturated chemical vapor; but instruments must be dried thoroughly.

efficiency. These same procedures and precautions apply to other items, such as air or water syringe tips and ultrasonic scalers. At all times manufacturer's directions must be followed to preserve the integrity of the instruments.

SURFACE DISINFECTION

Although the use of disposable covers is increasing, those surfaces that do not lend themselves to coverage must be cleaned and disinfected. When the large number of operatory surfaces that may become contaminated with saliva, blood, or exudate (bioburden) is considered, it is apparent that surface disinfection is a major factor in achieving asepsis in the dental office environment. Disinfection of environmental surfaces is actually a two-step procedure. An initial mechanical removal of gross organic proteinaceous debris (precleaning) is required. To accomplish this the surfaces are sprayed with a disinfectant and/or detergent, followed by application of an appropriate disinfectant, with adequate time allowed for the chemical to achieve disinfection. This process is referred to as spray/wipe/spray/wipe. The first spray is to remove the bioburden, and the second spray is to achieve disinfection after a period of time that is designated by the manufacturer. Table 8-7 lists representative disinfectants and the adverse effects involved with

each one. Since proteinaceous debris renders coated microorganisms more resistant to the effect of many disinfectants, surface precleaning is a mandatory step before chemical disinfection. A product that cannot penetrate and remove accumulated debris fails at the first step of surface asepsis. The use of a disinfectant that provides residual antimicrobial effect with repeated use is also desirable.

It is important to note that manufacturers recommend that their products be used on precleaned surfaces. Although separate surface cleaners and surface disinfectants may be employed, use of a chemical agent that accomplishes both functions during the two-step protocol provides a more efficient approach.

The dental professional must always be aware of the instruments and armamentarium that are used during dental treatment and often become contaminated: cement bottles, varnish, paper pads, amalgamators, and light curing units. The surfaces of these objects can also transmit disease from one patient to another. These objects should be disinfected the same as other surfaces before they are used with another patient.

Using paper pads to mix and transfer dental cements and materials to the oral cavity allows contamination of the pad at chairside. The use of overgloves when handling paper pads does not eliminate contamination, since the paper pad is usually used near the oral cavity to

TABLE 8-7   REPRESENTATIVE CHEMICAL DISINFECTANT TYPES

Disinfectant	Activity	Adverse features
Alcohol	Bactericidal and tuberculocidal; not sporicidal, limited virucidal activity	Denatures proteins, making it difficult to remove them from surfaces; denatured proteins protect bacteria from the effects of alcohol; rapid evaporation from treated surfaces
Chlorine dioxide	Rapid disinfection activity; can be used for sterilization with 6-hr exposure	Corrosive; activity greatly reduced in the presence of protein and organic debris; requires good ventilation
Glutaraldehyde	As 2.0%-3.2% immersion preparation, broad-spectrum antimicrobial activity; sporicidal after 10 hr exposure; long use life; surface disinfectant product available at 0.25% concentration	Very corrosive to skin and mucous membranes; allergenic with repeated exposures
Hypochlorite	Rapid-acting, broad-spectrum bactericidal, sporicidal, virucidal agent	Irritating to skin; corrosive; can degrade plastics
Iodophors	Rapid-acting, broad-spectrum disinfectant; residual antimicrobial activity remains on surface after drying	Corrosive to some metals; may discolor some surfaces; inactivated by hard water
Phenols	Broad-spectrum antimicrobial activity; effective in the presence of detergents	Can degrade plastics; irritating to skin and eyes; inactivated by hard water and organic debris
Quaternary amines	Effective against gram-positive bacteria; later generations, broader spectrum	May be inactivated by soaps and hard water; inactivated by organic debris

NOTE: Protective gloves should be worn when using disinfectant preparations.

transfer material into the mouth. The use of glass or plastic slabs is an alternative. Either of these can be immersed in cold disinfection for 10 hours to obtain a viable alternative. Small plastic dividers are found in the ends of certain radiography film packets and can be used easily for placement of cements and liners.

EQUIPMENT ASEPSIS

Dental equipment that is small and heat resistant should be sterilized. All other equipment must be covered or disinfected. Thus, infection control should be considered with the purchase of new equipment. Office design, traffic flow, construction materials, and fixtures are all elements that must be taken into account when implementing an asepsis regimen. The dental chair should be without cloth surfaces, seamless, and easily cleaned. Hoses on dental units should be smooth, without ribs or grooves, and should allow for easy disinfection. Other design features that minimize contact between hand and contaminated surfaces include dental chairs that are foot controlled; sink faucets that are foot, forearm, or electronically controlled; soap dispensers that are foot or forearm controlled; towel dispensers that dispense disposable paper towels without requiring touching of a release mechanism; waste containers that are plastic lined and recessed under cabinets beneath a countertop opening; an air circulation exchange system or single-room air filtration unit that reduces the amount of *airborne* microbes; and a floor covering, such as vinyl, that is constructed in a smooth and continuous manner, eliminating crevices that can trap debris.

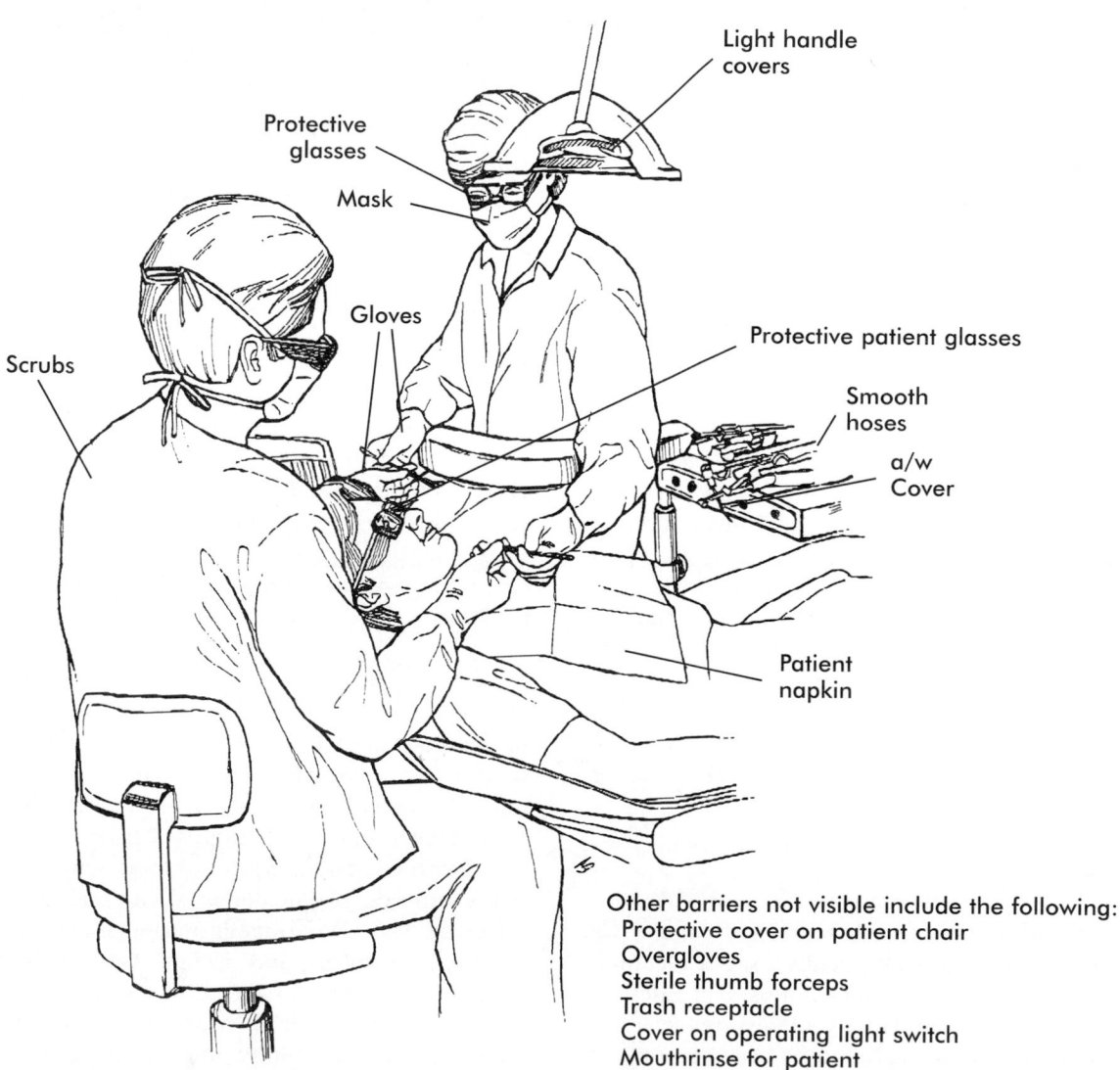

Light handle covers

Protective glasses

Mask

Scrubs

Gloves

Protective patient glasses

Smooth hoses

a/w Cover

Patient napkin

Other barriers not visible include the following:
Protective cover on patient chair
Overgloves
Sterile thumb forceps
Trash receptacle
Cover on operating light switch
Mouthrinse for patient

FIG. 8-13   Equipment covers and personal protection barriers used to eliminate cross-contamination.

COMMONLY USED BARRIERS

Barriers or coverings used to decrease the need for surface disinfection may include the following:

TREATMENT ROOM

Handle covers
On/off switch on operating light
Plastic bag over dental chair and adjustment buttons
Paper towel folded to cover working end of thumb forceps that is used to retrieve instruments from the mobile cabinet
Plastic tubing over hoses of unit (when accessible)
Plastic bag attached to mobile cabinet to catch debris
Overgloves to retrieve armamentarium or charts (Fig. 8-12)

RADIOGRAPHY TREATMENT ROOM

Plastic bag over radiographic head and position-indicating device
Plastic covering over on/off switch
Plastic covering over touch control panel
Plastic bag over dental chair
Covering over the area from which each dental film is retrieved if film is laid out on a surface before exposure, a covering placed under the films before use eliminates disinfection of the surface

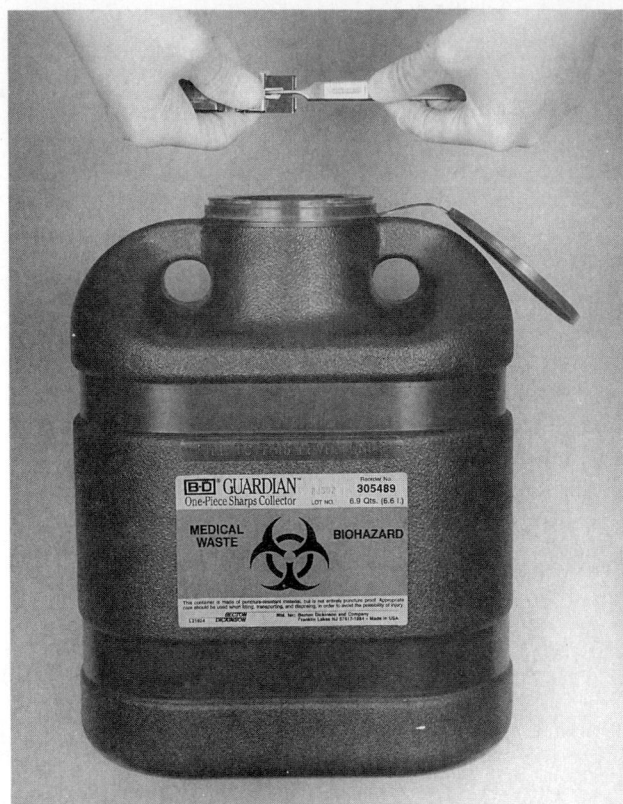

FIG. 8-14   Sharps container for designated *sharps.* (Courtesy of Becton-Dickinson Company, Franklin Lakes, New Jersey.)

Disposable barriers should be used whenever possible to avoid the necessity of excessive cleaning of both surfaces and equipment. Aluminum foil, plastic wrap, plastic bags, plastic-lined paper, or any other impervious sheeting can be used as a cover or barrier on equipment and surfaces (Box 8-11). For those equipment surfaces that cannot be covered, cleaning followed by disinfection is recommended. Certain coverings may be placed on light covers and other equipment in addition to the use of personal protective barriers pictured in Fig. 8-13. Some coverings on the surfaces may be reusable when placed in cold chemical for the time prescribed by the manufacturer's directions or can be disposed of after use. The elimination of any steps increases the risk of cross-contamination later.

DISPOSABLES

Items that are manufactured and identified for single use only or disposables, such as needles, saliva ejectors, prophylaxis cups and sealant, and composite brushes are not to be reused. The availability of disposable items continues to increase as manufacturers, distributors, and office personnel recognize their usefulness. Examples of recently marketed items include disposable prophylaxis angles, rag wheels, evacuation line traps, and HVE tips.

These products present lowered, cross-contamination risks, since they do not undergo recleaning and recycling, but they must be disposed of properly. This is especially important for needles and other sharps, which (1) should not be recapped by hand; and (2) should be placed in puncture-resistant containers for disposal (Fig. 8-14).

LABORATORY ASEPSIS

Impressions, prosthetic devices, and the instrumentation used in their construction generally require handling by multiple individuals, both in the dental office and in commercial dental laboratories. These items, contaminated with the patient's saliva, blood, and, in the case of old prostheses, plaque deposits, can serve as sources of infection. The ADA Councils on Dental Therapeutics and Prosthetic Services and Dental Laboratory Relations updated guidelines for infection control in dental laboratories in 1988. The ADA and the CDC have recommended that impressions, appliances, and other items that are removed from the mouth of a patient must be cleaned and disinfected before they are sent to the laboratory. Additionally, items received from the labora-

TABLE 8-8   GUIDE FOR SELECTION OF DISINFECTANT SOLUTIONS

	Glutaraldehydes[1]	Iodophors[2]	Clorine compounds[3]	Complex phenolics[1]
IMPRESSIONS				
Alginate	−	+	+	−
Polysulfide	+	+	+	+
Silicone	+	+	+	+
Polyether	+[4]	+[4]	+	+[4]
ZOE impression paste	+	+	−	?
Reversible hydrocolloid	−	+	+	?
Compound	−	+	+	−
PROSTHESES / APPLIANCES[5,6]				
Fixed (metal/porcelain)	+	−	−	?
Removable (acrylic/porcelain)	−	+	+	−
Removable (metal/acrylic)	−	+[7]	+[7]	−
Appliances (all metal)	+	−	−	?

Impressions/prosthesis should be rinsed under running water and then immersed for the time recommended for TB disinfection with the selected product. Thorough rinsing of impressions and prostheses under running tap water following disinfection is necessary to remove any residual disinfectant. (Courtesy Virginia A. Merchant, M.S., D.M.D., University of Detroit Mercy School of Dentistry, Detroit, Mich, 1993.)
[1] Prepared according to the manufacturer's instructions for disinfection.
[2] 1 : 213 dilution.
[3] 1 : 10 dilution of commercial bleach or prepared according to the manufacturer's instructions for disinfection.
[4] Use with caution. Consult manufacturer's recommendation.
[5] May also be ethylene oxide sterilized.
[6] Prostheses or appliances that have been worn by patients must be thoroughly cleaned before disinfection.
[7] Use minimal exposure time (10 minutes) to avoid damage to metal.

tory for delivery to a patient must be cleaned and disinfected before placement. All items must be disinfected according to product directions.

Materials and the instrumentation used in constructing dental prostheses pose special problems in maintaining an aseptic environment and in the delivery of a noncontaminated prosthesis to the patient. Many of these items may be damaged by exposure to heat or the chemicals may be used for disinfection. The use of barriers to prevent contamination, of separate materials for new devices and those previously inserted in the mouth and of unit doses of polishing materials, will minimize cross-contamination in the dental laboratory setting.

Disinfection of dental impressions and prostheses must be undertaken with caution to avoid distorting impressions and damaging the metal, porcelain, or acrylic surfaces of prostheses. Several groups of investigators have conducted studies to evaluate the effects of various disinfectant solutions on these materials. Table 8-8 presents recommendations for the disinfection of impressions and prostheses based on the results of several research investigations. Immersion is preferred over spraying when possible, since this ensures that all surfaces are adequately exposed to the disinfectant. Thorough rinsing under running tap water is essential both before disinfection to remove bioburden and after disinfection to remove any residual disinfectant.

Educating Patients about Infection Control Programs

Effective infection control must occur as a routine component of professional activity. The use of universal precautions in the management of all patients greatly minimizes occupational exposure to microbial pathogens by addressing the reality that most potentially infectious individuals are asymptomatic and therefore undiagnosed.

Procedures aimed at preventing the spread of infectious disease during dental treatment are also constantly being evaluated by the profession and an increasingly inquisitive public. The dilemma faced by dental practitioners was concisely summarized by Crawford (1987):

Discrepancies between *the ideal* and *the real* in dental asepsis provide fertile ground for rash statements of two kinds: "Sterilize everything! *versus* Do nothing, the mouth is a dirty place!" Both are expressions of compulsion, fear or frustration about a seemingly impossible dilemma. They may reflect the sentiment, "Go away; let me alone." Practical reality, of course, dictates that to prevent the possible spread of infectious diseases, dental professionals must be provided with inclusive, up-to-date information that can be utilized to develop an optimal program of asepsis.

When such a program has been implemented by the practitioner and auxiliary staff, the risk of disease transmission is significantly reduced.

BOX 8-12

MINIMUM DENTAL OFFICE INFECTION CONTROL PROGRAM

- Comprehensive medical history
- Hepatitis B vaccine
- Antiseptic mouthrinse
- Antiseptic handrinse
- Disposable face mask
- Disposable latex gloves
- Protective eyewear
- Clinic attire
- Rubber dam
- Sharps disposable container

- Sterilizable handpieces
- Ultrasonic cleaner
- Instrument packaging
- Heat sterilizer
- Sterilization monitoring
- Glutaraldehyde
- Surface cleaner
- Surface disinfectant
- Surface covers
- Waste disposal system

- *OSHA* poster

Much has been accomplished over the past 20 years in the clinical application of infection control techniques and procedures. Implementation and compliance with appropriate recommendations by many dental professionals and governmental organizations continue to have a major impact on the way dental treatment is provided in the 1990s. It is important to continue to remain current with developments as new information becomes available.

Box 8-12 presents 21 items that can be used to evaluate your own practice infection control program. Approach the task with a positive attitude, building on the strengths of your existing infection control procedures.

Substantial changes have been made, and our patients should be made aware of our professional efforts. Such communication of infection control measures to patients not only allays potential perceived fears, but also serves to reinforce patient confidence in the dental treatment that is being provided.

KEY POINTS

- In a dental office transmission of infection may occur through sources such as blood, saliva, nasal discharge, hands, clothing, and hair.

- Diseases can be transmitted by direct contact, indirect contact, or inhalation.
- Although HBV, HIV, tuberculosis, and other diseases pose risks for the health professional, it is well established that HBV remains the major occupational infection for the health professional.
- Universal precautions break the cycle of infection and eliminate cross-infection.
- Basic principles of an infection control program include patient screening, immunization, aseptic technique, personal protection, instrument sterilization, disinfection procedures, equipment asepsis, and dental laboratory asepsis.
- Regulatory agencies provide procedural guidelines for health professionals.
- Common sterilization techniques used in dentistry include steam under pressure, unsaturated chemical vapor, and dry heat.
- An effective infection control program must be a routine component of a dental practice and must be effectively communicated to all staff members and patients.

BIBLIOGRAPHY

American Dental Association: *Dental teamwork,* vol 7(1), Chicago, 1994, The Association.

Cottone JA, Geza TT, Molinari JA: *Practical infection control in dentistry,* Philadelphia, 1991, Lea & Febiger.

Crawford JJ: *Clinical asepsis in dentistry,* Mesquite, Tx, 1987, R.A. Kolstad.

Council on Dental Material, Instruments, and Equipment; Council on Dental Practice; Council on Dental Therapeutics: Infection control for the dental office and dental laboratory, *JADA* 116:241-248, Feb 1988.

Council on Dental Materials and Devices; Council on Dental Therapeutics: Infection control in the dental office, *JADA* 97(4):673-677, 1978.

Department of Labor, Occupational Safety and Health Administration: *Occupational exposure to blood-borne pathogens,* Instruction CPL2-244B, Dec 6, 1991.

Hopp JW, Rogers EA: *AIDS and the allied health professions,* Philadelphia, 1989, F.A. Davis.

Morbidity and Mortality Weekly Report: *Perspectives in disease prevention and health promotion,* 37:(24):1, June 24, 1988.

Personal communication, 1987.

U.S. Department of Health and Human Services, Centers for Disease Control and Prevention: *Recommended infection-control practices for dentistry,* 1993.

9 Dental Radiography

LEARNING OBJECTIVES

You will have mastered the material in this chapter when you can:
▶ Define the key terms
▶ Describe how x-ray photons are produced in a radiographic machine
▶ List and identify equipment components that limit and control excessive exposure to ionizing radiation in dentistry
▶ Define the ALARA concept
▶ List and identify procedures used to minimize exposure to ionizing radiation
▶ Observe the patient's reaction and modify the procedure to ensure patient comfort throughout the radiographic examination
▶ Answer patient safety questions or concerns based on knowledge, facts, and scientific data
▶ Describe the process by which radiographic images are created
▶ Describe the film placement and angle of projection used in the two major intraoral techniques (bisecting and paralleling)
▶ Differentiate between the types of radiographic films and how they are used in dentistry
▶ Select the appropriate film and correctly position it for all periapical and bitewing projections
▶ Define radiographic characteristics of density, contrast, geometric unsharpness, magnification, and shape distortion
▶ List the visual characteristics of an acceptable radiograph
▶ List and explain the quality control procedures necessary in dental radiography
▶ Evaluate radiographs for technical and diagnostic quality; determine if retake or additional radiographs are required for adequate diagnostic evaluation of the region of interest
▶ Given a radiograph of poor quality, identify and explain the cause and correction of errors
▶ Describe how dental radiographic film is developed
▶ Explain automatic and manual processing procedures
▶ Explain the process of film duplication used in dentistry
▶ Explain the legal factors involved in exposing, transferring, and retaining dental radiographs

KEY TERMS

Anode	Maximum permissible dose (MPD)
As low as reasonably	Milliampere (mA)
achievable (ALARA)	Occlusal radiograph
Atoms	Panoramic
Bisecting technique	Paralleling technique
Bitewing (BW)	Periapical radiograph (PA)
Bremsstrahlung	Position-indicating device (PID)
Cathode	Quality assurance
Cephalometric radiograph	Rad
Characteristic radiation	Radiation
Collimation	Radiation safety
Electrons	Radiograph
Energy	Radiology
Epilation	Radiolucent
Erythema	Radiopaque
Exposure	Rem
Filtration	Selective absorption
Gray	Sievert
Kilovolt peak (kVp)	Target
Kinetic energy	Tubehead
Matter	X-ray

Radiographs, visible images on a film, play such a vital role in diagnosing and managing care that it is difficult to imagine the practice of dentistry without them. One of the most important responsibilities of the qualified dental assistant is to expose, process, and mount dental radiographs. Learning to safely operate and maintain radiographic equipment is essential. Radiographic image quality directly contributes to the standard of care patients receive. For these reasons, federal law requires that states establish minimum educational and certification requirement for professionals who perform radiographic procedures. This chapter provides the background information necessary to produce diagnostic radiographs of the highest quality. It is the dental assistant's responsibility to practice perfect technical skills and to learn the specific legal requirements in the state.

History of Ionizing Radiation

A German physicist, Wilhelm Roentgen, discovered x-rays on November 8, 1895. The first radiograph (x-ray) ever made was of Wilhelm's wife Bertha. Wilhelm placed Bertha's hand on a photographic plate and directed x-rays toward it. When the plate was developed, an image of the bones of her hand appeared. It is said that Bertha was so frightened by this experience that she refused to return to her husband's laboratory. Bertha was not alone in her fear of x-rays; controversy concerning the use of x-rays spread almost as quickly as their discovery.

Scientists throughout the world began experimenting with x-rays. It was not long before the diagnostic value of x-rays was recognized. In 1896 Professor Edwin B. Frost of Dartmouth College diagnosed a fractured arm using x-rays. In that same year (January 1896), Dr. Otto Walkoff of Germany made the first dental radiograph. He placed a glass photographic plate covered with black paper and a rubber dam in his mouth and exposed it to 25 minutes of radiation. An exposure of this magnitude is incomprehensible by today's standards.

Edmund Kells, mentioned earlier in this text as being a significant contributor to the advancement of dental assistants, also made major contributions to dental radiography. Kells was the first dentist in the United States to use radiography. He conducted seminars and training programs in the application of radiography for dental diagnosis. Many of the principles Dr. Kells taught remain as standards of modern practice. For example, in an 1899 issue of *Dental Cosmos* he stressed the importance of keeping the film parallel to the teeth and at right angles to the x-ray beam. It was Dr. Kells who recommended using radiographs to ensure that endodontic wires did not extend beyond the tooth apex.

Unfortunately, Kells, like many scientists of his time, failed to recognize the harmful effects of radiation. It was common practice to focus the x-ray tube using the bones of the hands. Dr. Kells followed this practice of *setting the tube* for 12 years with no apparent damage. Then cancerous tumors developed on his hands and quickly spread to other parts of his body. Early in 1926 Kells's left arm was amputated. Later that same year, several fingers on his right hand had to be amputated. He developed radiation-induced cataracts and began to lose his eyesight. After enduring much pain and faced with the prospect of being a burden to his family, Kells committed suicide on May 7, 1928.

The discovery of x-rays not only significantly advanced the practice of dentistry, but also ranks as one of the most important scientific discoveries ever. Many scientists who contributed greatly to our understanding of the physical properties of x-rays remained unaware of the biologic consequences of the newly discovered energy. Careless and excessive x-ray exposures resulted in the death of many early x-ray pioneers. Although modern radiation protection practices originated from this unfortunate history, the consequences of excessive radiation exposures remain prominent in the public perspective. Dental professionals must be knowledgeable about x-radiation so that we can address patients' concerns and operate x-ray equipment safely and effectively.

Physical Properties of the Universe

To understand how x-rays are produced and how they interact with the human body, it is necessary to review some basic laws of physics. All things in the world around us can be classified as either matter or energy. Albert

TABLE 9-1   FORMS OF ENERGY

Energy form	Definition	Examples
Potential	Energy processed by matter by virtue of position	A guillotine blade pulled to its maximum height
Kinetic	Energy possessed by matter	A moving automobile, a turning windmill
Chemical	Energy released when molecular bonds are broken	An explosion, the act of metabolizing food
Electrical	Energy produced by moving electrons	Household electricity; an alternating flow of electrons that drives motors, operates appliances, etc.
Thermal	Energy associated with molecular motion	Kinetic energy of atoms; heat—the faster molecules move, the higher thermal energy they possess
Nuclear	Energy contained in the atomic nucleus	Nuclear power plants and atomic bombs
Electromagnetic	Energy moving through space	Radiowaves, microwaves, light, x-rays

Einstein is famous for discovering the interchangeability of matter and energy known as the theory of relativity. Einstein's mass equivalence equation, $E = mc^2$, describes the relationship of matter and energy where E is energy, m is mass, and c is the speed of light.

▶ Matter

Matter is anything that occupies space and has form or shape. Matter is the substance of which all physical objects are made. Matter has many forms, including solids, liquids, and gases. Matter is composed of **atoms** grouped together in specific arrangements called molecules.

▶ Energy

Energy is defined as the ability to do work. The seven fundamental types of energy are seen in Table 9-1. Electromagnetic radiation is the form of energy used in dentistry to make radiographic images. A constant amount of energy exists in the universe. Although energy can neither be created or destroyed, it can change form, thus maintaining total energy within the universe constant.

Atoms contain energy. The energy holding the nucleus together is called nuclear binding energy. The energy holding **electrons**, negatively charged particles, in their shells is known as electron binding energy. Inner shell electrons have greater binding energy than outer shell electrons. Nuclear and electron binding energies are characteristic for a given atom; the magnitude of these energies increases as the atomic number increases.

▶ Ionization

Electrons can be removed from an atom in a process called **ionization**. Enough energy to overcome electron binding energy must be absorbed by the atom for ionization to occur. Ionization results in the formation of an ion pair: a negatively charged free electron and the remaining part of the atom, now positively charged. The amount of energy required to displace outer shell electrons is less than that required to displace inner shell electrons. Ionization most frequently occurs in the outer electron shells. X-rays, however, can impart enough energy to an atom to displace inner shell electrons. When inner shell electrons are removed from an atom, the resulting ion is unstable. The remaining electrons in this unstable ion rearrange to fill the vacant inner shell, leaving the outer shell unfilled. **Characteristic radiation** is emitted from the atom when these electron rearrangements occur (Fig. 9-1). The energy of the characteristic radiation emitted is approximately equal to the difference in the electron binding energy between the shells.

Principles of Radiation

Although space appears empty, it is actually filled with electromagnetic radiation. The energy of this radiation ranges from low-energy radiowaves to high-energy gamma rays. The many types of electromagnetic radiation are grouped together and known as the electromagnetic spectrum (Fig. 9-2). Although visible light can be seen, it comprises less than 1% of the electromagnetic spectrum. We are unaware of the radiowaves surrounding us until a radio or television receiver intercepts them.

An important property of electromagnetic radiation is that substances selectively absorb, reflect, or transmit it, depending on their structure. **Selective absorption**, the ability of a substance to absorb or transmit x-rays is used to create dental radiographs.

▶ Bremsstrahlung Radiation

The transformation of kinetic energy to electromagnetic energy in an x-ray tube is known as **Bremsstrahlung radiation**. Bremsstrahlung is a German word that

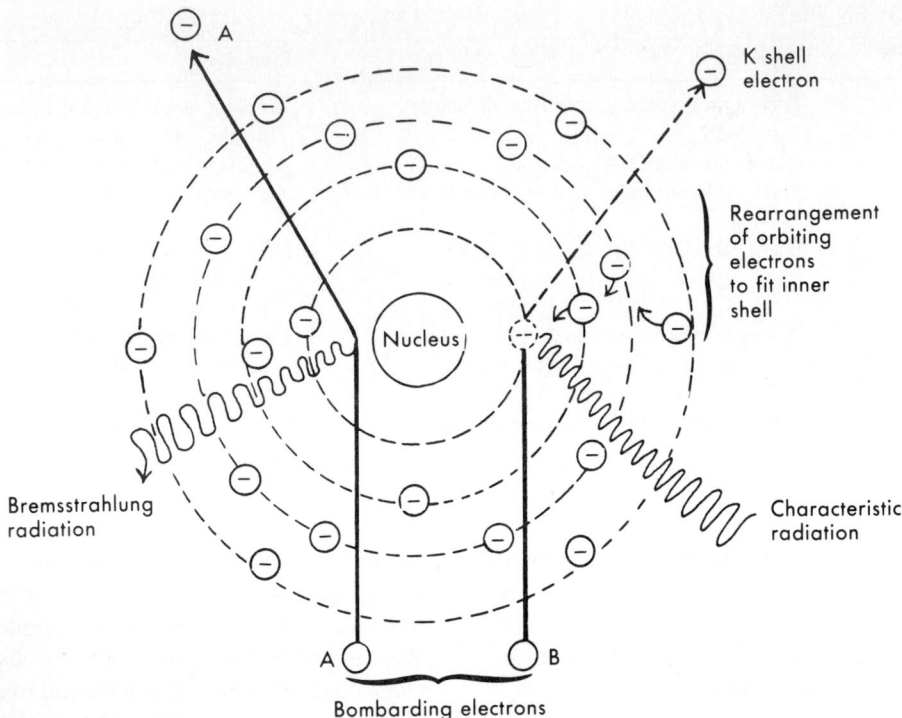

FIG. 9-1   Electrons colliding with a simulated tungsten atom forming Bremsstrahlung and characteristic radiation.

(From Frommer HH: *Radiology for dental auxiliaries,* ed 5, St Louis, 1992, Mosby.)

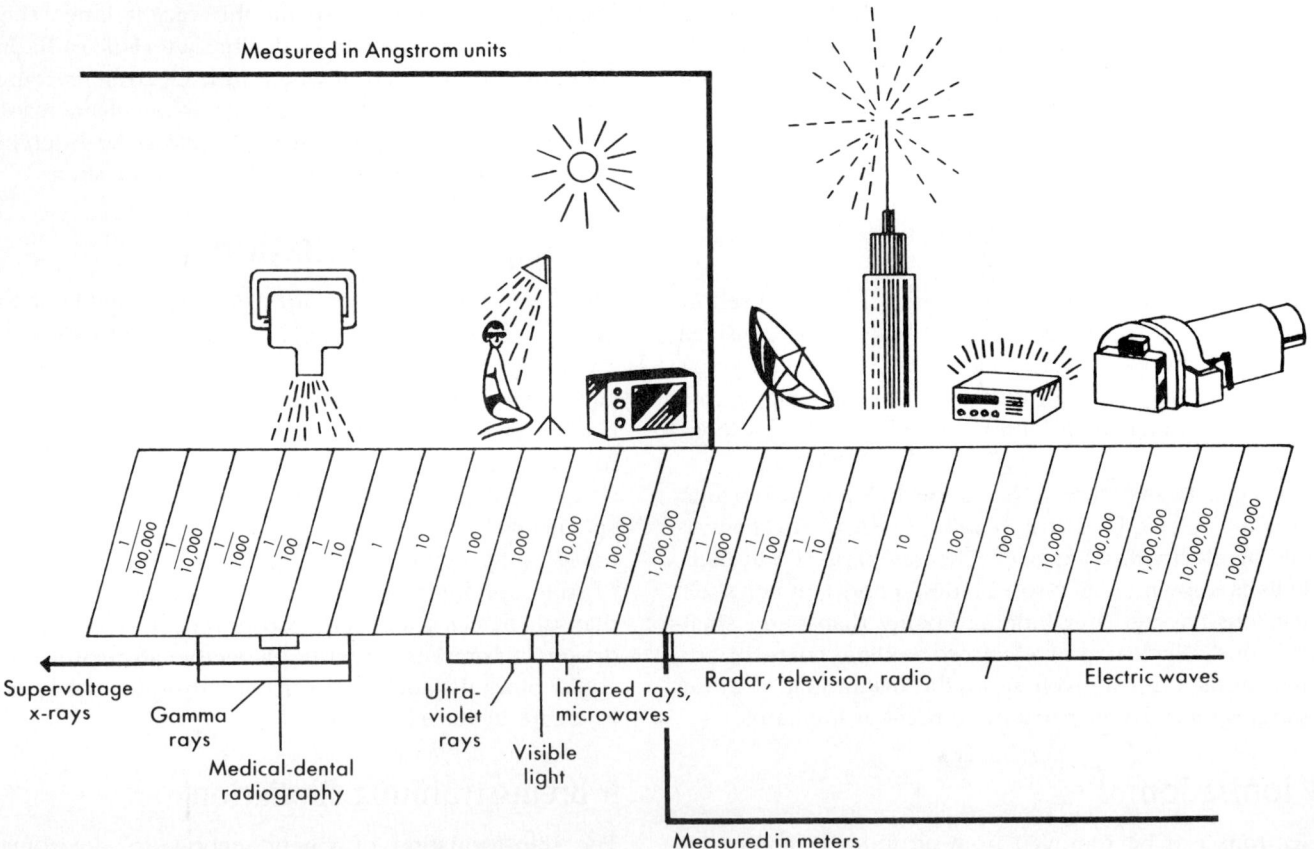

FIG. 9-2   Electromagnetic spectrum.

(From Frommer HH: *Radiology for dental auxiliaries,* ed 5, St Louis, 1992, Mosby.)

roughly translated means "braking radiation." This term was coined because radiation produced in the diode tube occurs when electrons are decelerated. The production of Bremsstrahlung radiation within the diode tube is, however, an inefficient process (see Fig. 9-1). Only about 1% of the electron interactions at the target actually result in x-ray production. Bremsstrahlung radiation occurs only when electrons strike the target close to a tungsten nucleus. The positive nuclear charge places an electrostatic force on the electron, causing it to decelerate suddenly, releasing enough energy to produce an x-ray photon. The majority (99%) of electrons striking the target dissipate acquired kinetic energy as heat. Dissipation of kinetic energy as heat occurs when electrons transfer some energy to orbital electrons in the tungsten target atom but do not cause ionization. Finally, some electrons interact with tungsten orbital electrons, imparting enough energy to ionize the tungsten target. As discussed earlier, when electrons displace inner shell electrons, characteristic radiation is produced. Thus, there are three major interactions of electrons with target atoms:

▶ Heat
▶ Bremsstrahlung radiation
▶ Characteristic radiation

Dental Radiographic Equipment

Radiographic equipment or x-ray machines are devices that use moving charges (electrons) to produce electromagnetic radiation. Laboratory electromagnetic radiation is designated as *x-rays*. A typical dental x-ray machine is illustrated in Fig. 9-3. An x-ray machine contains a tubehead, suspension arm, control panel, and power source.

The **tubehead** is the working part of the x-ray machine (Fig. 9-4). The *yoke* attaches the tubehead to a movable *suspension arm*. The tubehead rotates freely, allowing dental x-rays to be made from several directions and accommodating patients of different sizes and shapes. The tubehead is attached to the yoke by two *vertical connectors*. The *vertical connectors* allow adjustments in the vertical angle of the tubehead, while the yoke allows adjustments in the horizontal angle. The suspension arm is used to adjust the height of the tubehead independent of its vertical or horizontal position. The **position-indicating device (PID)**, the portion of the tubehead that emits the radiation, extends from the tubehead and directs radiation toward the patient. X-rays exit the machine from the PID only when the exposure switch is depressed.

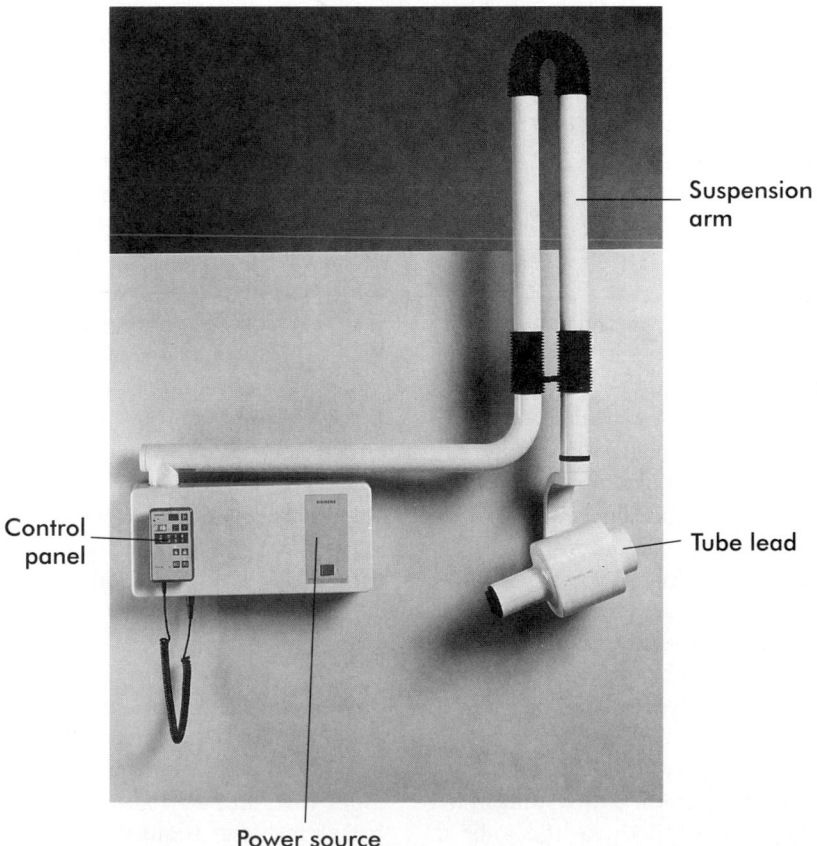

FIG. 9-3 **X-ray machine with tubehead, suspension arm, control panel and power source.**
(Courtesy of Pelton and Crane Company, Charlotte, North Carolina.)

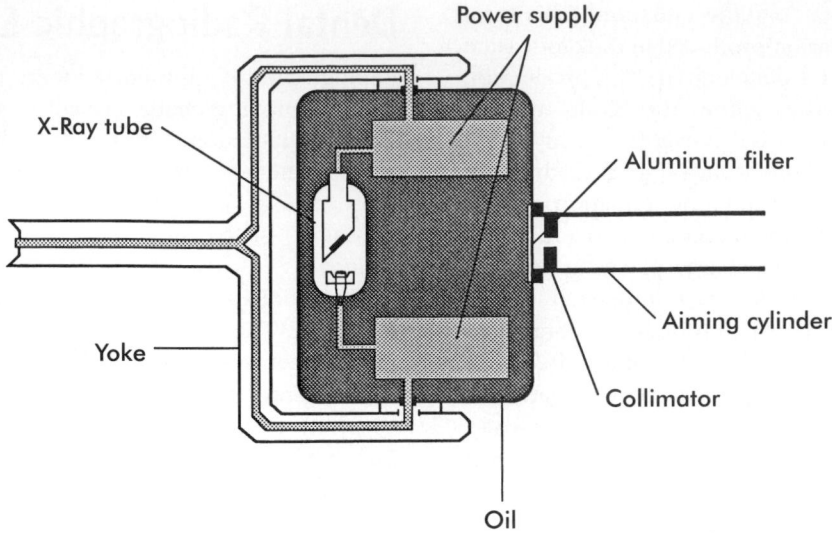

FIG. 9-4   Illustration of tubehead parts.

(From Goaz PW, White SC: *Oral radiology, principles and interpretation,* ed 3, St Louis, 1994, Mosby.)

Within the tubehead housing is a *diode tube.* The diode tube is the most important part of the tubehead because x-rays originate within this tube. A wire in the suspension arm connects the tubehead to the *control panel.* Power is supplied to the system through an electrical outlet.

The X-ray Tube

A closer view of the diode tube is seen in Fig. 9-5. The two main components of the diode tube are the **cathode** and the **anode**. The cathode provides a source of negatively charged particles (electrons). It contains a tungsten *filament* and a molybdenum *focusing cup.* When electrical current passes through the filament, electrons are given off by a process called thermionic emission, or heat production. The focusing cup further concentrates electrons into a cloud of charged particles. The **milliamperage (mA)** setting on the control panel regulates the amount of electrical current passing through the filament. Increasing the mA increases the number of electrons emitted by the filament. In many dental x-ray machines the mA is set by the manufacturer, usually between 7 and 10 mA. In other dental x-ray machines the mA can be changed by the operator.

The anode contains a copper *stem* and a tungsten **target**. When high voltage is applied to the tube, electrons are accelerated from the cathode toward the anode. These accelerating electrons contain kinetic energy, the energy of motion. When the electrons collide with the tungsten target, they stop suddenly. This sudden stop transforms the electron's kinetic energy into electromagnetic energy, thus producing x-rays. It is important to remember that the electron does not become an x-ray, but rather its **kinetic energy** is transformed to x-ray energy. The amount of kinetic energy acquired by electrons in the diode tube, depends on the peak **kilovoltage (kVp)**—the maximum amount of voltage that an x-ray machine is using—applied to the tube; when the kVp setting is high, the x-rays produced are more energetic and readily penetrate objects. Likewise, when the kVp setting is low, the x-rays produced are less energetic and more likely to be absorbed by objects. Because soft tissues absorb more x-rays when the kVp setting is low, federal law requires dental x-ray machines to operate at 50 kVp or higher. Dental x-ray machines are usually operated between 65 and 90 kVp.

Control Panel

The control panel of a dental radiographic machine contains an on/off switch with an indicator light, exposure button with indicator light and audible signal, timer dial, and kVp and mA selectors (Fig. 9-6).

Federal law requires the *exposure button* to be connected to an indicator light and audible signal. When the exposure button is depressed, the indicator light and

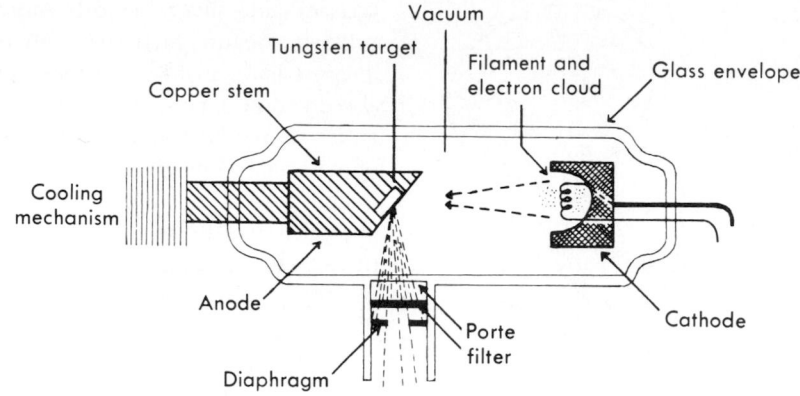

FIG. 9-5   X-ray tubehead has two main components, the cathode and the anode.

(From Frommer HH: *Radiology for dental auxiliaries,* ed 5, St Louis, 1992, Mosby.)

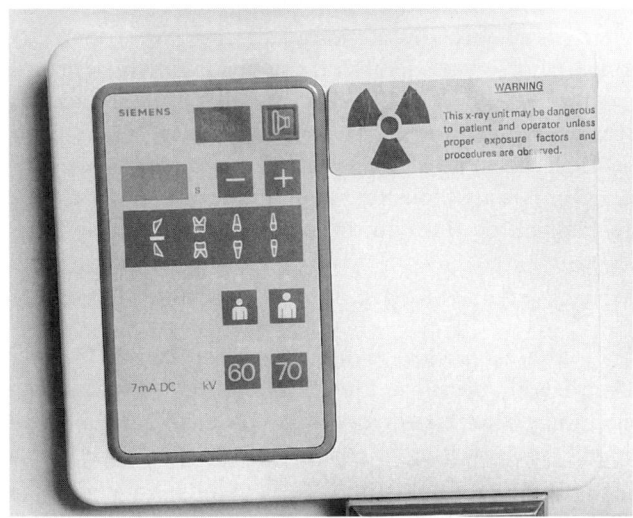

FIG. 9-6   Control panel of a radiographic unit.

(Courtesy of Pelton and Crane Company, Charlotte, North Carolina.)

audible signal are activated, signaling that x-rays are being produced. The exposure button must be a *dead-man* type. This means the switch operates only with continuous pressure.

The *on/off switch* controls electrical current to the radiographic machine. When the machine is turned on, an indicator light signals that x-rays can be generated.

The *timer dial* controls the number of impulses generated by the radiographic machine. The number of impulses produced is based on the cycle of electrical current available. For instance, if 60- or 70-cycle alternating currents are available, the number of impulses generated in 1 second would be 60 or 70 impulses. One impulse is equal to $\frac{1}{60}$ of a second. Most dental x-ray units do not use fractions for designation of x-rays emitted, but use impulses emitted. If a machine dial

is set for *16,* 16 impulses are emitted per second.

The exposure switch or button is located on the control panel. When the button is depressed, the circuit of electricity is completed, allowing the flow of electrons to occur and the x-ray process to continue.

The timer determines the length of time radiation is produced. Thus, like the mA, the timer also controls the number of x-rays produced, but not their energy. When the kVp and mA are preset (fixed) by the manufacturer, changing the timer is the only way to control x-ray output. For example, it may be necessary to increase exposure time slightly when duplicate (more than one film in a packet) film packets are used. Federal laws also regulate the accuracy of x-ray machine timers.

Collimation and Filtration

When electrons strike the anode their kinetic energy is transformed into electromagnetic photons (x-rays). X-rays are produced in many directions and of varying energies. To produce a useful beam of radiation, the x-rays must be collimated and filtered.

▶ Collimation

Collimation is the restriction in the size of the x-ray beam through the use of a lead shielding and diaphragms. The first step in constructing a useful beam of radiation is shielding the diode tube with a lead cylinder (see Fig. 9-4). This lead cylinder completely encases the tube except for a small opening, the window, or aperture. The lead cylinder completely absorbs x-rays, creating a beam of radiation at the window. The x-ray beam is further limited with an open-ended, lead-lined collimator. This collimator, also called the position-indicating device (PID), further restricts the diameter of the beam of

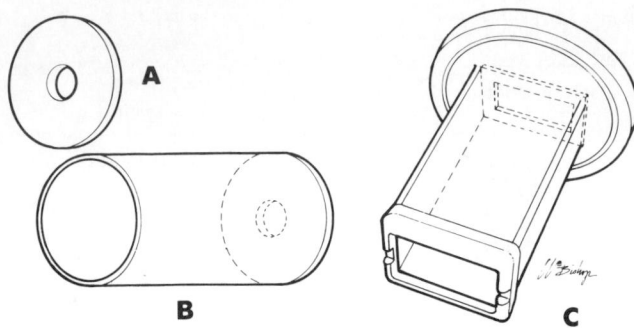

FIG. 9-7   *A,* Diaphram collimator. *B,* Tubular collimator. *C,* Rectangular collimator.

(From Goaz PW, White SC: *Oral radiology, principles and interpretation,* ed 3, St Louis, 1994, Mosby.)

radiation reaching the patient. The collimator is one of the most important ways patient exposure is kept to a minimum. The beam of radiation should be collimated so that it closely approximates the size of film used. Federal law requires the dental x-ray beam be no more than 2.75 inches in diameter. Using film holders, it is possible to limit a dental x-ray beam even more than is required by law. For example, rectangular collimators expose the patient to about half the radiation of round collimators (Fig. 9-7).

▶ Filtration

Remember that x-rays are produced at the target not only in all directions, but also at varying energies. Low-energy x-rays would be absorbed in the patient's soft tissues and contribute little to the radiographic image. These low energy x-rays can be preferentially removed from the beam with **added filtration**. Thus, added filtration selectively removes low-energy x-rays from the primary beam, reducing patient dose. Added filtration usually consists of a disk of aluminum placed at the window. Federal law requires 1.5 mm of added aluminum filtration when operating at 50 to 70 kVp and at least 2.5 mm of aluminum when operating above 70 kVp.

▶ Selective Absorption

An important property of electromagnetic radiation is that substances selectively absorb, reflect, or transmit radiation, depending on their structure. We use this selective absorption of radiation to create x-ray images, dental radiographs.

The amount of radiation absorbed by a substance depends on three aspects of its structure: effective atomic number, physical density, and thickness. Structures made up of atoms having large atomic numbers, such as

enamel and silver, absorb most of the x-rays in the primary beam. Structures made of atoms with an intermediate atomic number, like bones and dentin, absorb some x-rays, while many are transmitted. Finally, x-rays are readily transmitted through structures made up of material of low atomic number, like soft tissue and the dental pulp.

The human body selectively absorbs radiation. Structures that are physically dense (compact) absorb more radiation. For example, enamel, being denser than dentin, absorbs more x-rays. Cortical bone, which is more compact than medullary bone, absorbs more x-rays. On the other hand, cavities created by dental caries allow more x-rays to pass through. A large patient requires a higher mA setting to produce a dental radiograph because larger (thicker) anatomic structures will absorb more radiation.

Using Selective Absorption to Make Radiographs

When x-rays are directed toward the jaw, the teeth, bones, and soft tissue selectively absorb them, creating a pattern of *remnant* radiation unique for that individual. Because we cannot see this remnant x-ray pattern, we must use a receptor to collect it. In dental radiology the receptor is x-ray film. X-ray film detects the photons that are transmitted through the patient.

Transmission of X-ray to Film

X-ray film is a clear polyester sheet coated with a silver-halide *emulsion.* The film emulsion is sensitive to radiation. When x-rays strike the emulsion, silver atoms are released, creating an area of blackness. In areas where many photons strike the film, it becomes black; these black areas are called **radiolucent** areas. Remember that these black areas represent structures penetrated by x-ray photons. Areas where the film remains light are called **radiopaque**. Radiopacities correspond to tissues that have absorbed much of the radiation. Thus, silver amalgam fillings, which absorb a lot of radiation, are radiopaque (white), while cavities caused by dental caries are radiolucent (black). We count on the unique way a patient absorbs x-ray energy to make a diagnostic image.

Biologic Effects of Electromagnetic Radiation

Both patients and dental professionals are concerned about the absorption of energy required to produce a radiograph. How much electromagnetic energy can be safely absorbed by the human body? This is not an easy question to answer because the biologic effects of radiation are determined by several factors. These factors include the energy and amount of radiation absorbed, the length of time over which exposure occurred, the area of the body or the type of tissue irradiated, and environmental factors.

▶ High- and Low-Dose Effects

The most important determinant of biologic effect is the amount of radiation absorbed. Biologic effects can be classified into two categories based on the amount of radiation absorbed: *high-dose* and *low-dose* effects. High-dose effects occur when large amounts of radiation (>50 rem whole body) are absorbed, while low-dose effects occur when radiation exposures are minimal.

▶ High-Dose Effects

When tissues absorb high doses of radiation, biologic damage is predictable. Radiation damage in a biologic system is not seen immediately; the time it takes to develop is called the *latent period.* Specifically, the latent period is the time between exposure to radiation and clinical evidence of a harmful effect. When high doses of radiation are absorbed, harmful effects are seen after a short latent period (weeks or months). Thus, it is easy to relate these detrimental effects to absorption of radiation. High-dose effects are easily quantified and directly related to the amount of radiation absorbed.

The harmful effects produced by high doses of radiation also depend on cell type or tissue irradiated. When only a part of the body is irradiated as compared to whole body exposures, much larger doses of radiation are required to produce a response. Cells and organ systems also differ in sensitivity to radiation. Cells that are active and reproduce frequently are the most sensitive to radiation. Organ systems in which cellular turnover is infrequent are usually resistant to the detrimental effects of radiation (Table 9-2).

▶ Examples of High-Dose Radiation Effects

Because tumor cells have a rapid turnover, radiation therapy uses high doses of radiation to eliminate tumor cells preferentially. The common side effects of **epilation** (hair loss) and **erythema** (skin reddening) are examples of high-dose effects associated with therapeutic radiation. Initial x-ray machines were not built to modern standards; consequently, early radiation workers frequently suffered from the effects of high-dose radiation. Nuclear weapons dropped on Hiroshima resulted in 90,000 casualties and the radiation-induced death of 45,000 people. These weapons were so powerful that

TABLE 9-2 SENSITIVITY OF ORGANS TO HIGH-DOSE RADIATION

High sensitivity	Intermediate sensitivity	Low sensitivity
Lymphoid organs	Endothelial cells	Salivary glands
Bone marrow	Fibroblasts	Lungs
Testes	Growing bone	Muscle
Intestines	Growing cartilage	Brain and spinal cord

they ended a war and changed the way we think about radiation. Radiation accidents, such as occurred at the Chernobyl nuclear power plant, have resulted in many deaths. Media coverage of these events heightens public concern about all types of radiation. It is comforting to know that high-dose effects are not possible with modern dental x-ray machines using the amount of radiation required to produce a diagnostic radiograph.

▶ Low-Dose Effects

Low-dose effects, however, are a concern in diagnostic radiology. The detrimental effects associated with absorption of low doses of radiation include radiation-induced malignancies, local tissue damage, and genetic effects. Low-dose effects occur sporadically after a long latent period. In the past, concerns about low-dose radiation were focused on limiting exposure to reproductive organs. Low-dose exposures to somatic tissues were thought to be without risk. We now know that *any exposure* to radiation is *potentially* harmful.

Why were the detrimental effects of low-dose radiation not recognized earlier? Exposure to low-dose radiation increases diseases already present in a population. The probability that low doses of radiation will result in detriment is small. Thus, a small radiation-induced increase is difficult to notice when a naturally occurring incidence is large. Latent periods are long (years or decades), making it difficult or impossible to associate a specific radiation exposure to a specific effect. On an individual level, cause and effect cannot be measured because it is impossible to distinguish between radiation-induced and spontaneous disease. Finally, it is possible that other environmental factors (cocarcinogens) potentiate low-dose radiation, further confusing the relationship of low-dose radiation exposure to disease induction.

Epidemiologic research, examining large populations using sophisticated statistical analysis, must be employed to study the effects of low-dose radiation. Epidemiologic research of low-dose effects is difficult for a number of reasons. First, because the exact amount of radiation absorbed cannot be measured, it is usually estimated. Also, latent periods are long (10 to 35 years), so studies

TABLE 9-3   CRITICAL ORGANS

Tissue/organ	Low-dose effect
Hematopoietic	Leukemia
Thyroid gland	Neoplasia
Breast	Neoplasia
Salivary gland	Neoplasia
Gonads	Impaired fertility or mutations
Pregnancy	Fetal effects
Skin	Neoplasia
Lens of the eye	Cataracts

TABLE 9-4   TYPICAL ABSORBED DOSES TO CRITICAL ORGANS OF THE HEAD AND NECK ASSOCIATED WITH A 20-FILM, FULL-MOUTH SURVEY

	Circular collimators	Rectangular collimators
	(mrem)	(mrem)
Submandibular gland	287	41
Sublingual gland	867	373
Parotid gland	218	43
Bone marrow	1236	467
Lens of the eye	45	15
Thyroid gland	49	10

must extend over many years. The frequency of low-dose effects is so small that large populations must be examined to identify a significant radiation-induced increase. Often there are inadequate data regarding diagnostic dose levels, and effects in the diagnostic dose range are estimated from populations exposed to higher doses. When low-dose effects are studied in animals, it is not known with certainty that humans will respond similarly. Consequently, low-dose studies do not carry the same confidence as studies of high-dose effects. Nevertheless, there is overwhelming evidence that *any* exposure to radiation *conveys potential risk.*

While scientists continue to study low-dose radiation effects, certain facts are accepted as true in light of current knowledge. It is known that certain tissues are particularity sensitive to low levels of ionizing radiation. These organs are called **critical organs** (Table 9-3). It is important for dental professionals to learn the critical organs because radiation safety procedures are directed toward minimizing exposure to these highly sensitive organs. Low-dose radiation damage is cumulative over the lifetime of an individual. Even though the risk from low-dose radiation is minimal, any reduction in exposure is believed to result in additional risk reduction. Finally, it is believed the certain dental health benefit outweighs the potential risk of diagnostic radiation exposure.

Typical critical organ doses associated with dental radiographs are given in Table 9-4.

▶ Low-Dose Radiation Risk

Risk estimates are calculated because the harmful effects associated with dental x-rays cannot be proved or directly observed. Radiation-induced malignancy is one of the most important low-dose effects. Tissues at greatest risk of cancer induction following dental radiographs are the thyroid gland, salivary gland, female breast, brain, and bone marrow. The risk of radiation-induced cancer associated with dental x-rays is estimated as the number of excess cases per million persons irradiated per cSv (rem) per year (Table 9-5). These estimated risks are very small when radiographs are made using state-of-the-art techniques. The risk for radiation-induced malignancy is also small compared to the risk of spontaneously occurring malignancy. Cancer accounts for nearly 20% of all deaths in the United States; the estimated number attributable to low-level radiation exposure is a small fraction of the total. Nevertheless, it is important that dental professionals recognize the potential risk and use methods that minimize exposure while providing optimum diagnostic information.

Patients often ask how radiation-induced cancer risk compares to risks with which they are more familiar. The relative risks of mortality associated with other activities are found in Table 9-6. Dental professionals should address patients' concerns in a knowledgeable and confident way. Patients must be reassured that radiographic procedures have been selected to provide important diagnostic information and that optimum techniques are used to reduce risk to acceptable levels. The patient must be informed of the necessity of radiographs for meeting their specific dental health needs.

TABLE 9-5   PROBABILITY OF EXCESS FATAL CANCERS PER MILLION EXAMINATIONS*

	E Speed rectangular
Bitewings (4)	0.5
Panoramic	0.21
FMX	2.5

*Based on BEIR V, lifetime risks. Adapted from White SL: Assessment of radiation risk from dental radiography, *Dentomaxillofac Radiol* 21:118-126, 1992. There are approximately 512,680 deaths annually in the United States from all forms of cancer. The estimated, annual, worldwide fatality associated with dental radiography is 170 deaths. This estimate drops to 34 with E speed film and retangular collimation. (From *Monthly Vital Statistics Report NCHS* 40(10): Feb 1992.)

TABLE 9-6 ACTIVITIES INCREASING THE CHANCE OF DYING BY 1 IN 1 MILLION

Activity	Cause of death
TRAVEL	
150 miles by car	Accident
10 miles by bicycle	Accident
6 min by canoe	Accident
WORK	
10 days in a factory	Accident
1 hr in a coal mine	Lung disease
MISCELLANEOUS	
Smoking 1.4 cigarettes	Cancer, heart disease
Living 2 months with a smoker	Cancer, heart disease
Drinking 30 cans of diet soda	Chemical carcinogen
Drinking 0.5 liter of wine	Cirrhosis of the liver

◗ Radiographs During Pregnancy

Dental radiographs are considered safe for patients who may be pregnant. Radiography is avoided during pregnancy only when a fetus or embryo would be in or near the primary x-ray beam (such as lower abdominal or pelvic radiographs). For dental radiography the primary beam is limited to the head and neck region. The only radiation that a fetus or embryo is exposed to is secondary radiation. It has been recommended to avoid radiographs during the first trimester of pregnancy; this has been particularly true for weeks 2 through 6 of gestation. However, the final decision on radiographic exposure rests with the patient and her physician. Uterine doses for full-mouth intraoral radiography have been shown to be less than 1 mrem (even without a leaded apron in place). Uterine dose from naturally occurring background radiation during the 9 months of pregnancy is estimated to be about 75 mrem. Accordingly, there is no reason to postpone a properly justified dental radiographic examination because of pregnancy.

◗ Radiographs and Radiation Therapy

Dental radiographs do not present an additional risk for individuals who present with a history of radiation therapy to the head and neck region. Xerostomia frequently occurs following radiation therapy, resulting in a high risk for caries and other dental diseases in these individuals. Radiation therapy usually involves doses of more than 1000 rem, while diagnostic radiography results in doses of less than 1 rem. There is no reason to postpone necessary dental radiographic examination because of a history of radiation therapy.

The ALARA Concept

The National Council on Radiation Protection, a federal agency, establishes minimum radiation exposure limits. The guiding principle for protection from radiation exposure is known as the **ALARA concept (As Low As Reasonably Achievable)**. This principle means that when radiation is used, every available method for reducing exposure should be implemented to minimize potential risks and adverse consequences. When the ALARA concept is applied to patient exposures, it means that the maximum diagnostic benefit is provided with minimum exposure. When applied to occupational exposures, it means that diagnostic exposures should be completed without exposure to the operator.

The greatest amount of radiation to which an individual can be exposed in the work environment is called the *maximum permissible dose* (MPD). Currently the MPD is 2.5 cSv (rem) per year. It should be remembered that although a person can continue to work if exposed to less than 2.5 cSv (rem) in a year, no exposure should be the goal.

◗ The ALARA Concept Applied to Dental Radiography

The ALARA concept is widely practiced in dentistry. A summary of factors important to maintaining radiology practices resulting in the lowest exposure possible follows.

Collimation. The beam of radiation should be restricted so that the smallest volume of tissue possible is irradiated. Federal laws require the beam diameter be no more than 2.75 inches at the patient's face. Long, open-ended collimators (12 to 16 inches) are preferred because a smaller volume of the patient's face will be irradiated as compared to a shorter (8-inch) collimators. Pointed plastic cones should never be used because they increase the volume of tissue irradiated and the amount of scattered radiation absorbed in the patient's head and neck.

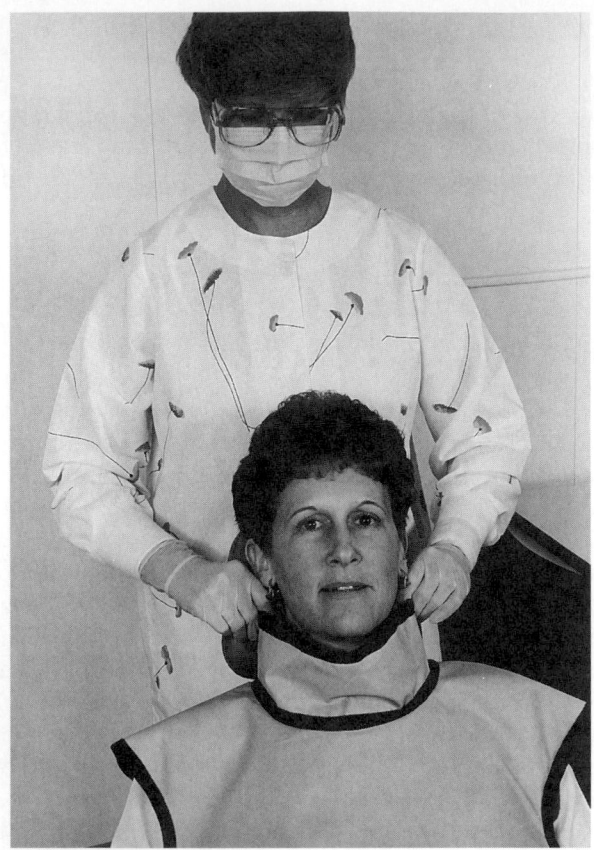

FIG. 9-8　Placement of the protective apron with thyroid collar on patient.

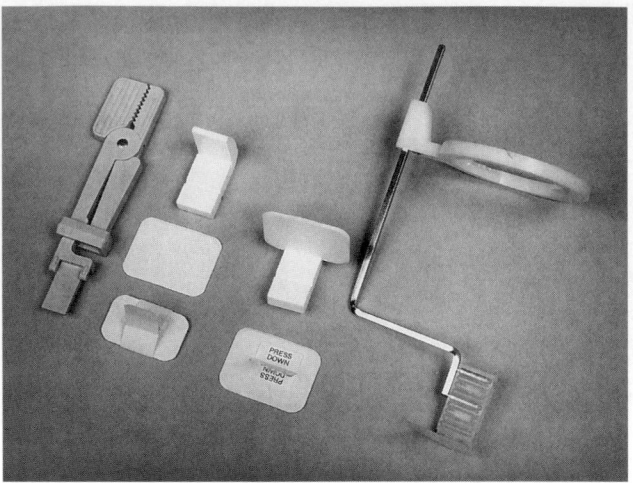

FIG. 9-9　Various film holders for periapical and bitewing projections.

Added Filtration. Filters selectively remove low-energy x-rays, which are absorbed in tissue and contribute little to the x-ray image. Aluminum filtration reduces patient exposures by as much as 57%. Federal laws require 2.5 mm aluminum filtration for operation voltages of 70 kVp or higher.

Equipment Factors. X-ray machines that operate below 60 kVp are not recommended. Low kVp x-ray machines result in absorbed doses almost twice as high as machines operating at 80 kVp. Electronic timers are preferred over mechanical timers because they more accurately reproduce short exposure times. Suspension arms should be stable and hold a position without movement or drift. Routine checks and a preventive maintenance program will ensure optimum equipment performance.

Film Selection. X-ray film varies in the amount of radiation required to make a diagnostic image. Film should be selected to give adequate diagnoses using the least amount of radiation, while quality images are obtained. *E* speed film is currently the most sensitive intraoral film commercially available, requiring about one half of the radiation of *D* speed film.

Leaded Apron and Thyroid Collar. Leaded aprons and thyroid collars reduce the possibility of exposure to critical organs outside the radiographic examination area (Fig. 9-8).

Optimum Processing and Dark Room Conditions. Processing conditions should be monitored and checked before patient films are developed. These procedures will decrease the number of retakes resulting from processing errors.

Film Holders. Film holders assist in x-ray tube placement and thus minimize retakes resulting from errors in projection. Film holders also allow a smaller beam diameter to be used. Examples of film-holding devices include bitewing tabs, Stabes, hemostats, XCP units, Snap-A-Ray, Intrax, and Precision paralleling devices. Several of these film holders are illustrated in Fig. 9-9.

Operator Shielding. Dental professionals may be exposed to radiation either from the primary beam, from leakage out of the tubehead, or from scattered radiation by the patient. Standing behind a protective barrier is the best way to prevent unnecessary exposure (Fig. 9-10). If standing behind a barrier or outside the operatory is not possible, the operator should be a distance of at least 6 feet from the x-ray tube. Operators should never hold the film, hold or stabilize the tubehead, or stand in the path of the primary beam. If a child or disabled person requires assistance during the exposure, a family member should be asked to help. Family members assisting in holding patients during radiographic procedures should be covered with leaded aprons and gloves.

Office Design. A properly designed office protects the

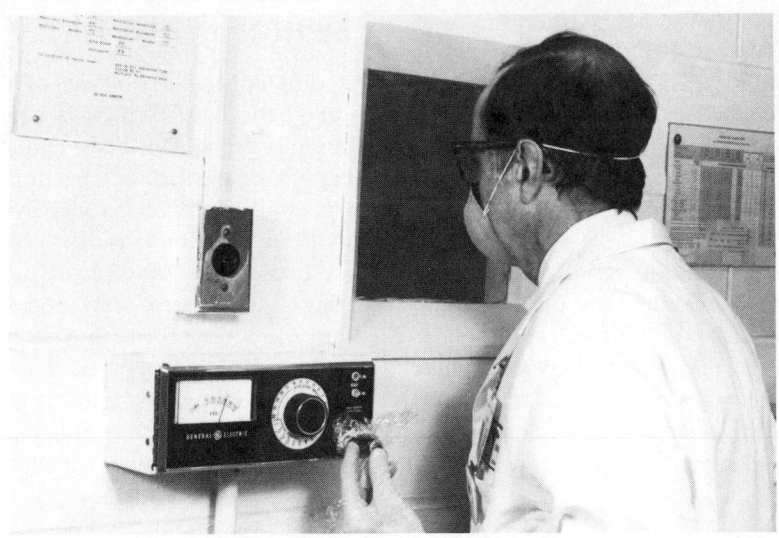

FIG. 9-10　Radiography operator behind protective shielding.
(From Frommer HH: *Radiology for dental auxiliaries*, ed 5, St Louis, 1992, Mosby.)

x-ray operator, patients, and staff in adjacent operatories and offices. Primary barriers are those walls intended to absorb radiation from the primary beam. Secondary barriers are intended to absorb secondary and leakage radiation. Appropriate barrier thickness is determined when x-ray machines are installed. Barrier requirements are determined for each x-ray unit and depend on maximum kVp, distance to the person to be protected, and occupancy factor of the areas adjacent to the x-ray machine.

Continuing Education. Dental professionals should continue to update knowledge and skills in radiology by taking continuing education courses. New discoveries and improved procedures in dental radiology are expected.

Patient Health History. As with all dental procedures, it is important to obtain a current health history on a patient. Information regarding other radiographic exposures, recent dental radiographic exposures, and current medical conditions are important factors evaluated when the need for radiographic exposure is assessed.

▶ Units of Measure

It is often necessary to quantify radiation. As in other systems of measurement, there is a move to use metric units. These units, called SI units (Systeme Internationale) and the corresponding traditional units are summarized in Table 9-7.

TABLE 9-7　SUMMARY OF RADIATION UNITS OF MEASURE

Quantity measured	Traditional unit	SI
Exposure	Roentgen	Coulomb/kg
Absorbed dose	rad	Gray
Equivalent dose	rem	Sievert

Exposure (Coulomb/kg; Roentgens)

X-rays cause the formation of ions in air. **Exposure** is defined as the number of ions produced by x-rays in a specific volume of air. Exposure is measured in units of coulombs per kilogram, or roentgens. One roentgen is approximately 2.58×10^{-4} coulombs/kg. Since only some of the x-rays emitted from the tube are absorbed by the patient, it is easy to see that exposure is always greater than the absorbed dose. Exposure and absorbed dose, however, are directly related. When exposure dose is high, the amount of radiation absorbed is also greater. Radiation exposure is easy to measure and consistent between individuals. Thus, exposure is the most frequently used measurement in radiation biology.

Absorbed Dose (Gray, rad)

The amount of radiation absorbed in tissues more accurately assesses biologic effects, but such measurements are not practical to make. Absorbed dose depends on individual characteristics of the irradiated tissue.

Absorbed dose is a measure of the energy imparted to a mass of tissue. An absorbed dose of 1 **gray (Gy)** is defined as the absorption of 1 joule/kg. The traditional unit is the **rad** (*r*adiation *a*bsorbed *d*ose). One gray is equal to 100 rad.

Equivalent Dose (Sievert, rem)

The unit used in radiation protection is dose equivalent, or sievert (Sv). This unit incorporates the quality factor (QF), which allows comparison of doses of different types of radiation. One **sievert** is equal to 1 Gy multiplied by the quality factor (1 Sv = Gy × QF). The traditional unit of dose equivalent is the **rem** (*r*ad *e*quivalent *m*an). One sievert is equal to 100 rem.

Dental X-ray Film

Radiographic film consists of a transparent plastic sheet, called the base, which is coated on both sides with a chemical emulsion. The emulsion contains silver halide crystals dispersed with gelatin. The exact composition of the emulsion silver halide crystals determines the sensitivity of the film to radiation or light.

Three types of film are used in dentistry: intraoral (direct exposure), extraoral (screen), and duplicating film. Direct exposure film is sensitive to radiation. Screen film is sensitive to a particular wavelength of light emitted by an intensifying screen. Duplicating film is sensitive to light emitted by a duplicating machine. Film speed specifies how responsive the film is to radiation. High-

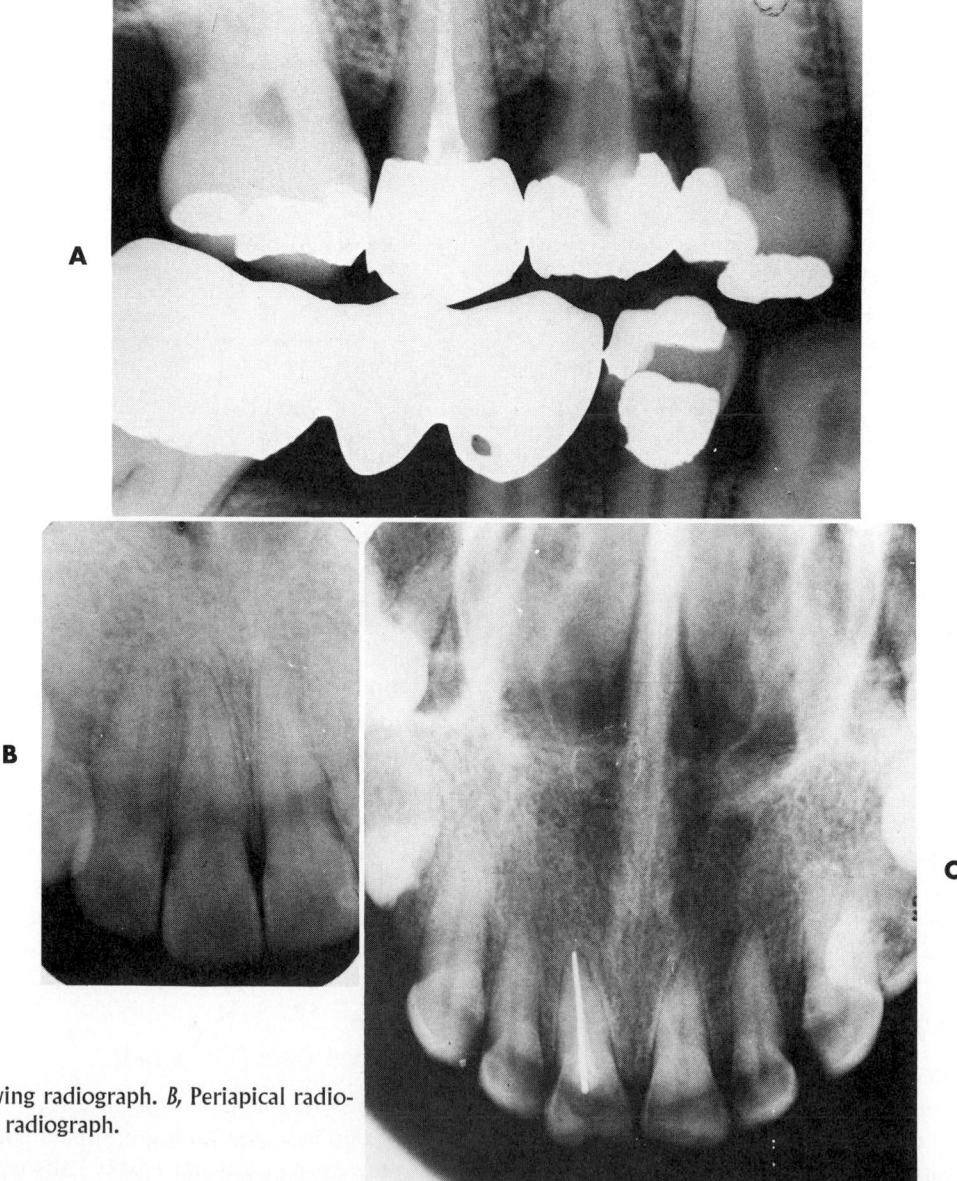

FIG. 9-11 *A,* Bitewing radiograph. *B,* Periapical radiograph. *C,* Occlusal radiograph.

BOX 9-1

APPLICATION OF RADIOGRAPHS

DENTAL TREATMENT PROCEDURE	COMMON RADIOGRAPHIC TECHNIQUE
Common operative	Bitewings, periapicals
Fixed prosthetics, partial	Periapicals, full-mouth series
Simple extractions	Periapicals, panoramic
Multiple extractions	Periapicals, panoramic
Additional maxillofacial procedures	Full-mouth series, panoramic
Dentures	Full-mouth series, panoramic
Endodontic treatment	Periapical
Periodontal treatment	Full mouth series
Orthodontic treatment	Panograph, cephalometric
TMJ treatment	Cephalometric, articular disk survey

---

speed (fast) film requires little radiation, while low-speed (slow) film requires more radiation.

Direct exposure film is used for periapical, bitewing, and occlusal exposures in the oral cavity. Extraoral radiographic procedures such as panoramic, cephalometric, and temporomandibular joint (TMJ) radiographs use screen film. Duplicating film is never used for patient exposures; instead, it is used to copy existing radiographs using special darkroom equipment.

1. **Bitewing** projections are radiographs depicting the crowns of maxillary and mandibular teeth and interdental alveolar crest (Fig. 9-11, *A*).
2. **Periapical** projections are radiographs depicting the majority of the crown, the apical portion of specific teeth, and the surrounding alveolar bone (Fig. 9-11, *B*).
3. **Occlusal** projections are radiographs depicting larger areas of an arch in one film compared to that seen in other intraoral films (Fig. 9-11, *C*).

Radiographic quality depends not only on exposure techniques, but also on the quality of processing and darkroom procedures. Process each type of film carefully following manufacturer's recommendations. Film should be stored so that it is protected from light, exposure to radiation, moisture, and extreme changes in temperature. Radiographic film has a shelf life and should be *rotated* so that the oldest film is used first. Patient radiographs should never be made using film past its expiration date.

▶ Intraoral Film Packets

Intraoral dental film is wrapped in a layered, light-tight paper or plastic packets (Fig. 9-12, *A*). The back of the film packet provides important information to the user (Fig. 9-12, *B*), including the following:

1. Location of the embossed dot
2. Side of the film that should be directed toward the PID

3. Speed of the film
4. Size of the film

Inside the packet the film is completely covered with black paper and a thin lead foil is positioned on the side opposite the image (Fig. 9-13, *A* and *B*). This lead foil absorbs any remaining x-ray photons and prevents exposure from stray or scattered radiation. The lead foil must always be placed away from the tooth being radiographed, while the *front* or white side of the film is placed toward the PID.

An orientation dot is usually embossed on the film packet. When the film packet is placed into the patient's mouth, the dot should be placed toward the occlusal or incisal edge of the tooth. Orienting the dot away from the apex ensures the image of the dot is not mistaken for an abnormality in the oral cavity.

Without the aid of the embossed dot, it would be impossible to know which side of the film should be viewed because a processed radiograph is transparent. The film packet is assembled so that the convex portion of the dot faces the *front,* or white surface. Placing the front surface of the film packet toward the primary beam also places the convex surface of the dot toward the primary beam. Consequently, when the processed radiograph is oriented with the convex surface of the dot up, the teeth are viewed from a facial orientation. The embossed dot is also used to identify the right or left side of the patient. When viewing processed radiographs from a facial orientation (dot convexity up), the mesial surface of teeth on the patient's right are located on the right side of the radiographic image, while the mesial surfaces of teeth on the patient's left are located on the left side of the radiographic image (Fig. 9-14, *A* and *B*).

Some film packets contain two pieces of film between the black paper lining. These two-film packets result in two identical radiographs. The two-film packets are used when it is anticipated that consultation regarding the patient's treatment may be required. It is important to

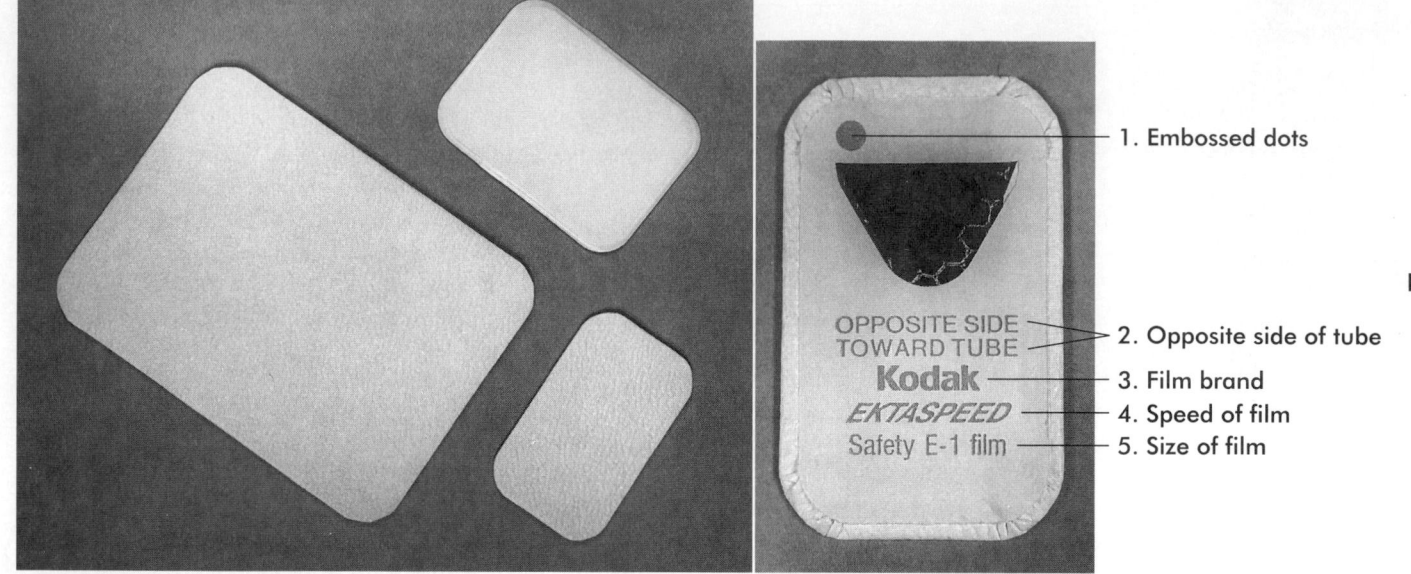

A

B

1. Embossed dots

OPPOSITE SIDE
TOWARD TUBE — 2. Opposite side of tube

Kodak — 3. Film brand

EKTASPEED — 4. Speed of film

Safety E-1 film — 5. Size of film

FIG. 9-12   *A*, Front of three intraoral film packets. *B*, Lingual side of intraoral film packet has film information: *1*, location of embossed dots; *2*, opposite side of the film is directed towards the PID; *3*, film brand; *4*, speed of film; *5*, size of film.

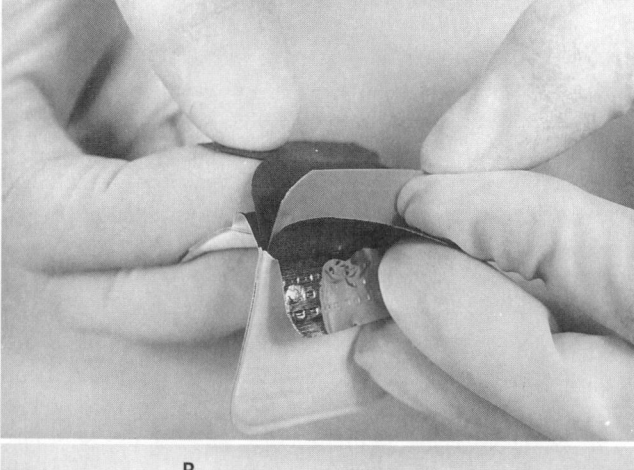

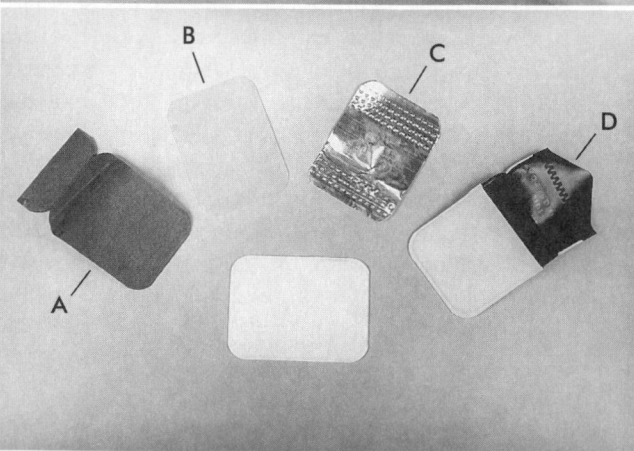

FIG. 9-13   Layer of the contents of a film packet, and parts of an intraoral film packet. *A*, Black paper; *B*, film; *C*, lead foil liner; and *D*, outer packet wrapping.

BOX 9-2

PATIENT WITH SPECIAL NEEDS

PATIENT WHO GAGS

Start taking the radiographs in the maxilla from the anterior to the posterior, since the posterior is the most responsive area to the gag reflex.

Position the film in the maxillary, allowing the teeth to rest on the film holder; do not have the patient move the film upward into the maxillary as the mandible closes.

Move the majority of the film holder toward the anterior so less material is toward the posterior of the patient's mouth.

Adjust the exposure settings and position the PID in the general area to be radiographed before the film is positioned.

Direct the patient to breathe through the nose and not the mouth.

The use of topical anesthetics placed in sensitive areas of the oral cavity may reduce gagging.

The tube shift method or buccal object rule technique may be necessary to obtain the third molar view.

SHALLOW OR NARROW PALATE

Change the film size to accommodate patient mouth size.

Place the film as parallel as possible to the teeth but it may be necessary to increase distance of the film from the teeth.

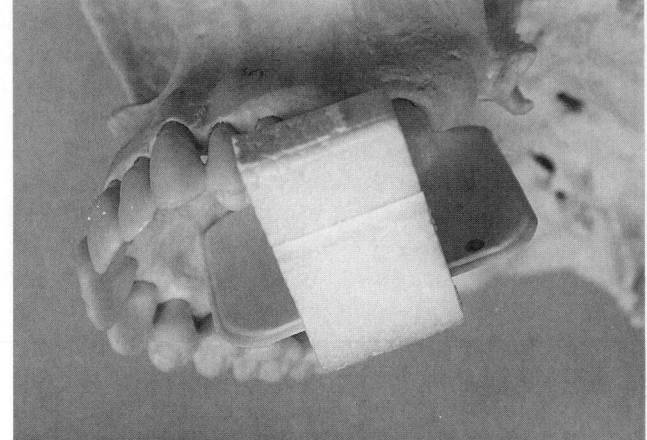

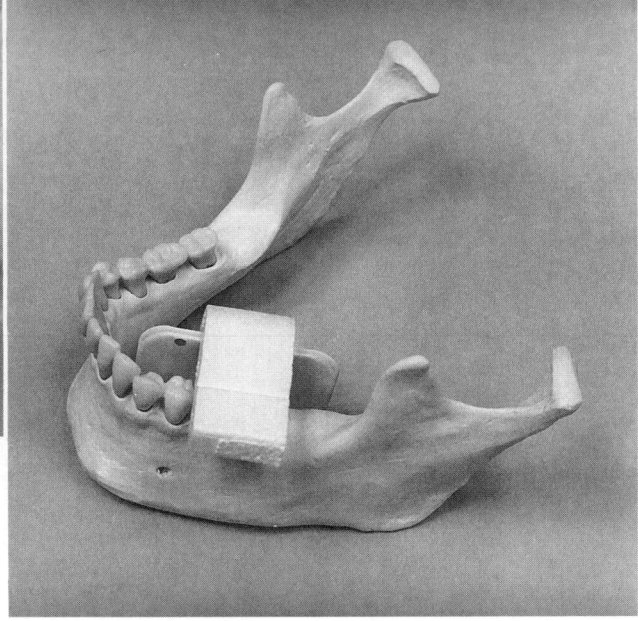

FIG. 9-14   *A,* Placement of bite block and film orientation in maxillary left quadrant. *B,* Placement of bite block and film orientation in the mandibular left quadrant.

It may be necessary to use the bisecting technique instead of the paralleling technique to achieve the required results.

TORI

Maxillary torus is not usually a problem, but if it is present, use an occlusal projection.

Mandibular tori/torus requires that the film be moved away from the lingual aspect of the teeth for patient comfort.

It may be necessary to change the film size.

DISABLED PATIENT

If the patient cannot remain still, a second person may need to be in the treatment room to assist the patient. A protective apron must be worn by this person, also.

The patient who is confined to a wheelchair may need to be radiographed while in the wheelchair.

The patient who cannot tolerate the procedure at all may need to receive sedation to accomplish this procedure.

LACK OF UNDERSTANDING DIRECTIONS

The assistant must determine why the patient is unable to understand directions. Is the person's hearing impaired? Is the patient able to speak?

If the person's hearing is impaired, but if he or she can read lips, be sure to pull the protective mask down to allow your lips to be seen.

Always talk to the patient while standing in front of him or her.

If the patient is unable to speak but can hear, provide a paper and pencil for communication.

TONGUE-TIED

If the paralleling technique is the technique of choice, it may be necessary to switch to the bisecting technique to obtain a diagnostic radiograph.

SPECIAL MANAGEMENT

If the patient presents a management problem, explain the procedure and the importance of obtaining diagnostic radiographs.

Use a firm and directive tone of voice and approach.

If the lack of cooperation stems from fear, especially when treating a child patient, explain the procedure in terms that the patient can understand; describe the x-ray unit as a camera and show examples of radiographs as pictures of the teeth; answer any questions that might arise.

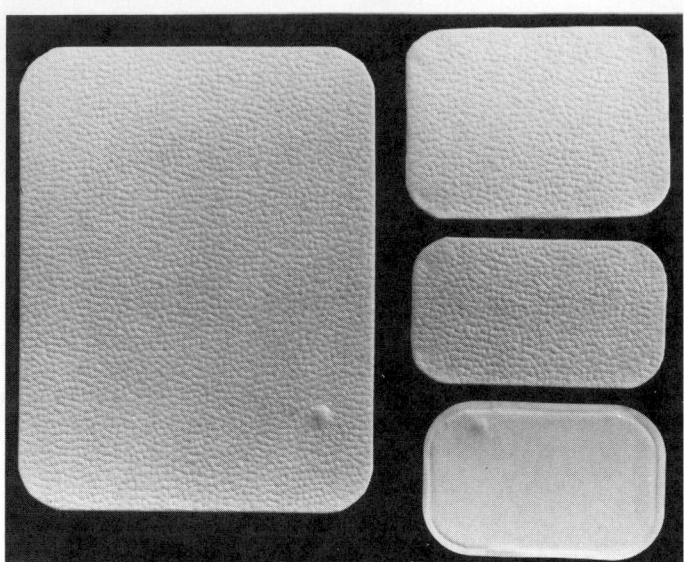

FIG. 9-15   Dental x-ray film is commonly supplied in various sizes. *Left,* occlusal film; *top right,* adult posterior; *middle right,* adult anterior; *bottom right,* child size in plastic wrapping.

remember to separate the two pieces of film before processing.

Intraoral film is available in five sizes: child #0, anterior #1, adult #2, large bitewing #3, and occlusal #4. The size of film used depends on the radiographic projection selected and the size of the patient's mouth. Intraoral film sizes are illustrated in Fig. 9-15.

Patient Management

A dental radiographic examination can be an uncomfortable procedure for the patient. It is essential that dental assistants employ an empathetic approach and practice some important patient management skills. As with any dental procedure a patient may be anxious or even uncooperative during a radiographic procedure. Approach the patient with a positive and confident attitude to gain trust and to decrease the patient's apprehension regarding your ability to complete the radiographic procedure. Individualize your technique, considering the unique needs of each patient. Some difficulties encountered when taking radiographs include patients who gag, who have a shallow or narrow palate, who have tori, who are tongue-tied, who do not understand directions, or who are uncooperative.

Handicapped, hospitalized, or bedridden patients may require specialized equipment and techniques to manage individual needs and achieve quality radiographs. In Box 9-2, patient management techniques are suggested to accommodate patients with special needs.

Intraoral Radiographic Techniques

The most common dental radiographs are intraoral projections. In intraoral radiography, film is selected and placed into the mouth, behind the teeth to be radiographed. The primary beam from the PID is then directed toward the teeth and the exposure is made. Two intraoral techniques are in common usage today.

▶ Bisecting Angle Technique

The **bisecting angle** technique was introduced in 1907 by Cieszynski. The accuracy of the bisecting technique is based on the geometric principle of isometry. This geometric principle states that two triangles are equal if they have one side in common. When the angle formed by the long axis of the tooth and the plane of the film is bisected, two triangles with a common side are created (Fig. 9-16, *A*). When the x-ray beam is directed perpendicular to the bisecting line, the length of the projected image is the same as its actual length. The resulting image has minimal distortion. The bisecting principle works well with single-rooted teeth but is not as successful for multirooted teeth. The bisecting method is technically difficult. Problems in conceptualizing the bisecting line result in incorrect projection angles. Errors in projection angle produce severely distorted radiographic images. Mastering the bisecting technique so that the tooth length is accurate is extremely important when radiographs are used in endodontic treatment.

▶ Paralleling Technique

In 1924, McCormack introduced a new intraoral radiographic technique designed to minimize distortion in the radiographic image. Because he recommended a 36-to-42-inch source-to-object distance, this radiographic method became known as the *long-cone* **paralleling** technique. The film is placed parallel to the long axis of the tooth, and the x-ray beam is directed at a right angle to the film. To place the film parallel to the tooth, it is necessary to move it a slight distance away from the crown (Fig. 9-16, *B*). Using film holders and smaller film packets in the anterior regions facilitates proper paralleling film placement. Radiographic images produced by the paralleling technique have optimum image characteristics and minimum distortion.

Full-Mouth Radiographs

The dentist will order radiographs necessary to make an appropriate diagnosis for an individual patient. When the

Text continued on p. 217.

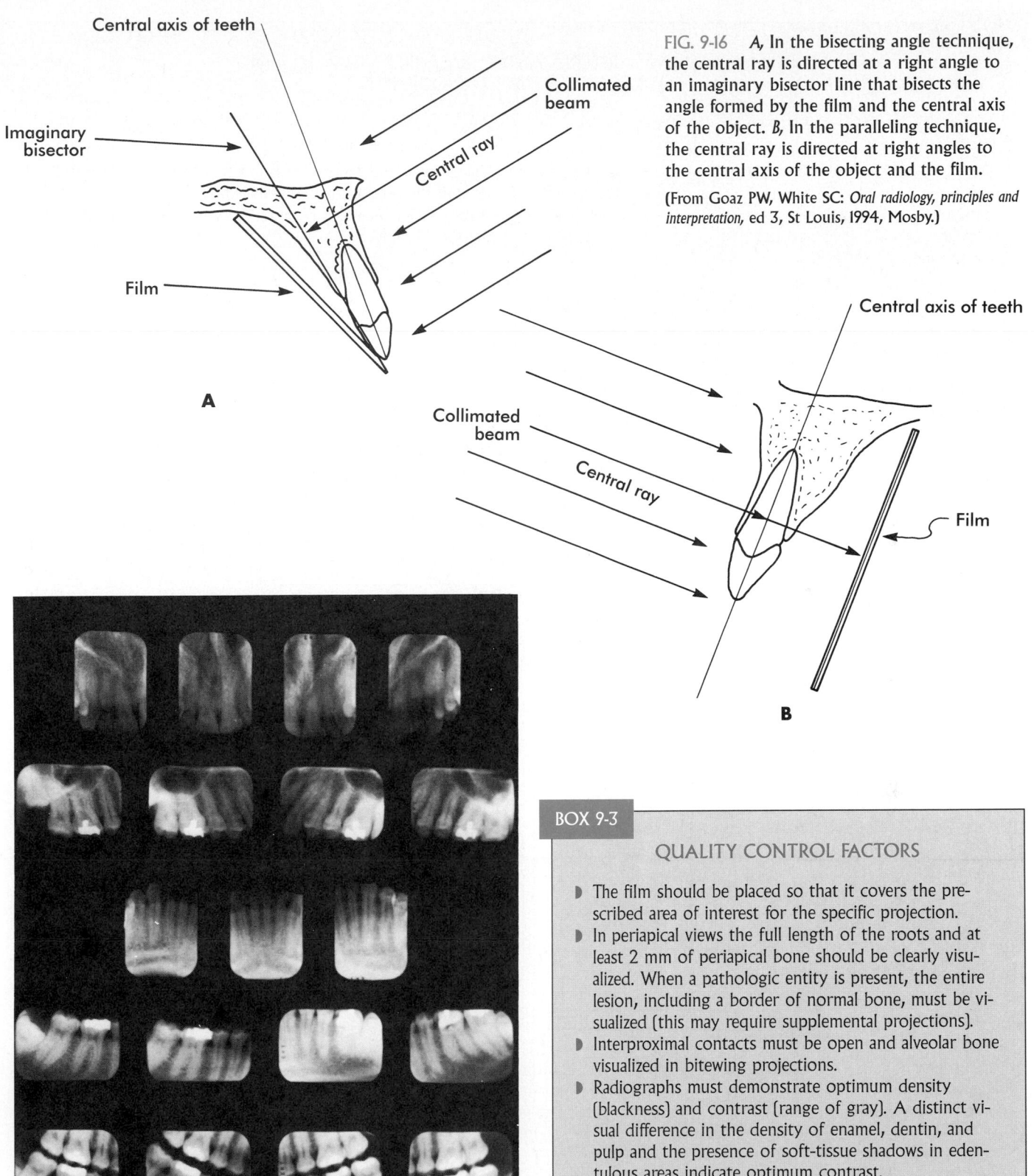

Central axis of teeth

Imaginary bisector

Collimated beam

Central ray

Film

A

FIG. 9-16   *A,* In the bisecting angle technique, the central ray is directed at a right angle to an imaginary bisector line that bisects the angle formed by the film and the central axis of the object. *B,* In the paralleling technique, the central ray is directed at right angles to the central axis of the object and the film.

(From Goaz PW, White SC: *Oral radiology, principles and interpretation,* ed 3, St Louis, 1994, Mosby.)

Central axis of teeth

Collimated beam

Central ray

Film

B

FIG. 9-17   Full mouth series of radiographs, including 15 periapicals and 4 bitewings.

BOX 9-3

QUALITY CONTROL FACTORS

▶ The film should be placed so that it covers the prescribed area of interest for the specific projection.

▶ In periapical views the full length of the roots and at least 2 mm of periapical bone should be clearly visualized. When a pathologic entity is present, the entire lesion, including a border of normal bone, must be visualized (this may require supplemental projections).

▶ Interproximal contacts must be open and alveolar bone visualized in bitewing projections.

▶ Radiographs must demonstrate optimum density (blackness) and contrast (range of gray). A distinct visual difference in the density of enamel, dentin, and pulp and the presence of soft-tissue shadows in edentulous areas indicate optimum contrast.

▶ Radiographs must be free of distortion caused by errors in vertical and horizontal angle of projection, improper film placement, or bending of the film.

▶ Radiographs must be free of processing errors.

BOX 9-4

FILM PLACEMENT CRITERIA AND STRUCTURES VISUALIZED IN INTRAORAL DENTAL RADIOGRAPHS

MAXILLARY CENTRAL-LATERAL INCISORS, PERIAPICAL
PROJECTION

Teeth. The contact between the central and lateral incisors is centered on the film. The entire crown and root of the central and lateral incisors, including apices, are fully depicted together with the interproximal alveolar crest of the adjacent central incisor and canine teeth.

Contacts open. The central ray is directed to open the contact between the central and lateral incisor.
Anatomic structures visualized. Floor of the nose, incisive fossa.
Film size. #1 or #2.

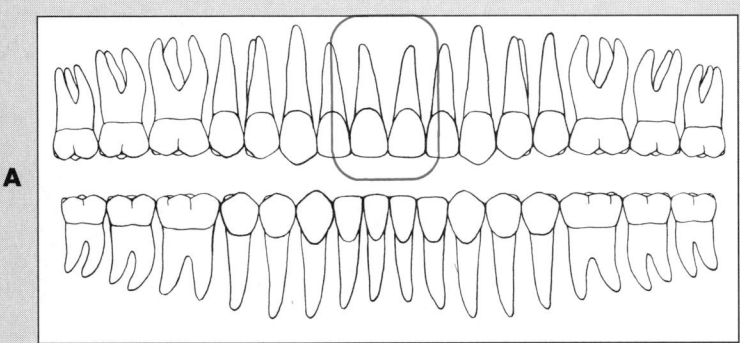

A

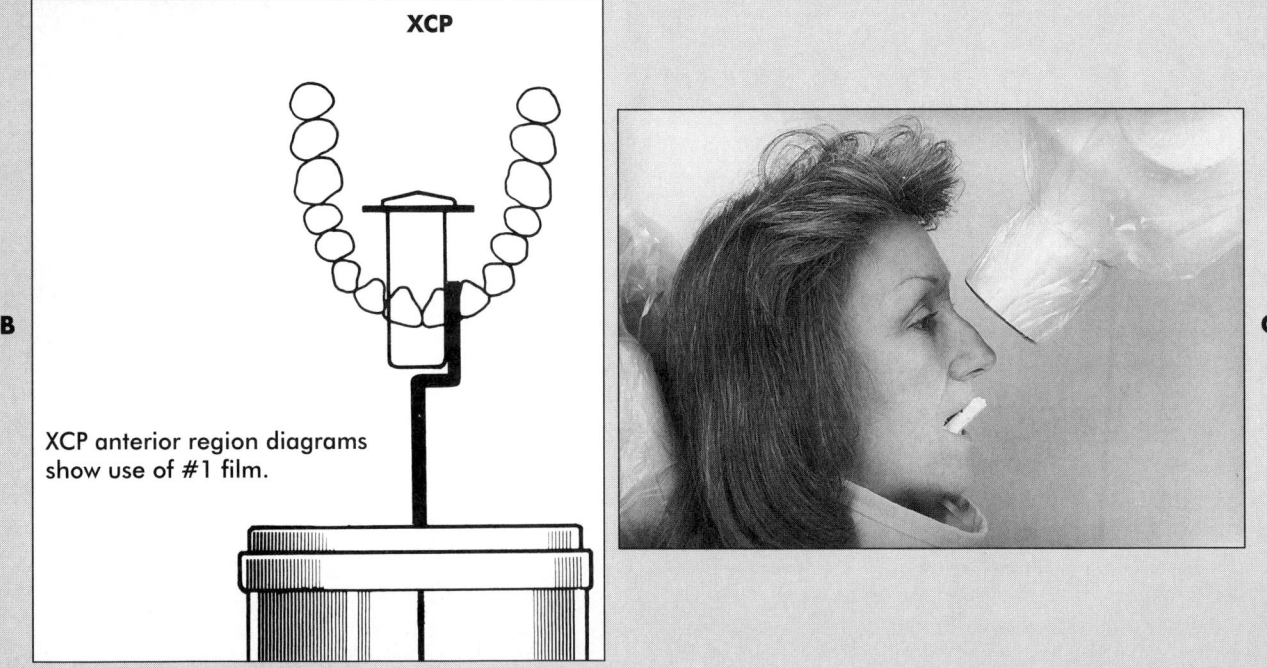

XCP

XCP anterior region diagrams show use of #1 film.

B

C

FIG. 9-18   *A,* Area to be exposed—maxillary central incisors, periapical projection. *B,* Film position in relation to teeth and PID. *C,* Film in holder positioned in maxillary incisor region on patient.

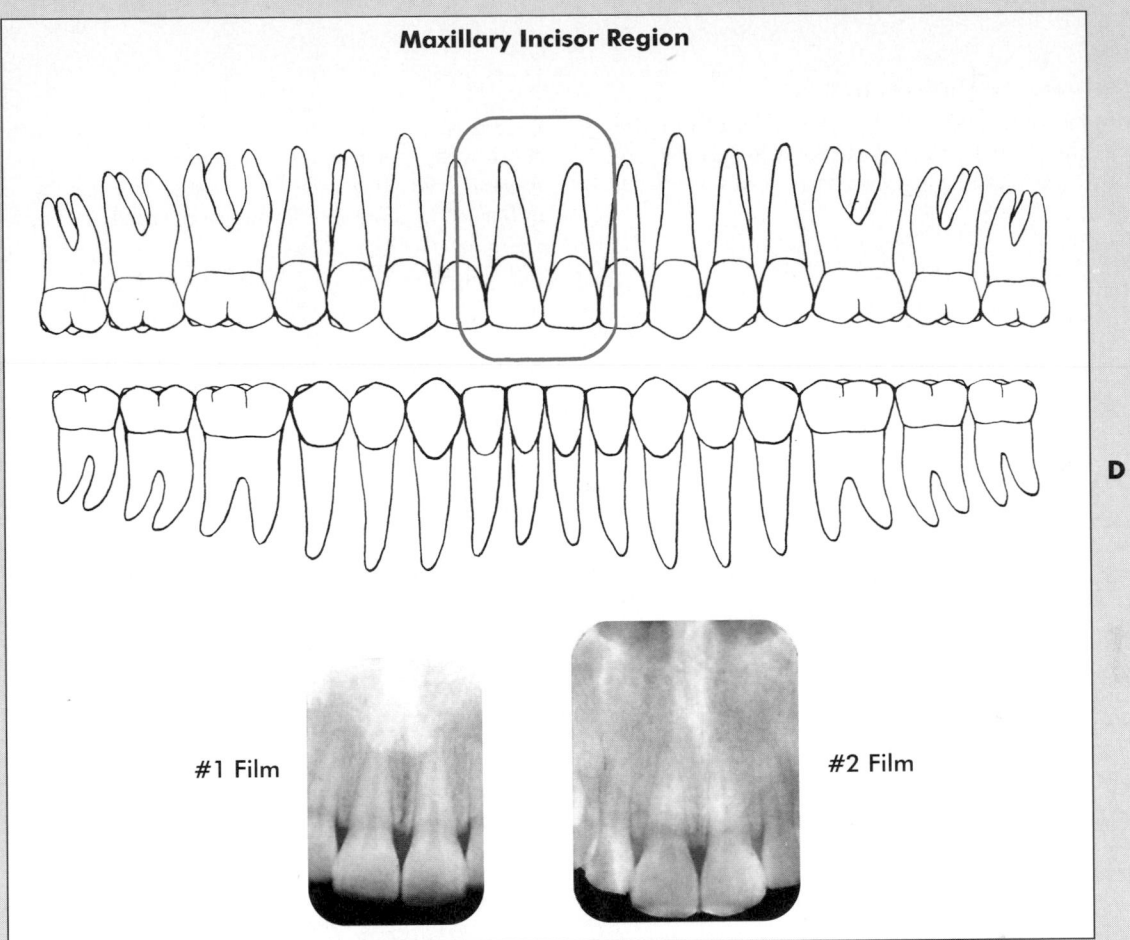

Maxillary Incisor Region

#1 Film

#2 Film

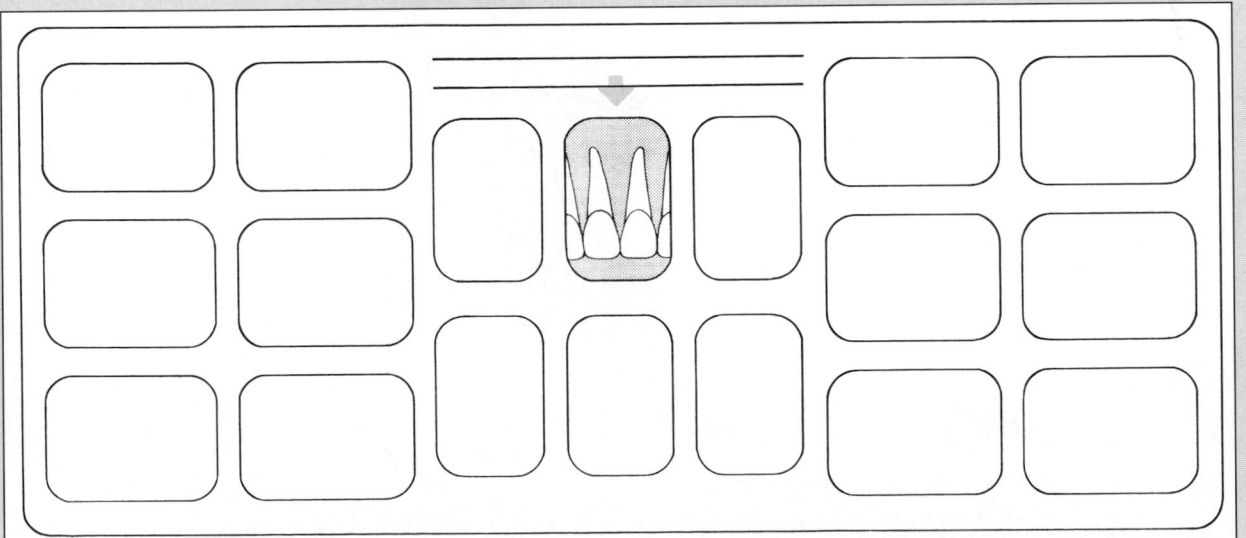

FIG. 9-18, cont'd.   *D,* Exposed film of area, reflecting section outlined in diagram above.
E, Film in mount.

Continued.

BOX 9-4, cont'd.

FILM PLACEMENT CRITERIA AND STRUCTURES VISUALIZED IN INTRAORAL DENTAL RADIOGRAPHS

MAXILLARY CANINE, PERIAPICAL PROJECTION

Teeth. The canine tooth is centered on the film. The entire crown and root of the canine, including the apex, is fully depicted together with the interproximal alveolar crest of the adjacent lateral incisor.

Contacts open. The central ray is directed to open the contact between the canine and lateral incisor.

Anatomic structures visualized. The *inverted* Y formed by the floor of the nose and the anterior wall of the maxillary sinus is often seen.

Film size. #1 or #2.

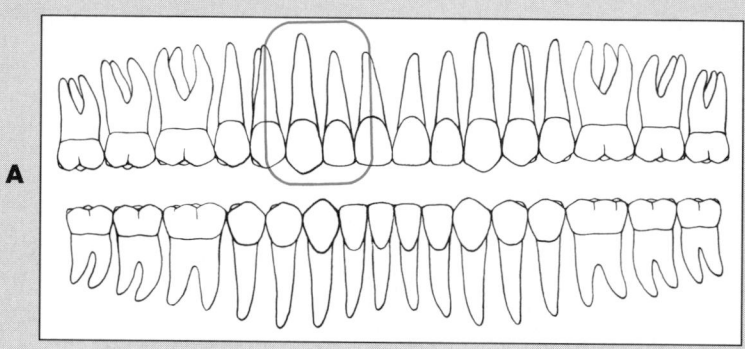

A

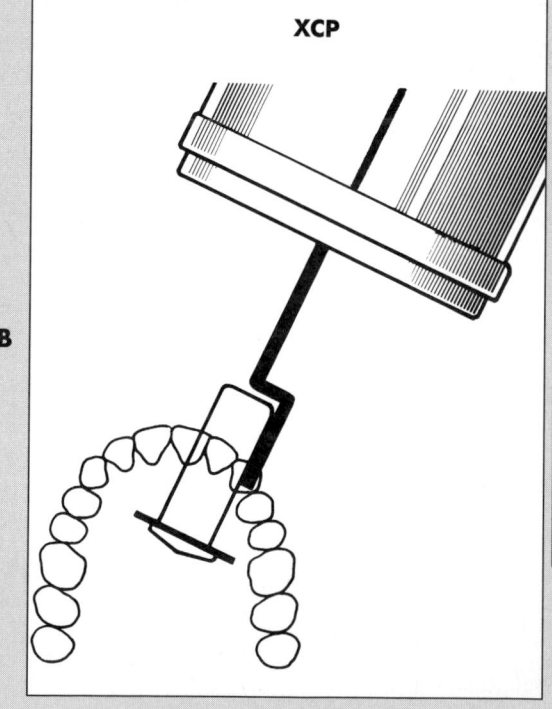

XCP

B

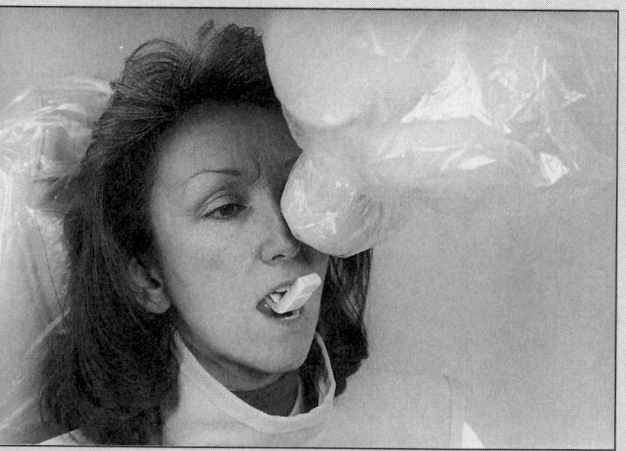

C

FIG. 9-19   *A,* Area to be exposed—maxillary canine, peri apical projection. *B,* Film position in relation to teeth and PID. *C,* Film in holder positioned in maxillary canine region of patient.

Maxillary Lateral Incisor Region

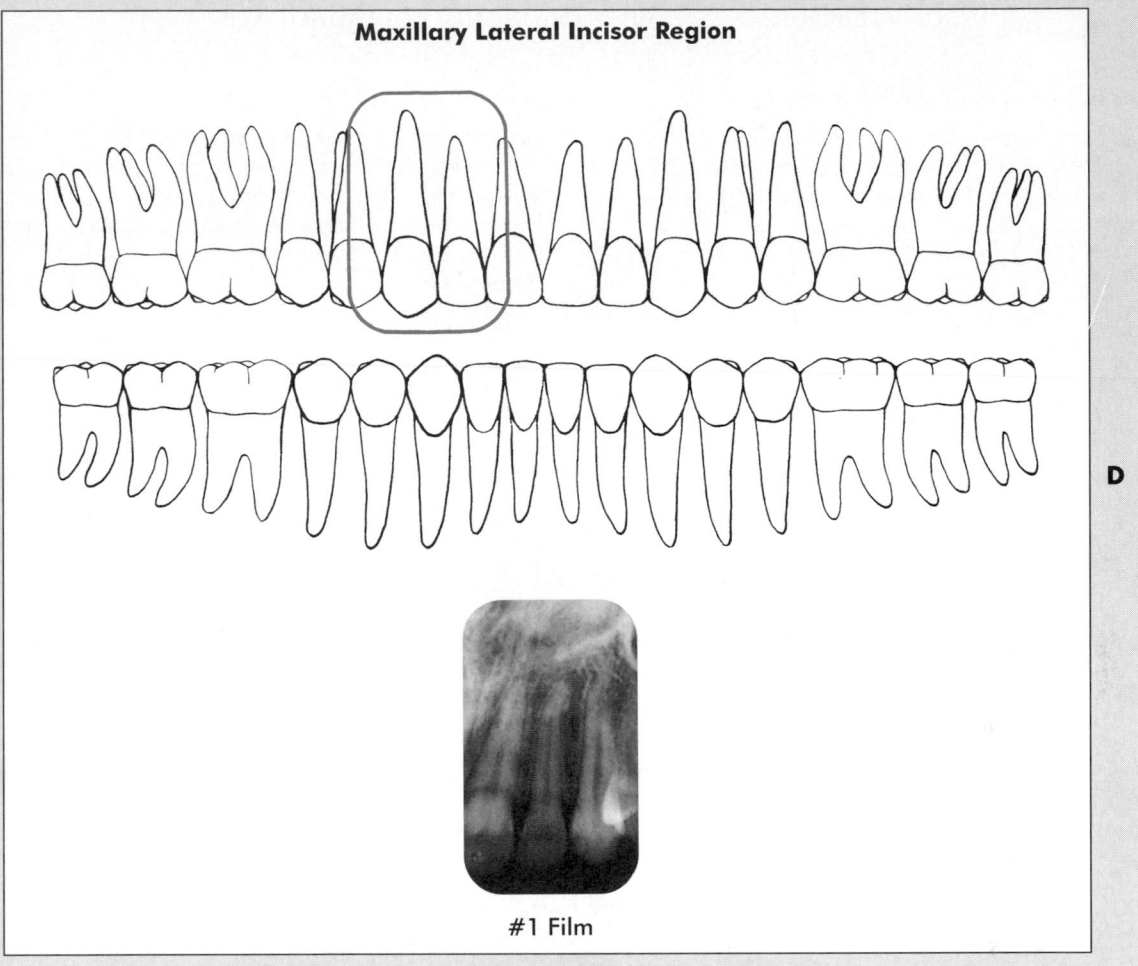

#1 Film

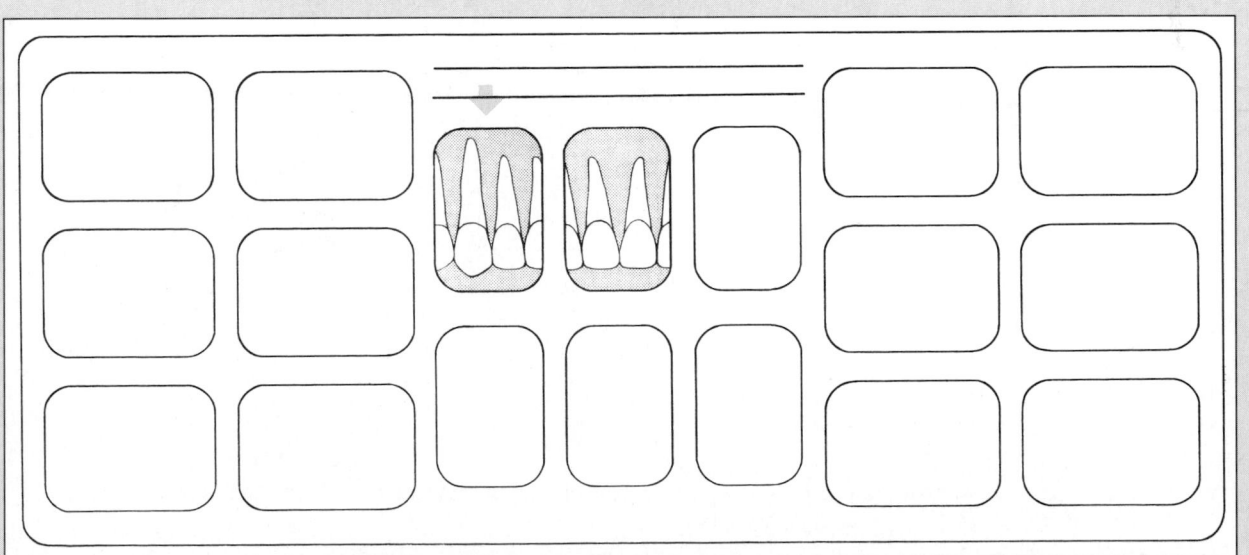

FIG. 9-19, cont'd. *D*, Exposed film of area, reflecting section outlined in the diagram above. *E*, Film in mount. The film is positioned on the left side of the patient's mouth, and the mounted film is for the opposite side, thereby presenting positioning for both sides.

Continued.

BOX 9-4, cont'd.

FILM PLACEMENT CRITERIA AND STRUCTURES VISUALIZED IN INTRAORAL DENTAL RADIOGRAPHS

MAXILLARY PREMOLAR, PERIAPICAL PROJECTION

Teeth. The distal surface of the canine crown and the entire crown and root of the first and second premolar, including apices, are visualized together with the interproximal alveolar crest of the canine and first molar teeth.

Contacts open. The central ray should be directed to open the contact between the first and second premolar and contact between the canine and the first premolar.

Anatomic structures visualized. The floor and anterior wall of the maxillary sinus are visualized.

Film size. #1 or #2.

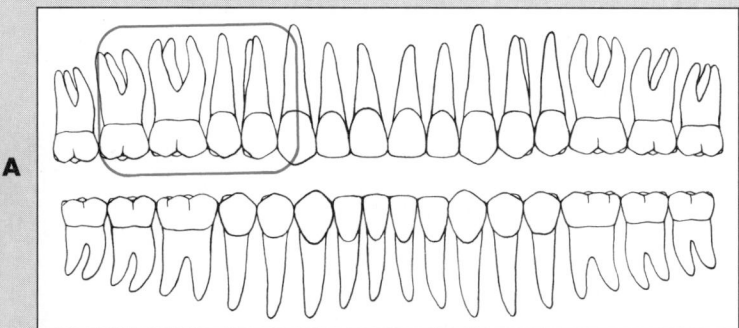

A

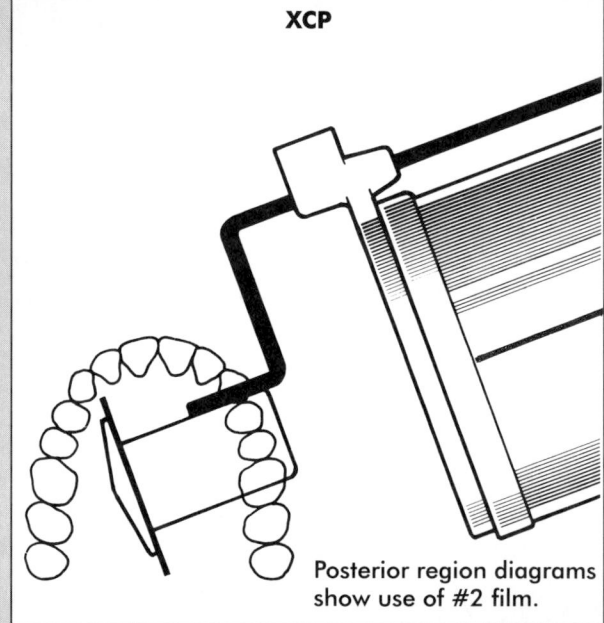

XCP

B

Posterior region diagrams show use of #2 film.

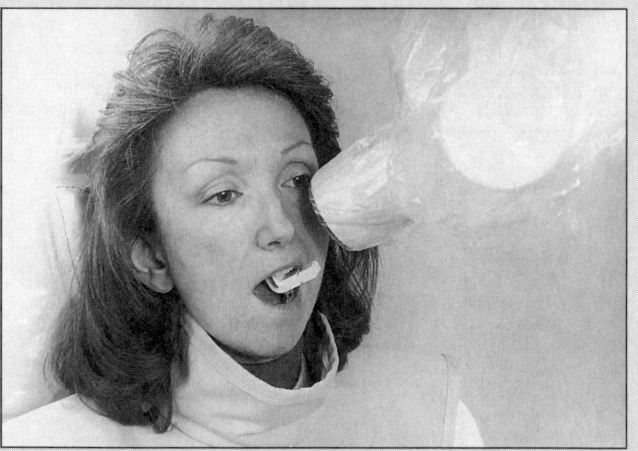

C

FIG. 9-20   *A,* Area to be exposed—maxillary premolar, periapical projection. *B,* Film position in relation to teeth and PID. *C,* Film in holder positioned in maxillary premolar region of patient.

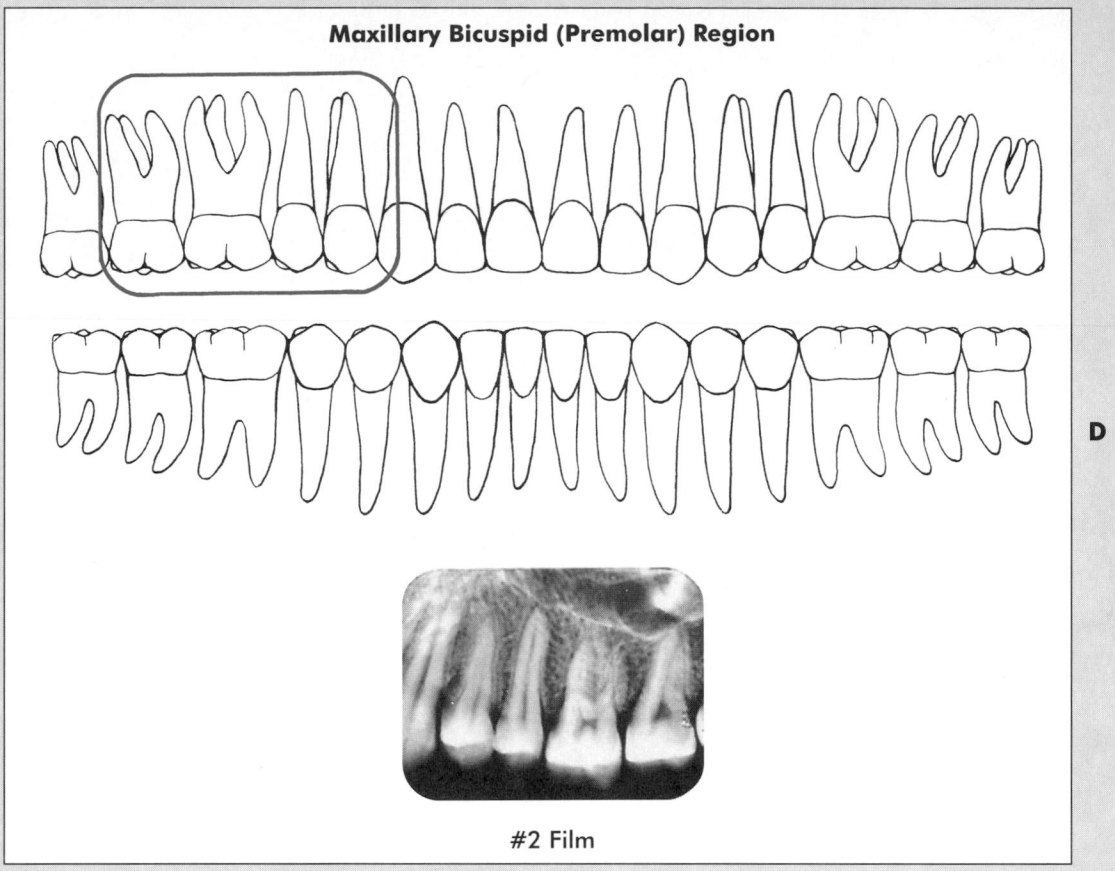

Maxillary Bicuspid (Premolar) Region

#2 Film

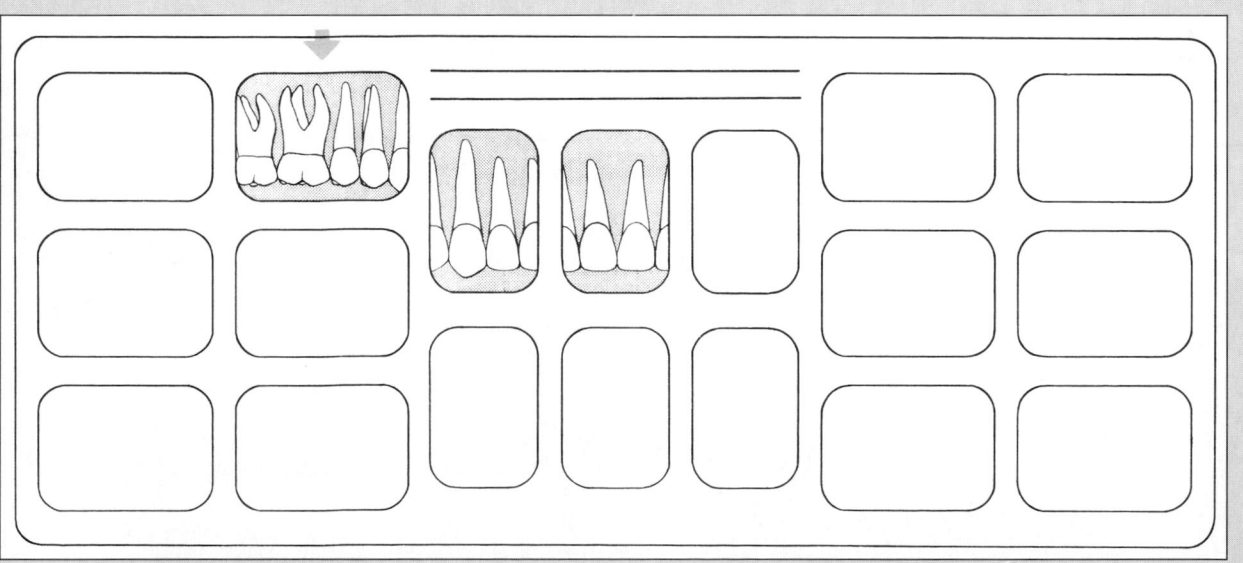

FIG. 9-20, cont'd.   *D,* Exposed film of area, reflecting section outlined in the diagram above. *E,* Film in mount. The film is positioned on the left side of the patient's mouth, and the mounted film is for the opposite side, thereby presenting positioning for both sides.

Continued.

BOX 9-4, cont'd.

FILM PLACEMENT CRITERIA AND STRUCTURES VISUALIZED IN INTRAORAL DENTAL RADIOGRAPHS

MAXILLARY MOLAR, PERIAPICAL PROJECTION

Teeth. The distal surface of the second premolar and the entire crown and root of the first, second, and third molars, including apices, are depicted together with the interproximal alveolar crest of the second premolar and the extent of the maxillary tuberosity.

Contacts open. The central ray should be directed to open the contact between the first and second molar. The contact between the distal aspect of the second premolar and the mesial of the first molar is usually open.

Anatomic structures visualized. The floor of the maxillary sinus, the maxillary tuberosity, and occasionally the hamular process of the sphenoid bone, and the coronoid process can be seen.

Film size. #2.

MAXILLARY DISTAL MOLAR, PERIAPICAL PROJECTION

Teeth. The distal portion of the first molar, the entire crown and root of the second and third molars, including the apices, are fully depicted, together with the full extent of the maxillary tuberosity.

Contacts open. The central ray should be directed perpendicular to the center of the film. Usually no contacts are open.

Anatomic structures visualized. The floor and posterior wall of the maxillary sinus, the maxillary tuberosity, often the malar eminence and the zygomatic arch, and occasionally the coronoid process and sigmoid process of the mandible can be seen.

Film size. #2.

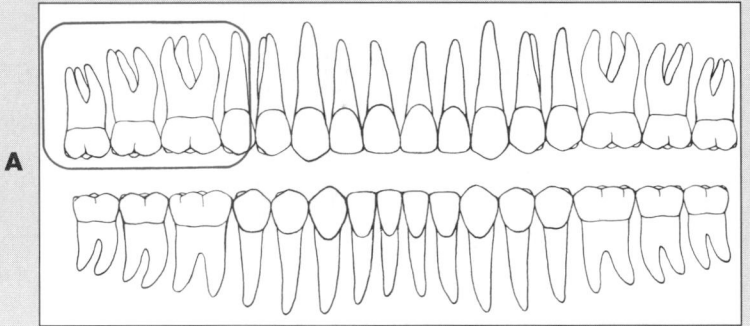

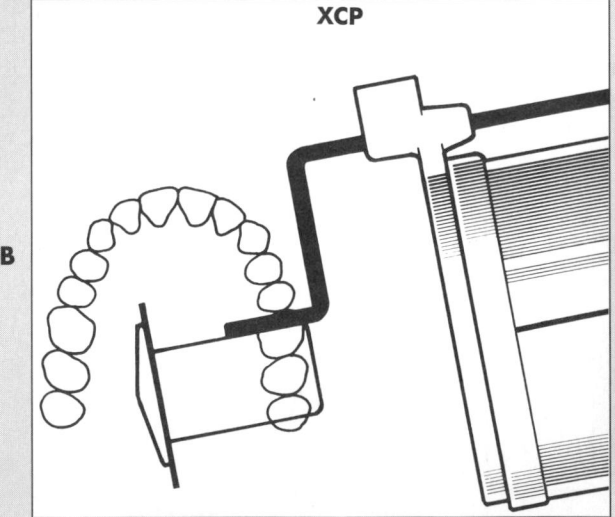

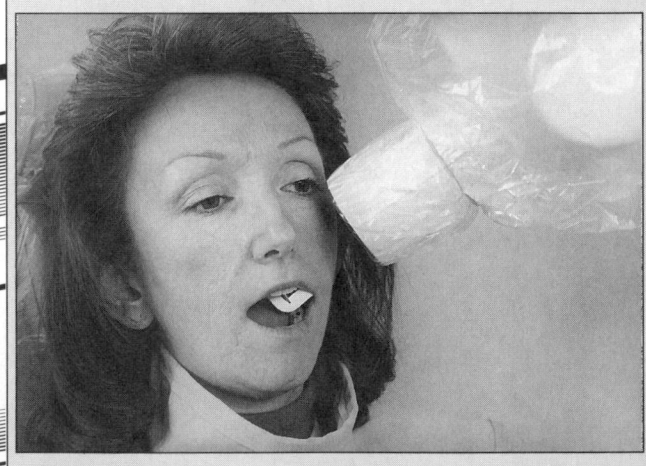

FIG. 9-21 *A,* Area to be exposed—maxillary molar, periapical projection. *B,* Film position in relation to teeth and PID. *C,* Film in holder positioned in maxillary molar region on patient.

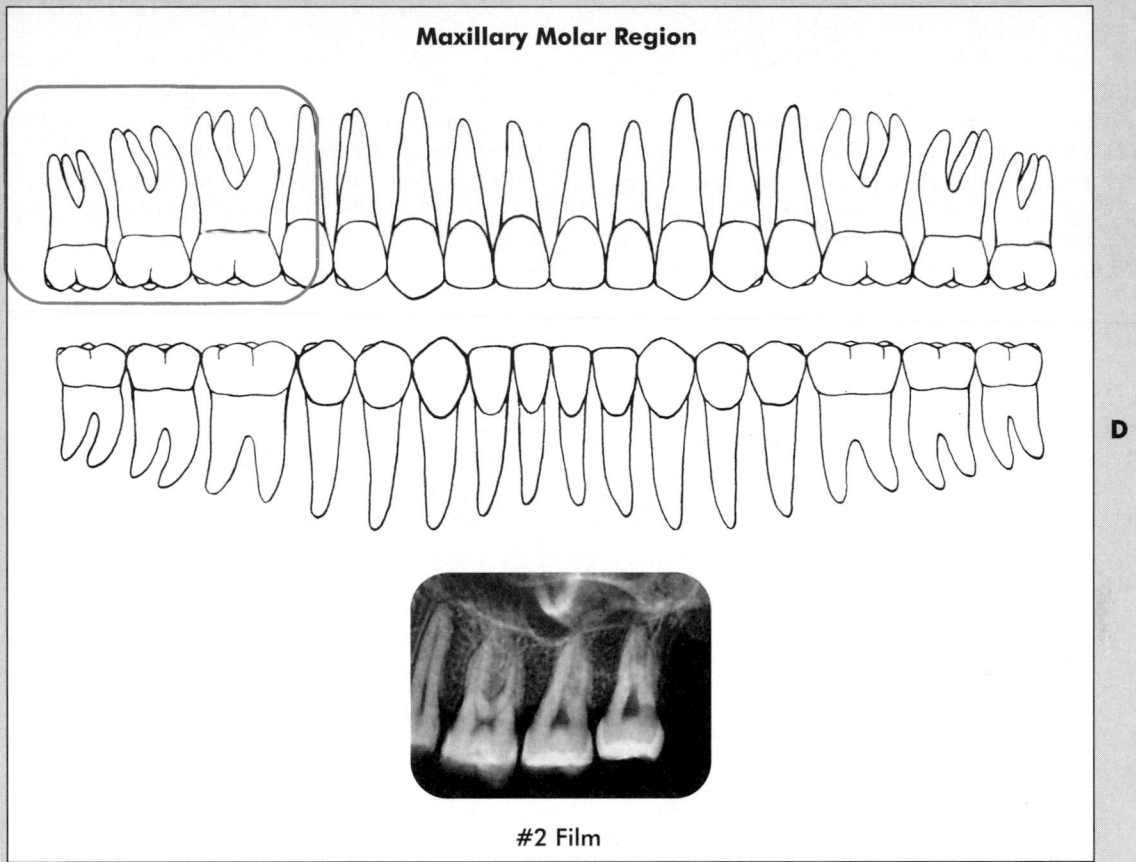

Maxillary Molar Region

#2 Film

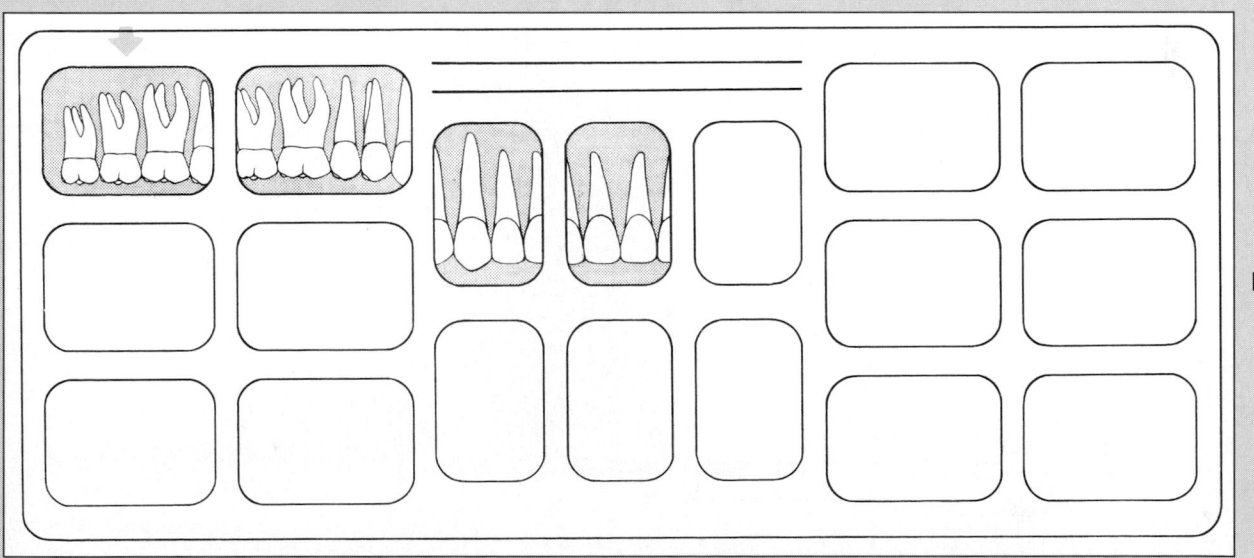

FIG. 9-21, cont'd.   *D,* Exposed film of area, reflecting section outlined in diagram above. *E,* Film in mount. The film is positioned on the left side of the patient's mouth, and the mounted film is for the opposite side, thereby presenting positioning for both sides.

Continued.

BOX 9-4, cont'd.

FILM PLACEMENT CRITERIA AND STRUCTURES VISUALIZED IN INTRAORAL DENTAL RADIOGRAPHS

MANDIBULAR CENTRAL-LATERAL INCISORS, PERIAPICAL
PROJECTION

Teeth. The contact between the central and lateral incisors is centered on the film. The entire crown and root of the central and lateral incisors, including apices, are fully depicted together with the interproximal alveolar crest of the adjacent central incisor and canine teeth.

Contacts open. The central ray is directed to open the contact between the central and lateral incisors.

Anatomic structures visualized. Occasionally the genial tubercles and/or the mental ridge or inferior border of the mandible can be seen.

Film size. #1 or #2.

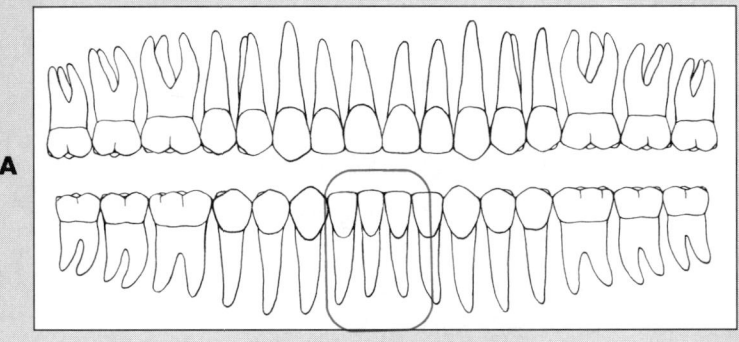

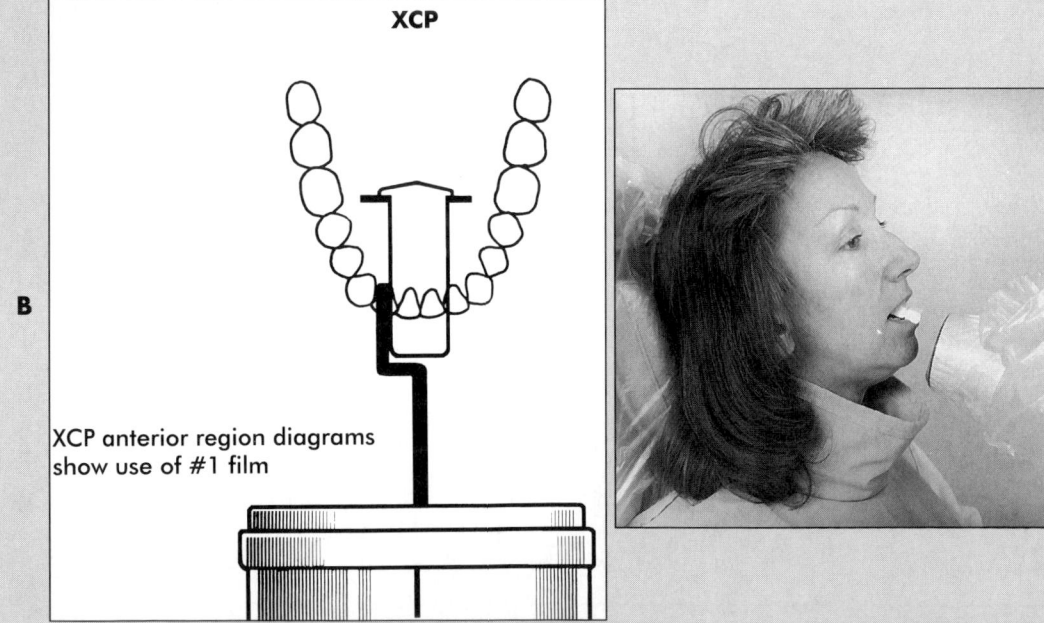

FIG. 9-22   *A,* Area to be exposed—mandibular central incisor, periapical projection. *B,* Film positioned in relation to teeth and PID. *C,* Film in holder positioned in mandibular central incisor area.

Mandibular Incisor Region

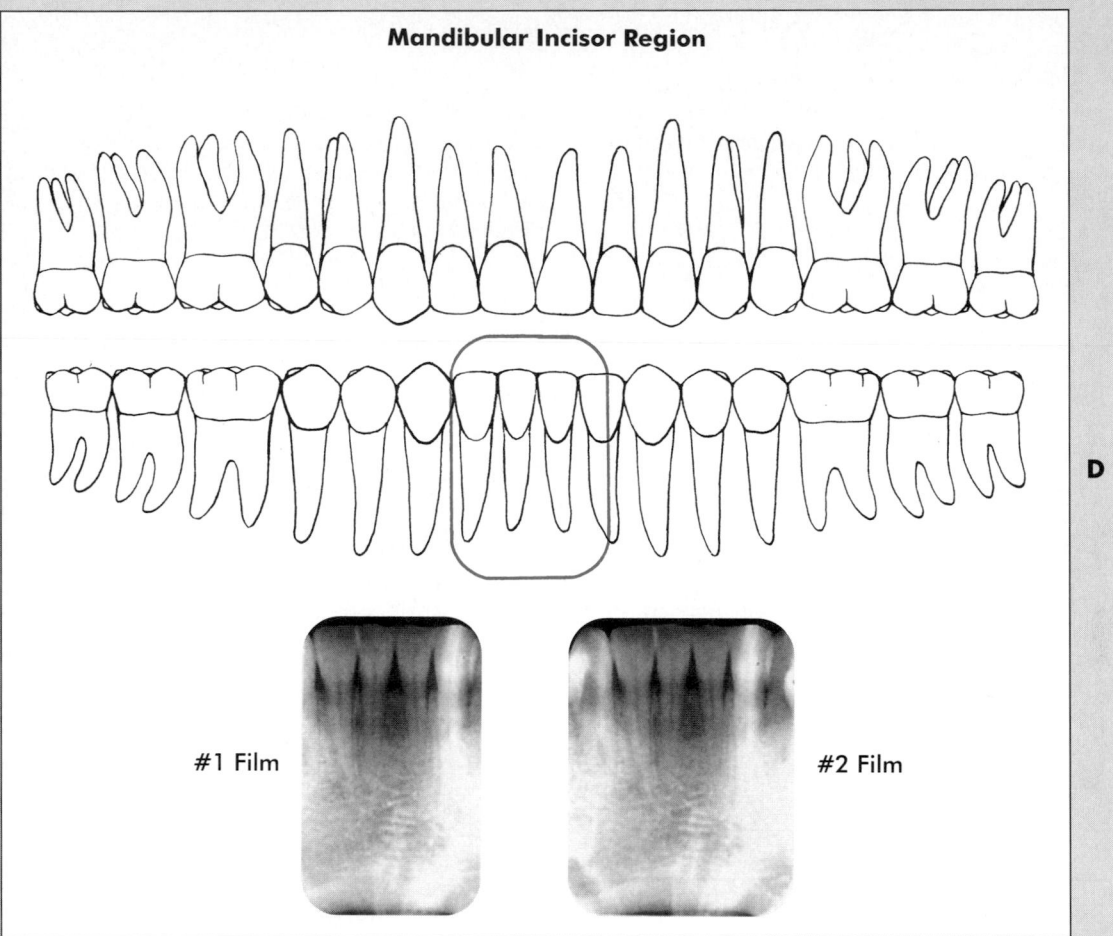

#1 Film #2 Film

D

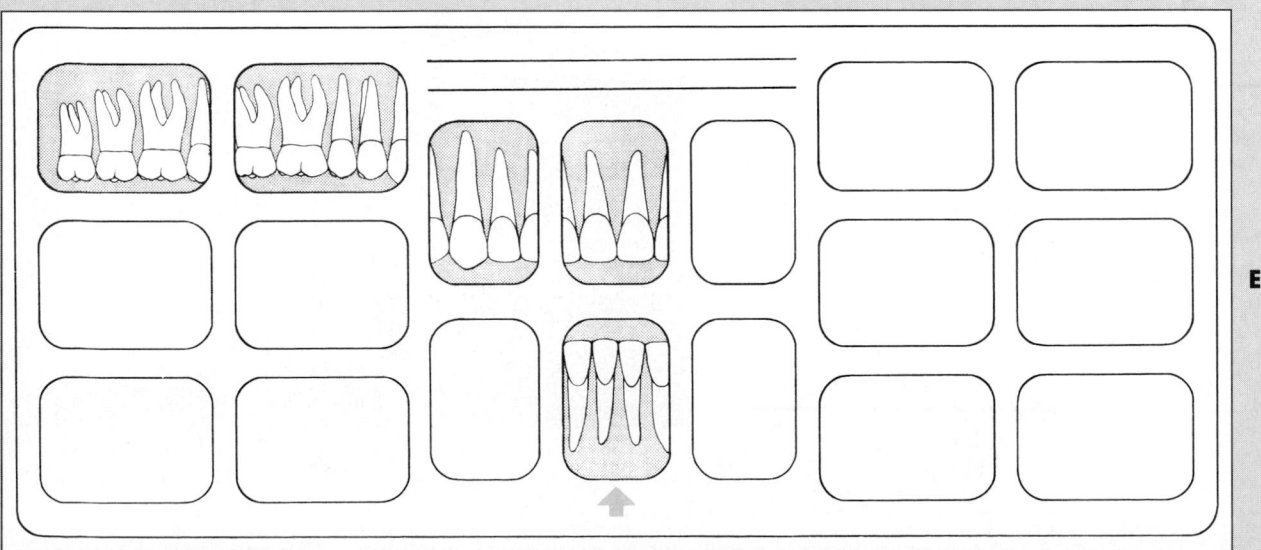

E

FIG. 9-22, cont'd.   *D,* Exposed film of area, reflecting section outlined in diagram above.
E, Film in mount.

Continued.

BOX 9-4, cont'd.

FILM PLACEMENT CRITERIA AND STRUCTURES VISUALIZED IN INTRAORAL DENTAL RADIOGRAPHS

MANDIBULAR CANINE, PERIAPICAL PROJECTION

Teeth. The canine tooth is centered on the film. The entire crown and root of the canine, including the apex, is depicted together with the interproximal alveolar crest of the adjacent lateral incisor.

Contacts open. The central ray is directed to open the contact between the canine and lateral incisor.

Anatomic structures visualized. The mental ridge and occasionally the lower border of the mandible are seen.

Film size. #1 or #2.

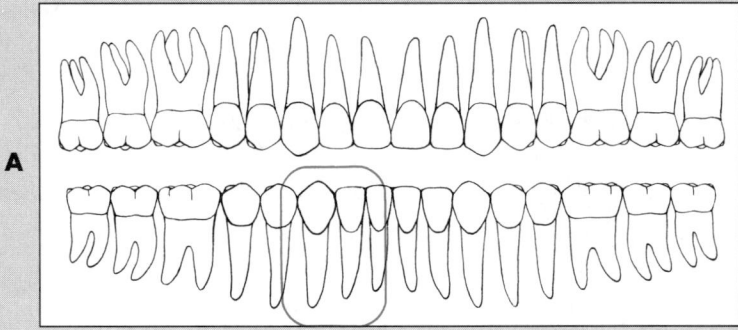

A

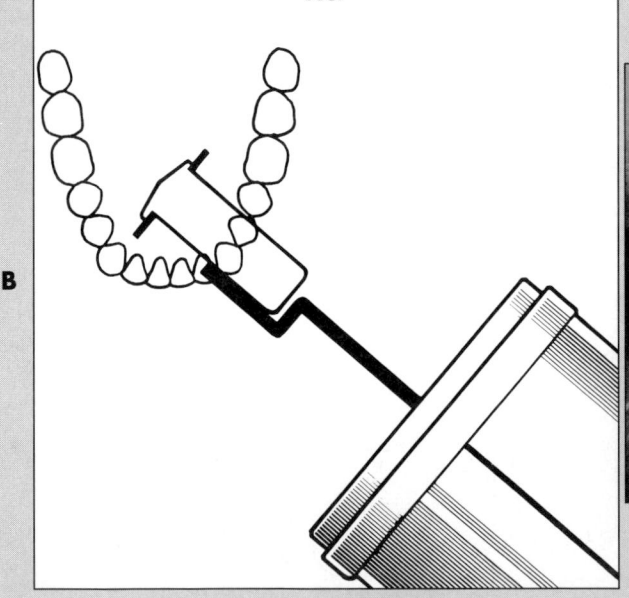

XCP

B

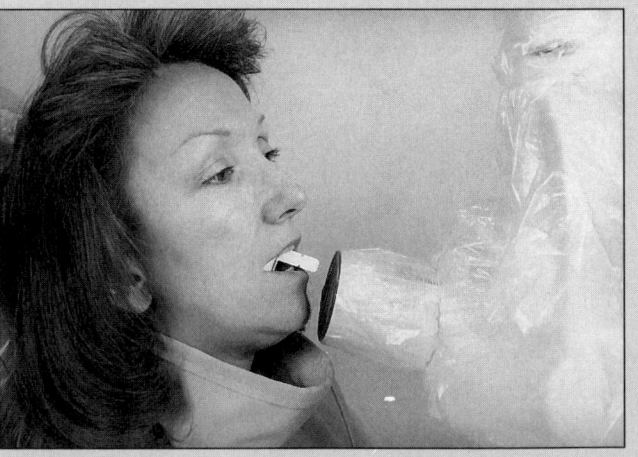

C

FIG. 9-23   *A,* Area to be exposed—mandibular canine, periapical projection. *B,* Film positioned in relation to teeth and PID. *C,* Film in holder positioned in mandibular canine area.

Mandibular Cuspid Region

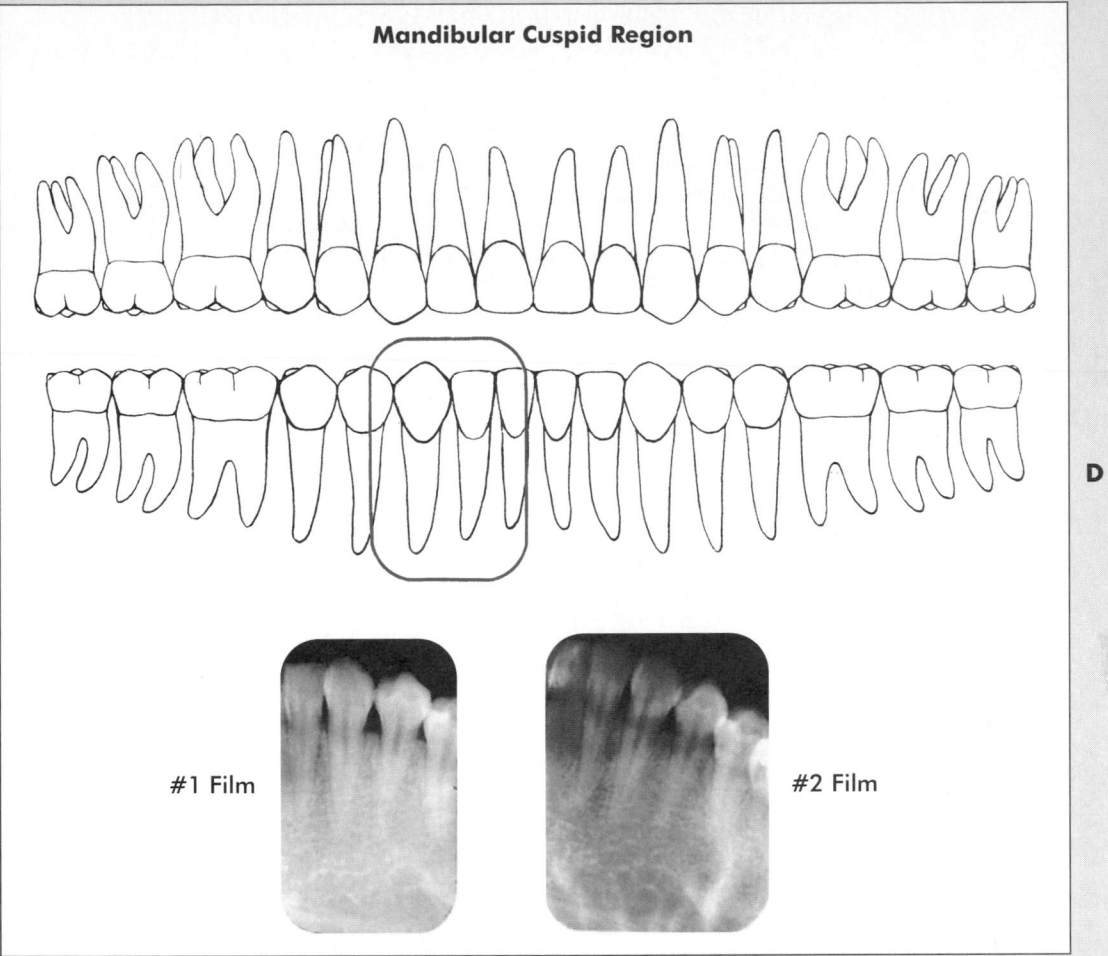

#1 Film #2 Film

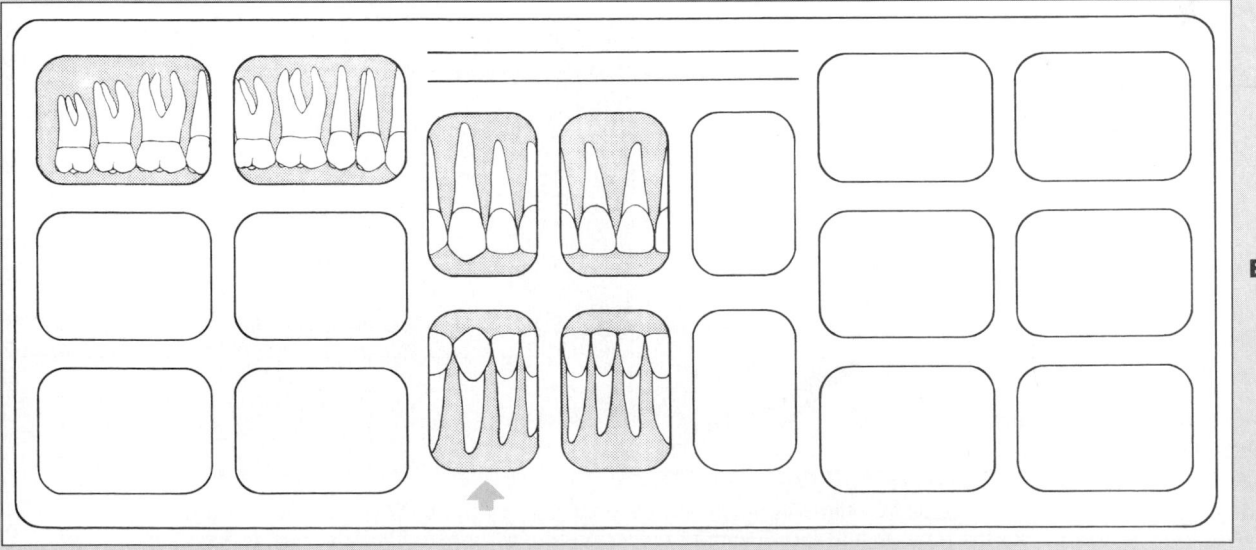

FIG. 9-23, cont'd. *D,* Exposed film of area, reflecting section outlined in diagram above. *E,* Film in mount. The film is positioned on the left side of the patient's mouth, and the mounted film is for the opposite side, thereby presenting positioning for both sides.

Continued.

FILM PLACEMENT CRITERIA AND STRUCTURES VISUALIZED IN INTRAORAL DENTAL RADIOGRAPHS

MANDIBULAR PREMOLAR PERIAPICAL PROJECTION

Teeth. The distal surface of the canine crown and the entire crown and root of the first and second premolar, including apices, are fully depicted together with the interproximal alveolar crest of the canine and first molar teeth.

Contacts open. The central ray should be directed to open the contact between the first and second premolar and the contact between the canine and the first premolar.

Anatomic structures visualized. The mental foramen and the mandibular canal are seen.

Film size. #1 or #2.

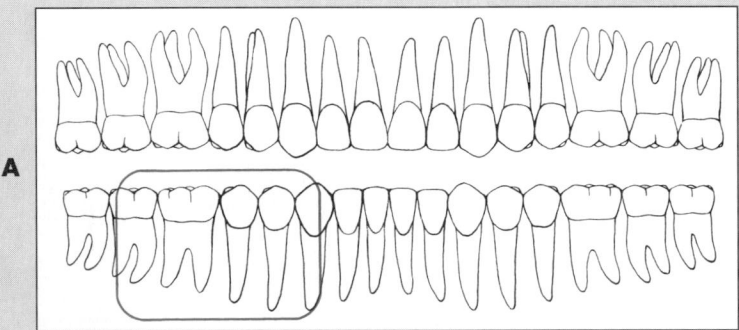

A

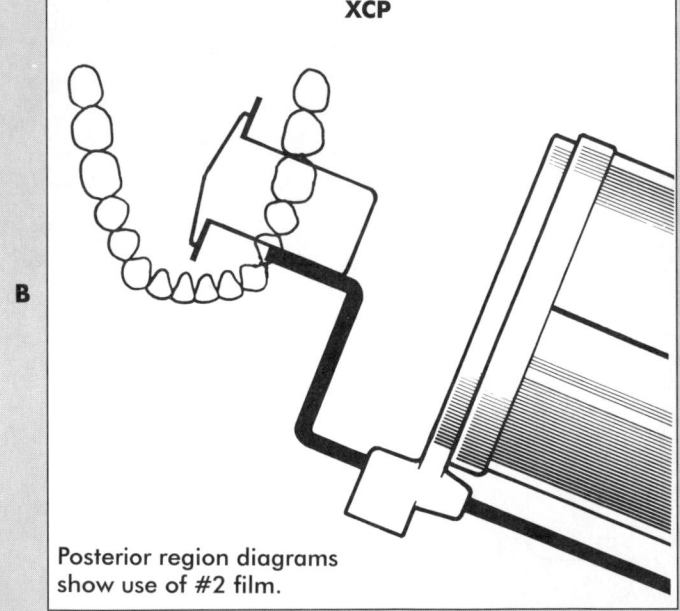

XCP

Posterior region diagrams show use of #2 film.

B

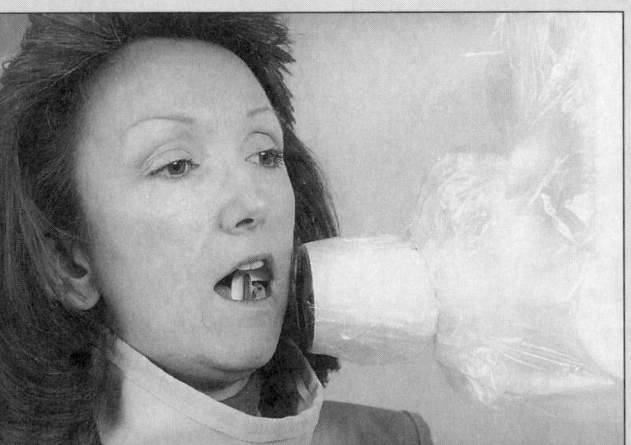

C

FIG. 9-24   *A,* Area to be exposed—mandibular premolar, periapical projection. *B,* Film positioned in relation to teeth and PID. *C,* Film in holder positioned in mandibular premolar area.

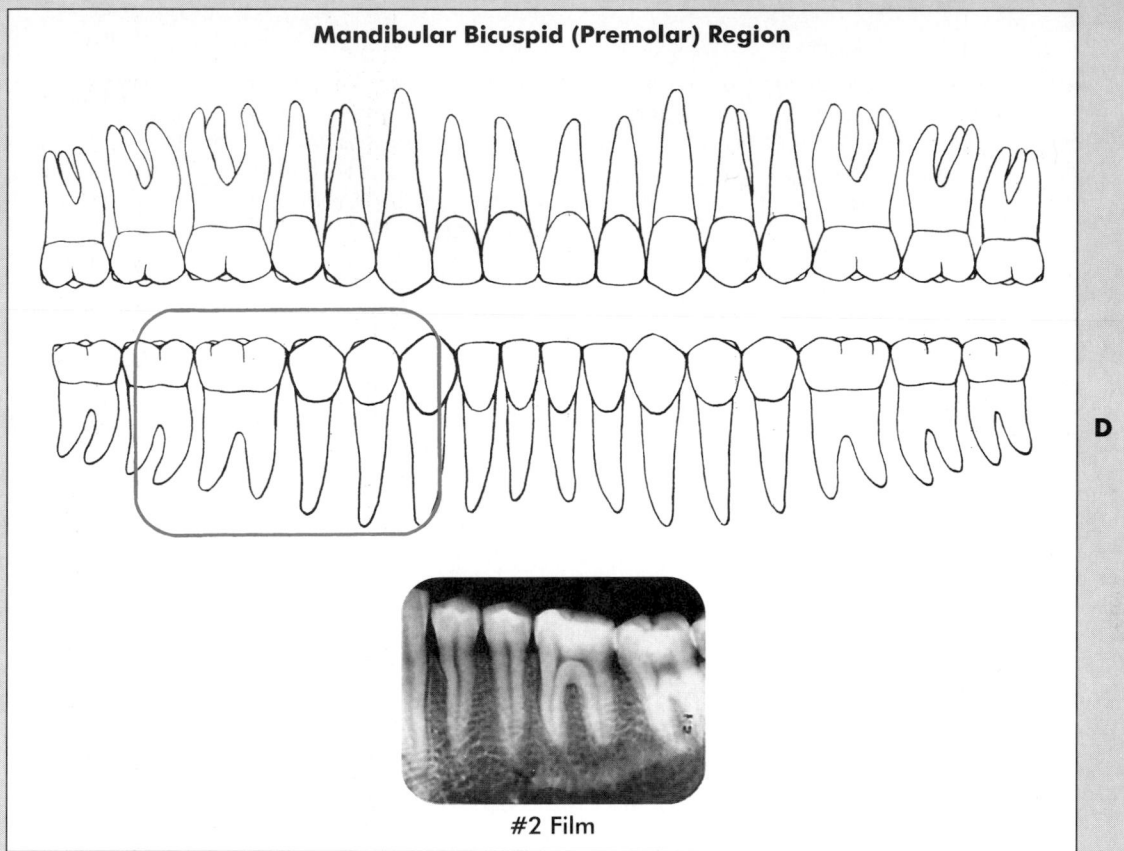

Mandibular Bicuspid (Premolar) Region

#2 Film

D

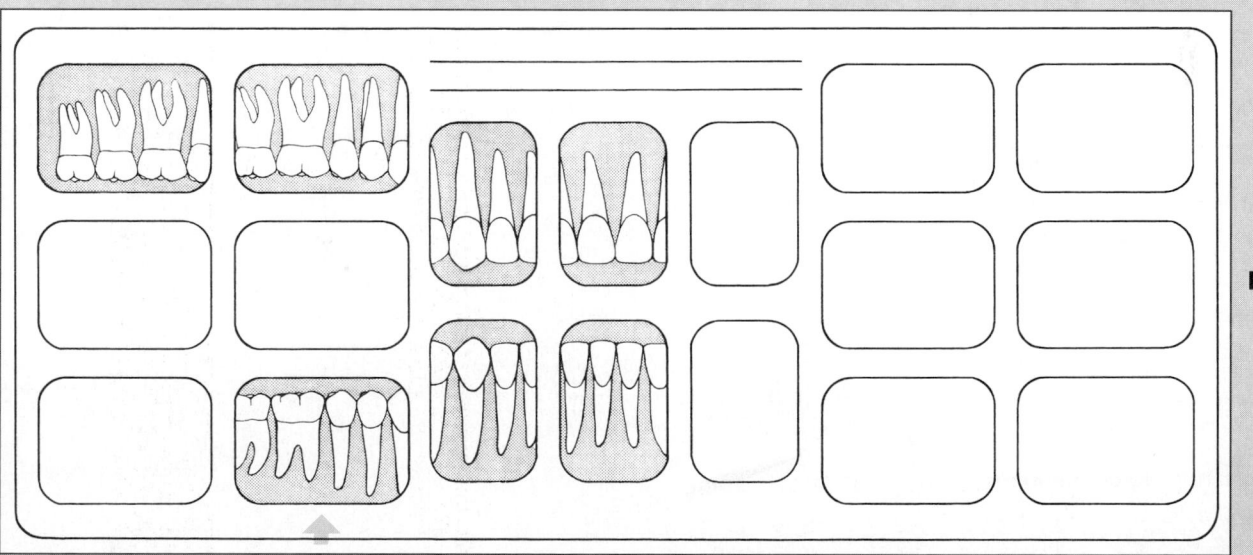

E

FIG. 9-24, cont'd.   *D,* Exposed film of area, reflecting section outlined in diagram above. *E,* Film in mount. The film is positioned on the left side of the patient's mouth, and the mounted film is for the opposite side, thereby presenting positioning for both sides.

Continued.

BOX 9-4, cont'd.

FILM PLACEMENT CRITERIA AND STRUCTURES VISUALIZED IN INTRAORAL DENTAL RADIOGRAPHS

MANDIBULAR MOLAR PERIAPICAL PROJECTION

Teeth. The distal surface of the second premolar and the entire crown and and root of the first, second, and third molars, including the apices, are fully depicted together with the interproximal alveolar crest distal to the third molar.

Contacts open. The central ray should be directed to open the contact between the first and second molar.

Anatomic structures visualized. The mandibular canal, the oblique ridge, the mylohyold ridge, and the anterior border of the ascending ramus are seen.

Film size. #2.

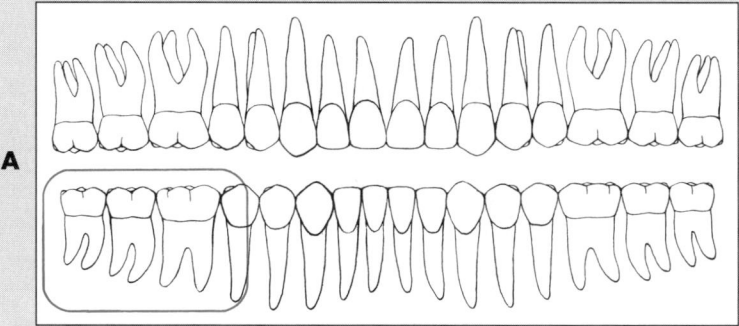

A

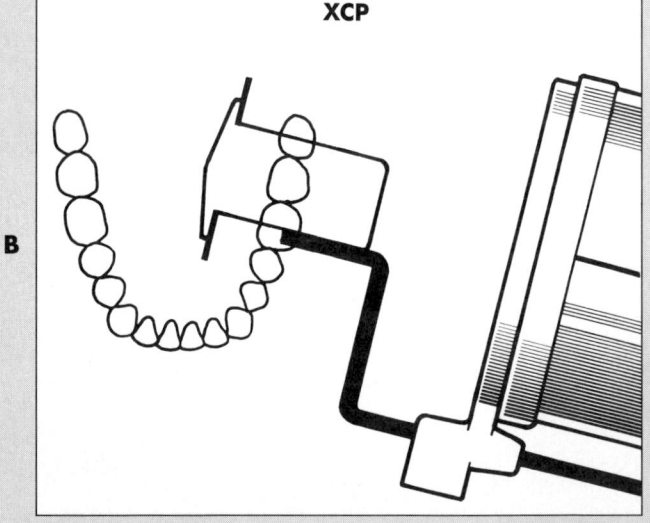

XCP

B

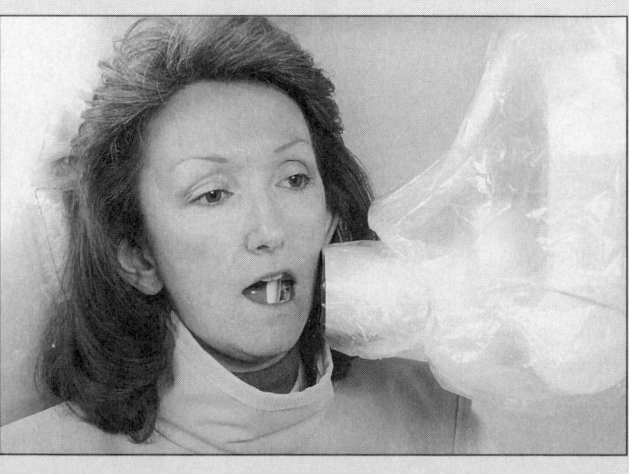

C

FIG. 9-25   *A,* Area to be exposed—mandibular molar, periapical projection. *B,* Film positioned in relation to teeth and PID. *C,* Film in holder positioned in mandibular molar area.

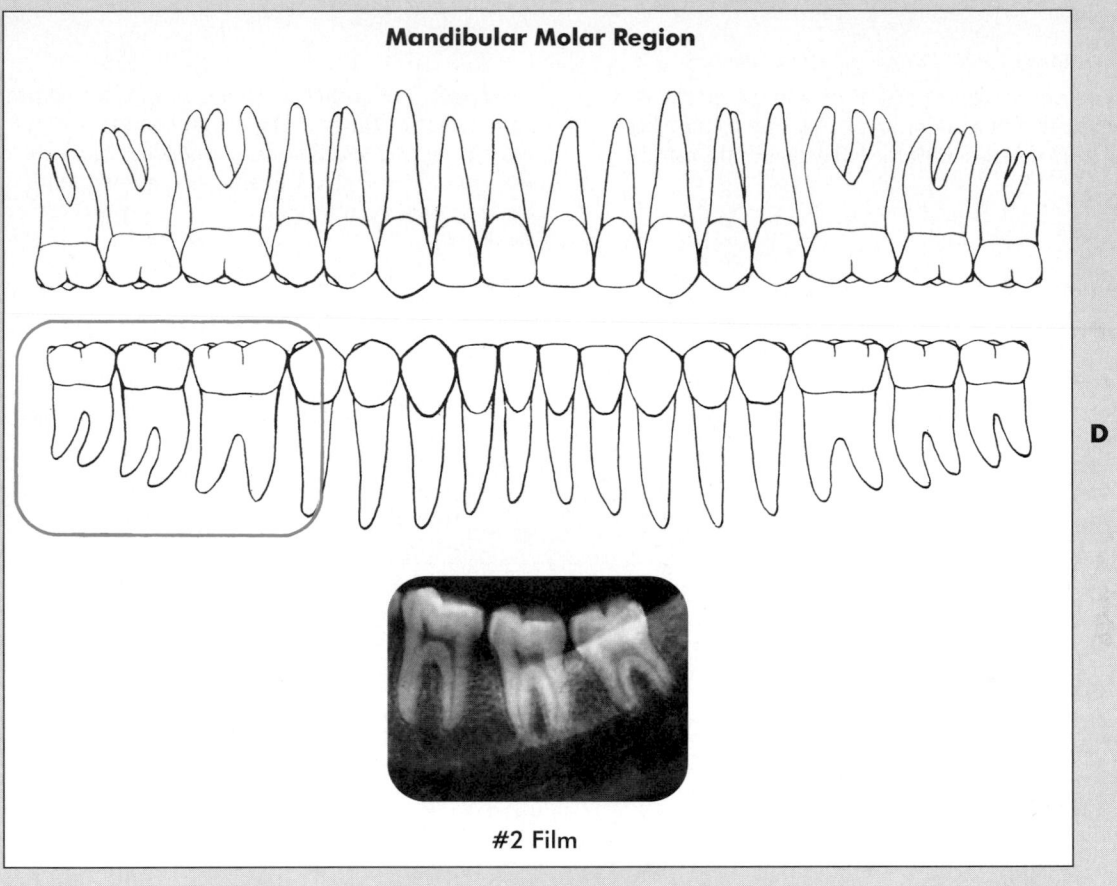

Mandibular Molar Region

#2 Film

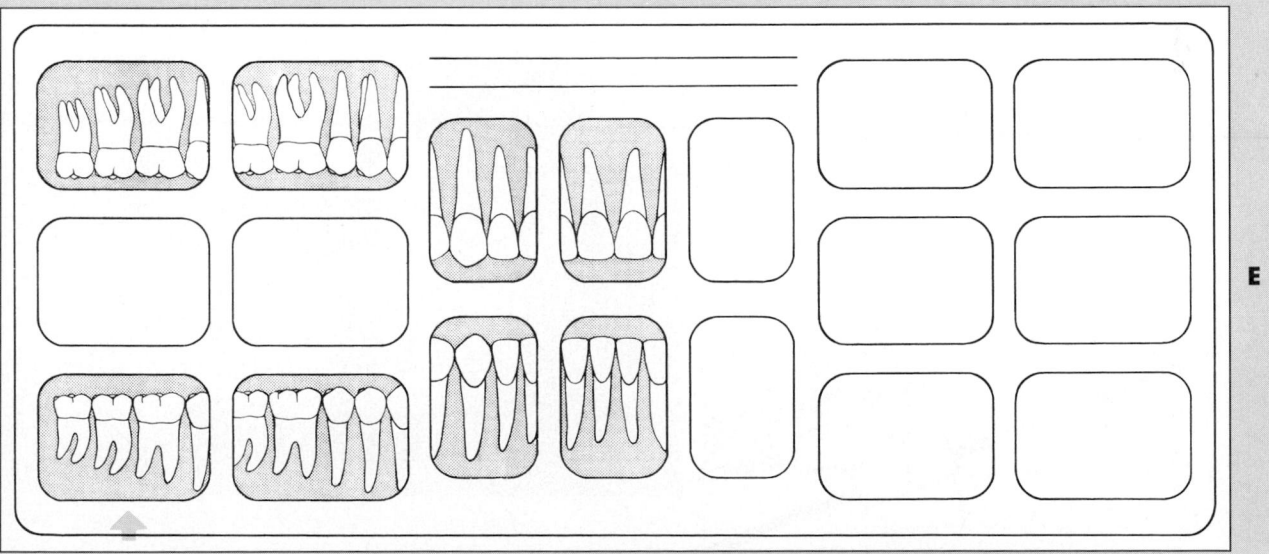

FIG. 9-25, cont'd. *D,* Exposed film of area, reflecting section outlined in diagram above. *E,* Film in mount. The film is positioned on the left side of the patient's mouth, and the mounted film is for the opposite side, thereby presenting positioning for both sides.

Continued.

BOX 9-4, cont'd.

FILM PLACEMENT CRITERIA AND STRUCTURES VISUALIZED IN INTRAORAL DENTAL RADIOGRAPHS

MANDIBULAR DISTAL MOLAR, PERIAPICAL PROJECTION

Teeth. The distal portion of the first molar and the entire crown and root of the second and third molars, including the apices, are fully depicted together with the full extent of the maxillary tuberosity.

Contacts open. The central ray should be directed perpendicular to the center of the film. Usually no contacts are open.

Anatomic structures visualized. The mandibular canal, the oblique ridge, the mylohyoid ridge, and the anterior border of the ascending ramus can be seen.

Film size. #2.

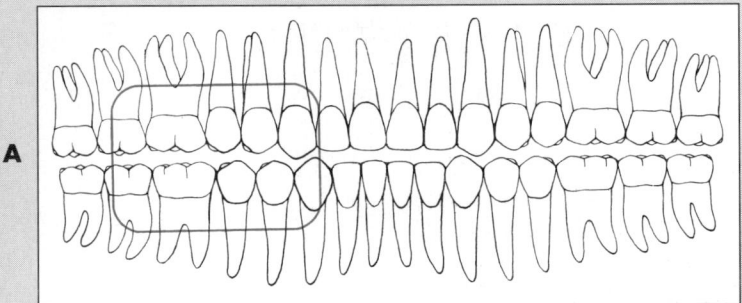

A

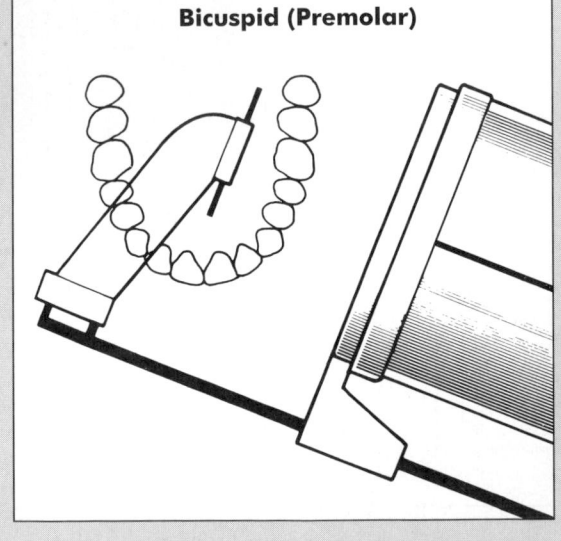

Bicuspid (Premolar)

B

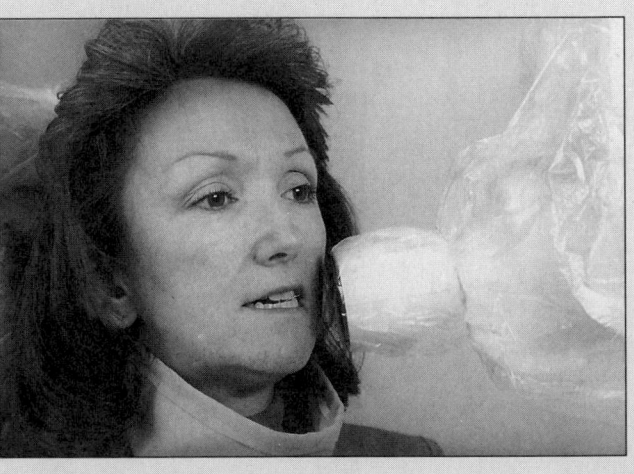

C

FIG. 9-26   *A,* Area to be exposed—premolar, interproximal projection (bitewing). *B,* Film positioned in relation to teeth and PID. *C,* Film in holder positioned in premolar area.

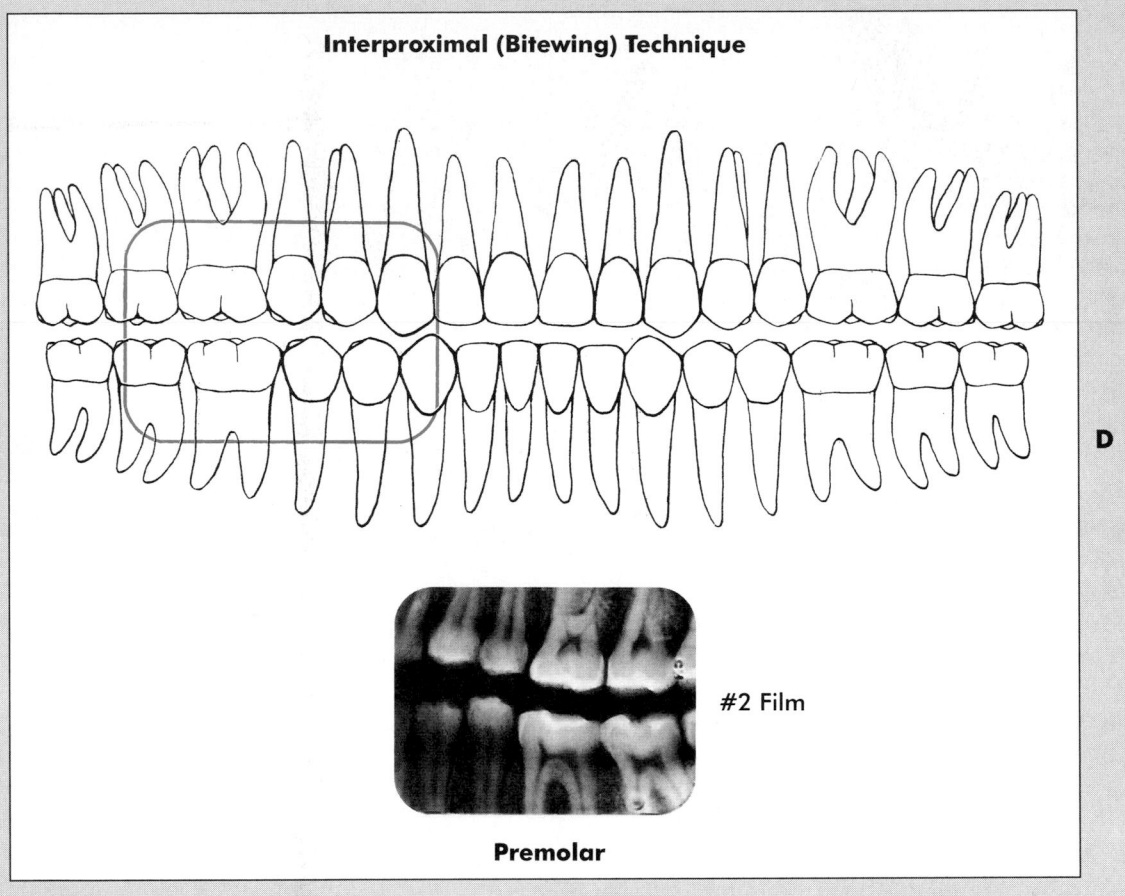

Interproximal (Bitewing) Technique

#2 Film

Premolar

D

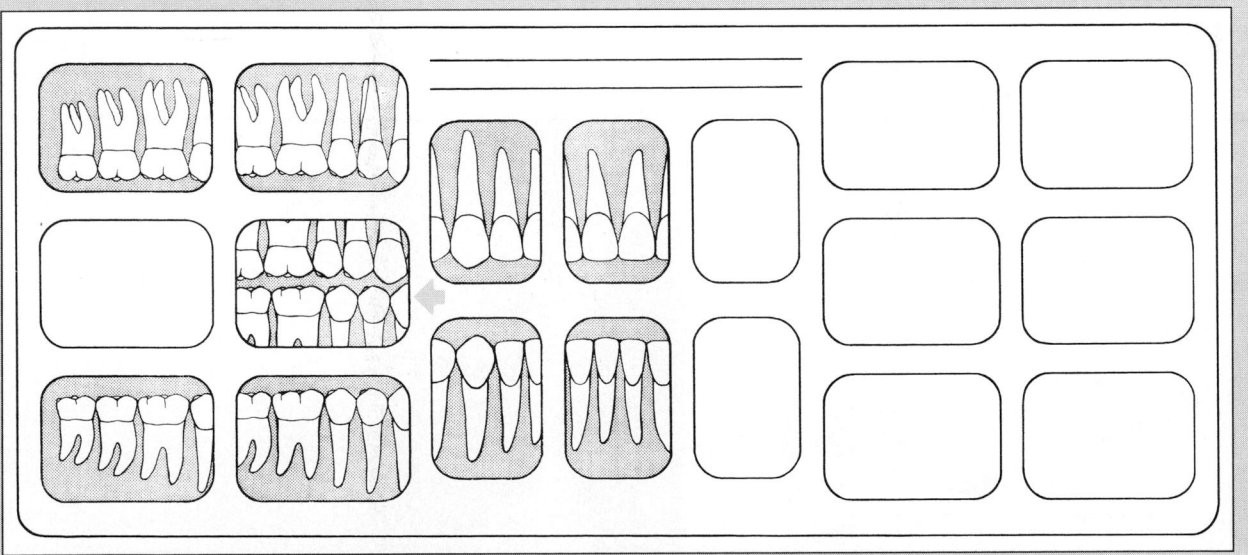

E

FIG. 9-26, cont'd.   *D,* Exposed film of area, reflecting section outlined in diagram above.
E, Film in mount. The film is positioned on the left side of the patient's mouth, and the
mounted film is for the opposite side, thereby presenting positioning for both sides.

Continued.

BOX 9-4, cont'd.

FILM PLACEMENT CRITERIA AND STRUCTURES VISUALIZED IN INTRAORAL DENTAL RADIOGRAPHS

HORIZONTAL PREMOLAR, INTERPROXIMAL PROJECTION (BITEWING)

Teeth. The distal coronal aspect of the canines and the crowns and crestal lamina of the first and second premolar are visualized as well as the interproximal alveolar crest distal to the canine and mesial to the first molar teeth.

Contacts open. The central ray should be directed perpendicular to the contact between the maxillary first and second premolars. The contacts open include the contacts between the canines and the first premolar and the contacts between the first and second premolars. Usually the contact between the first molar and the second premolar is open.

Anatomic structures visualized. The distal portion of both the maxillary and mandibular canines, the entire coronal aspects of the premolar teeth, and the mesial coronal surfaces of the first molars are seen, as are the crestal lamina and a portion of the intraradicular alveolar bone distal to the canine, mesial to the first molar and surrounding the premolar teeth.

Film size. #2 or #3.

HORIZONTAL MOLAR, INTERPROXIMAL PROJECTION (BITEWING)

Teeth. The distal aspects of the second premolar crowns and the crowns of the first and second molars are visualized as well as the interproximal alveolar crest distal to the second premolar and second molar.

Contacts open. The central ray should be directed perpendicular to the contact between the maxillary first and second molars. The open contacts include those between the first and second molars and those between the second premolar and first molar.

Anatomic structures visualized. The distal portion of both the maxillary and mandibular second premolar, the entire coronal aspects of the first and second molar teeth, and the mesial coronal surfaces of the third molars, if present, can be seen. Also, the crestal lamina and a portion of the intraradicular alveolar bone distal to the second premolar, mesial to the third molar and surrounding the molar teeth, are visualized.

Film size. #2 or #3.

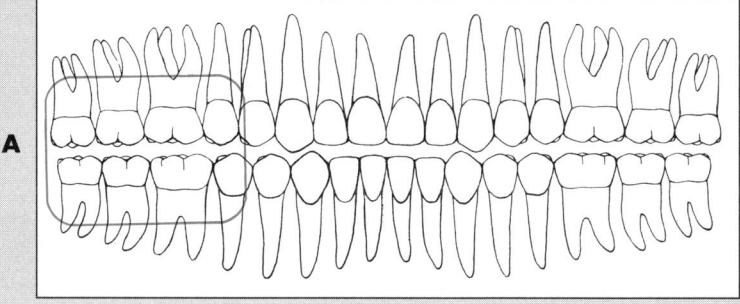

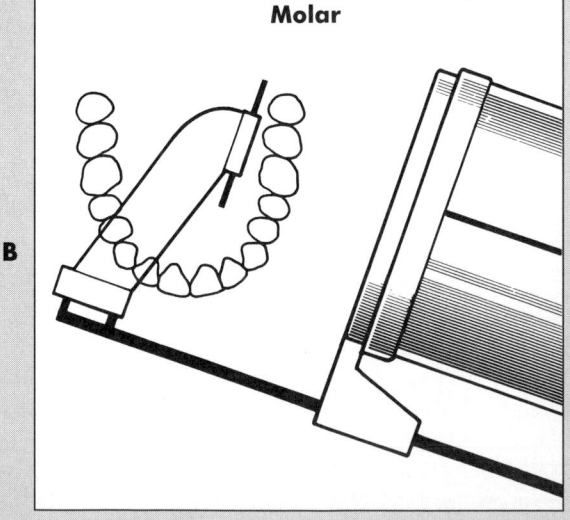

Molar

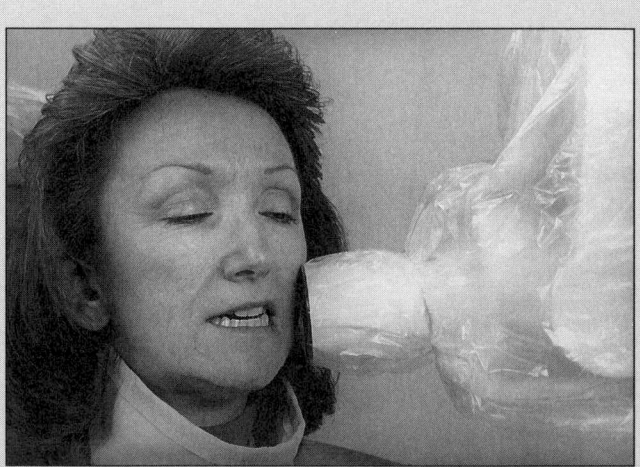

FIG. 9-27   *A,* Area to be exposed—molar, interproximal projection (bitewing). *B,* Film position in relation to teeth and PID. *C,* Film in holder positioned in molar area.

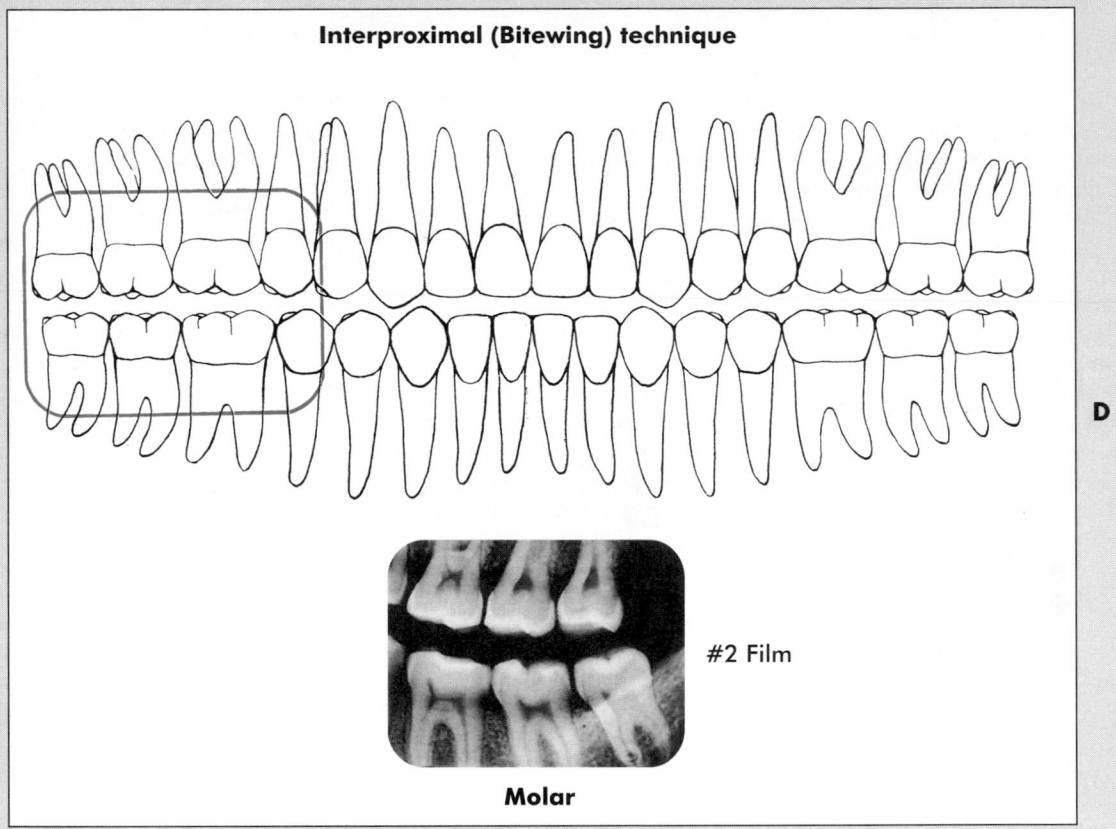

Interproximal (Bitewing) technique

#2 Film

Molar

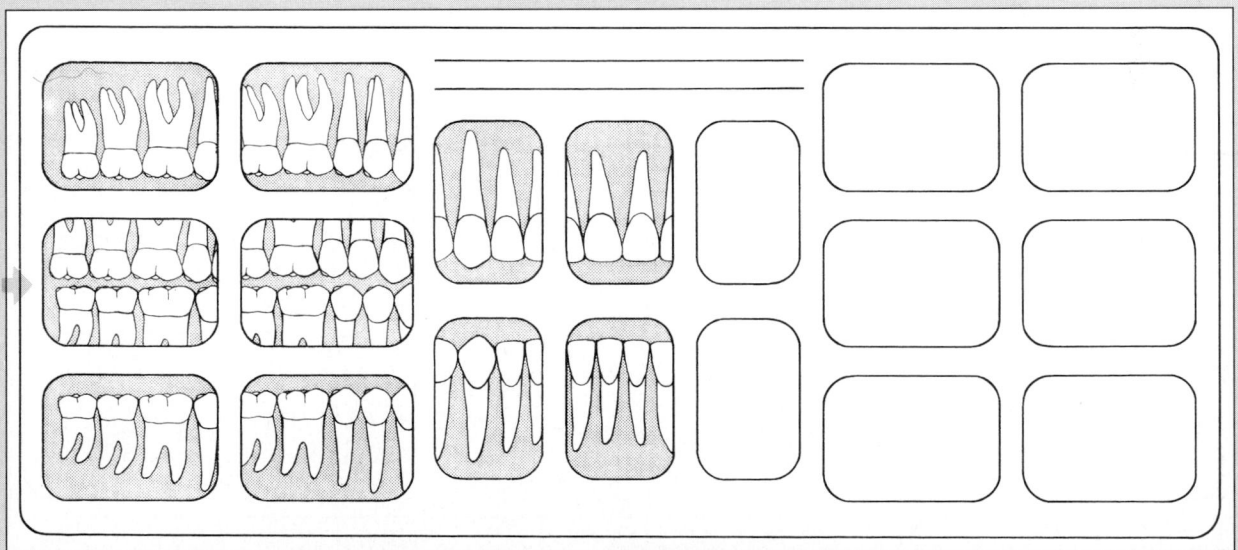

FIG. 9-27, cont'd.   *D,* Exposed film of area, reflecting section outlined in diagram above. *E,* Film in mount. The film is positioned on the left side of the patient's mouth, and the mounted film is for the opposite side, thereby presenting positioning for both sides.

Continued.

BOX 9-4, cont'd.

FILM PLACEMENT CRITERIA AND STRUCTURES VISUALIZED IN INTRAORAL DENTAL RADIOGRAPHS

VERTICAL PREMOLAR, INTERPROXIMAL PROJECTION (BITEWING)

Teeth. The distal coronal aspect of the canines and the crowns and crestal lamina of the first and second premolars, are visualized, as well as the interproximal alveolar crest distal to the canine and mesial to the first molar teeth.

Contacts open. The central ray should be directed perpendicular to the contact between the maxillary first and second premolars. The open contacts include those between the canines and the first premolar and those between the first and second premolars. Usually the contact between the first molar and the second premolar is open.

Anatomic structures visualized. The distal portion of both the maxillary and mandibular canines, the entire coronal aspects of the premolar teeth, and the mesial coronal surfaces of the first molar can be seen. The crestal lamina and a portion of the intraradicular alveolar bone distal to the canine, mesial to the first molar and surrounding the premolar teeth, can also be seen.

Film size. #1 or #2.

VERTICAL MOLAR, INTERPROXIMAL PROJECTION (BITEWING)

Teeth. The distal aspects of the second premolar crowns and the crowns of the first and second molars, are visualized as well as the interproximal alveolar crest distal to the second premolar and second molar.

Contacts open. The central ray should be directed perpendicular to the contact between the maxillary first and second molars. The open contacts include those between the first and second molars and those between the second premolar and first molar.

Anatomic structures visualized. The distal portion of both the maxillary and mandibular second premolar, the entire coronal aspects of the first and second molar teeth, the crestal lamina, and a portion of the intraradicular alveolar bone distal to the second premolar and the alveolar bone surrounding the molar teeth, including the furcation, can be seen.

Film size. #2.

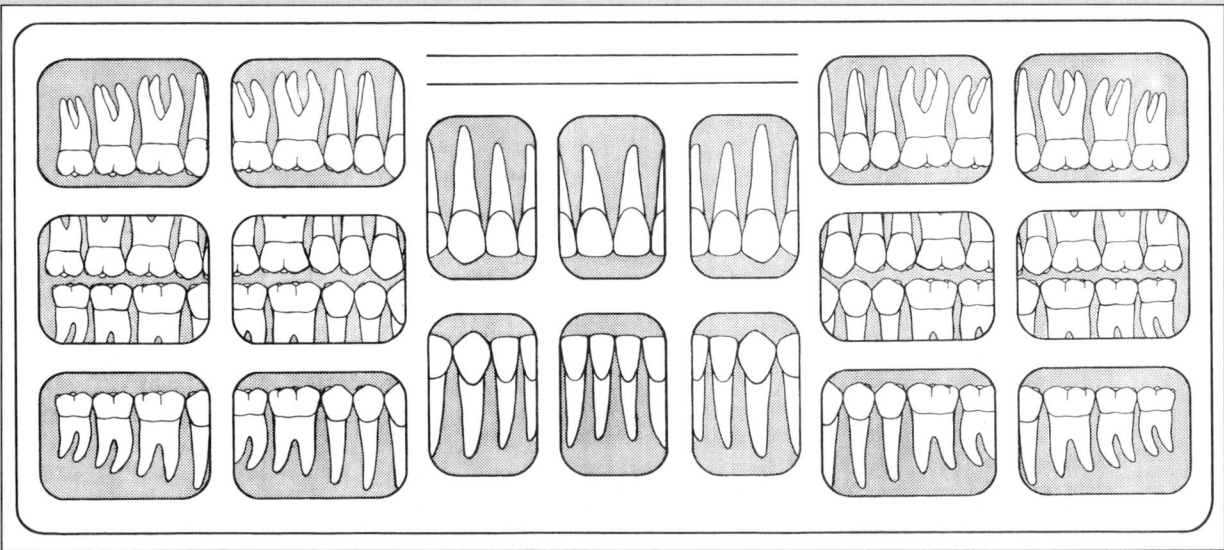

FIG. 9-28   Completed full series.

patient has extensive dental needs, a full-mouth series of radiographs is ordered. This series includes periapical radiographs to cover the apical area of all of the teeth or edentulous alveolar segments and bitewing radiographs to demonstrate the crowns and alveolar bone level, usually of the posterior region (Fig. 9-17). Panoramic, third molar, and occlusal projections are included when diagnostic criteria indicate the need for additional views. Interproximal (bite wing) radiographs are made on a horizontal projection unless the patient presents with moderate bone loss, indicating a need for vertical interproximal projections.

When the patient has less extensive dental disease, the dentist usually orders *selected periapicals,* that is, periapical radiographs for selected teeth or regions of the mouth. Bitewing radiographs are frequently ordered alone or together with *selected periapicals.* All radiographs should demonstrate optimum quality, considering the factors in Box 9-3.

The images projected on a film vary, depending on the number of radiographs taken in a series. A summary of common intraoral projections follows. The teeth and anatomic structures visualized in the projection together with the direction of the x-ray beam are summarized in Box 9-4.

Radiography for Edentulous Patients

Intraoral radiographs are usually required for the diagnostic evaluation of edentulous patients. Intraosseous pathosis may develop at any time, even though the teeth have been extracted and the patient has been wearing a prosthesis for some time. Many pathologic entities affecting the edentulous alveolus, including odontogenic cysts, tumors, and neoplasms, are more common in older individuals. Diagnostic evaluation of these diseases requires radiographic examination. Systemic diseases may also be manifested in the edentulous mandible. Other conditions such as residual root tips, infection, and foreign bodies require radiographic assessment. Finally, the clinical examination alone does not always provide sufficient information concerning the contour and character of the bone, anatomic features, and ridge relationships necessary for prosthetic diagnosis and treatment planning.

The dentist usually prescribes 10 to 14 periapical projections for the evaluation of edentulous patients. Obviously, bitewing exposures will not be necessary. Panoramic, occlusal, and lateral jaw radiographs are alternative projections used for edentulous patients.

Radiographic procedures for edentulous patients are similar to those used with dentate patients. Exposure times should be reduced by approximately 5% to achieve an appropriate density. All dental prostheses are removed before exposures are made. Either bisecting or paralleling technique can be used for edentulous periapical projections. Film placement, however, can be difficult. It is usually necessary to place cotton rolls in the space normally occupied by the crowns of the teeth. A modified bisecting technique must be used when the edentulous ridge is severely resorbed. Place the film against the ridge and direct the primary beam toward the center of the film at right angles to a line bisecting the angle formed by the long axis of the ridge and the film. A completed set of edentulous radiographs is shown as a 10-14 film series in Fig. 9-29.

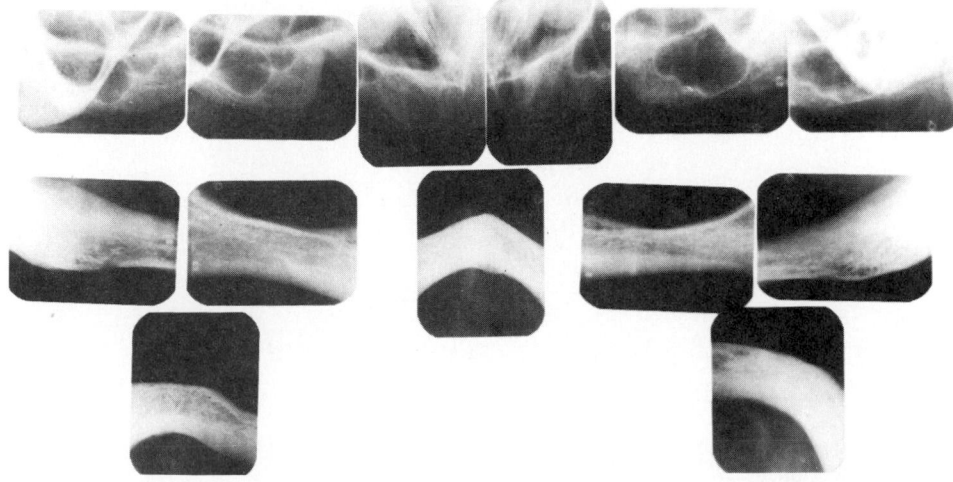

FIG. 9-29   Edentulous series of radiographs.

(From Frommer HH: *Radiology for dental auxiliaries,* ed 5, St Louis, 1992, Mosby.)

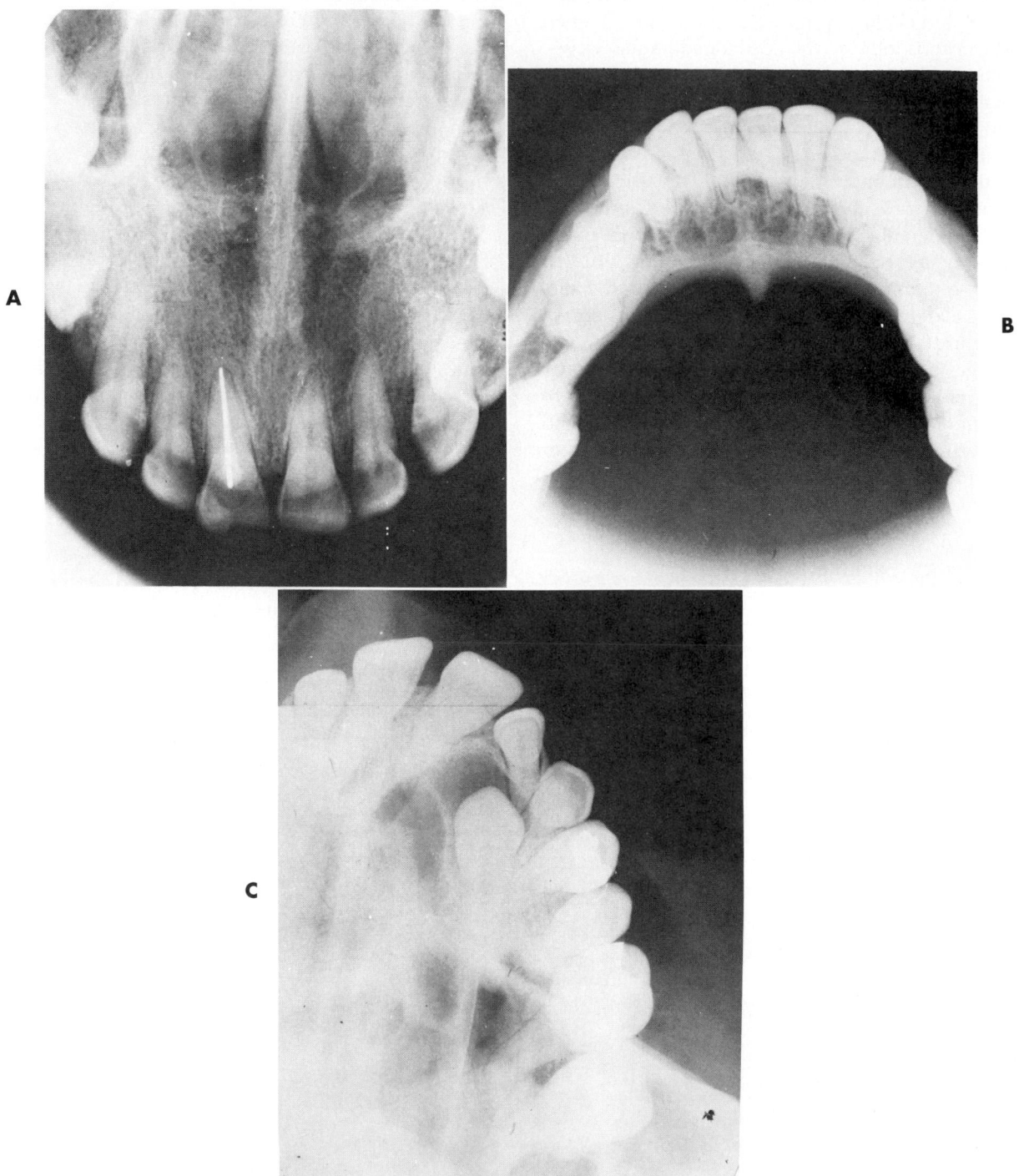

FIG. 9-30   *A,* Maxillary occlusal projection. *B,* Mandibular occlusal projection. *C,* Right-angle occlusal projection.

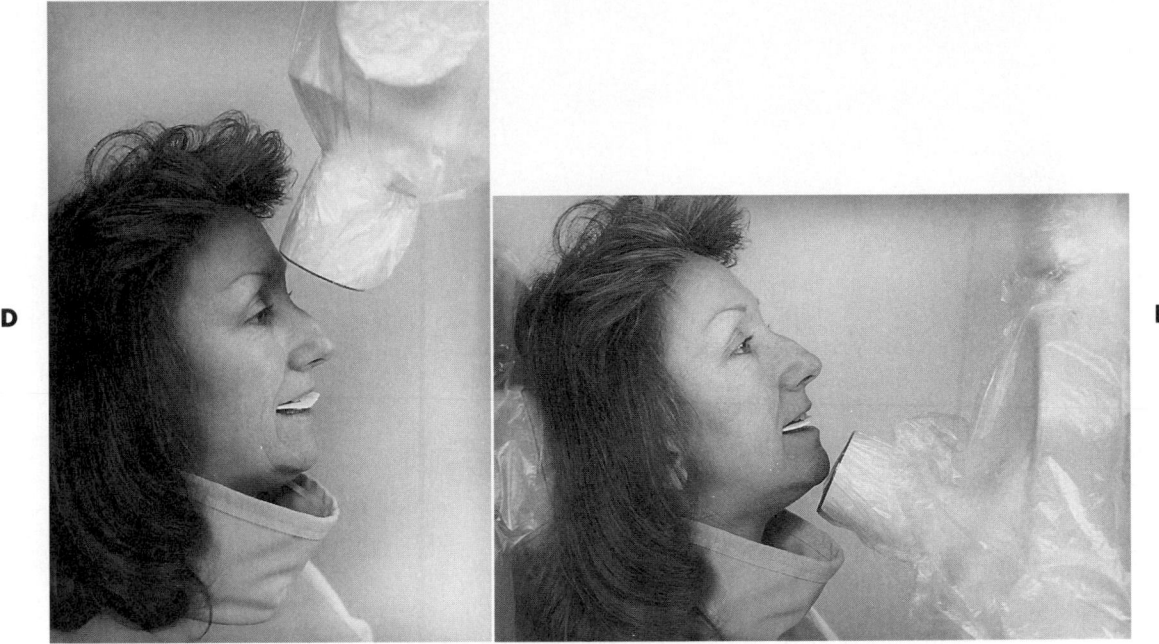

FIG. 9-30, cont'd.   *D,* Maxillary occlusal position on patient. *E,* Mandibular occlusal position on patient.

(From Frommer HH: *Radiology for dental auxiliaries,* ed 5, St Louis, 1992, Mosby.)

Occlusal Projections

Occlusal radiographic projections are used to obtain large areas of a single arch in one projection. The size of the film allows for increased field projection. An occlusal film packet is commonly 2 ¼ × 3 inches and may be a single- or double-film packet.

In addition to being useful in visualizing a large area of the arch, this type of exposure can be used for patients who find it difficult to open their mouths wide enough to accommodate the periapical film, as with a patient who has trismus or has experienced facial trauma. Common occlusal projections include maxillary occlusal technique, mandibular occlusal technique, right-angle projections, and lateral occlusal technique (Fig. 9-30, A through *E*)

▶ Procedure for Intraoral Dental Radiography

Several steps are required to complete the radiographic examination. These steps include the following:

1. Obtaining the prescription for the radiographs
2. Gathering the personal protection that will be necessary during the procedure
3. Preparing the treatment area, instruments, and required armamentarium
4. Complying with infection control techniques
5. Completing exposure procedures
6. Completing the processing procedures

Prescription and Examination

Patients are examined before radiographs are taken. The dentist selects the radiographs that are necessary, based on the individual needs of the patient. The procedure for the exposure of the radiographs may then be assigned to an auxiliary. If you are uncertain about the dentist's order, verify it before the patient is seated.

Personal Protection

Masks, gloves, and protective eyewear should be worn for all radiographic procedures. Using personal protection is necessary to safeguard against the transmission of disease. Although aerosols are not produced during radiographic procedures, saliva can be ejected from the oral cavity as the patient opens the mouth. Film placement frequently results in stimulation of the sublingual and submandibular glands, resulting in an exuberant projection of saliva as radiographic film is placed into or removed from the patient's mouth.

Surface Disinfection and Cross-Contamination

Place all items unnecessary to the procedure (supplies, equipment, and charts) outside the treatment room. Minimize surfaces touched by contaminated hands. Cover all surfaces, including countertops, tubehead, exposure button, and control panel (Fig. 9-31, *A* through *D*). Examples of surfaces covered include the tubehead

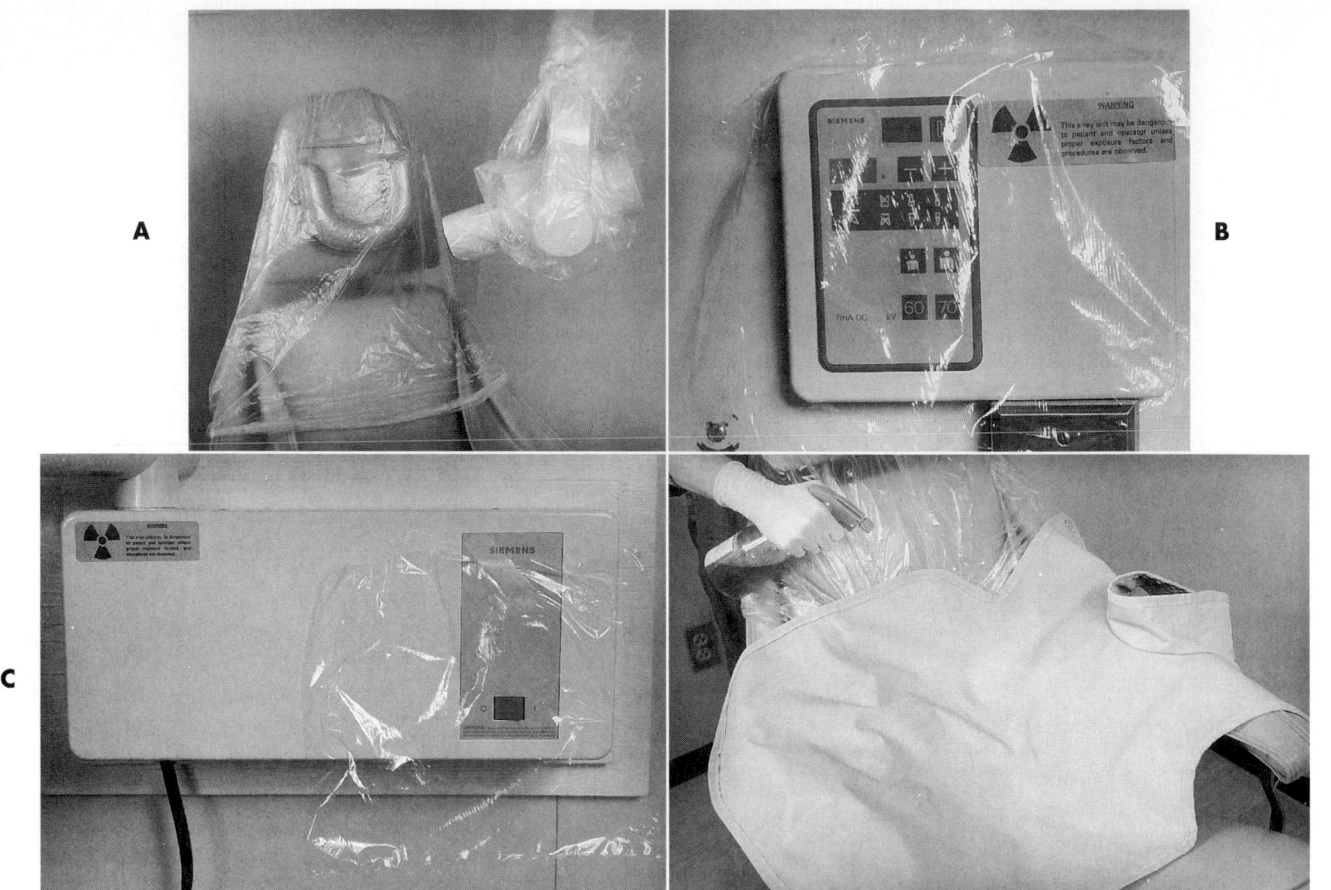

FIG. 9-31   *A,* **PID.** *B,* **Control panel.** *C,* On/Off switch. *D,* If surfaces such as the protective apron are not covered, they must be sprayed/wiped, sprayed/wiped.

and treatment chair; use clear plastic bags and plastic wrap over control panels and switch buttons. Any *touch or splash* surfaces not covered *must* be disinfected with an EPA-registered disinfectant.

Film Disinfection

Another procedure for avoiding cross-contamination in radiography is the practice of film disinfection and safe handling of that film. Common methods for film disinfection are as follows:

- ▶ Place each film in a clear plastic sleeve before patient contact (Fig. 9-32). After exposure remove the film from the sleeve while avoiding its contamination. Using care in opening the sleeve, allow the film packet to fall on a clean surface and dispose of the sleeves. Remove gloves, and wash hands before touching each film. These steps reduce cross-contamination.
- ▶ Remove all saliva from the exposed film and spray/wipe/spray/wipe each film for the recommended

period of time with an approved surface disinfectant. Film packets must be completely dry before removing the outer cover and processing the film. This method presents a potential for fluid contamination onto the unprocessed film.
- ▶ Process films using an infection control technique for the daylight loader processing unit as described in the following step-by-step procedures:

DAYLIGHT LOADER INFECTION CONTROL TECHNIQUES: STEP-BY-STEP PROCEDURE

1. Leave the treatment room with the exposed radiographs in a plastic cup.
2. If you are wearing treatment gloves from the radiographic procedure area, avoid contact with other objects (e.g., door knobs).
3. Place overgloves on the latex treatment gloves to avoid contamination of items. Another option is to remove the contaminated gloves, wash hands, and hold the plastic cup with the contaminated films, using a paper towel.

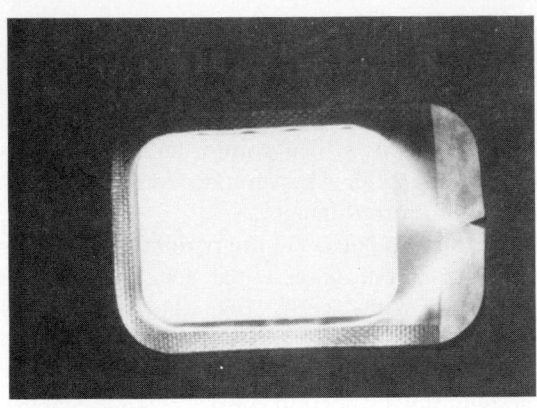

FIG. 9-32 Placement of film packet in protective plastic cover to avoid contamination of the film.

(From Goaz PW, White SC: *Oral radiology, principles and interpretation,* ed 3, St Louis, 1994, Mosby.)

4. Open the safety glass of the daylight loader, and place the cup inside. At the same time, place the anterior film holder in the daylight loader with the films if it is needed.
5. Close the safety glass of the daylight loader.
6. If your treatment gloves were removed or if you used overgloves, the safety glass will not require disinfection at a later time.
7. Place a new pair of latex gloves on hands.
8. Place both hands into the cuffs on either side of the daylight loader, making sure your arms are securely covered by the cuffs to avoid light leakage.
9. If overgloves are still on over contaminated treatment gloves, remove the overgloves inside the daylight loader, and proceed with the process.
10. Process all films; do not remove your hands from the daylight loader until all films are in the machine.
11. If it is necessary to remove your hands during processing, protect the films from exposure, and remove the contaminated gloves that were worn during processing inside the loader to avoid contamination.
12. Place all contaminated film packets inside the plastic cup or other holder.
13. Remove the treatment gloves inside out in the dayloader, and remove your hand from the cuffs.
14. Open the safety glass with another pair of gloves or a protective towel, and remove the cup with opened film packets and used gloves.

Setting Up

Mask, gloves, protective eyewear, and a paper cup, together with sufficient radiographic film, cotton rolls, bitewing tabs, and film holders to complete the process for a single patient, should be obtained before the procedure. Assemble film holders, and organize disposable supplies.

Instruments

When the radiographic examination is completed, film-holding devices should be scrubbed free of debris, dried thoroughly, and sterilized. Panoramic bite guides should be sterilized, disposed of, or covered with a suitable material.

Equipment Asepsis

The x-ray tubehead and control panel contain mechanical and electrical components that must be protected from excess moisture; however, this does not preclude disinfection of the x-ray unit after each patient procedure. If an uncovered equipment surface is touched, it must be disinfected. Moisten a paper towel with disinfectant. Starting with the least contaminated surfaces, wipe down areas of possible contamination. Do not spray the disinfectant directly on the tubehead or control panel. Wipe the surface dry with a paper towel, then reclean the surface with a fresh disinfectant-moistened towel, allow it to remain on the surface as recommended by the manufacturer, and wipe dry. NOTE: When you are disinfecting the tubehead and control panel and after you have used the second application of disinfectant, wipe the surface dry to protect the unit from excess moisture. Allow all other environmental surfaces to dry by evaporation.

Lead apron Wipe the lead apron clean and return it to the hanging rod. DO NOT FOLD! Folding the lead apron will result in breaks in the lead and decreased protective function.

Chair Disinfect any surface touched or splashed during the procedure, including the headrest, adjustment levers, and arms if they were not previously covered.

X-ray unit Take care when disinfecting the x-ray unit to avoid excess moisture leaking into the inner surface of the machine. Disinfect any uncovered surface that has been touched during the procedure, including the yoke, PID, tubehead, control panel, and exposure buttons.

RADIOGRAPHIC STEP-BY-STEP PROCEDURE

Preparing the Patient

1. Greet the patient in the reception area, check the patient's health history, and ask the date of the most recent dental radiographs. If radiographs were made by another facility, obtain the patient's permission to request previous radiographs.

2. Escort the patient to the treatment room. Seat the patient; adjust the occipital support so that the patient's head is comfortable and the occlusal plane is parallel to the floor.
3. Explain the x-ray procedure to the patient. If the patient is nervous, explain the safety precautions that are taken to prevent overexposure to radiation. Explain that radiographs are necessary to provide adequate, high-quality dental care.
4. Ask the patient to remove eyeglasses, dentures, or any other large objects around the head and neck. Drape the patient with a lead apron to cover the thyroid, spine, thorax, and abdomen.

5. Wash hands and put on gloves, mask, and protective eyewear.
6. Set kVp, mA, and timer, following recommendations for the radiograph you are taking. Make sure the patient's head is in a comfortable position and is immobile. Patient movement during an exposure creates a blurred image.
7. Place the film packet in the patient's mouth. Proper film placement is essential for successful radiographs. Visually verify that the film covers the intended area.
8. Position the tubehead, following guidelines for the radiographic projection you are making. Stabilize the

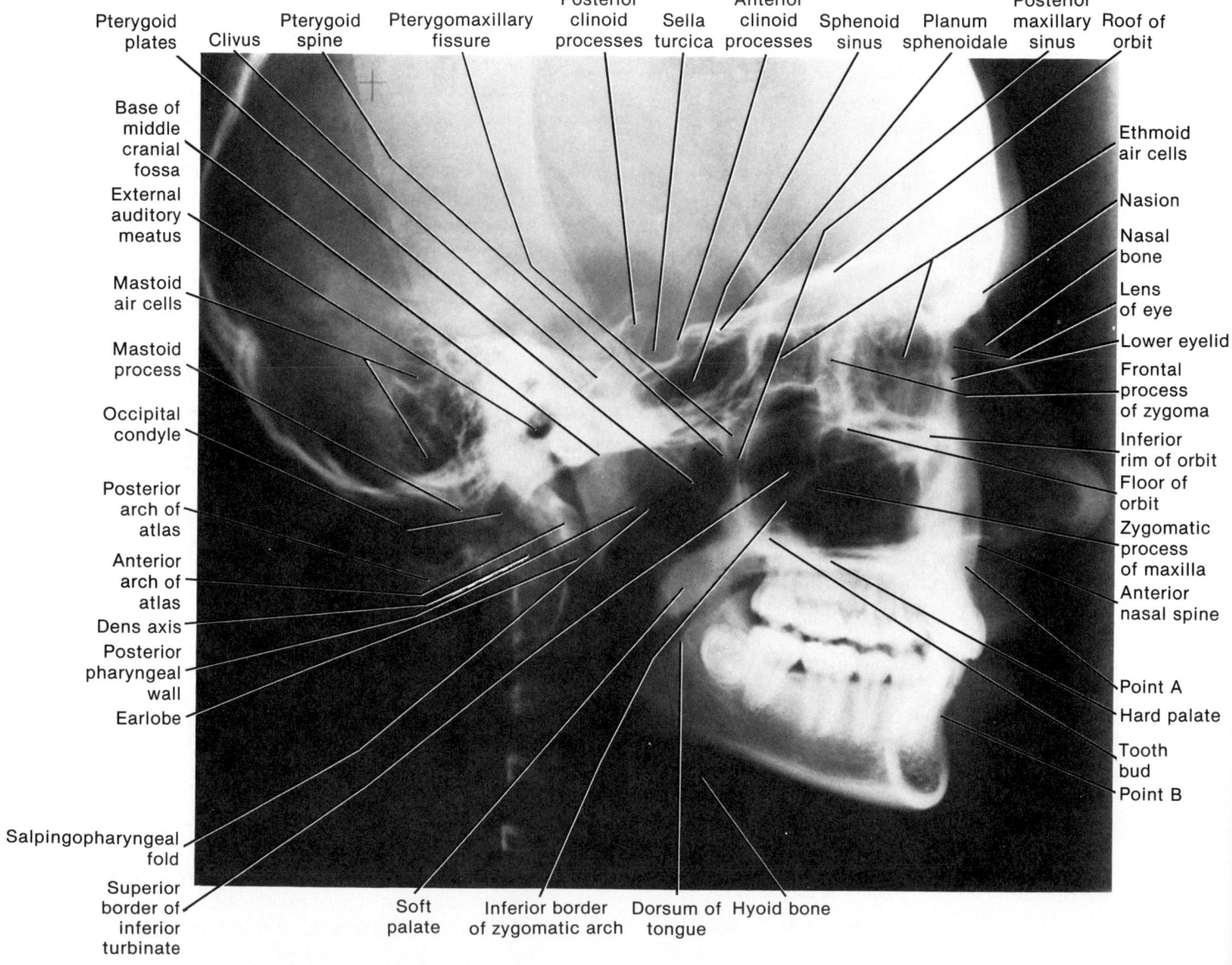

FIG. 9-33   Cephalometric projection of facial bones.

(From Goaz PW, White SC: *Oral radiology, principles and interpretation,* ed 3, St Louis, 1994, Mosby.)

tubehead, ensuring that all movement has stopped. Any movement of the tubehead during a exposure may create a blurred image.

9. Step behind the protective barrier, viewing the patient to verify position. Confirm exposure factors. Depress the exposure button, and continue to hold it until the audible signal has completely stopped. If the button is released too soon, the radiograph will be underexposed.

10. Remove the film packet from the patient's mouth, and place it in a paper cup outside the cubicle. (Do not leave the film packets in the cubicle; they will be exposed to scatter radiation.) When the procedure is completed, wipe the contaminated film packets *dry* with a paper towel, place them in an envelope or paper cup, and take them to the processing area. Each packet may be wiped dry after the exposure and then placed in a holding device until they are processed.

Extraoral Radiography

Radiographs of the maxillofacial area using film positioned outside the oral cavity are called extraoral projections. Extraoral radiographs are used when it is necessary to evaluate regions not covered by periapical films, when soft tissue injury or edema contraindicates intraoral film placement, to evaluate maxillofacial growth, to determine the relationship of facial bones to the skeletal base, and to assess the relationship of the mandible and maxilla.

Common types of extraoral radiographs include panoramic, cephalometric, lateral jaw, and temporomandibular joint projections.

Radiographs of the skull using a specialized head positioned are called cephalometric projections (Fig. 9-33). The lateral cephalometric radiograph is the most common cephalometric projection. Orthodontists use this projection to evaluate skeletal growth patterns, jaw relationships, and soft tissue profiles. Lateral cephalometric radiographs are usually ordered for diagnosis, during therapy, and at the conclusion of orthodontic treatment. Lateral cephalometric radiographs may also be necessary to evaluate patients receiving implants or other extensive restorative dental treatment.

Cephalometric analysis is the tracing of major anatomic landmarks depicted in the lateral cephalometric radiograph for diagnostic purposed. Through cephalometric analysis, the dentist determines appropriate treatment or assesses the progress of current therapy. Radiographs used for cephalometric analysis must be made with careful attention to detail; especially important is correct patient positioning.

The lateral jaw projection results in a radiograph of the entire mandible and maxilla (Fig. 9-34). This radiograph is often used for patients who are unable to tolerate intraoral film placement such as children, older adult, or handicapped individuals. Lateral jaw radiographs are also used to evaluate fractures of the mandible.

Oral surgeons and practitioners who specialize in the treatment of TMJ disorders rely on radiographs for the diagnostic evaluation of patients (Fig. 9-35). The TMJ is difficult to image because of its location within the cranial base. Specialized equipment or techniques are usually needed to produce a diagnostic radiograph for the TMJ.

Temporomandibular articulation survey is common to oral surgeons or other practitioners who specialize in TMJ disturbances. This type of radiography is more difficult to obtain, since it requires that the patient maintain a specific head position without any movement for an accurate image. Specialized imaging procedures, such as magnetic resonance (MR) are required to clearly define the articular disk. These specialized images are usually required when treating a patient with severe TMJ disturbances (Fig. 9-36).

Panoramic radiographs, first introduced in 1960, are becoming increasingly more common in all areas of dental practice. Panoramic radiography results in an image of both maxillary and mandibular alveolar processes, paranasal sinuses, and the TMJ on a single extraoral film (Fig. 9-37). Panoramic radiographs are

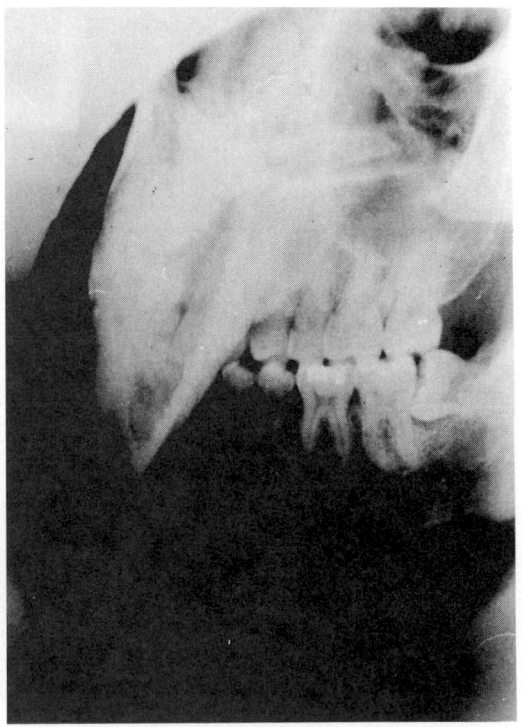

FIG. 9-34   Lateral oblique jaw projection.

(From Frommer HH: *Radiology for dental auxiliaries*, ed 5, St Louis, 1992, Mosby.)

usually prescribed when the diagnostic region of interest is extensive or falls outside the area normally covered by periapical projections. The oral surgeon finds this type of radiograph extremely helpful. A single periapical radiograph reveals limited information about the surgical site, while the panoramic film discloses a more complete view of the specific site and adjacent structures.

Tomographic radiography is an image *slice* that is created by moving the x-ray source and film (Fig. 9-38, *A* and *B*). The size, shape, and location of the image *slice* is determined by the path of movement.

Dental tomography is used in TMJ and implant imaging.

In computed tomography (CT) the x-ray source undergoes complex movements, and the radiographic attenuation is detected by sensitive electronic devices. These electronic signals are processed in a computer creating a detailed image of the internal anatomic structures of the patient. CT images can be projected on a monitor or printed on film.

The specific manipulation of the dental x-ray machines used for extraoral radiography is unique to each unit. It is necessary for the operator to follow the specific manufacturer's direction when operating extraoral radiographic machines.

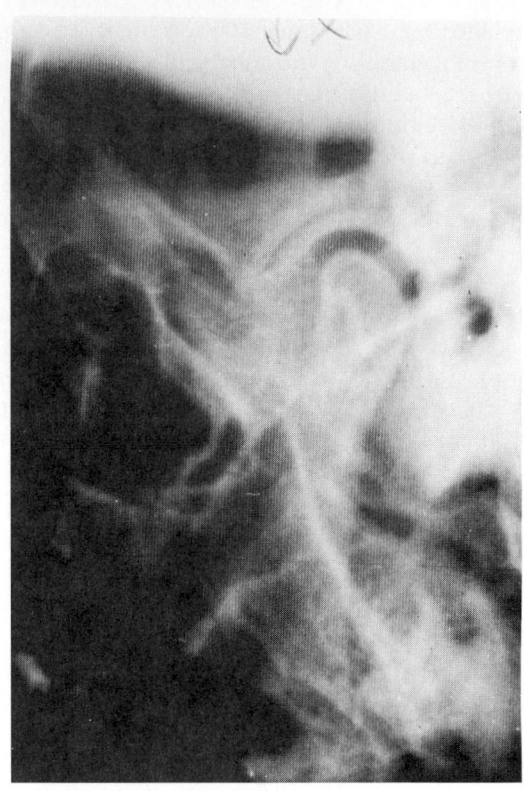

FIG. 9-35   Temporomandibular joint projection.

(From Frommer HH: *Radiology for dental auxiliaries,* ed 5, St Louis, 1992, Mosby.)

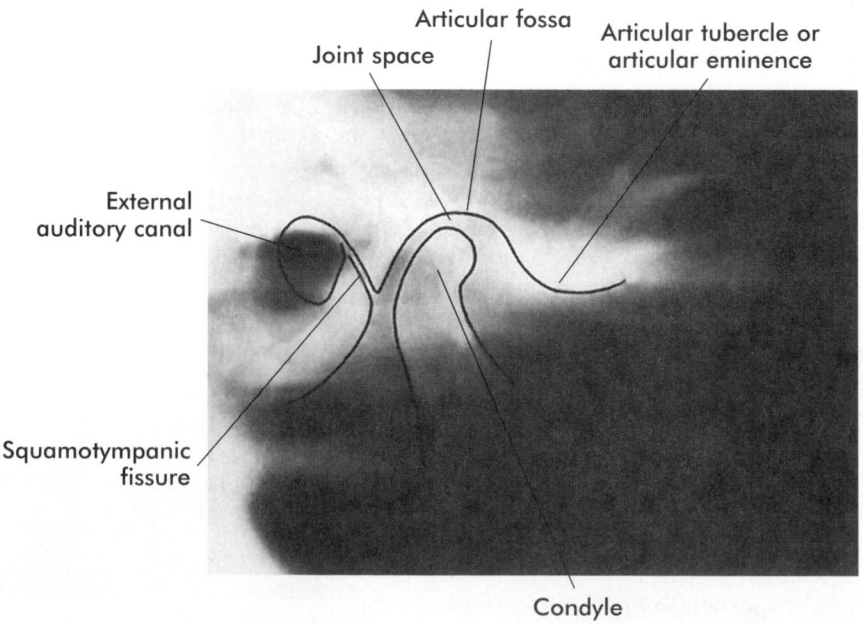

FIG. 9-36   Lateral aspect of TMJ.

(From Goaz PW, White SC: *Oral radiology, principles and interpretation,* ed 2, St Louis, 1987, Mosby.)

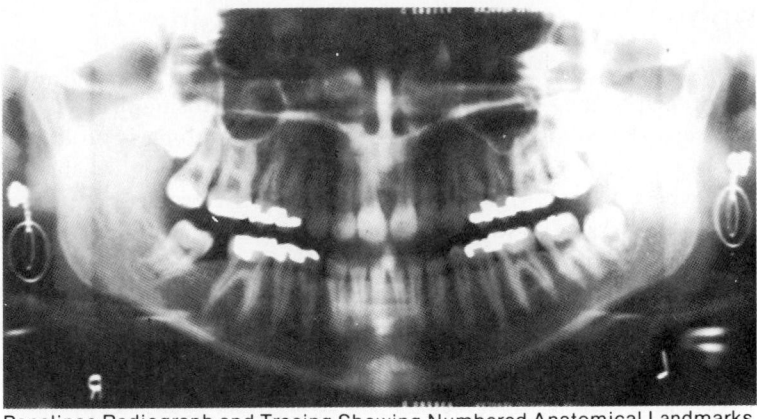

Panelipse Radiograph and Tracing Showing Numbered Anatomical Landmarks

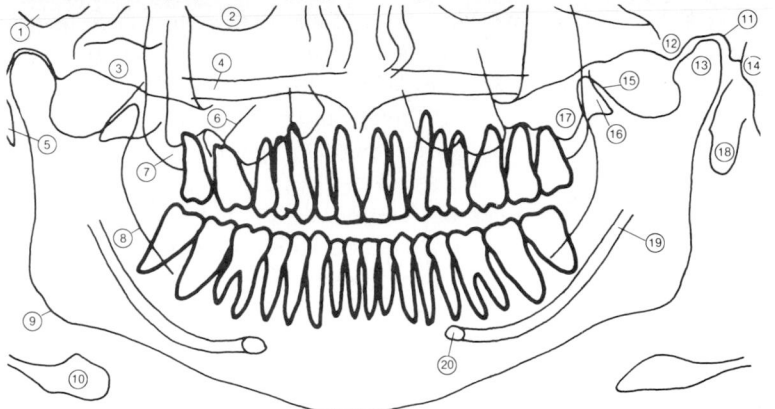

1. Middle cranial fossa
2. Orbit
3. Zygomatic arch
4. Palate
5. Styloid process
6. Septa in maxillary sinus
7. Maxillary tuberosity
8. External oblique line
9. Angle of mandible
10. Hyoid bone
11. Glenoid fossa
12. Articular eminence
13. Mandibular condyle
14. Vertebra
15. Coronoid process
16. Pterygoid plates
17. Maxillary sinus
18. Ear lobe
19. Mandibular canal
20. Mental foramen

FIG. 9-37   Panoramic radiograph.

(From Frommer HH: *Radiology for dental auxiliaries,* ed 5, St Louis, 1992, Mosby.)

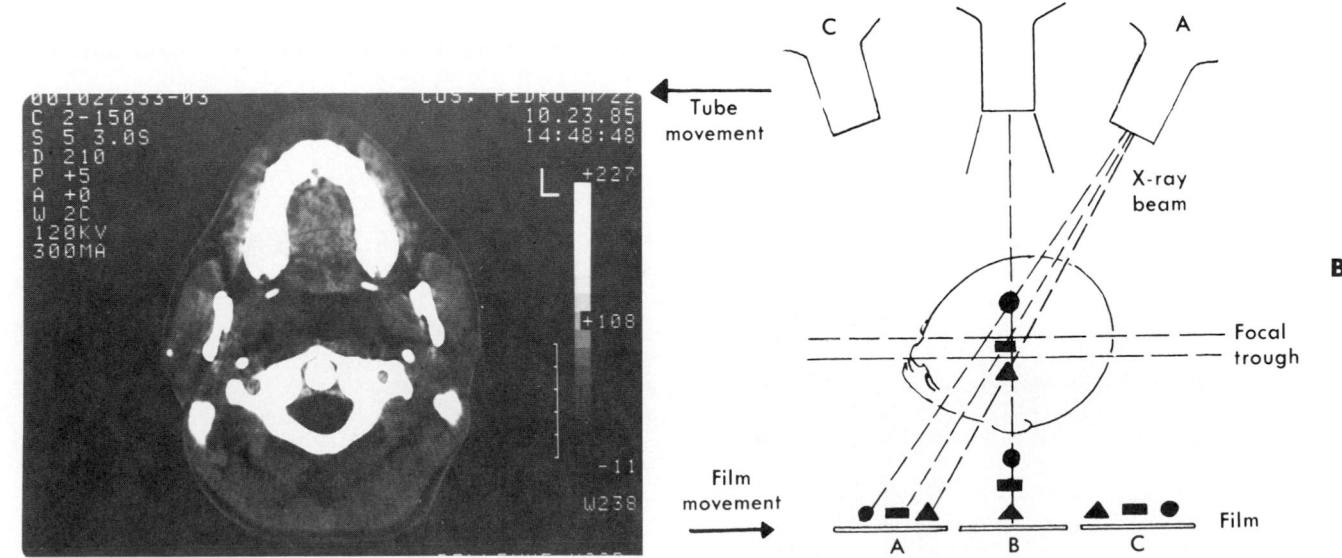

FIG. 9-38   *A,* CT scan of skull. *B,* Diagram illustrating the principle of tomography.

(From Frommer HH: *Radiology for dental auxiliaries,* ed 5, St Louis, 1992, Mosby.)

Processing Dental Radiographs

After radiographs have been exposed, the image is processed in much the same way a photograph is developed. There are five basic processing steps: developing, rinsing, fixing, washing, and drying. Consistent high-quality radiographs are produced only when processing is standardized. Processing times and temperatures must be carefully monitored. Host dental radiographs are developed in manual tank processors or in automatic film processors.

▶ Manual Processing

Processing tanks are used to manually develop, rinse, fix, and wash radiographs. A complete processing unit contains three separate tanks (Fig. 9-39). Two smaller tanks hold developer (usually on the left) and fixer (usually on the right). The large middle tank contains running water. Water is circulated continuously during film processing. The running water is controlled by an inlet valve and drain tube in the tank. Water temperature is controlled by hot and cold valves located on the wall above the unit. Because the water surrounds the smaller tanks, its temperature also controls developer and fixer temperatures. Film hangers are used to hold films for processing. Each film hanger is labeled to identify the films attached to it during processing (Fig. 9-40).

The time required for processing depends on the temperature of the solutions. Therefore an accurate thermometer is essential. Thermometers are either clipped to the inside rim of the developer tank or float in the solution. An accurate timer alarm is necessary to precisely time the various stages of film processing.

▶ Automatic Processing

Automatic film processors mechanically transport film through the developing, rinsing, fixing, washing, and drying cycles (Fig. 9-41). Automatic processing produces finished radiographs of uniform quality in 1 to 10 minutes, depending on the processor. Automatic processors located in the darkroom must be loaded under safelight conditions with the white light turned off. Processors may also be equipped with daylight loaders, thus eliminating the need for safelight conditions. When using a daylight loader, care must be taken to avoid contamination of the cuffs. Place contaminated films in a clean cup or towel, and enter the daylight loader wearing clean gloves. After films have been loaded into the processor, remove gloves and then remove hands from the daylight loader.

NOTE: Chemicals used in automatic processing are unique and contain special additives that control the thickness and stickiness of the film within a range of tolerance required for automatic processing. These chemicals are designed to reduce processing and transport times. *Never* substitute conventional (manual) processing chemicals for automatic processor chemicals.

▶ Manual Processing Procedure

Finished radiographs of high quality can be consistently achieved only when they are processed following standardized steps. Careful attention must be focused on the length of time and temperature of the solutions used.

MANUAL STEP-BY-STEP PROCESSING

1. Close and lock the darkroom door. Check solution levels, and replace or replenish if the levels are low. Gently stir the developer and fixer solutions, using a

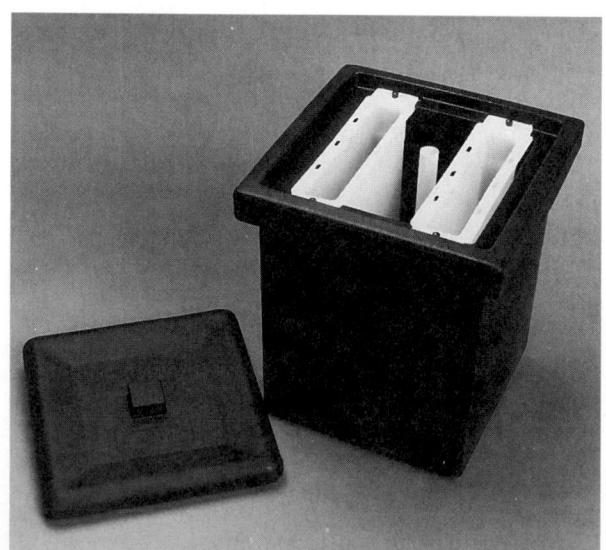

FIG. 9-39   Manual processing tanks.

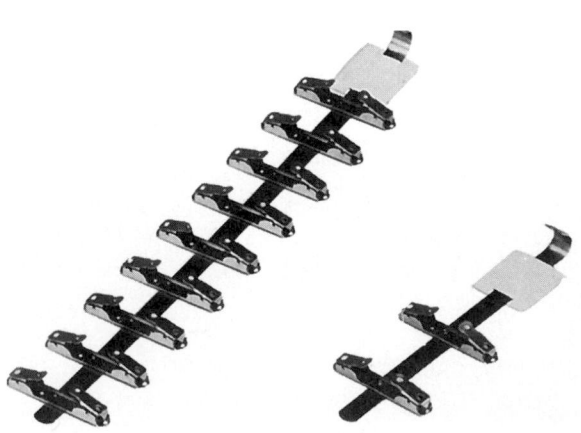

FIG. 9-40   Film hangers used to hold films during manual processing technique.

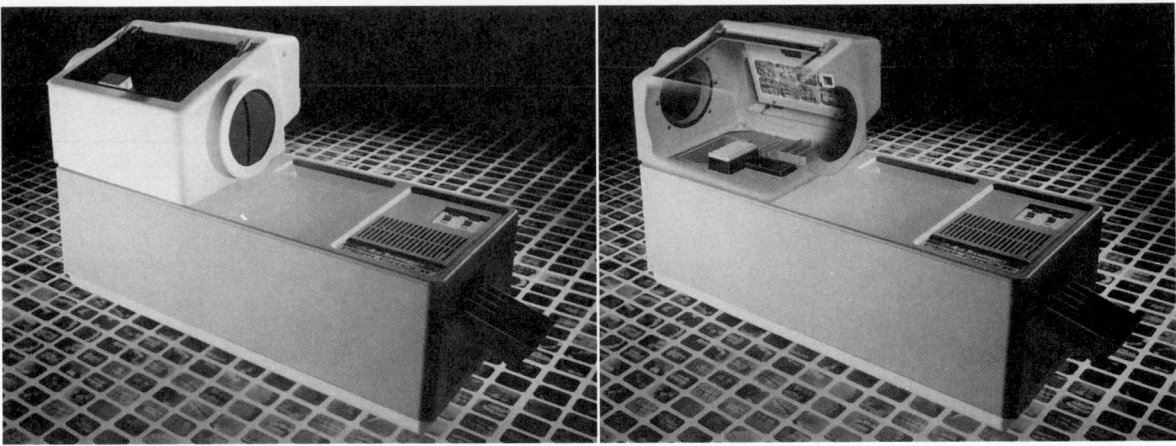

FIG. 9-41   Automatic processor system.

different stirring rod for each solution. (Stirring rods should be made of glass, plastic, or stainless steel, never wood.)

2. Check the thermometer, and determine the film-developing time, following the manufacturer's recommendations. Developing time depends on the temperature of the developer.

3. If the films are moist, dry each film with a paper towel before opening the film packets.

4. Select a film hanger, and place an identifying label on it. Turn off the room light, and verify that no outside or extraneous light is present in the darkroom. Illuminate the safe light.

5. Unwrap film packets, and remove the film slowly. Holding the film by the edges, attach the film to the hanger. Be sure to keep the film dry, and avoid smudging it with your fingers.

6. Place the film hanger in the developer solution. Agitate the hanger slightly to release air bubbles on the film surface, allowing optimum contact with the developer. Verify that all films are immersed completely in the developing solution. The films should not contact another film or the walls of the tank. Start the timer and replace the tank cover.

7. When the timer sounds, lift the cover and remove the film hanger from the developer. Rinse the films by agitating them for about 20 seconds in the water tank. Rinsing stops the action of the developer and prevents contamination of the fixer.

8. Place the film hanger into the fixing solution. Replace the tank cover, and set the timer for at least 10 minutes of fixing time. NOTE: If it is necessary, a brief inspection of the film can be made after 2 minutes of fixation. Be certain to return for complete fixing following this *wet reading.*

9. When the timer sounds, remove the film hanger from the fixer, and place the hanger into the water. The final wash requires a minimum of 20 minutes. NOTE: Incomplete washing will result in films that discolor with age.

10. Since the final step in film processing is drying, remove the film hanger from the water, and hang it on a drying rack. It is important to make sure the films do not contact other objects because wet films are easily scratched. Follow the manufacturer's instructions when using an electrical fan or a heated drying cabinet; avoid damage to radiographs by overheating.

▶ Manual Film Processor Maintenance

Processing Tanks

Keep tanks covered when they are not in use. Clean surfaces of the tanks and countertop with a damp sponge after each use. The tanks should be cleaned when solutions are replaced. Solution life is determined by how much they are used. Typically, solutions are changed every 2 to 3 weeks. Clean tanks with a gentle soap and soft bristle (nonmetallic) brush. Mineral deposits can be removed using a sponge and vinegar. Rinse the tanks thoroughly with clear water, removing all traces of soap.

Film Hangers

Clean hangers in a solution of ⅛ ounce sodium bicarbonate mixed in 1 gallon of water. Soak the hangers for ½ hour at 100° F to 125° F. Rinse the hangers completely, and allow them to dry.

AUTOMATIC STEP-BY-STEP PROCESSING

1. Check the solution level in internal replenishing tanks. If solutions are low, refill the tanks to the levels

recommended by the manufacturer. If the processor is not equipped with an automatic replenisher, add the recommended amount of replenisher to the developer and fixer tanks. Use separate cups for each solution. Add solution slowly, away from the drain and toward the center of the tank. Avoid splashing.

2. Turn the main water valve on. Check the drain hose to make sure that it is not obstructed and that it is inserted into the drain.

3. Observe the solutions in the internal tanks. A churning action indicates the circulating pumps are working properly. Depress the process switch to verify that the rollers are turning. Turn on the heating unit if it is available on the processor.

4. Replace the top cover of the processor and insert a cleaning film. Daily use of cleaning film helps to maintain rollers free of deposits. Purchased cleaning film is recommended. Alternatively, two processed clear panoramic, occlusal, or smaller films can be used.

5. When the processor ready light comes on, verify the accuracy of the temperature control setting by measuring the solution temperature using a hand-held thermometer.

6. Depress the process switch to begin automatic processing. Feed film lengthwise into alternating tracks to prevent overlapping. Allow at least 15 seconds between films. If films are fed into the processor too quickly, they will overlap, fail to dry adequately, or cause the roller transport to malfunction. Insert large films lengthwise, one at a time. Do not turn on the lights or open the darkroom door for at least 15 seconds after the last film is placed into the processor. NOTE: If #0 or #1 film is being processed, each film is placed in a slot in a film carriage device. Do not bend the film in the carriage because it must fit in the tracks of the processor. If #2 or #3 size films are processed, each is carefully placed in a separate track. Once the films are positioned, the lever is pulled to release the films onto the roller.

7. If the processor is not equipped with automatic replenisher system, activate the replenisher switch after processing 20 periapical and 5 panoramic films or 90 periapical films.

8. At the end of the day, turn the power switch to off, and shut off the water supply. Some processors may require the cover to be propped open for venting.

▶ Automatic Processor Maintenance

The processor must be checked daily to ensure optimum performance and equipment life. Additional weekly and monthly maintenance should be completed according to the manufacturer's specifications. Some general guide-

---

lines for maintaining automatic processors are listed in Box 9-5.

Daily Checks

Check and refill solution as needed in both the internal and replenisher tanks. Check solution temperature. Verify that circulating pumps and transport assemblies are working properly.

Process a cleaning film to minimize the accumulation of roller deposits. Check the drain hose for obstructions and to verify that it is inserted into the drain. Wipe up any spills on the cover and verify that the vent is not obstructed.

Weekly Maintenance

Remove and clean the roller transport assembly. Place the rollers in a large sink or plastic pan, and clean rollers with a brush or sponge under warm running water. Rotate the gears and rollers while cleaning. Use a separate brush or sponge for each rack. USE ONLY WATER.

Monthly Maintenance

Remove all roller transports, and completely drain the tanks. Check the drain tube, and replace it. Fill all tanks with water, and drain the tanks twice. Sponge the walls of the tanks, using a separate sponge for each tank.

Refill all tanks with water, and replace the cover. Turn the process switch on for approximately 2 minutes; this

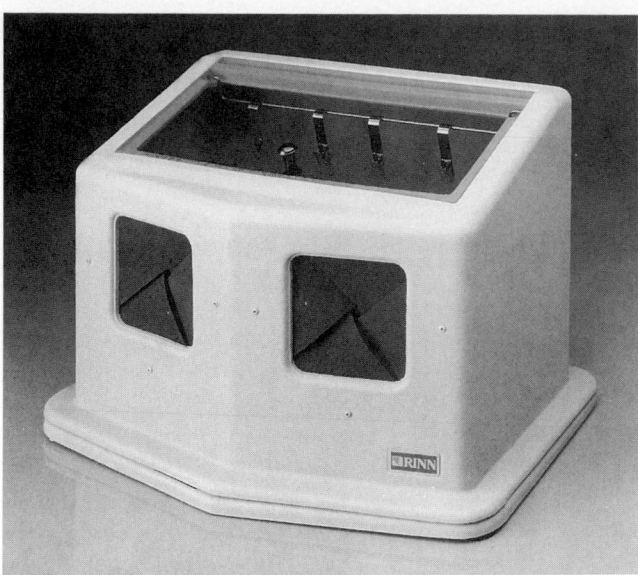

FIG. 9-42 **Rapid processing system.**

will allow the chemistry agitators to be flushed out. Turn the process switch off, remove the cover, and drain all tanks. Dry the tanks with a clean cloth or paper towel.

Place the racks in a large sink or plastic pan, and clean the rollers with a brush or sponge under warm running water. Rotate the gears and rollers while cleaning. Use a separate brush or sponge for each rack.

Three-Month Maintenance

Turn off the automatic replenisher. Remove all roller transports, and completely drain the tanks. Check the drain tube, and replace it. Fill all tanks with water, and drain the tanks twice.

Add mild soap to developer and fixer tanks, and add water to fill to ½ inch below the fill line. Add soap to the wash tank only if it is excessively dirty.

Insert roller transports into soap solution. Verify the automatic replenisher is off. Replace the cover, and turn the power and process switches on. Let the processor run with the racks in place for 10 to 30 minutes, depending on the degree of cleaning required. Occasionally wipe the rollers and drive gears above the solution level with a sponge while the processor is running. Turn the process and power switch off, remove the cover, and drain all tanks. Place the racks in a large sink or plastic pan, and rinse the rollers with a brush or sponge under warm running water. Rotate the gears and rollers while cleaning. Use a separate brush or sponge on each rack. All traces of soap must be removed to prevent contamination of the chemicals.

Clean the circulation agitators. Refill the tanks with water, and let the processor run for 1 minute. Drain and refill the tanks with water two more times. Dry the tanks with a clean cloth or paper towel.

▶ Rapid Processing

Rapid processing of radiographs is necessary when radiographs are made during endodontic or other operative procedures. Rapid processing systems use concentrated solutions often at high temperatures (Fig. 9-42). Film is agitated in the developer solution for 10 to 30 seconds, then is fixed for 1 to 2 minutes. Although the quality of radiographs developed in rapid processing solutions is adequate for endodontic working films, contrast and archival qualities are limited. Diagnostic radiographs should always be processed by conventional methods.

Mounting Radiographs

Although mounting intraoral radiographs is a relatively simple procedure, it requires knowledge of oral anatomy an tooth morphology. Care must be taken to avoid fingerprinting or smudging the radiographs. Handle radiographs by their edges with clean dry fingers. Radiographs are an important component of the patient record (Box 9-5).

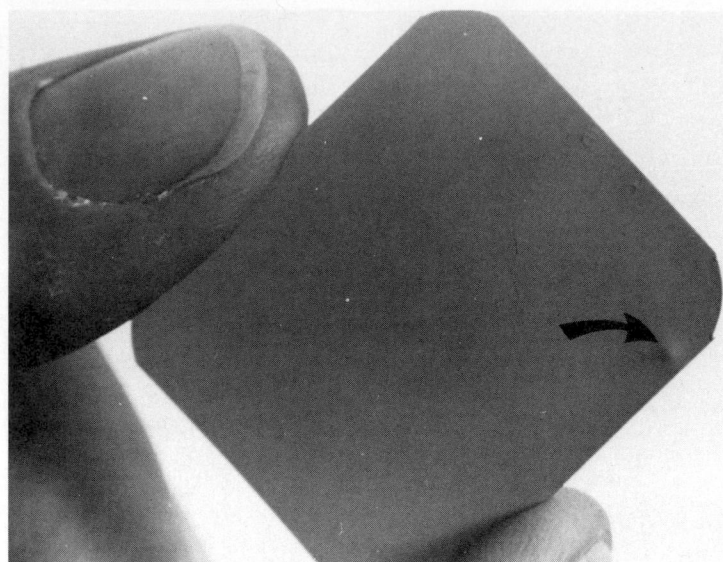

FIG. 9-43   Film dot. Raised side of dot (*arrow*) indicating tube side of film. This dot should also be oriented towards the incisal or occlusal surfaces.

(Illustrations from Goaz PW, White SC: *Oral radiology, principles and interpretation,* ed 3, St Louis, 1994, Mosby.)

▶ Identification Dot

Correct orientation of the processed radiograph is made possible by a small round embossed dot at the corner of each film. Before the radiographs are mounted and sorted, it is important to know from what aspect the radiographs will be viewed. Radiographs can be mounted for viewing in two ways: with the convexity of the dot up or with the convexity of the dot down. If the depressed or concave side of the embossed dot is toward the viewer, the radiographs are visualized from the lingual aspect as if inside the mouth looking out. In the second method of mounting, the radiographs are placed with the raised or convex side of the embossed dot toward the viewer. When the convexity of the dot is raised, the radiographs are viewed from the facial aspect. This method of mounting radiographs is recommended by the ADA. The primary advantage of mounting radiographs with the convexity of the dot up is that the radiographs are in the same orientation as the recorded chart, decreasing the likelihood of clerical errors.

The way a dentist views radiographs depends on previous training and preference. Most mounts are reversible and can be easily turned over for viewing. The most important aspect is to KEEP ALL THE DOTS IN THE SAME ORIENTATION and place the radiographs in the film mount so that right and left are correctly identified (Fig. 9-43).

Various anatomic and restorative landmarks can assist in identification during the radiographic procedure. Landmarks that can be identified in dental radiographs include (Figs. 9-44, *A* through *V* and 9-45).

STEP-BY-STEP MOUNTING PROCEDURES FOR RADIOGRAPHS

1. Arrange radiographs on a viewbox with the *dots* oriented in the same direction either up or out (convex) or down or in (concave).
2. Organize the radiographs according to anatomic areas. Arrange in groups of maxillary, mandibular, anterior, and posterior regions.
3. Position maxillary posterior radiographs with the crowns of the teeth toward the bottom edge of the mount. Identify mesial or distal anatomic landmarks to distinguish right from left. Premolar projections are mounted on the inside, while the most posterior landmarks are mounted toward the outside of the mount.
4. Identify maxillary anterior radiographs, and place them with the crowns of the teeth toward the bottom edge of the mount. Identify the right and left incisor projections, and place them with the central incisor toward the middle of the film mount. Orient the right and left maxillary canine projections, with the mesial structure toward the center of the film mount.
5. Identify the mandibular posterior radiographs, and arrange them with the coronal edge of the radiograph toward the top edge of the film mount. Place the molar projections toward the outside of the mount and the premolar projections toward the inside.
6. Arrange the mandibular incisor radiographs with the incisal edges directed toward the top of the film mount. Place the right and left central incisors toward

Text continued on p. 236.

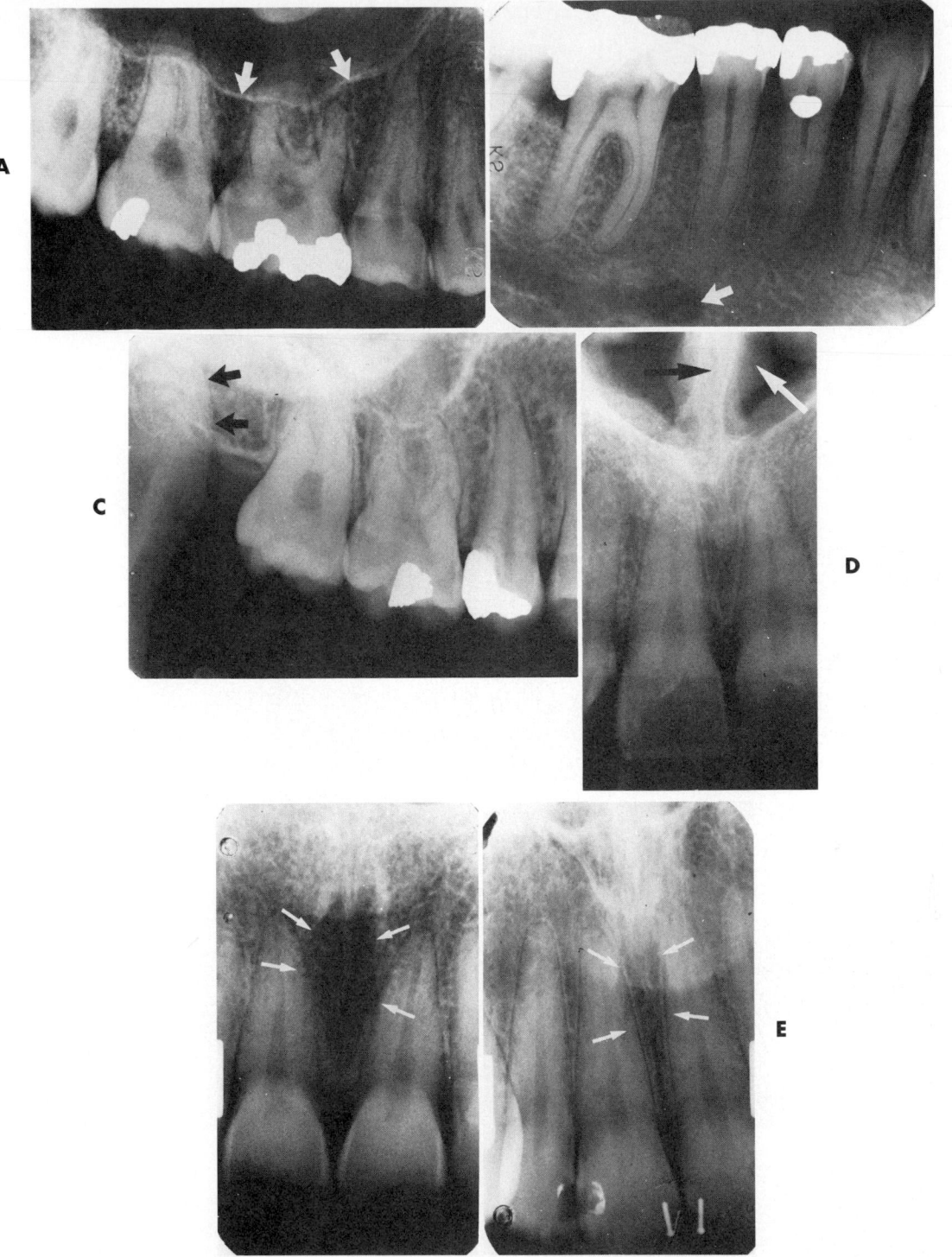

FIG. 9-44   *A,* The inferior border of the maxillary sinus (*arrow*) appears as a thin radiopaque line near the apices of the maxillary premolars and molars. *B,* The mental foramen (*arrow*) appears as an oval radiolucency near the apex of the second premolar. *C,* Coronoid process of the mandible (*arrow*) superimposed on the maxillary tuberosity. *D,* The nasal septum (*black arrow*) arises directly above the anterior nasal spine and is covered on each side by nasal mucosa (*white arrow*). *E,* The incisive foramen appears as an ovoid radiolucency (*arrows*) between the roots of the central incisors. Note its borders, which are diffuse but within normal limits.

Continued.

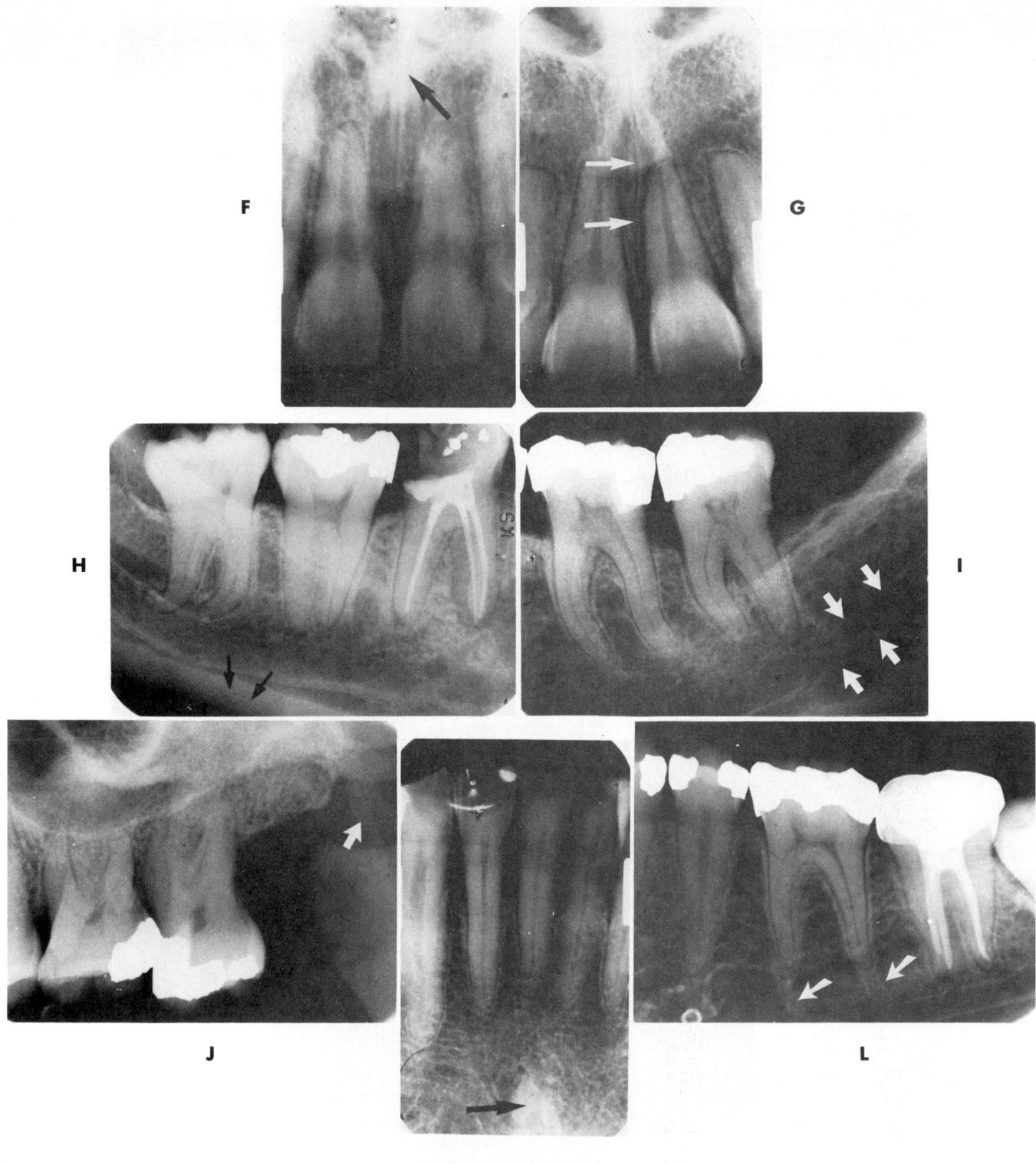

FIG. 9-44, cont'd.   For legend see opposite page.

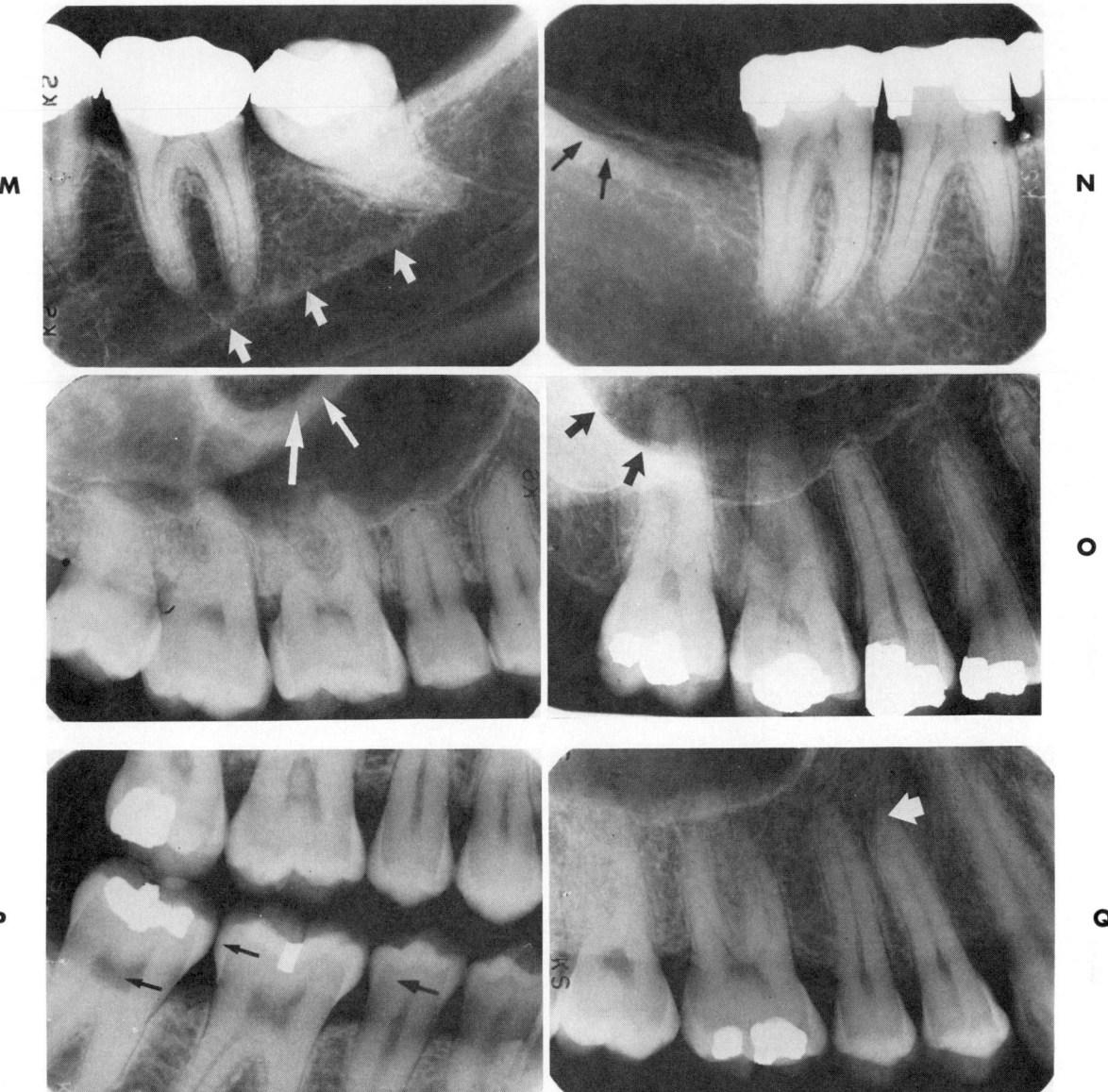

FIG. 9-44, cont'd. *F,* The anterior nasal spine is seen as an opaque V-shaped projection from the floor of the nasal fossa in the midline (*arrow*). *G,* The intermaxillary suture (*arrows*) appears as a curving radiolucency in the midline of the maxilla. *H,* The inferior border of the mandible (*arrows*) is seen as a dense broad radiopaque band. *I,* Mandibular canal. *Arrows* denote its radiopaque superior and inferior cortical borders. *J,* The hamular process (*arrow*) extends downward from the medial pterygoid plate. *K,* Lingual foramen (*arrow*), with a sclerotic border, in the symphyscal region of the mandible. *L,* Nutrient canals (*arrows*) demonstrated by radiopaque cortical borders, descend from the mandibular first molar. *M,* Mylohyoid ridge (*arrows*) running at the level of the molar apices and above the mandibular canal. *N,* External oblique ridge (*arrows*) seen as a radiopaque line near the alveolar crest in the mandibular third molar region. *O,* The zygomatic process of the maxilla (*arrows*) protrudes laterally from the maxillary wall. Its size may be quite variable: small with thick borders or large with thin borders. *P,* Teeth are composed of enamel (*arrow* on the first molar), dentin (*arrow* on the second premolar), pulp (*arrow* on the second molar), and cementum (usually not visible radiographically). *Q,* Although the root canal is not radiographically visible in the apical 2 mm of a tooth, anatomically it is present (*arrow*). *Continued.*

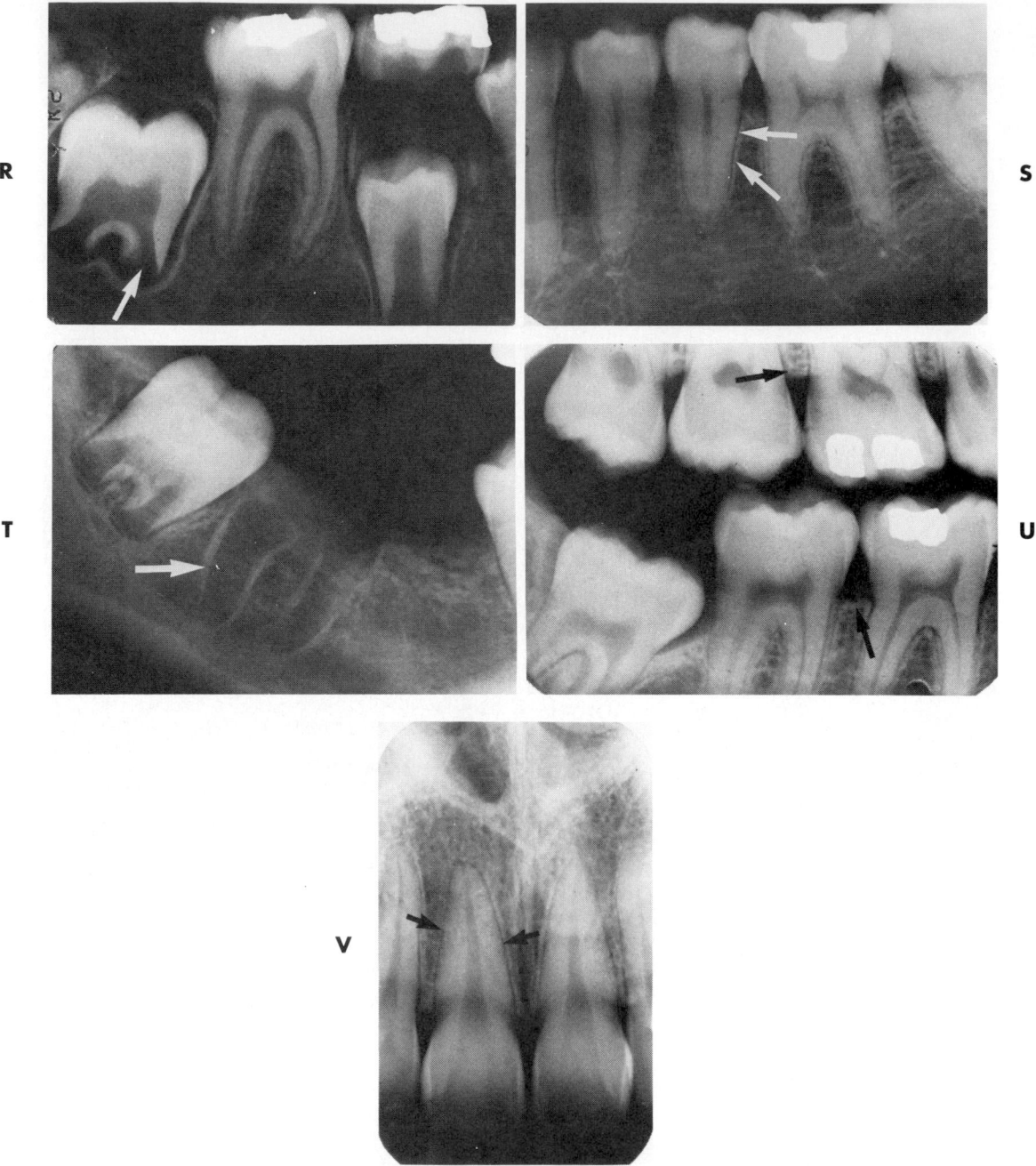

FIG. 9-44, cont'd. *R,* A developing root shown by divergent apex around the dental papilla (*arrow*), which is enclosed by an opaque bony crypt. *S,* The lamina dura (*arrows*) appears as a thin opaque layer of bone around teeth. *T,* The lamina dura (*arrows*) appears as a thin opaque layer of bone around a recent extraction socket. *U,* The alveolar crests (*arrows*) are seen as cortical borders of the alveolar bone. *V,* The periodontal ligament space (*arrows*) is seen as a narrow radiolucency between the tooth root and lamina dura.

(All illustrations are from Goaz PW, White SC: *Oral radiology, principles and interpretation,* ed 3, St Louis, 1994, Mosby.)

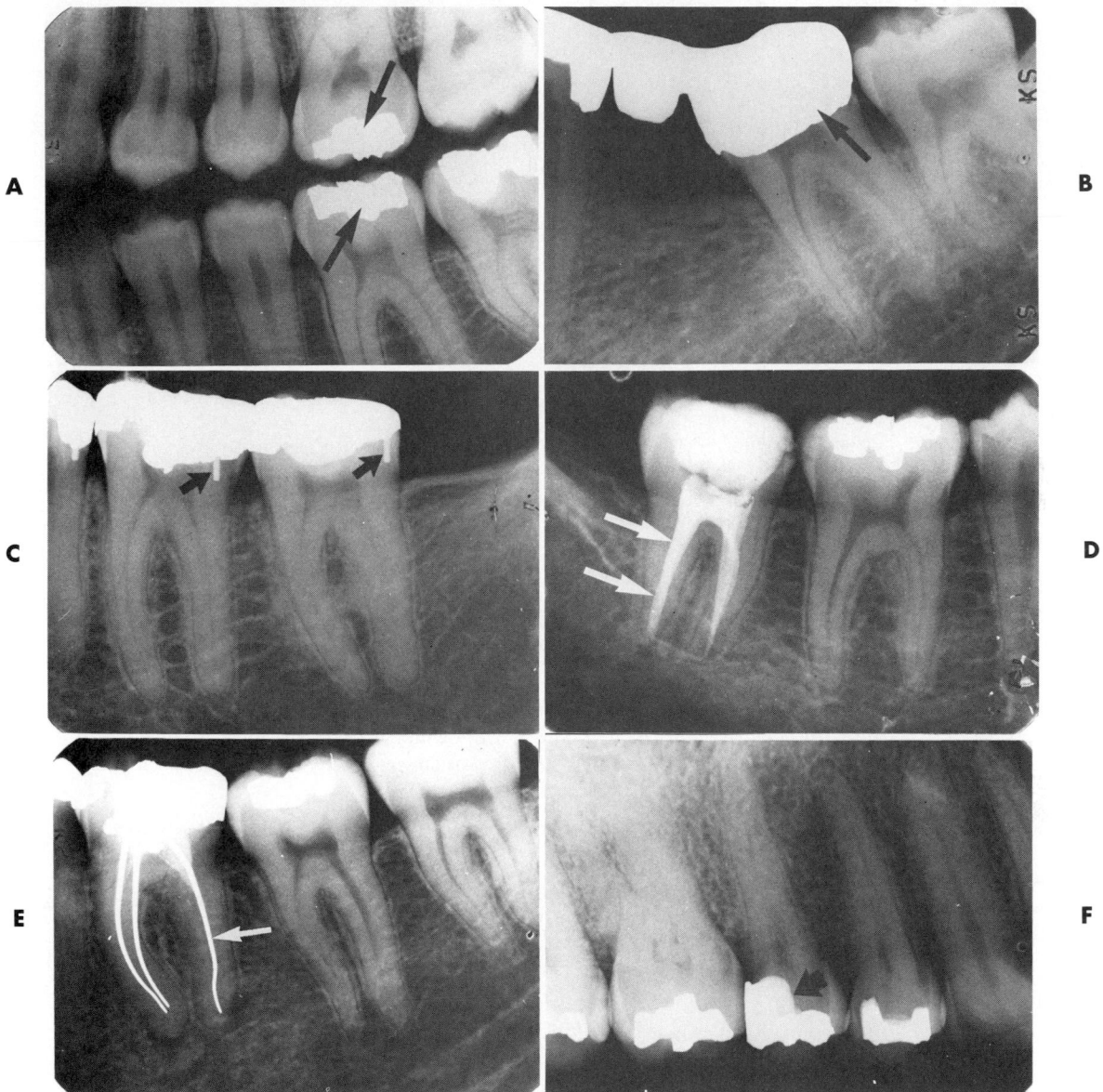

FIG. 9-45   *A,* Amalgam restorations appear completely radiopaque (*arrows*). *B,* A cast gold crown, appearing completely radiopaque (*arrow*), serves as the terminal abutment of a bridge. *C,* Stainless steel pins (*arrows*) provide retention for amalgam restorations. *D,* Gutta-percha (*arrows*) is a radiopaque rubberlike material used in endodontic therapy. *E,* Silver points (*arrow*) were used to fill the root canals in this patient. *F,* Base material (*arrow*) is usually radiopaque.

Continued.

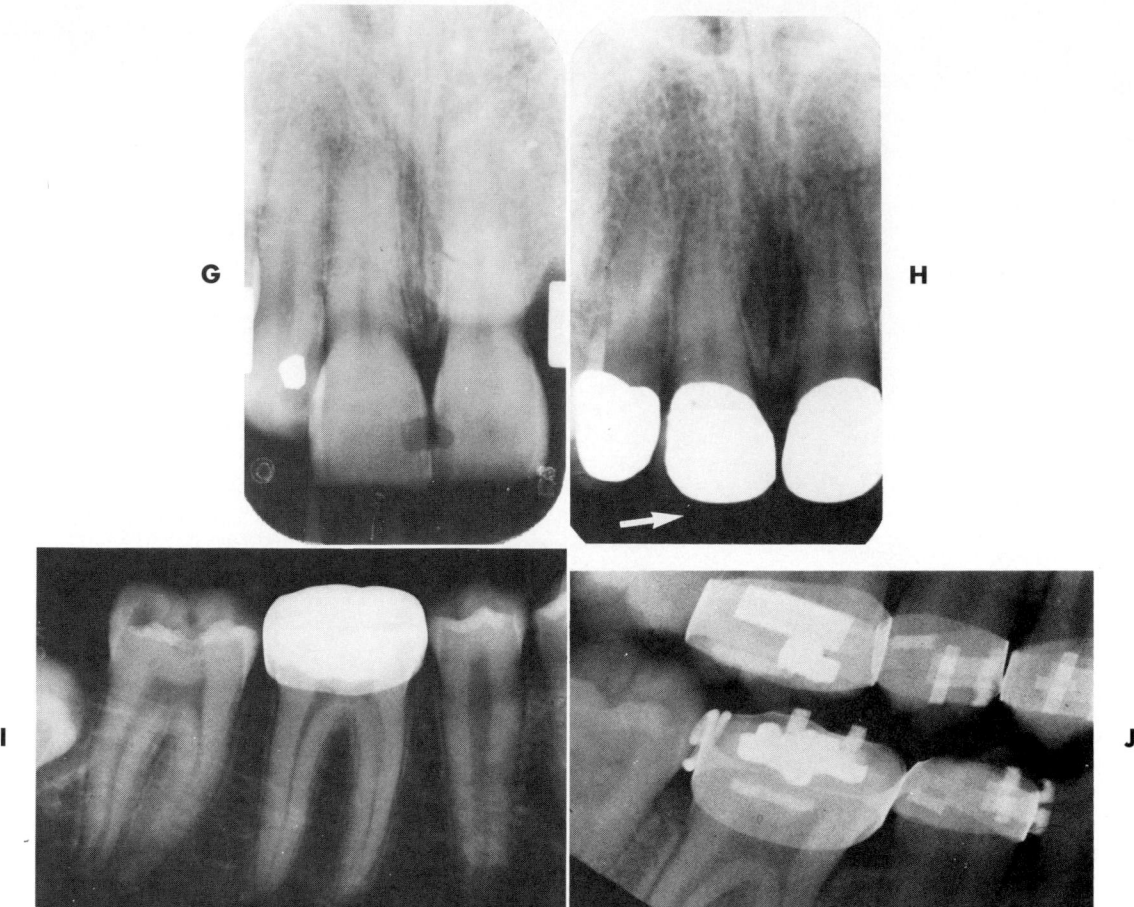

FIG. 9-45, cont'd.   *G,* Composite restorations may be radiolucent and may suggest caries but can be recognized by their well-demarcated border with dentin. *H,* Porcelain appears radiolucent (*arrow*) over a metal coping. *I,* Stainless steel crowns appear mostly radiopaque. *J,* Orthodontic appliances have a characteristic radiopaque appearance.

(All illustrations are from Goaz PW, White SC: *Oral radiology, principles and interpretation,* ed 3, St Louis, 1994, Mosby.)

the middle of the film mount. Orient the right and left maxillary canine projections with the mesial toward the center of the film mount.

7. Since the remaining four radiographs are the bitewing projections, orient these radiographs with the curve of Spee (occlusal plane between the maxillary and mandibular teeth) directed upward toward the distal. If the occlusal plane is flat, attempt to identify characteristics of the respective crowns. Frequently the bifurcation of the mandibular molars can be used as an aid in distinguishing mandibular from maxillary teeth. When the left and right projections are identified, orient them with the most mesial structures toward the middle of the film mount.

Common Errors in Intraoral Radiography

Several errors can occur during the radiographic process. These errors may include problems that include exposure, processing, and mounting techniques. Table 9-8 reviews several errors that may arise during radiography (Fig. 9-46).

Duplicating Radiographs

Radiographs frequently need to be reproduced. Radiographs may be needed for purposes other than that for

Text continued on p. 245.

TABLE 9-8 COMMON ERRORS IN INTRAORAL RADIOGRAPHY

Error	Result	Correction
EXPOSURE ERROR		
PID cutoff	Portion of the film is not exposed	Align the x-ray beam so the central ray is centered on the middle of the film (Fig. 9-46, *A*)
Film placement	Apex cutoff	Position film in film holder so ⅛ to ¼ inch of the film is positioned above the incisal or occlusal edge (Fig. 9-46, *B*)
	Necessary teeth are not visible on film	Move the film to the anterior or posterior to produce the correct image on the film (Fig. 9-46, *C*)
	Excessive space between occlusal planes of bitewing	Direct the patient to bite and hold the film in place (Fig. 9-46, *D*)
	Crown cutoff	Position the film in the film holder so that the incisal or occlusal edge of the film is not below the plane (Fig. 9-46, *E*)
Film reversal	Herringbone effect as radiation projects the image from the foil on the film	Always make sure the correct side of film is positioned near the image (Fig. 9-46, *F*)
Crescent marks or bent films	Black crescent-shaped marks or image is very distorted	Slightly roll film around finger to adapt the film for patient comfort (Fig. 9-46, *G*)
Overlapping	Interproximal contacts are not open	Horizontal angulation is brought as needed to the anterior or posterior, so the central ray is perpendicular to the film and the focal point (Fig. 9-46, *H*)
Blurred image	Lack of clarity on film	Instruct the patient to remain completely still during the procedure (Fig. 9-46, *I*)
Double exposure	Two sets of images on one film	Always be sure exposed film is placed separate from unexposed film (Fig. 9-46, *J*)
Light film	Low density or light images on film from underexposure	Check mA, time, or kVp for correct settings (Fig. 9-46, *K*)
Dark film	Dark, black films, creating inability to read images	Check mA, time, or kVp for correct settings (Fig. 9-46, *L*)
Clear film	No image on film	Film was not exposed (Fig. 9-46, *M*)
Elongation	Images on film are lengthened or elongated beyond actual size	Correct the vertical angulation so the central ray is perpendicular to the film and focal point during paralleling technique (Fig. 9-46, *N*)
Foreshortening	Images on film are shortened beyond actual size	Correct the vertical angulation so the central ray is perpendicular to the film and focal point during paralleling technique (Fig. 9-46, *O*)
Jewelry, dental appliance left in mouth	Superimposed or radiopaque images appear on the film	Always have the patient remove dental appliances and jewelry before procedure (Fig. 9-46, *P*)
PROCESSING ERRORS		
Fluoride artifacts	Black spots	Remove all remains of fluoride from hands before processing (if fluoride treatment and radiographs are planned for one appointment, expose radiographs first) (Fig. 9-46, *Q*)
Reticulation	Cracked, crazed appearance on film	Film is placed in high temperature processing and then cold temperature solution, causing a shrinkage and crazing of emulsion (Fig. 9-46, *R*)
Torn or scratched emulsion	Film base removed on film, reducing diagnostic value	Before films are dry, the emulsion is disturbed through contact with other films or hangers (Fig. 9-46, *S*)
Stained films	Stained areas, blotches	Work surfaces were wet or dirty during processing, disturbing the chemicals on the film (Fig. 9-46, *T*)
Discolored film	Brown staining	Film have not been fixed an adequate length of time (Fig. 9-46, *U*)
Light film	Low density of light images on film from underdeveloping	Check and correct for weak developing solutions, low developing time, or temperature of developing solutions (Fig. 9-46, *V*)
Developer cutoff	Straight line on films, radiopaque	Always check processing solutions to ensure tanks are full; never place films on top clips of film hangers (Fig. 9-46, *W*)
Clear film	Film has no image; emulsion is washed off	Do not leave films in water for more than 24 hours after fixing (Fig. 9-46, *X*)
Fogged film	Gray, unclear image contrast	Check for light exposure or improper film storage (Fig. 9-46, *Y*)
Static marks	Black streaks	Open film packets slowly to reduce static electricity (Fig. 9-46, *Z*)
Air bubbles	Radiopaque spots	Agitate film hangers in the processing solutions during placement in tanks (Fig. 9-46, *AA*)

Continued.

TABLE 9-8   COMMON ERRORS IN INTRAORAL RADIOGRAPHY—cont'd

Error	Result	Correction
AUTOMATIC PROCESSING ERRORS		
Overlapped films	Processing by the chemical is not complete	Films are fed into the machine too quickly and overlap during processing; more than one film is placed into the same slot (Fig. 9-46, *BB*)
Dirty rollers	Radiolucent markings or bands	Clean rollers regularly to remove residue (Fig. 9-46, *CC*)
Light leak	Dark or fogged film	Hands were moved in the daylight loader that allowed light leaks around cuffs; hands were removed from daylight loader and films were not in the machine or protected with a cover (Fig. 9-46, *DD*)

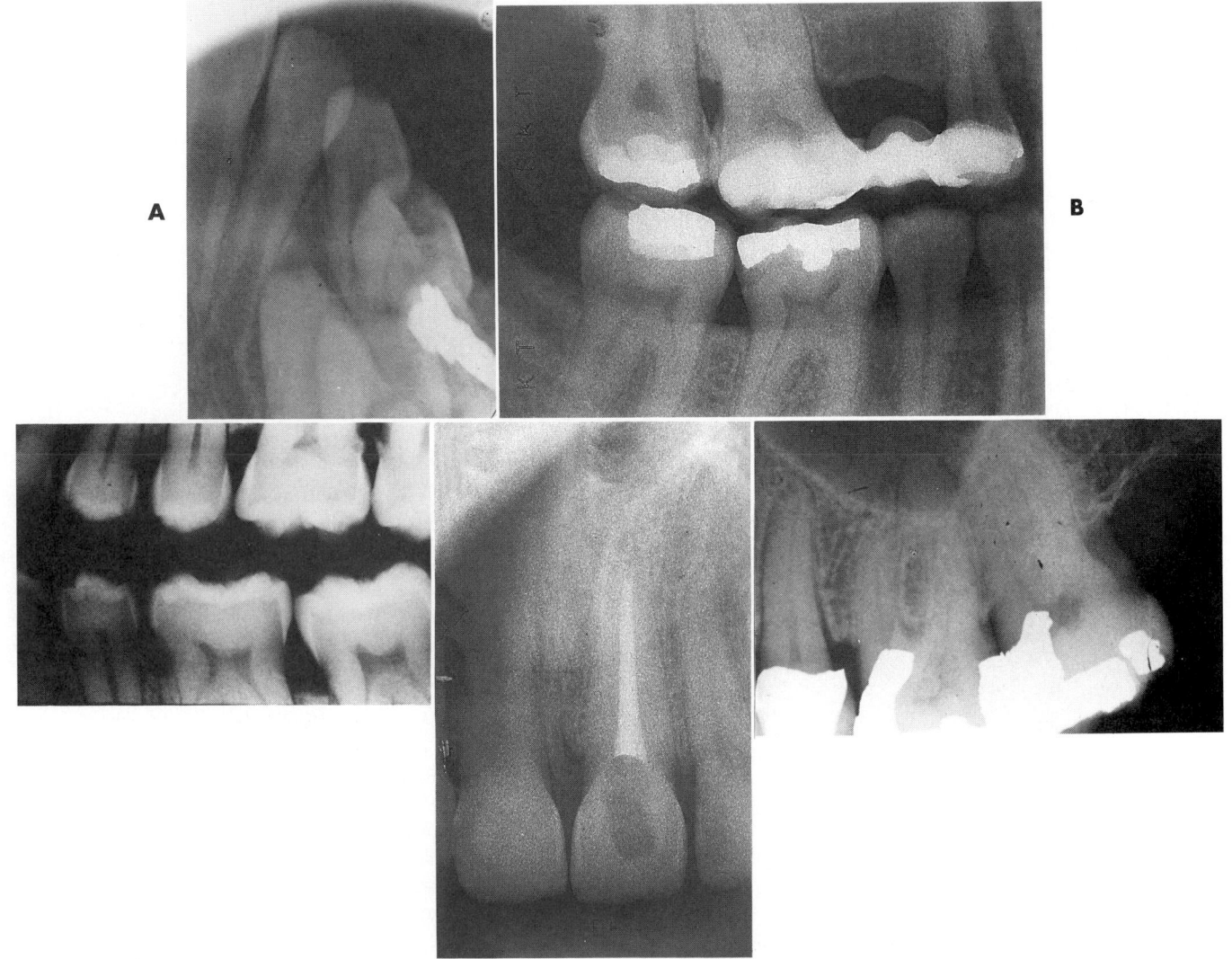

FIG. 9-46   *A,* Partial image caused by poor alignment of the tube head with the film. *B,* The apex of the third molar is not visible; to correct this error, move the film to the posterior. *C,* Necessary teeth are not visible in the radiograph. Move the film to the anterior. *D,* Gutta-percha is claylike material used in endodontic therapy. *E,* Gutta-percha may be used to visualize the depth of intrabony defects. This illustration fails to show the osseous defect without the use of the gutta-percha points.

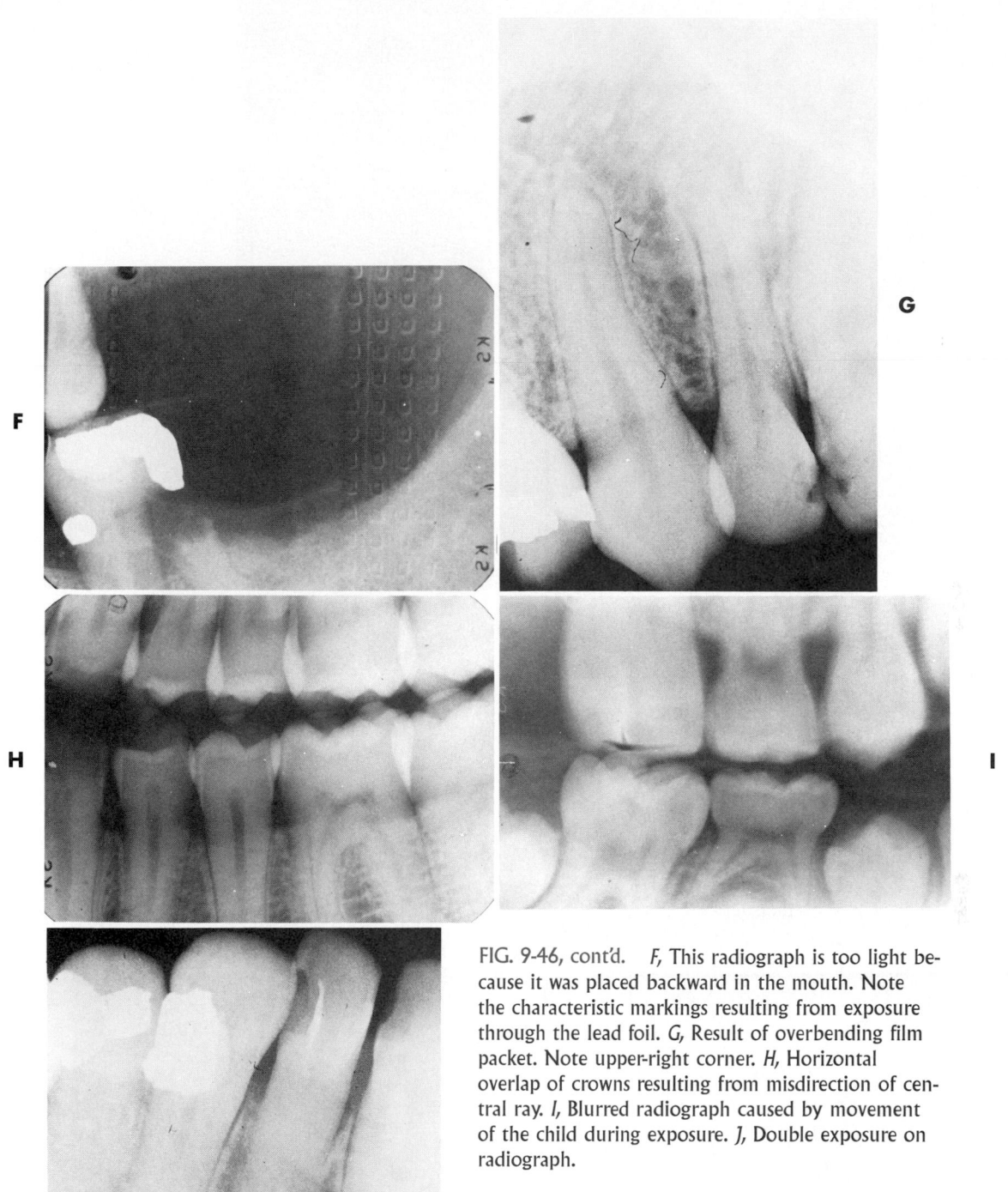

FIG. 9-46, cont'd.   *F,* This radiograph is too light because it was placed backward in the mouth. Note
the characteristic markings resulting from exposure
through the lead foil. *G,* Result of overbending film
packet. Note upper-right corner. *H,* Horizontal
overlap of crowns resulting from misdirection of central ray. *I,* Blurred radiograph caused by movement
of the child during exposure. *J,* Double exposure on
radiograph.

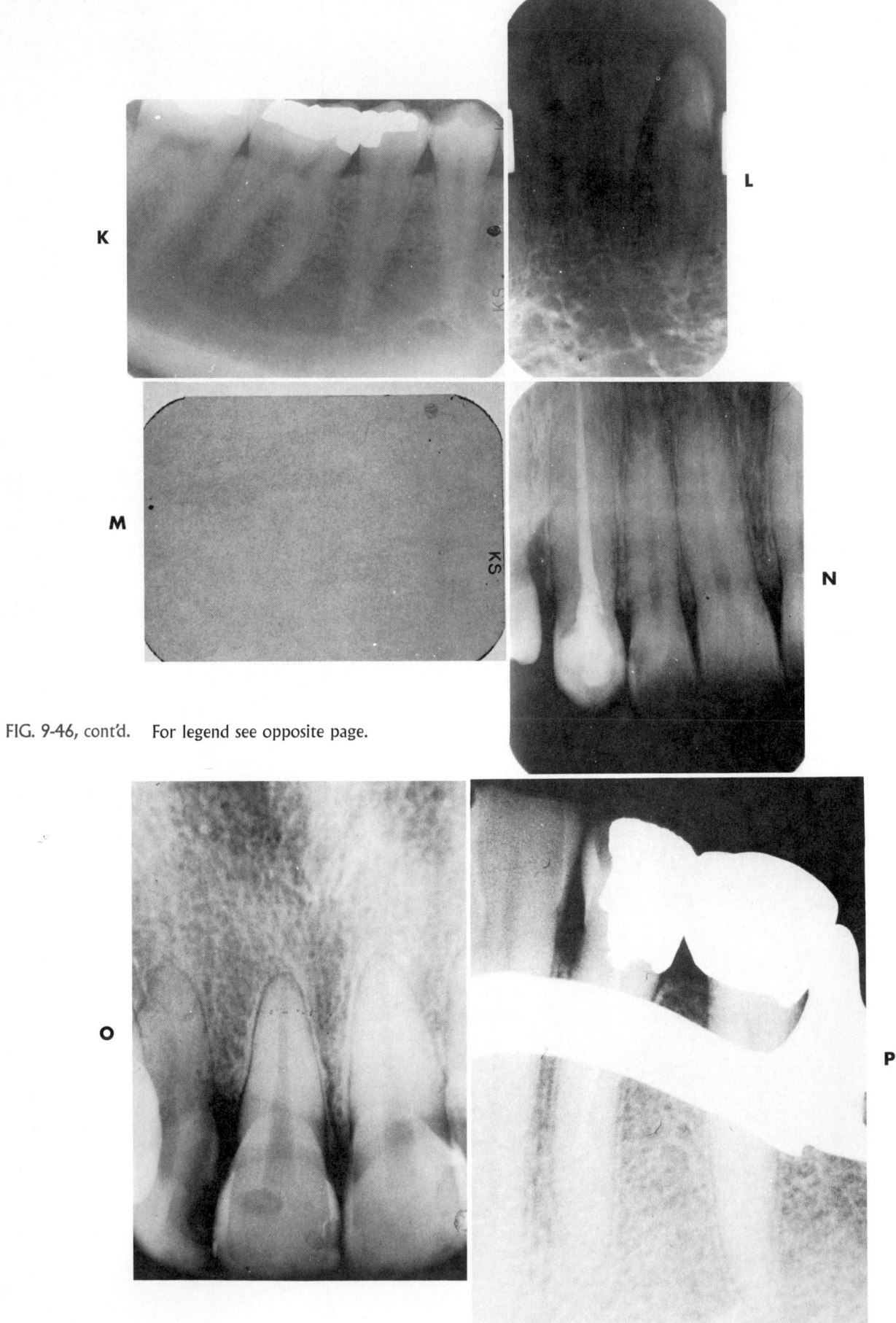

FIG. 9-46, cont'd.   For legend see opposite page.

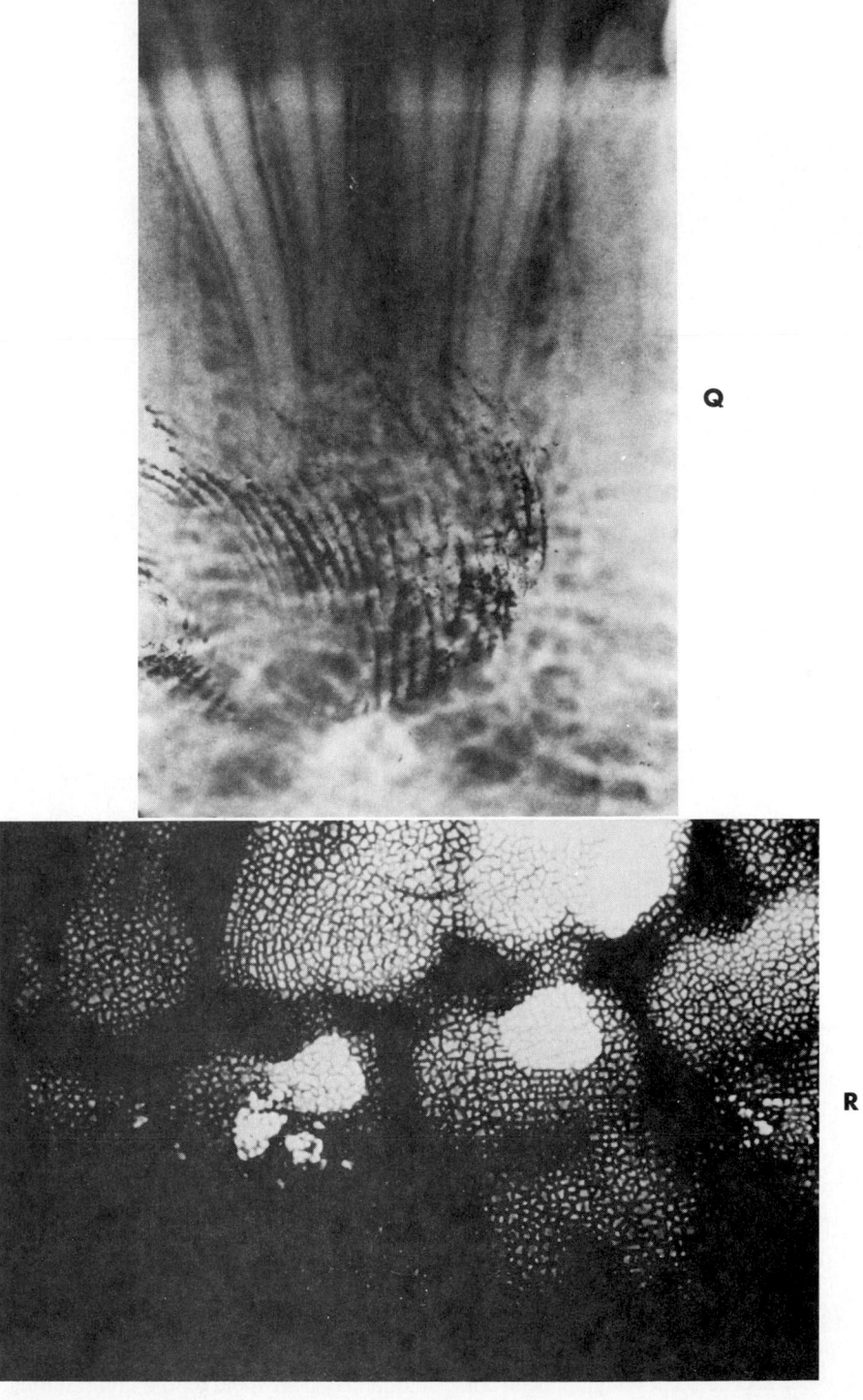

FIG. 9-46, cont'd.   *K,* The radiograph is too light because of inadequate processing or insufficient exposure. *L,* The radiograph is too dark because of overdevelopment or overexposure. *M,* Clear film. This can result from excessive washing or fixing or from an unexposed film. *N,* Elongated image. *O,* Foreshortened image. *P,* Patient's partial denture was not removed. *Q,* Fluoride artifact. Operator's fingertip contaminated by fluoride-touched film when stripping and placing film on hanger. *R,* Reticulation.   *Continued.*

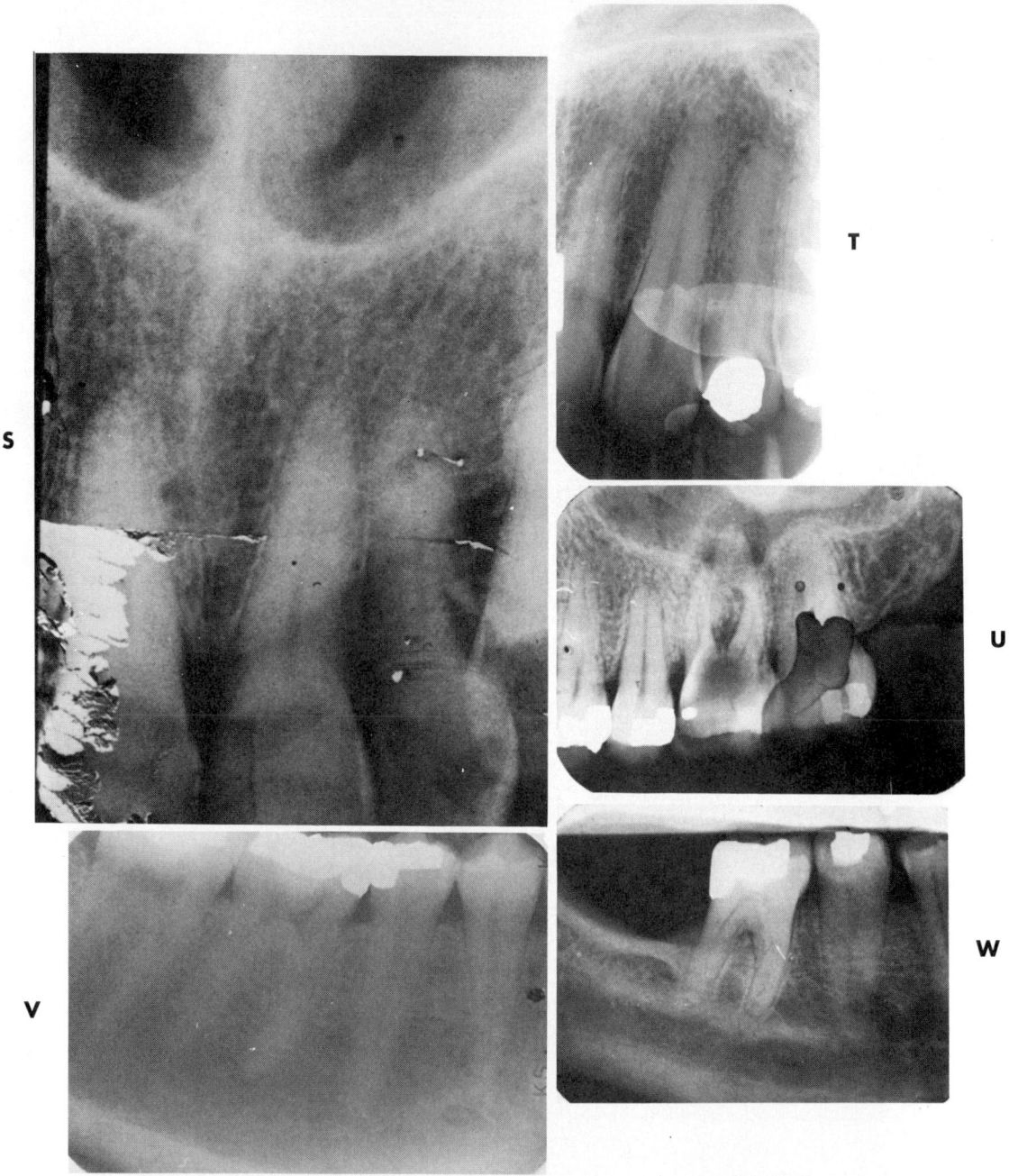

FIG. 9-46, cont'd.   *S,* Radiograph with torn emulsion. *T,* Light spots on the film resulting from contact with drops of fixer before processing. *U,* Stained radiograph. *V,* This radiograph is too light because of inadequate processing or insufficient exposure. *W,* Radiographs with developer cutoff.

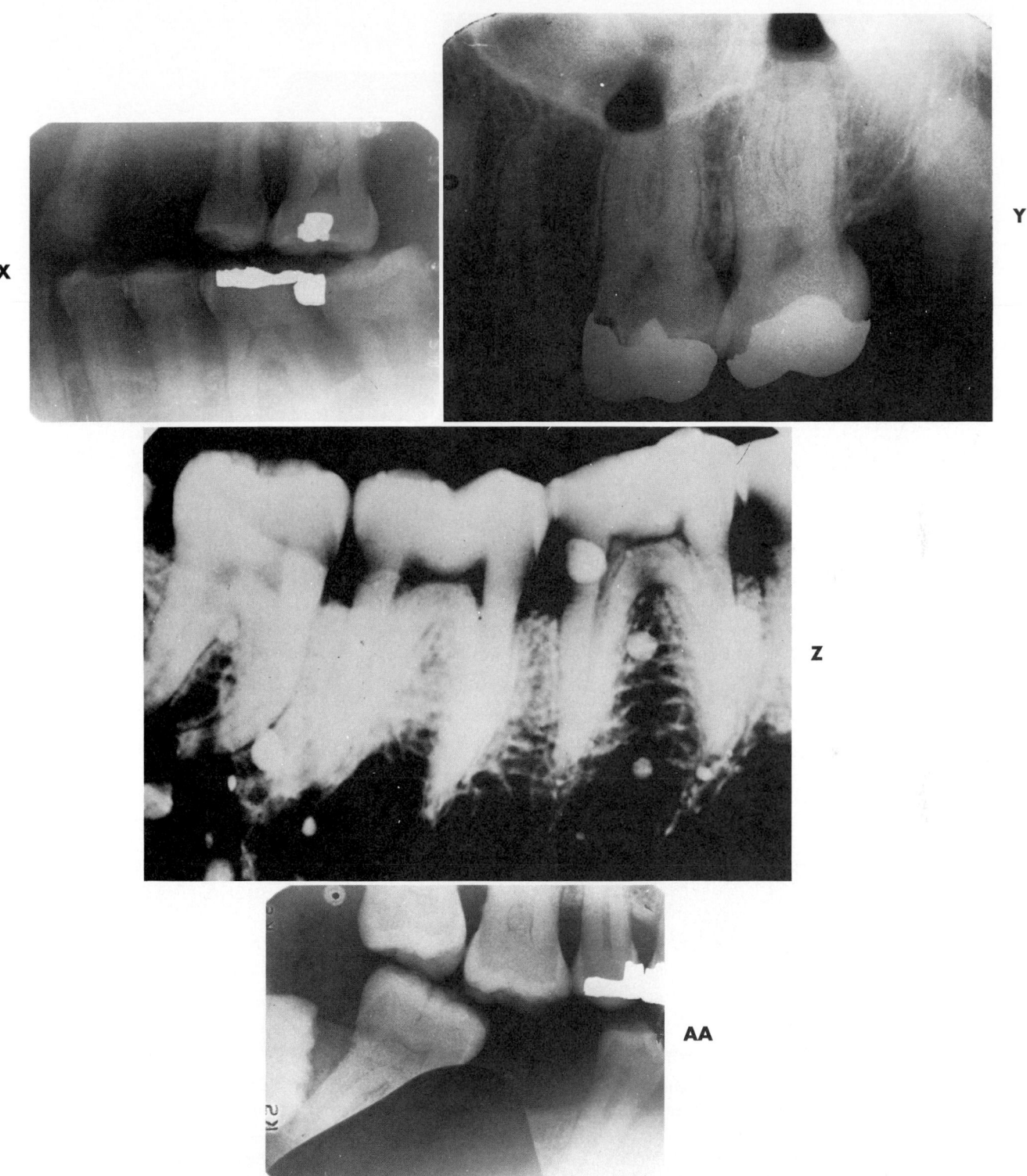

FIG. 9-46, cont'd. *X*, Fogged radiograph showing lack of image. *Y*, Periapical radiograph with static marks. *Z*, Artifact caused by air bubbles trapped on the film, preventing processing solution from touching film in the area. *AA*, Dark spot on the film resulting from contact with the tank wall during fixation.

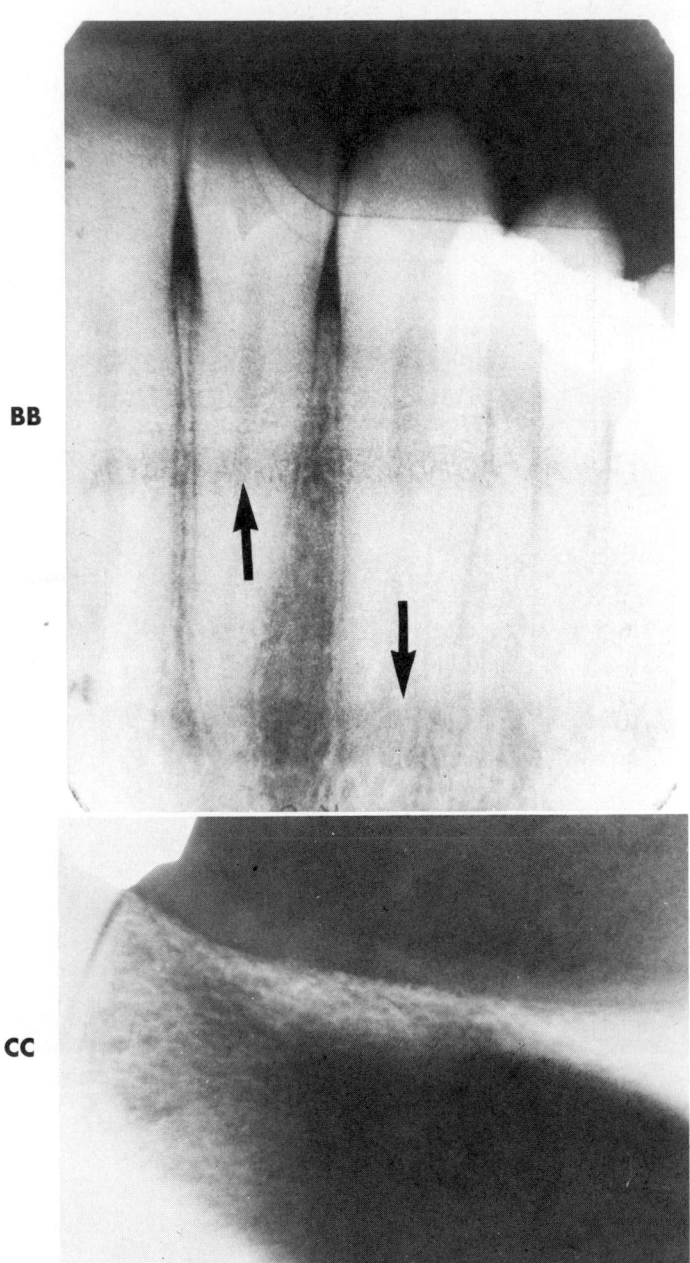

BB

CC

FIG. 9-46, cont'd.   *BB,* Bands of stain (*arrows*) from dirty rollers of automatic processor. *CC,* Artifact caused by light leak in daylight loader resembling a large pathologic area in bone.

(*A, E, F, H, I, K, L, T, V, X,* and *AA* from Goaz PW, White SC: *Oral radiology, principles and interpretation,* ed 3, St Louis, 1994, Mosby; *C, G, J, M, N, O, P, Q, R, S, U, W, Y, Z, BB,* and *CC* from Frommer HH: *Radiology for dental auxiliaries,* ed 5, St Louis, 1992, Mosby.)

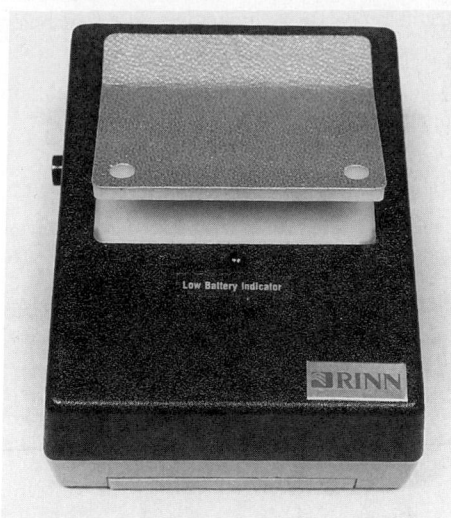

FIG. 9-47 Duplicating machine.

(Courtesy of Rinn Corporation, Elgin, Illinois.)

which they were originally exposed. Other sources that may need these radiographs include the following:

Insurance agencies

Dental specialists

Other general practitioners to which a patient may transfer

Court activities/malpractice suits

Forensic dentists

When insurance companies or other professionals require the patient radiographs, it is recommended that the dentist retain the original radiograph and provide the consultant with a duplicate copy.

Duplicating radiographs is simple and can easily be done in the dental office. Duplication is completed in the darkroom under safelight conditions. It requires a duplicating machine and a special type of duplication film (Fig. 9-47). Only one side of the duplication film is coated with emulsion; this side appears purple under the safelight. The original radiograph is placed on the duplicator glass with the viewing side up. The purple side of the duplication film is superimposed over the radiograph, and the duplicator light is turned on. The exposure time varies with the type of duplicator used. The exposure time also affects the density of the duplicate radiograph. Unlike radiographic film, shorter exposures increase the density (darkness), while a longer exposure lightens the duplicate radiograph. Duplicate radiographs are processed in the same way radiographs are processed.

DUPLICATION OF EXISTING RADIOGRAPHS: STEP-BY-STEP PROCEDURES

1. Place original radiographs and a sufficient number of duplicating film packets, corresponding in size to the original films, inside the daylight loader which houses the duplicating system.
2. Close the safety view glass.
3. Insert hand through cuffs of daylight loader, and open duplicator door within the unit.
4. Separate and lift the retainer plate from the duplicator door, and stabilize it.
5. Remove the duplicating film from the film packet, and place each film inside a section of the grid, with the lighter side of the film—the emulsed side—facing up.
6. On each duplicating film, place an original radiograph. Close the retainer plate, and squeeze it lightly to lock into the duplicating grid.
7. Close the duplicator door, and push firmly with both hands to activate the light source. NOTE: In some systems, if both door latches are not secure, the films may become blurry.
8. After the light source shuts off, open the duplicator door, and separate the retainer plate from the duplicating grid.
9. Remove the original films from the duplicating grid, set them aside within the daylight loader, and process the duplicating film through the normal manner in the automatic processor.

KEY POINTS

▶ Wilhelm Roentgen is attributed with discovering x-rays.

▶ Edmund Kells also made significant contributions to the area of dental radiography.

▶ X-rays are electromagnetic radiation used to create an image on photographic film.

▶ Electromagnetic radiation is the emission and propagation of energy through space or in a medium.

▶ A dental radiograph is a visible image produced on a radiation-sensitive film emulsion by exposing the film to radiation and chemical processing so that a negative is produced.

▶ An x-ray machine includes a tubehead, suspension arm, control panel, and power source. Within the tubehead is a diode tube, which is the most important part of the tubehead because x-rays originate within this tube. Wires in the suspension arm connect the tubehead to the control panel.

▶ Settings on the control panel include mA, kVp, timer and exposure controls. These controls determine the composition of the x-ray beam.

▶ X-rays are produced in many directions and of varying energies. To produce a useful beam of radiation, the x-rays must be collimated and filtered.

▶ Selective absorption depends on three factors: effective atomic number, physical density, and thickness.

▶ Factors related to radiation absorption of electromagnetic radiation include the energy and amount of radiation absorbed, the length of time over which exposure occurred, the area of the body and type of tissue irradiated, and environmental factors.

▶ The guiding principle for protection from radiation exposure is known as the ALARA concept.

▶ Units of measure include Roentgens, gray/rad, and sievert/rem.

▶ There are three types of x-ray film used in dentistry: intraoral, extraoral, and duplicating.

▶ The dental professional needs to develop an understanding for managing all types of patients.

▶ The two most common intraoral techniques are the bisecting and the paralleling techniques.

▶ Goals of film placement include correct teeth covered by the film, position of the PID, and patient management.

▶ Several steps are required to complete a radiographic examination; these include prescription and examination, personal protection, preparation of the treatment area, instrument and armamentarium preparation, infection control techniques, exposure, processing, and mounting procedures.

▶ Dental radiographs are developed through manual, automatic, and rapid processing techniques.

BIBLIOGRAPHY

DeLyre WR, Johnson ON: *Essentials of dental radiography for dental assistants and hygienists*, ed 4, East Norwalk, Conn, 1990, Appleton & Lange.

Frommer HH: *Radiology for dental auxiliaries*, ed 5, St Louis, 1992, Mosby.

Goaz PW, White SC: *Oral radiology, principles and interpretation*, St Louis, 1982, Mosby.

Miles DA, VanDis MV, Razmus TF: *Basic principles of oral and maxillofacial radiology*, Philadelphia, 1992, W.B. Saunders.

10 Pharmacology

LEARNING OBJECTIVES

You will have mastered the material in this chapter when you can:

▶ Define the key terms
▶ Give the definition for a drug
▶ Discuss current drug legislation
▶ Define the terms *trade name, generic name,* and *generic equivalent*
▶ List the sources of accurate drug information
▶ Define and discuss drug interaction, reactions, and effects
▶ List and discuss the types of drugs used in dentistry
▶ Describe the parts of a prescription
▶ Describe and discuss how to take or update a drug and allergy history
▶ Discuss the dental assistant's responsibilities for drugs used in dental practice
▶ Discuss the dental assistant's responsibilities when an emergency occurs
▶ Discuss important areas of patient education

KEY TERMS

Allergic
Analgesic
Anaphylactic
Angioedema
Antagonistic
Antibiotic
Antibody
Antigen
Antihistamine
Antineoplastic
Antiseptic
Barbiturate
Contraindications
Drug Enforcement Agency (DEA)
Food and Drug Administration (FDA)
Generic
Generic equivalent
Germicide
Hemostatic agent
Hypnotic
Illegal drug
Intradermal
Intramuscular (IM)
Intravenous (IV)
Legal drug
Narcotic
National Formulary (NF)
Nonprescription
Parenteral
Pharmacology
Physician's Desk Reference (PDR)
Prescription
Sedative
Subcutaneous (SC)
Synergistic
Topical
Trade name
Tranquilizer
United States Pharmacopoeia (USP)
Vasoconstrictor

The number of drugs used in dentistry is somewhat limited, but many patients seen by the dentist take drugs prescribed by a physician, as well as nonprescription drugs on an occasional or regular basis. Prescriptions and nonprescription drugs *have the potential* to affect certain dental procedures and surgeries. The dental assistant must be aware that *any* drug taken by the patient could have an effect on a dental procedure or a treatment prescribed or recommended by the dentist.

Many different types of drugs are available for prevention or treatment of medical, surgical, and dental disorders. There is no one way to classify drugs. Different references may list the classes or types in different manners. Table 10-1 is an example of how drugs may arbitrarily be divided into categories.

The rauwolfia derivatives are occasionally used in the treatment of hypertension and come from the Rauwolfia family of plants. It is believed that the use of this family of plants may have originated in India where the plant roots were chewed to relieve headaches.

Pharmacology Definition

Pharmacology is the study of drugs, including chemical formulas, uses, and positive and negative effects on all body structures. This definition of pharmacology includes facts about specific drugs, such as the following:

1. How the drug is metabolized (undergoes physical or chemical changes in the body)
2. How the drug is excreted from the body and the organ of excretion; for example, the kidneys, lungs, or bowel
3. Adverse (or side) effects
4. Appropriate dosage(s) or dose ranges
5. Method(s) of administration, for example, oral or intravenous
6. Contraindications for use, that is, situations or conditions, indicating that a drug should not be used or used with great caution in certain situations; for example, pregnancy, coronary artery disease, or a history of asthma
7. Warnings regarding serious and sometimes life-threatening adverse effects that may occur if the drug is administered, for example, drug excretion in breast milk, bone marrow depression, or impairment of kidney function
8. Improving methods of manufacture
9. Research
10. Continual updating of information

Pharmacology is an ongoing process involving the development of new drugs, reformulation or changes in the chemical formulas of current drugs, and collection of new information about specific drugs.

Drug Definitions

A **drug** is a natural or synthetic, legal or illegal, prescription or nonprescription substance (or chemical) that has the potential to produce a change in one or more functions of the body. This definition can also, with a few exceptions, be stated as *a drug is a substance not manufactured by the body.* An example of this exception is cortisone, a hormone produced by the body but also given in the treatment of certain medical and dental disorders or problems.

A **natural drug** is obtained from plant, animal, or

TABLE 10-1 TYPES OF PHARMACOLOGIC AGENTS

Type	More common uses	Examples of drugs*
Adrenergic agents	Hypotension, cardiac arrest, asthma, allergic reactions, certain cardiac dysrhythmias (irregular heartbeats), control of superficial bleeding, nasal congestion	epinephrine, ephedrine, isoproterenol (Isuprel)
Adrenergic blocking agents	Hypertension, certain cardiac dysrhythmias, glaucoma, angina	atenolol (Tenormin), propranolol (Inderal), nadolol (Corgard)
Cholinergic agents	Myasthenia gravis, urinary retention	bethanecol (Urecholine), pyridostigmine (Mestinon)
Cholinergic blocking agents	Peptic ulcers, preanesthetic sedation	atropine, L-hyoscyamine (Levsin)
Narcotic analgesics	Relief of moderate to severe pain	codeine, meperidine (Demerol), morphine, pentazocaine (Talwin), propoxyphene (Darvon)
Narcotic antagonists	Narcotic overdose, reversal of the depressant effects of narcotics	naloxone (Narcan)
Nonnarcotic analgesics	Relief of mild to moderate pain	acetaminophen (Tylenol), aspirin, ibuprofen (Advil)
Barbiturate sedatives and hypnotics	Sedation, sleep induction	phenobarbital (Luminal), secobarbital (Seconal)
Nonbarbiturate sedatives and hypnotics	Sedation, induce sleep	flurazepam (Dalmane), triazolam (Halcion)
Cardiotonics	Congestive heart failure, certain cardiac dysrhythmias	digitalis, digoxin (Lanoxin)
Antiarrhythmic drugs	Cardiac dysrhythmias (irregular heartbeats)	procainamide (Pronestyl), propranolol (Inderal)
Anticoagulants	Prevention of thrombi (blood clots)	heparin, warfarin (Coumadin)
Thrombolytic drugs	To dissolve newly formed thrombi	altepase (Activase), streptokinase (Streptase)
Antianginal agents	Prevention and treatment of angina	diltiazem (Cardizem), isosorbide (Isordil), nitroglycerin
Peripheral vasodilating agents	Nocturnal leg cramps, peripheral vascular disease	cyclandelate (Cyclan)
Electrolytes and electrolyte salts	Replacement of lost electrolytes	calcium carbonate, potassium chloride (Kaon)
Diuretics	Heart failure, hypertension, edema	chlorothiazide (Diuril), furosemide (Lasix)
Antihypertensive agents	Hypertension	captopril (Capoten), guanethidine (Ismelin)
Central nervous system stimulants	Drug-induced respiratory depression, treatment of narcolepsy and attention	doxapram (Dopram), methylphenidate
	Deficit disorders (children)	(Ritalin)
Insulin	Diabetes mellitus	
Oral hypoglycemic drugs	Diabetes mellitus	glipizide (Glucotrol), tolbutamide (Orinase)
Sulfonamides	Infections	sulfamethizole, sulfisoxazole (Gantrisin)
Penicillin	Infections	amoxicillin (Amoxil), ampicillin (Amcill), carbenicillin (Geopen), penicillin G potassium (Pentids)
Cephalosporins	Infections	cefaclor (Ceclor), cephalexin (Keflex)
Broad-spectrum antibiotics	Infections	erythromycin (E-Mycin), kanamycin (Kantrex), minocycline (Minocin), tetracycline (Sumycin)
Antifungal drugs	Fungal infections	fluconazole (Diflucan), flucytosine (Ancobon)
Antitubercular agents	Tuberculosis	capreomycin (Capastat), streptomycin
Leprostatics	Leprosy	clofazimine (Lamprene), dapsone
Antimalarial agents	Prevention or treatment of malaria	quinacrine (Atabrine), quinine (Quine)
Anthelmintic drugs	Helminthiasis	mebendazole (Vermox), thiabendazole (Mintezol)
Amebicides	Amebiasis	chloroquine (Aralen), metronidazole (Flagyl)
Antiviral agents	Virus infections	acyclovir (Zovirax), amantadine (Symmetrel)
Urinary antiinfectives	Urinary tract infections	cinoxacin (Cinobac), nitrofurantoin (Furadantin)
Topical antiseptics and germicides		chlorohexidine (Peridex), povidone-iodine (Betadine)
Anterior pituitary hormones	Anterior pituitary hormone replacement (failure to grow, ovulatory failure)	clomiphene (Clomid), somatropin (Humatrope)
Posterior pituitary hormones	Posterior pituitary hormone replacement (induction of labor, diabetes insipidus)	oxytocin (Pitocin), vasopressin (Pitressin)

*The drugs listed in this column may not be used for all of the uses listed under "More Common Uses."

Continued.

TABLE 10-1 TYPES OF PHARMACOLOGIC AGENTS—cont'd

Type	More common uses	Examples of drugs*
Glucocorticoids	Endocrine disorders, acute allergic states, skin diseases, asthma, rheumatic disorders	cortisone (Cortone), hydrocortisone (Cortef), prednisolone (Delta-Cortef), prednisone (Meticorten)
Mineralocorticoids	Partial replacement therapy for Addison's disease	fludrocortisone (Florinef)
Androgens	Male hormone replacement, inoperable breast cancer in females	fluoxymesterone (Halotestin), testosterone (Andro 100)
Anabolic steroids	Postmenopausal osteoporosis, metastatic breast cancer	nandrolone (Durabolin), oxymetholone (Androl)
Estrogens	Inoperable prostatic cancer, contraception, symptoms of menopause	chlorotrianisen (TACE), conjugated estrogens (Premarin), estradiol (Estrace)
Progestins	Amenorrhea, abnormal uterine bleeding, contraception	hydroxyprogesterone (Delalutin), norethindrone (Norlutin)
Oral contraceptives	Contraception	Ortho-Novum, Tri-Norinyl
Thyroid hormones	Hypothyroidism	levothyroxine (Levothroid), liotrix (Euthyroid)
Antithyroid agents	Hyperthyroidism	methimazole (Tapazole)
Oxytocic drugs	initiation of labor, uterine atony	ergonovine (Ergotrate), oxytocin (Pitocin)
Uterine relaxants	Management of preterm labor	ritodrine (Yutopar)
Abortifacients	Abort or terminate a pregnancy	dinoprostone (Prostin E2)
Antineoplastic drugs	Malignant diseases	busulfan (Myleran), cisplatine (Platinol), doxorubicin (Adriamycin), lomustine (CeeNu)
Anticonvulsant drugs	Convulsive disorders	diazepam (Valium), mephobarbital (Mebaral), phenytoin (Dilantin)
Antiparkinsonism drugs	Parkinsonism	benztropine (Cogentin), levodopa (Larodopa)
Psychotherapeutic drugs	Mental illness	alprazolam (Xanax), chlordiazepoxide (Librium), diazepam (Valium), haloperidol (Haldol)
Antihistamines	Allergic disorders	astemizole (Hismanal), diphenhydramine (Benadryl)
Bronchodilators	Bronchospasm, asthma	albuterol (Efedron), phenylephrine (Neo-Synephrine)
Antitussives	Relief of coughing	benzonatate (Tessalon), dextromethorphan (Mediquell)
Antacids	Neutralize or reduce acidity of gastric contents	aluminum carbonate (Basaljel), magaldrate (Riopan)
Antidiarrheals	Diarrhea	loperamide (Imodium), paregoric
Antiflatulents	Intestinal gas	simethecone
Digestive enzymes	Replacement of pancreatic enzymes	pancreatin, pancrelipase (Cotazym)
Emetics	Induction of vomiting in certain types of poisoning	apomorphine, ipecac syrup
Histamine H_2 antagonists	Ulcers	cimetidine (Tagamet), ranitidine (Zantac)
Laxatives	Constipation	bisacodyl (Dulcolax), mineral oil, polycarbophil (FiberCon)
Antiemetic drugs	Nausea, vomiting	diphenidol (Vontrol), perphenazine (Phenergan)
Heavy metal compounds	Gold—rheumatoid arthritis	auranofin (Ridaura)
	Silver—burns, eye infections	silver nitrate, silver sulfadiazine (Silvadene)
Heavy metal antagonists	Heavy metal poisonings	deferoxamine (Desferal Mesylate), edetate calcium disodium (Calcium Disodium Versanate)
Vitamins/drugs used in treatment of anemias	Vitamin deficiency	vitamin B_{12}
	Various types of anemia	folic acid, iron
Immunologic agents	Immunity to specific communicable diseases	diphtheria and tetanus toxoids and pertussis vaccine (DPT), measles vaccine (Attenuvax)
Anesthetic agents	Anesthesia (local, general)	enflurane (Ethrane), bupivacaine (Marcaine), thiopental (Sodium Pentothal)
Skeletal muscle relaxants	Acute, painful musculoskeletal conditions	carisoprodol (Soma)
Drugs used in gout	Gout	allopurinol (Zyloprim)
Nonsteroidal antiinflammatory drugs	Mild to moderate pain	ibuprofen (Advil, Motrin), flurbiprofen (Ansaid)

mineral sources. An example is digitalis, a drug that is obtained from a plant (purple foxglove) and used to treat certain types of heart disease. A **synthetic** drug is created (synthesized) by chemical manufacture. An example is glyburide (Micronase). Most natural drugs require some type of preparation during the manufacturing process before they can be used as drugs.

A **legal drug** is one that is approved by the **Food and Drug Administration (FDA)**. Examples of legal drugs are aspirin and penicillin. Sale and use of an **illegal drug** are against the law. Examples of illegal drugs are heroin and cocaine.

A **prescription drug** requires a written form completed and signed by a licensed physician, dentist, or veterinarian. This form, or prescription, is then filled, or dispensed, by a licensed pharmacist. Prescription drugs also may be kept in a dental office for use before, during, or after dental procedures. Prescription drugs commonly found in a dentist's office include diazepam (Valium), a tranquilizer, and mepivacaine (Carbocaine), a local anesthetic.

A **nonprescription** or over-the-counter (OTC) **drug** is any legal drug that may be purchased without a prescription. An example is aspirin, which is available under many brand names.

BOX 10-1

DRUG SCHEDULES AS DETERMINED BY THE DEA

SCHEDULE I (C-I)

High abuse potential and no accepted medical use (heroin, marijuana, LSD)

SCHEDULE II (C-II)

High abuse potential with severe dependence liability (narcotics, amphetamines, barbiturates)

SCHEDULE III (CIII)

Less abuse potential than schedule II drugs and moderate dependence liability (nonbarbiturate sedatives, nonamphetamine stimulants, limited amounts of certain narcotics)

SCHEDULE IV (C-IV)

Less abuse potential than schedule III drugs and limited dependence liability (some sedatives and antianxiety agents, nonnarcotic analgesics)

SCHEDULE V (C-V)

Limited abuse potential; primarily small amounts of narcotics (codeine) used as antitussives or antidiarrheals

---

Drug Legislation

The *Pure Food and Drug Act*, passed in 1906, was the first attempt by the government to regulate and control the manufacture, distribution, and sale of drugs. Before 1906 any substance could be called a drug, and no testing or research was required before placing a drug on the market. As a result, drug potency and purity were often questionable, and some drugs that were sold were even hazardous to human health.

The *Harrison Narcotic Act* of 1914 regulated the sale of narcotic drugs. Before passage of this act, any narcotic could be purchased without a prescription.

In 1938 Congress passed the *Pure Food, Drug, and Cosmetic Act,* which gave the FDA control over the manufacture and sale of drugs, as well as over food and cosmetics. Before the passage of this act some drugs, as well as foods and cosmetics, contained chemicals that were often harmful to humans. This law requires that these substances be safe for human use. It also requires that pharmaceutical companies must perform toxicology tests before a new drug is submitted to the FDA for approval. Following FDA review of the tests performed on animals, as well as other research data, approval may be given to market the drug. The Federal Trade Commission (FTC) controls and regulates the advertising of drugs.

The *Comprehensive Drug Abuse Prevention and Control Act* was passed by Congress in 1970. This act was written because of the growing problem with drug abuse. It regulates the manufacture, distribution, and dispensing of drugs that have the potential for abuse. Title II of this law, the *Controlled Substance Act,* deals with control and enforcement. The **Drug Enforcement Agency (DEA)** within the U.S. Department of Justice is the leading federal agency responsible for the enforcement of this act. Drugs under the jurisdiction of the Controlled Substances Act are divided into five schedules based on their potential for abuse and physical and psychologic dependence. These schedules are shown in Box 10-1.

Prescriptions for controlled substances must include the name and address of the patient and the DEA number of the licensed physician or dentist. Prescriptions for these drugs cannot be filled more than 6 months after the prescription was written or be filled more than 5 times. Under federal law, limited quantities of certain C-V (Schedule V) drugs may be purchased without a prescription, with the name of the purchases and the drug dispensed recorded by the pharmacist. An example of a C-V drug is cough syrup containing codeine, such as Tylenol with codeine elixir.

The Council on Dental Therapeutics

The **Council on Dental Therapeutics** is one of the councils of the ADA. One purpose of the council is to study, evaluate, and distribute information regarding dental therapeutic and cosmetic products, examples of which include toothpaste, toothbrushes, and mouthwashes. The Council on Dental Therapeutics also supports contact with related regulatory, research, and professional organizations.

If a product is approved by the ADA, a seal showing approval can be placed on the product by the manufacturer. Information regarding ADA approval is given to the public, as well as to members of the dental profession. The manufacturer may also mention ADA approval in advertising the product.

Trade Names and Generic Names

A **trade name** is the name a manufacturer gives to a product. When the trade name of a drug is printed or written, it is capitalized, for example, Lasix, the trade name for furosemide.

A **generic name** is the name of the drug other than the trade name. The term generic can be used to describe the chemical composition of the drug. An example of a generic name is furosemide. When a generic name is written or printed, it is not capitalized.

When a new drug is discovered or developed by a drug company, the drug is given a generic name and a trade name and the drug is patented. Following FDA approval for manufacture and sale, the drug can be manufactured and sold only by the company that owns the patent right. Patent rights last 17 years, after which time any company may legally manufacture the drug. An exception would be if the company that owns the patent decides to sell the patent rights to other drug manufacturers before the 17-year patent rights have expired.

Although all drugs have generic names, the term **generic equivalent** is usually used to mean a drug that is no longer under patent rights and is available from more than one company. In some instances, references simply use the term *generic* to indicate a generic equivalent drug. Although most generic equivalents are basically the same as their trade name counterparts, a few generic equivalents are known to meet a lower standard than the trade name drug, and this fact has been proven by research and documented in reliable references. Usually this difference is related to bioavailability (the ability of the drug to be absorbed and used by the body) of the drug, which, in some instances, can be extremely important.

The dentist decides, when using drugs that are stocked in his or her office, whether the drug should be purchased as a trade name or as a generic equivalent. The dentist also decides, when writing a prescription for a patient, whether the drug can be dispensed by the pharmacist as a generic equivalent or only as the trade name. This fact is noted on the prescription form.

Sources of Drug Information

There are several sources of information about drugs. The most commonly used source in a dental practice is the **Physician's Desk Reference** (PDR). Other references include *Facts and Comparisons*, drug package inserts, the **United States Pharmacopoeia** (USP), the **National Formulary** (NF), and drug textbooks. When it is necessary to obtain information about a specific drug, current drug references should be used.

▶ The *Physician's Desk Reference* (PDR)

This reference book is published yearly and provides periodic updates. The year of publication is printed on the spine of the book.

The front pages of the PDR contain color photographs of drugs for quick identification. Not all available drugs are included in the photo identification section. Behind the photo identification section is the index of all products contained in the PDR. The pink pages list the drug by trade or product name. The pale blue pages list drugs by category, for example, antibiotics or local anesthetics. The yellow pages list drugs by their generic and chemical names.

Most drugs in the PDR have a drug monograph, which is a complete listing of most known facts about the product. The subheadings in the drug monograph include the following:

Chemical description of the product
Clinical pharmacology
Indications and use of the drug
Contraindications to use of the drug
Warnings and precautions related to use of the drug
Adverse drug reactions
The recommended drug dosages
How the drug is supplied (e.g., tablets, vials for injection, or capsules)

The color of the drug and the product code number are usually included in the drug monograph. The information contained in a drug monograph is often identical to the drug information sheet that is packaged with most prescription drugs. Some older drugs may only be listed in the PDR and lack a drug monograph.

▶ Facts and Comparisons

Facts and Comparisons, a resource for drug information, is published yearly as a bound volume but is also available in a ringbinder looseleaf edition that is updated monthly by mailing supplements and changes to the subscriber. Many pharmacists use the looseleaf edition, since the monthly updated sheets make this reference more current than the PDR or the bound volume of *Facts and Comparisons*. Some dentists may also use this reference, especially oral surgeons or those prescribing a wide range of drugs to treat complicated dental problems.

❙ Drug Package Inserts

Many drugs are packaged with a product information sheet. The information contained in the drug insert is often, but not always, identical to the information contained in the PDR. Normally, drug package inserts are not given to the patient when a prescription is dispensed. However, some health professionals, when prescribing a drug, may include a notation on the prescription form, indicating that a drug package insert is to be given to the patient.

Some drug inserts are geared directly toward the patient and give detailed instructions for patient use. Examples of patient-oriented drug inserts are those for inhalers used in the treatment of asthma and the information sheets accompanying birth control pills. Drug inserts geared toward the patient are included with the prescription unless the health professional makes a notation on the prescription form to remove the drug package insert.

❙ *United States Pharmacopoeia* (USP) and the *National Formulary* (NF)

These two references are usually used by pharmacists or those involved in drug research. They include detailed information not as pertinent to the patient or prescribing professional as to the dispensing pharmacist.

❙ Textbooks

Occasionally a pharmacology textbook may be used to obtain information about a particular drug. Since textbooks may be several years old, current drug information may be not found in them. Drug textbooks are an excellent resource for obtaining general information on how a specific class or type of drug works.

Drug Actions, Interactions, Reactions, and Effects
❙ Drug Actions

Several factors influence drug action, and must be taken into account when a drug is prescribed by the dentist or used in the dental office.

AGE

The age of the patient may influence the action of a drug. Children almost always require smaller doses of a drug than do adults. Older adult patients may also require smaller doses, although this depends on the type of drug that is administered. For example, the older adult patient may be given the same dose of an antibiotic as a younger adult but may require a smaller dose of a drug that depresses the central nervous system, such as a tranquilizer or intravenous anesthetic like thiopental sodium.

WEIGHT

Drug dosages for children are often calculated on a weight basis; however, some drug dosages for the adult patient may also be calculated in this manner. When drug dosages are determined by the patient's weight in kilograms (kg) or pounds (lb), references list the dose as the amount of drug per kilogram or pound; for example, 5 milligrams per kilogram (mg/kg) or 2 milligrams per pound (mg/lb).

The dosages of some drugs are based on a weight of approximately 150 pounds, which is calculated as the *average* weight of men and women. In many instances the individual whose weight varies widely from the 150-pound average will benefit from the drug dose based on this average weight. Occasionally a drug dose may be increased or decreased because the patient's weight is

---

BOX 10-2

PREGNANCY CATEGORIES

Pregnancy Category A: Studies have not demonstrated a risk to the fetus in the first trimester (up to the third month of pregnancy), and there is no evidence of risk in the second (the third to sixth month of pregnancy) and third trimesters (the sixth to ninth month of pregnancy).

Pregnancy Category B: This category includes two distinctions. One is that animal studies have not demonstrated a risk to the fetus but no adequate studies on pregnant women are available. Animal studies have demonstrated an adverse effect, but adequate studies on pregnant women have not demonstrated a risk to the human fetus during the first, second, or third trimester of pregnancy.

Pregnancy Category C: This category includes two distinctions. One is that animal studies have shown an adverse effect on the fetus but adequate studies in humans are not available. There are no animal reproduction studies, and no adequate studies performed in humans.

Pregnancy Category D: There is evidence of risk to the human fetus.

Pregnancy Category X: Studies in animals and humans demonstrate fetal abnormalities, or reports indicate evidence of fetal risk.

significantly higher or lower than the average. An example of this is when thiopental sodium or a tranquilizer, such as diazepam (Valium), is used during dental surgery. Higher- or lower-than-average dosages may be necessary to produce the desired results in the patient who is significantly over or under the average weight.

GENDER

The sex of an individual may influence the action of some drugs. Women may require a smaller dose of some drugs than men because many women are smaller than men and have a different ratio of body fat to water than do men.

The use of any medication, prescription or nonprescription, carries a risk of causing birth defects in the developing fetus. The FDA has established five categories indicating the potential of a drug for causing birth defects. Information regarding the pregnancy category of a specific drug is found in reliable drug literature, such as the inserts accompanying drugs and approved drug references, including the PDR or *Facts and Comparisons*. The dentist should take into consideration the prescribing or use of a specific drug if the patient is pregnant (Box 10-2).

DISEASE

The presence of disease may influence the action of some drugs, and in some instances it may be an indication not to prescribe a drug or for reducing the dosage of a certain drug. In liver disease, for example, the ability to metabolize (creating a chemical or physical change in a drug) or detoxify (removing the toxic qualities of a drug) a specific type of drug may be impaired. If the average or normal dose of the drug is given, the liver would be unable to metabolize the drug at a normal rate. Consequently, the drug may be excreted from the body at a much slower rate than normal. The dentist may decide to use or prescribe a lower dose and lengthen the time between doses when liver function is abnormal.

 The drug belladonna, which can be extracted from a plant, was used as a liquid in the 15th century. The name of this drug was believed to have arisen from the fact that Italian women instilled a liquid form of the drug in their eyes to dilate the pupils—considered then a sign of beauty. In Italian, belladonna means *beautiful lady*.

ROUTE OF ADMINISTRATION

Drugs may be given by the following routes:
- Oral
- Subcutaneous
- Intramuscular
- Intravenous
- Respiratory (inhalation)
- Intradermal
- Topical

The term **parenteral**, meaning not in or through the digestive system, may also be used to describe the administration of a drug by the subcutaneous (SC), intramuscular (IM), intravenous (IV), or intradermal route.

Oral (PO) administration of a drug is the most frequent route of drug administration. Oral administration is relatively easy for most patients and rarely causes physical discomfort. This method of administration involves having the patient swallow a liquid, capsule, or tablet usually followed by a full glass of water.

A *subcutaneous* (SC) injection places the drug into the tissues between the skin and the muscle. Drugs administered in this manner are absorbed somewhat slowly. A volume of 0.5 to 1 ml is used for injection by this route. Larger volumes (e.g., over 1 ml) are best given as intramuscular injections. The sites for subcutaneous injection are the upper arms, the upper abdomen, and the upper back. Most subcutaneous injections are given in the upper arms.

An *intramuscular* (IM) injection is the administration of a drug into a muscle. Drugs given by this route are absorbed more rapidly than are drugs given by the subcutaneous route. In addition, a larger volume (1 to 5 ml) can be given at one site.

Intravenous (IV) administration is the injection of a drug directly into the blood by means of a needle inserted into a vein. Drug action occurs almost immediately. These drugs are usually given slowly over a period of a minute or more.

Drugs given by *inhalation* are quickly absorbed by the small blood vessels (capillaries and venules) that surround the thin-walled air sacs (alveoli) of the lungs. Drugs given by this route may be in the form of a gas or may be delivered by aerosol (a drug in solution that is dispensed by means of a mist). When a gas is given by inhalation, a mask is used to deliver the drug from its source, which is usually a metal cylinder containing the gas under pressure. Usually, drugs given by aerosol are contained in a small, pressurized canister to which an inert gas (which helps deliver the drug) and the drug have been added by the manufacturer.

The *intradermal* route of administration is the insertion of a drug under the top layer of the skin (epidermis). This route of administration is usually used for sensitivity testing; for example, the tuberculin test or allergy skin testing by an allergist.

The *topical* route of administration is the application of a drug to the skin surface or mucous membranes. Topical drugs may be in the form of ointments, lotions, liquids, gels, solids, or creams. In dentistry, topical anesthetics may be applied to the oral mucosa before injection of a local anesthetic.

Most topical drugs are not absorbed through the skin or mucous membrane and their action is to the skin and mucous membrane and not structures lying below the surface. A few topical drugs are absorbed through the skin. These drugs are applied topically for their systemic effects. An example of a topical drug that is absorbed through the skin is nitroglycerin, which is a drug used to treat angina (chest pain caused by coronary artery disease).

Intravenous administration of a drug produces the most rapid drug action. Next in order of time of action is the intramuscular route, followed by the subcutaneous route. Giving a drug orally usually produces the slowest drug action. Some drugs can be given only by one route, for example, antacids are only given orally. Other drugs are available as oral and parenteral drugs.

When drugs are used before or during a dental procedure, the dentist selects the route of administration based on many factors, including the desired rate and depth of action. For example, if the oral surgeon wants to produce a rapid drug effect, such as extreme sedation, during oral surgery, a tranquilizer, such as Valium, may be given intravenously. On the other hand, this same drug may be given orally as a tablet approximately 1 hour before a procedure to relax the patient and reduce anxiety. The intravenous administration of this drug produces effective and deep sedation, whereas oral administration usually produces relaxation and a reduction in anxiety.

▶ Drug Interactions

DRUG-DRUG INTERACTIONS

Some drugs interact with or interfere with the actions of other drugs. An example of one drug interfering with the action of another is the use of certain types of antacids, such as Maalox, at the same time tetracycline (an antibiotic used in the treatment of infections) is taken orally. The antacid may chemically interact with the tetracycline and impair its absorption into the bloodstream, thus reducing the effectiveness of the tetracycline.

Drug interactions can also be **antagonistic** or **synergistic**. Antagonistic drugs may interact with food, chemicals, or other drugs and produce opposing effects. An example of a beneficial antagonistic drug effect is the reaction of histamine with **antihistamine**. Antihistamines may be used to counteract (antagonize) the effects of histamine, which is a substance produced by the body as a natural **allergic** reaction response. Other antagonistic drug effects may not be beneficial. The administration of one drug that dilates blood vessels along with a drug that constricts blood vessels greatly reduces the effects of both drugs because the drugs are antagonistic to one another.

A synergistic drug effect may occur when a drug interacts with another drug (or drugs) and produces an effect that is *greater than* the sum of the separate actions of the two or more drugs. In other words, they end up working as an overdose of the individual drugs.

A synergistic drug effect is seen in the person who takes a **hypnotic**, a central nervous system depressant that induces sleep, along with alcohol—also a central nervous system depressant—at the same time or shortly before or after the hypnotic. As a result the action of the hypnotic is potentiated, or increased. The individual will most likely experience a drug effect that is greater than if either of these two agents were taken alone. On occasion a synergistic drug effect can be serious and even fatal.

DRUG-FOOD INTERACTIONS

Some drugs must be taken on an empty stomach, and some must be taken with food to achieve the best effect. Depending on the oral drug that is given, food may impair or enhance its absorption. When a drug is taken on an empty stomach, it will be absorbed into the bloodstream at a faster rate than it will be when taken with food in the stomach. Some drugs, especially those capable of irritating the stomach, can cause nausea, vomiting, or epigastric distress and are best taken with food or meals.

Manufacturers give directions in the package inserts regarding how the drug must be taken; approved drug references also give this information. When the drug is dispensed by a pharmacist, this same information is placed on the prescription label.

▶ Drug Reactions

ADVERSE DRUG REACTIONS

An adverse drug reaction is a symptom that is usually not desired when a drug is introduced to the body. Examples include nausea, vomiting, difficulty breathing, diarrhea, dryness of mouth, constipation, and headache. Almost all prescription and nonprescription drugs can potentially cause one or more adverse reactions, some of which may be severe and, on rare occasions, fatal. Usually, adverse reactions occur in few individuals, making many drugs relatively safe.

Individuals taking any drug may experience one or more adverse reactions to the drug. Adverse reactions, or side effects, may occur after the first dose or after several doses. Many adverse drug reactions occur without warning, but some adverse drug reactions are predictable. For example, drugs used in the treatment of cancer are toxic and are known to produce adverse reactions in most of the patients who receive them. These are predictable adverse reactions that cannot be avoided.

In some instances the adverse reaction may need to be tolerated because the drug is necessary for the treatment of a specific disease or disorder; examples include the antineoplastic drug used in the treatment of cancer. Many antineoplastic agents are extremely toxic; however, they are the only drugs available to treat cancer, and therefore the serious adverse reactions must be allowed to occur. In some instances the physician can minimize or treat some of the toxic effects of antineoplastic agents.

Sometimes adverse reactions can be controlled or nearly eliminated. For example, dryness of the mouth, although uncomfortable, may need to be tolerated by the patient who has an ulcer and is being treated with a drug that is known to cause this adverse reaction. Often drinking sips of cold water or allowing hard candy to dissolve in the mouth decreases this adverse reaction to a tolerable level.

Dryness of the mouth, xerostomia, can also evolve into mild to serious problems if the patient wears dentures. In this particular situation the patient's physician may need to reevaluate the patient's need for the drug, or the dentist may need to initiate a specific treatment or recommend the use of an agent that moistens the oral cavity, thereby partially or totally relieving the problem. This one example shows the need for medicine and dentistry to work together as members of the health team.

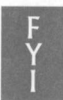

The Ebers Papyrus, an Egyptian recording of drug use, was written in 1500 BC and contained references to opium, castor oil, and squill (a plant that was once used as a diuretic).

DRUG ALLERGY

Drug allergy, or being allergic to a drug, is also called a hypersensitivity reaction. Allergy to a drug appears to occur after more than one dose of the drug is taken. When a drug allergy occurs, the individual has become *sensitized* to the drug; that is, the drug has become an **antigen**. An antigen is defined as any substance that stimulates the body to produce **antibodies**, which are specific protein substances manufactured by the body in response to contact with a specific antigen.

If the patient takes the drug after the antigen/antibody response has occurred, an allergic reaction will result, such as the allergy produced by ragweed pollen or *hay fever*. The ragweed pollen is the antigen, and the response of the individual to exposure to ragweed is an allergic reaction, which may include itching and watering of the eyes, increased nasal discharge, swollen nasal membranes, and sneezing.

Allergic reactions may be manifested by various signs and symptoms that are observed by the dentist or dental assistant or are reported by the patient. Examples of some allergic signs and symptoms include the following:

Itching

Various types of skin rashes

Hives (raised, red blotches on the skin)

Difficulty breathing

Asthmalike symptoms (difficulty breathing, wheezing accompanying each breath, tightness in the chest)

Cyanosis (blue coloration of the skin, nails, lips, tongue, oral mucosa membranes)

A sudden loss of consciousness

Swelling of the eyes, lips, or tongue

Allergic reactions to drugs can range from mild to extremely serious and some can be life threatening. Even a mild reaction can become serious if it goes unnoticed and the drug is given or taken again. This is why even the mildest allergic reaction must be detected early.

Some allergic reactions occur within minutes or even seconds after the drug is given. Other reactions may be delayed for hours or days. In many instances, allergic reactions that occur immediately are the most serious.

Another type of allergic drug reaction is an **anaphylactic** reaction, which usually occurs shortly after the administration of a drug to which the individual is sensitive or allergic. This type of allergic reaction is potentially life threatening and requires *immediate* medical attention. Symptoms of an anaphylactic reaction include the following:

Bronchospasm (difficulty breathing because of a narrowing of the bronchi or tubes that go to the lungs)

Extremely low blood pressure (also called anaphylactic shock)

Cyanosis

Dyspnea (shortness of breath, which is usually due to the severe bronchospasm)

Loss of consciousness

Convulsions

Cardiac arrest (complete cessation of the heartbeat)

All or only some of these symptoms may be present. Treatment is aimed at raising the blood pressure, improving breathing, restoring cardiac function, and treating other symptoms as they occur.

Angioedema, which is also known as angioneurotic edema, is another type of serious allergic drug reaction. It is manifested by the collection of fluid in subcutaneous tissues, which is evidenced by swelling. The areas that may be affected are the eyelids, lips, mouth, throat, hands, and feet, although other areas may also be affected. Angioedema can be life threatening when the mouth is affected because the swelling of tissues in this area may block the airway and asphyxia (insufficient intake of oxygen caused by an inability to breath or take in air) may occur. Any patient with swelling of any area of the body that occurs after a drug is given is closely observed for difficulty in breathing. The dentist is informed immediately if *any* signs of angioedema occur.

DRUG IDIOSYNCRASY

Drug idiosyncrasy is a term used to describe any unusual or abnormal reaction to a drug. It is any reaction that differs from the one normally expected of a specific drug and dose. For example, a patient may be prescribed a hypnotic drug to help sleep. Instead of falling asleep, the patient remains wide awake and shows signs of nervousness or excitement—a response that is different and unexpected for this particular drug. Another patient may receive the same drug and dose, fall asleep, and then after 8 hours find it difficult to awaken from sleep. This, too, is abnormal and is an unexpected response to the drug.

The cause of drug idiosyncrasy is not clear. It is believed to be due to a genetic deficiency wherein the patient is unable to tolerate certain chemicals, including drugs.

▶ Drug Effects

DRUG TOLERANCE

Drug tolerance is a term used to describe a *decreased* response to the dose of a drug, usually requiring an *increase* in dosage to give the desired effect. Drug tolerance may develop when certain drugs, such as narcotics and tranquilizers, are taken for a long period of time. An example of drug tolerance is the use of a hypnotic. For several weeks the patient is able to sleep using the prescribed dose. After several weeks, drug tolerance may develop and the patient may require more than the prescribed dose to sleep.

Drug tolerance is often seen in those using illegal drugs like heroin and cocaine, as discussed in the section that follows on substance abuse.

CUMULATIVE DRUG EFFECT

A *cumulative drug effect* may be seen in those with liver or kidney disease because these organs are the major sites for the breakdown and excretion of most drugs. This drug effect occurs when the body is unable to metabolize and excrete one (normal) dose of a drug before the next dose is given. Thus, if a second dose of this same drug were given or taken, some of the drug from the first dose still remains in the body. Because toxicity can occur with some drugs when too much of that drug is in the body, a cumulative drug effect may be seen. This situation may be serious, particularly with patients who have liver or kidney disease. These patients are usually given many drugs with caution because a cumulative drug effect may occur.

Substance Abuse

Substance or drug abuse has become a worldwide problem. The social and economic impact of drug addiction and abuse directly or indirectly affects every member of society. The Commission on Dental Accreditation recommends that all accredited dental and dental-related programs provide enrolled students with information regarding substance use, misuse, and addiction by means of classroom lectures.

It must be remembered that *any* patient seen by a member of the health team may be abusing drugs. This includes children, as well as adults of all ages. Substance abuse is not limited to purchasing an illegal drug on the street. Instead, substance abuse includes both legal and illegal drugs and may be seen in all age groups and all socioeconomic levels.

In many instances, substance abuse is a hidden problem. Patients seen by members of the health team normally do not admit to substance abuse. It is only with a careful health history, as well as observation of the patient, that a substance abuse problem may be suspected. Even then, many of those with a substance abuse problem are unable to realize that they are addicted until they are ready to admit that they have a problem.

▶ Terminology

The terms *drug* and *substance* often are used interchangeably. Substance abuse is the use of a natural or synthetic substance to alter mood or behavior in a manner that differs from its generally accepted use.

Substance abuse may be defined as the use of a drug or chemical to produce a change in mood or behavior in a way that departs from approved medical or social patterns.

Compulsive substance abuse is the need to use any drug or chemical substance repeatedly to produce the desired effect. The need to use a drug compulsively may be physical, psychologic, or both.

Physical dependency is a compulsive need to use a substance repeatedly to avoid mild to severe withdrawal symptoms and is the body's dependence on repeated administration of a drug.

Psychologic dependency is a compulsion to use a substance to obtain a pleasurable experience and is the mind's dependence on the repeated administration of a drug.

Drug tolerance is a need to increase the dose or the frequency of use to obtain the original or desired effect.

When an individual is physically or psychologically dependent on a drug, he or she craves the drug repeatedly. If the drug is suddenly withdrawn, symptoms of *drug withdrawal* occur, termed *abstinence syndrome*. Symptoms of the abstinence syndrome can range from mild to severe, depending on the drug(s) involved, the dosage used, the frequency of use, the length of time the drug has been used, and the individual.

Drug addiction may include the following:

▶ A compulsive desire or craving to use a drug or chemical
▶ An involvement with the drug to the exclusion of all other activities, such as work, recreation, family, or school
▶ A strong tendency to return to the drug after withdrawal
▶ Physical dependence
▶ An abstinence syndrome that produces moderate to severe physical reactions
▶ Detriments to society existing in the drug and its use, as well as in the user

Drug habituation may be defined to include the following:

▶ A desire to use a drug continually for the effects produced
▶ Little or no tendency to increase the dose
▶ No physical dependence, but rather a psychologic dependence
▶ When the drug is withdrawn, there is no true abstinence syndrome
▶ Any detrimental effect that exists is for the individual rather than society

Narcotics

Narcotics are substances that produce insensibility or stupor. Narcotic drugs are generally derived from opium. This category of drugs can relieve pain by suppressing the central nervous system to reaction.

▶ Heroin

Heroin (diacetylmorphine), a narcotic, is obtained from morphine, the principal alkaloid of raw opium, and is an illegal drug in the United States. It is the strongest and most addicting of all the opium derivatives, or opiates, and is not used in the United States as an analgesic. Physical addiction to heroin occurs rapidly, often within several weeks of frequent use; however, the time in which addiction will occur varies. Heroin addiction poses serious socioeconomic problems to individuals, families, and the community. The cost of a heroin drug habit is high and can deplete finances or require the user to engage in criminal activity to obtain money to support a drug habit. Continued use of heroin may result in other physical problems, such as malnutrition and physical neglect. Those using the drug intravenously (mainlining) may develop serious medical disorders. Septicemia, the presence of disease-producing bacteria in the blood, may develop if the needle, syringe, or equipment used to prepare the heroin for injection becomes contaminated. Hepatitis or AIDS can be transmitted from one individual to another when contaminated needles and syringes are shared among users. The occurrence of AIDS and hepatitis among intravenous drug users is increasing.

THE EFFECTS OF HEROIN

Heroin may be inhaled (sniffed) or injected subcutaneously (skin popping) or intravenously (mainlining). The desired effects on the user are euphoria and drowsiness. Mentally, there is an escape from reality. Other effects are those associated with the opiates, namely, loss of appetite, fixed pinpoint pupils, constipation, and a decreased pulse and respiratory rate. Continued IV use results in scarred veins with skin markings, also referred to as *tracks*.

HEROIN WITHDRAWAL

Signs of heroin withdrawal, or abstinence syndrome, are seen in Box 10-3.

Some heroin users accidentally or intentionally take or are given overdoses of heroin. Symptoms of overdose are as follows:

▶ Stupor
▶ Pinpoint pupils
▶ Nausea
▶ Vomiting
▶ Decreased pulse and respiratory rate
▶ Signs of shock
▶ Possibly coma

If the overdose is recognized and the individual is taken to a hospital, a narcotic antagonist, which will reverse the effects of the heroin, is administered. Other medical treatment is also instituted. Unfortunately, many cases of overdose are never treated, and the individual dies.

Heroin crosses the placental barrier. A child born of a mother addicted to heroin is also addicted to the drug and needs immediate treatment. Even after receiving treatment, many of these infants die.

▶ Other Narcotic Analgesics

Opiates, such as morphine, and other narcotics, such as meperidine (Demerol), are used less frequently than heroin as street drugs (i.e., drugs obtained from illegal sources). When heroin is unavailable, the heroin addict may attempt to obtain another narcotic by means of various techniques, such as stealing from drug stores or

BOX 10-3

SIGNS OF HEROIN WITHDRAWAL

Yawning
Perspiration
Tearing of the eyes
Increased nasal discharge
Gooseflesh
Abdominal cramps
Bone and muscle pain
Nausea
Vomiting
Diarrhea
Dilation of the pupils
Restlessness
Increase in body temperature
Increase in pulse and respiratory rate
Marked mental depression or despair
Intense desire for the drug
The symptoms of withdrawal usually begin when the next dose of heroin is due, reach a peak in 36 to 72 hours and gradually diminish in 4 to 5 days.

drug supply houses or faking pain when seeing a physician or dentist. The use of another narcotic instead of heroin may prevent withdrawal symptoms.

Addiction to *legal* narcotics, such as hydromorphone (Dilaudin), may occur in those receiving the drug while under the care of a physician, as in the case of a terminally ill cancer patient. Some also become addicted to a narcotic because of a physician's carelessness in prescribing the drug for a patient who does not have a terminal illness.

Individuals addicted to the opiates and other narcotics experience an abstinence syndrome similar to that experienced by the heroin user. They are also prone to the same dangers, such as hepatitis, septicemia, and AIDS, if materials for preparation and administration are shared with others.

Narcotics and the Terminally Ill

Terminally ill cancer patients who require repeated doses of a narcotic for pain eventually become addicted to the drug. Addiction in these patient is morally and legally acceptable.

Some terminally ill patients may not appear acutely ill but may still have a great deal of pain that must be controlled with a narcotic. These patients may be seen in the dentist's office for treatment of various dental problems, some of which may be associated with the patient's treatments for the cancer. The health history, and particularly the drug history, should reveal which drugs the patient is taking. A history of narcotic use in these patients is brought to the attention of the dentist.

Cocaine

Cocaine is an alkaloid obtained from coca leaves. Cocaine is highly addicting, and at the present time, its use is the number one substance abuse problem. Use of cocaine has created serious and sometimes deadly consequences that affect individuals, families, and the community. It still is occasionally used in medicine as a local anesthetic, but because of its widespread abuse, its use has been largely discontinued.

The Effects of Cocaine

Cocaine stimulates the central nervous system, producing marked euphoria and excitement. The powder form of cocaine is snorted (inhaled through the nose) or dissolved and injected intravenously. Crack, a purified form of cocaine with a crystalline or rocklike appearance, is smoked either by placing it in a pipe or by sprinkling it onto or mixing it with tobacco. Cocaine may be freebased, which reduces it to its purest form. It is smoked by sprinkling it onto a cigarette or inhaling it through a pipe. Freebasing produces a more immediate rush than when the substance is inhaled nasally. The heroin addict usually does not use cocaine as a substitute for heroin but may mix it with heroin and inject it intravenously to obtain a greater drug effect. This combination is called a *speedball.*

The Dangers Associated With the Use of Cocaine

Cocaine's danger lies in its ability to cause physical and psychologic dependency, as well as permanent damage to the nasal mucosa. The cost of a cocaine habit can reach astounding figures.

The individual using cocaine frequently can spend thousands of dollars a month to support a drug habit.

Signs and symptoms of acute cocaine toxicity include the following:

- Agitation
- Psychotic behavior
- Violent behavior
- Increased body temperature
- Seizures
- Irregular heartbeat
- Increase in blood pressure
- Respiratory failure
- Dilated pupils

In some individuals, acute toxicity can occur at any time and with any dose. There are times when acute

SIGNS AND SYMPTOMS OF COCAINE TOXICITY

Irregular heartbeat
Hypertension
Memory impairment
Personality and behavioral changes
Ulceration of the nasal mucosa
Perforation of the nasal septum (in those who inhale cocaine)
Needle marks along the pathways of veins (in those who use cocaine intravenously)
Loss of appetite with consequent weight loss
Psychosis
Hallucinations

SIGNS OF CHRONIC MARIJUANA USE

▶ Lack of interest in school, work, and other people
▶ Carelessness in personal hygiene and clothes
▶ Preoccupied appearance
▶ Lack of motivation
▶ Memory difficulty
▶ Passivity or apathy

toxicity can result in death. Signs and symptoms of chronic toxicity of cocaine are listed in Box 10-4.

Cocaine use results in physical dependence. In some people, dependence occurs rapidly, sometimes after using the drug once or twice. How soon physical dependence occurs appears to vary with the individual and pattern use. Use of this drug also results in psychologic dependency. Withdrawal usually is characterized by the following:

▶ Depression
▶ Psychosis
▶ Lethargy
▶ Restlessness
▶ Intense craving for the drug
▶ Inability to concentrate
▶ Irritability

Marijuana

Marijuana is classified as a hallucinogen, that is, a drug capable of producing a state of delirium characterized by visual and sensory disturbances that are bizarre and distorted. Marijuana belongs to a genus of plants called *Cannabis*. The substance or chemical that gives the hallucinogenic effect is a resin from the dried plant, tetrahydrocannabinol (THC). The resin extracted from the plant's flowers is call *hashish,* which is 5 to 10 times more potent than the more common variety.

▶ The Effects of Marijuana

Users of marijuana may experience various effects that appear to depend on the individual, as well as on the amount of THC in the marijuana. The user may experience any of the following:

▶ Euphoria
▶ Drowsiness

▶ Dizziness
▶ Lightheadedness
▶ Visual disturbances
▶ Sensory distortions
▶ Hunger (especially for sweets)
▶ Giddiness
▶ Hallucinations

On occasion other effects include the following:

▶ Panic
▶ Depression
▶ Nausea
▶ Vomiting
▶ Diarrhea
▶ Dryness of the mouth
▶ Inflammation and burning of the eyes
▶ Drop in blood pressure
▶ Rise in pulse rate
▶ Dilation of the pupils

Some individuals experience no drug effects, but this may be because the product they used contained fillers and little marijuana. The effects of the drug usually last 2 to 4 hours, but this is highly variable.

Marijuana is being used medically on a limited basis to lower intraocular pressure in those with glaucoma and in terminally ill cancer patients. Specific guidelines in dispensing the drug are required, and legal use of the drug is limited to research institutions or physicians who have applied for government approval of marijuana use in certain patients.

Psychotomimetic (Hallucinogenic) Drugs

A psychotomimetic drug produces an acute change in the perception of reality. Examples of drugs in this group are mescaline, lysergic acid diethylamide (LSD), 2,5-dimethoxy-4-methylamphetamine (DOM or STP), psilocybin, phencyclidine (PCP, angel dust), and dimethyltryptamine (DMT).

Use of these agents causes visual hallucinations and mood changes. The results are inconsistent and differ from person to person, and even within the same person, when the drug is taken under varying circumstances. Psychotic episodes may occur during and after use and may progress to periodic occurrences even when the drug is not being used. These events take place more frequently in those who have underlying emotional problems. Another problem that may occur for many years after use has discontinued is flashbacks, which are more common with LSD use. Flashbacks are brief episodes of the original sensations experienced during use of the substance. The frequency of flashbacks varies.

Although physical dependence on these drugs does not occur, the user can develop a psychologic dependence. There are no physical withdrawal symptoms if use of the substance is discontinued.

The Amphetamines

Amphetamine, dextroamphetamine, and methamphetamine are drugs intended for use as central nervous system stimulants and anorexiants (drugs that suppress the appetite). Because of the abuse potential of these drugs, their use in medicine in the treatment of obesity has declined. These drugs still have value in the treatment of some obese individuals and in those conditions or diseases requiring central nervous system stimulation. When medical use of these drugs is necessary, therapy is under the close supervision of a physician.

▶ Effects of the Amphetamines

Amphetamines produce euphoria, alertness, and a sense of excitation. The user appears talkative, restless, and excitable, may perspire freely, and the pupils may be dilated. Some use the drug to stay awake for long periods of time or to experience the euphoria produced by the drug. Others may use amphetamines when other illegal substances are not available, or when the drugs are of such a poor quality or strength that the expected effects are decreased.

The drug is usually taken orally, but it is also used intravenously to produce an instant euphoric effect that is greater in intensity than that produced by the oral route. Some individuals may use an amphetamine for several days, taking the drug every few hours. During this time the user is in a constant state of euphoria, excitement, and sleeplessness. The drug is usually discontinued because of exhaustion, confusion, or disorientation.

Some substance abusers are involved with more than one drug. Individuals using amphetamines may take a tranquilizer or barbiturate after several days of amphetamine use to reduce the effects produced by the amphetamine. Those using amphetamines may be belligerent and develop severe psychosis. Depression and

suicidal tendencies may occur when the drug is withdrawn. These drugs have addiction potential.

The Barbiturates and Nonbarbiturates

Barbiturate and nonbarbiturate drugs have their proper use in medicine but are also subject to abuse. Drug tolerance can develop in the chronic barbiturate user, and these drugs have physical and psychologic addiction potential when used for a period of time. Some of the nonbarbiturates have a low addiction potential but if used over a period of time, the result can be physical and psychologic addiction. An overdose of these drugs can result in convulsions, delirium, coma, and, in some instances, death.

When these drugs are subject to abuse or are used under a physician's supervision for a long period of time, they must *never* be suddenly discontinued. Instead, the dose must be slowly tapered over a period of time. When sudden discontinuation of a barbiturate occurs, there is an abstinence syndrome characterized by the following:

- ▶ Abdominal cramps
- ▶ Nausea
- ▶ Vomiting
- ▶ Weakness
- ▶ Tremors

In some persons, withdrawal from barbiturates can be more harmful physically than withdrawal from heroin.

Tranquilizers

As a group, tranquilizers have been subject to widespread abuse by those involved in substance abuse, as well as by persons who do not consider themselves *drug users.* When tranquilizers were first placed on the market, they were not believed to be physically addicting and were frequently prescribed by physicians for mild cases of anxiety and stress. Although tranquilizers have a definite use in medicine, they were and perhaps still are overprescribed by some physicians. Unfortunately, the overuse of tranquilizers has resulted in many individuals being physically addicted to these drugs.

Addiction to tranquilizers appears to occur fairly rapidly, although the time required to produce addiction often depends on the type of tranquilizer, the individual, and the tendency to increase the dose to produce the desired effect. Withdrawal, when it does occur, resembles barbiturate withdrawal, with the intensity of symptoms depending on the length of time that the drug was used and the dose that was most frequently used. Those experiencing withdrawal also experience extreme anxiety and nervousness and a strong desire to return to the drug.

Alcohol

Much has been written about alcohol abuse and alcoholism because it is a major problem. For various reasons, alcohol is subject to widespread abuse among all ages and socioeconomic levels. Malnutrition, physical disease, broken marriages, crime, loss of employment, and accidents resulting in injury or death are examples of the many problems associated with alcohol use. The chronic and even occasional alcohol user may additionally use other drugs, such as sedatives, tranquilizers, amphetamines, and cocaine. The combination of alcohol and any one of these drugs can produce a synergistic effect. Deaths have been reported with the use of alcohol alone with a CNS depressant, such as a barbiturate, nonbarbiturate, narcotic, or tranquilizer, because of the synergistic effect produced when any of these drugs are taken with alcohol.

Every year many people are killed by drivers who are under the influence of alcohol. Television commercials, newspaper and magazine articles, and raising the drinking age in some states are methods that are being used to discourage alcohol abuse. Groups have formed to encourage stricter laws for those convicted of driving while impaired, and businesses have developed programs aimed at helping the employee who is a compulsive drinker.

Alcohol is a potentially physically addicting substance. The time or amount of alcohol consumption required to produce physical addiction varies. Signs of physical withdrawal from alcohol usually appear within 12 to 72 hours, but may appear sooner in some individuals. These signs usually include the following:

- Tremors
- Weakness
- Anxiety
- Restlessness
- Excessive perspiration
- Nausea
- Vomiting

Seizures may occur in some individuals during the first 24 hours of withdrawal. Hallucinations, which are frequently terrifying, are often experienced. Recovery from withdrawal usually occurs within 5 to 7 days. During the period of alcohol withdrawal, or drying out, the patient should be under medical supervision.

Methods of Treating Substance Abuse

Methods for treating substance abuse vary, not only from drug to drug, but also in the methods that may be used for a specific drug. Physicians or drug rehabilitation centers will advocate one of many methods of treatment and claim good results. In some instances the individual addicted to one or more drugs or chemicals may need to try more than one treatment method to achieve results. In the treatment of substance abuse, success depends on the individual's desire to become drug free. If the individual is forced by parents, a spouse, or the court to enter a drug treatment program, there is less chance that treatment will be effective and that the individual will remain drug free for the rest of his or her life.

Narcotic addiction can be treated in clinics that aim to reduce or eliminate withdrawal symptoms. Methadone, a synthetic narcotic, may be used to wean the patient away from or to satisfy the craving for the narcotic to which he or she was addicted. Although addiction to methadone will occur, the patient can be gradually withdrawn from methadone after a period of time. Methadone withdrawal is less severe than withdrawal from heroin and other narcotics. Counseling and other types of support are provided during and after the treatment period.

Naltrexone (Trexan), a drug classified as a narcotic antagonist (e.g., a drug that antagonizes the effects of a narcotic), may be used in the treatment of addiction to one or more of the opiates. This drug is used to maintain an opiate-free state in those who have been addicted to an opiate. This drug is not given until the individual has been *without* an opiate narcotic for 7 to 10 days. The individual being treated must have gone through withdrawal before treatment with naltrexone is begun.

Naltrexone prevents or reverses the effect of the opiates. How this is accomplished is not fully understood. If the individual taking naltrexone on a daily basis attempts to take an opiate, he or she will not experience any of the narcotic's effects.

Addiction to other drugs, such as cocaine, tranquilizers, or barbiturates, may be treated by a physician, in individual clinics, or in public or private drug rehabilitation centers. Withdrawal from these drugs is necessary. Counseling and support therapy are important parts of treatment.

Chronic alcoholism, with or without a history of other substance abuse, may be treated by a physician or in public or private treatment centers. Alcoholics Anonymous (AA) is a support group that has done much to help the alcoholic attain and maintain an alcohol-free state. Just as important are the many support groups for *codependents,* those who are closely related or involved with the substance abuser.

Drugs Used in Dentistry

The types of drugs used in any one dental practice may vary, depending on the specialty of the dental practice.

▶ Analgesics

An **analgesic** is a drug that relieves pain and/or discomfort. This group of drugs may be divided into narcotic and nonnarcotic analgesics. An example of a narcotic analgesic is meperidine (Demerol). An example of a nonnarcotic analgesic is aspirin. An analgesic may be prescribed by the dentist for use after a dental procedure. The dentist may also recommend the use of an analgesic that does not require a prescription—for example, ibuprofen. Aspirin is usually not recommended for the relief of pain immediately after some dental procedures, such as extractions or periodontal surgery, since aspirin tends to lessen the ability of the blood to clot, thereby causing prolonged bleeding after the procedure.

▶ Antibiotics

An **antibiotic** is a drug used to prevent or treat an infection. These drugs work in various ways. Some have the ability to destroy specific microorganisms, whereas others slow or inhibit the multiplication of microorganisms, thus allowing the body's own defense mechanisms to control the infection.

The dentist may find it necessary to prescribe an antibiotic to prevent an infection; for example, an antibiotic may be needed by the patient who has lost the protective blood clot in the socket following a tooth extraction. The dentist may also prescribe an antibiotic to treat an infection of the oral cavity, such as an abscessed tooth.

Many different types of antibiotics are available. Penicillin and tetracycline are two examples of antibiotics. Each antibiotic can inhibit or destroy *specific* microorganisms. The dentist selects the antibiotic that will most likely treat a specific type of infection. If the patient fails to respond to treatment, the dentist may take a culture of the infected area, send it to a laboratory for culture and sensitivity studies, and then identify one or more antibiotics that will effectively control the infection. Culture and sensitivity studies take approximately 3 days from the time the culture sample has been received by the laboratory.

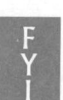 The antibacterial properties of penicillin were recognized in 1928, but it was not until 1941 that penicillin was used clinically in the treatment of infections.

▶ Tranquilizers

A **tranquilizer** is a drug that may be used to reduce anxiety and tension. While some patients are able to endure dental procedures such as a root canal or simple tooth extraction, others experience moderate to severe anxiety before the procedure. A tranquilizer, for ex-

ample, diazepam (Valium), may be given orally 30 to 45 minutes before a dental procedure to relax the patient and to reduce anxiety.

In some instances the oral surgeon may give diazepam orally 30 to 45 minutes before giving an intravenous anesthetic such as thiopental sodium (Pentothal). Diazepam may also be given intravenously to produce relaxation during a dental procedure.

 Mercury was used in the sixteenth century for the treatment of syphilis and remained in use for this sexually transmitted disease until the advent of antibiotics in the early 1940s.

▶ Barbiturates

In medicine, barbiturates are usually used as hypnotics or sedatives. A **hypnotic** produces sleep and is normally taken at bedtime. A **sedative**, which is usually taken during the day, produces sedation or relaxation. In dentistry, intravenous barbiturates may be used to produce unconsciousness during an oral surgery procedure such as the extraction of a third molar. Occasionally, the dentist may prescribe an oral barbiturate to be taken at bedtime for 1 or more days after extensive oral surgery.

▶ Nonbarbiturate Hypnotics

In many instances a nonbarbiturate hypnotic, for example, flurazepam (Dalmane), is sometimes preferred to the barbiturate hypnotics when the patient requires a drug to help sleep after extensive oral surgery. This group of hypnotics appears to cause fewer problems with excessive sedation the following morning and is also considered somewhat safer for older individuals.

▶ Antihistamines

Antihistamines oppose the action of histamine, a substance produced in response to injury or when coming in contact with antigens to which an individual is sensitive.

Antihistamines are used to treat allergies. In dental practice, these drugs are usually used to treat an allergic reaction to a drug or substance used during a dental procedure. The most commonly used drug is diphenhydramine (Benadryl). The injectable form of this drug is usually included in drug emergency kits.

▶ Vasoconstrictors and Topical Hemostatic Agents

A **vasoconstrictor** constricts blood vessels, primarily small arteries and capillaries. Constriction of small blood

TOPICAL HEMOSTATIC AGENTS

Absorbable gelatin sponge (Gelfoam): a gelatin-based sponge that can be cut to the desired size and placed on or in the bleeding area

Topical thrombin (Thrombinar): a substance that aids in the formation of a blood clot

Microfibrillar collagen hemostat (Avitene): aids in the clotting of blood; this product may be used in certain types of oral surgeries

Oxidized cellulose (Oxycel): aids in the formation of a blood clot; this product can also be cut to the desired size before being placed on or in the bleeding area

vessels helps reduce or stop bleeding that may occur during or shortly after the dental procedure. Local anesthetics containing a small amount of vasoconstrictor, such as epinephrine, may be used to control bleeding during a dental procedure. Epinephrine also prolongs the action of the local anesthetic by decreasing its rate of absorption because the blood vessels are constricted and therefore absorb the drug more slowly. Absorption of the anesthetic, with resultant excretion by the body, abolishes the local anesthetic effect. Use of a local anesthetic containing a vasopressor is not recommended if the patient has hypertension, high blood pressure, or a history of heart disease.

A topical **hemostatic** agent controls bleeding by methods other than vasoconstriction. Topical hemostatics that may be used in dentistry are found in Box 10-6.

▶ Adrenocortical Hormones

The adrenal gland manufactures the glucocorticoids and mineralocorticoids, which are collectively called adrenocortical hormones. The glucocorticoids and mineralocorticoids are essential to life. Glucocorticoids influence or regulate body functions, such as the immune response system; the regulation of glucose, carbohydrate, and fat metabolism; and control of the antiinflammatory response. Hydrocortisone and cortisone are the two major glucocorticoids produced by the adrenal gland. Prednisone and prednisolone are synthetic glucocorticoids.

Hydrocortisone may be used to treat emergency allergic reactions. On occasion the dentist may prescribe prednisone or prednisolone for a short period of time to reduce inflammation and swelling following certain types of oral surgeries.

▶ Antiseptics and Germicides

An **antiseptic** is an agent that stops, slows, or prevents the growth of microorganisms. A germicide is an agent

that kills bacteria. Examples of these types of drugs include benzalkonium (Zephiran), chlorhexidene (Hibiclens, Peridex), iodine, hydrogen peroxide, and povidone-iodine (Betadine). Chlorhexidene may be applied topically to the oral mucosa or used as an oral rinse. Iodine and povidine-iodine may be applied to the oral mucosa.

The Drug History

A complete drug history is an important component of the general health history. When a patient is first seen by a dentist, a complete health history, including a drug history, should be obtained. When appropriate, the patient should be asked if she is pregnant, as a pregnancy may indicate the need for a change in, or eliminate the use of, certain drugs before or during dental procedure. Since any prescription or nonprescription drug could have an effect on the developing fetus, dentists normally avoid prescribing any drug during a pregnancy. The components of a general health history are discussed in Chapter 24. A drug history should include the following two general areas.

Prescription Drugs. All prescription drugs that the patient is presently taking are entered on the dental record. It is also important to record any drugs that were prescribed for the patient by a physician or dentist within the past 6 months, even if the patient has discontinued use.

Although drugs taken in the past may not interfere with current treatments, procedures, or therapies, a history of past drug therapies could be important. An example of this is the prescribing of relatively high doses of an anticonvulsant for several months to prevent convulsive seizures following brain surgery. The drug may now be discontinued by the physician if the patient is presently complaining of gingival problems, which could be related to prior anticonvulsant drug therapy.

Nonprescription Drugs. All nonprescription drugs that the patient takes on a regular or occasional basis should also be entered on the dental record. Especially important is the use of aspirin, which may interfere with the blood's ability to clot, thus causing excessive bleeding after dental procedures, such as gingival surgery or extractions.

Any drug that the patient may be taking, as well as any current health problem, could affect the treatment of the patient in the dental office. A patient with arthritis may experience general discomfort while spending long periods in a dental chair because of this condition. Knowing this the dental assistant should attempt to make the patient as comfortable as possible and assist the patient when he or she is getting in or out of the dental chair.

The patient with arthritis also may be taking aspirin every day for a long period of time. If this is made known during the health history, the dentist is alerted to the fact that prolonged bleeding may occur following certain types of dental procedures, such as an extraction. When prolonged bleeding does occur, special treatment may be required.

Another example of the importance of a drug history involves the patient with treated or untreated high blood pressure. The history containing this fact may alert the dentist to avoid the use of epinephrine or drugs that are chemically similar to epinephrine; for example, norepinephrine and levonordefrin, in a local anesthetic. Epinephrine and its related compound can, even in small amounts, raise the blood pressure to unsafe levels in some individuals.

Sometimes patients do not know the exact name of the drug they are taking or do not understand why the drug was prescribed. Descriptions such as "the drug is for my heart" or "the doctors say I have bone problems" give little clues as to the name or type of drug or why the drug was prescribed. The patient should be asked to copy the name of the drug off the label of his or her prescription container and bring it to the office at the time of the next visit. The dentist should also be alerted to the fact that the patient is taking a prescribed drug but its name and purpose are unknown.

Some patients may give an unreliable drug history. Because a reliable drug history is important in the practice of dentistry, certain areas of the patient's general health history may need to be evaluated. If answers on the history require further investigation, the dentist may attempt to clarify or identify the patient's present drug history through further questions. The following areas of the general health history may identify those parts of the drug history requiring further understanding.

A History of Surgical Procedures. While some surgical procedures—for example, the removal of an appendix or appendectomy—are normally not applicable to dental care and do not present unclear areas in the drug history, other surgeries may be significant. A surgery, as well as the drug history, that could be relevant to dental practice is surgery performed for cancer. In this particular example, knowing that the patient has had treatment for cancer may require further investigation into other treatments the patient may have had recently. Patients who have recently had chemotherapy may have acquired problems with oral tissues, especially the gingival or oral mucosa, or may heal poorly after extractions of teeth.

A History of Past and Present Medical Disorders. Certain medical disorders are of major importance to the practice of dentistry. Some examples of these disorders are diabetes, cancer, heart disease, and epilepsy. Patients receiving drug therapy for certain medical disorders may be taking one or more drugs for the treatment or control of the disorder. As stated previously, some patients may have little understanding of their drug therapy. Knowing that the patient has a medical disorder and that this disorder may require drug therapy will possibly help clarify those areas of the drug history that require further explanation.

Other medical disorders may not be of direct importance but do help the dentist and the assistants treat the *whole* patient. An arthritic patient may experience difficulty holding a toothbrush, using dental floss, using a medication, or performing a treatment prescribed by the dentist. Knowing that the patient has a medical problem, as described in this example, directs the dentist, as well as the assistant and hygienist, to work with the patient in performing these activities.

Pregnancy. Patients who are pregnant should not take or be prescribed any drug unless the drug was prescribed for a specific circumstance by the patient's obstetrician. Most local anesthetics cross the placental barrier and thus potentially affect the fetus. The safety of local anesthetics in pregnant women has not been established. Etidocaine (Duranest), lidocaine (Xylocaine), and prilocaine (Citanest) are classified as Category B drugs. Bupivacaine (Marcaine), chloroprocaine (Nesacaine), mepivacaine (Carbocaine), and tetracaine (Pontocaine) are classed as Category C drugs. All of these drugs have the potential for crossing the placental barrier.

An Allergy History. When taking a general health history the patient should be asked if he or she has any allergies and if so what substances, if known, cause symptoms. Patients may be allergic to various substances, such as drugs, certain foods, and environmental substances like dust, animal dander, grasses, and trees. The patient should also be asked if he or she has a history of asthma or other breathing problems or if a problem was experienced when taking a particular drug. Sometimes patients have an allergic reaction to a drug but do not realize that the symptoms were those of an allergic reaction.

Patients with a history of one or more allergies may experience problems with drugs that are prescribed by the dentist; for example, local or parenteral anesthetics and antibiotics. It is most important that any allergy, including an allergy to drugs, be brought to the attention of the dentist before any dental procedure is begun.

A history of allergies should be entered in a prominent place on the patient's dental record when a patient has a known or suspected allergy to one or more drugs or has a history of an allergy to environmental substances. Various methods may be used to bring attention to this fact. Some office procedures may require color-coded tabs on labels or require labels that list the drugs or substances to which the patient is allergic. These labels

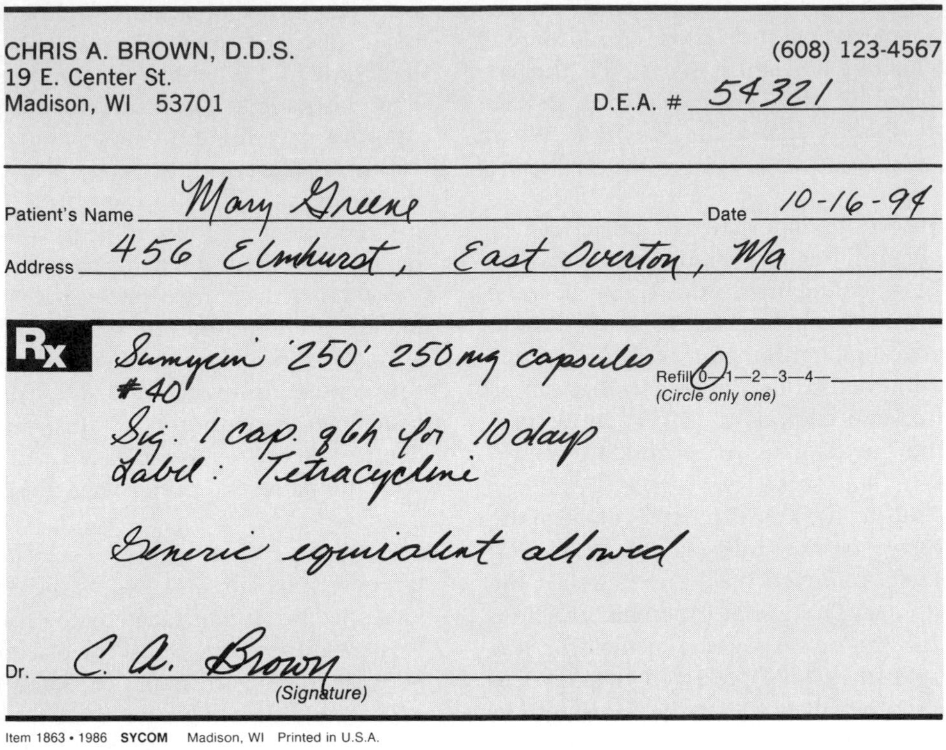

CHRIS A. BROWN, D.D.S.   (608) 123-4567
19 E. Center St.
Madison, WI   53701   D.E.A. # *54321*

Patient's Name _*Mary Greene*_____   Date _*10-16-94*_

Address _*456 Elmhurst, East Overton, Ma*_

Rx   *Sumycin '250' 250 mg capsules*   Refill 0—1—2—3—4—
          #40   (Circle only one)
          Sig. 1 cap. q6h for 10 days
          Label: Tetracycline

          Generic equivalent allowed

Dr. _*C. A. Brown*_____
              (Signature)

Item 1863 • 1986 **SYCOM**   Madison, WI Printed in U.S.A.

FIG. 10-1   Sample of a prescription.

or tabs are usually placed on the outside of the patient's record. If the patient's record is fully computerized with a viewing screen in each room of the office, a section of the record is usually reserved for allergies. The section displaying allergies may be presented in a color assigned to allergies or, if a monochrome screen is used, outlined or highlighted.

Health records, including a drug history, should be updated every 6 months. If visits to the dentist are longer than 6 months, the health history is updated at the time of the next visit. Should any new problems occur, they are brought to the attention of the dentist.

The abbreviations used in writing prescriptions, as well as examples of those that may be used in the patient's dental, are listed in Box 10-8.

Prescriptions

A prescription, as seen in Fig. 10-1, is a legal form, written and signed by a licensed physician, dentist, or veterinarian for the dispensing of drugs that are required by law to be sold only by prescription. Although some prescription forms may vary slightly in their content and order of presentation, a prescription usually has the parts listed in Box 10-7. The abbreviations used in writing prescriptions, as well as examples of those that may be used in the patient's dental record, are listed in Box 10-8.

▶ The Heading

The heading of the prescription is part of the printed form and contains the name, degree (M.D., D.D.S. or D.M.D., D.V.M.), address, and telephone number of the health professional writing the prescription.

▶ The Superscription

The superscription contains the date of the prescription and the patient's name, address, age, and gender.

▶ The Inscription

This part of the prescription contains the name of the drug, the dosage form, and the amount of the dose. An example of an inscription is as follows:
   ▶ Erythromycin 250 mg tabs
   ▶ (Erythromycin 250 milligram tablets)

Abbreviations are usually used when writing the inscription.

▶ The Subscription

The number of doses or the amount of the drug and, when applicable, directions for preparing the drug for dispensing are the components of the subscription section of the prescription. Some medications dispensed

PARTS OF A PRESCRIPTION

- Heading
- Superscription
- Inscription
- Subscription
- Signature
- Physician, dentist, veterinarian signature and DEA number
- Refill information
- Designation for filling with a generic equivalent

ABBREVIATIONS COMMONLY USED IN WRITING PRESCRIPTIONS

qd	daily
bid	twice a day
tid	three times a day
qid	four times a day
qh	every hour
q2h	every 2 hours
q3h	every 3 hours
q4h	every 4 hours
q6h	every 6 hours
ql2h	every 12 hours
stat	immediately
ac	before meals
pc	after meals
prn	whenever necessary, as needed
tabs	tablets
caps	capsules
liq	liquid
Sig	take
ml	milliliter
tsp	teaspoon

by the pharmacist must be specially prepared or compounded. Special preparations are the addition of certain materials or solutions to a drug and the mixing of two or more drugs. A subscription example would be as follows:

Dispense 30 (which may also be written # 30)

or

Dispense 500 ml

The number indicates the number that are to be placed in the prescription container and therefore applies to drugs available in solid form, such as tablets or capsules. When a liquid preparation is prescribed, the volume to be dispensed is entered in this area.

The Signature

The abbreviation *Sig* or *S* for signature, derived from the Latin word *Signum,* followed by specific directions indicates how the drug is to be taken. The word *signature* indicates that which is to be written or printed on the label of the prescription container. An example of the signature is as follows:

Sig: tabs I q6h

(write/print on the label "take one tablet every 6 hours")

The Label

By law, each prescription is labeled as to the contents. The health professional must indicate on the prescription form the desired label. Examples of labels follow:

Label: Betapen-VK 250 mg (trade name)

Label: penicillin V-K 250 mg (generic name)

The label of the container may also contain the dose, for example, 250 mg or 500 mg.

Refill Information

The health professional writing the prescription must indicate how many refills are allowed or if no refills are allowed.

Dispensing As Written or As a Generic Equivalent

The health professional must indicate whether the drug must be filled as written (when a trade name is written) or if a generic equivalent (if available) can be substituted.

Health Professional's Name and DEA Number

The health professional's name is signed on the appropriate line of the prescription. The DEA number of the health professional must be added if the prescribed drug is a controlled substance, for example, meperidine (Demerol) or codeine.

In some instances, preprinted prescription forms are made available to the dentist by the product manufacturer. These forms carry the name of the drug, the amount of the drug, and part or all of the signature, which contains the directions for use of the drug. Preprinted prescription forms, which still require a superscription and the health professional's signature, may be used for products such as oral rinses.

Recording the Prescription

In some dental offices it is the responsibility of the dental assistant to record on the patient's record all prescribed or recommended drugs. The dental assistant should record the following:

▶ The name and dosage of the prescribed or recommended drug; for example, tetracycline 250 mg capsules, or Advil 2 tablets q4h prn (2 tablets every 4 hours as needed) for pain or discomfort.

▶ If a prescription was written, the number of capsules or tablets or the amount of the drug by volume, for example, 15 ml or 500 ml, as stated in the subscription section of the prescription.

▶ The directions for taking the prescribed or recommended drug, for example, 1 tablet bid (twice daily) or 2 capsules q4h prn (every 4 hours as needed).

Drugs and the Dental Assistant's Responsibility

Dental offices may vary regarding the responsibilities required of the dental assistant. Some of the responsibilities that may be assigned to the dental assistant include checking the stock of drugs used in the office; checking all stock drugs for expiration dates on the drug container, bottle, or wrapper; and reordering stocked drugs.

Prescription and most nonprescription drugs sent from a manufacturer have an expiration date that is printed on the label of the container and/or outer packaging (box, sleeve, wrapper). The expiration date indicates the shelf life, or life expectancy, of the drug. Once the indicated date has passed, the drug could lose its potency, disintegrate, or undergo a chemical change that, in some instances, could be harmful. Drugs that have passed their expiration dates should not be used. Prescription drugs dispensed by a pharmacist usually do not have an expiration date printed on the label of the container.

All drugs used in a dental office are stored in a cool, dry place unless directed otherwise by the manufacturer or dentist. Drugs must be kept away from excessive heat or cold, direct sunlight, and excessive moisture. Drugs should not be stored next to or near sterilization equipment using steam under pressure. All covers or caps of drug containers should be closed tightly between uses because exposure to the air can cause deterioration of the drug.

When drugs are restocked, the new supply of drugs should be placed behind or below the present supply of drugs. Packaging is not removed until the drug is ready to be used. This is important because some drugs decompose and lose their effectiveness when exposed to light.

In addition to the responsibilities stated above, the dental assistant should be aware of some of the more common adverse reactions of the drugs used in the office. Patients receiving any drug in the office are observed before, during, and after administration of the drug. If a patient is left alone until a drug takes effect—for example, a local anesthetic—the dental assistant should check the patient every 3 to 5 minutes until the dentist enters the room and begins the procedure. The frequency of observation depends on the drug used, the health of the patient, and the condition of the patient before the administration of the drug. Patients who are extremely nervous and anxious about the procedure should be checked at more frequent intervals.

Another responsibility of the dental assistant is exercising care in handling needles and syringes when preparing a drug for administration. This is discussed in future chapters. Universal precautions when using sharp objects are discussed in Chapter 8.

If there is any question regarding the drug requested by the dentist before or during a procedure, the dental assistant should ask for clarification. The incorrect amount or strength of the drug could result in a drug reaction, as well as an increase or decrease in the action or expected result of the drug.

When preparing a drug for administration by the dentist, the label of the drug is checked twice to ensure accuracy. The drug is then placed on the mobile cabinet out of the patient's line of vision. Seeing a needle and syringe or other equipment used for the administration of a medication may frighten the patient and cause unnecessary anxiety.

During a dental procedure it is good practice to repeat the name of the drug when handing it to the dentist, for example, Xylocaine 2% (lidocaine) with 1:100,000 epinephrine. In some instances, it may be necessary to point out and name the drug or drugs that have been placed on the mobile cabinet before the dental procedure. The naming of drugs ensures accuracy and prevents drug errors. However, some dentists may feel that naming a drug before or during a dental procedure may result in patient anxiety.

The Patient's Dental Record

In addition to obtaining and updating the health history, the dental assistant may be responsible for recording the following drug information:

All drugs used or administered before, during, and after a dental procedure, for example, local anesthetics, tranquilizers, and fluorides; the name of the drug, the dose of the drug, and the route given are also noted on the dental record; when local anesthetics are used, the name of the anesthetic, as well as the percent and amount, are recorded; other drug dosages may be stated as volume, for example, 0.5 ml, or weight, for example, 500 mg

Prescriptions written by the dentist

The names or types of nonprescription drugs recommended by the dentist for use after a dental procedure, for example, acetaminophen (Tylenol) for discomfort

Drug samples given to the patient in the office to take immediately or at home, for example, samples of ibuprofen for discomfort or pain; the number of tablets or capsules given to the patient is also recorded on the patient's record

In some offices the dentist may record certain drugs administered, such as the short-acting general anesthetics and intravenous tranquilizers.

Emergencies

On occasion a patient may have a serious and even life-threatening adverse reaction to a drug or product used in dental practice. Patients may also experience situations such as an epileptic or convulsive seizure, a heart attack (myocardial infarction [MI]), fainting, angina (pain in the chest that may or may not radiate to the arm[s], jaw, back, or neck), or other medical problems requiring immediate attention by the dentist and assistant. Initial mild allergic reactions, such as moderate difficulty in breathing, fainting, lightheadedness, skin rash, hives, itching, and slight swelling of the lips and tongue require immediate treatment because these may become more serious in the minutes or hours after the initial mild reaction.

Most dental offices should have an emergency kit, as shown in Fig. 10-2, that can be used to treat serious and even life-threatening allergic drug reactions. Drugs contained in the emergency kit are usually in prefilled syringes, making them ready for immediate use. While these kits may vary with regard to contents, most contain some or all of the materials outlined here.

Epinephrine 1:1000. This drug is used to treat hypotension and other symptoms of an acute allergic reaction, primarily anaphylactic shock. Epinephrine raises the blood pressure, increases the heart rate, dilates the bronchi, and increases the amount of blood pumped by the heart with each heartbeat. The strength of epinephrine used for emergencies, that is, 1:1000, is greater than that used in local anesthetics.

During an emergency the dental assistant can loosen the cover over the needle of the prefilled syringe and hand it to the dentist, while at the same time *saying the name of the drug,* for example, "This is epinephrine 1 to 1000" (1:1000). Saying the name of the drug prevents errors in communication, which can occur during the management of an emergency situation. Great caution is exercised in administering epinephrine because it is a potent drug, even in small doses.

Ephedrine. This drug is chemically similar to, but not the same as, epinephrine and may be used to treat episodes of hypotension and asthma. Ephedrine raises the blood pressure, increases the pulse rate, and dilates the bronchi.

The names *epinephrine* and *ephedrine* are similar, which emphasizes the importance of saying the name of the drug. Epinephrine is many times more powerful than ephedrine. Ephedrine may be supplied in a prefilled syringe or an ampule, the top of which must be broken and the contents withdrawn.

Antihistamines. Histamine is released by certain body cells at the time of an injury or allergic reaction. The release of histamine results in dilation of blood vessels, and thus a drop in blood pressure and possibly a rise in the heart rate, localized swelling, itching, and redness. Severe allergic reactions accompanied by the release of large amounts of histamine may result in angioedema or an anaphylactic reaction.

Antihistamines counteract the effect of histamine and are used to treat allergic reactions such as hives, itching, and skin rash. An antihistamine may also be given after the administration of epinephrine to treat a life-threatening allergic reaction, such as angioedema or anaphylactic shock.

Usually diphenhydramine (Benadryl) is included in an emergency kit and may be given IV or deep IM. This drug may be supplied in a prefilled syringe or as a solution in a vial requiring removal of the drug with a needle and syringe before administration.

Diazepam (Valium). Diazepam, a tranquilizer, may be used for sedation, various forms of psychosis, anxiety, and convulsive seizures. In an emergency situation, diazepam may be used to treat convulsions that occur after overdose of a local anesthetic.

Patients with epilepsy, who are taking a prescribed drug to control their seizures, may have a seizure during times of stress or acute anxiety. Diazepam may be used to treat convulsions in such a patient.

A Bronchodilating Agent. This type of drug dilates the bronchi and therefore improves breathing when bronchospasm occurs. It may be used for the asthmatic patient experiencing an asthma attack, which may be a drug reaction or result from anxiety that occurs during or after a dental procedure, or for the treatment of an allergic reaction that is manifested by breathing difficulties. Bronchospasm caused by an adverse drug reaction is most likely to occur in those with a history of asthma. Examples of bronchodilators supplied in aerosol canister form are terbutaline (Brethaire), albuterol (Ventolin), and metaproterenol (Alupent).

These drugs are included in an emergency kit as aerosol inhalers. Illustrated and written directions for using the inhaler are included in the kit. The container must be seated firmly in the mouthpiece section of the inhaler by a downward motion and must be shaken several times before use. The patient is instructed to

RED

Stimulants - to combat respiratory depression
•Ammonia Inhalants

BLUE

Vasopressors - to combat falling blood pressures • Wyamine

YELLOW

Anti-allergic Drugs - to combat undue reactions to drugs such as penicillin, or to combat severe asthmatic attack
• Adrenalin (epinephrine)
• Aminophylline (bronchodilator)
• Benadryl (antihistamine)
• Solu-cortef (corticosteroid)

BLACK

Equipment • Airway
• Tracheotomy Needle
• Tourniquet • Syringes

WHITE

Combat nausea
• Tigan

DRUGS OF CHOICE EMPTY SLOT

GREEN

Depressants - to combat convulsions, etc.
• Diazepam

PURPLE

Vagal Blocking - to increase pulse rate
• Atropine

AQUA

Analgesics - to combat severe pain
• Talwin

ORANGE

Vasodilators - to increase blood supply to heart
• Amyl-nitrite Inhalants
• Nitroglycerin (nitrostat)

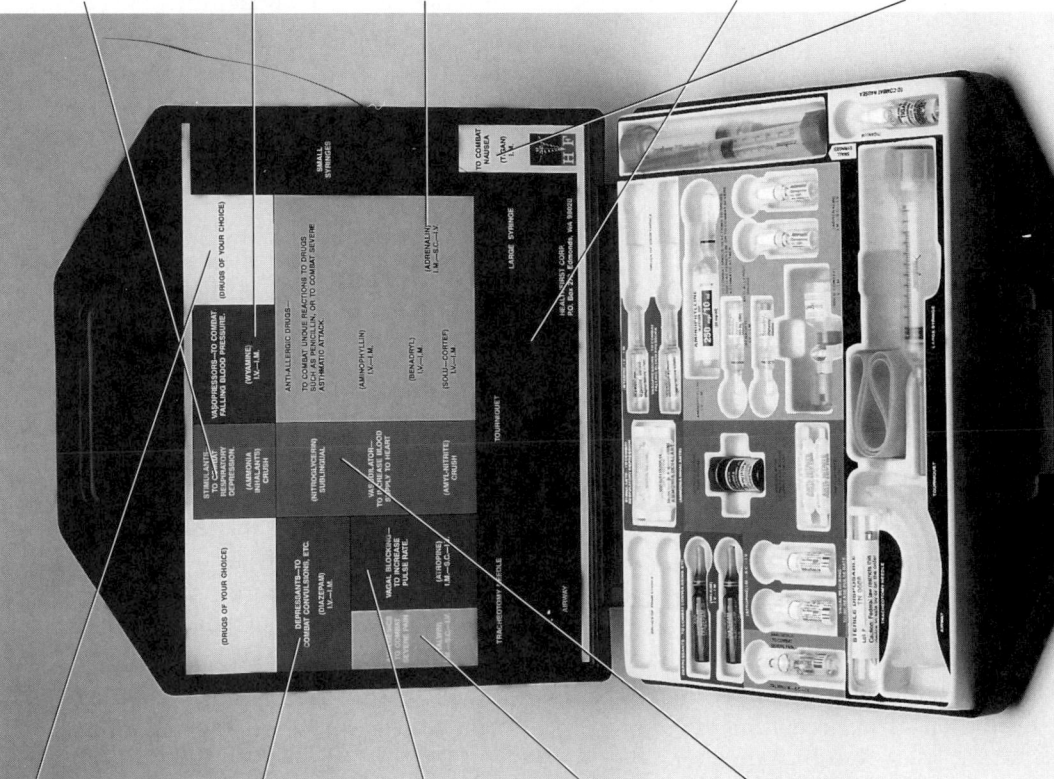

FIG. 10-2   Color-coded, emergency drug kit. (Courtesy of Health First Corporation.)

exhale, then place the lips around the mouthpiece and slowly inhale. As the patient inhales, the top container is pressed downward to deliver a measured dose of the medication. One full minute should elapse before a second inhalation is given.

Nitroglycerin. This drug is used to manage chest pain that occurs in those with a history of chest pain or angina caused by blockage in the arteries of the heart or pain resulting from a heart attack. The pain associated with the blockage of the heart's blood vessels is due to a lack of blood supply to the heart muscle.

Nitroglycerin is a potent vasodilator that especially affects the blood vessels of the heart. Dilating the blood vessels of the heart increases the blood supply to the heart's muscle, thereby relieving chest pain.

When supplied orally, the small tablet is placed under the patient's tongue and allowed to dissolve; when supplied in a vial, it is given IV by the dentist and must be removed from the vial with a needle and syringe immediately before administration.

Hydrocortisone. Hydrocortisone, an adrenocortical hormone, is used to treat severe allergic reactions once initial treatment has brought the symptoms of the reaction under control. This drug may be given IM or IV. Depending on the brand provided, the drug in the vial may be in powder or liquid form. The powdered form must be added to the liquid *provided with the vial* before the drug can be removed from the vial. Some brands use a container with the powdered drug in one half of the container and the liquid in the other half. The rubber-stoppered top is then firmly pushed down, and the liquid enters the area containing the powdered drug. The vial is rotated until all of the powder is dissolved and the solution is then withdrawn.

Intravenous Glucose. Glucose, a simple sugar, may be administered to the diabetic patient who has a hypoglycemic (low blood sugar) reaction. If the patient is awake and able to swallow, a glass of orange juice with sugar or water with 4 to 6 packages of sugar added may be given. If the patient is not responding or is too sleepy to swallow, the dentist must administer intravenous glucose.

Most diabetics are aware of an impending hypoglycemic reaction and are able to relate this fact to the dentist. Many carry a glucose product, such as Proglycem, which has been recommended by their physician. Use of a glucose product will most probably end the hypoglycemic reaction. If orange juice and sugar are not available in a dental office, the office could stock a small box of individual sugar packets, which can be added to water and given to the diabetic patient having a hypoglycemic

reaction. Sugar substitutes, such as NutraSweet, are of no value in the treatment of this reaction.

Ammonia Inhalers. Ammonia is used to stimulate respirations if the patient has fainted. This product is packaged in thin glass vials covered with a strong, woven fabric. The glass must be broken to release the ammonia vapors. To use this product, the fabric-covered vial is placed between several gauze sponges and broken. The easiest way to break the vial is to grasp it at both ends with the index fingers and thumbs. The broken glass will remain inside the tightly woven outer covering of the vial and the vial is waved back and forth under the patient's nose for a few seconds. Care must be taken not to hold it too close because it will burn the mucous membranes in the nose.

Additional Equipment. Tourniquets, sterile syringes, a mask for administering oxygen, and one or more oral airways to maintain an open airway may be included in an emergency kit. Additional drugs may also be added by the dentist or various manufacturers of emergency kits.

▶ The Dental Assistant's Responsibilities During an Emergency

The most important responsibility of the dental assistant is *recognition of an adverse drug reaction,* particularly those allergic reactions that require emergency treatment. If there is any doubt what adverse drug reactions may occur with the use of a specific drug in a dental practice, the dental assistant should ask the dentist to list or describe those reactions that could occur.

When an emergency occurs, the dentist is responsible for diagnosing the type of emergency and determining the drugs and the dosage to be used in the treatment of the problem. Since an emergency requires swift treatment, the dental assistant should be prepared to take the following steps:

▶ Bring the emergency kit to the room and open the kit

▶ Prepare the drug or drugs requested by the dentist by opening the package; some drugs require mixing before filling a sterile syringe with the dosage stated by the dentist; other drugs may be premixed in ampules and require filling a sterile syringe with the dosage stated by the dentist

▶ Prepare other materials, such as an oral airway or oxygen mask, by opening the package

After the emergency the dental assistant may be responsible for recording the drugs used in the emergency. Additional responsibilities of the assistant after the emergency may include replacing or reordering any drug taken from the emergency kit as soon as possible.

The contents of any kit should be checked monthly to be sure that all drugs and equipment are in place, that all drugs that were used have been replaced, and that any outdated drugs are discarded and the correct replacements ordered. Expiration dates for drugs are printed on the drug package. The dental assistant also should periodically review the printed information and instructions contained in the kit to remain familiar with its contents. When an allergic reaction occurs, actions taken by the dentist and the dental assistant must be swift and accurate.

Patient Education

In addition to the general areas of patient education, the dental assistant may be responsible for specific areas of patient education, such as the importance of (1) obtaining an accurate health history; (2) following the dentist's recommendations regarding the ingestion of prescription drugs; and (3) what nonprescription drugs may be used or should be avoided.

When a health history is taken or when the patient fills out a preprinted health history form, the patient should be told that it is necessary for the dentist to have full knowledge of a patient's health history, as well as a list of all currently used prescription or nonprescription drugs. The importance of this information can be made clearer to the patient if he or she is initially told the following:

▶ An *accurate* health history, including a drug and allergy history, is an important part of dental care.
▶ Drugs are often used or prescribed by the dentist.
▶ The dentist may decide to use a different drug or procedure because of information obtained during a health or allergy history.
▶ Certain medical conditions or diseases may require important changes in a dental procedure.
▶ Knowledge of all current prescription and nonprescription drug therapy helps the dentist treat the whole patient and may aid in the treatment of dental problems.

▶ Instructions Regarding Prescription Drugs

A prescription contains directions for taking a drug. This information is printed on the label of the container by the dispensing pharmacist. While most directions are clear and the dispensing pharmacist may remind the patient of certain facts, such as taking the drug 1 hour before meals or taking a drug with food, the assistant should also remind the patient that all directions written on the prescription label are followed. If the directions are not followed, the drug may fail to correct or control the problem for which it was prescribed.

▶ Instructions Regarding Nonprescription Drugs

Sometimes the dentist may recommend a nonprescription drug, such as ibuprofen, for mild pain or discomfort. The patient should understand that nonprescription drugs can be purchased without a prescription, including products such as aspirin, acetaminophen (Tylenol), ibuprofen (Advil), nonprescription bronchial inhalers such as epinephrine spray and antihistamines. The dentist may also advise the patient to avoid the use of certain nonprescription drugs, for example, aspirin, for a specified length of time before or after a dental procedure. The assistant should explain to the patient that the dentist's recommendations always should be followed and one drug should not be substituted for another. If the patient does not appear to understand the instructions given, the assistant must make the dentist aware of this problem.

Some patients use various nonprescription drugs to control or relieve the pain or discomfort associated with certain dental problems, such as abscessed teeth or ill-fitting dentures or bridges. Patients should be cautioned against certain practices, for example, the placing of an aspirin tablet on the gingiva, which can result in an acid burn of the oral mucosa. The greatest value of aspirin in the relief of dental pain is when the drug is swallowed.

Other practices, such as the topical application of certain nonprescription products for pain or discomfort, should be used only as temporary measures. The problem is best evaluated by a dentist as soon as possible. The danger in using these products for a relatively long period of time is a delay in treatment of more serious problems, such as oral cancer or abscessed teeth.

▶ General Instructions Concerning All Drugs

When a drug is prescribed, the dental assistant should review with the patient the importance of the prescribed drug and that it must not be stopped except on the recommendation of the dentist. This is especially important when an antibiotic is prescribed for an infection. Unless the *full* course of therapy is completed, some microorganisms may remain, and the infection could possibly return.

When use of a nonprescription drug is recommended, for example, acetaminophen, for pain or discomfort, the patient is instructed to read the drug label carefully and to follow the dosage and recommendations for use that are printed on the container. In some instances, the dentist may recommend a slightly higher or lower dose than is stated on the drug container. If this should occur, the dental assistant should remain with the patient to follow the instructions given by the dentist.

The patient is also advised to notify the dentist as soon as possible if any of the following should occur:

- The drug fails to relieve the problem for which it was prescribed; for example, relief of pain, reduction in swelling, or control of the symptoms of infection
- The drug causes problems that were not present before the drug was taken; for example, nausea, vomiting, diarrhea, itching, skin rash, or hives
- The problem for which the drug was prescribed or recommended becomes worse

KEY POINTS

- Pharmacology is the study of drugs, their chemical formula, uses, and positive and negative effects on the body.

- A drug may be natural or synthetic, legal or illegal, prescription or nonprescription and can be used to create a change in one or more body functions.

- Drug legislation was enacted as early as 1906 to regulate and control the manufacture, distribution, and sale of drugs. Today the FDA, FTC, and DEA—all federal agencies—are involved in the manufacture, regulation, and use of drugs in the United States.

- Council on Dental Therapeutics of the ADA studies, evaluates, and distributes information to the dental profession supporting the use of dental products.

- A trade name is the name given to the product by the manufacturer, and the generic name is the name of the drug other than the trade name.

- References that can be used by dental professionals regarding information about drugs include the PDR, *Facts and Comparisons,* inserts, USP, and the NF.

- Factors that influence drug action include age, weight, gender, disease, and route of administration.

- Drug interactions refer to the reaction of one drug to another or the reaction of drugs with foods. Drug interaction can be antagonistic or synergistic.

- Reaction to a drug can be negative and include an adverse reaction, such as vomiting, diarrhea, or headache; a drug allergy, angioedema, or an idiosyncrasy.

- Substance or drug abuse is a worldwide problem and the Commission on Dental Education recommends that all accredited dental/dental-related programs provide information to students regarding substance use, misuse, and addiction.

- The dental profession needs to be aware of the use, effects, and danger associated with the use of narcotics, psychotomimetics, amphetamines, barbiturates, nonbarbiturates, tranquilizers, and alcohol in treating dental patients.

- Drugs commonly used in dentistry include analgesics, antibiotics, tranquilizers, barbiturates, nonbarbiturate hypnotics, antihistamines, vasoconstrictors, adrenocortical hormones, antiseptics, and germicides.

- It is necessary to have a complete general and dental history of prescription and nonprescription drugs that a patient is taking for the dental team to provide safe dental care.

- A prescription is a legal form signed by the licensed dentist and is used for dispensing prescription drugs. This form includes a heading, superscription, inscription, subscription, sign, DEA number, and refill information. It is the responsibility of the dental assistant to record information on the patient's clinical chart regarding each prescription.

- A major responsibility of the chairside dental assistant is the recognition of adverse drug reactions, particularly those that require emergency treatment. It is important that emergency procedures be defined and the assistant be prepared to assist in all aspects of patient care.

BIBLIOGRAPHY

Neidle EA, Yagiela JA: *Pharmacology and therapeutics for dentistry,* ed 3, St Louis, 1989, Mosby.

Wingard L, Brody TM, Larner J, Schwartz A: *Human pharmacology: molecular to clinical,* St Louis, 1991, Mosby.

11 Dental Materials

LEARNING OBJECTIVES

You will have mastered the material in this chapter when you can:
- Define the key terms
- Explain the purpose of dental materials
- List the organizations responsible for establishing standards and specifications for dental materials
- Describe the properties of dental materials
- Identify the relationship of infection control and hazardous substances to dental materials
- Identify preventive dental materials
- Explain the function of preventive dental materials
- Describe the manipulation of preventive dental materials
- Identify direct restorative dental materials
- Explain the function of direct restorative dental materials
- Describe the manipulation of direct restorative dental materials
- Identify indirect restorative dental materials
- Explain the function of indirect and adjunct restorative dental materials
- Describe the manipulation of indirect restorative dental materials
- Identify and explain the sequence of use for finishing, polishing, and cleansing materials

KEY TERMS

Base
Compressive strength

Corrosion
Council on Dental Materials, Instruments, and Equipment
Deformation
Dimensional change
Direct
Ductile
Electrical properties
Exothermic reaction
Flow
Force
Galvanism
Hardness
Heavy body
Indirect
Light body
Luting
Malleable
Mechanical properties
Percolation
Primary consistency
Retentive properties
Secondary consistency
Shear strength
Solubility and sorption
Strain
Stress
Syneresis
Tensile strength
Thermal conductivity
Viscosity
Wettability
Yield point

The selection, manipulation, and handling of dental materials are important aspects of the dental assistant's responsibility in providing dental treatment. For the dental assistant the study of dental materials can present a complex experience that involves the basic concepts of chemistry and physics and requires following specific manipulation procedures outlined by the dental manufacturer. Virtually all phases of dentistry use dental materials during the course of treatment. Dental research, alone, does not develop the materials that are necessary to meet the needs of patients but relies on research provided through the work of the basic sciences in biology, chemistry, and physics, as well as the arts.

Dental materials are used to:

▶ Replace or restore tooth structure lost through trauma or dental caries
▶ Prevent the invasion of caries
▶ Replace soft tissues
▶ Take impressions of existing conditions or teeth prepared for a prosthetic device
▶ Finish, polish, and cleanse a restoration or prosthesis

Each type of dental material provides a means to assist in the development of a restoration or may be a portion of the restoration itself.

Council on Dental Materials, Instruments, and Equipment

The Council on Dental Materials, Instruments, and Equipment, a subgroup of the American Dental Association (ADA) in partnership with federal organizations, the Federal Specifications and Standards, and the National Bureau of Standards provides standards and specifications that all dental materials must meet. The Council ensures the safety and effectiveness of the materials, instruments, and equipment; encourages the development and improvement of materials, instruments, and equipment; coordinates national and international standardization programs and the evaluation of materials, instruments, and equipment; maintains a liaison with OSHA and other organizations to provide recommendations on materials, instruments, and equipment; and maintains a liaison with regulatory, research, and professional organizations. The subjection of dental materials to these guidelines provides the dental practitioner with dental materials that meet quality control standards.

The ADA through the Council on Dental Materials, Instruments, and Equipment developed a program that grants certification to certain dental materials and devices. Certification by this organization indicates that the manufacturer has verified that a specific product has met ADA specifications and has also followed ADA advertising and exhibition standards. Once the manufacturer's product has conformed with these specifications, the name is on a listing of all products that are certified. At any point a dental professional can determine whether a product is certified by the ADA by consulting the *Journal of the American Dental Association* for the current listing.

An acceptance program for products rates each as acceptable, provisionally acceptable, or unacceptable as determined through testing for safety and usefulness. The testing involves biologic, laboratory, or clinical evaluations to determine the level of acceptance.

Properties of Dental Materials

The selection and manipulation of dental materials are affected by various chemical and physical factors, including dimensional change, thermal conductivity, electrical properties, solubility and sorption, wettability, and mechanical properties. Other considerations in the selection of dental materials include being esthetically pleasing but not harmful to the patient or the oral tissues and the ease of manipulation of the material.

Dimensional Change

Changes in the dimension of a dental material are important to assure accuracy with certain materials. **Dimensional changes** occur during the chemical reactions that many dental materials undergo. The dimensions measured in recorded changes are in both length and volume. A good example of the importance of dimensional change is illustrated when an impression material is used for constructing a restoration such as a cast crown. The purpose of the impression is to create an exact duplicate of the prepared tooth. If, after the impression is taken, dimensional change occurs—either shrinkage or expansion—then the impression no longer replicates the detail and accuracy of the prepared tooth. The result will be a crown that does not fit the prepared tooth.

When dental materials are placed in the oral cavity, they are exposed to changes in temperature that result in dimensional changes of the material and different tooth structure. The temperature in the oral cavity is normally measured at 37° C (98.6° F), but may fluctuate from 5° to 60° C (41° to 140° F) as the patient breathes, eats, drinks, and chews. The amount of change or the linear coefficient of thermal expansion, when measured, is found to be different in various tooth structure and dental materials. This difference in expansion results in microscopic openings at the point of contact or at the interface, which is called microleakage. Microleakage creates an opening for carious activity to begin that can lead to the potential loss of a restoration (Fig. 11-1). Regular examination of restorations provides the operator with the opportunity to determine the existence of microleakage.

When a microleakage opening occurs, it sets up a situation where fluids present in the oral cavity penetrate the area of the opening. As the temperature in the mouth decreases and the opening enlarges, fluids flow into the opening. The increase of the temperature to normal forces the fluids from the opening. This in/out flow of liquid is referred to as **percolation**. This action of thermal expansion of the restorative material in the tooth can result in recurrent decay and irritation to the pulp.

Thermal Conductivity

Thermal conductivity is known as the rate of heat flow through a particular material. This is obvious in everyday life when hot coffee is placed in a metal cup and the heat is conducted through the metal. Place this same hot substance in an insulated cup and a barrier is set up so that the heat is not transmitted through the cup.

Certain materials are poor thermal conductors, meaning that heat and cold are not transported through the material. Enamel is a poor thermal conductor, while amalgam and other metals conduct the thermal change through the material more easily. This concept is important to remember when placing restorations in a tooth. For instance, if amalgam is placed in a cavity preparation, the potential of transmitting hot and cold to the pulp is possible. The placement of a cement base between the tooth and the amalgam restoration acts as a barrier or an insulation from the assault of temperature through ther-

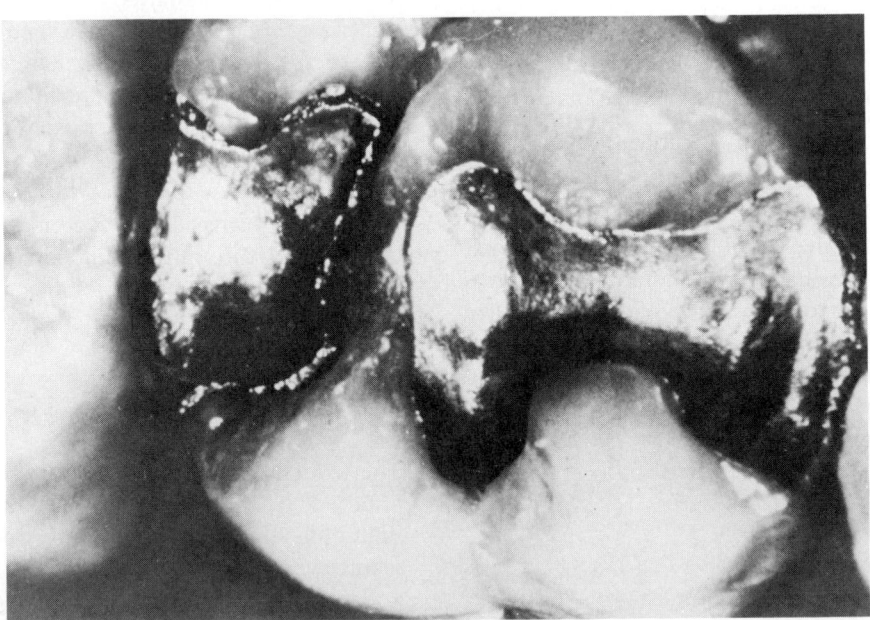

FIG. 11-1   Microleakage would likely occur around the margins of the restoration shown.

(From Craig RG et al: *Dental materials,* ed 5, St Louis, 1992, Mosby.)

mal conductivity. Without a barrier between the thermal conductor and the pulpal tissue, there is not a sufficient level of protection for the pulp. Dentin is considered a poor thermal conductor, but as dentin is removed during a cavity preparation, an insulating base must be placed under metallic restorations to protect the pulp.

▶ Electrical Characteristics

In this category, there are two properties or characteristics of dental materials that are important to the dental practitioner, and they both result in corrosion. **Corrosion** is a chemical reaction of nonmetallic elements with metal, which may result in the formation of corrosive products. An example of a corrosion product is rust that can develop on the surface of iron. Tarnish is sometimes mistaken for corrosion, but it is only the surface discoloration or change in the finish of the metal.

Corrosion reactions are classified as chemical or electrochemical corrosion. Chemical corrosion involves the direct contact of the metal and the nonmetallic substance, which causes a reaction. A common example found in the mouth would be that of silver sulfide. Certain foods, for instance, eggs, contain a large quantity of sulfur, which combines with other elements to corrode amalgam and other metallic restorations in the mouth. For sulfur to corrode amalgam, a chemical reaction creates silver sulfide, which attacks the amalgam surface.

Often when chemical corrosion occurs it is in conjunction with electrochemical corrosion that is the result of an electrical current in the oral cavity. Certain oral conditions must be present to be capable of creating and carrying electrical current in electrochemical corrosion. This means primarily that the fluids in the oral cavity must be good conductors of electricity or must be an electrolyte. Saliva, which contains salt, is an example of an electrolyte. Also two metallic restorations of different composition must be present to act as batteries and carry an electrical current through the saliva. The electrical current contacting two dissimilar metals is known as **galvanism** or galvanic action. This current contributes to the potential of disintegration, creating corrosion on a restored metallic surface. The galvanic action creates a roughness and pitting of the dental material.

Galvanic action may also result in galvanic shock. This same reaction can occur when a piece of aluminum foil or a fork comes in contact with a clasp of a retainer or partial denture or an existing metal restoration in the oral cavity. It is common practice to avoid placing dissimilar restorative materials in opposing teeth or in abutment teeth that have proximal surfaces which contact each other, so galvanic action does not occur. Corrosion may be the effect of galvanism when two dissimilar metals are placed as restorations next to each other.

▶ Mechanical Properties

Dental materials are continuously assaulted by forces in the oral cavity that push or pull on the material. **Mechanical properties** that affect dental materials include the tensile, compressive, and shear forms of stress and strain. The selection of a dental material is largely determined by the amount and type of **force** (an action against a material) that will be exerted on the material when it is placed in the mouth. Normally force is measured in pounds, but unless the location of the force and the direction it will be applied to a material are known, the information for selection of a material is limited.

The biting and chewing force of the teeth has been measured, and it has been determined that there is a decrease in biting force from the molars to the incisors. Biting force is approximately 130 pounds on molars decreasing to 40 pounds of force on the incisors. As teeth are lost and replaced by artificial ones, the force on the remaining natural teeth increases greatly. The same psi is distributed over less natural teeth, since artificial teeth can endure less stress.

STRESS

Force directed over a material creates resistance or **stress** within the material. This type of stress is realized when the biting force is applied to teeth and materials in the mouth. The following formula simulates the action of stress as a force:

$$\text{Stress} = \frac{\text{Force}}{\text{Area}} = \frac{F}{A}$$

If a wooden board is placed between two cement blocks and another cement block is placed in the middle of the board, this is considered a force or load that pushes downward on the board. The board with the weight of the block pushes upward to resist the downward force of the weight. This opposite and upward resistance is known as stress: the internal force of the board acting against the external force, resulting in stress of the board. This same situation is present in the mouth when biting force is exerted and the teeth resisting the downward action of this force create stress on the surfaces. Dental materials that can not resist these forces distort or fracture and fail as restorations.

STRAIN

Strain is another reaction to the push or pull of materials acted upon by force. Strain is seen on material when it deforms with stress. Stress and strain exist concurrently. The force on the materials creates deformation, movement, or change in shape. Certain materials that are deformed by strain will return to the original dimension after the load or the stress is removed. This is known as elastic strain. An example of this is a rubber band pulled apart to the point just before it breaks.

Elastic strain continues until the proportional limit or yield point is reached. At this point, additional stresses result in permanent deformation or plastic strain, preventing the material from returning to the original dimension. Using the rubber band as an example again, permanent deformation occurs when the rubber band is stretched to the point where it does not return to the same length. Strain is measured as follows:

$$\text{Strain} = \frac{\text{Change in length}}{\text{Original length}}$$

TYPES OF STRESS AND STRAIN

The three forms of stress are tensile, compressive, and shear. Often all three forms are found when stress is created that rises from a force on a material.

Tensile Stress

Tensile stress results when two forces are applied in opposite directions. An example of a force creating tensile stress would be a wire that is pulled by forces on each end in opposite directions. Biting force creates tensile stress because the action of biting tends to stretch a material in the mouth. When there is tensile stress, tensile strain is also present. The amount of stress that is necessary to pull a material apart is known as **tensile strength** (Fig. 11-2, A).

Compressive Stress

Compressive stress is formed when materials are compressed. **Compressive strength** is the amount of pres-

sure applied to cause a material to rupture. Columns on a building support and act against the weight of the structure, as well as on the base on which they rest, creating compressive stress (Fig. 11-2, B). The chewing forces on molar teeth are primarily compressive (crushing). Changes, either temporary or permanent, resulting from compressive stresses are called compressive strain.

Shear Stress

The creation of shear stress occurs when equal or opposite forces are applied against opposite planes. Sliding two surfaces parallel to each other back and forth, or in a twisting or rotating action, results in forces that create shear stress and strain. The cutting action of scissors (shears) depends on shear stress. An example of shear stress and strain might exist when restored molars are in occlusion and the patient is bruxing or grinding horizontally against cusps (Fig. 11-2, C). The point at which a material is destroyed through the action of two portions sliding over each other is **shear strength**.

As stated earlier, certain materials fail under the extreme forces that are applied in the oral cavity with the normal day-to-day activities of an individual. If a material fails, or reaches its **deformation** point, under tensile stress, the tensile strength of the material was inadequate; if this occurs under compressive stress, the compressive strength of the material was inadequate. It is important to know the type of forces applied to dental materials and whether the material is changed by any of these external actions. The materials selected for use in the oral cavity should be of a strength that does not fail under the normal forces of mastication. For instance, the compressive strength of zinc phosphate cement mixed to a base consistency is 10,000 to 17,000 psi, and a polymer modified zinc oxide–eugenol cement of the same consistency has a compressive strength of 8800 psi. There-

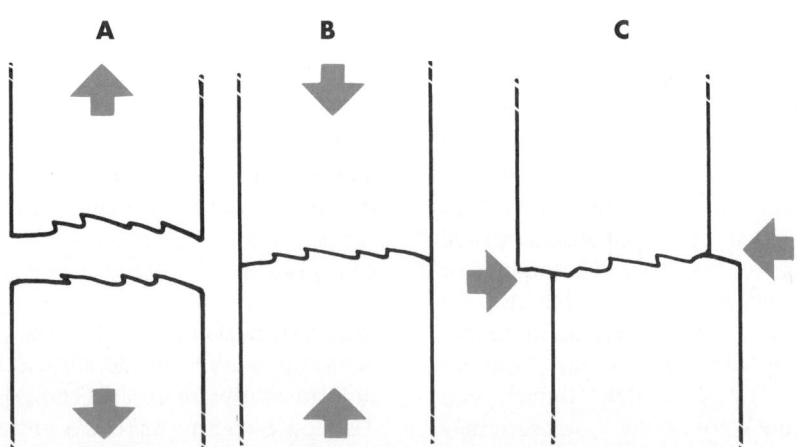

FIG. 11-2   Forces depicting results from: A, Tensile stress. B, Compressive stress. C, Shear stress.

fore, it is understood that zinc phosphate cement placed under a dental amalgam as an insulating base is more able to withstand compressive force than zinc oxide–eugenol. Obviously failure is less likely with the zinc phosphate base. However, as we will learn, other biologic properties must be considered when selecting which base material would be best.

▶ Hardness, Ductility, and Malleability

If a material can be dented or scratched, it will begin to show wear. **Hardness** tests are used to determine a material's resistance to scratching and denting. One such test for hardness used often in dentistry is Mohs scale, a test of scratch resistance. The scale of hardness values is provided in Box 11-1. Other hardness tests include the Knoop hardness test (a test which assigns a Knoop hardness number) and the Brinell hardness number system.

When forces on a material exceed the proportional limit, or **yield point**, permanent deformation occurs and the shape has been permanently changed. When reshaping or plastic deformation occurs, the material is ductile, malleable, or both. A **ductile** material can undergo forces of tensile stress without failing. A material under compressive stress that does not fracture is **malleable**. It is desirable to have certain metals that are ductile and can be formed into wire and others that are malleable and can be hammered or formed into a sheet of metal. An example of ductility is found with metals that have burnishability of margins, such as castings, to smooth the area that contacts the tooth surface. Box 11-2 illustrates malleability and ductility of metals common to dentistry in decreasing order of each.

▶ Flow

Flow, or slump and creep, is a type of undesirable permanent deformation. When a force is maintained as a constant, certain materials continue to permanently deform. Compressive stress that can cause flow is created during biting. The selection of a dental material may be based on the reaction of this material during compressive stress that results in flow.

▶ Solubility and Sorption

Other criteria in the selection of a dental material may be determined by solubility and sorption. **Solubility** is the rate at which a material dissolves in fluid. **Sorption** includes both absorption, the ability of the material to take in fluid as a solid, and adsorption, the concentration of molecules on the surface of a liquid or solid. The amount of both absorption and adsorption determines sorption. Certain dental materials are not selected for a purpose because of the solubility and sorption factors. For example, hydrocolloid impression materials are susceptible to sorption when immersed in water. The impression material imbibes the water, causing dimensional changes that affect the accuracy of the material.

▶ Retentive Properties

An important factor in the placement of a dental material is its **retentive property**, or the likelihood of the material to be retained in the tooth. This retention is also referred to as adhesion. Adhesion or retention may be achieved through the mechanical, physical, and/or chemical properties of the material. Physical adhesion must involve an electrostatic surface area between the tooth and the material and is not common to dentistry. A chemical adhesion is formed through a chemical bonding process whereby the material adheres to the enamel or dentin.

Mechanical retention is created through three different processes: undercuts, luting, and bonding. Undercuts are a primary means of retaining a restorative material. The cavity preparation is created in a geometric configuration that locks the restorative material in the preparation, as found in Fig. 11-3, *A* through *C*. Dental amalgam is placed

---

BOX 11-1

MOHS SCRATCH HARDNESS VALUES

HARDNESS	COMPARATIVE MATERIAL
10	Diamond
9	Corundum
8	Topaz
7	Quartz
6	Orthoclase
5	Apatite
4	Fluorite
3	Calcite
2	Gypsum
1	Talc

BOX 11-2

MALLEABILITY AND DUCTILITY OF METALS

MALLEABILITY	DUCTILITY
Gold	Gold
Silver	Silver
Aluminum	Platinum

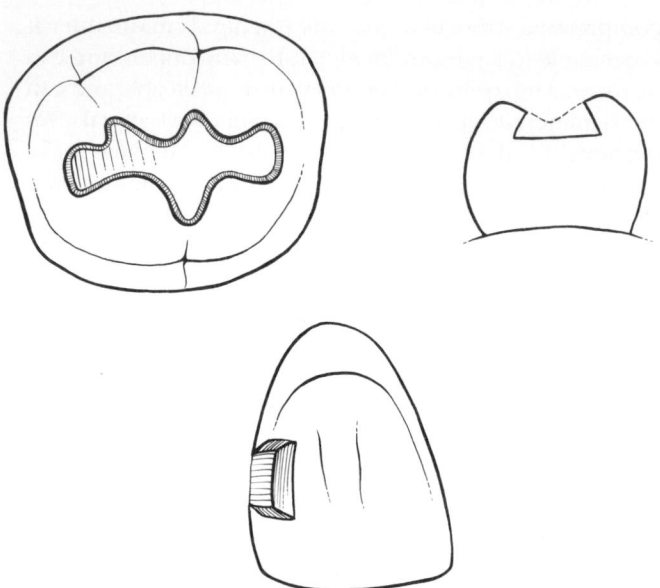

FIG. 11-3   Retentive cavity preparations designed to lock a restorative in place.

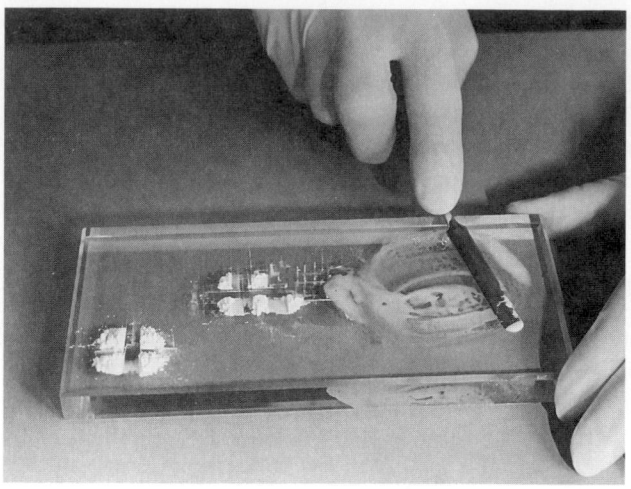

FIG. 11-4   Primary zinc phosphate cement mixed to illustrate capability of wettability.

in a cavity preparation designed as in Fig. 11-3, *A*, where the opening in the tooth is narrower than the internal area of the preparation.

Certain restorations, such as cast alloys in the form of a crown or inlay, are not placed in cavity preparations designed as just described. The opening at the surface of the preparation is larger than the internal portion of the preparation. Restorations of this form are retained by using dental cement that is mixed to a **luting** consistency, a thin, flowing thickness of material that is applied to the cast. The cement chemically and/or mechanically adheres to all surfaces of the restoration, thus retaining the restoration.

The last type of mechanical retention, bonding, is used predominantly with resin restorative materials. The enamel surface of a tooth is prepared through an acid etching process, often eliminating the need for gross removal of tooth structure to achieve retentive form. The etched surface has microscopic interstices or openings on the surface over which a fluid bonding material is placed. The bonding agent then chemically adheres to the material placed in the tooth.

WETTABILITY

The ability of a liquid to spread over a solid surface is considered **wettability**. This is an important property in applying certain materials, as in pit and fissure sealants. If the sealant material cannot be applied in a layer but rather beads up on the tooth surface, the material will fail because it leaves open margins and uneven surface areas. However, the high-energy solid of the enamel and the

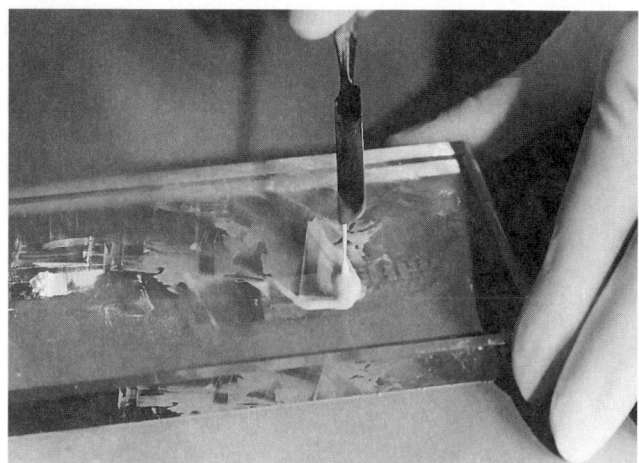

FIG. 11-5   Zinc phosphate cement mixed to a primary consistency or low viscosity as a luting agent.

low-energy liquid of the sealant material allow for good wetting characteristics (Fig. 11-4).

VISCOSITY

The term **viscosity** refers to the ability of a liquid material to flow. Generally speaking, viscosity is determined by the consistency of the liquid. If a liquid is of low viscosity or flow when it is placed on a surface, it is more likely to have good wettability. A material of high viscosity tends not to flow well and is of lower wettability. Many dental cements are mixed as luting agents to cement cast restorations in a preparation (Fig. 11-5). If a cement is mixed to a high viscosity, it does not adapt to the irregularities of the restoration and may not produce an acceptable seal or cementation of the cast restoration.

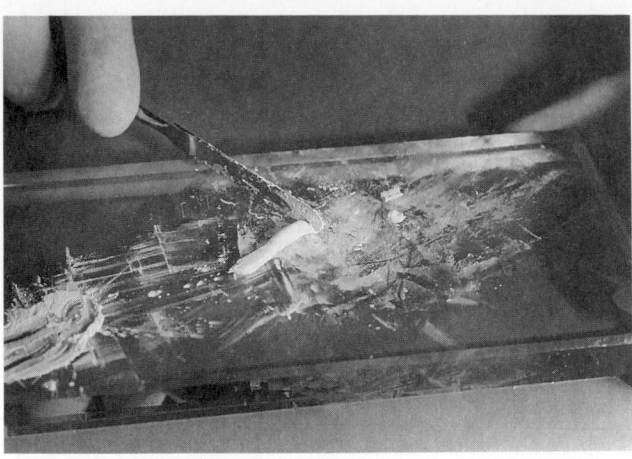

FIG. II-6 Zinc phosphate cement mixed to a secondary consistency or high viscosity as a cement base.

Cements mixed to the appropriate viscosity in these situations would be mixed to **film thickness**. Film thickness is appropriate for most cements to achieve the viscosity for appropriate adhesion in the cementation of restorations (Fig. 11-6).

Hazardous Substances that are Dental Materials

All individuals, dental professionals or otherwise, must be aware and concerned with the correct and safe management of hazardous substances. Dentistry involves the utilization of a variety of materials that are considered hazardous chemicals. The federal Occupational Safety and Health Administration regulates activity in the place of employment regarding the employees' right to know about hazardous substances. This regulation involves the employer providing the employee with information about hazardous chemicals in the work place. The employer must create a program that will inform employees of hazardous materials that applies to the specific work place. This program must include labeling of all materials, material safety data sheets, employee training, and record maintenance. Further information regarding maintaining material safety data sheet forms can be found in Chapter 8.

Preventive Dental Materials

Materials used in dentistry are developed for two major reasons: as preventive agents or to restore tooth structure. Preventive materials are those used to prevent disease or to protect tissue. Preventive materials most commonly used in dentistry include fluoride and pit and fissure sealants. Protective materials include mouthguards, splints, and periodontal dressings.

Early in the history of modern dentistry, G.V. Black proposed a concept, *Extension for Prevention*. The basic principle behind this concept was the removal of tooth structure in deeply pitted and fissured areas, usually when a restoration was placed, to avoid the potential of carious invasion and further damage to the tooth at a later time. Dentistry has taken this concept a step further and developed dental materials that prevent disease to the teeth and surrounding structures or protect the teeth from trauma. Materials used include fluoride gels, fluoride oral rinses, pit and fissure sealants, and mouthguards, splints, and periodontal dressings to protect tissues.

Fluoride

The element fluoride is found naturally in our environment and provides an anticarious effect when it is taken systemically during tooth formation or taken topically after eruption. Fluoride changes the crystalline structure of enamel, making it less soluble; topically it suppresses cariogenic bacteria in dental plaque and acts on the enamel to inhibit bacterial adhesion.

Studies have shown that when fluoridated water is consumed from birth, caries formation is reduced 50% to 65%. These percentages are also influenced by other fluoride-containing substances that are used regularly, such as dentifrices and oral rinses. Fluoride has also been added to some cavity liners to reduce sensitivity and secondary caries around a restoration.

The side effect of excess fluoride—mottled enamel—is actually the factor that stimulated studies in fluoride research. From this work it was determined that one ppm of fluoride in drinking water affords some protection against dental caries, while it prevents mottled enamel.

FLUORIDE ORAL RINSES AND DENTIFRICES

Fluoride can be provided through sources other than drinking water. Self-applied, fluoride-containing oral rinses and dentifrices supplement the process of caries reduction. Over-the-counter oral rinses have been shown to reduce caries when they are used on a regular basis.

Most dentifrices available for purchase contain fluoride. The use of fluoride-containing dentifrices in a fluoridated community has been found to be effective in reducing caries incidence. However, dentists still prescribe rinses and gels of high concentrations that are more effective for home use.

PROFESSIONALLY APPLIED FLUORIDE

The three types of topical fluoride applied in a dental office are sodium, stannous, and acidulated phosphate fluoride gels. Professionally applied topical fluoride has been found to be extremely effective in reducing caries incidence and sensitivity in teeth. Each of these fluorides is discussed in length in Chapter 26.

▶ Pit and Fissure Sealants

Fluoride use in the prevention of carious lesions is most effective on the smooth surfaces of teeth and least effective on the pits and fissures of teeth. The application of sealants to the pits and fissures has preventive results similar to those of fluoride. Sealants are thin layers of resin material placed on the pits and fissures of the occlusal surfaces of posterior teeth. Most sealants are composed of bisphenol A-glycidyl methacrylate (BIS-GMA), polymerized with a visible light source or via an organic amine, autocuring catalyst. The advantage to a BIS-GMA photopolymerizing sealant system is that materials need no mixing. The resin is polymerized with visible light. BIS-GMA sealants that are polymerized by an organic amine accelerator are found in two-step systems, which require the mixing of a monomer and benzoyl peroxide initiator with a monomer and 5% organic amine accelerator. Also, the working time is much more limited when using a base/catalyst system.

A distinct advantage of placing a sealant instead of a restoration is that no tooth structure is removed. The sealant creates a mechanical obstacle to any bacteria that attack the pits and fissures and try to break down the enamel, which would eventually result in a carious lesion. Sealants can be equated to varnish placed on a wood surface, sealing the porous layer of the wood from attack by outside substances.

The use of sealants was introduced to dentistry about 1965, but they have only recently garnered broader acceptance as a preventive treatment. The effectiveness of sealants is determined by the retention on the tooth surface and the reduction in carious activity.

Sealants are normally placed on noncarious occlusal surfaces of posterior teeth once they have erupted in the oral cavity. The normal life of properly placed sealants is 4 to 6 years, although some have remained effective as long as 10 years. Studies involving placement of sealants on teeth with carious lesions have reported that the number of active organisms left in situ, or in place, on carious dentin for periods of 5 years was less than at the time of sealant placement. From this it is suggested that sealing a carious lesion that is not extensive may be an acceptable form of treatment. The procedure for sealant placement is described in Chapter 26.

▶ Mouthguards

Often as you think of mouthguards, the vision of a burly football center comes to mind. Mouthguards are designed to protect the teeth and other oral structures from injuries that result from contact sports. Oral injuries may result from football, basketball, soccer, wrestling, hockey and lacrosse, but they may also occur during racquetball, squash, handball, baseball, and other physical activities. Injuries to the mouth are more often found in children or inexperienced individuals who participate in these activities.

A mouthguard is considered to be an effective preventive device to lessen or completely eliminate oral injuries. A patient can purchase stock mouthguards over the counter in a sports store that are then formed in the mouth, or they can have a mouthguard custom-made. Studies have not conclusively suggested that one way is preferable to another, but they promote the use of a mouthguard. Mouthguards can also be constructed for specialty situations, such as patients who are in complete orthodontic bands and brackets. The protection necessary in this circumstance may warrant fabrication of custom-made maxillary and mandibular mouthguards.

The preparation of a polyvinylacetate-polyethylene mouthguard is covered extensively in Chapter 40. A four-step method is used to fabricate the mouthguard: impression taking, pouring the model, fabricating the thermoplastic material on the model, and finishing the mouthguard.

OCCLUSAL BITE SPLINT

An occlusal bite splint is a device fabricated to aid in the treatment of patients with temporomandibular joint dysfunction or syndrome. The bite splint is designed to open the patient's bite and to reduce attrition of the teeth. A bite splint made of acrylic resin covers the occlusal surfaces and may or may not cover the incisal edges. The technique for fabricating this preventive appliance is similar to that used for a denture and will be discussed later in this chapter and in Chapter 37, *Removable Prosthodontics.*

PERIODONTAL DRESSING

Periodontal dressings are placed over periodontal surgery sites to protect the tissue from trauma. Dressings have been made of zinc oxide and eugenol, noneugenol materials, and light-cured synthetic materials. The purpose of the material is to protect a surgical site from trauma during eating and brushing the teeth. Periodontal dressing manipulation and application are discussed at length in Chapter 37, *Periodontics.*

Restorative Materials

Restorative dentistry encompasses a large percentage of time delegated to patient treatment. Its focus is the replacement of lost teeth or oral structures. This process is usually for the following purposes:

- To remove diseased tissue
- To produce an esthetically pleasing condition
- To restore function to the oral cavity

Two factors have plagued the dental practitioner in producing the desired results: the development of the appropriate dental material and the technology necessary to produce the restoration. As each of these areas has evolved over the years, restorative dentistry has progressed tremendously.

Restorative dental materials may be utilized in either direct or indirect restorative procedures. A **direct** restorative material protects tissue, stimulates growth of tissue, or replaces missing structures directly in the mouth. For example, a medication may be placed under a metallic restoration to protect the tooth from thermal reaction or to stimulate reparative growth in the tooth. A restoration, such as amalgam or composite, can replace tooth structure that has been lost to dental caries or trauma. Thus these materials are placed directly in the tooth to create the restoration.

An **indirect** restorative material is manipulated outside of the mouth to aid in the production of a final restoration or appliance. For instance, an impression material creates a negative of oral structures that can then be used to produce a model or positive reproduction of the structures. From this model, wax, gypsum, and gold can be used to create a restoration that is fabricated outside the mouth and then inserted in the oral cavity.

Factors that Affect Manipulation of Dental Materials

Various factors affect the manipulation of dental materials, including environmental conditions (temperature and humidity); presence of moisture; manipulating time; setting time; desired viscosity; and necessary armamentarium.

MANIPULATING TIME

Manipulating time is the time that is recommended by the manufacturer to completely mix the material. Exceeding the recommended manipulation time could reduce the amount of time that is needed to properly place the material, resulting in a less-than-desirable restoration, cement base, or impression.

SETTING TIME

Setting time refers to the amount of time it takes a material to harden. Two time periods are involved in the setting of dental materials. The first is the initial setting time, when the material has reached the stage where further manipulation is not possible or is difficult without distortion of the material. The final setting time of a material takes place later when the material has reached its complete hardness. The maximum strength of the material will have been reached at this stage.

Two terms that are frequently associated with manipulation time are **increased** and **decreased** setting time. To increase a setting time means to *lengthen* or extend the amount of time it takes for the material to set; to decrease the setting time means to *lessen* or shorten the amount of time required. Agents that increase or decrease setting time are often called retarders and accelerators, respectively.

MOISTURE

The presence of moisture from the material being manipulated or from an external source may decrease the setting time of the material. For example, when a zinc oxide–eugenol cement is mixed with a drop of water, the setting time is decreased because the material sets faster than the manufacturer's directions indicate; an exception to this is when an excess amount of moisture is used. Use of an excess amount of water, particularly with an alginate impression material, will increase the setting time because the mass of material becomes too thin. However, if the powder becomes contaminated by moisture during dispensing or storing, the reaction is usually quickened, resulting in a shorter setting time.

The introduction of moisture to the manipulation of a dental material decreases the setting time. This moisture can come from high humidity in the atmosphere, so many dental offices are air conditioned both for comfort and for humidity control.

Another factor involving moisture is the process of **syneresis.** Alginate impression materials are particularly susceptible to syneresis, which is a primary cause of loss of accuracy in such impressions. Syneresis is an agglomeration, a combining of agar and alginate molecules, that forces water from the alginate gel onto the surface of the impression. In addition to causing distortion on the impression, this exudate of material may cause distortion of the gypsum product that is placed in the impression.

If the alginate material is left exposed to the air, the water evaporates, causing shrinkage; if the material is immersed in water, it absorbs the water: imbibition. The absorption of water expands the material, causing distortion of the impression. A situation where 100% relative humidity is maintained controls the majority of distortion in alginate material. Because of syneresis and imbibition, alginate impressions ideally must be poured within 10 minutes of removal from the mouth.

TEMPERATURE

Temperature also affects the setting time of certain materials. In general, an increase in temperature decreases the setting time of material and may not allow enough time for manipulation and placement of the material before setting occurs. This temperature increase can come from the temperature of the room in which the material is mixed, may be added (as with the use of warm water to mix an alginate impression material), or may be generated by the material itself during a chemical reaction that produces exothermic heat.

Temperature can also affect the consistency of dental materials, such as waxes. In hot climates, such as the tropics, specialized waxes have been designed to compensate for the effect of temperature on the materials.

CONSISTENCY

Dental cements are often prepared to different consistencies. A **primary** or luting consistency is a cement that is less viscous and flows easily. Primary consistency is used to cement or lute crowns, bridges, inlays, and orthodontic bands in place. Usually a primary consistency results in the material being drawn into 1-inch string when the cement spatula is laid in the mass of material and is lifted from the cement (Fig. 11-7). The primary consistency has a greater wettability and can flow to provide a thin film thickness.

The **secondary consistency** of cement is more viscous, therefore the cement is thicker or tackier and may even be rolled into a mass or rope (Fig. 11-11). To obtain a secondary consistency, extra powder is added to the mix. This form of a dental cement is generally used as an insulating base under a restoration. The bulkier mass enables the operator to pack the material into the cavity preparation and provide a substantial base onto which the restoration can be placed. A dental cement mixed to secondary consistency or base consistency can withstand greater stress than one of primary consistency.

Other dental materials, such as impression materials, are mixed to different consistencies. The impression material mixed to a **light body** is thinner and may be placed in and extruded from a syringe on a prepared tooth surface to reproduce minute details in the preparation. A light body impression material can be mixed for a wash impression, which is a thin consistency of material placed and supported by the heavier material.

The **heavy body** material is much more viscous and is placed in a tray to be held. It does not necessarily provide the fine detail of oral structures that is obtained from the light body material, but it does achieve an accurate registration in the oral cavity. Certain impression materials have a putty consistency that is similar to the heavy body but is even thicker. This, too, is used as the heavy body material.

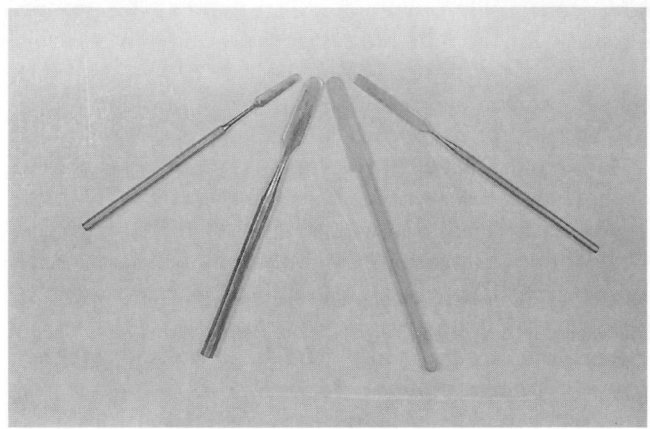

FIG. 11-7   Examples of various spatulas used to mix dental cements: 324, 326, 336, and resins spatula.

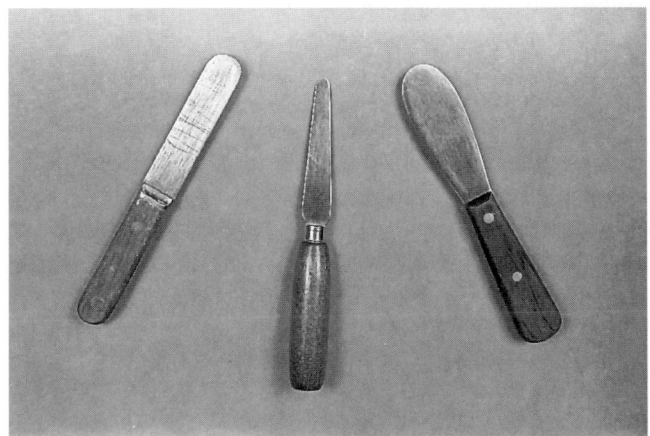

FIG. 11-8   Various other spatulas used to mix nonrigid impression materials.

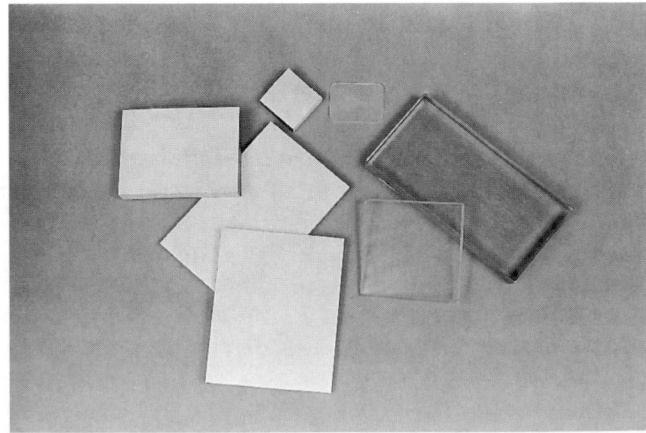

FIG. 11-9   Various mixing surfaces for cements and impression materials.

ARMAMENTARIUM SELECTION

The dental material manufacturers recommend special spatulas, measuring devices, and mixing surfaces on which to manipulate materials (Figs. 11-7 through 11-9). These suggestions should be followed to achieve maximum results. The dental assistant may be required to commit to memory the mixing times, proportions, and consistency of various dental materials. Two spatulas are common in mixing dental cements. A broad non-flexible spatula is used to mix most zinc oxide–eugenol cements; this heavier spatula is needed to properly incorporate the powder and liquid to enable the dental assistant to fold and pack the material with great force. A thin flexible spatula provides the rotary and crushing action needed to mix zinc phosphate cement. This thinner spatula provides more flexibility during manipulation of the cement.

Spatulas are also used in the manipulation of resin materials. The manufacturer often provides a plastic spatula with the kit of resin material. This spatula is usually slightly flexible to aid in the mixing of the material.

Impression materials have specially designed spatulas for the manipulation of catalyst and base. The spatula designed for mixing alginate materials is thin, flexible, and somewhat like a beaver tail in shape. This design allows for the proper manipulation of the alginate material, which requires broad crushing strokes against the material as it conforms to the shape of the rubber mixing bowl (Fig. 11-8).

Final impression materials require the use of a spatula that is heavier, stiffer, thinner at the tip, and narrower at the handle. This spatula allows for the incorporation of the base and catalyst with quick strong strokes.

Mixing surfaces may include a glass slab or paper pads made of treated, waxed, or plain material. Paper pads create a dilemma for the office concerned with eliminating the transmission of disease, since the sheets are on a tear off pad, which is difficult to disinfect. One option in lieu of a paper pad is the use of a plastic rectangular separator as found in the radiographic film package. The divider has a smooth rigid surface and works ideally for the manipulation of liners and some bases. The surface cleans easily, and the separator can be cold disinfected for an appropriate period of time. The use of overgloves during the mixing of the material eliminates potential cross contamination, but during placement of the material in the cavity preparation, it becomes more complicated, since contact with the oral cavity is made with hands, instruments, and the pad (Fig. 11-9).

A glass slab (a thick piece of smooth glass) is used to mix zinc phosphate cement to dissipate the heat that is generated during the manipulation of the material and to prevent it from setting too quickly. Many of the glass ionomer cements are mixed on a glass slab. Other cements, such as zinc oxide–eugenol, are mixed on wax pads to avoid the absorption of the liquid into a nonwaxed pad or to eliminate chasing the liquid on a glass slab. Most impression materials are mixed on treated or waxed pads, allowing for spatulation without ripping of the pad.

DISPENSING TECHNIQUES

Several suggestions should be followed when dispensing dental materials. Powder is always fluffed to avoid any settling of the chemical components; liquid is swirled for this same reason. If liquid is in a dropper, it should be dispensed into the bottle and the contents should then be swirled to obtain a homogeneous fluid before dispensing onto the mixing slab or pad. Always remember to recap the powder and liquid to avoid moisture contamination of each. Certain liquids are more viscous than others, making swirling more difficult. Each cement powder has a designated dispensing scoop, and many liquids have eyedroppers or are in bottles that are designed to dispense a regulated size of drop when pressure is applied to the sides. When liquid is dispensed from the eyedropper or the bottle, care is taken to hold each in a vertical position to ensure that the correct proportion of liquid is dispensed. Unused liquid or powder is not to be returned to the bottle.

CLEANING AGENTS

For some dental materials the proper cleaning agent is good old elbow grease, but for others, special substances have been designed to assist you. A solution of bicarbonate of soda is recommended for cleaning the materials that have debris from zinc phosphate cement, while orange oil solution is recommended for zinc oxide–eugenol cements. Polycarboxylate cements are particularly difficult to clean off instruments, but a solution of 10% sodium hydroxide assists in its removal. Many times an instrument can be cleaned before the initial set of the material occurs. The instrument can be easily cleaned of debris by wiping it off with damp gauze sponges.

Any alternative of the factors just discussed can increase or decrease compressive strength, film thickness, initial acidity, solubility, manipulation, and setting time. It is the dental assistant's responsibility to prepare and sometimes place dental cements in the oral cavity. A complete and thorough understanding of the function, manipulation, and application of these materials is necessary to meet this responsibility.

▶ Direct Restorative Materials

Direct materials are placed directly into the mouth to restore it to its natural anatomy. Direct restorative dental materials are used to replace tooth structures lost to carious lesions or trauma, as sedative treatment, and for cosmetic procedures. Direct restorative dental materials discussed in this chapter include cements, amalgam, gold, and esthetic restorative materials.

DENTAL CEMENTS

Dental cements are used for several reasons and in several specialties of dentistry. The dental assistant must have a working knowledge of the various dental cements and must prepare each for the specific requirements of the dental procedure. Cements are used as (1) luting agents for cementation of crowns, bridges, inlays, and orthodontics bands or brackets, and (2) as a temporary luting agent for temporary restorations, or as temporary itself, (3) as thermal insulating bases or liners, (4) for pulp capping, (5) for pulpal protection, (6) for root canal therapy, and (7) as surgical tissue dressings.

PULPAL PROTECTION

The protection of the pulpal tissues is a primary function of dental cements. Pulpal protection encompasses the use of cements to reduce or eliminate the trauma of thermal conductivity and as a buffer between the pulp and a metallic restoration when electrical conductivity occurs. Pulpal protection also includes covering dentinal and enamel openings that are exposed during the cavity preparation. The process of cutting enamel and dentin produces a thin layer of debris, called a smear layer, that provides minimal protection from chemical encounter; however, additional protection is often necessary. The form of pulpal protection is determined largely by the thickness of the dentin left in the cavity preparation after the carious lesion is removed. If the layer of dentin is too thin to withstand the force of stress and protect the pulp, a layer of dental cement is placed to relieve the situation. If most of the dentin remains, a dentin sealing agent may render adequate protection.

Cavity Liners and Varnishes

Cavity liners and varnishes are dental materials that provide no thermal insulation but are often necessary to create a protective barrier between dentin and the restorative material to protect the pulp. Cavity liners and varnishes are referred to as just liners, a term that may extend to include cement bases. In this chapter each type of dental material is presented individually.

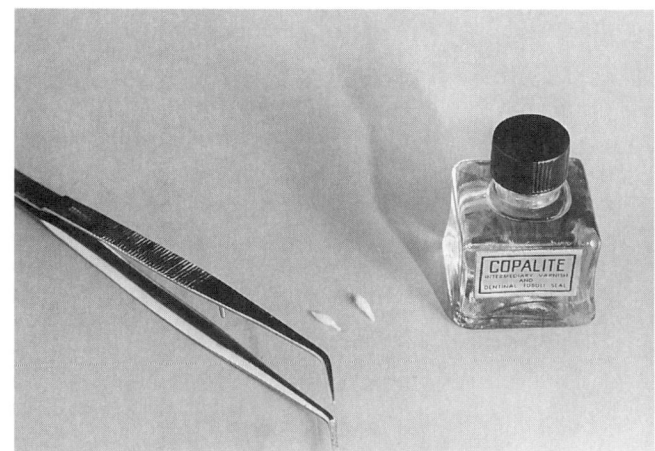 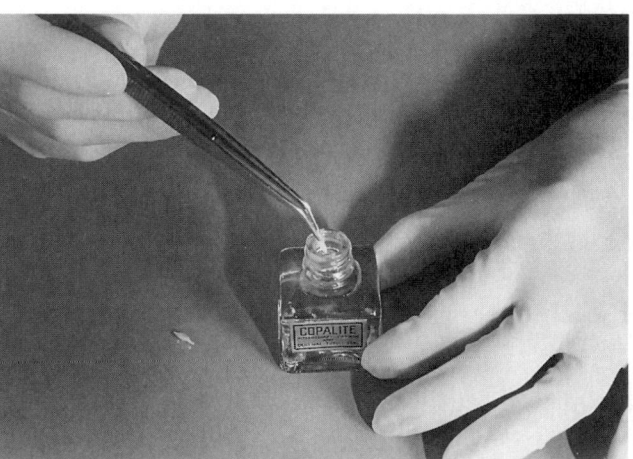

FIG. 11-10   A, Armamentarium for placment of liquid cavity varnish, cavity varnish, cotton pledgets, and cotton pliers. B, The cotton pledget is dipped into the varnish and applied to the cavity preparation. If a second applications is necessary, a second pledget and cotton pliers must be used to avoid cross-contamination of the varnish jar.

(Courtesy of Cooley and Cooley, Houston, Texas.)

CAVITY VARNISH

USE

Seal surfaces, particularly dentin tubules

COMPOSITION AND PROPERTIES

Solutions of resin in organic liquids
Provides protection from chemical and electrical stimulation

FACTORS TO BE CONSIDERED

▶ Dries quickly (5 to 30 seconds), and air dries in 5 to 15 seconds
▶ If left uncovered, liquid will evaporate, resulting in a thicker, darker solution
▶ Placing a small amount of varnish solvent reduces viscosity and lightens the varnish's color
▶ Not compatible with monomers of resin or composite restorations
▶ Use under therapeutic base (e.g., calcium hydroxide) negatively reduces the purpose of the base

ARMAMENTARIUM

Varnish
Cotton pliers
Cotton pledgets (small pieces of cotton pellet rolled tightly to absorb more liquid and for ease in application to the tooth)
Skubes

MANIPULATION

1. Place the cotton pledget into the cotton pliers.
2. Dip the pledget into the liquid and lightly dab it on a gauze sponge.
3. Apply the soaked pledget to the cavity preparation, covering all cut surfaces (Fig. 11-10).
4. If a second application is needed for maximum protective effect, you *must* use a second pledget and new cotton pliers to avoid contamination of the varnish.

CLEANING DIRECTIONS

Usually wiping the cotton plier end is sufficient cleaning until all instruments are processed for sterilization under appropriate circumstances.

CAVITY LINERS

Two types: calcium hydroxide and zinc oxide-eugenol (ZOE), with restrictive use of the latter under composite resin to avoid retarding the material

Usually set through a chemical reaction of two pastes being incorporated, when liner may release calcium hydroxide or ZOE

New forms are light cured and provide same benefits (Fig. 11-11, *A* to *C*)

ARMAMENTARIUM

Mixing surface
Instrument to mix and place material (e.g., ball applicator, spoon excavator, explorer) 2 × 2 gauze
NOTE: Manufacturer often provides paper pads for mixing and dispensing material; rectangular plastic dividers found in radiographic film packets also provide adequate mixing surface)

MANIPULATION

1. Dispense equal amounts, approximately 1 to 2 mm of catalyst and base, on mixing surface (Fig. 11-12).
2. Mix two pastes together until mixture is homogeneous or color and consistency are uniform.
3. Clean mixing instrument of cement and dip ball applicator, spoon excavator, explorer, or other instrument of choice into mix to cover end of instrument.
4. Pass instrument to operator, holding 2 × 2 gauze sponge in receiving hand and mixing pad in other hand under patient's chin so operator has access to cement liner.
5. After liner is placed, receive placement instrument, wipe off cement, and, if using the plastic divider, wipe it clean of cement. If paper pad used, tear the top sheet off and dispose of it.
6. NOTE: For newer cavity liners that are light cured (e.g., calcium hydroxides), placement is same, but there is no mixing and white light is applied to achieve set of the material (Fig. 11-13, *A* through *D*).

CLEANING DIRECTIONS

Can be removed from instruments simply by rubbing with a gauze sponge, even after cavity liner has set to final hardness

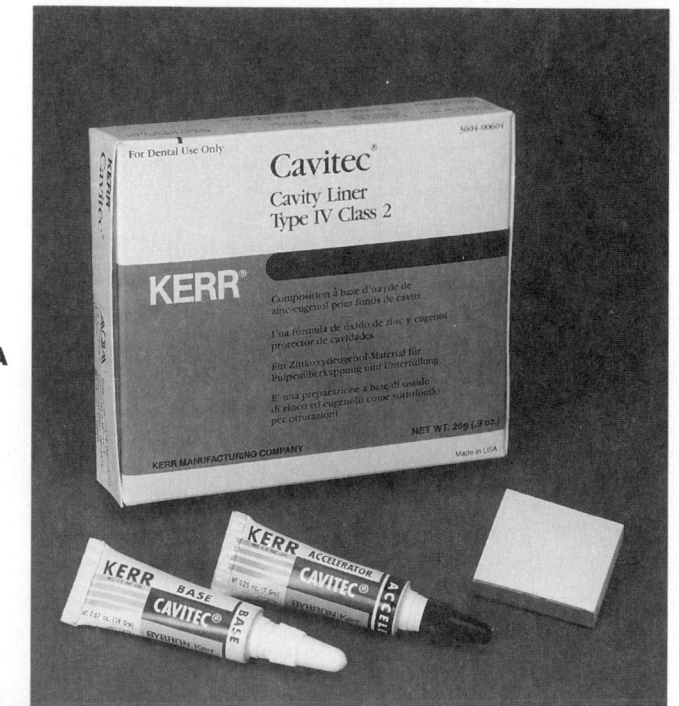

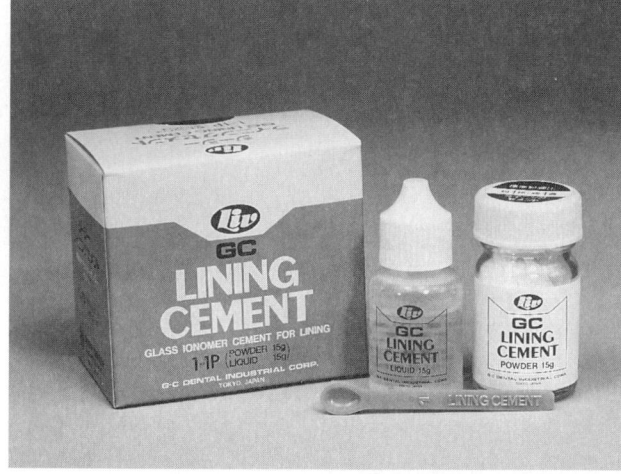

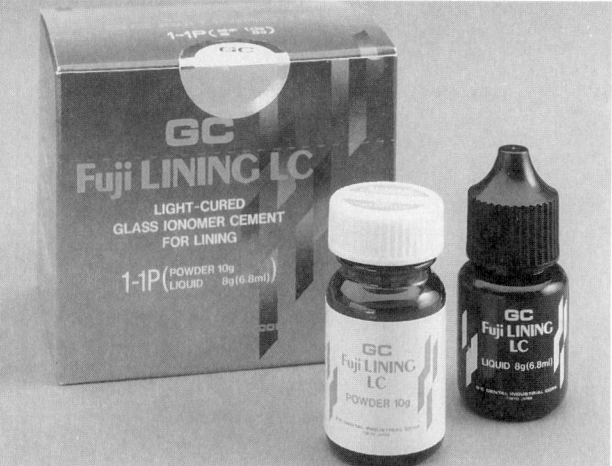

FIG. II-II   Various types of cavity liners.

(*A*, Courtesy of Kerr/Sybron Manufacturing, Romulus, Michigan. *B* and *C*, Courtesy of GC International, Scottsdale, Arizona.)

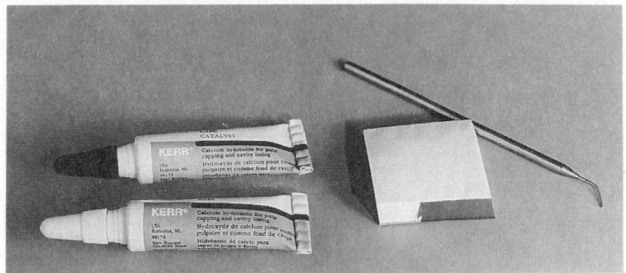

FIG. 11-12   Armamentarium for mixing a chemically cured cavity liner.

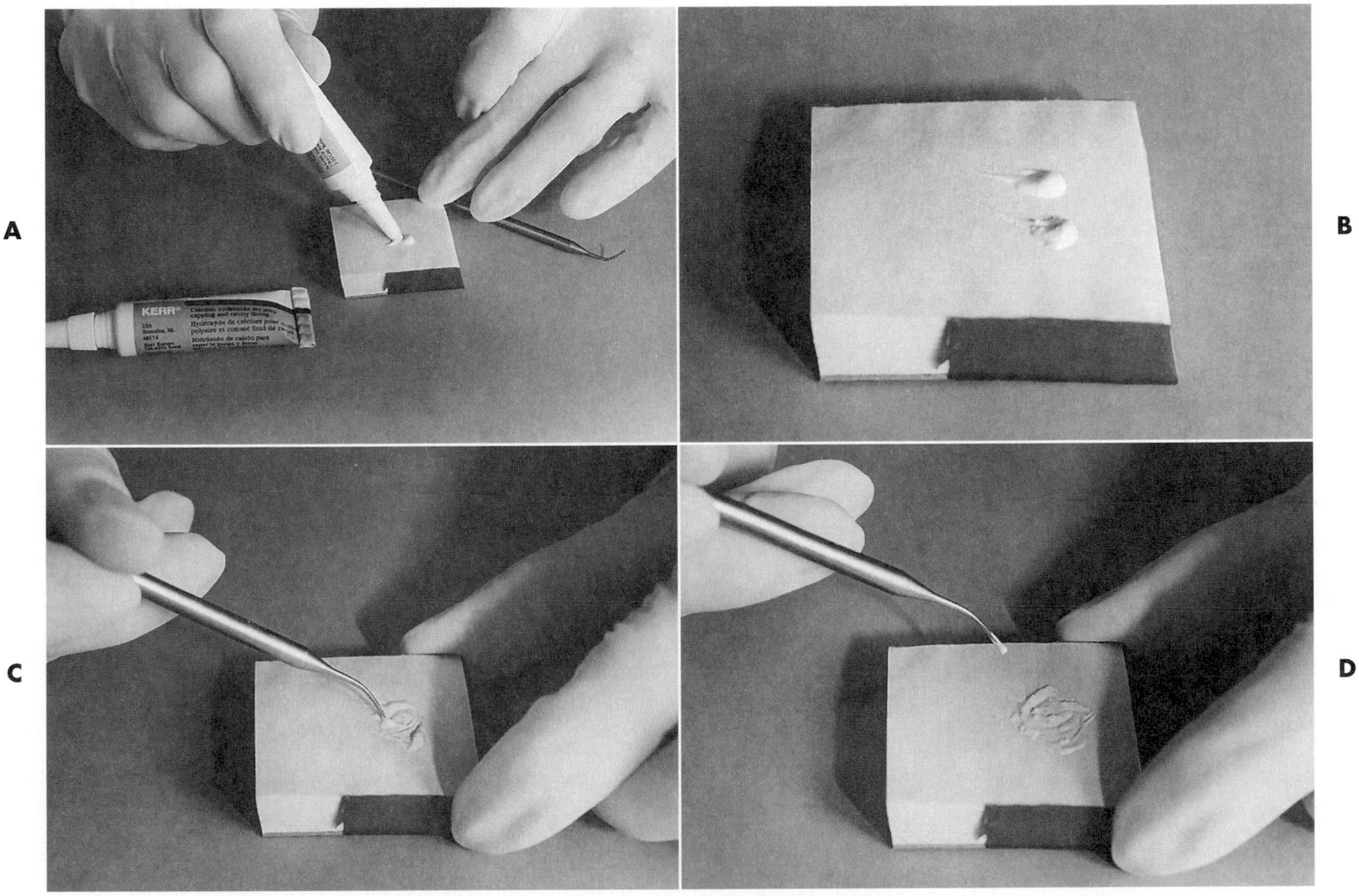

FIG. 11-13   *A,* The material is dispensed onto the mixing surface. *B,* Small equal amounts of the accelerator and base are dispensed. *C,* The base and accelerator are mixed to a homogeneous mass. *D,* The tip of the ball applicator is wiped clean and is redipped. A plastic divider from x-ray film packets can be used as a mixing surface that can be disinfected.

ZINC PHOSPHATE CEMENTS

USE

For cementation of crowns, bridges, inlays, orthodontic bands and brackets

As an insulating base

Sometimes as a temporary restorative material

COMPOSITION AND PROPERTIES

Combination of zinc oxide powder with magnesium oxide and pigments

Liquid consists of phosphoric acid in water buffered with aluminum and zinc ions to delay setting reaction

Can be prepared to primary or secondary consistency, depending on use

As powder and liquid are incorporated, an exothermic (heat-producing) reaction occurs, created by the alkaline powder dissolving in the acidic liquid

FACTORS TO BE CONSIDERED

▶ Extremely acidic and may irritate the pulp, so may need to have liner placed under it

▶ Viscosity affected by time and temperature

Mixing on cool glass slab increases working time, allowing proper incorporation of optimum amount of powder to achieve desired viscosity

During cementation of orthodontic bands, frozen slab method used to increase working time (when slab is cooled to 6° C, working time increases by 4 to 11 minutes and setting time in mouth decreases 20% to 40%, which allows orthodontic team to cement multiple orthodontic bands and brackets)

▶ Setting time also affected by use of higher powder-liquid ratio; recommended powder-liquid ratio should always be used

ARMAMENTARIUM

Glass slab

Flexible metal spatula

Measuring device

Timer

Cement placement instrument

Zinc phosphate powder and liquid (Fig. 11-14)

MANIPULATION

Primary consistency

1. Mix on a cool (70° F or 21° C) glass slab to dissipate heat from exothermic reaction and control setting time.
2. Swirl liquid and fluff powder.
3. Dispense powder and liquid in separate areas of slab as directed by manufacturer.
4. Divide the powder into 4 to 6 increments as directed by manufacturer.
5. Incorporate an increment of powder into the liquid using a rotating spatulation method over a broad area of the slab with the spatula face flat on the slab, crushing and incorporating all of the powder crystals completely.

6. Bring the mass together to introduce each instrument as described in the previous step. Before incorporating the last increment, test to see if the primary or luting consistency has been achieved by bringing the mass together and touching the spatula to the cement parallel to the slab surface, then lifting it upward to draw a string of 1 inch. If the cement string does not break before the length of 1 inch is met, the cement is mixed to primary consistency and is ready for application (Fig. 11-15, *A* through *C*).

Secondary consistency

1. Dispense a greater amount of powder at the beginning.
2. Follow the steps for primary consistency but place ⅕ of the mix in the corner of the slab to assist in initial retention while the secondary consistency is being placed.
3. Continue to incorporate the powder into the liquid mass using a folding and packing motion rather than a rotary one. Mix the powder into the cement until you achieve a homogeneous mass that can be rolled into a rope.
4. To roll the cement, cover the spatula with powder, lift the mass off the slab, and lightly remove from the spatula onto the slab.
5. Powder the spatula again and, with light pressure, roll the cement until it is of equal thickness, about 1 inch long.
6. If the operator prefers, cut the rope into small increments that can be easily managed for placement in the cavity preparation.
7. Transfer the placement instruments to the operator and hold the glass slab under the patient's chin so the operator has access to the cement.
8. Make extra powder available to the operator to dip the placement instrument in so that it does not adhere to the cement in the cavity preparation (Fig. 11-16, *A* through *C*).

CLEANING DIRECTIONS

Easily cleaned from the instruments and glass slab using bicarbonate of soda water.

Prepare a mixture ahead of time and make it available for dispensing in the operatory to ensure a more efficient cleaning process later.

HELPFUL HINTS

▶ While preparing the cement powder into increments, keep each mass separated completely so one is not contaminated when another is incorporated into the cement mass.

▶ Before incorporating each increment into the cement, bring the mass together.

▶ When you try to roll the mass of cement for secondary consistency, wipe excess cement on the spatula onto the slab and incorporate it all together.

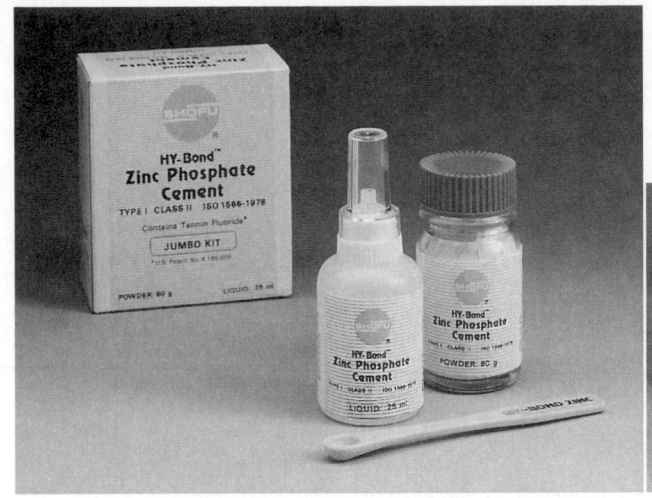

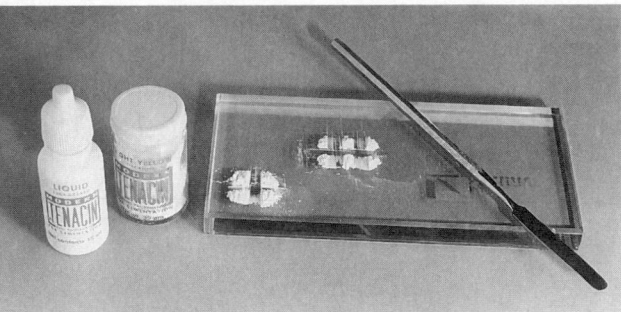

FIG. 11-14   *A* and *B,* Zinc phosphate armamentarium and powder dispensed into six equal increments in the center of the slab, with four increments in the upper corner.

(*A,* Courtesy of Shofu Dental Corporation, Menlo Park, California.)

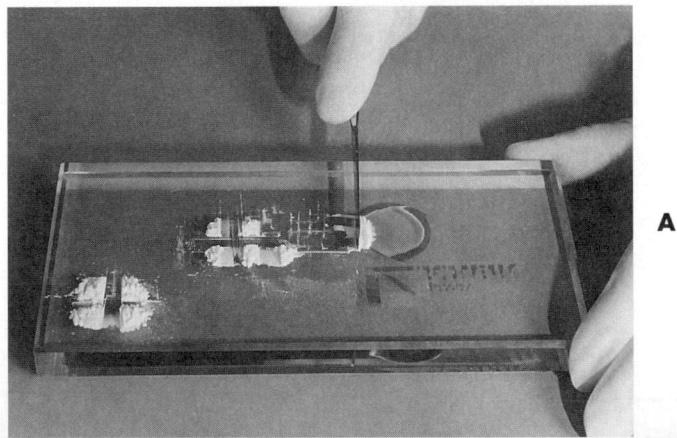

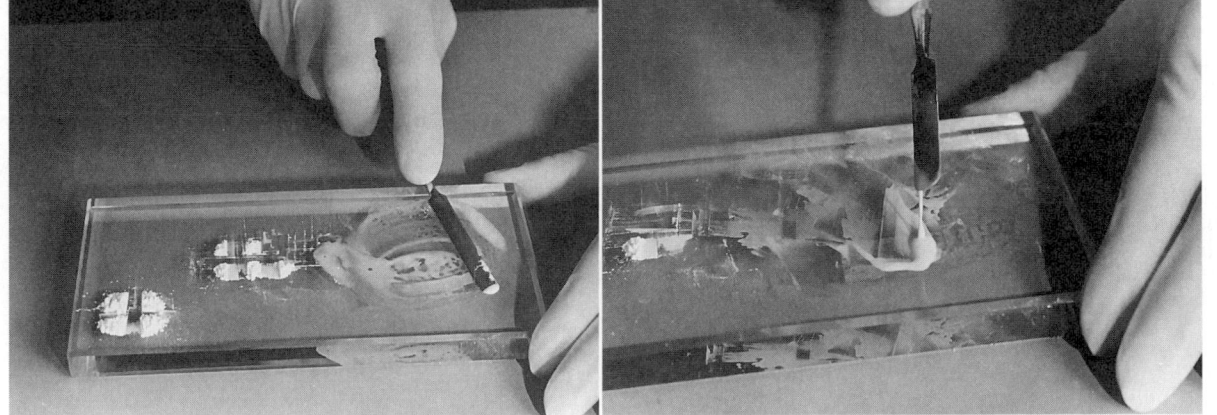

FIG. 11-15   *A,* Incorporate the first increment of powder into the liquid and mix for 15 seconds. *B,* Using rotary spatulation over a large area of the slab. *C,* At approximately the fourth or fifth increment, the mass is tested for primary consistency, resulting in a 1-inch string of cement off the spatula.

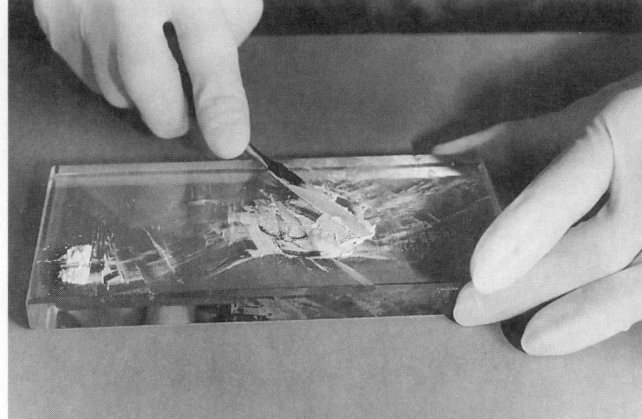

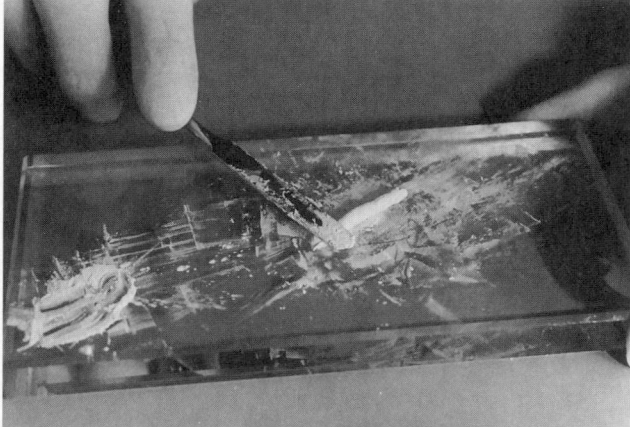

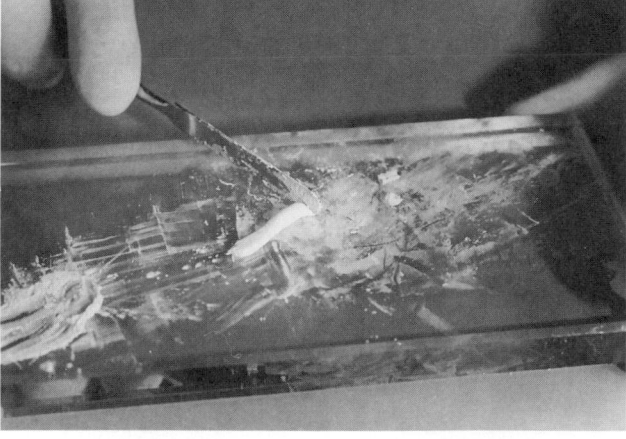

FIG. 11-16   *A,* Each additional increment is incorporated in the mass using a folding and packing motion. *B,* All the cement is brought together and rolled into a rope approximately 1 inch in length. *C,* The rope is cut into small increments for placement in the cavity preparation as a base.

ZINC SILICOPHOSPHATE CEMENT

USE

Type I, Cementing medium
Type II, Temporary posterior restoration
Type III, Cementing or luting medium and temporary posterior restoration

COMPOSITION AND PROPERTIES

Combination of zinc phosphate and silicate cements crossed to improve upon each cement's positive characteristics
Not widely used other than as a luting agent under porcelain restorations
Powder is a combination of silicate and zinc and magnesium oxides
Liquid is a phosphoric acid solution
Like zinc phosphate, highly acidic and requires a cavity varnish to protect the tooth

FACTORS TO BE CONSIDERED

▶ Many of the factors that are significant to zinc phosphate also pertain to zinc silicophosphate cements
▶ Not mixed on a broad portion of the glass slab but rather on a small area

ARMAMENTARIUM

Glass slab
Agate or stellite spatula
Measuring device
Timer
Cement placement instrument
Zinc silicophosphate powder and liquid

MANIPULATION

Procedure is similar to that of zinc phosphate cements.
1. Mix the cement on a cool glass slab (65° F or 18° C) to dissipate heat from the exothermic reaction.
2. Swirl liquid and fluff powder.
3. Dispense powder and liquid in separate areas of the slab as directed by manufacturer.
4. Divide powder into increments of ½, ¼, ⅛, and ⅛. Incorporate at 10-15 second intervals for 45-60 seconds.
5. To mix the material to primary or secondary consistency, follow the zinc phosphate directions.

ZINC OXIDE–EUGENOL (ZOE) CEMENTS

USE

Cementation of fixed prosthodontics
Sedative bases
Temporary restorations
Tissue packs
Root canal sealers

COMPOSITION AND PROPERTIES

Zinc oxide, rosin to reduce brittleness, zinc stearate to be a plasticizer, and zinc acetate for strength
Liquid consists of eugenol and olive oil as a plasticizer
To increase strength, methyl methacrylate polymer or alumina is added to the powder and ethoxybenzoic acid to the liquid (improved or fortified ZOE)
Many ZOE cements manufactured as two-paste systems [Fig. 11-17, *A* and *B*].

FACTORS TO BE CONSIDERED

▸ Great sedative or anodyne effects for tissues of the teeth, so if a tooth is sensitive, ZOE will be used to relieve discomfort

ARMAMENTARIUM

Parchment or waxed pad surfaces
Heavy, nonflexible spatula
NOTE: EBA with alumina cement is mixed on a glass slab with a flexible spatula
Timer
Measuring device
Cement powder and liquid
Cement placement instrument

MANIPULATION

Follow manufacturer's directions for specific incorporation of increments, time, and final result, depending on desired use.
1. Swirl liquid and fluff powder.
2. Dispense the amounts of each according to the manufacturer's directions.
3. Incorporate powder and liquid in increments or mix in mass together, using a folding and packing motion.
4. To wet all the powder particles, maintain an exacting pressure on the spatula tip.

Continued.

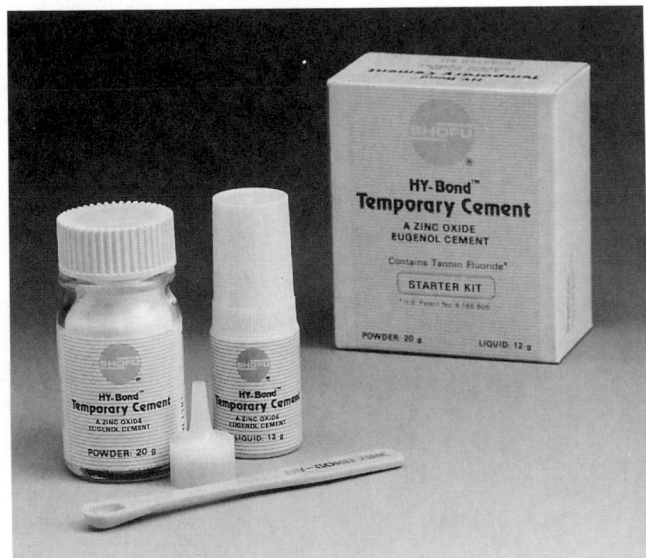
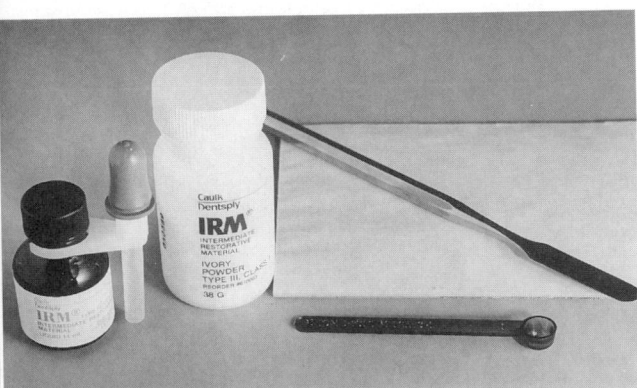

FIG. 11-17   *A* and *B*, Two examples of ZOE cements and armamentarium for mixing.

(*A,* Courtesy of Shofu Dental Corporation, Menlo Park, California. *B,* Courtesy of Dentsply International, York, Pennsylvania.)

ZINC OXIDE–EUGENOL (ZOE) CEMENTS—cont'd.

5. Mix powder and liquid to a homogeneous mass whether for primary or secondary consistency.
6. With certain ZOE cements (e.g., EBA) strop to achieve consistency (Fig. 11-18, *A* through *G*).

CLEANING DIRECTIONS

Easily cleaned by wiping the surfaces with gauze before set or by using orange oil solution. Do not use water for cleaning, and be careful of moisture contamination, which significantly reduces setting time.

HELPFUL HINTS

▶ If the combination seems too dry, apply more pressure to wet the mass and to make it more manageable and achieve the required consistency.
▶ The further your finger is placed down the spatula end, the greater the pounds per square inch of pressure.

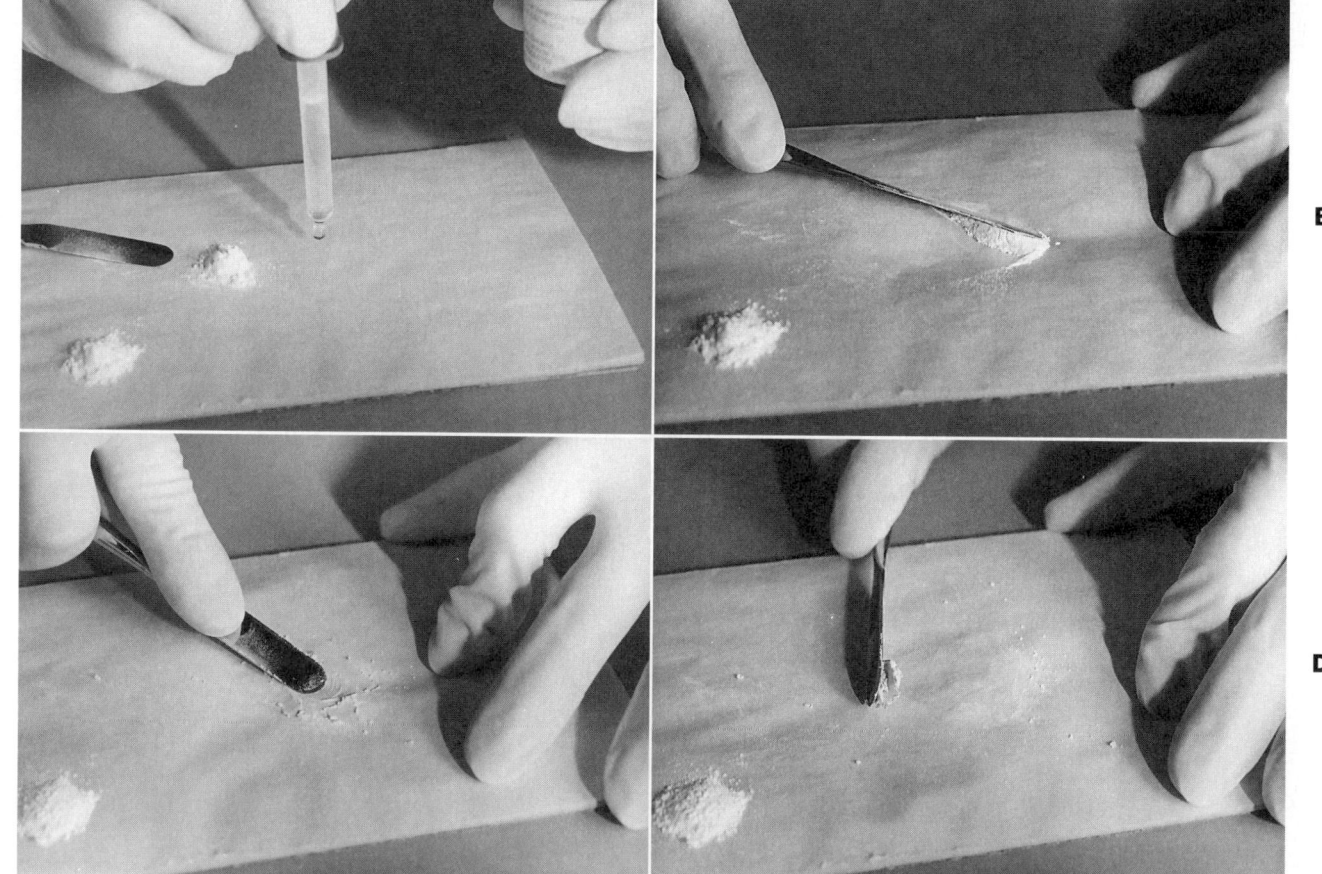

FIG. 11-18   *A,* The ZOE powder is dispensed first onto a parchment pad with extra powder in the corner. *B,* Immediately after the liquid is dispensed, the powder is drawn into it. *C,* Using force on the end of the spatula, wet all the powder. *D,* Bring the mass of mixed cement together at the end of the spatula.

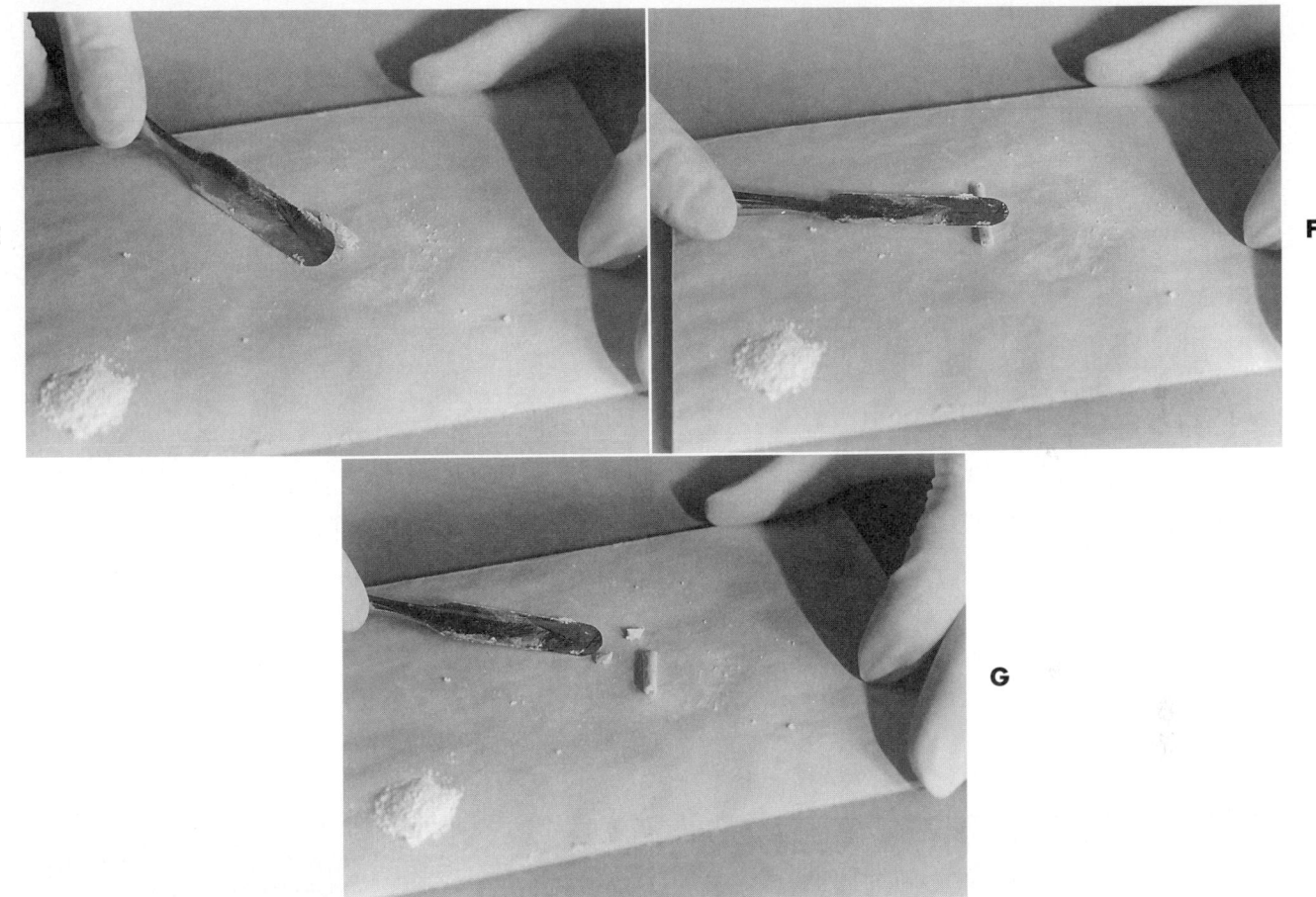

FIG. 11-18, cont'd.   *E,* Force the cement off the tip of the spatula. *F,* Roll the mass into a rope, using a light pressure. *G,* Cut the rope into small increments for placement in the cavity preparation.

POLYCARBOXYLATE CEMENT

USE

Luting agent for cementation of fixed prosthodontics
Insulating base

COMPOSITION AND PROPERTIES

Combination of zinc oxide powder and aqueous polyacrylic acid solution (used in place of phosphoric acid to reduce the acidity of the cement and the potential for pulpal irritation).

Setting time decreased or increased by warm and cold, respectively.

FACTORS TO BE CONSIDERED

▶ Usually mixed as quickly as possible
▶ May be mixed on a cooled glass surface to slow the chemical reaction
▶ Extremely adhesive to surfaces it contacts, so use of a paper pad may be preferred
▶ Typical working time 30 to 60 seconds and initial set reached in 3 minutes

ARMAMENTARIUM

Glass slab or paper pad
Flexible metal spatula
Measuring device
Cement placement instrument
Cement liquid and powder (Fig. 11-19, *A* to *B*).

MANIPULATION

Can be mixed to a luting consistency or to base consistency, with difference normally obtained by increasing the amount of powder incorporated into the liquid.

1. Fluff powder; swirling liquid is difficult due to extreme viscosity.
2. Dispense appropriate powder and liquid ratio for consistency of cement needed.
3. Incorporate all the powder into the liquid using a folding and packing motion, until all the powder is wetted.
4. Use broad stropping motion to develop primary consistency (Fig 11-20, *A* through *C*) or more folding and packing for secondary consistency.
5. A cement mixed to primary consistency will appear shiny; as it becomes dull, dry, and stringy, its ability to flow is diminished so it should not be used.

CLEANING DIRECTIONS

Sets quickly with extremely adhesive characteristic on the work surfaces, requiring quick action to remove it from the spatula and the slab or softening in a basic solution such as 10% sodium hydroxide.

HELPFUL HINT

▶ Use a paper pad to mix this cement, if possible, to eliminate extra work later.

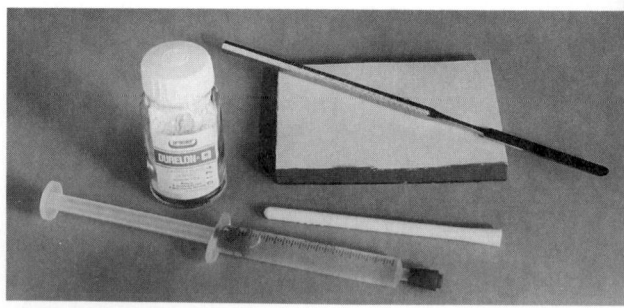
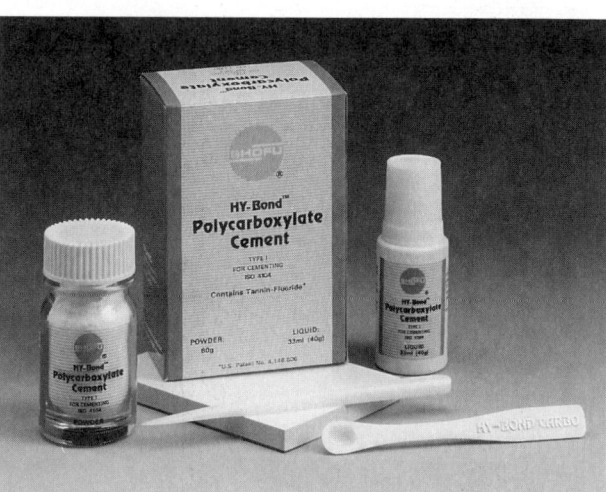

FIG. 11-19   *A* and *B*, Examples of carboxylate cements and armamentarium.
(*B*, Courtesy of Shofu Dental Corporation, Menlo Park, California.)

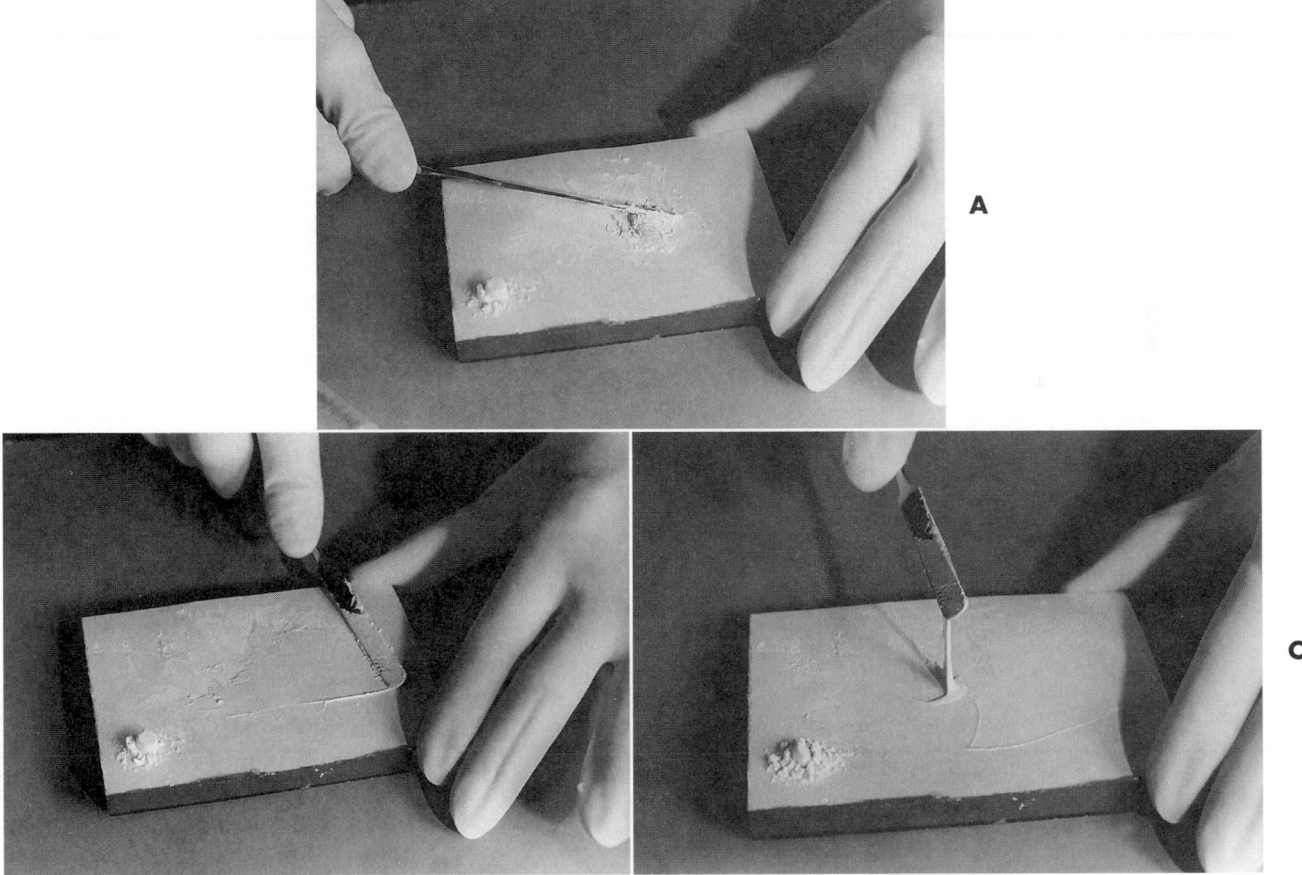

FIG. 11-20   *A,* The powder in the center is incorporated with the liquid. *B,* Once wetted, the cement mass is stropped. *C,* The homogeneous mix should result in a 1-inch string of primary consistency.

GLASS IONOMER CEMENT

USE

Supplied as Types I and II

Type I, Cementation of fixed prosthodontics, occasionally   pit and fissure sealant

Type II, Insulating bases, core buildup, and Class III and V restorations

COMPOSITION AND PROPERTIES

A recent hybrid that combines the better qualities of other cements

Glass ionomers are aluminosilicate-polyacrylate (ASPA)

Powder is a silicate porcelain

Viscous liquid is aqueous solution of polyacrylic acid

Cement releases fluoride ions intraorally, assisting in the reduction of secondary carious activity, an advantage over zinc phosphate

Glass ionomer cements, not as strong as zinc phosphate cements, and, if contaminated by water early in the setting process, may suffer cement failure

FACTORS TO BE CONSIDERED

▶ Glass ionomer cements bonded in place to aid in retention

▶ Many manufacturers supply products in preproportioned capsules to reduce the possibility of moisture contamination

▶ Because of moisture sensitivity, the cement must be mixed quickly

MANIPULATION

If the glass ionomer cement is to be bonded, prepare tooth surfaces through an acid-etching technique (described in Chapter 26 in the pit and fissure sealant procedure). The acid etching is completed just before manipulation of the cement.

1. Dispense the manufacturer's directed proportions of powder and liquid on a paper pad.
2. Divide the powder into halves or thirds and incorporate each increment into the liquid until it is uniform.
3. Include increments within 40 seconds, giving a homogeneous mix of cement.
4. The cement appears shiny for the ideal luting consistency; once the gloss is lost, the consistency becomes heavier.
5. If the cement is in a precapsulated form, use a capsule activator to enmesh the liquid and powder in the capsule.
6. Place the capsule in an amalgamator to triturate the liquid and powder to reach proper consistency.
7. Place cement in a Teflon syringe or capsule applicator and apply it through the use of either device, or remove it from the capsule and place it, using a plastic instrument.

CLEANING DIRECTIONS

Cleans easily from surfaces when wiped with gauze just after manipulation.

ARMAMENTARIUM

Glass slab or paper pad
Flexible metal spatula
Measuring device
Glass ionomer powder and liquid or amalgamator for preportioned capsules (Fig. 11-21, *A* through *E*)

A
B
C
D
E

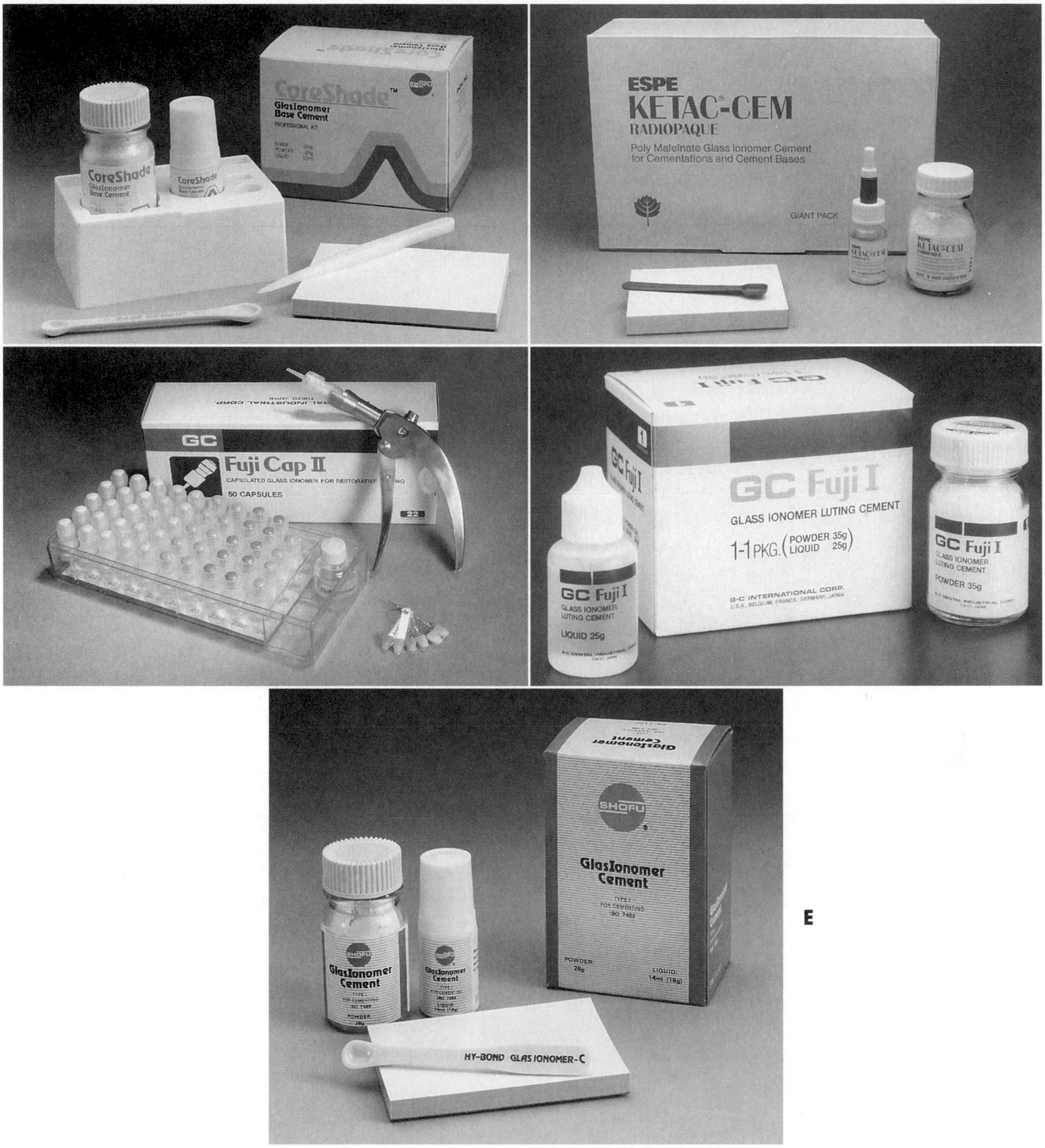

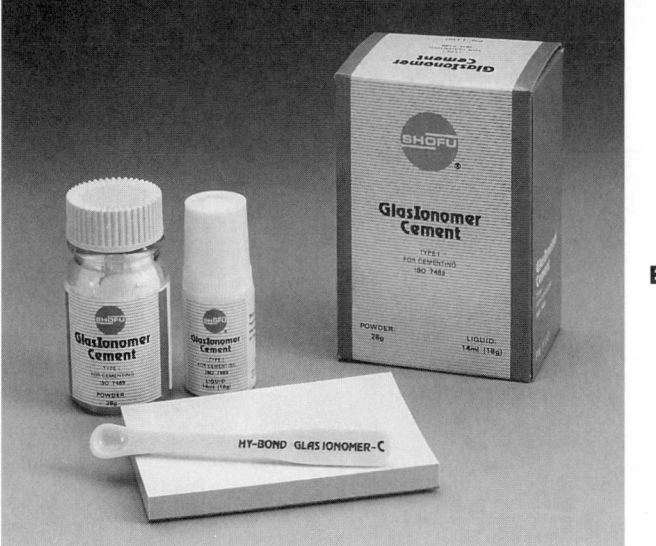

FIG. 11-21 *A* through *E*, Various types of glass ionomer cements.

RESIN CEMENTS

USE

Primarily luting agents for cast porcelain restorations
Bonding agents with enamel
Cementation of orthodontic brackets

COMPOSITION AND PROPERTIES

BIS-GMA- or BIS-GMA-like monomers without reinforced fillers
Resin cements have low viscosity, thus great flow capabilities during the initial period after manipulation, which can result in absorption into the dentin tubules causing damage.

FACTORS TO BE CONSIDERED

▶ Low viscosity of mix in early stages appeals in some circumstances
▶ Use is recommended primarily for luting of cast porcelain restorations

ARMAMENTARIUM

Paper mixing pad or dish
Flexible metal spatula
Both bottles of resin liquid
Disposable brush or syringe

MANIPULATION

The two components of this cement are in liquid form.
1. Dispense equal drops from both bottles of liquid.
2. Mix the two liquids together completely, and then either paint the cement on with a brush, or place it in a application syringe and apply it via the syringe tip.

CLEANING DIRECTIONS

Throw away disposable brushes and syringe tips.
Wipe the spatula clean immediately after mixing for ease of cleanup.
NOTE: Box 11-3 provides examples of several brand names of dental cements. This list is not indicative of all available products, but a sampling of dental cements.

BOX 11-3

BRAND NAMES OF COMMON DENTAL CEMENTS

CAVITY VARNISH

Copalite
Cavoline
Handi-Liner
Tubli-Seal
Copal with Fluoride
Varnal

CAVITY LINER

Cavitec
Kadon
Cavalite
Interface
Timeline

POLYCARBOXYLATE

Ceramco
Chemit
Durelon
PCA Cement
Tylok-Plus
Hy-Bond
Liv Cenera PC

ZINC PHOSPHATE

Ames Cement
S.S. White
Dicor
Flecks
Hy-Bond
Lee Smith
Tenacin
Zinc Cement

CALCIUM HYDROXIDE

Achatite
Dycal
Dropsin
Hypo-Cal
Hydroxyline
Life
MPC
Procol
Renew
Prisma VLC Dycal
Nu-Cap
Alkaliner
Preline

ZINC OXIDE–EUGENOL

E.B.A. Opoto with Alumina
Eucalyptol
Eugenol
Opotow
ZOE B&T
ZOE 2200
IRM
Fynal
Interval

RESIN CEMENTS

Comspan
Conclude
Resilute
Solo-Tach
Dual
Flexi-Flow
Resiment

GLASS IONOMER

Biocem
Ketac-Cem
Fuji-Ionomer

Glaslonomer
Shofu
BaseLine
Dentin Cement
Chelon-Silver
Ketac-Silver
XR Ionomer
Hy-Bond
EMKA
Ionoscem
Lining Cement
Vitrabond
Ketac-Fil
Core Shade

SILICOPHOSPHATE

Germicidal Kryptex
Fluoro-Thin

DENTAL ADHESIVES

Maryland Bridge Adhesive
Panavia
C&B Metabond
Dentin Bond
Scotchbond 2

TEMPORARY CEMENTS

Flow Temp
No Genol
Temp-Bond/ Temp-Bond NE
Buffalo Temporary Cement
Trial Cement
Tempak
Tem-Stik
Cavit
Cimpat
Neo-Temp
NOgenol
Proviscell
Temrex
ZOE-Plus
Freegenol

Dental Amalgam

An alloy is a substance that evolves from the combination of two different metals. Dental amalgam is an alloy with mercury as one of the metals combined with a mixture of silver, tin, copper, and zinc. Amalgam continues to be the most common restorative material placed in the oral cavity.

▶ Amalgam History

It is reported that amalgam was first used approximately 659 AD in China as a restorative material. The Chinese used arsenic to treat decayed teeth and then placed a *silver paste*. This paste was a triturated mass of 100 parts mercury, 45 parts silver, and 900 parts tin that produced something as solid as silver. In the West the introduction of silver amalgam was by two French brothers named Crawcour in 1833. This amalgam was known as Royal Mineral Succedaneum and was a combination of shavings from silver coins and enough mercury to produce a paste that was manageable. This crude material is a distant relative to the amalgam of today, but it provided the basis for experimentation and improvement.

The introduction of the Crawcour amalgam led to the first of the *Amalgam Wars*. The toxicity of mercury was known at this time, and the less-than-adequate amalgam restorations placed by the brothers instigated the American Society of Dental Surgeons to pass a resolution demanding that no member of the society use this alloy. This negative connotation associated with amalgam was somewhat dispelled through the work of G.V. Black, Elisha Townsend, and J. Foster, who improved the restorative material in the last half of the 1800s.

A second *Amalgam War* developed through the writings of Alfred Stock, a chemistry professor at Kaiser Wilhelm Institute in Germany who had experimented with mercury for years and subsequently had poisoned himself with the metal. His published papers decried the use of mercury in dentistry, and he garnered great support for his stand. However, an appointed committee from the Medical Department of the Charite Hospital in Berlin investigated and concluded the use of amalgam in dentistry was appropriate.

In recent history, dentistry has found itself perched on what could be called the *Third Amalgam War*. In the late 1970s, claims arose stating that mercury vapor was found after chewing in the breath of patients who had amalgam restorations. Several television shows created an intensified level of alarm in the profession of dentistry, but particularly in the dental consumer. A newly released report from the ADA Council on Dental Materials, Instruments, and Equipment, the Council on Dental Therapeutics, and the federal Food and Drug Administration has again allayed the fears regarding the use of dental amalgam. It is seen as an accepted restorative material and no data exist showing a direct hazard to humans from dental amalgams.

▶ Mercury Hygiene

Any groups that investigate dental amalgam realize that mercury in amalgam poses some hazards, but those who are affected are usually dental personnel who inhale mercury vapor. This fact reinforces the need for proper mercury hygiene procedures. Mercury contamination may result from exposure to mercury through the skin, inhalation of mercury vapor, and inhalation of airborne particles. To avoid the possibility of mercury contamination the ADA recommends the use of preproportioned single-use amalgam capsules, eliminating the need for mercury dispensers and possible accidents. All amalgam and mercury excess should be stored in an airtight container of radiographic fixer solution or other recommended solutions.

The use of water spray and high-velocity evacuation during the removal of existing amalgam restorations reduces the mercury vapors. Coverage of the operating team's faces with a mask and glasses and hands with gloves also reduces the possibility of contamination. The use of amalgamators with covers over the armature of the unit reduces the potential of airborne particles. It is also recommended that ultrasonic or pneumatic condensers not be used during the placement of amalgam, since this type of condenser can create aerosolized mercury.

The dental office must be well ventilated to include an exchange system for fresh air. Also, a yearly urine analysis of personnel should be conducted to monitor mercury exposure. If exposure is suspected, the office atmosphere should be monitored for mercury. An emergency spillage kit is required to be on site for unexpected accidents (Fig. 11-22). The floor covering of the office is

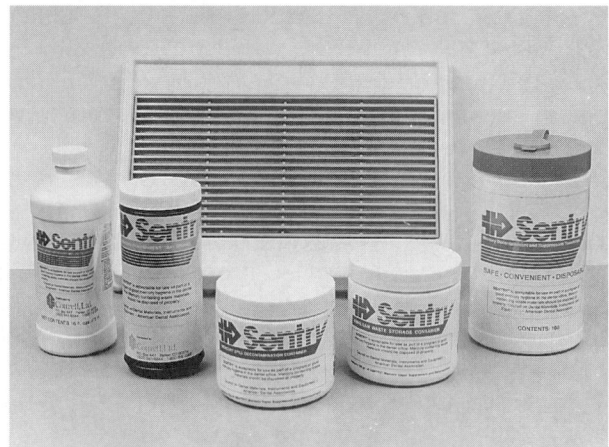

FIG. 11-22   Amalgam spill kit.

(Courtesy of Cottrell, Ltd., Parker, Colorado.)

MERCURY HYGIENE RECOMMENDATIONS

1. Follow recommended safety procedures for cleaning spilled mercury or mercury-contaminated surfaces.
2. Make sure that treatment rooms and the entire office have proper ventilation.
3. Store amalgam scrap in sealed containers, and cover them with the appropriate solutions.
4. Avoid heating mercury or amalgam.
5. Avoid direct contact with mercury. Do not handle it.
6. Dispose of mercury-contaminated items properly.
7. Use a precapsulated alloy to minimize the possibility of spilled mercury.
8. Use water spray and high-volume evacuation when removing amalgam to minimize vapors.
9. Enclose the capsule and amalgamator arms in a cover during trituration.
10. Monitor the office for atmospheric mercury on a yearly basis.
11. Monitor office personnel for mercury exposure on a yearly basis.

TABLE 11-1   COMPOSITION OF AMALGAM ALLOYS

Type of alloy	Component	Characteristic	Percent in alloy
Low copper	Silver	Luster, strength, durability, expansion	65 to 72
	Tin	Reduced expansion, strength, hardness; increased flow and workability	26 to 29
	Copper	High strength, low corrosion	2 to 7
High copper	Silver	Luster, strength, durability, expansion	40 to 70
	Tin	Reduced expansion, strength, hardness; increased flow and workability	0 to 30
	Copper	High strength, low corrosion	2 to 30

important in the effort of cleaning a mercury spill. Cleanup on any surface is difficult because mercury falling on hard surfaces spreads all over, but it can be easily picked up. However, carpeting contains the spill and also absorbs some of it, making removal all but impossible. The use of high-velocity evacuation or any form of vacuum system is not acceptable for mercury spills, since it creates a mercury aerosol. Box 11-4 summarizes these mercury hygiene recommendations.

▶ Mercury Toxicity

As an individual working in the dental profession, you should be aware of the effects of mercury intoxication. Contamination through mercury exposure results in various manifestations. Mercury level is measured by the amount and duration an individual is exposed to mercury vapors. The recommended safe mercury vapor level found in the air is 0.05 mg for a 40-hour week. An increase in this level could result in excess levels in the body.

Early indications of excessive mercury exposure include tremors and decreased levels of nerve conduction, brain-wave activity, and verbal skills.

Increased levels of toxicity could result in any of the following:
▶ Kidney dysfunction
▶ Irritability
▶ Depression
▶ Memory loss
▶ Minor tremors

▶ Various nervous system disorders
▶ Swollen gingiva
▶ Pronounced tremors

▶ Components of Alloys

The composition of alloys used for dental amalgam is regulated by ADA specifications, which basically state that the alloy is a combination of silver, tin, copper, zinc, gold, and mercury, with the last four in lesser amounts than the silver and tin. The actual percentages of each metal varies, but the permission for use of other metals must be requested through the Council on Dental Materials and Devices.

The type and quantity of each component of an alloy provide specific characteristics that are desired in an amalgam restoration. Table 11-1 provides specific information regarding these components. Alloys are classified as low copper or high copper alloys.

LOW COPPER ALLOY

Low copper alloy was the first to be developed and is used less often today than high copper alloys. Low copper alloys are supplied as spherical or as comminuted, either pulverized or lathe-cut particles. The shape of each of these alloy particles is different and distinct. Low copper alloys are found in combination with silver-tin alloys, which, when combined with mercury, react to form a weak tin-mercury phase. The phase is a recognized area in the mass that is inferior to the rest.

DENTAL AMALGAM

USE

Restore teeth to gain function and to relieve discomfort

Used most commonly in Class I, II, III restorations on molars and premolars

Used to restore the distal surfaces of cuspids, Class V, and modified Class VI preparations of teeth

FACTORS TO BE CONSIDERED

▶ A combination of alloy and mercury, which is a toxic element; therefore, great care must be taken in handling

▶ All OSHA and ADA recommendations followed to eliminate mercury contamination

NOTE: Since preproportioned amalgam capsules, with alloy and mercury in one capsule and separated by a thin diaphragm of plastic are recommended for use, only this type will be discussed in the manipulation step. Reusable capsules with removable metal pestles are still available, as are mercury dispensers or proportioners that allow for dispensing of a drop of mercury with a tablet of alloy (Fig. 11-23, *A* through *C*).

▶ Amalgam mixed to different amounts, depending on what is needed to complete a restoration; a single spill or mix of 600 mg of alloy is used with smaller preparations and often during restoration of a primary tooth; a double spill of 800 mg of alloy is used in larger preparations

▶ With a mechanical amalgamator (Fig. 11-24), alloy and mercury are triturated, mixed, for a specific time; amount of amalgam to be mixed and type of amalgamator are important factors

▶ Specific time and speed allotments are assigned for each type of alloy capsule with a particular amalgamator

ARMAMENTARIUM

Preproportioned amalgam capsule

Capsule activator

Mechanical amalgamator

Dappen dish or amalgam well

Amalgam carrier

Gun or syringe

Condenser

MANIPULATION

Place overgloves over examination gloves if they are contaminated to avoid contamination of the rest of the amalgam armamentarium.

1. Select a preproportioned capsule that is correct for the size of the preparation.
2. Activate the capsule by pressing hard on one end of the capsule on a hard surface or by using a capsule activator device (Fig. 11-25, *A* through *C*).
3. Set the mechanical amalgamator for the correct time and speed for use with the particular capsule.
4. Place the capsule securely in the armature of the amalgamator to ensure that it will not be thrown from the unit (Fig. 11-26, *A*).
5. Close the lid over the armature and capsule to ensure that no airborne particles will be propelled if the capsule is defective.
6. Set the timer for the correct time for the amalgam spill size (Fig. 11-26, *B*).
7. Press the activation button on the amalgamator to start the trituration (Fig. 11-26, *C* and *D*).
8. If the amalgamator is enclosed in a mobile cart, close the door to reduce noise next to the patient's head and to further reduce the possibility of airborne mercury particles.
9. Incorrect trituration times result in undermixed or overmixed masses of amalgam as seen in Fig. 11-27.
10. Remove the capsule from the amalgamator and, if suggested by the manufacturer, rap the end of the capsule on a hard surface to loosen the mass from the interior of the capsule.
11. Remove the overgloves.
12. Open the capsule and place the amalgamated mass in a dappen dish or an amalgam well (Fig. 11-28, *A*).
13. Load the amalgam carrier, gun, or syringe with amalgam, and pass the instrument to the operator for placement in the preparation (Fig. 11-28, *B*).
14. Exchange the carrier for a condenser of choice to condense or adapt the amalgam to the prepared surfaces of the tooth.
15. The goals of condensation are to apply equal pressure throughout the mass of material in the preparation to eliminate voids, compact the mass uniformly, and reduce excess mercury.
16. If the amalgam is of a type that can be polished at the placement appointment, then this may follow.

NOTE: The specific placement and carving of the amalgam is discussed in greater detail in Chapter 27.

CLEANING DIRECTIONS

Removed easily from working surfaces of instruments while it is soft and pliable (Fig. 11-28, *C*).

Once material has hardened, particularly in amalgam carrier, gun, or syringe, removal is difficult.

Regardless of the form of carrier that is used to transport the amalgam to the tooth, always check that all the amalgam is removed after the last increment is placed. If not, the instrument may be useless or need special attention to succeed in removing the hardened amalgam.

Place unused amalgam, silver alloy and mercury in manufacturer's scrap amalgam container or a container with fixer solution. Never place the unused amalgam in the trash, and never dispose of amalgam or mercury in any way other than through a licensed toxic waste contractor.

Continued.

HIGH COPPER ALLOY

High copper alloys used most often in dentistry are spherical, comminuted, or admixed, sometimes referred to as combination, particles. Of the spherical and comminuted, the latter is supplied in various sizes, including fine-cut and microcut. Since the admixed alloy is a combination of spherical and comminuted particles, the particles are spherical in shape as well as lathe-cut. High copper alloys do not have a tin-mercury phase like the low copper alloys, but form a copper-tin phase that provides the alloy with superior properties.

AMALGAMATION

Whether the amalgam alloy is of low or high copper content, each is combined with mercury to elicit a reaction. The introduction of mercury to the silver alloy creates a reaction called amalgamation. This reaction causes a hardening of the amalgam through solution and crystallization. Mercury, a fluid, contacts the alloy and wets the particles of powder. The absorption of the mercury by the particles creates phases of either silver-tin, gamma phase; silver-mercury, a gamma-1 phase; or tin-mercury, gamma-2 phase. The silver-tin alloy is considered a gamma phase when the particles have not yet reacted with the mercury.

To understand the process of amalgamation, which is a surface reaction, it is helpful to think of the silver-mercury phase, gamma, tied together by a combination of the gamma-1 and gamma-2 phases that form a matrix. The reaction of the gamma phase with gamma-1 and gamma-2 allows for no free mercury to be present in the amalgam restoration.

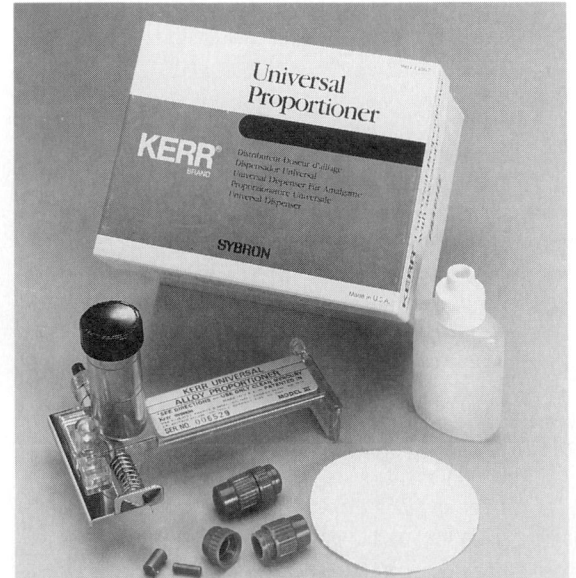

FIG. II-23   *A through C,* Various types of dental amalgam with proportioner, reusable capsules, alloy tablets and preproportioned capsules.

(Courtesy of Kerr/Sybron Manufacturing, Romulus, Michigan.)

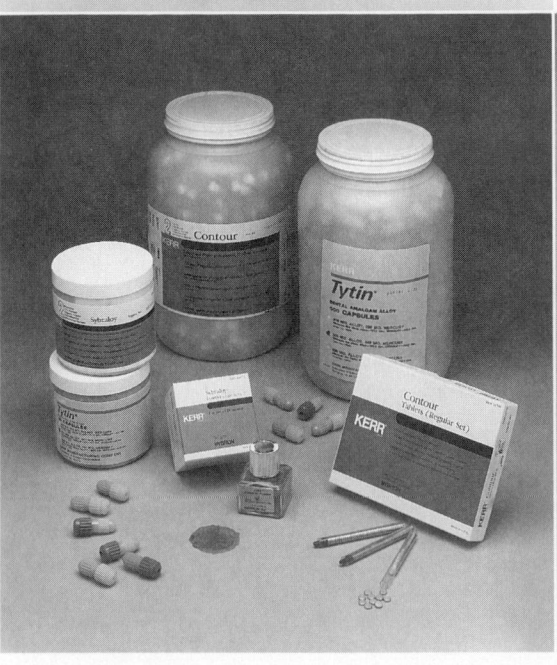

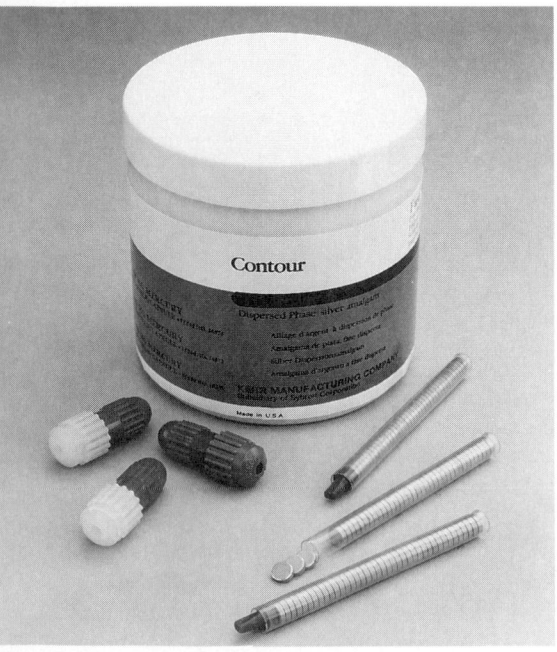

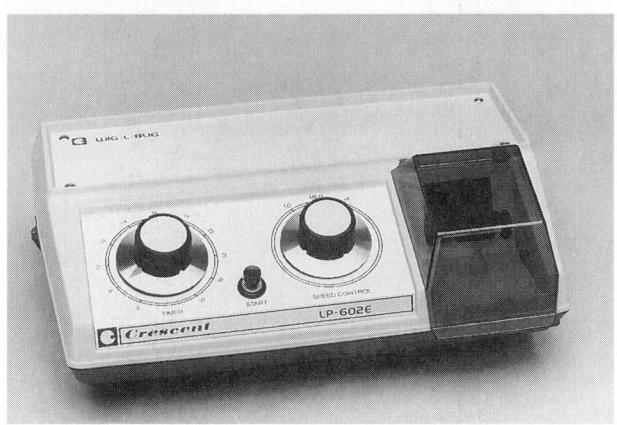

FIG. 11-24   Amalgamator with protective lid; timer and speed control.

(Courtesy of Crescent Dental Manufacturing Company, St. Lyons, Illinois.)

▶ Properties

The specific characteristics of the properties of dental materials were discussed earlier in this chapter. Amalgam displays many of the clinical properties addressed earlier. Amalgam undergoes dimensional change, specifically contraction and expansion, which is controlled by the techniques used during manipulation. An excess or incorrect trituration results in unwanted dimensional change. Contraction or expansion beyond the American National Standards Institute and the American Dental Association (ANSI-ADA) specifications may result in an amalgam restoration that pulls away from the margins of a cavity preparation. This situation may cause leakage to occur, or the amalgam may create sensitivity in a tooth. If expansion occurs, the amalgam may extend beyond the margins of the preparation.

Another dimensional change of concern with dental amalgam is creep, the change that takes place when the material is subjected to a constant load. Normal masti-

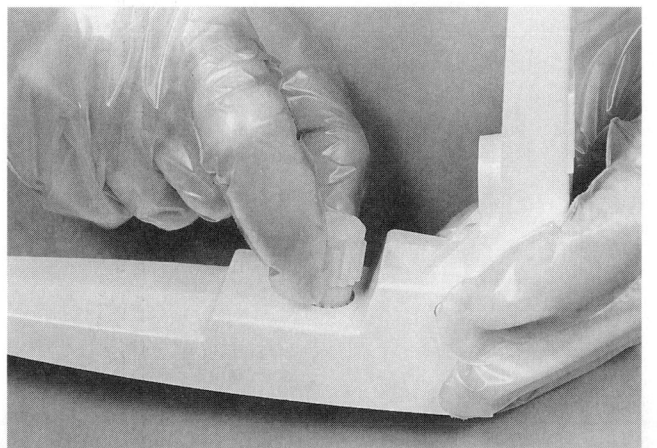

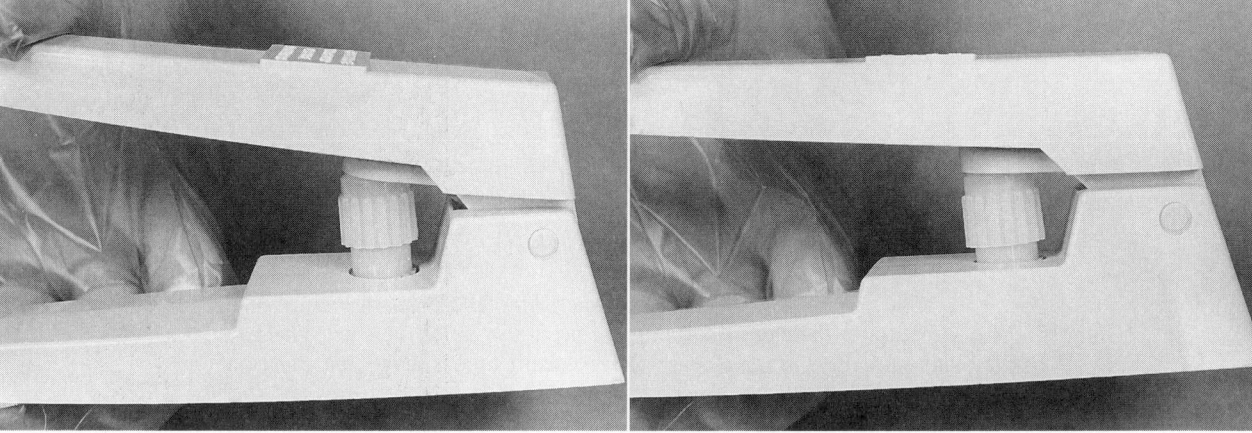

FIG. 11-25   *A,* The preproportioned capsule is selected and placed in the capsule activator with overgloved hands. *B,* The acitivator handle is compressed over the capsule to break the diaphragm that separates the alloy and the mercury. *C,* The compressed capsule compared to the one that is not yet compressed in Fig. 11-25, *B.*

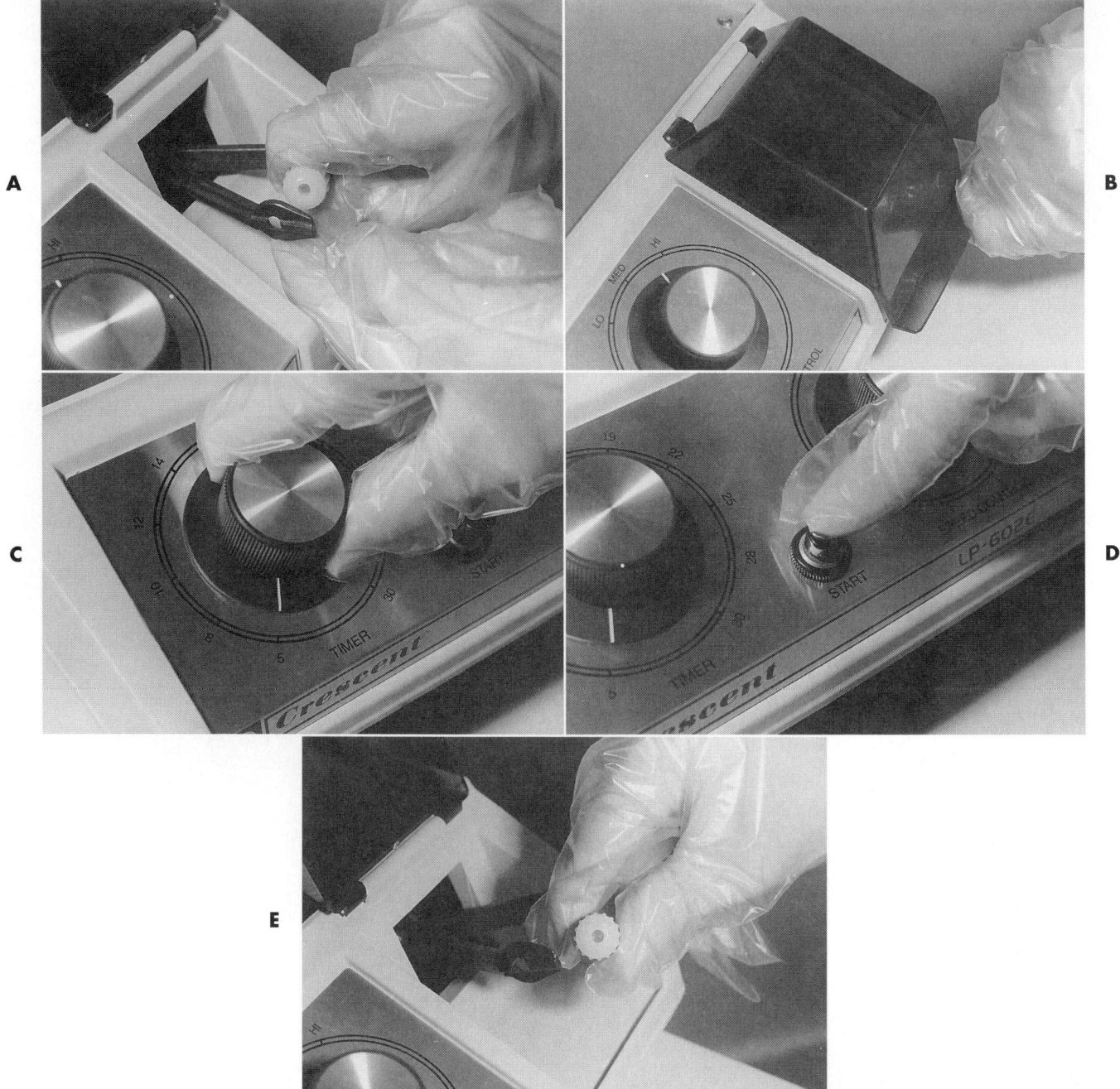

FIG. 11-26   *A,* Overgloves are kept over the treatment gloves, and the activated capsule is positioned in the armature of the amalgamator. *B,* The protective lid of the amalgamator is closed to avoid any mishaps with the capsule. *C,* The correct time is set on the amalgamator for the number of spills to be mixed. The speed control is positioned correctly, and *D,* the start button is depressed to begin amalgamation. *E,* After the amalgam is mixed, the capsule is removed from the amalgamator.

cation results in such a load force being applied to surfaces.

The strength of amalgam is affected by the three gamma phases being present in the correct configuration. The presence of voids created because of inadequate condensation decreases the strength potential of the restorative material. Thus the manipulation techniques employed during the placement of the amalgam restoration are extremely important. The compressive strength of the newer admixed and spherical high copper alloys is generally greater than that of the low copper alloys, spherical or comminuted.

Generally, the strength of amalgam alone is not adequate to withstand the forces applied during mastication. Thus, whenever possible, when an amalgam restoration is placed, the preparation should be designed so the remaining tooth structure sustains the forces rather than the amalgam.

As discussed previously, glass ionomer restorative materials are used in restorative dentistry. Glass ionomers containing silver alloys are often used in core buildups.

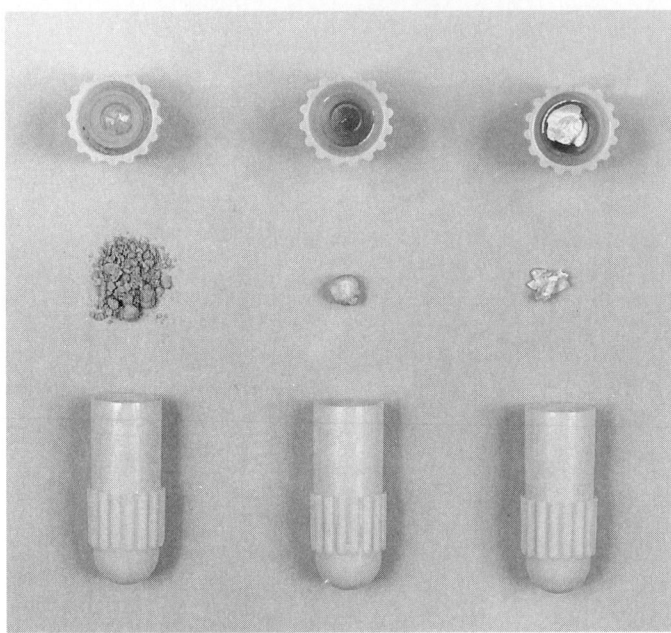

FIG. 11-27   Illustration of undermixed, correctly mixed, and overmixed amalgam.

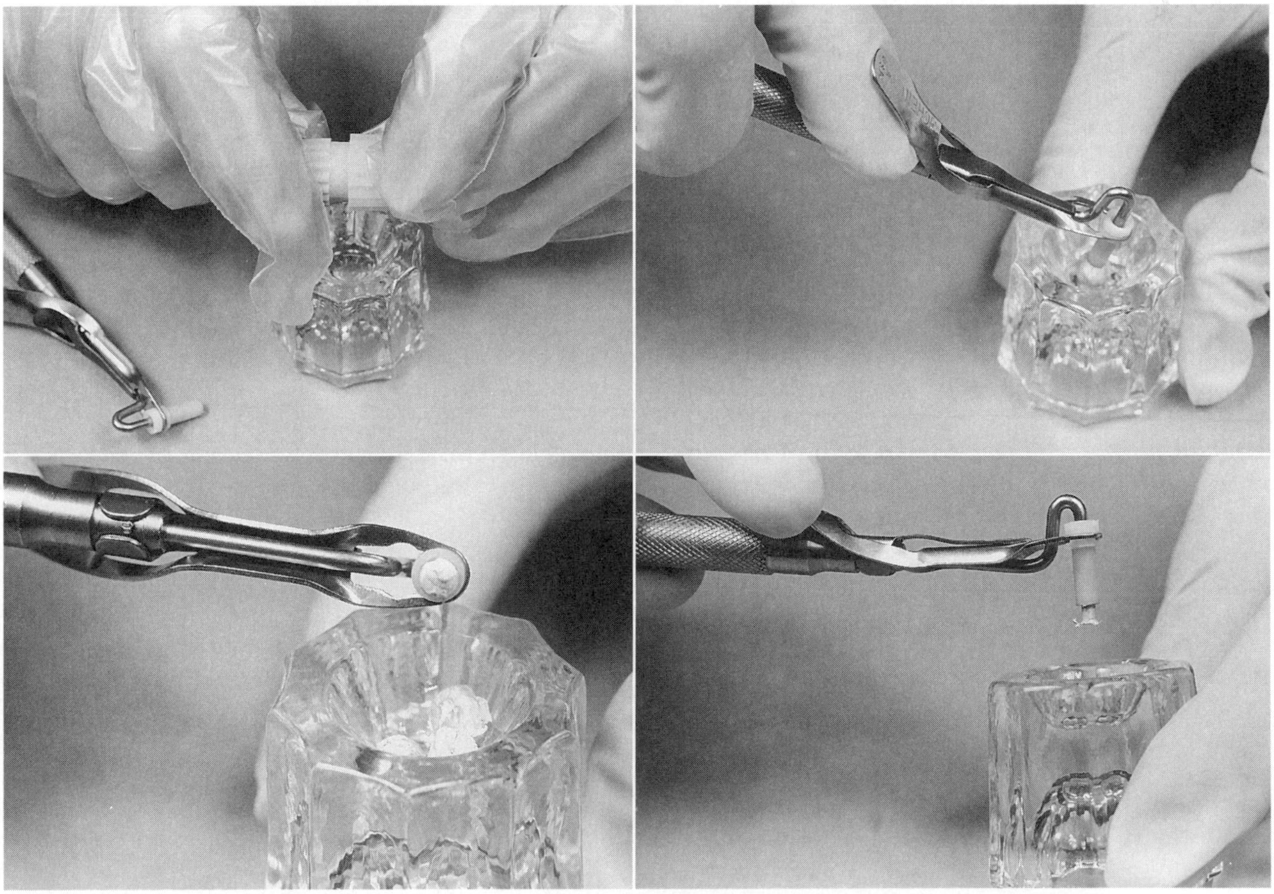

FIG. 11-28   *A,* The amalgam capsule is opened, and the amalgam is placed in a Dappen dish. *B,* The amalgam carrier is loaded while the finger is positioned under the lever of the carrier. *C,* Looking in the opening of the amalgam carrier it can be seen to be completely filled with amalgam. *D,* Excess amalgam must be completely removed from the carrier before it hardens.

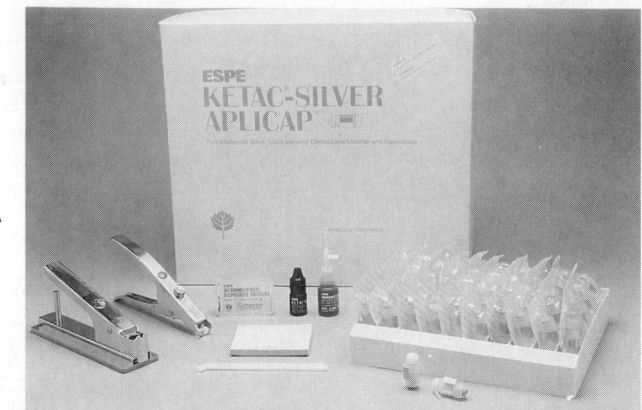

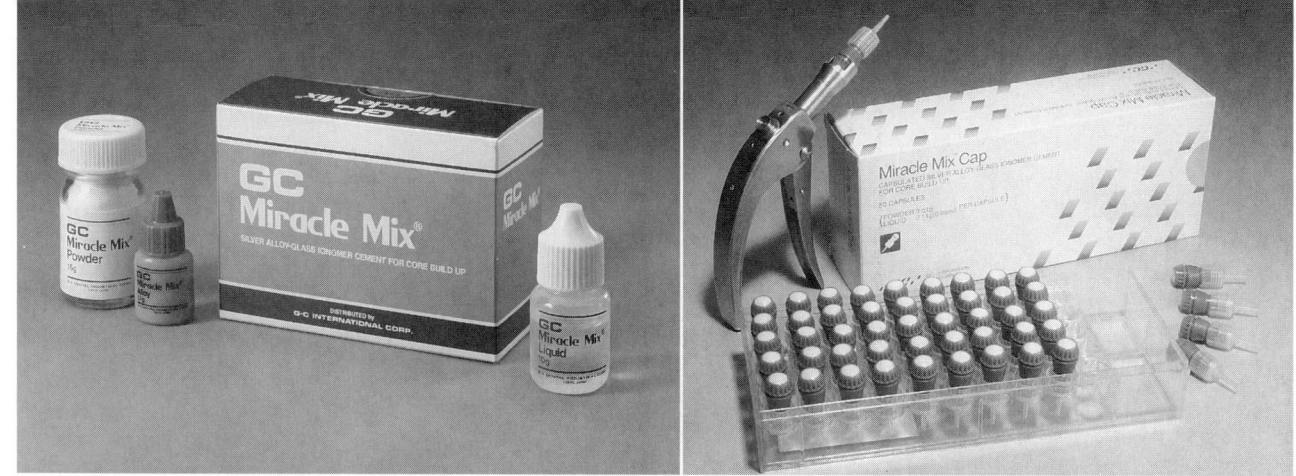

FIG. 11-29   *A* through *C,* Example of glass ionomers, with silver alloy for core build-up, and restorative material.

(*A,* Courtesy of Premier Dental Company, Morristown, Pennsylvania. *B* and *C,* Courtesy of GC International, Scottsdale, Arizona.)

A core is the buildup of tooth structure lost to carious activity or trauma to approximate the original tooth shape. The core is often covered by a cast restoration to maintain the integrity of the remaining tooth. Fig. 11-29, *A* and *B*, shows examples of various glass ionomers used for this purpose. Box 11-5 lists several different dental alloys.

Direct Esthetic Materials

Amalgam as a direct restorative material and in a plastic state can be placed and formed in a cavity preparation. Amalgam meets the needs of many patients, but does not meet the needs of a patient who requires an esthetic restoration, particularly in the anterior segment of the mouth. Esthetic restorative materials that are plastic, such as composite, and are placed in a single appointment reduce the cost of a restoration for a patient and eliminate time necessary to achieve esthetics with multiple treatment appointments, as with laminates or full-coverage restorations.

Throughout dental history the practitioner has tried to meet the patient's esthetic needs, which, during an ancient Egyptian era, meant the placement of precious gems in teeth. Today cosmetic dentistry plays a significant role in the type of dentistry provided to patients. The type and quality of esthetic restorative material have changed, and we are exposed almost daily to new and improved materials.

In past years, silicates and acrylic polymers were used as esthetic restorative materials and provided the groundwork for the more commonly used materials of today, specifically dimethacrylate polymers and ionomers. Silicates were used from the late 1800s until the 1970s. These material were highly soluble and discolored easily, resulting in restorations that deteriorated when exposed to invasive elements. Acrylic polymers with ceramic fillers provided reinforced capabilities and became popular as silicates were disappearing from use. As direct esthetic restorative materials, acrylic polymers were thought to be superior. But as time passed other undesirable characteristics appeared. Dimensional

COMMON BRAND NAMES OF DENTAL ALLOY

Contour
Dispersed Phase Alloy
Dispersalloy
Formula-T
Optaloy II
Permite-C
SDI Logic
SDI Permite
Sybraloy
Ternalloy
Tytin
Unison
Valiant Sure

changes occurred during the setting process, and as temperature changes took place in the mouth, percolation occurred at the margins. The dimensional change, lack of resistance to wear, and poor shade stability were compounded as recurrent decay occurred at the margins.

▶ Properties of Composite Materials

The physical and mechanical properties affecting the use of composites include some similar to the amalgam restorative material: compressive and tensile strength, thermal conductivity, hardness, and wear. Composites, however, differ in the polymerization shrinkage, water sorption, radiopacity, and coefficient of thermal expansion. Certain new hybrids or blends of composite materials provide many positive characteristics of each of these materials into one product.

The advantages of composites include the following:

▶ Development of the smaller particle (microfilled) resins has increased the compressive strength of the material.

▶ Thermal conductivity of these materials is lower because of the organic matrix that provides a thermal insulator.

▶ Increased quantity of fillers in composite restorative materials increases the hardness of the material, as well as increasing wear resistance and abrasion.

An important factor to consider when working with composite restorative materials is the polymerization shrinkage, caused by the high density of polymer formed around the oligomer. A plastic such as composite material is made up of monomers, a molecule of one part, and polymers, many parts. If a polymer is made of more than one type of monomers, it is called a copolymer. As the material polymerizes or begins to set, it shrinks and pulls away from the tooth structure, leaving an open margin where leakage occurs. A means of reducing polymerization shrinkage with the light-initiated composites is to place the material in the preparation in thin layers. A second method involves the development of a composite inlay on the prepared tooth or on a die, heated outside the mouth to allow for polymerization and to make the inlay more resistant to wear. After polymerization the inlay is cemented in place as with any other form of inlay.

As polymerization shrinkage affects the margin integrity of a composite, so does water sorption. The microfilled composites with a higher percentage of organic matrix are found to absorb more water than the conventional or fine particle composites. The absorbed water increases the potential for discoloration from water-soluble stains and the swelling of the composite in the preparation.

Radiopacity is caused by the existence of certain elements in the composite, such as barium, bromine, iodine, sirconium, strontium, zinc, and zirconium. Those composites that have any of these elements will have radiopacity, while those with any of the other fillers will not attenuate radiation. This fact is important in knowing that not all composites appear radiopaque on dental radiographs.

The coefficient of thermal expansion is another important factor determining the potential for marginal leakage of a composite restoration. The composite with a greater amount of organic matrix in the overall content exhibits a greater coefficient of thermal expansion.

▶ Polymer Dimethacrylates

Polymer dimethacrylates are composite or filled resin materials. The fillers are inorganic materials such as quartz, borosilicate glass, lithium aluminum silicate, barium aluminum silicate or barium fluoride, strontium, or zinc glasses. Each of these fillers is available in varying sizes: fine, irregularly shaped particles, microfine particles, and blends of the fine and microfine particle sizes. The filler material bonds with the matrix of an organic base, an oligomer, dimethacrylate or BIS-GMA, or urethane dimethacrylate (UDMA), making viscous liquids. Varying amounts and colors of inorganic pigments are added to provide diverse shade choice. These pigments range in shades and intensity from yellow to gray to white, opaque and translucent, to cover the spectrum of tooth colorings.

▶ Glass Ionomer Restorative Materials

The ionomer restorative materials are relatively new to dentistry as compared to amalgam as a restorative material. The use of ionomers has become more accepted and widespread as the application has become more diverse. As previously discussed in the dental cement segment of this chapter, glass ionomers are widely used as bases and luting agents in restorative dentistry. Ionomers are also used to restore particularly cervically eroded surfaces on teeth.

Ionomers are manufactured as a selection of shades of powder with a liquid. The powder consists of an aluminosilicate glass and is combined with a liquid of water, polymers, and copolymers of acrylic acid. In some instances certain products will have silver particles and fluoride ions added to this material. Glass ionomers have certain properties and improved characteristics: they bond to enamel and dentin, release fluoride ions into surrounding tooth structure, are biologically compatible and radiopaque, and the surfaces can be etched so that composites can be mechanically bonded to them.

Ionomer restorations have properties that are desirable in a restoration: the retention of ionomers in cervical areas is greater than that of composites, the composition of the material is similar to dentin and it bonds well to dentin, and the thermal coefficient of expansion is similar to dentin.

An important factor in the success of a glass ionomer restorative material is proper manipulation. Isolation techniques are inherently important to protect the material from saliva contamination, which results in a defective restoration. The manufacturer also recommends delaying final finishing and polishing for 1 day to achieve the ideal restoration.

▶ Manipulation

Manipulation and placement of glass ionomer restorative material is similar to the procedures with glass ionomer cement that are discussed earlier in this chapter. Composite packaging systems require different manipulation according to manufacturer's directions. These are discussed here.

▶ Packaging Systems

Initially most brands of composite restorative materials were autopolymerizing and packaged as two-paste systems or powder and liquid. Some are still found in this latter form. However, more common today is a single-paste, light-cure system with the composite in light-protected syringes or compules.

The two-paste system is contained in two jars, each of which includes 50% BIS-GMA and inorganic filler. The difference in the jars is that one contains the catalyst, a benzoyl peroxide initiator, and the other includes an organic amine accelerator. An equal amount of each is dispensed on a paper pad and mixed until homogeneous. The combination of the two pastes initiates the setting process, or polymerization (Fig. 11-30). The system may also be used with an acid etchant for preparing enamel

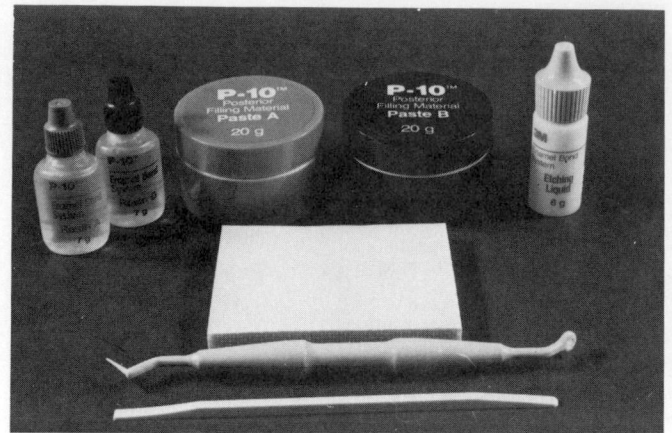

FIG. 11-30   Example of two-paste composite restorative materials.

(From Craig RG et al: *Dental materials,* ed 5, St Louis, 1992, Mosby.)

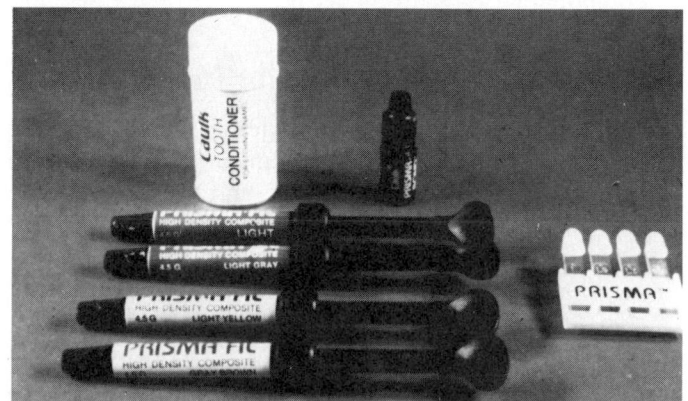

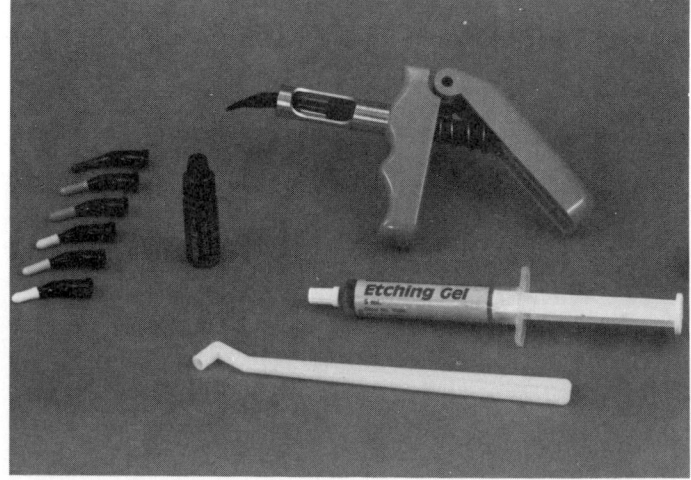

FIG. 11-31   *A* and *B,* Examples of single-paste composite restorative material.

(From Craig RG et al: *Dental materials,* ed 5, St Louis, 1992 Mosby.)

surfaces and a bonding agent for enamel and/or dentin to aid in the retention of the restoration.

The single-paste system that is photopolymerizing or photocuring is packaged by the manufacturer so that all the elements of the material are combined in a single dispensing device (Fig. 11-31). Again these materials are available in various shades to meet patient needs. The syringe compules have colored tips that correspond to the color of the material, while the material in the syringes is identified on an outside label. After the tooth is prepared, etched, and bonded, the desired amount of material is dispensed, placed in the preparation, and polymerized with a visible light unit.

▶ Plastics

Although some of the dental materials discussed previously in this chapter are referred to as plastics, this section will address plastics that are used predominantly in prosthetics. The types of plastics most common to dentistry are acrylic and rubber-reinforced acrylic. For the most part, acrylic plastic has been found to have greater use in dentistry because of the diverse properties

A

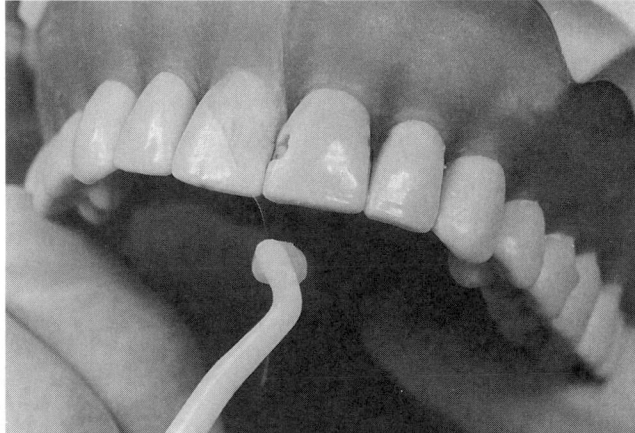

B

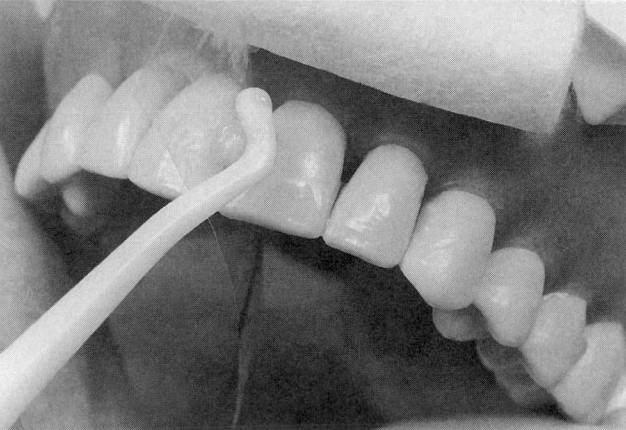

FIG. 11-32   *A* and *B,* Placement of composite with a Teflon plastic instrument.

TWO-PASTE COMPOSITE

USE

Esthetic restoration for Class I, III, IV, and certain Class V cavity preparations

FACTORS TO BE CONSIDERED

▶ The paste in the two jars should be stirred before use, since settling of the material may occur
▶ When using disposable mixing sticks, take care to use the opposite ends in each jar so as not to introduce the materials together, which may result in a chemical reaction
▶ Avoid contact of metal instruments with composite material because they may discolor the material

ARMAMENTARIUM

Two-paste system kit with material, disposable mixing stick, and plastic pad (If a paper pad is used, take care to avoid contamination of the pad)
NOTE: Acid etching and bonding material may be used in this or in the one-paste system; the technique and placement are discussed in Chapter 28, *Composites*
Placement instrument (e.g., Teflon plastic instrument or composite syringe with tip and plunger)

MANIPULATION

1. Perform shade selection.
2. Open jar containing the initiator, stir with the mixing stick, and dispense approximately one half of the size of the restoration.
3. Open the other jar, mix the material with the opposite end of the mixing stick, and dispense the same amount of material on the pad.
4. If the universal shade needs to be adjusted for the patient, combine the tinted material with the universal shade before it is mixed with the initiator.
5. Mix both materials for approximately 20 to 30 seconds, until the mix is homogeneous and the colors of the material are consistent.
6. The working time of the material is approximately 1 to 1 ½ minutes for mixing and insertion into the cavity preparation.
7. Either place the material by hand with an insertion instrument or with a composite syringe, which reduces the incidence of voids during insertion (Fig. 11-32).
8. Dispense a small amount of the material to be held between your fingers to simulate the heat generated in the oral cavity. This provides the operator with a guide to indicate when the material has reached a final set.
9. The material is set in approximately 5 minutes from initial mix. At this time complete the finishing and polishing steps.

CLEANING DIRECTIONS

Easily remove the material from the instruments before reaching a final set by use of a 2 × 2 gauze.

SINGLE-PASTE SYSTEM

USE

Same as for the two-paste system for esthetic restorations

FACTORS TO BE CONSIDERED

- Light sensitive; should only be dispensed as the material is used
- Visible light source is through a fiberoptic bundle or a fluid hose that emits an intense white or blue light that can damage the retina
- The team should wear protective eyewear and/or have shields on the light source or handheld, as seen in Fig. 11-33

ARMAMENTARIUM

Single-paste system

- Acid etching and bonding materials
- Shade guide buttons
- Visible light source
- Plastic placement instrument
- Protective eyewear (team and possibly patient)

MANIPULATION

1. In natural light, select the shade.
2. Perform the acid etch and bonding steps.
3. Dispense the selected shade from the syringe on a plastic slab or place the shade compule in the composite syringe.
4. Do not use the placement instrument to remove composite and place it on the tooth and then remove more material from the syringe. This action contaminates the material in the syringe.
5. If a compule is the source of the composite, it is intended for a single use only.
6. Place the material on the tooth and contour.
7. Hold the visible light source approximately 2 to 3 mm for 20 to 60 seconds. The time is determined by the light source unit, manufacturer's direction for the material, and the thickness of the composite material. Note that microfilled composites necessitate a greater period of exposure time compared to the fine particle
   composite, since the filler particles scatter the light more easily.
8. Check composite material for complete set and then complete the finishing process.

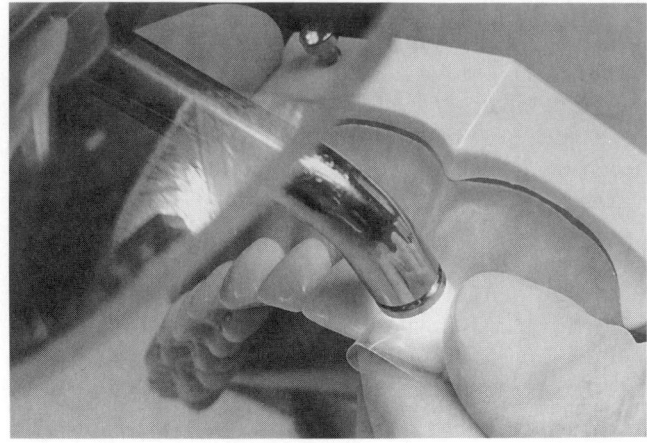

FIG. 11-33   Protective light shield on wand used during curing of light-activated plastics.

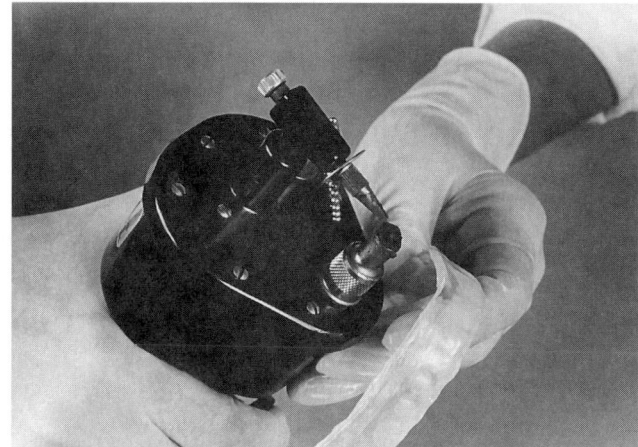

FIG. 11-34   Vinyl mouthguard material formed on model.

Usually the plastic used for the construction of denture bases is heat cured, while the material used for the other applications is self-cured plastic. As a heat-cured plastic the material has to be placed under pressure with heat to initiate polymerization. A self-cured, cold-cured, or chemically cured plastic begins to polymerize when the monomer and polymer are combined. As polymerization occurs, heat is released in an exothermic reaction. If an excess of heat is released during polymerization, the monomer, which has a high vapor pressure, can create porosity through the vaporization of the monomer. This factor makes it important to follow manufacturer's directions to avoid inconsistent mixtures of material, which may result in ill-fitting appliances and devices. In certain conditions, cross-linked polymers (high molecular weight polymers) may not be desirable as they tend to crack and craze in the mouth.

possible from soft and flexible to harder and more brittle (Fig. 11-34). These acrylic plastics are used to fabricate denture bases, temporary crowns and bridges, custom acrylic impression trays, and orthodontics appliances (Fig. 11-35, *A* through *E*).

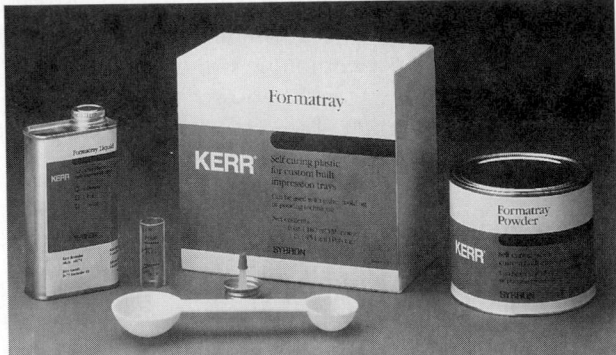

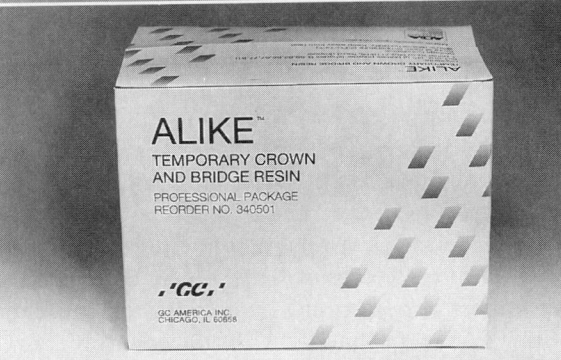

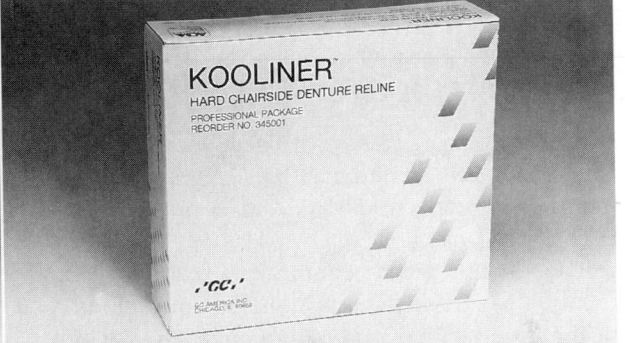

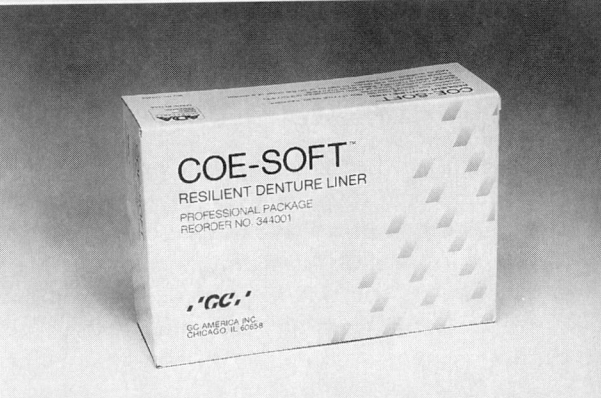

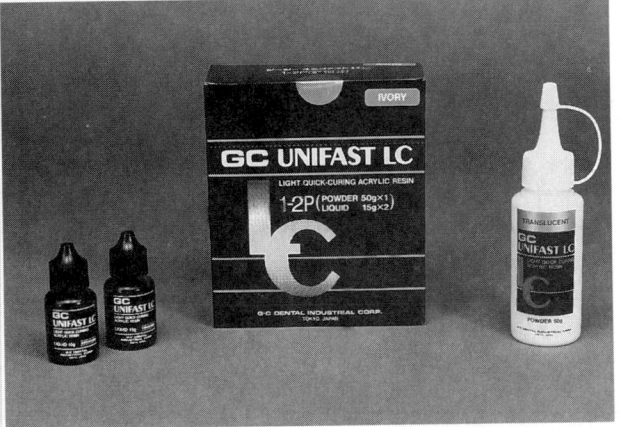

FIG. 11-35 *A* through *E*, Examples of various types of plastic acrylics used for temporary crowns and bridges, custom acrylic trays, and denture reline material.

(*A*, Courtesy of Kerr/Sybron Manufacturing, Romulus, Michigan. *B* and *E*, Courtesy of GC International, Scottsdale, Arizona.)

BOX 11-6

COMMON BRAND NAMES OF COMPOSITE AND IONOMER FILLING MATERIAL

COMPOSITE

Adaptic
Adaptic II
Centrix C-R
Command
Compolite
Compolite II
Composite
Concise
Coreform
Durafill
Durafill VS
Esthetic Design System
Estilux Posterior
Finesse

Fluorocore
Ful-Fil
Ful-Fil Sure-Pac
Heliobond
Heliolink
Heliomolar/Cavifil
Helio Progress
Heliocolor Progress
Herculite
Herculite XR
Isopast
Light Activated
Restorative
Love
Mastique

Microfil Composite
Miracle Mix
Miradapt
Natural Composite
Occlusin
Opalux
Pekalux PLT's
Posterior Light Cure Filling
Material
Prisma A.P.H
Profile/TLC
Silar
Silux Plus
Super C Composite

Valux
Visio-Dispers
Visio-Fil
Visio-Molar
Wunderfil

IONOMER

Chem-Fil II
Core Build-up Material
Fuji Glass Ionomer Type II
Glassic F
Glass Ionomer 6/2
Glass Ionomer 3/3
Ketac-Fil

The addition of compounds, such as oily organic esters, that do not interact with polymerization can improve the resistance to fracture of the acrylic plastics. However, these compounds can leach out over time as a result of using denture cleansers and other drying agents.

VINYL PLASTICS

Vinyl plastic is used in the construction of protective mouthguards and is composed of copolymers of vinyl acetate and ethylene. Other applications include usage as fluoride trays and other flexible appliances.

DENTURE BASE ACRYLIC PLASTICS

Most denture base acrylic plastics are heat accelerated; a few are chemically accelerated materials. The product is usually found in a powder and liquid, but is produced in gels, sheets, and blanks.

The powder of this plastic comprises predominantly polymer with peroxide that assists in the polymerization. These are combined with other components that provide translucency and color to allow for a plastic that resembles the patient's own tissue color for the denture base.

The majority of the liquid is monomer with hydroquinone, an inhibitor that retards any polymerization activity of the liquid during storage. Polymerization can occur through exposure to ultraviolet light, so the liquid must be packaged in light-resistant containers. The liquid may also contain a cross-linking agent to reduce cracks or crazing and an organic accelerator if the material is chemically accelerated.

The steps and techniques used in the fabrication of a denture base are varied and individual. The fabrication through the use of a dough-molding technique, considered one of the most common, will be described. It is helpful for the dental assistant to understand other techniques, so further research in specialized dental materials textbooks is advisable.

SOFT LINERS

The development and use of soft liners has been to aid the patient with residual alveolar ridge changes that cause ill-fitting dentures, which are uncomfortable and can irritate the tissue under the denture. Other uses include tissue treatment after surgery and obturators for defects in the palate.

Soft liners are either acrylic copolymers with plasticizers or copolymers. These acrylics can be processed through heat or at room temperature situations. Commercial over-the-counter materials are available for patients to perform home relining of dentures. As patients receive denture education, they should also be told the disadvantages of performing home relining. These materials may pose problems with the denture acrylic, resulting in further difficulties with the denture and possible problems with the oral structures.

PLASTIC DENTURE TEETH

Denture teeth may be made of plastic or porcelain; each has advantages and disadvantages. Plastic teeth have a greater resistance to breakage, create less noise during occlusion, and are easily brought to a comfortable finish after the grinding and polishing needed for adjustment takes place. Plastic teeth are also softer than porcelain teeth and are more susceptible to abrasion. Porcelain

---

STEP-BY-STEP PROCEDURE
DENTURE BASE FABRICATION USING
DOUGH-MOLDING TECHNIQUE

1. Introduce three parts powder to one part liquid, using a mixing jar that is closed.
2. Allow the material to stand. The solution step occurs as the materials now change from a gritty consistency to a doughy consistency.
3. Check the material to determine whether the solution process is complete (when the material can be separated by a wooden stick without flowing together again).
4. Place this material into a denture mold in a denture flask.
5. Construct a denture mold as discussed in depth in Chapter 31.

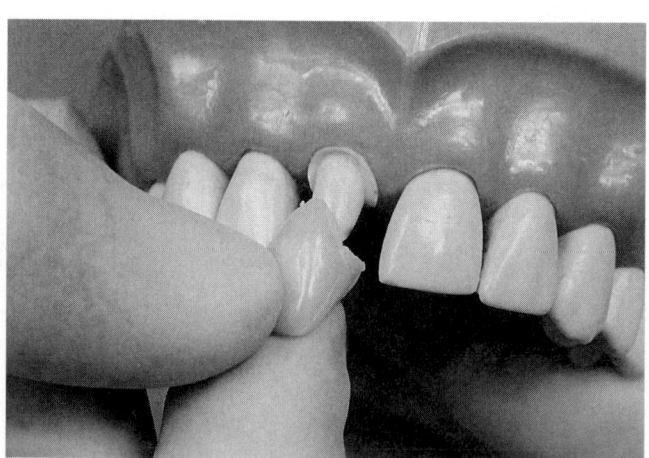

FIG. 11-36   Homogeneous mass of acrylic ready-to-use in the fabrication of a temporary restoration.

teeth are less able to accommodate the stress involved during occlusion.

Denture teeth made of plastic consist of acrylic and modified acrylic polymers. The material is similar to that of the denture base acrylic other than the difference in pigments placed in the acrylic. The density, color, translucency, and varying shade from the incisal edge to the cervical area can be controlled with the use of the pigments. A cross-linked polymer of greater strength is often used on the occlusal portion of the teeth to provide more resistance to force.

Plastic teeth are most often used where denture teeth oppose natural teeth, for patients with less than adequate ridge mass, and in areas where only low stress forces are applied. Porcelain teeth are usually preferred in areas where less stress is placed. This type of denture tooth is not usually placed to oppose natural tooth structure.

PLASTICS IN TEMPORARY CROWNS AND BRIDGES

Acrylics are also a common form of plastic used in the fabrication of crowns, bridges, and inlays. The acrylic polymer with the inert filler provides accurate and reliable reproductions of the plastic to act as a temporary or a provisional restoration until a permanent restoration is placed (Fig. 11-36).

The acrylic consists of a liquid and powder that are mixed into a homogeneous creamy mass that becomes rubbery in a few minutes. Acceleration of the polymerization can be accomplished through placement of the material in warm water. The step-by-step procedure for the fabrication of temporary restorations is described in Chapter 32.

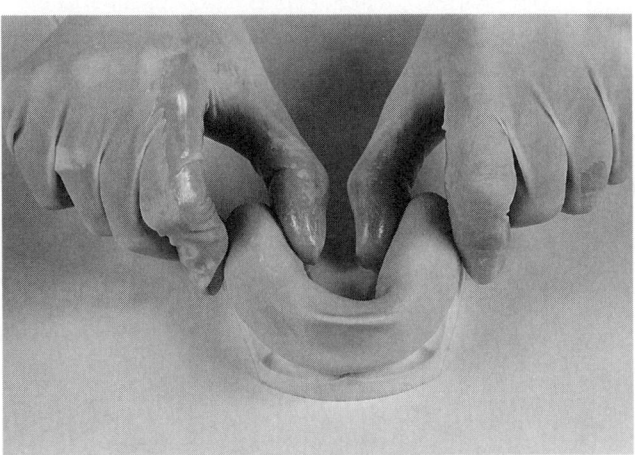

FIG. 11-37   Custom acrylic tray.

IMPRESSION TRAY PLASTIC

Acrylic with filler is necessary to fabricate rigid custom impression trays. The acrylic is manipulated in a fashion similar to that of the acrylic used in temporary restorations. The manufacturer's directions are followed, mixing the required amounts of powder and liquid together until there is a homogeneous mass. The material can be manipulated when the mix is divided with a wooden stick and does not flow together and when it has lost the glossy look it had when first mixed. The specific fabrication of impression trays is addressed in Chapter 40 (Fig. 11-37). Box 11-7 lists various plastic products.

Indirect Restorative Dental Materials

Indirect and adjunct restorative dental materials are used to fabricate a restoration or prosthesis outside the oral cavity. This restoration or prosthesis is placed in the

---

BOX 11-7

COMMON BRAND NAMES OF ACRYLICS/PLASTICS

Alike	Orthocryl
Coe-Comfort	Orthodontic Resin
Coe-Rect	Ortho-Jet
Coe-Soft	Perm
Coe Tray Plastic	Protemp
Cyano-Veneer	Recon
Denture Acrylic	Repair Material
Dura-Base	Reprodent
Duraloy	Repro-Therm
Duz-All	Rimseal
Fastcure	Silanit
Fastray	Snap
F-I-T	Softone
Flexacryl	Tab
Formatray	Tempo Cushion Treatment
4-Most	Temporary Bridge Resin
Grab	Tissue Conditioner
Hydrocryl	Total
Hygon	Tramix
Immediate	Tray Acrylic Material
Jet	Tray Mix Instant
Kooliner	Tray Resin
Lang's	Trim
Light Liner	Trim II
Lucitone	Tru-Kit
Lynal	Truliner
Minute Stain	Tru-Repair
Malloplast-B	Tru-Soft
	Viscogel Tissue Treatment

patient's mouth at a subsequent appointment. This category includes impression materials, waxes, gold, model and die materials, and porcelain.

FYI The first impression compound that could be softened in hot water and would harden when removed from the mouth was discovered by Charles Stent in 1857.

Impression Materials

Impression materials are used to reproduce, record, or register the relationship of the teeth and the oral conditions. Reproducing this relationship is usually a step in the process of providing a patient with a type of prosthesis or treatment as used in orthodontic care. The impression material is normally placed into an impression tray and then into the mouth while in its plastic stage. After setting to a rubbery stage, the tray, with the material still in place inside it, is removed from the mouth, providing a negative reproduction of the structure. The impression is then poured with a gypsum product in fluid form and allowed to harden to a set cast or model. The impression material is removed from the gypsum cast to expose a positive reproduction of the condition of the mouth. From this cast, orthodontic appliances, complete and partial dentures, cast restorations, temporary restorations, and temporary appliances are fabricated.

The different categories and physical properties of impression materials vary and provide today's operator with a plethora of options. Box 11-8 lists properties that encompass the ideals of an impression material.

Currently available are nine classifications of impression materials from rigid to flexible. A rigid impression material is used when undercuts or teeth in which the material can become trapped are absent: for a single prepared tooth or an edentulous impression. Flexible impression materials have more applications, including

reproductions of a single tooth, multiple teeth or a full mouth impression.

Rigid Impression Materials

The types of rigid impression materials commonly used are dental impression compound, impression plaster, and ZOE impression material.

▶ Dental Impression Compound

Dental compound is the common term used to describe all impression compounds regardless of purpose. However, dental impression compound, also known as impression compound, is manufactured in two types: tray compound and impression compound. Tray compound is supplied in cakes and is used as a preliminary impression and eventually as a tray to hold a final impression known as a corrective wash. The tray material does not provide an accurate impression of the tissue to fabricate a denture; thus a more accurate impression material is placed inside the dental compound and both are placed in the oral cavity to take a second impression (Fig. 11-38). The impression compound formed into a stick or cone may be used to obtain a final impression of a single tooth or for a *snap* impression that provides the operator an accurate assessment of margin definition and the draw of the prepared tooth.

▶ Properties

Dental compound is composed of 40% resins, 7% waxes, 3% organic acids, 50% fillers, and various coloring pigments. A unique characteristic of dental compound is its ability to be thermoplastic, meaning that it softens when heat is applied and rehardens as it cools.

BOX 11-8

CHARACTERISTICS OF IMPRESSION MATERIALS

1. Accuracy in clinical application
2. Ease in manipulation
3. Not toxic or irritating
4. Provides a pleasant odor, taste, and color
5. Economic
6. Provides dimensional stability
7. Maintains shelf life
8. Compatible with die and cast materials
9. Consistency in texture and wettability
10. Adequate mechanical strength to resist tearing or deforming

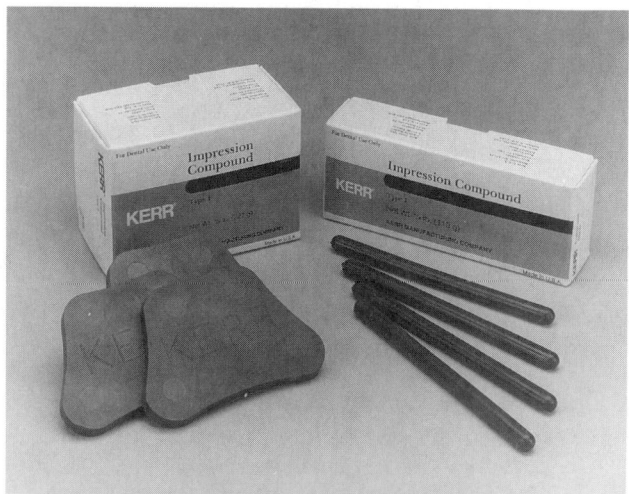

FIG. 11-38   Cake and stick impression compound.

(Courtesy of Kerr/Sybron Manufacturing, Romulus, Michigan.)

TABLE 11-2 ANSI-ADA SPECIFICATION NO. 3 OF DENTAL IMPRESSION COMPOUND

Compound	Flow	
	37° C	45° C
Impression (Type I)	Greater than 6%	Less than 85%
Tray (Type II)	Greater than 2%	70% to 85%

Dental compound is capable of flow at mouth temperature, which is approximately 37° C, but a temperature of 45° C is needed to obtain the flow that adequately records the tissues of the mouth. This temperature is not high enough to burn the oral tissues. The flow requirements of each of the materials is specified by the ANSI-ADA Specification No. 3 listed in Table 11-2. The higher flow requirement of the impression compound corresponds to the need to obtain an accurate final impression.

Dental compound is a poor thermal conductor that requires kneading during heating or cooling and adequate time to assure a uniform temperature is maintained throughout the material.

▶ Impression Plaster

Impression plaster (Type I gypsum) does not have the application it had in earlier dental practice to take impressions. The material is extremely rigid and fractures easily and could not be used in situations where undercuts existed. The material is used primarily to mount dental casts on articulators, since it sets quickly (3 to 5 minutes), although this has been modified by the introduction of inorganic salts.

▶ Zinc Oxide–Eugenol (ZOE) Impression Material

As with impression plaster, ZOE impression paste has been primarily replaced by rubber impression materials. The paste is packaged in two tubes, one containing zinc oxide, oils, and additives, while the other has eugenol, oils, resin, and additives. An equal amount of each of the contrasting colors of each tube is dispensed on an oil-resistant paper pad and mixed with a stiff spatula for 30 to 45 seconds, until there is a homogeneous mass. The mix is placed in a tray compound or an acrylic tray to obtain the impression. After the paste is mixed, it is

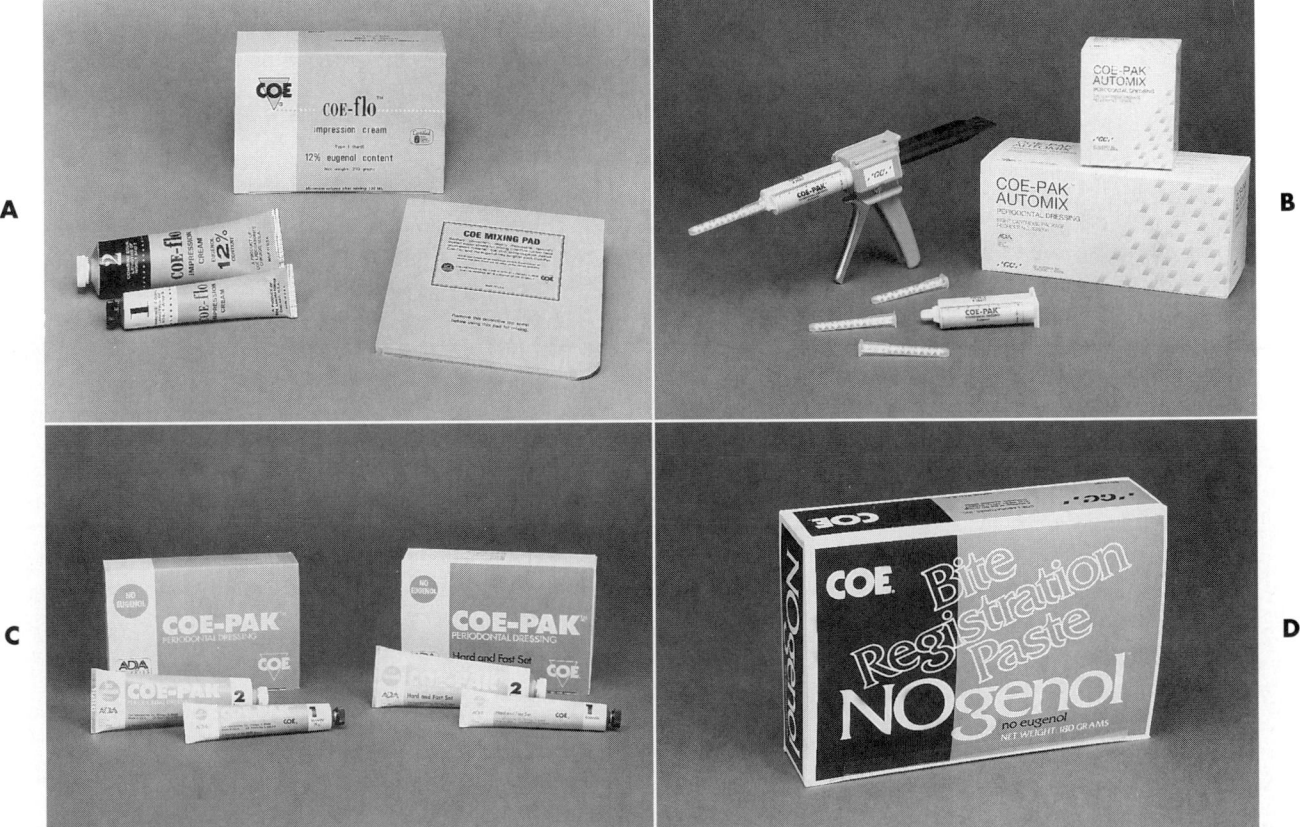

FIG. 11-39 *A through D,* Examples of several ZOE materials used as impression creams and periodontal dressings.

(Courtesy of COE/GC International, Scottsdale, Arizona.)

placed in an impression tray as a wash impression and then hardens to a brittle solid. The material sets in approximately 3 to 5 minutes (Fig. 11-39, A through C).

Alginate Impression Material

Alginate impression materials, also known as irreversible hydrocolloids, are probably used more often than any other single type of impression material in dentistry. Alginate materials are used to assist in the preparation of study models; in the fabrication of mouthguards, temporary restorations, orthodontic appliances, and custom impression trays; and as opposing models in fixed and removable prosthetics.

Reasons alginate impression materials are the materials of choice for these applications include the following:
  ▶ Low cost
  ▶ Easy to manipulate
  ▶ Flexibility in the set material
  ▶ Produces the necessary accuracy for the purpose

There are also disadvantages to the use of alginate impression material as follows:
  ▶ Susceptibility to atmospheric conditions
  ▶ Only used with gypsum products
  ▶ Provides limited definition of anatomy

Alginate material is a hydrocolloid, a colloid being a gluelike substance whose particles dispersed in a solvent (water) are somewhat uniform in distribution but fail to form a true solution. The powder of alginate contains sodium or potassium salt, calcium sulfate, sodium phosphate, diatomaceous earth or silicate powder, potassium sulfate or potassium zinc fluoride, organic glycol, and quaternary ammonium compounds. Key components to be aware of are the sodium phosphate,

---

ALGINATE

FACTORS TO BE CONSIDERED

▶ Susceptible to syneresis, so care must be taken to prevent dehydration of the impression by pouring it immediately

ARMAMENTARIUM

Flexible rubber bowl(s),
Broad-blade, flexible spatula
Alginate material
Water-measuring device
Powder-measuring device
Impression tray(s)

MANIPULATION

Supplied in bulk or in preproportioned packages of three measures of powder to be mixed with three measures of water.

For this example, alginate is in bulk form.

NOTE: Procedure for taking alginate impressions is discussed in Chapter 24, so the manipulation of the material alone will be reviewed in greater detail here.

1. Select and try-in maxillary and mandibular impression trays for accurate fit in the mouth.
2. Adjust the tray size with the use of wax ropes on the peripheral edge of the tray.
3. Mix the material for the mandibular impression first, which usually warrants the use of a smaller amount of water and powder than the maxillary tray.
4. Fill the water measure two-thirds full or to the second line on the device with room temperature water, as seen in Fig. 11-34, and place the water in a rubber bowl. (If hot water is used, the setting time is shortened.)
5. Fluff the powder to ensure that the powder has not settled, and carefully open the lid.
6. Dispense two even scoops of powder, slightly overfilling each and evened off with the spatula, in the second bowl, as seen in Fig. 11-40, A through C. (If the first scoop of powder is measured and placed in water as the second is readied, a reaction of the two can begin. Thus preparing all the powder before introduction to the water maintains the integrity of the mixture.)
7. Place the powder into the water rather than the reverse so that no powder is trapped in the bottom of the bowl, making manipulation more difficult.
8. Mix the two initially with a stirring action to wet all the powder crystals (Fig. 11-41, A through H).
9. Once the mixture is moistened, use a stropping action to continue mixing by placing the flat of the spatula into the material and working it around the bowl.
10. Turn the bowl in your hand to incorporate all the material in the mix, and use both sides of the spatula.
11. Mix for 1 minute for a normal-setting material and 30 to 45 seconds for fast-setting material, which results in a mixture that is homogeneous and creamy.
12. Bring the mass of material together and place in the impression tray.

NOTE: Proportions for a maxillary full arch impression would be a 3:3 ratio.

CLEANING DIRECTIONS

The material is easily wiped from the armamentarium before it has reached a final set.

If allowed to dry, remove by peeling or scraping it away.

which reacts with calcium ions, forming a calcium alginate and making the sodium phosphate a retardant. The calcium alginate that is formed when combined with water is called a hydrogel. Since this material cannot be transformed from this state once it has been reached, it is referred to as an irreversible hydrocolloid.

Agar Hydrocolloid Impression Material

As the first elastic impression material used in dentistry, agar hydrocolloid paved the way for newer and more efficient elastic materials to be developed. Agar hydrocolloid is also known as reversible hydrocolloid because of the material's ability to change from the gel to sol and back to the gel stage with minimal dimensional change. Even with this factor considered the time involved with the manipulation of the material, the special armamentarium, and the inability to be used with anything but gypsum dies have found more practitioners opting to use other elastic impression materials.

The syringe material is supplied in a syringe, syringe carpule, or cylinders in a jar, as seen in Fig. 11-42, while the tray material is in a collapsible tube. Each form of impression material contains agar; borax, for improved strength; potassium sulfate, to create a no-negative reaction situation, with gypsum products; benzoates, as preservatives; additives that aid flow of the material; flavoring; and water. Water, which is held in suspension by the agar gel, is the principal component of the impression material. As heat is applied, the suspension of agar and water is disturbed and the material becomes more fluid, going into the sol stage. As the hydrocolloid cools, it returns to the gel stage.

Since this material is currently not used to the extent it was in the past, the discussion of the armamentarium and manipulation will be dealt with differently than other materials in this chapter. To manipulate this material it is necessary to use a hydrocolloid conditioner with three separate temperature-controlled baths: a liquefying bath, a storage bath, and a tempering bath (Fig. 11-43). The tray material tube and the syringe material are placed in

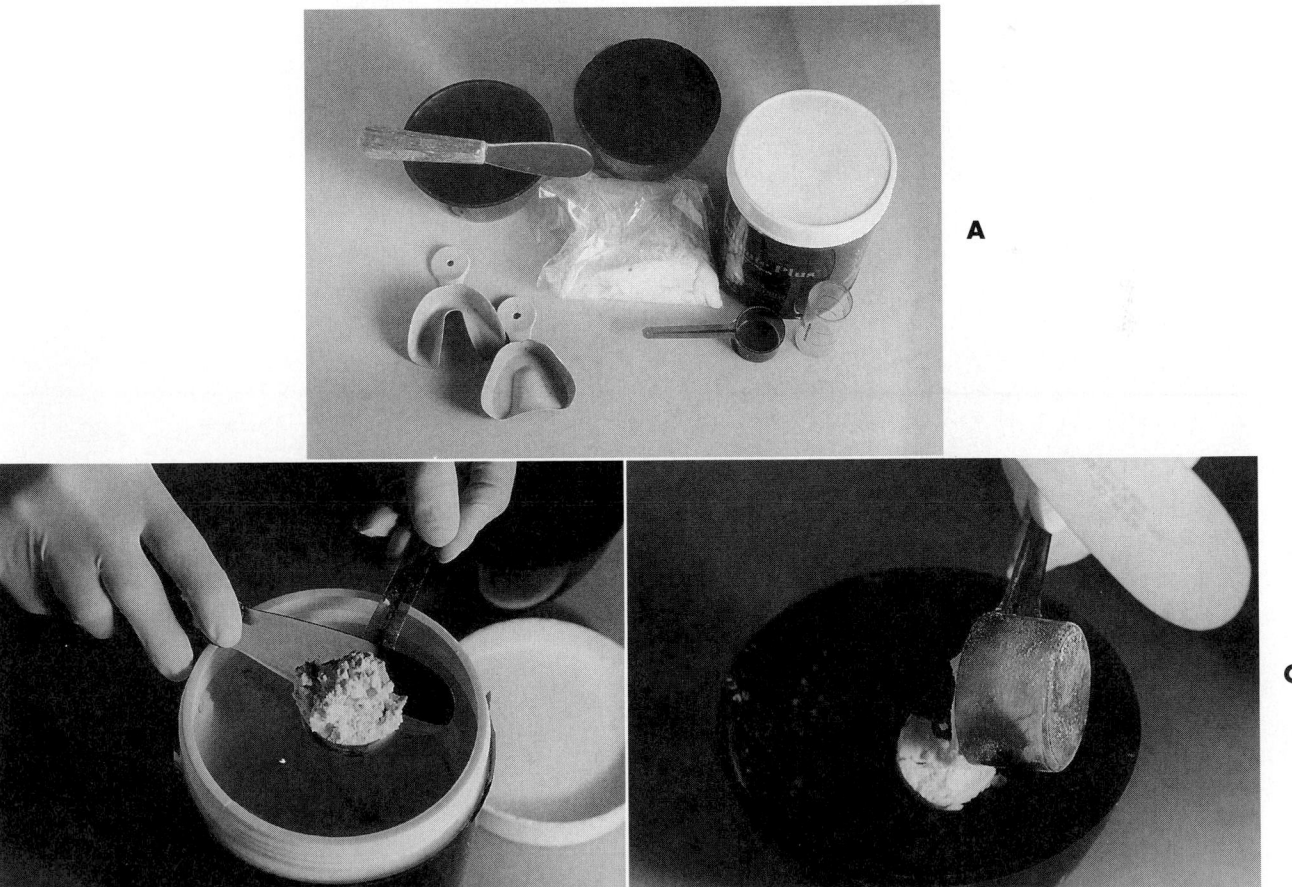

FIG. 11-40 *A,* The armamentarium for taking an alginate impression. *B,* Leveling off of scoops of alginate powder to ensure correct proportions. *C,* Dispensing powder into the water for mixing.

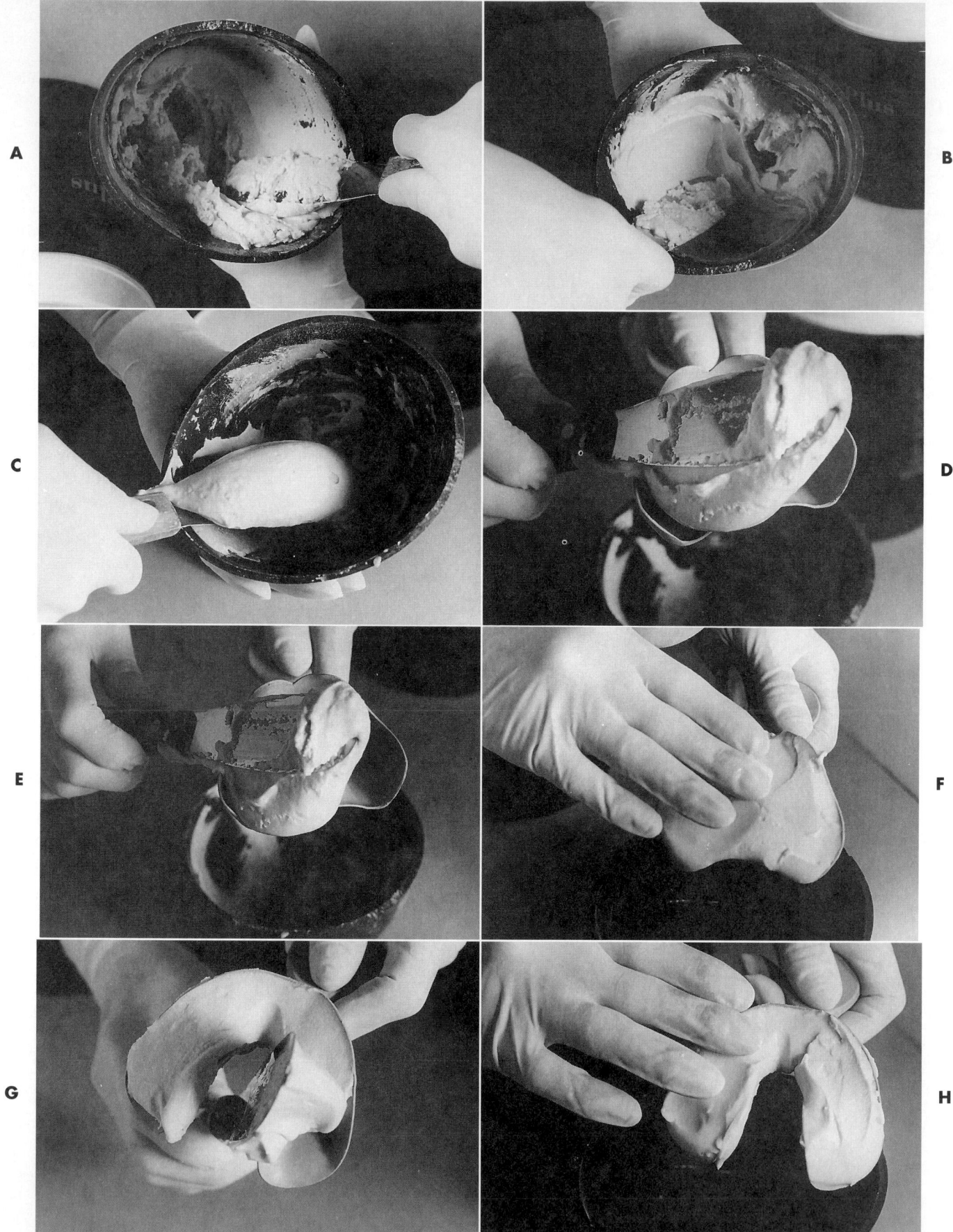

FIG. 11-41 For legend see opposite page.

◄ FIG. 11-41   *A,* The powder and water are incorporated. *B,* The mix becomes creamy. *C,* All the mass is lifted from the bowl with the spatula. *D,* The maxillary tray is loaded from one side across to the other side until the tray is full. *E,* Excess is removed from the posterior. The material is smoothed with wet fingers. *F,* The mandibular tray is filled similarly after another mixture of alginate is prepared. *G,* The material is loaded from one side of the tray to the other. *H,* When the tray is filled, the excess is removed from the tongue and posterior areas and smoothed with wet fingers.

FIG. 11-42   Agar syringe material.

(From Craig RG et al: *Dental materials,* ed 5, St Louis, 1992, Mosby.)

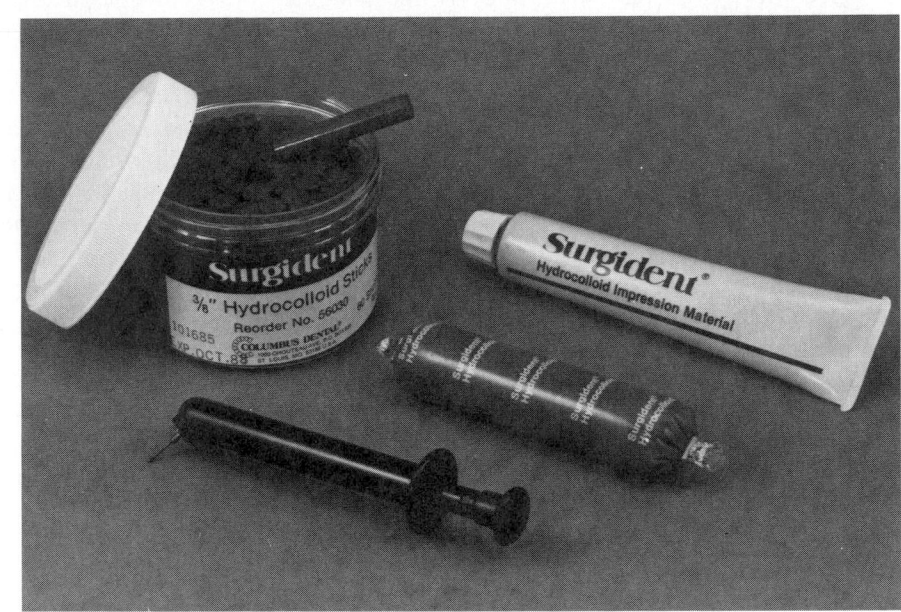

FIG. 11-43   Agar hydrocolloid conditioner.

(From Craig RG et al: *Dental materials,* ed 5, St Louis, 1992, Mosby.)

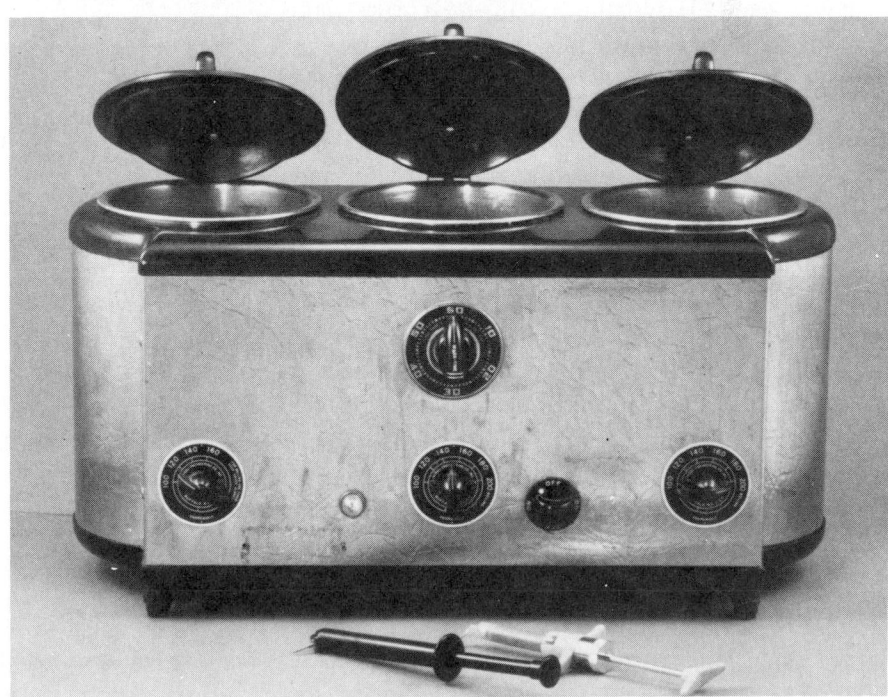

the liquefying bath of 100° C (212° F) for 10 to 15 minutes. The syringe material may also be boiled in water for 10 minutes and then placed in the storage bath, until it is ready for use. The materials reach the sol stage and are removed and placed in the storage bath of 60° to 66° C (140° to 150° F), which allows the material to remain in the sol stage for the length of time it is in the bath. Before the impression is taken the tray material tube is removed and squeezed into a water-cooled metal impression tray, then it is placed in the tempering bath with the syringe material to cool to 43° to 46° C (109° to 115° F) to avoid burning of the oral tissues.

Once the tray is tempered, the syringe material is removed and injected into the sulcus and around the preparation. The tray is removed, the outer skin that forms is removed, and the water hoses are connected. The operator places the tray in the mouth and water at 13° C (55° F) is turned on to flow through the hoses and tray to cool the material. It is also possible to spray water on the tray to assist in obtaining the return of the material to the gel stage. After the material has set or gelled, the impression is removed from the mouth, rinsed, and disinfected as described in Chapter 40. Storage of this material is not recommended; if storage is necessary, it should not exceed 1 hour in 100% relative humidity. This often will require in-office preparation of the die unless a professional laboratory is nearby.

Agar-Alginate Combination Impression

A technique using reversible and nonreversible hydrocolloid together is sometimes performed. This technique provides accuracy to the agar hydrocolloid throughout the anatomic portion of the impression and speed in manipulation of the alginate for the rest of the impression. The syringe hydrocolloid is prepared and placed on the tooth as in the hydrocolloid procedure, and the mixed alginate impression in a tray is positioned over it in the mouth. This combination gels the agar hydrocolloid quicker (3 to 4 minutes) through the cooling of the alginate and provides a more accurate and stronger impression than with the use of alginate or agar alone.

Rubber Impression Material

Three types of rubber impression materials are common to dentistry: polysulfides, silicones or polysiloxanes, and polyethers (Fig. 11-44, A through E). The rubber impression materials were the answer to the shortcomings of the alginate and agar materials. The first of the three developed was the polysulfide, a flexible material with good dimensional accuracy. Polysulfide impression material is of greater strength and tear resistance than agar

and alginate materials. Another asset of polysulfide is the ability to electroplate the material, allowing the fabrication of metal dies, as well as the ability to make epoxy models and dies. This material consists of predominantly organic polymers of the mercaptan group and reinforcing agents, titanium dioxide, zinc sulfate, copper carbonate, or silica.

Since polysulfides are less than desirable in odor, are difficult to mix, are long in setting time, may have deformation and moderate shrinkage after setting, and stain clothing easily, silicone rubber impression materials were developed to eliminate some of these problems. Silicones are either of the condensation or additive type. The condensation silicone contains a moderately low molecular weight silicone liquid, silica for reinforcement, tin organic ester suspension, and alkyl silicate. The consistency of the material varies with the percentage of reinforcing agent. Condensation silicone may undergo extensive dimensional change, so the manufacturers usually supply the material as a putty-wash system.

Addition silicone or vinyl silicone contains a low molecular weight silicone with vinyl group, reinforcing filler, and chloroplatinic acid catalyst, or it may have silane hydrogens with the filler depending on whether it is a two-paste or a two-putty system. The two putties are not to be mixed while wearing rubber gloves, since the rubber will retard the setting. The use of overgloves eliminates this problem. The addition silicone may also include palladium, a hydrogen absorber, to control hydroxyl, which forms hydrogen. Palladium allows the impression to be poured immediately. A negative factor involving addition silicone is the less-than-desirable wetting capability of gypsum products, which is resolved with the use of surfactants.

Polyether impression materials have less dimensional change and more favorable mechanical properties but are considered stiff and have shorter working times than other elastic impression materials. The material is composed of a moderately low molecular weight polyether, with ethyleneimine groups that react with sulfonic acid ester to create high molecular weight rubber. This material usually has less working time than other rubber materials.

▶ Manipulation and Consistency

Of the three rubber impression materials just discussed, several consistencies, weights, and techniques for manipulation are employed. These materials may be two-paste systems with light (syringe or wash), regular, heavy body (tray), or putty consistency. The light, regular, and heavy consistencies are usually supplied in two paste tubes, one a base and the other the accelerator or catalyst. Most impression materials are formulated to have contrasting colors of catalyst and base to assist in the

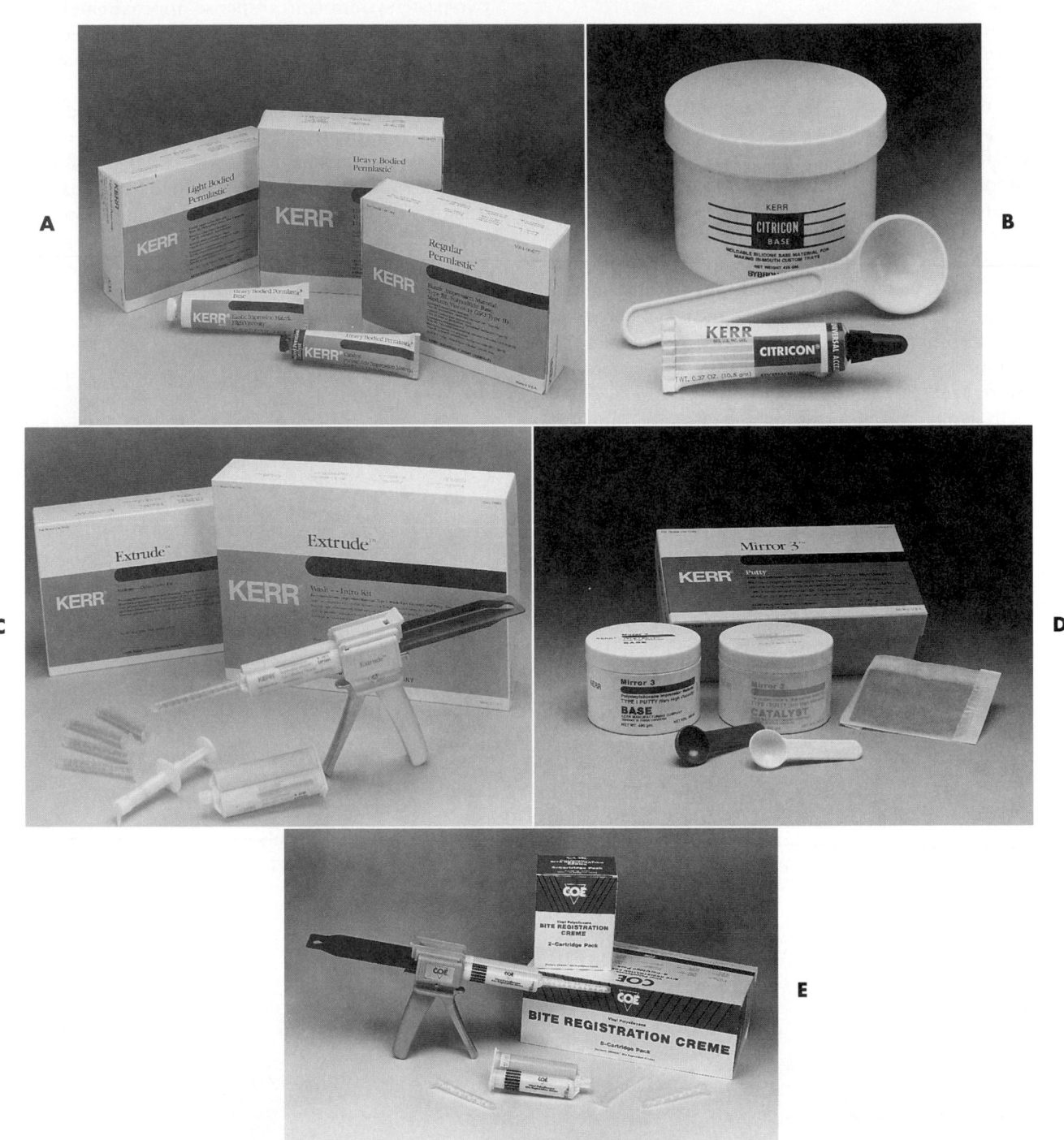

FIG. 11-44   *A* through *E*, Various types of elastic impression materials.

(*A–D*, Courtesy of Kerr/Sybron Manufacturing, Romulus, Michigan. *E*, COE/GC International, Scottsdale, Arizona.)

visual assessment of the homogeneous mix. Silicone impression materials may have the catalyst supplied as a liquid and putty consistency or have a liquid or putty catalyst.

The following is a generic description of the manipulation of each form of impression material without the specifics of the manufacturer's directions and time restraints. Some overlapping of technique is present in certain materials. To avoid repetition the steps in manipulation will be addressed once. Most manufacturers supply mixing pads with each package of material; the impression syringe and spatulas discussed earlier in the chapter may be used with any of these impression materials. Before any impression material is dispensed, the assistant must prepare all the armamentarium to reduce time at chairside and to make the procedure more comfortable for the patient. Rubber impression materials are formulated to be used with adhesive that is painted on the inside and the peripheral edge of the impression tray to help hold the impression material in the tray, particularly custom acrylic trays.

▶ Two-Paste System

A standard format for mixing impression material in the two-paste system is to dispense approximately 1 to 1½ inches of light-bodied catalyst on the pad and an equal length of the base material. Take care to dispense the materials so that they do not touch. The regular or heavy-bodied catalyst is dispensed on a second pad, with the length approximately twice that of the impression tray. The base is dispensed twice the length of the tray in an area separate from the catalyst. The box lists the step-by-step procedure for mixing the light-bodied material first and then the heavy-bodied material; Fig. 11-45, *A* through *C*, illustrates the preparation for the two-paste system.

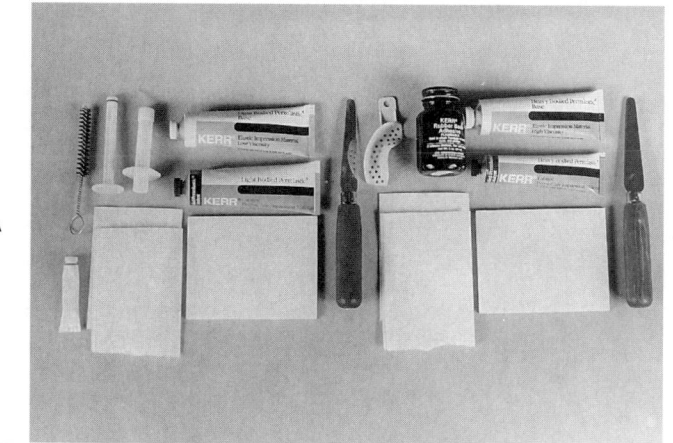

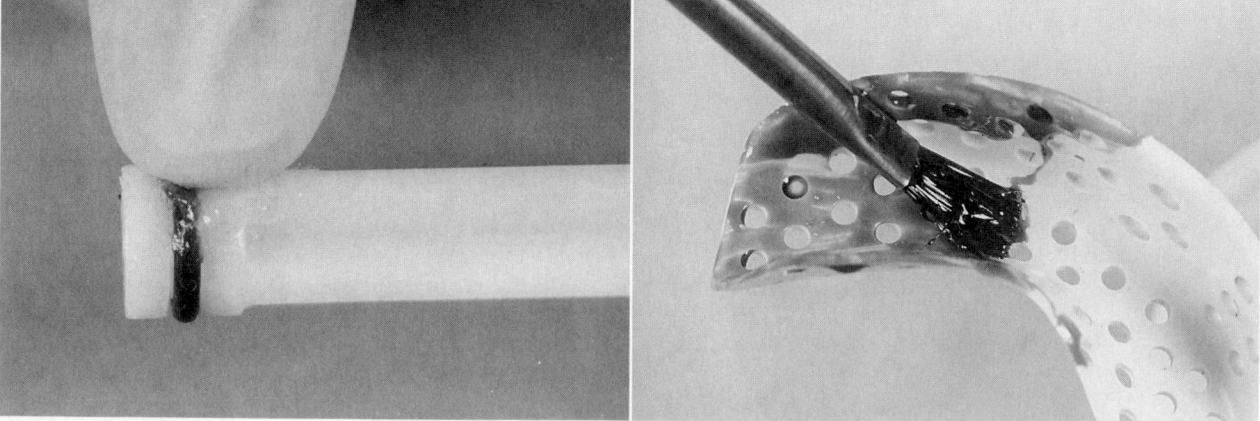

FIG. 11-45   *A*, Set-up of rubber base armamentarium. *B*, Lubricant on a tip of rubber base syringe plunger. *C*, Adhesive placed on stock impression tray.

STEP-BY-STEP PROCEDURE
TWO-PASTE SYSTEM FOR MIXING IMPRESSION MATERIALS

1. Place the spatula in a position to pick up all the catalyst with one motion and introduce it to the base (Fig. 11-46, *A* through *G*).
2. Mix the material until no streaks are seen, while holding the spatula in a vertical position.
3. Lightly press the spatula into the mixing pad to remove excess material, and wipe the rest of the impression material off of the spatula.
4. Take the spatula back to the material, and use a side-to-side stroke to continue to mix, forcing the spatula through the mix, and incorporating all the material. (Streaks will begin to appear as mixing begins again.) Turn spatula so that each side and the material on it is exposed to the mixture and incorporated.
5. Once the mix is homogeneous , bring it to the center of the pad.
6. Begin to load the syringe as shown in Fig. 11-41, pulling the material into the syringe through capillary action.
7. Once the syringe is filled, place the plunger into the end, force it into contact with the material, and dispense a small amount through the tip to ensure that there are no voids.
8. Pass the syringe to the operator for placement of the material on the tooth.
9. Begin to immediately mix the heavy-bodied material, repeating steps 1 through 5 (Fig. 11-47, *A* through *J*).
10. Place the material into the impression tray (usually a custom acrylic tray to reduce the amount of material necessary and to be assured of a good fit in the patient's mouth).

▶ Load the material into the tray by picking up the entire mix on the spatula at once.
▶ Load the tray starting from one side, placing the material into the opening and pulling it to the other side with a smooth stroke of the spatula.
▶ Do not move the spatula back and forth in the tray or introduce extra material from the mixing pad (this eliminates voids in the impression, which may require retaking the impression and repeating all the steps).
11. Pass the tray to the operator, positioning it over the syringe material.
12. Start a timer to record the time until the material is set.
13. Remove the impression after the material has set, using a steady force on the tray to pull it from the arch.
14. Check the impression for accuracy and detail and for the existence of voids.
15. Rinse it under water, and disinfect as recommended.

HELPFUL HINT

▶ A factor to remember when dispensing impression materials in collapsible tubes is that the manufacturer has prepared the tubes with different-sized openings and tubes.
▶ This ensures that as you dispense an amount of catalyst and base to equal lengths, you are also dispensing the proper configuration of the material. **Do not** attempt to dispense equal quantities of material, only equal lengths, to achieve the correct chemical and physical characteristics of the material.

STEP-BY-STEP PROCEDURE
PUTTY-WASH SYSTEM FOR MIXING IMPRESSION MATERIALS

This technique requires the impression be taken at two stages of the procedure. The putty material used in this system is extremely stiff and necessitates the use of the manufacturer's scoop to dispense properly.

1. Dispense the scoop of material on a paper pad, and use the spatula to make an indentation on the surface.
2. Dispense the catalyst in the indentation. (Usually the catalyst is liquid and the incorporation of the two is simplified by this technique.)
3. Mix the two with a spatula until homogeneous.
4. Mix the rest with the hands, since the catalyst is incorporated into the mix.
5. Place the putty in the impression tray, and pass it to the operator.

6. Rock the impression tray on the arch to create a space of 1 to 2 mm, which allows for the syringe material. (Some systems have cellophane spacer sheets that are placed between the teeth and the impression material and are removed after the material is set to allow room for the wash material that is used later.)
7. Once the material is set, remove the tray, and set it aside as the operator prepares the cavity preparation.
8. Mix the syringe material for the wash impression as in the two-paste system, and load it into the syringe.
9. Inject the material into the impression area and possibly the same area inside the tray impression.
10. Position the tray in the mouth, time it, allow it to set.

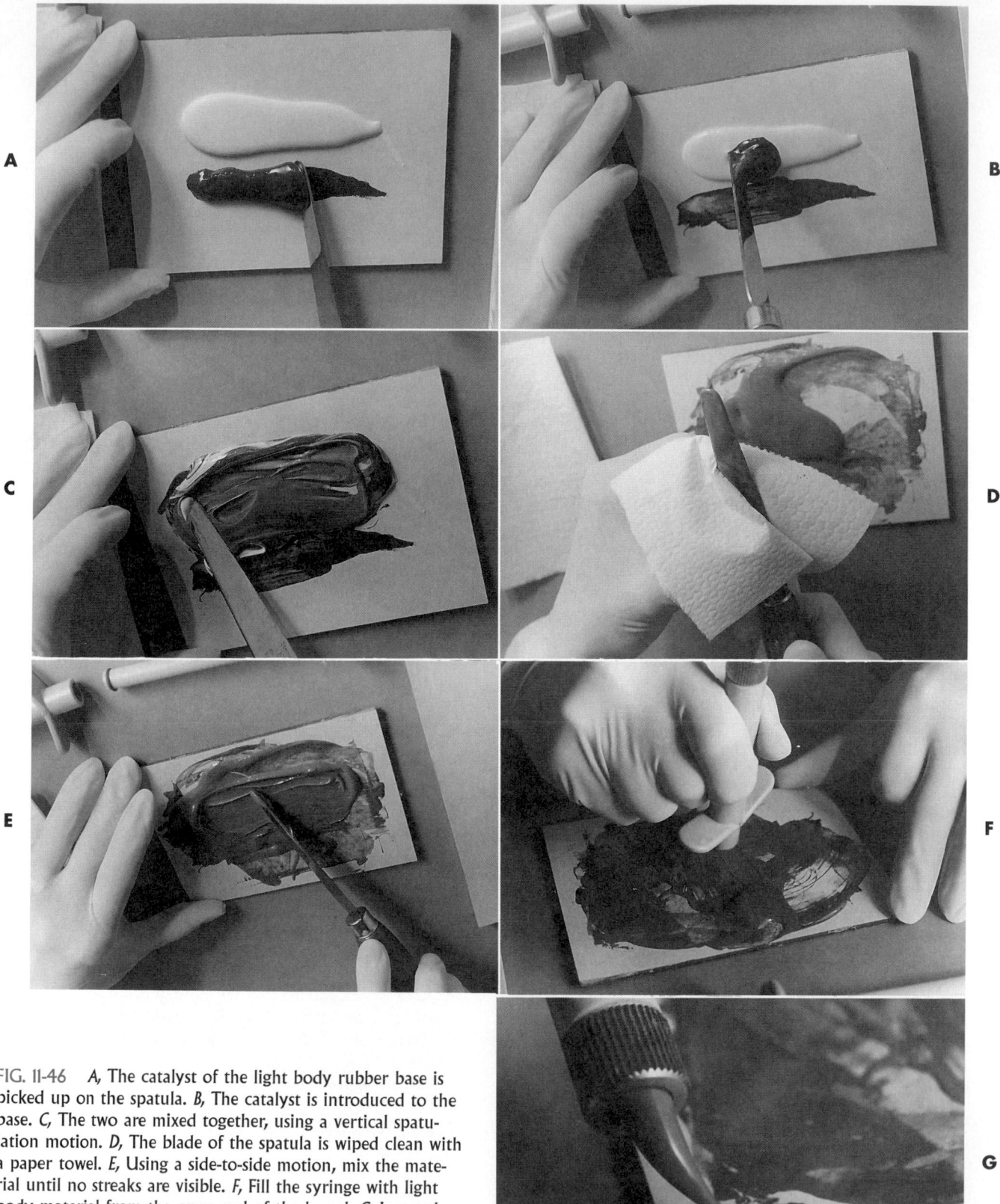

FIG. 11-46   *A,* The catalyst of the light body rubber base is picked up on the spatula. *B,* The catalyst is introduced to the base. *C,* The two are mixed together, using a vertical spatulation motion. *D,* The blade of the spatula is wiped clean with a paper towel. *E,* Using a side-to-side motion, mix the material until no streaks are visible. *F,* Fill the syringe with light body material from the open end of the barrel. *G,* Insert the plunger in the syringe and dispense a small amount out the tip to ensure that there are no trapped air bubbles.

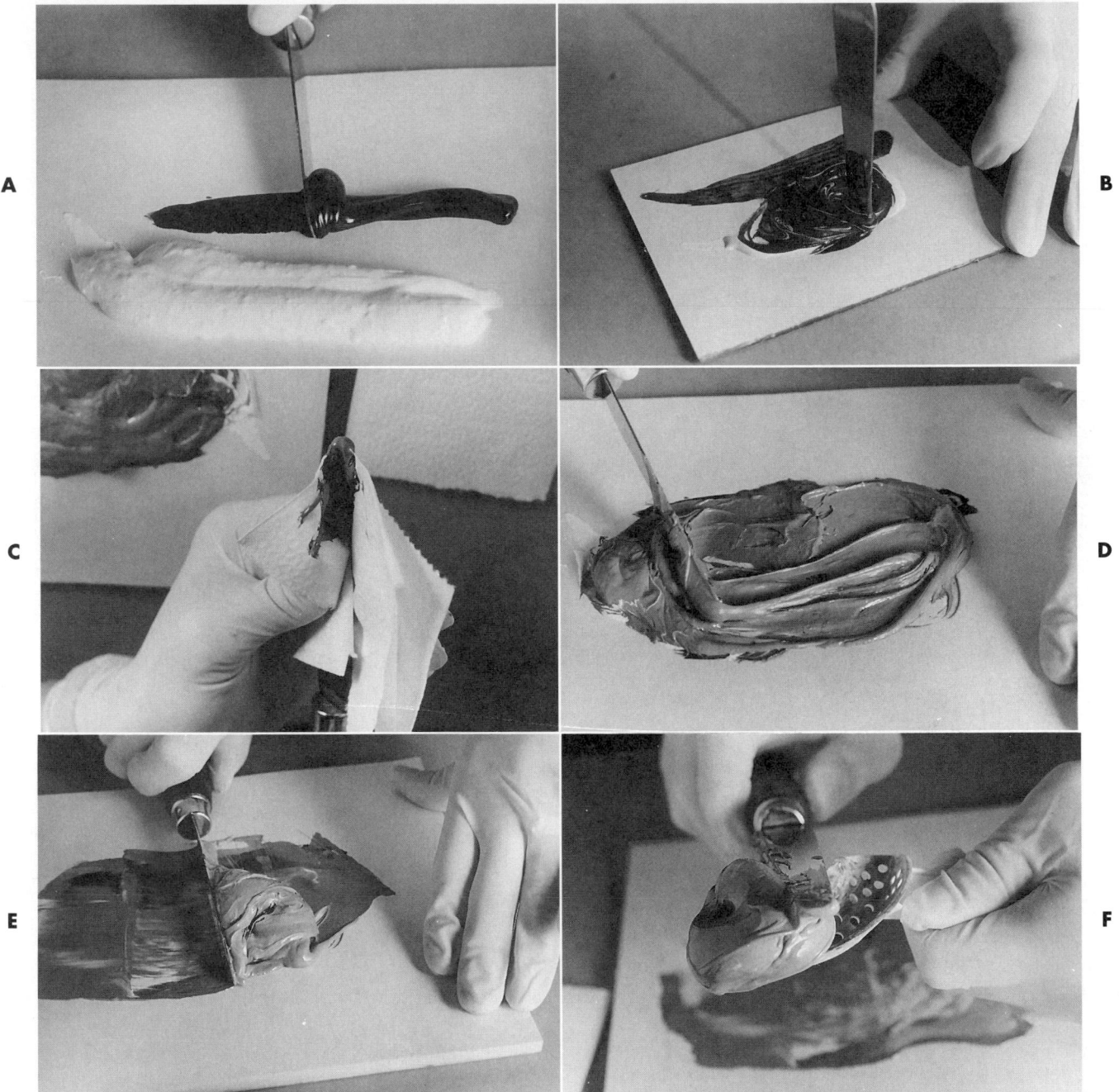

FIG. 11-47   *A,* Pick up the catalyst of the dispensed heavy body material. *B,* Incorporate the catalyst with the base, using a vertical spatulation. *C,* Mix the two until there are no visible streaks. Wipe the material off the spatula blade. *D,* Continue to mix the mass, using a side-to-side motion. *E,* Bring the mass together, and pick it all up on the spatula at once. *F,* Load the adhesive covered tray starting at one end.   *Continued.*

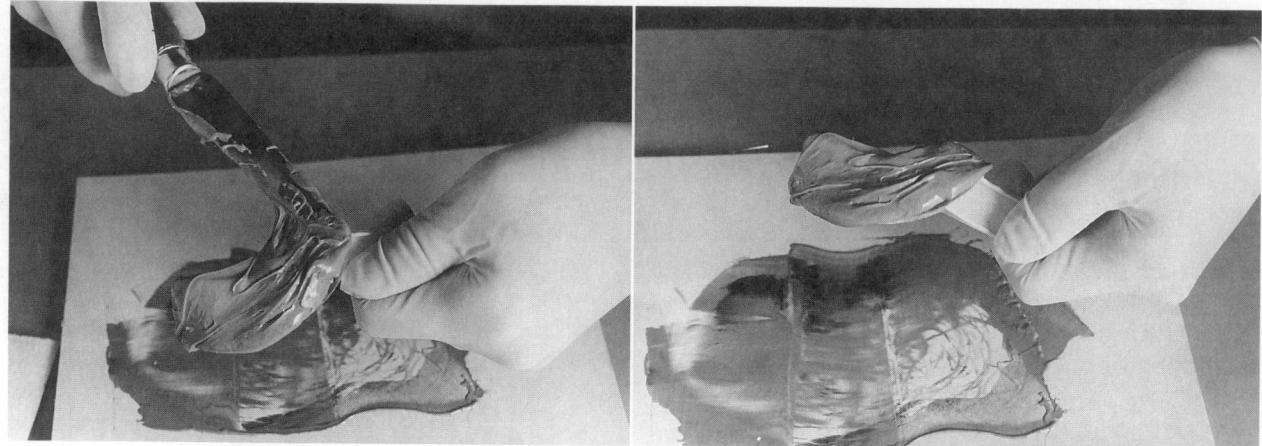

FIG. 11-47, cont'd.   *G,* Pull the material off the spatula in a continuous stroke to the other end of the tray. *H,* The loaded tray appears free of voids and strings of material.

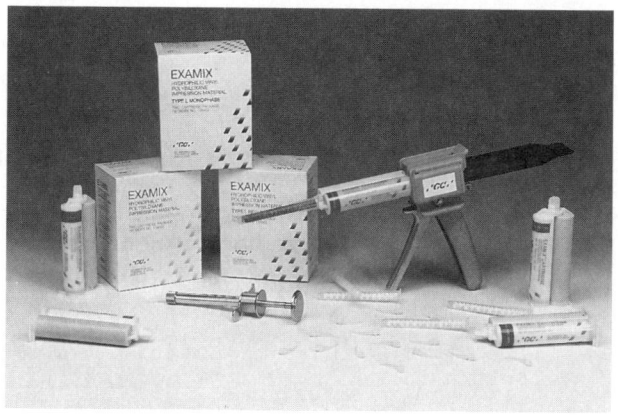

FIG. 11-48   Automix, self-mixing impression material system.

Many silicone impression materials have been designed to use an automatic mixing system that supplies light- and regular-bodied materials in small cartridges to be inserted into the end of a gunlike device shown in Fig. 11-48. The plungers on the gun are advanced, extruding catalyst and base in equal proportions that are mixed in the spiral attached to the cartridges. The material is advanced through the tip and is completely mixed as it is placed on the prepared tooth. The impression putty material is placed as described previously. Box 11-9 is a list of several impression materials.

Model and Die Materials

The impression is the first step in obtaining a reproduction of the mouth. Then that impression must be used to fabricate a model, cast, or die material to actually achieve a positive reproduction. The reproduction can be a

---

BOX 11-9

COMMON BRANDS OF IMPRESSION MATERIALS

AGAR HYDROCOLLOID	IRREVERSIBLE HYDROCOLLOID
Hydrocolloid Material	Alginate
Rubberloid	Coe-Alginate
Superbody	Jeltrate
	Jeltrate Plus
SILICONE	Kalginate
Absolute	
Accoe	POLYSULFIDE
Cinch-Vinyl	Coe-Flex
CutterFlex	Multi-Lastic
CutterSil	Neo-Plex
Detail	Omniflex
Exaflex	Permlastic
Express	Super-Flex
Extrude	
Fit-Checker	POLYETHER
Hydrosil	Genesis
Impra-mix/X	Impregum F
Imprint	Permadyne
Mirror 3	Polyjel NF
Omnisil	
Perfourm/C.D.	THERMOPLASTIC
Permagum	Adaptol
President	Compound Impression
Reflect	
Regisil	
Reprosil	

TABLE 11-3 SELECTION OF CAST OR DIE MATERIALS ACCORDING TO USE OF IMPRESSION

Cast/die material	Impression material
Gypsum material	Dental compound
	Agar hydrocolloid
	Alginate
	Zinc oxide-eugenol
	Polysulfide rubber base
	Silicone rubber base
	Polyether rubber base
	Impression plaster (if heavily coated with a separating solution)
Epoxy resin material	Polysulfide rubber base (with separator)
	Polyether rubber base
	Silicones (separator as necessary)
Electroplated copper	Dental compound
	Silicone rubber base
Electroplated silver	Polysulfide rubber base
	Polyether rubber base
	Addition silicone rubber base

model, which is generally used for case study or diagnostic purposes, or a cast, which is a working model of a reproduction to be used in the fabrication of an appliance or restoration. A cast is made from a material that is strong and able to resist wear and abrasion caused during the fabrication of the appliance or restoration. A cast is considered to be a reproduction of a quadrant or an arch, dentulous or edentulous, while a die is the replica of a one or more teeth, which is usually a removable portion of the cast.

The types of materials used to make reproductions from dental impressions are gypsum products, epoxy, and gypsum-plated metal. The use of any of the reproduction materials is precluded by the impression material and the reason for making the replica. Regardless of the type of material used, it should be accurate and have extremely little or no dimensional change to ensure the accuracy of the restorations and appliances made from the replicas. The type of cast or die material that is compatible and desirable with specific impression materials is categorized in Table 11-3.

Gypsum Products

Gypsum products can be used in all aspects of model, cast, and die fabrication because they are compatible with impression materials. A gypsum product may be a model plaster, dental stone, or improved dental stone (also called high-strength stone). The application or purpose of use of a model or cast is significant in selecting a material. All three materials are products of the gypsum mineral calcium sulfate dihydrate, which, during manu-

facturing, lose water and are converted to hemihydrates of calcium sulfate. The process of removing the water and producing the hemihydrate differs with each product, resulting in different chemical and physical characteristics. Thus model plaster is the least strong of the products, followed by orthodontic plaster, which has a small amount of dental stone added to model plaster. The next in increasing strength and resistance is dental stone, whose capabilities are less than those of improved stone.

The introduction of water to any gypsum product produces a chemical reaction that causes the hardening of the material. The amount of water necessary to mix these materials is greater than that necessary for the actual chemical reaction to occur. This water aids in wetting the calcium sulfate hemihydrate particles and flowing the material into the impression. It evaporates as the gypsum product sets during the exothermic reaction. The amount of the water needed is determined by the size, shape, and porosity of the particles. Plaster, which has larger and more porous particles, requires more water than the other gypsum products. The water/powder ratio for each is as follows:

Model plaster	$\dfrac{45 \text{ to } 50 \text{ ml water}}{100 \text{ powder}}$
Dental stone	$\dfrac{30 \text{ to } 32 \text{ ml water}}{100 \text{ powder}}$
Improved dental stone	$\dfrac{19 \text{ to } 24 \text{ ml water}}{100 \text{ powder}}$

PROPERTIES OF GYPSUM PRODUCTS

The properties of specific interest when working with gypsum products include the following:
- Setting times
- Detailed reproduction
- Compressive strength
- Tensile strength
- Resistance
- Dimensional accuracy

Each of these characteristics is important in determining appropriate applications for the various gypsum products.

The setting times to be considered with gypsum products are the initial and final setting times. The initial setting time includes the time to mix and manipulate the material. When the viscosity of the material increases and flow of the material is not possible, the initial set or working time ends. Another observable phenomenon is the visible loss of gloss of the material as the excess water on the surface of the gypsum is absorbed. The initial set usually occurs between 8 and 16 minutes from the time the water and powder are first mixed.

The final setting time is reached when the material is hard enough to be removed from the impression material with no distortion or fracture of the model. This time is usually 45 to 60 minutes after manipulation is started. It is indicated when the model feels cool and dry.

When a die is produced using a gypsum product, it is poured with improved stone. Ideally the stone is mixed in a vacuum mixer, vibrated thoroughly to remove any air bubbles in the material, and introduced and manipulated into the impression carefully. Because of the porosity of gypsum products, the quality of a die produced using these materials is less than desirable compared to epoxy or electroplated dies.

The compressive strength of gypsum products is closely related to the amount of water and thus the density of the material. Improved stone has greater compressive strength than dental stone or model plaster. Again, the tensile strength of model plaster is less than that of dental or improved dental stones.

The abrasion resistance and hardness of the surface of a gypsum product are also related to the compressive strength of the material. The improved or high-strength stone provides greater quality, but it is still less than that of epoxy or electroplated dies.

The dimensional accuracy of gypsum materials as they are manipulated and set decreases in percentage from model plaster, to dental stone, and finally to improved stone. Dimensional accuracy is critical in fabricating restorations. If the dimensional change is excessive, a wax pattern and eventually a cast restoration fabricated on a die of improved stone results in an oversized restoration. If shrinkage occurs, the die and restoration are undersized.

EXAMPLES OF USE

Since improved stone or Type IV stone has greater capabilities than the other gypsum products, its use is usually as a cast and die material in the fabrication of restorations. Type IV stone is the most costly of the three gypsum products. Type III gypsum, dental stone, has properties that fall between Types IV and II model plaster. It can be used for a working model or a study model that provides greater qualities. Type II model plaster is the weakest, least stable, and least costly of the products and is usually used in the fabrication of study models. Type I gypsum or impression plaster was discussed earlier in the chapter.

Plaster is generally selected for use with study models because of the ease of trimming the material as compared to dental stone or improved stone.

SPATULATION

Spatulation is the technique of mixing materials together to a homogeneous mass. In this case, gypsum powder is mixed with water. Certain factors during spatulation can cause variations in setting time and the expansion of gypsum products. If spatulation time or rate is increased, the setting time is shortened. The setting expansion may also be affected by the rate of spatulation. To avoid increased setting time and expansion, hand-driven or power-driven spatulators are often used. Vacuum mixing may also be used to reduce air bubbles and the possibility of voids in a pour.

It is possible to use mechanical devices to assist in the manipulation of gypsum products. One such device is a hand-driven mechanical spatulator. This is used when

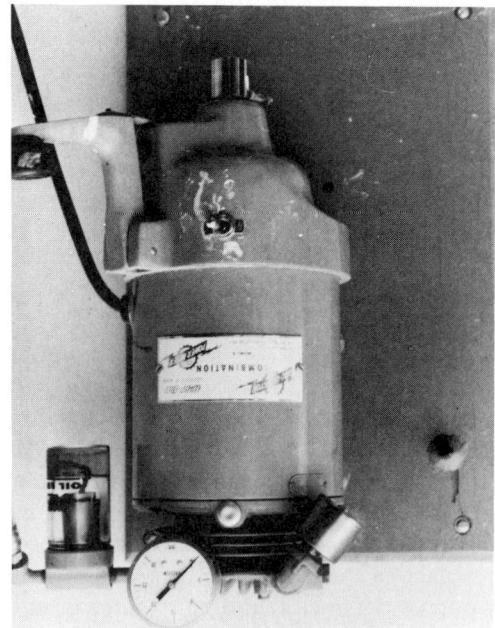

FIG. 11-49 Example of mechanical spatulation method.

(From Craig RG et al: *Dental materials,* ed 5, St Louis, 1992, Mosby.)

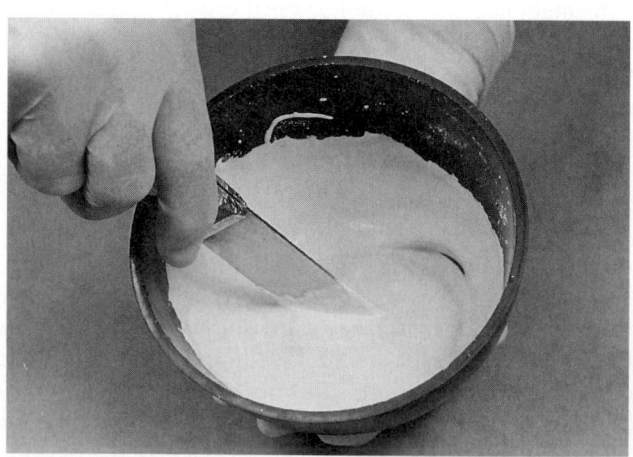

FIG. 11-50 Hand spatulation of plaster.

mixing small amounts of gypsum products, since the bowl of the spatulator is much smaller than others. Measure the water and place it in the bowl, then add the measured powder. The top of the spatulator has a crank handle and blades that are immersed in the gypsum and water as the top is sealed in place. Turn crank, approximately two revolutions per second, for a total of 1 minute, incorporating the water and powder together into a homogeneous mass.

Another mechanical spatulator is power driven with a vacuum attachment. The bowl with the water and powder is attached to the power-driven spatulator and mixed without using hand spatulation (Fig. 11-49). Both of these machines are designed to achieve the best

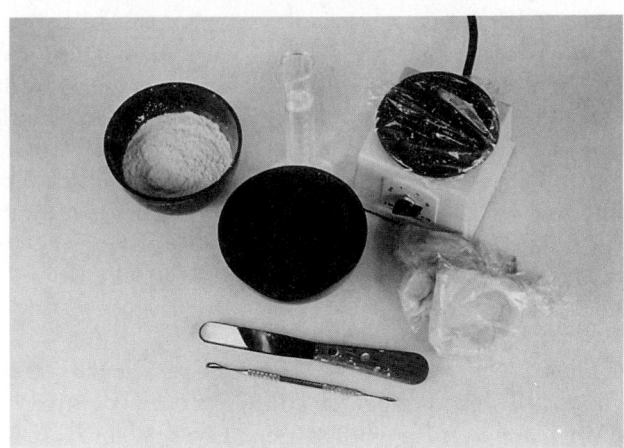

FIG. 11-51   Armamentarium for mixing gypsum and placing it into alginate impression.

possible characteristics of gypsum products and eliminate the potential for air bubbles.

Hand-spatulating gypsum materials are probably the most common means of manipulating the material, especially in a private dental office (Figs. 11-50 and 11-51). Whether the gypsum is model plaster or stone, the technique to achieve a homogeneous mass free of air bubbles and voids is the same.

▶ Stone Dies

Dies are replicas of the prepared tooth or teeth on which wax patterns are fabricated. By using the lost wax technique, these patterns are replaced and made into cast restorations. As stated earlier, dies can be fabricated from stone epoxy or through a metal-plating process.

If a die is to be fabricated, a small amount of improved stone is mixed to proper consistency and placed in the area of the prepared tooth and the abutment teeth. A small metal device called a dowel pin is placed vertically in the die material positioned on the prepared tooth and secured in place until the material is hardened. A separating solution is painted over the die with the dowel, dried, and then a second pour of either dental stone or model plaster is prepared and vibrated into the model to complete the cast.

After the second pour of gypsum has hardened, the impression is separated from the cast. The area in which the die is located is cut free from the rest of the cast and used to fabricate the wax pattern.

▶ Epoxy Dies

Epoxy dies are fabricated from a resin and a hardener that produces a stronger and more abrasion-resistant die than a stone die. Epoxy dies can be made from polysulfide, polyether, and silicone rubber impression materials.

GYPSUM

ARMAMENTARIUM

Flexible rubber bowl
Stiff-bladed spatula
Graduated cylinder
Measuring scale
Vibrator
Glass slab or other surface on which to place the model after it is poured (Fig. 11-51)

MANIPULATION

1. Prepare all the armamentarium.
2. Select the gypsum material of choice
3. Place the rubber bowl on the scale and set the tear.
4. Measure the appropriate amount of gypsum into the bowl.
5. Remove the bowl from the scale, measure cool water into the graduated cylinder, and place water in the rubber bowl.
6. Slowly pour the powder into the water, and allow it to settle for approximately 30 seconds to reduce the amount of air incorporated into the mix during spatulation.
7. Vigorously stir the mass with the spatula, wiping the insides of the bowl with the spatula to incorporate all the material
8. Mix for approximately 30 to 60 seconds, scraping the bottom and sides of the bowl and creating a homogeneous mixture. (The viscosity allows the material to flow through mechanical vibrations but maintains the approximate shape when placed in a mass.)
9. Place the bowl on the vibrator that is set at a moderate rate to force the trapped air to the surface of the mass.
10. Vibrate for approximately 1 minute until the air bubbles disappear (see Fig. 11-50).
11. The gypsum is ready to be placed in the impression as described in Chapter 40.

▶ Metal-Plated Dies

The production of metal-plated dies involves the use of an electroforming or electroplating process with an electric current and an electrolyte to form indirect dies for inlay, crown, and bridge restorations. The current can be supplied by a small dry cell battery or using a direct current power supply. The electrolyte or plating solution of acidic copper sulfate solution for copper plating or silver cyanide in an alkaline solution for silver plating is placed in a small container.

The anode from the power source is attached to either a piece of pure copper, if copper plating, or silver, if silver plating an impression (Fig. 11-52, *A* through *C*).

The anode and metal are placed in the plating solution and the surface of the impression that will be the metal-plated die is covered with a conductor of electricity for the copper plating or a silver powder for silver plating. The current creates a medium in the solution that allows the metal to be attracted and transferred to the area where the conductor of electricity is placed.

The impression is attached to a cathode lead wire and carefully immersed in the bath of solution, which is covered. The electrical current is established at 15 or 5 milliamperes to lightly cover the impression with a thin layer of the metal. Once covered, the current can be increased; the plating continues for 12 to 15 hours to produce a greater thickness of the metal. The metal-

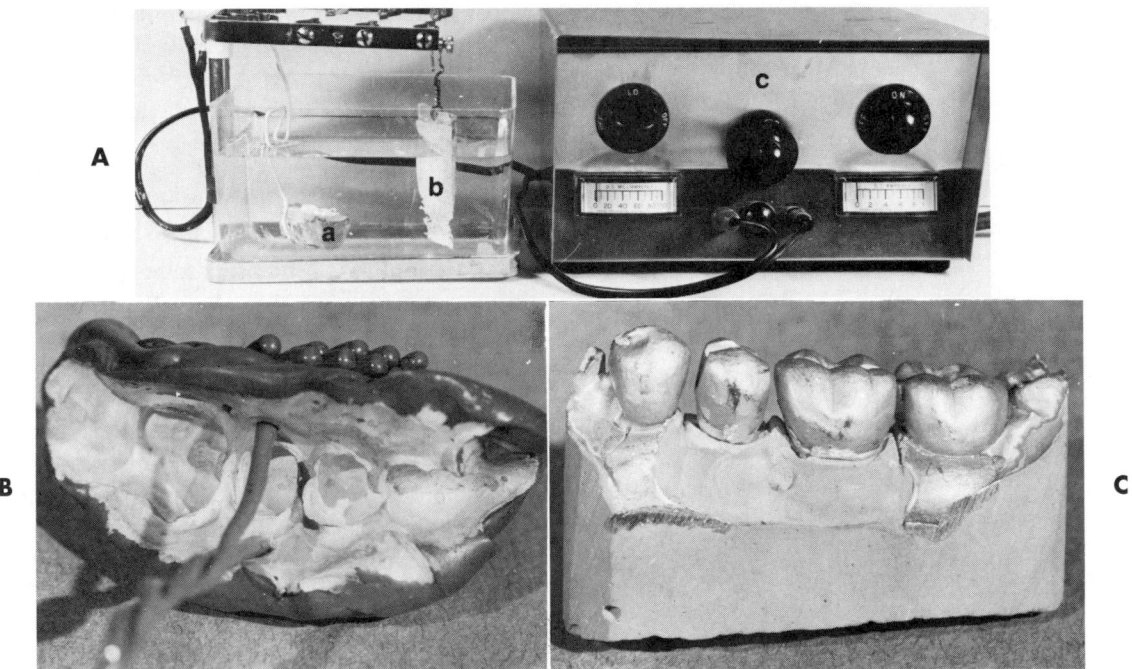

FIG. 11-52   *A* through *C,* Example of electroplating unit that produces a die of the impression.
(From Craig RG et al: *Dental materials,* ed 5, St Louis, 1992, Mosby.)

plated impression is removed from the solution, washed of any excess, and dried. The preparation of the cast is completed by placing a dowel in a medium of epoxy or plastic in the plated area of the die, allowing it to harden and pouring it with a gypsum product to create the rest of the cast.

When plating solutions are used, it is important to be careful, since they are usually poisonous and caustic to the skin and other tissue. Covering hands, clothing, face, and eyes is important in case of spillage and potential fumes.

▶ Investment Materials

Investment material is used in the process of obtaining a cast metal restoration during a lost wax technique. The investment is a ceramic material that can be molded into a form that withstands the procedure for producing an alloy cast. Investment material is a combination of refractory material, such as quartz, tridymite, or cristobalite, a binder material of calcium sulfate or a similar material, and a possible combination of sodium chloride, boric acid, potassium sulfate, graphite copper powder, or magnesium oxide. The exact composition is determined by the physical properties desired in the specific investment material.

The ADA specifies three different categories of investment materials appropriate for casting dental restorations. They are as follows:

Type I	Inlay, thermal
Type II	Inlay, hygroscopic
Type III	Partial denture, thermal

All investment materials undergo a certain amount of thermal expansion to allow for the shrinkage of the gold casting as it cools during the procedure. The expansion occurs as the investment material hardens after manipulation and during the heating of the material that is molded around the wax pattern. The temperature that a material must withstand to achieve ideal thermal expansion is 482° to 650° C (900° to 1200° F).

If the material is hygroscopic, it can be placed in contact with water to increase the expansion, thus reducing the need for higher temperatures during the burnout procedure (482° to 650° C). The procedure for manipulating investment material and producing a cast alloy restoration is described in Chapter 30.

Dental Waxes

Waxes are categorized into three groups: pattern, processing, and impression waxes. Among the many applications of waxes are making a wax pattern; boxing an impression; bite registration; attaching two objects that will be permanently attached with another material; try-in denture forms; bite rims; correction of impressions; and peripheral edge of an impression tray.

Waxes play an integral part in dentistry and are important to virtually all areas of the profession, but particularly in restorative dentistry. Dental waxes are composed of natural and synthetic waxes, gums, fats, fatty acids, oils, natural and synthetic resins, and pigments. Any of these substances are combined to achieve the physical characteristics that are needed in application of the waxes. These components include *paraffin,* a combination of petroleum and hydrocarbons for a high melting point, and *microcrystalline wax,* which is similar to paraffin but from a heavier oil, creating an even higher melting point. Other contents are *ceresin,* distillates from natural-mineral petroleum refining for greater hardness; *carnauba,* from esters, alcohols, acids, and hydrocarbons for hardness, brittleness, and high melting points; *candelilla,* a combination of paraffin hydrocarbons, free alcohol, acids, esters, and lactones to harden paraffin; and *beeswax,* an insect wax of esters to create a wax that is brittle but plastic at body temperature.

The ability of a wax to undergo thermal expansion is important when creating wax patterns. Since wax expands when exposed to heat and contracts when cooled, it is important for the manufacturer to provide the thermal limits of the product, since this may be a factor in the accuracy or inaccuracy of a final cast restoration. Flow, which is increased as the wax reaches its melting point or as load is increased, becomes important with respect to deformation. A wax used in the oral cavity may be required to have a low flow quotient to reduce the possibility of distortion.

With the lost wax casting procedure, no wax residue should remain in the mold space following burnout. This would cause a distortion in the final cast restoration. Also, as the wax is manipulated through heating and carving, residual stresses are caused. This stress can cause distortion and create an ill-fitting final cast restoration.

▶ Pattern Waxes

Pattern waxes include inlay, casting, and baseplate waxes (Fig. 11-53). These waxes are used to create a desired reproduction in wax that will become the shape of a metal casting or denture through use of the lost wax technique. With metal restoration the wax is placed on a die or cast model and invested, forming a mold of the wax pattern. The investment is heated, melting the wax and leaving a pattern inside the investment material that is replaced by the molten metal. In denture fabrication the eliminated wax is replaced with the denture base acrylic as described in Chapter 31.

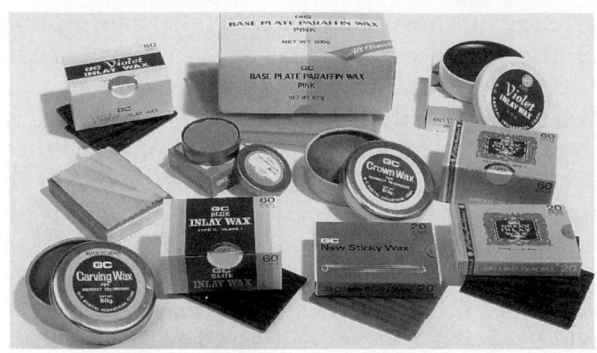

FIG. 11-53   Various pattern waxes.

(From Craig RG et al: *Dental materials,* ed 5, St Louis, 1992, Mosby.)

INLAY WAX

Inlay wax is particularly used in the fabrication of cast metal restorations through the creation of a wax pattern of the restoration. The wax is classified as Type I, used to form direct wax patterns in the mouth, and Type II, used to prepare wax patterns on dies. This wax is supplied in small sticks or premade shapes, in tins, or as bulk wax chunks.

CASTING WAX

Casting wax is used in the fabrication of a wax pattern of the metal framework for removable partial and complete dentures or other dental appliances. Sheets of this wax are also used by many practitioners to establish the occlusal clearance between a prepared tooth and the opposing tooth. The wax is supplied in thin sheets and ready-made forms and shapes that are slightly tacky in texture to assure the final position on a model.

BASEPLATE WAX

Baseplate wax is named from the original application for use as a rim of wax that is set on a baseplate tray for the establishment of the vertical dimensions of a denture. The wax rim then provides the contour of what will be the denture before setting the artificial teeth and processing. This wax is also categorized as Type I, a soft wax for creating contours; Type II, a wax of medium hardness for patterns used in the medium zones of weather; and Type III, a hard wax for patterns used in the tropical zones of weather. This wax may also be used to establish a bite registration on a patient to reflect the relationship of the teeth in one arch to those in the other.

▶ Processing Waxes

This type of wax is considered a utility or auxiliary wax in that it is used as an aid in the construction of restorations and appliances. The tasks performed with processing waxes make the process of creating final restorations and appliances easier.

BOXING WAX

Boxing wax is used in boxing an impression to create a form in which to pour a gypsum product. A utility wax rope is placed below the peripheral height of the impression; then a thin strip is formed around the rope and sealed in place by heating the edge of the wax. The gypsum material is placed in the impression and contained by the boxing wax.

STICKY WAX

Sticky wax is so named because when heated it is extremely sticky; as it cools, it becomes firm, not tacky, and somewhat brittle. It is used to assist in maintaining the position of two objects together: e.g., a denture that is fractured and is to be repaired with cold-cured acrylic. Sticky wax is used to hold the denture pieces in place during the placement of the acrylic. It is then easily removed when no longer needed.

UTILITY WAX

Utility wax is aptly named in that it serves utility functions. The wax is supplied in ropes, strips, and sheets. Common applications of utility wax include customization of a stock impression tray to capture all the anatomy in an impression, particularly the peripheral border, or to fill the palatal area of an impression tray for use with a patient who has a vaulted palate.

▶ Impression Waxes

A wax used to produce an impression of oral tissues must exhibit high flow and ductility.

CORRECTIVE IMPRESSION WAX

This wax is particularly popular in obtaining edentulous impressions in a situation with undercuts or making corrections in an edentulous impression. Since edentulous impressions always involve registration of areas that are undercut, it is necessary to use this wax together with another material to obtain an accurate registration of the edentulous arch. This wax can be warmed, flowed into a void or undercut area on an impression. When it is

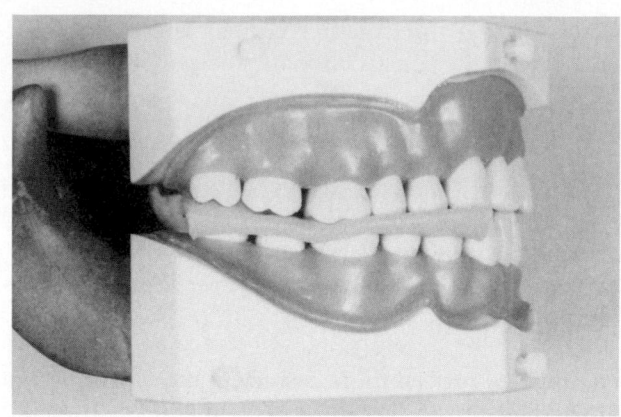

FIG. 11-54   Bite registration taken with an impression wax.

returned to the mouth, the wax flows to correct the void or undercut area in the impression.

BITE REGISTRATION WAX

As with the previously discussed baseplate wax, bite registration wax is used to reproduce the accurate articulation of the dental arches. The wax is supplied in preformed shapes of the arch to assist in positioning the wax over the teeth and to minimize the amount of wax necessary. This wax is susceptible to distortion and may be reinforced with metal between two sheets of the wax to assist in softening the wax and holding its shape once it has rehardened (Fig. 11-54).

Gold and Dental Alloys

Gold has been used for restorative purposes for many years. It was not until 1969 when the U.S. Federal Government lifted the regulations that maintained the price of gold that there was a substantial increase in the price of it. The cost factor stimulated the introduction of other alloys, such as palladium-silver, nickel, cobalt chromium, and nickel-chromium alloy, and lowered the content of gold alloy used in dentistry for restorative procedures. Still, the noble metals—gold, platinum, palladium, and iridium—are used predominantly for casting dental restorations. Silver is not considered a noble metal because of its tarnishability; however, it is present in small amounts in some casting alloys.

▶ Gold

Originally gold was used in its purest form, 24 karat (K), which is extremely soft, ductile, and malleable. Both karat and fineness are used to measure of the gold content of an alloy. Since pure gold is 24K, 50% gold is denoted as 12K. Pure gold is 1000 fineness (F); thus, if a metal is 12K, it would have a fineness rating of $1000 \times 0.50 = 500$ F.

The properties of pure gold allow it to be drawn into ropes and wires, ground into fine powder, and rolled into sheets of foil. Gold foil is used as a direct filling material in the mouth. During the procedure, gold foil must be annealed, which is a degassing of the gold surface by heat from an alcohol burner, to make the gold cohesive. Once cohesive, gold can be pressure welded to create an atomic bond between the layers of gold as they are condensed into the cavity preparation. Thus condensing the gold also strengthens it and hardens the surface.

The technique involved in the gold foil procedure is time consuming and may result in failure of the restoration if the material is not annealed properly, isolation is not maintained, and/or condensation is not performed properly. All these factors and more have resulted in fewer direct gold restorations being performed. Currently, gold is used more often as an alloy in cast gold restorations.

DENTAL ALLOY

Another desirable property that gold provides as a restorative material is that it does not oxidize easily. This lack of oxidization creates a surface that is high in luster and easy to maintain. Gold is also not soluble in sulfuric, nitric, or hydrochloric acids. The introduction of other noble metals and specific base metals, such as copper and zinc, forms alloys that exhibit properties that are ideal for many dental applications.

NOBLE METALS

Noble metals contain a minimum of 75% gold with the remaining metal derived from the platinum metal group. The properties held by the noble metals provide the characteristics of the alloys to meet their varied applications. Platinum has a high fusing point and is resistant to the corrosive oral conditions; it provides hardness and elasticity when it is added to gold alloys. Platinum in the form of foil is used for the framework in constructing porcelain-fused restorations. The metal restoration is not susceptible to melting when it is exposed to the temperatures necessary to fire porcelain. Platinum and porcelain also have a similar coefficients of thermal expansion. Therefore, as each is exposed to temperature fluctuations, the possibility of fractures is minimized.

Palladium is commonly a component of silver or gold alloys and has properties that are similar to platinum, but it is less expensive. When combined with gold, it lightens the alloy; when used with silver, it reduces tarnish and corrosion.

Iridium is added to gold alloys to reduce the grain. A fine-grained alloy is stronger and more ductile. The metal itself is very hard and brittle and has a high melting point.

BASE METALS

Base or nonprecious metals are combined with gold to improve properties for individualized applications of the alloys. One such base metal is indium. Indium does not tarnish in water or air and has a low melting point. This base metal can be used in place of zinc, particularly with patients who have a sensitivity to zinc.

Tin is high in luster and does not tarnish easily. This metal is relatively soft and has a low melting point. The application of tin is usually in conjunction with gold solder and specialized alloys. When tin is combined with palladium and platinum, it increases the hardness and brittleness. When tin is combined with copper, bronze is formed.

Zinc, combined with gold and platinum, increases the hardness and brittleness of the alloy. It also is a deoxidizing agent during the melting and casting of alloys, thus creating an alloy that is easier to cast.

Copper is combined with metals to increase hardness and strength and to enhance the quality of color of the alloy. Copper also assists in the heat treatment of the alloy—to use heat and cooling to harden or soften the material. Combining copper with zinc creates brass. Nickel in small amounts combined with gold alloys increases the strength and hardness of the alloy.

Gold alloys, for casting purposes, are classified by ANSI-ADA specifications as Type I, II, III, or IV. Each type of casting alloy has different properties that are necessary for various types of restorations produced for dentistry. The ADA specifies with the classification the following recommended applications for use in cast restorations.

TYPE I

Type I gold alloys are soft and are usually used in the fabrication of inlays that will be subjected to limited stress through mastication. This alloy is most often used with the direct method of making an inlay; thus it is used less often than the other types of alloys.

TYPE II

Type II alloy is of medium hardness and is used in all types of cast inlays and for certain posterior bridge abutments.

TYPE III

Type III alloy is harder and can withstand greater stress than Type I or II alloys. This makes the alloy useful for full crowns, certain three-quarter crowns and bridge abutments, and in the construction of precision-fitting inlays.

TYPE IV

A Type IV alloy is extra hard and of a strength to be used for partial dentures clasps, precision cast bridges, and three-quarter crowns.

▶ Solders

Soldering is a procedure necessary in the fabrication of many dental prostheses. In this technique, two metals are connected through a special low-fusing alloy. Solder selection depends on the type of metals that are to be fused. Thus, the content of solder varies, depending on the alloy. A gold solder containing a lower gold content with zinc and tin may be used or a silver solder designed to work with stainless steel and other metals. Usually a flux, a paste or powdered material, is placed on heated metal to remove oxidizations from the surfaces before soldering.

Finishing, Polishing, and Cleansing Agents

Fabrication of restorations and appliances and maintenance of existing prosthetics all require the use of finishing, polishing, and cleansing materials to achieve the ideal end product. Some of these materials are used intraorally, while others are only used extraorally. The materials may be in the form of a powder or a stick or may be mounted on a stone or mandrel, a disk, a point, a strip, or a wheel.

Before reviewing the materials used to finish, polish, or clean, it is necessary to understand the differences in their applications in dentistry. A material that is designated as a cleansing material is used to remove debris from the surface of an object, whether that object is a natural tooth or a prosthesis. A material that is considered a finishing agent removes excess material or structure from a prosthesis, while polishing materials are used to smooth roughened surfaces.

The materials used in a cleansing procedure are commonly dentifrices and prophylactic pastes used in home care and in professional procedures. These materials are of a small particle size, but if they are used inappropriately, it can lead to abrasion—the unnatural wear of a surface. Finishing and polishing materials are of a larger particle size and are designed as abrasives to complete the required steps in a sequence.

Four elements affect the rate at which something is finished: the particle size of the abrasive, the rate the abrasive moves over a surface, the pressure applied on the abrasive to a surface, and the hardness of the abrasive surface being finished. A coarser abrasive particle abrades the surface more quickly, as does greater pressure and speed of the abrasive on a surface.

Abrasives may be found in the following substances:

- Dentifrices that contain calcium carbonate, dibasic calcium phosphate dihydrate, anhydrous dibasic calcium phosphate, tricalcium phosphate, hydrated alumina, sodium metaphosphate, calcium pyrophosphate and silica
- Calcite or calcium carbonate
- Kieselguhr or siliceous materials from aquatic plants
- Pumice or siliceous volcanic glass
- Rouge or iron oxide powder
- Tin oxide or white powder
- Tripoli from North African rock or currently made from silica
- Zirconium silicate or a hard abrasive of small particles

Other abrasives are as follows:

- Aluminum oxide on paper or plastic disks in various grits,* reddish brown in color
- Cuttle, originally from bones of fish, now from quartz on paper or plastic disks in various grits, beige in color
- Sand, a quartz on paper or plastic disks in various grits, beige in color
- Garnet, a natural substance on paper or plastic disks in various grits, red in color
- Diamond chips imbedded in a matrix to create diamond points, disks, and stones, silver in color and hardest of the abrasives silicon carbide on paper or plastic disks in various grits, black in color

Various dental materials or surfaces found in the oral cavity require the use of different types of materials to cleanse, finish, and polish to obtain the desired final result. The following is a summary of common materials used to achieve these objectives.

Tooth structure—Use a dentifrice to clean and polish the surfaces of the teeth with a toothbrush or, professionally, use a prophylactic brush, cup, and paste.

Denture base—Remove soft debris with brush and dentifrice, hard deposits and stains through repolishing the denture with several alkaline substances, including perborates, hypochlorites, and peroxides, or dilute acids and abrasive powders and creams. May also soak the denture in a solution of 5% sodium hypochlorite and 3 parts water or 1 teaspoon hypochlorite and 2 teaspoons of a glassy phosphate (such as Calgon) in water. Follow the use of both soaking solutions by brushing and thorough rinsing.

---

*The grit of abrasive materials ranges from coarse to extra fine.

Composite—To minimize roughness and to reduce finishing and polishing, place Mylar matrix strips interproximally before inserting the material. Professionally, remove composite through the use of various grits of abrasive materials, starting with the coarsest and finishing with the finest. Examples of the instruments used include diamond stones, finishing burs, abrasive strips and disks, abrasive points, and polishing paste.

Amalgam—Place the material against a metal matrix band interproximally, condense it and carve it to the desired anatomic proportions, and then burnish it to smooth the surfaces of the restoration. To remove excess or roughened amalgam, use green stones, finishing burs, disks of adalox, silicon carbide and cuttle, soft brushing with silex or tin oxide, and finishing strips.

Gold—Finishing and polishing of cast gold alloy restorations is accomplished on the die when working with an indirect restoration. First, pickle the cast to remove oxidation, then polish proximal surfaces with a variety of devices: disks of sand, cuttle, crocus, burlew and cratex wheels, rag wheels with a slurry of pumice or radoff, sureshine, bendick, chamois, and rouge. Some of the processes are completed in the laboratory and others in the mouth. Take care to follow all methods of infection control, while going from the chairside with the restoration and back to the laboratory to use a polishing device, such as the rag wheel with rouge.

KEY POINTS

- Dental materials are used to replace tooth structure lost as a result of trauma or decay, prevent the invasion of caries, replace soft tissue, and make replicas of existing structures. Dental materials are also used to finish, clean, and polish various devices.
- The Council on Dental Materials, Instruments, and Equipment, an ADA subgroup, along with the Federal Specifications and Standards and the National Bureau of Standards establishes guidelines materials must meet.
- The properties of dental materials, such as dimensional change, thermal conductivity, electrical solubility, sorption, wettability and mechanical properties, affect selection and manipulation of a material.
- Several dental materials may be considered and designated as hazardous substances. These materials must be handled as directed by OSHA and other regulating agencies.
- Preventive dental materials, those used to protect tissue or as preventive agents, include mouthguards, splints, periodontal dressings, fluorides, and pit and fissure sealants.
- Restorative materials are primarily used to replace lost teeth and oral structures. These materials are divided into two categories: direct and indirect restorative materials.
- Several characteristics of restorative dental materials, direct or indirect, are similar. These include restrictions on dispensing the material, armamentarium used, and manipulation of the material.

▶ In the fabrication of restorations, appliances, and other devices, a final finish may require the use of finishing, polishing, and cleaning agents.

BIBLIOGRAPHY

Dentistry: an illustrated history, St Louis, 1985, Mosby.

Craig RG: *Restorative dental materials,* ed 9, St Louis, 1993, Mosby.

Craig RG, O'Brien WJ, Powers JM: *Dental materials properties and manipulation,* ed 5, St Louis, 1992, Mosby.

Food and Drug Administration: *Talk paper,* Rockville, Md, March 20, 1991, Public Health Service.

How finishing affects glass ionomers: results of a five-year evaluation, *JADA* 2:00-00, 1900.

UNIT III   THE BUSINESS OF DENTISTRY

12 Ethical and Legal Aspects of Dentistry

CHAPTER OUTLINE

LEARNING OBJECTIVES

You will have mastered the material in this chapter when you can:

▶ Define the key terms
▶ Explain the importance of ethics and law to dentistry
▶ Differentiate between the various types of law that affect the practice of dentistry
▶ Explain various types of consent
▶ Explain the effect of the good samaritan law on health care professions
▶ Describe the code of ethics of professional dental organizations
▶ Explain the importance of a state dental practice act
▶ Identify the function of a state board of dentistry

KEY TERMS

Abandonment
Assault
Assignment
Battery
Civil law
Consent
Credential
Defendant
Defamation of character
Dental practice act
Direct supervision
Ethics
Expert witness
Fact witness
Felony
Fraud
Implied consent

Informed consent
Invasion of privacy
Law
Lawsuit
Litigation
Malpractice
Misdemeanor
Negligence
Patient of record
Plaintiff
Respondeat superior
Standard of care
Stare decisis
Statutory law
Supervision
Tort
U.S. Constitution

Each day, dental professionals are faced with issues involving the legal requirements and voluntary standards in the delivery of dental treatment. The **dental practice act** of each state defines the legal requirements necessary to practice dentistry and the scope of dental practice. The legal standards for dental care are derived from both *common law (judicial decisions) and* **statutory law**, such as the dental practice act, which was enacted by a legislative body. Legal standards for dental care determined through common laws, such as the informed consent doctrine and the *reasonable man doctrine,* will be discussed later in this chapter. Legislative action in the form of each state's dental practice act establishes education, credentialing, and licensure requirements for the dentist and any dental auxiliaries recognized in that state's act.

 Kentucky was the first state to enact legislation to place the practice of dentistry under state regulation on February 6, 1868. New York and Ohio followed suit in the same year. Source: American Dental Association.

The dental professional is governed in practice not only by the dental practice act of each state and by the legal standards derived from common law, but also by the

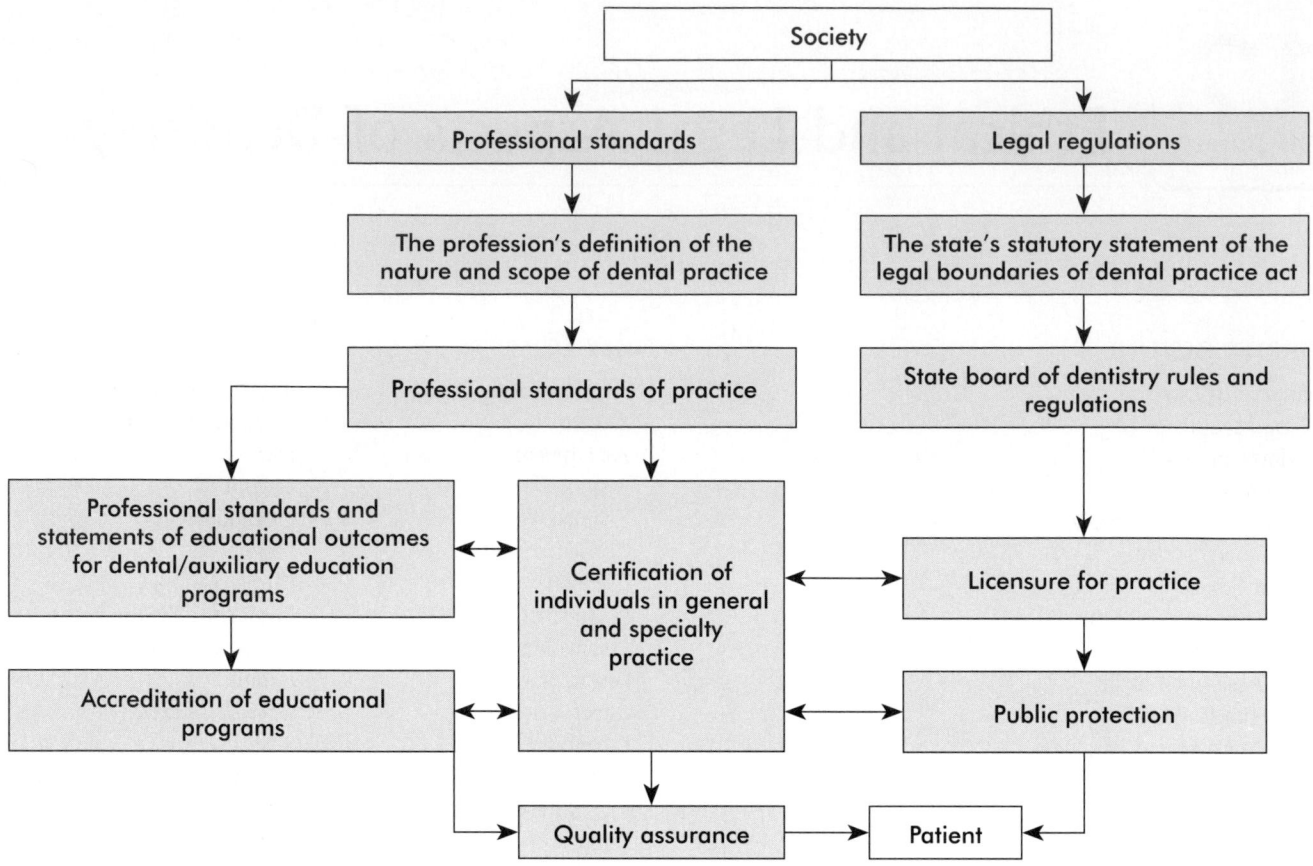

FIG. 12-1   Diagram of professional and legal regulations of dentistry.

voluntary standards, such as the principles of ethics that were developed and implemented by the dental profession itself. Both legal requirements and voluntary or professional standards are implemented for the protection of society and, ultimately, the patient. This process of regulation is illustrated in Fig. 12-1. The dental assistant practicing in a dental office today must understand the effect that law has on the dental practice and must be aware of how legal and ethical standards impact the performance of daily duties. Furthermore, each member of a professional organization should be familiar with that organization's code of ethics.

Membership in a professional organization is voluntary, and thus, the standards of these organizations are considered voluntary but are used as guidelines in peer review. Professional organizations continually reassess the functions of their standards and the qualifications of their members. The standards of professional health organizations reflect an assessment of the need for dental care and the public's expectations for dentistry. Examples of voluntary standards are illustrated in the professional code of ethics, standards for accreditation of

education programs, standards for credentialing, and standards of various service organizations.

Copies of the principles of ethics for any of the dental professional organizations may be obtained from their national offices. To obtain a copy of the state dental practice act, contact the state board of dentistry in your state.

Definition of Law

Law consists of enforceable rules governing relationships among individuals and between individuals and their society. This broad definition of law first requires the establishment of rules, such as constitutions, statutes, administrative agency rules, and judicial decisions. These rules are adopted with the desire that individuals will behave and conduct their affairs in the approved manner defined within the rules.

Over time, the body of laws established from customs or judicial decisions made in English and American courts has become known as *common law*. Also known as *case law,* common law makes up a predominant part of the everyday law we must follow. The cases that contribute to this law may involve court interpretations of a statute, regulation, or provision of the constitution. Such interpretations become part of the authoritative law and serve as precedents in particular jurisdictions. Common law is distinguished from **statutory law**, which is enacted by state and federal legislatures. In areas where legislation has not covered the relevant issue, the courts still refer to the common law. Differences in decisions vary between states.

Common law is based on the principle of *stare decisis,* or *let the decision stand.* For instance, when a decision has been made in a court of law, that decision becomes the rule to follow in future cases with similar circumstances. The case that first establishes the rule is referred to as the *precedent.* Court decisions can be changed, but only when a strong justification can be shown. The benefit of the doctrine of *stare decisis* is fairness. This doctrine prevents using one set of rules to judge one person and a different set of rules to judge another when the circumstances are similar.

The federal government and states have separate constitutions setting forth powers and limits for each level of government. However, the *U.S. Constitution* is the supreme law. *Constitutional law* involves cases that deal with interpreting the various provisions of the U.S. Constitution and addresses any powers and limits contained within it. Not all cases involve a constitutional issue or argument.

Administrative law is a body of law created by administrative agencies in the form of rules, regulations, orders, and decisions to carry out their duties and responsibilities. These laws can be enforced by the agencies outside the judicial process. A state board of dentistry is an administrative agency at the state level. The executive officers of an administrative agency perform specific functions, including enforcing laws within their agency. This body also has the power to make rules and regulations that conform to enacted laws, such as the state dental practice act. Rules and regulations adopted by this group are referred to as administrative laws.

Statutes are laws enacted by a legislative body. These laws must conform to state and federal constitutions. A dental practice act is an example of a statutory law.

▶ Classifications of Law

Law can be divided into two classifications: civil and criminal. **Civil law** relates to duties between persons or between citizens and their government. **Criminal law** deals with wrongs committed against the public as a whole. Criminal law is public law, whereas civil law is sometimes public and other times private. In a civil case,

one party tries to make another party comply with a duty or pay for damage caused by failure to comply with that duty. In criminal law, the government seeks to impose a penalty on the guilty person through fines or imprisonment.

▶ Crimes and Torts

A *crime* is a wrongdoing against society as a whole and is prosecuted by a public official. In most cases when a crime is committed, the intent is to do wrong. However, a person who breaks certain laws can be guilty of a crime whether there was intent or not. Criminal liability requires performing or committing a prohibited act with a specific state of mind showing intent on the part of the actor. In some cases the omission of doing an act can be a crime if the person has a legal duty to perform the act, e.g., failure to file a federal income tax return.

A crime can be classified as a **misdemeanor**: a less serious crime, punishable by a fine or imprisonment up to a year; or a crime can be classified as a **felony**: a more serious crime that is punishable by imprisonment for more than 1 year.

A **tort** is a civil wrongdoing. It is a breach of a legal duty owed by one person to another, and that breach must be the proximate cause of harm done to the complaining party. A tort is generally resolved through a civil trial with a monetary settlement for damages. Included in torts are the areas of assault and battery, infliction of mental distress, defamation, and fraud. Torts may involve an intentional or unintentional act of wrongdoing. An intentional tort means the one committing the tort intended to commit the act. Intentional torts for which a dental assistant could be held liable include assault and battery, defamation of character, invasion of privacy, and immoral conduct or fraud.

Unintentional torts involve a particular mental state. The failure to exercise a **standard of care**, treatment that the reasonable person would exercise in a similar circumstances, is an example of an element in an unintentional tort. If a dental professional had no intention of causing any harm through a particular act or failed to see that consequences or harm would occur through no action, negligence still could be alleged when someone suffers injury; the professional failed to live up to a particular standard of care. The questions to answer in determining whether an unintentional act of negligence has occurred are as follows:

1. Was there a duty to follow a standard of care?
2. Was this duty breached?
3. Did the plaintiff suffer injury?
4. Was that injury a direct result of that breach of duty?

These four elements make up the unintentional tort of negligence. Strict liability is an unintentional tort and relates to a person being held liable for personal actions

BOX 12-1

COMMON NEGLIGENT ACTS IN A DENTAL OFFICE

Abandonment
Burns
Mistaken identity
Foreign objects left in patients after surgical procedures
Defects in equipment
Failure to observe patient reactions and to respond appropriately
Medication errors
Drug administration errors
Failure to exercise good judgment
Failure to communicate
Loss of or damage to patient's personal property
Disease transmission

and for damages or injuries caused by these actions, regardless of the care they exercised.

Negligence is described as performance of an act that a reasonably prudent person under similar circumstances would not do; or negligence can be just the opposite: failure to perform an act that a reasonably prudent person would do under similar circumstances. **Malpractice** is usually considered negligence by professionals, but it can mean, in a broader sense, any wrongdoing by a professional. Malpractice can refer to *any* professional misconduct, evil practice, or illegal or immoral conduct and is not just limited to acts of negligence. While negligence involves unintentional acts, malpractice can be either unintentional or intentional. For example, immoral conduct is considered an intentional act of malpractice. Box 12-1 lists negligent acts that might occur in a dental office.

LITIGATION

Litigation involves the entire legal process encompassing a lawsuit, whereas the *lawsuit* itself is the legal action in a court. The person or party who initiates the lawsuit is the **plaintiff**, the injured party. The person being accused of the wrongdoing is the **defendant**.

During malpractice litigation the patient might be the plaintiff and the dentist or the person who is being sued is the defendant. It is likely that other individuals in the dental office, such as a dentist associate, dental assistant, or hygienist, might be named either as a party in interest to the legal proceedings, a defendant, a fact witness, or an expert witness. A **fact witness**, when placed under oath, can and must provide only firsthand knowledge testimony, not hearsay (rumor or speculation). In such testimony the fact witness describes what he or she saw

or did during a specific act. For instance, if the fact witness is being questioned about the administration of a local anesthetic for a patient, he or she may be asked if the dentist specified what type of anesthetic to prepare, if he or she then prepared the anesthetic and passed it to the dentist, how much anesthetic was administered to the patient, and what the patient's reaction was following the anesthetic administration. If the fact witness received only the directions and prepared the anesthetic for the setup but did not participate in its administration, only the initial questions can be answered. To describe any further action would be hearsay.

An **expert witness** is called to testify and explain to the judge and jury what happened based on the patient's record and to offer an opinion as to whether or not the dental care, as administered, met acceptable standards. Standards may vary by state. Often, a dentist may be called as an expert witness to testify in a malpractice litigation based on educational background and strong clinical expertise. An extensive knowledge of dental law and standards, as well as an understanding of malpractice liability, is beneficial in such cases.

The first state to license dental hygienists was Connecticut. The Connecticut Dental Law adopted in 1915 included an amendment to regulate the practice of the dental hygienist. This amendment served as a precedent for several states that adopted similar clauses. Source: American Dental Association.

▶ Dental Practice Act

The legal requirements necessary to practice dentistry, as well as the scope of that practice, are developed through legislative action within the state and then identified in the state dental practice act. This act defines the minimum educational standards, requirements for credentialing, and criteria for license revocation or suspension for a dentist, hygienist, and, in several states, the dental assistant. Other legal requirements are enacted by the government in the form of rules and regulations and, like the dental practice act, also regulate the practice of dentistry.

An example of a government agency making requirements that affect the practice of dentistry is the Occupational Safety and Health Administration (OSHA) blood-borne pathogen standards (see Chapter 8, *Infection Control*). The state dental practice act is not frequently changed. However, as changes take place in technology and the standards for dental care are modified, it can become necessary to add new rules and regulations to the state dental practice act. For instance, a dental practice act may define the delegation of duties assigned to a dental assistant. This definition may be rather broad, such as

A person may assist in rendering dental care to a patient under the supervision of a licensed dentist, excluding the diagnosing or prescribing for disease, pain, deformity, deficiency, injury or physical condition, or the cutting of the human teeth, alveolar process, gums, jaws or attendant tissue, the removal of accretion and stains including calcareous deposits, deep scaling, root planing, restoration of hard or soft tissue and the independent administration of anesthesia, analgesia or acupuncture and other procedures prohibited by rules promulgated by the board.

However, rules may be specifically enacted at a later date that regulate a specific section of the act in order to protect the public or to aid in delegation of duties to dental auxiliaries. In the dental practice act just described, rules were declared that specifically stated:

A dentist SHALL NOT delegate or assign the following functions to a dental auxiliary (dental assistant, registered dental assistant, or registered dental hygienist) unless authorized by the rules or the code:

1. Diagnosing or prescribing
2. Cutting of hard and soft tissues
3. Removal of accretions, stains, or calculus*
4. Deep scaling*
5. Root planing*
6. Any intraoral restorative procedure
7. Independent administration of anesthesia, analgesia, or acupuncture
8. Irrigation and medication of root canals, trying in cones, filing, or filling of root canals
9. Taking impressions for any purpose other than study or opposing models
10. Permanent cementation of any restoration or appliance

Rules in many dental practice acts specifically indicate the types of duties that can be performed by a dental assistant trained in an office setting, a certified or registered dental assistant (or other form of credential) and a registered dental hygienist. Frequently dental practice acts present rules in a *can do* or *cannot do* list format for easier interpretation of the tasks.

Many state dental practice acts define conditions under which a dental auxiliary can perform specific duties. Each state provides a list of definitions within the law, and the descriptive language may vary significantly from state to state. Examples of such terminology include assignment, patient of record, and supervision. **Assignment** commonly refers to the dentist assigning a specific procedure to a dental auxiliary that is to be performed on a designated patient of record. The physical presence of the dentist in the office or in the treatment room at the time the procedure is being performed will be defined in

this section of the law. **Patient of record** means a patient who has been examined and diagnosed by a licensed dentist and whose treatment has been planned by the licensed dentist. **Supervision** refers to the conditions under which a patient of record may be treated by an auxiliary and the protocol to be followed after the treatment is rendered. One type of supervision is referred to as **direct supervision**, which generally means the dentist has designated a patient of record on whom services are to be performed and has described the procedure to be performed. The dentist will examine the patient before prescribing the procedures to be performed and again on completion of the procedure. The dentist must be physically present in the office at the time the procedures are being performed.

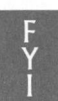 The first state to license dental assistants was Minnesota.

It is important to remember that the legal standards within a dental law are for the protection of the general public. The impetus for changes in these standards comes not only from the dental profession itself, often through the state board of dentistry and organized dentistry but also from the public consumer.

▶ State Board of Dentistry

The state board of dentistry is responsible for regulating the practice of dentistry in the individual states. Members of this board are commonly appointed by the governor of the state and generally include dentists, dental hygienists, and assistants in those states where assistants are licensed or credentialed by the board. Consumer members who have no relationship to dentistry may also be included. Membership on this board generally includes a cross section of the profession to obtain geographic, specialty, academic, and private sector representation.

Professional Standards

Over the last half century, dental assisting has taken several steps to ensure the competence of its practitioners—one of them being the process of credentialing. **Credentialing** is a generic term that refers to the ways in which a professional can ensure and maintain competence. The processes used in credentialing include accreditation, certification, and licensure.

Accreditation is the process by which an educational program is evaluated and recognized by an outside agency for having attained a predetermined set of standards. These standards are identified by the profession and educational peer groups. In dentistry the

---

*A registered dental hygienist is authorized to perform these functions under the appropriate supervision.

Commission on Dental Accreditation of the American Dental Association (ADA) is responsible for accrediting educational programs in dentistry, dental assisting, dental hygiene, and dental laboratory technology. When a program is accredited by the ADA, the program makes public its accreditation status. Such accreditation validates that the educational program has met a set of standards that satisfy the needs of the profession and the public. In many instances a criterion for obtaining a credential, such as certification or licensure, is contingent on successful completion of an ADA-accredited educational program. **National certification** in dental assisting is a voluntary procedure and may be achieved through the Dental Assistants' National Board (DANB), as described in Chapter 2. This process asserts that the person has met certain criteria that has been established by a nongovernmental association. **Licensure** is the credential granted to a candidate by the state after the candidate has met the necessary requirements to practice in the profession. Generally this license is granted after the person has met certain educational requirements and has completed some form of state testing.

Code of Ethics

Ethics is a branch of philosophy and consists of a systematic intellectual approach to the standards of behavior. Ethics in daily professional practice challenges a practitioner to differentiate between right and wrong. When someone asks a theoretical question, such as "How do I know what is good?" that person would be dealing with metaethics. A more utilitarian question the dental assistant might ask during daily work is "Am I doing what is right in this situation?" This question deals with a more practical application of ethics considered normative ethics; it also deals with morals and values. Morals are considered a more informal and personal commitment to a set of values. Values are the standards we use for making decisions that endure over a significant period of time. The behaviors expected of the dental professional are based on a set of standards developed from ethical considerations, and these determine what is acceptable.

Voluntary standards are shaped by personal morals and reflect the challenges and needs of society. Such standards were evident as early as the Hippocratic Oath in the sixth century B.C. As part of its existence, nearly every professional organization establishes some statement of ethical and professional conduct. Each organized group within the profession of dentistry, including the ADA, American Dental Assistants' Association (ADAA), and the American Dental Hygienists' Association (ADHA), has a code of ethics for its members. This code of ethics is based on moral principles that reflect concern and care for the patient.

▶ ADA Principles of Ethics

Dentistry as a profession enjoys the right of self-government that is based on its training and education. However, this right carries with it an obligation to maintain quality standards and to be responsible to your peers. This right of self-government does not allow a person to disregard professional standards or laws governing the practice of dentistry. The profession's primary goal is providing quality care to the patient in a competent and timely manner. The dental professional can maintain the quality of care through continuing education, training, and research. Additionally, the maintenance of a stringent code of ethics and professional conduct is essential to quality dental care. An overview of the ADA Principle of Ethics and Code of Professional Conduct is shown in Box 12-2.

▶ ADAA Principles of Ethics

Like the ADA, the ADAA has addressed the issue of ethics by preparing the following statement as the principles of ethics for its members.

Each individual involved in the practice of dentistry assumes the obligation of maintaining and enriching the profession. Each member may choose to meet this obligation according to the dictates of personal conscience based on the needs of the human beings the profession of dentistry is committed to serve. The spirit of the Golden Rule is the basic guiding principle of this concept. The member must strive at all times to maintain confidentiality and exhibit respect for the dentist/employer. The member shall refrain from performing any professional service which is prohibited by state law and has the obligation to prove competence prior to providing services to any patient. The member shall constantly strive to upgrade and expand technical skills for the benefit of the employer and the consumer public. The member should additionally seek to sustain and improve the local organization, state association, and the American Dental Assistants' Association by active participation and personal commitment.

Dental Assistant Liability

In the last 2 or 3 decades the need for liability insurance has become a major concern for the practicing dental assistant. As assignments for intraoral duties that involve direct patient care become more evident in state dental practice acts, the dental assistant's need for liability insurance will continue to increase. For years the **doctrine of** *respondeat superior* seemed the most applicable concept of liability for dental assistants who work in a dental practice. This concept holds an employer liable for the negligent acts of an employee when carrying out the employer's orders or when

BOX 12-2

OVERVIEW OF ADA PRINCIPLES OF ETHICS AND CODE OF PROFESSIONAL CONDUCT

PRINCIPLE #1

Service to the public

▶ Dentists may exercise reasonable discretion in selecting patients for their practice, but they shall not refuse to treat patients because of a patient's race, creed, color, sex, or national origin. Furthermore, it is recognized that each dentist has an obligation to provide care to those in need. Thus, a decision not to treat an individual because the person has AIDS or is HIV seropositive, based solely on that fact, is considered unethical.

▶ Dentists are obligated to protect the confidentiality of patient records.

▶ Dentists are encouraged to use their knowledge, skills, and experience to improve the dental health of the public by assuming leadership roles in the community. During such service dentists are expected to maintain or elevate the esteem of the profession.

▶ Dentists are obligated to make reasonable arrangements for emergency care for their patients of record. When such treatment is provided by another dentist, this dentist is expected to return the patient to his or her regular dentist.

▶ Dentists are obligated to protect the health of their patients by assigning to qualified auxiliaries only those duties that are legally delegable. Furthermore, dentists have the obligation to prescribe and supervise the work of all auxiliary personnel working under their direction and control.

▶ Dentists may provide expert testimony when necessary to arrive at a just and fair settlement of a judicial or administrative action. However, to accept a fee contingent on the favorable outcome of the litigation in exchange for such testimony is considered an unethical act.

▶ Dentists shall not accept or tender *rebates* or *split fees.*

▶ Dentists shall not represent the care being rendered to a patient in a false or misleading manner.

▶ Dentists shall not represent the fees being charged for providing care in a false or misleading manner. To overbill (i.e., increase a fee for a patient solely because the patient has insurance), submit claim forms with incorrect dates or procedural descriptions, or recommend and perform unnecessary dental services is considered unethical conduct.

▶ Dentists are obligated to inform a patient of the proposed treatment and any alternative treatment plans in a manner that will allow the patient to be actively involved in treatment decisions.

PRINCIPLE #2

Education

▶ All dentists as recognized professionals are obligated to keep their knowledge and skills current.

PRINCIPLE #3

Government of a profession

▶ Dentistry as a profession has an obligation to regulate itself. Dentists are obligated to make themselves part of a professional society and also to observe its rules of ethics.

PRINCIPLE #4

Research and development

▶ Dentists are obligated to make available the results and benefits of investigative results that will be useful in promoting or safeguarding the health of the public.

▶ With the exception of formal investigative studies, dentists have the privilege of prescribing, dispensing, or promoting only those devices, drugs, and agents whose formulae are available to the dental profession.

▶ Dentists may obtain a patent and copyright as long as it does not restrict research or practice.

PRINCIPLE #5

Professional announcement

▶ Dentists must represent themselves in a manner consistent with the esteem of the profession and must not misrepresent their training or competence through false or misleading information of any form.

▶ Dentists may advertise, but such advertisement should not communicate any false or misleading information.

▶ Since a patient may select a dentist based on a name, the use of a trade name that is false or misleading may be considered unethical.

▶ The ADA recognizes eight specialties in the profession: dental public health, endodontics, oral pathology, oral and maxillofacial surgery, orthodontics, pediatric dentistry, periodontics, and prosthodontics. A dentist who has met the educational requirements and standards for a specialty may select to announce the specialization with the use of the terms *specialist in* or *practice limited to* and shall limit the practice exclusively to the announced special area(s).

serving the employer's interest. This doctrine applies to an employee/employer relationship and is applicable only when a negligent act is committed within the scope of employment. This doctrine does not relieve the negligent employee of liability but opens the door for the injured person, commonly the patient, to sue another party. The employer, even if innocent except for the negligence of the employee, can be found liable because of this doctrine. The employer in this situation could subsequently sue the employee for negligence to recover any loss sustained.

A dental assistant's best legal safeguard is competent practice. However, with the increasing numbers of malpractice claims, it is wise for the practicing dental assistant to carry some form of liability insurance. This insurance may be obtained through the ADAA or by contacting either a local or state dental or dental assistant society. Obtaining a list of companies in the private sector within your geographic location is another source for liability insurance. You can also check with your employer to see if the employer's malpractice policy covers you. In an office where the dentist is incorporated, the corporation might cover all employees.

▶ Student Liability

Dental, dental assisting, and hygiene students are responsible for their own acts of negligence if these result in patient injury. In general, students are held to the same standards of care that would be used in judging the actions of licensed personnel. A student must assume the responsibility and be thoroughly prepared to accept a clinical assignment. Students must notify their clinical instructor or faculty member if they feel they are unprepared and could jeopardize the health of a patient. Furthermore, the student is responsible for being familiar with the policies and procedures of the school or clinical site. Although many schools may provide liability coverage for their students, there is no standardized procedure, and students should clarify such coverage with school officials.

▶ Risk Management Programs

A dental professional teaches preventive concepts to patients with a firm conviction that education will prevent future disease. This concept can be applied to the prevention of malpractice claims. Most dental societies, organizations, and institutions are taking an active role in risk management by providing educational opportunities such as seminars. Risk management programs primarily show where dentists have been found liable in the past and try to teach dentists how to avoid exposing themselves to such liability. Often, these programs accomplish this goal by reviewing real cases

where dentists have been successfully sued. This method has a great impact on the dentists and auxiliaries. Risk management programs aid the dental professional in identifying, analyzing, and dealing with risks in their dental office.

Risk management programs generally include information on operating safety, product safety, quality assurance, and waste disposal. Operating safety places emphasis on methods of operating an environment that ensures the safety of the patient, staff, and visitors. Product safety should update the dental team as to the safe use of current materials and equipment and how to evaluate and maintain these products. Quality assurance programs provide information about all systems used in the care of a patient based on an evaluation of these systems. Waste disposal programs update you about the most current methods for disposing of medical and dental wastes. Risk management education combined with competent practice can be the best insurance for the dental professional in avoiding situations that may prompt litigation.

Ethical and Legal Issues in Dentistry

Each day the dental professional is confronted with ethical and legal decisions. The basis for each of these decisions must change as laws and societal influence affect the delivery of dental care. As mentioned previously, the dental professional must constantly be aware of the changes taking place in laws affecting dentistry. Several issues persist in dental treatment, and these should be considered carefully as routine dental care is delivered. Many of these issues are addressed in dental laws, and others are covered in the principles of ethics. The following discussion provides the assistant with a practical understanding of various issues. These dilemmas are described for the purpose of promoting the process of critical thinking.

▶ Assignment of Duties

As described in the section on the state dental practice act, the assignment of specific procedures to dental auxiliaries is the responsibility of the licensed dentist. If a duty that is not legal within the state is assigned to the dental assistant, the dentist is liable for this illegal action. Furthermore, if a dental assistant performs a procedure that cannot be legally delegated to be performed by the assistant, the assistant is liable for such action. Often the employer/employee relationship creates conflict in such assignments. An assistant may feel that if the dentist assigns a task to perform, then it must be performed because the dentist is an authority figure and the assistant's job could be jeopardized if the assignment is not carried out. The assistant can be exposed to legal liability if he or she performs a task that cannot be legally delegated or if he or she performs a task that he or she is not qualified to do simply because the task was assigned by the dentist.

▶ Consent

Consent is the voluntary acceptance or agreement of what is planned or done by another person. To examine or treat a patient without consent constitutes unauthorized touching and makes the person committing the act guilty of battery as discussed below. Two forms of consent exist in the delivery of dental care: informed and implied.

INFORMED CONSENT

Informed consent is a concept that has evolved over the past 2 decades as courts and legislatures have demanded more disclosure on the part of the provider about the care given to a patient. The idea behind the concept of informed consent is that each adult of sound mind has the right to determine what can and cannot be done with his or her body. For a particular person to exercise proper judgment, he or she must be given information by the health care provider. The patient must receive enough information, in understandable language, about the proposed treatment to make an intelligent decision about whether or not to proceed with the treatment. Understandable language and sufficient information on which a sound decision can be made are only two elements that form the basis of informed consent. Moreover, the patient must have ample opportunity to ask questions and have them answered. In general, courts and legislatures have defined specific elements that describe informed consent.

1. Consent *must be* given freely.
2. Treatment and diagnosis *must be* communicated in understandable language.
3. Risks and benefits of the proposed treatment, estimate of success of treatment, prognosis if no treatment is elected, and alternative treatment plans *must be* given.
4. Rights of the patient to ask questions and have them answered *must be* part of informed consent.

An important point to remember about informed consent is that if these conditions are not met, the courts may conclude that the patient did *not* consent to the operation and therefore the doctor may be guilty of battery or negligence (depending on the individual state). Patients under the influence of alcohol, drugs, or severe stress may not have sufficient capacity to give consent for treatment. When treating a minor, only the

parent or guardian may grant consent. This excludes grandparents, babysitters, or siblings. The parents, however, may authorize another party to grant consent for treatment during their absence. Such authorization must be signed and dated before the treatment consent

---

BOX 12-3

IMPLIED DUTIES OWED BY THE DENTIST TO THE PATIENT

1. Use reasonable care in the provision of services as measured against acceptable standards set by other practitioners with similar training in a similar community
2. Be properly licensed, registered, and meet all other legal requirements to engage in the practice of dentistry
3. Obtain an accurate health (medical and dental) history of the patient before a diagnosis is made and treatment is begun
4. Employ competent personnel and provide for their proper supervision
5. Maintain a level of knowledge in keeping with current advances in the profession
6. Use methods that are acceptable to at least a respectable minority of similar practitioners in the community
7. Not use experimental procedures
8. Obtain informed consent from the patient before instituting an examination or treatment
9. Not abandon the patient
10. Ensure that care is available in emergency situations
11. Charge a reasonable fee for services based on community standards
12. Not exceed the scope of practice authorized by the license, nor permit any person acting under his or her direction to engage in unlawful acts
13. Keep the patient informed of his or her progress
14. Not undertake any procedure for which the practitioner is not qualified
15. Complete the care in a timely manner
16. Keep accurate records of the treatment rendered to the patient
17. Maintain confidentiality of information
18. Inform the patient of any untoward occurrences in the course of treatment
19. Make appropriate referrals and request necessary consultations
20. Comply with all laws regulating the practice of dentistry
21. Practice in a manner consistent with the codes of ethics of the profession
22. Use universal precautions in the treatment of all patients

Adapted from Legal considerations in sports medicine, *Dent Clin North Am* 35(4), October 1991.

BOX 12-4

IMPLIED DUTIES OWED BY THE PATIENT TO THE DENTIST

1. Cooperate in the care by following home care instructions, prescriptions, recalls, and any other reasonable instructions related to care
2. Keep appointments and notify the office should an appointment not be kept, or if the appointment will be delayed
3. Provide honest answers to questions asked on the history form and by the doctor and the office personnel
4. Notify the office staff or doctor of a change in health status
5. Pay a reasonable fee for the service if no fee is agreed on either in writing or orally
6. Remit the fee for services within a reasonable time

form is signed. Various consent forms are available and must be used during all invasive procedures. Chapter 14 illustrates an example of an informed consent form common in most general practices. Each specialty practice, such as endodontics and oral surgery, has forms designed for that specialty.

IMPLIED CONSENT

Other duties or actions that flow automatically from the relationship between the patient and the dental professional are referred to as **implied duties** or **consent**. These responsibilities work in two ways: those implied duties that the dentist owes to the patient and the duties that the patient owes to the dentist. When a dentist accepts a patient for treatment, this implies that he or she agrees to accept certain responsibilities for that patient's dental care. Likewise, if a patient agrees to accept treatment by the dentist, that patient is assuming certain implied responsibilities to the dentist. Boxes 12-3 and 12-4 list the implied responsibilities for each of these parties.

▶ Assault and Battery

Assault and battery is any unexcused, harmful, or offensive physical contact intentionally performed. The interest that tort law seeks to protect is the right to personal security and safety. The physical contact can be harmful or merely offensive (such as an unwelcomed kiss or hug), and physical injury does not have to occur. The contact can be made against any part of the body or anything attached to it, such as clothing, a purse, or a chair in which the person is seated.

Assault and battery consist of a common suit brought against health care professionals. **Assault** is the threat of touching another person without his or her consent, whereas **battery** is the actual carrying out of such a threat, such as the unlawful touching of a person's body. Both situations are considered intentional torts. When a child misbehaves in a dental chair and a dentist uses force and restraint without the consent of the parent or legal guardian, the dentist is opening the door to a potential battery lawsuit. Furthermore, inappropriate verbal comments that contain sexual connotations could be considered assault. The actual touching of the patient's body by the dentist in an area other than the oral cavity could be considered battery.

▶ Abandonment

Abandonment has been defined as the severance of a professional relationship with a patient who is still in need of dental care and attention without adequate notice to the patient. Although this legal concept primarily affects the dentist, the dental assistant should be aware of its existence and aid the dentist in making certain that no patient is abandoned in midtreatment.

Abandonment Dilemma #1

A dentist who has been in practice for nearly 20 years is suddenly diagnosed with malignant cancer. Many patients are in midtreatment stages; it appears that the dentist will be unable to resume work immediately. The future is uncertain for the dental practice.

Solution. In this case, arrangements must be made by the dentist and his or her family or staff to provide for treatment of the patients. This may involve hiring a dentist for the practice to provide professional coverage of the patients or establishing contact with referring dentists who are willing to accept the patients into their practices. The practice may ultimately need to be sold to another dentist. Patients should be informed of the transition and information on patient care transferred to the treating dentists in an efficient manner. When informing patients of such changes, they must be told where their dental records are located and be given a period of time, 30 to 60 days, to contact the office and have their records transferred elsewhere if they do not wish to be seen by the new dentist.

Abandonment Dilemma #2

A patient in the practice has been irritating. He or she has failed to keep appointments and gives no notification in advance for broken appointments. The dentist is distressed with this patient and states that the patient is no longer desired in the practice.

Solution. To refuse to treat this patient is abandonment. The patient must be informed in writing of the reasons the dentist is no longer able to treat him or her. A letter should be sent stating that if the patient needs a referral for a dentist in the geographic area, he or she may contact the local dental society (include the name, address, and phone number of the dental society). The letter should also include a statement indicating that the dentist is willing to provide emergency care, including treatment for pain and infection, for 30 days from the date of the letter. The letter should be sent by certified mail, with a return receipt requested. A copy of the letter and the returned receipt should be retained in the patient's record.

▶ False Imprisonment

Intentional confinement or restraint of a person's activities without justification is considered **false imprisonment**. It involves the interference with that individual's freedom to move without restraint. Confinement can be accomplished through use of physical barriers, physical restraint, or threat of physical force. Moral pressure or future threats do not constitute false imprisonment. The restraint must have been made without that person's consent or against his or her will.

An example illustrating a situation that could potentially prompt charges of false imprisonment in a dental office is the use of physical restraint on a pediatric patient. To use physical restraint, such as forcefully holding the child in a chair without the consent of the parent or guardian, could be interpreted as false imprisonment. Similarly, the restraint of a person in a treatment room by intentionally blocking the passageway or physically detaining him or her would be considered false imprisonment.

▶ Fraud

Fraud is a form of deception that is deliberately practiced to secure unfair or unlawful gain. One of the most common practices that constitutes fraud is obtaining fees by misrepresentation through third-party payments.

Fraud Dilemma #1

A patient has insurance coverage from July 1 of last year until June 30 of this year. After this time the patient will no longer receive insurance benefits. The patient has a maximum benefit coverage of $1000 for the year and to date has only used $300 of the benefit. Around the end of June the dentist determines that the patient needs to have a fixed bridge. The patient is informed of the fee for the bridge; after June 30 the services will not be covered by the insurance company, and the responsibility for

payment will be the patient's. The patient argues that the responsibility for payment is the dentist's, who should alter the treatment date for the bridge. The patient believes this is a legitimate request, since $700 is still available from the previous insurance benefit. The patient adds that in the future he or she will still bring business to the dentist.

Solution. Changing the date on an insurance claim form to indicate that the bridge was inserted on or before June 30 when the actual date of treatment is not until mid-July is considered fraudulent activity. Although the dentist and staff may make efforts to complete this patient's case before the June 30th deadline, a common solution is to explain to the patient that he or she is asking you to commit fraud. At this point, most patients will acquiesce and apologize.

Fraud Dilemma #2

A patient's dental fees are covered by two insurance carriers, thus requiring a coordination of benefits. After the claim forms are processed, a check is received from the primary carrier for the correct amount of money. However, when a check is received from the secondary carrier, the amount is in excess of the fee, and it appears the secondary carrier has paid as a primary carrier. Consequently, extra money has been received for this patient's dental fees. The assistant enters the fee correctly on the patient's financial record but then enters the entire check from the secondary carrier into the deposit, leaving an excess of funds in the dental practice account.

Solution. When the check was received from the secondary insurance carrier in excess of the correct payment, this insurance carrier should have been informed immediately. The correct way to handle this situation is to enter the check into the deposit, but then issue and return a check to the secondary insurance carrier for the amount of overpayment. Correspondence should accompany the check with all of the appropriate information concerning the overpayment.

▶ Records Management

Nothing can be more valuable to dental professionals in a potential litigation situation than adequate records. Although record keeping is discussed in other areas of this text, the importance of including complete and thorough information on a patient's record cannot be overemphasized. Not only should you record the exact date treatment occurred, the type of treatment performed, any materials used, whether or not complications arose, and any special notations about that treatment, but also note any unusual or unruly incidences created by the patient's comments or reactions. Initials of the treating operator(s) and recorder must be included in the patient record. Remember, good documentation lowers legal risks.

Documentation should also include special incidents that occur between patients, employee, and employer. Any employee reports must be retained in employee records. Such documentation might include episodes of accidental needle punctures and require a report, including the name of the employee, the patient being treated, and the date and time of the injury. Other incidents that may warrant documentation might include unusual behavior on the part of a patient or a verbal confrontation between staff members. *Thorough, accurate, and objective documentation* is your best defense in litigation!

▶ Defamation of Character

Defamation of character is the communication of false information to a third party about a person that results in injury to a person's reputation. Such communication can be verbal (slander) or written (libel). The false statement could be about a person's product, business, profession, or title to property. A dental professional should only make true statements about the dental care of patients and only to authorized persons, such as other health care providers.

▶ Negligence

Negligence is an act of omission or commission (neglecting to do something that a reasonably prudent person would do or doing something that a reasonably prudent person would not do). As stated earlier in this chapter, proving negligence requires proof that a deviation from the standard of care has occurred, and it is often necessary to provide expert testimony. To prove negligence, the plaintiff must show that (1) there was an obligation to provide care according to a specified standard; (2) there was failure to meet that standard; (3) this failure to meet the standard led to injury; and (4) there was in fact an actual injury to the patient.

Negligence Dilemma #1

A dentist has been treating a patient for over 25 years. During this period the patient has been seen by various hygienists for routine prophylaxis every 6 months. Over the years of treatment, the 60-year-old man has had various dental procedures performed, including a fixed bridge, several gold crowns, and some endodontic treatment. During the past 2 to 3 years the patient has complained about discomfort in the buccal region of the maxillary right quadrant. Each time the dentist has assured the patient that the patient has good looking teeth with no decay, and that the dentist would keep watch over the area in case something developed.

In February the patient was seen by a new dental hygienist, who recently graduated from a nearby hygiene program. During the procedure the hygienist seemed engrossed in humming to the music being played in the office, did little scaling or probing, and told the patient that he had a *neat* set of teeth. The patient told the hygienist that the discomfort in the maxillary right quadrant was increasing, and that he frequently experienced foul mouth odors. The patient questioned the hygienist whether the dentist could examine the area of discomfort more closely. The hygienist suggested telling the dentist the story.

When the dentist examined the patient, the patient again asked about the discomfort he was still experiencing. The dentist completed a visual examination and probed the teeth with an explorer. The dentist said the last x-ray examination taken nearly 4 years ago, had not indicated any problems. The dentist complimented the patient on the fine restorative dentistry in his mouth (done by this dentist over the past 25 years) and confirmed that everything looked okay.

In early March while vacationing in Florida the patient experienced severe discomfort in the maxillary right quadrant. He was seen by a dentist in the Florida area. The patient indicated that the last time dental radiographs had been taken was at least 4 years ago. After a thorough oral examination, including a periodontal examination and a complete series of radiographs, the patient was told that he had severe periodontal disease with extensive bone loss in the maxillary right quadrant. A treatment plan was outlined that included extensive periodontal treatment, home care, and some surgical procedures.

Solution. In this situation the dentist and the hygienist had an ethical obligation to provide timely and competent quality care. The dentist deviated from acceptable standards of care. Since the last radiographs had been 4 years previously and the patient was complaining about discomfort, a reasonably prudent dentist would have taken radiographs. The dentist only examined the teeth with an explorer and failed to examine the periodontal status of the patient. Furthermore, the dentist had an obligation to refer the patient for consultation to a person with special skills and knowledge in the area of periodontal disease if the dentist elected not to treat the patient.

In addition, all dental personnel have an obligation to keep their knowledge and skills current. Failure to listen to the patient's complaint and to explore the possible origin of the problem constitutes neglect.

▶ Invasion of Privacy

This type of tort, **invasion of privacy**, refers to the publishing, otherwise making known, or using information related to the private life and affairs of a person without that person's approval or permission.

Invasion of Privacy Dilemma #1

An insurance office employee contacts the dental assistant in an office to clarify information about a patient sent to them on a claim form. The insurance clerk asks for verification of data from the patient's chart, specifically the date of birth of the child patient and the father's name and Social Security number. The dental assistant offers to fax this to the insurance company. To save time the assistant simply transfers a copy of the entire patient record, including information about a communicable disease. The action taken by this dental assistant has now placed the patient's record in a setting the patient did not request or otherwise authorize. Thus the patient's privacy has been invaded.

Solution. The dental assistant should have requested that the incomplete insurance form be returned to the dental office or that a written request for clarification of information be made by the company. Only the information requested should have been provided to the insurance company, and a review of the claim form should have been completed to determine whether the information was part of the claim form that the patient had signed.

Invasion of Privacy Dilemma #2

An assistant was having difficulty collecting an account for the dental office. The patient had failed to make payments on an account balance of $3000 over the past 12 months. During a private conversation with the patient about the overdue account, the assistant was informed by the patient that the family business was about to enter bankruptcy, and the spouse had just been diagnosed with schizophrenia and was recovering from a serious alcohol dependency. Later, during a discussion with a friend who worked in a local business, the dental assistant shared the story about this patient, who was a well-known member of the community. Disparaging or damaging remarks about the patient and the personal information the patient had shared with the dental assistant were passed onto the assistant's friend. Later this story and the remarks made by the dental assistant were told to the patient and the source of information was definitely traced to the assistant.

Solution. Any information the patient gives to a member of the dental staff remains confidential within that office. No information about a patient is shared outside the office. When a patient requests a transfer of his or her records of dental treatment, a signed authorization to transfer *must* be completed by the patient.

Good Samaritan Law

In the last 2 to 3 decades, every state in the United States has passed some form of legislation that grants immunity for acts performed by a person who renders care in an emergency situation. This concept, called the *Good Samaritan* law, was considered necessary to create an incentive for health care providers to provide medical assistance to the injured in cases of automobile accidents or other disasters without the fear of potential litigation. This law is intended for individuals who do not seek compensation but rather are solely interested in providing care to the injured in a caring, safe manner, with no intent to do bodily harm. This law does not provide protection for a negligent health care provider who is being compensated for services.

Twelve Steps to Making Ethical Decisions

The dental assistant has much to consider when delivering care to the patient. During the treatment of each patient in the dental office, a dental assistant must keep in the forefront of his or her mind questions about the tasks being performed. Routinely ask yourself the questions in Box 12-5.

BOX 12-5

TWELVE STEPS TO MAKING ETHICAL DECISIONS

1. Is the task I am performing legally able to be delegated to me?
2. Do I have the necessary credential to perform this task?
3. Am I competent to perform this task, both physically and emotionally?
4. Am I performing this procedure in a safe working environment that meets the standards of OSHA?
5. Has the patient been informed about his or her treatment?
6. Am I respecting the patient's right to privacy and confidentiality?
7. Do I maintain complete and accurate records, and have I documented any special problems arising with patients, employees, and the employer?
8. Do I maintain professional liability insurance?
9. Do I participate in risk management programs?
10. Am I willing to compromise my standards for the lack of ethics or legal responsibility on the part of an employer or fellow employees?
11. Do I maintain current knowledge of changes in dental practice acts, occupational safety, and reporting methods?
12. Do I actively participate in my professional organization and contribute to community dental health?

KEY POINTS

▶ To practice competently a dental professional must not only have the knowledge and skills necessary to perform specific dental health care tasks but must adhere to a professional code of ethics and the dental practice act in the state where he or she practices.

▶ A crime is a wrongdoing against another person or the government that is generally punishable by a fine and imprisonment. A tort is also a wrong committed against another person or another's property. A tort may be intentional or unintentional. Malpractice and negligence are forms of torts. Torts are resolved in civil actions and generally result in a monetary award or settlement.

▶ The most common issues involving ethical and legal decisions in a dental office include assignment of duties, abandonment, fraud, assault and battery, invasion of privacy, character defamation, negligence, documentation, and consent for treatment.

▶ The dental assistant plays an important role in legal and ethical issues and should be acquainted with the consequences of each of these issues. Furthermore, dental assistants must assume responsibility for their actions, as well as protect themselves with malpractice coverage when applicable.

▶ Accurate record keeping can lower the risk of legal action. Keeping details of all aspects involved in the delivery of dental treatment is critical. Records should also be maintained about the people involved in the treatment and should include any unusual or unruly comments or actions.

BIBLIOGRAPHY

American College of Legal Medicine: *Legal medicine: legal dynamics of medical encounters,* St Louis, 1991, Mosby.

American Dental Association: *ADA principles of ethics and code of professional conduct,* Chicago, 1994, The Association.

Miller RL: *Business law today,* St Paul, Minn, 1991, West.

Northrop C, Kelly M: *Legal issues in nursing,* St Louis, 1987, Mosby.

Pollack BR: Legal considerations in sports dentistry, *Dent Clin North Am,* 35(4):00, October 1991.

Woodall I, Zorkowski P: *Legal, ethical and management aspects of the dental care system,* ed 4, St Louis, 1994, Mosby.

13 Human Relations in the Dental Office

LEARNING OBJECTIVES

You will have mastered the material in this chapter when you can:

▶ Define the key terms
▶ Explain human relations in dentistry
▶ Describe Maslow's hierarchy of needs
▶ Describe Carl Rogers' client-centered therapy
▶ Explain the concept of dentistry as a service profession
▶ Identify desirable characteristics in building relationships
▶ Describe relationship between communication and productivity
▶ Identify barriers to communication
▶ Recognize nonverbal cues
▶ Describe how to improve verbal images
▶ Define patient rights
▶ Explain staff management
▶ Describe professional etiquette

KEY TERMS

Client-centered therapy
Communication
Hierarchy of needs
Human relations
Nonverbal cues

People are central to the dental office, and *the most important people in the dental practice are the patients.* In a health care profession, it is not sufficient just to be able to perform sophisticated clinical procedures; it is also necessary to know how to interact with various behaviors. Studies have shown that 90% of the average employee's day involves interacting with others. **Human relations** is not just getting people to like you; it involves the ability to resolve unpleasant situations, to understand the reasons for another's reactions, or to rebuild a deteriorating relationship. All of the people with whom you will have contact in the office are different; they have different backgrounds, experiences, and needs. You need to treat each patient or staff person in the office as an individual and accept, understand, and work effectively together.

Psychology of Human Relations

Dental professionals must understand the needs of their patients and be concerned with each patient as an individual. With this concern for humanism in dentistry, it seems appropriate that you should be aware of the contributions of two humanistic psychologists: Abraham Maslow and Carl Rogers.

▶ Maslow's Hierarchy of Needs

Dr. Abraham H. Maslow has described a *hierarchy of needs* (Fig. 13-1) that aids in understanding how a person's needs motivate behavior. Maslow identified five basic levels of needs, ranging from basic biologic needs to complex social or psychic drives.

   1. *Physiologic or biologic.* These are physical needs for such things as food, water, and shelter that must be satisfied first or life won't last long enough to satisfy any of the social or psychologic needs. A

355

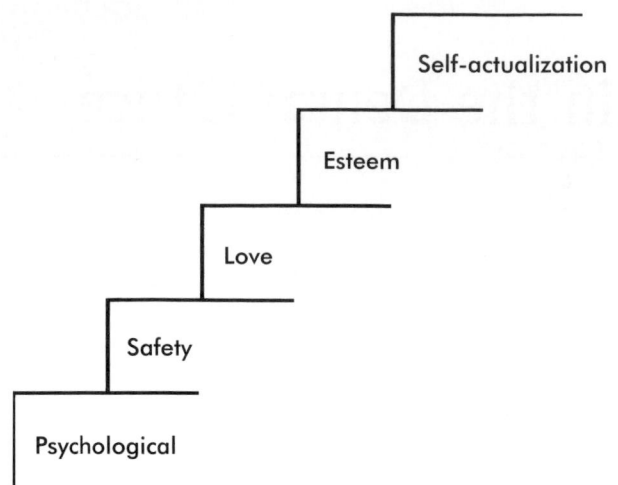

FIG. 13-1   Maslow's *Hierarchy of Needs.*

healthy, well-fed, and adequately housed person can advance to the next level of the hierarchy because of a sense of well-being.

2. *Safety or security needs.* Once the basic biologic needs are met, a person can advance to the next level on the hierarchy and explore the environment, just as a small child might explore his or her environment once food and comfort needs have been realized. At this level the person feels safe and free from danger, threats, or other deprivations. A nonthreatening job and a safe environment promotes a secure feeling and the person can advance to the next level on the hierarchy.

3. *Social or love needs.* Once a person is secure in his or her environment, the next level to attain involves social interaction. The poet John Donne wrote, "No man is an island, complete to itself." Donne realized that to be human meant to interact with people around you. Maslow, with this level on the hierarchy, realized that people need to interact with others who share similar beliefs and who provide positive reinforcement. This kind of love or social interaction gives the individual confidence to advance to the next level on the hierarchy.

4. *Esteem needs.* Interactions with others at the previous level will help generate further goals, such as higher self-esteem, better reputation, or additional recognition of peers. Typically, the self-satisfaction the individual realizes from achieving goals provides the impetus to establish new goals, thereby beginning the cycle over again.

5. *Self-actualization.* Self-actualized people are motivated by the need to grow. To fulfill this need the individual must have achieved self-esteem and have gained confidence. Maslow, later in life, expanded

his thoughts on the self-actualized person and explained that to achieve this level a person must be relatively free of illness; sufficiently satisfied, with regard to basic needs; using all capacities positively; and motivated by and committed to positive values. Often when a person reaches this level he or she, by teaching from his or her own past experiences, helps others achieve goals. It is possible that some people will never reach this level because they have not aspired to its recognition.

To relate this hierarchy to dentistry means to recognize the importance of getting to know your patients and associates. Before a dentist can motivate a patient to accept a certain type of dental treatment, it is helpful to know the level the patient occupies on the *hierarchy of needs.*

Consider this situation: A patient, who is a bank president and respected in civic activities and who has a warm, loving family and fine home, develops severe pain in the maxillary anterior area. The pain is sudden, sharp, and excruciating, making it difficult to eat and producing a great deal of swelling in the upper lip. This person may have dropped from perhaps a self-esteem level to the physiologic level. The dentist must satisfy this physiologic need immediately before attempting to suggest further treatment.

Setting up payment plans for a patient often exposes a conflict of needs. A patient must ensure that the basic needs for food, housing, and clothing are met, and yet a desire to meet social needs by improving appearance with some form of dental treatment also may be apparent. A conflict arises in the decision-making process when the patient is confronted with the conflict of how to satisfy all of these needs within a specified and perhaps limited income. The doctor and staff must make an effort to determine the patient's needs, realize the patient's potential conflict, and consider presenting an alternative treatment plan so that the patient has some options.

Maslow's hierarchy of needs not only applies to relationships with patients, it also can be applied to interactions among the staff. The dentist, assistant, and hygienist all have the same needs, and each is concerned, just as the patient, with security for today and in the future. Conflict can arise if a person becomes fixed at one particular level; the change in motivation may not be apparent, and others' perspectives may remain unchanged. This is evidenced often when a person has an interest in making money or in climbing socially without regard for other peoples' level of motivation.

Perhaps one of the best tenets in Maslow's theory is that an individual can choose his or her behavior. Although basic physiologic and environmental needs present strong influences, each individual can make alternative choices voluntarily.

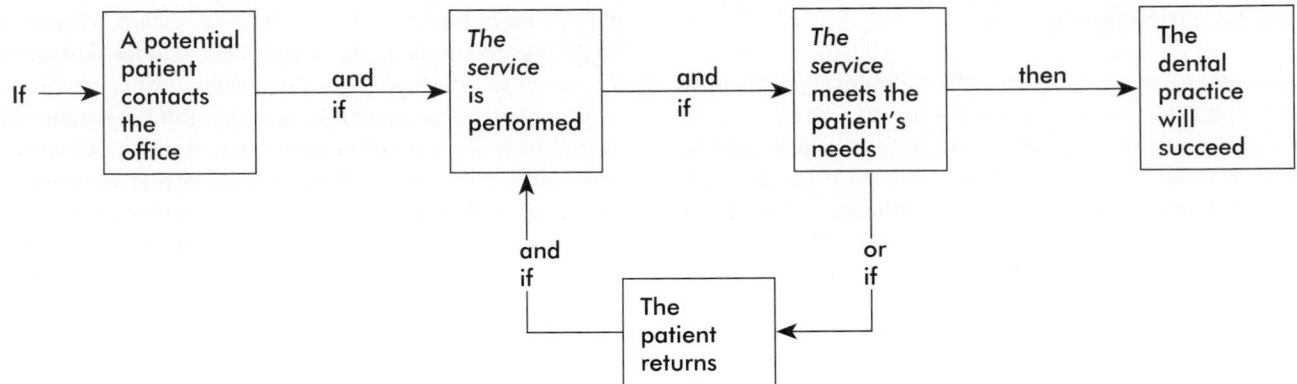

FIG. 13-2   The service concept applied to a dental practice.

▶ Rogers' Client-Centered Therapy

Carl Rogers, another humanistic psychologist, believed "that it is the client who knows what hurts, what directions to go, what problems are crucial, what experiences have been deeply buried." Rogers also suggests that the patient or other person must be accepted as a genuine person with a unique set of values and goals and that others must be treated with "unconditional positive regard."

Client-centered therapy assumes that patients know how they feel and what they want and have established their priorities. When applied to dentistry, this philosophy encourages the dental assistant to listen to the patient. Furthermore, this concept suggests that you must respect the patient as a human being, not just as a number, a case study, or a research project. The patient has needs, which should not be repressed or ignored.

These two concepts developed by Maslow and Rogers and in combination with each other, provide the groundwork for a humanistic, caring attitude that should be a prerequisite for all health care providers.

Dentistry as a Service Profession

Our society is no longer industrially oriented, but rather it is service-oriented, and dentistry certainly is an important health care service. The patient may be the focus of dental care, but the dental staff must constantly be aware that when the patient comes to the dental office to seek treatment and perhaps some type of restoration, which is a tangible product, the most important product the patient seeks is service. Only a patient who is satisfied with the services rendered will remain with the dental practice. Fig. 13-2 illustrates the many *Ifs* you will encounter in the retention of a patient to the dental practice. It is important to remember that the patient has choices: *if* the patient chooses to come to the office either because of a recommendation or because of a random

selection and *if* he or she is satisfied with the treatment and care, he or she may return. Furthermore, *if* at the return visit, the patient is still satisfied, he or she may continue to return; however, *if* dissatisfaction occurs at any stage of the service, the patient may opt not to return to the office.

The basis for patient retention is generally **communication**: the ability to understand and to be understood. A patient seldom leaves a dental practice because of dissatisfaction with the margins of a porcelain veneer crown. The patient may, however, leave because a staff member made it difficult to obtain a completed insurance claim form, was too busy to listen, made frequent errors on statements, or did not communicate the treatment plan in advance.

Desirable Characteristics for Building Relationships

It is difficult to identify a job today that does not include interaction with people. Whether the job is that of a teacher, janitor, astronaut, attorney, minister, secretary, or engineer, productivity is greatly enhanced by an ability to communicate. In fact, it is difficult to find any job today in which communication is not important. Eighty percent of people who fail at jobs did so not because of a lack of technical skills but because they did not relate well with people.

Generally, the patient's first contact in the dental office is with the dental assistant. Your attitude can give the patient a positive impression, or it may convince the patient to seek dental care elsewhere. Whether communicating with patients, staff, or friends, success depends on developing some basic *people skills.* These skills include self-confidence, genuineness, openness to experience, enthusiasm, assertiveness, integrity, honesty, an acceptance of others, the ability to be a good listener, and a willingness to be a team player.

Self-Confidence

Self-acceptance encourages self-confidence. A healthy mental picture of self accentuates positive attributes. To have self-confidence means to identify strengths and to build on them, accepting weaknesses for what they are and not dwelling on them. Self-confidence is the ability to believe that the job can be done and then doing it well.

A dental assistant with self-confidence assumes responsibility, adapts to change, is interested in the activities in the office, and provides input in decision making. For instance, a chairside assistant who is self-confident will anticipate the next step in a procedure and will determine the needed instrument or material without hesitancy, confident that he or she knows what is going on.

This same person is willing to take risks and is able to recommend changes in a routine or a procedure in the office, confident that the idea is worthwhile and merits consideration.

Genuineness

Being genuine means being yourself, being sincere, and being straightforward—important qualities when dealing with people in a health care profession. A genuine caring person is not afraid to reach out and touch someone. Placing a hand on the shoulder of a frightened patient or holding a child's hand when he or she expresses fear shows caring and displays a genuine concern for the other person's feelings. Put yourself in the patient's place and show the kind of concern you would like to receive.

A patient feels comfortable with a genuinely caring dental assistant and is likely to open up and share personal feelings. When a patient expresses depression, an assistant with genuine concern says "I'm sorry to hear you feel this way. Is there anything I can do to help you?" The patient may simply need a person to listen, a friendly smile, or a comforting pat on the shoulder.

Openness to Experience

A health care profession is no place to be close-minded. To be open to experiences means to be willing to try new techniques, to consider new ideas, to be willing to take a risk. Many people are afraid of change, and most people are afraid of the unknown. Being open means to be willing to accept new experiences; it means allowing something new to happen without tainting it with past prejudices or ideas.

Often staff members do not want to change the way things are done in the office, do not want to hire new people, and do not want to implement new technology. Consider this situation: You have worked in the same dental office for 8 years, and most of the staff members have developed good friendships. The doctor is male and has recently hired a new chairside assistant who also is male. Immediately being introduced, you feel suspicious of the new employee. As the weeks go by, he demonstrates that he is a capable and qualified assistant. You refuse to recognize his competence because of your past experiences and feelings that female dental assistants are more caring and dexterous at chairside. Openness to new experiences means accepting the present and not being committed to your past experiences. Openness is not easy and takes time, but it is essential for personal growth and for the growth of others.

Acceptance of Others' Backgrounds and Values

Each person's values are derived from his or her background and previous experiences. To accept others as worthy human beings without having a desire to change them to fit into a personal value system is to have acceptance of others. Accept others for whom they are—not for who you think they ought to be. Communication is often difficult when a person acts or appears *different* from a perceived norm. For instance, if a patient with a large facial birth defect visits the office, your attention may go to the birth defect, you may even stare at it. Your focus is on the defect and not on the patient. It is important in the health care profession to concentrate on the person and not on a particular disability.

Enthusiasm

Being enthusiastic means taking an interest in the work, being expressive, and leaving personal problems at home. To be enthusiastic does not mean to be phony or to be a constant chatterbox but to have a sincere interest in the work and the world in general. A dental assistant who is enthusiastic about the work is likely to read professional journals, seek knowledge about new technology or specific areas of interest, participate in community activities or professional organizations, and become an involved health care professional.

In working with patients, an enthusiastic dental assistant takes time to learn about the patient and his or her interests and has or finds answers for questions the patient may ask. An enthusiastic person is happy to get to work, enjoys sharing the experiences of others, appreciates good humor, and is not totally exhausted at the end of the day. An enthusiastic person has a positive outlook on life.

Assertiveness

To be assertive does not mean to be aggressive. An assertive person is bold and enterprising in a nonhostile manner. A dental assistant is often called on to assume new responsibilities and takes the initiative to get the job done. Consider this situation: The staff in the office where you have been employed for 3 years has been complaining about salaries—often among themselves at lunch time. Everyone feels awkward about discussing it with the doctor because no one is sure what to say. An assertive person will take the initiative to research salaries in the area that represent comparable responsibilities, determine the production and value of each of the staff, and present the data to the doctor in a nonthreatening manner. To be assertive often requires tact, initiative, and a willingness to take a risk.

▶ Integrity

A person with integrity is honest and lives by a code of ethics. To be honest the truth must be told, which is often difficult. It means we have to take the responsibility for our actions. Usually, we learn this lesson during childhood, but some adults continue to try to blame others for their own mistakes. Dentistry is no sanctuary for dishonesty. Dental assistants are often responsible for monies, business transactions, and records management. All of these activities require accurate and truthful records. To do otherwise sets the office staff up for unnecessary liabilities.

▶ Effective Listening

Listening is more than hearing. A good listener hears not only the facts but also the feelings that are behind the stated facts. Good listening is a combination of hearing a person's words and becoming involved with the person who is speaking. Sometimes involvement with your own problems, goals, or feelings or even a hearing loss can make it difficult for you to *hear* a particular communication. In a busy dental office, you may ignore what a person is really saying because you are too preoccupied with your work, with deadlines, or with future activities to listen effectively to a patient's needs. Often you hear only what you want to hear or have time to hear.

Sometimes, too, you forget to listen with your eyes. You need to see what the person is saying and look at the speaker when he or she is talking. When you observe a person's body language, you can notice facial expressions, gestures, and posture that can give clues to the person's feelings. Consequently, you can hear what a person is saying by observing the emotions that are displayed.

Reflective listening is the ability of the listener to absorb what has been said, reflect on it, and restate or paraphrase the feeling or content of the message in a way that demonstrates understanding and acceptance. This type of listening is beneficial to a health care professional

because both parties can interact to create a better understanding of the situation. The following is a scenario in a dental office that illustrates the point:

Patient:	I just don't know whether to have my front teeth bonded or not. My husband has always accepted me this way; but every time I have my picture taken, I always keep my mouth closed.
Assistant:	You have considered bonding, but sometimes feel you shouldn't have it done?
Patient:	Uh-huh.

The assistant has restated the basic statement of the patient. The message was in the assistant's own words and was not judgmental. When paraphrased on target, the speaker will generally respond in the affirmative. If not, the paraphrase needs to be restated until the message is received clearly.

Another example of this listening style and paraphrasing follows:

Dentist Employer:	I don't understand why we haven't been busy lately.
Assistant:	Do I hear you saying that you think we aren't working hard enough?
Dentists Employer:	No, I was just wondering if our recall system needs to be reviewed.

This conversation could have ended with the original statement of the dentist and the assistant huffing off and thinking that the opening statement contained a hidden meaning. Instead, the assistant queried the dentist to determine what the statement really meant and the true meaning of the statement was clarified.

At first, using these techniques may seem cumbersome or artificial. Try them, practice them, and soon you will realize the benefits of reflective listening. Good listening skills require that you try to understand a person before you speak. Such action results in improved relations with patients and staff and may result in fewer conflicts.

▶ Recognition of Others' Needs

All people need some form of recognition. Your colleagues within the office need friendship and recognition and desire to believe that they are valued for their contribution to the success of the team. This does not mean that you have to socialize outside the office. It simply means that you should be willing to work cooperatively to accomplish the objectives of the practice. The staff, as well as patients, have similar needs, as discussed earlier in Maslow's *Hierarchy of Needs.* To ignore another person's needs does not facilitate good interpersonal relations.

▶ Sense of Humor

A dental office can be a stressful setting for the staff who clamor to meet the demands of the daily schedule and the patient who is filled with fears of potential treatment. How you interpret a crisis situation, however, is more important. Consider the situation with a humorous eye and allow yourself to *lighten up.*

Take care to laugh at the situation and not at the people. Your patients and colleagues should not be made the brunt of a joke. Consider adding humor to the office with cartoons on the bulletin board, or, as one office staff has done, place a *whining* jar in the staff lounge with a label on it that reads, "Place all your whining and complaining in this jar and put a lid on it." Remember, humor softens conflicts and eases tension and perhaps is the best dosage of medicine that could be prescribed for any dental office.

Communication Skills

It is vital to efficiency that you work well with the patients, employer, and other staff members within the office and at the same time communicate effectively with people outside the office—other professional colleagues, suppliers, and members of the local community. Communication is the basis of human relations.

To succeed in your career, you must be a good communicator. Take a look at your own communication skills. Are there barriers you should avoid? Are there personal characteristics you need to develop or improve? Think about your communications with individuals with whom you have daily contact. Good communication takes time to develop, but it is the basis for success on the dental health team.

▶ Communication and Productivity

Since dentistry is a business, interpersonal communication must be understood in terms of productivity. Each member of the dental team is expected not only to maintain good human relations with patients and staff but also to be able to perform effectively and increase productivity. It is impossible to separate productivity from human relations. One cannot be substituted for the other. You will be expected to carry your share of the work load while maintaining good human relations with patients and staff.

Productivity is important to management; it is not just performing a task but includes the attitude of the employee and the environment in which the task is performed. Consequently, dentistry is faced both with a concern for productivity and with employee morale.

The two types of productivity on the dental team are individual productivity and group productivity. Each member of the dental team has a basic level of productivity that he or she can accomplish alone. This level of productivity may vary from day to day, depending on specific conditions, but the basic level of production is quite predictable. Fig. 13-3, *A,* illustrates the level of basic productivity for Assistant A. This productivity,

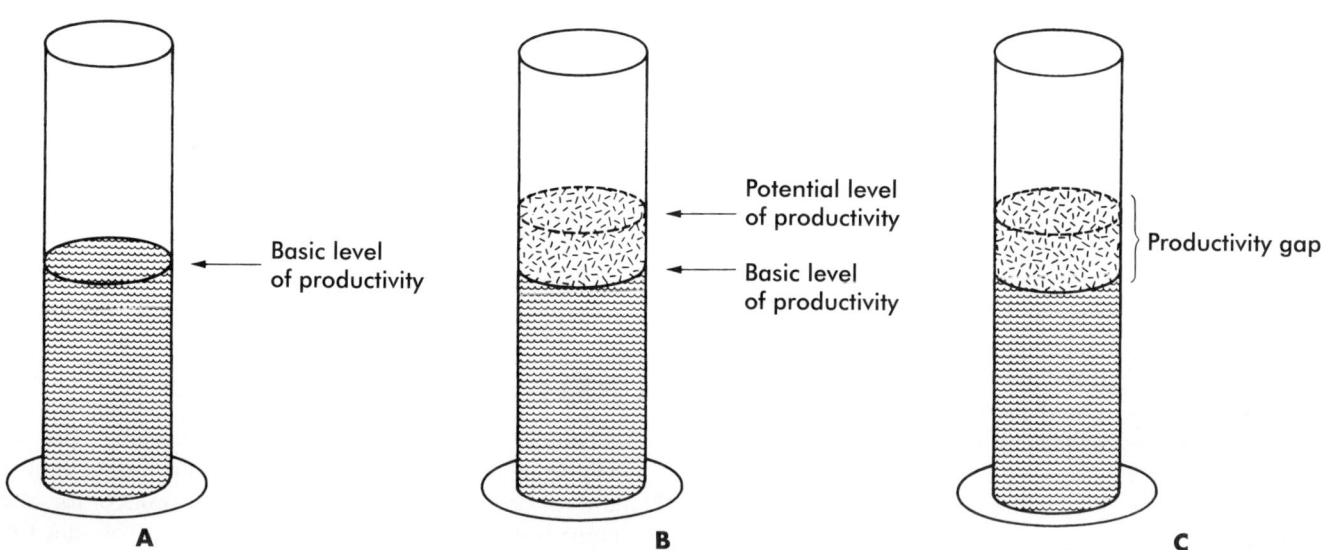

FIG. 13-3　*A,* Basic productivity of Assistant A. *B,* Potential productivity of Assistant A. *C,* Productivity gap of Assistant A.

however, is not the maximum or potential productivity of the assistant (Fig. 13-3, *B*). Most employees have a productivity gap (Fig. 13-3, *C*), which is the difference between their basic productivity and their potential productivity. Although it is likely that this productivity gap may not close completely, efforts should be made to narrow the gap as much as possible to maintain maximum productivity. This same procedure can be followed for each member of the dental health team (Fig. 13-4, *A*).

Group productivity, as shown in Fig. 13-4, *B*, diagrams each of the staff member's productivity into a group measurement. Group productivity is not simply the sum of each of the individuals's productivity, but rather the relationship of the team as they work together. It is possible to change any one of the staff members' individual productivity, depending on the interpersonal relationship of the group. Consequently the group productivity gap will change. For instance, the productivity gap could narrow or widen if a different staff member replaced an employee on the team.

It is important that each individual on the dental team try to close the gap between the basic production level and the potential production level. The doctor should also make a concerted effort to close the gap between the team's basic level of production and their potential level. To achieve the greatest potential level of productivity will require efforts on the part of the dentist to motivate the staff members by listening to their needs and suggestions, encouraging participation, and rewarding production and commitment through financial remuneration and benefit packages, as well as developing a pleasant working environment.

▶ Barriers to Communication

Perhaps the greatest potential for failure in communications are the roadblocks that a particular person sets up—roadblocks are barriers to a person's successful communication. Robert Bolton in his book, *People Skills,* divides barriers to communication into three categories:

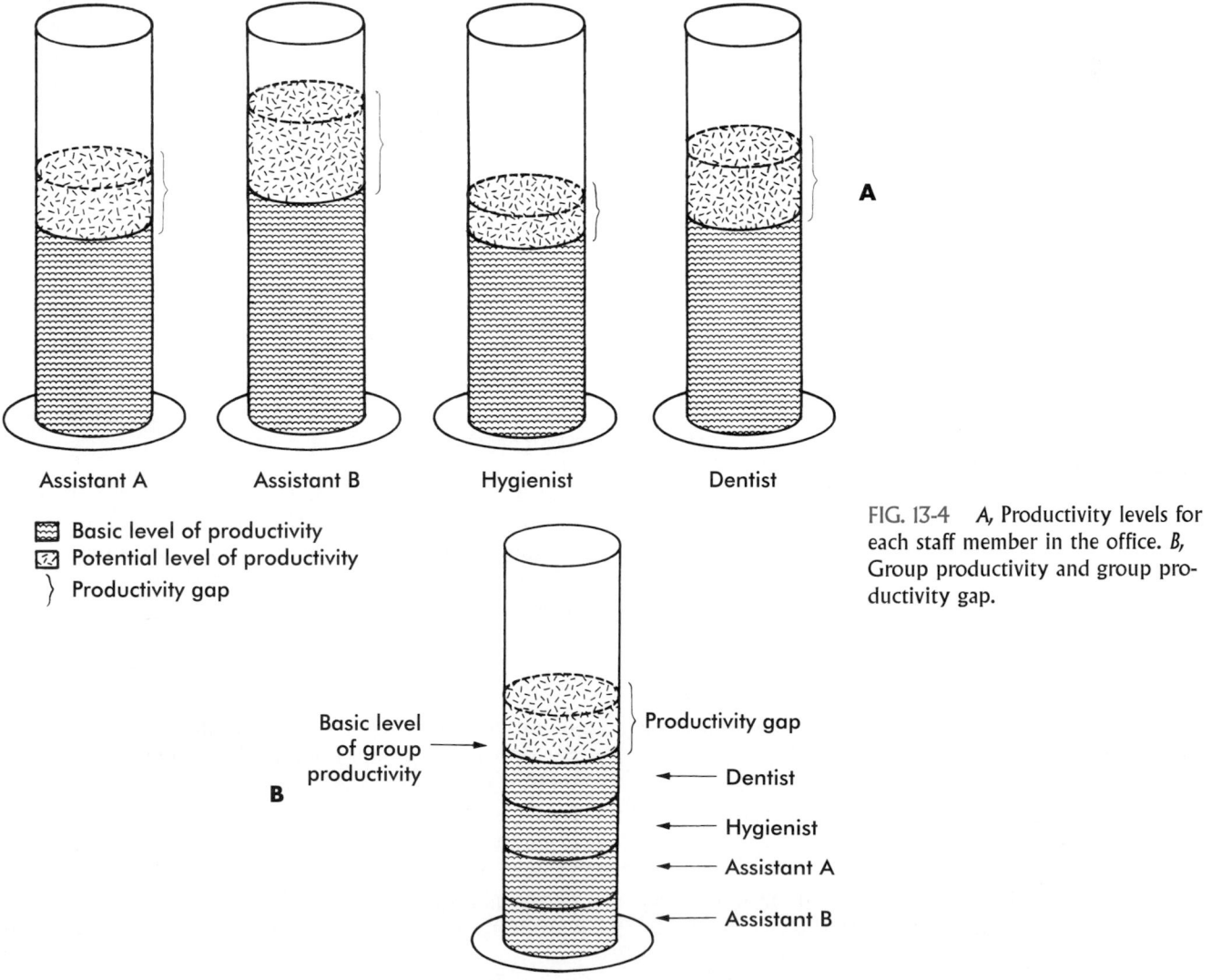

FIG. 13-4 *A,* Productivity levels for each staff member in the office. *B,* Group productivity and group productivity gap.

BOX 13-1

BARRIERS TO COMMUNICATION

JUDGING
1. Criticizing
2. Name calling
3. Diagnosing
4. Praising evaluatively

SENDING SOLUTIONS
5. Ordering
6. Threatening
7. Excessive or inappropriate questioning
8. Advising
9. Moralizing

AVOIDING THE OTHER'S CONCERNS
10. Diverting
11. Logical argument
12. Ignoring

judging, sending solutions, and avoidance of the other person's concerns (Box 13-1).

JUDGING

Judging as a barrier to communication includes criticism, name calling, diagnosing, and praising. Although at first observation some of these characteristics may seem to be positive attributes in communications, each poses potential dangers.

CRITICIZING

Many professional people believe that they must be critical and always look for ways to improve. This is evidenced especially in teaching, when the instructor tells students what is wrong with their work instead of what is right or good about the work. Employers believe that they must be critical of an employee or the employee may slack off and production will decrease. Likewise, patients may be told about the need to improve their health care, but are patients reinforced when they do well? The person being critical can often create an air of superiority or can lower the other person's self-esteem, which introduces a roadblock to good communication. Be cautious about being critical to avoid destroying the channel of communication.

NAME CALLING AND LABELING

Name calling and labeling people can have negative reactions in communications for both the sender and the receiver. Words or phrases such as *dope, nerd, nag, apple polisher,* or *the cherished one* present roadblocks and interfere with your ability to get to know another person or yourself. Take time to know your colleagues and patients, and listen to them and not to the labels that other people may have attached to them.

DIAGNOSING

Diagnosing is really a mind game. This roadblock is created when people try to diagnose what the other person means by particular actions or words. This problem can occur among staff members if one person attempts to analyze another person's behavior. Such a situation can have disastrous results in a small dental practice, and may require immediate action on the part of the office manager or dentist to prevent conflict among the staff.

PRAISING

Using praise as a gimmick to change a person's behavior is setting up a potential roadblock to communication. When someone offers praise with an ulterior motive, resentment can occur. Praise must be genuine and offered routinely—not offered just to have a favor returned. Often people are fearful of receiving praise and find it difficult to accept. For instance, when you compliment a person on a new piece of clothing, he or she may respond with an excuse to reject the praise by saying, "It was on sale" or "Thank you, it was a gift," as though they are apologizing for the praise. Expressing positive feelings toward patients and colleagues is important in interpersonal communication; however, the expression must be honest and not given with the intent of receiving something in return.

SENDING SOLUTIONS

The second category of Bolton's barriers to communication involves sending solutions to other people. These include ordering, threatening, moralizing, or inappropriately questioning another person. All of these can occur daily in a dental office.

ORDERING

To order simply means that one person tells another person what to do in a coercive, forceful manner. When such an approach is used, the staff person or patient who receives the order generally becomes resistant and resentful, which begins communication breakdown. Some individuals may become submissive and compliant, performing the task without any questions asked, while harboring resentment. In general, such orders will destroy a person's self-esteem. It is important to remember that in dentistry, a team approach is most effective, and participation in a team effort requires less of an authoritarian approach.

THREATENING

Threatening is often an action between a parent and a child, as expressed by the following: "If you don't behave, your privileges will be taken away." Threats produce the same type of negative results as orders. Sometimes, when you are at your wits' end with a patient who has a delinquent financial account, threats occur. The threat must be followed by an action, and generally, the action (usually a collection agency or other legal procedure) will result in a negative reaction from the patient. Had earlier and more positive action taken place, perhaps such unpleasant threats would have been avoided.

QUESTIONING

Excessive or inappropriate questioning can also be a barrier to communication. Questions obviously are necessary in patient care and staff interaction, but excessive questioning can foster negative reactions. For instance, when a staff member attends a professional meeting for which the employer has paid the fee and allowed the time to attend, it seems only appropriate that some communication should follow, but the following questioning and disinterested response seem inappropriate:

Dentist Employer:	Where was the meeting?
Assistant:	Downtown
Dentist Employer:	Were you on time?
Assistant:	Yes.
Dentist Employer:	What did you learn?
Assistant:	Not much.
Dentist Employer:	Was the speaker good?
Assistant:	I guess so.

The dentist was obviously interested in whether the assistant had acquired new information at the meeting. The assistant may have been resentful, however, about the specific questioning for details. Constant questioning seems common today, especially between parent and child, and when questioning is directed in an accusatory manner, people often become defensive. Perhaps the best approach for the dentist would have been to ask the assistant to describe the lecture and create a more positive atmosphere for discussion about the experience.

MORALIZING AND ADVISING

Other areas of concern are moralizing and advising. Some take great pride in attempting to solve other people's problems. A dentist may look in a patient's mouth and see evidence of treatment that appears substandard in quality. Before any statements are made, the dentist must understand the conditions under which the treatment was performed. This same attitude can exist with staff members of different backgrounds. A person who moralizes speaks with *shoulds* and *oughts:* this is what you *should* do or *ought* to do to change the way you are thinking. Moralizing creates anxiety, arouses resentment, and invites pretense among staff members and patients; it has no place in the dental practice. Advising comes easy for some people, and they may forget to consider the feelings of the person to whom they are offering the advice; it is often preceded by "I'll tell you what you ought to do ..." and then the advising person sounds off without fully understanding every facet of the problem. In a health care profession, where patients are in reality seeking advice, it is difficult to separate personal advice from professional advice; however, an opportunity to practice some active listening and perhaps offer the patient or colleague several options for consideration may arise. Respect your patient's or colleague's intelligence and believe that others have the ability to make a good decision.

AVOIDING A PERSON'S CONCERNS

Some people believe that the best way to deal with another person's concern is to avoid the problem. Some people purposely derail a conversation by diverting, applying logic, or ignoring the other person to avoid discussing a problem or to garner the attention for themselves.

DIVERTING

Diversion occurs frequently during a conversation when one person wants to switch the topic to a personal interest. If care is not taken, this situation can easily occur in a dental office. For instance, at chairside the conversation between the dentist, assistant, and patient could be as follows:

Patient	The pain in this tooth was excruciating last night. It was worse than when I....
Assistant	Speaking of pain, last night I fell over my son's skateboard coming out of our garage.
Dentist	Garage. Oh, goodness I'm glad you mentioned garage. My husband wants me to go look at a new garage door opener. Would you be sure and remind me to write that down when we finish here?
Assistant	Oh, yes, and you know, I have to go out to the mall and look for a wedding gift.

Whoa. What happened to the patient? Suddenly the patient's excruciating pain ended up at the shopping mall. Diversion of conversation can occur because people are not effectively listening to the other person. They want to divert the attention to themselves. Sometimes in dentistry the dentist thinks the only other person to talk to is the assistant once he or she begins to examine the patient's mouth. Take care to center conversations around the patient, listen to his or her needs, and involve the patient in the conversation. Sitting in a dental chair listening to other people's personal conversation is not enjoyable and does not lend to the professional atmosphere of the office.

APPLYING LOGIC

Some people may insist on resolving a problem only by logic. They may offer logical solutions to problems and not consider another person's feelings. When you are dealing with a person's discomfort, logic is sometimes not the only solution. Feelings should be the main issue in caring for another person, and since logic focuses on facts, it may be necessary to look beyond the facts to consider alternative solutions for a patient. A patient may come to the office with discomfort from a previously diagnosed condition. The dentist may have recommended that a cast metal crown be placed on the tooth. The most logical solution is to begin the preparation today and seat the casting in a couple of weeks, but the patient is uncertain about the financial situation and may want to delay the treatment; thus, the logical solution is not the practical solution, so alternatives must be considered. You need to listen to all of the patient's needs.

IGNORING

People may consider ignoring a problem to make it go away. Ignoring a problem can manifest itself in several forms in a dental office. When a patient enters the office, he or she expects to be recognized upon arrival; however, the staff may be busy talking together and may ignore the patient. The staff is too concerned with their discussion, and may hope that if they ignore the patient, he or she will go sit down in the reception room. This does not create a positive response from the patient, nor does it work for good public relations.

Similarly, ignoring a conflict with staff members can only result in the potential for greater hostilities to evolve. In general, to ignore a problem now will only lead to a more serious problem later. For improved communications it is best to face a situation, look at the potential resolutions, and take action. This action should result in improved relations between patient and staff.

Using Nonverbal Communication

Nonverbal cues are gestures that indicate a person's inner feelings without verbal communication. Nonverbal cues often indicate how a person is coping with these feelings. The dental office is one setting in which people display a myriad of nonverbal cues. These cues can happen when a doctor signals for an instrument exchange or when a complication develops in a procedure. A patient can display nonverbal cues (Fig.13-5, *A* and *B*) in the form of raised eyebrows or clenched hands to indicate fear; a menacing posture or hands on the hip can indicate disgust. An assistant can display caring and help to ease the situation by placing a hand gently on an elderly person's shoulder or by holding a child's hand to allay fear. It is a major responsibility of the assistant to recognize nonverbal cues, since the doctor's major focus is the oral cavity. If the patient appears to be in discomfort, the assistant must inform the doctor and question the patient about this discomfort. Sometimes words cannot describe the feelings of a person. Often words are not adequate to express what you see in the look of someone's face in the moment of anger, fear, or disgust. When a patient or staff member gives a cue of frustration or disgust, it must not be ignored. Ask the other person about his or her feelings. For instance, a person may be frowning a lot. You may ask, "Mrs. Brown, you seem upset. Is there something I have done or something I can help you with?" She may respond, "Yes, I hurried here for this appointment, and now I have to wait, and I just realized I forgot to bring my insurance claim form. I'm so mad at myself." Her problem may not be the potential of waiting; she may be annoyed with herself. Be objective and realize the person's reaction is directed at the situation, not at you. Offer the patient the opportunity to mail in the form or perhaps you have the necessary form in the office and can offer it to her.

Improving Verbal Images

A health professional has an obligation to allay fears and comfort patients. The most obvious way of accomplishing these tasks is to create a good image in the patient's mind. In a dental office you need to eliminate the use of words or phrases that conjure a negative thought. For instance, when you say, "This won't hurt," you have told the patient that the possibility of pain exists. However, if you say, "We will make you as comfortable as possible," or "You may feel this," you have let the patient know that you can provide comfort. Table 13-1 lists terms and phrases that are frequently used in a dental office. Try replacing these terms or phrases with the suggested ones to create a more positive environment. Also, use language the patient will understand when discussing his or her treatment.

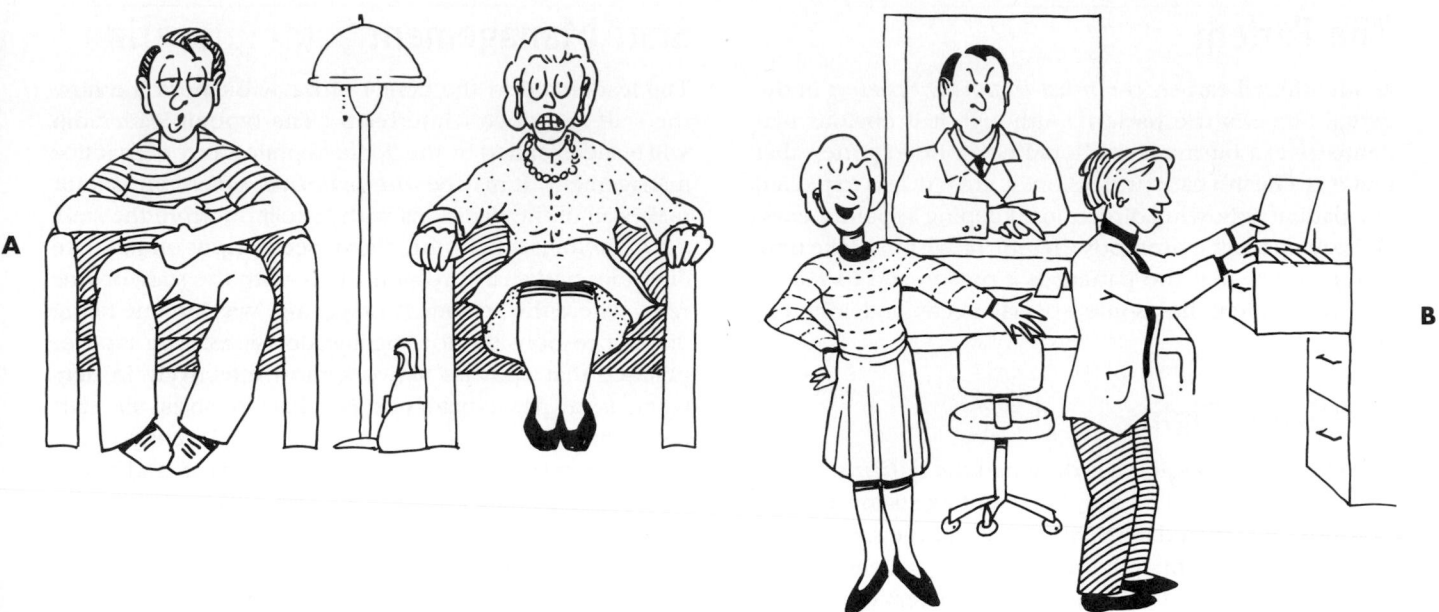

FIG. 13-5 *A,* A nonverbal cue of a patient demonstrating fear. *B,* A nonverbal cue of a patient demonstrating disgust or frustration because he or she is being ignored.

TABLE 13-1   SUGGESTIONS FOR IMPROVING VERBAL IMAGES

Avoid these phrases	Use instead
1. I don't know.	1. That's a good question. Let me check and find out.
2. We can't do that.	2. That may be difficult, but let me see what I can do. (Then find an alternative solution.)
3. You'll have to	3. Soften the phrase, saying, You'll need to, or Here's how we can help you with that.
4. This may hurt—or—You may have some pain.	4. Soften the phrase, saying, You will have some discomfort, or We will try to make you as comfortable as possible.
5. The doctor is at a convention. (This may denote a party atmosphere.)	5. Replace with, The doctor is at a seminar.
6. Old patient.	6. Former patient.
7. Spit.	7. Rinse your mouth.
8. Hatchet, hoe, chisel.	8. Soften by using instrument number; for example, T-1 or H-2.
9. Drill the tooth.	9. Prepare the tooth.
10. Pull the tooth.	10. Extract or remove the tooth.
11. Waiting room.	11. Reception room.
12. Shot.	12. Anesthetize or injection.
13. Would you like to come in? (Patient may say, No!)	13. Dr. Smith will see you now.
14. Filling.	14. Composite or amalgam restoration.
15. The girls.	15. The chairside assistant, hygienist, or office manager.
16. The doctor is tied up.	16. The doctor is with a patient.
17. Checkup or cleaning.	17. Examination or prophylaxis.
18. I want to remind you of your appointment. (People don't like to be reminded.)	18. I want to confirm your appointment.

The Patient

As mentioned earlier, the *most important person* in the dental office **is the patient**. Although it is obvious that dentistry is a business, it should never be forgotten that first it is a health care profession. A great deal is expected of a patient: following directions, keeping appointments, and paying the fee promptly. In return, we must take time to remember that the patient is a person and to realize that the patient has some special needs and inherent rights.

▸ Patients' Rights

The medical profession has designed the *Patients' Bill of Rights;* however, no formal document exists for patients in dentistry. It would be wise to consider the suggestions in Box 13-2 as potential rights of all dental patients. These suggestions are not to be considered barriers or punitive actions toward the dental profession but rather protection and courtesies for the patient.

BOX 13-2

PATIENT RIGHTS

1. Be treated with respect and consideration for his or her personal, medical, and dental needs
2. Be informed of all aspects of treatment
3. Be informed of appointment and fee schedules
4. Review of financial and clinical records
5. Obtain a thorough evaluation of needs
6. Be treated as a partner in care and decision making that is related to treatment planning
7. Receive current information, and be assured of quality treatment
8. Expect confidentiality of all records pertinent to his or her dental care
9. Be informed if the dentist participates in different third-party payment plans
10. Request and expect appropriate referrals for consultation
11. Be taught how to maintain good oral health for a lifetime
12. Receive treatment that will prevent future dental or oral disease
13. Expect continuity of treatment
14. Be charged a fair and equitable fee
15. Have appointment schedules and times maintained
16. Be treated by a staff of professionals who maintain good health and hygiene
17. Be respected for requesting a second opinion
18. Be respected as a human being who has feelings and needs

Staff Management

The leadership in the dental office will determine how the staff and doctor interrelate. The type of leadership will be determined by the doctor's philosophy of practice management. It may be *authoritative*, where the doctor makes all of the decisions with little input from the staff; *participatory,* where the doctor seeks input on practice decisions and shares responsibility with the staff; or *free rein*, where the attitude is easygoing, with no one being directly responsible for specific decisions. The type of practice that appears to work most effectively in dentistry is a participatory style that involves all staff members.

Human relations skills are as important in staff communication as they are with patients; essentially, there is no difference. With the staff, however, there is daily contact; therefore, courtesy and consideration are a prime necessity if the dental office is to function effectively. A caring attitude should exist even in situations that seem least important.

Conflicts with staff often arise from misinterpretation of responsibilities or over salaries. Before you begin work, an agreement should be made in writing regarding salary, and a well-defined salary and benefit scale should be established. In addition, responsibilities of each staff person should be well defined in the *Office Procedures Manual* (Chapter 14), and the concept of team dentistry should be emphasized. Each person should realize that everyone helps to make the practice successful.

Staff Meetings

Regularly scheduled staff meetings are necessary to maintain good communication within the office. An effective meeting serves as a forum for individuals to come together to solve problems, discuss achievements, evaluate effectiveness, and determine future goals. Many staff meetings are informal, are held in the employer's office, and consist of the dentist and a small staff. In larger practices the setting may be similar, but the structure may be a more formal one, involving a prepared agenda, with minutes that are distributed to each of the participants. In either situation the following basic rules should be followed to achieve an effective meeting:

1. Notify each staff person of the time, day, date, and location in advance of the meeting.
2. Obtain suggestions for agenda items from each staff member.
3. Determine the agenda, and prioritize items on the agenda.
4. Review accomplishments.
5. Determine goals and needs for change.
6. Maintain control of the meeting, not allowing it to turn into a session of complaints.

7. Review the outcome of the meeting, and provide minutes.
8. Begin and end on time.

Professional Etiquette

Webster defines etiquette as the forms, manners, and ceremonies established by convention, as required in society, as in a profession or official life. Professional etiquette is more than just manners, however; it also involves attitude. *An assistant may obtain a job because of excellent psychomotor or cognitive skills, but he or she may lose it because of the lack of effective skills.* More simply stated, an assistant may possess excellent clinical skills and have a wealth of technical knowledge but be sorely lacking in attitudinal and social skills. Thus this person is an undesirable employee. Having a good attitude means you possess initiative, display responsibility, work independently, anticipate a patient's or operator's needs, and operate as a team player with whom it is enjoyable to work.

Our society today has grown up eating in fast-food restaurants or eating take-out food in the living room, with little emphasis placed on the social graces that were prevalent in years past. It appears families spend less time together, and as a result there is less occasion for teaching manners or social etiquette. Possessing proper etiquette as a health professional is important to your success.

You will be attending professional meetings, seminars, and various dinner meetings during your career as a dental assistant. It is important that you take time to develop a good sense of proper etiquette. Invest some time in reviewing business etiquette texts and magazines to learn about appropriate dress, how to expand your vocabulary, and proper dining and social etiquette for the professional. You will find that the time spent on such endeavors will benefit you, and you will gain self-confidence in relating to patients of different educational and cultural backgrounds, as well as other professionals with similar or advanced educational background. It does not take an advanced college degree to be successful. It simply takes a little time to review basic skills and a little effort expended to prepare yourself for varying situations.

Our society survives on rules: traffic rules, construction codes, zoning rules; all the rules are made to enable us to survive in a world of automation, travel, and business. Manners are based on consideration for others, and in a profession such as dentistry, these are of major importance. Review Box 13-3 to identify suggestions for improving your professional etiquette in the office.

BOX 13-3

TIPS FOR PROFESSIONAL ETIQUETTE IN THE DENTAL OFFICE

- Use correct grammar; pronounce words correctly; expand your vocabulary.
- Do not interrupt another person during a conversation. If an emergency arises, excuse yourself before interrupting, state the message, and then close by apologizing for the interruption.
- Do not eat or drink in front of patients.
- Perform proper introductions for unacquainted people.
- Introduce yourself to patients; shake hands heartily to extend a warm welcome.
- If two people are engaged in a conversation, avoid standing within hearing range. If you wish to talk to one of them, leave the area and return later.
- Say "Thank you" when a person is helpful, has cooperated during treatment, or has complimented you.
- Send thank you notes for thoughtful acts or for gifts.
- Respect the space of your colleagues and do not interfere with their work.
- If the phone rings while you are talking to someone, excuse yourself to answer it. If a lengthy conversation is expected, ask the caller if you can return the call and complete the business with the person at hand.
- Avoid having friends drop in to talk.

KEY POINTS

- The major portion of a dental professional's working day involves interacting with people. Human relations requires a person to resolve conflicts, understand another person's reactions, and rebuild deteriorating relationships.
- Maslow's *hierarchy of needs* is a behavioral concept applied to motivating a person based on need. Human biologic needs must first be met before individuals can satisfy higher level needs, such as security, love, self-esteem, or self-actualization. It is vital for a health professional to understand the level of the patient's needs before proposing a treatment plan.
- Psychologist Carl Rogers developed a client-centered philosophy that can be applied to dentistry. Rogerian theory requires a clinician to accept the other person as a genuine person with his or her own set of values and goals who must be treated with respect.
- Dentistry is a service profession and requires that the patient be the central focus of all activity. To retain a patient in a dental practice the dental professional must be able to communicate effectively.
- Characteristics that lead to establishing sound relationships include self-confidence, acceptance of others' backgrounds and values, enthusiasm, assertiveness, integrity, and effective listening skills.
- Communication is the ability to understand and be understood. Communication relates directly to productivity. An individual's

productivity can be altered by the interpersonal relations with other members of the dental team. Similarly, group productivity is altered by the relationships of each person within the group.

▶ Barriers to communication, such as judging, criticizing, threatening, and name calling, inhibit successful human relations.

▶ A dental practice is a prime setting for the display of nonverbal cues. A dental assistant must be alert to these cues. If a patient gestures to indicate discomfort, the assistant must question the patient to allay further distress.

▶ A patient has many rights. These rights must be recognized and the patient treated with respect as a human being with feelings and special needs.

▶ Human relations skills do not stop with patients. They must extend to staff management. There really is no difference. Each day, each member of the dental health team must be treated fairly, with courtesy and consideration. Staff meetings should be arranged to determine office goals and objectives and as a forum to eliminate potential staff conflict.

▶ Professional etiquette requires a dental team member to display social graces, good manners, and communicate effectively in various professional and social situations.

BIBLIOGRAPHY

Albrecht K: *At America's service;* New York 1992, Warner.

Albrecht K, Zemke R: *Service America,* New York, 1990, Warner.

Bolton R: *People skills,* New York, 1986, Simon & Schuster.

Finkbeiner BL, Patt JC: *Practice management for the dental team,* ed 3, St. Louis, 1990, Mosby.

Glass L: *Say it . . . right,* New York, 1991, G.P. Putnam's Sons.

Mackoff B: *What Mona Lisa knew,* Los Angeles, 1990, Lowell House.

McConnell JV: *Understanding human behavior,* ed 6, New York, 1989, Holt, Rhinehart & Winston.

Mosley DC et al: *Supervisory management,* ed 2, Cincinnati, 1989, South-Western.

Sigband NB, Bateman DN: *Communicating in business,* Glenview, Ill, 1981, Scott, Foresman.

14 Business Office Procedures

LEARNING OBJECTIVES

You will have mastered the material in this chapter when you can:
▶ Define the key terms
▶ Explain the function of the dental business office
▶ Describe common telecommunications procedures
▶ Describe the effective use of an answering machine or service
▶ Discuss effective reception room techniques
▶ Identify appointment management
▶ Differentiate between clinical and financial records
▶ Identify the components of a clinical record
▶ Identify the components of an accounts receivable system
▶ Explain patient record transfer
▶ Describe the prevention of disease transmission from the treatment room to the business office
▶ Identify basic types of written communication
▶ Explain rules for letter writing
▶ Describe common recall systems
▶ Describe the importance of inventory control
▶ Explain the function of dental insurance
▶ Describe the components of an insurance claim form
▶ Explain basic insurance terminology
▶ Describe basic filing procedures
▶ Describe the use of computers and other automated equipment in a dental business office

KEY TERMS

Accounts payable	Fixed fee
Accounts receivable	Fraud
Appointment schedule list	Informed consent form
Capitation dentistry	Inventory control
Claim forms	Laboratory requisition
Clinical chart	Ledger card
Clinical record	Ledger card tray
Closed panel	Office policy
Code system	Predetermination
Coordination of benefits	Preferred Provider
Copayment	Organization (PPO)
Daily journal sheet	Primary carrier
Deductible	Recall system
Facsimile (FAX)	Receipt/Charge slip

Registration/Health questionnaire
Secondary carrier
Subscriber
Table of allowance
Telecommunications
Treatment plan
Unit
Update form
Usual, customary, and reasonable (UCR)

Dentistry is a business, as well as a health care profession. Therefore, while it is necessary to provide treatment for patients in a caring manner, it is also necessary to maintain maximum efficiency and production in order to make a profit.

The dental business office is the center for all activity in the office. A myriad of activities take place in this area. In addition to being the communications center, the business office is where appointments are scheduled; insurance claim forms are processed; and clinical, recall, financial, employee, and governmental records are maintained.

It is unreasonable to assume that in one chapter of text everything can be learned about managing a business office. Since this text is written primarily for the clinical dental assistant, the material presented is an overview of basic office procedures, with emphasis on the relationship between the business office and the treatment room. In this chapter you will learn basic skills in telephone and appointment book management, how to maintain various business records, inventory control, recall systems, and the basic tenets of insurance processing. For a more detailed description of business office procedures, a text such as *Practice Management for the Dental Team* is a good reference.

Telecommunication Systems

Telecommunications, communication by electronic or electric means as through radio, telephone, television, or computers, is no stranger to the dental profession. Today a dentist uses various telecommunications systems in the office. These may include a multiline telephone, cellular phone, pager, and facsimile (FAX).

▶ Telephone

The telephone is the most important instrument in the office. Most patients' first contact with the dental office takes place over the telephone. Since first impressions are so important, it is vital that the image presented to the patient relays a message that the doctor and the staff are concerned about the patient's dental health. It is vital to convey a feeling that the patient is the most important person in the office and that each member of the dental

---

BOX 14-1

SUGGESTIONS FOR IMPROVING YOUR TELEPHONE PERSONALITY

Be considerate.
Be attentive.
Be discreet.
Identify yourself.
Speak distinctly.
Use proper grammar.
Speak at a moderate rate.
Speak in a pleasant, normal voice.
Keep a smile in your voice.
Transfer calls pleasantly.
Take messages courteously and accurately.
Have writing implements accessible at all times.
Use a message pad to record complete information.
Ask questions tactfully.
Close the conversation politely.
Have emergency telephone numbers readily available.

---

staff wants to help resolve the patient's dental problems. Box 14-1 contains suggestions for improving telephone personality.

USING THE OFFICE TELEPHONE

Most offices today have telephones with multiple lines, with some form of push buttons (Fig.14-1). With the rapid development of new electronic equipment today, many variations of multiple line and hands-free systems that use head sets are available to dental offices. In most instances, when a multiple line phone is used to place an outside call, it is necessary to depress an unlighted line button and dial the number. To answer an incoming call, depress a flashing button. To answer another call while talking on one line, use the *hold* button. It is important to inform the person to whom you are speaking that you are going to place the call on *hold*. If he or she is unable to wait, ask if you may return the call; then the incoming call may be answered. If the second call continues for more than 40 to 60 seconds, return to the waiting first caller. The key to successful use of the *hold* button is courtesy—never let a caller wait for long periods of time on *hold*.

The salutation used on the telephone is the initial welcome to the office. The salutation should be short and include only basic information. A salutation such as, "Good morning" (or "good afternoon"); "Dr. Johnston's office; Miss Wilson (or Debbie) speaking," spoken in a slow, clear manner, will generally satisfy the attention span of most callers. A lengthier salutation such as "Good morning; Dr. Johnston's office; Debbie speaking; how may I help you?" says too much and will not be heard by the

BOX 14-2

RULES FOR INCOMING CALLS

Answer calls promptly.
Be certain you are answering the appropriate incoming line by depressing a flashing button.
Answer with a simple, cordial salutation.
Identify yourself.
Avoid placing a caller on *hold* for long periods of time.
Thank the caller for holding when necessary.
Record vital information on a message pad and confirm the message at the conclusion of call.
End the call with a courteous closure.
Allow the caller to hang up first before gently replacing the receiver.
Take any message that the doctor needs to receive immediately to the treatment area in written form, but do not discuss it in front of the patient being treated.

BOX 14-3

RULES FOR OUTGOING CALLS

Make calls only during acceptable business hours.
Determine that the call is placed at an appropriate hour for a particular time zone.
Be certain the phone number is accurate.
If the number is unknown, consult the telephone directory.
Have appropriate information available before placing the call (e.g., patient's record, doctor's notes, or appointment book).
Ascertain that the line to be used is available (depress only an unlighted button) before you place the call.
Make certain to listen for a dial tone before dialing.
Press buttons firmly but not too quickly.
When the call is answered, identify yourself and the doctor for whom you are calling.
State the reason for calling.
Be certain to repeat or confirm vital information at the conclusion of the call.
End the call with a courteous closure.
Allow the other person to hang up first, and then gently replace the receiver.

caller. All too often, after you have offered the salutation, a caller may ask, "Is this Dr. Johnston's office?" or "Who is this?" because he or she did not hear your message or because the message was delivered too rapidly. In an office setting where the telephone is answered for multiple dentists, a clinic name may be used or protocol should be established to ensure that the salutation is brief and yet acceptable to all dentists. A brief salutation makes the assistant's job of answering the telephone much easier. Basic rules that should be followed when making calls and receiving incoming calls are found in Boxes 14-2 and 14-3.

FIG. 14-1 **AT&T's** *SPIRIT* communications system was designed for businesses that need basic, easy-to-use telephone systems. The system offers a built-in speaker phone for convenience and the ability to answer intercom calls without touching the phone.

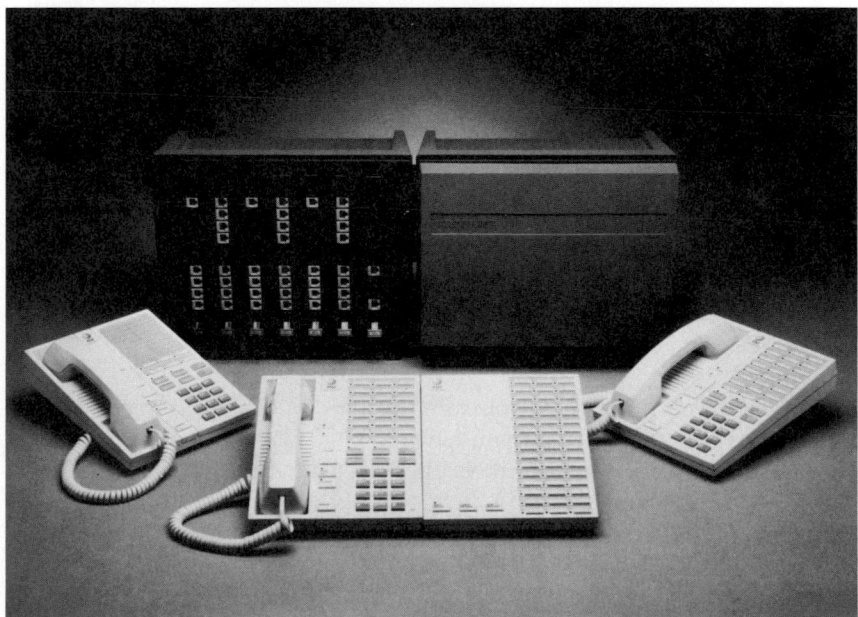

Establishing Acceptable Telephone Responses

One of the most difficult tasks to learn is how to respond to the many special situations that occur on the telephone. It is important that the doctor and staff develop some acceptable responses to patients' questions or to situations that occur frequently and that require some predetermined policy. A list of these responses kept near the telephone is especially helpful for the new assistant.

The New Patient

THE CALL

"I would like to make an appointment to have my teeth cleaned."

QUESTIONS TO ASK

"May I please have your name?"

"Have you seen the doctor previously?"

If the answer is "No":

"When was the last time you had a prophylaxis or a thorough dental examination? By whom were you referred?"

If the appointment is being made for a child:

"Who is the responsible party? What is the age of the child?"

If the child is covered by dental insurance:

"Please bring the necessary forms or verification of insurance coverage."

If the patient has never been to the office before, "Do you know where the office is located?"

BASIC CONCERNS

Avoid asking the person if he or she is an *old patient*. Be certain to obtain accurate and complete information about the patient, and make certain that appointments are scheduled within the insurance guidelines. When the patient is new to the practice, provide complete and exact directions to the office. Close the conversation with a cordial greeting to indicate that you are looking forward to meeting him or her.

Emergency Situation #1

THE CALL

"Hello, this is Mrs. Richter. I'm having some pain in a tooth and need an appointment."

QUESTIONS TO ASK

"Mrs. Richter, may I have the correct spelling of your first and last name? Your street address and phone number?"

"How long has it been since you were in the office?"

"What type of discomfort are you having?"

"Is it a sharp pain? Dull ache? Is there sensitivity to temperature or touch?"

"Where is the tooth that is bothering you?"

"How long has it bothered you?"

BASIC CONCERNS

You need to determine if this type of call is an emergency. If it appears to be, the patient should be seen as soon as possible. If, however, it can be determined that the patient is not experiencing severe discomfort or other systemic symptoms and is able to carry on routine daily activities, an appointment may be scheduled on another day in the near future.

Emergency Situation #2

THE CALL

(The caller in this situation sounds frantic.) "This is Mrs. Hernandez. My son Mark just fell off his bike and knocked out his front tooth.

QUESTIONS TO ASK

"Mrs. Hernandez, what is your son's name?"

"When did this happen?"

"How old is he?"

"Do you have the tooth?"

"How long will it take you to bring him into the office?"

BASIC CONCERNS

This situation requires remaining calm, reassuring the mother, and giving basic instructions about placing cold compresses on the site. It is important to remind the mother to obtain the avulsed tooth and secure it in a moist environment (i.e., place it in milk or back into the child's mouth). Telling the mother to bring the child in as soon as possible should be the primary issue. Do not worry about getting home and business phone numbers or some of the basic information. If the doctor is not in the office, refer the mother to the person covering for the doctor.

In the meantime, evaluate the daily schedule. If this emergency will cause a major delay in the schedule, contact patients who have appointments later to delay their arrival or reschedule the appointments. Do not tell these patients that you are behind schedule; inform them that there has been an unexpected emergency, and ask them to delay their arrival if possible. Patients generally appreciate your respect for their time.

Unidentified Person Requesting Fee Schedule

THE CALL

"How much does the doctor charge for a denture?"

QUESTIONS TO ASK

"Who is calling?"

"Have you been seen by the doctor before?"

BASIC CONCERNS

The major concern here is whether a patient is actually shopping around for the lowest fee. A policy must be established in the office for such calls. It is generally difficult to quote a fee on the telephone, since the conditions of the patient's mouth are unknown. Many doctors have addressed this problem by quoting fees for basic services, such as radiographs, initial examinations, and a basic prophylaxis. Any treatment beyond this scope would require an oral examination to determine the extent of treatment that is needed. It is important to remember that the patient is a consumer whose rights must be respected when the doctor establishes a policy for quoting fees.

A Patient Who Is Distraught Over a Billing Procedure

THE CALL

"This is Mrs. Schmidt. I just received my statement. The bill is wrong; it is too high, and I'm not going to pay it!"

QUESTIONS TO ASK

(Remain calm and positive, and, in a pleasant voice, respond as follows:)

"Mrs. Schmidt, I'm sorry there seems to be a problem. How may I help?"

"Mrs. Schmidt, what is the first name in which the account is listed?"

"What is the specific question on the account?"

BASIC CONCERNS

Two possibilities exist here: (1) The patient may be right, and an error may have been made on the statement—possibly an error on a ledger entry or incorrect information sent to the insurance company; and (2) a lack of communication between the patient and the doctor and staff regarding the fee. Successful management of such calls requires you *to not become defensive.* Do not make comments until you have had an opportunity to review the patient's records. Ask the patient to wait, or ask if you can return the call within a given time. If an error has been made, tell the patient that it will be corrected and send a corrected statement in the mail immediately. If a misunderstanding has occurred, clarify it with the doctor and present it to the patient in a nondefensive manner. Such incidents should be noted on the patient's clinical record, including the date and the action taken. Situations such as this can be avoided by having the patient sign off on the financial discussion before treatment. The safest action is *to inform before you perform.* Consequently, this will save many hours on the phone reexplaining the treatment plan and fees.

A Salesperson or Unknown Person Who Insists on Speaking to the Doctor.

THE CALL

"Hello, I want to talk to Dr. Smith."

QUESTIONS TO ASK

"May I say who is calling?"

"Dr. Smith is with a patient. How may I help you?"

"Is this call in regard to dental treatment?"

"If not, what may I say this call concerns?"

BASIC CONCERNS

This call may be from a new patient who wants an appointment, it may be a salesperson who wants to talk directly to the doctor, or it may be a personal call for the doctor. The important factor to remember is that a policy must be made in advance regarding such calls. It is vital that the doctor not be called to the phone for every request and that careful screening takes place. A frequent response to the caller who refuses to give an identity is, "The doctor is unable to return your call unless you can leave your name and state the nature of the call." With this, most persons will cooperate and give you a message. You may then give the information to the doctor for a decision on how to manage the return call.

▶ Answering Systems

Today, many offices use some form of answering machine or professional answering service when the doctor and staff are not in the office. Messages left on answering machines should be as caring and personable as possible with specific instructions as to what the patient should do in case of emergency and when the office will be reopened. If an answering service is used, one should be selected that will provide courteous, helpful, and prompt service. It is necessary to establish in advance how messages will be received, and the follow-up on these messages should be as prompt as possible.

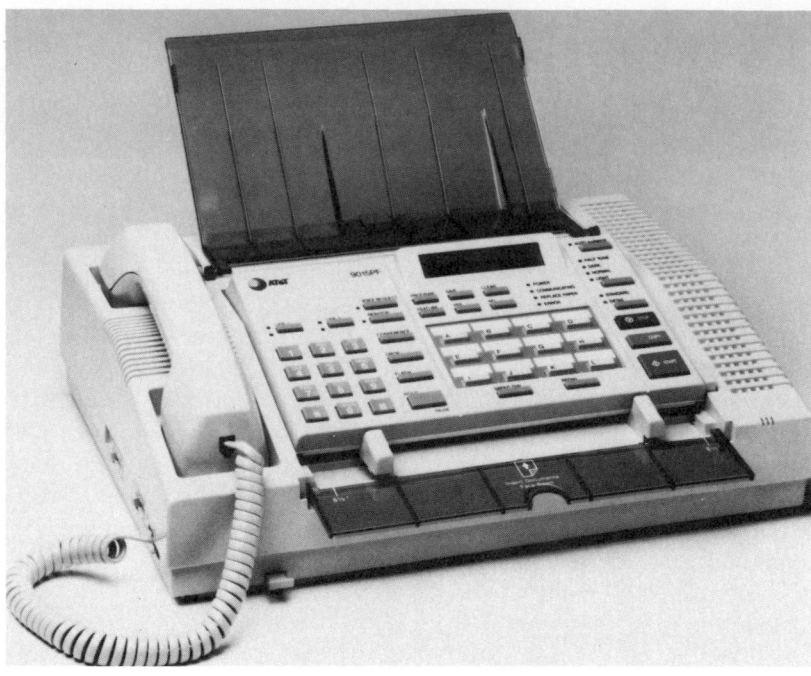

FIG. 14-2   **FAX** machine.

(Courtesy of AT&T.)

▶ Facsimile (FAX) Systems

At times, information must be transmitted immediately from the dental office to another site. Use of a **FAX** system, as shown in Fig. 14-2, is an electronic means of communicating information rapidly. The system operates like a photocopy machine that sends an image by wire. At the sending site the document is inserted into the machine and an image of the document is scanned over standard telephone lines. At the receiving end, a similar machine receives the transmitted copy. The message can be a handwritten one, a typewritten one, or a graph. The cost of transmitting a FAX message is similar to that of a long-distance telephone call because the message is transmitted through the telephone lines.

Reception Room Techniques

The gateway to the office, the reception room, is where the dental assistant meets and greets patients. The room should reflect the personality of the doctor and staff. This is not a waiting room, where people are expected to sit and wait for long periods of time. The room should exude the same warmth as a living room, where friends and family are received. The patient should be acknowledged on arrival in the reception room. A short friendly conversation can follow, and the patient can be told how long it will be before he or she is seen by the doctor or hygienist. The reception room must be kept neat and orderly at all times and be maintained at a comfortable temperature. It should be kept free of odors, and the reading materials must be kept current. Some helpful ideas that might enhance the reception room are shown in Box 14-4.

BOX 14-4

HELPFUL IDEAS FOR ENHANCING THE RECEPTION AREA

▶ Offer a wide range of reading material: books on sports, current events, homemaking, children, arts, architecture, health, gardening, or other special interests.
▶ Place magazine and/or book racks at two heights: one height for adults and one height for children.
▶ Place coat racks at two heights: one height for children and one height for adults.
▶ Install a rack with index cards and pens with a sign stating that they can be used to copy materials from magazines.
▶ Include a cookbook from a local organization.
▶ Make available an Etch-a-Sketch, coloring book, or other compact games for children.
▶ Post educational dental literature.
▶ Mount bulletin boards with special recognition of patients.
▶ Display name plates identifying staff members.
▶ Post a welcome sign or bulletin board announcing new patients/new staff for the day.

Appointment Book Management

The efficient management of the appointment book ensures a dental office that runs smoothly and is free of tension, and it precludes a waiting room that is full of disgruntled patients, who are experiencing lengthy delays.

▶ Appointment Book Features

Various appointment books are available for selection by the office staff. The color of appointment books reflects individual use. The style of an appointment book may vary in the following ways.

PAGINATION

A single day on each page makes for an inefficient method of entry. A week-at-a-glance appointment book (Fig. 14-3) allows all days of the week to be seen when the book is open. This is the preferred style in most offices today.

COLUMNATION

Each day of the appointment book may be divided into columns—from two to five, for use by multiple staff members. It is advisable to identify each person at the top of each column to avoid errors in scheduling.

BINDINGS

Variations may include notebooks with three to nine rings or those that are spiral bound. The spiral bound notebooks appear to last longer with repeated use.

TIME INCREMENTS

An increment of time is referred to as a **unit**. Most commonly, appointment books are provided with either 10-minute or 15-minute increments.

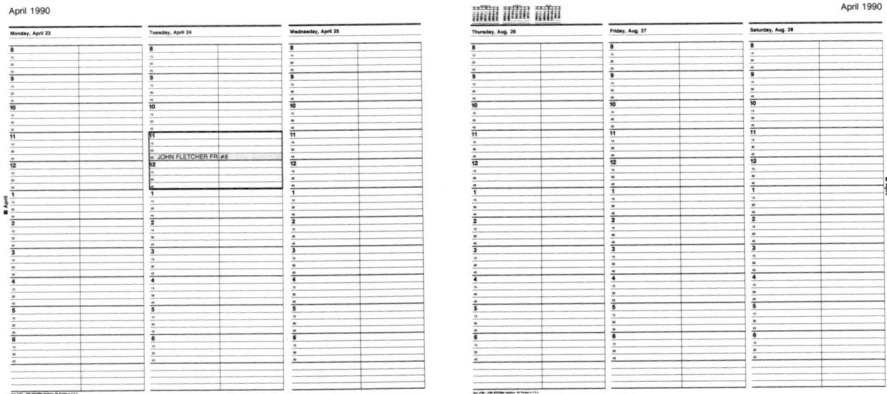

FIG. 14-3   **Week-at-a-glance appointment book.**

(Courtesy of Sycom.)

NOTATIONS/GRAPHICS

Most books are printed with months, days, dates, and time sequencing; however, those with blank pages may be purchased if desired. Most books include standardized national and religious holidays. When an appointment book is begun for a new year, the office manager goes through the book completely and outlines the matrix. The appointment book matrix is the blocking out of standard days off, special office closings, vacations, holidays, lunch hours, buffer times, and meetings that are routinely scheduled through the year. Fig. 14-4, *A* through *C*, includes examples of notations.

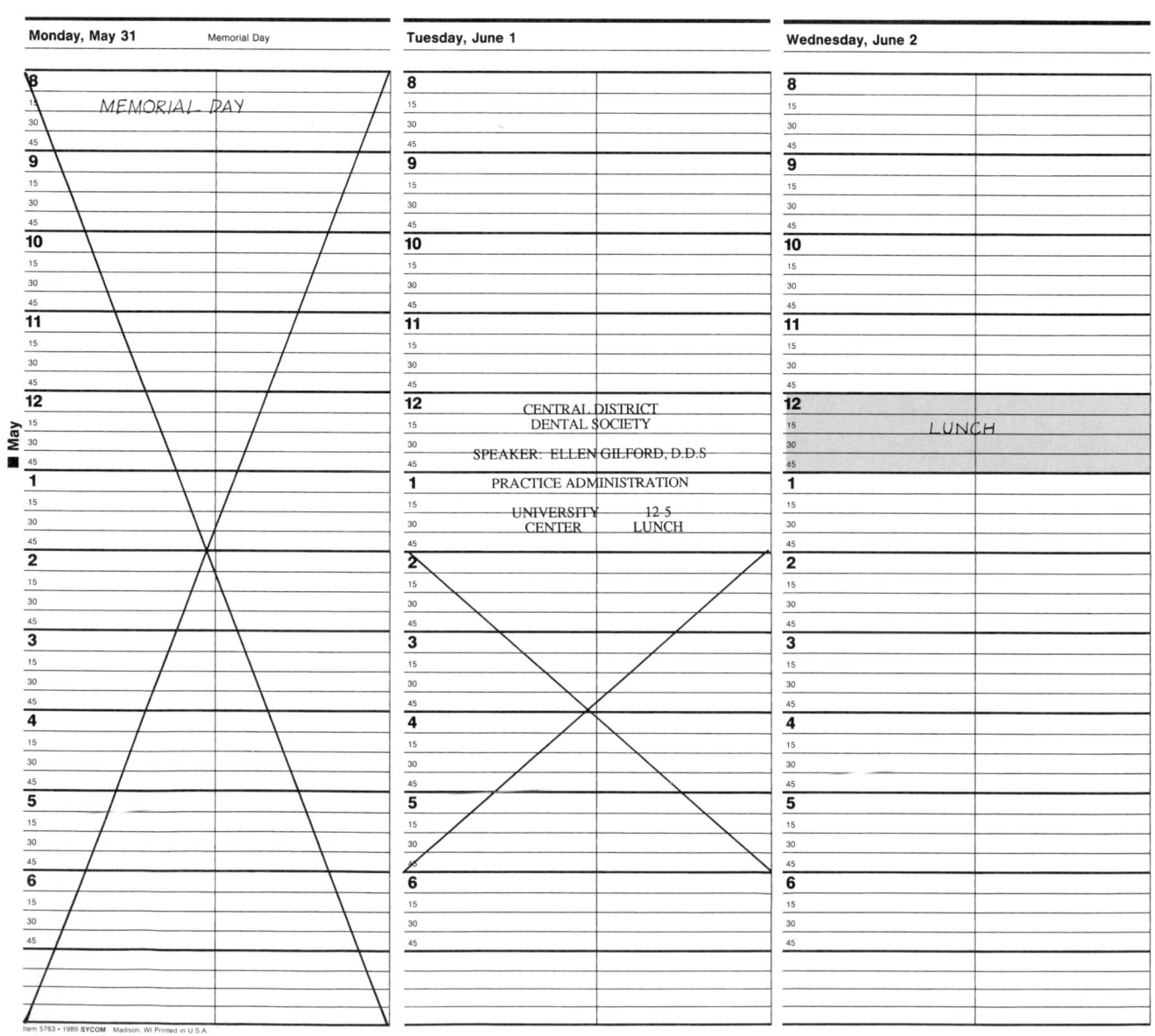

FIG. 14-4   Entries for an appointment book matrix. *A,* Notation of a holiday. *B,* Meeting. *C,* Lunch hour marked out with colored marker.

▶ Appointment Book Entries

To maintain consistency and eliminate potential problems, only one person should be responsible for the appointment book entries. All entries in the appointment book are done in *pencil* and the entry must be legible, complete, and accurate. The following information should be included with each entry and is shown in Fig. 14-5.

1. Patient's full name, with cross reference in case of duplication of names
2. Home and business phone numbers to confirm the appointment or to reach the patient in case of an emergency
3. Treatment to be done
4. Designation of the length of the appointment
5. Age of the patient, if the patient is a child
6. Special codes to denote a new patient, premedication, or laboratory status of a case

Box 14-5 displays examples of suggested codes that can be used to denote the special needs of patients. These codes provide a graphic notation beside a patient's name or appointment, as shown in Fig. 14-5.

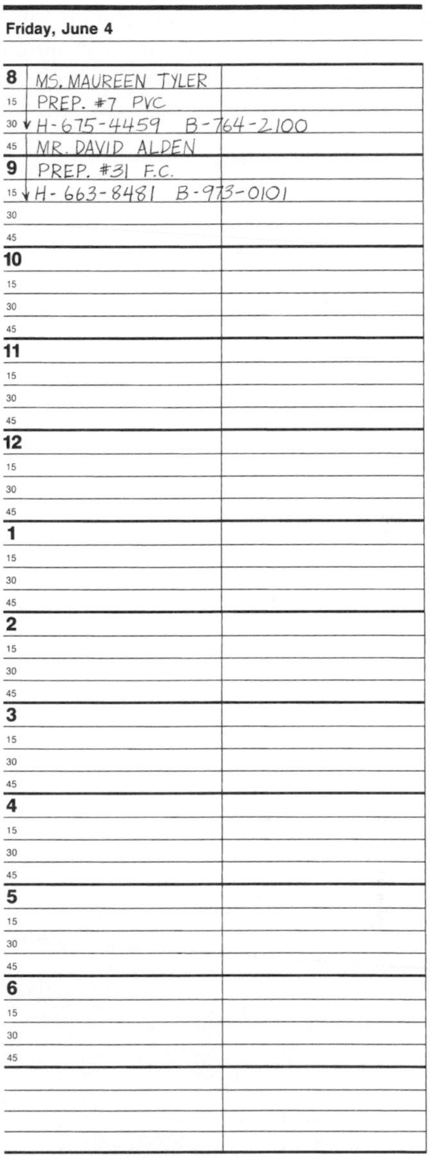

BOX 14-5

SUGGESTED APPOINTMENT CODES

N New patient
* Patient prefers an earlier appointment
B Business phone number
H Home phone number
L Case at laboratory
✔L Case returned from laboratory
PM Premedicate before treatment
✔ in red Confirmed appointment
↓ Length of appointment

Friday, June 4

8	MS. MAUREEN TYLER
15	PREP. #7 PVC
30 ✔	H-675-4459 B-764-2100
45	MR. DAVID ALDEN
9	PREP. #31 F.C.
15 ✔	H-663-8481 B-973-0101
30	
45	
10	
15	
30	
45	
11	
15	
30	
45	
12	
15	
30	
45	
1	
15	
30	
45	
2	
15	
30	
45	
3	
15	
30	
45	
4	
15	
30	
45	
5	
15	
30	
45	
6	
15	
30	
45	

FIG. 14-5 Appointment book entry, using symbols.

▶ Appointment Cards

An appointment card is given to the patient after the entry is made in the appointment book. The card is written in ink. The day, date, and time are clearly and accurately entered. Cards are made for single appointments (Fig. 14-6, *A* and *B*) or for a series of appointments (Fig. 14-7). Appointment cards come in a variety of colors and shapes but should always include the doctor's name, address, telephone number, and broken appointment policy. The opposite side of an appointment card frequently is used for patient education information.

▶ Appointment Schedule List

Each office should provide the office manager with an **appointment schedule list**, an outline of basic appointment sequencing, and the amount of time required for each given procedure. This sheet indicates the number of units for specific treatments. It can be laminated or placed in a celluloid folder to aid in appointment scheduling. An example of an appointment schedule list is shown in Fig. 14-8.

JOSEPH W. LAKE, D.D.S.
611 MAIN ST. S.E.   GRAND RAPIDS, MI   101-9575

M _____
HAS AN APPOINTMENT ON

DAY   MONTH   DATE

AT _____ A.M. _____ P.M.

THIS TIME IS RESERVED EXCLUSIVELY FOR YOU. 24 HOURS NOTICE IS APPRECIATED IF YOU ARE UNABLE TO KEEP YOUR APPOINTMENT.

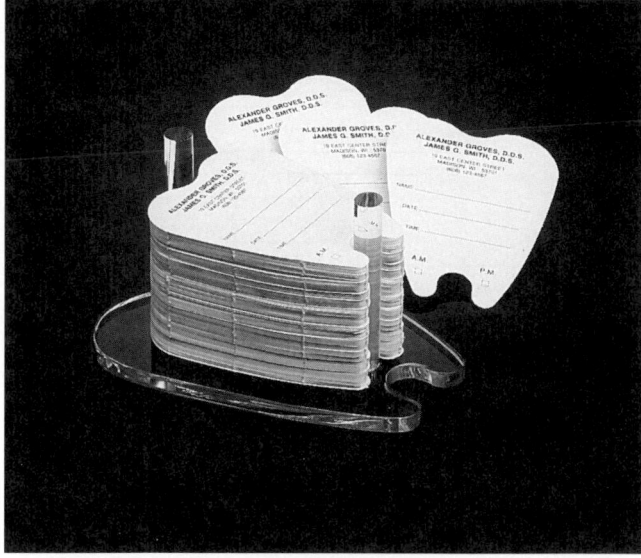

FIG. 14-6   Single appointment cards.
(Courtesy of Sycom.)

CHRIS A. BROWN, D.D.S.

19 EAST CENTER STREET
MADISON, WI 53701
TELEPHONE (606) 123-4567

M _____
HAS AN APPOINTMENT(S) ON

DAY   DATE   TIME

_____ _____ AT _____

_____ _____ AT _____

_____ _____ AT _____

_____ _____ AT _____

_____ _____ AT _____

_____ _____ AT _____

_____ _____ AT _____

24 HOUR NOTICE IS REQUESTED IF UNABLE TO USE APPOINTED TIME.

FIG. 14-7   Series appointment card.
(Courtesy of Sycom.)

TREATMENT	TIME NEEDED
Amalgam/Composite	
1 surface	1 u
2 surfaces	2 u
3 surfaces	2 u
4 surfaces	3 u
5 surfaces	3 u
6 surfaces	4 u

BONDING

One tooth	2 u
Two teeth	3 u
Three teeth	4 u
Denture Construction	
Initial impression	2 u
Final impression—2-3 days later	3 u
Bite relationship—3-4 days later	3 u
Try-in—4-5 days later	2 u
Insertion	
(If no changes in setup—1 week later)	
Nonimmediate	2 u
Immediate if surgery done out of office	2 u
Immediate if surgery done in office	6 u
Denture check	1 u
Denture—Partial	
Consult with doctor for schedule	
Denture Adjustment	Dovetail

Endodontics	Single root	Multiple root
1st—Opening—Filing	2 u	3 u
2nd—Culture (optional)	1 u	1 u
3rd—Final point—Sealing	2 u	3 u
Minimum of 48 hours between 2nd & 3rd appts.		

Extractions	
"Uncomplicated" single	2 u
2 or 3 "uncomplicated" extractions	3 u
Quadrant	4 u
Removal of sutures	Dovetail
Gingival Surgery	
Quadrant surgery	3 u
1 week later—dressing change	1 u
1 week later—dressing removal	Dovetail
Gold Restorations	
1-2 surface inlay	Prep—2 u
1 week to 10-day interval	Seat—2 u
3-4 surface inlay	Prep—2 u
1 week to 10-day interval	Seat—2 u
¾ crown or full crown	Prep—3 u
1 week to 10-day interval	Seat—2 u
Porcelain Veneer Crowns	
1 tooth	Prep—3 u
2 week interval	Seat—2 u
Prophylaxis	
Adult with doctor	2 u
Adult with hygienist	4 u
Child with doctor	1 u
Child with hygienist	2 u
New patient—schedule with hygienist for prophylaxis and with doctor for examination	2 u
Emergency	
Schedule according to nature; generally 2 u or utilize buffer as discussed	

FIG. 14-8 Appointment schedule list.

(From Finkbeiner BL, Patt JC: *Practice management for the dental team*, St Louis, 1991, Mosby.)

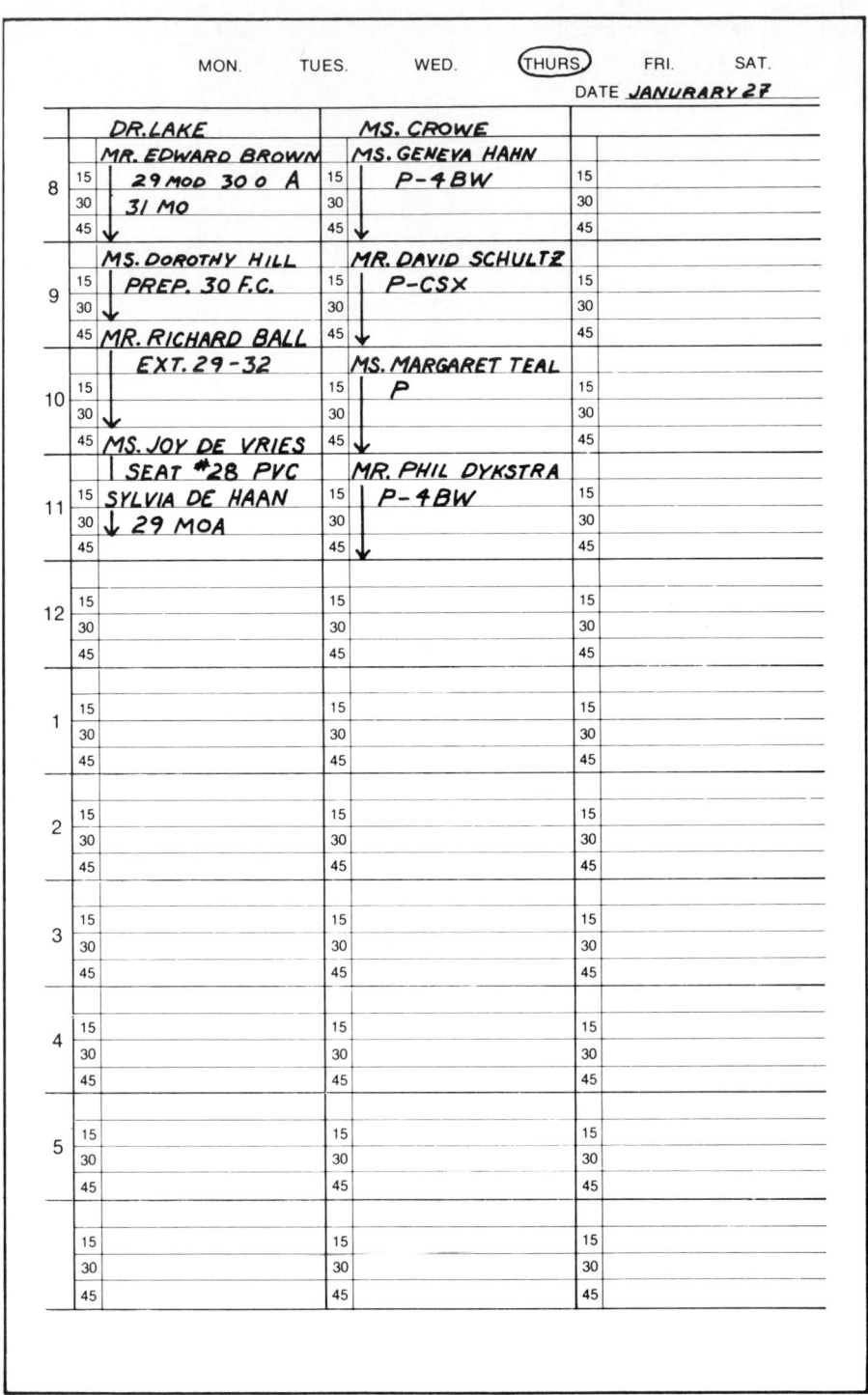

FIG. 14-9   Completed appointment schedule.

(Courtesy of Sycom.)

▶ Daily Schedule

Each day the office manager prepares a daily appointment schedule and distributes a copy to each treatment room, laboratory, private office, or other major area of activity. This may be printed or typed. This form should include the patient's name, treatment to be done, and other specific data as shown in Fig. 14-9. The office manager is responsible for updating this schedule during the day as changes take place, such as emergencies or cancellations.

Patient Records

It is the responsibility of each person in the office to maintain complete and accurate records for the clinical and financial activity of each patient. Well-maintained records can aid in patient treatment, provide verification of treatment for insurance and for the Internal Revenue Service, serve as evidence in malpractice suits, and even aid in identification of victims of crime or major disasters.

▶ Clinical Records

A **clinical record** is maintained for each patient and is actually a composite of many items that are most frequently maintained in a patient file folder, as shown in Fig. 14-10. The composite of such a record includes the following:

Registration / Health Questionnaire. These questionaires may be separate items or a combination form, as shown in Fig. 14-11. This form includes complete personal information about the patient and a thorough health history to aid in adequate patient treatment. The answers to questions on this form are kept in strict confidence by the staff. Care should be taken to obtain complete information without asking discriminatory questions. If the patient is a child, a special pediatric form must be completed by the parent or guardian, not by the child or baby-sitter (Fig. 14-12).

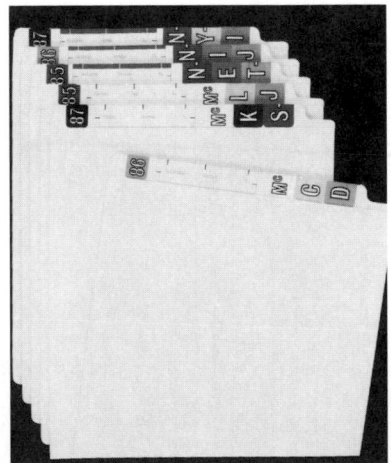

FIG. 14-10   File folders that use colored filing labels. (Courtesy of Sycom.)

HEALTH QUESTIONNAIRE

Name _____ Birthdate _____

Correct answers to the following questions will allow your dentist to treat you on a more individual basis, providing the care appropriate for your particular needs. Circle yes or no, whichever applies, in response to the following questions. Your answers are for our records only and will be considered confidential.

DENTAL

1. Are you having any discomfort at this time .... Yes No
2. Have you ever had any serious trouble associated with previous dental treatment? .... Yes No
   If so, explain
3. Does dental treatment make you nervous? No ____ Slightly ____ Moderately ____ Extremely ____
4. Date of last dental visit
5. Have you ever been treated for periodontal disease (gum disease, pyorrhea, trench mouth)? ..... Yes No
   If so, when?
6. How often do you brush?
   Brush is: Soft ☐ Medium ☐ Hard ☐
7. Do you have or have you ever had any of the following?

MOUTH
			TEETH		
Bleeding, sore gums	Yes	No	Loose teeth	Yes	No
Unpleasant taste/bad breath	Yes	No	Sensitive to hot	Yes	No
Burning tongue/lips	Yes	No	Sensitive to cold	Yes	No
Frequent blisters, lips/mouth	Yes	No	Sensitive to sweets	Yes	No
Swelling/lumps in mouth	Yes	No	Sensitive to biting	Yes	No
Ortho treatments (braces)	Yes	No	Food impaction	Yes	No
Biting cheeks/lips	Yes	No	Clenching/grinding	Yes	No
Clicking/popping jaw	Yes	No	If so, when		
Difficulty opening or closing jaw	Yes	No	Shifting in bite	Yes	No
			Change in bite	Yes	No

8. Do you use the following?
   Brush .... Yes No
   Dental floss .... Yes No
   Fluoride rinse .... Yes No
   Other

MEDICAL

1. Has there been any change in your general health within the past year .... Yes No
2. My last physical examination was on
3. Are you now under the care of a physician .... Yes No
   If so, what is the condition being treated
4. The name and address of my physician is
5. Have you had any serious illness within the past five (5) years .... Yes No
   If so, what was the illness
6. Have you been hospitalized or had an operation within the past five (5) years .... Yes No
   If so, what was the problem
7. Do you have or have you had any of the following diseases or problems
   a. Rheumatic fever or rheumatic heart disease .... Yes No
   b. Congenital heart disease .... Yes No
   c. Cardiovascular disease (heart trouble, heart attack, coronary insufficiency, coronary occlusion, high/low blood
      pressure, arteriosclerosis, stroke, etc.) .... Yes No
      1) Do you have pain in chest upon exertion .... Yes No
      2) Are you ever short of breath after mild exercise .... Yes No
      3) Do your ankles swell .... Yes No
      4) Do you get short of breath when you lie down, or do you require extra pillows when you sleep ... Yes No
   d. Artificial or replacement valves .... Yes No
   e. Pacemaker .... Yes No
   f. Allergy .... Yes No
   g. Sinus trouble .... Yes No
   h. Asthma or hay fever .... Yes No
   i. Hives or a skin rash .... Yes No
   j. Fainting spells or seizures .... Yes No
   k. Diabetes .... Yes No
      1) Do you have to urinate (pass water) more than six times a day .... Yes No
      2) Are you thirsty much of the time .... Yes No
      3) Does your mouth frequently become dry .... Yes No

Item 4054 • 10/88 SYCOM• Madison, WI Printed in U.S.A.   (over)

---

   l. Hepatitis, jaundice or liver disease .... Yes No
   m. Arthritis or inflammatory rheumatism .... Yes No
   n. Artificial or replacement joints, prosthetic .... Yes No
   o. Digestive system—Ulcers or stomach disorders (colitis) .... Yes No
   p. Kidney trouble .... Yes No
   q. Tuberculosis .... Yes No
   r. Persistent cough or cough up blood .... Yes No
   s. Immune System disorders (including AIDS, HIV, ARC) .... Yes No
   t. Venereal disease .... Yes No
   u. Other

8. Have you had abnormal bleeding associated with previous extractions, surgery, or trauma ..... Yes No
   a. Do you bruise easily .... Yes No
   b. Have you ever required a blood transfusion .... Yes No
      If so, explain the circumstances & when
9. Have you ever tested positive for the AIDS virus .... Yes No
10. Do you have any blood disorder such as anemia .... Yes No
11. Have you had surgery or x-ray treatment for a tumor, growth, or other condition .... Yes No
12. Are you taking any of the following:
    a. Antibiotics or sulfa drugs .... Yes No
    b. Anticoagulants (blood thinners) .... Yes No
    c. Medicine for high blood pressure .... Yes No
    d. Cortisone (steroids) .... Yes No
    e. Tranquilizers .... Yes No
    f. Antihistamines .... Yes No
    g. Aspirin .... Yes No
    h. Insulin, tolbutamide (Orinase) or similar drug for diabetes .... Yes No
    i. Digitalis or drugs for heart trouble .... Yes No
    j. Nitroglycerin .... Yes No
    k. Other medications
    l. If "Yes" to any of the above, state drug name, dosage and frequency
13. Are you allergic or have you reacted adversely to:
    a. Local anesthetics .... Yes No
    b. Penicillin or other antibiotics .... Yes No
    c. Sulfa drugs .... Yes No
    d. Barbiturates, sedatives, or sleeping pills .... Yes No
    e. Aspirin .... Yes No
    f. Iodine .... Yes No
    g. Codeine or other narcotics .... Yes No
    h. Other
14. Do you use any tobacco products .... Yes No
    If so, how much per day and what
15. Do you use any alcohol products .... Yes No
    If so, how much per day/week/month and what
16. Do you use any caffeinated products (coffee, tea, chocolate, etc.) .... Yes No
    If so, how much per day and what
17. Do you have any disease, condition, or problem not listed above that you think I should know about ... Yes No
    If so, explain
18. Are you employed in any situation which exposes you regularly to x-rays or other ionizing radiation ... Yes No
19. Are you wearing contact lenses .... Yes No
20. Are you experiencing stress or pressure in your work or at home .... Yes No

WOMEN
21. Are you pregnant .... Yes No
22. Do you have PMS or problems associated with your menstrual period .... Yes No
23. Are you taking birth control or hormone therapy .... Yes No

Remarks:

To the best of my knowledge, all of the preceding answers are true and correct. If I ever have any change in my health or change in my medication, I will inform the dentist at the next appointment.

Signature of Patient _____ Date _____

Signature of Dentist _____ Date _____

FIG. 14-11 Patient health questionnaire.
(Courtesy of Sycom.)

CHILD'S REGISTRATION AND HISTORY

Child's name _____

Date _____

Nickname _____ Age _____ Birthdate _____

Residence address _____

City _____ State _____ Zip _____

School _____ Grade _____

Father's name _____

Mother's name _____

Father employed by _____ How long _____ Home phone _____ Bus. phone _____

Mother employed by _____ How long _____ Home phone _____ Bus. phone _____

Person financially responsible (if other than parent) _____

Relationship to child _____

Address _____ City _____ State _____ Zip _____ Phone _____

Father's Social Security number _____ Driver license no. _____ State _____

Mother's Social Security number _____ Driver license no. _____ State _____

Father's birthdate _____ Mother's birthdate _____

Credit card name _____ No. _____ Expiration date _____

When dental insurance coverage name of carrier _____

Secondary insurance coverage, if any _____

Whom may we thank for referring you _____

What is child's favorite: sport _____ toy _____ hobby _____ person _____ fictional character _____

DENTAL HISTORY

	Yes	No
Date of last visit to a dentist _____		
For what service _____		
Does your child brush teeth daily _____	☐	☐
Do you assist child with tooth brushing _____	☐	☐
How often _____		
Is dental floss used _____	☐	☐
How often _____		
Are disclosing tablets used _____	☐	☐
Is fluoride taken in any form _____	☐	☐
Do you desire complete dental service for the child _____	☐	☐
Has child complained about dental problems _____	☐	☐
Any unhappy dental experiences _____	☐	☐
Any injuries to mouth - teeth - head _____	☐	☐
Any mouth habits - thumbsucking, nail biting, mouth breathing, nursing bottle habits, pacifer, etc. _____	☐	☐
Child's attitude to dentistry _____		
Any unusual speech habits _____	☐	☐
Summary: (for doctor's use) _____		
Any lost teeth _____	☐	☐
Have missing teeth been replaced _____	☐	☐
Orthodontic appliances worn now or ever been _____	☐	☐

Item 1022 • 12/89 SYCOM ™ Madison, WI Printed in U.S.A.

Child's physician _____ Address _____ Phone _____

Date of last physical examination _____ Results _____

	Yes	No
Is child under care of physician now _____	☐	☐
Does child have good physical coordination _____	☐	☐
Is child receiving any medication or drugs _____	☐	☐
Are there any emotional problems _____	☐	☐
Is there any excessive bleeding when cut _____	☐	☐
Summary: (for doctor's use) _____		
Has child ever been hospitalized _____	☐	☐
Has child ever had surgery _____	☐	☐
Is there any allergy to penicillin or other drugs _____	☐	☐
Are there other allergies: food - pollen - animals - dust - other _____	☐	☐

Has child any history of or difficulty with any of the following:

— Anemia — Chronic sinus — Hearing — Mastoid — Thyroid
— Asthma — Convulsions — Heart — Measles — Tuberculosis
— Bladder — Diabetes — Kidney — Mononucleosis — Venereal disease
— Cerebral Palsy — Epilepsy — Liver — Mumps — Other
— Chicken pox — Fainting — Malignancies — Rheumatic fever

Summary: (for doctor's use)

Please describe any current medical treatment including drugs, pending surgery, recent injuries or any other information I should be aware of that we have not discussed. _____

May we request release of your child's medical records for our reference _____

This information was discussed with and given by _____

Relation to child _____

Yes ☐ No ☐

FIG. 14-12 Pediatric patient health questionnaire. (Courtesy of Sycom.)

Update Form. This form is used for a patient's return visit after an absence from the office and will update a patient's address, insurance, and employment changes, as well as provide information about changes in a patient's health status (Fig. 14-13).

Clinical Chart. Personal information and health data are transferred to this record. As with the other forms in this record, information on this document is confidential. Each time a patient is treated, the nature of the treatment, medication, anesthesia, and other data are recorded on this chart, along with the date of entry. Initials of the treating dentist or auxiliary should be recorded. Any information about conversations with a patient or recommendations for treatment should be recorded and dated. Often patients may forget about a discussion the doctor had with them, and such documentation will provide legal evidence if needed. An example of a chart and a data entry is shown in Fig. 14-14.

■ PERSONAL INFORMATION UPDATE ■

Name _____ Date _____

1. Has your name changed since your last visit here? ____ yes ____ no
   If yes, what was the old name? _____
   What name do you use for health insurance if different than above? ____
   _____

2. If you have a new or different address since your initial visit here, please indicate below:
   _____
   _____
   _____

   Please indicate if any apartment # or P.O. Box # _____

3. Has your marital status changed? ____ yes ____ no

4. Has your telephone number changed? ____ yes ____ no
   Please indicate your correct telephone number _____

5. Has your employment changed? ____ yes ____ no
   Please indicate your new employer name and address:
   _____
   _____
   _____

   New employer telephone #: _____

6. Have you changed health insurance companies? ____ yes ____ no
   If yes, please indicate your new health insurance carrier and address.

   Primary _____   Secondary _____
   _____   _____
   _____   _____
   Group Nos. _____   Group Nos. _____
   Subscriber Nos. _____   Subscriber Nos. _____

7. Who is responsible for this bill? _____

8. Signature _____

Thank you for your assistance.

Item 4595 • 11/88 SYCOM® Madison, WI Printed in U.S.A.

HEALTH HISTORY UPDATE ■

Patient: _____ Date: _____

1. Have there been any changes in your health since your last visit?
   _____
   _____

2. Have you recently required other health services? _____
   If yes, nature of care _____

3. Physician's name: _____

4. Have you been hospitalized since your last visit? _____
   If yes, nature of problem _____

5. Any new illnesses? _____
   _____

6. Are you taking any medication(s) now? _____
   To treat: _____
   Name & dosage: _____

7. Do you have any new allergies or reactions to any medications or drugs?
   _____

8. Women only: Are you pregnant? ____ If yes, due date: _____

9. Any other new diseases, conditions or problems you think we should know
   about? _____
   _____

Patient Signature: _____

Doctor Signature: _____

Form 4051 • 3/88 SYCOM® Madison, WI Printed in U.S.A.

FIG. 14-13   Patient update form. *A,* Personal information. *B,* Health history update.
(Courtesy of Sycom.)

PATIENTS NAME DYKSTRA, MR. FRED

BILLING NAME same as above

ADDRESS 31 Highland Way N. E.
Grand Rapids, MI 49504

FINANCIAL ARRANGEMENT

1 - 2 - 3 - 4 - 5

DATE	SERVICES	CHARGES	PAID	BALANCE
1/22/—	18^{2-5} PREP., DYCAL, CAT, VAR, $ZnPO_4$, AMAL.			
1/24/—	9^{1-4} PREP., CAT, PIN MINIKIN, $ZnPO_4$, COMP.			
2/1/—	BROKEN APPT.			

FORM C - 103 - C

FIG. 14-14 Clinical chart illustrating various data entries.

Laboratory Requisitions. Most states require that a copy of written instructions accompany each case sent to a commercial laboratory. This form is also a mechanism for indicating special precautions that need to be taken when handling the contents of a laboratory box. A copy of this form is retained in the patient's record as evidence that a licensed dentist has prescribed the specific laboratory procedure.

Informed Consent Forms. This form is signed by a patient or parent of a minor child to grant permission for the administration of anesthetic or other specified procedures (Fig. 14-15, *A* and *B*).

Letters. Copies of all letters sent to or concerning a patient become part of the clinical record and may become evidence in a malpractice suit.

Radiographs. Radiographic films are stored in a patient's record. Each mounted set of radiographs should be labeled with the patient name, date of exposure, and the doctor's name. If copies of the radiographs are transferred to another office, a notation is made on the record that notes the date of transfer and to whom the films were sent. A request for such transfer must also be included in the record.

Postal Receipts. If radiographs or copies of other information are sent from a patient's record to another office, they should be sent by certified mail. A receipt is kept in the record as proof of transfer of the materials.

▶ Financial Records

Two types of financial records exist in the dental office: accounts receivable and accounts payable. The **accounts receivable** records are used for patient transactions, including debits or charges for services and credits or payments on a patient account, resulting in the accounts receivable balance, or the amount the patient owes the practice. The **accounts payable** system is the recording of all transactions that the doctor pays out (e.g., salaries, supplies, rent, and utilities). Although the business manager may be responsible for writing checks, the accounts payable system is commonly managed by the office accountant. However, the accounts receivable system is the responsibility of the dental assistants, and both the business and clinical assistants should be familiar with the system used in the office.

CONSENT TO TREATMENT ■■■■■■■■■■

CHRIS A. BROWN, D.D.S.
19 E. Center St. — Madison, WI   53701
(608) 123-4567

Date _____

I was informed by the above named doctor(s) of the risks, possible alternative methods of treatment, and possible consequences involved in the treatment by means of:

_____

_____   **A**

_____

for the relief of _____

_____

Understanding this, I hereby authorize the above named doctor(s) or whomever s/he (they) may designate, to administer such treatment to

me (or _____   _____)
                    Name of Patient if Minor

Signed _____
           Patient or Person Authorized to Consent for Patient

Witness _____

Date _____

Form 4554 • 3/86   **SYCOM**   Madison, WI   Printed in U.S.A.

FIG. 14-15   *A,* Informed consent form.

(*A* courtesy of Sycom.)

PATIENT NAME: DATE:

ORAL SURGERY CONSENT

The oral surgery procedure to be performed has been explained to me and I understand what is to be done, the type of anesthesia to be used, and the possible complications, if any, that may be encountered. I realize the doctor cannot guarantee the result of any surgical procedure. The more common complications are pain, infection, swelling, bruising and discoloration, and temporary or permanent numbness and tingling of the lip and chin, or in extremely rare cases, the tongue. Sinus complications, which may include an oral antral fistula (or opening into the sinus from the mouth), may occur with removal of upper teeth.

Circle: A) Extractions
         B) Removal of impacted teeth
         C) Removal of cyst or tumor
         D) Other_____

I CONSENT TO THE PERFORMANCE OF THIS PROCEDURE

Signed _____   Date _____

Witness _____

SEDATION CONSENT

B

Sedation refers to the use of selected medicines in order to help a patient relax, decreasing anxiety and excitement. In the oral surgery office, these medications are most commonly administered through an intravenous injection in the arm, forearm, or hand. This allows rapid onset of action as well as providing for adjustment of dosage depending on patient response. Typically, acute sedative effects will last for 30 minutes to several hours providing relaxation for the patient during the oral surgery procedure. **Because of this, in order to have this type of sedation, a responsible adult, who can drive, must accompany the patient to the procedure.** After the procedure has been completed instructions for postoperative care are given both to the patient and to the accompanying adult. These include written instructions. The sedated patient should not drive a motor vehicle or operate machinery until at least the following day.

Since there can be significant interaction between sedative medicines and other medicines the patient may be taking, it is very important that the doctor be told of **all** medications (including over the counter drugs such as aspirin and cold preparations) that the patient is taking. The doctor should also be told about any allergies or unusual reactions the patient may have had to other drugs, especially general anesthetics.

A bruise and some soreness may develop at the injection site. Typically, this bruise will turn various colors before disappearing. The soreness often responds to the application of cold during the first 48 hours and later the application of moist heat as needed. Rarely nerve damage and weakness may result.

I HAVE READ THIS AND UNDERSTAND ITS CONTENTS

Signed _____   Date _____

Witness _____

FIG. 14-15, cont'd.   *B,* Oral surgery consent form.

FIG. 14-16   *A*, Standard ledger card.
B, Computerized ledger/statement form.

(*A* courtesy of Creative Systems.)

JOSEPH W. LAKE, D.D.S.
611 MAIN ST., S.E.
GRAND RAPIDS, Mi 49502
PHONE 101-9575

Mr. Tom Smith
18280 W. Ten Mile Road
Southfield, Michigan 48075

DATE	FAMILY MEMBER	DESCRIPTION	CHARGE	PAYMENTS	ADJ.	CURRENT BALANCE
		BALANCE FORWARD →				30.00
1/8/—	MR	D	75—			105—
1/12/—	MRS	RCT	50—			155—
1/12/—	MR	D	50—			205—

FORM NO. 51-4555-L

AM—Amalgam Filling   EXT—Extraction   NC—No Charge   PF—Porcelain Filling
BR—Bridge   FA—Failed Appointment   NT—Nerve Treatment   PRO—Prophylaxis
CN—Crown   FMS—Full Mouth Survey   OV—Office Visit   RCT—Root Canal Treatment
CR—Complete Restoration   FT—Fluoride Treatment   P.C.A.—Previously Charged   ROA—Received on Account
D—Denture   G—Gold Inlay   on Account   SM—Space Maintainer
DR—Denture Repair   GT—Gum Treatment   PD—Partial Denture   X—X-Ray
EX—Examination

THIS IS A COPY OF YOUR ACCOUNT AS IT APPEARS ON YOUR LEDGER CARD

STATEMENT DATE   10/25/—

AMOUNT DUE   856.00

JOSEPH W. LAKE D.D.S.
611 MAIN STREET S.E.
GRAND RAPIDS MI   49502
616-101-9575

ACCOUNT NO   4A1E

R M ANDREWS
16657 DIANA
HOUSTON TX 77062

AMOUNT PAID $_____

PLEASE RETURN THIS PORTION WITH YOUR REMITTANCE
RETAIN THIS PORTION OF STATEMENT FOR YOUR RECORDS

DATE MO	DAY	NAME	CODE	DESCRIPTION		
				PREVIOUS BALANCE		0.00
8	18	BOB	0120	PERIODIC ORAL EXAMINATION		8.00
9	2	RON	2162	AMALGAM-FOUR SURFACE (PERM)		80.00
				PAYMENT, THANK YOU	50.00	
9	2	RON	2790	FULL GOLD CROWN		150.00
9	2	JUDY	1330	ORAL HYGIENE INSTRUCTION		8.00
9	2	RON	2750	PORCELAIN WITH GOLD CROWN		440.00
9	2	RON	2750	PORCELAIN WITH GOLD CROWN		220.00
						856.00

CURRENT AMOUNT	AMOUNT 30 DAYS PAST DUE	AMOUNT 60 DAYS PAST DUE	AMOUNT 90 DAYS OR OVER PAST DUE	PLEASE PAY LAST AMOUNT
856.00				

▶ Accounts Receivable

A patient's financial record is as important as his or her clinical record. This record is a ledger card and is kept separate from the clinical record; it is generally maintained for each family or responsible person. Therefore, all financial activity for each member of a family, either charges or payments, is maintained on one file or ledger card (Fig. 14-16, *A* and *B*).

Financial records provide protection for the dentist and patient, information for insurance and tax purposes, and data for practice analysis audits. The office manager or a member of the business office is responsible for recording all of the business transactions.

▶ Financial Record Features

The type of financial record used in an office is determined by the type of bookkeeping system implemented. The two most common bookkeeping systems used today are the peg board (a write-it-once system) and a computer software program. Regardless of which system is selected, the components of each will provide the same documentation. In a peg board system, ledger cards for each patient and day sheets are produced every day. In a computerized system these data will be stored on the computer disks or drives and hard copies can be made as needed. Of course, backup of these computer files must be done routinely. Each system will provide the following:

▶ A **code system** that is to be used to denote specific treatment or payments in an abbreviated form; these codes may appear on the ledger card, statement, and/or the patient receipt (Fig. 14-17)

▶ A **daily journal sheet** will provide a listing of all activity for the day, including patient treatment and receipts (Fig. 14-18)

▶ A patient **ledger card**, shown in Fig. 14-16, *A* and *B,* contains all of the financial information for each patient or family; most ledger cards are made out in the name of the person responsible for paying the account; at the end of the month a photocopy or computer copy of the ledger card is sent to the responsible person as a *statement* or request for payment (Figs. 14-19 and 14-16, *B*)

▶ A **ledger card tray** is used to store ledger cards; these cards are filed in alphabetical order and generally divided into two categories: active (with debit or credit balances) and inactive (with no balances and/or currently not under treatment); in a computer system the records are stored on a hard drive, and a backup disk is made routinely and stored outside the office

▶ A **receipt/charge slip** is given to the patient at the end of the procedure to indicate charges and payments; several styles exist, such as the basic two-part form that is shown in Fig. 14-20, which may serve as a fee slip and a receipt, or the form in Fig. 14-21, which is often referred to as a super bill, since it includes the fee slip and receipt in addition to listing the American Dental Association insurance codes

FIG. 14-17 Ledger card with codes.
(Courtesy of Creative Systems.)

DATE	FAMILY MEMBER	DESCRIPTION	CHARGE	CREDITS		CURRENT BALANCE
				PAYMENTS	ADJ.	
		BALANCE FORWARD ⟶				75 –
9/17/—	MRS.	2 AM	20 –	50 –		45 –
9/19/—	MR.	CN	125 –			170 –
10/10/—		ROA		100 –		70 –

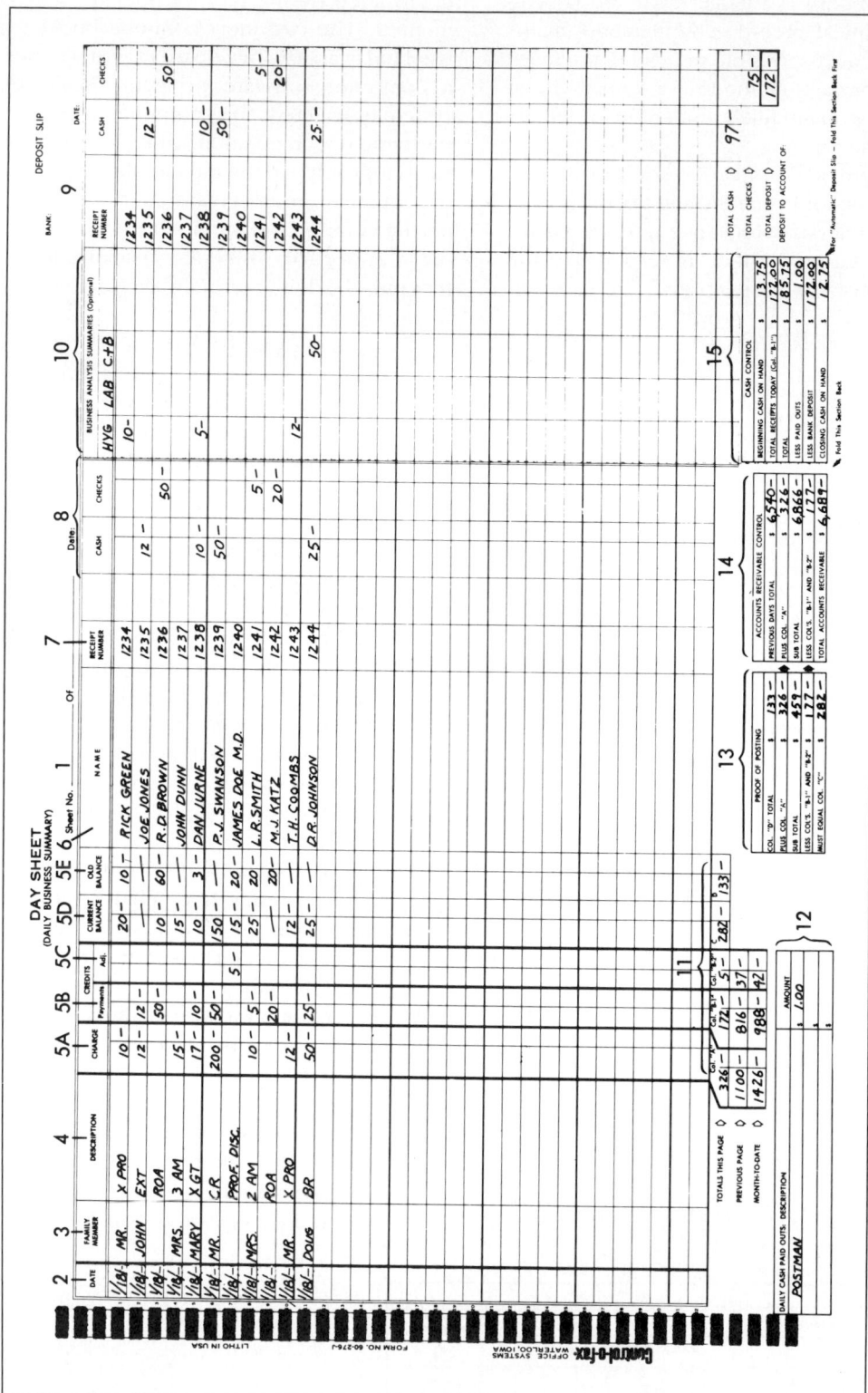

FIG. 14-18   Completed daily journal sheet from peg board.
(Courtesy of Creative Systems.)

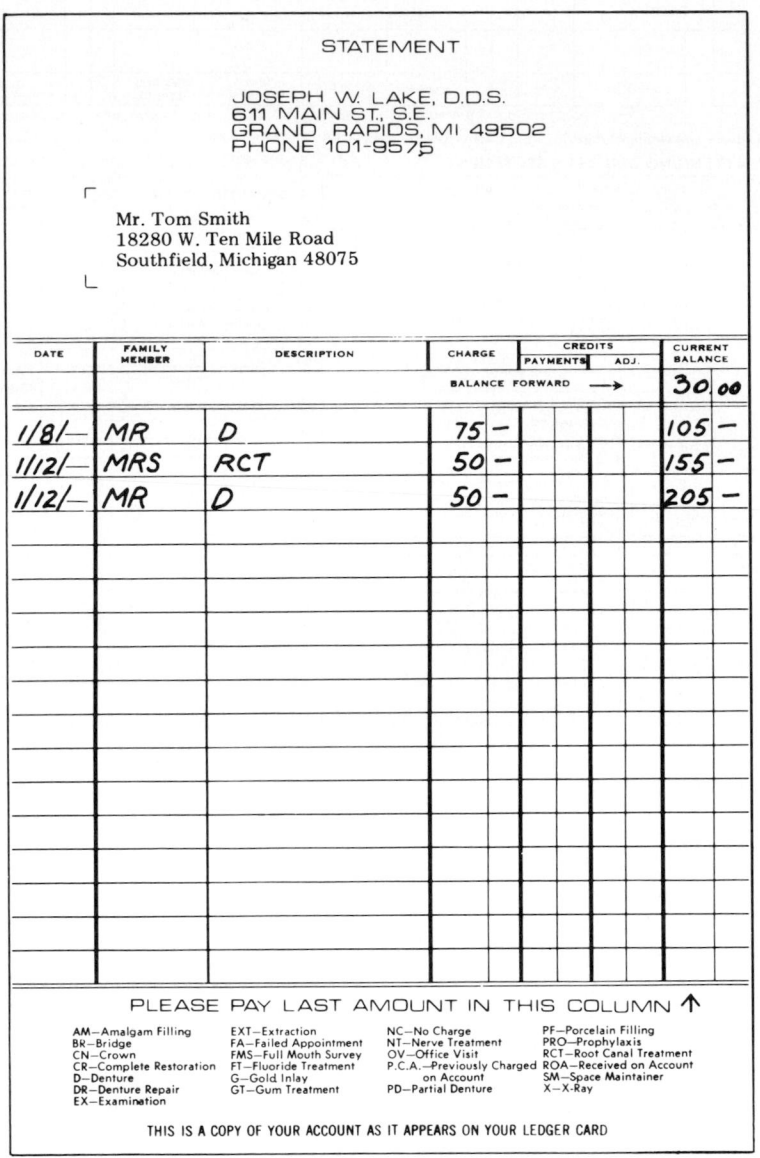

FIG. 14-19   Patient statement with codes.

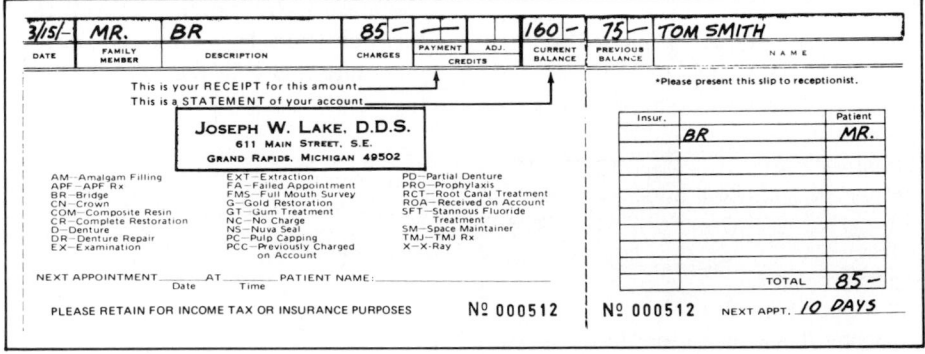

FIG. 14-20   Two-part receipt/charge slip for pegboard.

(Courtesy of Creative Systems.)

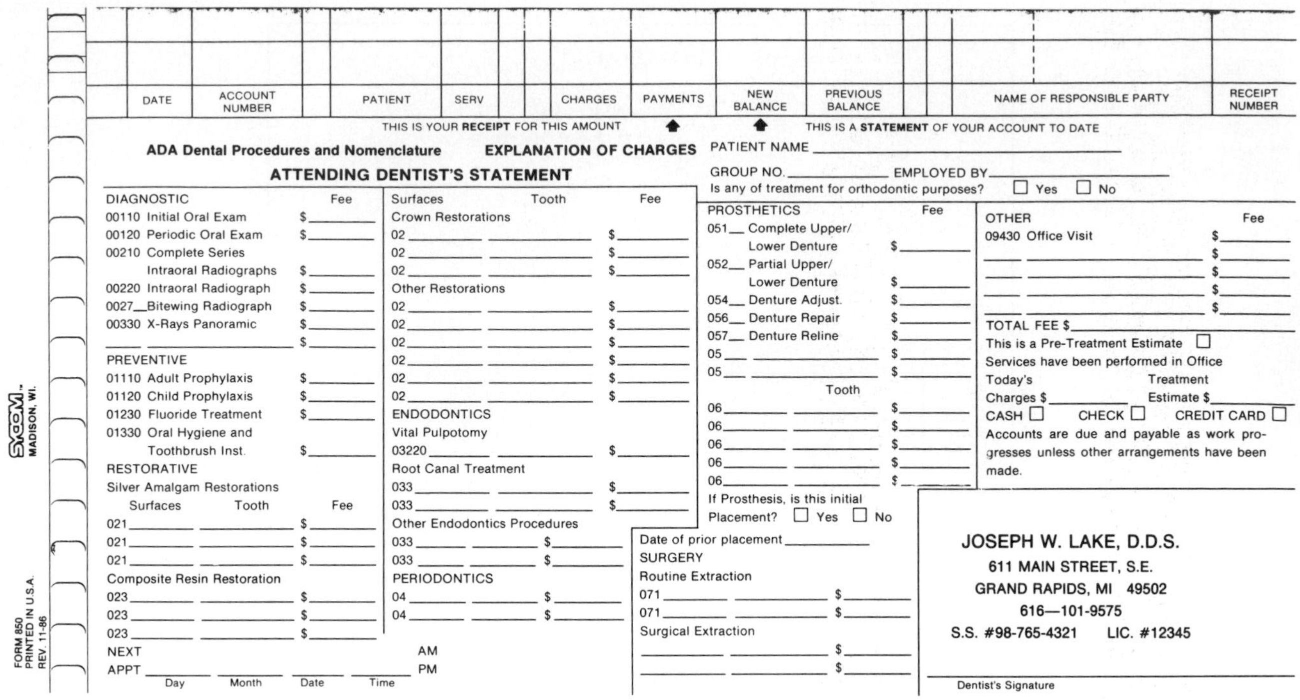

DATE	ACCOUNT NUMBER	PATIENT	SERV	CHARGES	PAYMENTS	NEW BALANCE	PREVIOUS BALANCE	NAME OF RESPONSIBLE PARTY	RECEIPT NUMBER

THIS IS YOUR **RECEIPT** FOR THIS AMOUNT ⬆ ⬆ THIS IS A **STATEMENT** OF YOUR ACCOUNT TO DATE

ADA Dental Procedures and Nomenclature **EXPLANATION OF CHARGES** PATIENT NAME ____

ATTENDING DENTIST'S STATEMENT

GROUP NO. ____ EMPLOYED BY ____
Is any of treatment for orthodontic purposes? ☐ Yes ☐ No

DIAGNOSTIC Fee
00110 Initial Oral Exam $____
00120 Periodic Oral Exam $____
00210 Complete Series Intraoral Radiographs $____
00220 Intraoral Radiograph $____
0027__Bitewing Radiograph $____
00330 X-Rays Panoramic $____
____ ____ $____
PREVENTIVE
01110 Adult Prophylaxis $____
01120 Child Prophylaxis $____
01230 Fluoride Treatment $____
01330 Oral Hygiene and Toothbrush Inst. $____
RESTORATIVE
Silver Amalgam Restorations
Surfaces Tooth Fee
021____ ____ $____
021____ ____ $____
021____ ____ $____
Composite Resin Restoration
023____ ____ $____
023____ ____ $____
023____ ____ $____
NEXT APPT ____ ____ ____ ____ AM PM
Day Month Date Time

Surfaces Tooth Fee
Crown Restorations
02____ ____ $____
02____ ____ $____
02____ ____ $____
Other Restorations
02____ ____ $____
02____ ____ $____
02____ ____ $____
02____ ____ $____
02____ ____ $____
02____ ____ $____
ENDODONTICS
Vital Pulpotomy
03220____ ____ $____
Root Canal Treatment
033____ ____ $____
033____ ____ $____
Other Endodontics Procedures
033____ ____ $____
033____ ____ $____
PERIODONTICS
04____ ____ $____
04____ ____ $____

PROSTHETICS Fee
051__ Complete Upper/ Lower Denture $____
052__ Partial Upper/ Lower Denture $____
054__ Denture Adjust. $____
056__ Denture Repair $____
057__ Denture Reline $____
05__ ____ $____
05__ ____ $____
Tooth
06____ ____ $____
06____ ____ $____
06____ ____ $____
06____ ____ $____
06____ ____ $____
If Prosthesis, is this initial Placement? ☐ Yes ☐ No
Date of prior placement ____
SURGERY
Routine Extraction
071____ ____ $____
071____ ____ $____
Surgical Extraction
____ ____ $____
____ ____ $____

OTHER Fee
09430 Office Visit $____
____ ____ $____
____ ____ $____
____ ____ $____
____ ____ $____
TOTAL FEE $____
This is a Pre-Treatment Estimate ☐
Services have been performed in Office
Today's Charges $____ Treatment Estimate $____
CASH ☐ CHECK ☐ CREDIT CARD ☐
Accounts are due and payable as work progresses unless other arrangements have been made.

JOSEPH W. LAKE, D.D.S.
611 MAIN STREET, S.E.
GRAND RAPIDS, MI 49502
616—101-9575
S.S. #98-765-4321 LIC. #12345
Dentist's Signature

SYCOM. MADISON, WI.
FORM 850 PRINTED IN U.S.A. REV. 11-86

FIG. 14-21 Modified single receipt/charge slip used as superbill.
(Courtesy of Sycom.)

BOX 14-6

RULES FOR ENTERING DATA ON FINANCIAL RECORDS

- Always use ink, not pencil. Remember these are permanent records.*
- Use good penmanship. Do not attempt to use fancy letters.*
- Keep columns of figures straight.*
- Use well-formed figures.*
- Place decimal points correctly.
- Do not erase. If an error occurs, draw a straight line through it and write the correct figure above it.*
- Enter all charges and payments as soon as the patient leaves the treatment room.
- Make certain that for each patient who is listed in the appointment book an entry has been made on the day sheet.
- Check math carefully.
- Store records in a fireproof file.
- Make a backup of the computer file.
- Retain backup computer files at an out-of-office site.

* Applies to a peg board system.

Principles of Financial Record Keeping

Whether a computerized bookkeeping system (Fig. 14-22, *A*) or a peg board system is used (Fig. 14-22, *B*), some basic rules should be followed. Remember that all patient records are legal documents and each record requires neat penmanship, accuracy, and thoroughness in making entries. If they are prepared by hand, financial records are always written in ink and no erasures are made to the entries. Financial records are subject to review by the patient, as well as the Internal Revenue Service. Box 14-6 contains suggestions for maintaining accurate financial records.

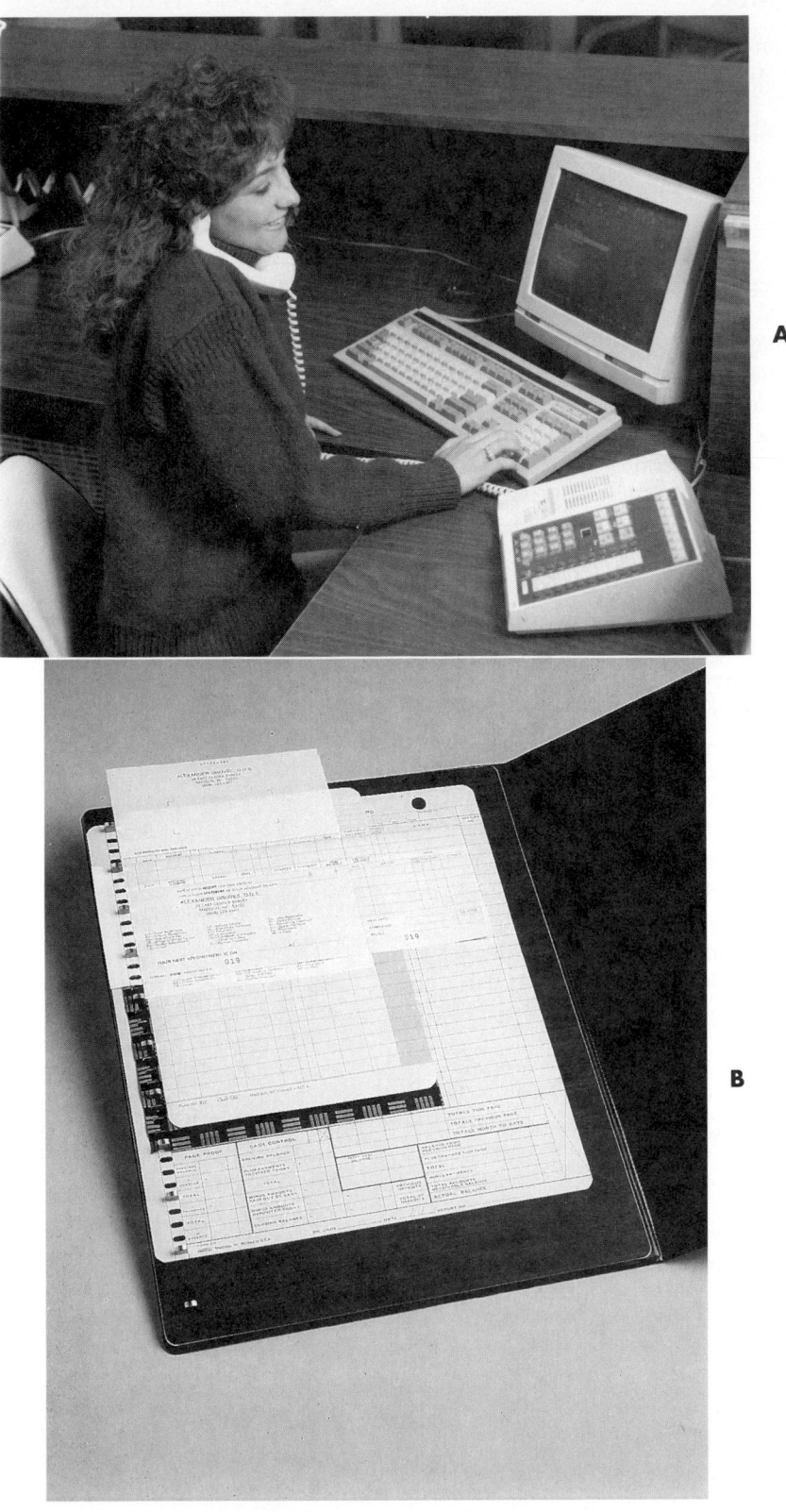

FIG. 14-22 *A,* Computerized bookkeeping system. *B,* Assembled peg board.
(*B,* courtesy of Sycom.)

▶ Accounts Payable

The previous section described the management of accounts receivable. **Accounts payable** is the process of disbursing monies in the office. Some of the banking responsibilities an assistant may encounter include the following:

- ▶ Check writing
- ▶ Endorsing and depositing checks
- ▶ Maintaining an accurate bank balance
- ▶ Endorsing and depositing monies
- ▶ Reconciling bank statements

Various checks may be used, including personal, certified, cashier's, money order, traveler's, bank draft, or voucher checks. An assistant should become familiar with the types of checks received and written in the office and understand the function of each.

Writing checks is commonly done by the assistant. these may be payroll checks or checks that are written as payment of bills incurred by the practice. The checks may be produced manually or through a computer payroll software package. In either case the assistant should be familiar with the step-by-step procedure for check writing, as illustrated in Fig. 14-23. The business assistant may sign checks if a power of attorney form has been signed and the signature appears on a signature card that is filed with the bank.

Once the check has been written, an entry must be made manually in the check book or entered in the computer program to indicate the check number, date, payee, amount of the check, purpose of the check, and the new balance. Statements from which the checks have been paid are then transferred to paid files with appropriate documentation to indicate the date, the check number, and that the payment was made.

Records Transfer

For various reasons it may be necessary to transfer a patient record or some portion of it to another doctor or agency. It may be necessary to transfer radiographs or test results to a specialist for consultation or to an insurance company for predetermination of a patient's eligibility for services. This can only be done by written consent of the patient or the patient's legal representative, since this record is privileged and confidential information (Fig. 14-24).

The original record is retained in the office, and only a copy of that part of the record specifically requested is transferred. In the case of radiographs a duplicate set may be sent. It is also recommended, when possible, that the materials be mailed in a manner that will provide a return receipt for the sender. A reasonable clerical fee, consistent with local practice, may be charged for furnishing these records.

FIG. 14-23   How to write a check: *1*, Date the check. *2*, Type or write the name of the person or firm to whom the check will be payable. *3*, Enter the amount of the check (in figures) opposite the dollar sign. *4*, Write the amount of the check (in words) under *pay to the order of* line. Start as far to the left margin as possible. *5*, The bottom line is for the signature and should be signed as it appears on the bank signature card. *6*, Memo line to record what the payment is for.

(Courtesy of American Bank Stationery.)

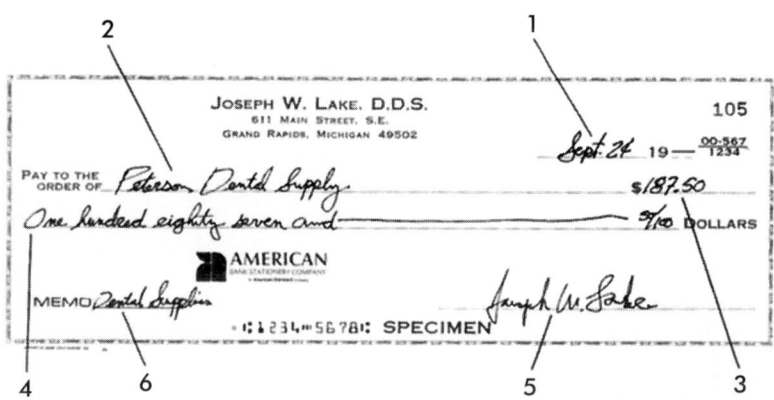

Treatment Plans

A **treatment plan** is like a road map that describes or outlines the needs of the patient and the recommended treatment for restoring the patient's mouth to good health. Generally this plan (also described in Chapter 24) is presented to the patient by using an assortment of visual aids that may include the patient's diagnostic models, radiographs, and diagrams or other visual aids to describe the needed treatment. Commonly, the doctor presents the treatment plan to the patient and then refers the patient to the office manager to make payment arrangements. At times, the patient may be unsure of the need for the recommended treatment; here the dental assistant becomes a vital component to patient education. The assistant may reexplain, in other terms, why the patient needs this treatment. Sometimes patients are apprehensive about asking the doctor questions and feel more comfortable asking the assistant additional questions. Therefore, before the doctor's presentation the assistant must thoroughly understand the patient's needs, as well as the procedures that are being recommended.

Preventing Disease Transmission in Records Management

Transporting records from the dental treatment room can be an unsafe procedure if care is not taken. All staff in the office, both in the business office and in the clinical areas, must have a thorough knowledge of the use of barrier techniques for the prevention of disease transmission, as discussed in Chapter 8.

The safest way to avoid disease transmission from the treatment room via patient records, of course, is not to take the records into the room. This can be done by arranging a records observation area outside each treatment room. However, some dentists believe that this is impractical. Thus, the alternative to this method might include one of the following:

1. Only touch or write on the record after treatment gloves are removed
2. Wear overgloves when touching the record
3. Enter and review all data on a monitor and protected keyboard in the treatment room.

The latter suggestion provides the ability to have barrier coverings that can be discarded or disinfected.

RECORDS RELEASE

CHRIS A. BROWN, D.D.S.
19 E. Center St. — Madison, WI 53701
(608) 123-4567

Date of request _____

My permission is granted to Dr. _____

to disclose to _____
complete information concerning the medical findings and treatment of

_____
Patient

from _____ to _____
Date · Date

I release Dr. _____
from any laws related to disclosure of confidential or privileged information.

Signature _____
Patient or Person Authorized to Consent for Patient

Address _____

Witness _____ Date _____

Form 4559 • 3/86 **SYCOM** Madison, WI Printed in U.S.A.

FIG. 14-24   Record release form.

(Courtesy of Sycom.)

Written Communication

Many forms of written communication are created in the business office each day. The written word is sometimes more difficult to present, since you do not receive immediate feedback from the reader and you must rely on the reader's interpretation of your words.

BASIC Cs OF CORRESPONDENCE

To write letters that create good public relations, familiarize yourself with the *Basic Cs of Correspondence:* rules for effective letter writing:

1. *Correctness.* Be certain all data are correct. Check details carefully. Use a dictionary to obtain the correct spelling of difficult words and technical terms. Be thoroughly familiar with basic rules of grammar. Do not guess.
2. *Clarity.* Do not try to be a literary genius. Use language that your reader will understand, and be certain each statement cannot be misinterpreted.
3. *Conciseness.* Be brief. Do not include lengthy sentences and meaningless phrases. The reader should not have to wade through a lot of jargon to arrive at the intended message.
4. *Completeness.* Be certain to include all data that the reader needs to make a decision or take action. A lack of information may delay a reaction you expect from the reader.
5. *Consideration.* Make the recipient of your letter feel important. Place emphasis on the reader's needs, not those of the office.
6. *Cheerfulness.* Be sincere and natural in your letters. Write the letter as though you were talking with the person, and avoid phrases you would not ordinarily use in conversation.
7. *Courtesy.* Good public relations requires good manners. Do not make derogatory statements.
8. *Carefulness.* Be neat in your letter writing. A messy letter, full of smudges, gives an office a poor image. Be certain your typewriter is clean, and be careful to eliminate the need for erasures.

From Finkbeiner BL, Patt J: *Practice management for the dental team,* ed 3, St Louis, 1991, Mosby.

▶ Business Letters

Several forms of written communication have been discussed earlier in records management, but no piece of written communication is more important for the image of the office than the business letters transmitted from the office. The most common letters produced in the office are letters of welcome to the office, referral to another dentist, thank you letters, birthday or congratulatory letters, recall notices, letters of request for information, or collection letters for delinquent accounts.

Regardless of whether a letter is produced on an automatic typewriter, on a sophisticated memory typewriter, or through the use of a word processing package on a computer, certain basic rules should be followed:

- ▶ The letter should be free of grammatical and keyboard errors. Use a dictionary or spelling check function on the computer to correct spelling.
- ▶ Use language that the reader can understand, and make the letter *you* oriented rather than *I* oriented.
- ▶ Be brief and concise. Do not use lengthy sentences that introduce multiple ideas.
- ▶ Demonstrate consideration and courtesy to the reader. Display the same manners in the written message that would be forthcoming in person.
- ▶ Write the letter as if talking to the person.
- ▶ Maintain patient confidentiality, and provide information only to authorized sources for whom you have written consent.
- ▶ Be complete and accurate in the information included. Be certain that all of the information is included and that none of the statements can be misinterpreted.
- ▶ Display neatness by avoiding smudges, erasures, or unclear copies.

A letter with a clear sharp image that is well formatted, technically correct, and thoughtfully presented will create a positive image for the office. The business staff should create a series of letter samples for various situations, which allows them to easily produce an original letter with relative ease. Figs. 14-25 through 14-28 are samples of a several common letters that might be sent from an office.

FIG. 14-25   General *thank you* letter to a patient.

JOSEPH W. LAKE, D.D.S.
611 Main Street, S.E.
Grand Rapids, MI 49502
616—101-9575

September 15, 19——

Ms. Marsha Meyer
2492 Plymouth Road
Escanaba, MI 49829

Dear Ms. Meyer:

I would like to take this opportunity to thank you for your confidence in referring your friend, Mrs. Judy McKay and her children Debbie and Rick, to my office for treatment.

My staff and I are pleased to learn of your satisfaction, and we will make every attempt to justify the confidence you have shown in us during the treatment of Mrs. McKay.

Thank you again for your expression of confidence.

Sincerely,

Joseph W. Lake, D.D.S.

db

JOSEPH W. LAKE, D.D.S.
611 Main Street, S.E.
Grand Rapids, MI 49502
616—101-9575

September 15, 19——

Daniel R. Perry, D.D.S., M.S.
2495 Packard Road S. E.
Grand Rapids, MI 49506

Dear Dr. Perry:

I am referring Frank Wiard, age 12, to you for an orthodontic examination. Mrs. Wiard will be calling your office for an appointment. Frank appears to have a Class II malocclusion with crowding of the mandibular anteriors.

Enclosed you will find a complete series of radiographs which were taken on September 11, 19——.

I will look forward to your diagnosis and assistance with this case.

Sincerely,

Joseph W. Lake, D.D.S.

db

Enclosure

FIG. 14-26   **Referral letter to an orthodontist.**

FIG. 14-27   Collection letter to a patient.

JOSEPH W. LAKE, D.D.S.
611 Main Street, S.E.
Grand Rapids, MI 49502
616—101-9575

November 5, 19—

Mr. Marvin Beattie
1407 Colorado Street, N.W.
Grand Rapids, MI 49505

Dear Mr. Beattie:

Your account of $210.00 is over 90 days past due. If you are unable
to pay this account in full, perhaps we can help you in making arrangements to take care of this account.

Please contact us before November 15, 19— at 5:00 p.m.

Sincerely,

Deborah L. Benson, R.D.A.
Business Assistant

JOSEPH W. LAKE, D.D.S.
611 Main Street, S.E.
Grand Rapids, MI 49502
616—101-9575

November 26, 19—

REGISTERED

Mr. Marvin Beattie
1407 Colorado Street, N.W.
Grand Rapids, MI 49505

Dear Mr. Beattie:

Since we have not heard from you regarding your account of $210.00
from August 1, 19—, please be informed that it will be necessary to
transfer this account to a collection agency.

This account must be paid in full by Friday December 1,19— to avoid
such legal action.

Sincerely,

Deborah L. Benson, R.D.A.
Business Assistant

FIG. 14-28   Follow-up collection letter to a patient.

◗ Office Procedures Manual

This manual is a step-by-step description of common procedures within the office. The manual is specifically designed for the office staff. It serves as a training manual for new staff and as a reference manual for the entire staff. A typical table of contents for such a manual is shown in Box 14-7.

TABLE OF CONTENTS
FOR A PROCEDURAL MANUAL

Statement of purpose or objective of the manual
Statement of philosophy of the practice
Office communication
Staff policies
Job descriptions
Employment policies
Salaries and benefits
Office records
Infection control policies
Emergency procedures
Clinical procedures
Inventory system
Recall system
Professional organizations
Credentialing processes

Adapted from Finkbeiner B, Patt J: *Practice management for the dental team,* St Louis 1990, Mosby.

◗ Office Policy

This form of written communication is designed for the patient. An **office policy** outlines office procedures and the philosophy of the doctor and introduces the staff functions. It can also provide a mechanism for education. This form is generally presented to a new patient at his or her first visit to the office and informs the patient of the doctor's and patient's responsibilities. The form may be prepared on office letterhead, or it may be a sophisticated brochure that welcomes the patient to the office.

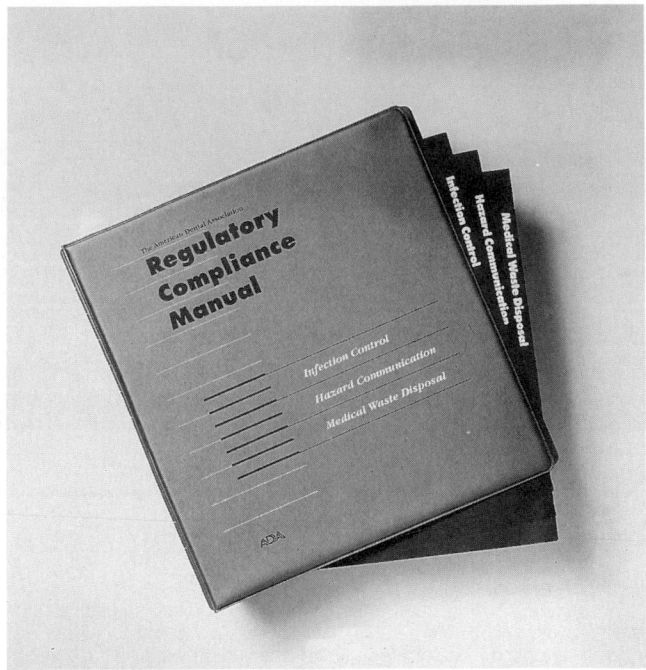

FIG. 14-29   Regulatory Compliance Manual.
(Courtesy of American Dental Association.)

◗ Regulatory Compliance Manual

This form of written communication can be created in the dental office, with the use of the Regulatory Compliance Manual from the American Dental Association (ADA), which serves as a reference manual for all staff members (Fig. 14-29). This reference manual identifies information on all regulations relating to infection control, hazard communication, training procedures, and medical waste disposal. The doctor and each staff member should review this manual and all updates to ensure that the Occupational Safety and Health Administration (OSHA) guidelines are being followed thoroughly.

◗ Newsletters

A newsletter is an excellent marketing tool for a doctor to incorporate into the practice (Fig. 14-30). Mailing newsletters regularly updates patients about activities in the practice, provides an opportunity for dental education, and serves as a form of professional advertising.

'BY WORD OF MOUTH'

Dental Health News For The Patients Of: John W. Farah, D.D.S., Ph.D.   No. 23
                                           John Shamraj, D.D.S.

Orthodontics: A Balancing Act

Some people are born to have a perfect face and dazzling smile. Those of us who choose our parents with careful attention to facial structure definitely have an advantage in this area. For the rest of us, today's dentistry often has a great deal to offer. In many situations, Orthodontic treatment can help with the development of balance in facial bones and teeth. The Orthodontic balancing act will result in a smile to feel good

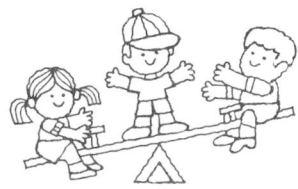

about plus teeth that can last a lifetime.

Imbalance: Imbalances can be caused by:

- ◆ size of teeth (too small or too large)
- ◆ muscular habits: such as thumb sucking, clenching or grinding, and improper swallowing
- ◆ missing teeth
- ◆ improper nutrition
- ◆ hereditary growth patterns of facial bones

These imbalances can cause many problems, including:

- ◆ uneven tooth alignment (crooked teeth)
- ◆ difficulty in chewing
- ◆ inability to clean teeth properly
- ◆ speech impairment

- ◆ mouth breathing
- ◆ TMJ syndrome (headaches or related symptoms)
- ◆ uneven growth of facial bones, which will affect the shape and appearance of the face

All of these factors work together in determining the shape of the growing face.

Balance: Balancing your smile and facial structure with Orthodontics will:

- ◆ increase self confidence with a beautiful smile
- ◆ improve the health of teeth, gum tissue and bones
- ◆ improve chewing, speech, and breathing
- ◆ guide the development of bones and teeth in harmony with the growing face

The muscular balance of the head, neck and shoulders can also be affected by the structure of the jaws and teeth. The muscles of this entire area all work together in speech, posture, chewing and swallowing. Any imbalance in the structure or alignment of the jawbones can cause muscle

See **Orthodontics,** page 2.

INSIDE

The Temporary Tooth

Several dental procedures require the placement of a temporary plastic tooth while the patient is waiting for the final cap to be received from the laboratory. Sometimes these temporaries look and feel great and the patient will exclaim "wow, this looks great. Do I really need to come back?"

As nice as the temporary tooth might look, yes, you do need to come back, hopefully, not before the final tooth is ready. The temporary tooth is just that, "temporary." The material used for the temporary tooth is not very strong; therefore, it may break. It's not to say that all temporaries are going to crack, but if you love popcorn, eat lots of carrots, enjoy chewing gum, or grind your teeth at night, you may be calling us to let us know you broke your temporary or it fell out. Don't panic. There is no need for

alarm. Call our office and we can have you come in to make a new temporary.

Simple reminders for avoiding an unnecessary trip to the dentist before your permanent tooth is ready:

❶ Avoid flossing or floss carefully around the area where the temporary is placed.
Many times the floss will catch on the material and it may "pop off."

❷ Avoid chewing gum.
Because this restoration is temporary, you can expect that we will use a temporary cement to keep it affixed to the tooth. Chewing gum will stick to the temporary and sometimes pull it off the tooth.

❸ Avoid chewing sticky or very hard foods in the "temporary" area, or chew only softer food in this area. ■

Orthodontics, *from page 1.*

stress. This can lead to headaches, chronic fatigue, dizziness, hearing problems, and many other symptoms. These problems can develop over many years before symptoms appear. Adult orthodontic care is often directed at correcting these types of problems.

Although Orthodontic patients are commonly children, patients range in age from 6 to 60 years. Approximately 25 percent of all Orthodontic treatment is performed on adult patients.

During Orthodontic treatment remember that proper brushing and nutrition are essential to keeping healthy teeth and gums. The Orthodontic braces in the mouth can easily trap food and if you

are improperly brushing and flossing your teeth, this may result in decay upon removal of the appliances. You may want to try rinsing your mouth regularly to assist in food removal near the braces.

The science of Orthodontics has come a long way since the days when only 13-year olds sported a metallic smile. Braces can be nearly invisible, and many problems can be intercepted before they become severe. Orthodontic care can often improve your smile, your facial appearance, your health, and your entire quality of life.

If you have questions or concerns about the alignment of your teeth or your child's teeth, ask us and we will let you know if Orthodontics can help you. ■

FIG. 14-30   Newsletter from a dental office to a patient.

(Courtesy of Drs. John W. Farah and Diane Charney.)

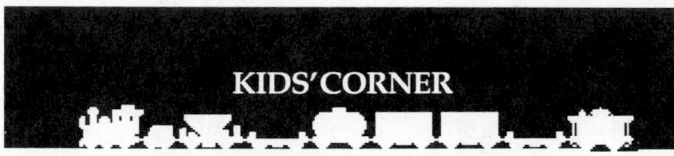

KIDS'CORNER

Baby Bottlers Beware

If you use a bottle of milk or juice to comfort a fussy baby or let the baby have a bottle at nap time or at bedtime, you may be putting your child at risk for serious, early tooth decay called baby-bottle syndrome. Baby-bottle syndrome is most likely

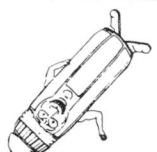 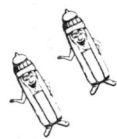

caused by the frequent exposure of the teeth for long periods of time to liquids containing sugars and/or acids. These sugars, contained in milk, juice, soda, or other sweetened beverages, cause the bacteria that are present in the plaque in your child's mouth to thrive. In the process, the bacteria produce acids that attack the tooth enamel.

Not only should you be concerned about what you put in your child's bottle that causes baby-bottle syndrome, but how often and for how long the child's teeth are exposed to the decay-causing acid attack. Each time your child drinks a sugared liquid, acids attack the child's teeth. During sleep, the flow of saliva

decreases and the liquids from the bottle pool around the child's teeth increasing the chances for decay.

Primary teeth are important teeth. Children need them to chew their food, speak clearly and look good to themselves and their friends. The primary teeth also help to reserve space in the jaw for the permanent teeth.

Remember: Baby's teeth are susceptible to decay as soon as they appear in the mouth. By the time decay is noticed, it may be too late to save the child's teeth.

✔ If your child needs a bottle to fall asleep, try using water or half-water/half-juice, thereby reducing the amount of sugar left on your child's teeth.

✔ Make sure your child is receiving the fluoride needed for decay-resistant teeth. If your water supply does not contain the right amount of fluoride, ask your dentist how your child should get the fluoride supplement he/she needs.

✔ Start dental visits when your child is three years of age.

If you suspect that your child has dental problems, give us a call and we'll schedule an appointment right away. ■

FOR YOUR HEALTH

Preventing Food Poisoning
S H I G E L L O S I S

Shigellosis, a type of food poisoning, is on the rise! This food-borne disease can be spread easily unless efforts are made to prevent it. We are often infected with the disease when hands are not properly washed after using the toilet or when contaminated food is eaten.

Food poisoning has become a major problem in day-care centers, where both children and child-care workers may neglect to wash their hands after using the toilet or before

handling food. A child-care worker, for example, may change an infected child's diaper and then, without washing hands thoroughly with soap and running water, handle food consumed by other children. Also, an infected child with contaminated hands may touch the hands, mouths, toys or food of other children. In addition, the disease is spreading among nursing homes

See **Food Poisoning**, page 4.

Food Poisoning, *from page 3.*

and other health- care institutions.

The infectious bacteria can remain living in our intestinal tract for months, long after symptoms have gone, and can infect others even one month after recovery. Infected people can transmit the disease to others if personal hygiene is lax.

Foods most commonly associated with transmission of food poisoning include salads, like potato, tuna, shrimp,

macaroni and chicken. Typically, the ingredients start out free of the bacteria but become contaminated when handled or mixed by an infected person.

Symptoms:

stomach upset diarrhea
fever headache
vomiting

Symptoms typically last five to six days, but can last as long as three weeks. ■

Congratulations!!!

Babies...
Sylvia and **Tony Lang** have a new baby girl born in April.
Leguietta and **David Folk** have a new son D.J
Francisco and **Maria Sturla** have a new son.
David and **Susan Anderson** had a boy in November 1991 – Kyle Theodore.
Nair and **Eduardo Matsuo** had a baby girl in February – Karen Hiromi.

Weddings:
Rick Bricault and **Debra O'Connell** married on March 29, 1992.
Marge Hagene got married on April 11, 1992.
Leslie G. Muscott and **Don Adiska** tied the knot on April 11, 1992.

● Congratulations to eight-year-old **Teo Ahlbrandt** for winning 1st place in the State of Michigan Children Chess Championship for kids 10 years and younger.

● **Laurie Venable**, our Assistant for seven years, is moving to Midland. Her husband was transferred. We will all miss Laurie and wish her the best.

Continuing Education:
Dr. Farah will be lecturing on New Materials and Techniques to:
 ● Santa Barbara Dental Society in California (June 18)
 ● Degussa Dental Products, Frankfurt, Germany (August 13)
 ● Stark County Dental Society in Canton, Ohio (September 2)
 ● 3M Dental Products "Future 2000", Minnesota (September 16–20)

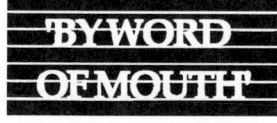

BULK MAIL
U.S. POSTAGE
PAID
Permit No.
Ann Arbor MI

ADDRESS CORRECTION REQUESTED

FIG. 14-30, cont'd. Newsletter from a dental office to a patient.

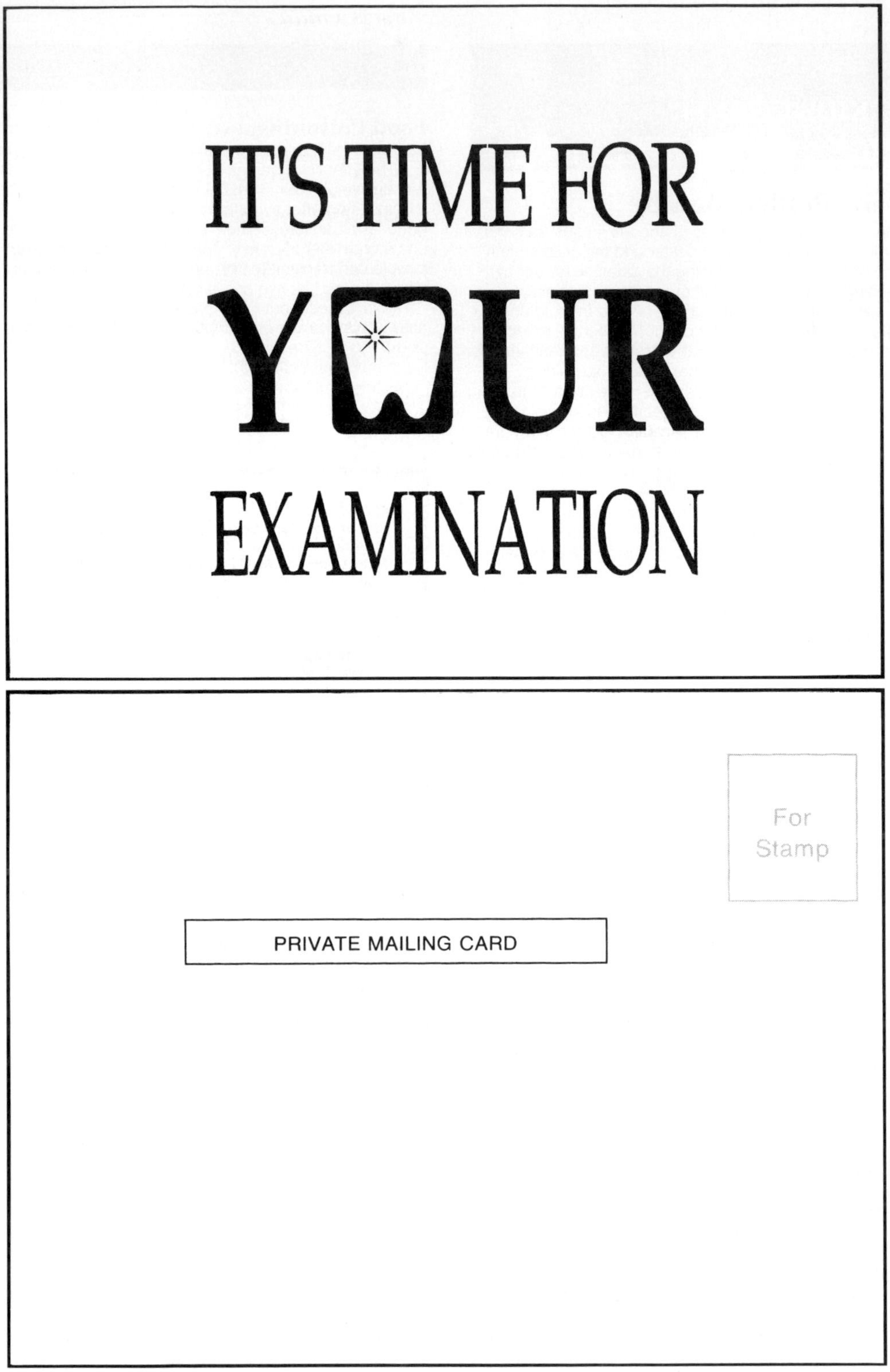

IT'S TIME FOR YOUR EXAMINATION

A

For
Stamp

PRIVATE MAILING CARD

FIG. 14-31   *A,* Sample of a recall card sent to patients.

Recall Systems

A **recall system** is a preventive program that recalls patients to the office. A patient is recalled to the office for various reasons, including denture checks, orthodontic development status, periodontal evaluation, or an endodontic treatment follow-up. The most common reason, however, is for an oral prophylaxis. Patients are placed on a recall system in accordance with the conditions in the mouth. The most common recall times are 3, 4, or 6 months.

◗ Types of Recall Systems

There are three basic systems of recall in an office. The first is a *mail system*, where notices are sent to a patient to inform him or her of the need for an appointment (Fig. 14-31, *A*). This appears to be the most common method of recall because it places the responsibility on the patient to contact the office, and the patient will generally receive the mail regardless of when he or she arrives home. The second system is a *telephone system* that requires that each patient who is due for an appointment be called by the business staff to schedule an appointment. The telephone system is used frequently since many patients have answering machines, which increases the possibility that the patient will receive the message. The third system is an *advanced appointment system*, whereby the patient makes the appointment at the time of departure from the office and a card is mailed several weeks before the appointment for confirmation. Each of these systems has obvious benefits and disadvantages, as noted in Table 14-1. Probably the best system for any office is a combination of all three. It appears, however, that the mail system is the most popular.

TABLE 14-1   COMPARING RECALL SYSTEMS

Type of system	Advantages	Disadvantages
MAIL SYSTEM	Places responsibility on the patient	Patient may ignore the notice
		Postage is costly
	Message will be waiting for patient at home	Not certain the message was received
		May not receive a response from patient
TELEPHONE SYSTEM	Immediate response, either positive or negative	May not receive an answer or will need to leave the message on the answering machine
	Personal contact can be a practice building tool	May disturb the person
		Time consuming for a large practice
ADVANCED APPOINTMENT SYSTEM	Minimal cost involved	Patient may not know future plans or schedule
	No time required to implement	Appointment book is filled months in advance
		May forget the appointment

Adapted from Finkbeiner B, Patt J: *Practice management for the dental team,* ed 3, St Louis, 1990, Mosby.

J   F   M   A   M   J   J   A   S   O   N   D

NAME _____   BUSINESS TELEPHONE _____

ADDRESS _____   RESIDENCE TELEPHONE _____

RECALL DATE	TREATMENT NOTES

B

FIG. 14-31, cont'd.   B, Sample of a recall file card maintained in the office.

(A and B courtesy of Sycom.)

▶ Maintaining a Recall System

The success of any recall system depends on the effectiveness of its implementation. It is necessary to educate the patients regarding the value of routine recall, to notify them of the need for an appointment, and to follow-up on patients who are negligent in making appointments. Also, a recall system is the lifeline of a practice—it keeps the patients coming back. If the recall system is neglected, soon the patient load in the appointment book begins to diminish.

Each of the systems described requires some form of recall management. Recall file cards can be purchased from dental stationery suppliers (Fig. 14-31, B). These recall cards are filed in a monthly file, and each month one of the systems is activated. After the patient is seen for a prophylaxis, the card is advanced to the next recall time. Care should be taken to make certain that appointments are consistent with a patient's insurance coverage. Failure to schedule appointments in compliance with the patient's insurance coverage may result in nonpayment by the insurance company. Such action may place unexpected financial responsibility on the patient.

Inventory Control

Inventory control in a dental office refers to the method of keeping track of the number and amount of dental instruments and materials. Records for inventory of supplies are maintained in the business office. Three types of supplies are used in an office: *capital items,* which are large, costly items, such as a typewriter or dental chair; *expendable items,* which are disposable or are consumed after each use, such as cotton rolls, dental cements, local anesthetic, or stationery; and *nonexpendable items,* which are reused but not of major cost, such as syringes, spatulas, or rubber bowls.

Good inventory control ensures that when a supply is needed, it is available. Nothing is more frustrating than being ready to perform a procedure and not having the necessary dental material available to do so. Maintaining an effective inventory system requires that everyone in the office accept responsibility for implementation of the system. Frequently, a file for capital equipment is maintained separately and includes information on the date of purchase, the model numbers, and a record of maintenance of the equipment. Expendable supplies require that the staff determine the rate of use, the amount that is needed at all times, the available storage, the amount of capital available for purchases, and the shelf life of the material. A projected budget is needed for supply purchases and to maintain a system for ordering supplies. A manual system may be used, but inventory management is a good application for the computer.

The general procedure for obtaining supplies is to complete an order list or purchase order, place the order with the dental supplier, and receive the materials. When the supplies are received in the office, each supply is checked off the packing slip or invoice to ensure that all the supplies are correct and are in the package. At the end of the month the invoices are cross referenced with the supplier's statement and a check is written for payment. If a supply is not available, it is placed on back order for a later delivery. If a product is returned, a credit slip is sent to the office and the account is credited for the proper amount.

Dental Insurance

Today's dental business office is deluged with paperwork. The insurance **claim form**, a statement of services, dates of service, and itemization of fees, represents a major portion of this activity. The filing of claim forms is a benefit to the patient as it provides payment for dental care.

The Council on Dental Care Programs of the ADA has worked closely with representatives of insurance companies in an effort to maintain a quality dental care system for patients and the profession. Many of the forms and administrative procedures have been a direct result of this committee's work.

Dental insurance involves the following four parties:

1. *Patient:* the person who is receiving the treatment; this person may be the subscriber to the insurance or may be a spouse or dependent child
2. *Group:* sometimes a union or organization that has negotiated dental insurance as a benefit
3. *Carrier* or insurance company: the company that distributes the money to the provider for services rendered
4. *Dentist:* the provider of the dental services

▶ Types of Prepaid Dental Plans

Three basic types of insurance programs are common to dentistry today: usual, customary, and reasonable fee (UCR); fixed fee; and table of allowances.

Usual, Customary, and Reasonable Fee (UCR). This plan, which is used by many dental service corporations, is based on the usual, customary, and reasonable fees of the dentist. The usual fee is that fee which is *usually* charged for a specific service by an individual dentist. A *customary* fee is a fee that is usually charged by dentists of similar training and experience for the same service within a specific and limited geographic area or socioeconomic level of society. A fee is *reasonable* when it meets the above two criteria or can be justified because of special circumstances that pertain to a particular case.

Fixed Fee. In this type of coverage a fixed fee is established for service rendered. Fixed fee coverage is often federally supported. Dentists who participate in this type of program must accept the fees listed on a fee schedule from the responsible agency as the total fee and cannot charge the patient an additional amount.

Table of Allowance. This program provides a table of allowances that fixes a dollar amount as the benefit for each individual's dental service. The patient is responsible for any difference between the dentist's fee and the amount provided for in the table of allowances.

In addition to the traditional fee for service programs listed, several alternative dental delivery systems are available today, including capitation, closed panel, and preferred provider organization systems.

Capitation Dentistry. The **capitation dentistry** system is based on the concept that the dentist assumes the risk in delivering dental care rather than a third party, such as the insurance carrier. The dentist is paid a fixed fee, per capita per month, which entitles members of a group to a specified set of services. Regardless of the number of patients treated or the cost of the services rendered, the dentist receives the fixed fee and is not paid for individual services rendered. Two of the most common capitation programs operating today are the closed panel and Individual Practice Association (IPA) system.

Closed Panel Dentistry. In a **closed panel** system the group contracts with a clinic for the delivery of dental care to its members. Covered individuals must receive dental care from a clinic dentist or pay for the services themselves. Dentists working in such a clinic are generally salaried. In the IPA system a group may contract with a clinic, with partnership, or with individual practitioners for the delivery of dental care to its members. When a covered individual selects a dentist in this system, typically, he or she must continue treatment with this same dentist for a specified time, generally a contract year.

Preferred Provider Organization. Another system available to patients is the **Preferred Provider Organization** (PPO) model. In this system an individual practitioner or clinic may contract with a group purchaser of benefits to provide dental service at a lower cost than is usually offered. The dentist thus becomes a preferred provider. In return for this, the purchaser publicizes the agreement to the group, which could result in additional patients for the dentist. A PPO is frequently offered as an additional benefit to supplement an existing dental program. Subscribers are not required to receive dental care from a preferred provider, but the lower out-of-pocket cost often is an incentive.

It is impossible in this comprehensive clinical text to make you insurance literate within the space provided. The staff person who is responsible for insurance must spend a great deal of time to develop a basic knowledge of insurance systems and to become familiar with procedures for completing the claim forms used by the many different carriers. The following discussion provides you an overview of some of the basic procedures in dental insurance management and a cursory review of terminology and insurance claim forms.

Working with insurance claim forms requires that a dental assistant understand basic insurance. Box 14-8 lists terms likely to be used during common insurance transactions.

INSURANCE TERMINOLOGY

Approved services All services covered under a dental plan

Audit of treatment An administrative or professional review of a dentist's treatment plan or of the dentist's reimbursement claims for services performed

Birthday rule This rule is implemented in the coordination of benefits when the patient is a dependent; dependents are covered as primary under the plan of the parent whose birthday (month and day) occurs earlier in the calendar year

Certificate of eligibility An identification card or document that verifies the individual is covered by a particular group, provided the eligibility requirements continue to be met

Claim form A statement listing services rendered, date of the services, and itemization of the fees; the completed and signed form serves as a request by the dentist for payment of benefits by the carrier

Commercial carrier A corporation that contracts with groups of consumers to administer dental care plans; it is a profit-making organization, with a group of stockholders

Contract year The period of time (usually, but not necessarily, a calendar year) for which a contract is written; it could also be a fiscal year

Copayment The amount or percentage of the total approved amount that the subscriber is obligated to pay; this is not to be confused with the deductible amount

Deductible amount This is the portion or percentage that the subscriber must pay before the plan's benefits begin; this may be a yearly or a one-time amount

Dental service corporation A legally constituted organization that contracts with groups of consumers to administer dental care plans on a prepaid basis; these groups are sponsored by state dental societies and are nonprofit organizations

Dependents Those persons, generally a spouse and children, who receive benefits of a subscriber covered by a dental plan

Effective date The date the contract goes into effect and from which benefits are afforded

Eligible individual A person entitled to benefits under a dental plan

Exclusion Dental services not provided for under a dental plan

Maximum benefit The maximum dollar amount a dental plan will pay toward the cost of dental care incurred by an individual or family in a specified period, whether a calendar year or a contract year

Member The employee who represents the family unit in relation to the prepayment plan

Nonparticipating dentist A dentist who has not entered into an agreement with a service corporation or agency and has not agreed to the rules and regulations of the board of directors of the corporation

Participating dentist A dentist who has an agreement to render care to a member and dependents under the rules and regulations promulgated by a board of directors or agency

Predetermination/preauthorization A proposed treatment plan submitted for verification of eligibility and identification of covered benefits and plan allowances, limitations, and exclusions

Primary carrier The dental plan that covers the patient as the employee (1) when the patient is the male employee or his dependent children; or (2) when the patient is the female employee

Secondary carrier The plan covering the patient as a dependent when the patient is the spouse or dependent child of the employee covered by the primary carrier

Subscriber The employee who represents the family unit in relation to the prepayment plan

▶ Working with Claim Forms

To become proficient in the management of claim forms you will need to attend one of the many workshops provided by the various carriers. The ADA has provided a standardized form that may be purchased by the office, or the patient may obtain an ADA-approved form from his or her employer. The form is divided into two parts: the top part is a request for general information about the patient and/or subscriber; the bottom part of the form requests information about the dentist and includes a listing of services rendered for the patient.

The ADA standardized form (Fig. 14-32) is relatively easy to complete. However, it is important that the information be thorough and accurate. Shortcuts or incomplete information only results in rejection of the claim form by the insurance company. Such errors delay payment and make it necessary to resubmit the claim form with the correct information. Something as simple as the wrong birth date or inserting a patient's nickname instead of the proper name can result in the claim form being returned. Before you complete a claim form, review it thoroughly and be certain you understand the information required for each of the spaces provided.

ATTENDING DENTIST'S STATEMENT

CHECK ONE:

☐ DENTIST'S PRE-TREATMENT ESTIMATE

☐ DENTIST'S STATEMENT OF ACTUAL SERVICES

CARRIER NAME AND ADDRESS

PATIENT SECTION

1. PATIENT NAME	2. RELATIONSHIP TO EMPLOYEE	3. SEX	4. PATIENT BIRTHDATE	5. IF FULL TIME STUDENT
FIRST M.I. LAST	☐ SELF ☐ CHILD	M Ⓕ	MM DD YYYY	SCHOOL CITY
Lynn Carey	☒ SPOUSE ☐ OTHER ____		11 20 52	

6. EMPLOYEE/SUBSCRIBER NAME AND MAILING ADDRESS
Ronald I. Carey
2750 Wyoming S.E.
Grand Rapids, MI 49502

7. EMPLOYEE/SUBSCRIBER SOC. SEC. NUMBER
123-45-6789

8. EMPLOYEE SUBSCRIBER BIRTHDATE
MM DD YYYY
9 18 52

9. EMPLOYER (COMPANY) NAME AND ADDRESS
General Motors
Grand Rapids MI
49506

10. GROUP NUMBER

11. IS PATIENT COVERED BY ANOTHER PLAN OF BENEFITS?
DENTAL X
MEDICAL ____

12-A. NAME AND ADDRESS OF CARRIER(S)
Metropolitan
14600 Walton Blvd.
Rochester MI

12-B. GROUP NO.(S)
8330

13. NAME AND ADDRESS OF EMPLOYER
Jones Electric
Grand Rapids MI
33304

14-A. EMPLOYEE/SUBSCRIBER NAME (IF DIFFERENT THAN PATIENT'S)

14-B. EMPLOYEE/SUBSCRIBER SOC. SEC. NUMBER
383-10-1789

14-C. EMPLOYEE/SUBSCRIBER BIRTHDATE
MM DD YYYY
11 20 52

15. RELATIONSHIP TO PATIENT
☒ SELF   ☐ PARENT
☐ SPOUSE ☐ OTHER ____

I HAVE REVIEWED THE FOLLOWING TREATMENT PLAN. I AUTHORIZE RELEASE OF ANY INFORMATION RELATING TO THIS CLAIM. I UNDERSTAND THAT I AM RESPONSIBLE FOR ALL COSTS OF DENTAL TREATMENT.

▶ Lynn Carey   DATE 9-2-94
SIGNED (PATIENT, OR PARENT IF MINOR)

I HEREBY AUTHORIZE PAYMENT DIRECTLY TO THE BELOW NAMED DENTIST OF THE GROUP INSURANCE BENEFITS OTHERWISE PAYABLE TO ME.

▶ Ronald L. Carey   DATE 9-2-94
SIGNED (INSURED PERSON)

DENTIST SECTION

16. DENTIST NAME
CHRIS A. BROWN, D.D.S.

17. MAILING ADDRESS
19 E. Center St.

CITY, STATE, ZIP
Madison, WI 53701

18. DENTIST SOC. SEC. OR T.I.N. 123-45-6789
19. DENTIST LICENSE NO. 1111
20. DENTIST PHONE NO. (606) 123-4567

21. FIRST VISIT DATE CURRENT SERIES 9-2-94
22. PLACE OF TREATMENT OFFICE HOSP. ECF OTHER
23. RADIOGRAPHS OR MODELS ENCLOSED? NO YES HOW MANY?

24. IS TREATMENT RESULT OF OCCUPATIONAL ILLNESS OR INJURY?	NO	YES	IF YES, ENTER BRIEF DESCRIPTION AND DATES.
25. IS TREATMENT RESULT OF AUTO ACCIDENT?			
26. OTHER ACCIDENT?			
27. ARE ANY SERVICES COVERED BY ANOTHER PLAN?			
28. IF PROSTHESIS, IS THIS INITIAL PLACEMENT?			(IF NO, REASON FOR REPLACEMENT)
			29. DATE OF PRIOR PLACEMENT
30. IS TREATMENT FOR ORTHODONTICS?			IF SERVICES ALREADY COMMENCED ENTER: DATE APPLIANCES PLACED MOS. TREATMENT REMAINING

IDENTIFY MISSING TEETH WITH "X"

FACIAL

UPPER RIGHT — PERMANENT — LEFT
LOWER — PRIMARY

FACIAL

32. REMARKS FOR UNUSUAL SERVICES

31. EXAMINATION AND TREATMENT PLAN - LIST IN ORDER FROM TOOTH NO. 1 THROUGH TOOTH NO. 32 - USE CHARTING SYSTEM SHOWN.

TOOTH # OR LETTER	SURFACE	DESCRIPTION OF SERVICE (INCLUDING X-RAYS, PROPHYLAXIS, MATERIALS USED, ETC.) LINE NO.	DATE SERVICE PERFORMED MO. DAY YEAR	PROCEDURE NUMBER	FEE	FOR ADMINISTRATIVE USE ONLY
		1	10 5 94	00	110	
		2	10 5 94	00	210	
19	Med	3	10 12 94	02	160	
16		4	10 12 94	07	220	
27		5	10 28 94	06	750	
28		6	10 28 94	06	240	
29		7	10 28 94	06	750	
9		8	10 19 94	03	310	
9		9	10 28 94	02	750	
		10				
		11				
		12				
		13				
		14				
		15				

I HEREBY CERTIFY THAT THE PROCEDURES AS INDICATED BY DATE HAVE BEEN COMPLETED AND THAT THE FEES SUBMITTED ARE THE ACTUAL FEES I HAVE CHARGED AND INTEND TO COLLECT FOR THESE PROCEDURES.

____ SIGNED (DENTIST) ____ DATE ____

TOTAL FEE CHARGED	1950⁰⁰
MAX. ALLOWABLE	
DEDUCTIBLE	
CARRIER %	
CARRIER PAYS	
PATIENT PAYS	

Form 4048 • 7/86 **SYCOM** Madison, WI Printed in U.S.A.

FIG. 14-32 ADA standardized claim form.

(From Finkbeiner BL, Patt JD: *Practice management for the dental team,* St Louis, 1991, Mosby.)

TABLE 14-2 INDEX TO MOST FREQUENTLY REQUESTED PROCEDURE CODES*

Procedure	Procedure code	Procedure	Procedure code
Acid etch bridge	06200 series for pontic 06545 for each retainer	Gross scaling (no root planing)	01110 (as part of prophylaxis)
Alveoplasty	07300 series	Home fluoride treatment	09630, by report
Alloplastic implant	07993	(when fluoride provided by treating dentist)	
Amalgam core (no crown placed)	02161	Hydroxylapatite implant	07993-07994
Base, restorative	02999, by report	Identification disk	09999, by report
Bite plane	07880	Implants	03460; 05973-05976; 07993-07994
Bite wings	00272-00275		
Blade (ramus) implant	05974	Nightguard	09940
Bleaching (any tooth)	03960	Nitrous oxide	09230
Bonded bridge	06999, by report	Occlusal adjustment	09951-09952
Bonding		Occlusal orthotic appliance	07880
Esthetic	02960-02962	Occlusal radiograph	00240
Restorative	02300 series	Odontoplasty (per tooth)	09951, by report
Bone graft	04261-04262	Overdenture	05860-05861
Bruxism appliance	09940	Partial dentures	05211-05281; 05820-05821
Cantilever bridge	06200 series for pontic; 06700 series for retainer	Panoramic radiograph	00330
Cephalometric radiograph	00340	Periapical radiograph	00220-00230
Ceramic substrate crown	02740	Pins (per tooth, in addition to restoration)	02951
Composite restorations			
Anterior	02330-02335	Pit and fissure sealants	01351
Posterior	02380-02387	Porcelain laminate veneer (laboratory)	02962
Composite core (no crown placed)	02387	Precision attachment	
Composite crown (strip crown)		Fixed appliance	06950
Anterior	02335	Removable appliance	05862
Posterior	02382; 02387	Preventive resin restoration	02300 series
Copings (for overdentures)	05860-05861, by report	Pulpectomy	03300 series
Crown lengthening		Ramus blade implant	05974
Surgical (bone)	04260	Radiographs	00210-00340
Nonsurgical (tissue)	04211	Recontouring, per tooth	09951, by report
Dentures		Ridge augmentation	07993
Complete	05110-05120	Root canal therapy	03300 series
Immediate	05130-05140	Space maintainers	01510-01550
Overdenture	05860-05861	Splints	
Partial	05211-05281	For periodontal purposes	04320-04321
Disking, per tooth	09951, by report	For treatment of TMJ disorders	07880
Electrosurgery, per tooth	04211	Stainless steel crowns	02930-02931
Emergency treatment for pain	09110	Strip crowns	02335; 02382; 02387
Enamelplasty, per tooth	09951, by report	Study models	00470
Equilibration	09951-09952	Temporary crown	02970
Extractions		Temporary restoration	02940
Nonsurgical	07110-07130	TMJ appliance	07880
Surgical	07210-07250	TMJ examination	00110; 00120
Fiberotomy	07291	TMJ radiograph	00320; 00321
Flipper	05820-05821	TMJ splint	07880
Fluoride treatments		Ultrasonic scaling	01110 (as part of prophylaxis)
For home use	09630, by report		
In office	01201-01205	X-rays—see Radiographs	
Glass ionomer restorations	02300 series or 02999, by report		
Grafting			
Bone	04261-04262		
Tissue	04270-04271		

*This report was approved by the Council in January 1987.
From Finkbeiner BL, Patt JG: *Practice management for the dental team,* ed 3, St Louis, 1991, Mosby.

Code on Dental Procedures and Nomenclature

The Council on Dental Care Programs has approved a list, *Code on Dental Procedures and Nomenclature,* which has been designed to identify standardized procedures and services. An index to the most frequently requested procedure codes is shown in Table 14-2. A service is given a 5-digit number. The first digit, a zero throughout the series, denotes the service as dental rather than medical; the second digit denotes the category of service; the third designates the class of a specific procedure; the fourth denotes the subclass of the procedure; and the fifth digit has been provided for expansion of the code as necessary. All codes within a single category are in a specific number series; for example, all diagnostic procedures are listed in the series 00100-00999. If a patient were having a complete series of radiographs the code would be 00210 and could be broken down as follows:

0 Dental service

0 Diagnostic service

2 Radiographs

10 Intraoral—complete series

In a different situation, the patient might have a code of 00274. The first 3 digits would refer to the same as the first patient, but the last 2 digits (74) refer to a different type of radiography code. The 7 refers to bite-wing and the 4 indicates the number of radiographs. Each office should have a current listing of these ADA codes to help in completing the forms.

Coordination of Benefits

Coordination of benefits (COB) is a situation that arises when patients are covered by more than one dental plan. Therefore, it becomes necessary to coordinate these benefits. This situation, referred to as the primary-secondary rule of payment, requires the assistant to observe the following few basic rules:

▶ The employee, retiree, or surviving spouse is covered as primary under his or her own dental program.

▶ Dependents are covered as primary under the plan of the parent whose birthday (month and day) occurs earlier in the calendar year. If the parents' birthdays are identical, the **primary carrier**, the carrier responsible for payment, will be the one who has covered the child for the longer time.

▶ Dependents whose parents are divorced or legally separated are covered as follows:

1. The natural parent with custody (except in 5)

2. The spouse of the natural parent with custody

3. The natural parent without custody

4. The spouse of the natural parent without custody

5. If the divorce decree places financial responsibility on one parent, that parent's plan is primary over any other plan; the preceding is then used to determine the remaining order of payment

▶ When a COB occurs between carriers in two different states, the birthday rule is often used, but individual plans should be reviewed to determine the primary-secondary rule in this situation.

Payment Voucher and Check

Some insurance companies provide a payment voucher with the check (Fig. 14-33). The voucher describes the payment in a detailed description that facilitates the posting to the patient account. If a company does not provide such a voucher, it is more difficult for the assistant to determine for whom and for what a payment was made when he or she enters the payment on a patient's financial record.

It is vital to the financial activity of the office that insurance claim forms be processed in an efficient timely manner. The suggestions in Box 14-9 may be helpful in meeting these goals.

BOX 14-9

HELPFUL HINTS FOR PREPARING CLAIM FORMS

1. Be accurate.
2. Maintain an extra supply of claim forms on hand.
3. Type all data on an electric typewriter or use a computer software package to generate forms.
4. Answer *all* questions completely, providing details when required. If a question does not apply, insert *NA* for not applicable.
5. Obtain the most current information on each type of insurance that the patients carry and become familiar with the provisions of each policy. Regularly attend workshops sponsored by various carriers to update your knowledge of insurance procedures.
6. Establish a list of contact persons, phone numbers, and addresses for each of the carriers used in the office.
7. Maintain complete and current information on each patient and update regularly.
8. Be certain to send claim forms to the appropriate carrier and the correct branch office.
9. When necessary, obtain prior authorization before treatment is begun.
10. Be certain the doctor and patient have signed the form before mailing.
11. Retain a copy of the completed form for the office.
12. If required, include copies of radiographs or periodontal charting and be certain each is well identified with both the patient's and the doctor's name.
13. Set aside a specific time to work on claim forms and to review the status of previously submitted forms.

Delta Dental Plan of Michigan
P.O. Box 30416
Lansing, Michigan 48909-7916

CLAIM PAYMENT
VOUCHER

Check No.: 215100

Issue Date: 11-11-

Patient: Lynn
Relationship Code: 2   Date Of Birth: 11-20-52

Receipt Date: 11-02-
Contract/SSN No.: 123456789
Group No.: 83300029
Claim Document No.: 331502735
DDS Lic. No.: 0007378 MI
701000003PD

Name ●   Ronald Carey
Address ●   2750 Wyoming, S.E.
Grand Rapids, MI 49502

Tooth No. or Letter	Surface	Date of Service	Procedure Code	Submitted Amount	Approved Amount	Approved Code	Allowed Amount	Allowed Code	% Co-Pay	::	Patient Payment	Delta Payment	Processing Policies
		10-05-83	00110	10	10	0	10	0	100		0.00	10.00	
		10-05-83	00210	35	35	0	35	0	090		3.50	31.50	
19	MOD	10-12-83	02160	40	40	0	40	0	090		4.00	36.00	
16		10-12-83	07220	60	60	0	60	0	090		6.00	54.00	
27		10-28-83	06750	300	300	0	300	0	050		150.00	150.00	
28		10-28-83	06240	300	300	0	300	0	050		150.00	150.00	
29		10-28-83	06750	300	300	0	300	0	050		150.00	150.00	
9		10-19-83	03310	140	140	0	140	0	090		14.00	126.00	
9		10-28-83	02750	300	300	0	300	0	090		30.00	270.00	

Predetermined On
Claim Number: _____

Code Definitions On
Reverse Side

507.50	977.50	
TOTAL	TOTAL	
977.50	14.66	962.84
MAXIMUM USED TO DATE	R & D WITHHOLD	NET AMOUNT

Name ●   Dr. J. Lake
Address ●   611 Main St., S.E.
Grand Rapids, MI 49502

MI-620-34SM (2-83)

- -

Delta Dental Plan of Michigan
P.O. Box 30416
Lansing, Michigan 48909-7916

PAYABLE THROUGH
AMERICAN
BANK & TRUST COMPANY
LANSING, MICHIGAN

74-67
724

Check No.: **215100**

Issue Date: 11-11-

Void After 90 Days

Amount
$ ***962.84

Not To Exceed $2,000.

Pay   Nine Hundred Sixty Two Dollars and 84 Cents

To The
Order Of ●   Dr. J. Lake
●   611 Main St., S.E.
Grand Rapids, MI 49502

VOID

_____
Authorized Signature

⑆ 215100 ⑆ ⑆072400670⑆   12 50 10 9⑈

FIG. 14-33 Payment voucher and insurance check.

▶ Preventing Fraud in Insurance Payments

Fraud can be defined as deceit, trickery, or double dealing, but no matter how it is defined, fraud is cheating. As much as we may wish to deny it, fraud does exist in dentistry. Special effort must be taken to maintain accuracy and honesty at all times. The following actions constitute fraud and should be avoided by the dentist and the staff:

- ▶ Padding fees
- ▶ Billing before completion of treatment
- ▶ Predating or postdating claim forms
- ▶ Falsely listing treatment that was rendered
- ▶ Not working within the contract

Filing Systems

Five basic methods of filing are used in most dental offices, including alphabetic, geographic, numeric, subject, and chronologic—methods that apply alphabetic procedures (except for the numeric). In an alphabetic system the arrangement appears in sequence from A to Z.

Major equipment and record styles are a choice of the dentist, with input from the business assistant. A common file system, the open shelf style with a file folder index that uses a color code system, is popular today. Consultation with a dental office designer and a dental stationery supplier will prove advantageous when selecting new equipment and filing supplies.

Computer Applications

Computers have gained wide recognition in the dental business office today (see Fig. 14-22, *A*). It is vital that anyone working in a dental office today have some basic understanding of microcomputers for entering clinical data at chairside and for financial transactions in the business office. Software packages or program instructions are available for many of the common procedures discussed in this chapter, including word processing, accounts receivable, accounts payable, recall, inventory control, and practice analysis.

▶ Hardware Components of a Computer

Regardless of the type of computer selected for the dental business office, each should be capable of performing the basic operations, including (1) input; (2) processing; (3) output; and (4) storage. Fig. 14-34 graphically illustrates these components.

INPUT

The keyboard is the most common method of entering data into the computer. The keyboard includes the traditional alphabetic keys in addition to a numeric pad, cursor control keys, and specialized function keys.

PROCESSOR

The processor (CPU) is the *brain* of the equipment. Depending on the type of software package that is being used the processor receives the data from the input device and directs the computer to perform a specific set of tasks. The amount of data that can be stored in the processing unit depends on the main memory of the system.

OUTPUT

The output device is commonly the printer. If you need a hard copy (paper copy) of a patient record or financial statement, the computer is directed to print a copy. Most

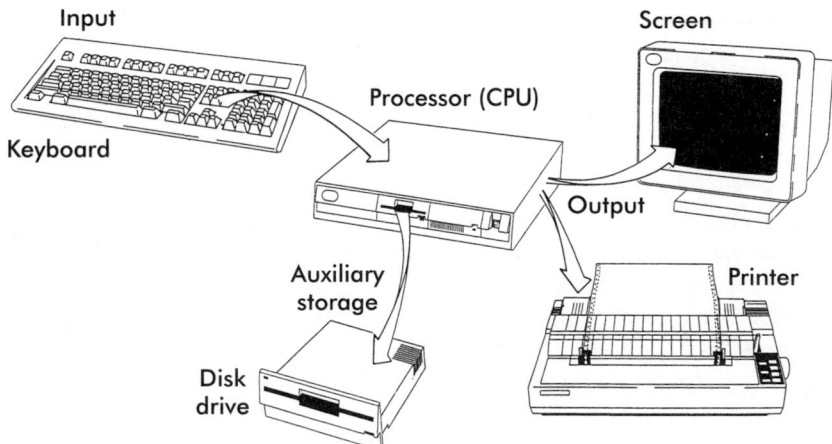

FIG. 14-34   Graphic illustration of computer hardware components.

(From Finkbeiner BL, Patt JC: *Practice management for the dental team*, St Louis, 1991, Mosby.)

offices today are using laser printers because they provide sharp copies, are relatively inexpensive, and are quiet to operate. Another output mode is the display terminal or monitor, which allows the information to be displayed (soft copy) for review.

DATA STORAGE

The storage medium of the computer may be a floppy disk or a hard disk. The hard disk is a fixed disk that is sealed in an enclosure and is permanently mounted in the disk drive. It contains rigid metal disks that are coated with magnetic material that makes them suitable for recording and storage. A hard disk storage is usually measured in millions of characters or megabytes, whereas floppy disk storage is usually measured in thousands of characters. A floppy disk is a thin flexible plastic disk that is enclosed in a protective jacket; it quickly allows the user to interchange data or software. Floppy disks are produced in two common sizes, 3½ or 5¼ inches. Because of the greater amount of memory and the faster access, the staff in most dental offices prefer the hard disks. To protect records in a dental office a hard disk will commonly need to be backed up routinely on a floppy disk or on magnetic tape.

The use of computers in clinical dentistry is rapidly expanding to include cephalometric tracings, charting, entering clinical data at chairside, and dental imaging and evaluation in diagnosis.

KEY POINTS

▶ Dentistry is a business, as well as a health care profession. Not only must treatment be provided in a caring manner, it must be efficient and productive to create a profit.

▶ Telecommunication systems in the office include telephones, FAX machines, cellular phones, pagers, and computers. The dental assistant in the business office assumes responsibility for the effective utilization of each of these.

▶ To gain confidence in telephone communication, it is wise to establish a policy for a salutation, responses to routine situations, and rules for making and receiving calls. Some form of answering machine or service should be provided with responsibilities defined for receiving and responding to messages.

▶ The reception room is the gateway to the dental office. This room becomes a place to greet patients and creates the initial image for the office. Each staff member should assume responsibility for keeping this area neat, comfortable, and free of odors, as well as maintaining current reading materials.

▶ Effective appointment book management lays the groundwork for a smoothly run office that is free of tension and lengthy delays. A week-at-a-glance style appointment book allows for easy review of future scheduling. One person should manage this book, make neat and complete entries in pencil, and use a predetermined schedule list to ensure appropriate scheduling for various treatment. Adjunct appointment materials include daily schedules, appointment cards, and a list of common codes for data entry.

▶ Two types of legal records are maintained for patients: clinical and financial. A clinical record verifies the date and type of treatment performed, a collection of diagnostic data, consent forms, laboratory requisitions, and other confidential materials specific to an individual patient. A financial record is verification of charges, debits, and credits for an individual or family.

▶ When records are transferred from one office to another site, written consent, with specific directions, must be obtained from the patient. Original records are retained in the office and duplicates sent. Verification of records transfer should be retained in the patient record.

▶ Transferring records from a treatment room to the business office must be done in a manner to prevent disease transmission. This can be done by only touching the records after treatment gloves are removed, using overgloves, or entering data on a protected keyboard in the treatment room.

▶ Many forms of written communication are produced in a dental office, including letters, procedural manual, office policy, newsletters, compliance documents, and recall notices. Each piece of written communication should follow standard business principles.

▶ A recall system in a dental office is a lifeline for the practice. This system recalls patients to the office for routine prophylaxis, denture checks, or orthodontic, periodontic, or endodontic evaluation. Three types of recall systems are common: mail, telephone, and advanced appointment.

▶ An inventory system ensures that current dental instruments and materials, as well as other supplies, are always available for use.

▶ Dental insurance claim management represents a major portion of activity in the business office. Many types of programs are available; and a business assistant must become familiar with insurance terminology, codes on dental procedures, and nomenclature and must maintain a thorough understanding of claim form management.

▶ Computers are widely used in dental practices today for word processing, accounts receivable and payable, recall, appointment control, inventory, and practice analysis. Familiarity with the components of a computer and with the ability to use common dental software packages ensures the business of the practice, maintains currency, and increases productivity.

BIBLIOGRAPHY

Christensen GJ: *A buyer's guide to dentistry*, St Louis, 1994, Mosby.

Fulton, PJ: *General office procedures for colleges*, ed 10, Cincinnati, 1994, Southwestern.

Finkbeiner BL, Patt JC: *Practice management for the dental team*, ed 3, St Louis, 1990, Mosby.

Weber RD: Dental records: ownership and access, *Mich Dent Assoc J* 69:00, Nov-Dec, 1987.

UNIT IV PRECLINICAL SKILLS

15 Four-Handed Dentistry

LEARNING OBJECTIVES

You will have mastered the material in this chapter when you can:

▸ Define the key terms

▸ Explain the concept of advanced functions in relation to four-handed dentistry

▸ Describe the benefits of four-handed dentistry

▸ Identify the principles of motion economy

▸ Identify the classification of motions

▸ Describe six-handed dentistry

▸ Describe the function and styles of preset trays

▸ Define and explain the application of color coding

▸ Explain positive phrases for implementing four-handed dentistry

KEY TERMS

Classification of motion
Color coding
Ergonomics
Four-handed dentistry
Motion economy
Preset trays
Six-handed dentistry
Supine position
Work simplification

The keystone to a successful dental practice, **four-handed dentistry**, is a chairside technique that involves four hands working together simultaneously to provide treatment to the oral cavity. This concept evolved in the 1950s and dramatically changed the practice of dentistry. Before this time, dentists practiced in a standing position at chairside, which caused unnecessary physical stress in an already highly demanding profession. In the 1990s **ergonomics**, the concept of adapting the environment to the worker, became the term for increased efficiency by design.

Research done in the 1940s indicated that a dentist who used one dental chair and worked with a chairside assistant could provide treatment to 33% more patients than a dentist who worked alone. It was further shown that with additional dental chairs and two full-time, well-qualified chairside dental assistants, the dentist could provide care to approximately 75% more dental patients. This chapter will define the *why* of four-handed dentistry and illustrate the concepts and advantages of practicing four-handed dentistry. In subsequent chapters the *how* of four-handed dentistry will be described. These chapters will thoroughly describe the basic skills and procedures that are required to practice the concepts of four-handed dentistry, including seating the patient and operating team, exchanging instruments, and evacuating the oral cavity. Later, basic dental procedures will be presented using these concepts.

Benefits of Four-Handed Dentistry

The benefits of four-handed dentistry are many but can generally be divided into three basic categories: increase in patient comfort, reduction in operator and assistant fatigue, and increase in productivity.

Four-handed dentistry increases patient comfort. One method that is used involves seating the patient in a **supine position**: the patient lies on the back with the face upward and with the arms and body well supported (Fig. 15-1). Other methods of increasing patient comfort include the use of high-velocity evacuation (HVE) and fiberoptic handpieces. HVE quickly removes debris, saliva, and other fluids from the mouth. The use of high-speed fiberoptic handpieces provides patient comfort and increases the operator's visibility. When the

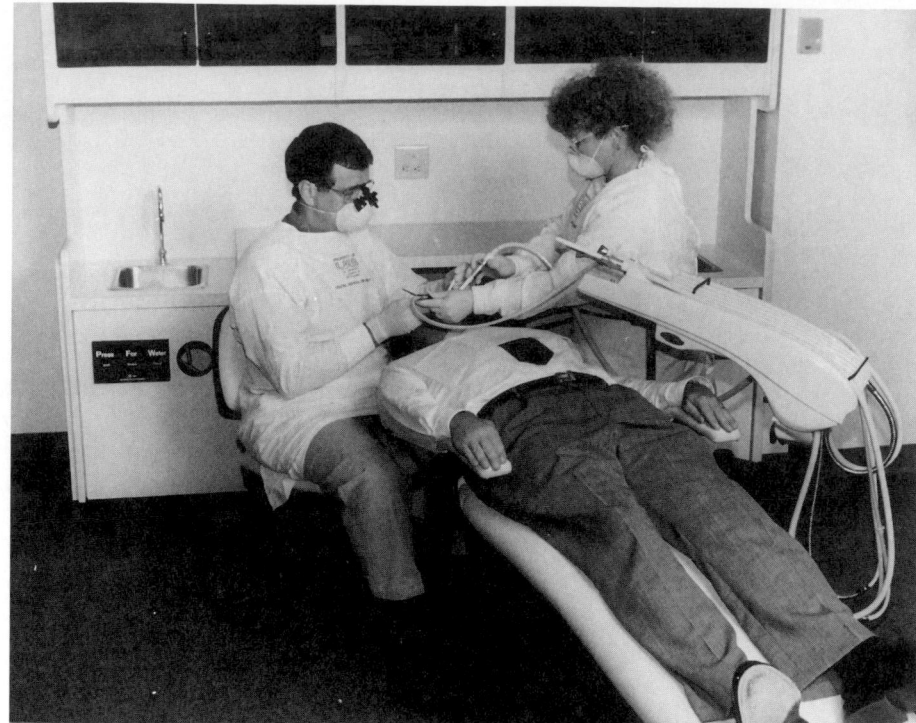

FIG. 15-1   Ergonomically correct position at chairside. Patient is placed in a supine position and the operating team has balanced posture.

(Courtesy of Health Science Products, Birmingham, Alabama.)

patient is comfortable and the need to stop in midprocedure to empty the mouth of fluids and debris is eliminated, the procedure can flow smoothly and efficiently.

Four-handed dentistry reduces fatigue for the operating team. Because the dentist and assistant are seated with their bodies well supported, unnecessary motions (bending and reaching) are eliminated and visibility is improved. In Fig. 15-1 the operating team is positioned in a balanced posture. Their bodies are well supported, using ergonomically designed operating stools. By adhering to the principles of motion economy, the dentist and assistant are able to practice more comfortably. Body fatigue occurs when either the dentist or the assistant is standing, straining, or bending to observe the operating site. Once negative factors are removed, efficiency can be increased.

Four-handed dentistry increases productivity. When fatigue is reduced, the physical and mental stamina of the dental team is maintained for longer time periods, efficiency is increased, and the dental team is able to provide more treatment for more people.

Four-handed dentistry is much like a medical team performing an operation. The only differences in medicine are the greater number of team members needed and the use of different terminology. In dentistry the assistant and dentist work together as *the team,* performing a treatment procedure— *the operation*—for a patient positioned in the chair—*the operating table.* This team performance, using four hands together to treat the patient, requires the knowledge and skill of the dentist to perform the treatment with the qualified assistant anticipating the sequence of the procedure and the instrumentation that will be needed. The assistant must always be ready to meet patient and operator needs as they arise, as well as to perform various intraoral duties that are delegated by dental law.

▶ Advanced Functions

An adjunct to four-handed dentistry is advanced or expanded functions. These intraoral duties are delegated to an assistant or hygienist. The dental practice act in each state specifies which duties may be delegated and the conditions under which the duties may be performed. In the 1970s the government expanded the use and management of dental auxiliaries. Thus, a great deal of research preceded the changes in dental practice acts that delegate specific advanced functions to the dental assistant or hygienist. Appendix A is a listing of legal

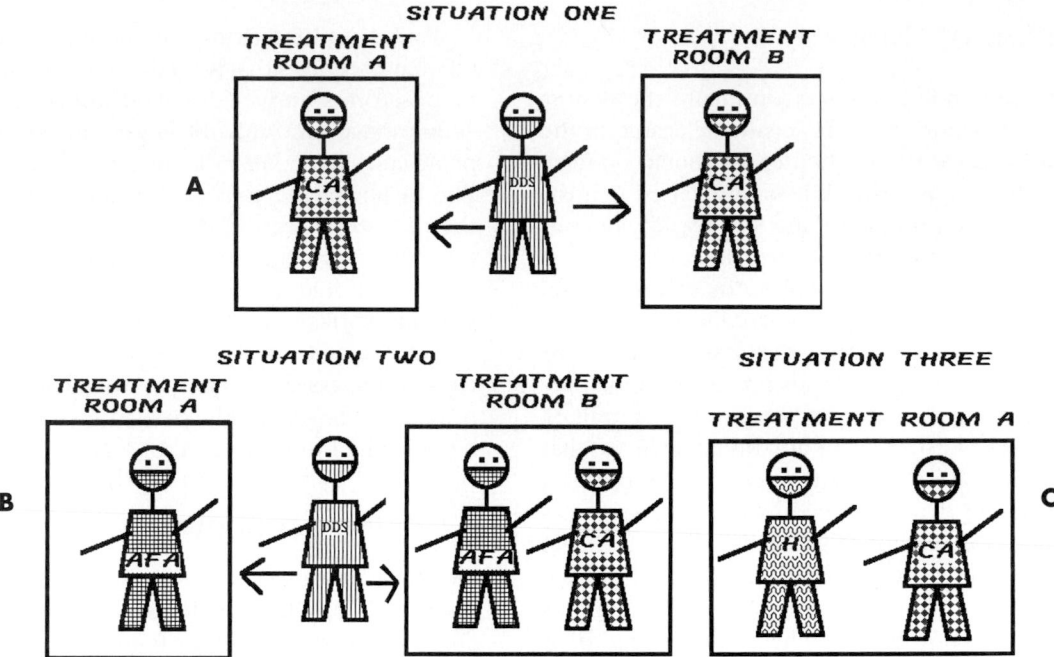

FIG. 15-2   *A,* The dentist works with a chairside assistant in Room A. When the treatment is completed, the dentist moves to room B with a new chairside assistant or the assistant from Room A follows to Room B. Another staff person dismisses the patient in Room A. *B,* At a point in treatment, the dentist leaves the patient to an advanced functions assistant. This could be the original chairside assistant who was assisting the dentist or it could be another assistant. The advanced function assistant could work alone, as in treatment Room A, or with a chairside assistant as in Room B. *C,* A dental assistant assists the dental hygienist.

(Courtesy of Charles Finkbeiner, Ann Arbor, Michigan.)

advanced functions for each auxiliary in each state. Laws change so rapidly that you should refer to the latest documents provided by your state.

Many scenarios will occur each day that require the use of four-handed dentistry or advanced functions. These situations will allow an auxiliary to perform the maximum delegable duties as shown in Fig. 15-2. First, a chairside assistant could assist the dentist in Treatment Room #1 during anesthesia administration. At the conclusion of this procedure, the dentist could go to Treatment Room #2 and be assisted by another assistant, or the first chairside assistant could go to Treatment Room #2. In Treatment Room #1 the chairside assistant, who has the proper qualifications or credentials, could assume the role of an advanced functions assistant or remain at chairside to assist an advanced functions assistant. The final scenario is that of the hygienist and assistant working together. This combination could improve patient comfort, reduce stress and strain on the hygienist, and increase productivity.

Basic Concepts of Four-Handed Dentistry

Four-handed dentistry is based on the premise that a qualified chairside assistant always works with the dentist as a team to provide quality care to as many patients as possible, with reduced stress for the patient and the staff. Four-handed dentistry was intended not to create an *assembly line* type of production, but rather to reduce time and motion and to relieve the stress caused by bending and standing in the same position for a long time. The following text discusses the basic concepts of four-handed dentistry that have been tested through research and are well accepted by the profession today and form the foundation for any sound four-handed or advanced-functions practice. It is not possible to implement only one or two of these concepts; each depends on the other for success.

❯ Delegation of Duties

To practice four-handed dentistry optimally, the dentist must delegate all duties that are legally delegable in the state to a qualified assistant. The dentist should perform those duties that require the skills of a licensed dentist, such as diagnosis, cutting hard and soft tissue, administering anesthesia, and other irreversible procedures. Duties that do not require the skill of the dentist should be performed by a qualified dental auxiliary.

Research conducted by both private and government agencies indicates that many duties previously done only by the dentist can be skillfully performed by trained dental auxiliaries. Results from all studies indicate that dental auxiliaries can, with the proper training, perform selected reversible dental procedures at an acceptable level of quality. Delegation of duties is necessary if the dentist expects to provide more treatment to more patients. Therefore, the term *operator* in situations described in the text from this point forward may refer to either the dentist, the assistant, or the dental hygienist, depending on the specific task being performed and the legal assignment of the duty within the state.

❯ Advanced Planning

The success of four-handed dentistry is predicated on the fact that the patient has had a prophylaxis and a complete oral and radiographic examination and that the doctor has reviewed the patient's record and arranged for sequential appointments to complete the treatment. Advanced planning places treatment in a logical sequence and aids in determining effective delegation of duties for effective utilization of the dental auxiliaries. Such planning becomes critical in an advanced functions practice where scheduling the personnel is vital to time management. An example of such planning can be demonstrated in the scheduling of a patient for an amalgam restoration. The first phase of the appointment involves anesthesia administration by the dentist; then rubber dam placement by an auxiliary; followed by the cavity preparation by the dentist, using a chairside assistant; and the placement and carving of the amalgam by an advanced functions auxiliary, who will then remove the rubber dam. Final articulation check is done by the doctor. At first, such an appointment seems fragmented, but with advanced planning, such an appointment can run smoothly.

❯ Seating the Operating Team

Four-handed dentistry is *sit down* dentistry. This ergonomically sound way to practice dentistry uses the skills of a well-qualified dental assistant, while employing basic work simplification techniques.

Work simplification, a method of making work more efficient, requires that both the operator and the assistant be positioned on well-designed stools; the patient is in a supine position, with the nose and knees on the same plane and the maxillary arch, perpendicular to the floor. The height of the chair is typically 1 to 2 inches above the operator's legs, thus allowing the head portion of the patient's chair to rest nearly in the operator's lap. The assistant should be in line with the oral cavity and the working surface is positioned over the assistant's legs. The dental unit, with all its instruments, should be as close to the assistant and operator as possible. A detailed procedure for seating the patient and operating team will be described in Chapter 17.

❯ Motion Economy

Motion economy is a concept that eliminates or minimizes the number and length of the motions used at chairside. Early studies in four-handed dentistry at the University of Alabama identified specific principles of motion economy. A close look at the list in Box 15-1 quickly tells the dental assistant that great emphasis is placed on the organization of equipment and materials at chairside and that it is advisable for the assistant to consider how best to arrange the instruments or material to avoid wasting time and energy.

BOX 15-1

PRINCIPLES OF MOTION ECONOMY

- ❯ Minimize the number of instruments to be used for a procedure.
- ❯ On a preset tray, position the instruments in the sequence that they will be used.
- ❯ Position instruments, materials, and equipment in advance whenever possible.
- ❯ Place instruments and materials on a mobile cart as close to the patient as possible.
- ❯ Place the patient in a supine position.
- ❯ Provide work areas that are 1 to 2 inches lower than the elbow.
- ❯ Use operating stools that provide good posture and body support.
- ❯ Minimize the number of eye movements.
- ❯ Reduce the length and number of motions.
- ❯ Use body motions that require the least amount of time.
- ❯ Use smooth continuous motions, and avoid distracting zigzag movement.

BOX 15-2

CLASSIFICATION OF MOTIONS

Class I	Movement of the fingers only, as when picking up a small cotton pellet
Class II	Fingers and wrist motion, as used when transferring an instrument to the operator
Class III	Fingers, wrist, and elbow, as when reaching for a handpiece
Class IV	The entire arm and shoulder, as when reaching into the mobile cart
Class V	The entire torso, as when turning around to reach for equipment on the fixed cabinetry

Classification of Motion

Motion economy refers to the way energy can be conserved and strain on the body, reduced by refining specific motions. To understand motion economy, it is necessary to classify common motions used at chairside. Motion can be classified into five categories, according to the length of the motion, as shown in Box 15-2. Think about your daily activities and imagine how you could lessen motions and thus conserve energy.

Conservation of motion often may require you to *rearrange* equipment and materials so that they are placed closer to you. Other times you may need to *plan ahead* to ensure that all materials are prepared in advance so that you do not have to move about to obtain the materials you need. You may even need to *reorganize* a procedure to eliminate unnecessary steps. Think about a hospital operating room scene, and realize how all the materials are within easy reach. The staff doesn't scurry about or reach into drawers. The same readiness should exist in a dental treatment room.

Six-Handed Dentistry

Sometimes, an extra pair of hands is needed at chairside to aid in completing treatment for a patient. **Six-handed dentistry** refers to the use of another assistant to come to chairside and perform tasks to assist the operator, the assistant, or both. Six-handed dentistry could apply to any of the following situations:

- Retracting oral tissues—During an operative or surgical procedure when the chairside assistant is busy evacuating blood and saliva and passing instruments, it may be impossible to retract soft tissues

from the operative site. The third pair of hands is used to retract the tissues or pass instruments to provide the operator better visibility and access to the operative site.

- Controlling a patient—A medically or physically compromised patient may be unable to control his or her movement. To complete the necessary treatment, a third pair of hands may be used to control the patient's movement and avoid potential injury to the staff or patient. Similar control or restraint may be necessary in managing patients with behavioral problems. Take care in all restraint situations not to use force and to ensure that such restraint is discussed with the primary caregiver (parent or legally responsible person) and consent given before its use.

- Preparing dental materials—When the operator is completing multiple preparations for extensive prosthetic treatment, it may be necessary to prepare several mixes of an impression material to avoid its setting during insertion. Therefore, while the chairside assistant is passing materials and maintaining a dry field, the third set of hands can be preparing additional impression material.

Use of Preset Trays

A **preset tray** is an accumulation of instruments or armamentarium (assorted materials and equipment) that is identified for a specific procedure and placed in sequence of use on a specially designed tray. These trays are timesaving and are used for most of the common procedures in dentistry. They were developed as a direct result of time and motion studies. Before the use of preset trays, the assistant had to open and close many drawers to obtain the armamentarium needed for any procedure. Not only did this waste time and motion, but the assistant was also likely to forget an instrument and have to search for it in midtreatment, thus delaying the procedure. Preset trays play a major role in preventing cross contamination, since instruments from the cabinetry are seldom needed during a procedure, which would present the potential for cross contamination.

The tray and/or instruments can be **color coded** (specially colored or marked with colored tape or rings) for a specific procedure. For instance, a tray for an amalgam procedure may be color coded blue and the instruments on the tray will be placed in the order of use, beginning with the explorer and mirror for the initial examination; then the instruments used for cavity preparation, cavity medication, amalgam insertion, amalgam carving; and finally the finishing instruments. By returning instruments to the proper location on the tray after each use during the procedure, the dental assistant can maintain instrument organization. For every procedure, additional instruments or materials will be needed, such as anesthesia, cements, or amalgam. The preset tray, however, cuts down considerably on preparation time.

Today, trays come in various styles, each with particular features that can be adapted to a variety of dental practice needs. Most of these trays satisfy the basic criteria for preset trays, which include the following:

▶ The ability to be sterilized (preferably with the cover on) and stored as a single unit

▶ The ability to hold a minimum number of double-ended instruments and adjunct supplies for a specific procedure

▶ Specifically colored trays for given procedures, or a color code tape that is affixed to the tray

Trays are available in many styles, as shown in Fig. 15-3, A through C. The trays may be constructed of plastic or metal and are supplied in a variety of colors to aid in color coding for specific procedures. A tray insert (Fig. 15-4) can be used as a barrier technique in infection control. Most trays not only provide grooves for common instruments, but also include specially designed areas for burs, cotton pellets, and other auxiliary items that may be needed during the procedure. At the time of sterilization the instruments are processed together as a unit, either on the preset tray, in an ultrasonic tray (Fig. 15-5), or in a sterilizing bag. If the latter methods are used, these instruments can remain stored until the tray is later assembled at chairside. A concept shown in Fig. 15-6 has been designed to ensure that all the instruments remain with a specific tray from the time they are used with a patient, through the cleaning and sterilization process, and until they are used again with another patient.

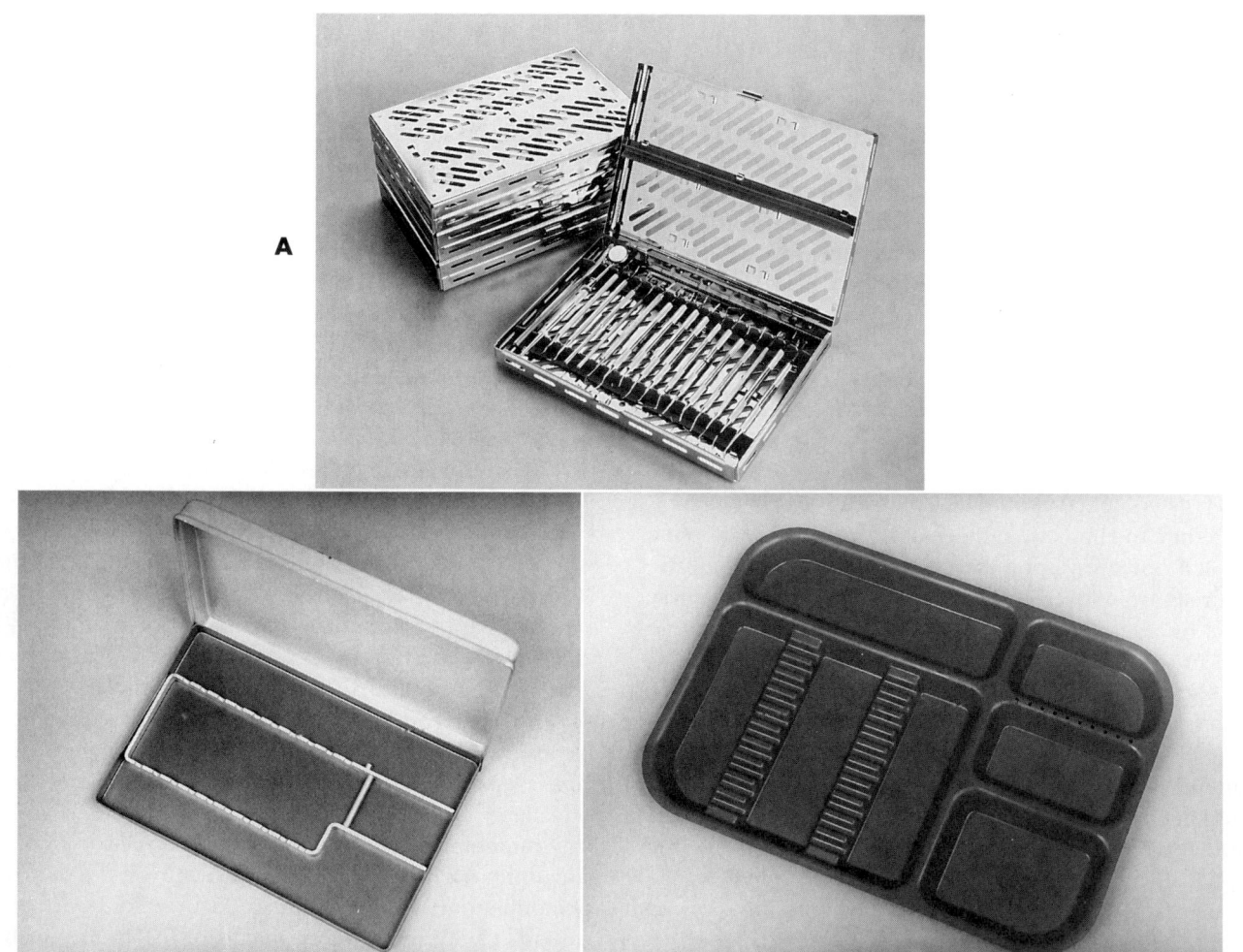

FIG. 15-3 Three styles of common preset trays. *A,* Instrument tray that can be placed in ultrasonic device and sterilized. *B,* Metal tray with insert that can be sterilized. *C,* Plastic tray that can only be disinfected.

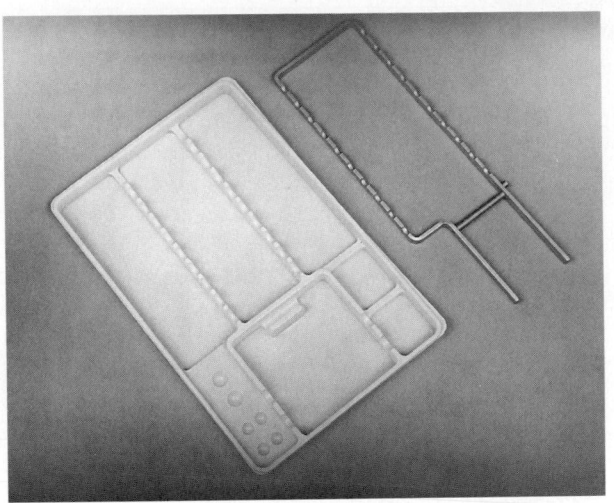

FIG. 15-4   Sterilizable and disposable tray inserts, which aid in maintaining an organized tray.

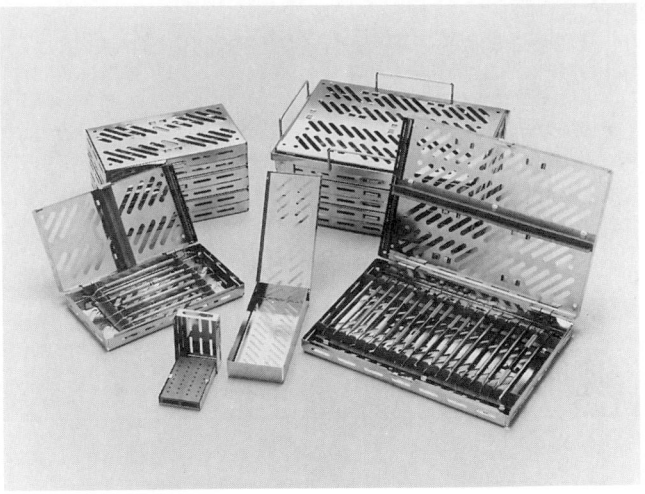

FIG. 15-5   Instruments are prepared for processing in an ultrasonic tray as a unit.

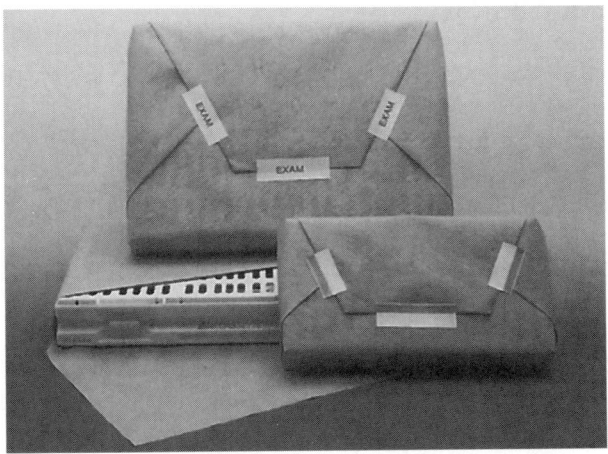

FIG. 15-6   The tray shown in this photo can be processed through cleaning and then sterilized. Note cloth wrapping and coding to aid in maintaining sterility and identification.

Color Coding for Location

Most offices use some form of color coding that aids in identifying the storage location for instruments that are not part of a specific tray setup. Extra instruments, used for special situations in a procedure, may be taken from a mobile cart. These instruments may be color coded to ensure that they will be returned to the proper room and location within the room. Color coding can range from the simple (instruments are coded with a colored tape for a specific room location) to the more complex, with multiple markings on an instrument to indicate room, drawer, and location within a drawer. The instruments shown in Fig. 15-7 are coded with a pressure-sensitive tape and plastic rings that can be sterilized as the instrument is sterilized.

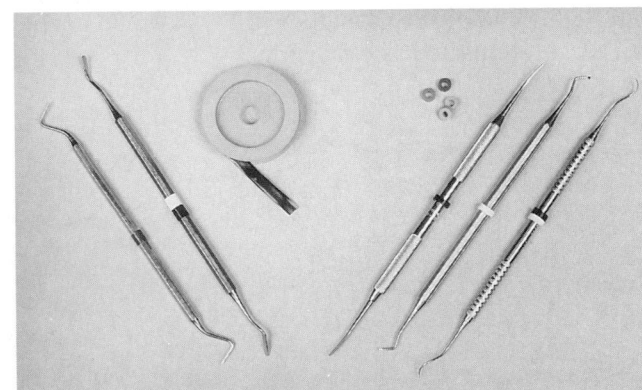

FIG. 15-7   Pressure-sensitive tape *(left)* and rings *(right)* on instruments aids in relocating instruments for later use.

BOX 15-3

STRESSFUL PHRASES THAT RESIST CHANGE

"It costs too much!"
"We tried it and didn't like it."
"It wouldn't work in this kind of practice."
"No one in this area does that."
"We do not have enough instruments."
"We do not have enough space."
"It takes too much equipment."
"Our patients would not like it."
"It sounds like a production line."
"This practice is not big enough."

BOX 15-4

POSITIVE PHRASES THAT INSPIRE CHANGE

"It sounds as if it has merit."
"Let us start a new trend."
"That is interesting..."
"That is a great idea!"
"I have faith in you."
"I am glad you brought that up."
"We should try it."
"Good work!"
"It just might create a better environment."
"Things are beginning to improve."

Implementing Four-Handed Dentistry

Four-handed dentistry is the keystone to a successful productive practice. If this is true, then why doesn't every dentist use it? The answer could be lack of motivation, lack of knowledge that such a concept exists, lack of experience, resistance to change, or a combination of any of these reasons. A good attitude is necessary to encourage the staff to undertake a change to incorporate the concepts of four-handed dentistry into the practice. It may take time to bring about the change, but the practice of four-handed dentistry is worth the effort. Box 15-3 lists phrases that are often used to resist change. These phrases destroy ideas and creativity. Try using the phrases in Box 15-4 to encourage the staff and start the change process.

When the concepts of four-handed dentistry are implemented by the dental team, not only are the previously described benefits realized, but also an *esprit de corps* (a spirit of enthusiasm in the group) is developed within the dental team. This enthusiasm creates a feeling of satisfaction and a sense of responsibility in the staff, confirming that they have contributed to the patient's treatment and that without them the task would not have been accomplished as efficiently.

KEY POINTS

▶ Four-handed dentistry is a chairside technique that involves four hands working together simultaneously to provide treatment to the oral cavity. This concept increases patient comfort, reduces operator and assistant fatigue, and increases productivity.

▶ By design, ergonomics, the concept of adapting the environment to the worker, increases efficiency.

▶ Advanced functions is an adjunct to four-handed dentistry, allowing specific duties to be delegated by law to a dental assistant.

▶ To successfully practice four-handed dentistry, the dentist must delegate to qualified assistants all legally delegatable duties; plan treatments in advance; seat the patient in a supine position, with the dental team using ergonomically sound concepts; and use motion economy.

▶ Preset trays provide for all instruments and materials to be placed sequentially on a tray identified for a specific procedure. This concept saves time and motion and aids in preventing cross contamination.

▶ Color coding of trays and instruments ensures return of instruments to the proper location. Options for coding include colored trays, pressure-sensitive tape, or rings.

▶ Successfully implementing four-handed dentistry involves a positive attitude and the use of phrases that create a spirit of enthusiasm in the staff and acceptance by patients.

BIBLIOGRAPHY

Pollack R: Ergonomics: efficiency without strain, *Dental Team,* Sept, Oct 1993; ADA.

Robinson GE et al: Four-handed dentistry: the whys and wherefores, *J Am Dent Assoc* 78(2):305-309, 1969.

Robinson GE et al: *Four-handed dentistry manual,* ed 6, Birmingham, 1990, University of Alabama School of Dentistry.

Sharma PS, Kuster CG: Basic principles of four-handed, sit-down dentistry and effective utilization of a chairside dental assistant, *J Wisc State Dent Soc* 50(6):252-254, 1974.

Waldman HB: The reaction of the dental profession to changes in the 1970s, *Am J Public Health* 70(6):619-624, 1980.

16   The Dental Suite

LEARNING OBJECTIVES

You will have mastered the material in this chapter when you can:
- Define the key terms
- Identify the factors that determine dental office design
- Describe the basic floor plan of a dental suite
- Explain the function of each room in the dental suite
- Describe the arrangement of a dental treatment room
- Describe the basic features of dental equipment used in four-handed dentistry
- Describe office care and maintenance procedures
- Explain the use of an office evaluation form

KEY TERMS

Air/water syringe	Handpiece
Bracket table	High-velocity evacuation (HVE)
Business office	Laboratory
Curing light	Mobile cabinetry
Cuspidor	Patient chair
Dental stool	Preset trays
Dental unit	Radiography processing area
Electrosurgery unit	Reception room
Eyewash	Recovery room
Fixed cabinetry	Treatment room
Foot control	Ultrasonic scaler

A well-designed and well-maintained office has a direct effect on the credibility of the practice. Regardless of the type of equipment or the proficiency of the staff's technical skills, the patient forms an image of the practice from the environment. Important to the patient is the comfort of the surroundings and whether the office is clean, neat, and reflects a current style. The dentist and staff, who seek to produce quality dentistry, must take care to look like a quality team. Designing a functional and esthetically pleasing office is a complicated process that reflects the personal and professional needs of the dentist and includes input from patients, staff, the architect, the builder, and the decorator. The following discussion outlines the concepts of office design, describes the rooms common to most dental suites, and presents ideas that could be incorporated into each of these areas. The last part of this chapter discusses the dental treatment room and basic equipment for use in four-handed dentistry.

Basic Concepts of Office Design

The dentist is faced with the following questions when attempting to achieve a quality office design:

▶ What image do I want to create?

▶ Which office design is appropriate for my type of practice?

▶ Which equipment will be most efficient and yet be cost effective?

▶ How can I create an attractive, comfortable office for patients and staff and maintain an efficient traffic flow?

▶ How can I stay within a budget?

▶ How often will it be necessary to redecorate?

There is no *right* answer to all of these questions. The design of an office depends on the personality and practice philosophy of the doctor or doctors, the number of patients, the number and type of staff members, the amount of available capital, and the type of practice. There are some basic concepts that should be considered by the dental staff in designing an office that is to be used for the practice of four-handed dentistry.

First, traffic patterns should be given primary consideration in the office design. Unnecessary movements create confusion, inefficiency, and tension, as well as increase the potential for cross-contamination. Proper traffic flow eliminates unnecessary activity. Second, flexibility should be built into the office. Modular units

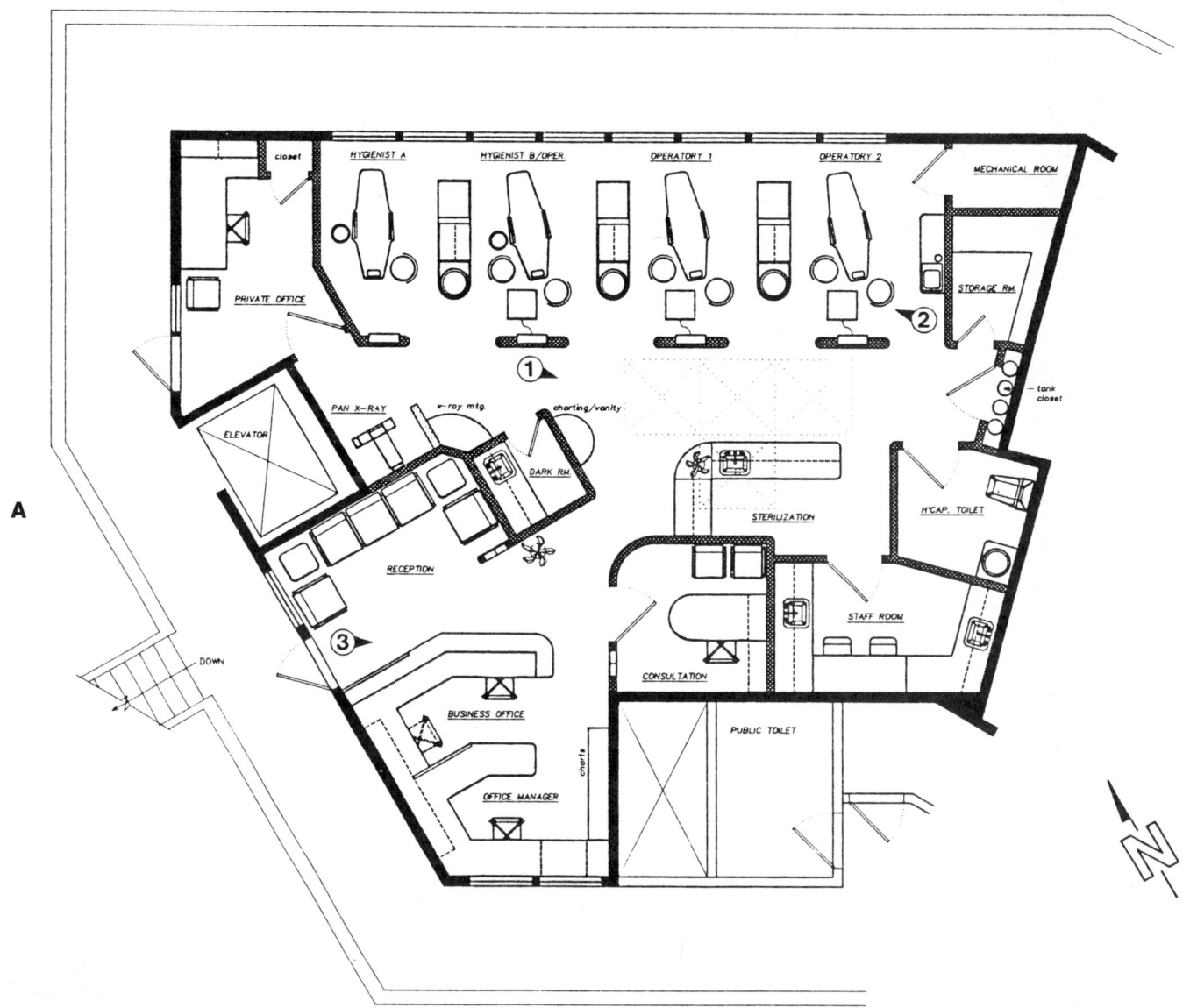

FIG. 16-1   *A,* An irregular-shaped dental suite that uses the concept of openness. The isolating impact of doors between the clinical and business areas has been removed, yet privacy and separation of these areas is provided for patients by the use of modular dividers.

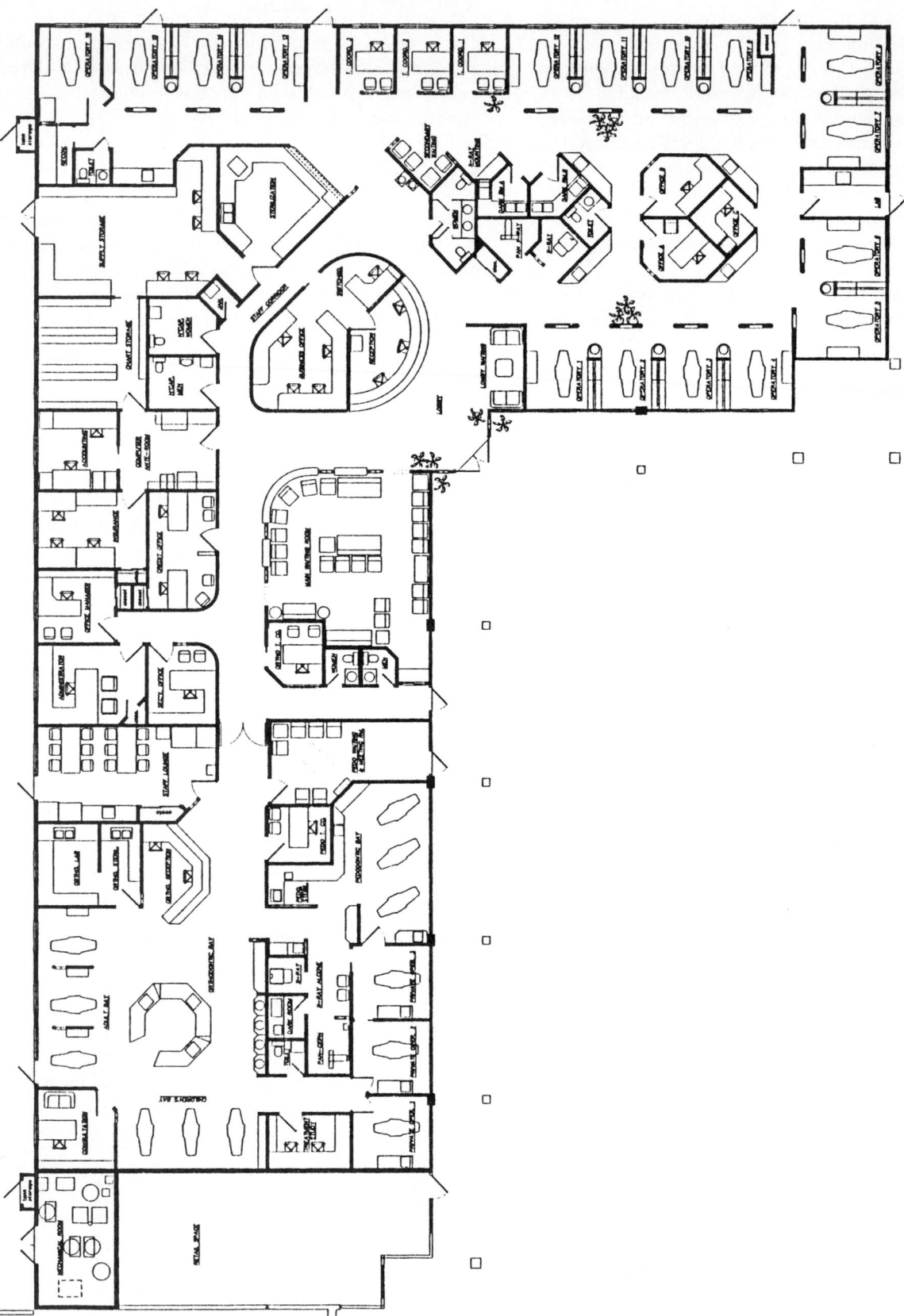

FIG. 16-1, cont'd. *B*, A large group of dental practitioners use this spacious office for patient and staff comfort. The office suite includes an open concept and multireception areas; it also provides patient privacy.

(*A* and *B* courtesy of Design for Health, Mitchell Goldstein, Santa Cruz, Calif.)

Continued.

that are designed for flexibility and for future growth are available, especially in business systems.

In many new buildings, efforts have been made to provide walls that can be moved, again allowing for flexibility as the practice grows and changes. Third, comfort for the patient and staff must be a priority. Comfort helps to eliminate patients' fears and to reduce staff tension. Openness in the environment is a relatively easy way to create a more relaxed atmosphere. It may be necessary to eliminate walls, create curves in the design, add different lighting or skylights, or include dimensional effects in wall coverings.

It could be said that there are as many floor plans as there are dentists, and yet in all of these floor plans there would be some basic similarities. Fig. 16-1, A through C, shows examples of several floor plans; each provides a different style and yet functions effectively for the dentist for whom it was designed. Today, much emphasis is placed on openness, specifically, the elimination of doorways and walls—a concept that provides a nonrestrained feeling for the patient and staff.

The Dental Suite

The dental suite is a composite of many rooms, offices, and hallways; each has a specific purpose, and yet all interrelate to provide an efficient, comfortable working environment.

▶ Reception Room

The reception room (Fig. 16-2, A through C) is the first room the patient enters; it creates the initial impression of the office. This room must be pleasant, be free of clutter, and provide comfortable furnishings. The room should be furnished with seating that is comfortable for a variety of patients and yet be able to accommodate various numbers of patients. Observe the reception area frequently to straighten magazines and remove debris. This room should be fresh and odor free. If windows cannot be opened, a ventilation system can be installed to move air through the dental suite. A suitable exhaust system should also be in place to dispose of fumes that are created by some dental materials. It is important that the decor in this room, as well as the others, receive periodic attention. A dentist doesn't spend time in the reception room; therefore, it becomes the responsibility of the entire dental staff to be attentive to the appearance of the reception room. Decor changes frequently, and routine redecorating should be considered for this room every 4 to 5 years to keep its style fresh and current.

c

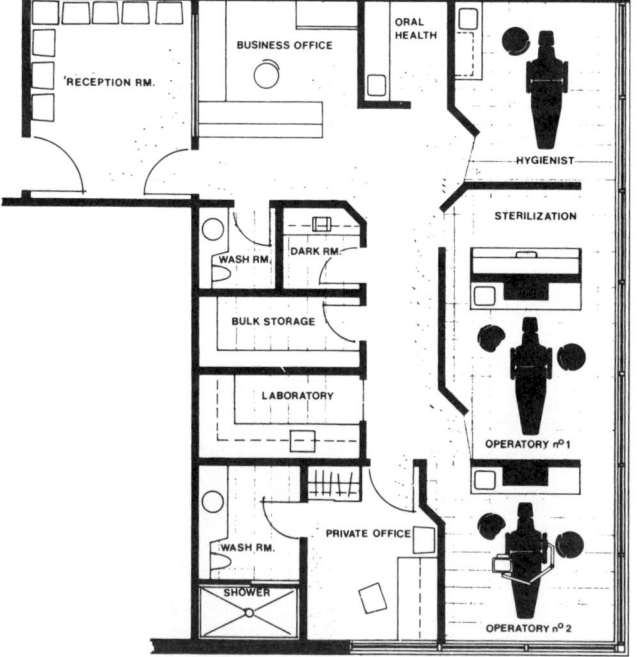

FIG. 16-1, cont'd.   C, A small office designed for efficiency and patient comfort includes all basic rooms and yet provides openness.

(C courtesy of Health Science Products, Birmingham Ala.)

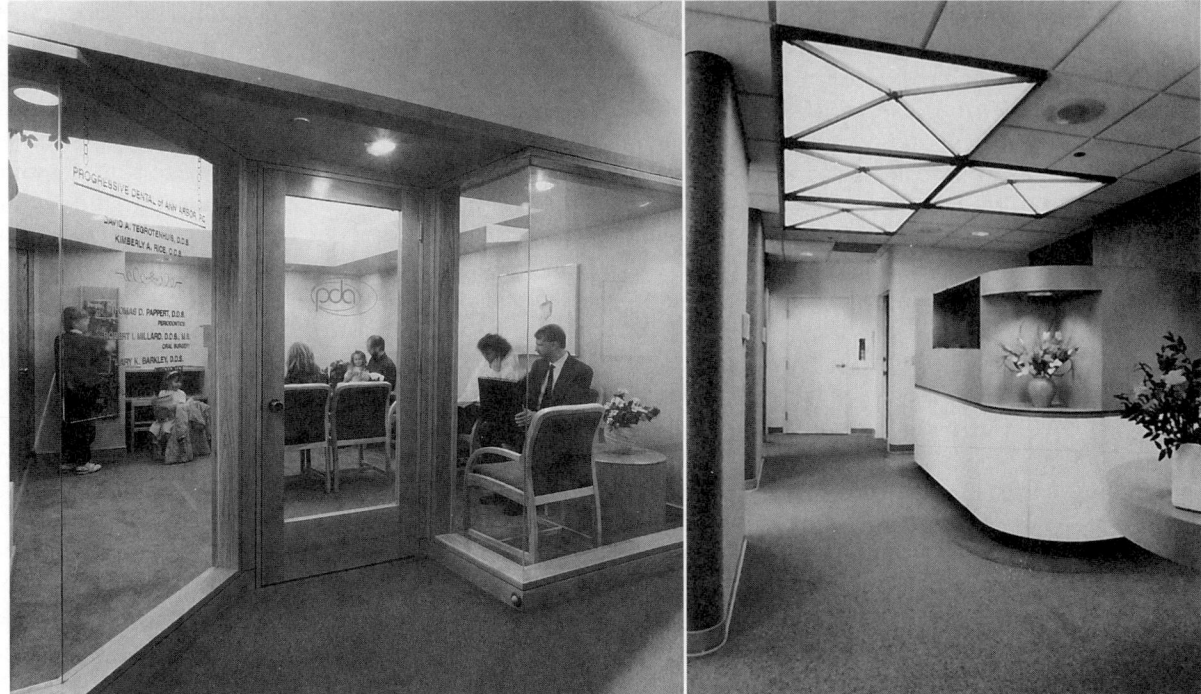

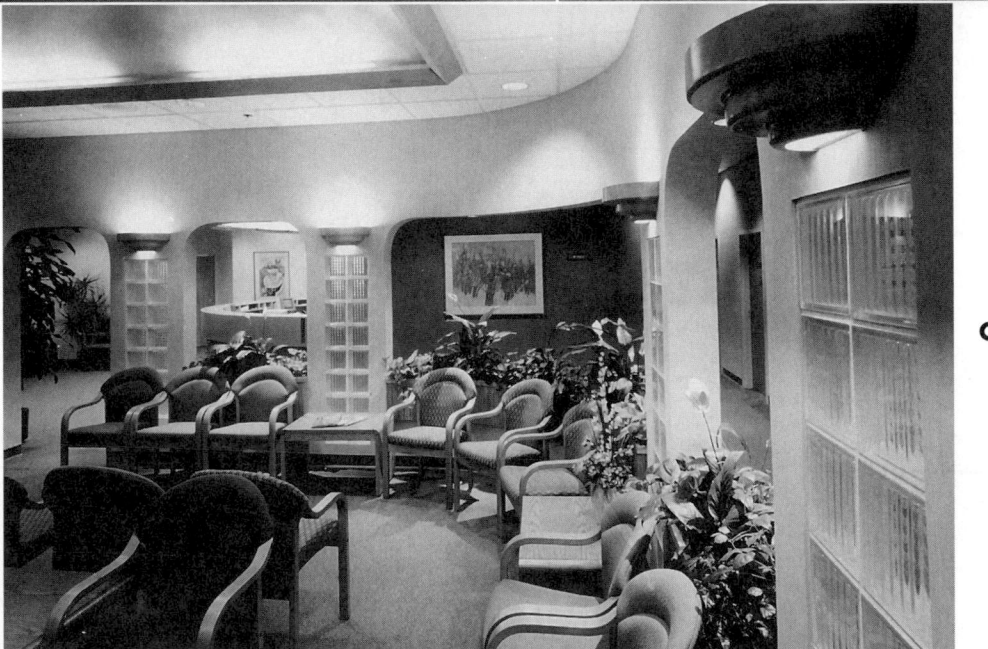

FIG. 16-2   *A,* Reception room within a professional building provides openness, adequate seating, children's play area, and appropriate signage on the hallway door. *B,* Hallways should be well lighted, wide enough for wheelchair access and yet maintain comfortable design lines. *C,* A larger practice may need more seating for patients. Lines used in architectural design emit a soft, open feeling to patients.

(*A* courtesy of Kimberly Rice, D.D.S., Ann Arbor, Mich., Progressive Dental of Ann Arbor; *B* and *C* courtesy of Designs for Health, Mitchell Goldstein, Santa Cruz, Calif.)

▶ Business Office

Adjacent to the reception room is the hub of the office, the **business office** (Fig. 16-3), where all business activities occur and where records are maintained. The business assistant should be able to greet patients as they enter the office and yet easily return to work at an area free from interruptions by patients in the reception area. Adjacent to, or within, the business office an area should be available for personal conversations with patients or for private telephone business.

All patient records are maintained in the business office. Therefore, one or more computer terminals are housed in this area for use in word processing and records management, as well as several filing cabinets for storage of hard copies of patient records. The patient should pass through the business office on arriving and again on leaving. This allows the office manager to update patient information, clarify financial arrangements, and make future appointments for the patient. A counter about 44 inches high and 12 to 15 inches wide provides the patient with an area on which to write (Fig. 16-4) and desk privacy is still maintained for the assistant.

▶ Dental Laboratory

Generally, a small **dental laboratory** is part of the suite. This room houses equipment that is used for extraoral work, such as finishing a crown or bridge, adjusting a denture, pouring impressions, trimming models, or making custom acrylic trays within the office. Many doctors send detailed laboratory work to a commercial laboratory; however, a laboratory within the dental office is always needed. A doctor may include a large laboratory in the office and hire one or more laboratory technicians. Obviously the caseload of the office would need to justify such a space allocation. In any situation the laboratory should have a good exhaust system, with adequate ventilation for the variety of dental materials that may be used in this area. Some offices combine this area with the sterilization area. In other facilities the laboratory may be a separate room.

▶ Sterilization Area

The *sterilization area* (Fig. 16-5, *A* through *C*) is vital in any dental office today. This area should be located near the dental treatment rooms, and should be well ventilated. Equipment found in the sterilization area is discussed in Chapter 8.

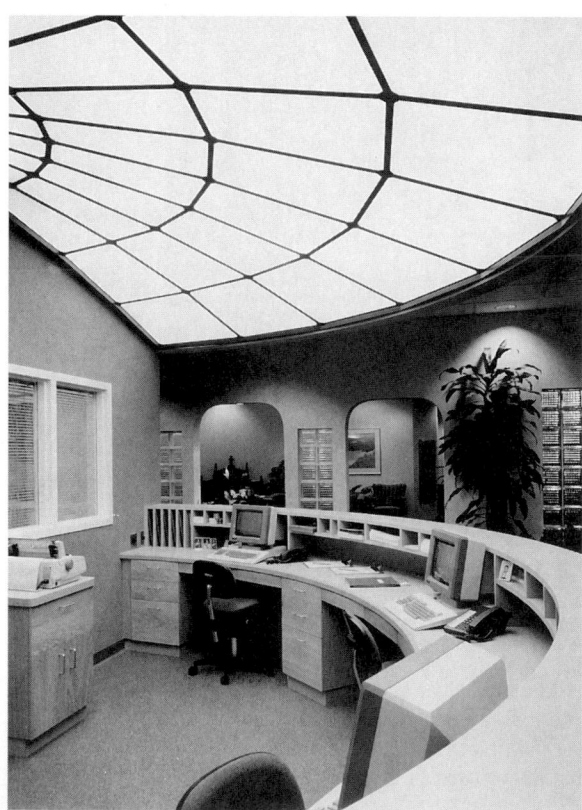

FIG. 16-3   The business office adjacent to the reception room provides adequate desk space, lighting, filing area, comfortable seating and direct access to computer and telecommunication systems.

(Courtesy of Designs for Health, Mitchell Goldstein, Santa Cruz, Calif.)

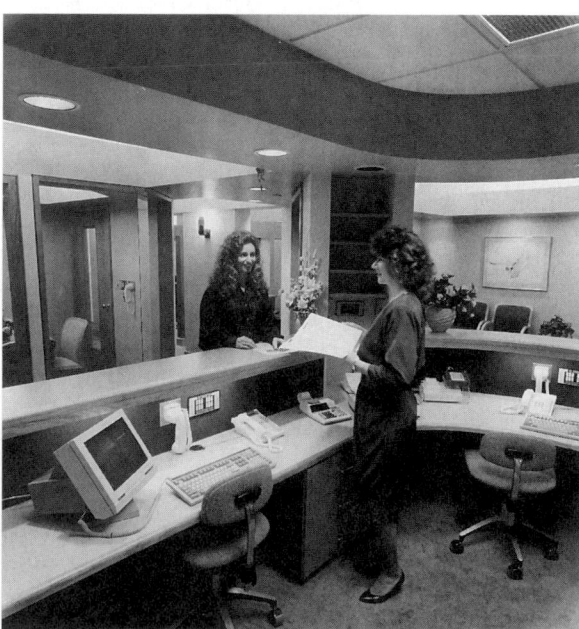

FIG. 16-4   Counter space in the business offices provides a patient with a comfortable position for business transactions.

(Courtesy of Kimberly Rice, D.D.S., Ann Arbor, Mich.)

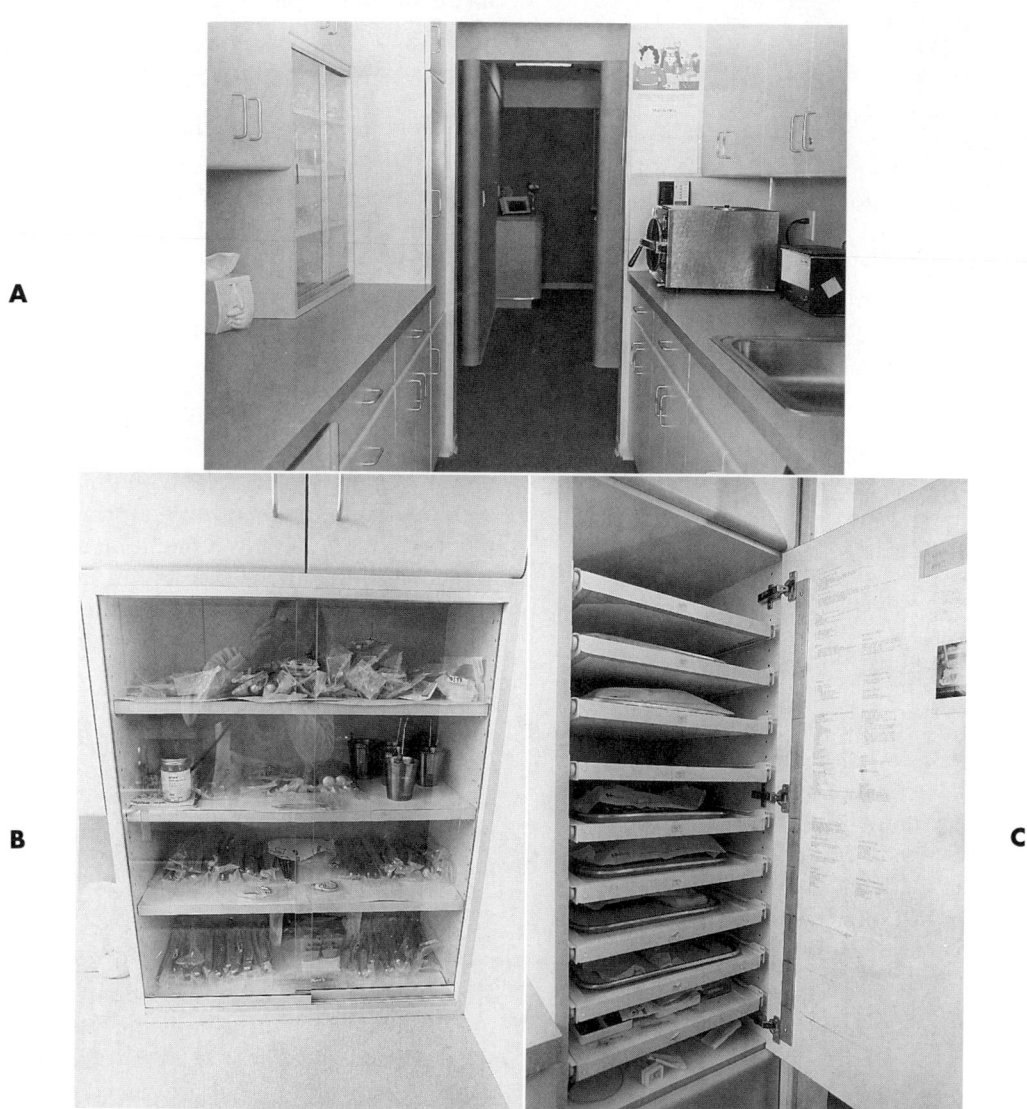

FIG. 16-5   *A,* Sterilization area within a dental suite. *B* and *C,* Sterilization storage areas. (Courtesy of Helen Zylman, D.D.S., Ann Arbor Mich.)

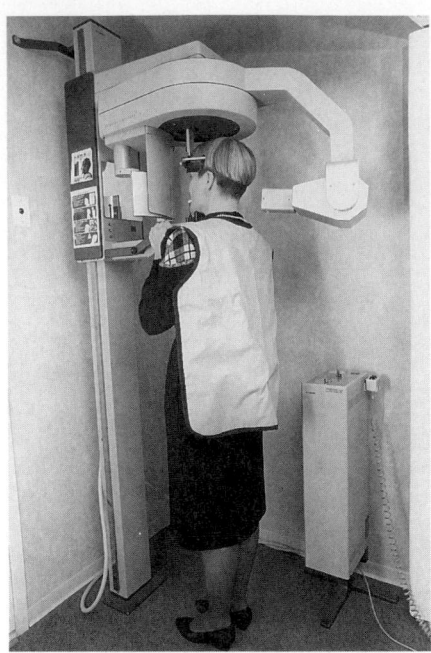

FIG. 16-6   Panoramic radiography unit within a dental office. (Courtesy of Helen Zylman, D.D.S., Ann Arbor, Mich.)

Radiography Rooms

Radiography rooms are specifically designed for exposing dental radiographs. In some offices, radiographic equipment for intraoral exposures is within the treatment room. However, larger units (Fig. 16-6) for panoramic radiography require separate rooms. Regardless of the type of room, specific guidelines are established by the state department of health for equipment location, lead lining, and other protective features.

Radiography Processing Area/ Darkroom

A *radiography processing area/darkroom* is included in most offices for developing dental radiographs. With the use of automatic processors in many offices, this room has taken on a new look. It may be part of the laboratory, treatment room, sterilization area, or it may be a designated area for processing and mounting, if a darkroom is not required. However, if the traditional processing tanks are used, it will be necessary to have a small darkroom. Regardless of which type of processing is done in the office, it will be necessary to have an area set aside for mounting radiographs. This could be a small counter area with film viewers available.

Doctor's Private Office

The look of the doctor's private office varies from doctor to doctor. It may be an elaborately furnished room or it may be furnished more conservatively. This room is generally intended for private study and consultation. In some instances this office is used by staff for private conversations with patients regarding financial arrangements or other confidential discussions.

Insurance Room/ Area

An insurance room/area has become a popular room, since the person responsible for claim forms needs privacy to complete the forms and to carry on private conversations on the telephone. This room is generally one of the sites for a computer terminal.

Patient Education/ Oral Hygiene Area

A patient education/oral hygiene area is common in many offices. It may take on a different look, depending on the type of office. For instance, in an orthodontic office it may be in an open area with mirrors where young patients can be easily observed practicing oral hygiene. In a periodontic office, it might be a private area where adults can have more privacy. In any situation, it will generally include visual aids and an area for demonstration of oral hygiene procedures.

Recovery rooms are sometimes required in an oral surgery office for patients to recover following general anesthesia. These rooms are minimal in size and furnishings, since they are not used for long periods of time. Some surgeons opt to have the patient remain in the treatment room, where instruments, materials, and monitoring devices are more accessible.

Other Rooms

Storage rooms are desirable, but not all offices can afford the space for this. Care should be taken when allocating space for storage that it is a dry, cool area that will not damage the supplies that are stored there. Sometimes a small refrigerator is placed in this room or the staff lounge to provide storage for dental materials that require a cool environment.

A *rest room* for patients should be provided that is easily accessed from the reception room. It is wise to avoid having a rest room for patients in the inner office, thereby eliminating undue traffic. The rest room should be maintained regularly. A separate rest room for the office staff is advisable.

A *staff lounge* is sometimes considered a luxury, while in other areas it is a necessity if no eating facilities are nearby. Eating and drinking should be confined to the lounge area out of view of patients and away from areas of possible patient contamination. Frequently the staff will gather in the laboratory or sterilization area to eat and talk. This is not an acceptable area because of the potential for patient contamination. A lounge provides a place for the staff to go for a break when time permits. This area should be kept clean and neat, and care should be taken not to make it a salvage area for old equipment and out-of-date materials.

The Dental Treatment Room

The dental treatment room or operatory is where all of the clinical activity takes place. Before four-handed dentistry can be practiced, the function of the dental treatment room, which type of equipment is appropriate, and the reasons for placing equipment in specific locations must first be understood. Two major types of treatment rooms exist: one is used primarily for dental

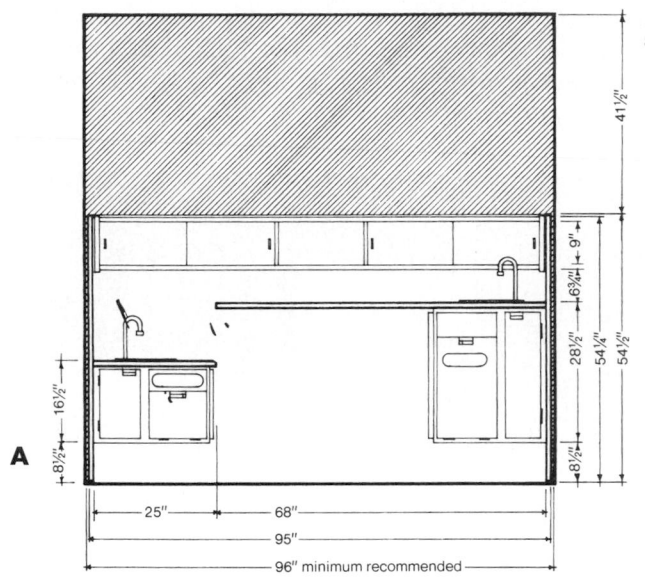

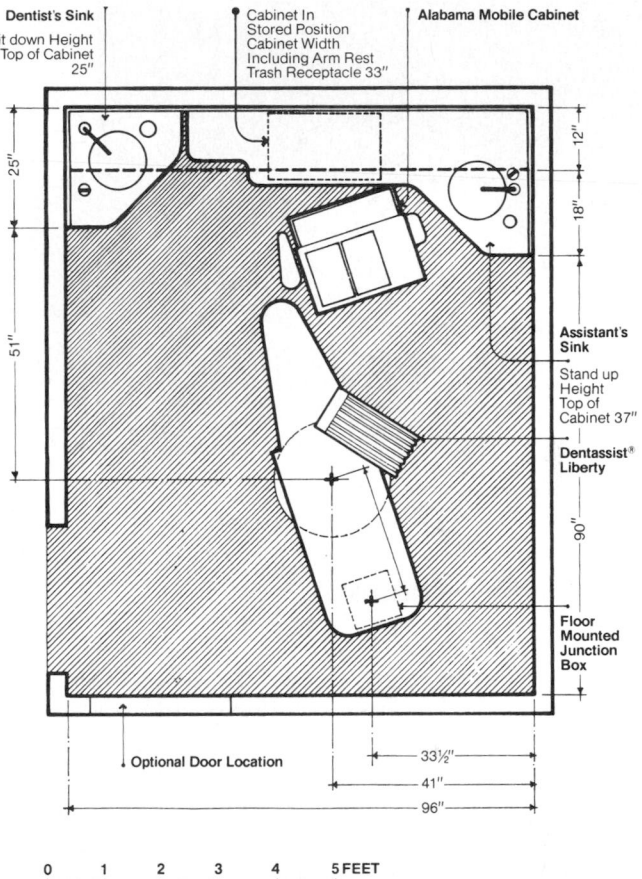

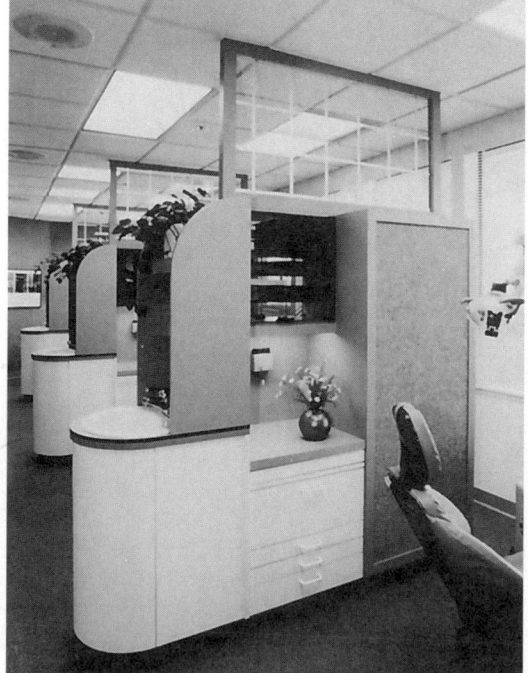

FIG. 16-7 *A*, Treatment room arranged for use in four-handed dentistry concepts. The room includes a dental chair, two sinks with fixed cabinetry, transthorax dental unit, two operating stools, mobile cabinet, and operating light (not shown). *B*, Room dividers can separate rooms to provide function and privacy.

(*A* courtesy of Health Science Products, Birmingham, Ala; *B* courtesy of Designs for Health, Mitchell Goldstein, Santa Cruz, Calif.)

hygiene and the other is where all other patient care takes place. Many variations of these rooms exist, depending on the number of auxiliaries and dentists on staff and whether employment is full-time or part-time. Typically the treatment room should not be smaller than 8 feet × 10 feet (Fig. 16-7, *A*). The room may be designed as a separate unit or in a bay concept, as shown in Fig. 16-7, *B*. This size permits for convenient placement of all equipment and provides for adequate walk-around space.

Any smaller room creates congestion, and too large an area obviously is wasteful. When possible, two room entrances can help create an efficient traffic floor plan for patients and staff. To simplify procedures, all rooms used for hygiene or operative treatment should be arranged and equipped identically. Other rooms in the dental suite may be carpeted, but the dental treatment room and the sterilization areas should not be carpeted because of potential contaminant hazard.

The two basic types of treatment room arrangements today are rear delivery and side delivery (Fig. 16-8, *A* through *C*). Emphasis in the following discussion will be on the selection and placement of equipment for use in a treatment room that is designed for four-handed dentistry.

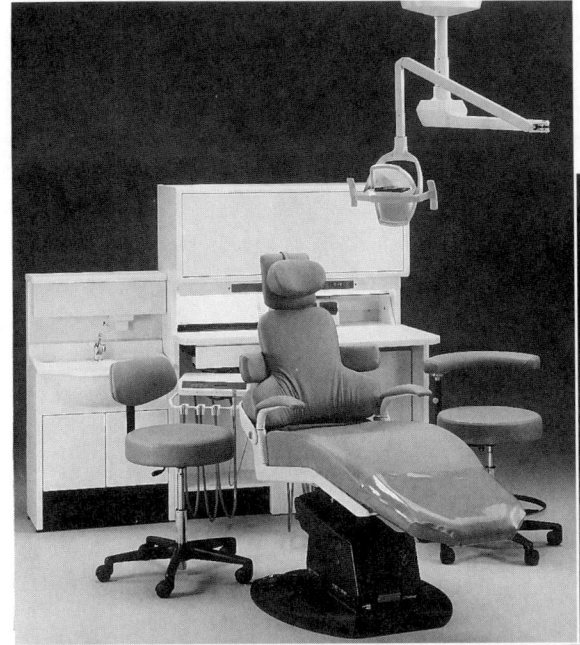

A

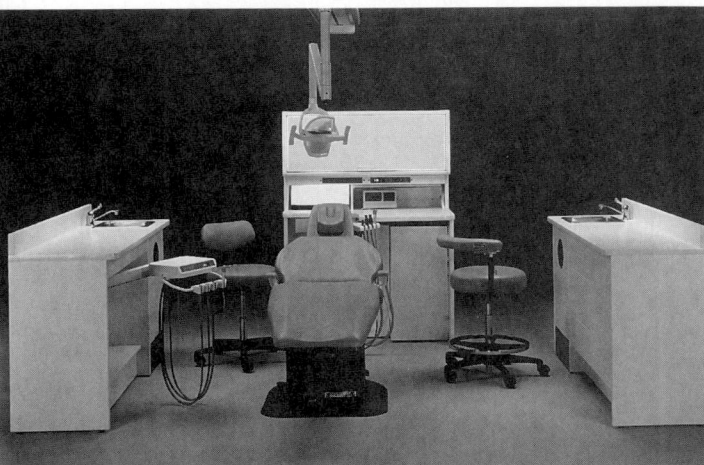

B

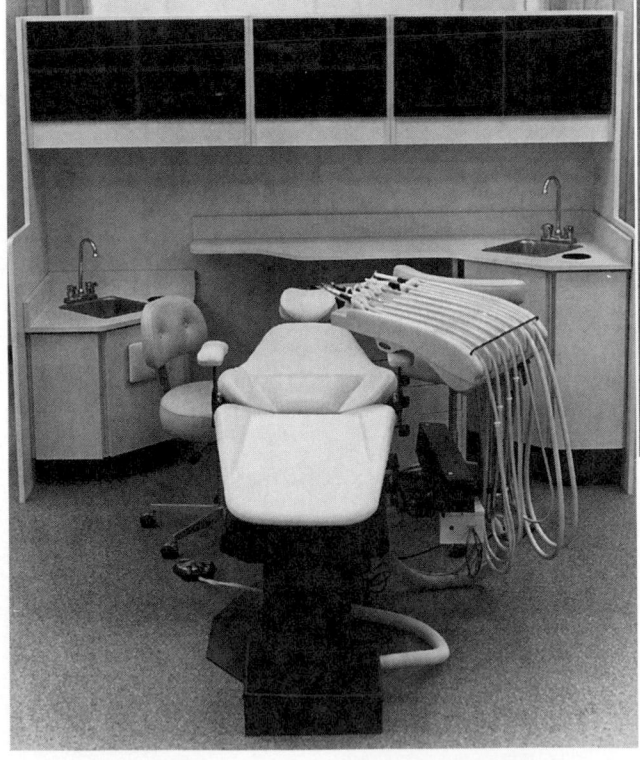

C

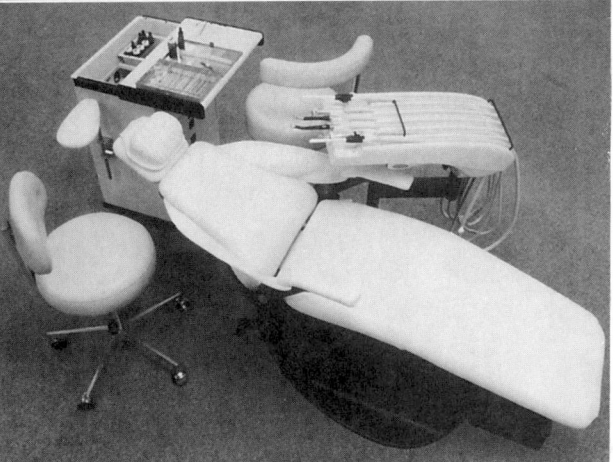

D

FIG. 16-8　*A*, A rear-delivery system places the unit behind the patient chair. *B*, A combination of side / rear delivery shows handpieces on the operator's side and air / water and HVE hoses at the rear of the chair. *C*, This treatment room is arranged for a right-handed operator using a transthorax unit along the side of the dental chair (front view). *D*, A superior view of the transthroax unit in place.

(*A* and *B* courtesy of Pelton Crane; *C* and *D* courtesy of Health Science Products [HSP].)

Basic Dental Equipment

Early dental equipment was designed for a standup method of dental care delivery. Originally the dentist stood at chairside and most of the time practiced alone, reaching for instruments from a bracket table and for handpieces and water syringes from an extension on a dental unit (Fig. 16-9). When use of an assistant at chairside came into existence, the assistant was also in a standing position (Fig. 16-10). The equipment still came out of the unit, which caused the assistant to have to turn the entire body to reach for handpieces. The instruments remained on the **bracket table**, a small glass or metal tray that extends off the arm of the dental unit, also making it necessary for the assistant to reach. The first major changes came when both the assistant and doctor were seated; however, the equipment design still caused undue stress and strain on both parties. Over the last 30 to 40 years, major design changes have occurred. Today the operator and assistant can be seated comfortably in balanced posture, with the patient in supine position and the equipment and materials easily accessible to the assistant, as shown in Fig. 16-11. With the use of mobile cabinetry and specially designed dental units, instruments such as the handpieces, a/w syringe, and high-velocity evacuation (HVE) hoses are at the assistant's fingertips, allowing the operator to maintain focus on the field of operation and to reduce reaching and straining.

Regardless of the brand of equipment chosen, the selection and placement of dental equipment should follow these general guidelines:

- Position equipment for the patient's easy access to the dental chair.
- Provide comfortable seating for patient, operator, and assistant.
- Eliminate the need for the operating team to twist, turn, or reach.

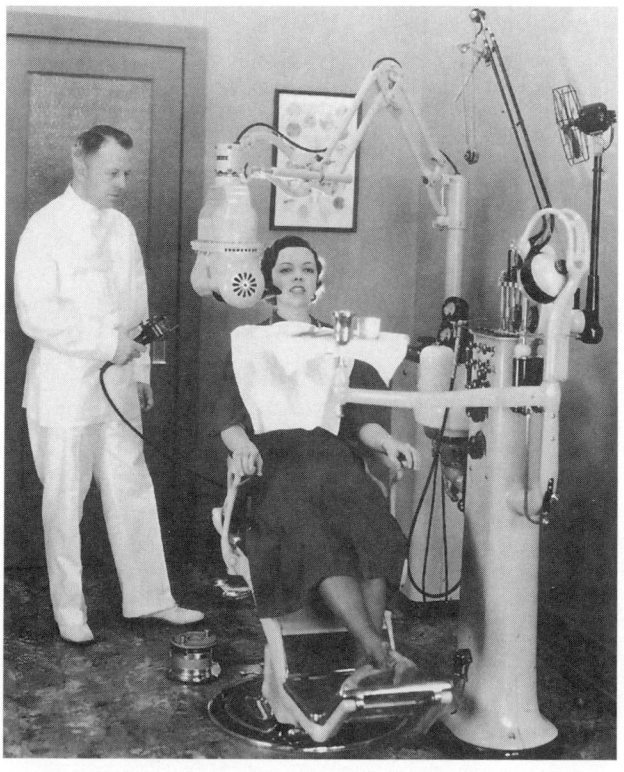

FIG. 16-9 A dentist working alone without an assistant.

(From Ring ME: *Dentistry: an illustrated history,* St Louis, 1985, Mosby.)

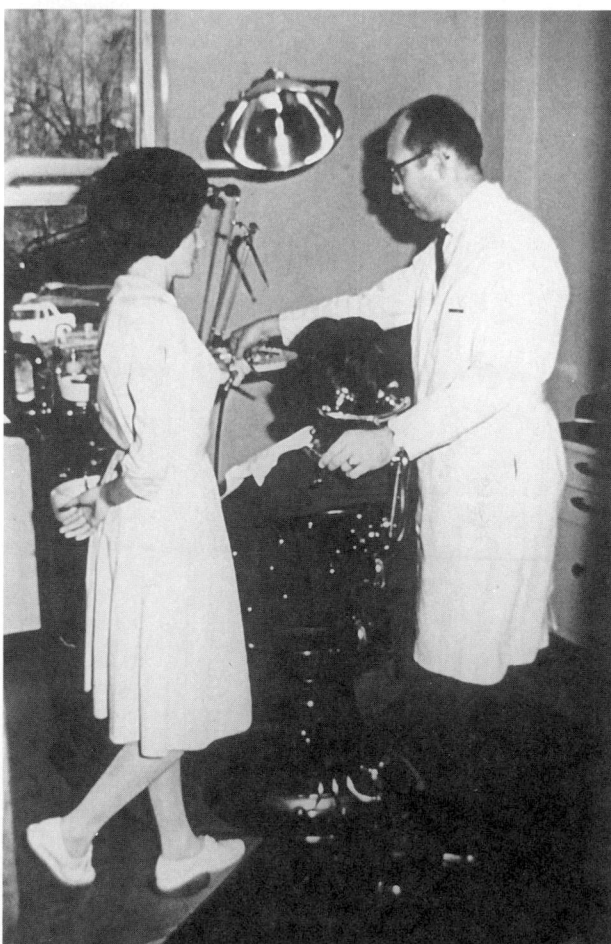

FIG. 16-10 A dental assistant standing at chairside.

(Courtesy of University of Alabama, School of Dentistry, Birmingham, Ala.)

▶ Use aseptic-style hoses that eliminate tension and pullback.

▶ Eliminate the need for the doctor's eyes and hands to leave the site of operation.

▶ Position handpieces so that the assistant can easily pass them to the operator.

▶ Eliminate tubing that touches the patient.

▶ Transfer instruments only within the transfer zone.

▶ Provide for easy use of the HVE hose and a/w syringe simultaneously.

The basic equipment (Fig. 16-12) for four-handed dentistry includes the dental chair, the dental unit, the foot control, the dental light, the assistant's stool, the operator's stool, the assistant's sink, the operator's sink, the mobile cabinetry, and the fixed cabinetry. Specific criteria for this equipment and its components are listed in Box 16-1.

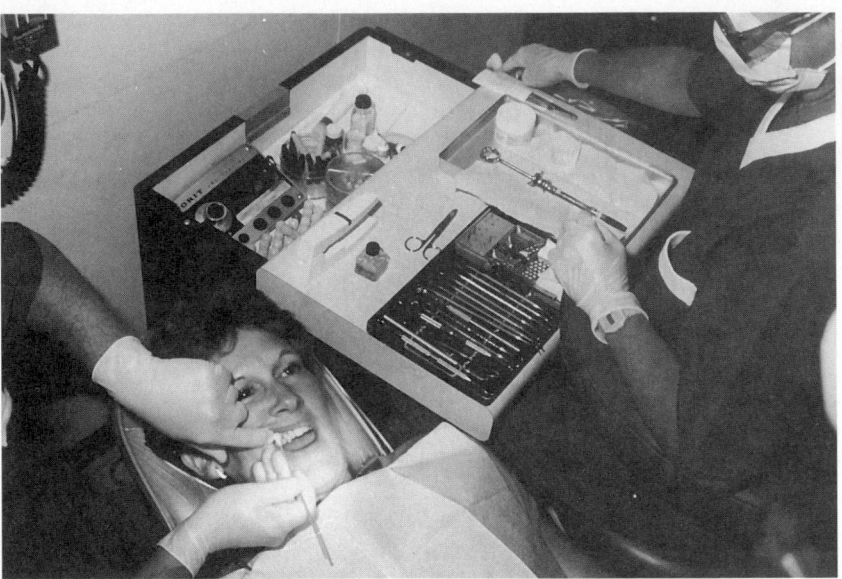

FIG. 16-11 Four-handed dentistry being practiced using modern equipment.

FIG. 16-12 A treatment room furnished with basic equipment.

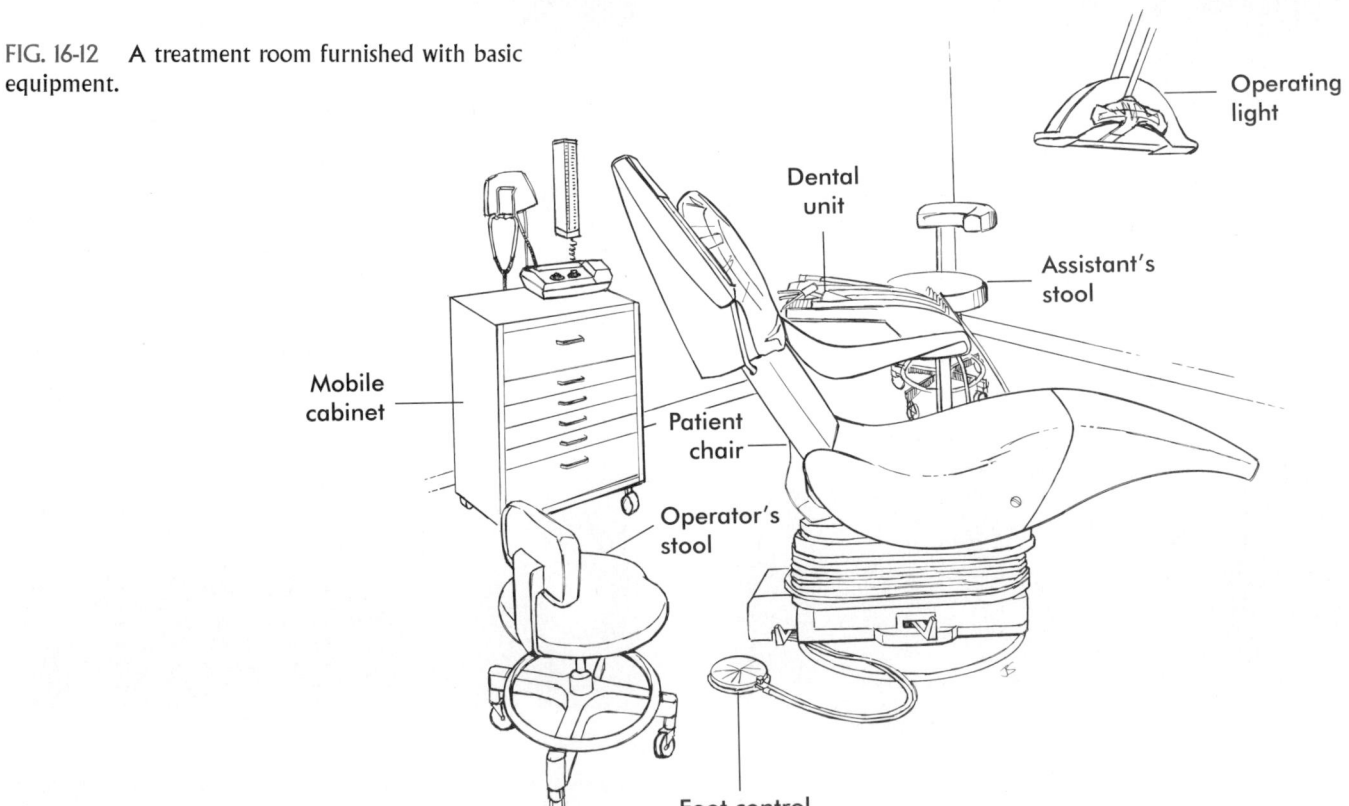

CRITERIA FOR EQUIPMENT USED IN FOUR-HANDED DENTISTRY

PATIENT CHAIR

Thin, narrow back
Adequate body and arm support
Adjustment buttons on both sides
Able to be placed into supine position
Free of protrusive devices on back
Easily cleanable (not fabric)
Aseptic control option

DENTAL UNIT

Adjusts vertically
Independent of chair movement
Hosing is smooth and easily retractable
Able to withstand rigorous daily use with minimal repairs
Accessible to right- or left-handed operator

HVE SYSTEM

Hoses are lightweight, smooth, and flexible
On/off button is easily controlled with one hand
Waste empties directly into the sewer system
Trap for separation of solid materials is available
Adaptable for saliva ejector use

AIR/WATER SYRINGE

Lightweight
Easily operated
Provides air, water, and aerated spray separately
Provides graduated air and water flow
Tip is easily rotated and angled
Autoclavable tips are easily removed and replaced
Able to accept disposables or protective tip covers

HIGH-SPEED HANDPIECES

Easy to use
Hoses are smooth and flexible
Provides a range of speeds
Locking mechanism for hoses
Removable for sterilization
Two handpieces are desirable

SLOW-SPEED HANDPIECES

Easy to use
Hose is smooth and flexible
Provides a range of speeds
Locking mechanism for hose
Removable for sterilization
Accepts a variety of attachments

CURING LIGHT

Easy to use
Hose is smooth and flexible

FOOT CONTROL

Easily activated with foot pressure
Accessible to right- or left-handed operator
Chip blower option

DENTAL STOOLS

Broad stable base, with four or five casters
Flat or contoured well-padded seat
Seat is easily adjustable
Back and abdominal support adjusts vertically and horizontally

OPERATING LIGHT

May be mounted on ceiling, wall, or chair
Easily adjustable by operator or assistant
Easy to maintain
Adjustable intensity

ROOM LIGHT

Diffused
Includes natural daylight

MOBILE CABINETRY

Unit is easily moved and stable
Provides easy access to instruments and materials
Adequate work surface
Movable work surface that can be positioned over the assistant's lap
Provides adequate storage space

FIXED CABINETS

Wall cabinets located for maximum floor space and easy cleaning
Allows minimal storage

SINKS

Two sinks
Knee, foot, or automatic controls for liquid soap dispensers
Faucets are motion controlled or operable without the use of hands
Eyewash connected to a sink near treatment area

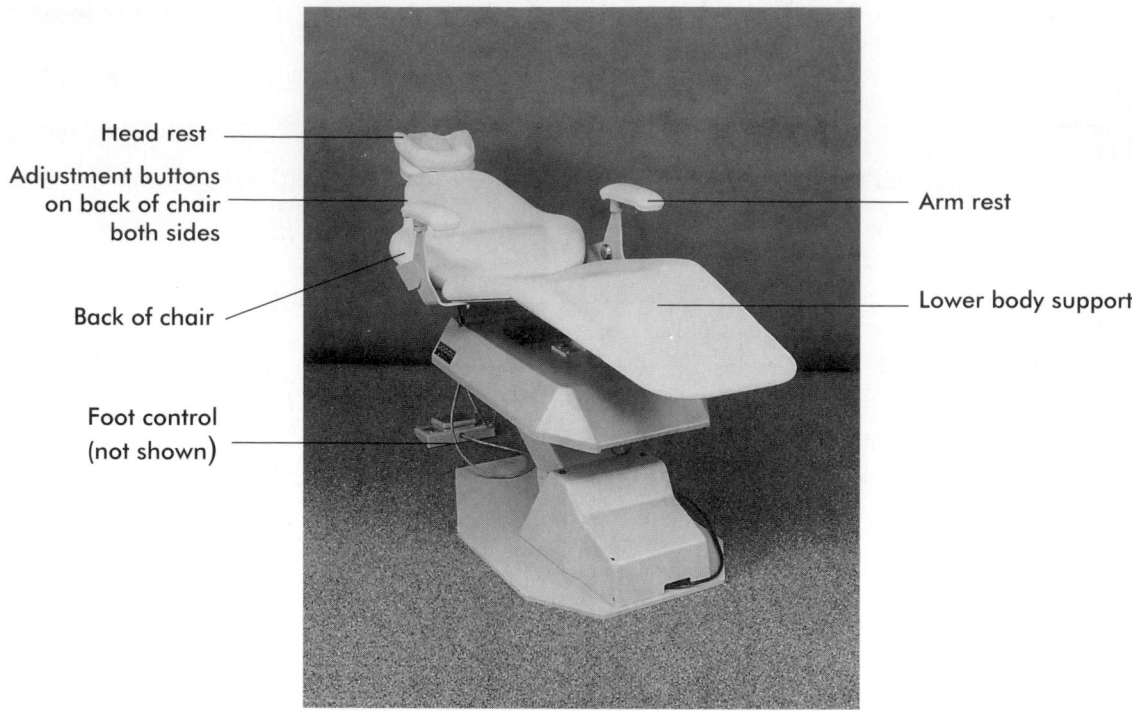

Head rest

Adjustment buttons
on back of chair
both sides

Back of chair

Foot control
(not shown)

Arm rest

Lower body support

FIG. 16-13   Patient chair with various parts identified.
(Courtesy of Health Science Products.)

▶ Dental Chair

The **patient chair** (Fig. 16-13) supports the patient and is the site around which all clinical activity takes place. The chair should have a thin, narrow back and provide complete body and arm support for the patient when it is placed in supine (patient is lying on the back) position. Separate controls for elevation, tilting of the seat, and lowering of the backrest should be available for both the operator and the assistant. The chair in Fig. 16-14 is an example of an aseptic chair. Only one button needs to be pressed, and the patient is automatically placed into the supine position, thus eliminating various adjustments to the chair. This adjustment button may be on the side of the chair back or on a foot control on the floor. In addition, the chair should also provide for rotation. The upholstery on the chair should be easily cleanable and made of a nonporous material according to the Occupational Safety and Health Administration (OSHA) standards.

Chair placement is primary to the location of other equipment in the room. As previously shown in Fig. 16-7, *A*, the chair has been placed diagonally so that when the patient is placed in the supine position, the head of the chair will be about 36 inches from the corner wall. This position allows adequate space for the assistant's stool and cabinetry and provides barrier-free access to the chair.

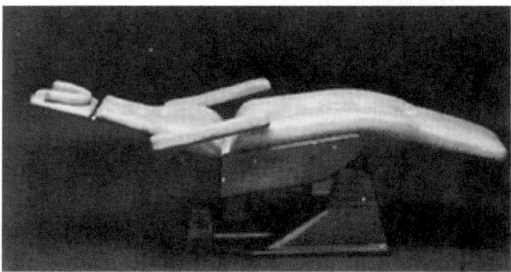

FIG. 16-14   An aseptic chair. The ultimate dental chair achieves new levels of engineering excellence, yet it is economically affordable. It provides the ultimate in function, quality, patient comfort and offers ideal direct vision for the doctor and assistant. The chair is fully automatic with all-steel construction, ergonomic design, premium upholstery and offers a dual four-way foot control for disease control.

(Courtesy of Health Science Products.)

▶ Dental Unit

The **dental unit** is the workhorse of the dental treatment room and must be durable enough to withstand rigorous daily use with minimal repairs. The dental unit houses all of the dynamic instruments that the dentist uses during most operative procedures. The dental unit should adjust vertically and yet be independent of the vertical movement of the chair. Energy to the dental unit comes from electricity and from an air compressor that is stored outside the treatment rooms, often in a central mechanical area in the building. The hosing for the handpieces should be smooth and should provide easy extension to any distance, along with an easy return to the permanent position on the unit. Each dental unit may house different equipment according to the needs of the dentist. Fig. 16-15 represents components that are typically found on many dental units.

The dental unit is located on the left side of the chair for a right-handed operator and on the opposite side for a left-handed operator, as in Fig. 16-16, *A* and *B*. The unit should not occupy space that is needed by the assistant nor should it interfere with the patient's access to the chair. The unit is located so that all instruments from the unit are within the transfer zone: close to the patient's mouth, but placed so that it will not interfere with instrument passing.

On the right side of the photo in Fig. 16-15 are the first two devices: the **high-velocity evacuation (HVE)** hoses. One is used by the assistant for high-speed evacuation of fluids from the patient's mouth. The second can serve as a backup if the other hose is dropped, or, with an attachment as shown in Fig. 16-17, it can serve as a saliva ejector to be placed in the patient's mouth for slow removal of fluids. Text in Chapter 21 will describe the proper placement and use of these devices in the mouth. Criteria for an efficient HVE system requires that the hoses be lightweight and flexible and not collapse when used, as well as have smooth surfaces for easy cleaning and disinfection. The design of the on/off button should allow the assistant to turn the unit on and off with one hand. Wastes from the HVE system drain directly into the sewer system. A trap for the separation of solid materials, such as amalgam or cement pieces, should be in the operatory and should include an infection control filter.

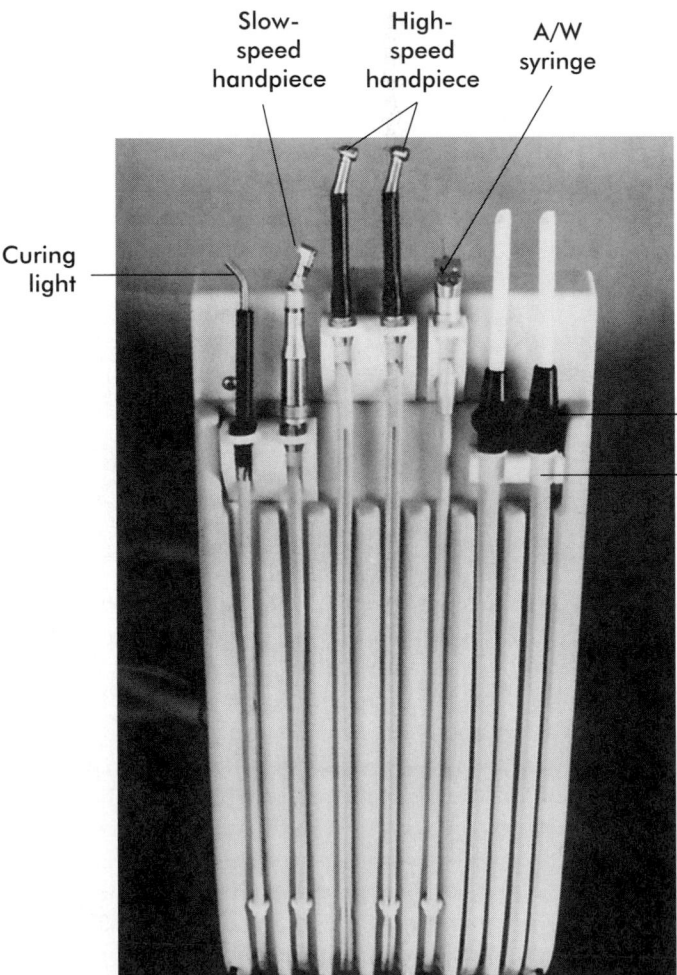

FIG. 16-15 **Dental unit with various components identified.** (Courtesy of Health Science Products.)

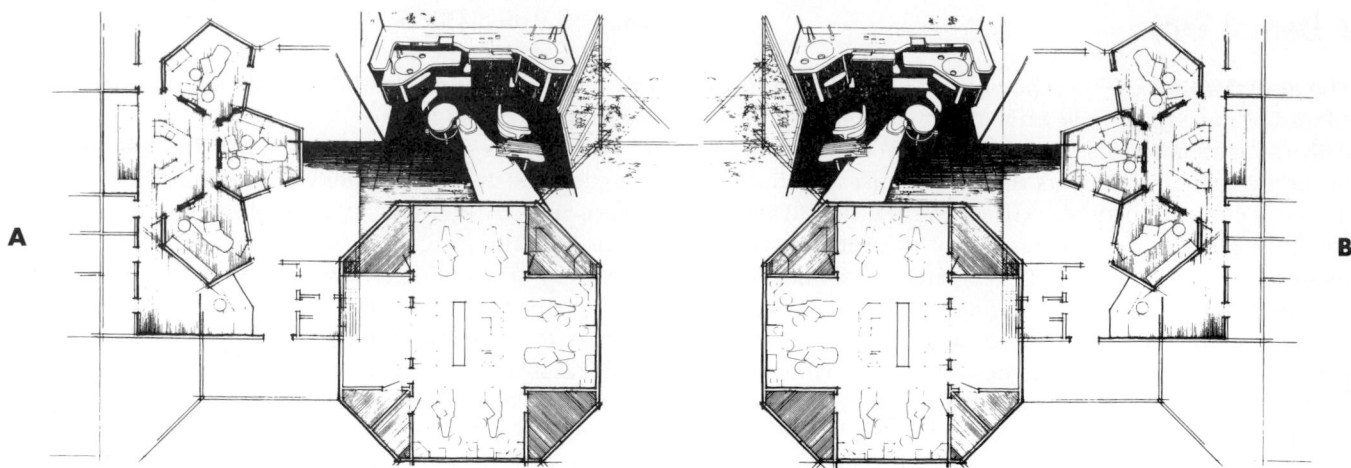

FIG. 16-16   A, Arrangement of a dental suite for (a) right-handed dentist and (b) left-handed dentist.

(Courtesy of Health Science Products.)

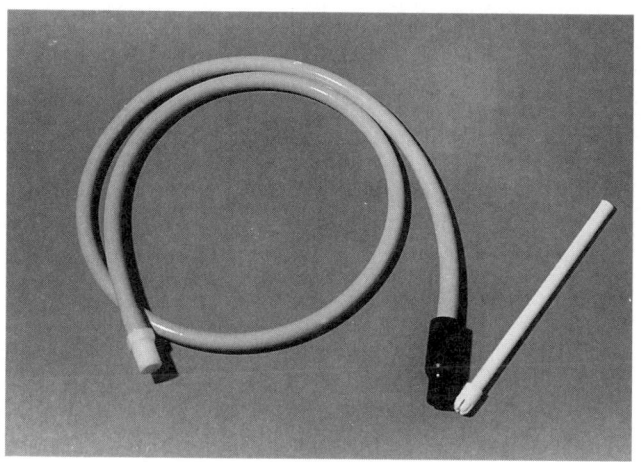

FIG. 16-17   Saliva ejector hose.

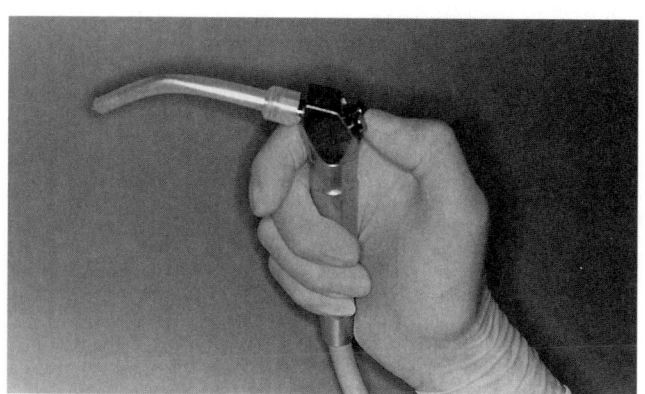

FIG. 16-18   Air/water syringe.

Air/Water Syringe

The next instrument on this unit is the **air/water syringe** (triplex syringe). This device provides three functions: air spray, water spray, and aerated spray (a combination of air and water). The a/w syringe should be lightweight and easily operated (Fig. 16-18), provide for graduated air and water flow, and provide an autoclavable tip that is easily removed and replaced. The tip should be angled and easily rotated in the barrel of the syringe.

High-Speed Handpieces

A high-speed **handpiece** provides the operator ultra speed at 250,000 rpm or above to easily prepare a tooth to specific shapes to receive a restoration. With two handpieces on the unit the dental assistant is able to prepare the dental burs (small cutting devices attached to the head of the handpiece) in advance to eliminate delays in the procedure for bur changes. The second handpiece also ensures a backup in case the first handpiece needs repair. Style and options for these handpieces vary greatly and are discussed in detail in Chapter 19. Basic criteria, however, require that these handpieces be flexible, easy for the operator to use, and easily removed for sterilization procedures.

Slow-Speed Handpieces

The **slow-speed handpiece** is used when slower speeds are needed, as in the removal of carious tooth structure or for polishing teeth during an oral prophylaxis. Special attachments and dental burs can be attached to this handpiece. A handpiece should provide a range of speeds and be sterilizable. An adequate number of slow-speed handpieces should be available to avoid delays in a procedure.

Curing Light

The **curing light** uses ultraviolet or another light source to activate and cure dental materials. Although this light is conveniently placed on the unit, it is not uncommon to find the light as an independent piece of equipment that is brought to the treatment area when needed. The use of the curing light is described in greater detail in Chapter 28.

The unit that has just been described includes the traditional devices found on most dental units today. Other options are available for a unit, including ultrasonic scalers, electrosurgery units, or even a cuspidor. The following provides a description of these devices, which are illustrated during use in later chapters.

Ultrasonic Scaler

An **ultrasonic scaler** can be attached to the unit. This device is used in prophylaxis and periodontal treatment or for other areas of operative dentistry. Small tips placed on the handpiece are activated electronically, causing a vibratory action that removes calculus and other debris from the teeth.

Electrosurgery Unit

An electrical device that generates energy from high-frequency current to enable the dentist to cut soft tissue within a confined area is referred to as an **electrosurgery unit**. Various electrode tips are available for use in removing, contouring, incising, or coagulating tissue.

Cuspidor

A **cuspidor** is a small sink that is attached to the unit into which a patient empties fluids from the mouth. Although many units are still supplied with a cuspidor, it is an unsanitary, time-consuming device and has no function in sit-down, four-handed dentistry. This device has been replaced by the use of an HVE system; it may be found on older units, or it may be used if an operator is working alone.

Foot Control

The **foot control** is the device found on the floor (Fig. 16-19, *A* and *B*) near the chair that the operator activates with foot pressure to operate all of the handpieces on the unit. Many styles provide a chip blower option, which allows the doctor to provide bursts of air to the area being treated. In addition, a foot control is available for the aseptic chair. The foot control should be placed in position for operator use and yet out of the way of the patient's entrance to the chair.

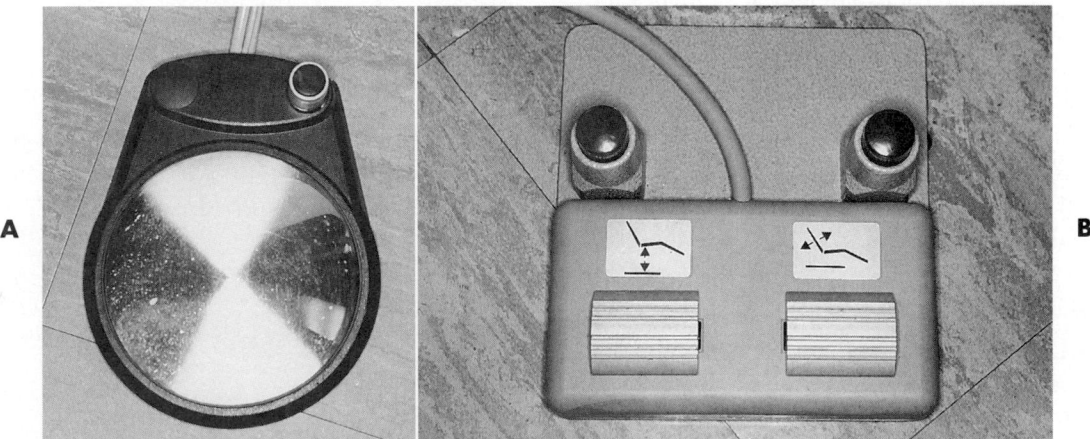

FIG. 16-19 *A,* Foot control to activate handpieces. Chip blower in upper right provides short bursts of air. *B,* Foot control for aseptic chair.

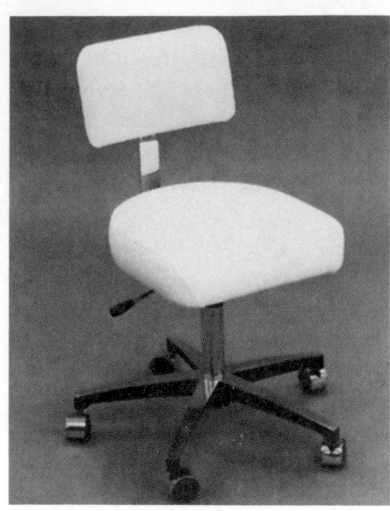

FIG. 16-20   Operator's stool.

(Courtesy of Health Science Products.)

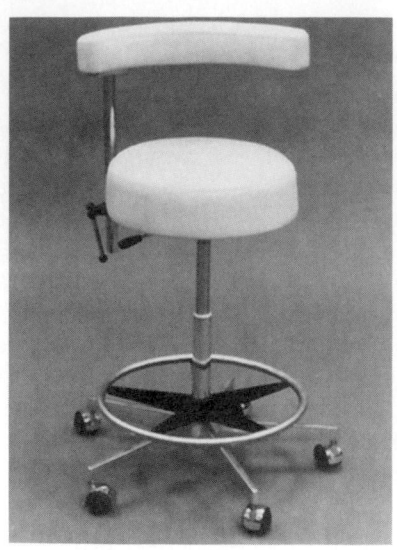

FIG. 16-21   Assistant's stool.

(Courtesy of Health Science Products.)

▶ Dental Stools

Dental stools are required to seat the operator and the assistant. It is wise to invest in a quality stool, since much time is spent seated at chairside. Although the stools may have some similarities, several differences between the operator's and the assistant's stools should be noted.

The **operator's stool** (Fig. 16-20) should have a broad, stable base. The seat should be well padded and may be flat or contoured. It should adjust from 14 to 21 inches in height and have a back support that adjusts vertically and horizontally. The operator's stool goes on the right side of the chair for a right-handed operator and on the opposite for the left-handed operator, as previously shown in Fig. 16-16, *A* and *B*.

Both the operator's and assistant's stools should have five casters for stability (Fig. 16-21). The seat of the assistant's stool should adjust to a height of 27 inches and have an adjustable front and left side body support that will prevent unnecessary bending, which can result in back pain. A stool that adjusts the height by foot pressure is desirable because it allows the assistant to make height adjustments without moving from the stool. The assistant's stool is placed on the side of the chair opposite the dentist, as previously shown in Fig. 16-16, *A* and *B*.

▶ Lighting

Lighting in the treatment room comes from two sources: the general room light and the operating light. Room light should be diffused to avoid shadows and should be color balanced to simulate natural daylight as closely as possible. This latter characteristic aids in the shade selection of many tooth-colored restorations. The light should be operable by either the assistant or the operator and must provide an intensity that lights the patient's mouth adequately. Heat from the lamp should be directed away from the mouth. Fig. 16-22 illustrates a common light used today.

The operating light may be mounted on the ceiling or wall or attached to the chair. The ceiling mount is the preferred style; if a chair mount is used, it should not interfere with the assistant's access to the unit nor should it take space from the assistant's work area. When the patient is in the supine position, the light must be placed so that illumination is directly over the patient's mouth.

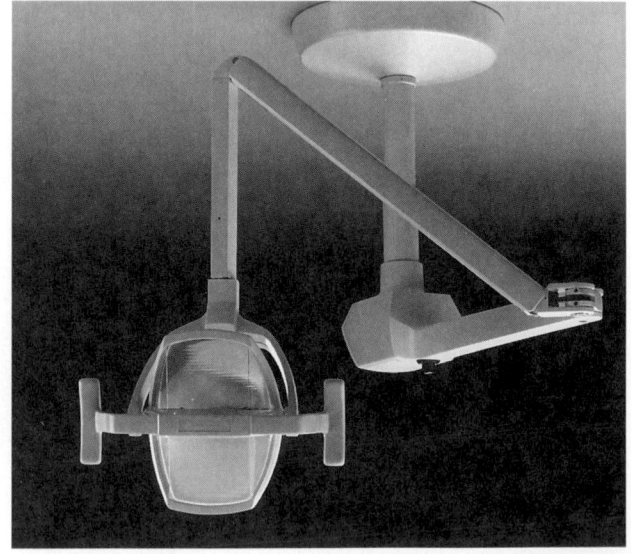

FIG. 16-22   Light.

(Courtesy of Pelton and Crane Company.)

Cabinetry

Cabinetry is necessary in the treatment room to provide work and storage areas. The two most common types are mobile and fixed cabinetry.

Mobile Cabinetry

The **mobile cabinet** is the lifeline for supplies and materials used by the assistant during treatment. A mobile cabinet should provide easy access to all instruments and materials: a well-type storage area in the top that permits the assistant to obtain supplies without bending or stretching, a work surface over the assistant's lap that is at or near elbow height, and an area for a waste receptacle. The mobile cabinet shown in Fig. 16-23 meets all of these specifications. Note that this particular model has a top that moves toward or away from the assistant, allowing the assistant to have a convenient work area directly over the lap area. When the top of this cabinet is opened, the assistant has access to commonly used materials, such as cotton rolls, gauze, and anesthetic (Fig. 16-24). An alternative style is the model shown in Fig. 16-25, which has a top that moves from left to right.

The mobile cabinet is placed to the left of the patient's head for a right-handed operator and the opposite side for a left-handed operator, as previously shown in Fig. 16-16, *A* and *B*. When a procedure begins, the assistant is seated and the mobile cabinet is moved into position, with the front of the cabinet close to the assistant's knees and its top pulled forward or moved to the side as close as possible to the field of operation, without interfering with the doctor's arm. The top of the mobile cart is used as a work surface to hold a tray setup or to hold individual instruments. Consumable supplies can also be organized on this surface. When it is not in use, the top of the mobile cabinet is closed, and it is returned to a storage area.

This cabinet must be restocked daily with supplies. To neglect restocking the cabinet means that a procedure may be halted at a crucial moment so that the material can be obtained; this is not productive.

FIG. 16-23 Mobile cabinet with top that moves to back. Arm rest for operator optional.

(Courtesy of Health Science Products.)

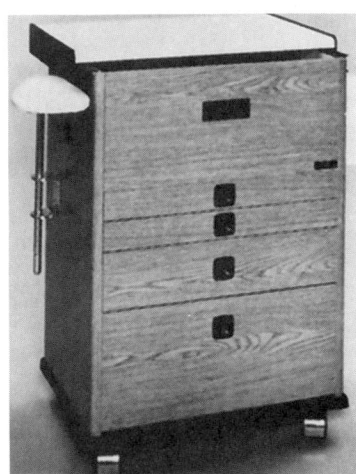

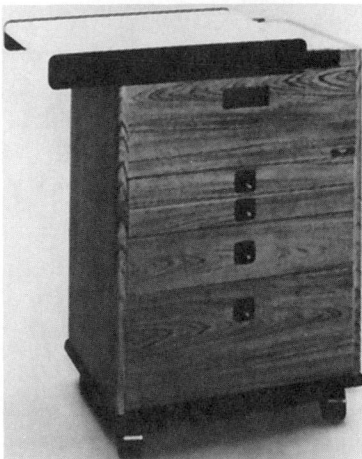

FIG. 16-25 Alternative mobile cabinet design with top movable from left to right.

(Courtesy of Health Science Products.)

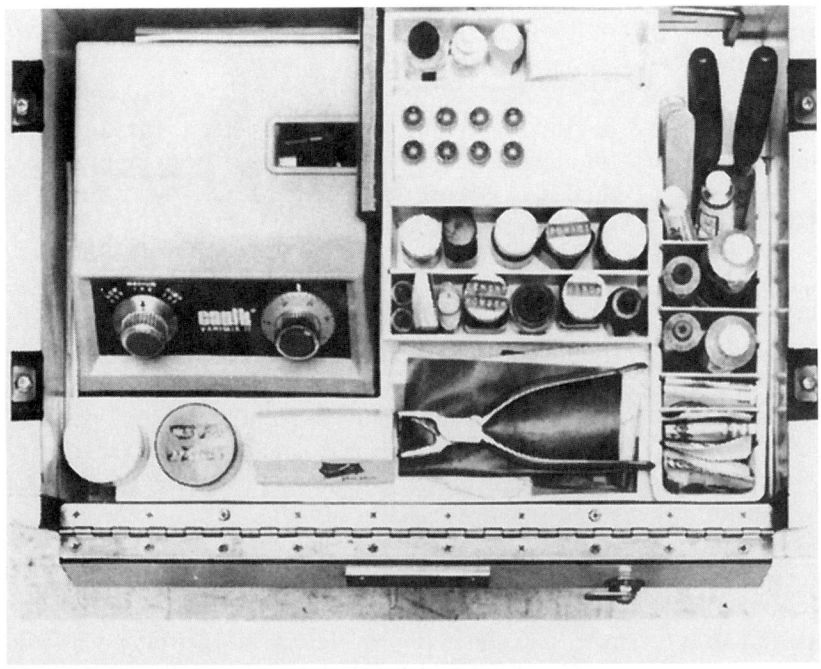

FIG. 16-24 Typical deep well and medication tub setup.

(Courtesy of Health Science Products.)

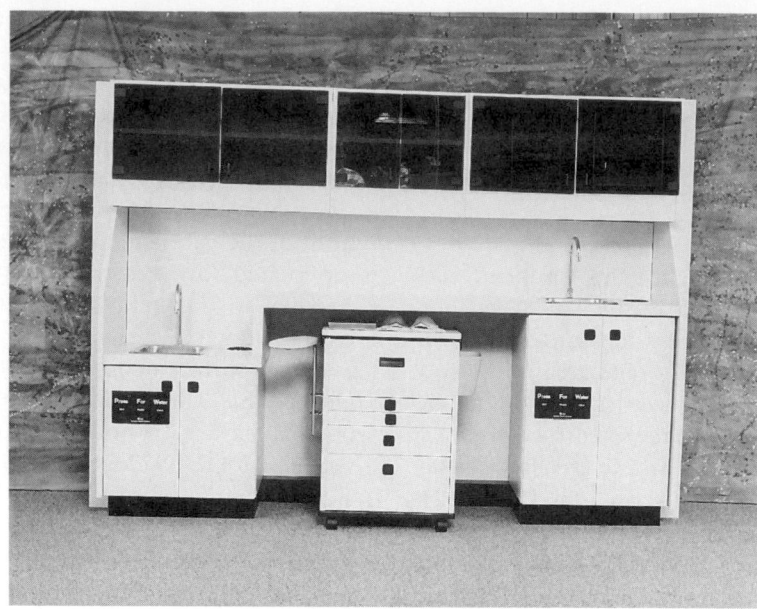

FIG. 16-26   Location of two sinks in fixed cabinetry. Sinks are knee activated.
(Courtesy of Health Science Products.)

▶ Fixed Cabinets and Sinks

Fixed cabinetry, generally used for the placement of sinks, must be kept to a minimum in a treatment room. Wall-hung cabinets provide more floor space and make cleaning easier. Two sinks are located in the treatment room—one for the assistant, and one for the doctor. To eliminate the potential for cross-contamination, knee or foot controls should be used to turn faucets on and off. Liquid soap dispensers and disposable towels are placed near the sink, and a waste receptacle is located nearby that is adequate in size and easy to empty without cross contamination.

Fig. 16-26 indicates a convenient location of sinks in the corners of the room. The assistant's sink is generally at a standup height, but the operator may opt for a sink at a sitting height.

▶ Emergency Equipment / Supplies

OSHA requires that an eyewash and emergency kit be available in the dental office. A medical emergency kit and oxygen should also be part of the office's emergency equipment. Safety warning signs should be posted to indicate the location of the eyewash, oxygen, and emergency kits. The oxygen tank and medical kit must be examined regularly to ensure readiness and currency of drugs.

▶ Eyewash

An **eyewash** system must be installed that enables a staff member to immediately flush the eyes when they have come into contact with a potentially hazardous material.

▶ First Aid Kit

A first aid kit is equipped with basic first aid supplies. A small compact unit such as this model can be hung in a central location or in the dental laboratory where it is easily accessible.

▶ Medical Emergency Kit

In the event of an office medical emergency, it will be necessary to have oxygen and a supply of emergency drugs. Most kits contain common emergency needs, such as a ventilating mask and common emergency drugs, to aid the patient between the call for medical assistance and the arrival of help.

▶ Alternative Equipment Placement

This discussion has provided a basic overview of the major dental equipment that is found in most dental treatment rooms. However, other types of dental equipment and alternative placement patterns may be used effectively in a four-handed dentistry practice. Each of the foregoing units and chairs is representative of equipment that is used in dentistry today. In most instances, these units and chairs satisfy the criteria for equipment selection listed on p. 432.

Equipment Maintenance

Just as a dentist recommends an oral prophylaxis as a preventive procedure for a patient, a dental manufacturer recommends routine maintenance of dental equipment to avoid major repairs. Maintenance of equipment can be categorized as daily or periodic.

▶ Daily Care

Daily equipment maintenance is the routine care done by the assistant and is separate from disinfection, sterilization, or the use of barrier techniques as described in Chapter 8. This care includes chair cleaning to remove aerosol contamination from all surfaces or debris that might collect in the seams of the chair. Regular attention should also be given to the chair base by using a manufacturer's suggested cleaner. Care of the sinks is important. At all times they must be kept immaculately clean and free of medicaments, blood, or other debris.

The towel dispenser and soap container should be restocked regularly and the waste receptacle should be emptied as often as necessary to avoid an untidy appearance.

Periodic care is done by the assistant at weekly or monthly intervals and includes tasks such as cleaning the omniclave/autoclave, changing rubber rings in the a/w syringe, or changing solutions in a radiographic processor. A supply of replacement parts that are frequently used must be maintained by the assistant. Such items include bulbs for the lights, O rings for the a/w syringe, and chucks for the handpieces. It would be wise to inventory equipment with replacement parts and be certain that these parts are always available in the office.

Periodic care also includes annual or biannual care provided by a service representative from a local dental supply company. This extensive care includes the preventive maintenance of internal wiring and hoses to major equipment. Failure to maintain dental equipment can only result in unexpected repairs and delays in patient treatment.

Routine Office Care

Everyone in the office should assume responsibility for maintaining a clean, organized working environment. No one clamors to do housekeeping duties; however, general pickup, dusting, and straightening of the office are necessary activities that must be done each day. Many offices make provision, sometimes through an outside agency or person, for general housekeeping duties. Each day, routine duties are performed in opening and closing the office. Special assignments based on the daily schedule should be made to ensure that all tasks are completed and that everyone shares in the responsibility.

▶ Daily Office Preparation

Reception Room

Opening the office each day requires that all access areas are unlocked, lights turned on, magazines rearranged, and all areas dusted thoroughly. Take time to sit where the patients sit and observe that all areas have a neat and welcoming appearance.

Business Office

In the business office all of the files should be unlocked, patient records should be pulled and then placed in chronologic order, and daily schedules should be posted in the appropriate rooms. Turn on communication systems and other automated equipment, check answering machines or the answering service, and organize the work areas.

Radiographic Processing Area

The radiographic processing area will require that the water in the manual/automatic tanks be changed and adjusted to the correct temperature. Turn on the equipment. If radiographs remain from the previous day, process and mount them.

Treatment Room

Preparation of the treatment room requires routine housekeeping duties, if not previously done. Change into clinical attire, and perform the OSHA startup routine described in Chapter 8. Turn on the equipment, and position it for patient entry; prepare records outside the treatment area; remove perishable dental materials from the refrigerator; and set up the armamentarium for the first patient. Do an overview of the day's patients to ensure the availability of appropriate trays and the readiness of any laboratory work that is needed for these patients.

Sterilization Area

In the sterilization area preheat sterilizers where appropriate and prepare new ultrasonic and disinfectant solutions. Remove instruments that may have been in solutions for sterilization over night. This area needs to be well organized for the day's activities.

▶ Office Closure

At the end of the day, office closure is as important as was opening the office. Emphasis at closure is placed on safety and security of the office. Equipment that is not turned off can present potential hazards, and unsecured areas can invite vandalism. Often, closing tasks will be rotated among staff members, depending on individual schedules.

Reception Room

In the reception area all access areas are to be locked, the lights turned off; debris picked up, and magazines rearranged.

Business Office

Various activities must take place in the business office to complete closure for the day and to prepare for the following day, including the following:

▶ Send designated cases to the laboratory, with a completed requisition
▶ Ascertain that laboratory work has been returned for the next day's patients
▶ Complete the daily bookkeeping entries
▶ Complete banking activities
▶ Confirm appointments, pull records, and prepare the daily schedule for the following day
▶ Turn off the automated equipment
▶ Turn on the answering machine/service
▶ Lock the files

Radiographic Processing Area

Remove all radiographs from processing units or tanks and turn the automatic processor off. If a manual tank is used, be certain to turn off the safe light and any water lines that are going to the tank.

Treatment Room

The treatment room requires special attention, but nothing significantly different from the opening proce-dure. Turn all equipment off; return all perishable dental materials to the refrigerator; remove all armamentarium from the room; and perform the OSHA end-of-day procedures. Remove clinical attire and, if possible, shower.

Sterilization Area

Sterilize all instruments, and arrange preset trays. Empty the solutions from the containers where possible, and pick up and organize the area for the next day.

On-Going Tasks

Some tasks may not be done daily but must be done periodically to ensure safe and efficient operation, including the following:

▶ Changing radiographic solutions
▶ Cleaning/defrosting the refrigerator
▶ Cleaning sterilizing units
▶ Changing disinfectant solutions
▶ Contacting a licensed waste removal service to transport hazardous wastes/sharps
▶ Sharpening instruments
▶ Restocking supplies
▶ Checking inventory

Office Evaluation

To ensure that the office has an appearance of quality, the dentist and staff must make a special effort to observe the external and internal areas of the office regularly. Once every 1 to 2 months, imagine that you are the patient and evaluate the office with a critical eye beginning as you enter your parking space. Once you are inside the office, sit where the patients sit and look at what they see at each visit. Using a checklist like the one shown in Fig. 16-27, determine if each of the areas is adequate in size, neat in appearance, clean, and shows no signs of wear or need for repair or maintenance. This evaluation could be used in a staff meeting to discuss office improvements. If several people in the office all identify an area as needing improvement, these areas should be taken care of as soon as possible.

OFFICE EVALUATION FORM

Check off your evaluation of each of the following areas in the columns provided. E = Excellent condition, A = Adequate condition, or NI = Needs improvement.

	E	A	NI
1. Parking facilities			
2. Appearance of the building			
3. Cleanliness of the exterior of the building			
4. Interior and exterior signage			
5. Signage on door of suite			
6. Appearance and smells of reception room			
7. Office furniture			
8. Location of signs, books, and magazines			
9. Interior hallways, walls, and floors			
10. Appearance of the reception desk			
11. Lighting			
12. Cleanliness of the treatment rooms			
13. Use of universal barrier techniques			
14. Equipment in good working order			
15. Temperature and humidity control			

FIG. 16-27   **A form used to evaluate the appearance of the dental office.**

KEY POINTS

▸ A dental office suite is a composite of many different rooms, each with a specific function. The design of an office should reflect the personality of the dentist, should be comfortable and esthetically pleasing, should meet patient and practice needs, should promote efficient traffic flow, and should provide flexibility.

▸ The dental treatment room is where all clinical activity takes place. This room should be no smaller than 8×10 feet and be designed for the placement of basic dental equipment, including a patient chair, unit, fixed and mobile cabinetry, two sinks, operator and assistant stools, and a dental light.

▸ Selection and placement of dental equipment must consider OSHA guidelines and the basic concepts of time and motion as applied to four-handed dentistry.

▸ Routine and periodic care of dental equipment is important to ensure safe operation and maximum performance. Replacement parts, such as bulbs and chucks for handpieces, should be readily available.

▸ Periodic evaluation of the office suite, both external and internal, aids in maintaining a professional image of the office and reducing maintenance costs.

BIBLIOGRAPHY

Chasteen JE: *Essentials of clinical dental assisting*, ed 4, St Louis, 1990, Mosby.

Combs R: *Openness provides privacy, efficiency: dental economics*, Jan 1992, Pennwell.

Robinson GE, et al: *Four-handed dentistry manual*, ed 6, Birmingham, 1990, University of Alabama School of Dentistry.

17

Seating the Patient and Operating Team

LEARNING OBJECTIVES

You will have mastered the material in this chapter when you can:

▶ Define the key terms

▶ Explain the concept of *see ability* in dentistry

▶ Identify the zones of activity at chairside

▶ Describe the preparation of a treatment room before seating a patient

▶ Explain and demonstrate the process for seating a dental patient for treatment in any area of the oral cavity

▶ Explain and demonstrate the positioning of the assistant and operator for treatment in any area of the oral cavity

▶ Describe the procedure for dismissing a patient

▶ Explain and describe the aseptic techniques used during the setup, treatment, and dismissal of the patient

▶ Identify special needs of patients during the seating and dismissal procedures

KEY TERMS

Assistant's zone	Operator's zone	Supine
Direct vision	See ability	Transfer zone
Indirect vision	Static zone	Zones of activity

In the previous chapters the concepts of four-handed dentistry were examined, as well as the selection and placement of dental equipment. In this chapter the first steps in the application of the basic concepts of four-handed dentistry, seating the patient and operating team, will be applied. Before any treatment procedure can begin, the treatment room must be prepared and the patient must be seated. The operating team is then seated in a balanced posture that will provide efficiency and reduce stress during the procedure. The actual seating of the patient begins with the initial greeting in the reception room and continues through the process of positioning the patient and the operating team comfortably. This procedure is repeated many times during the day and eventually becomes routine. Each time this procedure is performed, the dental assistant must demonstrate a sincere degree of enthusiasm, interest, and confidence to instill in the patient a belief that he or she must be the most important person to be seen today.

See Ability in Four-Handed Dentistry

In the early 1950s the University of Alabama researched four-handed dentistry. A concept, *See Ability in Four Handed Dentistry,* was developed as a result of this research and provided general guidelines for positioning the patient and operating team when treating various areas of the oral cavity (Table 17-1).

The purpose of *see ability*, an ergonomic concept, is to change the environment to enhance the visibility of the operating team. To accomplish this objective may require changing or repositioning the equipment, the patient, or the dentist and assistant to maximize visibility for the dental team when treating any area of the oral cavity. From the suggested guidelines for *see ability* several principles can be identified that will aid in positioning the dental team to provide maximum comfort and efficiency.

▶ Chairside Zones of Activity

All treatment revolves around the patient's mouth; the area around the mouth is divided into four **zones of activity**: operator's zone, assistant's zone, transfer zone,

447

TABLE 17-1   GENERAL GUIDELINES FOR EFFECTIVE FOUR-HANDED DENTISTRY

Area of operation	Vision	Operator's position*	Patient's chair position	Head position
MAXILLARY RIGHT POSTERIOR				
Buccal	Direct	9:00	Backrest horizontal	Straight, chin elevated slightly
Occlusal	Direct	9:00	Backrest horizontal	Chin elevated maximally, head straight
Occlusal	Indirect	11:00	Backrest horizontal	Straight, chin elevated slightly
Lingual	Direct	9:00	Backrest horizontal	Turned toward operator, chin elevated
MAXILLARY ANTERIOR				
Labial	Direct	11:00	Backrest horizontal	Straight, chin elevated slightly
Lingual	Indirect	11:00	Backrest horizontal	Straight, chin elevated slightly
MANDIBULAR ANTERIOR				
Labial	Direct	11:00	Backrest horizontal	Straight or turned slightly toward operator or assistant
Lingual	Direct and indirect	11:00	Chair seat lowered maximally, chair back elevated	Straight or turned slightly toward operator or assistant
MANDIBULAR RIGHT POSTERIOR				
Buccal	Direct	10:00	Seat lowered and backrest elevated slightly	Straight or turned slightly toward assistant
Occlusal	Direct	9:00	Seat lowered and backrest elevated slightly	Turned slightly toward operator, chin lowered slightly
Lingual	Direct	11:00	Backrest horizontal	Turned toward operator maximally, chin elevated slightly
MAXILLARY LEFT POSTERIOR				
Buccal	Direct	9:00	Backrest horizontal	Turned toward operator, chin elevated slightly
Occlusal	Direct	9:00	Backrest horizontal	Chin elevated maximally, head turned slightly toward operator
Occlusal	Indirect	11:00	Backrest horizontal	Turned toward operator
Lingual	Direct	9:00	Backrest horizontal	Turned toward assistant, chin elevated slightly
MANDIBULAR LEFT POSTERIOR				
Buccal	Direct	11:00	Backrest horizontal	Turned toward operator
Occlusal	Direct	10:00	Backrest horizontal	Straight, chin elevated
Lingual	Direct	9:00	Seat lowered and backrest elevated slightly	Turned slightly toward assistant

*NOTE: The assistant's position remains the same between 2 and 4 o'clock in all situations.
Adapted from University of Alabama School of Dentistry, Birmingham, Ala.

and static zone. In Fig. 17-1 these four zones are illustrated using the patient's head as the face of a clock. The **operator's zone** extends from 7 to 12 o'clock for a right-handed operator and from 1 to 4 o'clock for a left-handed operator. The operator is able to move about within the zone of activity to improve visibility. For instance, the 12 o'clock position would allow the operator to work on the labial surface of the maxillary anterior teeth and use direct vision, while the operator could use direct vision by moving to the 8 o'clock position when working on the occlusal surface of mandibular right posterior tooth (Fig. 17-2).

The **assistant's zone** is from 2 to 4 o'clock for a right-handed operator and 8 to 10 o'clock for a left-handed operator. This area is the assistant's domain. Nothing in this area should interfere with the assistant's access to instruments on the mobile cart or to the handpieces on the dental unit. The movable top of the mobile cart is

Retraction	Operator's fulcrum	HVE tip parallel to tooth surface
Left index finger	Handpiece head on left index finger	Lingual
Left index finger	Left index finger	Lingual
Right third finger	Buccal surfaces of right posterior teeth	Lingual
Left index finger	Left index finger	Lingual (distal tooth being treated)
Left index finger	Occlusal surfaces of right premolar teeth, or incisal surfaces of anterior teeth	Lingual (incisal edge)
Assistant retracts with left index finger	Occlusal surfaces of right premolar teeth	Lingual (incisal edge)
Operator retracts lower lip with thumb and index finger	Buccal surfaces of lower right premolar teeth	Lingual
Operator retracts tongue with back of mirror	Buccal surfaces of lower right premolar teeth	Labial
Left index finger	Labial surfaces of lower anterior teeth	Lingual
Left index finger assistant retracts tongue with mirror	Labial surfaces and incisal edges of lower anterior teeth	Lingual
Operator retracts tongue with mirror	Labial surfaces of lower anterior teeth	Lingual (distal to tooth being treated)
Left index finger	Anterior incisal edges	Buccal (distal to tooth being treated)
Left index finger	Occlusal surfaces of right premolar teeth	Buccal
Assistant retracts with left index finger	Occlusal surfaces of right premolar teeth	Buccal
Assistant retracts with left index finger	Labial surfaces of lower anterior teeth left index finger stabilizes; handpiece head	Buccal
Left index finger or mirror	Labial surfaces of lower anterior teeth	Buccal (distal to tooth being treated)
Operator retracts tongue with mirror Assistant retracts buccal tissues	Labial surfaces of lower anterior teeth	Buccal
Operator retracts tongue with mirror Assistant retracts buccal tissues	Labial surfaces of lower anterior teeth	Buccal

brought into the assistant's zone (over the lap) on the upper edge of the arc and the dental handpieces from the unit extend into the zone at the lower edge of the arc.

The **transfer zone** is the area around the patient's mouth where instrument transfer occurs. The transfer zone extends from 5 to 8 o'clock for a right-handed operator or 4 to 7 o'clock for the left-handed person. This area should be used only for transfer of instruments and materials to and from the patient's mouth. Because the transfer zone is specifically designated for instrument transfer, the operator will be able to keep hands and eyes on the field of operation without wondering from which direction the next instrument will come.

The static zone is the zone of least activity. It extends from 12 to 2 o'clock when working with a right-handed operator or 10 to 12 o'clock for a left-handed operator. Instruments or equipment that are used infrequently, such as a curing light or sphygmomanometer, and the assistant's cart when not in use, may be stored in this area.

Care should be taken by both members of the team to avoid interfering with the activities of the other person within the designated zones. The operator should not interfere with the assistant's domain: the preset tray, instruments on the mobile cabinet, or handpieces. The assistant likewise should not interfere with the operator's vision or operative site.

To enter into the other person's zone of activity violates the smooth flow of activity and will likely require unnecessary movement, interference with the procedure, and the operator's refocusing on the site.

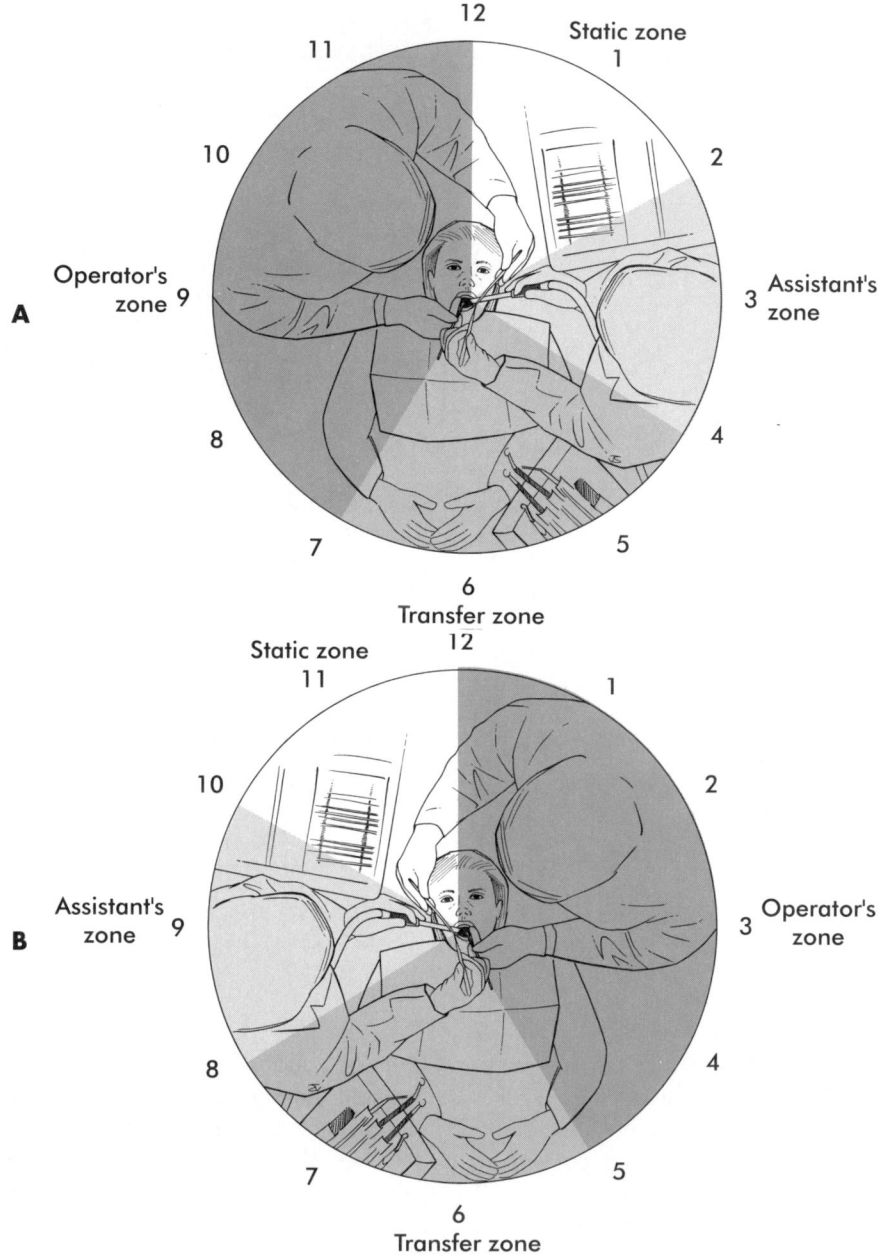

FIG. 17-1   *A,* Zones of activity for a right-handed operator. *B,* Zones of activity for a left-handed operator.

▶ Patient Head Mobility

The patient can change position to increase the visibility of the operating team for any operative site. Often a dentist or an assistant will stretch or strain to see the operative site without asking a patient to move his or her head. The team forgets that the patient is mobile and can move or change head position to improve the team's visibility. A good example of the need to have the patient turn the head occurs when a right-handed operator is working on the lingual surface of a mandibular left molar (Fig. 17-3, *A*). If the patient is asked to turn toward the assistant, the operator, who is seated in the 9 o'clock position, can look directly into the cavity preparation, thereby eliminating the need to strain and lean across the patient. Fig. 17-3, *B* illustrates the result of this concept.

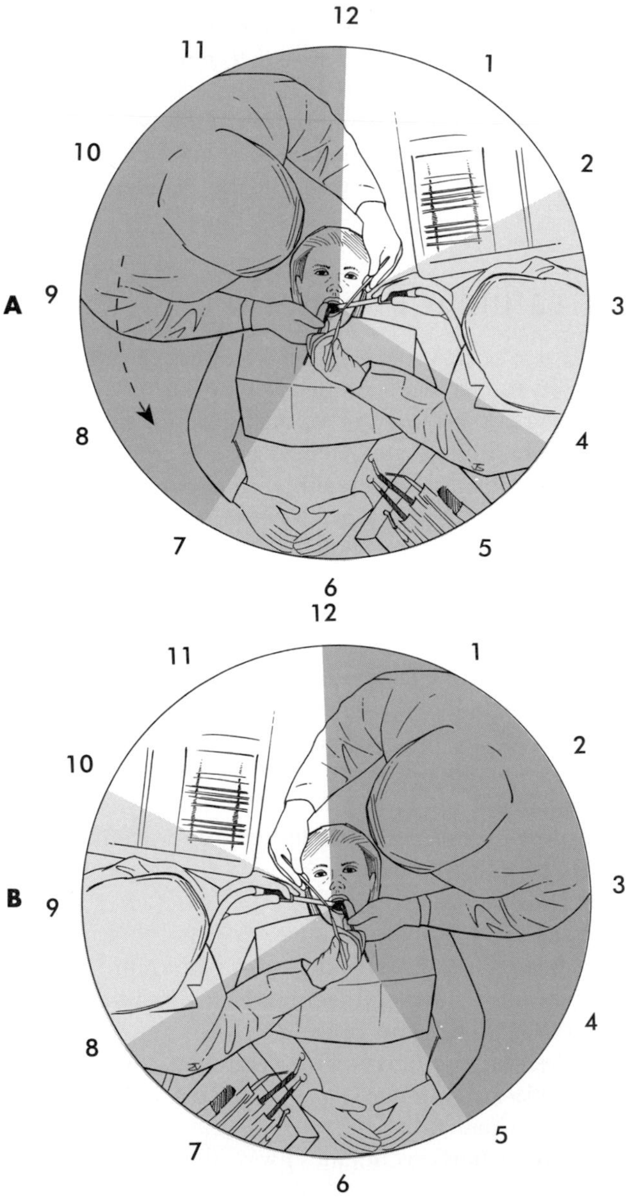

FIG. 17-2 *A,* The right-handed operator is at the 11 o'clock position for treatment on the maxillary anterior. *B,* The left-handed operator is at the 1 o'clock position for treatment in the same area.

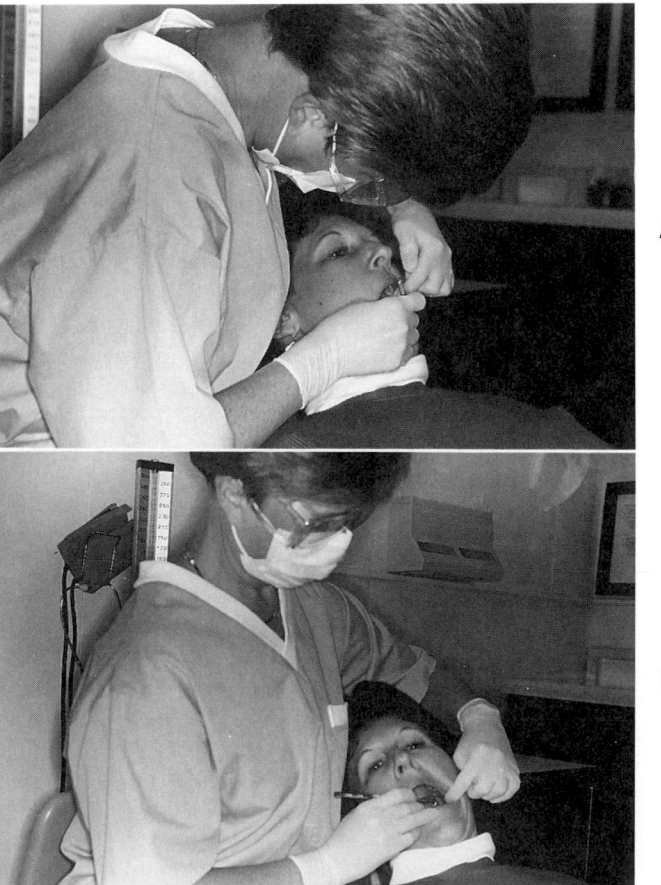

FIG. 17-3 *A,* Operator bending over patient to see buccal surface of #19. NOTE: The incorrect position will cause undue fatigue over long periods of time. *B,* Operator's position is improved when the patient's head is turned toward the operator to eliminate bending.

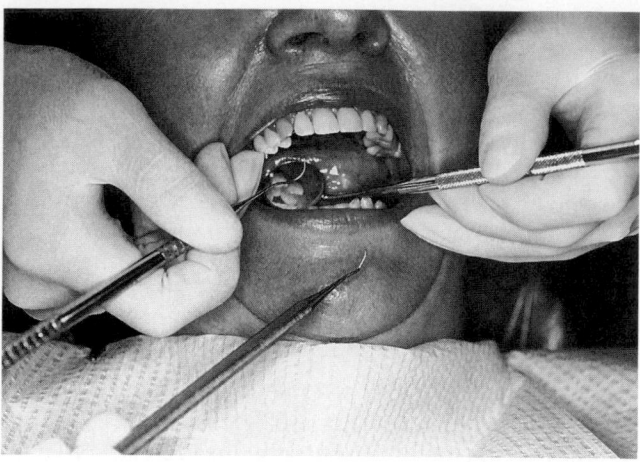

FIG. 17-4 The use of indirect vision on #4 allows the operator to maintain a comfortable position.

Direct versus Indirect Vision

The operator must use two forms of vision: direct and indirect. **Direct vision** occurs when the operator is looking directly into the cavity preparation or treatment site. **Indirect vision** requires the operator to look into a mirror to observe the area. The use of indirect vision eliminates the need for the operator to bend over to view the operative site. To treat the occlusal surface of tooth #2, even with the patient in a supine position, would require the operator to bend over. The use of a mirror will allow the operator to be seated with balanced posture and to observe the operative site satisfactorily in the mirror (Fig. 17-4). Table 17-1 offers suggestions for the use of direct vs indirect vision in many areas of the mouth.

Patient Positioning

The patient is seated and is then placed in a **supine** position, with the knees and nose on the same plane. Essentially the patient lies flat, as though on an operating table. Once the patient is in the supine position, the operator can lower the chair until the patient's head is centered over the operator's lap. The operator should not have to reach up with the arms or bend over to work in the patient's mouth. Occasionally, lowering the chair base and raising the back of the chair will enhance the operator's visibility; this is especially true when the work is being done on the mandibular arch. Visibility can be improved when this change is made. Special needs of patients may require a more upright position, especially when treating patients with emphysema or other upper respiratory ailments.

Operator Positioning

The operator's chair position changes in relation to the area of the mouth that is being treated. A change in the position of the operator within the zone of activity can greatly improve visibility and reduce back and neck strain caused by bending and leaning. In Table 17-1, positions for specific areas of the mouth are recommended.

Assistant Positioning

The assistant's chair position remains the same regardless of the treatment site. Although the zone for the assistant extends from 2 to 4 o'clock, when he or she assists a right-handed operator the assistant remains relatively stationary regardless of the quadrant being treated. To see more clearly in the mandibular arch, it is possible to raise the stool slightly, but it seldom will require movement back and forth within the zone of activity.

Pretreatment Preparation

The final success of a procedure can be directly correlated to advanced preparation. If all of the armamentarium is positioned in an organized manner, if the barrier techniques are in place, if records are placed in a safe and visible location, and if the patient and the operating team are positioned for maximum comfort and visibility, only an unexpected complication in the clinical procedure can deter the possibility for success. Such preparation can be compared to planning an extensive automobile trip. Before the trip all systems in the car must be readied: the tank must have a full tank of gas, the spare tire must be in good repair, and the road maps and directions to the final destination must be accessible. Organization and preplanning will ensure success in either situation.

A typical routine for completing any procedure will require the following:

- Prepare the treatment room
  - Disinfect all exposed surfaces
  - Arrange preset tray and armamentarium
  - Set up records and radiographs
  - Place barrier coverings
  - Position equipment and armamentarium
- Provide an antimicrobial oral rinse for the patient
- Seat the patient
- Prepare barrier techniques for patient and operating team
- Seat the operating team
- Position the operating light
- Perform the clinical procedure
- Dismiss the patient
- Return records to the business office

▶ Remove armamentarium and barrier techniques
▶ Clean and disinfect and/or sterilize the armamentarium and exposed surfaces

▶ Preparing the Treatment Room

Before the patient enters the treatment room, the dental assistant prepares the area for the designated treatment. After the dismissal of the preceding patient remove all of the armamentarium and clean and disinfect the treatment room. At this point, preparation for a new patient begins. The use of preset trays and the organization of the room before the patient's entry can do much to minimize patient apprehension. Review the patient records, and bring the radiographs and any necessary models to the treatment area. Place the radiographs and chart in a position that is away from the treatment area to avoid contamination. A good place for the chart is outside the treatment room, perhaps on a hanging shelf, as in Fig. 17-5.

All of the equipment is positioned as shown (as suggested in Chapter 16), and the barrier techniques are in place. At this point the traffic area to the dental chair is made ready for the patient by clearing away the foot controller, operator's stool, operating light, and any hoses that may obstruct the patient's entry to the chair.

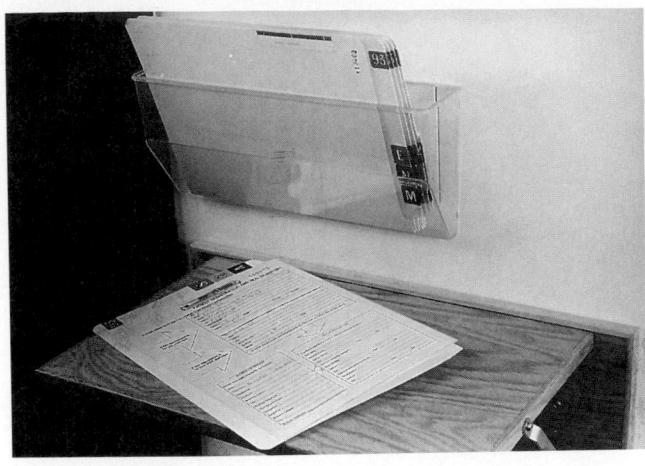

FIG. 17-5   The patient chart is placed outside the treatment room on a hanging shelf.

Position the chair seat at a normal seating level, about 15 to 18 inches off the floor, raise the arm rest, and tilt the chair back about 15 degrees from vertical to a comfortable seating position. This position will allow the patient easy and comfortable entrance into the chair. See Fig. 17-6 for the appearance of the room before seating the patient.

Chair arm
raised

Operating
light raised

Dental unit
to side

A

Operator stool
out of way

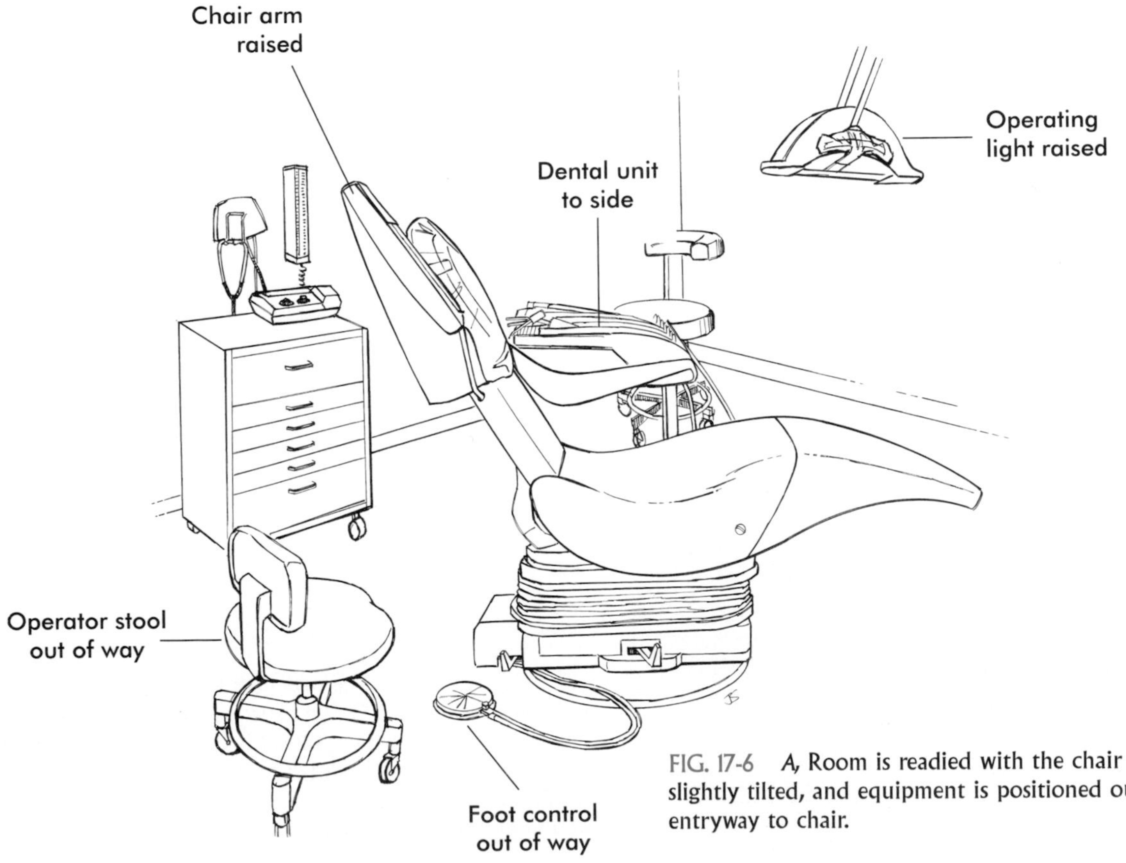

FIG. 17-6   *A*, Room is readied with the chair arm up; chair is slightly tilted, and equipment is positioned out of the patient's entryway to chair.

Foot control
out of way

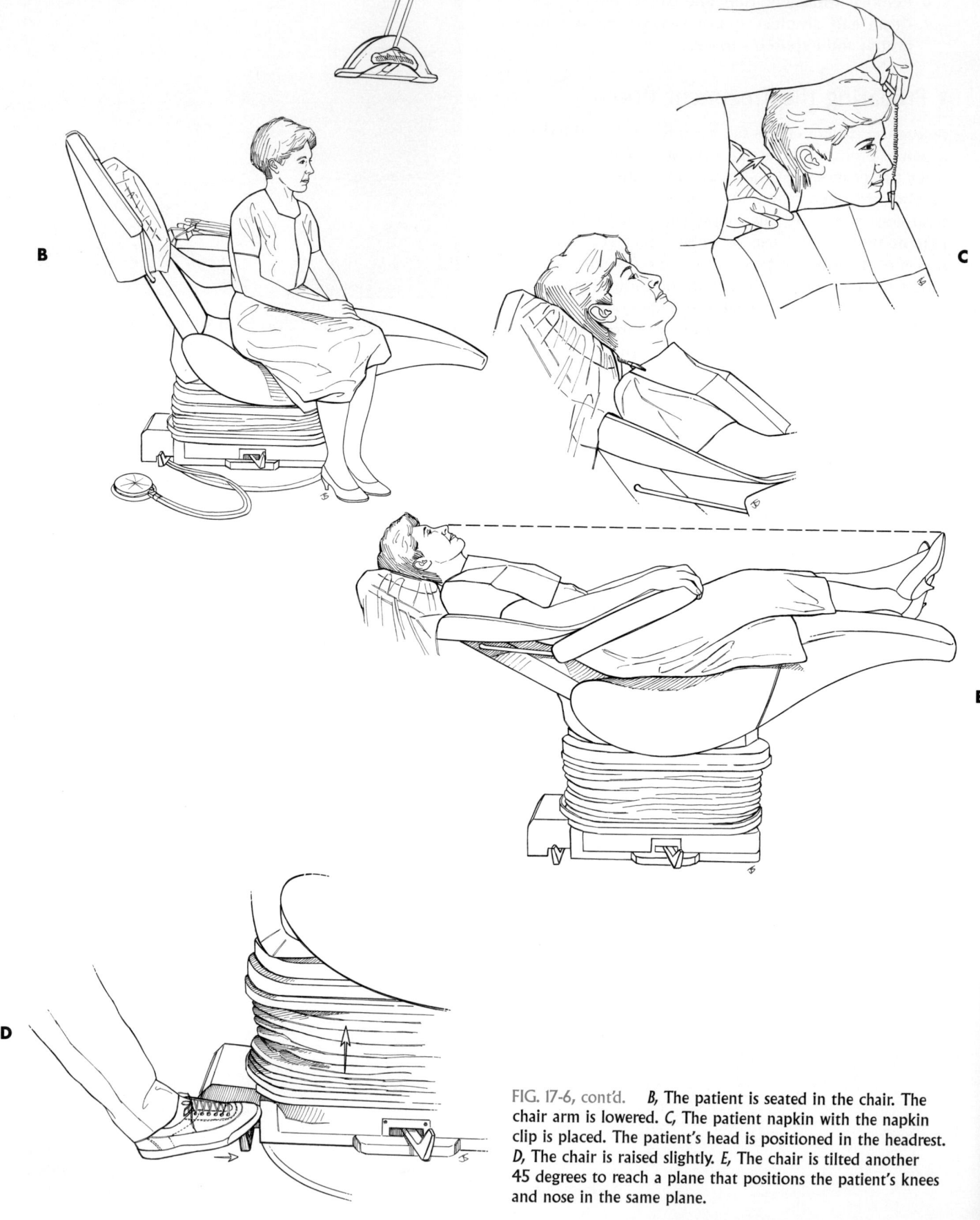

FIG. 17-6, cont'd.   *B,* The patient is seated in the chair. The chair arm is lowered. *C,* The patient napkin with the napkin clip is placed. The patient's head is positioned in the headrest. *D,* The chair is raised slightly. *E,* The chair is tilted another 45 degrees to reach a plane that positions the patient's knees and nose in the same plane.

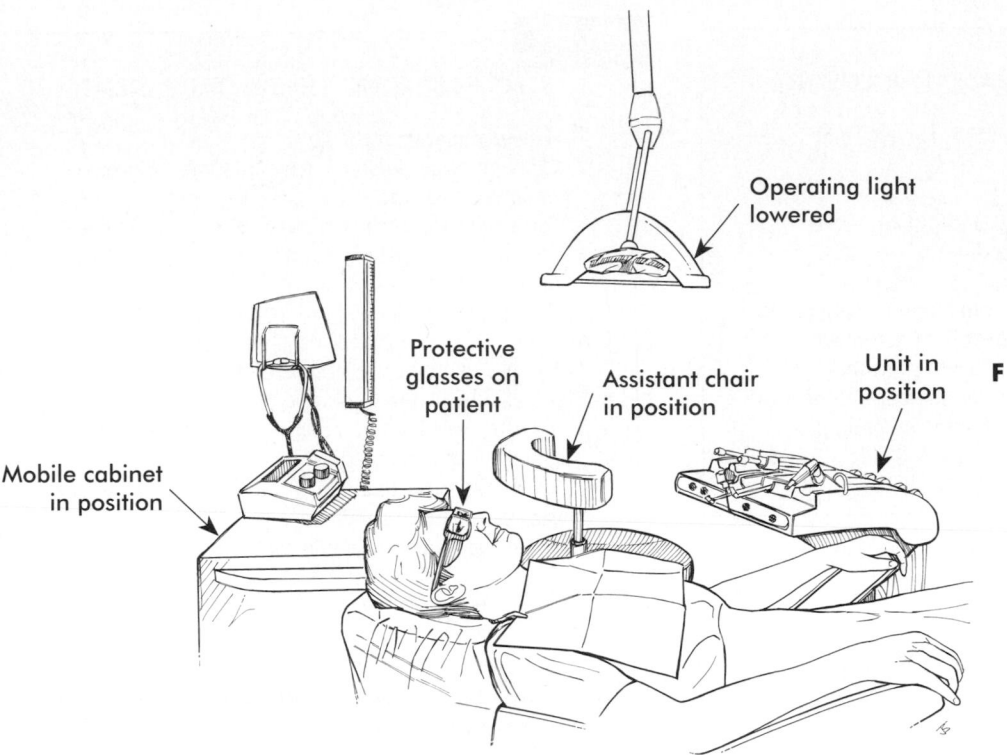

FIG. 17-6, cont'd.   *F,* The operating light, unit, assistant's stool, and mobile cabinet are positioned. Protective glasses are provided for the patient. *G,* The operating team is positioned with the light focused for the appropriate arch, and the assistant is 4 to 6 inches higher than the operator. The operator's arms and thighs are parallel to the floor and both team members have balanced posture.

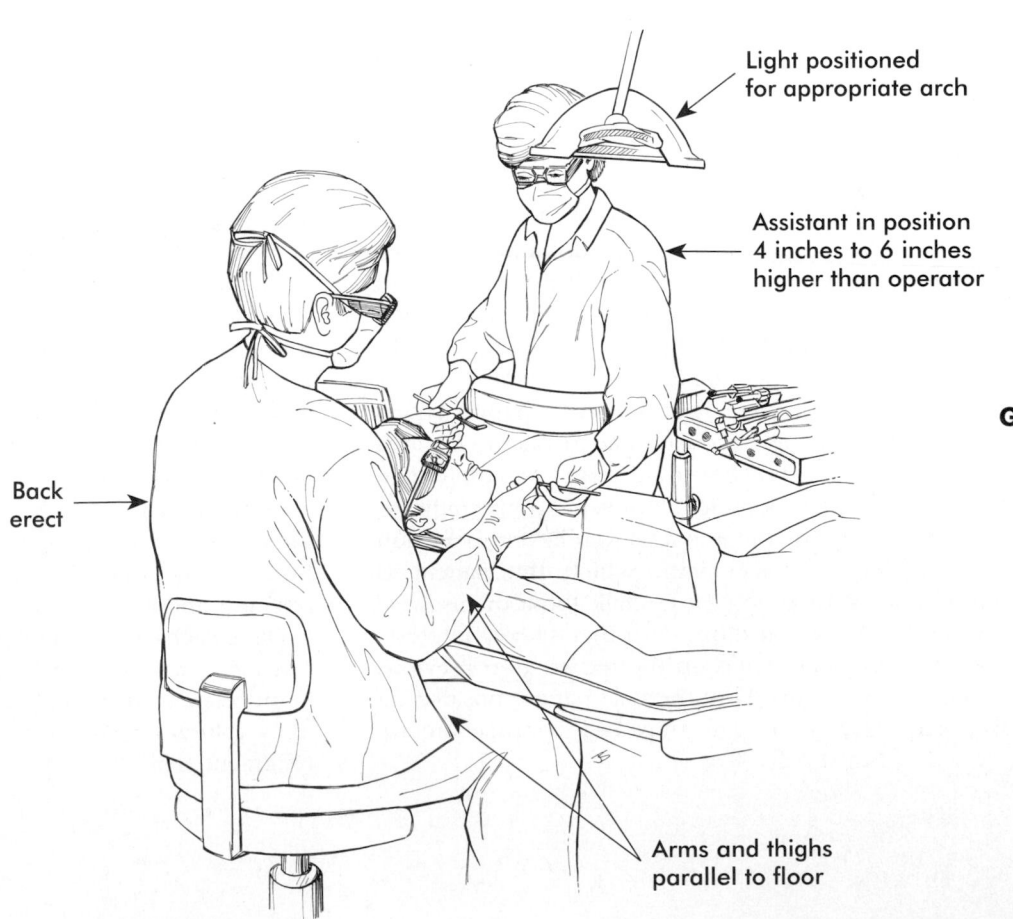

Gloving and Ungloving Before and After Treatment

The preparation for and dismissal of the patient are prime times to consider the application of universal precautions in infection control. Follow the general rules identified in Box 17-1 for gloving and ungloving. In addition, the *Stop and Think* messages will alert you to stop and think whether universal precautions are in place before and after each clinical procedure throughout the remainder of this textbook.

Seating the Patient

This activity actually begins in the reception room when the patient is requested to come into the treatment area. When you enter the reception room to notify the patient that you are ready to see them, you should state the patient's name, and when he or she answers, introduce yourself and inform the patient that you are now ready to begin. It is a good idea to inform the patient which treatment room you will be using. For instance, "Mr. Richards, we are going to be in treatment room three" or "the second door on your right." When the patient enters the room, thoughtfully step back and gesture to the area where you wish him or her to be seated or simply state "You may be seated." A patient at this point may indicate some apprehension, and it is wise to relieve this tension by discussing a subject with which the patient is comfortable. Most people like to talk about themselves, their family, work, vacations, or other special interests that may have been noted on the record after previous appointments. At this point the final patient positioning takes place (Fig. 17-6). The steps in this procedure are outlined in Box 17-2.

On many chairs it is possible to eliminate several of these steps simply by touching a single button that places the patient automatically into a supine position. Regardless of the type of chair that is used, avoid sudden, jerky motions and explain changes in chair positioning to the patient as they occur. Ultimately the patient must be positioned so that the knees and nose are on the same plane and the maxillary arch is perpendicular to the floor. Although this procedure may appear basic, special courtesies should be extended along the way, including offering a tissue to a female patient to remove lipstick to avoid smudging it during the procedure; placing a longer style apron to protect clothing during an extensive procedure or impression taking; and placing partial or full dentures in a protected area.

Positioning the Operating Team

In Chapter 15, emphasis was placed on sit-down dentistry and the importance of motion economy. Properly seating the operating team is one of the most important procedures in preserving motion economy and in preventing operator/assistant fatigue. Appropriately positioning the team so that the equipment and armamentarium are as close to the operative site as possible will eliminate the need to turn the body or reach for instruments and supplies. The list of criteria shown in Box 17-3 identifies the objectives for seating both the operator and the assistant (Fig. 17-6).

Once each of the members of the team is seated, the operator can position the patient for treatment in the appropriate arch, the light can be turned on, and a mirror and explorer are passed to the operator to examine the treatment area.

CRITERIA FOR POSITIONING THE OPERATING TEAM

OPERATOR

1. The stool is adjusted to allow the operator's feet to rest firmly on the floor and to provide adequate support for the back
2. The thighs should be parallel to the floor.
3. The patient's chair is lowered so that the chair back is nearly in the operator's lap over the thigh area
4. The operator should be able to move freely in the operator's zone of activity.
5. The patient's head is positioned so that the mouth is as close as possible to the operator's elbow.
6. Elbows should be close to the side of the body.
7. Lower arms are nearly parallel to the floor.
8. Shoulders are parallel to the floor.
9. Back is straight.
10. Neck is not bent or strained.
11. Distance from the operator's eyes to the patient's mouth should be no less than 14 inches.

ASSISTANT

1. The stool is positioned as close to the patient's chair as possible.
2. The front edge of the stool should be nearly even with the patient's mouth to ensure that the assistant is in line with the patient's oral cavity.
3. Legs are parallel to the side of the chair and are facing the direction of the patient's head.
4. Feet rest on the rim of the stool and are parallel to the floor.
5. The body support is positioned to come around the left side and to support the assistant's torso when it is leaning forward, thereby reducing stress on the back and neck.
6. When seated the assistant's eye level should be 4 to 6 inches higher than the operator's eye level. In general the assistant's eye level should be just over the top of the operator's head, (approximately 4 inches, when the work involves the maxillary; the eye level should be slightly higher for working on the mandibular arch.
7. Position the stool before positioning the mobile cabinet.
8. Position the mobile cabinet directly in front of the assistant's knees and as close to the chair as possible.
9. Avoid excessive bending or extending the arms to reach for materials or instruments.
10. Maintain a relatively straight back and neck.

▶ Positioning the Light

Most dental operating lights are designed to illuminate the mouth when placed 3 to 5 feet away from the operative site. If the lights are placed too closely they can interfere with vision and inhibit easy movement in the transfer zone, as well as create unnecessary heat. When the operator is working on the mandible, the light is raised to a higher position so that its beam can be tilted down toward the mandibular teeth. For the maxilla the entire light can be lowered and the beam can be aimed more parallel to the floor.

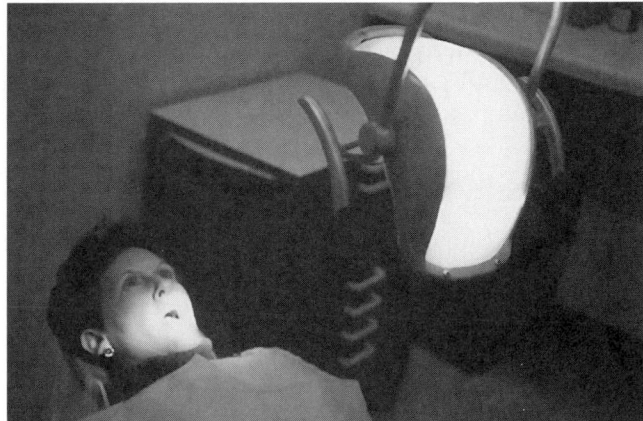

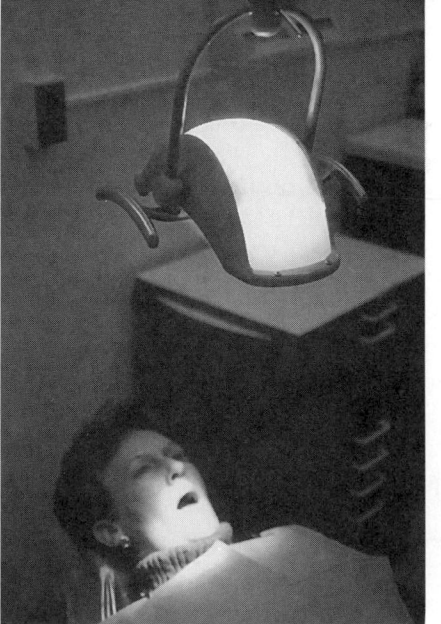

FIG. 17-7　*A,* The light is positioned for the maxilla. *B,* The light is positioned for the mandible.

When the light is positioned, lower the beam and then raise it into the oral cavity. If the light is positioned too high, it will be necessary to lower it, causing the beam to pass over the patient's eyes when it is adjusted to the proper position. It is wise to position the light and then turn on the beam for final adjustment (Fig. 17-7). The position of the assistant and the operator should not interfere with the path of the light. Avoid leaning over the patient because this will obstruct the light and increase fatigue.

The assistant must be observant during the procedure to detect any potential for patient or operating team discomfort; frequently glance around the zones of activity. If the operator or the assistant must lean over, if the arms are raised needlessly, or if the visibility is not good, pause for a few seconds. Suggest to the operator that the team or the patient needs to be repositioned, and if necessary reposition the light. To continue to work in a stressful position will cause body fatigue and will ultimately make the practice unpleasant. Pause for only a few seconds during a procedure to adjust position, and turn the unpleasant stressful position into a more comfortable productive situation.

◗ Dismissing the Patient

When the treatment is completed, postoperative directions are given and the patient is dismissed. The following steps are used for this procedure:

1. Turn off the operating light
2. Move the unit out of the way.
3. Raise the backrest slowly in short increments to a comfortable sitting position.
4. Tilt the chair forward.
5. Lower the chair base.
6. Return any personal items previously removed.
7. Allow the patient to remain seated to reestablish equilibrium.
8. Raise the arm of the chair.

Once again, special courtesy should be extended by directing the patient to the rest room to check appearance or freshen up; by leading him or her back to the business office to make payments or future appointments; by helping with a coat or sweater, and by thanking the patient for being cooperative during the treatment.

Seating Patients with Special Needs

Not every patient is able to be seated in the routine manner because of special needs. Special attention should be given to the young patient; to older adults; to those who use a wheelchair, crutches, or a walker; and to the blind or hard of hearing. In general, most of these patients will require some extra time and explanation as

you proceed to seat them. For special situations the following suggestions may be helpful.

◗ Older Adult Patients

Older adults frequently need some assistance into the treatment room. If their pace is a little slower, take time as you escort them to the treatment room. You may need to help them as they get into or out of the chair. Once they are seated, place canes or walkers out of the way and inform patients about what you are doing so that they will not worry. Also, take care as you change chair position because the patient may resist being placed in a completely supine position. Again, explain what you are doing to help reduce stress. As you dismiss older adult patients, allow them to remain in the chair longer to be certain that their equilibrium is well established and, again, aid them with their personal items and help them to put on a coat or sweater, if necessary.

◗ Pregnant Patient

A pregnant patient may find it uncomfortable to be positioned in a supine position or to sit for long periods

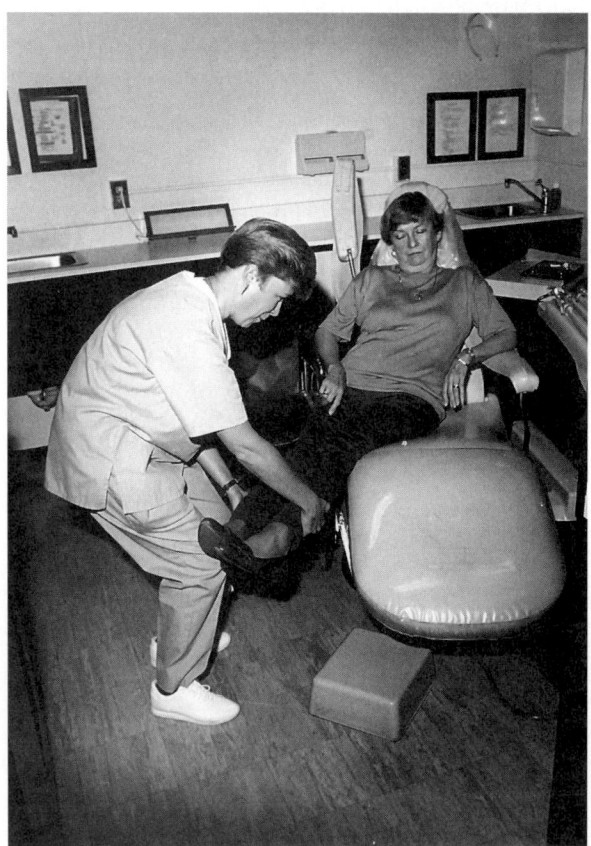

FIG. 17-8 **Single person transfer of a patient from the wheelchair to the dental chair.**

of time without an opportunity to change position. Indicate to the patient your plan to place her into a supine position and offer to modify this position to ensure her comfort.

▶ Sensory-impaired patients

A patient who is blind or who has a hearing problem presents a different type of concern. Frequently this person will be escorted to the office by a friend or family member who plans to aid with communication. It is important to remember to allow the patient to be as independent as possible. A blind patient communicates through other senses, such as touch, hearing, and taste. Therefore, it is helpful to explain what you are doing, let the patient feel the materials being used, and explain if there might be an unpleasant taste from medicine that is being used.

A patient with a hearing problem sometimes has less obvious needs. The patient may smile or nod and appear to understand out of politeness. It is important to establish the best communication possible: stand directly in front of the patient; lower your mask; establish direct eye contact, being sure to have his or her attention; and speak slowly and distinctly. It is recommended that words not be over enunciated but speak normally because the patient may be lip-reading.

A patient who has a physical impairment may require some help into the dental chair. This is especially true with a patient in a wheelchair. Fig. 17-8 illustrates a method of transferring a patient from the wheelchair to the dental chair with relative ease. A patient with some mobility may require only that you support the chair or aid in moving his or her legs to the chair. Other situations may require that two staff members transfer the patient: one person is responsible for the upper body, and the other supports the lower body (Fig. 17-9). In either situation do not strain yourself when aiding the patient. If it is necessary to bend over, do so from the knees, making certain the patient is well supported before the transfer takes place. It is important to remember that a patient who has a physical disability is usually still capable of understanding what is said to him or her. Do not make the mistake of ignoring and possibly insulting the patient by directing your remarks to the person who has escorted the patient to your office.

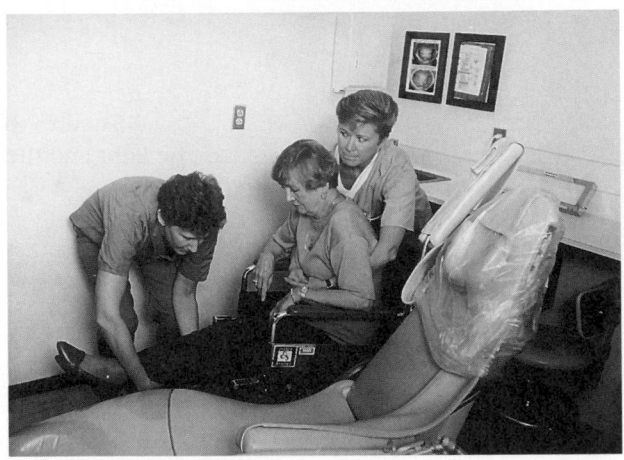

FIG. 17-9 Two staff members transferring the patient. One is responsible for the upper torso region and the other, for the lower body.

KEY POINTS

▶ The concept of *see ability* changes the environment for the dental health team by repositioning the patient, dentist, or assistant to enhance visibility.

▶ Treatment at chairside revolves around the patient's mouth, an area that can be divided into zones of activity. These include the operator's zone, assistant's zone, transfer zone, and static zone. These zones take their position from the face of a clock, using the patient's head as the focal point.

▶ All basic dental equipment should be positioned before seating the patient. Universal precautions are implemented and the patient is placed in a supine position with the light, unit, and mobile cart positioned appropriately and with the dental team seated in balanced posture.

▶ Not all patients can be placed in a supine position. The chair position may need to be modified for the older adult, the physically impaired, the pregnant patient, or the patient with systemic diseases that would contraindicate a supine position.

BIBLIOGRAPHY

Four handed dentistry manual, ed 6, Birmingham, 1990, The University of Alabama.
Holm-Pedersen P, Loe H: *Geriatric dentistry,* St. Louis, 1986, Mosby.
Yemm R, Drummond JR, Newton J P: *Color atlas and textbook of dental care for the elderly,* St. Louis, 1993, Mosby.

18 Basic Dental Instruments

LEARNING OBJECTIVES

You will have mastered the material in this chapter when you can:

▶ Define the key terms
▶ Identify the parts of a dental instrument
▶ Explain the G.V. Black instrument nomenclature
▶ Classify dental instruments according to use
▶ Identify and explain the function of basic dental instruments
▶ Identify and describe basic hand cutting instruments
▶ Identify and describe supplementary instruments and armamentarium common to most dental procedures
▶ Explain the process of instrument sharpening

KEY TERMS

Binangle	Instrument number
Blade	Monangle
Cone socket handle	Shaft
Cutting edge	Shank
Double ended (DE)	Single ended (SE)
Handle	Triple angle
Instrument formula	

Instruments are the primary domain of the chairside dental assistant. The dental assistant is responsible for assembling and maintaining the sequence of instruments on the preset tray; exchanging instruments during treatment procedures; and sterilizing, ordering, maintaining, and sharpening instruments. Most dental instruments used in treatment today are either hand instruments that require manual effort to operate or rotary instruments, which are placed in some type of electronic handpiece.

In this chapter, basic hand instruments that are common to most dental procedures will be described in detail, and in the following chapter, handpieces and rotary devices will be reviewed.

A myriad of instruments are available for the many procedures performed daily in a dental office. The choice of a specific instrument and its style is the responsibility of the dentist. This choice is dictated by the ease of access to the treatment site and is often influenced by the dental school attended or the region of the country in which the dentist practices. Each dentist will have *favorite* instruments for a particular procedure and, unfortunately, for the dental assistant, the dentist may even have a special name for the instrument that does not coincide with the name designated by the manufacturer. This obviously can cause confusion when instruments are ordered from a supply company. Instrument identification can be further complicated by the fact that many instruments have multiple purposes or different names. Perhaps one of the most common examples of this situation is the #7 wax spatula. The instrument is basically a laboratory instrument as illustrated in Chapter 40, but many dentists like to use it as a periosteal elevator during periodontal surgery because of its delicate blade. Obviously, instruments can be interchangeable in their function; however, the dental assistant must be aware of the proper name and manufacturer's number when the instrument is ordered.

In this chapter, emphasis will be placed on dental instruments used in basic clinical dental procedures, common hand cutting instruments, and the maintenance of these instruments. In each of the specialty chapters, such as oral surgery and endodontics, instruments unique to those specialties will be described in detail.

Instrument Design

Dental instruments may be made of stainless steel, Teflon, or plastic and are supplied as **single-ended (SE)**, with one working end, or as **double-ended (DE)** instruments, with two working ends (Fig. 18-1). The use of a double-ended instrument will allow the operator to use the instrument twice without exchanging it. The working end of the instrument may be designed to provide a right and a left, meaning that one end of the instrument can be used on the right side of the tooth and, by reversing the instrument in the hand, the opposite end can be used for the left side of the tooth. Some instruments are designed to be used on the mesial or distal surfaces of the teeth. In other instruments, such as an amalgam carver, each end may be designed to provide two distinct cutting or carving shapes. By using double-ended instruments the number of instruments necessary for a procedure is reduced, as well as the amount of time and motion needed for an instrument exchange. Thus, double-ended instruments are desirable in four-handed dentistry. Some instruments, however, are more commonly supplied in a single-ended version, such as mirrors or scalpels. In the case of the mirror the double end would interfere with the operator's holding position, while a scalpel would pose safety risks.

▶ Instrument Components

The basic parts of an instrument include the handle or shaft, shank, and blade (Fig. 18-2). At the terminal end of the blade is the working end of the instrument, which may be a bevel terminating into a cutting edge, a nib, paddle, beaks, or other specialized shapes.

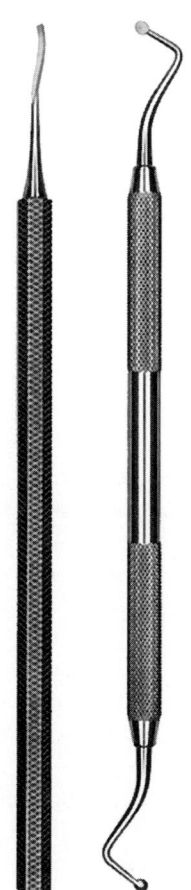

FIG. 18-1 *A,* A single-ended (SE) instrument has one working end, and *B,* a double-ended (DE) instrument has two working ends.

(Courtesy of Hu-Friedy.)

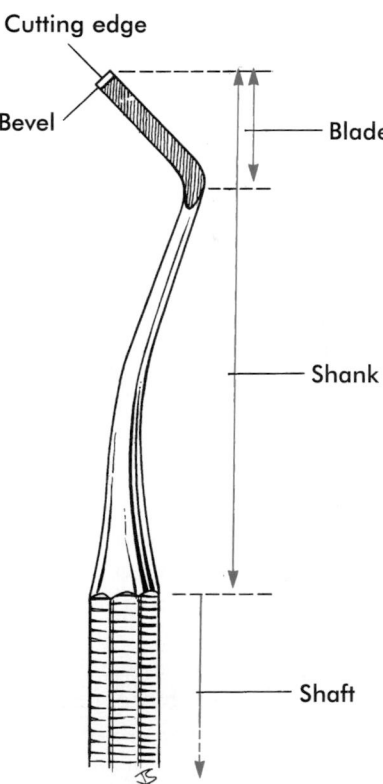

FIG. 18-2 Basic parts of an instrument.

HANDLE OR SHAFT

The **handle** or **shaft** of an instrument is the portion by which the instrument is held. It may be smooth, ribbed or knurled, wide or narrow, round or square, or cut into shapes like an octagon. Most handles are mounted to the shank of the instrument, but a few instruments are designed with **cone socket handles** that allow for the working ends to be replaced.

The cone socket concept is most commonly found in dental mirrors and scalers, where the working end of the instrument can be replaced when it becomes scratched, damaged, or dull (Fig. 18-3). The same concept is used in the design of the pen probe that is a sterilizable combination of a pen and periodontal probe (Fig. 18-4). The design allows for improved infection control procedures by reducing cross-contamination. Some instruments, such as the mirror, have a ruler calibration within the handle (Fig. 18-5). This enables the operator to check measurements of devices being used in the mouth during specific treatment.

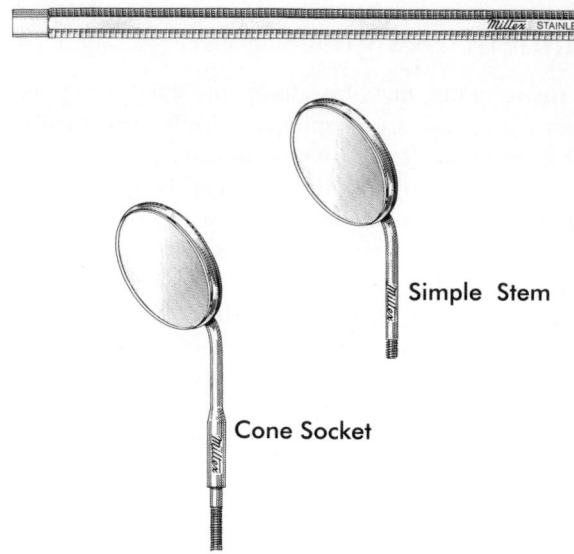

FIG. 18-3   *A,* The cone socket handle allows mirror face to be replaced, retaining the handle. *B,* The difference between a simple stem mirror and a cone mirror.

(Courtesy of Miltex.)

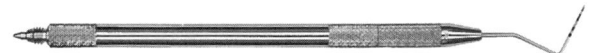

FIG. 18-4   Example of a pen probe.

(Courtesy of Hu-Friedy.)

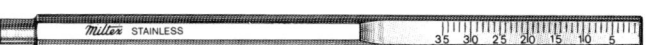

FIG. 18-5   A cone socket hand with millimeter calibrations for cone socket mirror.

(Courtesy of Miltex.)

SHANK

The **shank** is the part of the instrument that extends from the handle to the working end of the instrument. The shank of an instrument is often angled to provide access to various areas of the mouth. The final angle of the shank is the actual working end. In hand cutting instruments, this last angle is called the blade, terminating in a cutting edge. In other instruments, this final angle of the shank may be a specialized shape. Shanks of instruments may be straight, with no angles; **monangle**, with one angle; **binangle**, with two angles; or **triple angle**, with three angles in the shank. Examples of each of these shank styles are shown in Fig. 18-6.

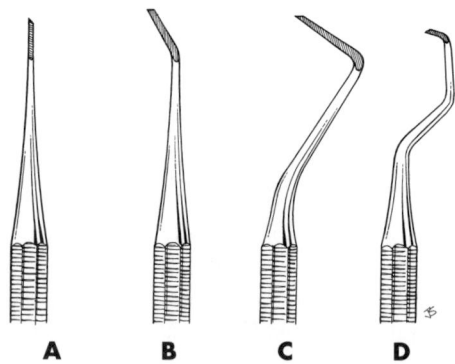

FIG. 18-6   *A,* Straight shank. *B,* Monangle shank. *C,* Binangle shank. *D,* Triple angle shank.

BLADE

Most hand cutting instruments and scalers have a final angle off the shank of the instrument that is the **blade**. At the terminal end of the blade is the **cutting edge** or working end of the instrument. In a hand cutting instrument, such as a chisel or hatchet, a bevel extends at an angle off the end of the blade and terminates in a sharp cutting edge (see Fig. 18-2).

Some instruments, such as cotton pliers and hemostats, have beaks that extend off the handle and do not have a blade. Other instruments that are not used for cutting will have working ends, which are referred to as tips, nibs, or points. These working ends may be smooth, serrated, or sharp and are designed in various shapes. The ends of several instruments are shown in Fig. 18-7. The plastic instrument has a nib shape at one end and a paddle shape at the opposite end to enable the operator to insert dental materials into a cavity preparation. An explorer has sharp points to detect anomalies in a tooth, whereas a spoon excavator has a rounded, curved blade that enables the operator to easily remove soft carious material from a tooth. The condenser has a flat surface to aid in condensing amalgam, the carver has rounded or pointed ends to create anatomy in the amalgam restoration, while a burnisher may have a rounded surface that can be used for smoothing margins of a restoration. Note also that the condenser on the right has a triple angle configuration that enables it to be used as a *back action* condenser, meaning that the instrument can be used to condense amalgam into a distal surface from the posterior to the anterior.

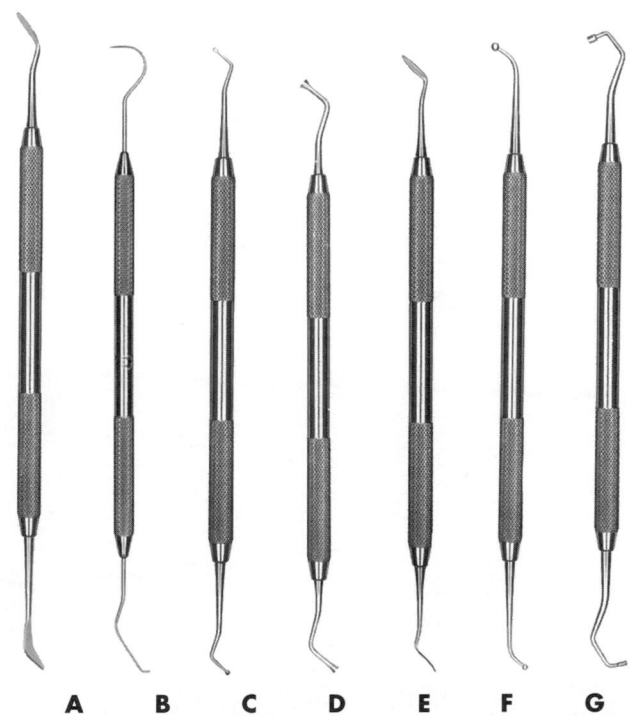

A   B   C   D   E   F   G

FIG. 18-7   Tips of an instrument. *A,* Plastic instrument has nib and paddle shape working ends. *B,* The explorer has sharp points. *C,* A spoon excavator has a rounded curved blade. *D,* A condenser has a flat surface. *E,* A carver has curved or pointed ends. *F,* A burnisher has rounded surfaces. *G,* This condenser has a triple angle shank to be used as a *back action* condenser.

(Courtesy of Hu-Friedy.)

Instrument Nomenclature

Instruments are basically named for their function. For instance, amalgam condensers condense amalgam into a tooth, an explorer explores the anomalies of a tooth, and a periodontal probe probes the depth of the gingival sulcus. However, instrument nomenclature involves more than just the instrument name. Two other factors that are involved include the instrument formula and the manufacturer's number.

▶ Black's Instrument Formula

G.V. Black, one of the early pioneers in operative dentistry, designed an **instrument formula** that de-scribes the dimension and angulation of a hand instrument. This formula is typically applied to all hand cutting instruments that have cutting edges. The basic instrument formula consists of three units, each with a measurement based on the metric system. The instrument formula is stamped on the handle by the manufacturer for each of the basic cutting instruments. For the instrument in Fig. 18-8, a binangled hatchet, a three-number formula is imprinted: 10-6-12. These numbers specifically describe the dimensions of this instrument as follows:

10 = The width of the blade in tenths of millimeters; thus, the width of this blade is 1 mm

6 = The length of the blade in millimeters; thus, the length of this blade is 6 mm

12 = The angle of the blade in relation to the long axis of the handle or shaft in degrees centigrade; thus, the angle of this blade is 12 degrees

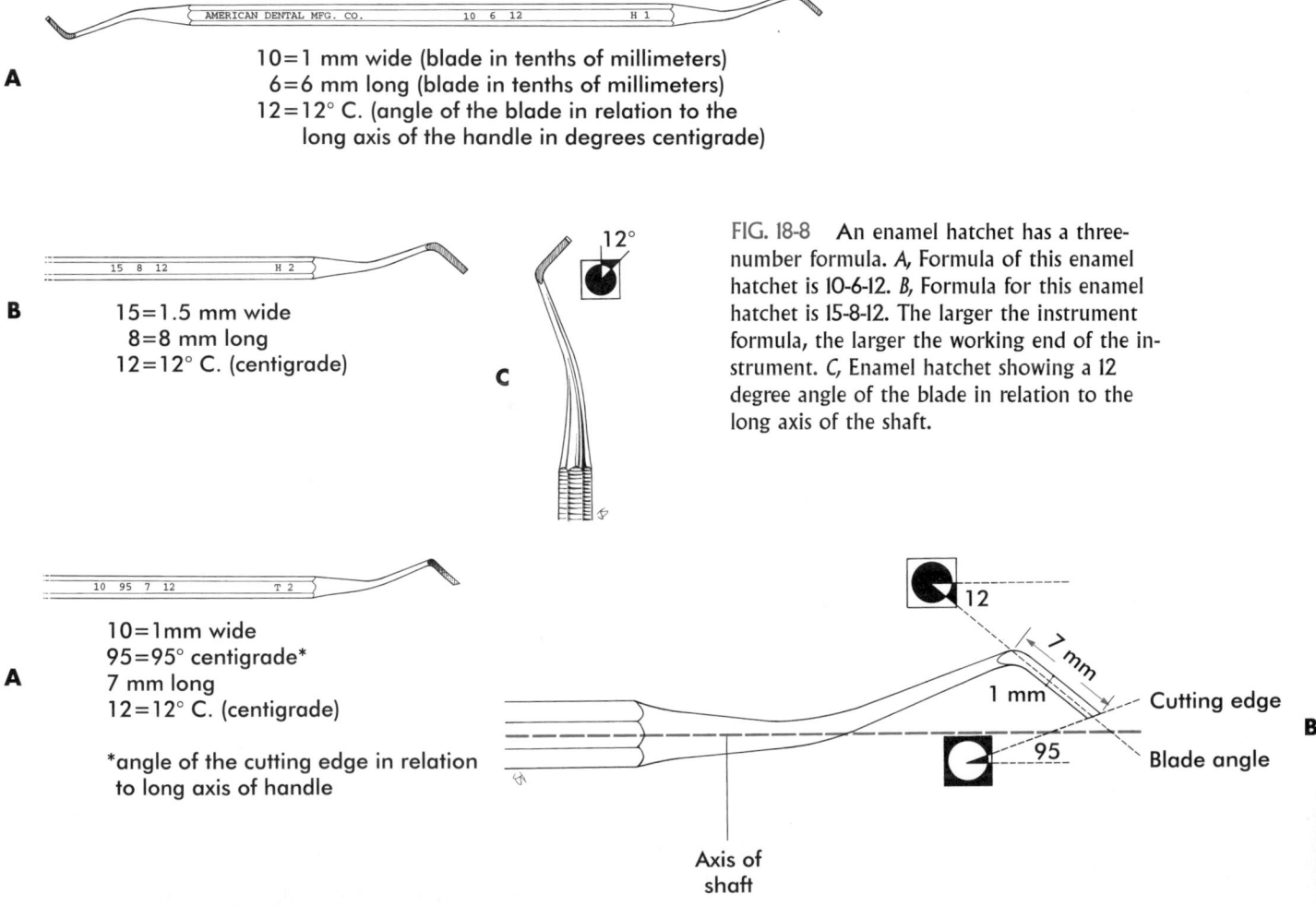

A

AMERICAN DENTAL MFG. CO.   10 6 12   H 1

10=1 mm wide (blade in tenths of millimeters)
6=6 mm long (blade in tenths of millimeters)
12=12° C. (angle of the blade in relation to the long axis of the handle in degrees centigrade)

B

15 8 12   H 2

15=1.5 mm wide
8=8 mm long
12=12° C. (centigrade)

C

12°

FIG. 18-8   An enamel hatchet has a three-number formula. *A,* Formula of this enamel hatchet is 10-6-12. *B,* Formula for this enamel hatchet is 15-8-12. The larger the instrument formula, the larger the working end of the instrument. *C,* Enamel hatchet showing a 12 degree angle of the blade in relation to the long axis of the shaft.

A

10 95 7 12   T 2

10=1mm wide
95=95° centigrade*
7 mm long
12=12° C. (centigrade)

*angle of the cutting edge in relation to long axis of handle

B

12

7 mm

1 mm   Cutting edge

95   Blade angle

Axis of shaft

FIG. 18-9   *A,* A distal gingival margin trimmer with a four-numbered formula 10-95-7-12. The additional number is placed in second position to denote the angle of the cutting edge. *B,* The 95 degree angle of the cutting edge is shown in relationship to the long axis of the shaft.

Two hand cutting instruments—the angle former and the gingival margin trimmer—have a four-number formula. Each of these instruments has a cutting edge that is at an angle to the blade. The additional number in the formula is used to describe the angle of the cutting edge in degrees centigrade in relation to the long axis of the handle. This additional number is placed in second position in the formula. Thus, the distal gingival margin trimmer, shown in Fig. 18-9, has the formula 10-95-7-12; the number 95 designates the angle of its cutting edge. In Fig. 18-10 the enamel hatchet with a straight cutting edge that has a three number instrument formula is compared with the gingival margin trimmer, with its angled cutting edge and four number formula.

The importance of learning an instrument formula can best be realized when sharpening dental instruments. Specific angles of cutting edges must be maintained.

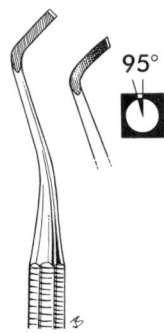

FIG. 18-10   The straight cutting edge of an enamel hatchet is compared with the angled cutting edge of a gingival margin trimmer.

Understanding this relationship will aid in restoring an accurate cutting edge to the instrument. Understanding the instrument formula will also aid in ordering replacement instruments. If the dentist wants a specific instrument and the dental assistant orders a new instrument from a different manufacturer, it may be necessary to request the instrument by its formula rather than number to obtain the exact instrument, since the manufacturer may use a special numbering system unique to its production.

▶ Instrument Number

The dental manufacturer provides an **instrument number** on each dental instrument that identifies the instrument for that manufacturer. The number correlates with the formula. Typically the higher the number, the larger the instrument size. In the case of hand cutting instruments, a correlation exists between the instrument number and the instrument formula. For instance, in Fig. 18-11 the *H-1* enamel hatchet has an instrument formula of 10-6-12 and the *H-2* has a formula of 15-8-12. With the *H-2* the length and width are both larger than the *H-1*.

Letter abbreviations are frequently used by manufacturers in the instrument number to indicate the name of the instrument. For instance, the *H* in the instrument *H-1* indicates that the instrument is a hatchet. Some of the following letters are used to quickly identify hand cutting instruments:

B   = Burnisher
BB   = Ball burnisher
CP   = Cavity preparation (some form of hand cutting instrument)
GF   = Gold foil
H   = Enamel hatchet
C or
CHI = Chisel
T   = Gingival margin trimmer
PLG = Plugger

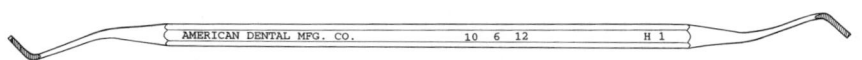

A

10=1 mm wide (blade in tenths of millimeters)
6=6 mm long (blade in tenths of millimeters)
12=12° C. (centigrade; angle of the blade in relation to the long axis of the handle in degrees centigrade)

FIG. 18-11   The instrument number correlates to the instrument formula. *A,* The H1 enamel hatchet has a formula 10-6-12, and *B,* the H2 15-8-12. The H2 is longer and wider than the H1.

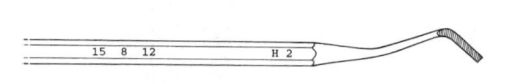

B

15=1.5 mm wide
8=8 mm long
12=12° C. (Angle of blade)

Classification of Dental Instruments

Another of G.V. Black's major contributions to operative dentistry was the classification of dental instruments. He classified instruments into six categories according to their function or use: cutting (hand and rotary); condensing; plastic; finishing and polishing (hand and rotary); isolation; and miscellaneous. Since many changes have taken place in the twentieth century, the list in Box 18-1 is a modification of these classifications representative of hand instruments commonly used in operative dentistry today. Technology moves at such a rapid pace that it is possible new categories can soon be added to this list. This classification should enable the assistant to review instruments according to their function and then identify them according to their physical characteristics.

Table 18-1 provides a descriptive overview of each of the instruments in each of these six categories. For any dental assistant the task of learning all of the dental instruments in the office seems overwhelming at first; however, this table, combined with a review of manufacturer catalogs and actual visualization of instruments in action will make this task easier.

▶ Examination Instruments

We have added the category of examination instruments to designate instruments used specifically for examining the teeth and oral tissues. Examination instruments may be used to examine the tooth or other structures during an initial oral diagnosis or after placing a restoration.

The explorer, mirror, and cotton pliers are three instruments that are basic to every dental procedure. These instruments are generally the first three instruments in sequence on most preset trays. The explorer and mirror are frequently used simultaneously during the examination of a tooth. Other examination instruments include the periodontal probe, an Expro, and the articulating paper forceps.

EXPLORER

An **explorer** is used to detect irregularities in the tooth or restorative surface, detect calculus or other anomalies during a scaling procedure, and aid in detecting carious lesions in the tooth surface. This instrument is most commonly a DE instrument, but it is also supplied as an SE instrument. The working ends of this instrument may be tapered, right angled, shaped like a shepherd's hook or a cow's horn, or may be any combination of these various shapes. The variations in shape aid the operator in gaining access to the various areas of the mouth. Each operator will have favorite explorers for various procedures, and the dental assistant should become familiar with the application of the various explorers that the operator may use. Fig. 18-12 illustrates several varieties of explorers. It is common today to find explorers with tip ends that are made of graphite for use with resin materials. The use of graphite eliminates marring or discoloring the restoration.

MIRROR

The **mouth mirror** is used to provide indirect vision; to provide indirect illumination to improve vision in the posterior of the mouth; and to retract the cheek, lip, and tongue (Fig. 18-13). Dental mirrors come in a variety of sizes ranging from ⅝ inch to 2 inches (Fig. 18-14).

Mirrors are provided in disposable styles, single or double sided, and are either flat surface, concave (providing magnification), or front surface, which has a reflecting surface on the front of the lens rather than on the back to eliminate ghostlike images. Nondisposable mirrors come with attached or cone socket handles.

BOX 18-1

CLASSIFICATION OF HAND INSTRUMENTS

EXAMINATION INSTRUMENTS

Explorer	Articulating paper forceps
Mirror	Probes
Cotton pliers	

CUTTING INSTRUMENTS

Angle former	Gingival marginal trimmer
Chisel	Hatchet
Excavator	Hoe

INSERTION/CONDENSING INSTRUMENTS

Plastic instrument	Condenser
Placement instrument	Gingival cord packer
Amalgam carrier	

CARVING INSTRUMENTS

Anatomic	Smooth surface

FINISHING AND POLISHING

Burnishers	Amalgam files
Orangewood stick	Knives
Finishing strips	

ADJUNCT

Thumb forceps	Pliers
Scissors	Spatulas
Dappen dishes	Matrices
Napkin chains	

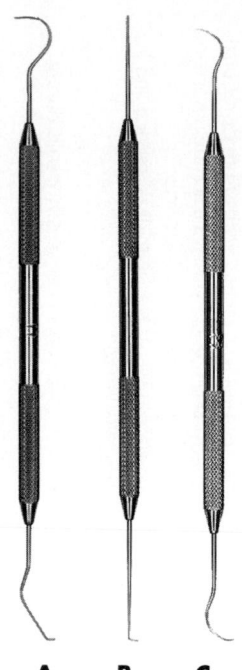

A   B   C

FIG. 18-12   *A,* Right angle shepherd's hook explorer. *B,* Right angle explorer. *C,* Cowhorn explorer.

(Courtesy of Hu-Friedy.)

TISSUE/COTTON PLIERS OR FORCEPS

Tissue forceps or cotton pliers are used to hold onto materials when transporting them from one place to another. Three types of pliers common to operative dentistry include the cotton or dressing pliers, articulating paper forceps, and thumb forceps (Fig. 18-15). The first two forceps are used intraorally, whereas the thumb forceps is used extraorally and is described in detail later in this chapter.

The standard cotton pliers or dressing pliers are used to transport materials into and out of the oral cavity. These instruments are used frequently during a cavity preparation to dry the cavity with cotton pellets, to transport medication on a cotton pellet to the preparation, or to carry other materials to the site. These pliers are supplied with serrated or smooth beaks, with or without a groove in the beak, and with plain or locking handles. The tips may be monangled or binangled.

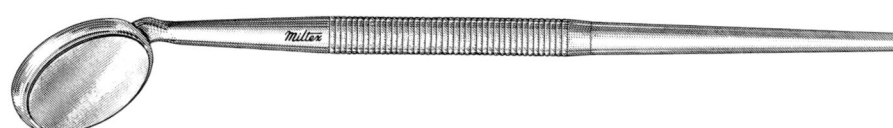

FIG. 18-13   Basic sterilizable front surface fiberglass dental mirror used for indirect vision, retraction, and illumination.

(Courtesy of Miltex.)

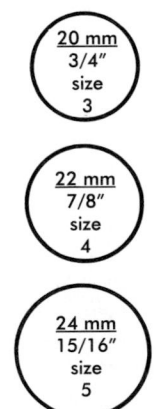

FIG. 18-14   Mirrors come in a variety of sizes.

(Courtesy of Miltex.)

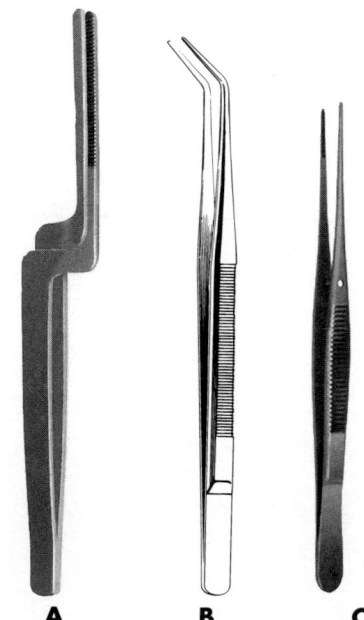

A   B   C

FIG. 18-15   *A,* Articulating paper holder. *B,* Cotton pliers. *C,* Thumb forceps.

(Courtesy of Hu-Friedy.)

TABLE 18-1 INSTRUMENT CLASSIFICATION*

Instrument/device	Physical characteristics	Function
EXAMINATION INSTRUMENTS		
Explorer	DE or SE: Sharp pointed working end; common shapes cowhorn, right angle, and shepherd's hook; graphite tip available / Endodontic explorer has elongated working ends; Expro is combination explorer and periodontal probe	Detects tooth anomalies; checks margins of restorations; detects calculus
Mirror	SE: Disposable or nondisposable; regular or cone socket handle; single or double sided; flat or concave face; width 7/8 to 2 inches / Ruler calibration on handle available	Indirect vision; indirect illumination; retraction of cheek, lips, tongue
Tissue/cotton/pliers	SE: Serrated or smooth beaks, pointed beaks; locking or nonlocking; angled beaks	Grasp oral tissues; transfer materials into and out of oval cavity
Articulating paper forceps	Groove in center of beak for grasping endodontic points / SE: Locking pliers; beak parallel to handle	Grasps and holds articulating paper for insertion into oral cavity
Probe	DE or SE: Pointed working end; calibrated in mm of various combinations / May have color-coded mm markings; Expro is combination of explorer and periodontal probe	Measure depth of gingival sulcus
CUTTING INSTRUMENTS		
Angle former	DE or SE: Modification of a chisel; supplied in right and left; cutting edge at angle to blade; commonly beveled on side of blade, as well as on end	Defines line angles, places retention in dentin and bevels on enamel margins in cavity preparation
Chisel	DE or SE: Standard or reverse bevel; cutting edge is at right angle to plane of instrument; Wedelstaedt chisel has curved blade	Planes and cleaves enamel and dentin walls during cavity preparation
Excavator	DE or SE: Spoon-shaped blade that is rounded; wide range of sizes; curved blade	Removes soft carious debris from cavity preparation; places cavity medication; inverts rubber dam into gingival sulcus
Gingival marginal trimmer	DE or SE: Instrument supplied as mesial for distal; each has a right and left end; angled cutting edge; curved blade	Places bevel at mesial or distal cervical and pulpal margins
Hatchet	DE or SE: Paired right and left; cutting edge in same plane as the instrument	Prepares retention, sharpens internal line angles, and smooths internal cavity walls during tooth preparation
Hoe	DE or SE: Cutting edge at right angle to blade; blade at nearly right angle to handle; commonly triple angle shank	Creates retention form in dentin; used with pull action
CONDENSING/INSERTION INSTRUMENTS		
Plastic instruments	DE or SE: Plastic or metal; tip ends have various shapes—round, flat, or paddle-like; special modifications	Place composite restorative material or dental cements into cavity preparation

Instrument	Description	Function
Amalgam carrier	DE or SE: Mini to large end; plastic or metal; metal or Teflon ends; carrier or gun style; retrograde for endodontic filling	Transports amalgam to cavity preparation
Condenser/plugger	DE: Smooth or serrated ends; flat or concave; square or ovoid ends; plain or tapered ends; monangle, binangle or triple angle shank	Condenses amalgam into compact mass; removes excess mercury; adapts amalgam to cavity walls
Gingival cord placement instruments	DE: Thin blade; resembles condenser; plain or serrated tip end	Place gingival retraction cord into gingival sulcus
Placement instrument	SE: Small ball burnisher type working end; shorter handle than traditional instruments; delicate working end	Places cavity medications
CARVING INSTRUMENTS		
Anatomic	DE: Disk or claw-like end; rounded or spoon shape	Recreate anatomic form in occlusal surface of amalgam restoration
Smooth surface	DE: Flat, elongated knifelike blade	Contour buccal, lingual, and proximal surfaces of amalgam restoration
FINISHING AND POLISHING		
Burnishers	DE or SE: Flat, pointed or circular rounded ends	Burnish or polish hardened metallic surfaces and cavosurface margins, refine anatomy
Orangewood stick/points	Sticks, pegs, or points; soft splinter-proof wood	Sticks or pegs aid in seating restoration such as crowns, bridges, or inlays; soft points used to polish teeth
Finishing strips	Linen or metal; extra fine to coarse grit; narrow to wide width	Polish or finish interproximal tooth or restorative surfaces
ADJUNCT INSTRUMENTS		
Thumb forceps	Straight beak	Aids in maintaining aseptic working area; transfers materials to operative site from clean area; used extraorally only
Scissors	Many variations: Straight or curved; sharp or blunt tips; suture, surgical, tissue, bandage, crown and collar	Cut tissue, sutures, or a variety of materials
Dappen dish	Metal or glass; single or double ended; concave ends	Holding device for medicaments and various dental materials
Napkin chain	Alligator-like beaks for holding; metal or plastic	Hold patient napkin in place; holds materials
Spatulas	Various shaped blades: Flat, curved, or pointed; narrow or wide; flexible or rigid; all metal or combination metal blade with wooden or plastic handle	Mix plaster or cements; carve wax or porcelain
Matrix	Plastic, celluloid, or metal strips; various widths; curved or straight; modifications in shapes	Provides missing wall when placing restorative material

*The instruments are displayed throughout the chapter.

ARTICULATING FORCEPS

The **articulating paper forceps** has one primary purpose and that is simply to hold articulating paper. This forceps is supplied with smooth or serrated beaks and a handle that, when depressed, enables the assistant to place a piece of articulating paper into the beaks. When pressure is released from the handle, the articulating paper is firmly held by the beaks. This feature enables the dental assistant to place the paper in and remove it from the mouth several times without readjusting the position of the paper. This is especially helpful during an examination of the occlusion that requires repeated use of the articulating paper.

PERIODONTAL PROBE

The **periodontal probe** is used to measure the depth of the gingival sulcus or periodontal pockets. Various styles of probes are illustrated in Fig. 18-16. The working end of each of these probes is calibrated in millimeters at varying intervals to facilitate the reading of depth measurements. Periodontal probes are available in a variety of calibrations, including 1-2-3-5-7-8-9-10, 3-6-8, 3-6-9-12, 3-5-8-10, or even 3.5-5.5-8.5-11.5. Periodontal probes are often given the name of a dental school or of the person who developed the probe, such as the University of Michigan's O probe or the Merrit, Naber, Goldman-Fox, or Cattoni probe. Many companies now provide color-coded tips that enhance the readings. The color coding is durable and does not wear down, chip, flake, or fade during routine sterilization processes.

EXPRO

An Expro is simply a combination instrument of the various features of an explorer and a periodontal probe. Fig. 18-17 illustrates several Expro combinations. The operator may use one end of the instrument as an explorer and the opposite end as a periodontal probe.

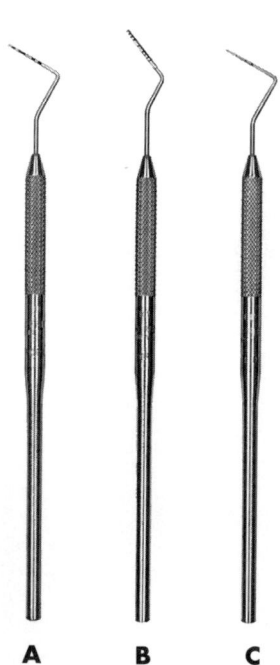

FIG. 18-16   *A* through *C,* Various styles of periodontal probes.

(Courtesy of Hu-Friedy.)

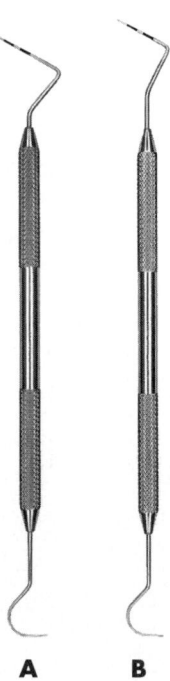

FIG. 18-17   *A* and *B,* Two styles of Explorer-probe Expro instruments.

(Courtesy of Hu-Friedy.)

❱ Hand Cutting Instruments

The **hand cutting instruments** are used for cutting or removing hard tooth tissue. The functions of these instruments generally include shaping cavity walls, floors, and line and point angles during cavity preparation by planing, cleaving, or laterally scraping the tooth structure. These instruments may also be used to remove carious tooth tissue. Hand cutting instruments typically include angle formers, chisels, hatchets, spoon excavators, and gingival margin trimmers. In recent years, rotary instruments have gained wide use in cutting tooth tissue during cavity preparation, and consequently some dental schools rely less on teaching the use of hand cutting instruments during basic restorative dentistry.

ENAMEL HATCHET

Commonly called a hatchet, this instrument is used primarily to prepare retentive areas, sharpen internal line angles, and smooth internal cavity walls. The cutting edge of this instrument is in the same plane as the instrument.

This instrument is paired *right* and *left,* with the blades beveled on opposite sides to form the cutting edges. In a DE instrument, one end is *right* and the opposite end is *left.* If SE instruments are to be used, both a right and left hatchet would be required to complete the pair. During a cavity preparation the operator will need to use both ends of the instrument to plane or cleave the enamel and dentin walls of both sides of a cavity preparation. Fig. 18-18 illustrates how this instrument might be positioned to smooth the internal walls on both sides of the cavity preparation. To determine the correct side of the instrument, hold the instrument in a pen grasp with the working end of the instrument positioned to be used on the mandible. If the cutting edge is to the patient's left, that side of the instrument is the *left* end of the instrument; if the cutting edge is to the patient's right, that end of the instrument is the *right* end of the instrument. Since the operator will reverse the ends of the instrument during use, the dental assistant does not need to give special attention to which end is passed first.

FIG. 18-18   Enamel hatchet positioned in cavity preparation. The enamel hatchet in *A* is being used to remove underminded proximal enamel on the right side. *B,* Left side of the mandibular, right first premolar. The instrument is used first on one end, then reversed in the operator's hand for the opposite side.

(From Sturdevant CM: *The art and science of operative dentistry,* ed 2, St Louis, 1985, Mosby.)

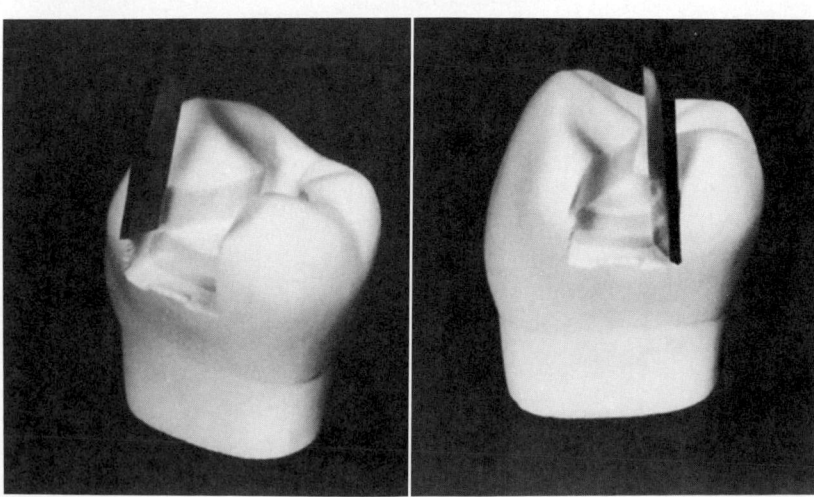

A   B

CHISEL

The **chisel**, like the enamel hatchet, is used to plane and cleave the enamel and dentin walls of the cavity preparation. However, unlike the hatchet, the chisel has a cutting edge that is at a right angle to the plane of the instrument. Common chisels are monangled or binangled. A popular chisel, the Wedelstaedt chisel, shown in Fig. 18-19 has no sharp monangle, but rather a curve in the blade.

Unlike the enamel hatchet, which has a right and left end, the chisel has a standard and reversed bevel. In a DE instrument the end that has the cutting edge distal to the shaft is the *reverse* or *contra-beveled* end and the end with the cutting edge nearest or mesial to the shaft is the standard end, as in Fig. 18-20. The chisel is used by the operator with a push action.

HOE

A hoe is actually a chisel whose blade is at nearly a right angle or greater than 12.5° C, as shown in Fig. 18-21. A chisel is used with a push action, but the hoe is used with a pull action, like that of a garden hoe. A hoe functions to create retentive form in dentin.

ANGLE FORMER

The **angle former** was described earlier as one of the instruments with a four number instrument formula. It has a cutting edge that is sharpened at an angle to the axis of the blade. This instrument is a modification of a chisel, with an angled cutting edge. The angle former is supplied as a *right* and *left* and takes its identification from the location of the acute cutting angle, as illustrated in Fig. 18-22. The angle former is used to define line angles, place retentive form in dentin, and aid in placing bevels on enamel margins. In offices where cohesive gold restorations are placed, this instrument will be used frequently to provide retention in these particular cavity preparations. Commonly this instrument is beveled on the sides, as well as the end, providing three separate cutting edges. This is a characteristic also found in chisels and hoes.

GINGIVAL MARGIN TRIMMER

The **gingival margin trimmer** is used primarily to place bevels at the cervical cavosurface margins when preparing a tooth to receive an amalgam and certain types of cast gold inlay restorations. As the angle former is a

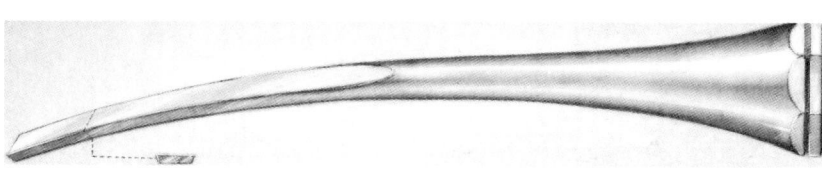

FIG. 18-19   Wedelstaedt chisel.

FIG. 18-20   *A,* The chisel has a standard and reverse bevel; the standard end is shown in *A. B,* The reversed end of the chisel is shown here. The opposite end is the standard end.

(From Sturdevant CM: *The art and science of operative dentistry,* ed 2, St Louis, 1985, Mosby.)

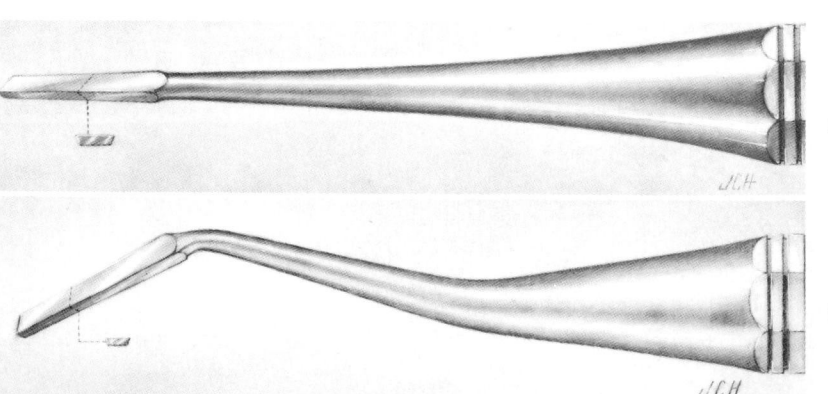

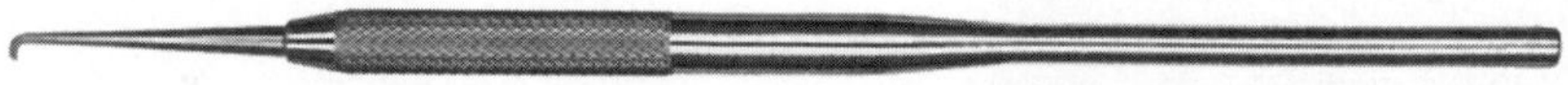

A

B

FIG. 18-21   Dental hoe.

(Courtesy of Hu-Friedy.)

modification of the chisel, the gingival margin trimmer is a modification of the enamel hatchet. Like the enamel hatchet, this instrument has a *right* and *left* end.

There are two distinct differences between the enamel hatchet and the gingival margin trimmer. First, the gingival margin trimmer is doubled planed, that is, it has a curved blade. The second difference is its angled cutting edge. This comparison was made with the enamel hatchet, in Fig. 18-11, when the two types of instrument formulas were discussed. The angled cutting edge of the gingival margin trimmer provides for the placement of bevels at the mesial or distal cervical margins. This feature requires that the cutting edge be angled either for the mesial or distal margins. Conse-

quently, a single DE instrument will be either a *mesial* or *distal* trimmer. The mesial trimmer has an acute angle of the cutting edge nearest the shaft, and the distal trimmer has the acute angle of the cutting edge farthest or distal to the shaft, as shown in Fig. 18-23. It is important for the assistant to learn the difference between these two instruments, as only the appropriate instrument will be passed to the operator, depending on the location of the cavity preparation. For instance, in a cavity preparation on 29MO, the mesial trimmer would be passed, on 29DO, the distal trimmer would be used, and if 29^{MOD} were being treated, both trimmers would be used. Fig. 18-24, *A* and *B*, illustrates the gingival margin trimmer being used in a cavity preparation.

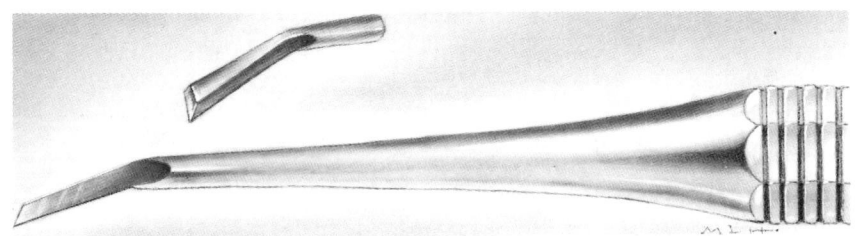

FIG. 18-22   An angle former.

(From Sturdevant CM: *The art and science of operative dentistry*, ed 2, St Louis, 1985, Mosby.)

FIG. 18-23   *A*, Mesial gingival margin trimmers. *B*, Distal gingival margin trimmer.

(Courtesy of Hu-Friedy.)

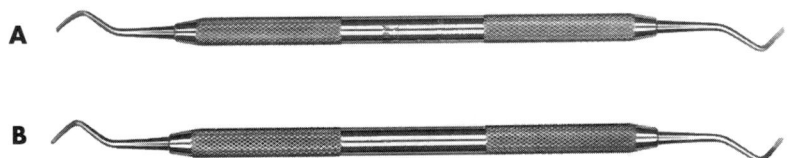

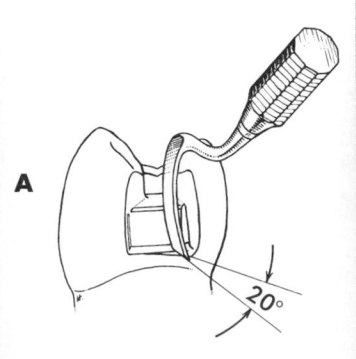

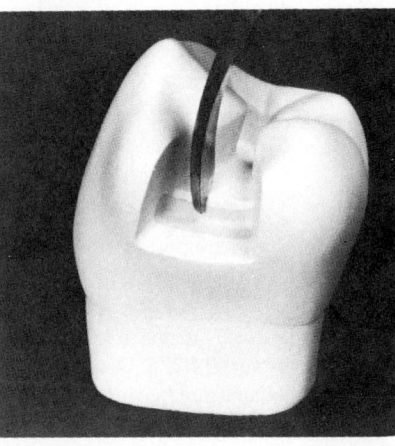

FIG. 18-24   Gingival margin trimmer being used in a cavity preparation. *A*, Sharp angles of the linguogingival and buccogingival corners are rounded with a rotational sweep of gingival margin trimmer. *B*, Beveling the axiopulpal line angle with a gingival margin trimmer.

(Courtesy of Sturdevant CM: *The art and science of operative dentistry*, ed 2, St Louis, 1985, Mosby.)

SPOON EXCAVATOR

The **spoon excavator** has the distinction of being unlike all of the other cutting instruments in that it has a rounded cutting edge and consequently does not fit neatly into the G.V. Black instrument formula. The primary function of the excavator is for removal of soft carious debris from the tooth, but its use extends far beyond its original design. This instrument can be used for carving amalgam and wax patterns, placing cavity medication, and inverting rubber dam material into the gingival sulcus. Most dental manufacturers make a wide range of sizes and designs, ranging from a most delicate instrument to one that could be used for gross removal of amalgam during a carving procedure (Fig. 18-25).

▶ Condensing/Insertion Instruments

Condensing/insertion instruments are most frequently used to insert dental restorative materials into the cavity preparation. Commonly these instruments are used to place amalgam, composite, or dental cements into the tooth. Those used to place amalgam include the amalgam carrier, which transports the material to the cavity preparation, and the condensers or pluggers, which then are used to condense the material into the preparation.

PLASTIC INSTRUMENTS

Plastic instruments are used to insert composite restorative materials or dental cements. They are called plastic instruments because they are used with plastic or moldable materials. Although they are referred to as plastic instruments because of their function, these instruments are made of plastic and metal. Typically the ends of plastic instruments are shaped with flat, paddle-like blades or nibs (Fig. 18-26).

FIG. 18-26   Example of a plastic instrument.

AMALGAM CARRIER

The **amalgam carrier** may be an SE or a DE instrument and is supplied as a standard carrier or an amalgam gun (Fig. 18-27). The ends of this instrument vary in size from a mini end to a large end. The larger the end opening, the more amalgam can be transported to the cavity preparation. Many operators prefer a DE instrument with variably sized ends. The assistant's primary responsibility is to load the instrument with amalgam, place it into the prepared tooth, and make certain no amalgam remains in the tip end to harden.

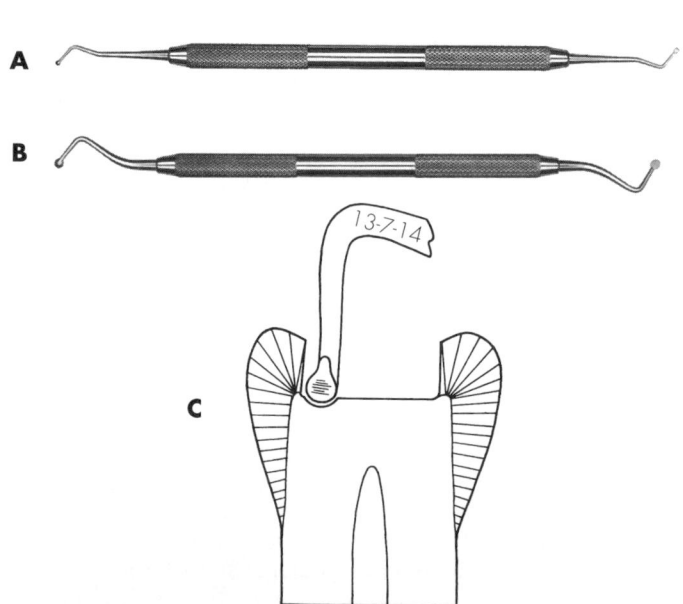

FIG. 18-25   A, A small delicate spoon excavator. B, Larger spoon excavator. C, Spoon being used in a cavity preparation.

(A and B courtesy of Hu-Friedy; C from Sturdevant CM: *The art and science of operative dentistry,* ed 2, St Louis, 1985, Mosby.)

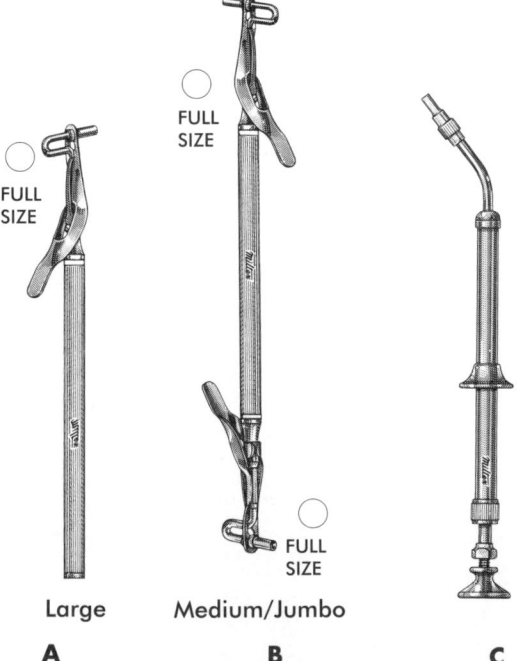

FIG. 18-27   Various amalgam carriers. A, Single-ended amalgam carrier 71-52. B, Double-ended amalgam carrier 71-64. C, Amalgam gun/syringe 71-92.

(Courtesy of Miltex.)

CONDENSERS OR PLUGGERS

Condensers or **pluggers** are used to adapt the amalgam to the cavity walls, condense the amalgam into a compact mass, and aid in removing excess mercury from the mass. A wide range of condensers are available, since so many variables exist in gaining access to the preparation. Manufacturers have designed condensers with concave ovoid shapes to condense amalgam into a Class V preparation and even a back action condenser that allows the operator to easily condense amalgam into a distal surface on the tooth, pushing from the posterior to the anterior (or from the back to the front).

The tip end of the condenser/plugger may be smooth or serrated; flat or concave; round, square, or ovoid in shape; and the shank may be monangled, binangled, or triple angled; and may be tapered or plain. Several of these variables are shown in Fig. 18-28.

PLACEMENT INSTRUMENT

A placement instrument, such as a calcium hydroxide placer, is often considered a plastic instrument, since it is used to place a cavity liner. This small ball-burnisher–type instrument is often used to place cavity liners in the prepared tooth. An example of this instrument is shown in Fig. 18-29. It is especially useful because it is small, is easy to use to mix a paste type liner, and can be passed to the operator for easy placement of the liner.

GINGIVAL CORD PLACEMENT INSTRUMENT

The **gingival cord placement** instrument is used when placing gingival retraction cord into the sulcus around the tooth before taking a final impression. The tip ends of these instruments are generally thin for easy access to the sulcus and may be plain or serrated. Fig. 18-30 illustrates this instrument being used to place retraction cord.

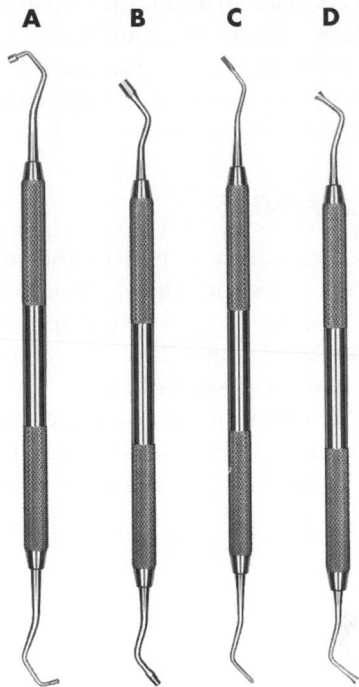

FIG. 18-28   Various amalgam condensers. *A*, Back action, triple angle shank. *B*, Serrated. *C*, Ovoid. *D*, Smooth surface amalgam condenser.

(Courtesy of Hu-Friedy.)

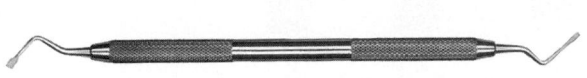

FIG. 18-29   Placement instrument.

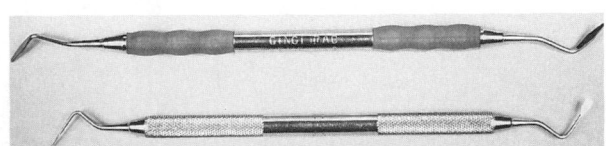

FIG. 18-30   Gingival cord placement instruments.

(Courtesy of Hu-Friedy.)

▶ Carving Instruments

Carving instruments, whether being used to carve amalgam or wax, generally are classified into two categories: anatomic and smooth surface carvers. The anatomic carvers place anatomy, pit, and fissures into the occlusal surface, while the smooth surface carvers remove the excess from the mesial, distal, buccal, and lingual surfaces of the tooth and contour these surfaces to normal anatomic shape.

ANATOMIC CARVERS

The cleoid-discoid carver is one of the most popular anatomic carvers; it is sometimes classified as a spoon excavator because it has a spoonlike shape. Typically, the cleoid end is clawlike and the discoid end is more rounded, resembling a disk (Fig. 18-31). This instrument is a widely used instrument for recreating anatomic grooves in the occlusal surface of an amalgam restoration and may also be used for burnishing inlay margins.

SMOOTH SURFACE CARVERS

Like the anatomic carvers, an abundance of designs of **smooth surface carvers** is available. Among the oldest and most popular are the Wards, Hollenback, and Walls carvers (Fig. 18-32, *A* through *C*). Each of these has a flat, elongated knife-like blade that is used to contour the buccal, lingual, and proximal surfaces.

Like many other instruments designed by dental schools and pioneers in restorative dentistry, many variations exist in anatomic carvers, including the Woodson, Andrews, Hollenback, and Tanner, as well as interproximal style carvers as shown in Fig. 18-32, *D* through *F*.

▶ Finishing and Polishing Instruments

Finishing and **polishing instruments** are used to smooth, burnish, and polish restorations. Finishing and polishing instruments can be manual or rotary. As new restorative materials are developed, this category of instruments continues to expand.

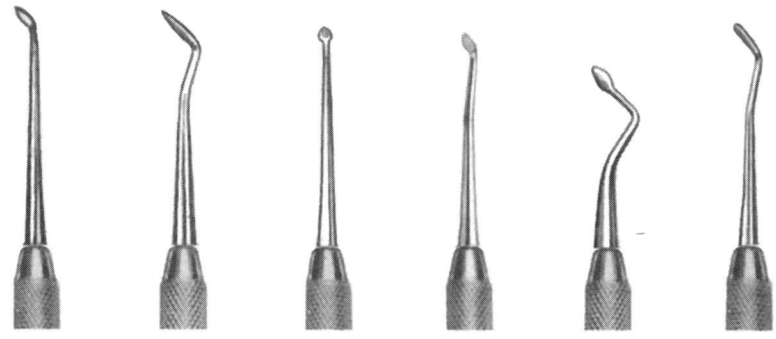

FIG. 18-31   Various cleoid discoid carvers.
(Courtesy of Hu-Friedy.)

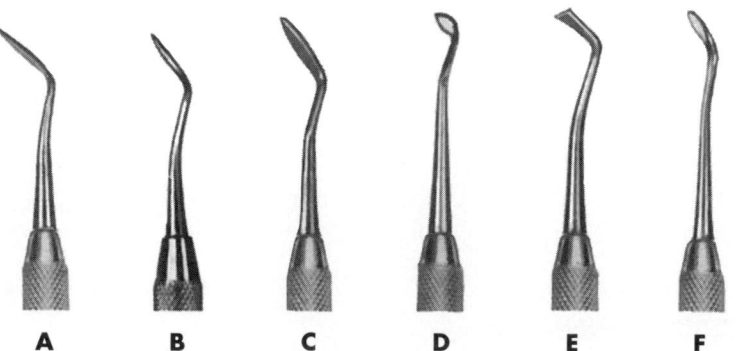

A   B   C   D   E   F

FIG. 18-32   Variations in smooth surface carvers. *A*, Ward's. *B*, Hollenback. *C*, Wall's. Variations in anatomic carvers. *D*, Andrew's. *E*, Hollenback. *F*, Tanner.
(Courtesy of Hu-Friedy.)

❱ Burnishers

A **burnisher** is an instrument that is shaped with rounded edges and is used to burnish or polish and work harden metallic surfaces, such as amalgam or gold. Several popular shapes include the straight, ball, T-ball, football, beaver-tail, or fishtail burnisher, as shown in Fig. 18-33. Burnishers may be SE or DE instruments; many of the basic burnishers are found in combination with each other as DE instruments.

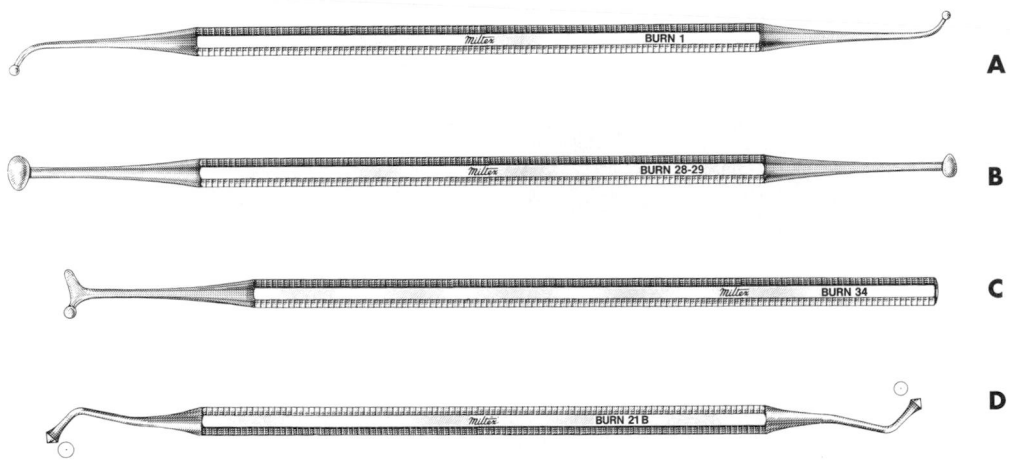

FIG. 18-33   Various burnishers. *A,* Ball. *B,* Football. *C,* T-ball/beavertail. *D,* Anatomic. (Courtesy of Miltex.)

ORANGEWOOD POINTS OR STICKS

Orangewood points or sticks serve multiple purposes in dentistry. They may be used to check occlusal relations or to aid in seating a crown or bridge (Fig. 18-34). The soft wood makes it a desirable device for intraoral use because it does not splinter and can withstand great pressure. A variation of the orangewood stick is an orangewood point that can be used in a porte polisher. The soft orangewood makes it a desirable device for polishing teeth because it is soft, resists splintering, and creates a highly polished tooth surface.

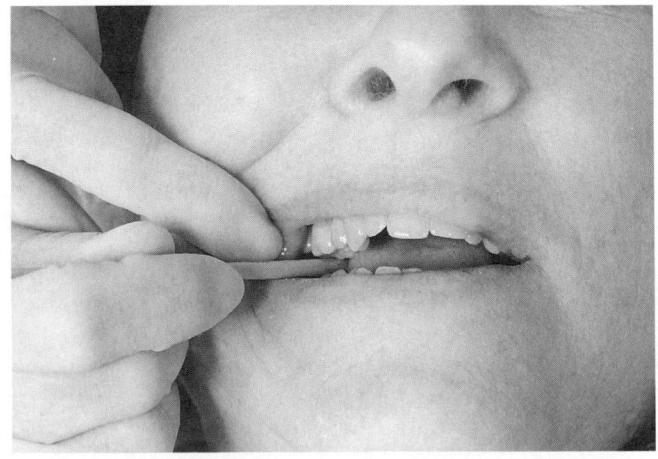

FIG. 18-34   Orangewood stick being used in the mouth.

FINISHING STRIPS

A **polishing strip** is a ribbonlike piece of linen of varying lengths and widths on which one side has some form of abrasive particles of grit bonded to it. These strips are especially helpful in contouring and polishing proximal surfaces of various types of restorations (Fig. 18-35). To avoid abrading the restoration when inserting this strip at the interproximal, each strip is designed with a nonabrasive area at the midpoint.

A similar strip is a lightening or separating strip which is made of steel with an abrasive on one side (Fig. 18-36). This heavy duty strip is used to open rough or improper contact of proximal restorations or to begin the reduction of proximal excess in amalgam or cohesive gold restorations.

AMALGAM FILES

Amalgam files are supplied in various sizes and shapes and are designed with a tip end that has numerous ridges or teeth on the cutting surfaces. They are used to smooth or reduce metallic restorations. The delicate tip of most designs makes this a useful instrument in removing excess amalgam or gold at gingival margins. The Rhein and Wedelstaedt trimmers are popular examples of this instrument (Fig. 18-37).

KNIVES

Gold, amalgam, and composite **knives** (Fig. 18-38) are designed with angular, knifelike cutting edges for use in trimming excess filling material. Supplied as an SE or DE instrument, these knives work effectively in hardened restorative material but require caution when used to remove the excess material.

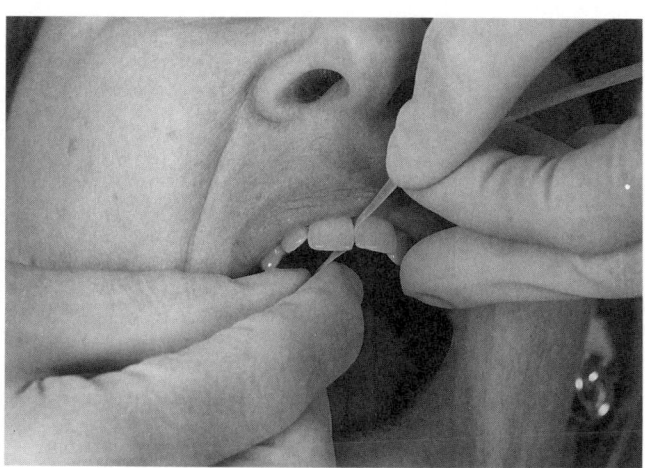

FIG. 18-35   Linen strip being used to polish interproximal surface.

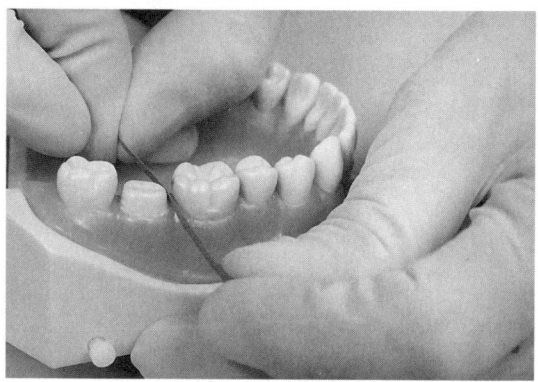

FIG. 18-36   Lightning strip.

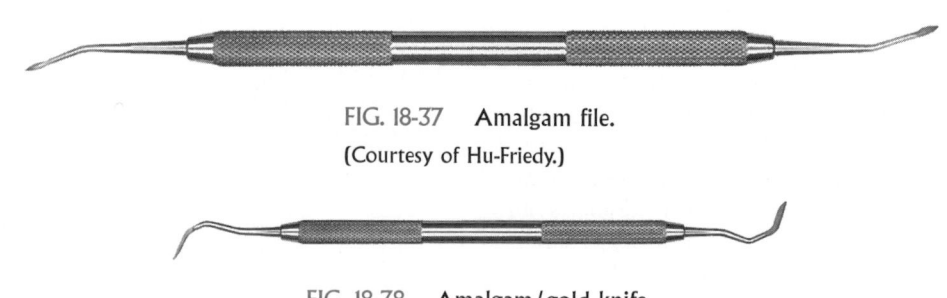

FIG. 18-37   Amalgam file.
(Courtesy of Hu-Friedy.)

FIG. 18-38   Amalgam/gold knife.
(Courtesy of Hu-Friedy.)

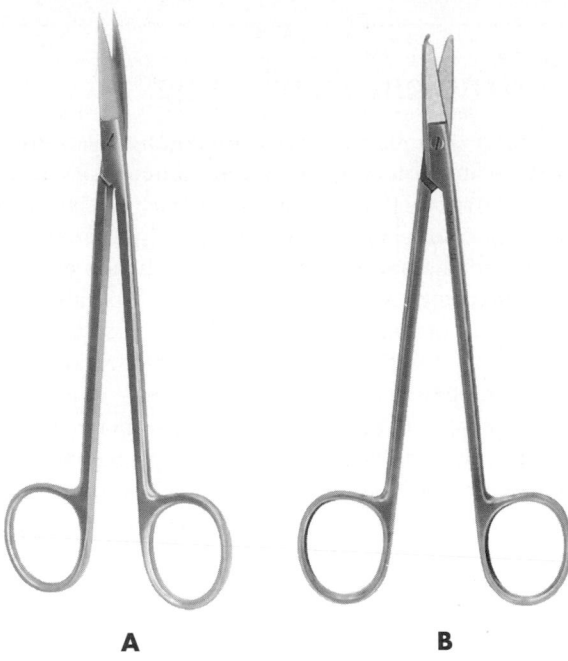

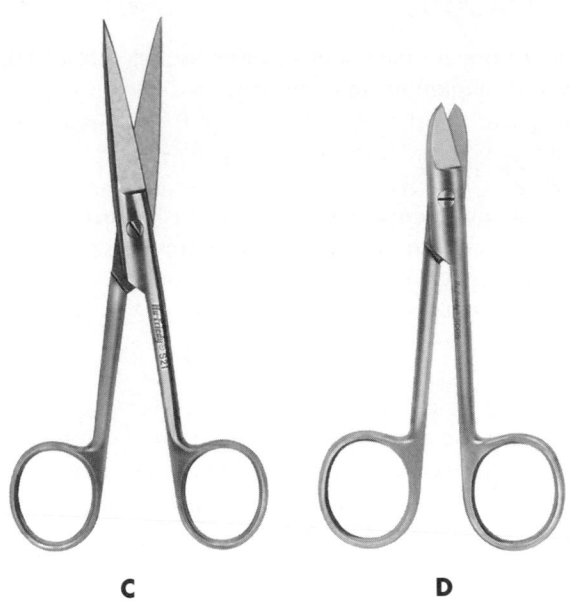

A   **B**   **C**   **D**

FIG. 18-39   Various styles of scissors. *A*, Curved. *B*, Suture. *C*, Surgical. *D*, Crown and collar.

(Courtesy of Hu-Friedy.)

▶ Adjunct Instruments

A variety of adjunct instruments are available in dentistry today. It is impossible to introduce all of them, but in this chapter the dental assistant will be introduced to many of the basic instruments familiar to most dental practices.

THUMB FORCEPS

The **thumb forceps** was mentioned earlier in this chapter when discussing the basic types of forceps that are used in dentistry. The thumb forceps is used outside the oral cavity, most commonly to enter a cabinet to retrieve an instrument for use on the tray setup. The thumb forceps shown in Fig. 18-15 is straight and has no angled beaks; thus, it would not be conveniently used in the mouth.

SCISSORS

The various categories of **scissors** include (Fig. 18-39) tissue scissors, with fine delicate beaks; suture scissors, with special beak configurations for cutting a suture; bandage scissors, with a beak for grasping tape; crown and collar scissors, with blunted beaks that are designed to cut metallic crowns and other devices during routine operative dentistry. Take special care to avoid interchanging the use of these instruments, since scissors specifically designed to cut soft tissue should maintain the sharp cutting edge and not be dulled by cutting other substances.

DAPPEN DISHES

The **dappen dishes** are small holding devices that are made of metal or glass, as shown in Fig. 18-40. Their primary function is to hold medicaments or solutions, such as disclosing solution or polishing paste. A modification of a dappen dish, called an amalgam well, is designed with a weighted nonslip base and is used for handling amalgam while filling an amalgam carrier (Fig. 18-41).

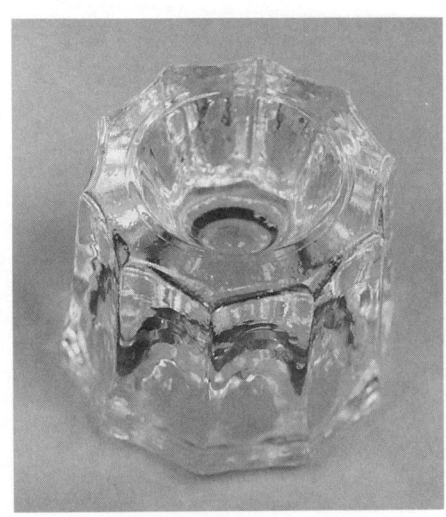

FIG. 18-40   Glass dappen dish.

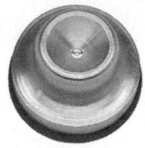

FIG. 18-41   Amalgam well.

(Courtesy of Hu-Friedy.)

NAPKIN CHAINS

Napkin chains are basic devices that are used to attach a protective napkin around the patient's neck.

SPATULAS

In the chapter on dental materials, various **spatulas** were introduced for mixing various dental materials. Here, the most common styles—cement, plaster or gypsum, and impression spatulas—are presented.

Cement Spatulas

Cement spatulas are single ended and most commonly made of stainless steel. They include small and large flexible spatulas that are used for mixing cements that require a rotary type action and a larger, more rigid spatula that is used with dental cements which require greater force in mixing and a folding and packing action (Fig. 18-42, *A*).

Impression and Laboratory Spatulas

Impression and laboratory spatulas are used to mix impression materials. An assortment shown in Fig. 18-42, *B*, illustrates the difference in these spatulas compared with the cement spatulas. In general, these instruments are bulkier and have wider blades, which may be rigid or flexible. The broader, flexible spatulas enable the assistant to easily mix alginate impression material in a flexible rubber bowl. The more rigid spatulas can be used for mixing impression materials on paper pads or for mixing gypsum material in the laboratory.

MATRICES

A **matrix** is a device that is used during a restorative procedure to replace a missing proximal wall or tooth structure. The two basic styles that are commonly used are made of metal or celluloid. Two styles of metal matrices include the circumferential and the noncircumferential, shown in Fig. 18-43. In Chapter 27 the various applications of these matrices are described in detail. The application of the celluloid matrix is described in Chapter 28.

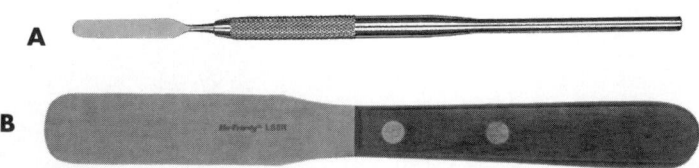

FIG. 18-42 *A,* Cement spatula. *B,* Plaster spatula.
(Courtesy of Hu-Friedy.)

Instrument Sharpening

Using a dull instrument in the oral cavity can damage tissues and potentially create an unnecessary accident. A dull instrument requires excess force to be applied when cutting enamel and dentin and risks potential damage to the hard and soft tissues. Dull, roughened cutting edges on instruments do not allow the operator to make efficient cuts on the tooth or, in the case of a scaler, do not allow for thorough removal of hardened calculus. Chisels, hatchets, spoon excavators, gingival margin trimmers, and scalers are all instruments that should receive routine sharpening. When an instrument is not cutting effectively, it should receive prompt attention.

Learning to sharpen instruments is another important task for a dental assistant, which can be assigned to a tickler/reminder file and can be done on a day when patients are not scheduled in the office. Regular and routine sharpening of instruments can ensure safety during the use of any of these cutting instruments.

Various devices are available for use in sharpening instruments, including an electric oscillating instrument sharpener (Fig. 18-44), an assortment of flat, conical, or cylindric stones (Fig. 18-45) in various grits, and similar types of mounted stones (Fig. 18-46) for use in a handpiece. A sharpening oil is applied to the surface of most of these stones to prevent frictional heat, which could temper the metal. The oil also aids in washing away metal particles (Fig. 18-47).

To become proficient at instrument sharpening will take some time and experience. It is not possible in this brief discussion to provide techniques for sharpening each of the cutting instruments and scalers, but hopefully this discussion will whet your appetite for practicing this skill.

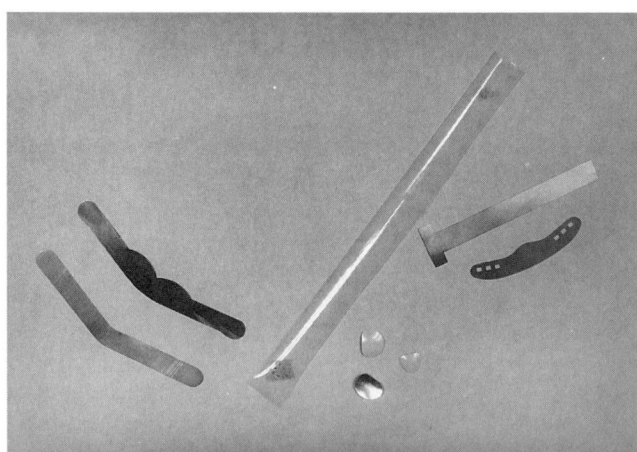

FIG. 18-43 Assorted matrices.

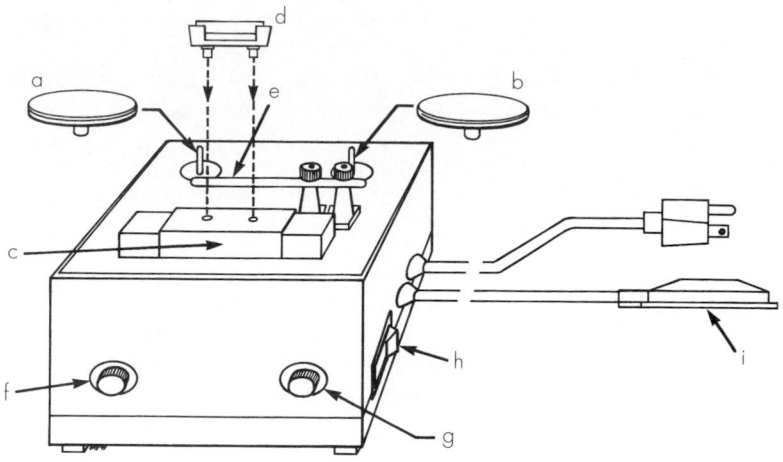

FIG. 18-44   Electronic instrument sharpener.

(From Sturdevant CM: *The art and science of operative dentistry,* ed 2, St Louis, 1985, Mosby.)

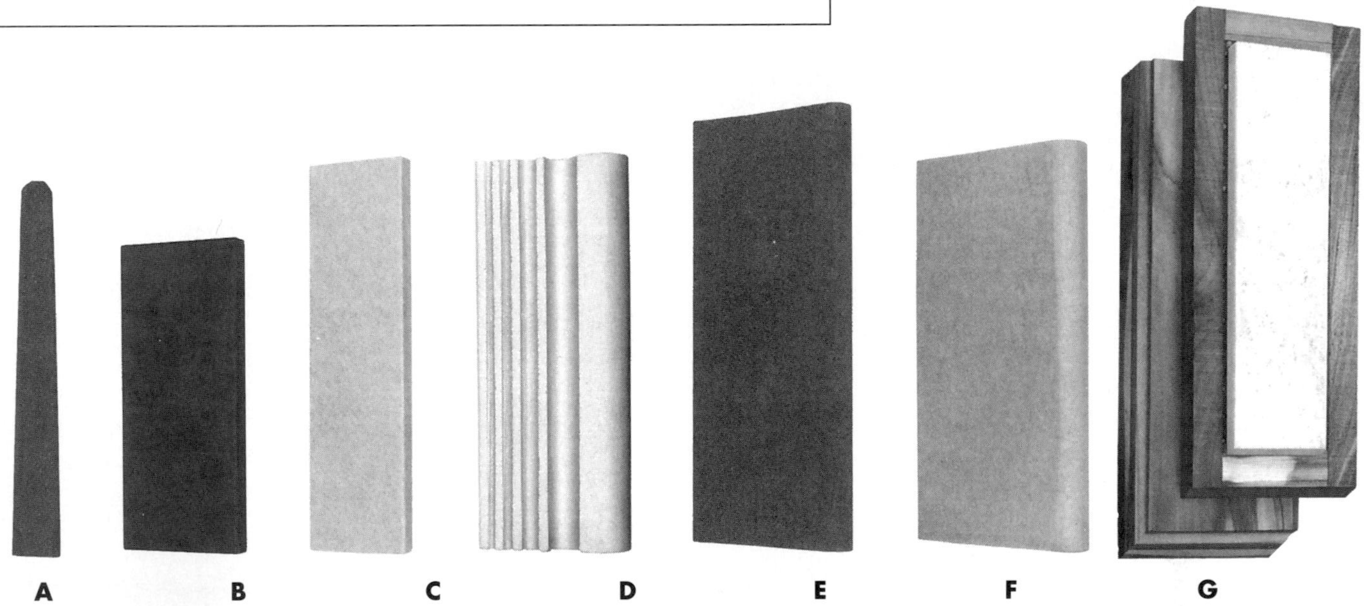

A   **B**   **C**   **D**   **E**   **F**   **G**

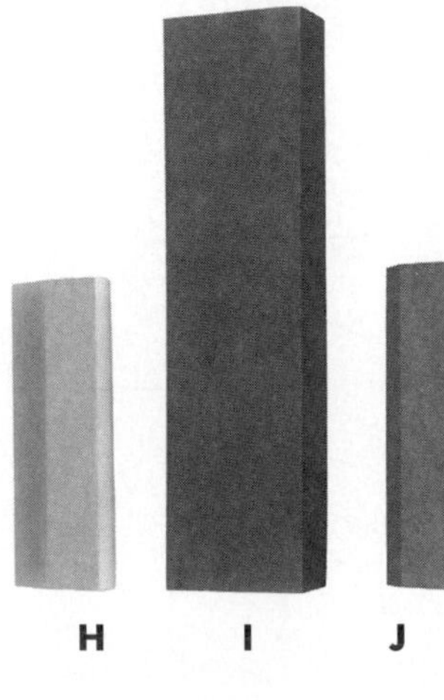

FIG. 18-45   *A* through *J,* Assorted sharpening stones.

(Courtesy of Hu-Friedy.)

H   **I**   **J**

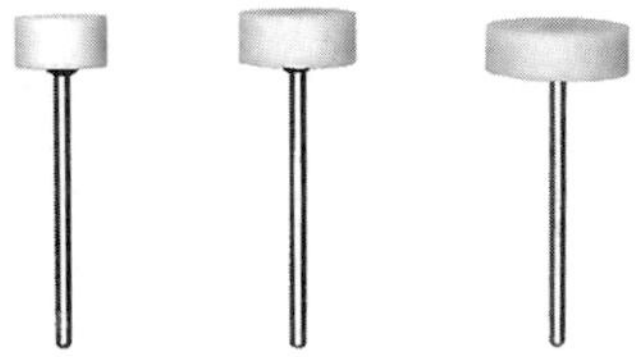

FIG. 18-46   Assorted mounted sharpening stones.

(Courtesy of Hu-Friedy.)

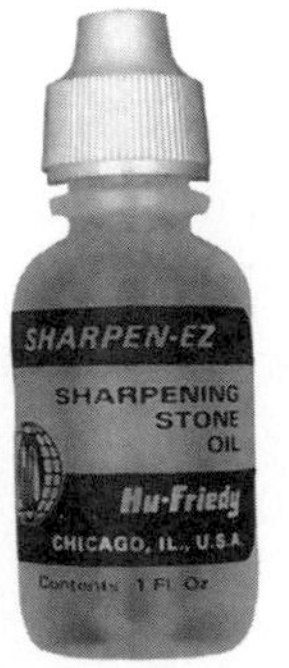

FIG. 18-47   Sharpening oil.

(Courtesy of Hu-Friedy.)

BOX 18-2

METHOD FOR SHARPENING INSTRUMENTS

HAND SHARPENING

1. Instruments and sharpening stones must be sterile when sharpening the instruments to avoid cross contamination. At the conclusion of the sharpening procedures, these devices are sterilized before returning them to their appropriate storage areas.
2. Examine the blade contours. Hold the blade at eye level and observe the angle of the cutting edge from the side. The use of magnifying loupes will help in evaluating the condition of the cutting edge.
3. The cutting edge must have an angle acute enough to cut but not so acute that the blade is weakened and will break. Cutting angles of most hand cutting instruments are about 50 degrees, as compared to instruments with more acute angles, such as razors or scalpel blades that are used to cut soft tissue (Fig. 18-48).
4. A dull instrument has been created if the thin cutting edge breaks away in tiny metallic fragments when it is used against rough enamel. After repeated use the cutting edge becomes rounded or flattened and is no longer efficient. A dull edge can be observed usually by holding the blade to reflect light. A dull instrument will produce sharp lines or catches in the light.
5. To sharpen the instrument on a flat stone, a couple of drops of sharpening oil are placed on the stone. The oil is spread evenly over the surface (carefully, with your fingers or with a 2 × 2 gauze sponge) to create a light film.
6. To recreate the sharp edge on the cutting instrument, metal must be removed evenly from the beveled surface so that it remains flat and the angle of the cutting edge is maintained.
7. An instrument like a chisel is placed on the stone (Fig. 18-49). The bevel is placed flat against the stone and pressure is applied to the instrument to move it across the length of the stone. This is done in one direction, as shown in Fig. 18-50. On the return stroke, no pressure is applied.
8. As the blade moves across the sharpening stone, the direction must be straight and steady with even pressure applied to the beveled surface. Avoid rocking or tilting the blade back and forth. This will alter the contour and will prevent obtaining a sharp cutting edge. Fig. 18-51 illustrates errors in placement of the blade on the stone, resulting in incorrectly sharpened edges.
9. Test the blade for sharpness by placing the blade on a plastic test rod at about a 45-degree angle, with the cutting edge pressing into the rod (Fig. 18-52). If the cutting edge pierces the rod, it is sharp; if it glides over the rod, it is still dull.
10. When the desired sharpness is achieved, the instrument can be wiped free of the oil and fragments with a gauze that has been saturated in alcohol. Other instruments can continue to be sharpened. At the conclusion of all sharpening, the stone is wiped free of debris and oil and the stone and instruments are sterilized.

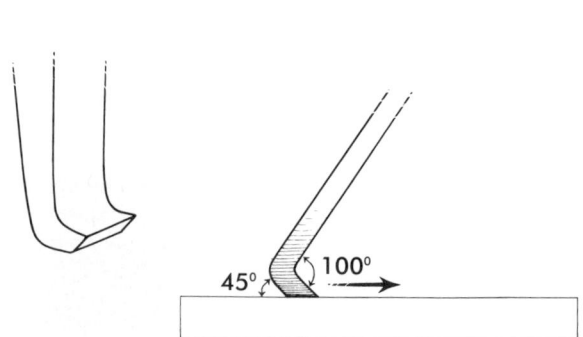

FIG. 18-48   Cutting angle of most hand cutting instruments is approximately 45 to 50 degrees.

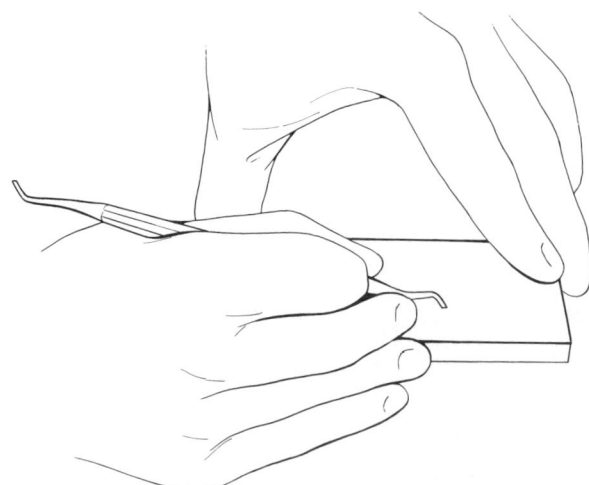

FIG. 18-49   A hand cutting instrument is placed on the stone for sharpening.

Rules for Instrument Sharpening

The design of each instrument will dictate the method of sharpening (Figs. 18-48 through 18-52). However, several basic suggestions should be followed when sharpening most instruments (Box 18-2).

The use of an oscillating instrument sharpener takes away some of the worry about angulation. The machine is designed with preset guides for various cutting angles. Many of these machines come with wax-impregnated wheels that eliminate the need to apply oil to the wheel (Box 18-3).

ALTERNATIVE HAND METHODS

Free hand sharpening, using mounted stones, is frequently employed when sharpening scalers (Fig. 18-53). In skilled hands, such stones can be used to sharpen hand cutting instruments. The most difficult task in using this method is maintaining a flat surface.

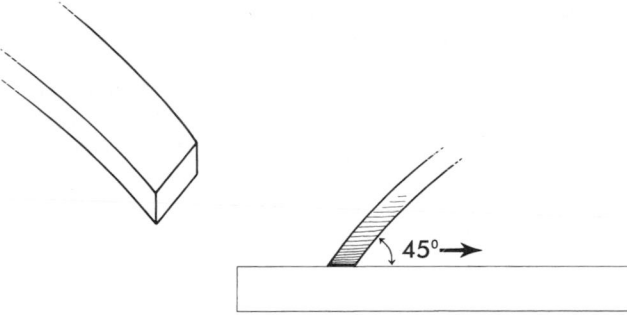

FIG. 18-50 The bevel is pressed against the stone and pressure is applied in one direction to move across the length of the stone. On the return stroke no pressure is applied.

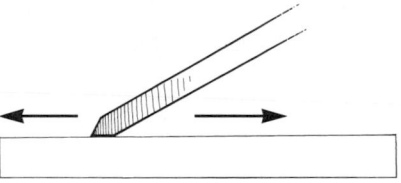

FIG. 18-51 An instrument should not be tilted or rocked back and forth; this will alter the contour and prevent obtaining a sharp cutting edge.

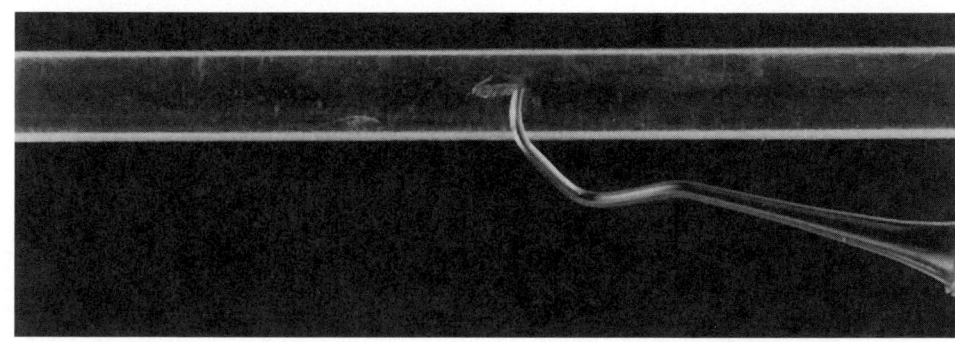

FIG. 18-52 The sharpness of the blade can be tested by placing the blade on a plastic test rod at about a 45-degree angle.

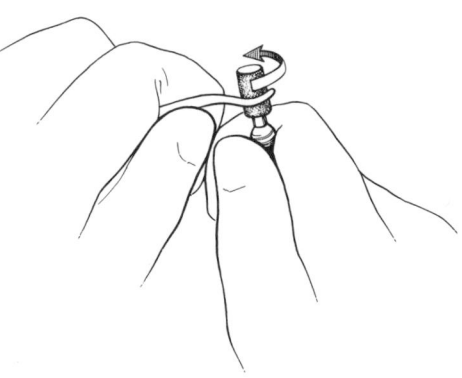

FIG. 18-53 Free hand use of mounted stones in sharpening.

(From Sturdevant CM: *The art and science of operative dentistry,* ed 2, St Louis, 1985, Mosby.)

KEY POINTS

▶ Dental instruments are made of stainless steel, Teflon, or plastic and are supplied as single ended (SE) or double ended (DE) instruments. The components of a dental instrument include the handle, the shank, and the blade, which terminate into the cutting edge or working end.

▶ Hand cutting instruments are given an instrument formula that was devised by G.V. Black. This formula designates the width, length, and angle of the blade and cutting edge. In addition, a manufacturer's number is given to each instrument, which, in the case of hand cutting instruments, correlates to the instrument formula.

▶ Basic dental instruments can be classified into six categories: examination, hand cutting, condensing/insertion, carving, finishing/polishing, and adjunct instruments.

▶ Instruments with sharp edges need periodic sharpening to prevent dullness of the instrument from causing tissue damage. Instruments, such as chisels, hatchets, gingival margin trimmers, spoon excavators, and scalers, can be sharpened manually or with an automatic sharpener. Each procedure requires special guidelines and practice to gain an understanding of the process.

BIBLIOGRAPHY

Charbeneau GT: *Principles and practice of operative dentistry,* ed 3, Philadelphia, 1988, Lea & Febiger.

Sturdevant CM et al: *The art and science of operative dentistry,* ed 3, St Louis, 1994, Mosby.

U.S. Department of Health, Education and Welfare: *Instrument sharpening: project Acorde,* Washington, DC, 1979, Quercus.

Woodall IR: *Comprehensive dental hygiene care,* ed 4, St Louis, 1993, Mosby.

19 Rotary Instruments

LEARNING OBJECTIVES

You will have mastered the material in this chapter when you can:

▶ Define the key terms

▶ Describe the function of rotary devices used in dentistry today

▶ Explain the use of a water coolant system in conjunction with dental handpieces

▶ Differentiate between various types of handpieces

▶ Identify the various shapes, sizes, types, and functions of common rotary devices

▶ Describe the maintenance of handpieces

KEY TERMS

Bur	High speed
Chuck	Low speed
Contra-angle	Mandrel
Disk	Revolutions per minute (rpm)
Fiberoptic	Rotary
Finish	Shank
Flutes	Stone
Handpiece	Torque

The term **rotary** when applied to cutting instruments used in dentistry refers to a large group of devices, such as burs, stones, or disks that rotate on an axis to cut, polish, abrade, and burnish tooth tissues and restorative materials in and out of the oral cavity. A **bur** is made of metal and fabricated into a variety of shapes. A **stone** is a device made of abrasive materials impregnated in a matrix and formed into various shapes. A **disk** is a flat paper, plastic, or metal surface impregnated with different abrasives.

The alarming word *drill* has no place in the vocabulary of a dental professional, since the connotation is one of potential discomfort to the patient. Unfortunately, early dental history used this term widely to describe most rotary devices used in the last century. Today, the term **handpiece** denotes the electronic device used to provide rotary action when used in conjunction with various attachments. The handpiece enables the operator to expeditiously cut, polish, and abrade tooth tissue; cut bone; and polish and burnish all types of preventive and restorative materials.

Handpiece Development

The hand cutting instruments described in the previous chapter were among the earliest instruments used in cavity preparation. Today, with improved technology in the use of rotary devices, many hand cutting instruments have been laid aside in favor of the more efficient rotary instruments. It was not until 1858, however, when Isaac Singer's treadle-driven sewing machine was invented that the stimulus was created to fashion rotary instruments in dentistry. J.B. Morrison designed a foot treadle *drill* in the 1870s, and by 1872 the first electric powered *drill* was developed by a mechanic of the S.S. White Company, George F. Green (Fig. 19-1).

After World War II, great strides were made in the development of dental handpieces based on an air turbine concept. This development brought dentistry out of the belt-and-pulley era and into the air-driven handpieces, which made dentistry a more comfortable experience for the patient and increased efficiency for the dentist.

Speeds of most handpieces continued to be at or below 100,000 **revolutions per minute (rpm)** until 1957 when

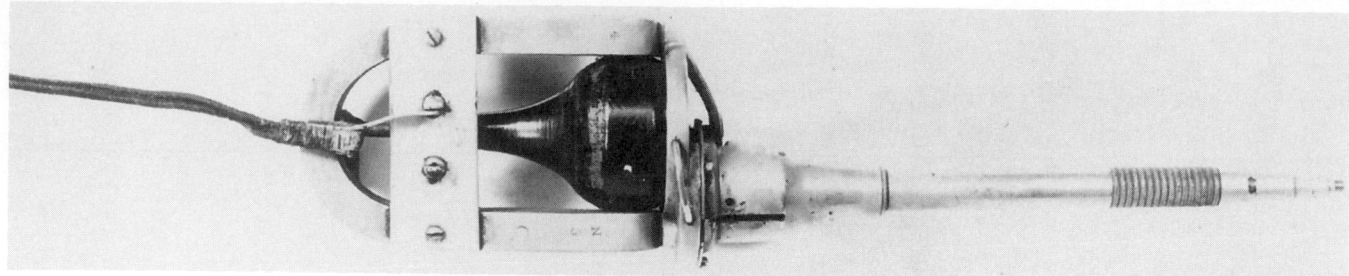

FIG. 19-1   First electric powered drill developed by George F. Green of the S.S. White Company.

(From Ring ME: *Dentistry: An illustrated history,* St Louis, 1985, Mosby.)

the S.S. White Company developed the Borden Airotor, which propelled the rpm to 300,000. For a dentist the ultra speed handpiece created new dimensions in speed and efficiency. Since then, few advances have been made in handpiece design except for the development of **fiberoptics**, which, when incorporated into a handpiece, increases the visibility of the operative field. Today the slower belt-and-pulley engine, if used, is dedicated primarily to laboratory use.

The assistant's role in the use of rotary devices includes the preparation of the handpiece and the appropriate attachments for use during operative and surgical procedures, sterilization, maintenance, and ordering. The assistant will also use the slow-speed handpiece for a variety of laboratory procedures and for certain advanced functions in those states where it is legally delegable.

Low-Speed versus High-Speed

Two speeds of handpieces are available in dentistry today. The low-speed or conventional handpieces typically operate under 30,000 rpm, and the high-speed or ultra-speed handpieces operate from 30,000 to 600,000 rpm. Today most handpieces are activated by air passing over a variety of gears and turbines.

▶ Low-Speed Handpieces

Low-speed handpieces are used when the concern is for the creation of frictional heat or to avoid removing tissue at a rapid speed. Low-speed devices can generally be used without a water coolant. However, it may be necessary for the dental assistant to intermittently spray air on the site to remove debris. The exception would be when the caries removal is near the pulp, where air could desiccate or dry the pulpal tissue and create pain for the patient. At other times, when a dentist is holding a metal casting in the hand and grinding the restoration, frictional heat can be created. Short spurts of air that are sprayed from an a/w syringe by the assistant can make the procedure more manageable for the operator. Most common

---

BOX 19-1
APPLICATIONS OF LOW-SPEED HANDPIECES
▶ Polishing teeth during a prophylaxis procedure
▶ Removing stains from teeth
▶ Refining cavity preparations after the tooth has been opened and shaped with a high-speed handpiece
▶ Removing soft carious material from the tooth during cavity preparation
▶ Making an occlusal adjustment of natural tooth or a restoration
▶ Making a smooth cut on a tooth with a disk
▶ Smoothing or burnishing a tooth with a stone or disk
▶ Polishing a restoration
▶ Grinding and finishing acrylic or metal on a prosthesis

applications for the use of low speed handpieces would include the list in Box 19-1.

A low-speed handpiece can be used at chairside or in the laboratory. Typically a low-speed handpiece can be distinguished from a high-speed handpiece on a dental unit by its size. Low-speed handpieces are more streamlined today, but since these handpieces are often used with some form of **contra-angle**, an attachment used to accommodate the placement of rotary devices, they are generally bulkier. Low-speed handpieces used in the dental laboratory are often attached to a single arm and electric engine as illustrated in Chapter 40.

STYLES OF LOW-SPEED HANDPIECES

The primary variations in low-speed handpieces are in size and speed. Most manufacturers produce a standard and shorty or mini handpiece. Low-speed handpieces are available with a single speed ranging from 0 to 6 to 10,000 rpm or with multiple speeds whose range extends from 0 to 6 to 10,000 to 30,000 rpm. Multiple-speed handpieces will be supplied with an adjustment button that allows speeds to be easily changed. Low-speed hand-

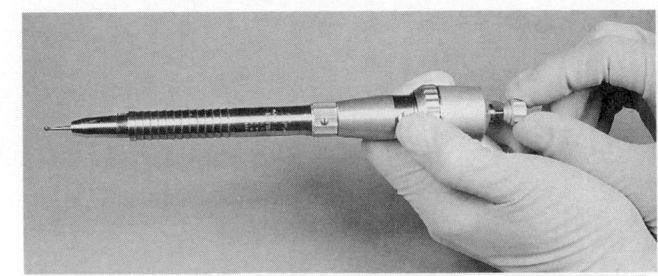
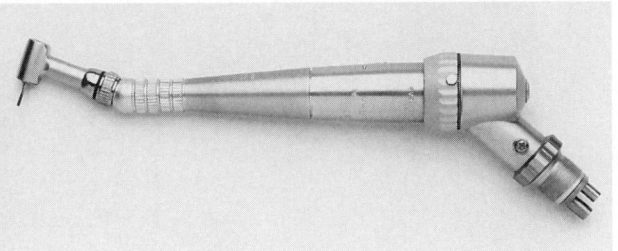
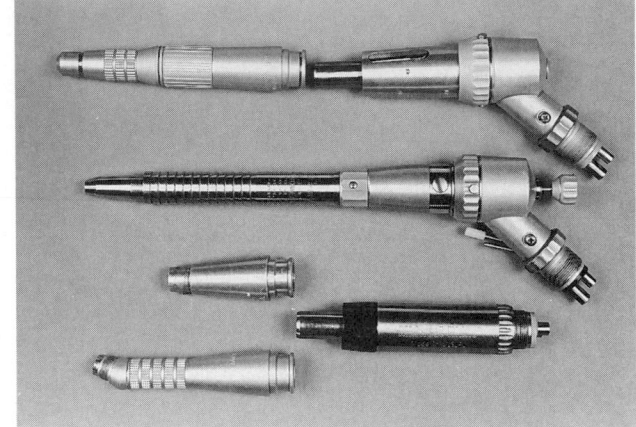

FIG. 19-2 *A,* Low-speed straight handpiece, with a straight shank bur. *B,* Low-speed handpiece, with a contra-angle and bur in place. *C,* Assorted low-speed handpieces with attachments.

pieces are also equipped with the ability to operate in a forward or reverse mode, allowing the operator to burnish margins on a restoration. Low-speed handpieces are often referred to as *straight* handpieces, since this is the basic shape of the device, until some form of angle is placed on it to make it a right or contra-angled instrument (Fig. 19-2, *A* and *B*). Assorted styles of low-speed handpieces are illustrated in Fig. 19-2, *C.*

▶ High-Speed Handpieces

High-speed handpieces are used primarily for rapid cutting of hard tissues. High-speed handpieces are ready to be used with only a bur added, and they never require the addition of an angle (Fig. 19-3, *A*). Various high-speed handpieces are shown in Fig. 19-3, *B.* New bur styles, however, have made this device useful in fine **finishing** of composite restorations. High-speed handpieces traditionally have lacked **torque,** the ability to rotate, when excess pressure is applied. Most high-speed handpieces operate most efficiently when light pressure is applied. All high-speed handpieces are designed with water coolant systems and optional features, including lasers and fiberoptics.

STYLES OF HIGH-SPEED HANDPIECES

In Chapter 16 a brief description was given for various handpieces. Unlike the low-speed handpieces, the high-speed handpieces are designed with a contra-angled configuration within the handpiece. The only attachment made to a high-speed handpiece is the bur. The primary variation in high-speed handpiece design is its size. Most manufacturers produce a standard and a pediatric style. The latter handpiece has a shorter head, which provides for easier and safer access to the small opening of a child's mouth or for difficult-to-reach areas in the adult mouth.

WATER COOLANT SYSTEM

A **water coolant** is used with these handpieces to reduce frictional heat created by the high speed. The water coolant system is designed within the handpiece, allowing for an automatic flow of water when the handpiece is activated. The concept used in most designs allows the water spray to hit the bur as it rotates on the tooth (Fig. 19-3, *A*). This concept may be referred to as the *washed field* technique, since not only does it serve to cool and protect the tooth but it also washes away the debris in the operative field as the bur rotates. The use of high-speed handpieces with a water coolant contributed to the expansion of four-handed dentistry. Without the use of oral evacuation by a dental assistant, the abundance of water associated with the use of the high-speed handpiece would be prohibitive.

FIBEROPTICS

High-speed handpieces also can provide the operator with increased visibility of the work area through the use

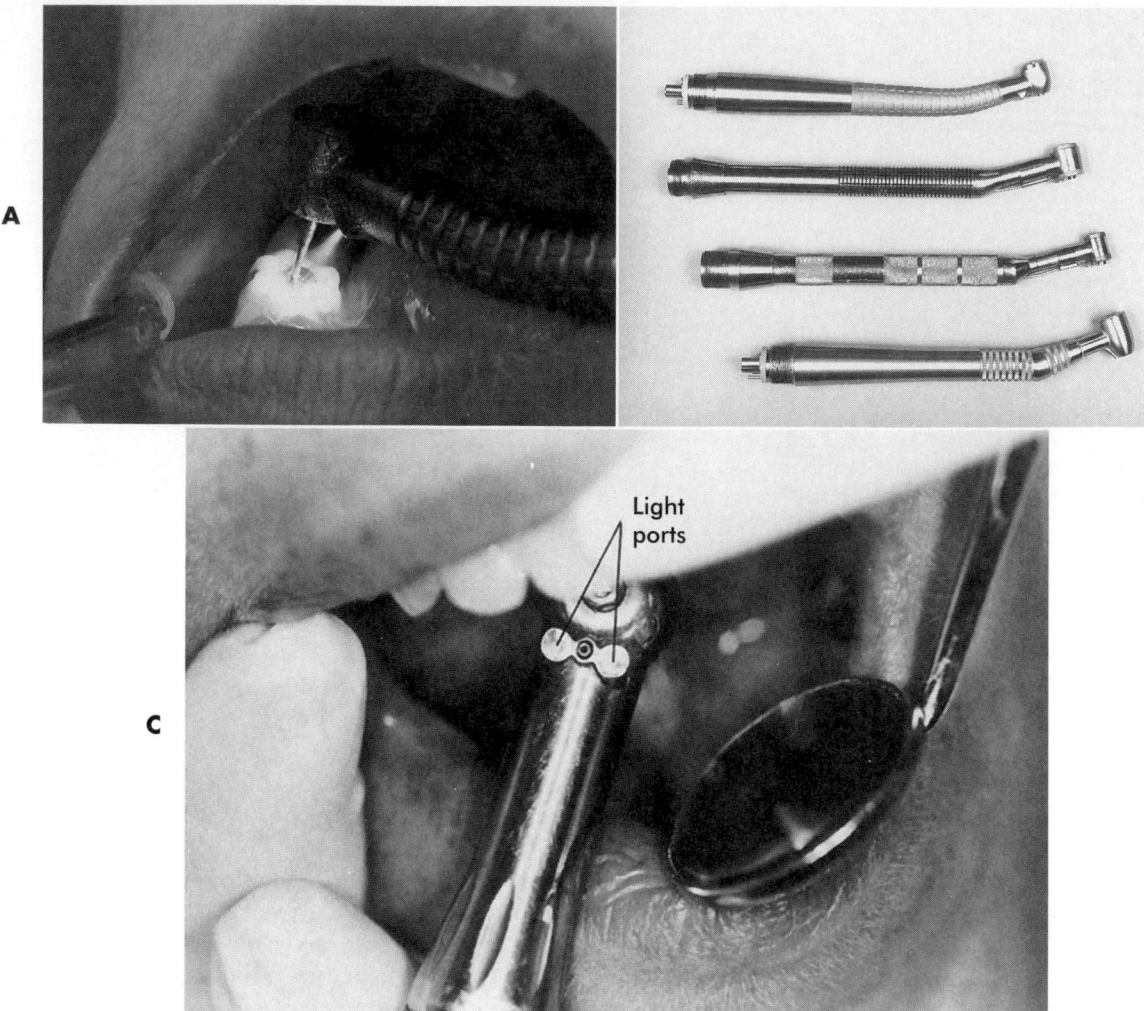

FIG. 19-3   *A,* Bur attached to a high-speed handpiece, showing water coolant and fiberoptic light source on the bur. *B,* Various types of high-speed handpieces. *C,* Close-up of light ports on high-speed handpieces.

(From Chasteen JE: *Essentials of clinical dental assisting,* St Louis, 1989, Mosby.)

of fiberoptic light sources. Fiberoptic handpieces have flexible materials of glass or plastic within the unit. These materials allow the light to be reflected off the wall or the side of the fiber, providing increased visibility in the oral cavity. A close-up of the high-speed handpiece, showing the water coolant and fiberoptic parts, is seen in Fig. 19-3, *C.*

LASERS

The use of lasers in dentistry is expected to expand in the future. Currently, laser units are used in dentistry for surgical procedures, particularly periodontal surgery. The use of laser units reduces the amount of blood loss and potential tissue trauma. Dental lasers allow the tissue to be cauterized during excision or removal, and thus

reduce healing time and discomfort for the patient in some circumstances.

Although the use of lasers for dental care is limited at this time, researchers continue to develop the application of use to other areas of dentistry.

BOX 19-2

APPLICATIONS OF HIGH-SPEED HANDPIECES

- Cut/prepare tooth tissue to receive some form of restoration, such as amalgam, composite, or gold casting
- Section a tooth for surgical removal
- Remove faulty restorations
- Finish restorations, using specialized burs

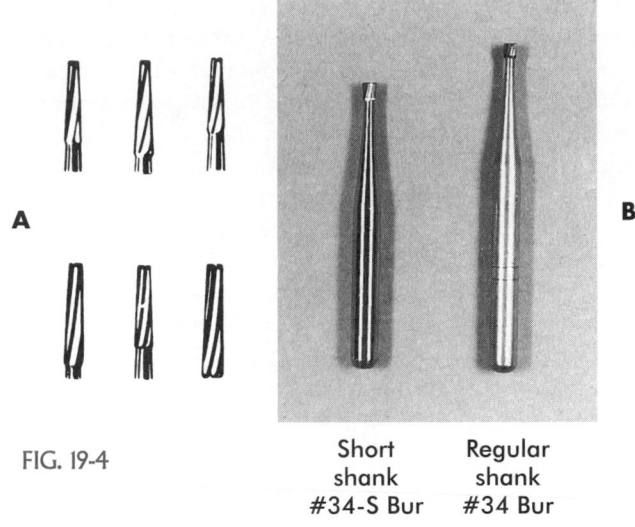

FIG. 19-4

Short
shank
#34-S Bur

Regular
shank
#34 Bur

Comparison of burs. *A,* Long and regular cutting surfaces. *B,* Short and regular shanks.

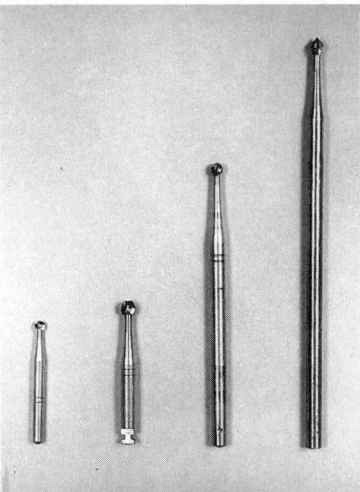

Friction
grip
(FG)

Latch
type
(RA)

Handpiece
(HP)

Handpiece
(HP)
Longer
shank
surgical
bur

FIG. 19-5   Photo of 3 shanks of burs and surgical bur.

High-speed handpieces are used primarily for the purposes listed in Box 19-2.

▶ Symbols and Terminology

Various symbols and terminology are related to the use of rotary instruments, and since the assistant is responsible for the preparation and ordering of these devices, it is important to understand this language.

On any package that contains a rotary device a symbol can be found that indicates some special design of the instrument. The symbol often follows the bur or stone number. In addition, most catalogs describe special functions of rotary instruments, and to determine which to order, be familiar with these terms. Symbols and terminology commonly used include the following:

L — Long cutting surface. A bur with the number #169L would provide a longer cutting surface, allowing the operator to cut a greater length of tissue. This is especially helpful when a preparation extends below the gingiva (Fig. 19-4, *A*).

S — Short shank. The cutting surface of this bur is the same size as standard burs, but the length of the **shank,** which is the part that attaches to the handpiece, is shortened to allow the bur to be used in difficult access areas (Fig. 19-4, *B*).

FG — Friction grip. These burs are shorter shanked and are used only in handpieces and contra-angles with some type of **chuck** that will hold them in place by friction.

RA — Right angle. This style of rotary device, whether it is a bur, stone, or disk, will have a small latch at the base of the shank. When it is placed into a

latch-type contra-angle, it will be at a right angle to the head of the angle.

HP — Handpiece. Burs with this designation will have longer shanks and are used only in a straight handpiece. The three basic shanks are illustrated in Fig. 19-5.

Mounted versus unmounted — When a rotary device is referred to as being mounted, it means that the **stone** or **disk** is permanently mounted to a shaft or mandrel. An unmounted stone or disk must be attached to a mandrel or a shaft for use. When a mounted disk or stone becomes dull, the entire device is discarded. When an unmounted disk or stone becomes dull, only the disk or stone is discarded and the mandrel is retained (Fig. 19-6, *A* through *C*).

T & F — Trimming and finishing. These burs and stones are designed in a shape and style that can be used in finishing and trimming tooth surfaces or restorations.

FF — Fine finishing. These burs and stones are designed with a more delicate cutting edge or have a finer grit for use in fine finishing of margins and various types of restorations.

Abrade — To abrade a tooth or restorative material means to wear or cut away by friction. To use a stone or bur in a rotary action on a tooth is to abrade it.

Burnish — Burnishing is a process related to polishing, smoothing, and abrading. This process is commonly accomplished during the polishing of gold. It

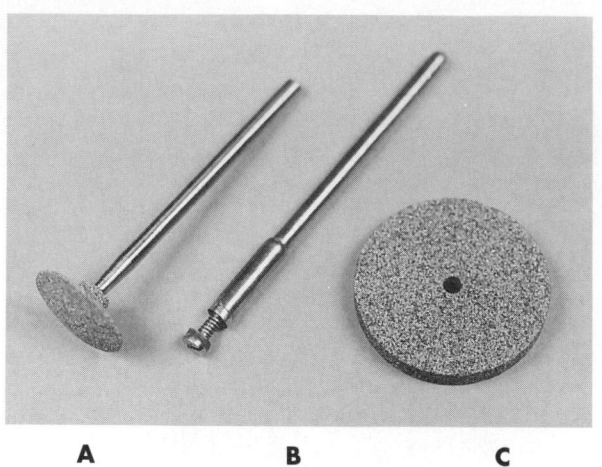

FIG. 19-6   A permanently mounted stone, *A;* screw type mandrel, *B;* and unmounted stone, *C.* All can be mounted together.

is common to burnish the margins of a metal casting, which is the action of smoothing the margins and is not a process of removing significant amounts of tooth or restorative material.

Polish — To polish is to make a tooth or restorative material smooth and glossy, giving luster to the surface. Polishing can be accomplished with brushes, stones, disks, and rubber points and wheels, often in conjunction with a polishing agent.

Finish — Finishing is not unlike burnishing and polishing. It generally refers to removing excess restorative material from the margins and contours of a restoration to ensure a smooth line of demarcation between the cavosurface margin of the preparation and the restoration.

Attachments

A handpiece is a highly sophisticated piece of equipment. Without this single device a dentist would be sorely handicapped performing most dental procedures. However, for a handpiece to function effectively, some type of device must be attached to it. These attachments include angles, burs, stones, disks, and mandrels. An overview of the basic rotary instruments and attachments is shown in Table 19-1.

▶ Angles

Common types of angles used in dentistry include the prophylaxis angle or right angle, the contra-angle, the Auto Klutch Chuck angle, or an endodontic head contra-angle.

PROPHYLAXIS ANGLE

A prophylaxis angle is sometimes referred to as a right angle because the head of the angle is at a right angle to its shaft. The most popular types of prophylaxis angles are the snap-on and the screw types. The snap-on prophylaxis (prophy) angle uses snap-on types of rubber cups; the screw type can accept rubber cups or brushes that are designed with small screws at the back for easy attachment. Disposable prophy angles eliminate the necessity to sterilize this device. A contra-angle described in the next section can also be used with a latch-type shank prophylaxis cup. See Fig. 19-7, *A* and *B,* for examples of common prophylaxis angles.

CONTRA-ANGLE

A contra-angle is attached to a low-speed handpiece to accommodate the placement of rotary devices in the handpiece. A contra-angle is an instrument with one or more offset angles of such a degree that the end of the instrument is kept within 3 mm of the axis of the shaft. The design of a contra-angle allows the operator to gain access to all surfaces of the posterior teeth (Fig. 19-8). Contra-angles are available as friction grip (FG) or latch-type styles (Fig. 19-9). The friction grip contra-angle holds only FG shanks, which are held in place by friction. The latch type, just as named, holds the rotary device in place with a small latch on the back of the head. Most auxiliary devices, including disks, burs, stones, mandrels, and even prophy cups and brushes, are available with shanks for use in either style contra-angle.

AUTO KLUTCH CHUCK ANGLE

The **Auto Klutch Chuck Angle** is specifically designed to be used for the insertion of threaded pins as described in Chapter 27. The specialized feature of this device allows the operator to place a small pin into the angle, and through rotation, embed the pin into the dentin of the tooth. The Auto Klutch Chuck Angle automatically stops when the pin has reached the final depth of insertion (Fig. 19-10).

ENDODONTIC ANGLE

It is important that a rotary device used in endodontics can be controlled to avoid extending an instrument too far into the canal. Therefore, the specially designed endodontic angle allows only a quarter turn with an alternating rotating head.

▶ Burs

Burs are considered the workhorse of rotary devices in dentistry. Burs are designed to cut tooth tissue and bone,

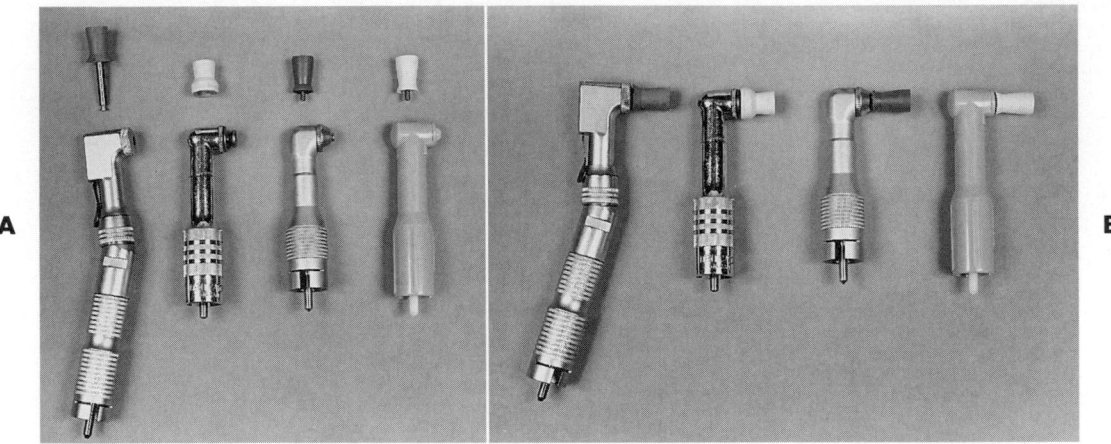

FIG. 19-7   *A,* Three types of prophylaxis angles and latch type contra angle, with appropriate prophylaxis cups for each. *B,* Cups attached to each of the angles shown in *A.*

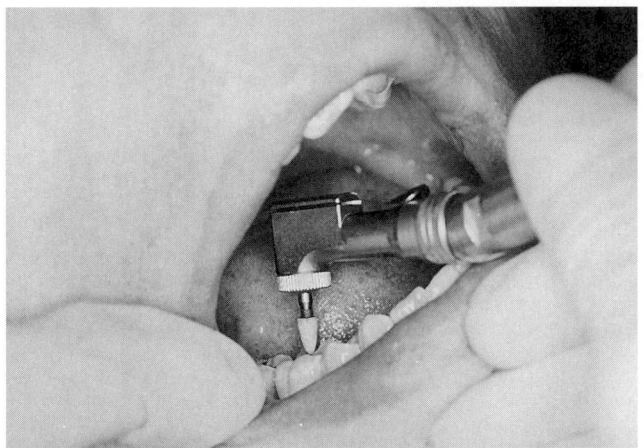

FIG. 19-8   Latch-type contra-angle with a stone attached that is being used in the posterior of the mouth.

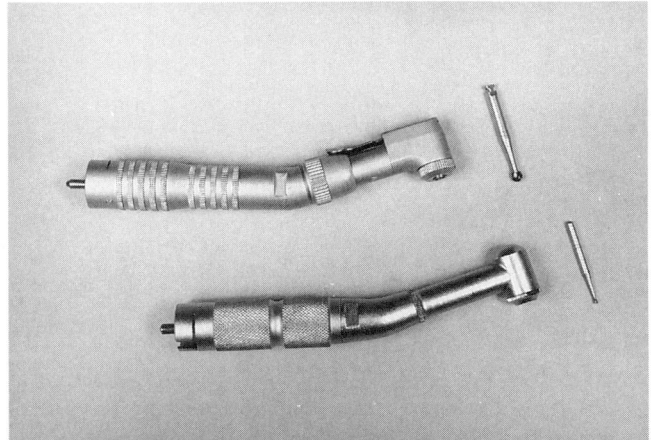

FIG. 19-9   Friction grip and latch type contra-angles, with appropriate burs.

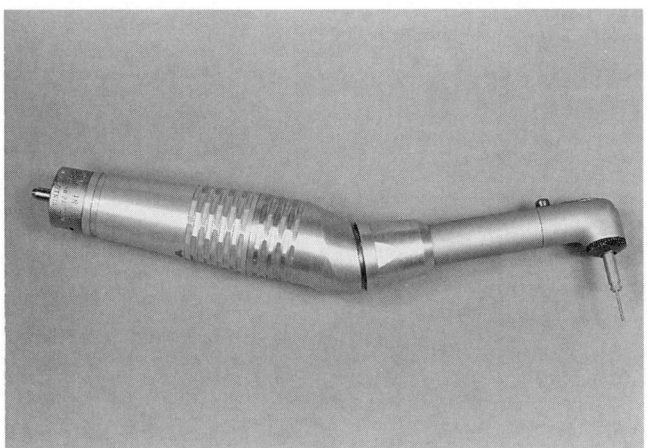

FIG. 19-10   Auto Klutch Chuck Angle, with a retention pin attached for insertion into a pin hole.

(Courtesy of Whaledent International, New York, New York.)

TABLE 19-1 COMMON ROTARY INSTRUMENTS AND DEVICES

Name	Common series no./shape	Shanks	Intraoral/ extraoral use (IO/EO)	Purpose
Round burs	¼ to 8	RA, HP, FG	IO/EO*	Cutting tissue, cavity preparation
Inverted cone burs	33½ to 39	RA, HP, FG	IO/EO*	Cutting tissue, cavity preparation
Straight fissure—plain cut	55 to 64	RA, HP, FG	IO/EO*	Cutting tissue, cavity preparation
Straight fissure—cross cut	556 to 564	RA, HP, FG	IO/EO*	Cutting tissue, cavity preparation
Tapered fissure—plain cut	169 to 172	RA, HP, FG	IO/EO*	Cutting tissue, cavity preparation
Tapered fissure—cross cut	699 to 708	RA, HP, FG	IO/EO*	Cutting tissue, cavity preparation
Pear	½P to 4P	FG	IO/EO*	Cutting tissue, cavity preparation
End-cutting	956 to 959	RA, HP, FG	IO	Endodontic opening
				Placing bevels or shoulders in anterior crown preparations and endodontic opening
Wheel	14	RA, HP, FG	IO	Gross reduction of incisal/occlusal surfaces
Finishing burs	Round	RA, HP, FG	IO/EO	Finish and polish restoration
	Needle	RA, HP, FG	IO/EO	Finish and polish restoration
	Bullet	RA, HP, FG	IO/EO	Finish and polish restoration
	Flame	RA, HP, FG	IO/EO	Finish and polish restoration
	Cone	RA, HP, FG	IO/EO	Finish and polish restoration
	Taper	RA, HP, FG	IO/EO	Finish and polish restoration
	Egg	RA, HP, FG	IO/EO	Finish and polish restoration
	Pear	RA, HP, FG	IO/EO	Finish and polish restoration
Orifice bur	Flame	RA	IO	Prepare openings in tooth
Diamonds	Shapes are similar to finishing burs with a variety of different identifying numbers	RA, HP, FG	IO/EO	Preparation of teeth
Mounted green stone	Cone, cylinder, flame, inverted cone, knife-edge, round-edge, round, tapered cylinder, wheel	RA, HP, FG	IO/EO	Abrasive points used to finish and polish

Mounted white stone	Cone, cylinder, flame, inverted cone, knife-edge, round-edge, round, tapered cylinder, wheel	RA, HP, FG	IO/EO	Abrasive points used to finish and polish
Heatless stone	Unmounted wheel		EO	Used on devices to reduce heat during application
Moore's mandrel/snap-on		RA, HP, FG	IO/EO	Mount for snap-on finishing and polishing disks
Screw-type mandrel		RA, HP, FG	IO/EO	Mount for disk, wheels with pin hole opening
Snap-on disks with various abrasive substances	$3/8, 1/2, 5/8, 3/4$ inch disks with snap-on openings	Mount to RA, HP snap-on mandrel	IO/EO	Polish and finish surfaces
Lightening disk	$3/8, 1/2, 5/8, 3/4$ inch pin hole–opening disk	Mounted on screw-type mandrel RA, HP, FG	IO/EO	Usually used to place a slice on a tooth or preparation
Carborundum/separating/Jo-Dandy disk	$3/8, 1/2, 5/8, 3/4$ inch pin hole–opening disk	Mounted on screw-type mandrel RA, HP, FG, or premounted	EO	Used in laboratory to finish stone die before creating wax pattern; cuts metal casting
Rubber polishing wheel		Mounted on screw-type mandrel RA, HPG, or premounted	IO/EO	Used as soft or hard rubber to polish restorations
Polishing points		RA, HP, FG	IO/EO	Polish and finish surfaces of teeth and restorations
Rubber/polishing cup	Conical	RA, screw, snap-on	IO	Polish coronal surfaces
Bristle brushes	Conical, wheel, straight	RA, screw, or snap-on, mounted or unmounted	IO/EO	Polish teeth, restorations, and appliances

*When this bur is used extraorally, it will likely be an HP shank.

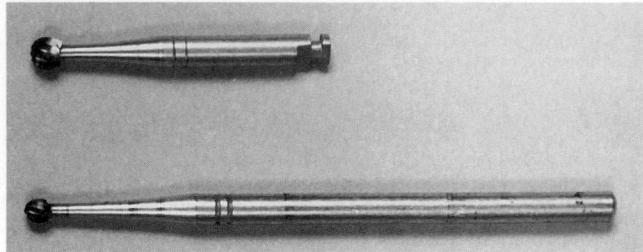

FIG. 19-11   Two parts of a bur, a shank, and the working end. Rings on an RA or HP bur indicate tungsten carbide.

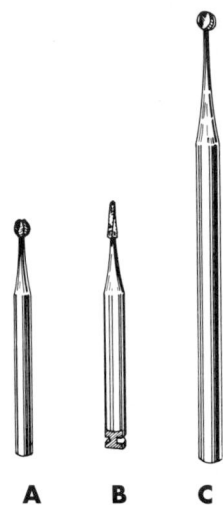

FIG. 19-12   Different styles of shanks on rotating cutting instruments. *A,* Friction grip (FG). *B,* Latch (RA). *C,* Handpiece (HP).

(From Chasteen JE: *Essentials of clinical dental assisting,* St Louis, 1989, Mosby.)

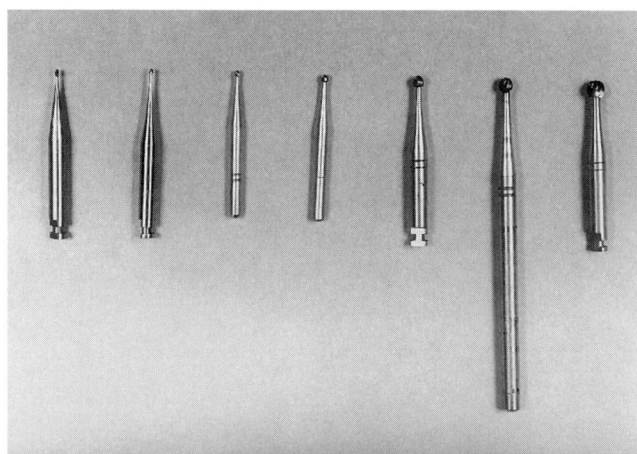

FIG. 19-13   A variety of round cutting burs.

to remove soft carious material from the dentin, to burnish margins of restorations, to cut restorative materials, and to polish and finish restorations. Burs are made of steel or tungsten carbide and can be categorized by shape into traditional and specialty burs. The use of tungsten carbide has increased because the hardness of the carbide gives it a longer life. Traditional burs are used primarily in cavity preparation, whereas specialty burs provide fine finishing and trimming and perform uncommon tasks, such as placing special cuts on teeth during tooth preparation for a fixed prosthesis.

The two identifying parts of every bur are the shank and the working end or head. These two parts are connected by the neck of the bur (Fig. 19-11). Burs, stones, and mandrels are manufactured with three different shanks: friction grip (FG), latch-type or right angle (RA), and straight handpieces (HP) (Fig. 19-12).

BUR SERIES

A series number is the range of sizes in which a specific bur shape is available. For instance, one of the shapes, a round bur, has a series number of ¼ to 10 with some manufacturers. The smaller the number of the series, the smaller the size of the bur. Each operator has favorite burs in each series and may not want to stock all of the burs in every series. Many operators like to use only the ½, 1, 2, 4, and 6 in the round bur series (Fig. 19-13). As you work in an office, you will become acquainted with the various burs that should be stocked routinely.

TRADITIONAL BURS

Traditional burs can be categorized into the six basic shapes, as listed in Box 19-3.

Other bur shapes are available and include end cutting (956 to 957), straight dome (1156 to 1158), tapered dome (1169 to 1172), straight dome—cross cut (1556 to 1558), and tapered dome—cross cut (1700 to 1702).

BOX 19-3

TRADITIONAL BURS

▶ Inverted cone (series 33 ½ to 39 or 43)
▶ Round (¼ to 10)
▶ Straight fissure—plain cut (55 to 64)
▶ Straight fissure—cross cut (555 to 564)
▶ Tapered fissure—plain cut (169 to 172)
▶ Tapered fissure—cross cut (699 to 708).

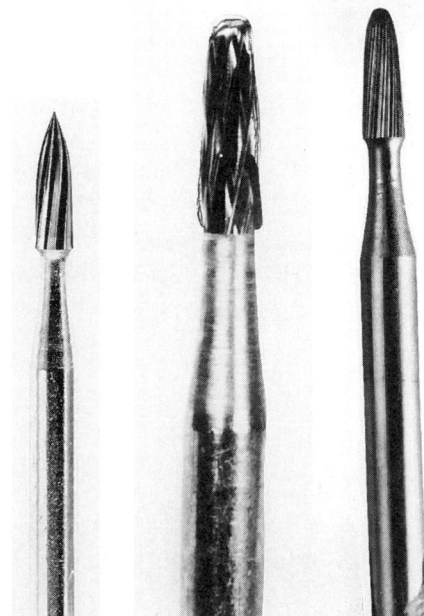

A (top row labels): A B C D E F G H I J K L

	Round			Inverted cone			Plain straight fissure		Crosscut straight fissure		Plain tapered fissure			Pear shape		Crosscut tapered fissure		End cut	Round-nose straight fissure
Friction grip	¼	½	1	33½	34	35*	55	56	555	556	169	169L	170	330 331L / 331		699 700* / 699L			1057
	2	4	6	37	37L		57	57L	557	558	170L	171	171L	332 333L / 332L		701	701L	957	1557
Right angle and straight handpiece	1	2	3	4 33½ 34 35 36			57	58	557	558	170					700	701		
	5	6	7	8 37 38 39			59		559	560	171					702	703		

B

C

Fine crosscut straight dome	Trimming and finishing needle	Crosscut taper dome	Fine finishing bullet

FIG. 19-14   *A,* Basic shapes of burs. Six traditional burs *A* through *F;* basic shapes of traditional cutting burs; round, inverted cone, straight fissure-plain cut, straight fissure-cross cut, tapered fissure-plain cut, tapered fissure-cross cut. Also illustrated are *G* through *L* wheel shape, round end fissure-plain cut and round end fissure-cross cut burs. *B,* Common bur styles, illustrating variations in size. *C,* Specialty burs: straight dome. Trimming and finishing (T&F) needle, taper dome, and fine finishing (FF) bullet.

(*B,* from Chasteen JE: *Essentials of clinical dental assisting,* St Louis, 1989, Mosby. *C* courtesy of Midwest Dental Products Corporation, Des Plaines Ill.)

SPECIALTY BURS

Since dental manufacturers are always creating new bur designs, it is difficult to cover all of the burs designed for special cutting. However, several burs have gained popularity in various phases of operative and surgical dentistry. Many of the standard shapes are also designed for trimming and finishing (T & F) and fine finishing (FF) characteristics (Fig. 19-14, *A* through *C*).

Typically the difference between a cutting bur and a finishing bur is the number of flutes in the working end. The more **flutes**, or cutting surfaces, on a bur, the greater the polishing capability. For instance, the round burs used for cutting, trimming, and fine finishing are seen in Fig. 19-15. The fine finishing burs are often referred to as plug finishing burs. Many manufacturers have retained the series number for the burs but have added extra digits to differentiate between the cutting and finishing burs. For instance, the round bur series for finishing burs in one company is 9004 to 9008; the last digit is the traditional series number.

Not only do these finishing burs have changes in the flute design, but also the shapes can vary beyond the standard shapes. For instance, the crown and bridge chamfering bur is designed for finishing the chamfer line during crown or bridge preparation; the concave interproximal bur is for finishing interproximal surfaces with pronounced concavity; and a needle-shaped bur provides a sharp point for gaining access to cervical finishing (Fig. 19-16).

A surgical bur is another classification of specialty burs. These burs are generally designed with longer shanks and special heads to cut bone and section teeth more aggressively than the traditional burs (Fig. 19-17).

DIAMONDS

Diamond rotary instruments can be categorized as stones or burs; their primary function is for tooth reduction in operative dentistry. They are used widely for preparing fixed prostheses, for tooth contouring in occlusal adjustments, and for osseous and gingival contouring in periodontal surgery. Diamonds are supplied in a variety of shapes and grits; because they are strong tools, they have a long life and are efficient cutting devices (Fig. 19-18).

Many diamond burs or stones are created for special operative procedures. Among these are the double inverted cone diamond that is used to rapidly cut out old amalgam from a tooth preparation; the gross reduction diamond that is used for rapid tooth reduction; the depth

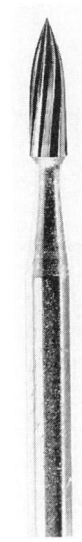

Trimming and
finishing
needle

FIG. 19-16   Specialty finishing bur.

(Courtesy of Miltex.)

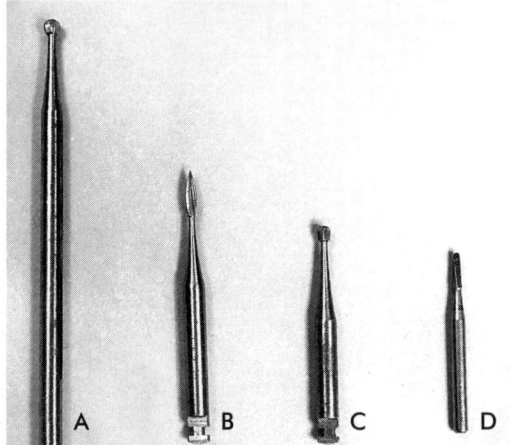

FIG. 19-15   Comparison of different polishing burs. *A,* FG needle-shaped finishing bur. *A,* HP Round finishing bur. *B,* Flame-shaped (orifice) finishing bur. *C,* RA round finishing bur. *D,* Tapered, dome-shaped finishing bur. Note the difference in the number of flutes on the round burs in *A* and *C,* compared with the flutes of the round burs in Fig. 19-13.

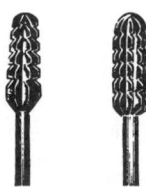

FIG. 19-17   Surgical bur with a longer shank and specialized head to cut bone and section teeth.

(Courtesy of Hu-Friedy.)

marking stone that is used for making depth cuts on the enamel of teeth that are being prepared for restorations, such as laminates; and the gingival curettage diamonds that are used for gingival contour during periodontal surgery.

Rubber Abrasive Points and Disks

A plethora of rubber points, disks, and wheels, are available in dentistry today. A point, just as named, is a

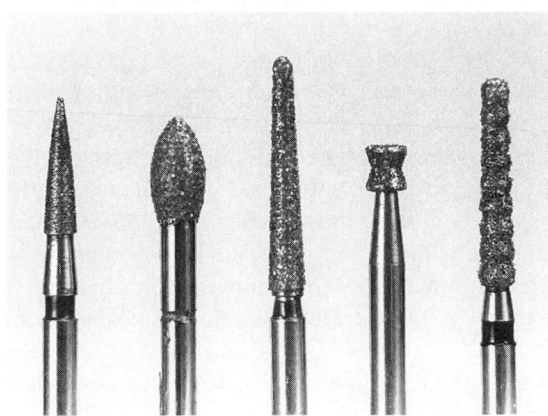

FIG. 19-18   A variety of diamond cutting burs.

(Courtesy of Midwest Dental Products Corporation, Des Plaines, Ill.)

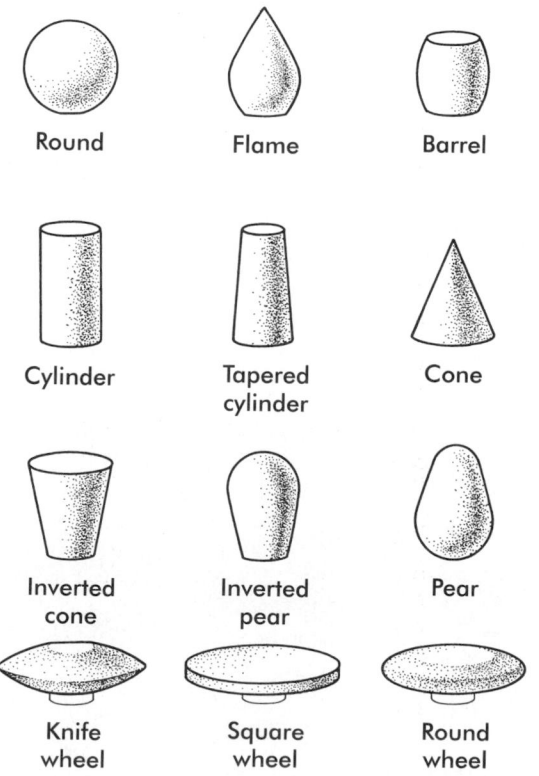

| Round | Flame | Barrel |

| Cylinder | Tapered cylinder | Cone |

| Inverted cone | Inverted pear | Pear |

| Knife wheel | Square wheel | Round wheel |

FIG. 19-19   Common shapes of points and stones.

device that terminates in a point and enables the operator to polish anatomic pits and fissures. Rubber abrasive disks are made with some form of abrasive, such as carborundum or other material that is impregnated into the rubber medium. The shapes of these devices can vary from one manufacturer to another but often include the standardized shapes illustrated in Fig. 19-19. Many companies today have designed specialized polishing points and disks for finishing composite restorations, such as the kit shown in Fig. 19-20.

Mandrels

A **mandrel** is a shaft onto which some type of disk, stone, or rubber device is placed. A screw-type and Moore's mandrel are available for various attachments. Each of these mandrels is provided with the three previously identified shanks: FG, RA, and HP (Fig. 19-21).

Disks

Disks are thin, flat circular objects made of metal, paper, or plastic that are used to polish, cut, or smooth teeth or restorative materials. Disks come in a variety of sizes ranging in diameter from 3/8 inch to 7/8 inch. Most disks are designed with some form of abrasive matrix on the cutting surface that can be provided in various grits from extra fine to extra coarse.

The cutting surface of disks may be on the edge or on one or both sides of the disk. When the abrasive is on one side of the disk, the side with the abrasive is referred to as the face of the disk. The assistant will attach a disk to a mandrel, either face in or face out. When placed on a mandrel *face in,* the disk can be used predominantly on the distal of the tooth; when it is placed *face out,* it can be used on the mesial surface (Fig. 19-22). The following

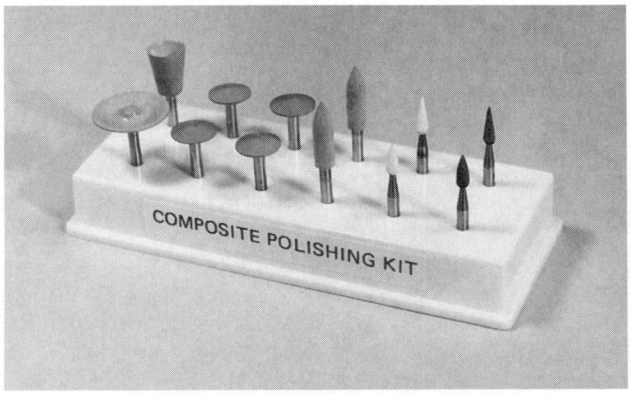

FIG. 19-20   Manufacturer's kit for specialized purposes, such as finishing composite and amalgam restorations.

(Courtesy of Shofu Dental Corporation, Menlo Park, Calif.)

are examples of some of the most common disks used in dentistry today.

Jo-dandy is the trade name of a popular disk that is made of carborundum and is used as a separating disk; it cuts or sets apart one structure from another. These disks are relatively inexpensive, are fragile, and, with little pressure, can break easily. Although

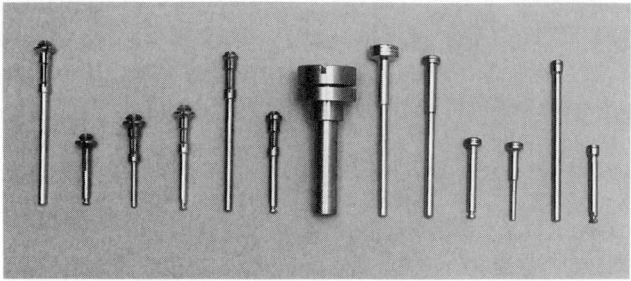

FIG. 19-21 Mandrels used to hold disks, points, or stones are available in FG, RA, or HP shanks.

(Courtesy of E.C. Moore, Dearborn, Michigan.)

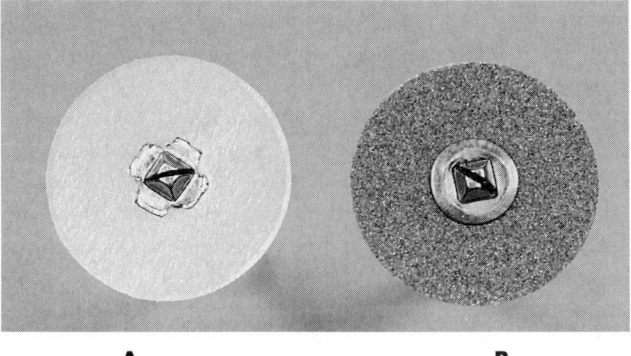

A　　　　　**B**

FIG. 19-22 Example of a paper disk placed *A,* face in, and *B,* face out.

(Courtesy of E.C. Moore, Dearborn, Michigan.)

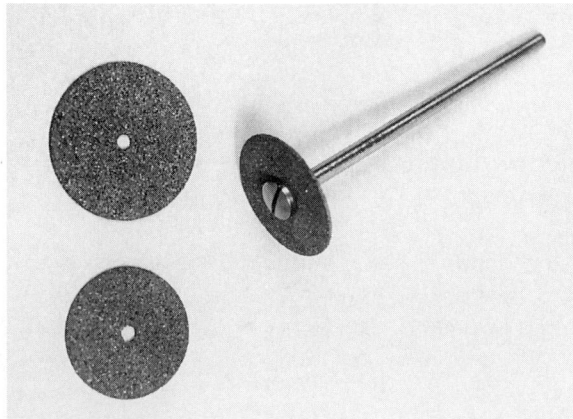

FIG. 19-23 Jo-Dandy, or carborundum, disk is impregnated with abrasive materials on both sides of the disk.

(Courtesy of E.C. Moore, Dearborn, Michigan.)

their use is primarily limited to the laboratory to cut and finish gold castings, they can be used intraorally with caution (Fig. 19-23).

Diamond disks are made of steel onto which diamond chips have been bonded. This type of disk is used to cut tooth tissue; it is made of diamond chips and cuts rapidly (Fig. 19-24).

Lightning disks are made of steel and are used to cut tooth tissue. They are used as a separating disk intraorally on tooth tissue. With a quick glance at a lightening disk you may confuse it with a diamond disk, but it can be differentiated by its flexibility and its duller appearance.

Paper/disposable (sandpaper, cuttle, garnet) These disks are made of paper, are flexible, and use sandpaper, particles of garnet, adalox, emery, or cuttle as the abrading medium. They are widely used in all types of finishing and polishing (Fig. 19-25).

Disks are supplied mounted or unmounted. Many of the diamond disks are permanently mounted on a mandrel and the others are commonly unmounted. With the exception of the Moore's disks, the disks can be

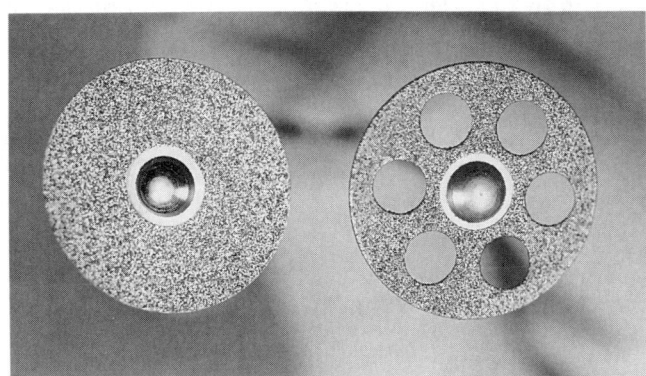

FIG. 19-24 Diamond disks are designed with diamond chips impregnated in a matrix. They are used to remove tooth structure.

(Courtesy of E.C. Moore, Dearborn, Michigan.)

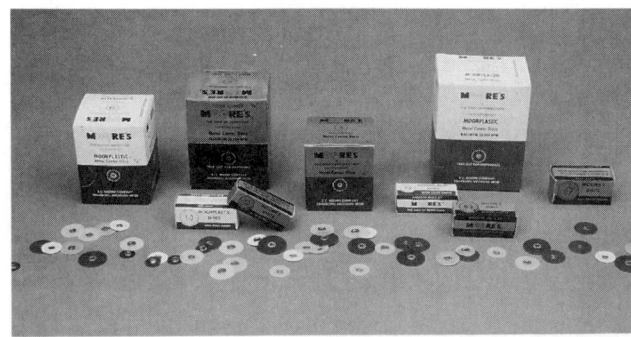

FIG. 19-25 Moore's paper disks are provided in a variety of sizes, grits, and materials.

(Courtesy of E.C. Moore, Dearborn, Michigan.)

attached to a screw-type mandrel. Although there is a pin-style Moore's disk, the most widely used Moore's disk is the brass center disk. The brass center disk fits only on a Moore's mandrel, which can be easily identified by its split head (Fig. 19-25).

The use of any disk presents a potential hazard for the patient and special attention must be given to ensure that the patient's tongue and cheek are retracted to avoid contact with the disk. It may be necessary to use a large mirror for retraction if a rubber dam is not in place.

▶ Stones

Stones, like disks, are designed to abrade and finish teeth and restorative materials. Stones are available as mounted or unmounted devices and are produced in a myriad of shapes; they are sized similarly to disks (see Fig. 19-24).

An *Arkansas* stone is a fine-grained stone that is used primarily to sharpen instruments. (See Chapter 18 for instrument sharpening.)

Heatless stones are gray-green stones that are made of silicon carbide and are used for polishing metallic restorations. The heatless characteristic allows the operator to grind on the restoration without creating frictional heat.

Colored stones, such as garnet (red), black, green, white, and gray, are made of various substances that are often impregnated in rubber. Each of these colored stones can be used for specialized restorative materials or tooth tissue (Fig. 19-26).

Acrylic stones and burs are large bulky devices that are used to cut and polish acrylic denture base material. The large acrylic burs remove the bulk of material from a full or partial denture, after which the prosthesis will need to be polished (Fig. 19-27, *A* and *B*). The stones, on the other hand, are able to reduce the denture base, while giving a smooth finish.

▶ Supplemental Components

To place and remove many of the attachments to a high-speed handpiece, it is necessary to use a *bur tool or device.* Each manufacturer provides such a device when a handpiece is purchased. It is wise to purchase additional bur tools in order to have a sterile bur tool for each setup. The physical characteristics of each of these devices will vary according to the design of the handpiece; however, most of them are small metallic devices with an assortment of prongs that fit into the head of the handpiece and are used to tighten and loosen the bur (Fig. 19-28).

Perhaps one of the most vital and needed back-up devices is a **chuck.** Most chucks are made of metal. The majority of high-speed handpieces are designed with a chuck in the head of the handpiece as a retentive device.

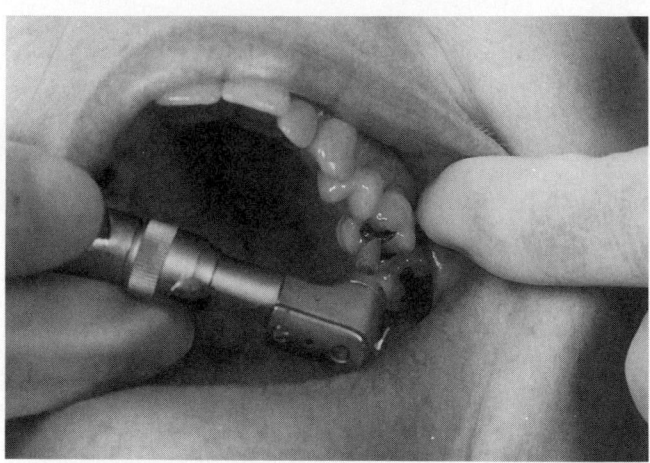

FIG. 19-26   Abrasive point attached to a low-speed handpiece that is used to polish an amalgam restoration.

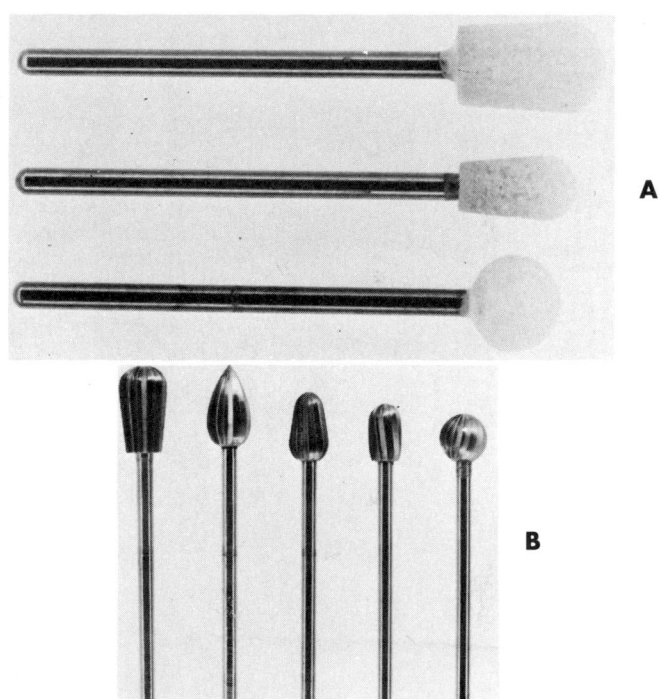

FIG. 19-27   *A,* Large acrylic stones. *B,* Acrylic burs are used to cut and polish acrylic.

(From Chasteen JE: *Essentials of clinical dental assisting,* St Louis, 1989, Mosby.)

In most handpieces the routine for bur usage is to insert the bur, secure it in place with a bur tool, use the bur, and then remove the bur with the bur tool. Obviously, this procedure can be modified, depending on the manufacturer's design, and in some instances bur tools may not even be needed.

If you are careless in removing burs, the chuck can be removed and, because of its size, easily lost. A bur should

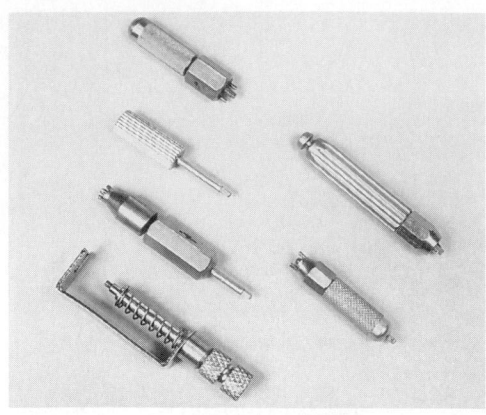

FIG. 19-28 Various types of bur tools.

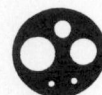

5-Tube
Fiber optic
connection

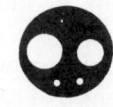

Midwest 4-tube
connection

3-Tube
connection

2-Tube
connection

FIG. 19-29 Hose connections to handpieces; from two to five holes, depending on the number of tubes from the main hosing to the handpiece.

(Courtesy of Midwest Dental Products Corporation, Des Plaines, Ill.)

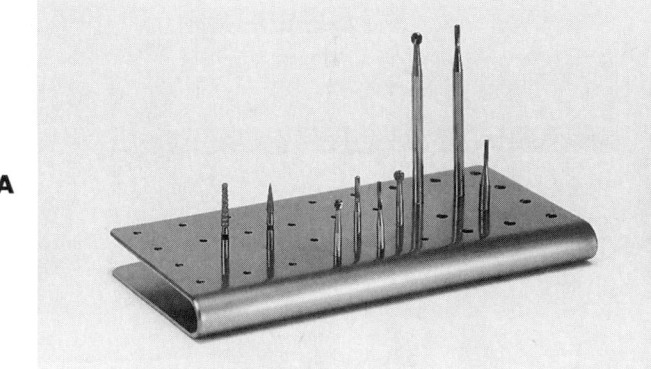

A

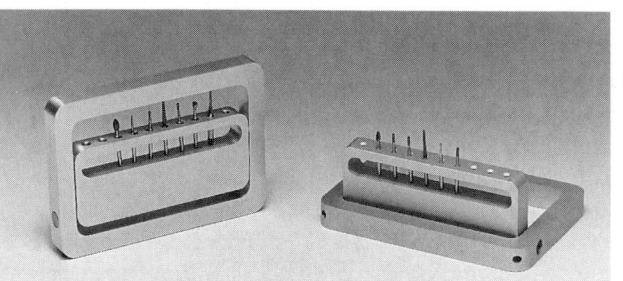

B

FIG. 19-30 A and B, Two examples of bur blocks used to hold and organize burs.

(Courtesy of Midwest Dental Products Corporation, Des Plaines, Ill.)

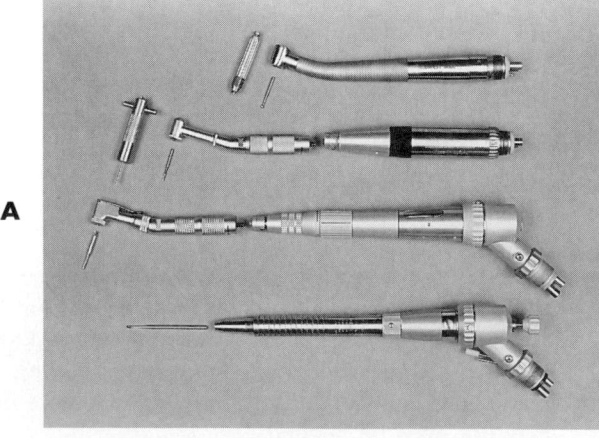

A

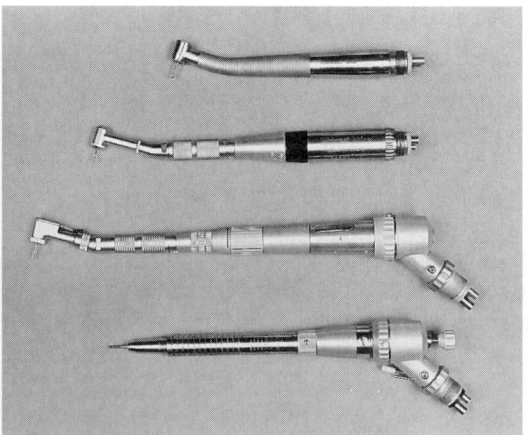

B

FIG. 19-31 A and B, Several different handpieces, with and without attachments and/or burs.

be loosened from the handpiece, grasped in the fingers, and pulled out of the head of the handpiece. After removing the bur, look at the handpiece to ensure that the chuck has remained in place. When a chuck is lost from a handpiece, it renders the handpiece inactive until the chuck is replaced.

A **hose connector gasket** is another device that is necessary for back-up on all high-speed handpieces. The gasket at the rear of the handpiece provides a tight seal between the handpiece and the hose. Gaskets will vary for different handpieces in the number of tubes going from the main hosing to the handpiece. Commonly, the number of holes varies from 2 to 5, as shown in Fig. 19-29.

Preparation of Rotary Devices

Every preset tray for any operative or specialty procedure has the necessary armamentarium for the procedure. Burs, when needed, are part of this setup. The burs will likely be in a bur tray or holder in sequence of use (Fig. 19-30, *A* and *B*). It is the responsibility of the dental assistant to assemble the burs onto the appropriate handpiece in sequence of use. It is necessary that the assistant understand the operator's preferred sequence of use during any clinical procedure. Typical examples of handpieces and the assembled armamentarium for use are illustrated in Fig. 19-31, *A* and *B*. Steps for the procedure of preparing rotary devices are shown for the straight handpiece when it is used alone, the low-speed handpiece used with a variety of attachments, and the high-speed handpiece with bur placement (Figs. 19-32 through 19-35). Assembly may vary with different manufacturers' equipment, but this description is generic to most handpieces. Box 19-4 is a checklist to use when preparing and using rotary devices.

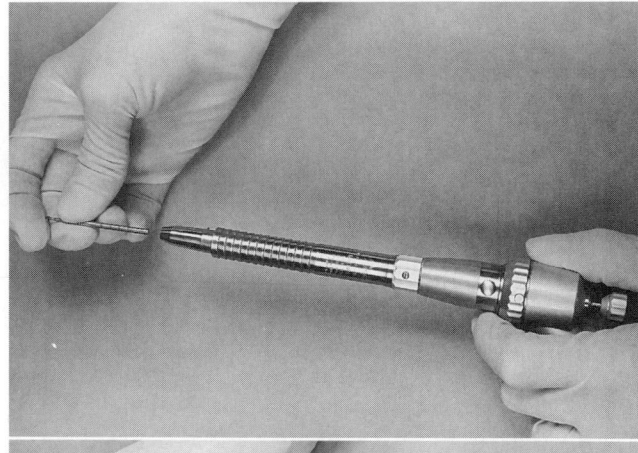

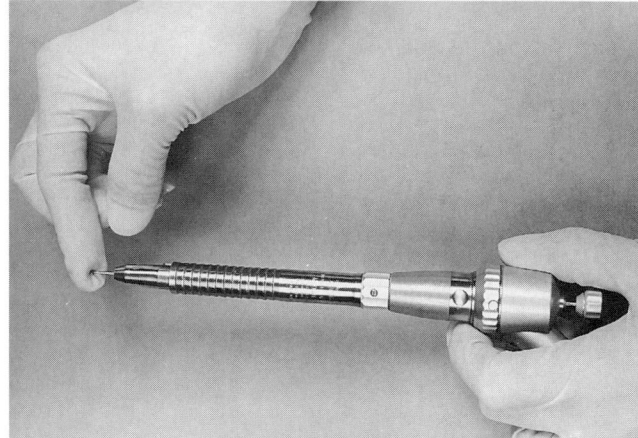

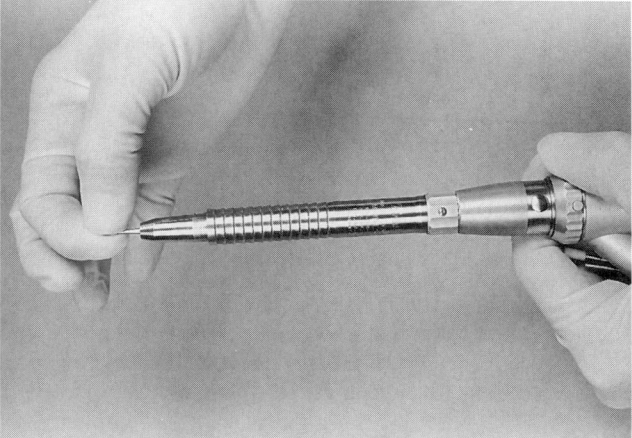

FIG. 19-32 Assembly of a low-speed straight handpiece. *A,* The straight handpiece bur is placed into the opening. *B,* After the bur is positioned, the buttons and knobs on the handpiece are tightened. *C,* The bur is checked to be certain it is secure in the handpiece.

BOX 19-4

CHECKLIST FOR USING ROTARY DEVICES

1. Are all of the rotary devices and attachments that are to be used for this procedure at chairside on the mobile cabinetry?
2. Have these devices been sterilized before use on this patient?
3. Is the attachment, such as a contra-angle, bur, or stone, securely in place for use by the operator?
4. Has the appropriate handpiece been turned *on* and is it in position to be used?
5. After the procedure has been completed, have all of the rotary devices been removed from the handpieces?
6. Are the chucks still secure in the handpieces?
7. Have the angles, burs, and handpieces been sterilized properly after each patient?

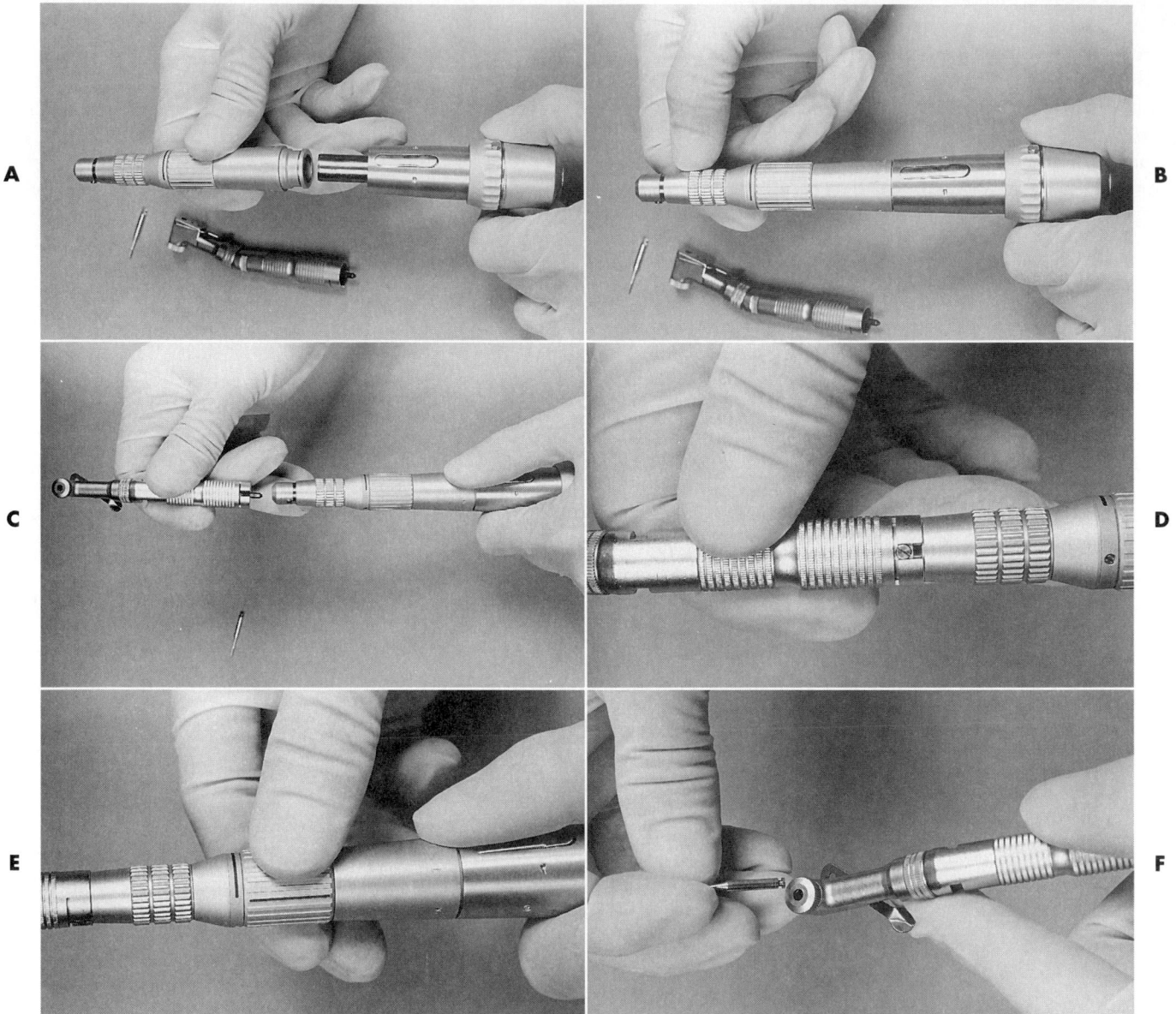

FIG. 19-33   Assembly of a low-speed handpiece with a RA contra-angle. *A,* The straight hand-piece attachment is centered over the motor of the low-speed handpiece. *B,* The straight at-tachment is positioned. *C,* The RA contra-angle is positioned onto the straight handpiece. *D,* The opening of the contra-angle is positioned over the screw of the straight handpiece. *E,* The swivel arm (note dark lines) is positioned to form a *T* that secures the contra-angle. *F,* The latch of the contra-angle is opened for placement of the bur.

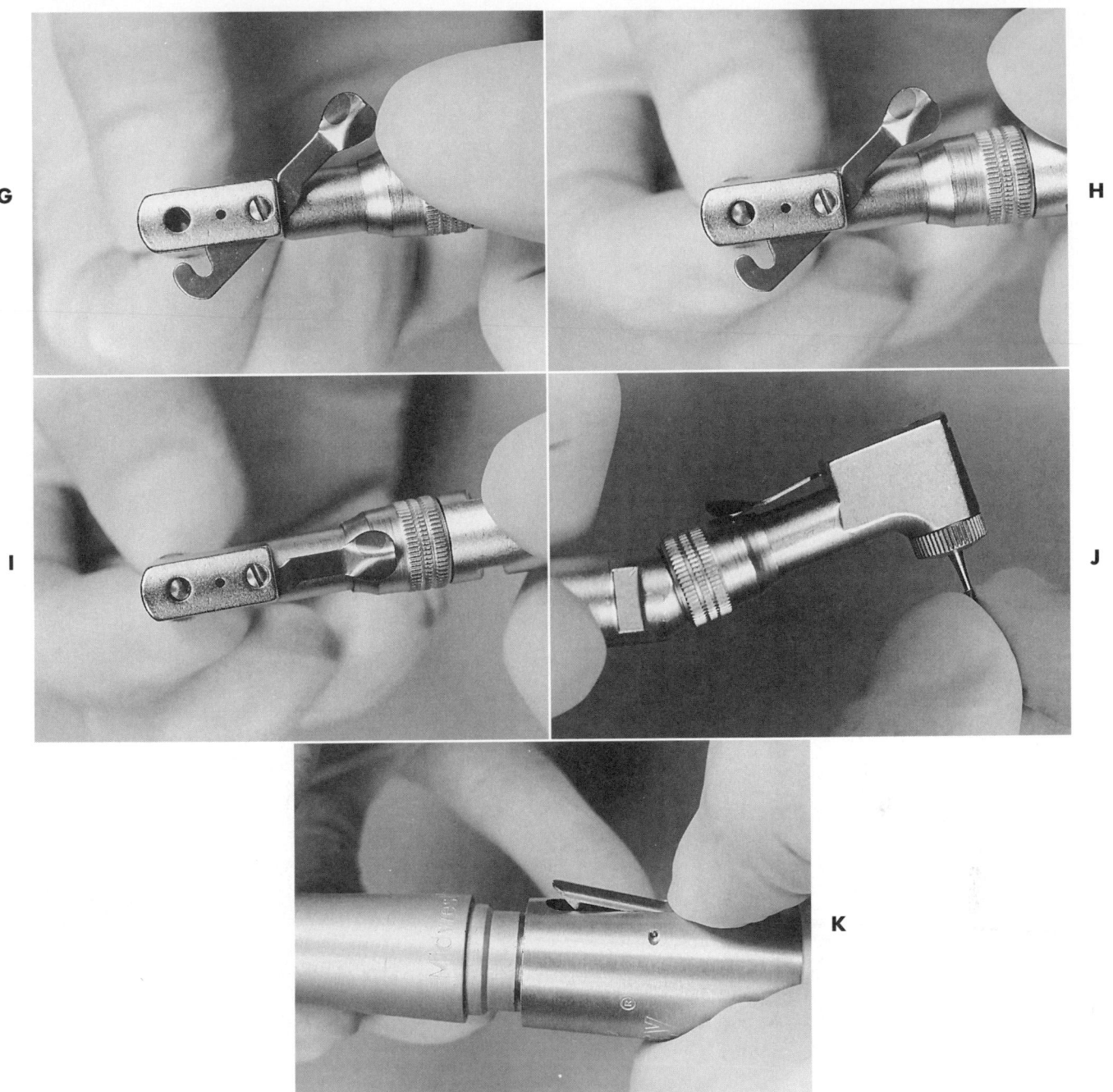

FIG. 19-33, cont'd.   *G,* The RA bur may stop before it is completely seated in place. *H,* Twisting the bur until it can be seen in the rear of the angle ensures that the bur is in position correctly. *I,* The latch is turned to lock the bur in place. *J,* The bur is tested by gently pulling on it to ensure its security. *K,* This style handpiece provides a latch for easy removal of the straight handpiece attachment. NOTE: Following these steps in reverse makes disassembly easy.

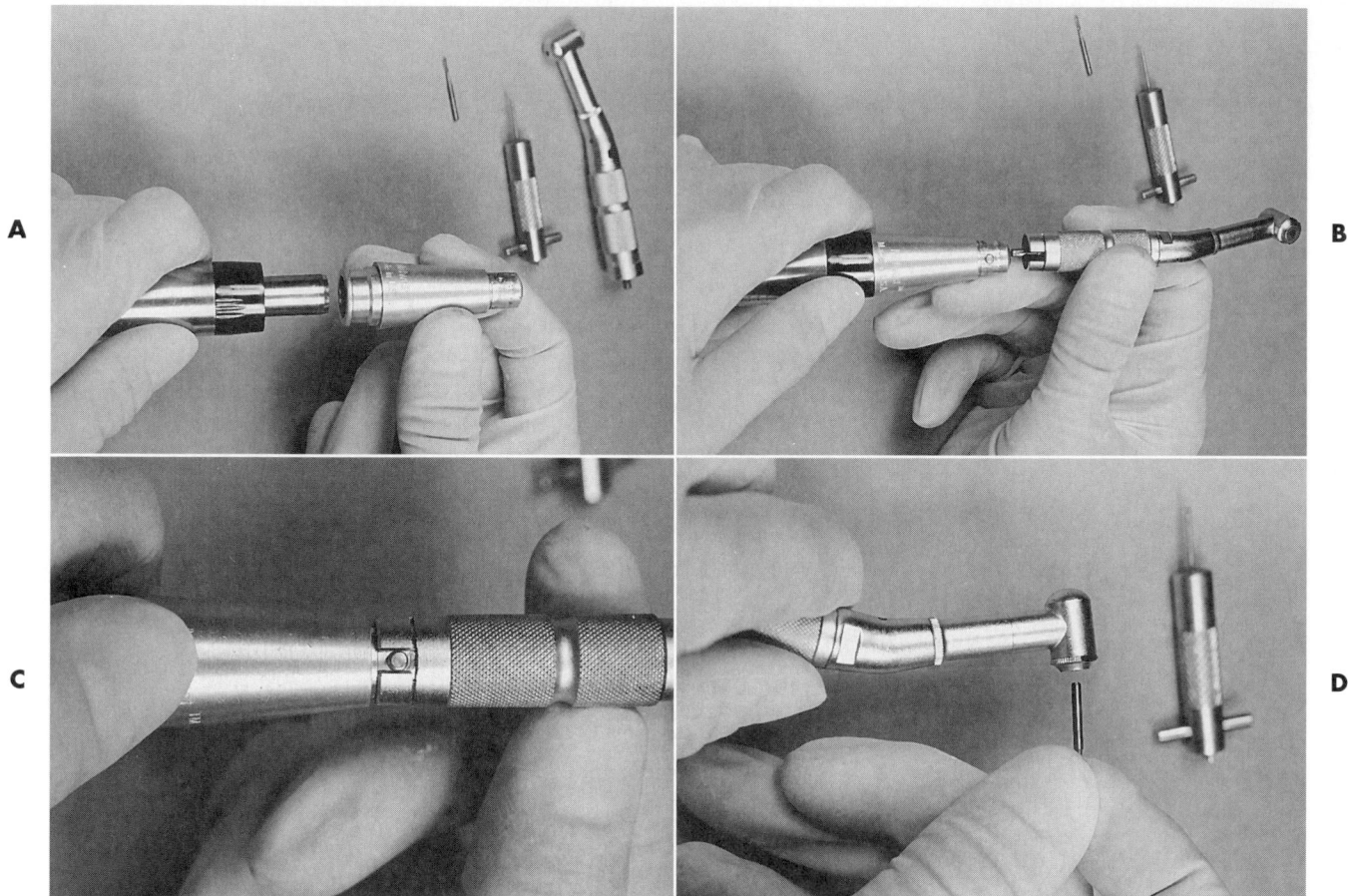

FIG. 19-34   Assembling a low-speed handpiece and an FG contra-angle. *A,* The low-speed attachment is made to the motor. *B,* The FG contra-angle is positioned over the straight hand-piece. *C,* The FG angle opening is positioned over the nub of the handpiece. *D,* The FG bur is placed in the angle and is tested to make sure that it is secure.

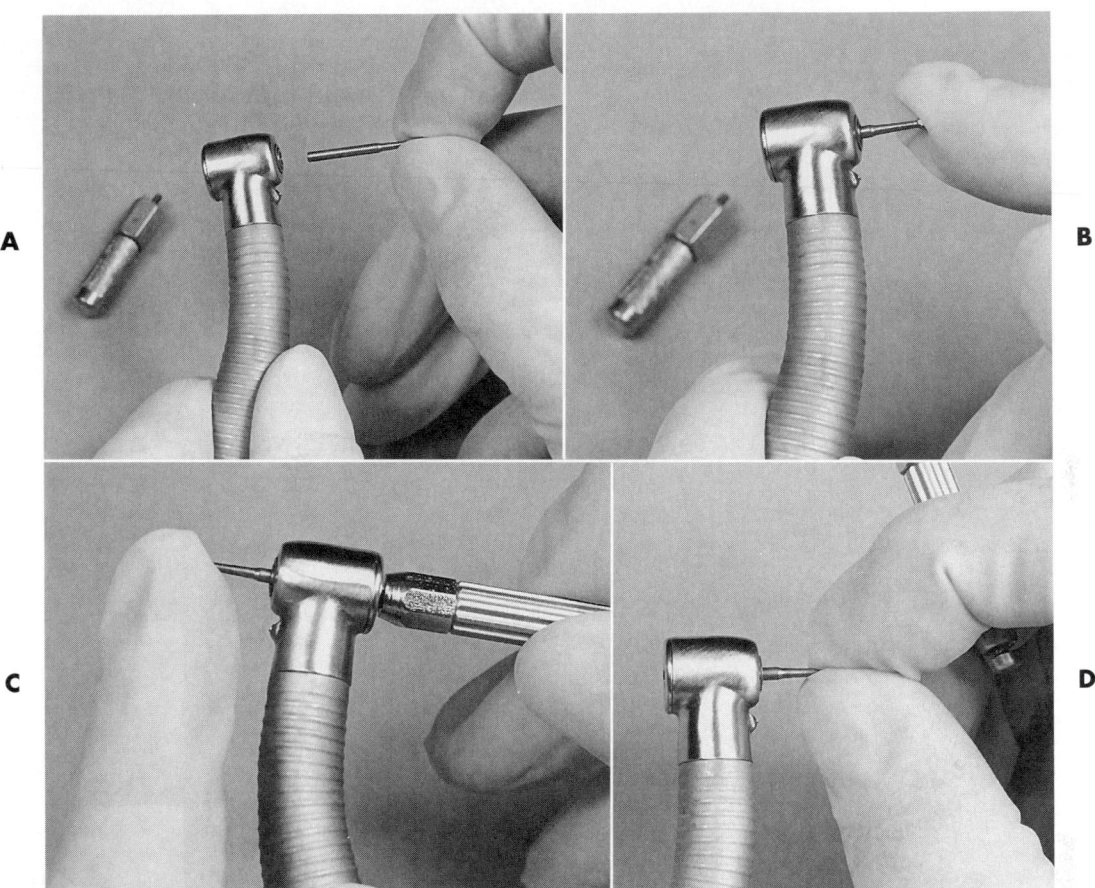

FIG. 19-35   Assembly of high-speed handpiece. *A,* The FG bur is positioned to be placed in the high speed handpiece. *B,* The bur is placed completely in the head of the handpiece. *C,* The bur tool is placed in the back of the handpiece and is turned clockwise to tighten the chuck around the shank of the bur. *D,* After it is tightened the bur is checked to make certain that it is secure.

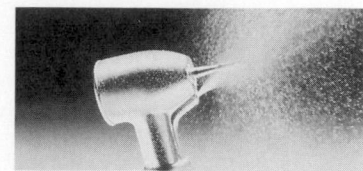

Scrub External Surface

All Products: Remove bur or prophy cup. Using a sponge, scrub and rinse external surface under hot tap water.

Dry

All Products: Thoroughly dry using gauze, paper towel or air syringe.

Pre-Clean Internal Surfaces

High Speed Handpieces: Spray with Spray-A-Day+® into: (1) drive air tube: for 1-2 secs. (lever down), and (2) chuck (lever up).

Midwest Angles: Disassemble and spray with Spray-A-Day+ into: (1) backend of angle head, (2) chuck, (3) both ends of sheath, and (4) both gears on gear and shaft assembly. Reassemble.

Midwest Triple-Seal* Angles and Low Speed Motors: Go directly to **Bag and Cycle**.

Expel Lubricant/Cleaner

High Speed Handpieces and Midwest Angles: Insert bur. Run for 30 seconds or longer to expel internal debris and excess lubricant/cleaner. Remove bur.

Clean Fiber Optics

High Speed Handpieces: Clean fiber optic surfaces, on both ends of the handpiece, using a cotton swab wet with isopropyl alcohol.

Bag and Cycle

All Products: Insert handpiece, angle or attachments into sterilization bag. Load into autoclaving/chemiclaving device. Cycle following sterilizer manufacturer's recommendations. Do not exceed 275°F (135°C).

Lubricate

High Speed Handpieces: Lubricate with Spray-A-Day+ into: (1) drive air tube: for 1-2 secs. (lever down), and (2) chuck (lever up).

Midwest Angles: Disassemble and lubricate with Spray-A-Day+ into: (1) backend of angle head, (2) chuck, (3) both ends of sheath, and (4) both gears on gear and shaft assembly. Reassemble.

Midwest Triple-Seal Angles: Spray with Spray-A-Day+ into backend of sheath.

Low Speed Handpieces: Place two (2) drops of Tru-Torc® Conditioner into: (1) drive air tube, and (2) inside nose of motor.

Expel

All Products: Insert bur or prophy cup. Run for 30 seconds or longer to expel excess lubricant/cleaner.

* Triple-Seal is a registered trademark of Young Dental Corporation.

Handpiece Maintenance Procedures

HIGH SPEED HANDPIECES	LOW SPEED ANGLES	LOW SPEED MOTORS
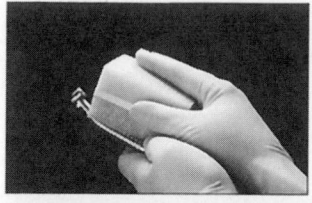	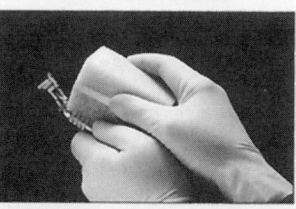	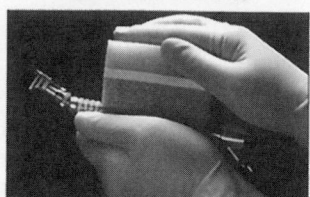
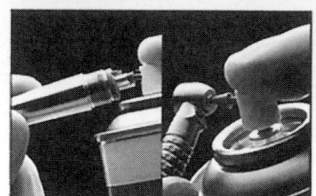	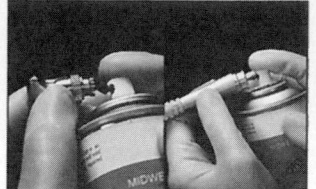	Low Speed Motors do not require internal cleaning prior to sterilization cycle
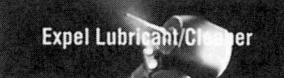 Expel Lubricant/Cleaner	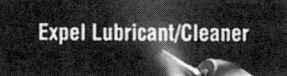 Expel Lubricant/Cleaner	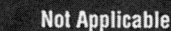 Not Applicable
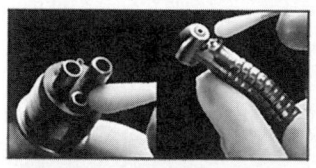	Not Applicable	Not Applicable
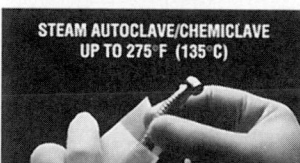 STEAM AUTOCLAVE/CHEMICLAVE UP TO 275°F (135°C)	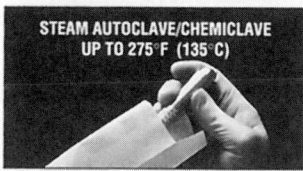 STEAM AUTOCLAVE/CHEMICLAVE UP TO 275°F (135°C)	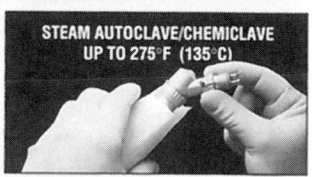 STEAM AUTOCLAVE/CHEMICLAVE UP TO 275°F (135°C)
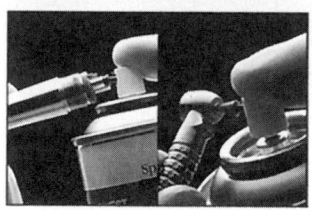	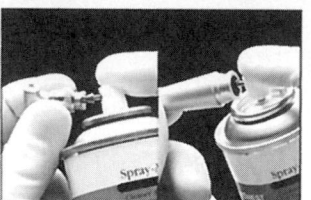	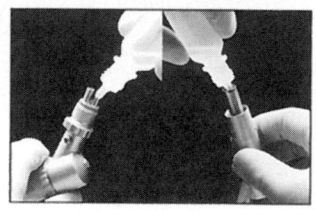

Weekly Maintenance Procedures

HIGH SPEED HANDPIECES

Ultrasonically clean handpiece head, without bur, for 1 minute in Midwest Handpiece Cleaner. If Power Lever® Handpiece, make sure lever is down. Remove and allow to air dry for 10 minutes.

Continue with Maintenance Procedures on left, beginning with **Bag and Cycle.**

LOW SPEED ANGLES

Disassemble and ultrasonically clean for 1 minute in Midwest Handpiece Cleaner. Remove and allow to air dry for 10 minutes.

Midwest Angles: Continue with Maintenance Procedures on left, beginning with **Bag and Cycle.**

Midwest Triple-Seal Angles: Apply small amount of Midwest Lubricating Grease on gears inside head. Spray with Spray-A-Day+ into front end of sheath, and both gears on gear and shaft assembly. Reassemble and continue with Maintenance Procedures on left, beginning with **Bag and Cycle.**

SHORTY® AIR MOTORS

Place one (1) drop of Tru-Torc Conditioner: (1) on each side of forward/reverse valve, (2) on outer surface of nose; and (3) on motor latch.

Wipe air motor clean (using alcohol, if preferred). Continue with Maintenance Procedures on left, beginning with **Bag and Cycle.**

RHINO XP® AIR MOTOR

Weekly Maintenance not required on Rhino XP Air Motors.

FIG. 19-36   For legend see opposite page.

Care of Rotary Devices

Each handpiece in the office represents a sizable investment for a dentist, and since it is primary to nearly every treatment procedure, the care and maintenance become a major responsibility.

Because the handpiece also is in direct contact with oral fluids, blood, and aerosol spray, it becomes a major vehicle for transmission of disease. Other than disposable prophylaxis angles and some disks, no other way exists to eliminate disease transmission other than to sterilize the handpiece. In recent years, manufacturers have made great strides in developing handpieces that can be sterilized. Cost is still a major concern for practitioners. Since most dental units house a minimum of two handpieces, even in an average dental practice it is conceivable that at least 4 to 6 low-speed handpieces and 8 to 10 high-speed handpieces are needed to ensure sterile handpieces for the minimal turnover of patients.

The procedure for the care and maintenance of dental handpieces varies with each manufacturer. Examples of a step-by-step procedure for maintaining a high-speed handpiece and maintaining a low-speed handpiece and contra-angles are found in Fig. 19-36.

KEY POINTS

▸ The ability to create a cavity preparation has evolved from the use of only hand cutting instruments, to rotary devices with less than 100,000 rpm, and further to modern handpieces that provide 600,000 rpm and laser capability.

▸ Handpieces are usually categorized as low and high speed. Low-speed handpieces are commonly used to polish teeth and restorations; refine cavity preparations; remove carious material; adjust occlusion; and grind, finish, and burnish structures. High-speed handpieces commonly cut tooth structure, remove defective restorations, finish restorations, and section teeth during extractions.

▸ All high-speed handpieces have water coolant systems to protect oral structures and may have fiberoptic or laser capability.

▸ The dental assistant must have a basic working knowledge of the symbols and terminology of rotary instruments to order and prepare the devices in handpieces. The long cutting surfaces, short shank, FG, RA, and HP shanks, mounted versus unmounted, ability to finish, abrade, burnish, and polish are features of rotary devices that provide a variety of functions.

▸ A high-speed handpiece will only accept an FG shank device, whereas a low-speed handpiece will accept all shanks of devices, as well as all angles.

▸ Traditional cutting burs are classified by a specific series number and are also known by a basic shape: inverted cone, round, straight fissure—plain cut, straight fissure—cross cut, tapered fissure—plain cut, and tapered fissure—cross cut.

▸ Besides cutting burs, other rotary devices are specialty burs, diamonds, points, disks, mandrels, and stones.

▸ The maintenance of handpieces and rotary devices according to manufacturers' directions is necessary to maintain function and decrease operating costs in a dental practice.

BIBLIOGRAPHY

Carter L, Finkbeiner BL, Yaman P: *Dental instruments,* St Louis, 1981, Mosby.

Charbeneau GT: *Principles and practice of operative dentistry,* ed 3, Philadelphia, 1988, Lea & Febiger.

FIG. 19-36　Step-by-step procedure for maintaining high-speed and low-speed handpieces and contra-angles.

(Courtesy of Midwest Dental Products Corporation, Des Plaines, Ill.)

20 Instrumentation and Exchange

LEARNING OBJECTIVES

You will have mastered the material in this chapter when you can:
- Define the key terms
- Explain the importance of instrument exchange in four-handed dentistry procedures
- Describe various instrument grasps
- Identify the basic types of instrument exchanges used at chairside
- Explain the step-by-step procedure for common instrument exchange procedures
- Describe and demonstrate how to maintain a fulcrum rest
- Describe and demonstrate the use of basic hand and rotary instruments
- Identify the responsibility of the dentist and the dental assistant during instrument exchange

- Explain various safety precautions that should be implemented during instrument exchange

KEY TERMS

Fulcrum
Hidden transfer
Instrumentation
Instrument exchange
Modified pen grasp
Palm grasp

Palm-thumb grasp
Pen grasp
Reverse exchange
Signal
Two-handed exchange

Instrumentation is the actual use of either rotary or basic hand instruments. Unlike the norm in past decades the modern dental assistant uses instruments for a variety of procedures both intraorally, while performing advanced clinical functions, and extraorally, in laboratory procedures. **Instrument exchange** is the process of transferring instruments and materials to and from the operator, within the transfer zone, at the precise moment of need.

Instrument Exchange

Instrument exchange or transfer is the first of the basic skills a chairside dental assistant must learn to increase efficiency and to reduce stress during routine dental treatment. Efficient instrument transfer can accomplish the following:
- Enable the operator to maintain vision on the field of operation
- Save time and motion for the operating team
- Reduce stress and strain on the operating team

When an instrument exchange is used in conjunction with the oral evacuator and the a/w syringe, the operator can ensure that the operative site will always be clean and the next instrument always ready for use.

Just as a surgical nurse is an asset to the surgeon during critical moments in a hospital operating room, the chairside dental assistant becomes vital to the efficiency in the dental treatment room. The value of the dental assistant depends on the efficiency with which the instruments and materials are made available to the operator. This chapter provides the basic information to develop one of the most valued chairside skills. Combined with the skills that will be learned in the next three chapters, the assistant will develop the foundational skills that are needed to become an efficient chairside assistant.

Importance of Chairside Efficiency

Before any of the basic skills at chairside are learned, the dental assistant must realize how important he or she will be to the success of the procedure and must develop a sense of anticipation for the operator's needs. The assistant's job at chairside is multifaceted and includes the following:

- Maintaining a clear, dry field of operation
- Retracting tissues that interfere with the operator's view of the treatment site
- Anticipating the operator's next need
- Passing the next instrument at the moment of need
- Observing patient needs and vital signs
- Preparing materials or medicaments when needed
- Maintaining infection control procedures

The tasks just listed seem relatively easy to learn. Anticipation, however, although most vital, may be more difficult to achieve. To learn to anticipate the operator's needs requires a thorough understanding of the procedure, full concentration focused on the treatment at hand, and an alert maintenance of a state of readiness. With today's technology, patient and operator's needs, and regulations on infection control, a dentist simply cannot work at chairside alone and maintain productivity and efficiency. Therefore, a well-educated dental assistant, who quickly learns chairside skills, becomes a necessity rather than a luxury at chairside.

Instrument Grasps

To understand how to transfer an instrument to the operator, it is necessary to understand how the instrument is held in the operator's hand. Several different instrument grasps may be used by the operator, depending on the type of instrument or the area of the mouth that is being treated. The most common methods of holding an instrument include pen grasp, modified pen grasp, palm grasp, and palm-thumb grasp.

Pen Grasp

The **pen grasp** allows the instrument to be used in a position that is common to the use of a pen or pencil. This is a comfortable, natural grasp for most operative instruments. When this grasp is used, the operator simply holds the hand in a position as though to receive a pen or pencil (Fig. 20-1, *A*) and the assistant places the instrument into the operator's hand (Fig. 20-1, *B*).

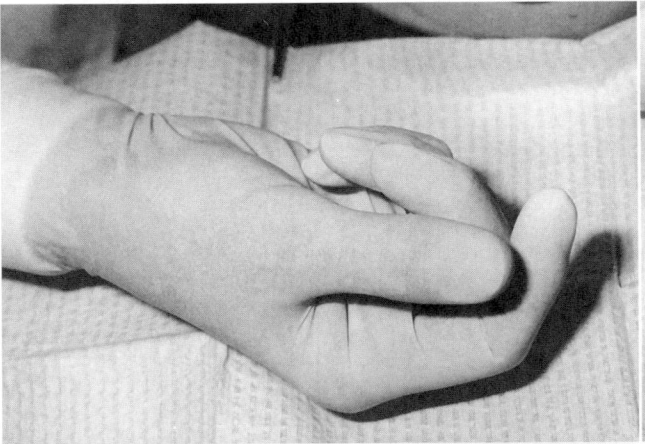
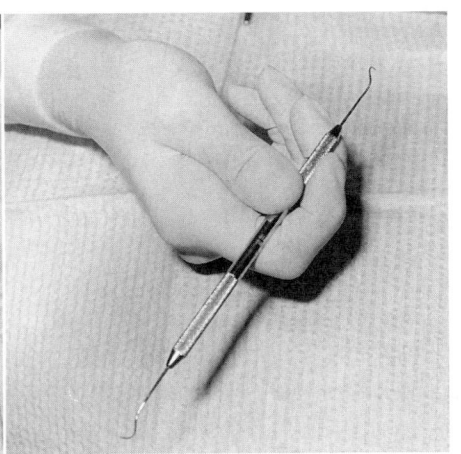
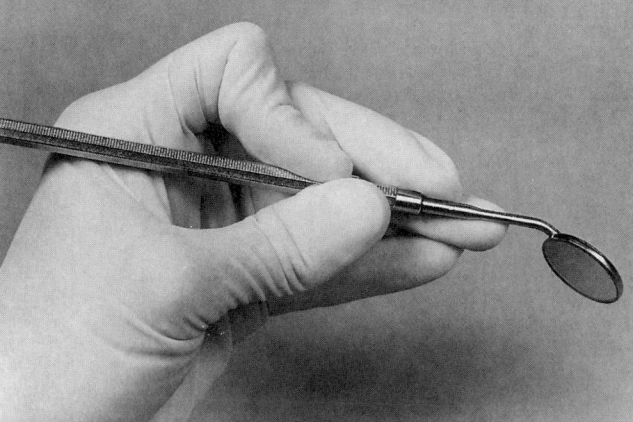

FIG. 20-1 *A*, The pen grasp. This grasp requires that the operator hold the hand in a position to receive an instrument, as if a pen or pencil were to be used. *B*, Once the assistant has delivered the instrument to the operator's hand, it is held in a pen-like position. *C*, The modified pen grasp provides more strength and stability in some procedures by using the middle finger for additional support.

◗ Modified Pen Grasp

The **modified pen grasp** is similar to the one just described, except the operator uses the pad of the middle finger on the handle of the instrument (Fig. 20-1, *C*). The simple pen grasp may not be stable enough when performing tasks in the oral cavity. The modified pen grasp is more comfortable to some operators, provides more strength and stability in some procedures, and may result in more comfort to the patient.

◗ Palm Grasp

The **palm grasp** is used for large bulky instruments. This grasp requires the operator to turn the hand back and open the palm to receive the instrument (Fig. 20-2, *A*). Once the instrument is in the palm, the operator can have a firm grip on it (Fig. 20-2, *B*). This grasp is commonly used for surgical forceps, rubber dam clamp forceps, or the a/w syringe.

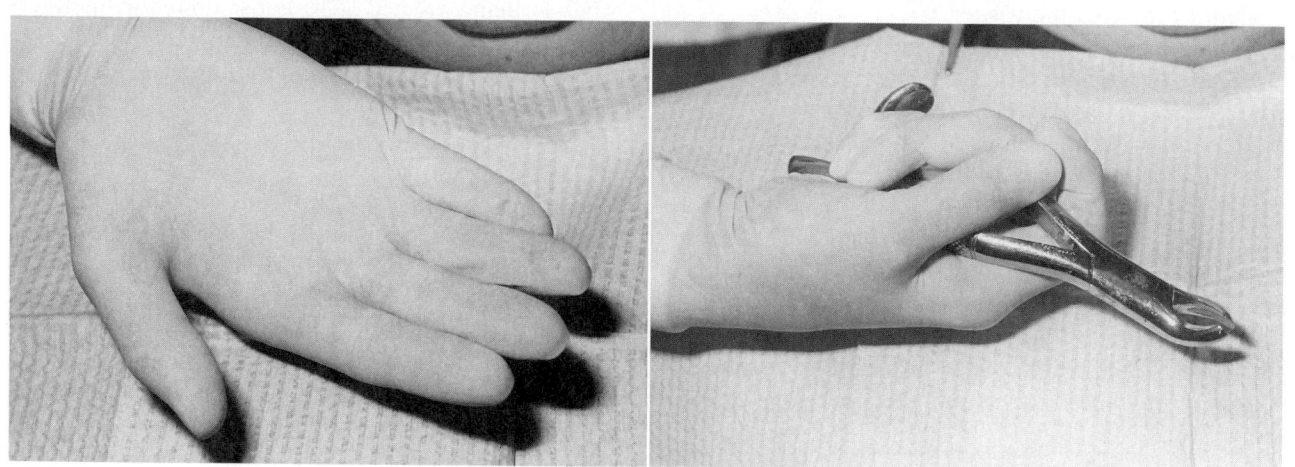

FIG. 20-2 *A,* Palm grasp. This grasp requires that the operator turn the hand back and open the palm to receive the instrument. *B,* Once the assistant delivers the instrument to the operator, it can be grasped firmly in the palm.

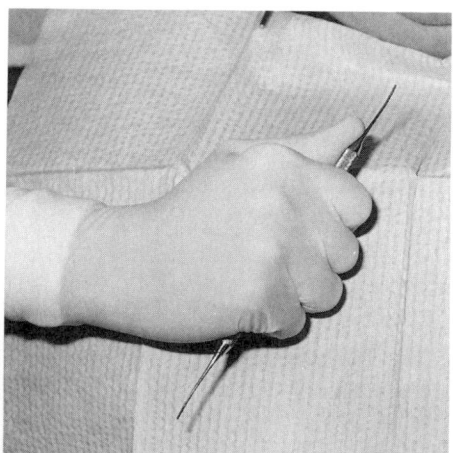

FIG. 20-3 Palm-thumb grasp. This grasp requires the operator to hold the instrument in a vertical position with the bulk of the instrument held in the palm; the thumb is used as a fulcrum on the instrument to provide stability.

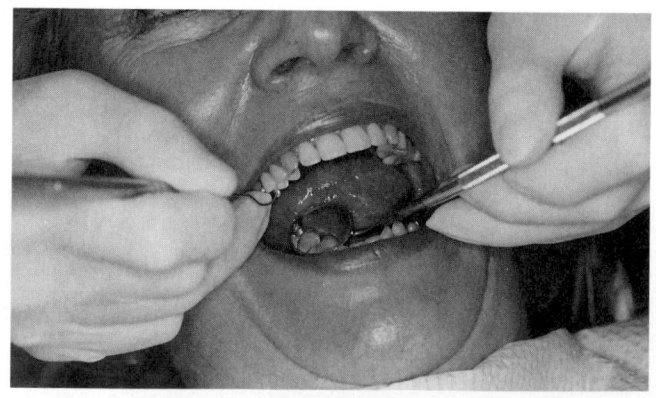

FIG. 20-4 Operator uses the small and ring fingers to maintain the fulcrum.

◗ Palm-Thumb Grasp (Thumb-to-Nose Grasp)

A **palm-thumb grasp** (Fig. 20-3) is used with instruments that require a more vertical movement, such as a Wedelstaedt chisel. In this situation the instrument is placed in the operator's palm and the thumb is used as a fulcrum on the instrument to provide stability when the instrument is used in a pushing action. This same grasp is often used by the assistant when holding the high-velocity evacuation (HVE) tip.

While using an instrument with any of these grasps, the operator must maintain a *fulcrum*. A fulcrum is the point on a tooth or the nearby tissue where the operator's hand is stabilized to allow the instrument to be used more comfortably and effectively. The use of a fulcrum is also a safety measure to avoid slippage of the instrument, which could result in injury to the patient. Commonly a doctor uses the little and ring fingers to maintain the fulcrum, as shown in Fig. 20-4.

Common Instrument Exchange Methods

Instrument exchange is one of the earliest skills developed in four-handed dentistry. Several modifications have taken place from the original methods, but the basic premise that four hands are always at work is still the primary objective of instrument exchange. To accomplish an efficient exchange, the instrument must be positioned for the arch that is being treated and the operator must be able to grasp the instrument in a normal holding position without unnecessary hand movement, while keeping the eyes on the field of operation. If a double-ended instrument is being used, the appropriate end must be placed into the working position. The basic instrument exchanges used in dentistry include the two-handed, single-handed, and hidden syringe methods.

◗ Two-handed Exchange

In a **two-handed exchange** the assistant picks up the used instrument with one hand and delivers a new instrument with the opposite hand (Fig. 20-5). This exchange requires more movement and limits efficient use of the HVE and a/w syringe. Although this method is not the preferred exchange in most common operative procedures, it is well suited for oral surgery. The palm grasp is a natural exchange for surgical forceps and elevators, which require that the operator's entire hand be used for grasping the tooth. The same grasp is used for rubber dam forceps, illustrated in Chapter 22.

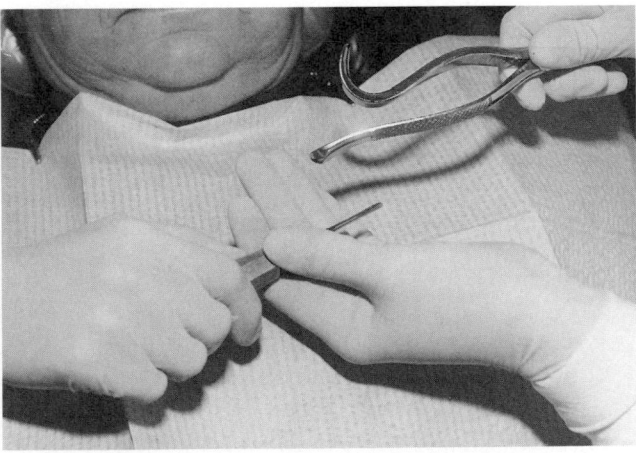

FIG. 20-5   Two-handed exchange. This exchange requires that the assistant pick up the used instrument with one hand and transfer the new instrument with the opposite hand.

◗ Single-Handed Exchange

In a **single-handed exchange**, two areas of the assistant's passing hand are used: the delivery portion and the pickup portion. The delivery portion of the hand includes the thumb and first two fingers, and the pickup portion includes the third and small finger, as illustrated in Fig. 20-6. This technique allows the assistant to take the used instrument from the operator with the pickup portion of the hand and deliver the new instrument with the delivery portion of the same hand. The assistant's opposite hand is free for retraction or for oral evacuation (Fig. 20-7).

In single-handed exchange, three areas of the instrument are considered (Fig. 20-8). The working third is the part of the instrument that must be ready to use once it is delivered to the operator; the middle third includes the handle on which the operator rests the hand; and the assistant's third is the nonworking part of the instrument held in the delivery portion of the assistant's hand. When using a single-ended instrument, such as the cotton pliers, there is only one working end. With a double-ended instrument, such as an explorer, a spoon excavator, or other hand-cutting instrument, the assistant's end and the working end may be interchangeable.

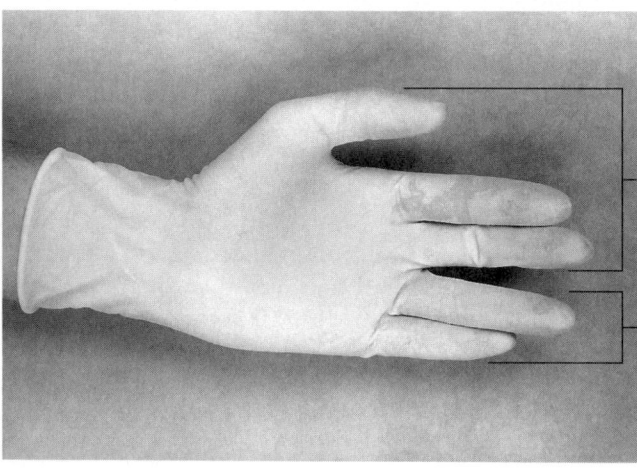

FIG. 20-6   The area of the exchange hand is divided into two parts—the delivery portion, which includes the thumb and first two fingers, and the pickup portion, which includes the third and small finger.

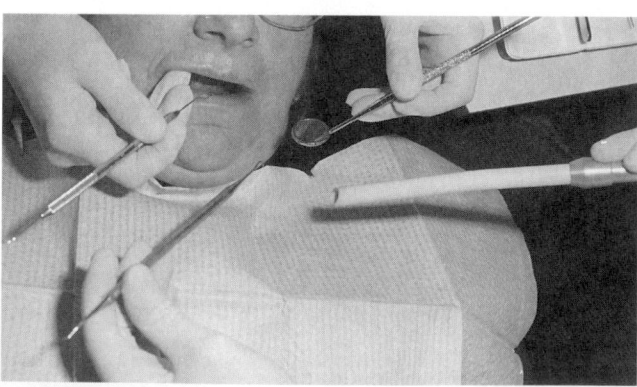

FIG. 20-7   Single-handed exchange. The assistant transfers an instrument with one hand and uses the opposite hand for retraction or oral evacuation.

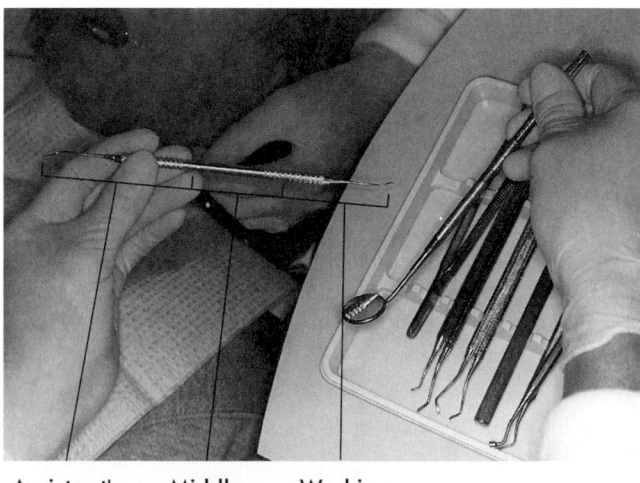

FIG. 20-8   The area of an instrument is divided into three parts—the working third, the middle third, and the nonworking third, which is held in the delivery portion of the assistant's hand.

▶ Hidden Syringe Technique

The **hidden syringe technique**, a special technique that is used to hide an instrument or device from the patient's view, is reserved primarily for the transfer of the local anesthetic syringe to the operator. In the first part of such a procedure the single-handed transfer can be used to exchange 2 × 2 gauze sponges, topical anesthetic, or an explorer (Fig. 20-9). During the actual transfer of the syringe, the two-handed transfer must be used, while the operator receives the syringe in a palm grasp position, as shown in Fig. 20-10. The syringe is *hidden* from the patient's view, hence the name of the exchange. This technique can be performed in the transfer zone or behind the patient's head in order to be hidden from the patient's sight. This procedure is described in detail in Chapter 23.

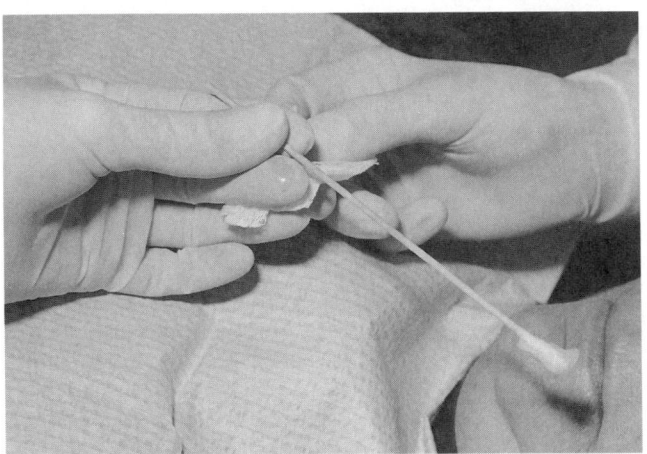

FIG. 20-9   A single-handed transfer can be used in the first phase of the hidden syringe technique to exchange a 2 × 2 gauze for a cotton tipped applicator.

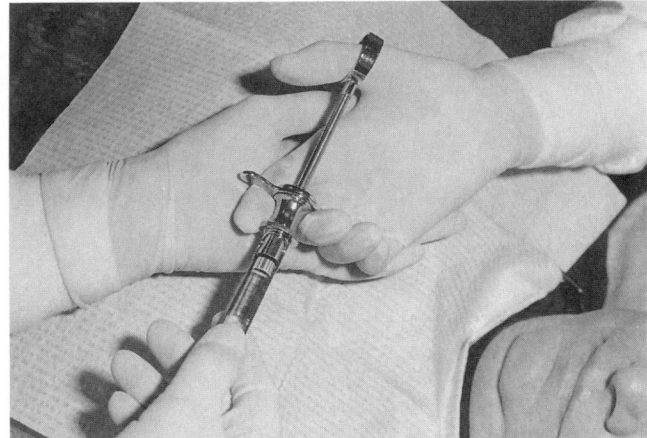

FIG. 20-10   The actual transfer of the syringe requires a two-handed transfer, which stabilizes the operator's hand while he or she passes the syringe. The syringe is *hidden* out of the patient's view.

Team Responsibilities in Instrument Exchange

For effective instrument exchange to take place, both clinicians must be committed to the concept of instrument exchange and be willing to assume specific responsibilities. Both the operator and the assistant must be concerned about safety and proper infection control techniques during the exchange of all instruments and materials. See Boxes 20-1 and 20-2 for suggested responsibilities of the assistant and operator. In addition, it is vital that safety precautions be followed for the protection of all concerned (Box 20-3).

BOX 20-1

OPERATOR'S RESPONSIBILITIES DURING INSTRUMENT EXCHANGE

▶ Develop a standardized routine for basic dental procedures.
▶ Confine movements to the oral cavity and transfer zone.
▶ Maintain a fulcrum in the oral cavity.
▶ Avoid removing instruments from the preset tray.
▶ Develop a nonverbal signal denoting a need for instrument exchange.
▶ After the signal is given for an instrument exchange, place the used instrument in a position that will enable the assistant to easily parallel the new instrument without twisting the hand.
▶ When necessary, give advance distinct verbal direction to communicate a need for a different instrument. This should be done in plenty of time so as not to disrupt the flow of the procedure.
▶ Maintain eyes on the operative site.

BOX 20-2

ASSISTANT'S RESPONSIBILITIES DURING INSTRUMENT EXCHANGE

▶ Develop a thorough understanding of the procedure.
▶ Maintain instruments in sequence of use.
▶ **Anticipate** the need for the next instrument.
▶ Be alert to any change in the procedure, and be ready to modify the sequence of instruments when necessary.
▶ Position the instrument for the proper arch—up for maxillary, and down for mandibular.
▶ Maintain the next instrument in readiness close to the transfer area before the operator's signal.
▶ Follow a safe standardized exchange procedure.
▶ Use a positive pressure transfer that ensures the operator knows that the instrument has been delivered and need not look up from the site of operation.
▶ Remove debris from the used instrument before returning it to the tray or to the operator for use again.
▶ Keep preset tray and work area free of debris and disarray.

BOX 20-3

SAFETY PRECAUTIONS FOR THE OPERATOR AND ASSISTANT

▶ When movement takes place outside the mouth, do it only in the transfer zone.
▶ Follow a safe, standardized exchange that allows a secure pickup and delivery of the instrument.
▶ Maintain firm control of the instrument at all times.
▶ Avoid tense movement.
▶ Deliver the instrument with positive pressure to the operator to ensure that it is in place.
▶ Observe patient movement, especially during syringe or sharp instrument transfer, to avoid contacting the patient with an instrument.
▶ Do not lay instruments or material on the patient napkin.

Step-by-Step Procedure for Single-Handed Transfer

Since the single-handed procedure is so widely used, it is described in a step-by-step procedure in the following discussion. The exchange can be divided into three basic stages: *instrument preparation, instrument pickup,* and the actual *instrument exchange.* Instrument exchange should flow smoothly from anticipation, to operator signal, approach, and retrieval, and finally to delivery. The description in the following step-by-step procedures for exchanging instruments is written for use with a right-handed operator. When a left-handed operator is working, use the reverse hands, and the equipment will be placed on the opposite side of the chair.

STEP-BY-STEP PROCEDURES INSTRUMENT EXCHANGE

INSTRUMENT PREPARATION

Efficient instrument exchange begins with instrument preparation.

1. Assemble instruments and armamentarium before seating the patient.
2. Use a preset tray with instruments assembled in sequence of use. Instruments may be placed on this tray at chairside from a sterile package.
3. Place tray on left side of cart as close to the patient as possible.
4. Place tray in vertical (Fig. 20-11) or in horizontal (Fig. 20-12) position with nonworking end close to the transfer hand.
5. Place auxiliary equipment, such as anesthesia, isolation materials, or cements, nearby on the mobile cart (Fig. 20-13).
6. Use the left hand for instrument exchange and the right hand for evacuation, retraction, and the a/w syringe.

INSTRUMENT PICKUP

Once the instruments are in position and the patient and operating team are seated, the following instrument exchange can begin:

1. Pick up the instrument at the nonworking third of the unit with the thumb and first finger (Fig. 20-14, *A*).
2. Rest the instrument on the middle finger, with the working end in position for the correct arch.
3. Maintain the instrument in this holding position near the transfer zone, until the operator gives a signal for exchange.

INSTRUMENT EXCHANGE

Instrument exchange then takes place in the following manner:

1. While maintaining a fulcrum, the operator signals for the exchange by moving the instrument from the tooth and bringing it outside the mouth (Fig. 20-14, *B*).
2. Parallel the new instrument with the instrument in the operator's hand.
3. Pick up the used instrument between the ring and middle fingers (Fig. 20-15, *A*). The depth at which the instrument is picked up will vary with the assistant's ability to return the instrument to the delivery portion of the hand.
4. Tuck the used instrument toward the palm (Fig. 20-15, *B*) and deliver the new instrument securely into the operator's hand.
5. Reposition the used instrument to the delivery portion of the hand. This is done by using the tip of the thumb to roll the instrument from the palm up to the ring finger, until it is above the first knuckle. Then fold the index and middle fingers under the handle of the instrument to return to the original delivery position, between the thumb and first finger (Fig. 20-15, *C* through *F*). When the fingers are wrapped around the instrument, take care to avoid puncturing the latex gloves.
6. If the instrument is to be used again, retain the delivery position. If not, return it to the proper position on the tray setup (Fig. 20-15, *G*)

▶ NOTE: An alternative method of repositioning the instrument is the *baton.* This method allows the assistant to flip the instrument from the pickup position to the delivery position without rolling the instrument. This method may require that the instrument be flipped twice to return it to the original working end. With this method, take care not to flip the instrument out of the hand and cause an injury to the patient or the operator.

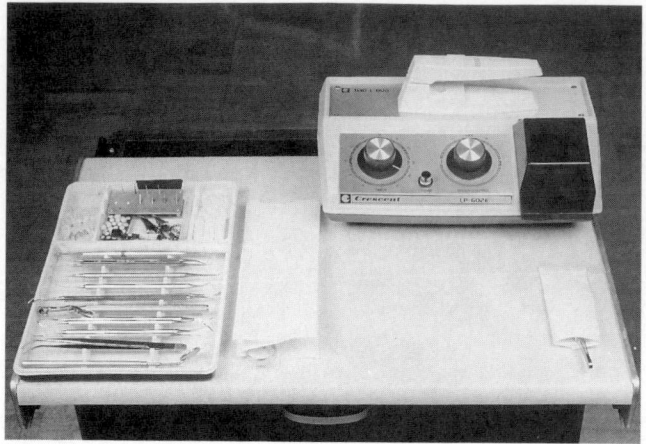

FIG. 20-11   The instruments are placed in position vertically on the mobile cabinetry, with the instruments in sequence from bottom to top.

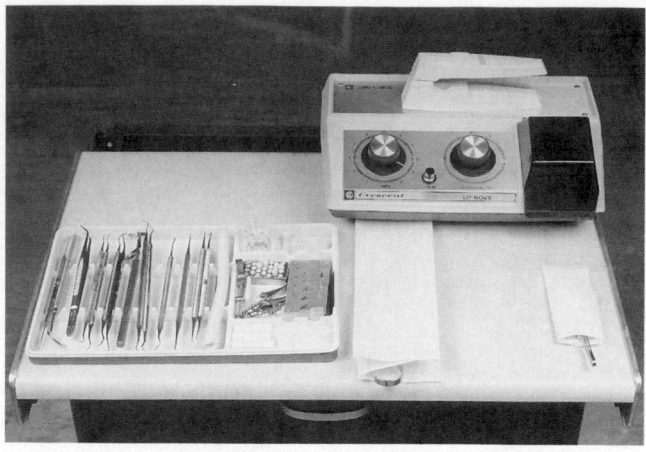

FIG. 20-12   Horizontal positioning of the instrument tray, with the sequence of instruments from left to right.

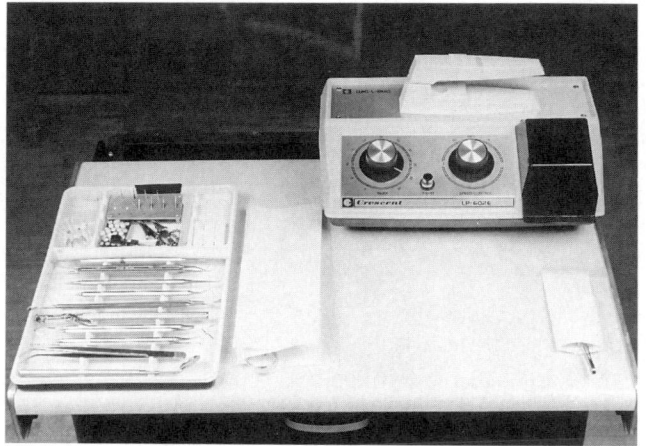

FIG. 20-13   The tray setup is positioned on the mobile cart with the auxiliary equipment, such as anesthesia and the amalgamator.

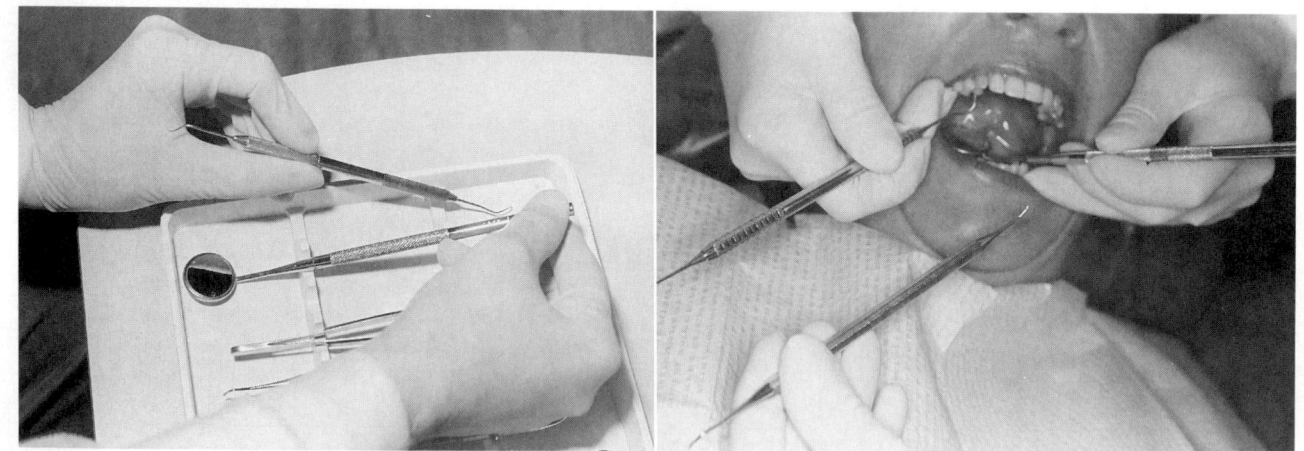

FIG. 20-14   *A,* Pick up instrument, with the thumb and first finger at the nonworking third of the instrument. *B,* Rest the instrument on the middle finger, making certain that the working end is positioned for the correct arch.

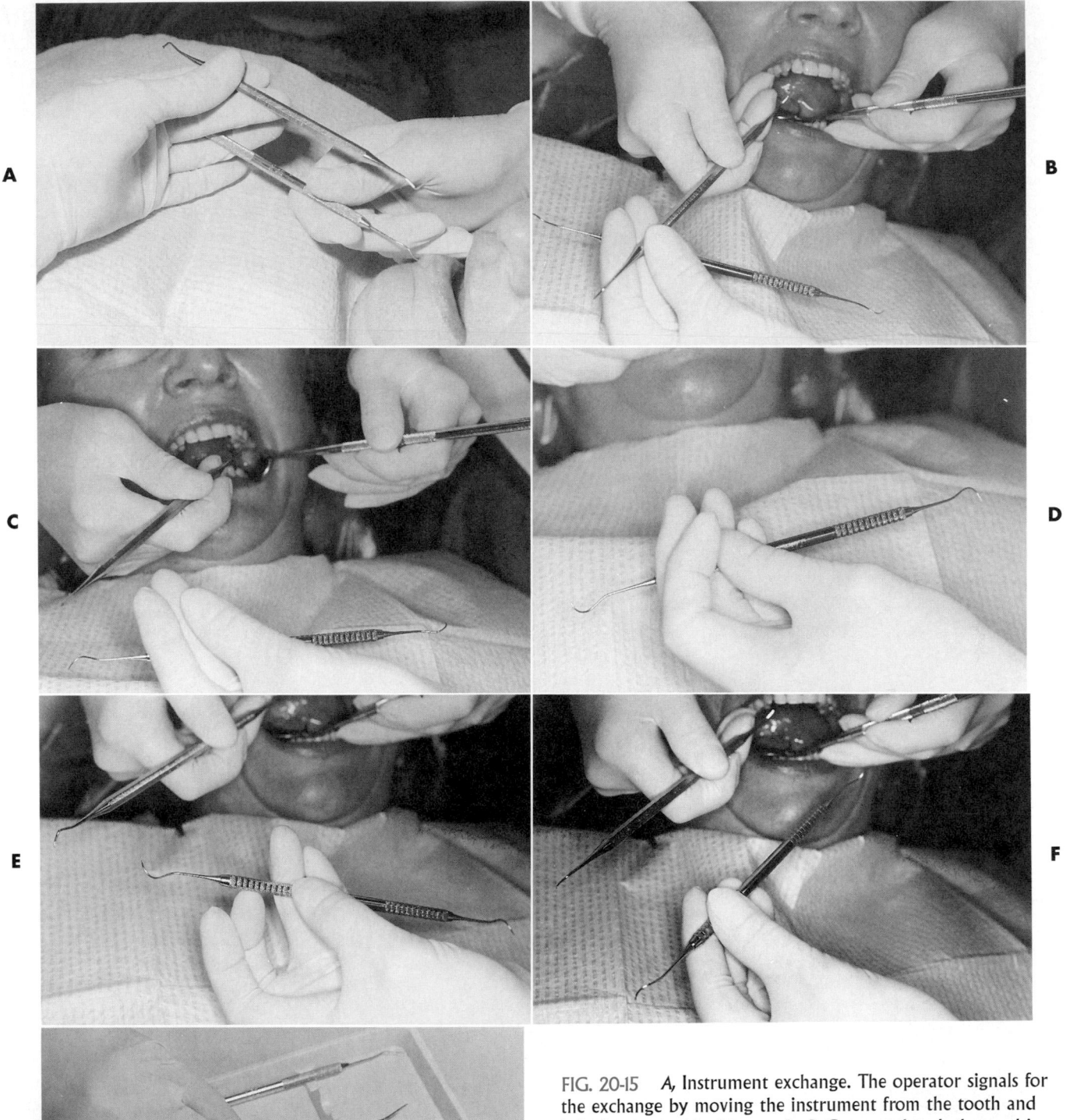

FIG. 20-15   *A,* Instrument exchange. The operator signals for the exchange by moving the instrument from the tooth and bringing it outside the mouth. *B,* Grasp and tuck the used instrument toward the wrist, and deliver the new instrument into the operator's hand. *C* through *F,* The operator returns to the mouth with the new instrument. Use the thumb to roll the instrument from the palm up to the ring finger, until it is above the first knuckle. Take care to avoid puncturing the gloves. Fold the index and middle fingers under the handle and return the instrument to the holding position. *G,* If the instrument will not be reused, it is returned to the proper position on the tray setup.

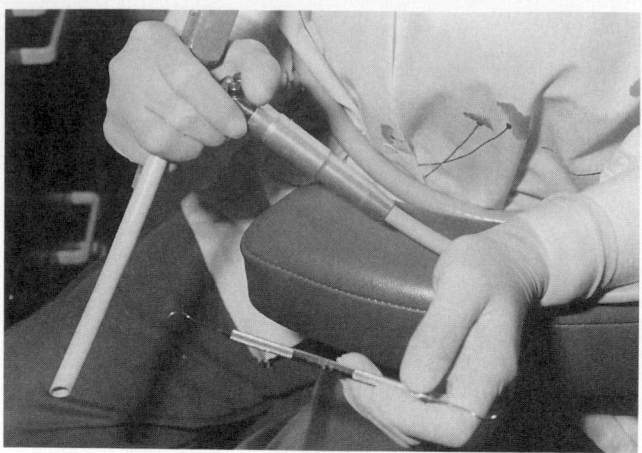

FIG. 20-16   When the a/w syringe and the HVE tip are used, the assistant places the a/w syringe in the right hand to free the other for an instrument exchange.

Procedure for Single-Handed Transfer

Instrument exchange does not occur as a separate activity. The assistant is performing several tasks at one time: exchanging instruments, evacuating oral fluids, maintaining a clear dry field, observing the patient's needs, noting changes in the operative procedure, and anticipating the operator's future needs. The assistant will be using the oral evacuator in the right hand, the a/w syringe in the left hand, and transferring a new instrument to the operator with the left hand. To do this the assistant removes the oral evacuator from the oral cavity, transfers the a/w syringe to the right hand with the oral evacuator, as shown in Fig. 20-16, and exchanges the instrument. The transfer of the a/w syringe to the right hand eliminates the need to replace it on the unit, which would create unnecessary movement and delay in the procedure.

TEAM APPROACH
Instrument Exchange

OPERATOR	ASSISTANT
	Assemble instruments in sequence of use
	Place on mobile cart
	Place instrument tray as close to patient as possible
	Using the left hand, pick up the explorer at the third of the instrument nearest to you, and with the right hand pick up the mirror by the nonworking end of the handle
	Position instruments into the delivery portion of the hands
Bring both hands into the transfer zone	Move hands with instruments into the transfer zone
Position hands to receive mirror and explorer in a pen grasp	Deliver both instruments with a firm motion
Position in oral cavity	
Signal for an exchange by lifting instrument from treatment site with right hand while maintaining fulcrum	Pick up instrument to be transferred with left hand at the third of instrument nearest you
	Position instrument in delivery portion of hand
	Move hand to transfer zone
Bring instrument out of mouth into transfer zone	Parallel new instrument with used instrument
	Pick up used instrument with the pickup portion of hand
	Tuck used instrument into palm
	Deliver new instrument
Grasp new instrument and return to treatment site	Roll instrument back to end of fingertips and reposition in delivery portion of hand
	Retain instrument in this position if to be used again
	Return instrument to original position on tray, if not to be used again

Modifications for Special Instruments or Situations

Many special situations arise that require an alternative instrument exchange. Some instruments or materials may be too bulky, may be small, may have an unusual design, or may require a special position to transfer them to the operator.

◗ Dental Mirror and Explorer

During the initial transfer to the operator, a mirror and explorer are passed simultaneously. For a right-handed operator the explorer goes into the right hand and the mirror goes into the left hand. The mirror is placed on the tray with the handle away from the assistant, as in Fig. 20-17, *A*. When the operator is ready to receive these instruments, the assistant picks up the explorer with the left hand as previously described and picks up the mirror from the handle end with the right hand. The assistant moves into position, the operator opens both hands, and the instruments are delivered simultaneously and with significant positive pressure, as in Fig. 20-17, *B*. Future exchanges of the mirror are generally confined to the completion of the procedure or to times when it is not needed for retraction or indirect vision. The exchange of the explorer will remain the same as other instruments.

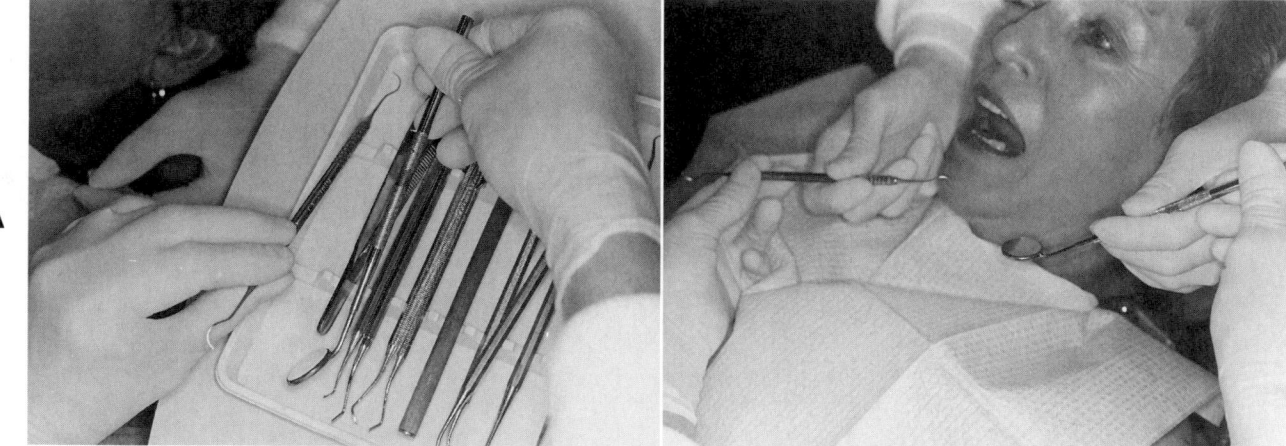

A **B**

FIG. 20-17   *A,* When the dental mirror and the explorer are passed, the assistant must pick up the mirror from the handle end with the right hand and pick up the explorer with the left hand. *B,* The mirror and explorer are delivered simultaneously.

▶ Scissors

Scissors require the operator to change finger position for reception. Since the operator's fingers must fit into the finger rings on the scissors, it is necessary for the operator to turn the receiving hand outward and spread the fingers open to receive the scissors. To prepare to pass the scissors, the assistant picks up the scissors with the left hand (Fig. 20-18 *A*) and opens the handles slightly with the right hand (Fig. 20-18, *B*). When the operator signals for the exchange, the assistant holds the scissors in the hinged area near the beak end and parallel with the operator's instrument, placing the curve according to the arch being treated. The assistant picks up the used instrument, and the operator places the thumb and first or second fingers into the finger rings of the scissors (Fig. 20-18, *C*). The scissors are returned with the beaks toward the assistant and the normal exchange resumes (Fig. 20-18, *D*).

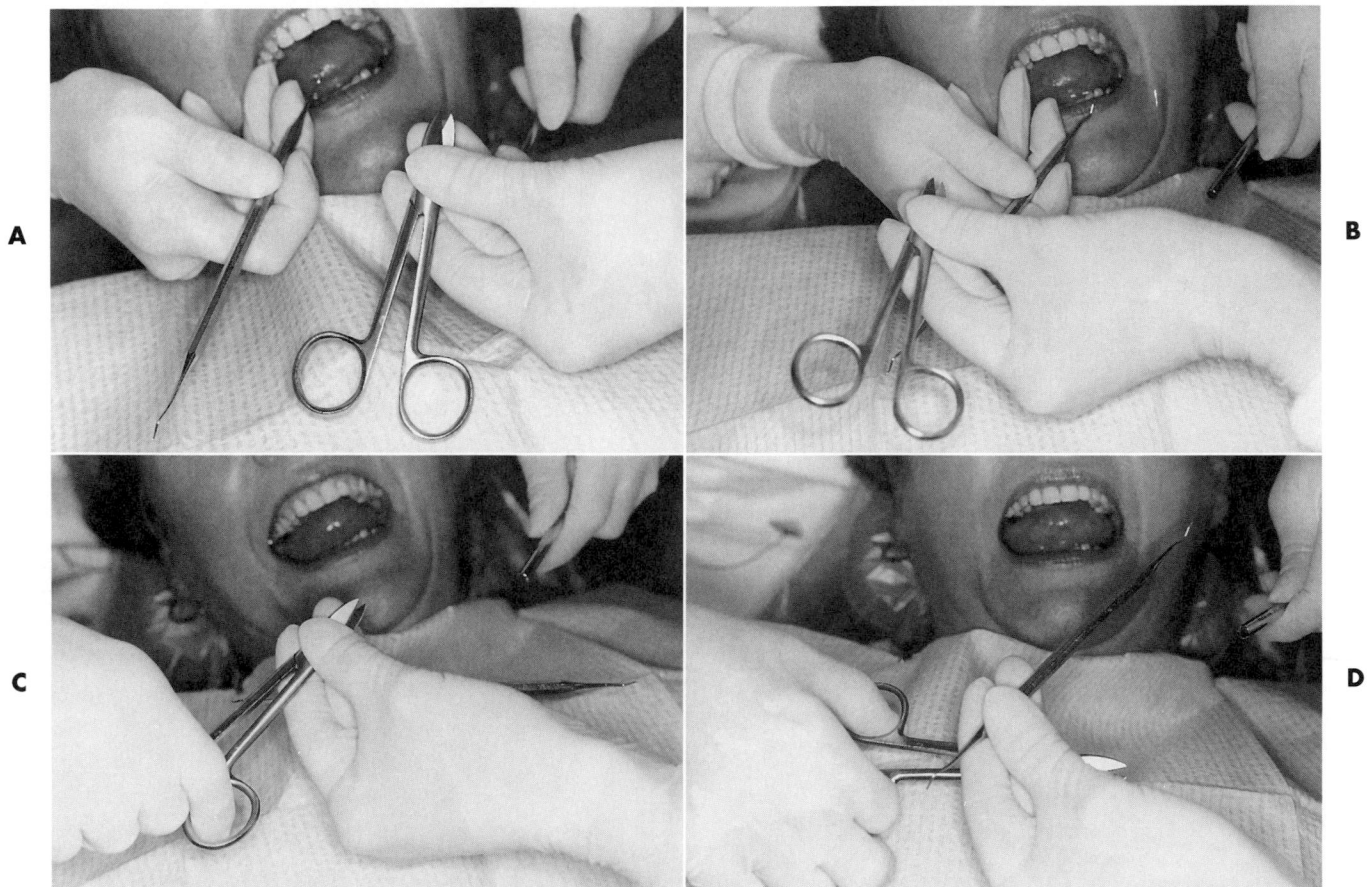

FIG. 20-18   *A*, Pick up the scissors with the left hand, open the handles slightly and parallel the scissors with the operator's instrument. *B*, Pick up the used instrument. *C*, The operator places the thumb and first or second finger into the rings of the handles. *D*, The scissors are returned with the beaks pointing toward the assistant, and the normal exchange resumes.

Tissue Forceps (Locking and Nonlocking)

When tissue pliers or forceps are used, they generally have some material between the beaks such as a cotton pellet, articulating paper, or wooden wedge. Obviously the objective is to transfer the forceps with the material to and from the mouth without dropping the contents out of the forceps. Locking pliers provide stability to the device being transferred. When a nonlocking pliers is used, the material is placed securely in the beaks before transfer. To transfer a tissue forceps requires some modifications. The assistant holds the forceps with the left hand, inserts the material to be transferred (Fig. 20-19, A), and then grasps the forceps at the back end, firmly holding the beaks closed and positioning the instrument parallel with the instrument that is being exchanged; and the transfer takes place (Fig. 20-19, B). The return of the forceps to the assistant differs from other instruments. The assistant will receive the working end of the forceps in the palm of the hand (Fig. 20-19, C) to eliminate potential dropping of the contaminated contents from the forceps. Two situations may exist (Fig. 20-19, D). First, the operator may want to return the used forceps and not receive a new instrument. This is a relatively simple procedure. The assistant opens the palm of the hand and grasps the working end of the instrument with the contaminated material, discards the contaminated material into the appropriate waste receptacle, and returns the forceps to the tray. Second, the operator may wish to exchange the used cotton forceps for a new instrument, perhaps an explorer. In this situation, the explorer is positioned parallel with the forceps, the assistant receives the working end of the used forceps in the receiving part of the hand, firmly tucking the beaks into the palm, and then places the explorer into the operator's hand. This situation requires that the assistant have a firm grip on the forceps to deliver the new instrument.

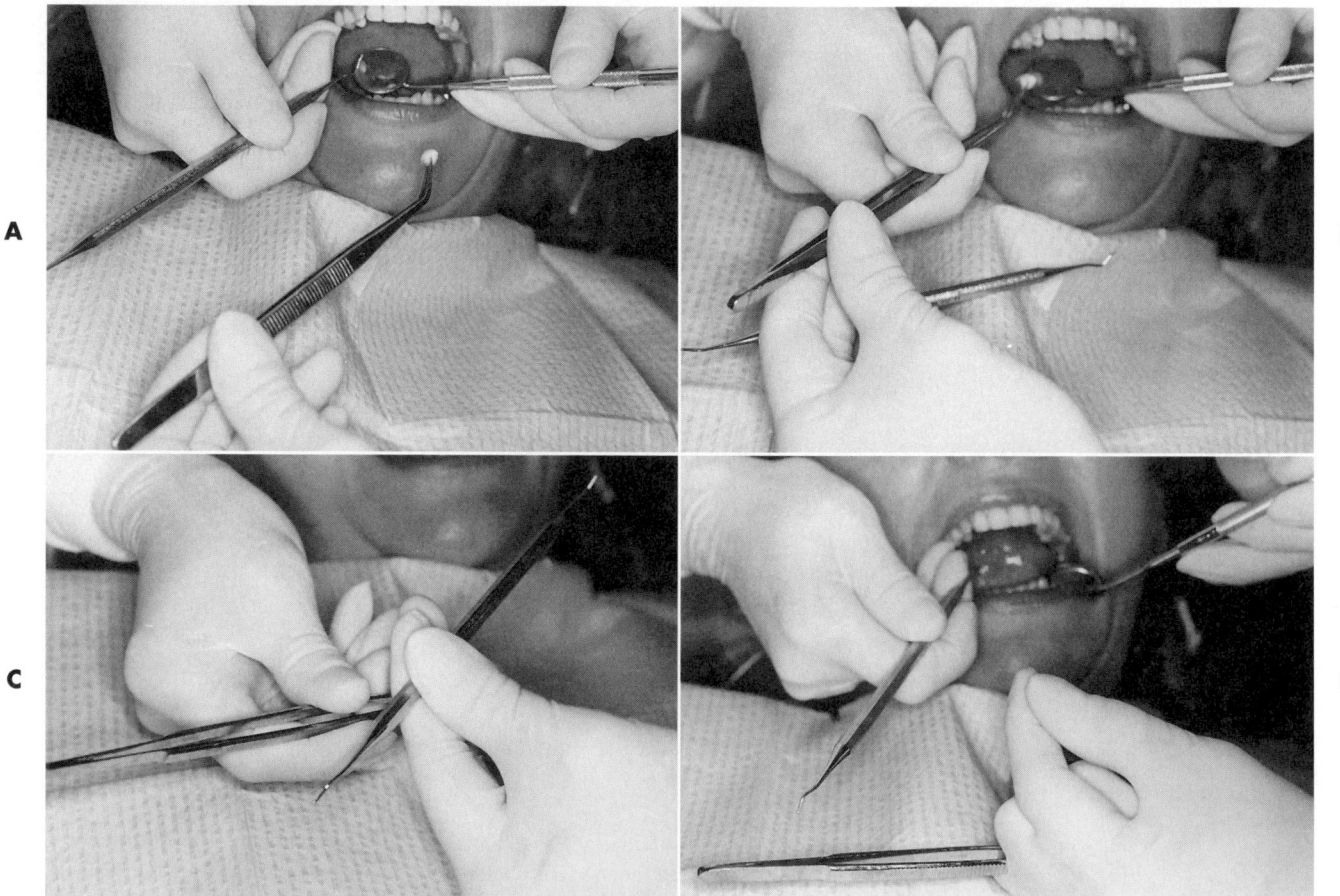

FIG. 20-19   A, The material is inserted into cotton forceps by grasping the forceps at the nonworking end. The forceps are parallel with the used instrument that is to be exchanged. B, The instrument is exchanged. C, When the used forceps is returned, the working end of the forceps is grasped in the palm of the hand to eliminate the potential of dropping the contaminated contents. D, The instrument is not rolled back into position, but rather the assistant discards the material from the forceps and returns the instrument to the tray.

▶ Dental Handpieces

Handpieces, although bulkier than the basic hand instruments, can be passed with the single-handed technique. After the handpiece is removed from the unit (Fig. 20-20, *A*), it is paralleled (Fig. 20-20, *B*). When the finger signal is given for the exchange, the used instrument is picked up, tucked (Fig. 20-20, *C*), and the handpiece is delivered (Fig. 20-20, *D*). The return of the handpiece to the assistant's pickup portion of the hand is done in the same manner as it is done with other instruments. This procedure may seem slightly cumbersome at first, but with repeated use it will become comfortable. Some units require that guide stops be placed into a holder before the handpiece is passed to the operator. If this is not done, there will be tension or pull on the handpiece, which may require the operator to have to stop before proceeding to use the handpiece. When transferring handpieces take care to avoid placing the cords on the patient's chest or face. Before the handpiece is returned to the unit, release the guide stops.

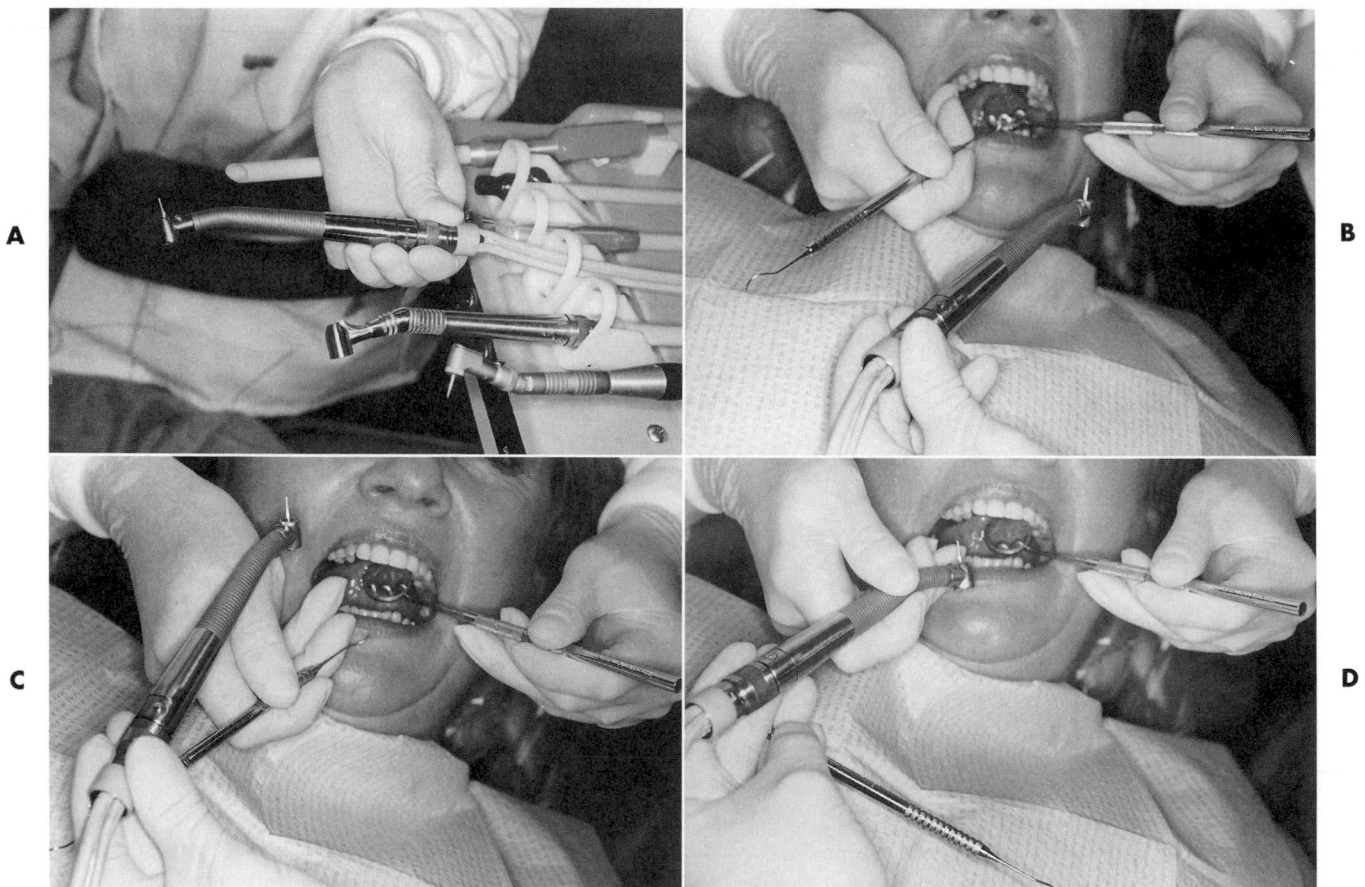

FIG. 20-20   *A,* The handpiece is retrieved from the unit in a manner similar to an instrument being retrieved from a tray. *B,* The handpiece is parallel after the finger signal is given for the exchange. *C,* The used instrument is picked up and tucked. *D,* The handpiece is delivered to the operator.

REVERSE EXCHANGE

Typically, when handpieces are used, the assistant prepares the burs in the handpieces in sequence of use. The handpiece nearest the assistant is the first to be used. To maintain maximum efficiency the operator should complete all the cutting or shaping activity with the bur before progressing to the next bur. Exchanging one handpiece for another is done just as any other exchange is done. At times, however, the operator may need to return to a previously used handpiece; to do this requires a **reverse exchange**. This exchange is necessary to eliminate the tangling of hoses on the unit, which would require unnecessary movement or delay in the procedure. A reverse exchange is done by placing the new handpiece in the pickup portion of the hand, receiving the used handpiece in the delivery portion, and delivering the new handpiece to the operator, as shown in Fig. 20-21, *A* through *C*.

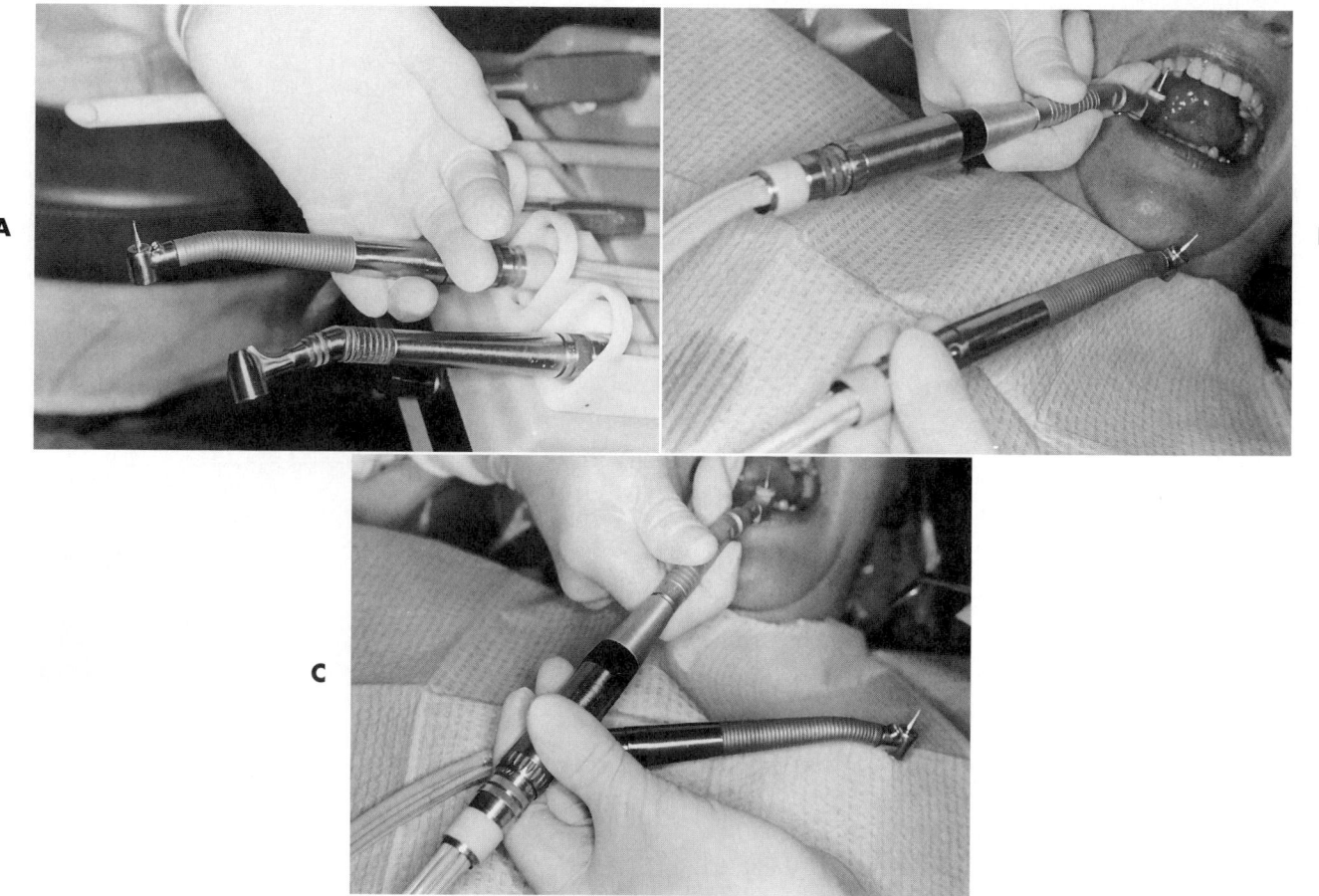

FIG. 20-21   *A,* For a reverse exchange, place the new handpiece in the pickup portion of the hand. *B,* Parallel the new handpiece with the used handpiece. Receive the used handpiece in the delivery portion of the hand, and deliver the new handpiece to the operator. *C,* Reposition handpiece for reuse, or return it to the dental unit.

▶ Air/Water Syringe

Despite the bulky size of the **a/w syringe**, it is relatively easy to exchange (Fig. 20-22, *A* and *B*). The assistant grasps the tip of the a/w syringe in the delivery portion of the hand, positions the tip parallel (as closely as possible) to the used instrument, retrieves the instrument to be exchanged, and transfers the syringe so that the operator can grasp the handle. The assistant retrieves the a/w syringe by grasping the tip and then delivers the new instrument. Paralleling of the new instrument is not easily done during this exchange (Fig. 20-22, *C*).

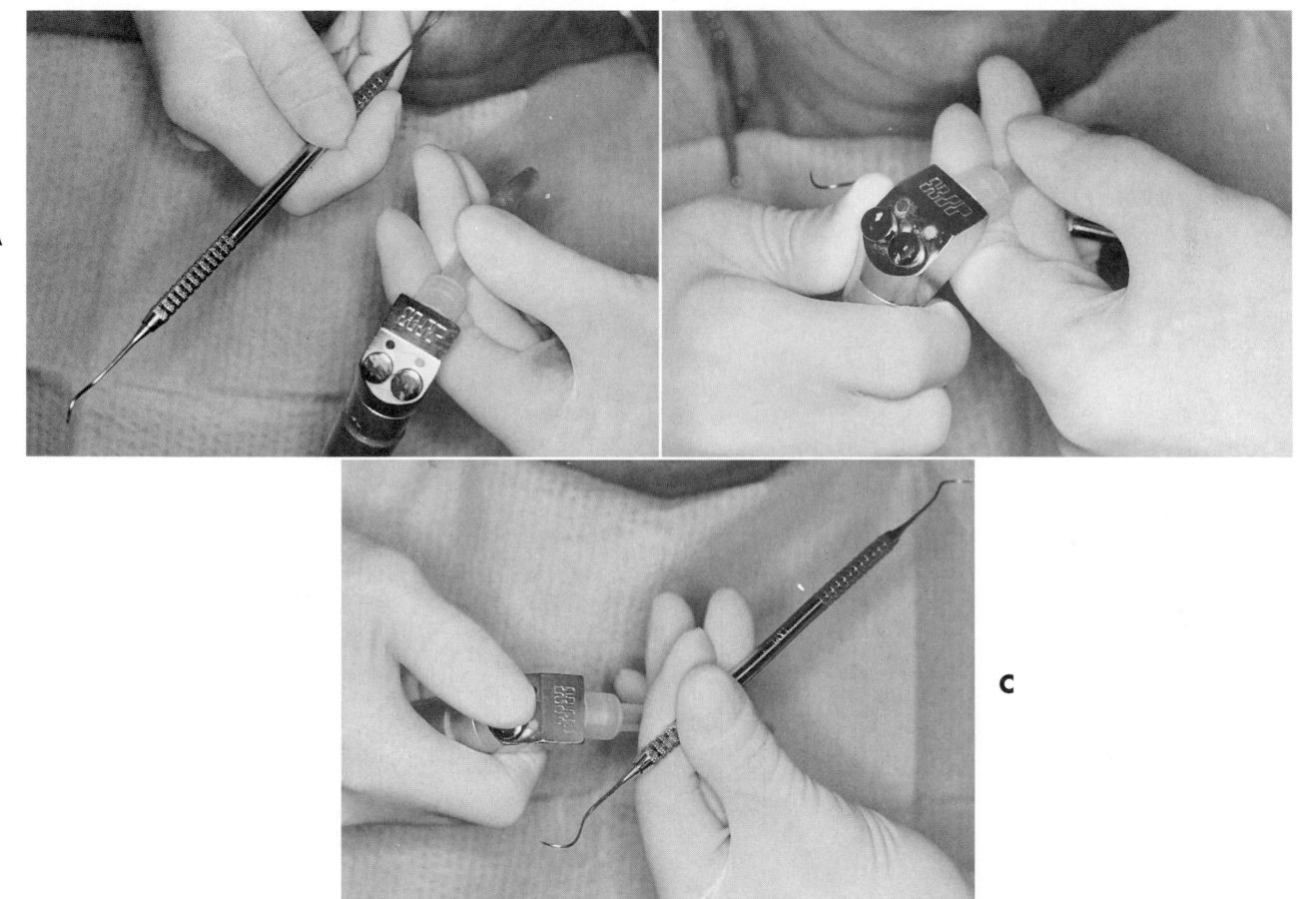

FIG. 20-22   *A,* Grasp the tip of the a/w syringe in the delivery portion of the hand and parallel the tip as close as possible to the used instrument. *B,* Retrieve the instrument that is to be exchanged, and transfer the syringe so that the operator is able to grasp the handle. *C,* When the a/w syringe is exchanged for another instrument, the tip is grasped in the pickup portion of the hand.

◗ Dental Cement

Dental cements present several concerns. The instrument that is used to insert the material is passed in a single-handed pass (Fig. 20-23, *A*). The assistant holds the dental cement in its prepared state, on a pad or a cement slab, under the patient's chin and in the transfer zone for the doctor to pick up with the packing instrument. The mixing slab with the material can be held in the right hand, and the left hand can wipe the excess material from the instrument with a 2 × 2 gauze sponge (Fig. 20-23, *B*). The pad or cement slab will need to be held with finger support beneath it because the operator will exert downward pressure when picking up the cement. It will be necessary to wipe off the instrument during this procedure, and this can be done with the opposite hand.

SMALL ITEMS

Items, such as cotton rolls, 2 × 2 sponges, or cotton-tipped applicators, are treated just as any other hand instrument (Fig. 20-24, *A* and *B*). The items are passed with the delivery portion of the hand and can be retrieved with the pickup portion. Since these items may be saturated with oral fluids, take care to discard them in the waste container on the mobile cabinetry.

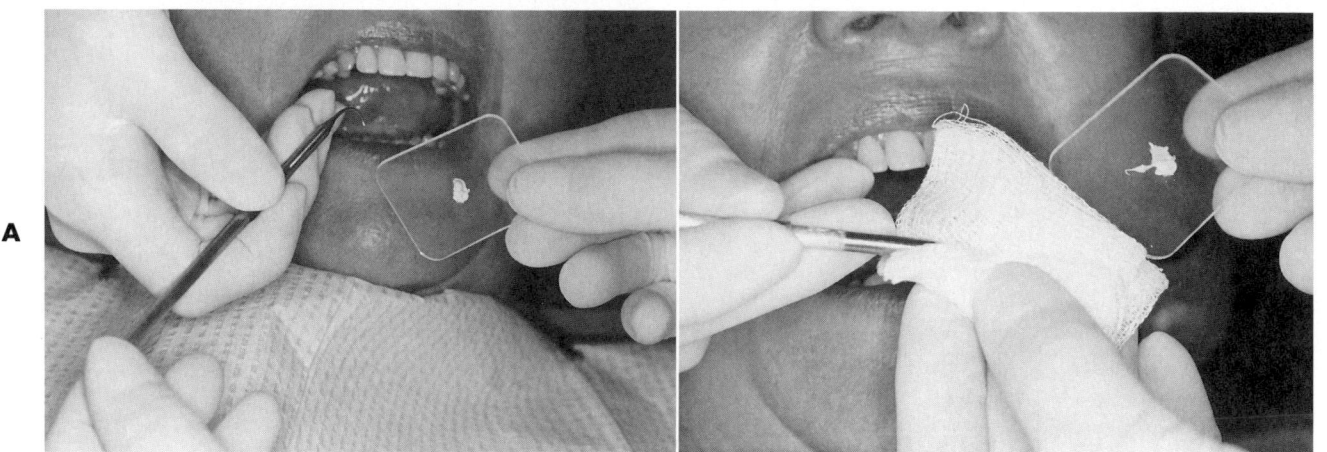

FIG. 20-23 *A,* The instrument used to insert the material is passed in a single-handed pass, and the dental cement is held in its prepared state under the patient's chin in the transfer zone. *B,* The mixing slab is held in the assistant's right hand and with the left a 2 × 2 gauze is used to wipe excess material from the instrument.

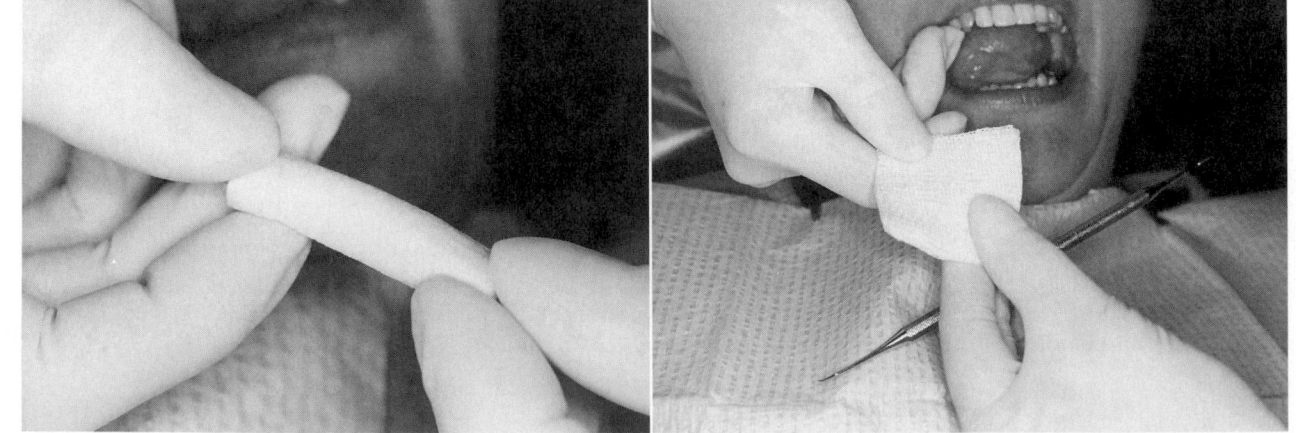

FIG. 20-24 *A,* Cotton rolls can be passed with the delivery portion of the hand. *B,* When a 2 × 2 gauze sponge is transferred, it is held near the instrument to be exchanged.

Instrumentation

In the earlier part of this chapter, emphasis was placed on the exchange of instruments from the assistant to the operator. In the latter portion of this chapter the process of using basic instruments, such as the mirror, the explorer, and the operating rotary handpieces for the purpose of advanced functions, both intraorally and extraorally, will be described. The transition from chairside assistant to operator can be relatively smooth if some basic suggestions are followed. Actually, the grasps described earlier remain the same but now the emphasis is placed on using the basic instruments intraorally. Just as it takes time to become proficient in instrument exchange, it will take time to gain proficiency in the operator position.

▶ Use of the Dental Mirror

The actual use of the mirror was described in Chapter 18. It was noted that the mirror not only provides indirect vision, but also aids in illuminating the area and provides retraction of the cheeks, lips, and tongue. The mouth mirror is the primary instrument used for visual examination, an advanced function in many states. Without the use of a mirror, unnecessary stress and strain would be required to visually observe many areas of the mouth. For instance, in the posterior of the mouth the operating light can be directed onto the mirror and the lingual surfaces of the maxillary teeth, the maxillary tuberosities, the lingual tonsils, and the palate can be seen more readily.

The dental mirror is held in the hand opposite the working hand. For the right-handed operator it will usually be held in the left hand. This allows the explorer or another instrument to be used in the working hand. Grasp the mirror with the thumb, middle finger, and index finger of the left hand as though you were holding a pen. This is the standard pen grasp (Fig. 20-25, *A*). To use the modified pen grasp, assume a comfortable working position, place the *pad* of the middle finger (instead of the side) against the shank of the mirror. The thumb and index finger should be opposite each other at the junction of the handle and the shank of the mirror. The handle will rest against the hand at any point beyond the first joint of the index finger, giving stability to the mirror (Fig. 20-25, *B*).

In the chairside role the assistant is skilled in using direct vision. As the operator, it is necessary to orient the mind and eye to using a dental mirror for indirect vision. Remember, everything in the mirror is a reflection, and the hand instrument seen in the mirror's reflection must be coordinated with the image the eye sees. The mirror is carried into the mouth, while using the small and next finger to retract the cheek. The mirror is placed, the light is positioned for adequate illumination, and the tooth or tissues are reflected into the mirror by moving the mirror back and forth until a complete and clear image is obtained. Often, it will be necessary to turn the wrist to gain access to specific areas. This is especially true when examining some of the posterior maxillary areas or the mandibular lingual aspect.

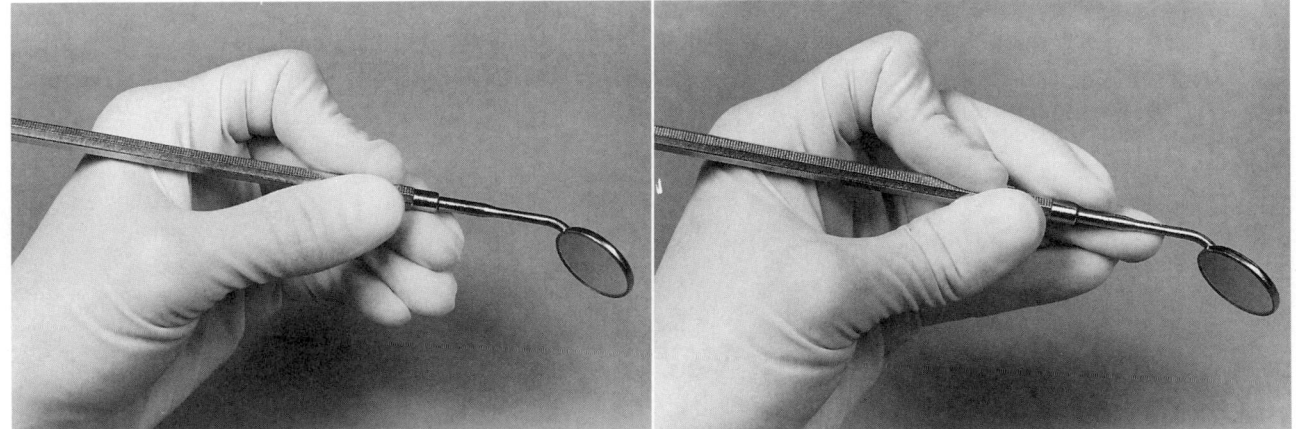

A   **B**

FIG. 20-25   *A*, The mirror is grasped, using a standard pen grasp. *B*, The mirror is grasped using a modified pen grasp.

▶ Use of the Explorer

The actual use of the **explorer** and other basic hand instruments intraorally varies with each state. However, whether the explorer is used intraorally or extraorally, it is important for the assistant to achieve this manual skill. The explorer must be held with a light but firm pen or modified pen grasp in the right hand for a right-handed operator and the opposite for the left-handed operator. When an exploratory stroke is used, the instrument must be held lightly to ensure maximum tactile sensitivity. A fulcrum (finger rest) should be maintained on teeth that are close to the working area or site that is being explored (Fig. 20-26). When the work area is on posterior maxillary teeth, it may be necessary to use an alternative rest, such as the mandibular teeth on the opposite arch. When these areas are explored, it is not uncommon to use an extraoral hand rest on the mandible to gain access to distal surfaces of the maxillary second and third molars, especially when a straighter shanked explorer is used.

For the dental assistant the use of the explorer may include checking and marking the cervical margins of

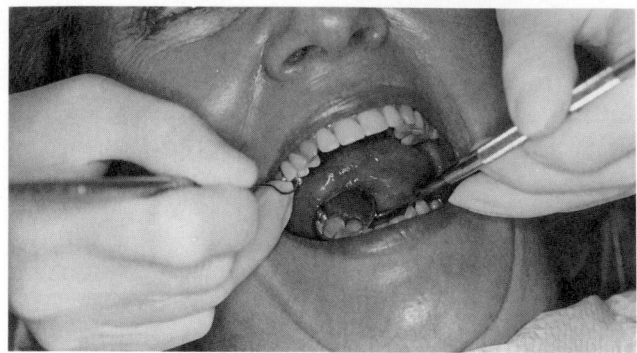

FIG. 20-26   A fulcrum is maintained on the teeth that is close to the working area.

A   Vertical

B   Oblique

C   Horizontal

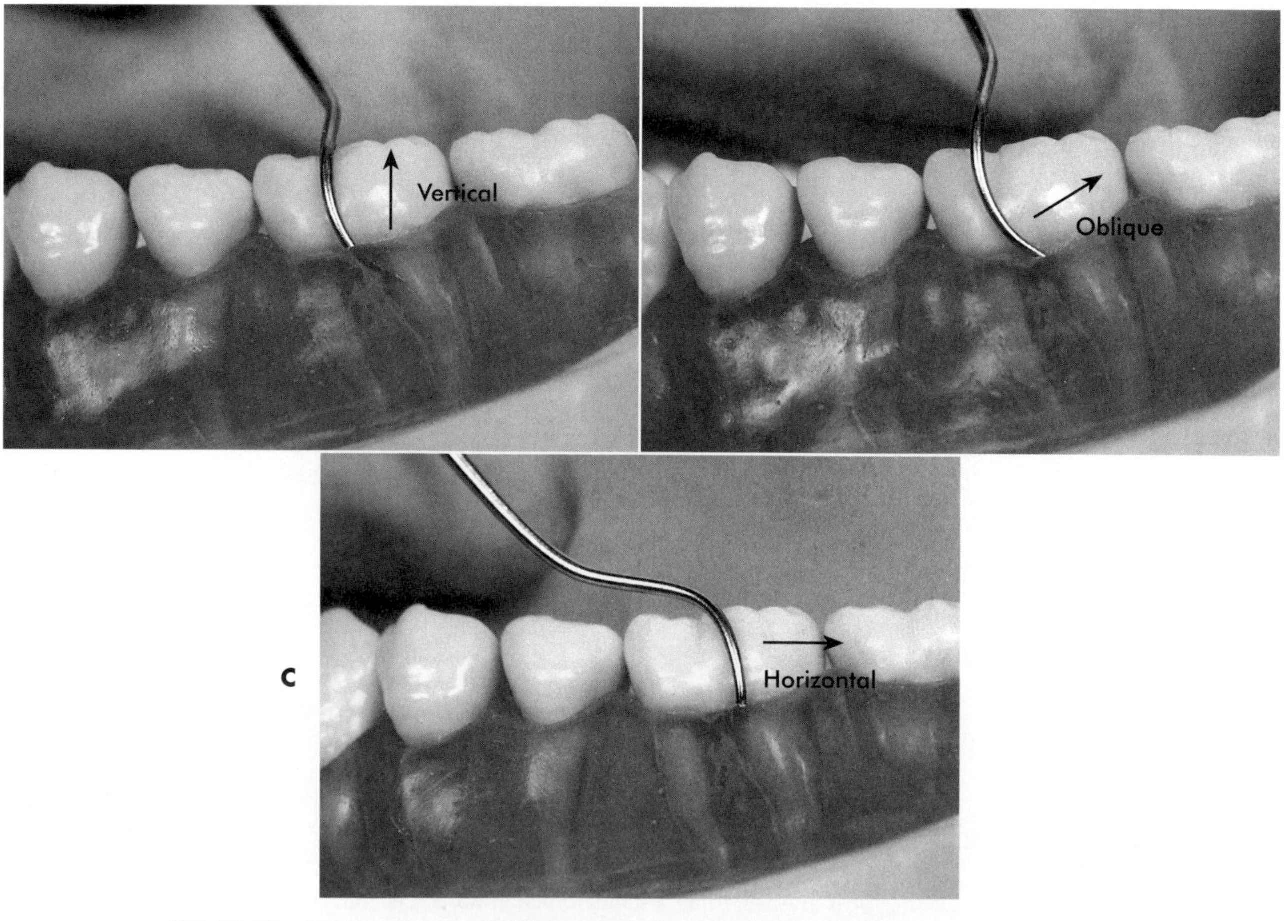

FIG. 20-27   The explorer used in three different positions: vertical, oblique, and horizontal.

temporary crowns, checking the hardness of a pit and fissure sealant, contouring a periodontal dressing, or removing supragingival cement, an intraoral temporary, or a piece of rubber dam at the interproximal surface. During each of these tasks it is necessary to adapt the explorer to the tooth to accurately detect anomalies. The explorer is used in three different positions: *vertical, oblique,* and *horizontal* (Fig. 20-27). These positions follow the contours of the teeth, and each one enables the operator to detect anomalies from a different perspective. For instance, if the margins of a temporary crown are being examined with the *vertical stroke,* unnecessary bulk or roughness could be detected. If the tip becomes caught on the cervical margin of the crown, this area will require modification or recontouring to avoid its being an irritant to the gingival tissues. The *horizontal* and *oblique stroke* will aid in defining contours. The tip of the explorer can also be used to mark a metal crown when it is too long and needs to be relieved at the cervical margin.

To use the explorer effectively, grasp the handle of the explorer in the operating hand in a modified pen grasp, with the middle finger on the shank of the instrument to increase tactile ability. The explorer is a sharp instrument that is capable of puncturing tissue if it is not well controlled. When the explorer is held properly, the operator has maximum tactile sense, as well as complete control of patient and operator safety. Practice manipulating the explorer by grasping it as previously described; slowly rotate the instrument in a clockwise direction, between the thumb and the opposing index and middle fingers. Continue this rotation until the instrument is turned approximately 180 degrees; then roll the handle counterclockwise to its original position. This activity will enable the assistant to simulate the actual use of the explorer as it is rotated into various positions on the tooth.

Use of Rotary Instruments

Handpieces are typically more bulky instruments, and, like the mirror and other hand instruments, dexterity in their use promotes safety. Many of the legally delegable duties that require the use of handpieces are performed outside the mouth; yet the assistant needs to understand the use of these devices for intraoral procedures where they are delegable.

The differences that exist between the use of a handpiece and hand instrument include the following:

- Irreversible damage can be created more commonly by misuse of a handpiece than by misuse of a hand instrument.
- The maintenance of a fulcrum when using a handpiece is similar to that of hand instruments; however, the handpiece rotates and can potentially cause damage to surrounding tissues or materials.
- The handpiece should not be activated until it is in the oral cavity.
- Handpieces are activated by energy through the use of another device, such as a foot control, and have varying speeds.
- To function, a handpiece requires that some type of attachment be added to the working end, such as a bur, a disk, or a polishing cup.
- Bulkiness of the handpiece requires it be held with a firm grasp to maintain control.

To use the handpiece, hold it in a palm-thumb or pen grasp. Either of these grasps provides the opportunity for the operator to maintain a fulcrum, intraorally or extraorally, when using the handpiece (Fig. 20-28). Establish the fulcrum, turn on the handpiece, and place the working end on the surface that is to be treated. Exercise caution when using the handpiece to avoid exerting excess pressure. Excess pressure or the speed of the handpiece may remove more structure than is required, may create heat that can damage the tooth or other structures, or may result in damage to the handpiece.

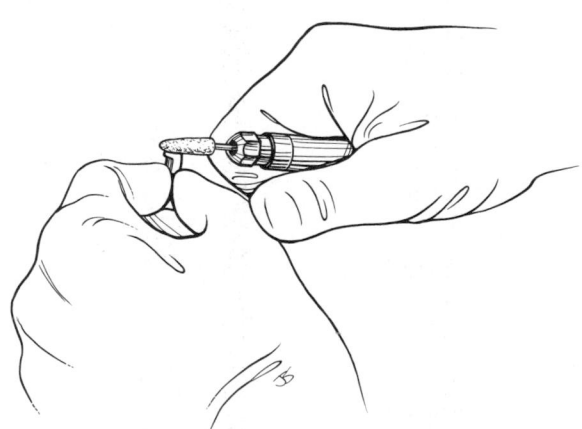

FIG. 20-28 Using a rotary instrument, while maintaining a fulcrum.

KEY POINTS

▶ The basic grasps that are used during instrument exchange include the pen, the modified pen, the palm, and the palm-thumb grasps. Instruments can be exchanged by using the single-handed, two-handed, or hidden syringe technique.

▶ Each member of the dental health team must assume responsibility for safe and efficient instrument exchange during a procedure.

▶ A step-by-step procedure for the commonly used single-handed transfer includes three basic stages: instrument preparation, instrument pickup, and instrument exchange.

▶ Several situations require an alternative instrument exchange. Instruments such as dental mirrors, scissors, tissue forceps, and handpieces will require a modification in the procedure.

▶ With advanced functions the dental assistant needs to make a smooth transition from chairside assistant to the role of operator. Consequently, the assistant should also become proficient in the various grasps that are employed by operators.

BIBLIOGRAPHY

Four-handed dentistry manual, ed 6, Birmingham, 1990, The University of Alabama.

Woodall IR: *Comprehensive dental hygiene care*, ed 4, St Louis, 1993, Mosby.

21 Oral Evacuation Systems and Techniques

LEARNING OBJECTIVES

You will have mastered the material in this chapter when you can:
- Define the key terms
- Explain the function of a high-velocity evacuation system
- Explain how the HVE system can aid in reducing aerosols in a dental clinical environment
- Differentiate between the use of an HVE system and a saliva ejector
- Identify the armamentarium used with an HVE system
- Explain the basic rules for oral evacuator tip placement
- Describe the placement of an evacuator tip for any given operative or surgical site
- Describe the procedure used in a complete mouth rinse
- Describe the use of the a/w syringe in maintaining a clear operating field
- Describe the routine care of the HVE system.

KEY TERMS

High-velocity evacuation (HVE)
Low-volume evacuation (LVE)
Oral evacuation
Saliva ejector
Suction
Svedopter

One of the primary duties of a clinical dental assistant is the removal of fluids, saliva, and materials from the oral cavity during routine operative and surgical procedures. **Oral evacuation**, the process of removing fluids and materials from the mouth, provides comfort to the patient and allows the operator to work in a clear operative field. The use of the oral evacuator also removes much of the aerosol spray created by the handpiece so that it does not exit through the patient's mouth onto the operating team. This obviously provides greater safety for the team. The two devices used in dentistry for oral evacuation are the **high-velocity evacuation (HVE)** system or oral evacuator, which is used to remove large volumes of fluid and debris from the mouth rapidly, sometimes referred to as **suction**; and the **low-volume system** known as the **saliva ejector**, which removes liquid slowly from the mouth but is not capable of picking up solid debris.

Saliva Ejector

The earliest method of removing fluids from the mouth was the cuspidor, which required the patient to empty fluids from the mouth into this small sink-like structure (Fig. 21-1). Later the low-volume saliva ejector became the popular device for removing these fluids. Although this method is still useful in several treatment situations, the choice for rapid removal of large volumes of fluids and debris is the HVE system. Indications for the use of a saliva ejector are as follows:

▶ During an oral prophylaxis
▶ When the operator is working alone
▶ When a patient resists the use of the suction
▶ When a patient salivates heavily under the rubber dam
▶ With the addition of an appropriate device, it retracts the tongue

> The saliva ejector was developed in 1882. This development made it possible to keep teeth dry during treatment and to eliminate the practice of stuffing the patient's mouth with cotton napkins or *bibulous paper*.

The saliva ejector presents several disadvantages for use in four-handed dentistry. It is a slow-speed device that requires the tip to be immersed in the oral fluids before it can function. The saliva ejector cannot remove debris, such as amalgam or cement pieces, from the mouth, nor can it remove large volumes of fluid; it is not easily placed in all areas of the oral cavity.

Although stainless steel saliva ejectors are available, disposable plastic tips are more common. These tips are flexible and can be bent for easy placement in the mandibular arch (Fig. 21-2). Plastic saliva ejectors are relatively inexpensive and are discarded after each use.

High-Velocity Evacuation System

A high-velocity evacuation (HVE) system for the removal of saliva, water, and materials from the oral cavity is a natural adjunct to sit-down, four-handed dentistry. In four-handed dentistry when the patient is placed in a supine position for treatment, it becomes impossible for the patient to comfortably raise up and empty fluids that are in the mouth into a cuspidor.

The high-velocity evacuator system makes it possible to pick up fluids and materials without bringing the tip of the evacuator in contact with the fluid. To be most effective the tip opening must be placed parallel with the surface of the fluid. The use of the HVE system eliminates the use of a cuspidor and results in more comfort to the patient, a clear field of operation for the dentist, and increased infection control for the operating team.

> Dr. Edmund Kells invented the suction pump in the late 1800s, making it possible to rapidly aspirate fluids during surgery. This discovery evolved later into the development of high-velocity evacuation.

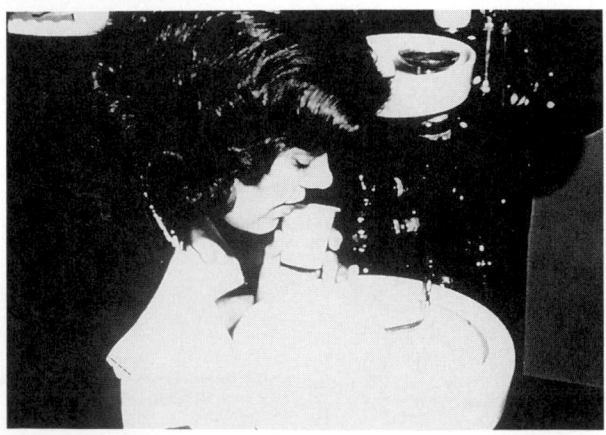

FIG. 21-1   Patient emptying the mouth into a cuspidor.
(Courtesy University of Alabama—School of Dentistry, Birmingham.)

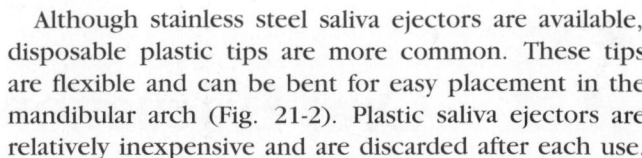
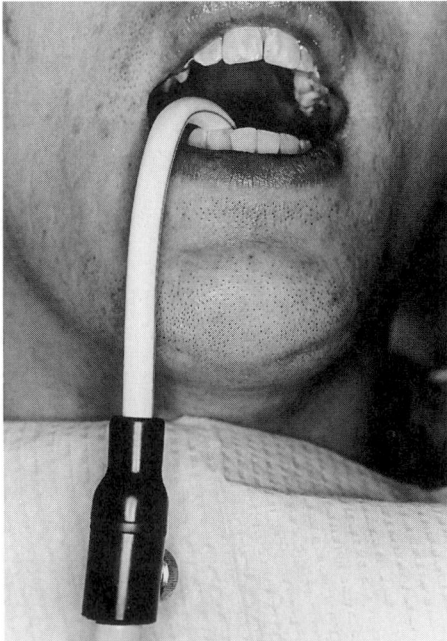

FIG. 21-2   Saliva ejector in place in the patient's mouth.

Choosing an HVE Tip

The tip that fits into the oral evacuator hose is the primary instrument used in oral evacuation. The procedure will dictate the type of tip to be used. The two basic types of tips are surgical or operative.

▶ Surgical Tip

This smaller tip is more site specific than the standard operative tip. For instance when the operator is extracting a tooth or cutting soft tissue in a restricted area and no water spray is being used, it is necessary to concentrate on removing blood, tissue, or other debris from this site (Fig. 21-3). Because the opening is narrow, this smaller tip may clog frequently when evacuating blood and tissue, and it will be necessary to clear the tip with some sterile water or saline solution.

▶ Standard Operative Tips

These tips are used more frequently in general dentistry and are available in a variety of shapes. They are made of metal or plastic and are supplied with an angled or a straight shaft. These tips vary in design and size of openings and may be disposable or sterilizable.

METAL VERSUS PLASTIC TIP

Obviously, the metal tip is more durable and can be sterilized; however, the disadvantages are that it cannot be used during electrosurgery and a coldness is created by air constantly running through the tip. This coldness may cause discomfort to a tooth that is not anesthetized or to nearby soft tissues. The plastic tip eliminates this problem, but some plastic tips are not strong enough for use as a retraction device. When a plastic tip is chosen, select one that is stiff and has an adequate length— approximately 6 to 7 inches, a length that will easily reach the operating field. Plastic tips are available in both sterilizable and disposable styles.

ANGLED VERSUS STRAIGHT SHAFT

Evacuator tips with a bend in the shaft seem to be more common than straight tips. Perhaps this is because the bend allows the assistant to maneuver the tip with greater ease, while the lips, cheeks, and tongue are retracted during placement of the tip.

▶ Optional Designs

Manufacturers have created a myriad of tip designs, some with merit and others without. Tips that display the flange and the spoon shape are illustrated (see Fig. 21-5). The concept behind these designs is to enhance retraction and to follow the contour of the mouth. Such designs may constrict the volume of fluids the tip is able to pick up or may deter access to debris in the mouth. Further, sharp edges on the tips may cause discomfort to the patient.

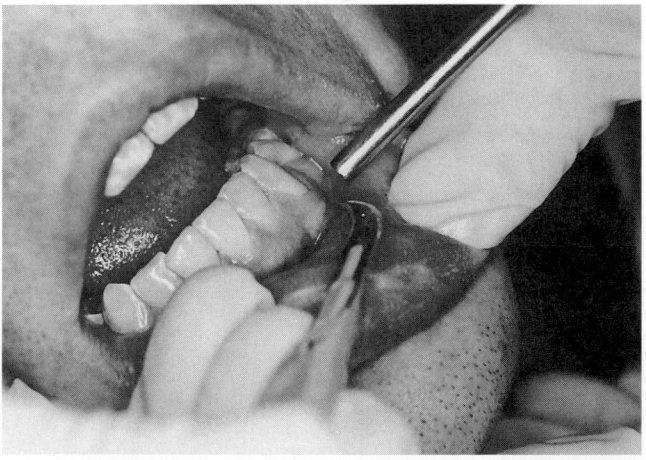

FIG. 21-3   Surgical tip in use during a procedure.

▶ Auxiliary Evacuator Devices

In addition to the standard oral evacuator tips, auxiliary equipment is available. An adapter may be attached to the HVE hose, and into this adapter a saliva ejector may be attached. This setup may be used as a traditional saliva ejector, or it can be used by the patient during an oral prophylaxis. If it is used in the latter manner, water is sprayed into the mouth, the patient rinses and then inserts the saliva ejector to withdraw fluids.

A **svedopter** can be used in the adapter or on the saliva ejector hose (Fig. 21-4, *A*). It serves as a saliva ejector and also provides retraction of the tongue. This device is supplied with three sizes of flange tips (Fig. 21-4, *B*). The svedopter is especially helpful when a disk or bur is used in the mouth to protect the tongue from potential injury. It can also be useful with small children who have active tongues. Care must be taken when placing the svedopter to avoid irritating the delicate tissue on the floor of the mouth. A disposable version of this device is a hygroformic (Fig. 21-5). The major disadvantage of this device is its limited retraction ability.

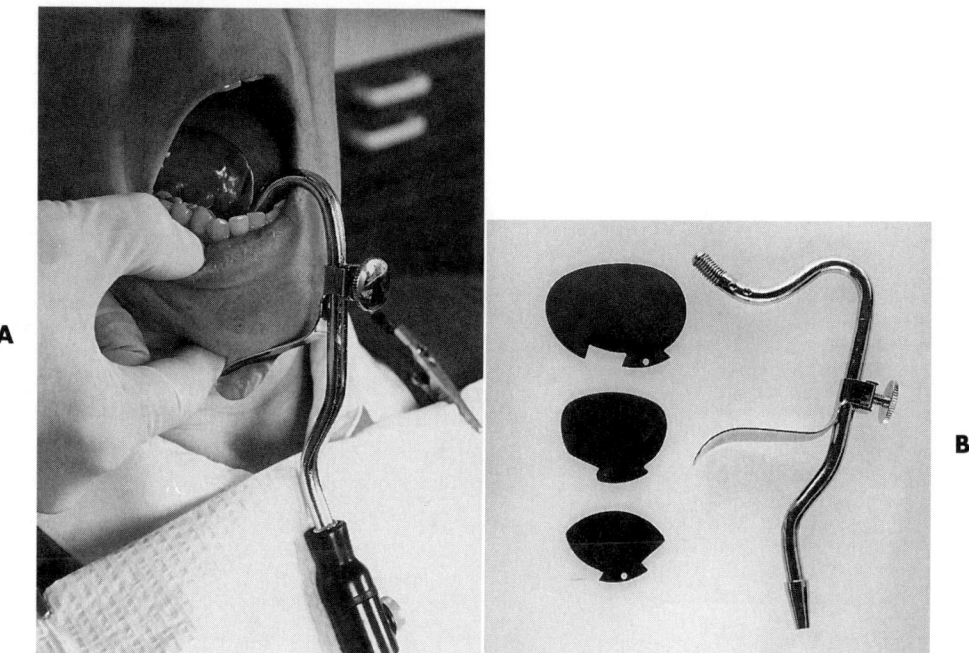

FIG. 21-4   *A,* Svedopter in place. *B,* Svedopter with variously sized flange tips.

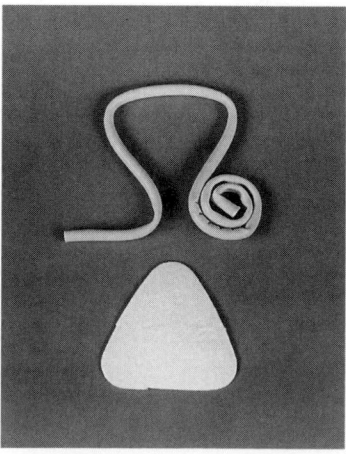

FIG. 21-5   Hygroformic and celluloid wafer.

Using the Oral Evacuator Tip

Successful oral evacuation is dependent on a few simple rules as discussed in the following situations.

▶ Selecting

Select the appropriate end of the evacuator tip. One of the most popular tips is designed with the tip ends beveled for use in either the anterior or posterior areas of the oral cavity (Fig. 21-6, *A* and *B*). Note the bend in the tip. To place the tip into the hose for posterior use, hold the bend toward you. In this position the open end of the tip will be visible (Fig. 21-7, *A*). The opposite end of this tip is used for anterior placement. When it is held with the bend toward you, the open end will not be visible (Fig. 21-7, *B*).

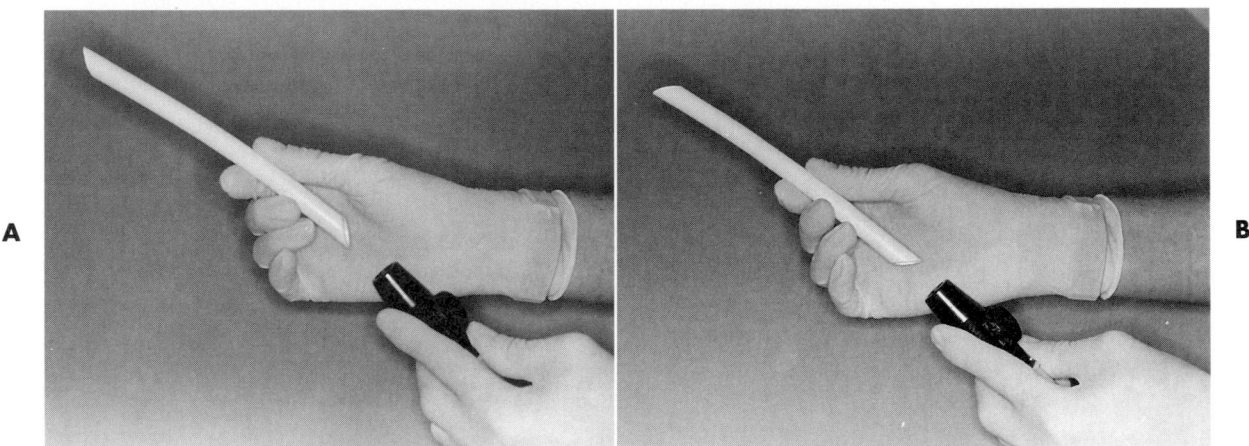

FIG. 21-6   *A,* and *B,* HVE tip, with beveled ends.

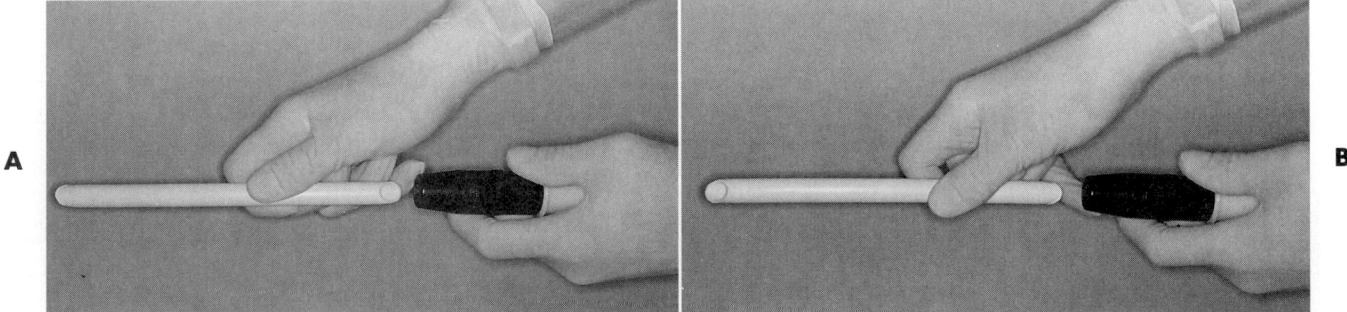

FIG. 21-7   *A,* Open end of tip visible for posterior areas. B, Open end not visible for use in the anterior.

▶ Grasping

The most common grasps used during placement of the HVE are a thumb-to-nose or pen grasp (Fig. 21-8, *A* and *B*). The thumb-to-nose grasp allows you to retract oral tissues and provide greater stability when retracting the lips, tongue, or cheeks (Fig. 21-8, *C*). For this reason, when you are working in the posterior area of the mouth in an operative procedure, this grasp is the most efficient, since it causes less strain on your hand and provides greater control of tissues.

When you are working in the anterior of the mouth or in a surgical procedure, the pen grasp is frequently used, since lip retraction may be done by the operator or with your free hand. A pen grasp is most effective when a surgical evacuator tip is used.

▶ Holding

When you are working with a right-handed operator, use the right hand to operate the oral evacuator (Fig. 21-8, *D*). *This technique is reversed for a left-handed operator.* When the tip is used in the right hand, the left hand is used for the a/w syringe and for passing instruments. The a/w syringe is held in the left hand, until the operator signals for a new instrument. At this time the evacuator can be removed from the mouth, the triplex syringe tip is transferred to the right hand, and it is grasped by the free fingers. A new instrument is transferred to the operator with the left hand. You should practice oral evacuator placement with both hands when first learning the technique to gain proficiency for working with a left- or a right-handed operator.

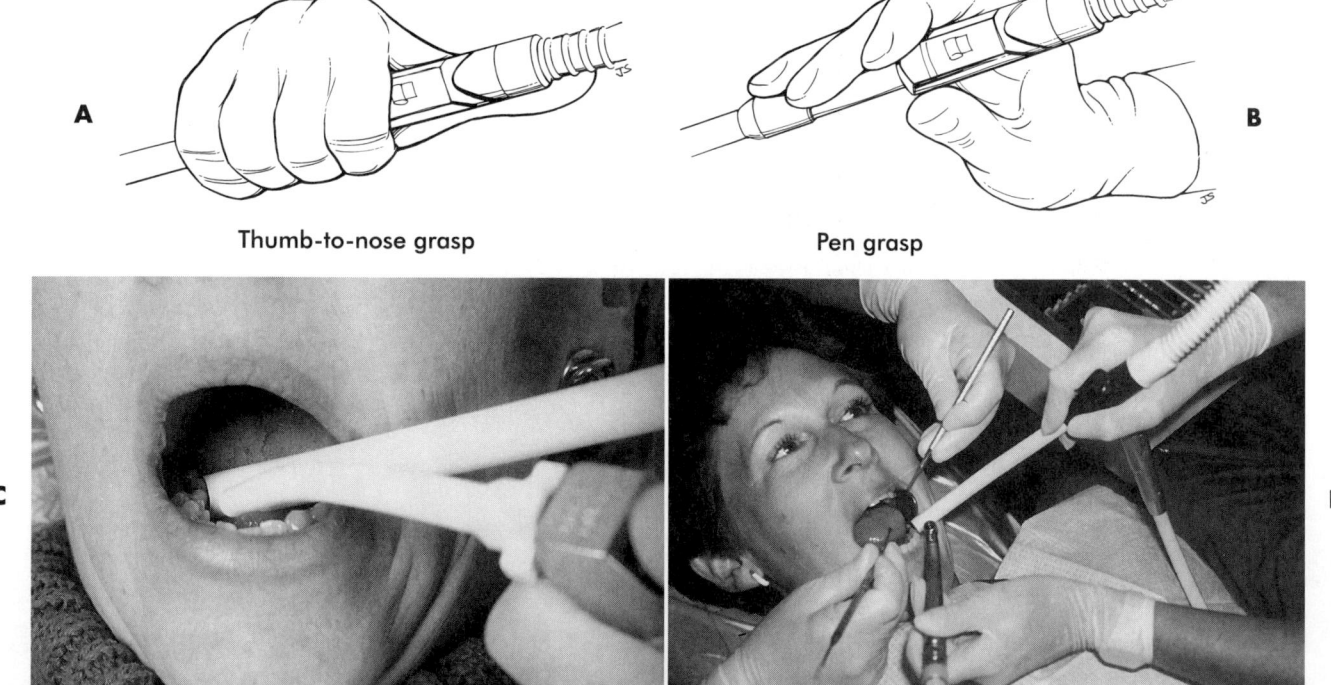

A, Thumb-to-nose grasp   **B,** Pen grasp

FIG. 21-8   *A,* Thumb-to-nose grasp. *B,* Pen grasp. *C,* Using the thumb-to-nose grasp aids in retracting the tongue. *D,* Transferring a new instrument with the left hand, while HVE is held in right hand. The a/w syringe is transferred to the right hand during the exchange.

Timing

Place the evacuator tip before the operator places the handpiece and/or the mirror. The evacuator tip needs to be positioned before the operator places the handpiece or the operator may have to reposition the handpiece.

PATIENT EDUCATION TIP

Most patients today are acquainted with the use of an oral evacuator in the mouth; however, if a patient has not been accustomed to having fluids removed in this manner, he or she may be somewhat resistant. Explain to the patient that this device will help to quickly remove large volumes of water that enter the mouth from high-speed handpieces, and demonstrate how the device works. Explanation and demonstration usually satisfy most patients. For small children who are new to the office, the use of the oral evacuator can be a fun experience. You may demonstrate the use of the tip to the child by turning it on, letting the child feel the tip end, and then compare it to a vacuum cleaner.

Placing

Place the tip as close to the tooth as possible. Unlike the saliva ejector, which must be immersed in fluids, the oral evacuator tip can pull fluid into the tip from a short distance. Therefore, the tip should be placed as close to the tooth being treated as possible so that as the water falls from the tooth, it is picked up immediately.

Place the edge of the evacuator tip even with or slightly above the occlusal or incisal edge of the tooth. The handpiece provides a stream of water that acts as a coolant and washes the tooth during the preparation. The objective of the evacuator is to pick up the water and any debris that may be present after the tooth is rinsed. Take care not to place the tip directly beside the handpiece because you may draw the fluid from the handpiece before it has cooled or rinsed the tooth.

Place the tip near the tooth surface closest to the assistant. For instance when you are working on the right side of the mouth, the tip is placed on the lingual surface and will aid in retracting the tongue. When you are working on the left side of the mouth, the tip is placed on the buccal surface and will aid in retracting the cheek. This rule is reversed for a left-handed operator.

When the handpiece is being used on the surface nearest the assistant, place the evacuator tip slightly distal to the surface that is being treated. In a cavity preparation on the buccal surface on the left side of the mouth or on the lingual surface on the right side of the mouth the tip may interfere with the placement of the handpiece. To avoid this situation move the tip distal to the preparation. This position may create a slight inconvenience, but the fluids can still be picked up adequately.

A patient's comfort is always the major concern of the assistant. When you first learn to use an oral evacuator tip, the procedure may seem cumbersome. The rules that have been presented are reviewed in Box 21-1. Suggested tips for oral evacuation are listed in Box 21-2 and may benefit you to avoid discomfort to the patient.

BOX 21-1

RULES FOR ORAL EVACUATOR PLACEMENT

▶ Select the appropriate end.
▶ Use a thumb-to-nose or pen grasp (Fig. 21-9, *A* and *B*).
▶ When you are working with a right-handed operator, the assistant operates the oral evacuator with the right hand and the left hand is used for a left-handed operator.
▶ Place the evacuator tip before the operator places the handpiece and/or mirror (Fig. 21-9, *C*).
▶ Place the tip as close to the tooth as possible (Fig. 21-9, *D*).
▶ Keep the edge of the evacuator tip even with or slightly above the occlusal or incisal edge of the tooth (Fig. 21-9, *E*).
▶ Place the tip near the tooth surface closest to the assistant (Fig. 21-9, F_1 and F_2, right-handed; 21-9, F_3 and F_4, left-handed).
▶ When the handpiece is being used on the surface nearest the assistant, place the HVE tip slightly distal to the tooth being treated (Fig. 21-9, *G*).

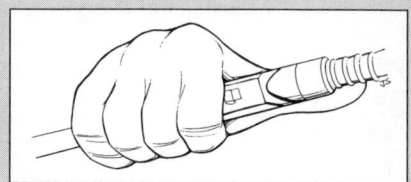

A

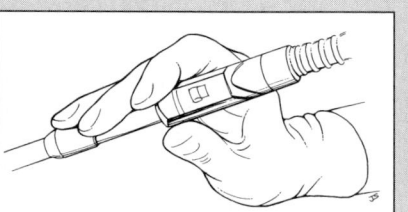

B

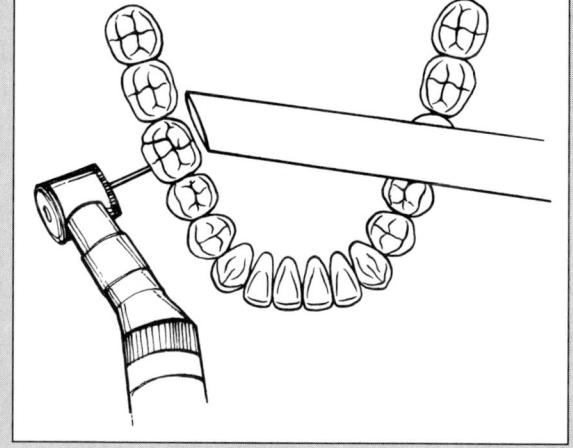

C

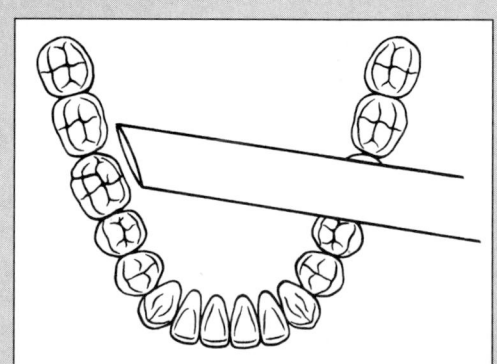

D

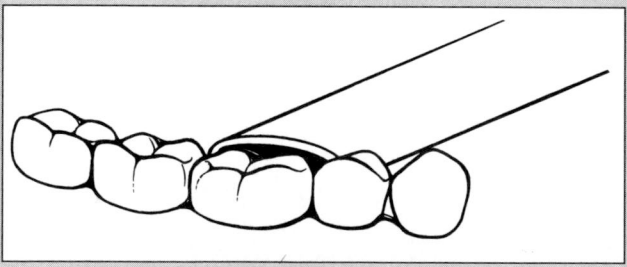

E

FIG. 21-9

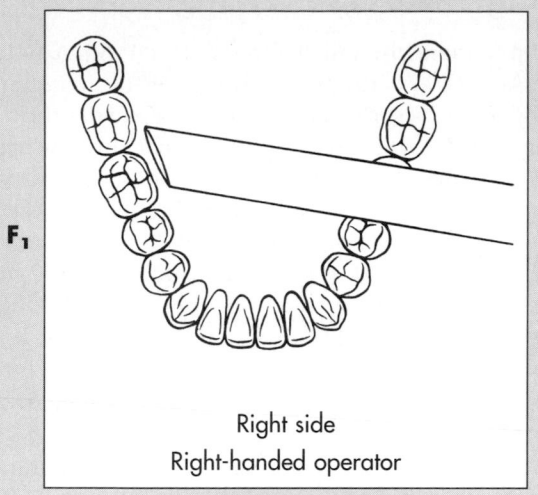

F₁

Right side
Right-handed operator

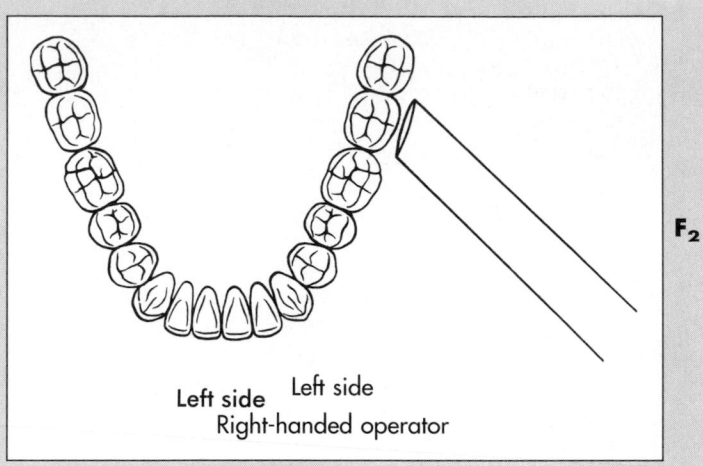

F₂

Left side
Left side
Right-handed operator

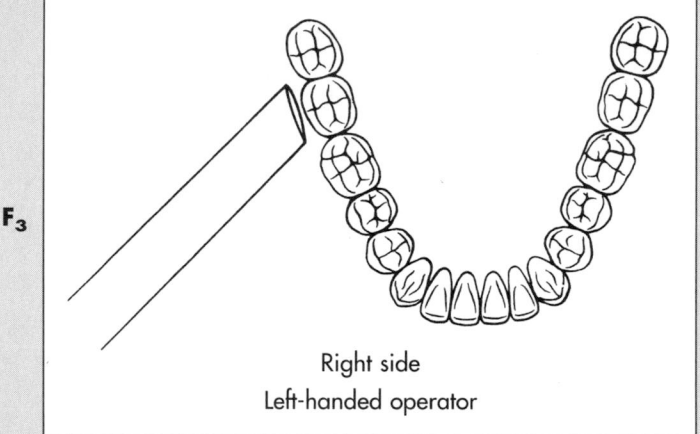

F₃

Right side
Left-handed operator

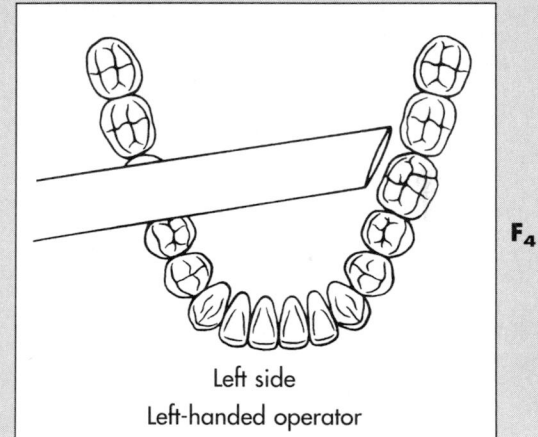

F₄

Left side
Left-handed operator

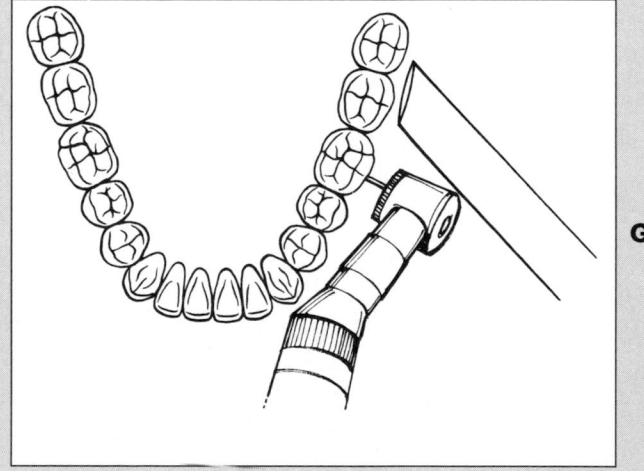

G

FIG. 21-9, cont'd.

SUGGESTIONS FOR ORAL EVACUATOR USE

1. Place the tip securely into the hose to avoid accidental dislodgment.
2. Minimize the noise of the HVE system by turning on the evacuator completely.
3. Turn the angle of the tip opening parallel to the buccal or lingual plane of the teeth to avoid contact with soft tissue.
4. Avoid contact with soft tissue when the tip is initially placed in the mouth by entering toward the midline where the opening is greater; then concentrate on specific placement.
5. Avoid cold temperature discomfort to sensitive or nonanesthetized teeth by using a plastic HVE tip.
6. If a tip falls on the floor, replace it with a clean one and pick up the dropped tip at the end of the procedure.
7. Clean a surgical tip frequently by dipping the tip into a cup of sterile water or saline solution to avoid clogging.
8. Avoid quick and sudden movement of the tip. This can be distracting to the operator and potentially dangerous to the patient.
9. Avoid contact with the soft palate and pillar areas to eliminate potential gagging.
10. Remove the tip whenever possible to allow the patient to close and swallow. This avoids overdrying the mouth and will give the patient a break from the constant noise in the mouth.
11. Observe fluids and debris collecting in other areas of the mouth, and remove them intermittently.
12. When a complete mouth rinse is performed turn the tip so that the back of the tip (side opposite the tip opening) lies on the lateral surface of the tongue or cheek.
13. Keep the evacuator tip turned on at the end of the procedure for a short time to ensure that all fluids are drawn into the system and do not remain at the hose opening.
14. Avoid saying "oops" or "I'm sorry," or gasping when you grasp tissue with the HVE tip. Such reactions do not build patient confidence.
15. Avoid contact with sublingual tissues since they can be more susceptible to injury than other oral tissues.

Using the A/W Syringe

To supplement the effectiveness of oral evacuation it is necessary to use the a/w syringe with maximum efficiency. The a/w syringe is used to rinse and dry the tooth. It was noted earlier in Chapter 16 that the a/w syringe provides three forms of spray: air only, air and water (aerated spray), or water only. When using the a/w syringe the tip is turned in the direction of the arch, up for the maxilla and down for the mandible (Fig. 21-10, *A* and *B*). When the operator stops the handpiece during a cavity preparation, rinse the tooth by using the aerated spray followed by a spurt of air to thoroughly clean and dry the tooth. You can also use the a/w syringe to clean and dry the mirror. When the operator is working on the maxillary arch, the water mist from the handpiece naturally falls onto the mirror, interfering with the operator's vision (Fig. 21-10, *C*). Spray air intermittently on the mirror to keep it dry. If the mirror becomes foggy, use a quick aerated spray, and then dry with air.

▶ Positioning the Oral Evacuator Tip and Air/Water Syringe

Once the techniques for use of the a/w syringe and oral evacuator have been practiced separately, it is time to coordinate these two tasks in actual clinical activities. From the patient's chart, determine the location of the treatment, and then apply the various rules stated earlier. Table 21-1 identifies several locations of treatment and provides an overview of evacuator tip placement and the use of the a/w syringe.

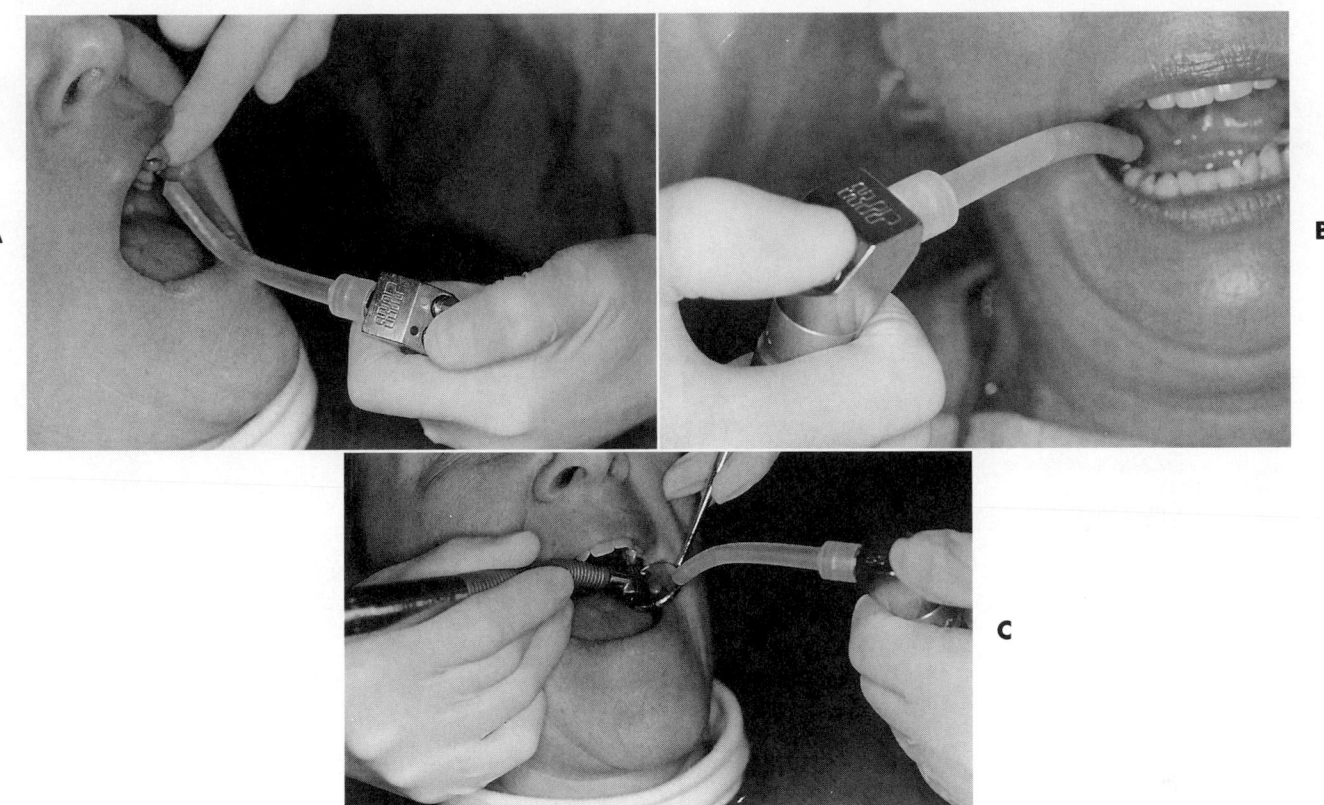

FIG. 21-10 *A,* A/w syringe tip turned for use in the maxillary arch. *B,* A/w syringe tip turned for use in the mandibular arch. *C,* Air spray placed on mirror.

TABLE 21-1 POSITIONING THE EVACUATOR TIP AND A/W SYRINGE

Handpiece placement	Evacuator tip placement
2^{MOD}	Lingual of #2, AOM*
8^L	Facial of #8, AOM
12^B	Buccal surface slightly distal to #12, AOM
14^L	Buccal of #14, AOM
15MO	Buccal of #15, AOM
18^L	Buccal of #18
18^B	Buccal surface slightly distal to #18
20^{MOD}	Buccal of #20
24^F	Lingual of #24
25^L	Facial of #25, AOM
29^{MOD}	Lingual of #29
30^L	Lingual surface slightly distal to #30
31^B	Lingual of #31

*AOM refers to placing air on the mirror.

BOX 21-3

MAXIMUM EFFICIENCY TIPS FOR A/W SYRINGE

1. Turn the tip in the direction of the arch: up, for the maxilla, and down, for the mandible.
2. To thoroughly cleanse the site, place the tip directly over the opening of the preparation when a cavity preparation site is flushed.
3. Be assertive in cleansing a site. Don't hold the tip too far away. Place the tip within ¼ inch, and press firmly on the buttons to cleanse the area.
4. Quickly move the syringe tip into an area to be cleaned; flush, evacuate, and move the tip out of the area quickly.

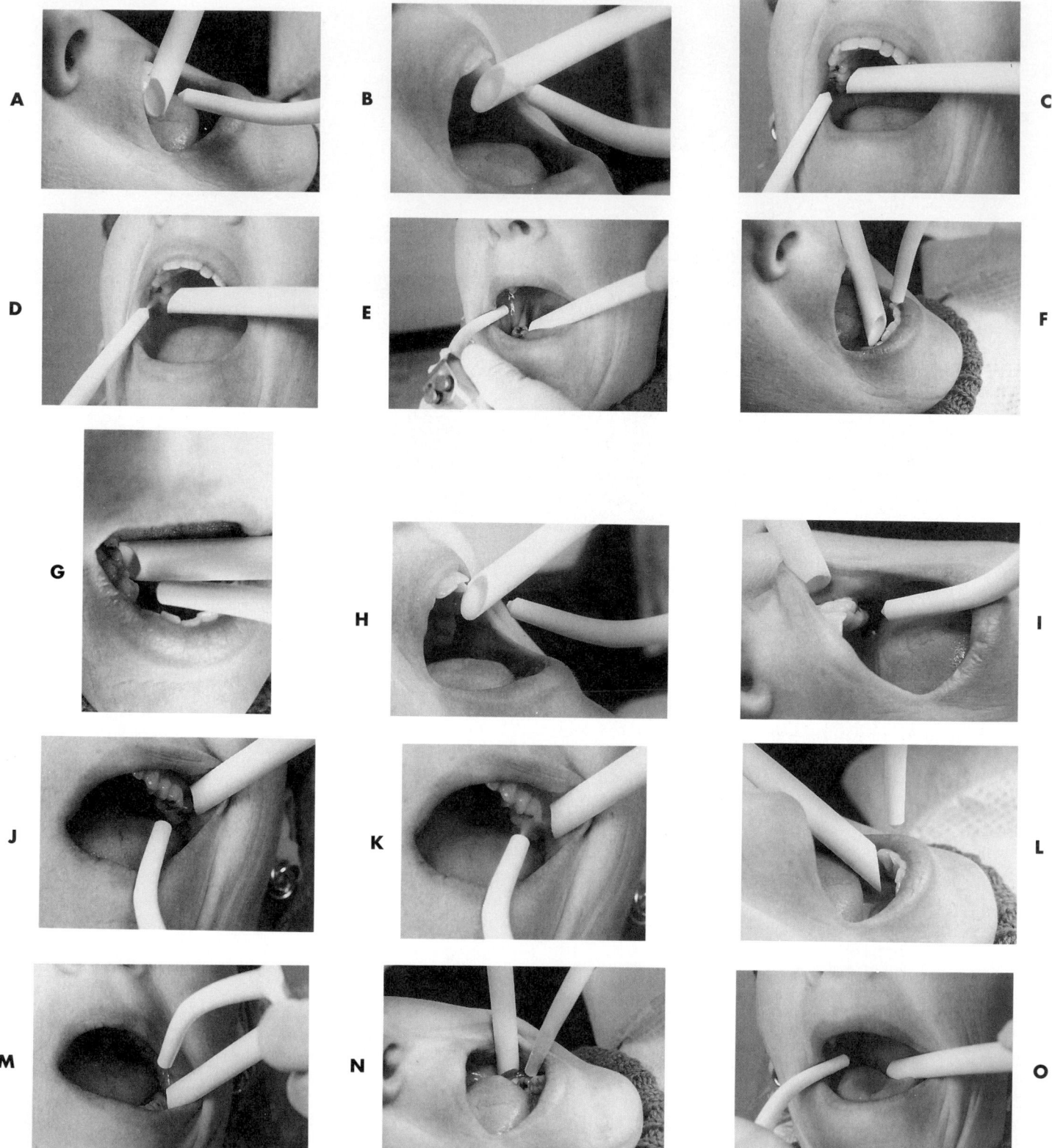

FIG. 21-11   *A through O.* (See box on opposite page for legend.)

TWO-HANDED MOUTH RINSE PROCEDURE

A, Begin on the patient's right side at #8. Turn the triplex syringe tip toward the maxillary arch. Place the suction tip on the lingual surface near the incisal edge. *B,* Spray an air/water combination to avoid splatter. (A solid spray of water will result in splash back.) *C,* Continue distally, using both devices simultaneously. When you reach the cuspid area, move the evacuator tip completely to the lingual surface. With the left hand use the triplex syringe, and retract the cheek. *D,* Spray water on occlusal surfaces forcing water spray to wash the entire tooth. It may be necessary to spray toward the buccal or lingual surfaces when debris remains, especially when you are removing a substance like polishing paste. *E,* Observe the floor of the mouth and the posterior pillar areas to pick up any accumulation of fluids. *F,* When all of the maxillary right quadrant has been completed, move to the mandibular arch, and begin with tooth #25. *G,* Turn the tip in the direction of the mandible. Repeat steps 3 through 9 in the same manner—except that this time, the evacuator tip can aid in retracting the tongue. *H,* When the mandibular right quadrant has been rinsed thoroughly, ask the patient to turn toward you and begin the maxillary left quadrant at #9. *I,* Place the tip on the labial surface near the incisal edge and continue distally as was done for the opposite side. *J,* On the left side, when the cuspid is reached, move the tip to the buccal surface, and use the oral evacuator to retract the cheek. *K,* Continue to the molar region. Spray water on the occlusal to flush all tooth surfaces. *L,* When the maxillary left side is rinsed thoroughly turn the tip of the triplex syringe to the mandibular position. *M, N,* and *O,* Begin at tooth #24 and progress distally following steps 3 through 9 once again. At the conclusion of the complete mouth rinse, wipe any water spray from the patient's face with the napkin, and thank the patient for cooperating during the procedure.

Performing a Complete Mouth Rinse

At the end of any procedure a patient needs to have the mouth refreshed and you need to ensure that no debris remains in the oral cavity. A complete mouth rinse may be done by the assistant alone or as a four-handed technique with the operator. The following sequence offers an easy step-by-step procedure for the two- or four-handed method. In either method, begin on the anterior of the maxillary arch on the side opposite the assistant and continue to the distal of the arch. Proceed to the mandibular arch on the same side, and conclude by picking up excess water in the pillar area. Then ask the patient to turn toward you, and rinse the maxillary and mandibular arches on the opposite side of the mouth in the same manner. The following describes the technique for a full mouth rinse done two-handed by the assistant (Fig. 21-11).

▶ Four-Handed Mouth Rinse Procedure

This procedure is preferred because it can be done more efficiently. However, the demands on the dentist's time may dictate the use of the two-handed procedure.

The same steps are followed, except that it is the operator who uses the a/w syringe and is able to aid in retraction of the cheek and tongue. The assistant is able to retract the lips, cheek, and/or tongue with the free hand, thereby gaining greater access to the vestibular areas.

TEAM APPROACH
Oral Evacuation—Four-Handed

OPERATOR	ASSISTANT
Direct patient to turn toward operator	
	Pass a/w syringe with tip toward maxilla
Retract cheek	
	Turn on HVE
Grasp a/w syringe	Position HVE near incisal edge
Begin at maxillary right central incisor	
Direct water spray toward incisal edge	
Continue toward distal, spraying the occlusal surface	Move HVE tip to lingual surface following movement of a/w syringe
	Move HVE tip to pillar region to pick up excess water
Turn a/w tip toward mandible	
Continue to retract cheek	
Begin at midline of mandibular right central incisor	Position HVE on mandibular anterior lingual surface
Spray water toward incisal edge	
Continue toward distal, spraying the occlusal surface	Move HVE tip to lingual surface following movement of a/w syringe
	Move HVE tip to pillar region to pick up excess water
Direct patient to turn toward assistant	
Repeat identical procedure for left side	Repeat identical procedure for left side
	Wipe off extraoral region around mouth if moist with napkin or 2 × 2

Maintaining the HVE System

Remove the evacuator tip after completion of each mouth rinse procedure, and disinfect the hoses. Keep the system turned on after treatment so that the fluids completely drain into the system.

At the end of the day the following procedure is initiated:

1. Always wear utility gloves, masks, and protective glasses when cleaning the system.
2. Flush the system with a premixed, antimicrobial solution that is placed in a rubber bowl or other appropriate container. Flush thoroughly for 2 to 5 minutes using 1 or 2 quarts of solution.
3. Remove and replace disposable traps in the evacuator trap cup (Fig. 21-12).
4. Remove and replace disposable screens in the saliva ejector hose (Fig. 21-13).
5. If heavy metals are found in the disposable trap the materials are discarded in the heavy metals waste receptacle. If not, the debris is discarded in the biohazard waste receptacle. Always follow the EPA laws and recommendations within your state.

KEY POINTS

▶ Oral evacuation is an integral part of four-handed dentistry today. Successful oral evacuation is dependent on the assistant's ability to have concern for the needs of both the patient and the operator, to select the appropriate devices, and to place the evacuator tip in a location that is safe and yet removes fluids and debris with maximum efficiency.

▶ Efficient placement of the HVE tip can be obtained by selecting the proper tip end, by using the appropriate grasp, by placing the angle of the bevel end parallel to the buccal or lingual surfaces, by placing the tip as close to the tooth as possible, and by placing the edge of the tip even with or slightly above the occlusal or incisal edge.

▶ A low-speed system, the saliva ejector, has limited use in four-handed dentistry and is primarily used during an oral prophylaxis or as an adjunct to the HVE system.

BIBLIOGRAPHY

Finkbeiner BL: *Oral evacuation placement module 4-DEN 110,* Ann Arbor, Mich, 1992, Washtenaw Community College.

Robinson GE, McDevitt EJ, Sinnett, GM, Wuehrmann AH: *Four-handed dentistry manual,* ed 6, Birmingham, 1991, University of Alabama, School of Dentistry.

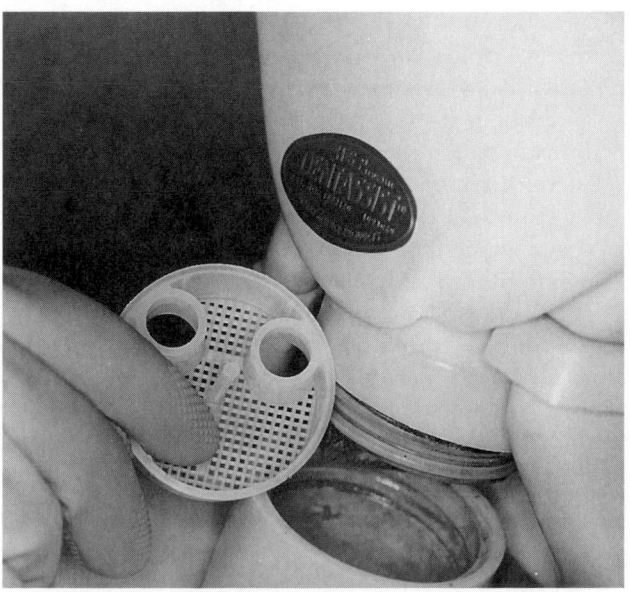

FIG. 21-12 Disposable traps in evacuator trap cup.

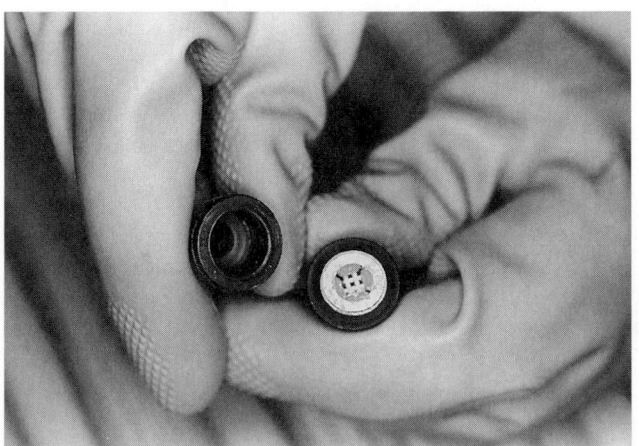

FIG. 21-13 Disposable screen in saliva ejector.

22 Isolation Materials and Applications

LEARNING OBJECTIVES

You will have mastered the material in this chapter when you can:

▶ Define the key terms

▶ Explain the purpose of isolation techniques in dentistry

▶ Identify the armamentarium used in different isolation procedures

▶ Describe the step-by-step procedure in rubber dam isolation

▶ Explain the importance of rubber dam isolation in today's dentistry

▶ Describe techniques in rubber dam isolation to accommodate the less ordinary oral situation

KEY TERMS

Cellulose wafer
Clamp
Clamp forceps
Cotton roll holder
Frame
Gingival retracting clamp
Isolation
Ligature
Napkin
Rubber dam
Rubber dam stamp
Septum
Template
Winged/wingless clamps

Isolation—its purpose and the materials and techniques used to maintain a clear dry field in the oral cavity in which to work—is introduced in this chapter. **Isolation** means to set apart from others or to place something by itself. In dentistry, isolation is used during a treatment procedure to separate a specific tooth, a group of teeth, or a region in the mouth.

Purpose of Isolation

The following are the primary objectives of isolation:

▶ Maintain a dry field
▶ Retract soft tissue
▶ Prevent materials from falling into the oral cavity
▶ Aid in infection control techniques by decreasing aerosol sprays from the oral cavity
▶ Reduce potential contamination to the tooth
▶ Provide a visual contrast between tooth structure and rubber dam material
▶ Provide patient management
▶ Increase patient comfort
▶ Increase success of restorations by providing a dry operative field

The question to ask yourself before each procedure is "Which of the isolation procedures is the most efficient and the safest for the patient and for the operating team?" It then becomes your responsibility to be the advocate for a system that is efficient and that promotes maximum safety for everyone. Of the various types of isolation: rubber dam, cotton rolls, cellulose wafers, svedopters, hygroformics, and mouth props, the rubber dam meets all of the objectives. This procedure may require more time and effort initially, but as the assistant gains expertise the benefits of rubber dam will soon be realized by the operating team and the patient (Box 22-1).

BOX 22-1

OBJECTIVES OF ISOLATION

Maintain a dry field
Aid in infection control
Eliminate materials falling into the patient's mouth
Aid in retraction of soft tissues
Improve visibility
Improve patient management
Promote efficiency

Isolation in Specialty Procedures

The decision to isolate teeth is determined by the particular procedure that is to be used. The following situations illustrate how rubber dam use can be adapted to meet special needs.

Endodontic procedures—Isolate a single tooth: the tooth receiving the treatment. With single-tooth isolation, contamination of the surgical site is reduced if not eliminated, which is important to successful endodontic treatment.

Pediatric procedures—Isolate only the teeth that are involved in the operative treatment—usually two or three teeth. With young children the use of rubber dam can increase safety because youngsters may have active tongues or may move suddenly, thereby creating the potential for injury to soft tissue when high-speed handpieces or other instruments are used.

Restorative procedures on anterior teeth—Isolate the anterior segment of the arch, incisors, cuspids and first and second premolars.

Restorative procedures on posterior teeth—Isolate the tooth being treated and one tooth posterior and two teeth anterior to that tooth. Another option is to isolate the tooth that is being treated, as well as the tooth posterior to it, and include all teeth anterior to the opposite central incisor or even cuspid.

Rubber Dam Isolation

Rubber dam isolation is one of the earliest methods of isolation. Its use dates back over a hundred years. Rubber dam isolation was common in the past, and its use as an isolation technique has gained a resurgence because it is the only isolation technique that provides a barrier in infection control. The use of rubber dam reduces contamination from the patient's oral cavity and consequently is recommended by the American Dental Association (ADA) and many other organizations as an acceptable source of infection control.

In 1864 Dr. Sanford C. Barnum, a dentist in New York, invented the rubber dam while treating a lower molar that was inundated with saliva. Exasperated, he punched a hole in a thin sheet of oilskin, placed it over the tooth, and attached a little rubber ring around the neck of the tooth; thus rubber dam was created.

Inexperienced persons may believe that the use of rubber dam requires more time and equipment during a procedure than other techniques; however, when rubber dam technique is performed by an experienced dental team, its use can actually save time. Though placement and removal of rubber dam are often a legally delegated auxiliary responsibility, it is most efficiently placed as a four-handed procedure. The procedural description in this chapter will be presented as a four-handed task.

The Rubber Dam Armamentarium

The armamentarium used for the rubber dam isolation technique varies according to the type of procedure that is being performed and the individual operator's preference.

Rubber Dam Material

The **rubber dam material**, a latex material into which holes are punched for teeth to be exposed during the treatment procedure, is used to isolate a tooth or teeth. This material is supplied in a roll from which pieces are cut or in precut sheets 4 inches × 4 inches, 5 inches × 5 inches, and 6 inches × 6 inches. The latex materials are manufactured in colors such as dark green (to provide contrast with oral structures), pastels, and a light beige. Rubber dam material has different weights or gauges that vary from thin, to medium, to heavy, and even to extra heavy or special heavy (Fig. 22-1)

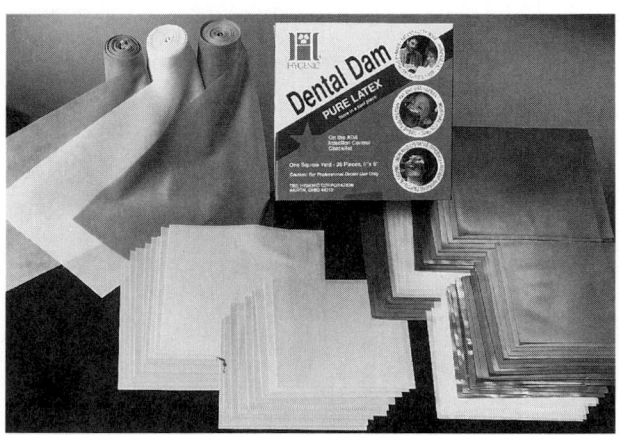

FIG. 22-1   Rubber dam material in rolls; precut and in various colors.

(Courtesy of Hygenic.)

Rubber dam material has a limited shelf life and will tear easier as it ages. Complete and current stock should be maintained, and the oldest stock should always be used before the newer inventory.

Rubber Dam Stamp and Pad or Template

The **rubber dam stamp and pad or template** provides a guide for punching holes in the rubber dam for teeth that are to be exposed or isolated. The **rubber dam stamp,** a rubber stamp with images of a dental arch and tooth positions, is placed on an **inked pad**: a standard ink pad with colored ink applied. The stamp is then placed on the piece of dam material. The stamp establishes markings on the dam for an ideal tooth configuration of the primary and permanent dentition.

The **template** is a 6-inch × 6-inch piece of plastic with holes, which can be placed over or under the rubber dam material to make markings. A pen is placed in the holes to mark the rubber dam material at the location to be punched. Either of these devices works with an ideal tooth arrangement. However when teeth are out of alignment or are malpositioned in the oral cavity, the operator must evaluate the position of the holes in the rubber dam material and adjust the holes to compensate for malalignment (Fig. 22-2). If a study cast is available, the rubber dam material can be placed over the teeth in the arch and marked, working as a template or guide for the position of the teeth.

Rubber Dam Frame

The **rubber dam frame/holder** is used to hold and position the rubber dam material over the oral cavity.

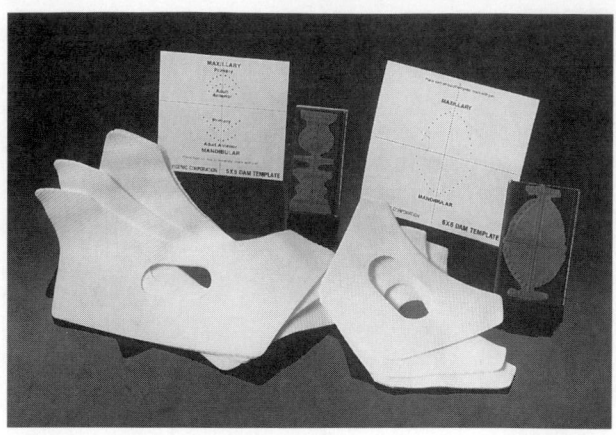

FIG. 22-2   Rubber dam stamp, template, and napkins. (Courtesy of Hygenic.)

Several designs have prongs that provide points onto which the stretched material can be secured on the frame (Fig. 22-3, *A* and *B*). The most common styles include the Young's frame, which is made of metal or plastic, with the plastic being the ideal frame to be used during endodontic treatment. The Young's frame has an additional style that secures the rubber dam with an anterior pouch to collect fluids. The E-Z Ray frame is designed for use when radiographs are needed because this frame can be easily manipulated. Another style of frame is the Hygienic frame, which is larger, more bulky, and plastic; it is often used in endodontic treatment. The Woodbury frame is strikingly different from the other frames; it is metal, with a cloth holder that wraps around the back of the patient's head. Certain products are available that have a disposable frame built in the piece of latex.

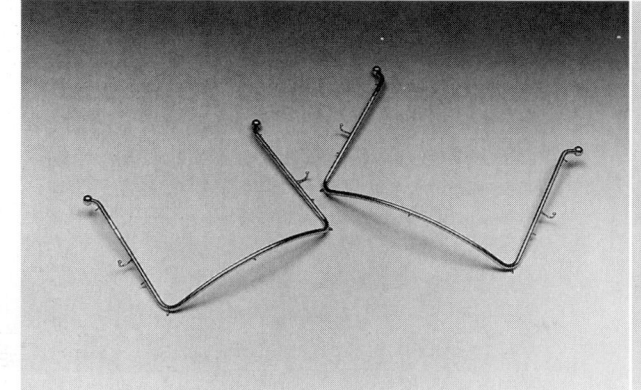

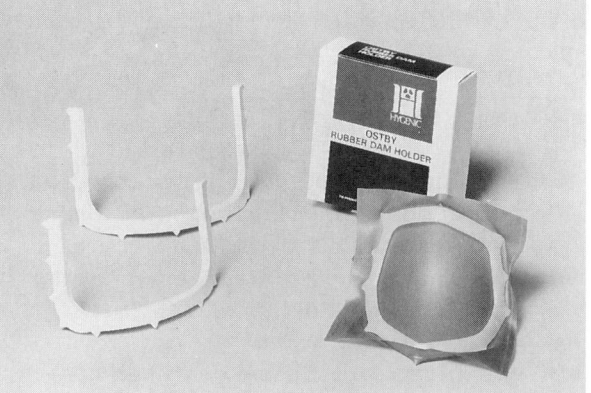

A   **B**

FIG. 22-3   *A,* Young's rubber dam frame. *B,* Two forms of plastic rubber dam frames. (Courtesy of Hygenic.)

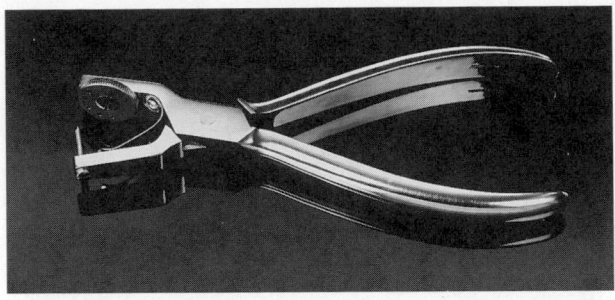

FIG. 22-4   Rubber dam punch with five-hole turntable.
(Courtesy of Hygenic.)

Rubber Dam Punch

The **rubber dam punch** is a forceps-like device that has a movable circular turntable at one end with holes of various sizes. The size of the hole used depends on the size of the tooth to be exposed through the rubber dam. Either five or six holes are on each turnplate, with the small holes intended for primary teeth and permanent mandibular incisors; hole No. 2 is for the permanent maxillary incisors; hole No. 3 is for the permanent canines and premolars; hole No. 4 is for the permanent molars; and hole No. 5 is for the clamped permanent molar tooth or bridge abutment teeth. Opposite the turntable is a punch point that is forced through the rubber dam when the arms of the punch are brought together (Fig. 22-4).

Rubber Dam Clamps

Rubber dam clamps anchor the dam to the tooth to avoid movement and slippage of the rubber dam material during treatment. The rubber dam clamps vary in size and shape to conform to the area where they will be placed (Fig. 22-5, *A*). Clamps are supplied with wings or without wings. The wings are projections at the clamp's jaw that attach to the rubber dam material to secure the clamp in the punched hole. The parts of the rubber dam clamp are illustrated in Fig. 22-5, *B*.

Clamps are designed for use in specific areas, teeth, or procedures. An example is the Ferrier #212 clamp, which may be used on anterior teeth or for a Class V restoration that is placed in the anterior or posterior teeth (Fig. 22-6, *A*). Other clamps are specifically for incisors, cuspids, premolars, or molars. Occasionally, the gingival

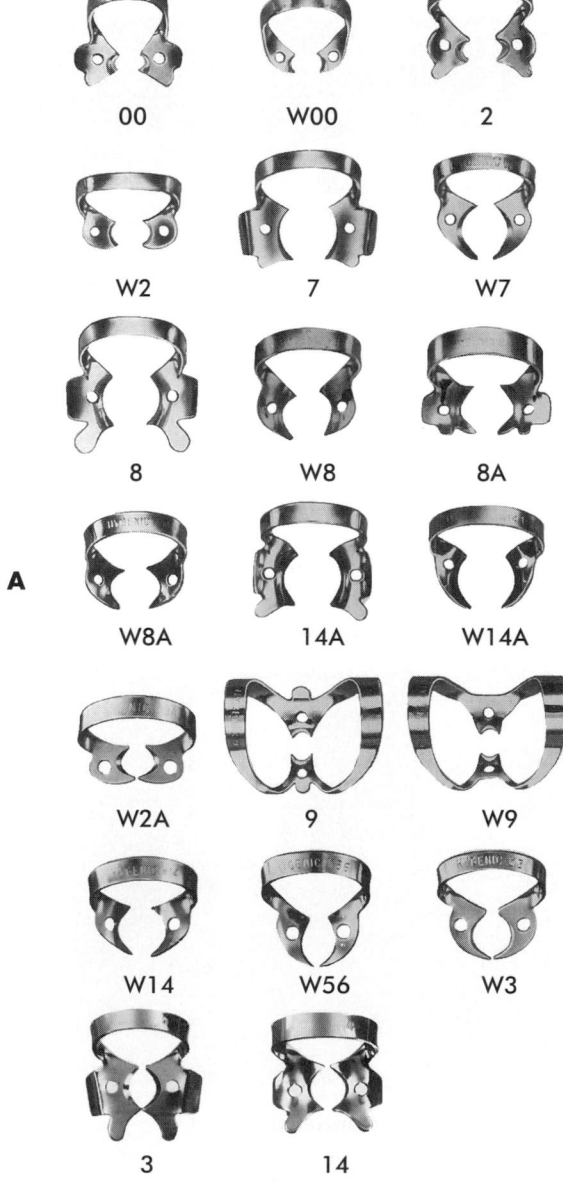

A

00 W00 2
W2 7 W7
8 W8 8A
W8A 14A W14A
W2A 9 W9
W14 W56 W3
3 14

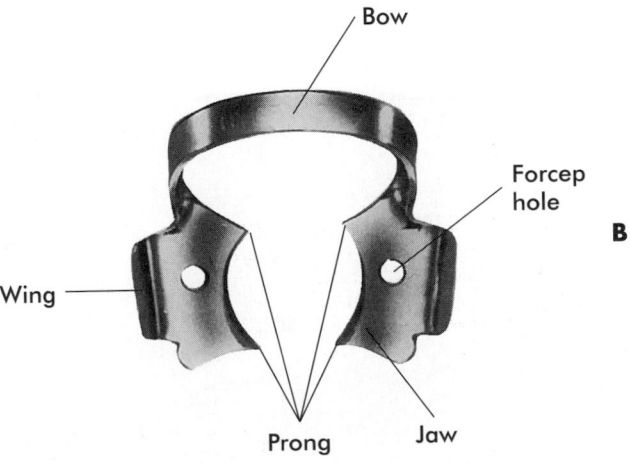

Bow
Forcep hole
B
Wing
Prong Jaw

FIG. 22-5   *A,* Variety of rubber dam clamps. *B,* Molar clamp from above chart identifying the bow, jaws, wings, and hole opening for forceps.

(*A* Courtesy of Hygenic.)

tissues need to be forced away from the cervical area of the tooth to gain access to a particular surface. The gingival retracting clamp is designed to assist in this action. The jaws of the clamp extend down toward the cervical area retracting the gingival tissues (Fig. 22-6, *B*). Certain other clamps are of smaller design and are used in pediatric situations. The shape and design of clamps vary greatly to meet the needs in isolation.

▶ Rubber Dam Forceps

The **rubber dam forceps** is used to place rubber dam clamps on the tooth/teeth to stabilize or anchor the rubber dam in the oral cavity (Fig. 22-7). The prongs on the beaks of the forceps fit in holes or grooves on the clamp to stretch the clamp to fit over a tooth. Once the clamp is positioned, the prongs are lifted from the clamp's holes and removed from the clamp that is now stabilized on the tooth.

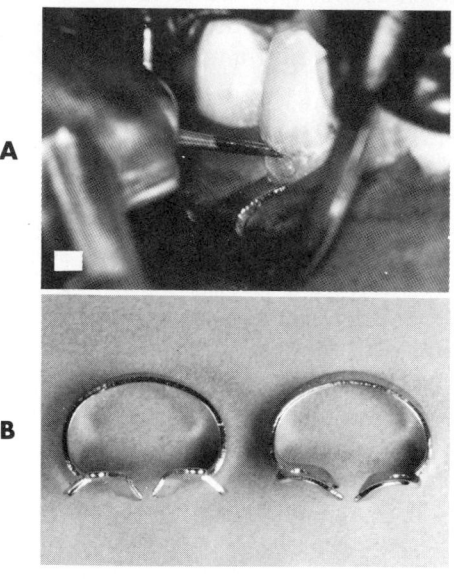

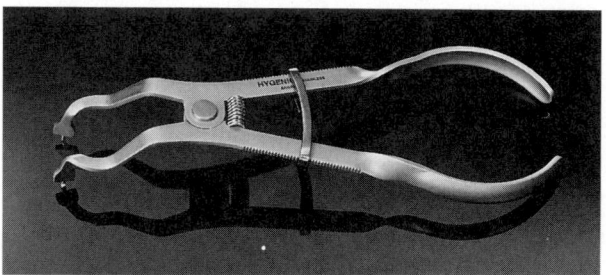

FIG. 22-7   Rubber dam forceps with the crossbar in the middle of the handle.

FIG. 22-6   *A,* Ferrier 212 clamp used on anterior teeth. *B,* Gingival retracting clamps.

(Sturdevant CM et al: *The art and science of operative dentistry,* ed 2, St Louis, 1985, Mosby.)

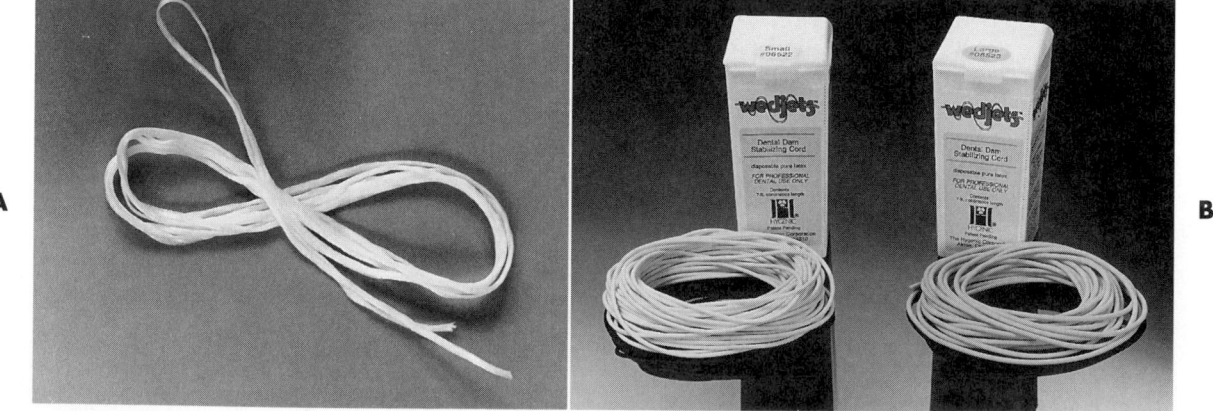

FIG. 22-8   *A,* Figure 8 of waxed floss. *B,* A prefabricated rubber stabilizing material/Wedjet.

(*B* courtesy of Hygenic.)

Ligatures

Ligatures are devices used to ligate or anchor the portion of the rubber dam material that is not stabilized by the rubber dam clamp. Ligatures for anchoring the rubber dam material may include the following:

- A piece of dental floss that is tied around the circumference of the tooth that is exposed on the most anterior tooth
- A piece of dental floss that is doubled in thickness and placed interproximally on the surface farthest from the clamped tooth. For instance, if teeth #27, #28, #29, and #30 are exposed and the clamp is on tooth #30, the ligature would be placed on the mesial of #27
- A corner of the rubber dam that is cut and placed interproximally next to the tooth that is exposed on the most anterior tooth
- A premanufactured material, such as a Wedjet, is placed interproximally at the most anterior tooth that is isolated (Wedjets can also be used in place of a clamp when placed around the neck of the tooth) (Fig. 22-8, *A* and *B*)

The patient can aspirate the rubber dam clamp during dental treatment, which is an occurrence a dental professional must prevent. A piece of dental floss is tied to the rubber dam clamp and acts as a safety precaution. The dental floss is connected to the clamp at the time the clamp is tried on the tooth and during the entire isolation procedure. If the clamp loosens at any time, it can be retrieved by grasping the length of floss attached to the bow of the clamp (Fig. 22-9).

Rubber Dam Napkin

The **rubber dam napkin** is placed between the rubber dam material and the patient's skin to avoid chafing and discomfort. It is also helpful in absorbing saliva during and after the isolation procedure.

Additional Items

Several additional items are needed to place the rubber dam; some of these are optional, depending on the individual treatment situation.

Dental floss
Lubricant
Pen (if template is used)
Crown and collar scissors
Choice of instrument to invert the rubber dam material
    FP1
    Beavertail burnisher
    Spoon excavator
Saliva ejector and adapter hose if necessary
Alcohol or Bunsen burner (optional)
Stick impression compound (optional)
Matches (optional)

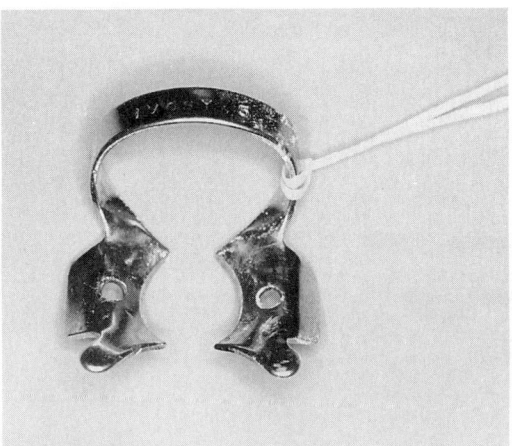

FIG. 22-9 A piece of floss looped through the bow of the clamp acts as a safety precaution for retrieving a clamp that may become dislodged.

The Rubber Dam Procedure

With the use of rubber dam isolation comes the need for patient education. Children usually experience apprehension when visiting a dental office, and an explanation of steps in the procedure provides comfort. When the procedure is explained to children, the rubber dam can be described as a raincoat or a slicker—an analogy the child can understand. An adult patient can be instructed in the various positive aspects that the rubber dam technique can provide, such as not having to swallow as often and no debris falling in the mouth.

Some preparation of the rubber dam armamentarium can be completed before the patient is seated in the treatment room. Complete preparation would be ideal to reduce chairside time; however, this is not always possible. The rubber dam material can be selected, stamped, punched, and placed on the rubber dam frame if the alignment of the patient's teeth is known. If tooth alignment has not been determined, these steps must wait until the patient is in the treatment room and seated. The following procedural description discusses the preparation of the rubber dam for the isolation of a quadrant.

PUNCHING THE RUBBER DAM

1. Punch the rubber dam once clearance to the interproximal areas is achieved (Fig. 22-10). Use the rubber dam stamp if available.
   a. If the template or study casts are not used, the holes could be punched after a thorough observation of the mouth allowing for any malpositioned teeth.

As each hole is punched, material is left between the holes. This material is **the septum,** the portion of the rubber dam that must slip between the teeth. The ideal amount of rubber dam between the edges of the holes is 3 to 3.5 mm. In the anterior segment of the mouth, particularly the mandibular anteriors, the septum may be reduced in size to allow for the small size of the teeth and the curvature of the arch.

2. Avoid punching the holes too far apart since this creates excess bulk of material interproximally and can make it difficult to invert the rubber dam material.
   a. Punching the holes too close together stretches the holes, and the rubber dam does not cover all the gingival tissues.
   b. The closeness of the holes does not allow for the inversion of the rubber dam, a step that creates a completely isolated area for performing operative procedures (Fig. 22-10).

EXAMINATION OF THE TREATMENT AREA

1. Escort the patient into the prepared treatment room, and seat him or her.
2. Ask the patient to rinse thoroughly with an approved oral rinse to reduce microbes in the oral cavity.
3. Inspect the oral cavity for the alignment of the teeth.
4. Floss the patient's teeth at this time to evaluate the contact areas before the rubber dam is applied.
   a. An extremely **tight contact** could cause difficulty as you try to the pass rubber dam material through the interproximal contact.
   b. If contacts are too tight, a wooden wedge can be placed interproximally, for approximately 5 minutes, to force the teeth apart.
   c. After this time the wedge is removed and the contact is checked for clearance.

NOTE: *Uneven contacts,* rough interproximal surfaces, need to be evaluated as the floss is passed through the interdental area. If heavy calculus exists on surfaces that are to be isolated, removal of the calculus is advised before the rubber dam is placed. If the calculus is not removed, complete isolation may not be possible because inversion of the rubber dam would be difficult. Overhangs might also be found on the interproximal surfaces of restorations and will need to be removed. The removal of overhangs can be accomplished by using a lightning strip (a metal strip with abrading grit adhered to one side), a Bard-Parker scalpel, or a diamond point on a handpiece to gain access to the interproximal area. If calculus or overhangs need to be removed, the assistant would be responsible only for flossing the teeth; a dentist will make alterations in the structures in the oral cavity.

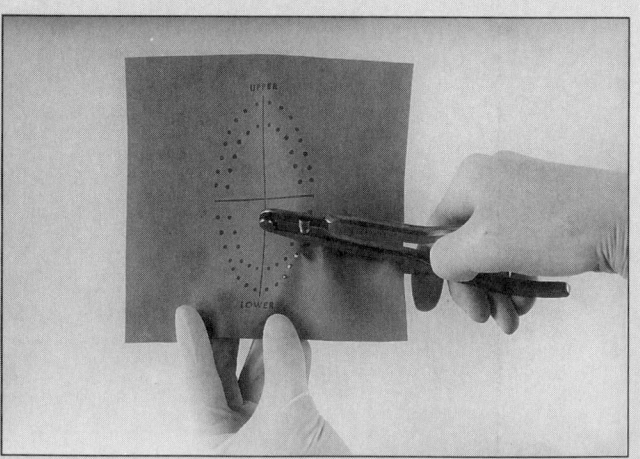

FIG. 22-10　Punching the rubber dam.

PUNCHING THE RUBBER DAM—cont'd.

c. The curve of the dental arch is another consideration when punching the rubber dam. If the rubber dam is punched so that the arch is too close together, the results are folds and stretching of the rubber dam toward the anterior of the mouth. If the rubber dam is punched so the arch is further apart and has less curve, the results are folds and stretching of the dam towards the lingual (Fig. 22-11).

d. The holes on the turntable of the rubber dam punch vary in size and allow the operator to select the size that corresponds with the size of the tooth (Fig. 22-12).

It should be noted when the treatment involves the mandibular teeth and before the holes are punched in the rubber dam, the holes should be positioned so that they allow at least 1½ inches to 2 inches of extra material inferior to the most anteriorly punched teeth. When treating maxillary teeth the holes should be positioned to allow 1½ inch to 2 inches of material superior to the most anteriorly punched teeth (Fig. 22-13).

1. Observe the common rules for hole punching:

a. For endodontic treatment only the tooth (teeth) being treated is exposed.

b. In operative treatment at least one tooth anterior and one tooth posterior to the tooth (teeth) being treated is exposed.

c. An alternative method for punching the rubber dam is to expose more teeth—even an entire quadrant or segment.

NOTE: The number of holes punched will vary with the type of procedure and the personal preferences of the operator.

Occasionally, a piece of dam material will not be completely punched or cleanly cut from the dam. The hole is visible but a tag of the material remains in the opening. This tag must be removed by repositioning the punch over the hole and cutting the material again, or it can be pulled out with the fingers, leaving the hole intact. If this tag is not removed, it is difficult to invert the rubber dam around the exposed tooth and may lead to tears in the rubber dam material during placement. Some assistants find it easier to force the prong of the punch further through the dam to avoid leaving a tag.

NOTE: Without care being taken for the steps just discussed, it makes no difference how well the rubber dam is placed, it simply will not function as it was intended: as a tight moisture sealed unit. Complete isolation can only be achieved when leakage of any oral fluids is eliminated from the treatment area.

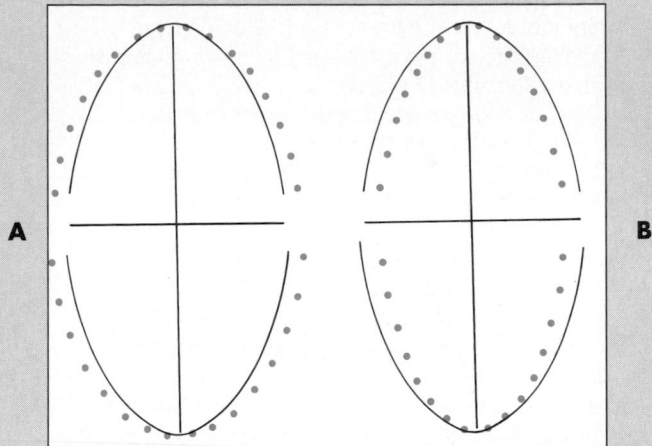

FIG. 22-11 Properly punched rubber dam for *A,* maxillary arch, and *B,* mandibular arch.

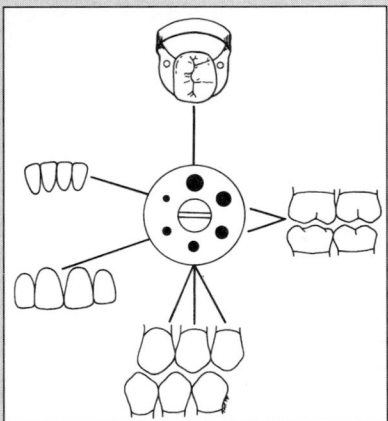

Cutting table on the rubber dam punch, illustrating the size of the hole in relation to various teeth.

(Sturdevant CM et al: *The art and science of operative dentistry,* ed 2, St Louis, 1985, Mosby.)

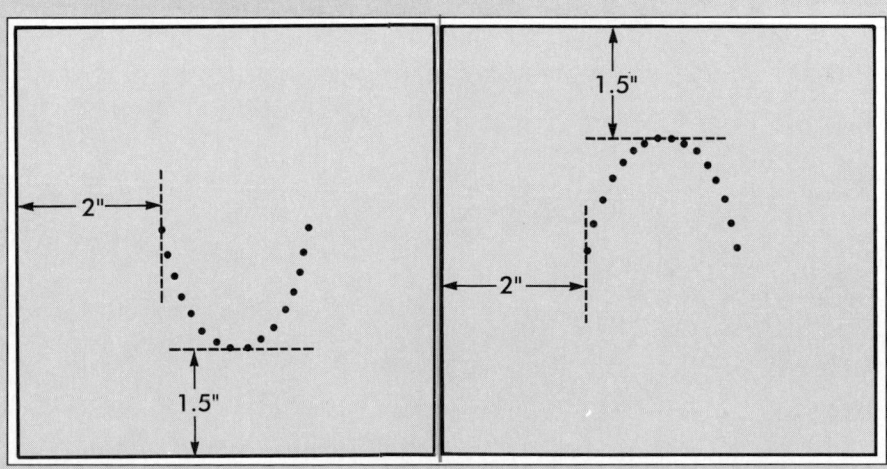

A and *B,* The position of the holes for maxillary and mandibular placement.

1. Always place a ligature on the selected clamp as a safety measure before trying it in the oral cavity.
   a. The ligature is a piece of dental floss that is approximately 16 inches in length.
   b. It is doubled over, and the looped portion is fed through the bow of the clamp.
   c. The free ends of the floss are threaded through the loop and pulled tightly to secure it on the bow of the clamp.
   d. The floss is positioned on the buccal side of the clamp so that it will be out of the operator's way during the procedure.
2. Place the clamp on the tooth posterior to the tooth being treated.
   a. It is possible to place the clamp on the tooth receiving treatment if it is the most posterior tooth in the quadrant.
   b. Access to the tooth may be less than desirable and alternative isolation techniques, such as cotton roll isolation, may be necessary.
3. Position the rubber dam forceps beaks in the hole openings of the rubber dam clamp. Grasp the forceps handles together, stretching the opening of the clamp wider.
   a. The crossbar of the clamp forceps is pulled closer to the handles and locked on the teeth of the handles.
   b. This enlarges the clamp opening, causing the spring action in the forceps to be stabilized (Fig. 22-14).
   NOTE: If the treatment procedure is in the maxillary arch, the operator usually positions the hand palm up to receive the forceps and clamp. The assistant passes the forceps and clamp so that they are directed toward the patient with the handles in the operator's palm.
4. If the operator positions the receiving hand with the palm down, pass the forceps and clamp with the beaks and cervical of the clamp face down.
5. If the operator's hand is positioned with the palm up to receive the forceps and clamp, pass the forceps with hands clear of the handles and the beaks of the forceps and the cervical of the clamp facing up.
   a. In this situation the operator is able to position the receiving hand on the forceps and turn the forceps over and place the clamp on the tooth to test the fit (Fig. 22-15, A and B).
6. Position the lingual points on the clamp first as a clamp is placed and then slide the buccal points down into place as is illustrated later during the placement of the rubber dam.
   a. The clamp should not impinge on the oral tissues or push the tissues down unless it is a gingival retracting clamp.
   b. The clamp should be stable, and not rock back and forth or side to side. If the clamp is not stable a second or third clamp should be tested, until one fits correctly.
   c. After repeated use, rubber dam clamps may lose tension. This occurs when the metal of the clamp has been stressed beyond the yield point and does not return to the original shape. These clamps are useless and should be discarded.
   d. After the appropriate clamp has been selected, the forceps and clamp are passed back to the assistant.

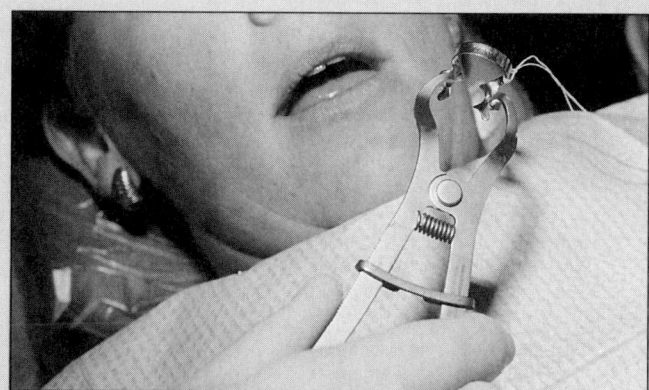

FIG. 22-14   The clamp opening is enlarged by pulling the crossbar of the forceps toward the handles to lock it in place.

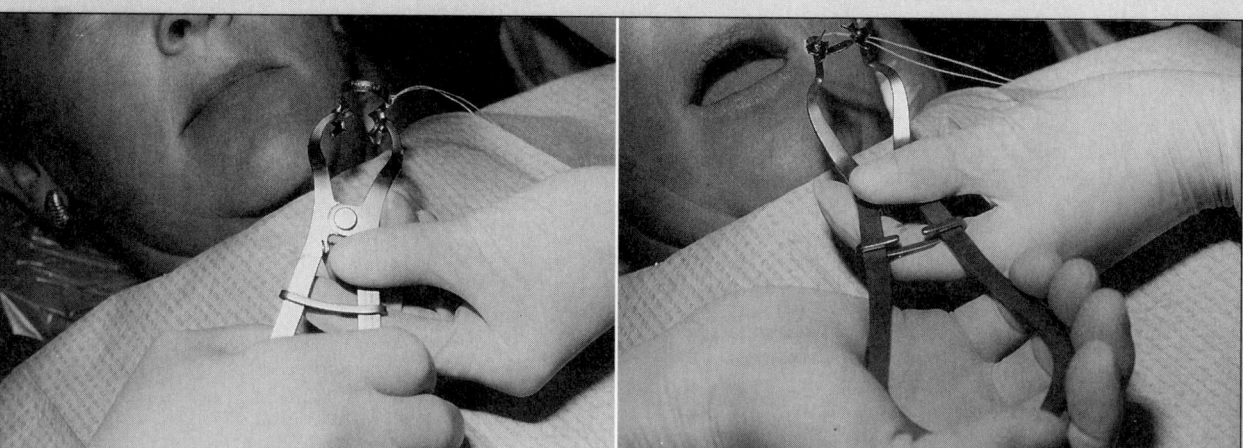

FIG. 22-15   *A,* The clamp and forceps are passed for placement in the mandibular arch, and *B,* for the maxillary arch.

ASSEMBLING THE RUBBER DAM

At this point the steps of assembly may vary, depending on the operator's preference to use winged or wingless clamps.

1. Assemble the frame and rubber dam material while the operator tests the clamp.
2. Lay the rubber dam material flat on a surface and position the Young's frame over or under the rubber dam material.
3. Pick up the two pieces of equipment as one unit, positioning both thumbs on the frame, while the rest of your hands support the assembly.
   a. More specifically, one hand holds the frame and material in place, while the other pulls the rubber dam material over the prongs of the frame.
   b. The prongs do not have to poke through the material but should hold the material in place on the frame.
   c. The same is done to the opposite side of the frame, and then the lower part of the dam is attached to the frame (Fig. 22-16).
   d. When the dam is secure on the frame it should be taut but still have enough flexibility to be molded when placed in the oral cavity.
   e. With the frame on top of the rubber dam, the descending layers are as follows: the frame, the rubber dam material, the patient napkin, and finally, the patient's skin.
   f. If the frame is placed below the rubber dam material, the order is: rubber dam material, frame, patient napkin, and patient's skin.
4. Remove the clamp from the rubber dam forceps and place it in the rubber dam material that is attached to the frame.
5. Position the projection of the jaws (the wing) on one side of the clamp in the most posterior tooth hole opening.
   a. When this is done the wing is under the rubber dam material.
   b. The hole opening is stretched, and the wing on the other side of the clamp is carefully forced into the enlarged hole (Fig. 22-17, *A* through *C*).
   c. At this point exercise care since it is easy to tear rubber dam material, especially if it is old.
   d. When both wings are under the dam, the rest of the clamp, the bow and the jaws, are still on the upper surface of the rubber dam with the points exposed under the rubber dam material.
6. Place the beaks of the rubber dam forceps in the clamp forceps holes and secure in position as previously described, thereby completing the assembly (Fig. 22-18).

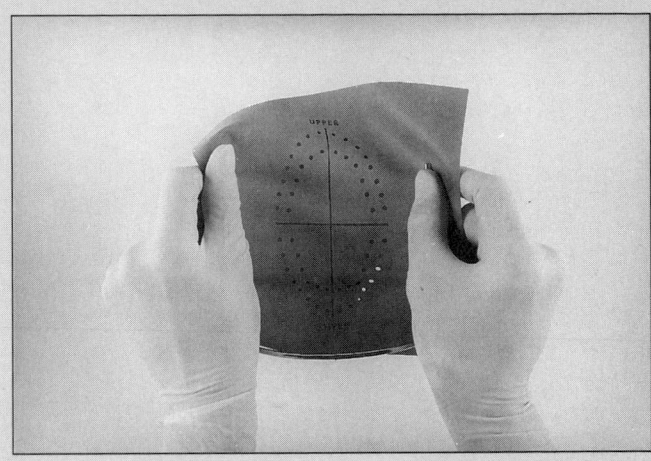

FIG. 22-16 **The rubber dam is attached to the prongs of the frame.**

7. Choose one of several options when the operator has selected to use a wingless clamp, since the rubber dam procedure varies from the winged clamp procedure.
   a. The following several options are open to the operator during placement:
      ▶ Place the clamp before the rubber dam material
      ▶ Place the clamp after the rubber dam material
      ▶ Attach the rubber dam material to the frame and then over the clamp
      ▶ Place the rubber dam material over the clamp when it may not be attached to the frame, and then attach the frame
8. Position the clamp on the tooth first and pull the rubber dam, with or without the frame, over the clamp and tooth.
   a. Once the clamped tooth is isolated, the rest of the teeth are exposed through the hole openings.
   b. Some operators may prefer to position the punched dam over the teeth that are to be isolated before the clamp is placed. With this technique the rubber dam clamp is positioned on the tooth after the rubber dam material is pulled over the crown of the tooth.
   c. Another option in rubber dam isolation is to not use the clamp when the rubber dam is stabilized on the teeth that are being isolated.

Continued.

ASSEMBLING THE RUBBER DAM—cont'd.

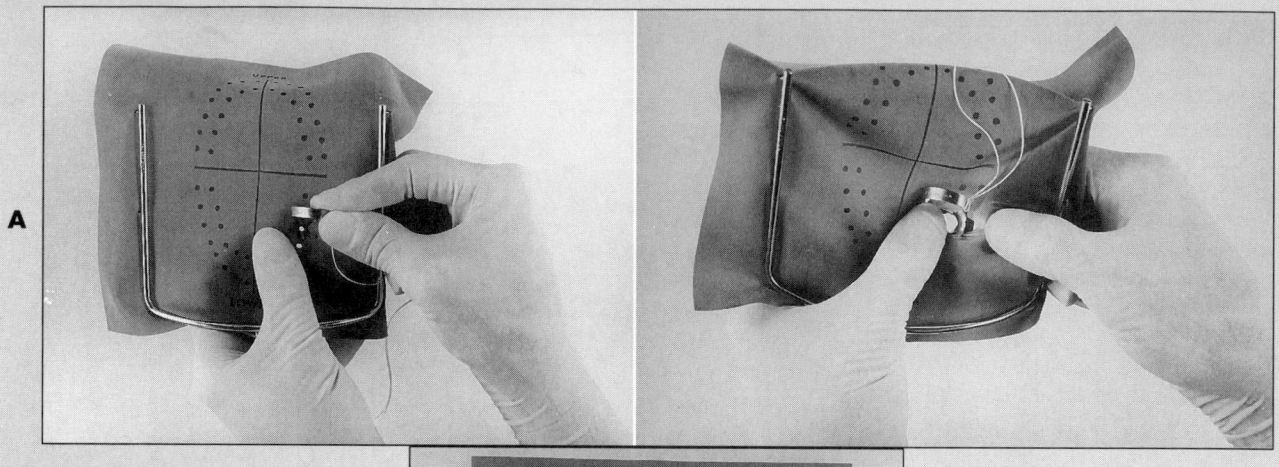

FIG. 22-17   A and B, The clamp is placed on the rubber dam with the wings holding it in place. C, Clamp secure in rubber dam.

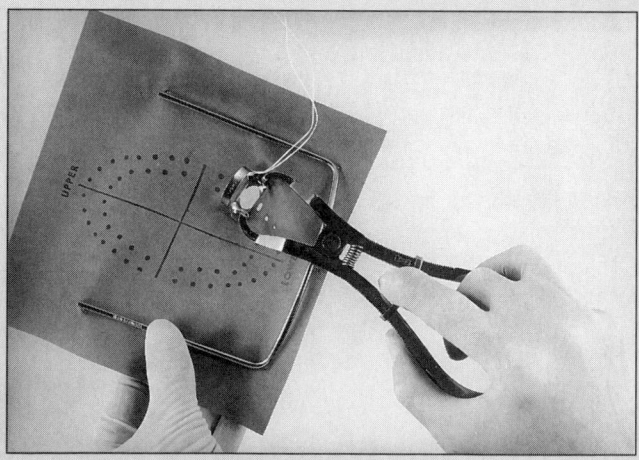

FIG. 22-18   Rubber dam forceps positioned in clamp holes.

PLACING THE RUBBER DAM ASSEMBLY

1. Evaluate access to the interproximal spaces after the rubber dam has been assembled.
   a. This is accomplished by passing floss through each contact to ensure clearance.
   b. If the floss freely passes through the contact, it is likely that the rubber dam material can be passed through the contact.
2. Pass the assembly to the operator as a single unit.
   a. The assistant's hands are now free from the handles of the forceps, which is positioned under the dam in the area of the forceps end, the clamp, and the upper edge of the material and frame.
3. Help guide the assembly into place and stabilize the frame to avoid injury to the patient (Fig. 22-19, *A* and *B*).
   a. The rubber dam assembly is positioned so that the clamp is over the most posterior tooth.
4. The operator carefully sets the lingual jaw of the clamp onto the tooth first (Fig. 22-20, *A* through *C*).
5. The operator widens the clamp opening and slides the clamp down as the buccal jaw of the clamp contacts the tooth surface.
   a. Since the clamp was previously tested for fit, it should not cause any discomfort for the patient.
6. The operator lifts each side of the clamp forceps from the holes in the clamp and returns the forceps to the assistant.
7. The operator checks for stability of the clamp on the tooth by using a finger placed on the clamp.
   a. If the clamp is not stable it may be necessary to retrieve the forceps and reposition the clamp.
8. The operator proceeds to isolate the remainder of the teeth by stretching the material over each tooth.
   a. It is necessary to use a piece of dental floss to assist in securing the remainder of the rubber dam material.
   b. A prepared piece of waxed dental floss that is approximately 16 inches in length can be wrapped around two fingers into a lasso that is twisted into a figure eight for easy use.
   c. The free ends of the floss can be freely grasped and unwound, reducing the possibility of the floss being tangled.

NOTE: If unwaxed floss is used it may easily fray. A piece of floss left loose in a treatment area may become tangled with other instruments.

9. Wrap the floss with an excess on one hand and less on the other.
10. Hold the floss securely, usually by using the forefingers or the middle fingers of both hands and pass it into the interproximal contacts (Fig. 22-21).
11. Work the floss down the mesial surface of one tooth and the distal surface of the other.
    a. The floss is passed through the contact and then pulled off of the hand with the least amount of floss.
    b. The floss is then removed from the sulcus area by pulling free of the teeth.
    c. If the floss is pulled back up through the contact, the dam material may come with it and the placement of the floss into the sulcus must be repeated.
    d. As the septum of the rubber dam material is forced down between each consecutive tooth with the floss, the assembly becomes more stable.

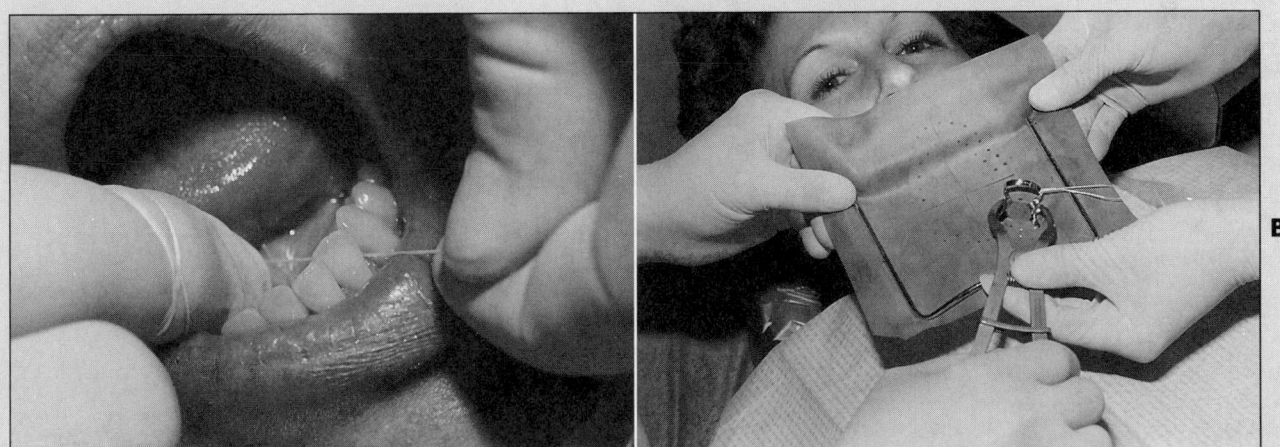

FIG. 22-19 *A,* The proximal contacts are checked. *B,* The completely assembled rubber dam is passed to the operator.

Continued.

PLACING THE RUBBER DAM ASSEMBLY—cont'd.

12. Position the anterior ligature on the mesial surface, once the most anterior tooth is isolated (Fig. 22-22).
    a. The anterior ligature is a corner of dam material that can be stretched thin like a rubber band and pulled into the mesial contact or twisted in a *bow tie* and placed into the interproximal space.
    b. Other alternatives to anchor the anterior portion of the rubber dam material include a doubled piece of floss thick enough to hold the dam in place, commercially produced ligature, a piece of floss looped around the tooth, tied on the buccal surface in a double knot, and then cut to remove any excess.

13. The operator removes the dam material from the wings of the clamp by hand or with the instrument of choice.
    a. Initially the wings of the clamp helped to stabilize the clamp in the hole opening of the dam material, but now the rubber dam must be removed and placed under the wings to achieve complete isolation.
    b. The material snaps down under the clamp and fits snugly around the cervical of the tooth.

14. The operator positions the forceps in the clamp openings if any gingival tissue is exposed, and slightly lifts the points of the clamp away from the tooth.

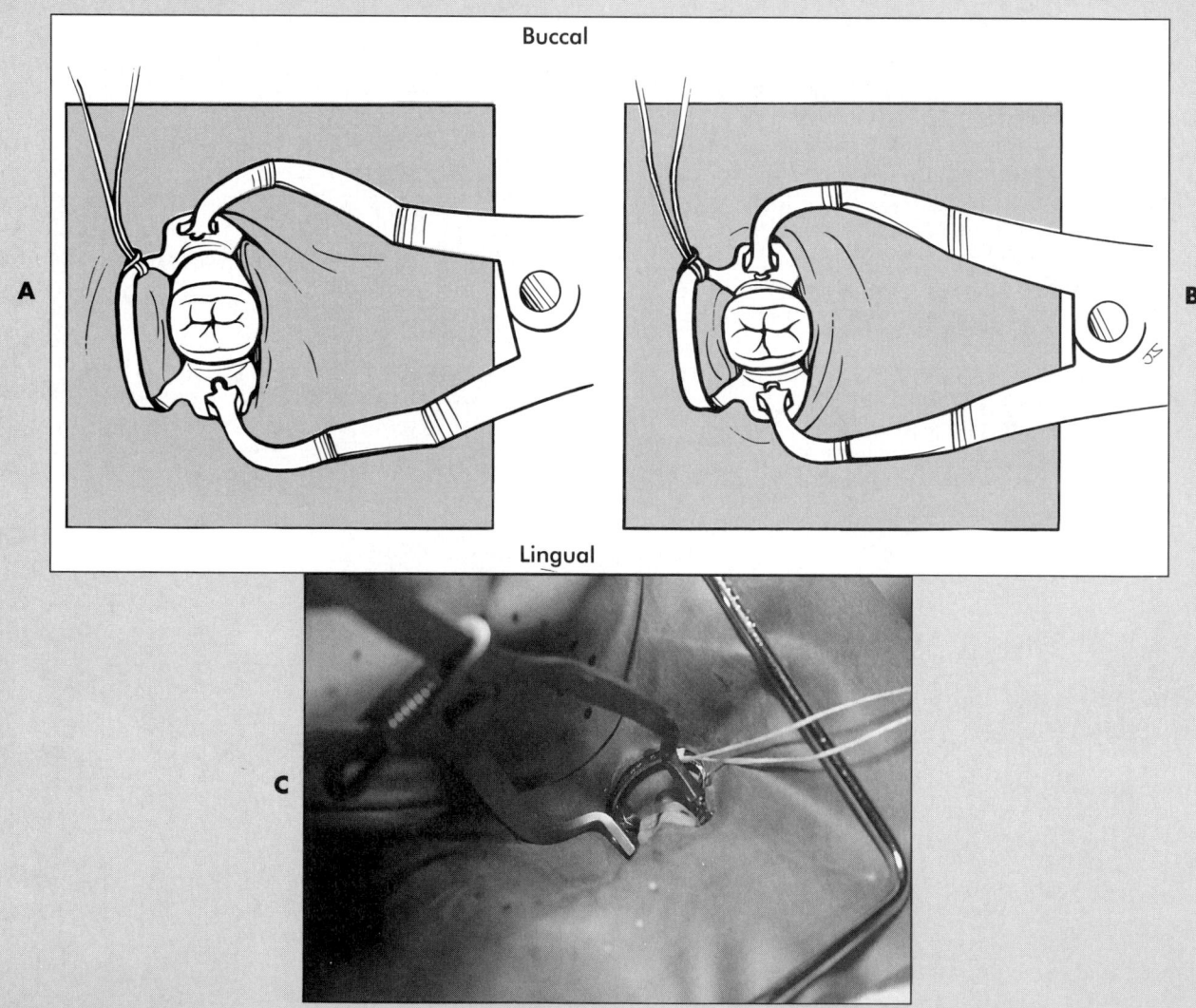

FIG. 22-20   *A,* The enlarged clamp is positioned by placement of the lingual jaw first. *B,* The buccal jaw is positioned after the lingual jaw. *C,* The clamp positioned on the tooth. The operator checks the clamp for stability on the tooth.

PLACING THE RUBBER DAM ASSEMBLY—cont'd.

a. The dam material will slide against the cervical of the tooth, and the clamp is repositioned, thereby avoiding placement of the points on the dam material.

b. Important: the dam might be secure, but the rubber dam material does not provide complete isolation at this point.

15. The operator uses an FPI, beavertail burnisher, spoon excavator, or other instrument to invert the rubber dam material.

a. Inversion, sometimes referred to as tucking, involves turning the edge of the rubber dam's hole that surrounds the tooth into the free gingival sulcus.

b. This step provides a seal that stops moisture from leaking into the operative area.

16. Blow air with the a/w syringe on the surface where the instrument is positioned to help turn the material into the sulcus (Fig. 22-23, *A* and *B*).

a. This procedure helps to secure the dam in the sulcus and forces any fluid from the hole opening.

b. The dam material is inverted on the buccal and lingual of all teeth isolated except the clamped tooth.

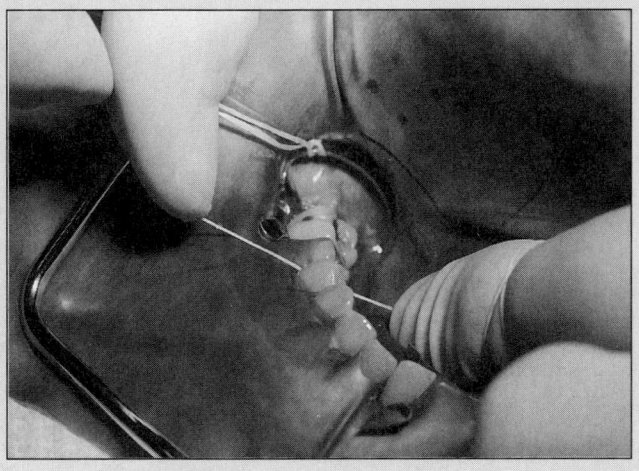

FIG. 22-21   Each proximal contact is flossed, moving the floss from the cusp tip to each side of the sulcus.

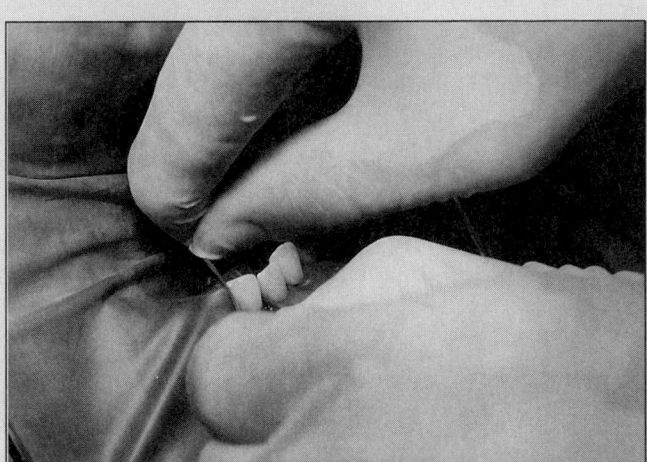

FIG. 22-22   A ligature formed from rubber dam material is placed in the anterior.

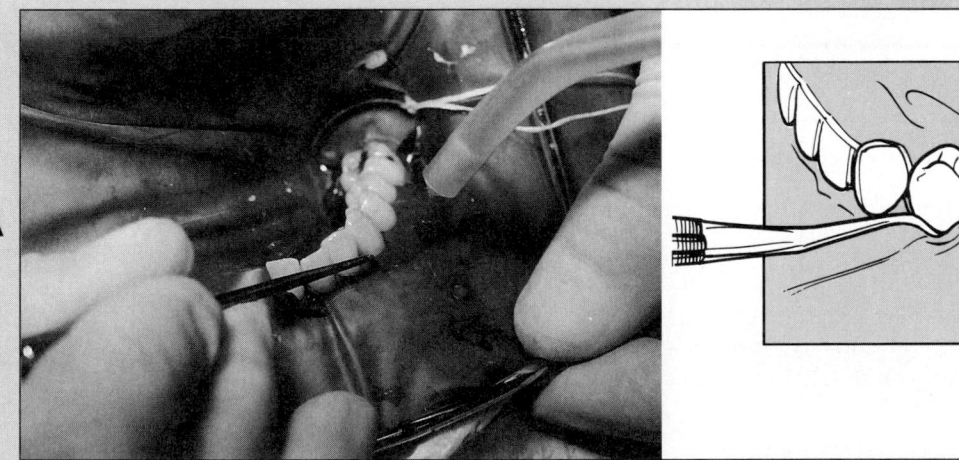

A   B

FIG. 22-23   *A* and *B,* The assistant dries the tooth as the operator inverts the rubber dam into the gingival sulcus.

PLACING THE RUBBER DAM ASSEMBLY—cont'd.

17. Place the rubber dam napkin under the dam material once the assembly is stable.
    a. The napkin provides the patient a buffer from the latex material, which can cause increased perspiration and chafing.
    b. Some operators prefer to place the napkin before the assembly, but the napkin might slip out of position if it is placed at this time.
    c. Another important reason the napkin is used between the patient's tissue and the dam material is that some people have latex allergies. It is important to ask a patient if he or she has a latex allergy before placement of the rubber dam. If the patient is aware of such an allergy, rubber dam material should not be used.
    d. If the rubber dam material blocks the patient's nose, it may be necessary to remove excess material by cutting an opening to breathe (Fig. 22-24).

NOTE: Any time a patient has anything in the oral cavity, increased saliva production takes place. Even though the patient can physically swallow with a rubber dam in place, he or she often feels that they cannot or should not.

18. Place a saliva ejector under the dam in the mandibular arch as soon as the rubber dam assembly is completely in place.
    a. If a quadrant in the mandible is isolated with rubber dam, the saliva ejector is placed opposite the quadrant that is receiving treatment.
    b. The saliva ejector relieves the patient of the need to swallow and provides comfort during the operative procedure.
19. The criteria for clinically acceptable rubber dam placement are shown in Box 22-2.

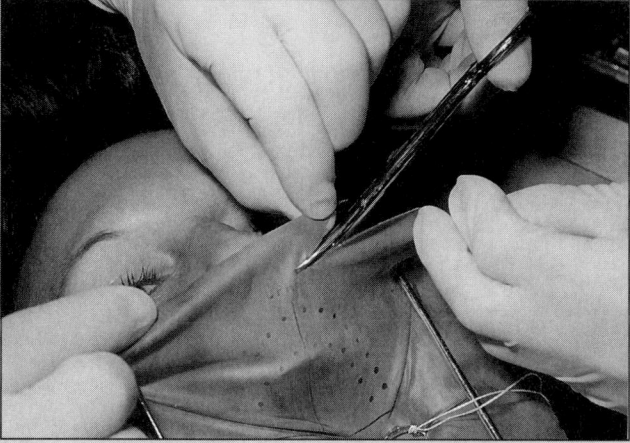

FIG. 22-24   **An opening for the nose is created to allow the patient to breathe easier.**

BOX 22-2

CRITERIA FOR CLINICALLY ACCEPTABLE RUBBER DAM PLACEMENT

Floss on the bow of the clamp towards the buccal or facial side
Clamp is stable on the tooth
Holes are punched in the correct location
Clamp is placed in the correct hole
Orientation of the rubber dam assembly (no folds in material)
Rubber dam material is completely inverted
Each tooth has either a seal through the inversion or is ligated
No soft tissue trauma
Rubber dam napkin or other protection is placed
Saliva ejector is in place

REMOVING THE RUBBER DAM ASSEMBLY

Once the operative procedure has been completed and debris, such as fluids and amalgam scrap, is evacuated from the dam surface the rubber dam assembly is removed. The steps run almost in reverse of placement.

1. Remove the saliva ejector.
2. Remove the ligature, either by stretching it and pulling it through the contact or by using scissors to cut the buccal surface of the tied dental floss and pulling it from the buccal surface with cotton pliers.
3. Roll the dam over a finger and stretch the interseptal dam away from the teeth.
4. Use curved crown and collar scissors with the beaks pointed away from the tissues, and cut along the line of interseptal material that the operator has pulled away (Fig. 22-25).
    a. Since the dam was stretched by the operator, it often snaps free of the interproximal space when it is cut.

REMOVING THE RUBBER DAM ASSEMBLY—cont'd.

b. If the rubber dam material still lies in the interproximal space, it is cleared from the buccal or lingual surface.

5. Pass a rubber dam clamp forceps to the operator, and place the forceps in the holes of the clamp.

   a. The clamp is expanded and lifted off the tooth (Fig. 22-26, *A* and *B*).

   b. The clamp should be free of the rubber dam when the clamp and forceps are passed to the assistant who receives them by cupping both in the palm of the hand.

   c. Occasionally the clamp pops free of the clamp forceps and cupping can avoid the clamp flying out of the mouth and causing injury.

6. The operator lifts the frame and dam material as a unit from the oral cavity and passes it to the assistant.

7. Remove the rubber dam napkin and wipe any debris from the patient's face.

8. Place the rubber dam and frame on the top of the mobile cart, and remove the frame to examine the dam for missing pieces.

9. Lay the material flat on the surface, and reposition the cut pieces of rubber dam material (Fig. 22-27).

   a. If a piece of material is missing, it might be in the patient's mouth.

   b. By repositioning the material the assistant can direct the operator to check a certain interproximal space.

   c. If, on inspection, the operator observes the piece of dam material in the mouth, it can be removed with an explorer or with floss.

   d. The piece of dam must be removed or it will cause tissue trauma to the area.

The team completes a full mouth rinse on the patient. During rubber dam placement a patient's saliva may become viscous and a refreshing rinse of the oral cavity is a courtesy to the patient.

See the *Team approach: four–handed rubber dam application* box for assistance in understanding how your actions will synchronize with the operator's actions.

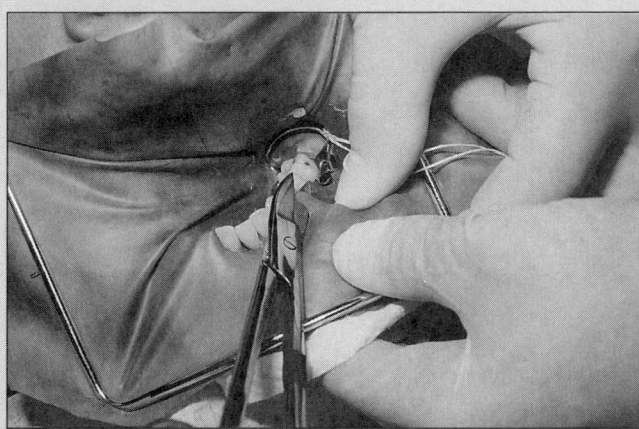

FIG. 22-25　The interseptal material is cut between each tooth to assist in the removal of the rubber dam.

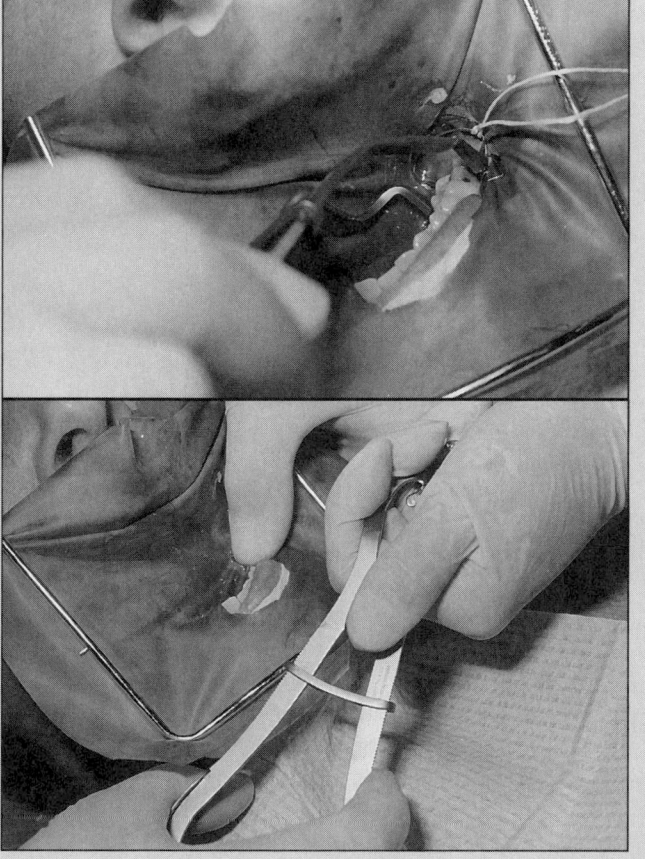

FIG. 22-26　*A,* The clamp is removed from the tooth with the forceps. *B,* The forceps and clamp are returned to the assistant.

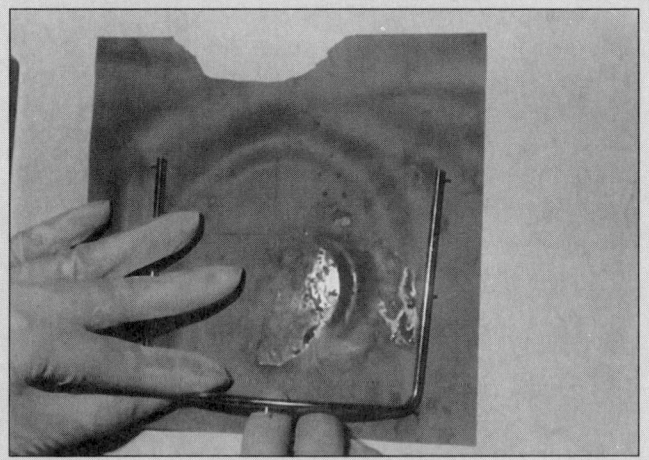

FIG. 22-27　The assistant lays the rubber dam material on a flat surface to check for missing pieces.

TEAM APPROACH
Four-Handed Rubber Dam Application

OPERATOR	ASSISTANT
	Select clamp, and attach floss to ligature
	Try in clamp
	Assemble rubber dam
	Floss interproximal contacts to determine clearance
	Pick up entire assembly
	Leave handle of forceps free for operator to grasp
	Pass to operator
Grasp handle and side of assembly	
Position clamp over most posterior tooth	Stabilize frame to avoid patient injury
Open jaws of clamp	
Position lingual jaw of clamp onto tooth	
Position buccal jaw of clamp onto tooth	
Lift forceps out of clamp holes	
Return forceps	Grasp forceps
Using fingers, check stability of clamp	Return forceps to mobile cart
If not stable, retrieve forceps and reposition clamp	
Begin to stretch punched holes over remaining teeth	Wrap floss around one finger of each hand*
	Assist in securing the remaining rubber dam between teeth
	Work floss down the mesial of one tooth, then down the distal of adjacent tooth
	Continue to floss between remaining exposed teeth, until septum of dam is forced down between each tooth
	Ligate mesial of most anterior tooth
	Place napkin under dam
	Pass spoon excavator or other instrument to invert dam
Retrieve instrument to invert the rubber dam	
Place instrument on dam at cervical buccal and turn edge of dam into sulcus	Turn a/w tip to appropriate arch
	Spray air at site of inversion
Continue on buccal surface, until all dam is inverted	Follow operator to complete inversion on buccal, then move to lingual
Move to lingual, and repeat process	Continue to spray air, until all dam is inverted
Ask patient to turn to improve vision as needed	Cut excess dam from nose area if needed
	Place saliva ejector if needed

*If it is more convenient for the operator to floss the contacts and the assistant to hold the dam, the tasks can easily be reversed.

Variations in Rubber Dam Placement

Circumstances of dental treatment will often warrant a change from that which is ordinary or normal. Variations in rubber dam isolation may be needed to accommodate circumstances such as missing teeth or fixed prosthetics.

▶ Missing Teeth

If the rubber dam assembly is placed in a quadrant where one or more teeth are missing, the procedure for preparation and placement is adjusted. If the teeth are missing and have not been replaced by a fixed bridge, no holes are punched for those teeth. Missing teeth that have been replaced by fixed bridges change the procedure. Holes are punched for the teeth that are present in the oral cavity, not for the pontic/pontics. The dam material is cut with scissors between the abutment teeth and across the septa of the pontics. The rubber dam assembly is positioned as described. In the area of the pontic the material is pulled under the soldered area to the buccal surface. The two cuts of the dam material are pulled and held together. A needle with suture material or floss is used to sew the pieces together (Fig. 22-28, *A* through *C*). Once the rubber dam material has been sewn and released, it snaps back under the pontic, providing a snug fit. The rest of the placement proceeds as previously described. The removal of the dam material must include the cutting of the floss that rests under the pontic.

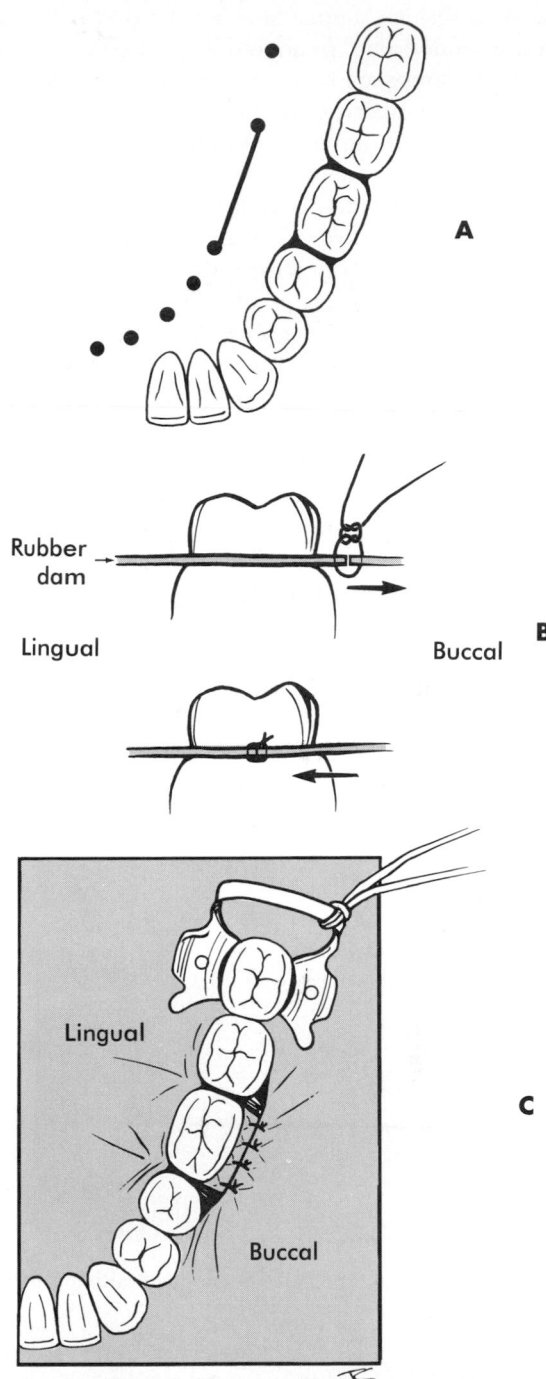

FIG. 22-28 *A,* When the rubber dam is placed over a bridge, a hole is not punched for the pontic, but rather the holes adjacent to the pontic are punched, and a cut is made between those holes to fit the material over the pontic. *B,* The rubber dam is pulled under the pontic to the buccal area, sutured, and allowed to slide back into place. *C,* The sutured rubber dam isolation for the bridge.

Use of an Anterior Clamp

Another variation in rubber dam placement involves the use of anterior clamps. Anterior clamps are commonly used in endodontic treatment and anterior restorations. Anterior clamps are relatively unstable compared to posterior clamps because the points that contact the tooth are not as broad, however, they can become more stable when impression compound is used. The rubber dam material is positioned over the anterior segment of the mouth, from premolar to premolar or possibly from cuspid to cuspid. The operator places a Ferrier #212 clamp on tooth #9. During clamp placement the assistant lights the alcohol torch and begins to heat the end of a stick of impression compound. Dip a finger in a bowl of cold water and mold the compound to a point. The compound is passed to the operator who places it on the clamp bow on both sides and on the incisal edge of the tooth (Fig. 22-29). The material is hardened immediately by forcing water spray from the a/w syringe over the compound.

Once the material hardens it provides stability to the clamp. Some operators may opt to position a clamp on a premolar or molar. For instance, in a case when an anterior clamp might be placed on #8, a premolar clamp is placed on #5 to provide a stable field of work. When the clamp is removed, the compound easily breaks away from the tooth and the clamp.

Other Isolation Materials

Rubber dam isolation is not the only alternative to ensure a clear, dry work area in the oral cavity. Other materials and devices are used for various situations. These include **cotton rolls**, alone or with **cotton roll holders**; **cellulose wafers**; **svedopters**; **hygroformics**, as well as **rubber dam**. Whatever type of isolation is used in a dental office, it is evident that successful isolation can provide a clear operative field for the dental team, reduce stress, and provide patient comfort during many procedures.

Cotton Rolls

The use of cotton rolls as a means of isolation in the oral cavity is common. Cotton rolls are easy to place and remove and require a minimal amount of time to use; however, they, as well as the other types of isolation, do not provide the same level of isolation and protection as rubber dam.

Cotton rolls are precut and preshaped rolls of cotton fibers that are placed in the vestibules and under the tongue to absorb the saliva flow. Cotton rolls vary in length, width, and absorbency. A cotton roll may be placed as a single unit to contain saliva flow, or they may be placed in plastic or metal devices called cotton roll holders or garmers. When the operator works on the maxilla, a single roll of cotton is generally placed near the site that is being treated. The cotton roll holders are only

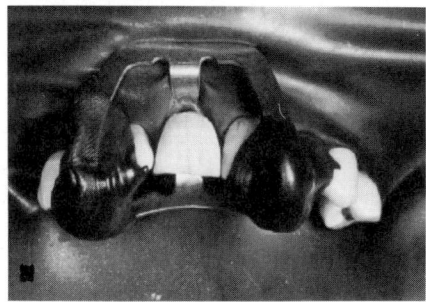

FIG. 22-29   An anterior clamp stabilized with dental compound.

(Sturdevant CM et al: *The art and science of operative dentistry,* ed 2, St Louis 1985, Mosby.)

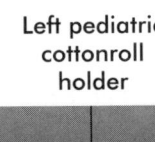

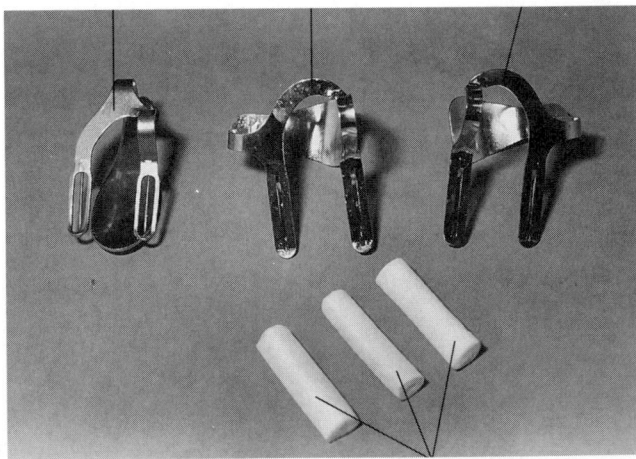

Left pediatric cottonroll holder   Left adult cottonroll holder   Right adult cottonroll holder

Three cotton rolls, two for holder, and one for maxillary parotid area

FIG. 22-30   Pediatric- and adult-sized cotton roll holders.

used on the mandible, for the right or left side of the mouth, and for either pediatric or adult patients (Fig. 22-30). When this holder is used, a cotton roll is placed on the lingual and buccal sides. When the holder is in place, as it is in Fig. 22-31, a *hump*, the curved anterior portion of the holder, goes over the anterior teeth and the clamp of the holder under the chin to secure the placement. An additional cotton roll placed on the maxillary vestibule is often necessary when working on the mandible to restrict saliva flow from the parotid duct that empties into the site.

▶ Cellulose Wafer

Cellulose wafers are triangular pieces of an absorbent, processed layered cotton that is placed in the vestibule near the maxillary arch. Like the cotton roll it is used to absorb saliva that is produced by the parotid gland. When a wafer or cotton roll is used, the cotton must be saturated with fluid before removing it from the mouth. If it is not saturated with fluid, the oral mucosa may be traumatized when the cotton is removed because the cotton may adhere to the oral mucosa (Fig. 22-32).

▶ Svedopters and Hygroformics

Svedopters and hygroformics are devices used to remove fluids from the oral cavity during a procedure. Each has to be immersed in the oral fluids to remove the fluids, and both devices are able to retract the tongue. The hygroformic is less effective for retraction of the tongue than the svedopter. It is made of plastic and is flexible, while the svedopter is made of metal and has blades of various sizes that attach to retract the tongue.

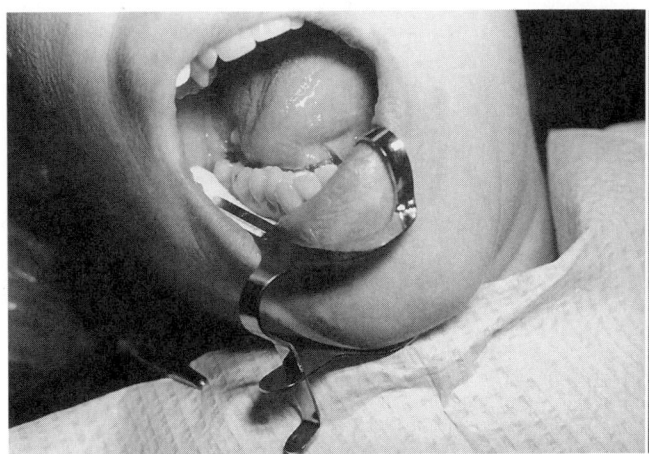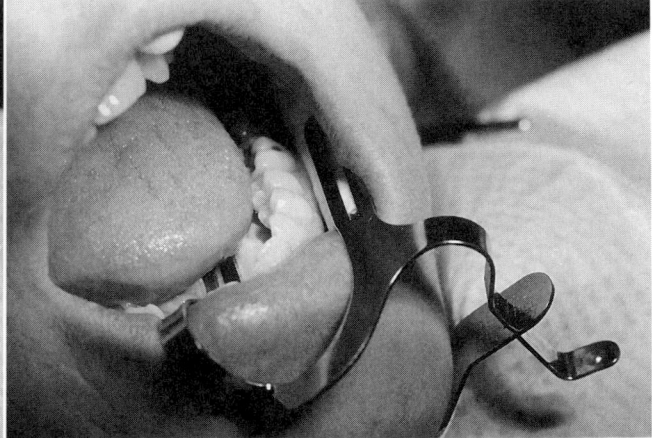

FIG. 22-31   A cotton roll holder positioned in the patient's mouth.

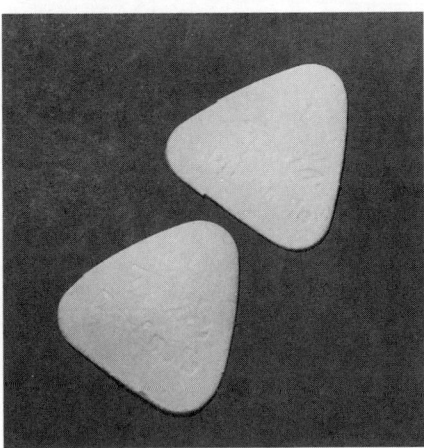

FIG. 22-32   Cellulose wafers used in place of cotton rolls to isolate an area and to absorb fluids.

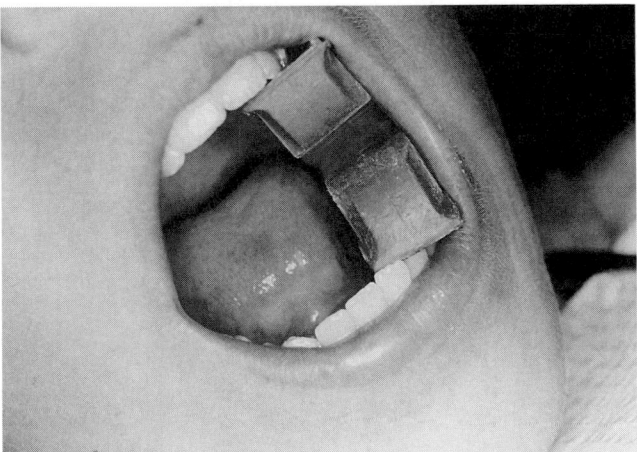

FIG. 22-33   A mouth prop is an auxiliary device used to assist the patient and operating team for access into the oral cavity.

▶ Mouth Prop

Occasionally, a patient may have difficulty keeping the mouth open during dental treatment. A mouth prop positioned in the posterior as illustrated in Fig. 22-33 allows the patient to bite on the device, while not straining to maintain an adequate work area for the operator. Mouth props are sized from small to large and may be disposable or sterilizable.

KEY POINTS

▶ Isolation is used in dentistry to separate a specific tooth or region in the mouth during a treatment procedure.

▶ Isolation can maintain a dry field, retract soft tissue, prevent materials from falling in the mouth, provide infection control, aid in patient management and comfort, as well as promote success of a restoration.

▶ Rubber dam, which is one of the oldest methods of isolation, is most efficiently applied as a four-handed procedure. Rubber dam is the method of isolation that satisfies all of the major objectives.

▶ Other armamentaria that meet some of the objectives include cotton rolls, cellulose wafers, svedopters, and hygroformics.

BIBLIOGRAPHY

Barton RE, Matteson SR, Richardson RE: *The dental assistant*, ed 6, Philadelphia, 1988, Lea & Febiger.

Schwarzrock SP, Jensen JR: *Effective dental assisting*, ed 6, Dubuque, Iowa, 1982, WC Brown.

Siwinski J: *Hygenic dental dam procedures manual*, ed 4, Akron, Ohio, 1984, Hygenic.

23 Topical and Local Anesthesia

LEARNING OBJECTIVES

You will have mastered the material in this chapter when you can:

▶ Define the key terms

▶ Describe the purpose of anesthesia

▶ Explain the different types of topical and local anesthesias and indications for use

▶ Describe the types of anesthesia and their application in dentistry

▶ Explain the components of local anesthesia and the effect of each on the human body

▶ Identify the parts of a local anesthetic carpule/cartridge, needle, and syringe

▶ Describe the procedure for assembly and disassembly of the anesthetic syringe

▶ Identify types of syringes used in dentistry

▶ Explain the technique for syringe transfer

▶ Explain the accepted safety guidelines regarding the use of sharps

KEY TERMS

Amide
ASA Physical Status Class
   System
Infiltration
Local anesthesia
Lumen

KEY TERMS—cont'd

Carpule
Cartridge
Conscious sedation
Contraindication
Ester
Field block
General anesthesia

Nerve block
Nitrous oxide
Pain
Paresthesia
Periodontal ligament injection
Topical anesthesia

Principles of Pain Control

All dental professionals would like to believe that dentistry is completely painless; however, some patients are likely to tell a different story. The practice of dentistry can be an invasive process, and dental pain may result from a procedure. The dentist is responsible for providing the patient with comfortable dental treatment, which usually indicates the use of some form of anesthesia.

The International Association for the Study of Pain defines **pain** as "the sensory and emotional experience associated with actual or potential tissue damage." Pain can be a perception of uncomfortable stimuli and the response to that perception. It is estimated that 50% of individuals who seek some form of medical care do so as a direct result of experiencing pain. Pain can be acute or chronic and can be treated with a form of analgesic that is discussed in Chapter 10.

The sensation of pain occurs when pain receptors, or nerve endings that warn of harmful changes in the body's environment, such as a rise in blood pressure or temperature, transmit impulses to the central nervous system (CNS). The CNS interprets the signal and produces the perception of pain. Anesthesia eliminates the pain experience by interrupting the transmitted impulse. Anesthesia is "the absence of normal sensation, especially sensitivity to pain." The goals in the relief of pain and anxiety are to control patient actions, to maintain vital signs, and to create a positive memory of dental care.

Anesthesia is administered by several methods, depending on the level of pain or anxiety relief that is sought for the patient. In dentistry, anesthesia is provided in the following forms from the least invasive to the most invasive:

- Topical anesthesia—an application of a substance to the tissues that creates loss of feeling on the surface
- Local anesthesia—placement of a substance by injection at a site that creates a loss of sensation to one part of the body
- Conscious sedation—anesthetic agent used to produce a sedative effect while the patient remains conscious
- Inhalation anesthesia—an anesthesia produced by the respiration of an anesthetic agent without loss of consciousness
- General anesthesia—an anesthetic agent that creates a state of unconsciousness with absence of sensation over the entire body

This chapter will concentrate on topical and local anesthesia, while Chapter 34, *Oral Surgery,* will examine the other forms of anesthesia and the application of conscious sedation and general anesthesia. Chapter 10 discusses the types of drugs used in achieving certain types of anesthesia and analgesia.

> Evidence exists that the Inca civilization used resin from a particular tree to treat gingival disease. They heated the plant root, and, when it was hot enough to glow, they placed it on the gingival tissue on both sides of the tooth and let it cool. Essentially the tissue was burned away, and new tissue was regenerated. Anesthesia or relief from pain for this procedure was provided by having the patient chew on leaves from a coca bush.

Anesthesia can range from a localized tissue numbness to complete sedation. The indicators for the selection of relief for a patient are as follows:

- Anxiety or fear
- Medical history
- Physical inability to receive dental treatment
  Gagging
  Pain threshold
  Inability to sit for long periods of time
- The level of invasive procedure to be performed

Dental treatment can be provided comfortably for a patient with the use of topical, local anesthesia, and/or conscious sedation nitrous oxide. In some instances, dental care requires the use of general anesthesia. These situations are not common in general dentistry and require an individual who has at least one year of specialized training to administer general anesthesia. For this reason, more practitioners use conscious sedation as an alternative to general anesthesia.

Local Anesthesia

Local anesthesia is the direct administration of an anesthetic agent to tissues—particularly oral mucosa—to block the sensation of pain. The reduction in neural sensation achieves the desired effects of a local anesthesia and reduces or eliminates pain. Two ways to administer local anesthesia are by topical application or by injections in tissues. Local anesthesia is also referred to as regional anesthesia, depending on the types of nerves that are affected by the anesthetic. Placement of anesthesia on the nerve endings disrupts the sensation of pain that results during the cutting of living tissues in the course of dental treatment. Local anesthesias are used to anesthetize tissues and structures in the oral cavity. Various types of common local anesthetics, dosages, and contraindications are found in Table 23-1.

Topical Anesthesia

The simplest of local anesthetics is **topical anesthesia**, which provides a surface analgesia by the application of a substance. Several forms of topical anesthesia are applied by using a cotton-tipped or another type of applicator. The liquid form, or spray, is applied to the oral tissues in a metered dose of 10 mg. Fig. 23-1 shows examples of some of the topical anesthetics available.

Application of topical anesthesia is a procedure that may not be performed in every office. In some states,

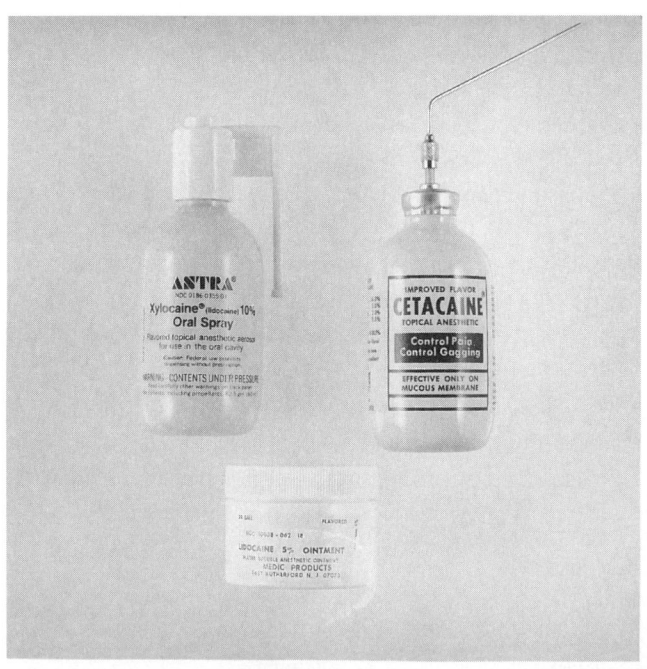

FIG. 23-1   Various types of topical anesthesia.

TABLE 23-1 PHARMACOLOGY OF DENTAL ANESTHESIA/ANALGESIA

Substance	Chemical composition	Primary function	Common dosages	Brand names	Duration (min.)	Contraindications	Hazards
Mepivacaine	d, 1-N-methyl-pipecolic Acid-2,6, dimethylanilide	Local anesthesia	1:20,000	Carbocaine with Neo-Cobefrin	100	Pts. with history of malignant hyperpyrexia Heart patients	Biting of oral tissues
Lidocaine	Diethyl 1 to 2, 6 dimethylacetanilid	Local anesthesia	1:50,00 1:100,00	Xylocaine Octocaine	100	Same as above	Same as above
Benzocaine	Ethyl aminbenzoate	Topical anesthesia	As indicated	Hurricaine	15 to 30		Localized irritation; allergic reaction
Nitrous oxide		Conscious sedation	35% to 40%		10 to 15 after delivery	Pregnancy (for repeated exposure) Pt. with mental or physical inability to communicate Pt. with respiratory problems	50% administration may cause general anesthesia
Barbiturate	Malonylurea	Conscious sedation, primary CNS depressant	50 to 100 mg	Nembutal	2-4 hrs. IV	Pts. with cardiovascular, renal, hepatic system impairment	Respiratory depression resulting in death
Narcotic	Opiate	Conscious sedation, primary CNS depressant	8 to 16 mg	Morphine		No operating motor vehicles, tools or ingesting alcohol and drugs	Bradycardia

This chart is a sampling of available anesthesia agents. It is not all inclusive for use, contraindications, or potential hazards. It is the dentist's responsibility to know the pharmacology of these and any other drugs that a patient may take.

placement of topical anesthesia is a legally delegated responsibility of the dental assistant and/or hygienist. Topical anesthesia is placed on mucosal tissues and acts on the particular nerve endings that are located there to relieve the sensation of pain and to reduce the possibility of psychogenic response. This procedure is associated with the dental injection that often causes discomfort for the patient. Many patients claim that they would not mind going to the dentist if they did not have to have an injection. Topical anesthetic that is placed on the oral mucosa before the injection helps to relieve discomfort. Topical anesthesia is also placed on the oral tissues to relieve the gag reflex before impressions and radiographs are taken.

ADMINISTRATION

The assistant prepares the anesthesia as indicated on a cotton-tipped applicator and sets the material aside on the tray setup. The mucosal tissues at the site of the injection are dried with a 2 × 2 gauze. The topical anesthesia is applied and left at the injection site for 60 to 90 seconds. When surface anesthesia of the mucosal tissues has been achieved, the dental injection is given.

DRUG REACTIONS

Topical anesthesia application may result in an adverse drug reaction. Two types of reactions have been observed: (1) an allergic reaction to certain ingredients of the anesthesia that presents as erythema—a diffused redness of the tissues—or as angioedema—a swelling of the mucous membranes; and (2) an overdose reaction that is caused by the quick absorption of the anesthesia through the mucous membranes, which eventually results in an increase in local anesthesia blood level.

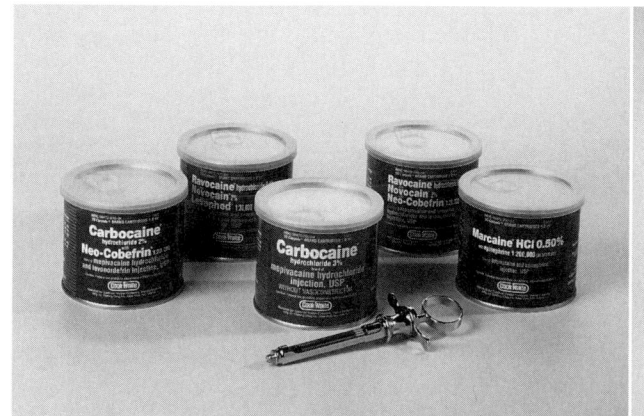

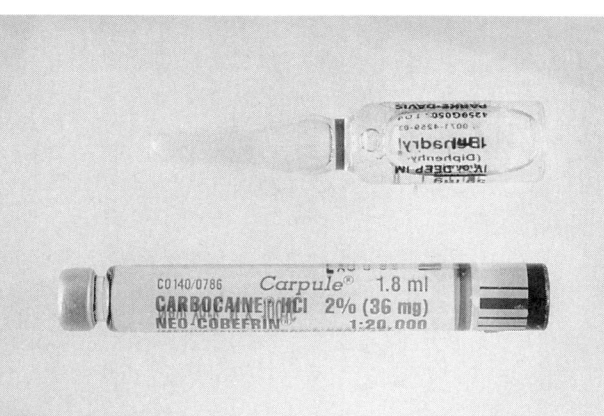

FIG. 23-2   *A through C,* Injectable local anesthetics in carpule/cartridge and ampule form.
(Courtesy of Eastman Kodak, Inc., Rochester, New York.)

▶ Injectable Anesthetics

Local **injectable anesthetics** used in dental care are either **amides** or **esters**, which are types of compound chemicals that are used in anesthesia. Common accepted amides are lidocaine, mepivacaine, and prilocaine; esters are procaine, tetracaine, and propoxycaine. If a sensitivity to a drug of one group exists, the other can be substituted. Of these local anesthetics, lidocaine is usually the most accepted for use in dental treatment.

ADMINISTRATION

The local anesthetics are available in liquid form in premeasured carpules, or cartridges, and in ampules as illustrated in Fig. 23-2, *A* through *C*. The form selected depends on the operator's choice; however, in general dentistry the carpule or cartridge form is the one most commonly used.

Any of the local anesthetics may contain a vasoconstrictor, which constricts blood flow at the site of injection. The benefits of a vasoconstrictor are that it increases the duration of the anesthetic in the injection site and that it lowers the systemic toxicity of the drugs by slowing the absorption of anesthetic into the cardiovascular system.

DRUG REACTIONS

Vasoconstricting anesthetics have also been found to cause overdose reactions, as do the topical anesthetics. An increased blood level of vasoconstrictors may result in systemic reactions, such as seizure activity or central nervous system depression, and extreme levels of vasoconstrictors may negatively affect the cardiovascular system.

Common vasoconstrictors used in dentistry are Neo-Cobefrin and epinephrine, in a concentration of 1 part vasoconstrictor to 50,000 parts of anesthesia solution (1:50,000) or as 1:100,000 or 1:200,000. By constricting the blood vessels at the site of injection, the duration of anesthesia is increased by the delayed absorption of the solution in the tissues. A vasoconstrictor also decreases the amount of blood in the injection site. The use of a vasoconstrictor increases pain control, which often coincides with the elimination of an exaggerated stress response. Pain causes stress in the body, which in turn causes a release of catecholamines, epinephrine or norepinephrine, in the cardiovascular system. At most levels of release little effect on cardiac output is observed from the release of catecholamines.

The American Society of Anesthesiologists adopted a standard for referencing the physical classification of patients known as the **ASA Physical Status Classification System**. This classification provides the operator with a benchmark of categorizing patient medical risk. Initially, the classification was designed to be used with patients receiving general anesthesia; however, it also has been used for all patients undergoing surgery.

If the ASA rating shown in Box 23-1 is used, the patient who is contraindicated for dental treatment, such as those with an ASA IV rating, would be the least likely candidate for use of a vasoconstrictor. However, because of the known natural interaction of catecholamines without adverse reactions, most patients can receive an injection of a vasoconstrictor for normal dental treatment.

If the use of epinephrine is contraindicated, the drug of choice would then be a local anesthesia without a vasoconstrictor. The use of a nonvasoconstrictor anesthetic would result in reduced duration of the anesthetic and increased bleeding. When anesthesia is used, a complete and updated health history is crucial. Complications resulting from the use of any drug with a patient is an experience that no dental professional wants to encounter. The checking and rechecking of the health questionnaire before the preparation of dental anesthesia is a necessity.

BOX 23-1

ASA PHYSICAL STATUS CLASSIFICATION SYSTEM

ASA I — Patient without systemic disease
ASA II — Patient with mild systemic disease
ASA III — Patient with severe systemic disease, limiting activity
ASA IV — Patient with incapacitating systemic disease that is a threat to life
ASA V — Patient not expected to survive 24 hours with or without surgery
ASA E — Emergency operation, the E precedes the number to designate status

Types of Injections

Three common forms of injections are performed in dentistry—**infiltration**, **field block**, and **nerve block**. A less common form would be the **periodontal ligament injection** or intraligamentary injection.

▶ Infiltration Anesthesia

An **infiltration** injection of anesthesia is the process of depositing anesthesia solution into tissues, allowing time for the absorption of the solution by the many terminal nerve endings at the site. The terminal nerve endings absorb the solution, thereby suppressing the pain impulse. This type of anesthesia is usually used when a single tooth is designated for treatment or when a biopsy, gingivectomy, or other tissue surgery is planned.

▶ Field Block Anesthesia

Infiltration and field block anesthesia are sometimes considered interchangeable. **Field block** anesthesia consists of the deposit of anesthetic solution near a major terminal nerve. This usually involves the deposit of anesthetic solution at the apex of a tooth. The apex is completely encircled with anesthesia. This anesthetizes the major terminal nerve branch or smaller terminal nerve endings that transmit the sensation of pain to the brain.

▶ Nerve Block Anesthesia

Nerve block anesthesia is most commonly used in the mandibular arch, with the deposit of anesthetic solution near the inferior alveolar nerve. The innervation, or stimulation of a part through the action of nerves, allows the blockage to prevent the transmission of pain or sensory signals to the central nervous system. During innervation, the tongue, lip, cheek, gingiva, and teeth are anesthetized. After the pain signal to the brain is blocked, dental treatment can be performed without discomfort to the patient (Fig. 23-3, *A* through *C*).

Nerve block anesthesia is the only effective local anesthesia in the mandibular arch. The density of the bone in the mandibular posterior teeth does not allow penetration of the solution to the terminal nerve branches and the apices. Occasionally, the field block technique is used on the mandibular anterior teeth or even premolar areas of some patients depending on the anatomic structures of the patient. A field block would provide the necessary level of anesthesia without involving adjacent structures that would be anesthetized during a nerve block.

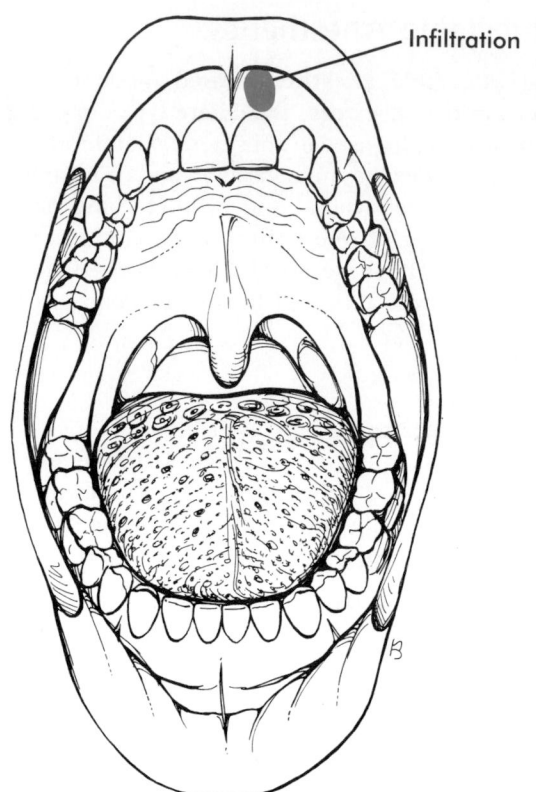

FIG. 23-3   Common examples of anesthesia injections. *A*, Infiltration.

▶ Intraligamentary Injection (Periodontal Ligament Injection)

The **periodontal ligament** technique of local anesthesia involves the injection of anesthetic solution under pressure into the periodontal membrane of a specific tooth. The procedure is a type of infiltration technique and an aspirating syringe or a periodontal ligament syringe is available for this technique (Fig. 23-4).

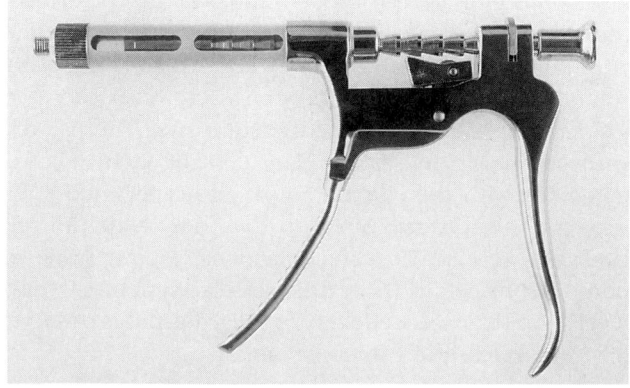

FIG. 23-4   Intraligament injection syringe used for anesthetizing periodontal ligaments.

(Courtesy of Miltex.)

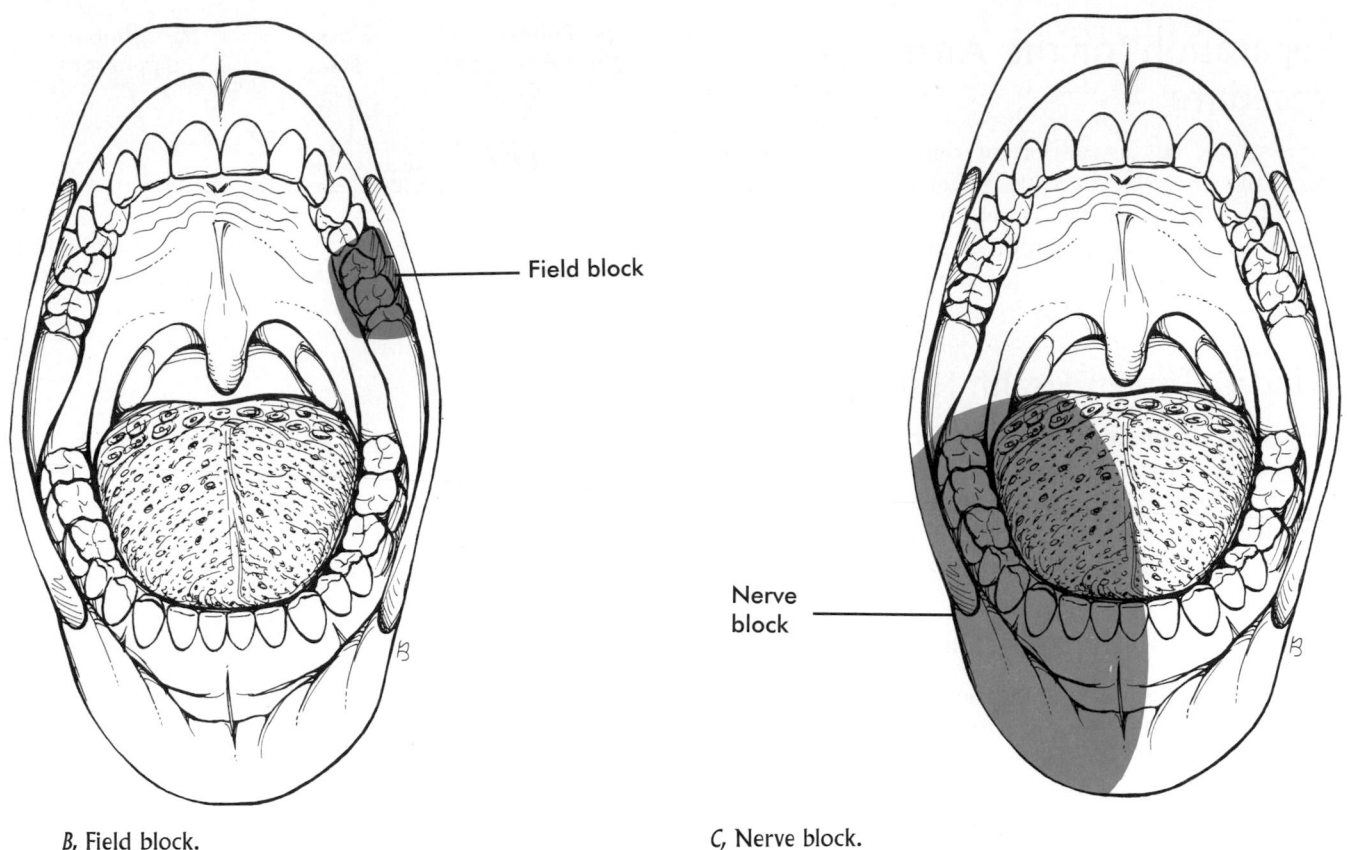

B, Field block.

C, Nerve block.

Special Concerns for the Administration of Local Anesthetic

The concerns that are present when a vasoconstrictor is used with certain patients has already been mentioned. The injection of a vasoconstrictor into a blood vessel is of equal concern during a dental procedure. The injection of local anesthesia into a blood vessel can result in complications in vital organs, particularly the heart.

DURATION

The injection of anesthetic solution produces a lack of sensation, the desired effect under which to perform dental treatment. But the patient must be cautioned about the duration of the anesthesia and about the possibility of injuring themselves during this time by biting the tongue, lip, and cheek; once the anesthetic effect subsides, the pain will return. When a child is treated, the parents or caregiver must be informed of this situation.

TOXICITY

Toxicity—the degree to which an anesthetic solution can be poisonous—is a concern when working with dental anesthetics. Even though the types of anesthesia used in dentistry have a positive record, complications need to be noted on the patient's medical history with respect to toxic reaction or to the symptoms that result from the use of an anesthetic solution. The toxic reaction is related to the amount of drug in the blood that affects the central nervous system, the respiratory system, or the circulatory system. The reaction to toxicity depends on a number of factors, including the following:

- The compound of the solution used
- The amount of solution used
- Rate of injection
- Rate of absorption of the solution
- Age of patient
- Physical characteristics of patient

Another complication that can result from an injection of local anesthetic is **paresthesia**, the sensation of numbness that is experienced after the effect of the anesthesia is exhausted. Paresthesia is usually caused by trauma to nerve tissues, hemorrhage near the nerve sheath, or contamination of the anesthetic solution. The paresthesia usually resolves itself within 6 to 8 weeks after the onset, but damage can be permanent.

Preparation for the Anesthetic Procedure

The assistant has an important role when he or she selects the prescribed anesthetic agent and the needle, assembles the anesthetic syringe, and assists during transfer and administration of the anesthesia. Before the anesthesia is administered, the patient's health history is examined.

▶ Update Patient Health History

The patient is required to complete or update a medical history record before beginning any treatment. The dental assistant and the operator are responsible for checking the patient's record for health conditions that would warrant the use of a nonvasoconstrictor anesthesia.

▶ Selection of the Anesthesia Carpule

In the following discussion the patient is to have treatment on tooth #28. The patient has no **contraindications** (reasons to prohibit the use of a drug) that alert the assistant to use a nonvasoconstrictor anesthetic. The assistant is directed to select 2% lidocaine **carpules** or **cartridges**, glass containers that hold anesthetic solution, as the anesthetic agent. Fig. 23-5 illustrates the contents of an anesthesia carpule, with which the assistant should be familiar. The contents of anesthetic solution is printed on each vial.

The assistant removes the carpule from the container and checks the type of anesthesia, the concentration, and the expiration date. The carpule should also be examined to determine if it is safe to use.

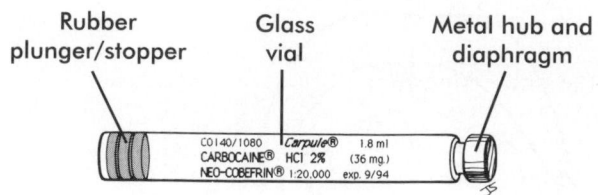

FIG. 23-5   Common parts of an anesthetic carpule, including the metal hub, the diaphragm, the glass vial, and the plunger or rubber stopper.

If any the situations just mentioned are evident, the carpule should be discarded and another carpule selected. The anesthetic carpule has the following main components (Fig. 23-5):

▶ Metal hub with a rubber diaphragm into which the hub end of a needle is inserted
▶ Center rubber stopper or plunger that is penetrated by the harpoon of the syringe
▶ Glass vial, which houses the anesthetic solution

The rubber stopper has been color coded in the past, but recently manufacturers have replaced the color-coded stoppers with color-coded bands for identification purposes. Some operators prefer to have the anesthesia carpule or cartridge warmed before use. This can be accomplished by placing the carpule or cartridge in a heating device before it is assembled with the syringe.

▶ Selection of the Anesthetic Needle

Many designs of anesthetic syringes and injection needles are available in dentistry. Today, however, the most important consideration is in selecting a needle that is disposable and then disposing of the needle in a *safe* manner. The majority of injection needles that are available are supplied in sterilized package form.

Needles are supplied in two lengths 1 inch and 1⅝ inches, and the selection of the needle depends on the operator's choice and the area that is to be anesthetized. Generally, a long needle, 1⅝ inches, is selected for use

---

INSPECTION OF ANESTHETIC CARPULES

▶ Is the diaphragm or rubber plunger free of cracks or tears?
▶ Is the solution clear and free of discoloration?
▶ Are there cracks in the glass container?
▶ Is the carpule completely filled with solution?
▶ Is the type of solution selected appropriate anesthesia based on the patient's medical history?
▶ Are there any air bubbles in the carpule?
▶ Has the expiration date lapsed?
▶ Have you rechecked the type of anesthetic to be used with this specific patient?

BOX 23-2

BENEFITS OF DISPOSABLE NEEDLES

▶ The presterilized needle is used only once for patient safety.
▶ The risk of needle punctures during a sterilization procedure is eliminated with disposal of the needle.
▶ Since the needle is for a single-use injection, it is always sharp.

during a nerve block or for the mandibular injection. The longer needle allows the operator to gain access to the site of injection. During an infiltration or field block the choice is usually a short needle: 1 inch (Fig. 23-6, *A* and *B*). An exception to this rule could be the selection of a needle for the maxillary premolar, cuspid, or incisor area. In this situation the operator may opt to select a long needle in order to access the infraorbital nerve.

Another factor to be considered during needle selection is the diameter or gauge of the needle. The smaller the diameter of the needle, the larger the gauge number. Likewise, the larger the diameter of the needle, the smaller the gauge number. The normal range of needle gauge used in dentistry is 25 gauge to 30 gauge. The 30-gauge needle is smaller in diameter than the 25-gauge needle, as shown in Fig. 23-7.

A smaller gauge needle is often used in the infiltration and field block methods of injection, so a selection might be a 30-gauge, 1-inch needle. A needle selection for a nerve block, which requires a stronger and often longer needle, might be a 25- or 27-gauge, 1⅝-inch needle. An operator may select any combination of needle lengths and gauges, and it is the assistant's responsibility to be aware of the operator's preference when the anesthetic syringe is prepared. The assistant always consults with the operator to determine the specific needle and anesthesia to use.

PARTS OF THE DISPOSABLE ANESTHETIC NEEDLE

The most common type of disposable anesthetic needle is manufactured with a plastic sheath cover that serves as a protective shield. One section of the protective cover is clear and the other may or may not be color coded to coordinate with the gauge of the syringe. The longer needle is obvious when a 1-inch and a 1⅝-inch needle are compared. The clear cover protects the hub end of the needle, which attaches to the hub of the syringe. The other protective section of plastic covers the injection end of the needle. The needle itself has a hollow center called a **lumen**, which terminates in a beveled end. The lumen allows the anesthetic solution to pass from the carpule/cartridge into the patient's tissue.

▶ The Anesthetic Syringe

In some offices the anesthetic syringe is packaged in a bag for sterilization. Other items used during local anesthetic administration may be included in the package. Examples of these items are: cotton-tipped applicators, 2 × 2 gauze sponges, and paper towels.

The most common form of syringe found in dentistry today is the metal or nonmetal aspirating syringe. The aspirating syringe provides the operator with several advantages: (1) the ability to aspirate, which allows the plunger of the syringe to be pulled back to determine where the needle has been positioned in the tissue; if it has been placed in a blood vessel, blood will be aspirated or drawn back into the carpule, and the operator can withdraw and reposition the needle; and (2) the needle and carpule used with this style of syringe can be discarded.

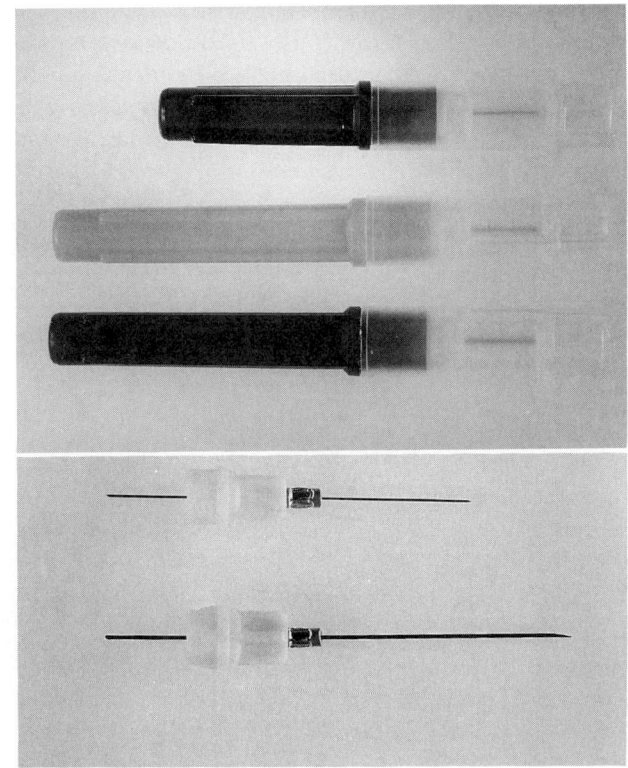

FIG. 23-6   *A,* Anesthetic needles, with protective cover. *B,* Needles without protective covers to illustrate differences in the 1 inch and 1 ⅝-inch length

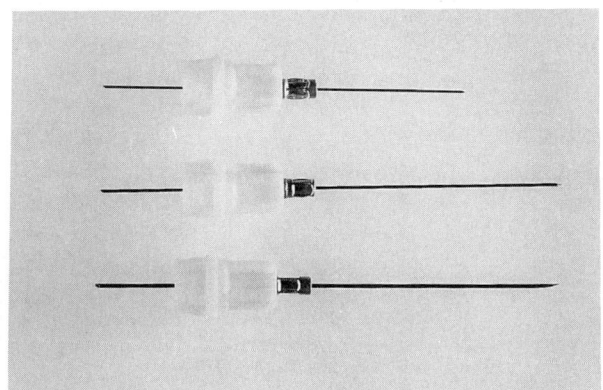

FIG. 23-7   Examples of 30g, 27g, and 25g needle diameters.

THE PARTS OF THE ASPIRATING SYRINGE

Thumb Ring. The circular ring is found at the top of the syringe and allows the operator to apply force during the injection and to aspirate. This ring can become loosened, and care should be taken to ensure that the thumb ring is attached securely to the plunger.

Finger Grip and Bar. The fingers that are not in the thumb ring are positioned on the finger grip and bar to provide the operator with stability during the injection.

Piston or Plunger. The rod that is attached to the thumb ring provides the force to the plunger of the carpule/cartridge that in turn forces the anesthetic solution into the needle.

Harpoon. The triangular end of the piston/plunger, the harpoon, engages the carpule plunger by penetrating the rubber and setting itself in the plunger. The harpoon is set in the carpule plunger to enable the operator to aspirate with the syringe; the harpoon allows the thumb ring and piston to be pulled back with the carpule plunger attached.

Syringe barrel. The body of the syringe holds the anesthetic carpule or cartridge in place. If the syringe has an opening on the side, it is considered a breech-loading syringe. The plunger and harpoon of the syringe are located in the center of the barrel.

Hub end of syringe. A metal threaded end rests at the end of the syringe. It is secured to the syringe by a threaded area, and the outer tip is threaded to attach the anesthetic needle to it. Take care to ensure that the hub is securely threaded and flush with the barrel, thereby avoiding any leakage of anesthetic solution during the injection (Fig. 23-8, *A* and *B*).

Other types of anesthetic syringes include the nonaspirating and the Luer-Lok forms. The type of anesthetic syringe used in dentistry depends on the procedure and on the operator's preference. The Luer-Lok style of syringe, for example, is often used in oral surgery offices to draw medications from ampules.

BOX 23-3

ANESTHETIC SELECTION CHECKPOINTS

Checkpoint #1 — When patient record is examined
Checkpoint #2 — When the anesthetic solution is examined
Checkpoint #3 — Before assembly of the syringe

Assembly of the Anesthetic Syringe

Before the syringe is assembled, the materials that are selected, the needle and the anesthetic carpule, should be checked for correctness. The anesthetic should be checked three times before it is used: when the patient record is examined, when the solution is selected, and when the syringe is assembled.

The sterilized syringe and hub are checked to see if the fit is snug against the barrel of the syringe. The hub can become loose when a previously used needle has been removed. The plunger is also checked to ensure smooth movement inside the barrel, to avert difficulty during the injection when the solution passes from the carpule into the patient's tissue. The thumb ring should also be securely attached to the plunger, since it is a threaded end and can become loosened.

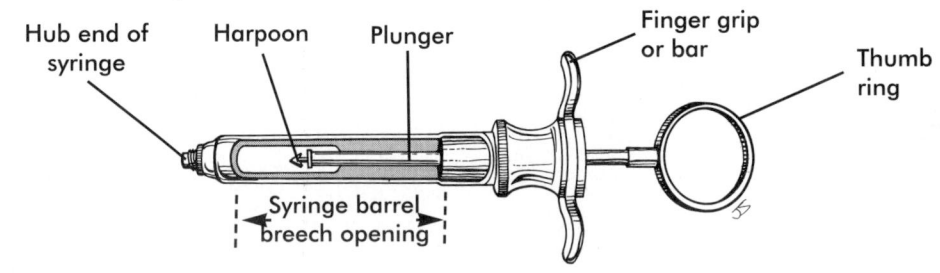

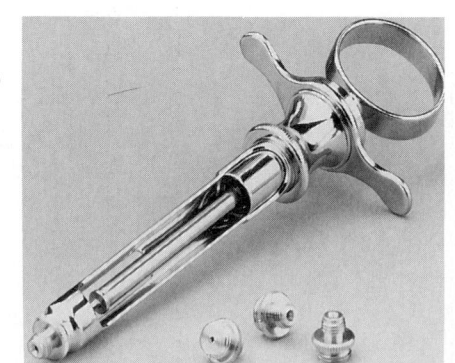

FIG. 23-8 *A* and *B*, Parts of the aspirating anesthetic syringe include the thumb ring, finger grip or bar, plunger, harpoon, barrel, and hub.

ASSEMBLYING THE ANESTHETIC SYRINGE

STEP A

1. Pick up the injection needle, and break away the clear protective cover, taking care not to touch the needle.
2. To avoid contamination of the needle, *do not remove the opposing protective cover* until the operator is ready to administer the anesthesia.
3. Hold the needle end protective cover, and carefully feed the hub end of the needle on a parallel plane into the hub end of the syringe (Fig. 23-9).
4. Do not screw the needle on at an angle, but continue to keep the hub ends parallel to each other as you twist the needle into place creating threads in the plastic needle hub. A plastic hub needle that is threaded at an angle will not have a snug fit between the two hubs, resulting in leakage of the anesthetic solution during injection (Fig. 23-10, *A* through *C*).
5. If the needle hub is metal, thread it onto the needle with the existing threads.
6. Loosen the protective cover of the injection end of the needle, but do *not* remove it. (The plastic of the sheath will sometimes be tightly fused to the hub of the needle; to loosen it now avoids the need to do so during syringe transfer.)

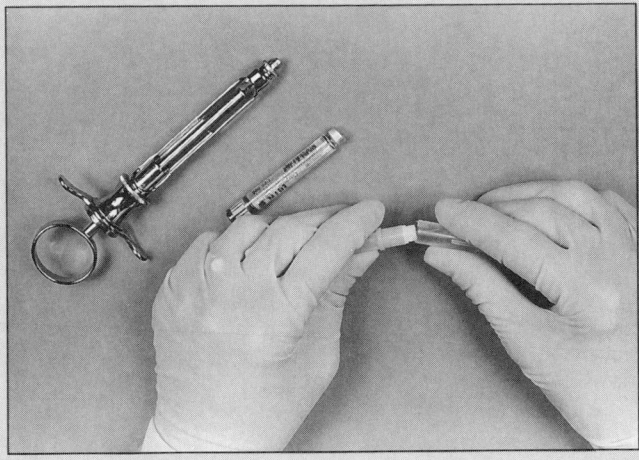

FIG. 23-9   The protective cover for the syringe's needle is removed and fed into the hub end of the syringe.

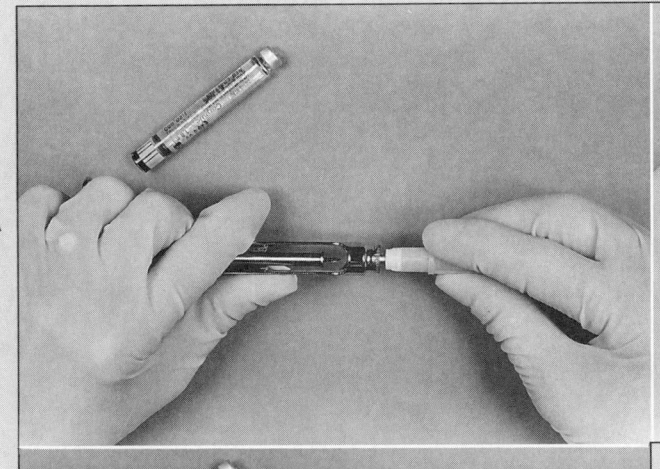

A

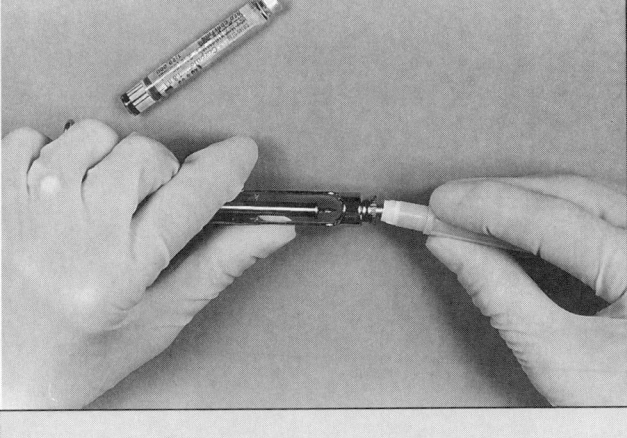

B

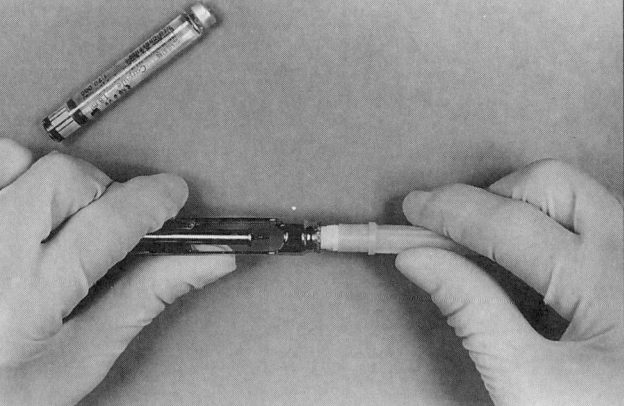

C

FIG. 23-10   The anesthetic needle is attached. *A*, Correctly positioned needle. *B*, Incorrectly positioned needle. *C*, The final position of the needle is securely in place.

Continued.

ASSEMBLYING THE ANESTHETIC SYRINGE—cont'd.

7. Always leave the cover that is on the injection end of the needle in place until you place the syringe into the operator's hand. This step may also be completed after the carpule is positioned (Fig. 23-11).

8. After the needle is placed, check to see that the hub end of the needle is visible through the syringe's hub end or breech opening to ensure that the anesthetic solution can flow through the needle. If you cannot see the hub end of the needle, it may have bent during placement; if this occurs, the assistant removes and discards the needle and replaces it with another needle. If the assistant does not check to be sure the needle is through the hub, the

anesthetic solution cannot flow through the needle because there is no opening.

STEP B

1. Position a hand on the thumb ring area of the syringe, and pull back on the piston/plunger of the syringe to increase the opening of the breech area (Fig. 23-12). If you try to position the carpule in the breech-loading area of the syringe without pulling back on the plunger, the carpule will not fit into the barrel (Fig. 23-13, *A* and *B*).

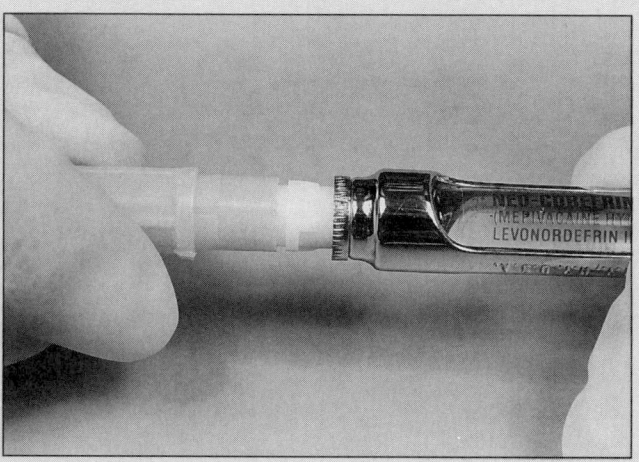

FIG. 23-11   Loosened protective cover without removal from the needle.

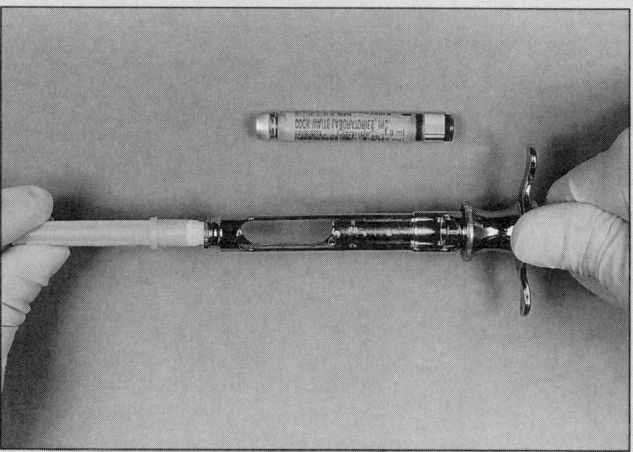

FIG. 23-12   The assistant pulls back on the plunger of the syringe, increasing the size of the breech opening.

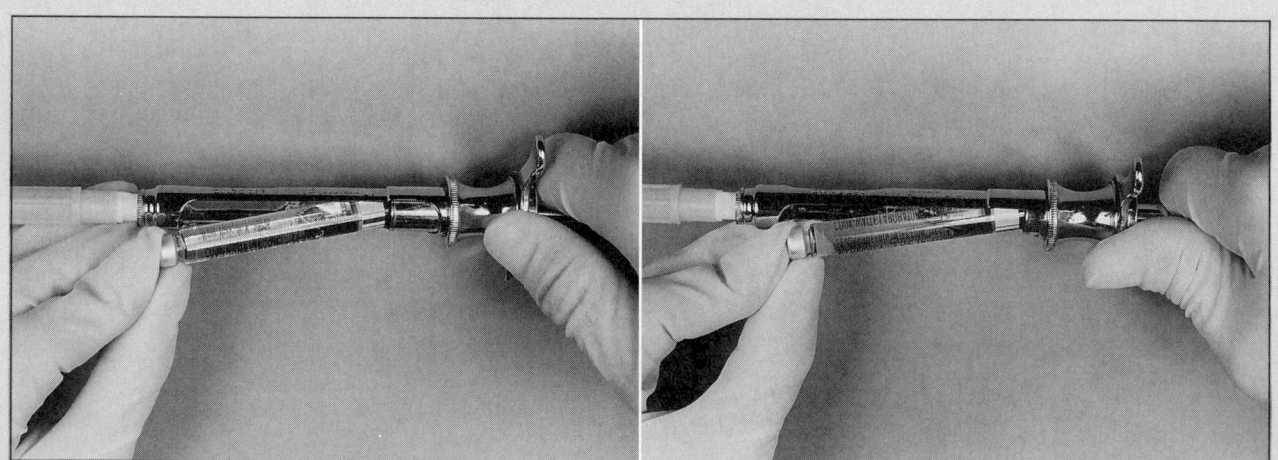

FIG. 23-13   *A,* Positioning the carpule without enlarging the breech opening does not allow the carpule to be placed. *B,* The opened breech allows for the proper carpule placement. The carpule is forced into the hub end of the needle as the spring action plunger is released. This allows penetration of the hub end of the needle into the diaphragm first, and then contact is made with the harpoon.

2. Hold the syringe, which has a spring action in the finger grip area, and force the breech opening to enlarge it, allowing for the placement of the carpule.

STEP C

1. Place the preselected anesthetic carpule in the breech side of the syringe so that the metal diaphragm of the carpule is near the needle and the plunger end of the carpule is near the harpoon of the syringe.
2. Carefully load the carpule into the breech opening and release the plunger allowing force on the carpule, as it is pushed into the needle. This action engages the needle into the carpule.

STEP D

1. Cup a hand around the breech of the syringe, and firmly rap the opposing hand against the thumb ring to engage the harpoon in the carpule (Fig. 23-14). The harpoon of the syringe is firmly set in the plunger of the carpule.
2. To ensure that the harpoon and the carpule plunger are engaged, hold the assembled syringe in a vertical position and place a slight forward pressure on the thumb ring. Initially the plunger in the carpule will move forward, forcing a small amount of anesthesia from the carpule.
3. With the thumb in the thumb ring, draw back on the plunger to create an aspirating action. If the harpoon is properly engaged in the rubber plunger, the needle will draw air bubbles into the carpule.
4. Remove the air bubbles by keeping the syringe in a vertical position, and force the air bubbles out by slightly pressing on the thumb ring until all bubbles are expressed (Fig. 23-15). If bubbles do not develop in the carpule, the harpoon is not engaged completely, and the procedure must be repeated.
5. The anesthetic syringe is prepared for the anesthetic procedure.

6. Place the syringe on the tray setup or on a separate tray. Cover the syringe to prevent the patient's seeing the device.

NOTE: Should the exposed needle end touch anything at any time before the actual injection, the needle and anesthetic carpule must be replaced.

STEP E

1. Prepare the topical anesthetic before the injection, if it is used by the operator.
2. When the gel, paste, or cream form of topical anesthetic is used, dip a cotton-tipped applicator into the anesthetic and place it with the anesthetic setup to be used shortly. The dipped applicator can also be placed in the clear protective sheath of the syringe end of the needle to avoid smearing topical anesthetic on other surfaces.
3. If spray anesthetic is used, it is positioned on the mobile cart and ready for application. Some operators may opt not to use any topical anesthetic.

ALTERNATIVE METHOD OF PREPARATION

It is possible to assemble the anesthetic syringe through a variation in the above mentioned steps. The following is the sequence of assembly:

1. Place the carpule in breech-loading area as described through the extension of the opening.
2. Engage the harpoon into the rubber plunger of the carpule using firm hand pressure only.
3. Screw the needle into the hub of the syringe as described and continue with the rest of the sequence as previously mentioned.

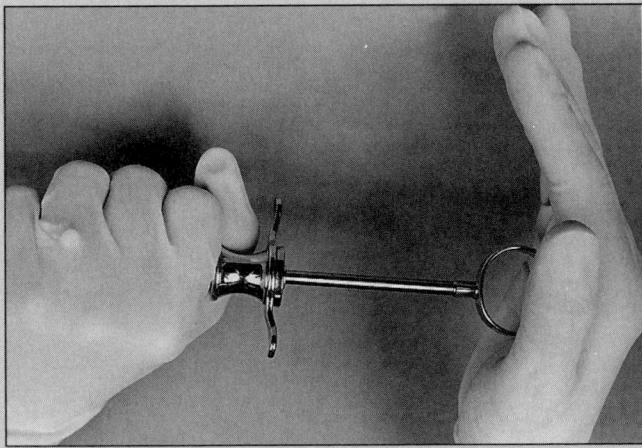

FIG. 23-14 **The assistant cups one hand around the breech area of the syringe and firmly raps the thumb ring with the palm of the opposite hand.**

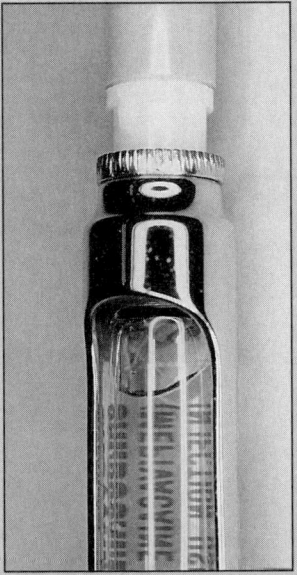

FIG. 23-15 **Place the syringe vertically, forcing the air bubble to the needle end of the carpule, and place force on the thumb ring, pushing the air bubble through the needle.**

CRITERIA FOR ANESTHETIC SYRINGE PREPARATION

- Select correct anesthesia for individual patient.
- Select correct needle length for treatment area.
- Check carpule for expiration date and for lack of bubbles.
- Secure syringe hub.
- Secure thumb ring.
- Check plunger to ensure free movement.
- Place needle securely.
- Insert carpule in correct position.
- Engage harpoon for aspiration.
- Loosen needle cover slightly.
- Turn breech side of syringe toward operator's vision.
- Do not

  Remove the protective cap before transfer

  Incorporate bubbles in carpule

  Use a two-handed recapping

  Express excess solution into protective cover

  Puncture protective cover when needle has been bent

  Unscrew the syringe hub when removing the needle

Hidden Syringe Transfer Technique

The *hidden syringe technique* is an accepted method of instrument transfer during local anesthesia administration. This technique reduces the patient stress and anxiety that frequently occurs during the anesthetic procedure. Most patients do not like to see the syringe before or during anesthetic injections; this transfer method keeps the syringe out of the patient's sight.

The anesthesia syringe is prepared and is placed under a paper towel with the topical anesthetic and 2 × 2 gauze. Ideally the anesthetic armamentarium can be placed on a lid of a preset tray, and after anesthesia administration the entire setup is placed aside and away from the working area (Fig. 23-16). If a tray lid is not used, the setup is set inside a paper towel.

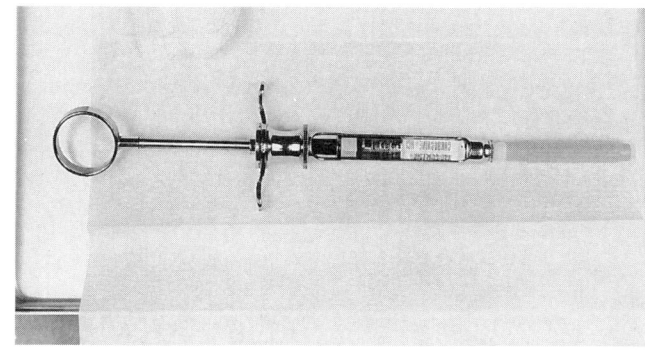

FIG. 23-16   Anesthesia armamentarium.

HIDDEN SYRINGE TRANSFER TECHNIQUES

STEP A

1. Assist the operator as he or she describes the procedure to the patient and tells the patient that a local anesthesia will be administered. If the patient is a child, the procedure will need to be explained in terms that the child can understand. For instance, a light pinch of the arm can demonstrate the feeling that the child will have in his or her mouth during the injection; an analogy is to compare the feeling that is created by anesthesia with the feeling of a child's foot falling asleep when he sits on it or compare the way the injection will feel to the sting of a mosquito bite. The patient needs to be educated so that he or she is not alarmed by the unexpected.
2. Assume a caring role to allay any possible fears while the operator positions the patient's head to gain the best visibility at the injection site.
3. Pass a 2 × 2 gauze sponge to the operator to dry the oral mucosa at the site of injection (Fig. 23-17, *A*).

4. The operator exchanges the gauze sponge for the cotton-tipped applicator that has been dipped in topical anesthetic (Fig. 23-17, *B*).
5. The operator applies topical anesthetic to the site, which remains there for at least 60 to 90 seconds.

STEP B

1. Dispose of the applicator after the operator returns it to you (Fig. 23-17). Pick up the syringe in the right hand to pass it to the operator.
2. If it is preferred, use the left hand to lift the operating light closer to the patient's eyes or ask the patient to close the eyes.
3. The operator retracts the oral tissues with the left hand and positions the right hand, palm up, below the patient's chin, while still maintaining eye contact in the oral cavity. If the operator's eyes shift to follow the delivery of the syringe, the patient may look down and become frightened (Fig. 23-17, *D*).

HIDDEN SYRINGE TRANSFER TECHNIQUES—cont'd.

4. Rest the left hand under the operator's right hand to steady the two together. With the right hand, carefully move the syringe below the patient's chin and place the thumb ring over the operator's thumb (Fig 23-17, *E*).

5. The operator wraps at least two fingers around the finger rest securely. The barrel of the syringe is laid into the operator's palm and the breech side of the syringe is turned toward the operator. The breech opening must face the operator so that he or she can see the movement of the plunger, any blood that might be aspirated, the rate of injection and the amount of anesthesia being injected.

6. Remove the protective cover on the needle with the right hand, and clear the left hand from the site (Fig. 23-17, *F*). The protective cover is laid in the lid of the tray, with the opening pointed toward the assistant; or the assistant can place the sheath in a manufactured recapping device.

7. The release of the operator's hand is a signal that the injection can begin. As the operator administers anesthesia, gently place the left arm over the patient to prevent any attempts by the patient to move toward the operator during the injection. This step is important when you are working with children because their first reaction is to grab out at what is causing discomfort.

8. Observe the patient's reactions during the injection, unusual flutters of the eyes, change in skin color, undue perspiration, or anguish. The assistant can see problems the operator cannot since the operator is concentrating on the oral cavity and the injection. If problems arise, such as the patient's eyes fluttering, or change in facial coloring, the assistant should discretely inform the operator.

9. The operator draws back on the plunger to ensure that the injection needle is not positioned in a blood vessel. During the anesthesia injection the operator may jiggle the patient's cheek (Fig. 23-17, *G*). This may serve to distract the patient, although its purpose is to stretch the injection site tautly to ease the needle's passage through the tissue.

STEP C

1. The operator completes the injection and removes the syringe from the patient's mouth (Fig. 23-17, *H*).

2. Hold a 2 × 2 gauze between the thumb and index finger of the left hand. Retrieve the syringe from the operator with the right hand; carefully clear the needle; grasp the barrel of the syringe, and pass the gauze sponge to the operator (Fig. 23-17, *I*).

3. Do not recap the needle by using the two-handed technique. OSHA guidelines require that a recapping device or a single-handed technique be implemented. The single-handed technique involves laying the needle sheath on a surface (as was described) with the opening facing the assistant. The contaminated needle is placed deep in the opening of the cover (Fig. 23-17, *J*), and the cover is then positioned the rest of the way with the opposite hand holding the syringe (Fig. 23-17, *K*).

4. The operator uses the 2 × 2 gauze to absorb any anesthetic fluids or blood that has leaked from the injection site and returns it to the assistant.

The anesthetic syringe should remain intact throughout the entire procedure because additional injections may be needed to maintain patient comfort. If, during the procedure, the operator needs an additional anesthetic carpule, the syringe transfer is the same. The assistant recaps the syringe using the described technique. The thumb ring is forcefully pulled back on the syringe to disengage the harpoon from the rubber plunger. The carpule is pulled back toward the thumb ring to disengage it from the needle and the carpule is lifted out of the opening. A second carpule is placed and the harpoon is engaged, using the previously described procedure.

As soon as the treatment is completed, an entry of services rendered is placed on the patient's permanent record. Pertinent information that involves the treatment is entered, including the type and amount of anesthesia administered.

The step-by-step procedure just described reflects a right-handed operator at chairside. With a left-handed operator the hands would simply be reversed but the technique would remain the same.

STEP D

1. After the treatment is completed, disassemble the syringe in the sterilization area.

2. Remove the carpule by pulling back on the thumb ring, disengaging the harpoon, and lifting the carpule from the breech opening.

3. Remove the needle with the cover in place from the syringe hub and dispose of the needle and carpule in a sharps container (Fig. 23-18). Some people prefer to remove the needle before the carpule, but the needle on the end of the surface provides air flow into the carpule. When the needle is removed first and the carpule later, a suction in the carpule will sometimes occur causing the glass to explode. After the anesthetic syringe is disassembled it is sterilized according to the practices of the dental office.

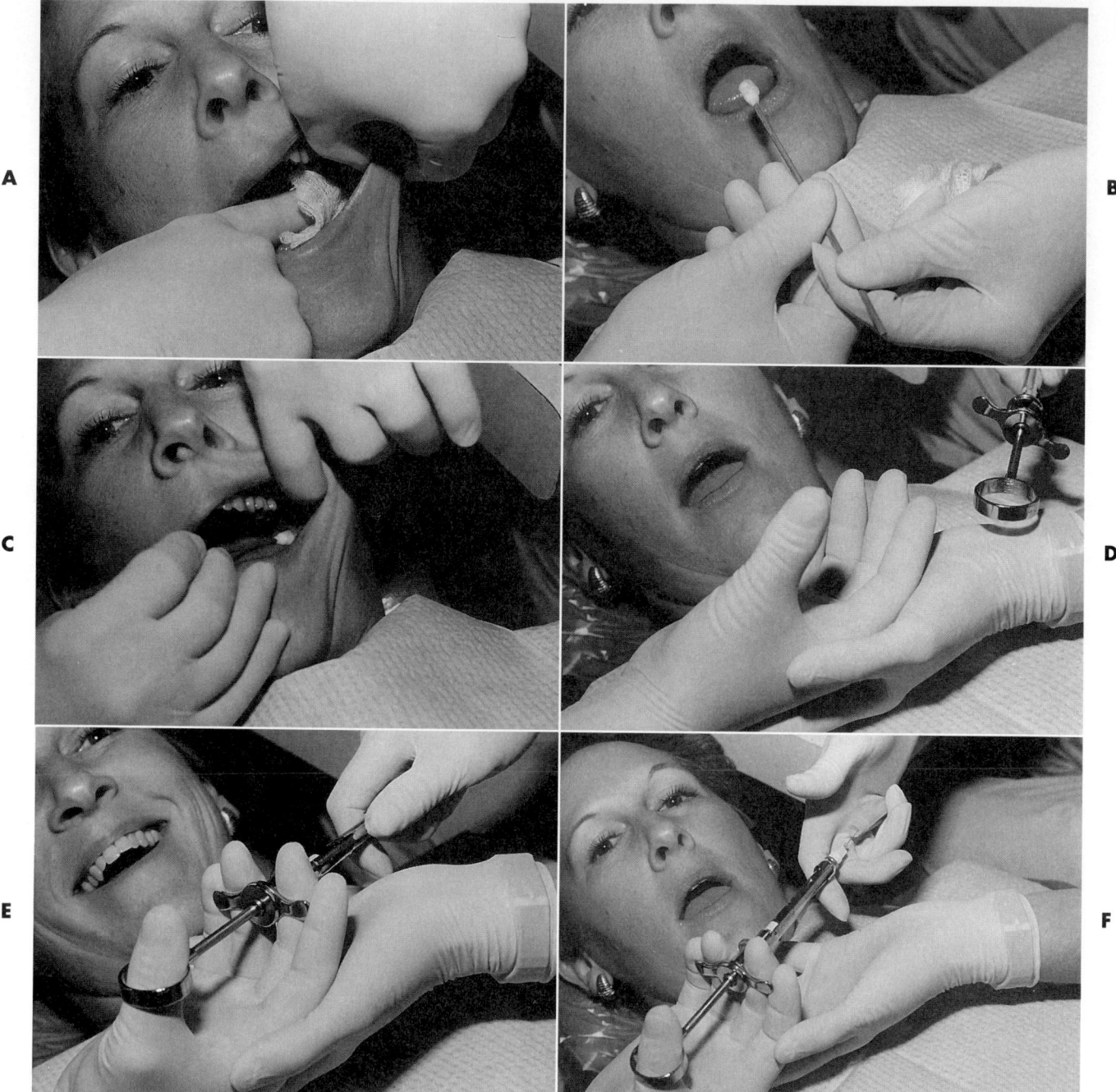

FIG. 23-17   *A,* The dental assistant passes the operator a 2 × 2 gauze. The oral mucosa is
dried at the injection site. *B,* The dental assistant receives the gauze and passes the cotton tip
applicator that has been dipped in topical anesthetic to the operator. *C,* The topical anesthetic
is placed on the oral mucosa at the injection site for 60 to 90 seconds. *D,* The operator positions a hand under the patient's chin before receiving the syringe. *E,* The assistant's left hand
rests under the operator's hands, steadying the two hands, while the syringe is passed with
the right hand. *F,* The operator's thumb is positioned in the thumb ring, while the fingers are
securely positioned on the finger rest. The assistant turns the breech opening to face the
operator and removes the needle cover.

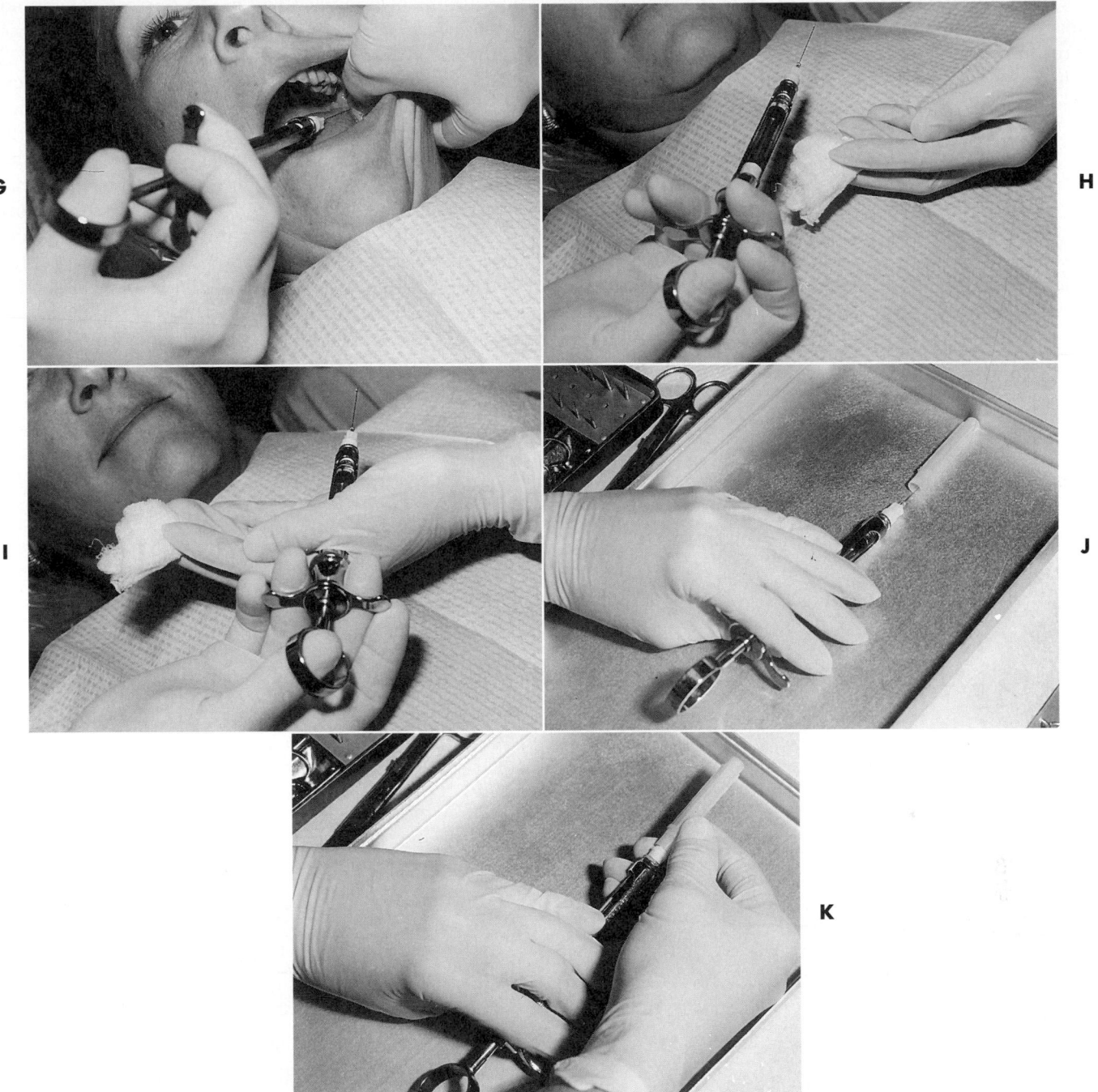

FIG. 23-I7, cont'd.   *G,* The operator places the injection needle in the tissue and gently draws back on the plunger to ensure that the needle is not in a blood vessel. *H,* The assistant positions the left hand nearby with a 2 × 2 gauze. *I,* As the operator removes the syringe from the oral cavity, the assistant grasps the syringe by the barrel and passes the 2 × 2 gauze to dry the injection site. *J,* The single-handed technique is used to recap the needle. The needle cover has been placed on the preset tray cover, and the assistant uses a one-handed scoop technique to place the needle inside the cover. *K,* Once the needle is placed deep in the protective cover, the assistant can use both hands to securely position the cover in place.

This procedure for administration of anesthesia uses the hidden syringe transfer technique. Another technique used during the administration of anesthesia is the rear delivery system. This system is more often used in a situation where the patient is extremely anxious; examples of this would be in an oral surgery or in a pediatric dentistry setting.

This procedure also emphasizes the one-handed scoop technique that is OSHA approved for the recapping of the anesthetic syringe. Instead of this technique, various types of needle guards are available for use in place of covering the needle with the protective sheath (Fig. 23-19); each of these has been designed to avoid needle sticks and to meet OSHA regulations. The technique, the device selected, and OSHA requirements involve careful consideration of all members of the dental team. If a member of the operating team has sustained a needle stick, the incidence must be recorded and all regulations as outlined by OSHA must be followed.

The importance of the role of the dental assistant in local anesthesia administration may be overlooked. Think for a moment how vital you are to this procedure and realize the consequences that could result if you are not alert and conscientious in performing these tasks. A life-threatening situation could arise if the wrong anesthetic is prepared and injected. If the syringe is not prepared correctly, the operator may not realize it until the injection has begun. As a result the syringe must be removed and reassembled necessitating an additional injection for the patient. To provide safety and comfort to the patient and operator during this invasive procedure, the dental assistant is required to have knowledge of the patient's history, to be able to assemble the necessary armamentarium, and to transfer the armamentarium to the operator. This is not enough, however; the dental assistant must also be observant of patients' reactions, anticipate emergency needs, and display a calm, caring manner.

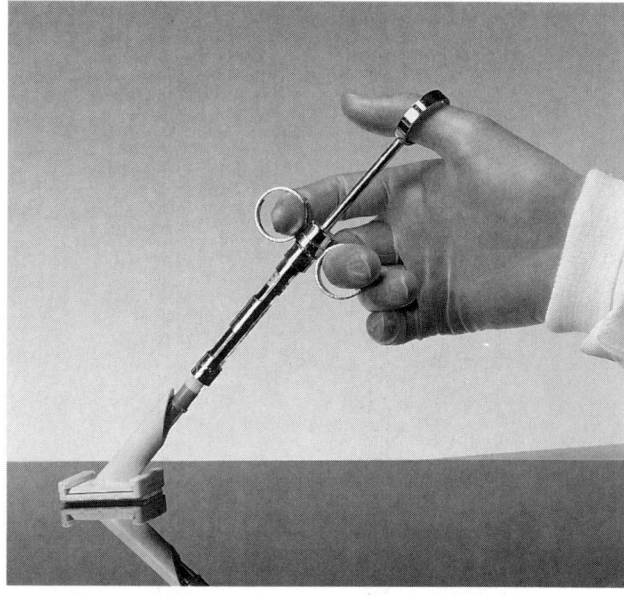

FIG. 23-19   Example of an approved recapping device.

(Courtesy of Palco/Palermo Dental Manufacturing, Stratford, Connecticut.)

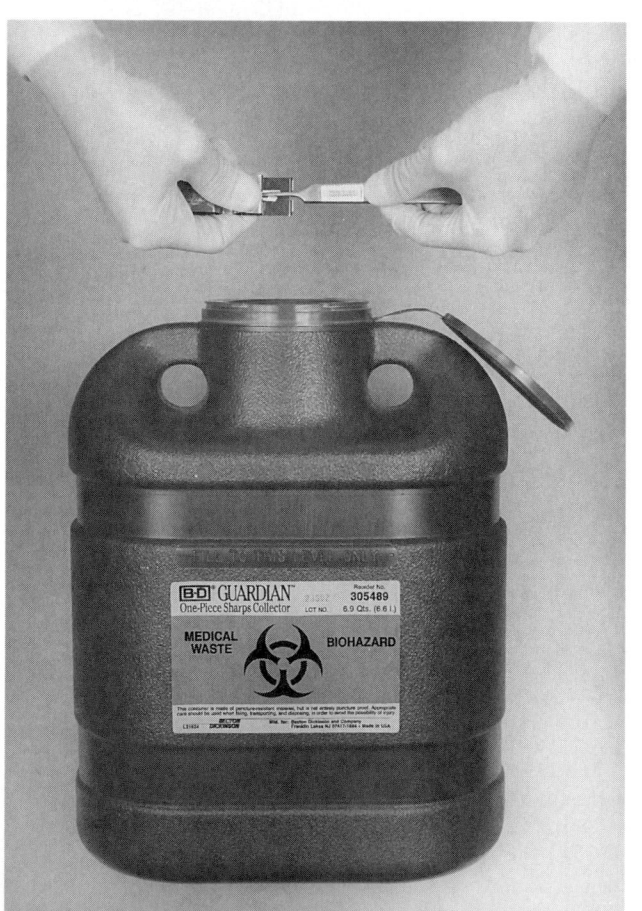

FIG. 23-18   Sharps container for needles and other devices, as designated by OSHA guidelines.

(Courtesy of Becton-Dickinson, Franklin Lakes, New Jersey.)

TEAM APPROACH
Four-Handed Hidden Syringe Technique

OPERATOR	ASSISTANT
	Assemble armamentarium
	Place on mobile cart out of patient's view
	Pass 2 x 2 gauze
Dry site with gauze	Pick up applicator with topical anesthetic
Return 2 x 2, receive applicator	Exchange applicator for 2 x 2 gauze
Place topical anesthetic	Discard 2 x 2 gauze
Return applicator	Receive and discard applicator
Wait for topical anesthetic effectiveness	Pick up syringe
	Loosen protective cover slightly
	Hold syringe in right hand
Position right hand in the transfer zone	Stabilize operator's right hand with left hand
	Position thumb ring over thumb and lay barrel of syringe into palm of operator's hand
Place thumb into thumb ring and place fingers on to grip	Turn breech opening so that operator can observe carpule
	Withdraw protective covering
	Release operator's right hand
	Move hand out of position
Move syringe to oral cavity	
Make injection	Place left arm over patient's torso area, if needed, to avoid patient making sudden movement (hold hand of young child, if necessary)
	Observe vital signs, nonverbal cues
	Grasp 2 x 2 gauze in receiving portion of hand (note reverse position in this transfer)
Return syringe (observe location of needle for safe transfer)	Observe location of needle for safe pick up
	Grasp syringe by barrel
	Pass 2 x 2 gauze
Receive 2 x 2 gauze	Return syringe to mobile cart
Wipe injection site	Recap with single hand or recapping device
	Transfer setup to fixed cabinetry, if desired
Return 2 x 2 gauze	Receive 2 x 2 gauze, discard
	Pick up a/w syringe in left hand and HVE hose in right hand
	Turn a/w nozzle to appropriate area, and turn on HVE
Retract tissue	Transfer a/w syringe
Receive a/w syringe	
Spray water at injection site	Evacuate fluid from the mouth
Return a/w syringe	Receive a/w syringe

KEY POINTS

▶ The dental team strives to provide dental care to a patient without the patient's experiencing any sensation of pain. Topical anesthesia, local anesthesia, conscious sedation, nitrous oxide, and general anesthesia are types of anesthesia that are used to block perception of normal sensation and to interrupt the sensation of pain.

▶ Local anesthesia involves the use of topical anesthesia and injectable anesthesia. The local topical anesthesia is applied to mucous membranes to relieve sensation, while an injectable anesthesia is administered through infiltration, field block or nerve block injections. Periodontal ligament injections are also used in certain circumstances and are not as common as the other local anesthesia techniques.

▶ An anesthetic carpule is composed of a glass vial, a rubber plunger, and a metal hub, which has a rubber diaphragm. Pertinent information regarding the components, the amount, and the percentage of the anesthesia is included on the outside of the glass vial.

▶ The anesthesia needle has a protective cover on the hub end and on the needle end of the syringe needle. The hub end is attached to the hub of the anesthetic syringe. Other parts of the syringe include the barrel with a breech opening, a plunger with a harpoon at one end and a thumb ring at the other, and the finger grip.

▶ The assembly of the anesthetic syringe involves the selection of the correct anesthesia and needle, the correct placement of the needle on the syringe to avoid leakage or blockage, and the correct placement of the carpule to ensure easy flow of the anesthesia during injection and aspiration.

▶ The hidden syringe transfer allows the operating team to have a fluid exchange of the anesthetic syringe and ensures that the patient will not become alarmed at the sight of the syringe.

BIBLIOGRAPHY

Anderson KN, Anderson LE, Glanze WD, editors: *Mosby's medical, nursing, & allied health dictionary,* ed 4, St Louis, 1993, Mosby.

Bennett CR: *Monheim's local anesthesia and pain control in dental practice,* St Louis, 1984, Mosby, pp. 125-183.

Dejong RH: *Local anesthetics,* St Louis, 1993, Mosby.

Little JW, Falace DA: *Dental management of the medically compromised patient,* ed 3, St Louis, 1988, Mosby.

Malamed SF, Sheppard GA: *Handbook of medical emergencies in the dental office,* ed 4, St Louis, 1993, Mosby.

UNIT V BASIC CLINICAL PROCEDURES

24 Oral Diagnosis

LEARNING OBJECTIVES

You will have mastered the material in this chapter when you can:

- Define the key terms
- Describe the process of oral diagnosis
- Describe the importance of a complete personal and medical history
- Explain the need to update a patient's personal and medical history
- Describe the procedure for obtaining vital signs
- Describe the use of consent forms, radiographs, laboratory studies, study models, and photographs in clinical evaluation
- List the data necessary for a complete dental clinical examination
- Describe an extraoral examination
- Describe an intraoral examination
- Identify common abbreviations and symbols used in charting a dental examination
- Explain the step-by-step procedure for obtaining diagnostic impressions
- Describe common laboratory reports
- Explain the development of a treatment plan
- Describe the process of case presentation

KEY WORDS

Adventitious	Occlusion
Blood pressure (BP)	Patient history
Clinical examination	Prognosis
Clinical record	Pyrexia
Dental history	Sphygmomanometer
Diagnosis	Stethoscope
Diagnostic models	Stridor
Diastole	Systole
Dyspnea	Temperature, pulse, and
Hypertension	respiration (TPR)
Hypotension	Treatment plan
Hypothermia	Vital signs
Medical history	

A **clinical record** is an accumulation of data that is gathered from a clinical, radiographic, and photographic examination. From these data the dentist determines a **diagnosis**. A diagnosis is the translation of the data into an organized, classified definition of the conditions present. In some instances, treatment may be necessary before arriving at a final diagnosis. The process of diagnosis is the legal responsibility of the dentist only, and though it may appear that the dentist makes a diagnosis quickly, it is arrived at through observation, logical and systematic thinking, and experience. To arrive at a diagnosis, the dentist must rely on the most complete and accurate data, including past and present history, existing symptoms, and conditions.

Oral diagnosis is seldom just the identification of a single disease in the mouth, but rather it is a disclosure of conditions of an oral or a systemic nature that will require treatment or management. The dentist should be concerned about the patient's total health, the relation of the oral cavity to the patient's general systemic health, the effect of systemic health on the management of the patient's oral conditions, and the patient's self-image. A diagnosis need not be negative. It can be a confirmation of good oral health, healthy tissues, and the absence of disease. Modern dentistry places emphasis not only on the control of disease, but also on the prevention of disease.

A patient is concerned for the future and what will occur with the conditions in his or her mouth when treated or the consequences of these conditions if they remain untreated. Therefore, the dentist makes a **prognosis**: the foretelling of the probable course of disease. For instance, if the patient has severe gingivitis the dentist can explain that with a thorough oral prophylaxis, good home care, and routine follow-up examinations, the prognosis can be favorable. However, if the condition is left untreated, it can develop into periodontal disease, which, if it is neglected, can ultimately lead to tooth loss. The patient's prognosis is based on the existing conditions in the patient's mouth and on scientific knowledge.

This chapter describes each phase of the oral diagnosis procedure and explores the data collection process for each of these phases. A brief description of various business forms, including the components of a clinical record, was given in Chapter 14. In this chapter the mechanics of using these forms are described as the process of oral diagnosis evolves.

Examination Process

To collect data about a patient is an ongoing process. Typically a patient visits the dental office as a new patient who seeks complete and thorough treatment for conditions that he or she may or may not be aware exist, as an emergency patient for treatment of a specific or chief complaint, or as a returning patient of record for continuing care. Each of these situations requires some type of clinical and radiographic examination, a review of the medical history, and a diagnosis. Regardless of the course of treatment the patient may need, the most complete and accurate information must be obtained to enable the dentist to obtain an accurate diagnosis.

The phases of oral diagnosis focus on the patient's personal, medical, and dental history: the clinical examination; radiographic, photographic, and diagnostic mod-

els; laboratory tests; and the diagnosis. A diagnosis is seldom made after the review of a single phase of history. Each phase provides the dentist with different but interrelated information, and when all are combined, they contribute to the final diagnosis.

▶ Dental Assistant's Role

The dental assistant plays an integral role in the collection of data for a clinical record by performing the following:

1. Obtaining a patient history
2. Exposing, processing, and mounting radiographs
3. Obtaining and recording vital signs
4. Obtaining preliminary impressions for study models
5. Taking photographs
6. Recording clinical data
7. Charting oral conditions
8. Completing laboratory requisitions
9. Transferring the patient to a laboratory or physician for follow-up studies or care
10. Obtaining laboratory results
11. Preparing a clinical record for review
12. Preparing materials for case presentation

▶ Patient History

A **patient history** is a personal document of specific information about the patient, and it requires that each person who comes in contact with this record must maintain the highest degree of confidentiality. The dentist must learn as much as possible about the patient's history to provide the most thorough dental treatment. To do this it is necessary to develop a sense of trust and confidence between the patient and the dental team.

PERSONAL

The **personal history** about a patient is obtained from a registration/questionnaire form. The patient must give his or her complete legal name, address, phone number, employment, social security number, physician's name and address, name of the person responsible for payment, spousal and family member information if applicable, occupation, and information about insurance, as well as a contact person in case of an emergency. This personal information will aid in routine business activities, such as billing and insurance claim filing, and will serve as legal identification of the patient.

MEDICAL

A patient's **medical history** is a collection of data provided by the patient about his or her general health; it is an important means of preventing medical emergencies. Some of the procedures that are performed and drugs that might be prescribed in a dental office can be potentially fatal for patients who may have systemic diseases (known or unknown), who may be taking drugs, or who may have special sensitivities. The dentist has a moral, legal, and ethical responsibility to learn as much as possible about the patient's medical history before treatment is provided. When the dental assistant initially presents the questionnaire to the patient to complete, it is important to inform the patient of the need for complete and accurate information and to explain how it relates to his or her dental care.

To protect the dentist from potential litigation and to protect the well being of the patient, it is vital that a complete medical history be obtained from the patient before treatment begins. An in-depth health questionnaire, completed and signed by the patient and updated at least annually ensures the dentist's commitment to this objective (see Figs. 14-11 and 14-12). After the patient completes the questionnaire, the dental assistant reviews it thoroughly to confirm that all questions have been answered. In addition, it is wise to carry on a dialogue with the patient to clarify any questions and to develop an understanding of the patient's medical history. When it is necessary, the dentist should clarify with the patient's primary physician any medical history or the patient's use of certain drugs or treatment that might pose contraindications to dental treatment. Once the dentist has consulted with the patient's physician, this should be noted in the patient record.

The health questionnaire includes information about the patient's past systemic diseases, injuries, operations, or allergies. A thorough drug history, as discussed in Chapter 10, should be included to determine which medications the patient may have recently taken or may be taking now. The questionnaire includes most of these categories of questions. A patient may wonder why certain questions are asked, since some questions may seem unrelated to dental care. The dental assistant must understand how certain diseases or illnesses affect dental care. A detailed discussion on the effect that changes in a patient's general health and various diseases have on the delivery of dental treatment is provided in Chapter 25.

When a patient has confirmed any of the questions on the health questionnaire, the patient must be queried to determine when the disease or change occurred, the extent of the illness or change, the prescribed treatment or medication, and the present status of the condition.

DENTAL

A patient's **dental history** provides information about previous treatment and dental experiences and is often a component of the health questionnaire. Some dentists prefer to use a separate questionnaire; this is common

practice in several specialties, such as pediatric dentistry. Information that is important to obtain should include the following:

1. Frequency of dental visits and an oral prophylaxis
2. Past experiences or reactions with local anesthetics and other intraoral agents
3. The dates, nature, and length of time of past specialty treatment, such as periodontal therapy and including subgingival curettage, gingival surgery, or occlusal adjustments; orthodontic treatment, and any appliances still being worn; endodontic therapy, such as root canal fillings or an apicoectomy; surgical procedures, such as extractions or other treatment that has been performed inside or around the oral cavity
4. Placement of fixed bridges, including the insertion dates and any complications that were experienced
5. The use of removable dental prostheses, and if and when these appliances have been adjusted or relined
6. The use of bite splints or other oral appliances, including the type and the reason for use
7. The attitude of the patient toward past dental treatment and experiences

▶ Clinical Examination

The **clinical examination** begins with general observations of the patient as early as he or she enters the treatment area and continues through the thorough examination of the extraoral tissues, the intraoral tissues, the soft and hard tissues, the periodontium, and the teeth and their occlusal relationship.

The clinical examination is one of the most important services that can be performed for a patient in the dental office, and it is initiated after the patient completes the medical and dental history. This type of examination is repeated at subsequent visits when the patient is seen for the routine prophylaxis. A thorough extraoral and intraoral examination can often save a patient's life through the early detection of lesions that occur in the tissues of the face, neck, and oral cavity. Many oral lesions begin innocently and may go undetected by the patient until the lesion has advanced to a dangerous stage.

Typically, the patient is seated comfortably in an upright position, and the dentist reviews the history; then the dentist and the patient discuss the contents of the history. The dental assistant records data from the examination and provides appropriate instruments that will be needed during the procedure. In the following description, each phase is described in a step-by-step procedure, beginning with general observations about the patient and concluding with the charting of common oral conditions.

GENERAL DIAGNOSTIC SIGNS

▶ Is there any facial asymmetry, such as a drooping eyelid, bulging eyes, or drooping lip?

▶ Is the skin color appropriate for the patient, or is there a grey pallor, yellowed skin or eyes, or redness on the skin? Is the skin drawn and glossy, or is it dry?

▶ Does the patient appear alert or withdrawn? Is the patient aware of the questions you are asking? Does the patient seem anxious?

▶ Are there obvious breath odors, and if so, can they be traced to a source?

▶ Is the patient ambulatory? Does he or she seem to be flexible when moving about?

▶ What is the reaction of the pupils? Are they dilated?

▶ What do the patient's nails look like? Are the nail beds discolored? Is there evidence of nail biting?

▶ Does the patient seem able to use his or her hands, or are the hands crippled, or do they appear arthritic?

▶ Does the patient display a reaction to stimuli?

GENERAL OBSERVATIONS

Several factors aid in evaluating a patient's general health. Each factor can be assessed by observing the patient when he or she is escorted to the treatment room and seated and by carrying on a normal conversation with the patient. Note on the record any abnormal conditions the patient may have, such as facial pallor, a slow or difficult gait, an offensive breath odor, or dilation of the pupils. While you are interacting with the patient, observe for diagnostic signs that are listed in Box 24-1.

Any information that needs to be relayed to the dentist can be written in a note rather than verbalized; hearing it may cause undue alarm to the patient. Later, questions about the patient's general health may help to explain the visual observations. Appropriate comments that relate to the patient's dental care may be entered on the patient's record at the conclusion of the appointment.

VITAL SIGNS

Assessment of a patient's vital signs is important in oral diagnosis and in the delivery of treatment to a patient. **Vital signs**, known as cardinal symptoms because these measurements are indicators of vital functions that are necessary to sustain life, include **temperature (T)**: the degree of heat of a living body; **pulse (P)**: the rate of blood traveling through the arteries; **respiration rate (R)**: the rate of oxygen intake (or **TPR**); and **blood pressure**: pressure in the arteries at the height of pulse wave (or **BP**).

Changes in a patient's TPR or BP may be an indication of actual or future problems that a patient may experience. Since the TPR and BP are measurements of functions of life, any alteration in normal body function can be observed in these measurements.

Normally, a patient is seen in a dental office biannually—an appropriate time to collect data. More frequent measurement of vital signs may be necessary if health problems exist.

A patient may not understand the need for the dental professional to assess temperature, pulse rate, respirations, and blood pressure before dental treatment. Therefore, it is the dental assistant's responsibility to inform the patient that treatment includes the whole of the person and not just a part. If a patient does not seek regular medical examinations, the health assessment provided in the dental office could be the first indication of a problem, and the patient can be directed to a physician.

Temperature

Body temperature measures the amount of heat within the body. A normal body temperature registers approximately 98.6° F or 37° C. Various factors, such as exercise, excitement, the process of digestion, infection, cold, shock, and drugs, may effect the level of body temperature. Temperature may vary with a patient's age and with the time of day. Adults often have a lower temperature in the morning and a higher temperature later in the day. An infant's or small child's temperature may normally be higher than an adult's temperature.

A temperature reading is obtained by using a thermometer that is covered with a disposable sheath or by using a disposable thermometer. If the design of the thermometer is a traditional glass type or a digital readout type, a plastic protective sheath is placed on the bulb end of the thermometer to ensure sterility. A more modern design of thermometer, an electronic monitoring system, is found commonly in hospital, in surgery settings, or in the home.

A normal temperature of 98.6° F indicates no obvious physical problems. Fluctuations of 0.5° F to 1.0° F are still considered within normal limits. An elevated temperature, known to the layperson as fever or **pyrexia**, is usually an indication of an illness. **Hyperpyrexia** is a high fever—usually above 105.8°. When a temperature reaches 110° F, a person's survival is rare, since the high temperature damages the respiratory center. A subnormal temperature, **hypothermia**, is often a result of trauma; however, each abnormality in temperature may be a protective measure for the body. A body temperature below 93° F may be life threatening and may result from being in cold water or from being buried in snow. Often it is impossible to obtain vital signs at subnormal temperature range, and if confronted with a hypothermic

---

BOX 24-2

TO OBTAIN A BODY TEMPERATURE

The oral registration of a patient's temperature is assessed with an electronic thermometer.

▶ Wash and glove.
▶ Determine that the patient has not eaten, smoked, drunk, rinsed or brushed the teeth within the last 15 minutes.
▶ Place a protective disposable sheath over the stem of the thermometer.
▶ Hold the tip near the high graduated numbers of the thermometer.
▶ Turn on the electronic readout.
▶ Place the tip with the sheath under the patient's tongue, and ask the patient to hold it in place for approximately 25 to 30 seconds.
▶ Listen for the sound of the electronic signal, which indicates that the temperature has registered on the electronic readout.
▶ Read the temperature with the plastic sheath in place.
▶ Turn off the thermometer probe.
▶ Remove the plastic sheath.
▶ Remove the protective gloves, and wash your hands.
▶ Record the data in the patient's clinical record.

WHEN A CLINICAL GLASS THERMOMETER IS USED

▶ Wash and glove.
▶ Wipe the thermometer with a disinfectant-saturated wipe.
▶ Shake down the mercury toward the bulb by holding the opposite end with the thumb and forefinger and snapping the wrist once or twice.
▶ Place the thermometer under the tongue, as in the previous procedure, and ask the patient to hold it stationary for approximately 3 to 4 minutes.
▶ Remove the thermometer, and hold it parallel to the floor at eye level.
▶ Slowly turn the thermometer until you can see the exact point at which the mercury is registered.
▶ Wipe the thermometer with a disinfectant-saturated gauze.
▶ Remove the gloves, and wash your hands.
▶ Record the information on the clinical record.
  NOTE: The registration is not in tenths of degrees other than 98.6° F.

TABLE 24-1   TERMS RELATED TO PULSE AMPLITUDES

Definition of pulse	Description
Normal	Pulse is easily felt and requires moderate pressure to disappear
Absent	No pulse can be felt, even when extreme pressure is applied
Thready	Pulse is difficult to feel; slight pressure causes it to disappear
Weak	Stronger than thready pulse; when slight pressure is applied, it may disappear
Strong	A pounding pulse that does not disappear with moderate pressure

---

the arteries of the body. This action creates vibrations in the arterial system that can be felt through touch. The areas where the vibration or pulse can be easily felt include the temporal region and the mandibular, carotid, femoral, and radial arteries.

The number of times the heart beats and forces a pulsation of blood is the pulse rate, and this fluctuates with a person's age, weight and size. An infant's pulse rate normally falls between 120 to 140 beats per minute. An adult's pulse rate is approximately 60 to 80 beats per minute. A female's pulse rate is usually slightly higher than that of a male.

Fluctuations in Pulse Rate

Usually a pulse rate is slower when a person is at rest and when he or she first awakes. Factors that cause increased fluctuations in pulse rate are pain, anger, fear, stress, and the element of surprise. Physical activity, increased heat, an elevated body temperature, decreased blood pressure, and disease that causes lowered oxygenation of the blood supply can cause changes in the pulse rate. The quality of the pulse or its amplitude can be described in terms of its fullness and strength. Terms that describe pulse amplitude are illustrated in Table 24-1.

Occasionally, a pulse rate cannot be accurately determined with the radial measurement. An option is to measure the apical pulse, particularly if the radial pulse measurement indicates an irregular, thready, or rapid pulse. The apical pulse rate is the most accurate measurement of the pulse because it is registered at the source of the pulse: the heart. The apical pulse rate is registered through the use of a warmed stethoscope that is placed at the apex of the heart, between the fifth and sixth ribs and slightly below the left nipple. The pulse rate for this position is counted for 1 minute, and then it is recorded. Other sites where the pulse can be detected are illustrated in Fig. 24-1.

person, a health care worker should attempt to warm the hypothermic victim and continue resuscitation efforts.

Pulse Rate

With each contraction of the left ventricle of the heart, a wave of blood is forced into the aorta and then through

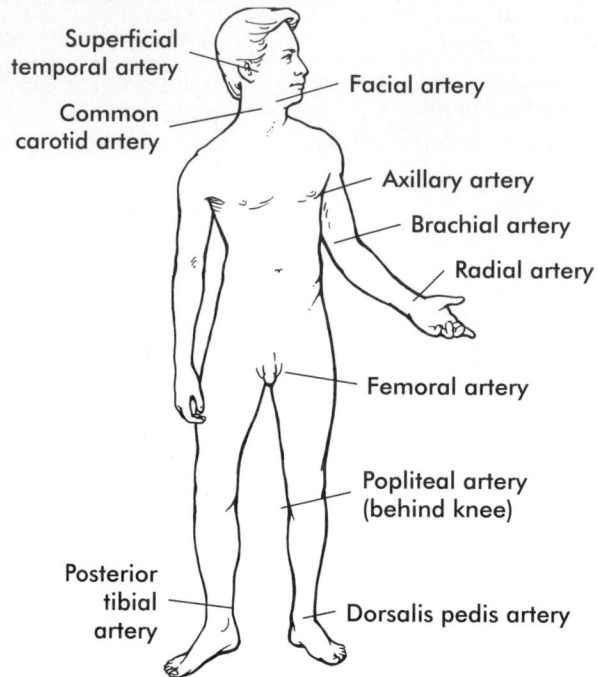

FIG. 24-1   Sites where a pulse can be detected.

(From Thibodeau GA, Patton KT: *Anatomy and physiology*, ed 2, St Louis, 1993, Mosby.)

Respiration Rate

Respiration is inhaling oxygen into the lungs and exhaling carbon dioxide from the lungs. Often a person is not aware of respiration activity, since the exchange of oxygen and carbon dioxide occurs through no voluntary effort on the part of the person. An individual can control respiration to maintain normal activities, such as talking and singing.

Normal respiration rate for an adult is 14 to 18 respirations per minute; a female's respiration rate is faster than is a male's. An infant's respiration rate is approximately 40 counts per minute, and a child's rate is 25 to 30 counts per minute. The pattern of respiration may vary from a slow, regular rate, to a normal, fast, or patterned one as shown in Table 24-2, which illustrates the nature of respiration rhythm.

A variety of terms are used to describe breathing sounds and the nature of respirations. Typically, respirations are noiseless, but certain sounds have been identified to describe noisy respirations or stertorous breathing (snoring sound). **Stridor** is a term used to describe a harsh, high-pitched sound that is heard on inspiration when the upper airway is narrow. This sound is not unusual in children with croup. **Dyspnea** is the term used to describe difficulty in breathing, which, in some, may be a temporary condition, such as in a runner

BOX 24-3

TO OBTAIN A PULSE RATE

Under normal conditions in a dental office, a patient's pulse rate would be assessed in the radial artery of the wrist.

▶ Palpate the artery on the medial surface and thumb side of the wrist.
▶ Place the patient's arm in an extended position, with the palm up; provide support.
▶ Place two or three fingers on the radial artery and radius bone, until the pulsing blood is felt. If excess force is placed or if the thumb is used, the sensation of contraction and expansion of the blood through the artery cannot be felt.
▶ Use a watch with a second hand or with a digital second counter to count the pulse for 15 seconds.
▶ Multiply the number of pulses by four to determine the minute rate of pulsations. The pulse can also be counted for 30 seconds and multiplied by two for the minute rate.
▶ Record the patient's pulse rate in the clinical record. If you are uncertain of the rate, take a second reading.

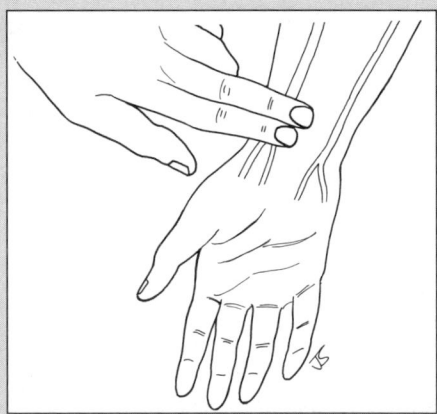

FIG. 24-2   Palpation of the artery to obtain a pulse.

who gasps for air at the end of a race or in a person who may be gasping for breath after quickly running up stairs. In some patients, breathing is difficult; for example, patients who are obese, who have emphysema, or who have some type of heart disease may experience difficulty with breathing. **Adventitious** sounds are abnormal sounds, and although they are often not heard, the sounds are evident with a stethoscope. Common breathing sounds are identified in Box 24-4.

A dental assistant should not only be aware of the specialized types of breathing, but also should be alert to the signs of breathing difficulties that indicate a patient's life is in jeopardy. Two cardinal signs are cyanosis (blueness) and the Cheyne-Stokes respiration: when the patient breathes deeply and rapidly for approximately 30 seconds, stops breathing for 10 to 30 seconds, then repeats the cycle. In this situation the patient is usually not cyanotic. The respirations are slow and shallow at first, then they grow faster and deeper and gradually taper off, until they stop entirely. Cheyne-Stokes respirations are critical symptoms and usually precede death in cerebral hemorrhage, uremia, or heart disease.

TABLE 24-2 TYPES OF BREATHING

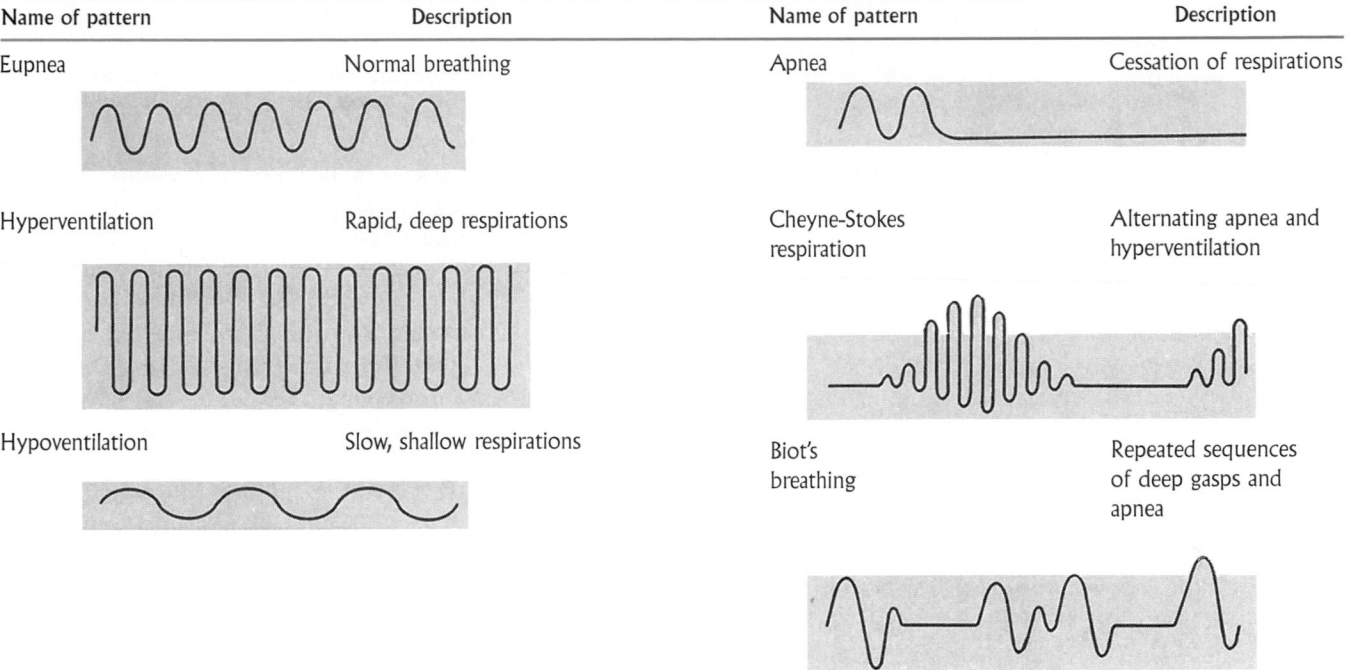

Name of pattern	Description	Name of pattern	Description
Eupnea	Normal breathing	Apnea	Cessation of respirations
Hyperventilation	Rapid, deep respirations	Cheyne-Stokes respiration	Alternating apnea and hyperventilation
Hypoventilation	Slow, shallow respirations	Biot's breathing	Repeated sequences of deep gasps and apnea

From Thibodeau GA, Patton KT: *Anatomy & physiology*, ed 2, St Louis, 1993, Mosby.

BOX 24-4

COMMON BREATHING SOUNDS

- **Rales or crackles** are intermittent sounds that are caused by moisture in the respiratory passage; these often sound like air-filled rice cereal after milk is poured over it.
- **Rhonchi or gurgles** are continuous, low-pitched sounds that occur when air moves through narrowed passageways in the lungs that contain an accumulation of secretions. These sounds may occur during inhalation but are commonly heard during expiration or during both. The sounds may change with coughing.
- **Wheezing** is a high-pitched sound that occurs during respiration when air is forced through narrow respiratory passages. Wheezing is often heard in patients with asthma.
- **Friction rub** is a grating noise that occurs when two structures rub across each other, occurring when membranes are dry and the pleura of the lungs rub against each other.

BOX 24-5

TO OBTAIN A RESPIRATION RATE

Respiration rate fluctuates when body temperature increases with exercise, pain, excitement or when diseases of the respiratory system are present.

- Continue to maintain the same position that is used to assess the pulse rate.
- Try to obtain the measurement when the patient is unaware of your actions. Often a patient breaths abnormally when a breathing measurement is taken.
- Count the number of respirations with the rise and fall of the patient's chest as a single respiration.
- Count the respirations for 30 seconds; then multiply the number by two for the minute rate of respirations.
- If the rates are abnormal, count a second time to confirm the first number.
- Record the information in the patient's clinical record.

Blood Pressure

Blood pressure is the force that the heart places on the blood against the arterial walls. The highest pressure registered, or the top number, is the systolic pressure, or the systole. The **systole** occurs when the greatest force is placed on the arterial walls as the heart beats. Between the beats is the time when the least force is placed on the arterial walls, and it is called the diastolic pressure or **diastole**. The difference between the two is known as the **pulse pressure**, which is an indication of the amount of blood that is forced through the heart between contractions.

In a dental office the blood pressure is usually monitored *indirectly* with the use of a **stethoscope** and a **sphygmomanometer**. A stethoscope is the instrument placed against the patient's chest to hear the heart and lung sounds. A sphygmomanometer is the device used to actually measure the blood pressure indirectly. The use of the manual system may be replaced by an automatic/ digital sphygmomanometer which eliminates the use of the stethoscope (Fig. 24-3). The automatic system is especially useful in surgery, since it is possible to place the cuff around a patient's arm; an automatic reading can be obtained at periodic intervals without interrupting the procedure or disrupting the aseptic techniques that are used during surgery. A *direct* monitoring of blood pressure is determined by placing a probe directly into a blood vessel or into the heart. This latter technique is not normally practiced in a dental office and is used during critical care of a patient.

When a normal blood pressure is registered, 120/80, the higher number—120—is the systolic pressure and the lower number—80—is the diastolic pressure. Blood pressure varies according to the patient's age, gender, and the time of the day; exercise, stress, emotion, body position, and whether a meal has been ingested also

affect the reading. Normal blood pressure can have a systolic measurement up to 140 mm Hg, with 140 to 159 mm Hg considered as borderline hypertensive; any higher reading is isolated systolic hypertensive. Normal blood pressure shows a diastolic reading under 85, with 85 to 89 mm Hg as the high end of normal, 90 to 104 mm Hg as mildly hypertensive, 105 to 114 mm Hg as moderately hypertensive, and 115 mm Hg and above as severe hypertension.

Hypertension is an elevated blood pressure for a sustained period of time; this is a problem found in great numbers in the general public. On occasion, when a patient's blood pressure is registered during a dental visit, an elevated blood pressure reading may be the patient's first awareness of the problem. The blood pressure can be taken again to determine if it is still elevated and whether the patient should be directed to seek a physician's care. A patient may react to the *white coat syndrome* when the blood pressure is taken before treatment. A second reading after treatment is completed might show a normal reading, leading the dental professional to believe the elevated pressure could have been caused by stress and anxiety.

Hypotension is a condition that involves below-normal blood pressure. Hypotensive patients register a systolic blood pressure reading of approximately 90 to 115 mm Hg for an adult. This condition can be the result of illness, blood loss, vomiting and diarrhea, burns to the body, or certain medications. At the completion of dental

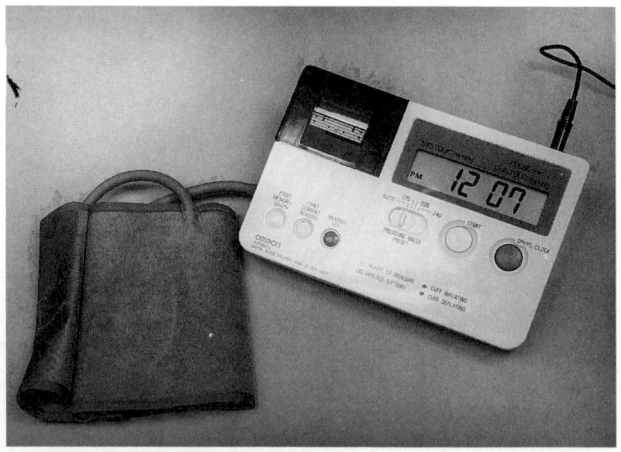

FIG. 24-3   Automatic/digital oximeter registering blood pressure and pulse.

TABLE 24-3   KOROTKOFF SOUNDS

Phase	Description
Phase I	Characterized by the first appearance of faint but clear tapping sounds that gradually increase in intensity; the first tapping sound is the systolic pressure
Phase II	Characterized by muffled or swishing sounds; these sounds may temporarily disappear, especially in a hypertensive patient; the disappearance of the sound during the latter part of Phase I and during Phase II is called the auscultatory gap, which may extend to a range of 40 points; failing to recognize this gap may result in underestimating systolic pressure or overestimating diastolic pressure
Phase III	Characterized by distinct loud sounds as the blood flows relatively free through an increasingly open artery
Phase IV	Characterized by a distinct abrupt muffling sound, with a soft blowing quality; this is considered to be the first diastolic figure
Phase V	The last sound heard before a period of continuous silence; the pressure that correlates with the last sound is the second diastolic figure

BOX 24-6

TO OBTAIN A BLOOD PRESSURE (FIG. 24-4)

▶ Describe the procedure to the patient; explain that the cuff may be tight around the arm for a short period of time.

▶ Have the patient remove or loosen any constricting clothing that might interfere with the reading.

▶ Seat the patient comfortably in a chair with the arm supported and with the palm up or lying down.

▶ Position yourself so that you are at eye level with the manometer.

▶ Remove all air from the cuff by opening the valve and forcing the air out.

▶ Wrap the cuff around the arm over the brachial artery and slightly above the elbow; secure the cuff in place with the Velcro end. The width of the cuff should be roughly the diameter of the patient's arm. Cuff sizes vary for newborns, infants, children, adults, large adults, and the thigh. Incorrect sizes can distort readings.

▶ Place the stethoscope over the site where the pulse of the artery is felt (Fig. 24-5).

▶ Pump the air bulb of the manometer to force air into the bladder of the cuff. The mercury should rise to approximately 20 mm Hg above an expected systolic pressure for this patient.

▶ Open the air valve of the manometer, allowing the air to escape slowly.

▶ Visually and mentally record the number at which the first heartbeat is heard (systolic pressure).

▶ Continue to release air through the cuff gradually, until the heartbeat can no longer be heard, and again make a visual and mental record of this number (diastolic pressure).

▶ Release the remaining air from the cuff, and remove the stethoscope and cuff from the patient's arm.

▶ Record the information on the patient's clinical chart.

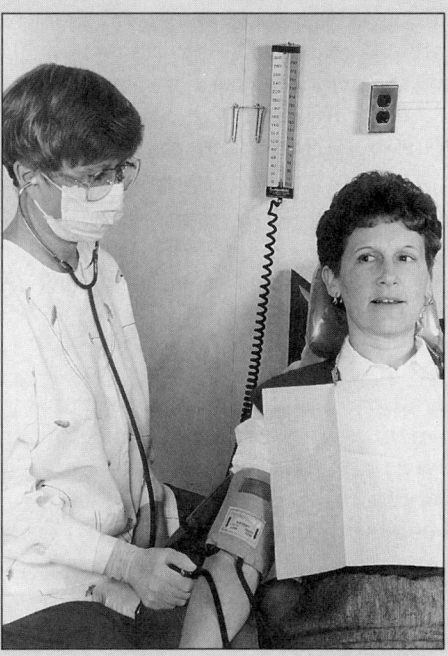

FIG. 24-4　The dental assistant is shown obtaining a blood pressure reading, using the mercury manometer.

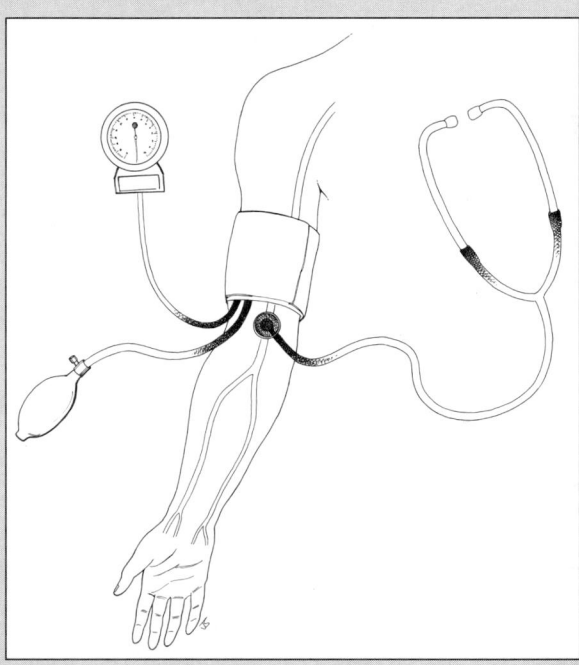

FIG. 24-5　A schematic drawing, illustrating placement of the stethoscope and sphygmomanometer.

treatment on a hypotensive patient, the patient may experience a feeling of lightheadedness as the dental chair is brought to an upright position. The lowering of the patient's head toward the knees for a few minutes will normally restore the flow of blood to the brain and result in the patient feeling normal.

Indirect blood pressure is obtained through the use of a sphygmomanometer, a cloth-like bladder device, with two tubes attached: one tube is attached to a rubber bulb and the other, to a manometer. The first tube with the bulb forces air into the bladder when it is pumped. A valve opens or closes the force of air. The **manometer** is a device that encloses the mercury in a glass tube that has markings to register the blood pressure. An **aneroid manometer** is a device with a dial that is attached to the cloth cuff. Obtaining a blood pressure with an aneroid manometer reads blood pressure less accurately than does a mercury manometer.

To obtain an accurate recording of a blood pressure, the clinician must use two senses at one time: sight and hearing. The sounds heard through the stethoscope when blood pressure is measured are referred to as Korotkoff sounds and are described in Table 24-3. Listen for the first heartbeat through the stethoscope and mentally record that number as it is observed on the manometer. The second sound (absence of a heartbeat) is the second recording. The two sounds—the first rush of blood through the constriction of the cuff and the normal not-as-noticeable flow of normal blood—are known as Korotkoff sounds. The first sound that is heard is the systolic reading and the second sound is the diastolic reading. To obtain an accurate blood pressure with a mercury manometer, use the steps in Box 24-6.

> Once all of the vital signs have been obtained, they can be entered on the patient's records as follows:
> 12/10/94 TPR 98.6, 76, 16; BP 120/80

Special Considerations When Obtaining a Blood Pressure

Several factors should be considered when obtaining an accurate blood pressure. They include the following:

1. Movement of stethoscope, operator, or patient will create inaccurate sounds.
2. Stethoscope and manometer should be maintained regularly to ensure that no breaks or leaks are present in the tubes, bag, or valves.
3. If stethoscopes are shared, be certain that the ear tips are cleaned and disinfected.
4. Make sure the patient is seated comfortably and that the operator is positioned to observe the manometer clearly.
5. The bladder of the cuff should be completely empty of air before using.
6. Repeated attempts to obtain a blood pressure in the same limb may cause false readings.

▶ Charting Oral Conditions

The charting of oral conditions is a form of dental shorthand. A variety of symbols (Table 24-4) and abbreviations (Table 24-4, *B*) are used to indicate specific conditions that exist on the teeth and on the supporting structures of the mouth. The use of symbols makes it easy to look at a dental chart and to identify easily conditions that exist in the mouth, without reading a detailed narrative.

Table 24-5 lists symbols that are commonly used for a variety of conditions that exist in a patient's mouth. In some areas alternative suggestions have been made, since there are many options. This table represents commonly used symbols; however, each dental specialty area may have symbols that are unique to the specialty. Some dentists may use symbols that work effectively for them, while other dentists may prefer the use of color (e.g., yellow for gold, blue for amalgam, red for composite) to denote different types of restorations. No particular system is right or wrong; however, charting symbols need to be identified and used consistently by all members of the staff within the office.

EXTRAORAL EXAMINATION

The extraoral examination observes for asymmetry, lesions, swellings, or discoloration. Data collection begins at this point. It is an important task that requires good listening skills, attention to detail, and a high degree of accuracy. Portions of this examination may be performed by the dental assistant in some states. Regardless of who collects the data, the collection and recording must be thorough and accurate.

Data that are collected during this phase of the examination are obtained by observation or palpation. Observation is a visual inspection; it is the act of noting size, shape or contour, and color of tissues. Palpation is to use the sense of touch to denote consistency, whether the tissue is soft, firm, hard, or nodular, and to denote tenderness in tissues when they are palpated.

To palpate external tissues, the operator's fingers will be used on the outer surfaces of the face and neck or one or two fingers may be placed on the inside of the oral cavity, depressing on a finger that is held in an opposing position outside the mouth. Palpation is a gentle but firm tactile pressure.

STOP AND THINK

At the beginning of this procedure

1. Are all *universal barrier techniques* being used?
2. Is the armamentarium available and prepared for use?
3. Are the instruments arranged in sequence of use?
4. Am I prepared for alternative treatment plans?
5. Is the necessary equipment turned on and ready to operate?

TABLE 24-4, A

Term	Symbol	Term	Symbol
Abscess		Composite restoration	
Amalgam restoration		Defective restoration	DEF
Beginning furcation involvement		Diastema	
Bonding		Extraction	
Bridge		Extrusion	
Caries		Fistula	

Continued.

TABLE 24-4, A

Term	Symbol	Term	Symbol
Food impaction		Missing (radiographically confirmed) CNP-clinically not present-when not radiographically confirmed	
Fracture		Missing crown	
Furcation involvement		Mobility	M-2
Hypersensitivity		Open contact	
Maryland Bridge		Overhand (D-distal surface)	OH-D
Cast metal crown (Gold crown)		Partially erupted	PE

TABLE 24-4, A

Term	Symbol	Term	Symbol
Pocket depth	ML-5 mm / L-6 mm	Root canal	
Porcelain crown		Rotated	
Porcelain fused to metal		Sealant	PFS / ← dM
Porcelain inlay		Shifted	
Post and core		Unerupted tooth	U
Recession		Vitality	V-6

TABLE 24-5   SUGGESTED CHARTING ABBREVIATIONS

Abbreviation	Term	Abbreviation	Term
@	at	I & D	Incision and drainage
a, am, ag	Amalgam	IA	Incurred accidentally
amp	Ampule	IH	Infectious hepatitis
amt	Amount	IM	Intramuscular
anes	Anesthesia	imp	Impression
appl	Applicable, application, appliance	IMP	Impacted
		inj	Injection, injury
approx	Approximate	inop	Inoperable, inoperative
BF	Bone fragment	IV	Intravenous
BP	Blood pressure	lab	Laboratory
Br	Bridge	lac	Laceration
BW	Bite-wing radiograph	lat	Lateral
Bx	Biopsy	ling	Lingual
C	Composite	liq	Liquid
carbo	Carbocaine	LLQ	Lower left quadrant
caps	Capsules	LN	Lymph node
cav	Cavity	LRQ	Lower right quadrant
CC	Chief complaint	M, mes	Mesial
CM	Cast metal	mand	Mandibular
cond	Condition	max	Maximum, maxillary
CSX	Complete series x-rays	MDR	Minimum daily requirement
cur	Curettage	med	Medicine, medical
CV	Cardiovascular	mg, mgm	Milligram
CVA	Cerebrovascular accident	MO	Mesioocclusal
D or DV	Devital	MOD	Mesioocclusodistal
dbl	Double	mo	Month
DEF	Defective	MS	Multiple sclerosis
Dg or Dx	Diagnosis	narc	Narcotic
DM	Diagnostic models	nc	No change, no charge
DMF	Decayed, missing, and filled	NCP	Not clinically present
DO	Distoocclusal	neg	Negative
DOB	Date of birth	norm	Normal
DR.	Doctor	occ, occl	Occlusal
EMT	Emergency medical treatment	OH	Oral hygiene
est	Estimate, estimation	OHI	Oral hygiene instructions
evac	Evacuate, evacuation	opp	Opposite
eval	Evaluate, evaluation	P	Pulse
ext	Extract, external	PA	Periapical
FBS	Fasting blood sugar	path	Pathology
FH	Family history	Ped	Pediatrics
FLD	Full lower denture	PO, postop	Postoperative
FMS	Full mouth series	preop	Preoperative
FMX	Full mouth x-ray	prep	Preparation, prepare for treatment
FR or frac	Fracture	prog	Prognosis
frag	Fragment	Px, Pro, Proph	Prophylaxis
frec	Frequent, frequency	R	Respiration
FUD	Full upper denture	R_x, RX	Take (thou) recipe
G	Gold	RC	Root canal
GF	Gold foil	req	Requisition
GI	Gold inlay	resp	Respiration
ging	Gingiva, gingivectomy	RHD	Rheumatic heart disease
HBP	High blood pressure	ROA	Received on account
Hx	History	SBE	Subacute bacterial endocarditis
		Sig	Write on label l

TABLE 24-5   SUGGESTED CHARTING ABBREVIATIONS—cont'd.

Abbreviation	Term	Abbreviation	Term
sol	Solution	TMJ	Temporomandibular joint
stat	Immediately	Tr.P	Treatment plan
stim	Stimulate, stimulator	URI	Upper respiratory infection
surg	Surgery, surgeon	ULQ	Upper left quadrant
Sx	Symptom	URQ	Upper right quadrant
T	Temperature	VD	Venereal disease
tab	Tablet	wh	White
TAT	Tetanus antitoxin	wnd	Wound
TB	Tuberculosis	x	Times, such as 4x = 4 times; x-ray
TBI	Toothbrush instructions	xyl, xylo	Xylocaine
temp	Temperature	YOB	Year of birth
TLC	Tender loving care	yr	Year
TPR	Temperature, pulse, respiration		

CONDUCTING AN EXTRAORAL EXAMINATION

1. Observe facial symmetry (Fig. 24-6, *A*). Irregularities, such as drooping eyelids or lips, may be associated with some form of weakness in the musculature or other systemic conditions. For instance, prominence of the eyeballs and an enlargement in the neck may indicate that the patient has a severe thyroid condition; a cyst, such as the branchial facial arch cyst, may be causing the asymmetry in Fig. 24-6, *B*.

2. Inspect the skin of the face and neck. Note any lesions, swellings, or discoloration (Fig. 24-6, *C*). Presence of jaundice, a yellowness of the skin, may be a sign of liver disease or the retention of broken down red blood cells. These conditions can contraindicate the use of some drugs. Severe bruises about the head and face area may indicate abuse. Abuse is discussed in a later chapter. The dental professional is required to assume a legal and ethical responsibility for reporting observations of abuse.

3. Inspect the nails. This can be done in comparison with the operator's nails (if those are healthy) to distinguish the difference. Bluish color of a nail bed may indicate a chronic or acute problem with circulation, while pallor may indicate anemia. Rounded clubbing of the fingers may also indicate the presence of systemic diseases. A close observation of the nails may indicate lesions caused by nail biting habits.

4. Observe the hands. The creases in a healthy person's hands retain a normal pigmentation. The vascular bed is close to the surface in the hands and the lack of hemoglobin is evidenced by a lighter color.

5. Examine the lymph nodes. Criteria for this examination include *size and shape.* Most nodes are approximately the size and shape of a kidney bean; *mobility:* lymph nodes are freely mobile; *single or multiple:* most nodes are commonly found singly and even in groups they can be identified as separate entities; when the nodes are multiple or coalesced, it is a sign of a disease process; *tenderness* is a sign that an inflammatory process has invaded and produced tenderness.

   Begin in the *submental area,* and, with fingers opposing each other, try to trap the lymph node against muscular or connective tissue near the bone or between the fingers (Fig. 24-6, *D*). Then proceed to the *submandibular* (Fig. 24-6, *E*) and the *carotid region* (Fig. 24-6, *F*). When the nodes are examined in the parotid region, the parotid should not be prominent. The preauricular nodes are above the parotid region but are not accessible to palpation. Have the patient turn so that access can be made to examine the nodes in the *jugular chain* along the sternocleidomastoides muscle (See Fig. 24-6, *G*). Run a finger along the side of the muscle to examine these nodes.

   Examination of the lymphatic system in the head and neck area is important because the vessels of the oral cavity and face drain through these areas, and any evidence of swelling or tenderness in this area may indicate an infection or the presence of a tumor.

6. Examine the TMJ. Place a finger tip anterior to the tragus of each ear and ask the patient to open wide. Any tenderness, popping, clicking, or other abnormality in the opening, such as excessive lateral movement, should be noted. These symptoms may indicate problems with the patient's occlusion or TMJ (Fig. 24-6, *H*).

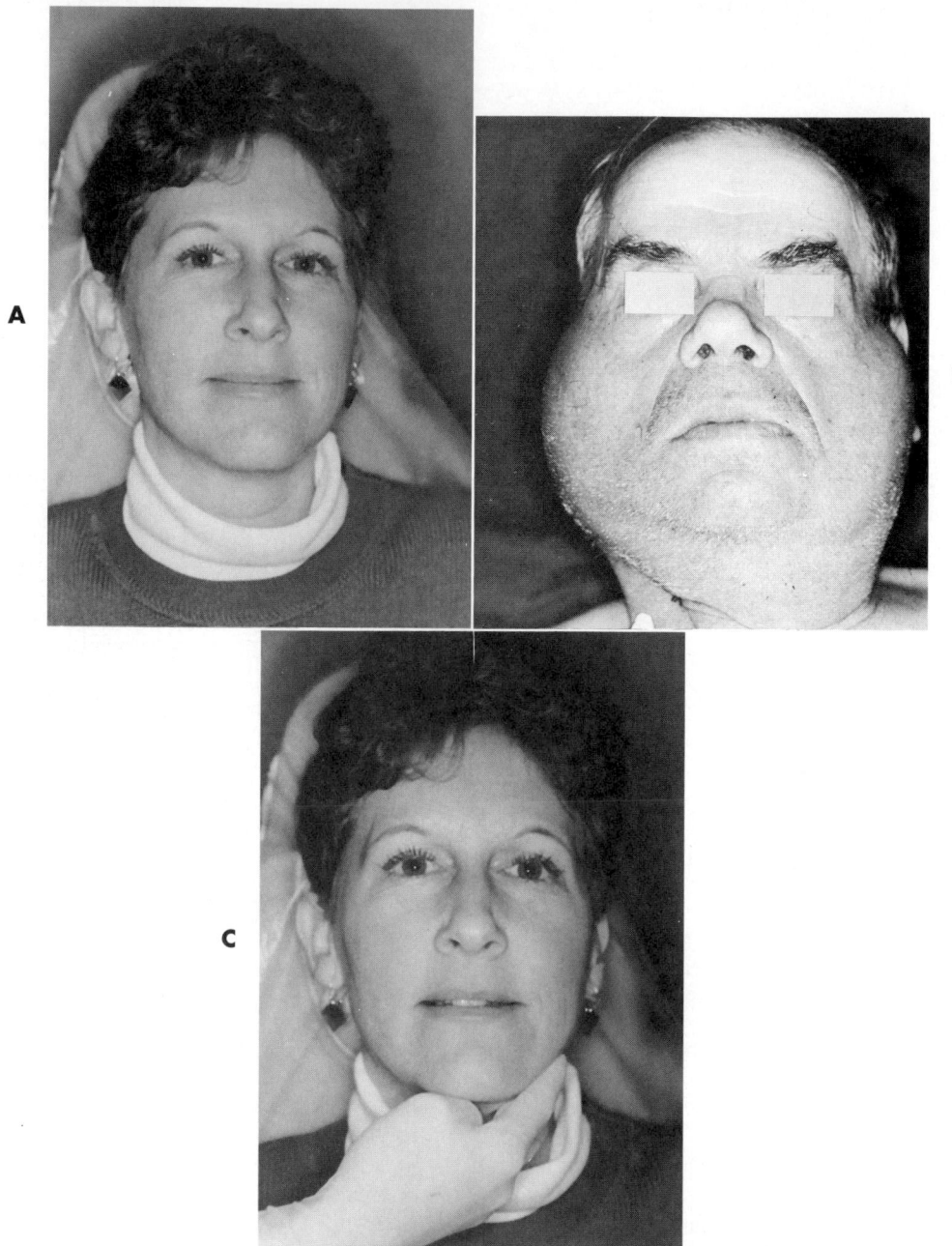

FIG. 24-6   *A,* Symmetry of face. *B,* Asymmetry of face. *C,* Inspect and palpate the neck.
(From Wood NK, Goaz PM: *Differential diagnosis of oral lesions,* St Louis, 1991, Mosby.)

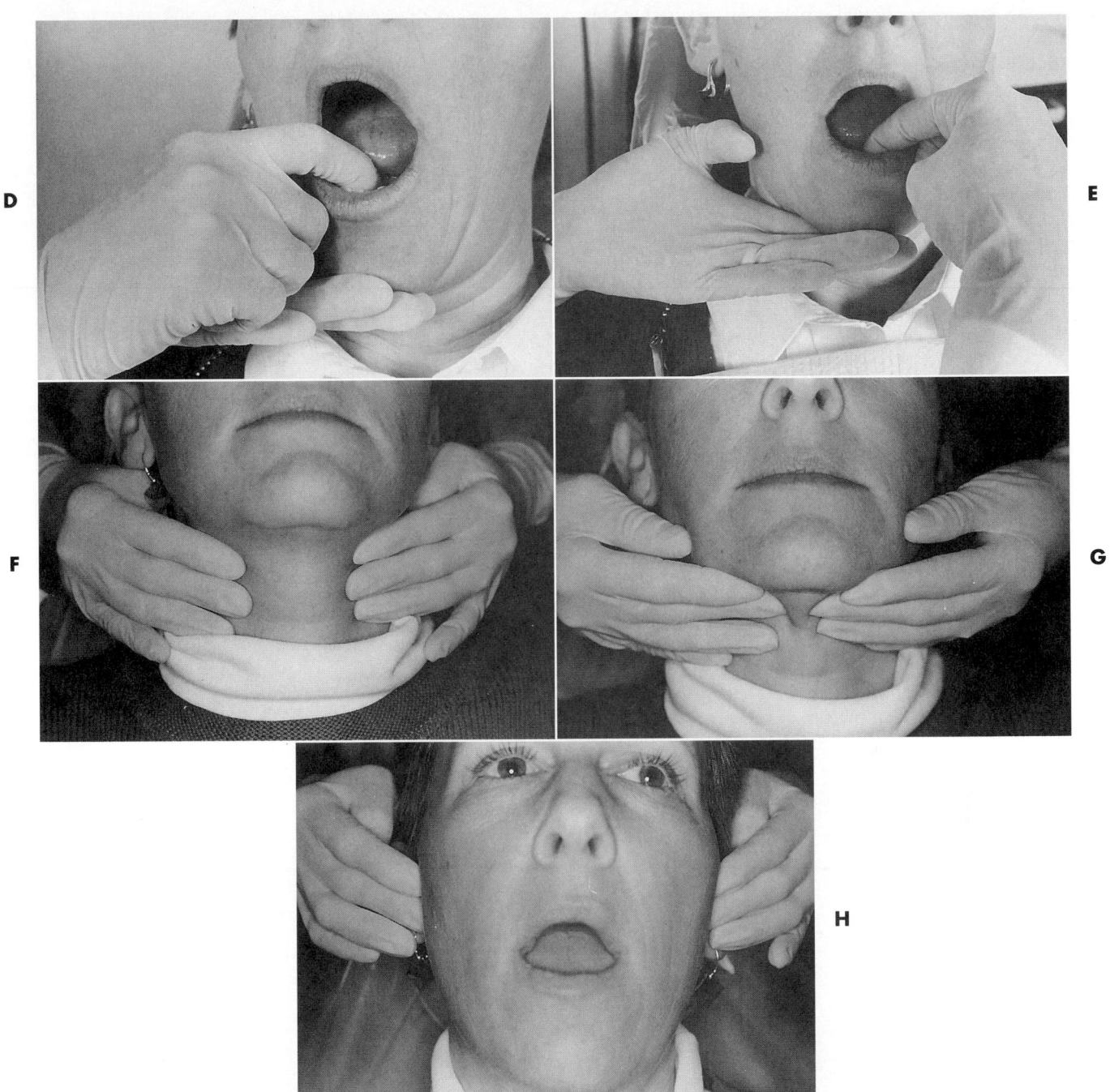

FIG. 24-6, cont'd.   *D,* Submental glands. *E,* Submandibular glands. *F,* Palpate carotid region. *G,* Examine jugular chain along sternocleidomastoid. *H,* Palpate TMJ area.

INTRAORAL EXAMINATION

The intraoral examination is divided into three phases: the soft oral tissues; the periodontium; and the teeth and their occlusal relationship. As with the extraoral examination both visual inspection and palpation are used in this examination. Once again, when intraoral tissues are inspected, the visual emphasis should be on size, shape or contour, and color; palpation should identify the consistency and the tenderness of tissue. Several factors should be considered when intraoral tissues are examined; these are listed in Box 24-7.

At this point in the procedure the patient should be placed into a supine position. The preset tray for this procedure provides the basic instruments for all phases of the intraoral examination.

Armamentarium includes the following (Fig. 24-7):

▶ Explorer
▶ Mirror
▶ Cotton pliers
▶ Periodontal probe
▶ Articulating paper
▶ 2 × 2 Gauze
▶ Napkin/napkin chain
▶ a/w Syringe tip
▶ Articulating paper forceps, optional
▶ Dental floss or tape
▶ Patient's chart or examination sheet
▶ Pencils, lead and colored (optional)

BOX 24-7

INTRAORAL TISSUE EXAMINATION

▶ Tissue integrity of covering tissues; the epithelium over the surface should be intact
▶ Degree of keratinization will vary in different parts of the oral cavity
▶ Sense of touch will indicate consistency and whether tissue is soft, firm, hard, or nodular
▶ Sense of touch will indicate tenderness; if a mass is found, if it is mobile or if it is fixed to surrounding tissue
▶ Bilateral palpation can compare one part to another
▶ Anatomic consideration; does the anatomy compare or differ to its bilateral counterpart and does it deviate from the normal?

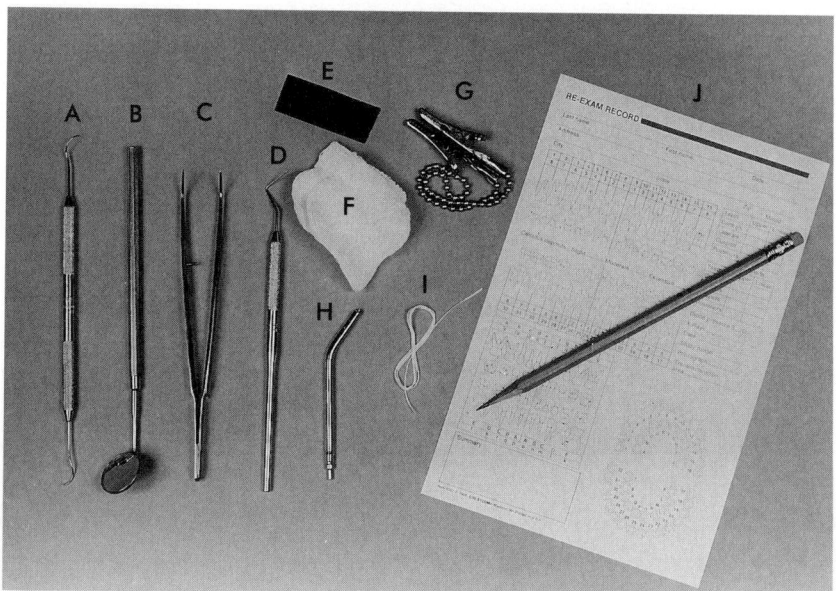

FIG. 24-7   Armamentarium for an oral examination includes the following: *A,* explorer; *B,* mirror; *C,* cotton pliers; *D,* periodontal probe; *E,* articulating paper; *F,* 2 × 2 gauze; *G,* napkin chain; *H,* a/w syringe tip; *I,* dental floss; *J,* chart and pencil. Optional: articulating paper holder.

SOFT TISSUE EXAMINATION

The first phase of the intraoral examination begins with the examination of soft tissues. The dental mirror may be used to improve vision or for retraction, while the operator performs the following:

1. Examine the upper and lower lips. Lipstick should be removed if it is worn by the patient. Once the lipstick is removed, the residue of lipstick may still mask color changes or lack of change. Look for a well-defined line of demarcation between the vermilion border and the skin. The folds or lines of the lip should be evident at right angles to the vermilion border. When the lip is palpated it should be supple and the vermilion border should be a distinctive and uniform color that is different from the rest of the labium (Fig. 24-8, *A*). Any abnormalities, such as opaque areas on the lip, loss of deep creases, thinning of surface tissue, or loss of line of demarcation between lip and skin, should be noted. Any areas of increased keratinization or scaly patches should be noted. These may be herpetic lesions, small cancers on the lip, or basal cell carcinoma. Until these areas have been diagnosed, the color and character of the lesion should be noted on the patient record (Fig. 24-8, *B*).

2. Inspect the vestibular regions, the frenum, and labial mucosa. Retract the mandibular lip, and expose the mandibular labial mucosa (Fig. 24-8, *C*). Redness in this area may indicate a smoking habit. Tiny elevations that indicate the nests of salivary glands will be evident. Similarly, the maxillary lip is raised, and the labial mucosa in this area is examined (Fig. 24-8, *D*). In both arches the base of the frenum should be well away from the gingival margin.

3. At this time the lips should be palpated to determine consistency and presence or absence of firmness, which might be associated with the underlying salivary beds. Any tissue discoloration, lesions, edema, lip or cheek habits, or undue stress on the frenum is noted. Evert and inspect the labial mucosa by palpating the lips between the thumb and forefinger. Any tenderness, swelling, or masses may be an indication of an infection or of small tumors.

4. Examine the buccal mucosa on both sides of the oral cavity, from the maxillary vestibule to the mandibular vestibule, by retracting the cheek and palpating the tissue. Parotid papilla and nests of labial salivary glands should be evident. Observe the buccal mucosa for the presence of Fordyce spots or linea alba. Identify the characteristics of the tissue and the relationship of the superior and inferior buccal frena to the gingival margins (Fig. 24-8, *E*).

5. Palpate each cheek between the thumb and forefinger to determine the presence of tenderness or of small tumors (Fig. 24-8, *F*).

6. Palpate the parotid salivary glands. Any swelling or tenderness is noted. These symptoms may indicate infection, blockage, or the presence of tumors in these glands (Fig. 24-8, *G*).

7. Progress to the posterior of the arches, using a mouth mirror to examine the maxillary tuberosity and retromolar pad areas. Observe any tissue irritation or tooth eruption in these areas (Fig. 24-8, *H*).

8. Inspect the hard palate, including anterior landmarks, such as the rugae and incisive papillae. Smokers may have increased tissue keratinization in this area. Palpate the entire hard and soft palate with the mid- or forefinger to detect swellings that might indicate an infection in this area or small tumors of the minor salivary glands. When the hard palate is palpated, there should be a continuity of the underlying bone. Tori also may be evident in this region and may go unnoticed unless the region is palpated (Fig. 24-8, *I*).

9. Continue to examine the soft palate posteriorly. When the soft palate is depressed with a finger, an underlying nodular-like area should be apparent. Depress the dorsum of the tongue to increase vision to the soft palate, uvula, and tonsils. By pressing on the tongue with the face of the mirror and asking the patient to say *ah*, these tissues will be better viewed. Inflammation of the tonsils, if they are present, can be observed, and lesions may be evident on the tip of the uvula, such as a neoplasm or a papilloma (Fig. 24-8, *J*).

10. Examine the dorsum of the tongue. Ask the patient to stick out the tongue. It is grasped with a 2 × 2 gauze. The dorsal surface is inspected, and the tongue is moved laterally to inspect both sides for the presence of lesions (Fig. 24-8, *K*). Smokers may have an increase in the length of the filiform papillae and discoloration of the dorsum of the tongue. Glossitis or geographic tongue may be observed. Ask the patient to raise the tongue to inspect the ventral surface for the presence of tumors (Fig. 24-8, *L*).

11. Examine the floor of the mouth. In the anterior portion of this area the lingual caruncle and sublingual folds are evident on both sides. A mirror can be used for retraction of the tongue to examine the color of the tissue.

12. Palpate the lingual aspect of the mandible. This is a location where mandibular tori may be evident. Run a finger along side-to-side to trap soft tissues

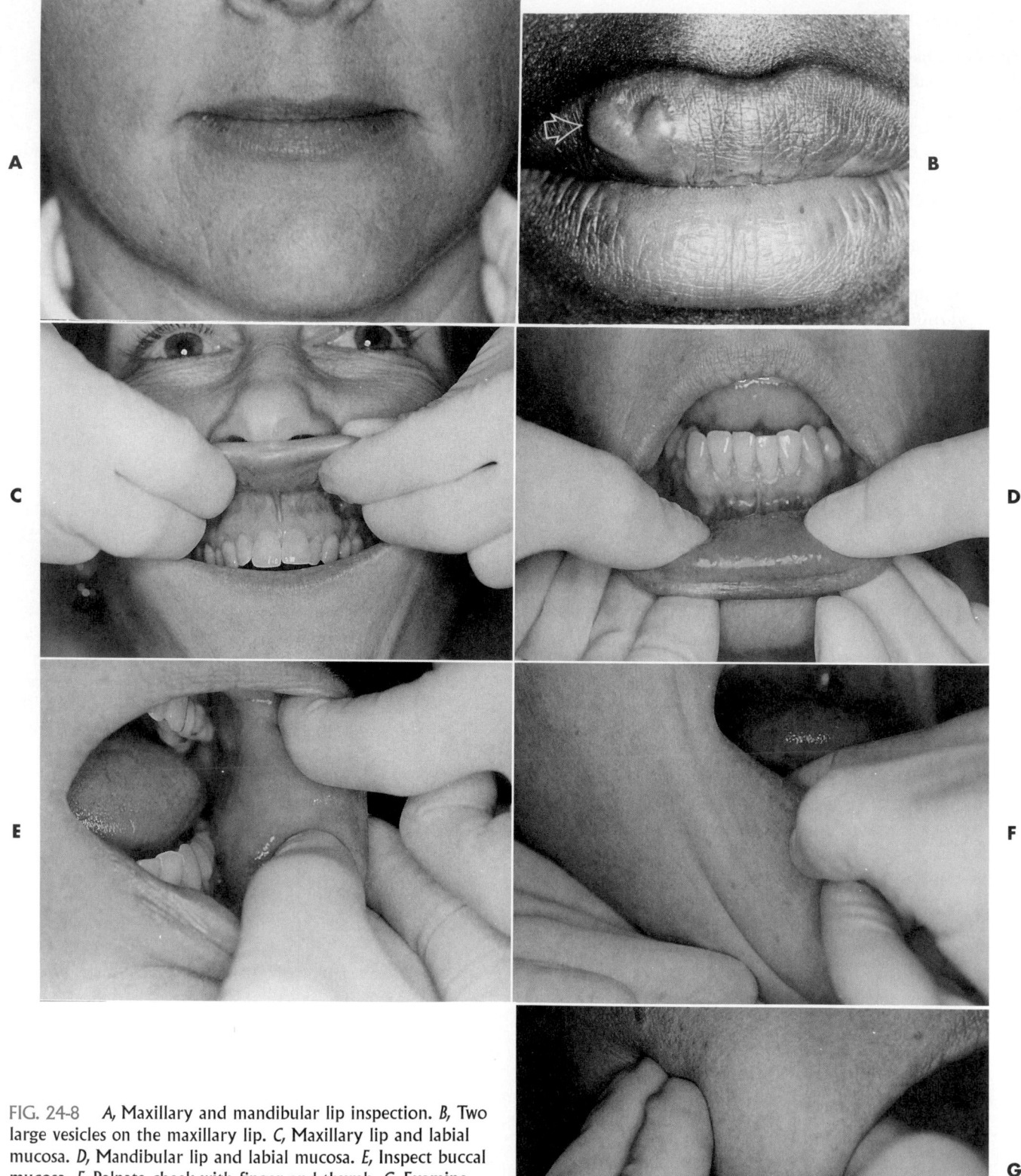

FIG. 24-8   *A,* Maxillary and mandibular lip inspection. *B,* Two large vesicles on the maxillary lip. *C,* Maxillary lip and labial mucosa. *D,* Mandibular lip and labial mucosa. *E,* Inspect buccal mucosa. *F,* Palpate cheek with finger and thumb. *G,* Examine parotid area.

(*B* from Wood NK, Goaz PM: *Differential diagnosis of oral lesions,* St Louis, 1991, Mosby.)

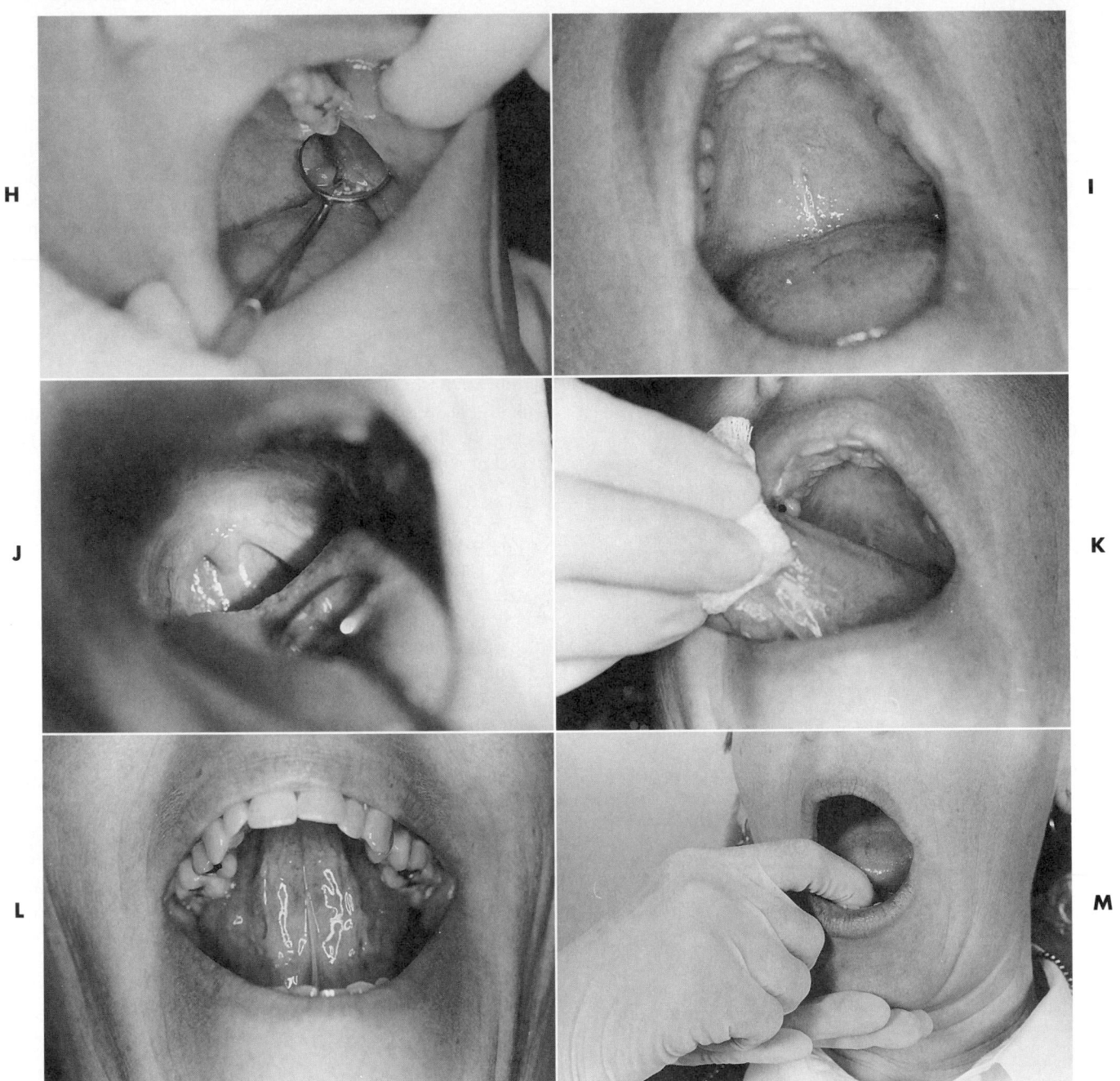

FIG. 24-8, cont'd. *H,* Maxillary tuberosity area. *I,* Examine hard palate. *J,* Examine the soft palate and uvula. *K,* Inspect dorsum and sides tongue. *L,* Inspect ventral surface of tongue. *M,* Palpate the sublingual aspect of the mandible.

with an intraoral finger and extraoral hand. In this area are the submandibular glands and the sublingual gland, though the latter is not palpable as an isolated mass (Fig. 24-8, *M*).

13. Check secretions of the salivary glands. Dry off the ductal openings of Wharton's duct, apply pressure under the anterior of the mandible and look with a mirror at the lingual surface under the tongue. Press upward with light pressure to empty the duct. Proceed to the parotid orifice and dry the site with a 2 × 2 gauze. With light pressure to the cheek, stroke the area to stimulate saliva flow from the duct.

A typical charting of the soft tissue examination would be recorded on the patient's examination sheet.

TABLE 24-6   TERMS COMMONLY USED TO DESCRIBE CONDITIONS OF THE PERIODONTIUM

Term	Meaning
Localized	The condition is confined to one area, to one tooth, or to a small segment of teeth
Generalized	Evident throughout most or all of the mouth
Slight	Beginning evidence or early stages of the condition
Moderate	Significant amount of progression, but not to the advanced stage
Severe	Most advanced stage
Bulbous	Enlarged, swollen, and rounded
Blunted	Receded, not sharp, rounded
Cratered	Crater-like depression in the center of the papillae
Normal, healthy	Tissues are dense and fibrous; in Caucasians the tissue will be uniformly pale pink; areas of pigmentation, from light to dark brown, may occur in various skin colors or races
Soft, spongy	Tissues are swollen and contain fluid
Stippled	Tissues contain many tiny indentations, a healthy condition
Bleeding	When gently probed, tissues bleed
Recession	Margin of gingiva located apical to the CEJ
Cleft	Narrow slit-like recession that occurs where margin tissue is destroyed
Red	This is erythema and indicates early or acute inflammation
Bluish purple	This is cyanosis and indicates an inflammation of chronic, well-established nature

Periodontium Examination

This phase of the oral examination includes assessment of the tissues that support the teeth: the gingivae, cementum, periodontal ligament, and the alveolar and supporting bone. The alveolar and supporting bone evaluation requires the use of dental radiographs, while the other tissues are evaluated visually and with the use of a periodontal probe and mirror. The operator will use a variety of terms to describe the conditions of the periodontium and accumulations of accretions. The assistant should be familiar with descriptive terms that are used to identify the location, severity, color, shape, or form of the periodontium. Table 24-6 lists key terms that are commonly used to describe these conditions. Additionally, the dental assistant should have an awareness of the clinical characteristics of healthy and unhealthy gingival tissues. Table 24-6 provides an overview of the most common clinical characteristics of the gingival tissues. Fig. 24-9 depicts several shapes and forms of the periodontium. During the periodontal examination the following findings are recorded in the patient's chart:

1. General health of the gingivae and notation of any signs of inflammation
2. Location and amount of plaque and calculus
3. Lack of attached gingiva
4. Presence and depth of periodontal pockets
5. Presence of furcation involvement, where pockets exist in multirooted teeth
6. Mobility of teeth
7. Position of teeth
8. Effect of existing restorations on gingival health

The periodontal probe and mouth mirror are the primary instruments that are used in this phase of the examination. The mouth mirror is used for indirect vision, illumination, and retraction, while the probe aids in determining the presence of periodontal pockets or furcation involvement. Data from this examination are recorded during each of the phases of the examination.

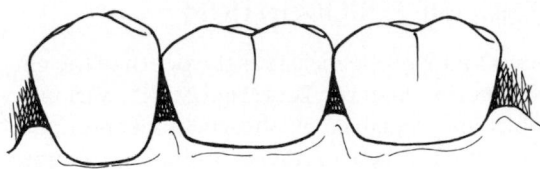

Blunted

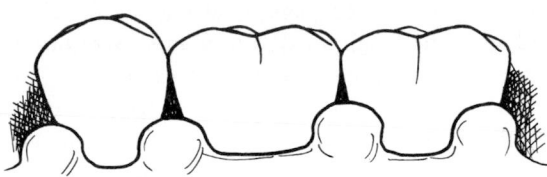

Bulbous

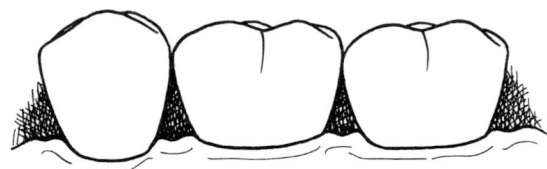

Cratered

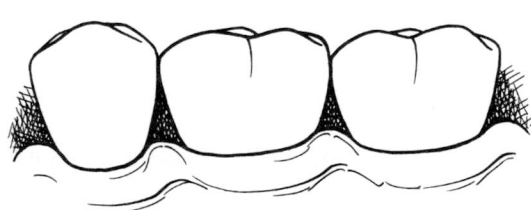

Rolled

OBSERVING GINGIVAL HEALTH

1. Visually observe the buccal gingiva by retracting the cheek with the mirror. Note changes in color, form, and texture throughout the segment.
2. Use the periodontal probe to gently press against the attached gingiva (Fig. 24-10), the gingival margin, and the interdental papilla to determine the firmness of the tissue.
3. Probe the interdental papilla area to identify the presence of inflammation or bleeding.
4. At sites of gingival recession, measure the depth of the recession from the gingival margin to the CEJ.

Continue this process around other segments of the mouth. Findings from this phase of the examination would be recorded on the patient's record.

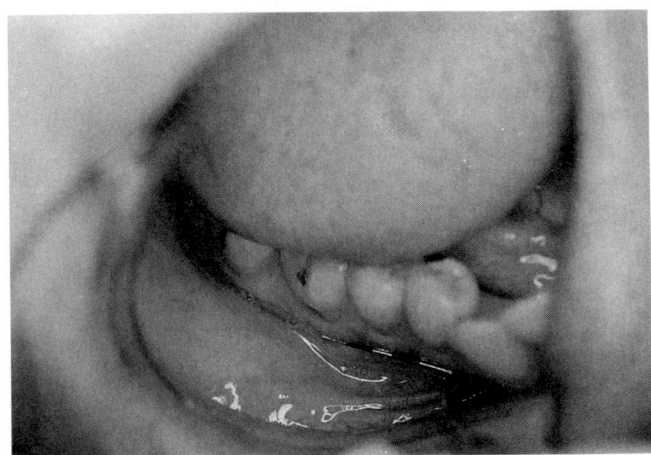

FIG. 24-10　Probe pressed against attached gingiva.

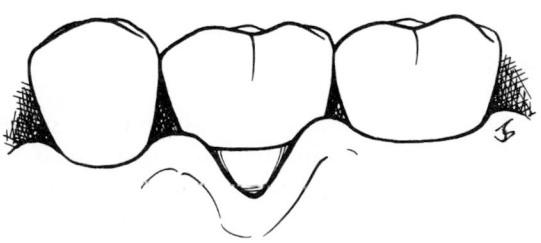

Cleft

FIG. 24-9　Several shapes of the periodontium.

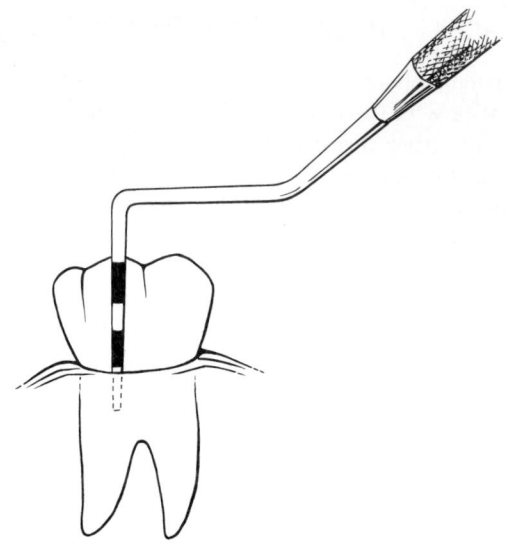

FIG. 24-11   The probe is placed into the gingival sulcus to measure the depth of the periodontal pocket.

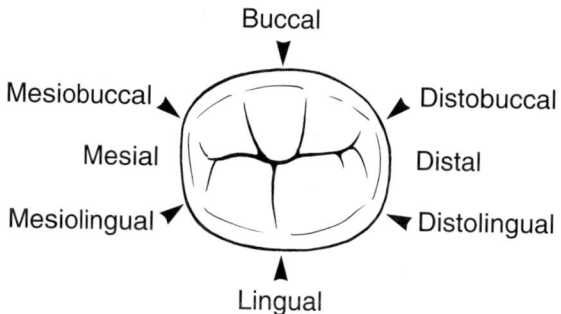

FIG. 24-12   Six points of periodontal measurement: distobuccal, buccal, mesiobuccal and distolingual, and lingual and mesiolingual.

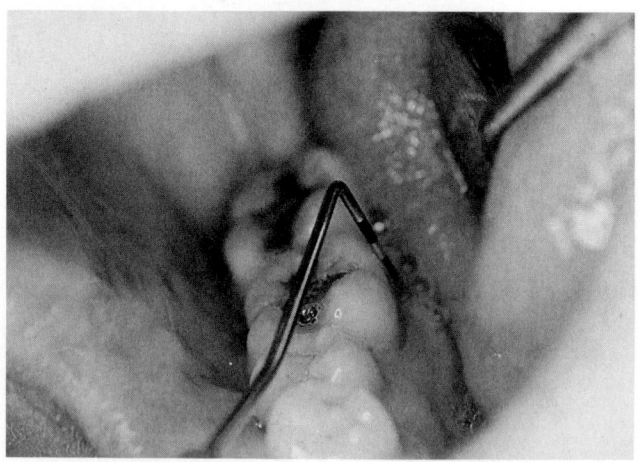

FIG. 24-13   Use of probe on tooth.

PROBING THE PERIODONTIUM

The periodontal probe measures the depth of the gingival sulcus or periodontal pockets (Fig. 24-11). Various types of probes are available, as shown in Chapter 18. The working end of each of these probes is calibrated in millimeters to facilitate in reading depth measurements. Periodontal probes are available with varying millimeter readings: 3, 6, 9, and 12 mm; 1, 2, 3, 5, 7, 8, 9, 10 mm; and 3, 6, 8 mm, or the probes are noncalibrated, as in a probe that is specifically designed for examinations of furcations. Probes are also available with alternate colored bands to designate depth. Some operators prefer the color-coded probe for increased visibility.

Measurements are recorded at six points on each tooth—three from the buccal (distobuccal, buccal, and mesiobuccal) and three from the lingual surface (distolingual, lingual, and mesiolingual) as shown in Fig. 24-12. The assistant records these data as the operator probes the periodontium to identify the presence of periodontal pockets. The operator actually *walks* the probe around the tooth, beginning at the distobuccal area and continuing around to the mesiobuccal area (Fig. 24-13). The measurements for each area are recorded (Fig. 24-14) in numeric form or in graphic form. This procedure is continued around the arch on the buccal aspect, and then the operator transfers to the lingual aspect before proceeding to the opposite arch. A healthy periodontium is one that can be probed at 2 to 3 mm. In most cases only measurements that deviate from the normal are recorded.

An alternative to manual periodontal probing is the automated system shown in Fig. 24-15. This system provides highly accurate and repeatable periodontal measurements by using a probe with constant pressure. The system requires only a single operator and records, stores, and prints a periodontal examination automatically.

During periodontal probing the operator may encounter bleeding, sensitivity, calculus, or saliva. Therefore, the assistant must observe the probing sites regularly and use the HVE tip as needed to remove fluids and debris. Frequently the operator may request that a specific site be dried thoroughly with air to improve visibility or to gain access to the gingival sulcus.

PROBING THE FURCATION

When a periodontal pocket extends apically and severe bone loss occurs in multirooted teeth, often the furcation area becomes involved. Examination of the furcation is necessary to determine the degree of involvement. The straight periodontal probe, a special furcation probe, or even a curet scaler can be used to determine if bone still fills the area between the roots. A furcation is charted as shown in the symbols in Table 24-4, *A*.

DETERMINING MOBILITY

Bone loss from periodontal disease can create tooth mobility as a result of progressive loss of the periodontal attachment. The operator will determine the degree of mobility by exerting force in a buccal-lingual direction. Each tooth is tested in a systematic method, generally beginning in the maxillary right quadrant, proceeding to the maxillary left quadrant, from there to the mandibular left, and concluding on the mandibular right. Mobility is charted as shown in the symbols in Table 24-4, *A* and may be classified as the following:

+ mobility	Movement that is barely discernible
I mobility	Movement from buccal to lingual totaling 1 mm
II mobility	Movement from buccal to lingual totaling 2 mm
III mobility	Movement from buccal to lingual totaling 3 mm

▶ Teeth

Much information needs to be recorded about the teeth. The symbols described in Table 24-4, *A* are especially helpful in this phase of the examination. All existing restorations, missing teeth, malpositioned teeth, dental caries, or other anomalies that exist on the teeth are recorded at this time. The operator may dictate the information, while the assistant records it on an examination sheet. The operator uses the mirror and explorer for this phase of the examination. The explorer aids in probing and examining all surfaces of the teeth. At this point the assistant may change from a lead pencil to a colored pencil if the office uses a color-coding system to denote different restorations. Note these pencils may be packaged and sterilized and should receive the same infection control care at the end of the procedure as other instruments receive.

The operator will typically begin in the maxillary right or left tuberosity area and progress to the tuberosity area on the opposite side of the arch, describing any abnormalities as each tooth is examined. The operator then drops down to the mandibular arch and continues examining around to the opposite side of the mouth. For instance, conditions illustrated in Fig. 24-16, *A*, might be described in the following manner:

#1 is missing
#2 has mesioocclusal caries
Food impaction between #3 and #4
Diastema between #8 and 9
#9 has mesial caries
#12 is rotated distally
#13 is missing
#14 is shifted mesially
#15 is partially erupted
#17 needs to be extracted
#18 has a beginning furcation
#19 has furcation involvement
#20 has a defective distoocclusal amalgam
#23 has mesiofacial caries
Between #26 and #27, there is an open contact
#28 is hypersensitive
#31 has cervical buccal caries
#32 is hypererupted

The three charts in Fig. 24-16, *B* through *D*, show examples of oral examinations that were completed for three different patients who had a variety of oral conditions. The codes used in these charting exercises are from Table 24-4, *A*.

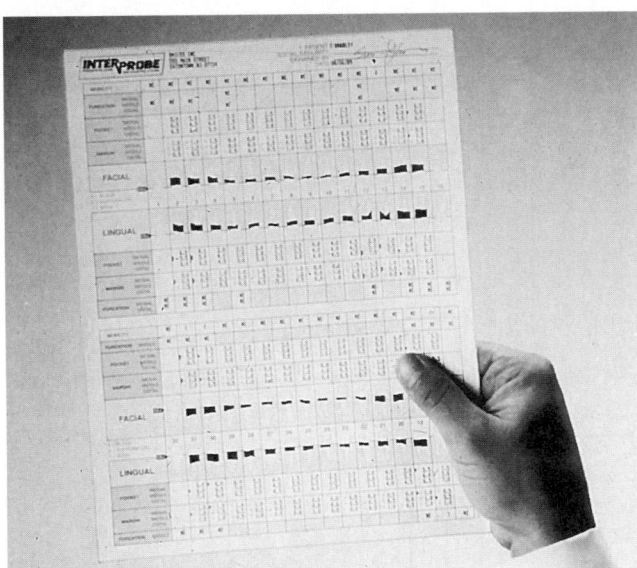

FIG. 24-14 Numeric and graphic entries of probing on a chart.

(Courtesy of Interprobe.)

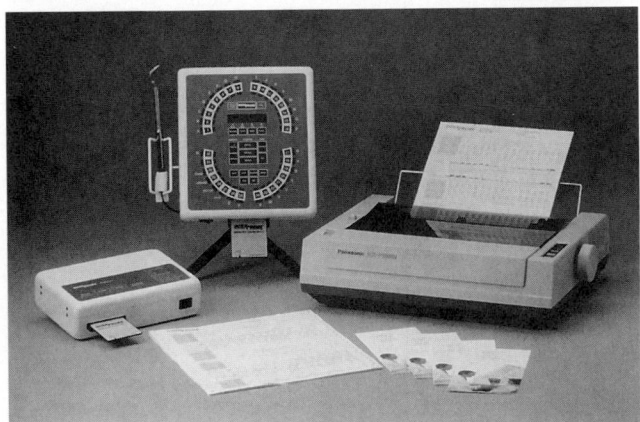

FIG. 24-15 Interprobe system, including main unit with automatic probe, printer, and chart.

(Courtesy of Interprobe.)

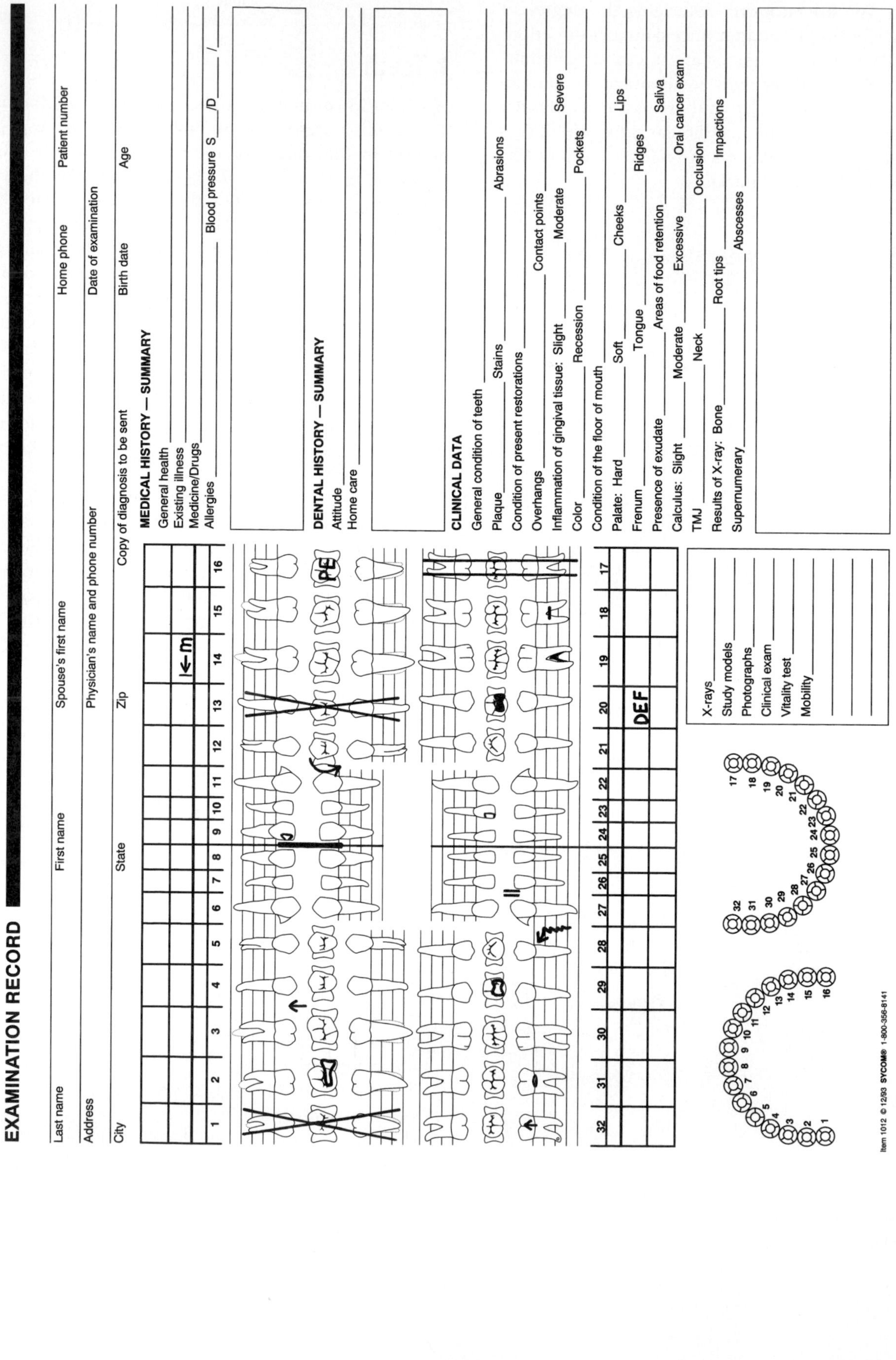

EXAMINATION RECORD

Last name ___ First name ___ Spouse's first name ___ Home phone ___ Patient number ___

Address ___ Physician's name and phone number ___ Date of examination ___

City ___ State ___ Zip ___ Copy of diagnosis to be sent ___ Birth date ___ Age ___

MEDICAL HISTORY — SUMMARY

General health ___

Existing illness ___

Medicine/Drugs ___

Allergies ___ Blood pressure S___/D___ /

DENTAL HISTORY — SUMMARY

Attitude ___

Home care ___

CLINICAL DATA

General condition of teeth ___

Plaque ___ Stains ___ Abrasions ___

Condition of present restorations ___

Overhangs ___ Contact points ___

Inflammation of gingival tissue: Slight ___ Moderate ___ Severe ___

Color ___ Recession ___ Pockets ___

Condition of the floor of mouth ___

Palate: Hard ___ Soft ___ Cheeks ___ Lips ___

Frenum ___ Tongue ___ Ridges ___

Presence of exudate ___ Areas of food retention ___ Saliva ___

Calculus: Slight ___ Moderate ___ Excessive ___ Oral cancer exam ___

TMJ ___ Neck ___ Occlusion ___

Results of X-ray: Bone ___ Root tips ___ Impactions ___

Supernumerary ___ Abscesses ___

X-rays ___

Study models ___

Photographs ___

Clinical exam ___

Vitality test ___

Mobility ___

1	2	3	4	5	6	7	8	9	10	11	12	13	14	15	16
32	31	30	29	28	27	26	25	24	23	22	21	20	19	18	17

Item 1012 © 12/93 SYCOM® 1-800-356-8141

FIG. 24-16 Four separate charts completed for a variety of charting situations. *A*, See text narrative.

EXAMINATION RECORD

Last name _____ First name _____ Spouse's first name _____ Home phone _____ Patient number _____

Address _____ Physician's name and phone number _____ Date of examination _____

City _____ State _____ Zip _____ Copy of diagnosis to be sent _____ Birth date _____ Age _____

Blood pressure S___/D___/

MEDICAL HISTORY — SUMMARY

General health _____
Existing illness _____
Medicine/Drugs _____
Allergies _____

DENTAL HISTORY — SUMMARY

Attitude _____
Home care _____

CLINICAL DATA

General condition of teeth _____
Plaque _____ Stains _____ Abrasions _____
Condition of present restorations _____ Contact points _____
Overhangs _____
Inflammation of gingival tissue: Slight _____ Moderate _____ Severe _____
Color _____ Recession _____ Pockets _____
Condition of the floor of mouth _____
Palate: Hard _____ Soft _____ Cheeks _____ Lips _____
Frenum _____ Tongue _____ Ridges _____
Presence of exudate _____ Areas of food retention _____ Saliva _____
Calculus: Slight _____ Moderate _____ Excessive _____ Oral cancer exam _____
TMJ _____ Neck _____ Occlusion _____
Results of X-ray: Bone _____ Root tips _____ Impactions _____
Supernumerary _____ Abscesses _____

X-rays _____
Study models _____
Photographs _____
Clinical exam _____
Vitality test _____
Mobility _____

Item 1012 © 12/93 SYCOM® 1-800-356-8141

FIG. 24-16, cont'd. *B*, Tooth #2 has a full coverage gold crown; #4 has an MOD amalgam; #6 is discolored; #7 has a periapical abscess; #8 has a distal incisal fracture; #9 has a porcelain crown; #11 has a labial fistula; #12 has Class II mobility; #14 has a MOD porcelain inlay; #16 is partially erupted; #18 has an occlusal amalgam; #19 has a buccal cervical amalgam; #20 has a pit and fissure sealant; #22 has a vitality of six; #24 has a facial laminate; #25 has a facial laminate; #27 has a buccal cervical composite; #29 has a post and core, cast metal crown; #30 has a fractured crown.

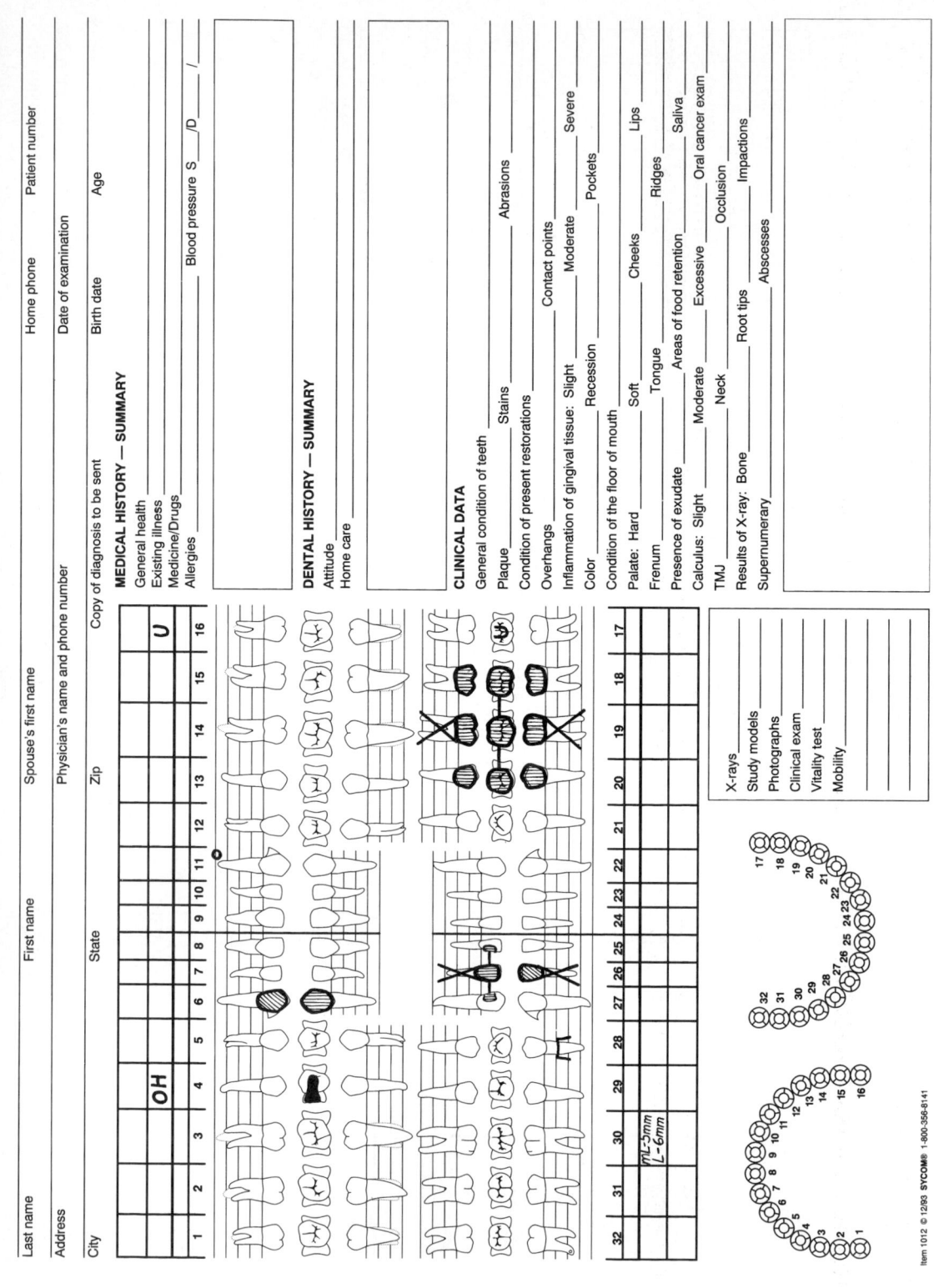

FIG. 24-16, cont'd.   C, Tooth #4 has a DO amalgam with overhang; #6 has a porcelain fused to metal crown; #11 has a labial fistula; #16 is unerupted; #17 is unerupted; #18 is a distal abutment for 3 unit bridge, full coverage gold; #19 has a gold pontic; #20 has a mesial abutment, gold crown; #25 has a mesiolingual abutment for Maryland bridge; #26 has porcelain fused to metal pontic; #27 has a distolingual abutment for Maryland bridge; #28 has recession; #30 has a periodontal pocket mesiolingual 5 mm and lingual 6 mm.

EXAMINATION RECORD

Last name   First name   Spouse's first name   Home phone   Patient number

Address   Physician's name and phone number   Date of examination

City   State   Zip   Birth date   Age

Copy of diagnosis to be sent

MEDICAL HISTORY — SUMMARY

General health
Existing illness
Medicine/Drugs
Allergies   Blood pressure S____ /D____ /

DENTAL HISTORY — SUMMARY

Attitude
Home care

CLINICAL DATA

General condition of teeth
Plaque _____ Stains _____ Abrasions _____
Condition of present restorations
Overhangs _____ Contact points _____
Inflammation of gingival tissue: Slight _____ Moderate _____ Severe _____
Color _____ Recession _____ Pockets _____
Condition of the floor of mouth
Palate: Hard _____ Soft _____ Cheeks _____ Lips _____
Frenum _____ Tongue _____ Ridges _____
Presence of exudate _____ Areas of food retention _____ Saliva _____
Calculus: Slight _____ Moderate _____ Excessive _____ Oral cancer exam _____
TMJ _____ Neck _____ Occlusion _____
Results of X-ray: Bone _____ Root tips _____ Impactions _____
Supernumerary _____ Abscesses _____

X-rays _____
Study models _____
Photographs _____
Clinical exam _____
Vitality test _____
Mobility _____
_____

16 15 14 13 12 11 10 9 8 7 6 5 4 3 2 1

17 18 19 20 21 22 23 24 25 26 27 28 29 30 31 32

17 18 19 20 21 22 23 24 25 26 27 28 29 30 31 32
16 15 14 13 12 11 10 9 8 7 6 5 4 3 2 1

Item 1012 © 12/93 **SYCOM**® 1-800-356-8141

FIG. 24-16, cont'd. *D,* The maxillary arch is covered by a complete denture. Tooth #18 has an MO amalgam; #18, 22, and 29 have buccal and lingual partial clasps; the lingual bar extends from #21 through #29; partial denture replaces teeth #19 through 21 and #30 through 31; #32 is clinically not present.

▶ Occlusion

The manner in which the maxillary and mandibular teeth contact is referred to as **occlusion**. The relationship of the two arches as they occlude (close together) is included as part of the oral examination. The operator evaluates how the patient opens, closes, and laterally moves the arches to determine if any abnormalities exist. Factors that affect proper occlusion include the relationship and size of the arches to each other; premature contact; teeth that are rotated, hypererupted, unerupted or crowded; occlusal relationships, including crossbite, overjet or overbite. Such abnormalities can cause damage to the periodontium or the temporomandibular joint, or they can create increased wear patterns on the teeth.

EXAMINING THE OCCLUSION

The operator asks the patient to gently close the arches together, and the patient brings the dental arches together in a normal position: centric position. Often, when a patient is directed to close in centric or normal position, he or she may find it difficult to close in this position or may want to bring the anterior teeth together in an end-to-end relationship. The operator may need to ask the patient to relax and bite on the *back teeth*. The operator may have observed the patient's occlusion earlier in the examination, so there will be an awareness of the proper occlusion before it is checked.

Articulating paper or marking paper is placed between the arches, and the patient is directed to bite down and slide from side to side. This action marks the surfaces of the teeth that are in improper articulation or gives evidence of interference that could cause occlusal trauma.

Through examination the operator determines whether the patient has normal; Class I; Class II, Division 1 or 2; or Class III occlusion. The factors that determine the classification of occlusion and malocclusion are discussed in Chapter 35. The clinical examination is combined with photographs, radiographs, and study models to determine the patient's occlusion. Any deviations from normal occlusion may prompt the operator to refer the patient to an orthodontist for further examination and consultation.

Radiographic Examination

The radiographic examination is a common reliable diagnostic aid for evaluating the tissues in a patient's mouth, especially those tissues not visible to the naked eye. The intraoral examination is effective in determining anomalies and carious lesions in areas visible to direct examination. The visual and tactile examination used to detect caries is adequate in most areas, but in areas of limited access, particularly the interproximal surfaces of the teeth, the quality of such an examination is restricted by the close contact points of the teeth.

In a radiographic examination, the use of bitewing radiographs aids in diagnosing interproximal caries and determining the level of the bone, the periapical radiograph illustrates the entire tooth and its supporting tissues, while extraoral radiography provides the dentist a view of the teeth in relationship to other head and neck anatomy.

▶ Interpretation

The interpretation of radiographs for the purpose of diagnosing requires a thorough understanding of radiographic anatomy found on bitewing, periapical, occlusal, and extraoral radiographic films. The ability to determine normal from abnormal structures is necessary when radiographs are evaluated. Knowledge of the type, location, size, and radiographic image of each structure is important when normal anatomic landmarks and abnormal structures are viewed and evaluated.

Dental radiographs used in conjunction with the thorough intraoral examination allow the dentist to complete the examination.

Although it is the responsibility of the dentist to diagnose, it is vital for the assistant and hygienist to realize the importance of their roles in the radiographic examination. The auxiliaries will be responsible for producing the radiographs. Consequently, a thorough knowledge of proper radiographic techniques, necessary anatomic detail, and proper processing techniques is vital to the success of creating a diagnostically acceptable set of radiographs.

BOX 24-8

RADIOGRAPHIC EXAMINATION

1. Evaluate the enamel or dentin for evidence of dental caries or other abnormalities. The periapical radiograph in Fig. 24-17 illustrates a carious lesion on the mesial of the mandibular right first molar.
2. Determine the integrity of existing restorations on the radiograph. The amalgam restoration on tooth #29 illustrates the presence of an overhang on the distal (Fig. 24-18).
3. Examine the periodontal tissues for bone loss in the area of the root or for hypercementosis. Fig. 24-19, *A*, illustrates bone loss on the mandibular anterior teeth and 24-19, *B*, illustrates bone loss between #18 and #20.
4. Examine the pulp chamber and canals for size, position, integrity, or decomposition of the tissues (Fig. 24-20, *A* is normal; Fig. 24-20, *B* is abnormal).
5. Examine the lamina dura. A healthy lamina dura is represented by a 1 to 1.5 mm radiopaque line beginning at the CEJ and surrounding the root of the tooth and separated by a fine, black radiolucent line, which is the periodontal ligament space, as shown in Fig. 24-21, *A*. When inflammation extends into the alveolus, the crest of the lamina dura becomes indistinct and fuzzy, as shown in Fig. 24-21, *B*.
6. Examine for the existence of calculus. Calculus appears radiopaque in a radiograph. Heavy interproximal calculus resembles a spur or a bulbous lump, as in Fig. 24-22.

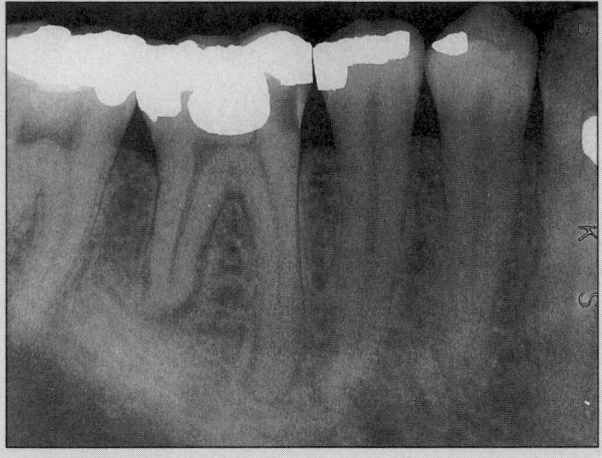

FIG. 24-17   Dental caries on a radiograph.

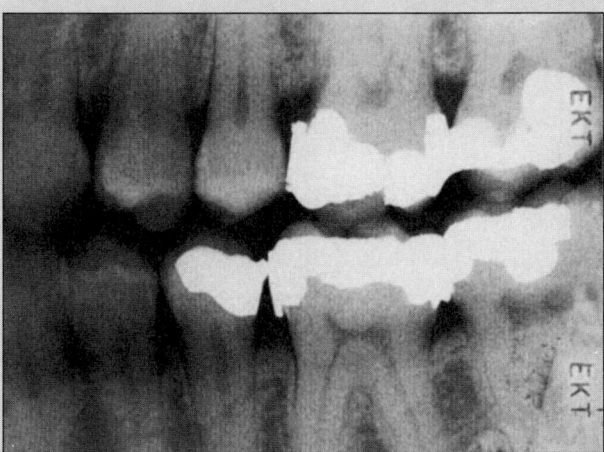

FIG. 24-18   Radiograph of an overhang on amalgam restoration.

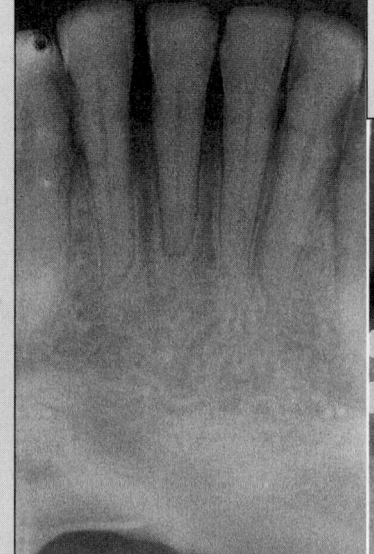

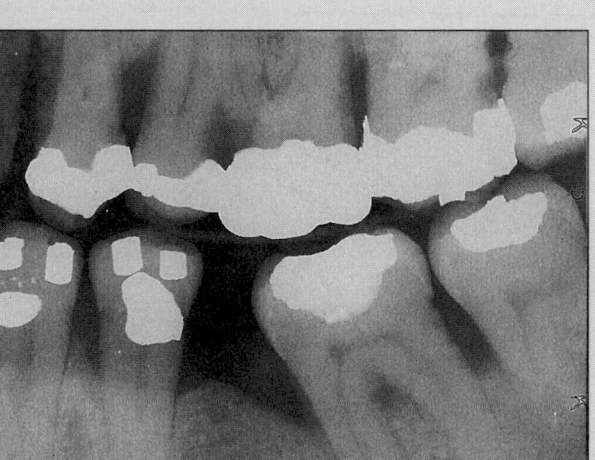

A

B

FIG. 24-19   *A* and *B*, Bone loss on radiograph.

Continued.

Box 24-8

RADIOGRAPHIC EXAMINATION—cont'd.

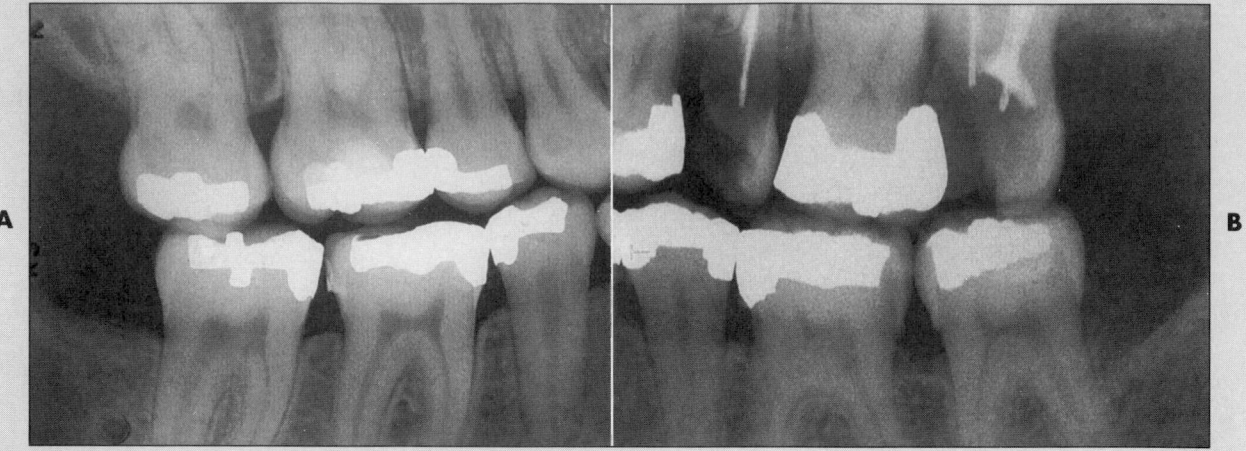

FIG. 24-20   Constriction of pulp canal. *A,* Normal, *B,* Abnormal.

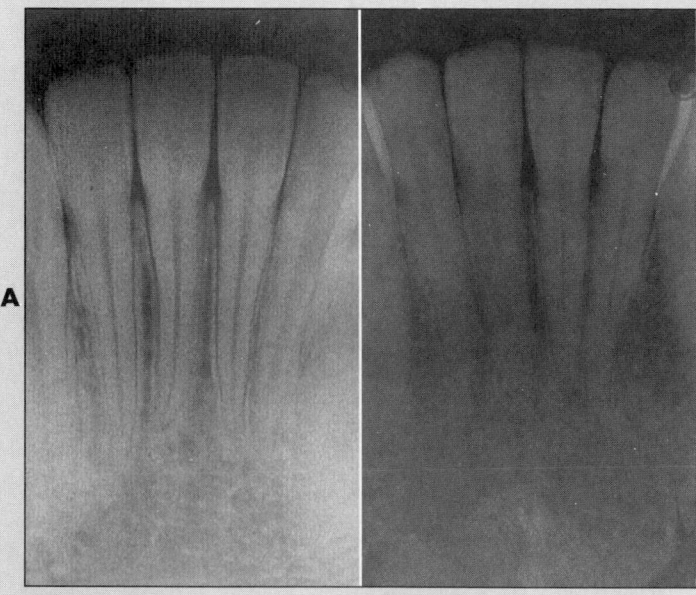

FIG. 24-21   *A* and *B,* Healthy and unhealthy lamina dura in radiograph.

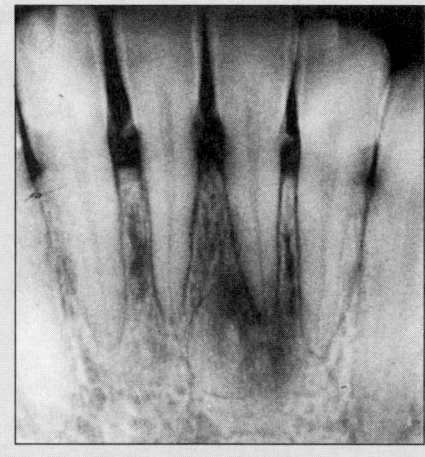

FIG. 24-22   Calculus present on a radiograph.

(From Wood NK, Goaz PM: *Differential diagnosis of oral lesions,* St Louis, 1991, Mosby.)

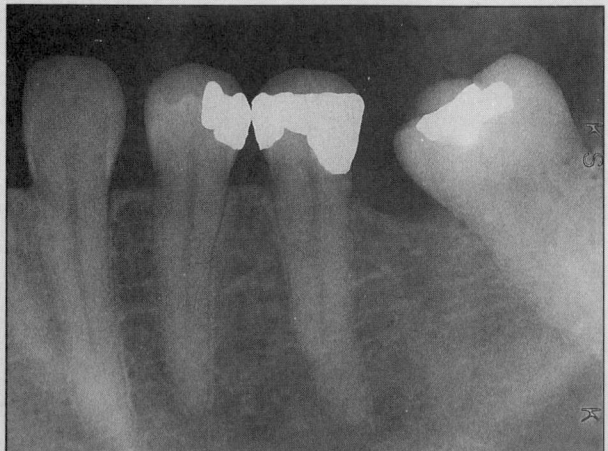

FIG. 24-23   Horizontal bone loss on radiograph.

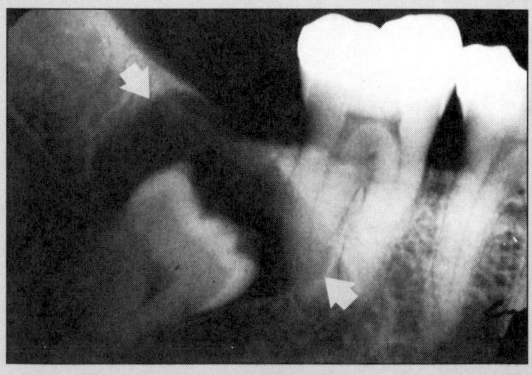

FIG. 24-24   Cyst on radiograph.

(From Goaz PW, White SC: *Oral radiology: principles and interpretation,* St Louis, 1994, Mosby.)

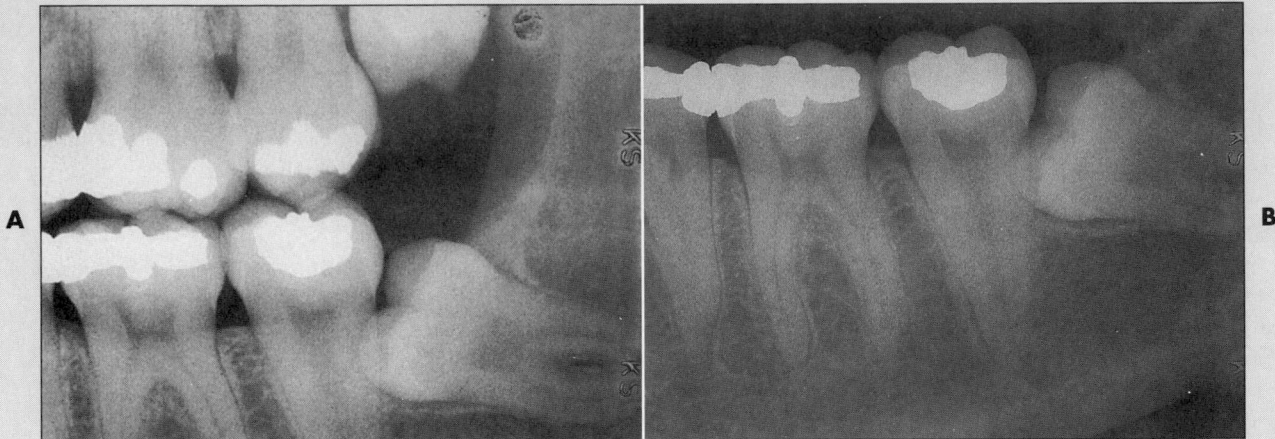

FIG. 24-25   *A* and *B*, Unerupted tooth on radiograph.

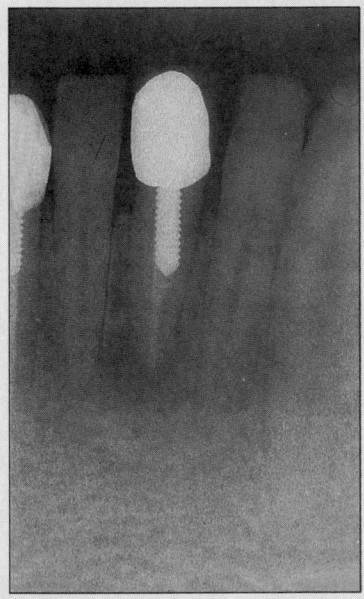

FIG. 24-26   Endodontically treated tooth.

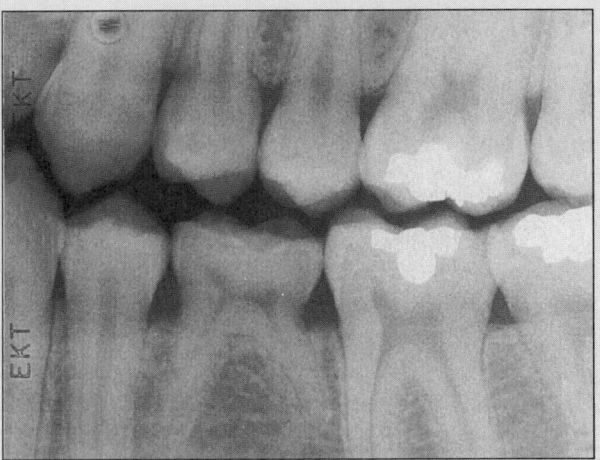

FIG. 24-27   Retained primary tooth.

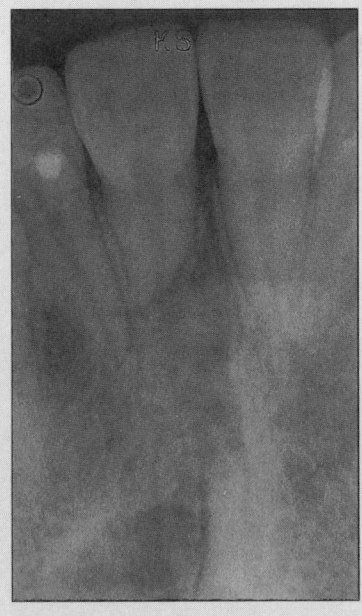

FIG. 24-28   Resorbed root caused by orthodontic treatment on radiograph.

7. Examine the alveolar bone for horizontal bone loss (Fig. 24-23) and for various levels of periodontal disease, including interdental bone loss in the posterior regions or furcation involvements.

8. Evaluate the alveolar process for the presence of cysts, tumors (Fig. 24-24), unerupted teeth (Fig. 24-25, *A* [bitewing] and *B* [periapical]), endodontically treated teeth (Fig. 24-26), or other anomalies, such as concrescence, dens invaginatus, dilaceration, gemination, fusion, enamel pearls, cleft palate, or retained primary teeth (Fig. 24-27).

9. Identify the resorption of roots caused by trauma or orthodontic treatment (Fig. 24-28) or other foreign bodies that can be observed through radiographs.

Photographic Examination

Photography has become a valuable component of a clinical record. A chart provides a symbolic annotation of the oral conditions in the patient's mouth; study models present replicas of the teeth and adjacent structures; and radiographs provide assessments of caries, restorations, and underlying tissues; only clinical photography provide a visual image that illustrates color, shape, and texture of tissues and conditions in the oral cavity.

Intraoral photography has become a significant part of comprehensive dental care, with limitless applications to any phase or specialty of dentistry. An orthodontist may use before and after photographs to illustrate the profound change that has taken place during the treatment period. The hygienist or periodontist may use photographs to differentiate between healthy and unhealthy tissue, while a prosthodontist is able to explain, with a series of photographs, the process of constructing a fixed bridge or other prosthetic device. In each of these situations photography can be used not only for patient education, but also as a motivational tool that actually allows the patient to gain a more personal role in the procedure.

Many dentists use photography to promote the practice. New forms of dental imaging and cosmetic imaging have proven successful as educational tools and as practice builders. Photography can be an excellent public relations tool, and it is not uncommon to see school, newspaper, or special event photographs of patients posted on bulletin boards or in photo albums in many dental offices. This makes the patient feel important, and it can serve as a marketing tool for the office.

The extent to which intraoral photography is used in the office depends on the dentist's and the staff's personal interest, which varies from general practice to specialty practice. Photographs provide various options for use, including the following:

- Diagnosis
- Patient education and motivation
- Research
- Case presentation
- Patient identification
- Peer review
- Dental and community education
- Public relations and marketing

◗ Photographic Equipment

Photographic equipment can be categorized into traditional still photography, intraoral imaging, or cosmetic imaging.

TRADITIONAL PHOTOGRAPHY

The selection of the camera and its attachments is generally done by the dentist. The choice can range from a simple Polaroid camera to a complex intraoral camera, with a macro lens and a ring light (Fig. 24-29, *A* and *B*). Accessories for intraoral photography are relatively simple cheek retractors and mirrors. Cheek retractors are supplied in metal or plastic, are single or double ended, and are used to retract the lips and cheeks to improve

FIG. 24-29   *A,* Polaroid-style camera for intraoral photography. *B,* Traditional 35 mm camera with light ring for increased light source for intraoral photography.

(Courtesy of Lester A. Dine, Inc.)

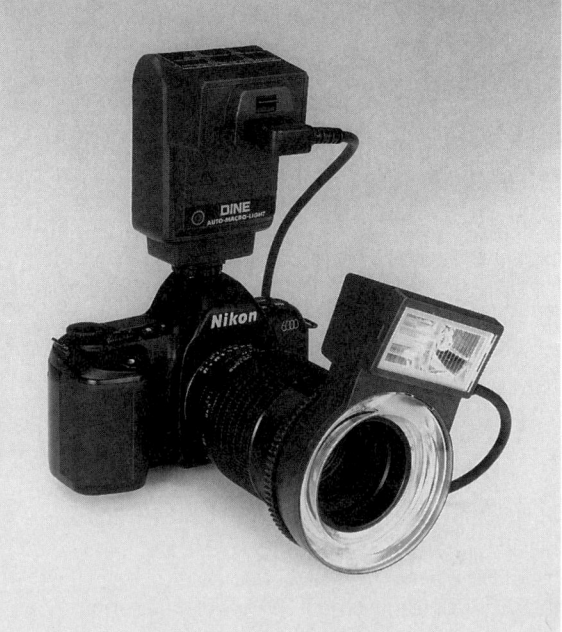

visibility of the teeth and intraoral tissues. Fig. 24-30 shows the plastic cheek retractor. The patient or assistant holds the cheek retractors, and the exposure can be made. If a mirror is used to illuminate the area or to photograph the occlusal of the maxillary teeth, a second pair of hands may be needed. Regardless of the type of camera or the complexity of the auxiliary equipment, the benefit of intraoral photography can not be underestimated. The reality of "a picture is worth a thousand words" is evident when the patient observes the before and after pictures upon completion of extensive dental treatment.

INTRAORAL IMAGING

This type of system allows the dentist to show a patient the precise oral pathology in high detail, with magnification ranging up to 38 times the actual size. This concept, illustrated in Fig. 24-31, can visually illustrate existing conditions to a patient on a monitor at chairside and can also provide a hard copy in full color prints. The prints can be made of an individual area or a composite print.

COSMETIC IMAGING

Cosmetic imaging provides the patient with a *before* and *after* visual of existing conditions, such as a fractured tooth; then specialized computer action generates a visual appearance of the way the tooth will look when it is repaired with a particular restoration. This is discussed and illustrated in greater detail in Chapter 31.

The Perspective Dental Imaging System provides a modular approach to intra-oral imaging. Start with a Basic System that includes the Camera-Handpiece/ Processor and color monitor and then add the components that best suit your needs for... • Diagnosis ▶ Treatment plan presentations • Patient education ▶ Insurance submissions • Risk management ▶ Practice marketing • Video records • Consultations ▶ Education and tracking treatment progression.

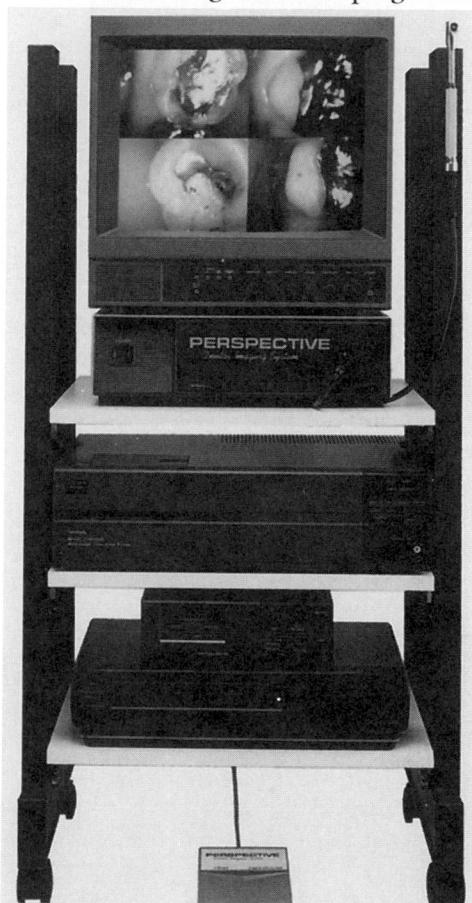

The optional Mobile Cart (19"W x 18"D x 36"H) is designed to be an adjustable system platform that can be moved from room to room while taking up the minimum amount of valuable floor space.

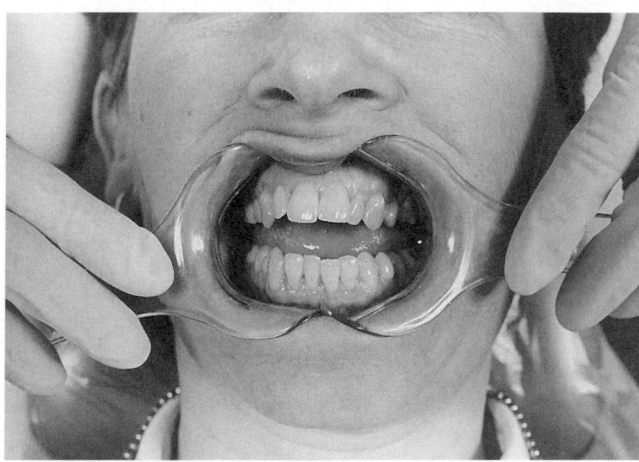

FIG. 24-30 Plastic cheek retractors.

(Courtesy of Lester A. Dine, Inc.)

FIG. 24-31 Intraoral imaging system.

(Courtesy of Dentsply International.)

Obtaining Diagnostic Impressions

One of the final steps in accumulating data for a patient is to obtain a set of alginate impressions, which are used to construct diagnostic or study models. These **diagnostic models** are three-dimensional, positive reproductions of the patient's teeth and alveolar processes. From these diagnostic models, which are generally made of plaster, the dentist is able to observe and analyze the position of the teeth, evaluate the occlusal relationships, and examine the size and shape of the alveolar processes.

The dental assistant is responsible for taking the impressions, pouring them in plaster, and trimming the casts to specifications. The finished set of models must be diagnostically acceptable and must provide an esthetic and artistic exhibit for use during case presentation.

The steps in making the alginate impressions include the following:

Assembling the armamentarium
Selecting and preparing the appropriate sized trays
Preparing the patient
Mixing the alginate

ASSEMBLING THE ARMAMENTARIUM
(Fig. 24-32)

Before impressions are taken, the following materials should be assembled in the treatment room:

2 rubber bowls
Water graduate
Water about 70° F
Powder measuring device
Flexible alginate spatula (Kerr 11R)
Alginate powder
Utility wax, rope, and sheets
Baseplate wax, or bite wafer wax
Disinfectant
Paper towels
Plastic bag
Barrier techniques

▶ Selecting and Preparing the Trays

Trays are supplied in a variety of sizes: small, medium, and large; are solid or perforated; are made of plastic or metal; and are disposable or sterilizable (Fig. 24-33). Choosing the appropriately sized tray to fit a patient's mouth is often a process of trial and error. Look at the arch, select a tray, and try it in the patient's mouth, until one tray fits. Some general guidelines should be followed to obtain the best results. For a maxillary arch select a tray that:

▶ Completely covers the maxillary tuberosity
▶ Covers the anterior teeth so that the incisal edges are in contact with the flat arch portion of the tray at least 3 to 4 mm anterior to the raised palatal portion of the tray
▶ Has enough width in the molar region to allow 4 to 5 mm distance between the widest and most apical portion of the alveolar process in the molar region

It is often wise to add rope wax to the anterior flange area to help force some of the alginate into the deepest portion of the anterior vestibule (Fig. 24-34). In addition, if a patient has a high palatal vault, place a small amount of utility wax in the palatal region to eliminate potential voids (Fig. 24-35).

The tray for the mandibular arch should:

▶ Cover all of the teeth and retromolar pad area
▶ Allow for centering the teeth labially and lingually in the tray

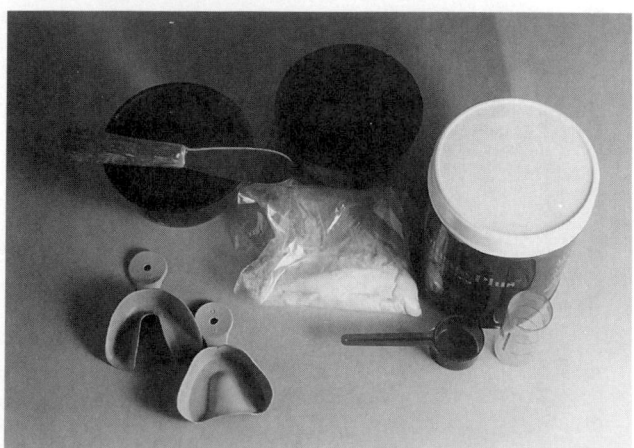

FIG. 24-32   Armamentarium for taking an alginate impression.

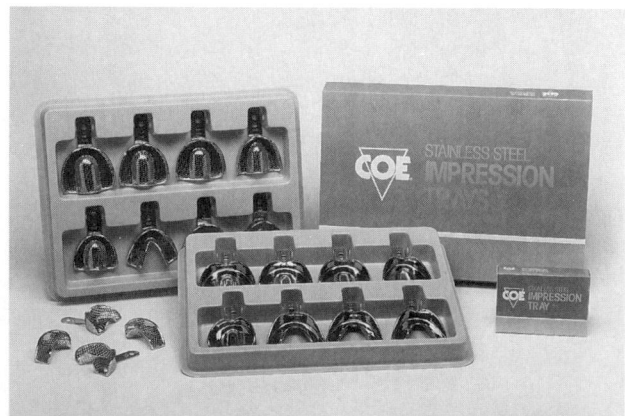

FIG. 24-33   Variety of alginate impression trays.
(Courtesy of G.C. America, Chicago Il.)

▶ Have a wax rope extension placed on the anterior labial flange to allow the alginate to flow deeply into the labial vestibule as the impression is seated in the mouth.

▶ Preparing the Patient

Before the impression is taken, briefly describe the procedure to the patient. Explain the technique, the consistency of the material, and the length of time the process will take. During the procedure, demonstrate caring for the patient by positive reinforcement and by thanking him or her for being cooperative. The patient should be seated in an upright position with the eye to ear plane parallel to the floor.

▶ Mixing the Material

Chapter 11 illustrates the mixing technique for alginate impression material. Disposable packets often are desirable because they save time and eliminate the potential for contaminating bulk material when the alginate powder is measured. The premeasured packets come

supplied with the equivalent of three scoops of powder. If bulk material is used, a general rule to follow for dispensing the material is as follows.

	Small Powder:water	Medium Powder:water	Large Powder:water
Maxillary	2:2	2:2	3:3
Mandibular	2:2	2:2	3:3

Measure the water into the bowl, add the powder, and mix according to the directions in Chapter 11. To fill the mandibular tray, pick up the material with the spatula and load one side of the mandibular tray, bringing the top layer of the material around to the opposite side (Fig. 24-36). Force the material firmly into the tray to avoid creating bubbles. When the tray is filled evenly, smooth the surface with a moist finger. The impression is taken as described in the following procedure.

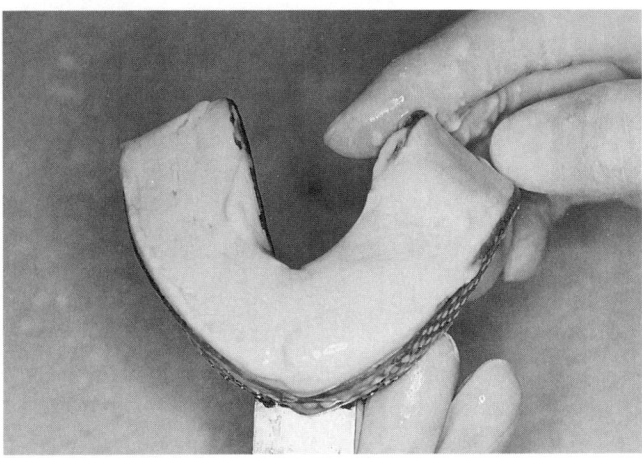

FIG. 24-36   The mandibular impression tray is filled with alginate and is smoothed.

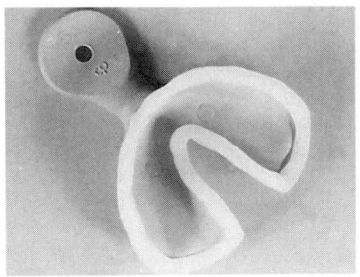

FIG. 24-34   Wax extension is placed to aid in obtaining all anatomical structures in the impression.

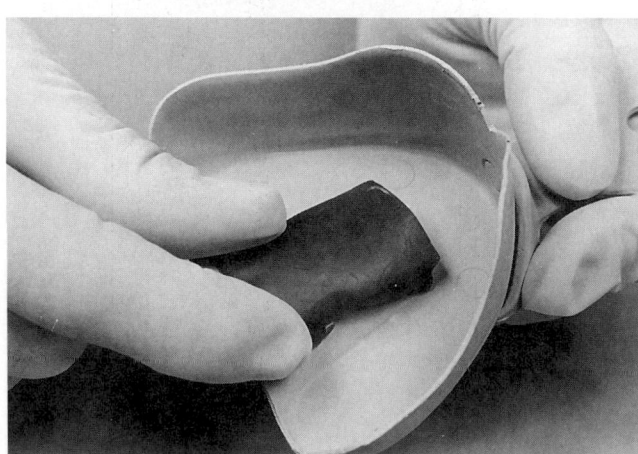

FIG. 24-35   Palatal area of maxillary tray is built up with utility wax.

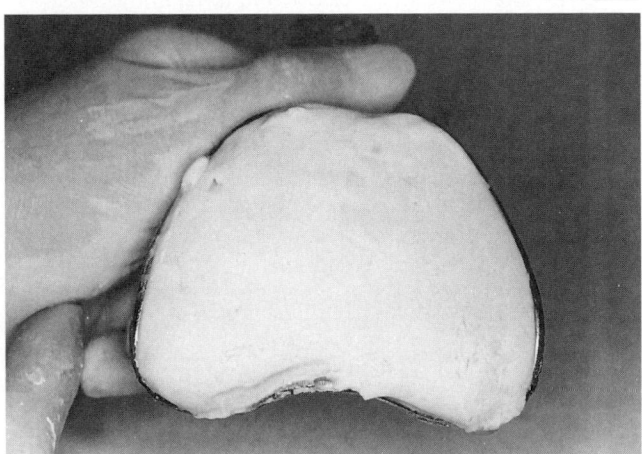

FIG. 24-37   The maxillary impression tray is filled with alginate. The filled tray is smoothed on the alginate surface.

To load the maxillary tray, pick up all of the material with the spatula and lay it on the tray, with the bulk of the material in the anterior portion of the tray (Fig. 24-37). With a moist finger, smooth the surface of the material and, if desired, make a small indentation in the material at the site of the teeth.

▶ Taking the Impression

The mandibular impression is taken first. For a patient who anticipates the potential of gagging, the positive experience of taking the mandibular impression can allay the difficulty of taking the maxillary impression where the gag reflex is present. It is wise to practice the movements of inserting the tray before the actual impression procedure occurs.

CRITERIA FOR A CLINICALLY ACCEPTABLE ALGINATE IMPRESSION

Once the impression has been obtained, it should be examined to ensure that it replicates the oral tissues accurately. Check to see that the impression meets the following criteria:

1. The impression should be free of voids, air bubbles, and tears.
2. All peripheral borders should be clearly defined.
3. Anatomic areas should be clearly defined, including coronal portions of teeth, rugae, frena, retromolar pads, tuberosities, palate, and sublingual areas.
4. Impression material should have a uniform thickness without showing exposed tray surfaces.

The impressions are then disinfected and wrapped for 15 to 20 minutes (Fig. 24-40, *A* and *B*) before pouring with a gypsum product. The procedure for pouring the impression is discussed in detail in Chapter 40.

Supplementary Tests

Although extensive medical laboratory tests are not used routinely in a dental office, occasionally such tests are ordered directly or through consultation with the patient's physician. Test results that might be used in

---

BOX 24-9

OBTAINING A MANDIBULAR ALGINATE IMPRESSION (FIG. 24-38)

1. Stand in front of the patient.
2. Ask the patient to open the mouth slightly; too wide an opening will cause tension on the cheeks and will make it difficult to insert the tray.
3. Slowly rotate the tray into the mouth.
4. With the free hand grasp hold of the lower lip and continue to insert the tray completely.
5. Seat the posterior of the tray first.
6. Be sure the teeth are centered in the tray, then seat the tray slowly but firmly in place. Take time in doing this to ensure proper seating.
7. Seat the tray until 1 to 2 mm of the alginate separate the teeth from the tray.
8. Hold the tray in place until the alginate is set.
9. When the alginate is set, break the peripheral seal gently, and remove the tray with a quick snap.
10. Examine the impression to ensure that all anatomy and associated structures have been imprinted in the impression. If not, it may be necessary to repeat the process. NOTE: Refer to criteria for a clinically acceptable alginate impression.
11. If the impression is acceptable, rinse it under running water, shake off the excess water, spray it with an acceptable disinfectant, wrap in a paper towel, and store it in a small plastic bag for 15 minutes.

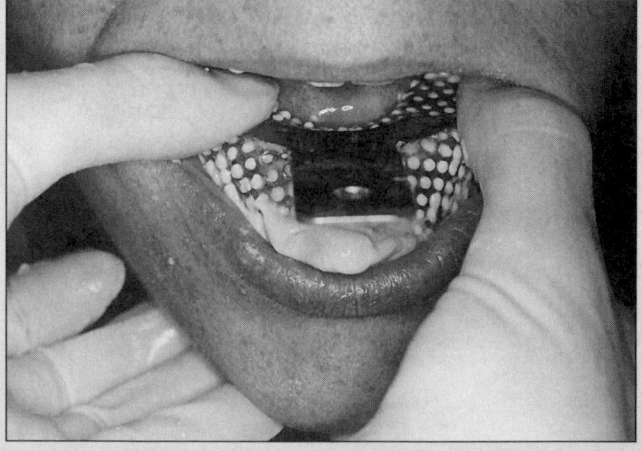

FIG. 24-38   The mandibular alginate impression is positioned in the arch with the tongue out of the way.

OBTAINING A MAXILLARY ALGINATE IMPRESSION (FIG. 24-39)

1. Stand behind or to the side of the patient.
2. Slowly rotate the tray into position, making certain that the tray is centered in the mouth.
3. Seat the posterior of the tray first.
4. Hold onto the upper lip with the free hand and pull it up and out of the way of the anterior portion of the tray.
5. Slowly but firmly seat the tray.
6. Seat the tray until 1 to 2 mm of space separate the incisal edges of the tray surface from the teeth.
7. When the impression has set, break the peripheral seal gently and then remove it with a quick snap.
8. Repeat steps 9 and 10 as described in Box 24-9.

NOTE: To ensure complete and accurate registration of tooth anatomy, a small amount of impression material may be placed on the occlusal surfaces by hand.

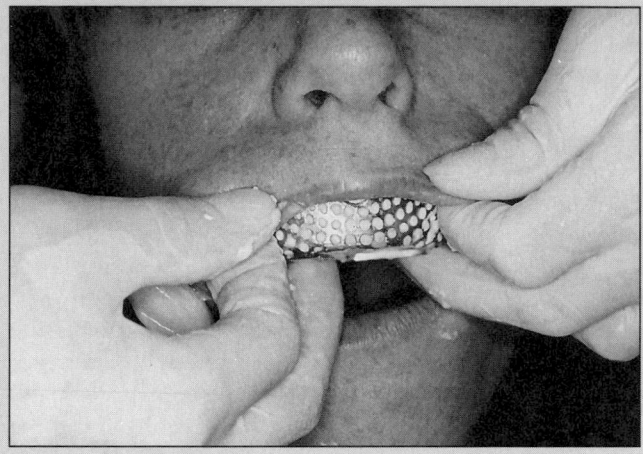

FIG. 24-39 A maxillary alginate impression is placed in the arch. The maxillary lip is lifted and positioned outside of the tray.

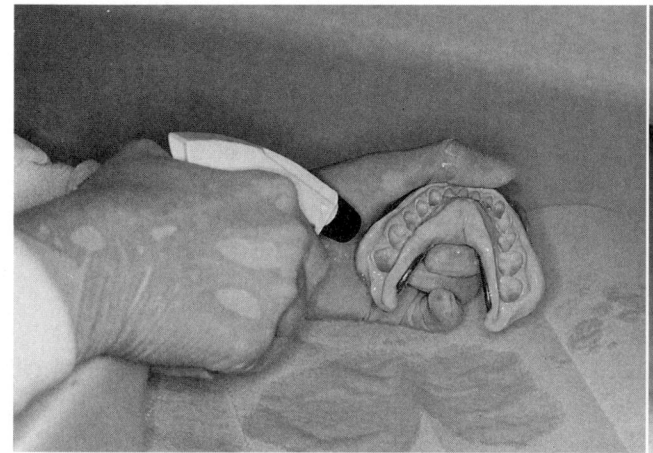

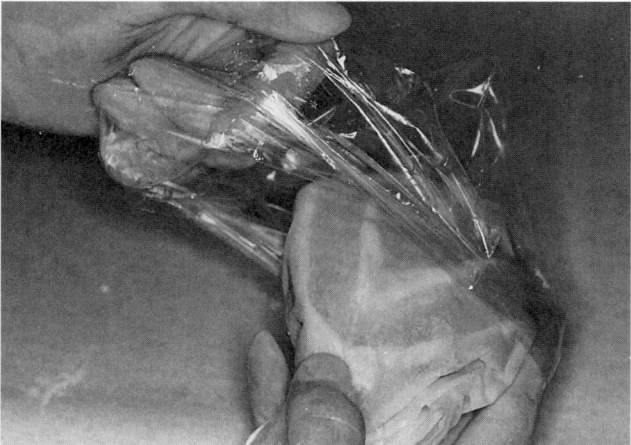

FIG. 24-40 *A,* The impression is sprayed with an approved disinfectant. *B,* The impression is wrapped in a disinfectant-moistened towel and placed in a plastic bag for at least 10 minutes.

diagnosis or during a patient's dental treatment might include the following:

- Vitality, thermal, or percussion tests are done in the dental office and may be used to indicate the physiologic condition of the pulp. These tests are described in detail in Chapter 33.
- Antibiotic sensitivity tests are used to determine the effectiveness of a specific antibiotic on a certain strain of bacteria that is causing a patient's illness.
- Caries activity tests are used to determine the

potential effectiveness of a preventive program that has been recommended for a patient, particularly the restriction of carbohydrate intake.

- Biopsy reports or exfoliative cytology are used for the detection of disease.
- Blood tests are used to indicate glucose levels for diabetic patients, to assess bleeding time for patients on blood thinning medication, or to provide white cell blood counts that may identify the presence of infection.

Case Presentation

Once all of the diagnostic data have been collected, the material is prepared for the dentist's evaluation. When it is assembled, this material will include the following:

▶ Complete medical and dental history
▶ Thorough oral examination with current findings
▶ Mounted radiographs
▶ Summary of laboratory tests
▶ Trimmed set of diagnostic models
▶ Developed photographs

The dentist will interpret the clinical data, determine a diagnosis, and recommend a prescribed **treatment plan**. A treatment plan is a recommended course of care for a patient and includes a sequence of appointments. The dentist must be careful to consider how the recommended treatment plan will be accepted by the patient. Often the dentist will ask himself or herself several questions in preparation for the case presentation with the patient.

1. Does this treatment plan satisfy the needs for which the patient presented himself or herself to the office initially? The patient may have identified a specific need "to have something done about the discolored tooth in the front of my mouth," and the dentist has not included this need as a first priority. If the patient's expressed need is not addressed, he or she may lose interest in a proposed treatment plan.

2. Have priorities been established to provide for emergency care, prevention, and long range dental care? It may be necessary to treat conditions for patient's that are painful, before progressing even to preventive care. A patient's oral hygiene may need improvement before future restorative or periodontal surgical procedures can be scheduled. The dentist's personal philosophy may enter into prioritizing treatment appointments.

3. What is the best method for presenting this diagnosis and treatment plan so that the patient has a thorough but accurate understanding of the needs and treatment procedure? Will a video, a series of photographs, models, or graphs be effective? Should the case presentation include the spouse or other responsible persons? If such persons are not included, can the patient convey the information satisfactorily to other family members? The patient may agree to pursue a treatment plan, but a spouse, as the person responsible for payment, may not understand the nature of the treatment.

4. Are alternative treatment plans available for the patient? If the plan requires extensive treatment— several crowns, fixed bridges, or extensive surgery—is there an alternative plan that the patient might consider that could extend the treatment time? Can short- and long-range treatment plans be considered? Is this feasible? What are the alternatives and the consequences of these alternatives?

The primary purpose of case presentation is to assess the patient's needs, to develop a treatment plan that will satisfy those needs, and to establish a contractual relationship between the patient and the dentist for treatment. This relationship, or informed consent, is the legal reason for the case presentation. A formal contract can be signed by the patient for the protection of both parties.

The conditions in a patient's mouth need to be explained in accurate and understandable terms. The patient needs to be informed of the risks involved and of the consequences of not proceeding with the treatment as it has been described. The process should take place in a nonthreatening environment that promotes discussion and allows the patient to ask questions. This type of environment can create a relationship of understanding, trust, and cooperation.

If during the consultation the patient hesitates or indicates a disinterest in the treatment plan it may be necessary to question the patient about his or her concerns. The patient may elicit real concerns regarding the cost of the treatment or a fear of the treatment; or he or she may not clearly understand the need for such a treatment plan. In this situation more clarification may be needed and a caring attitude can be used to reassure the patient that treatment is a team effort that involves commitment on the part of the dentist and the dental office staff, as well as on the part of the patient.

Once the case presentation has been completed and the patient has accepted the proposed treatment plan, the dentist will provide the dental assistant with the treatment schedule. Appointments and payment arrangements are then completed by the business office assistant.

KEY POINTS

▶ A clinical record includes an accumulation of clinical, radiographic, and photographic examination data from which a dentist can determine a diagnosis.

▶ A thorough dental examination includes a patient's personal, medical, and dental history; a clinical, radiographic, and photographic examination; and diagnostic models and laboratory tests. From these data the dentist makes a diagnosis and designs a treatment plan.

▶ The clinical examination is one of the most important services provided to the dental patient. This examination includes general observations, vital signs, and complete extraoral and intraoral examinations. During this procedure the dental assistant plays a vital role in the collection and recording of data.

▶ The use of symbols, terminology, and abbreviations is necessary during the charting procedure. A complete and accurate recording must be maintained to ensure comprehensive treatment and patient identification.

▶ The dental assistant must assume responsibility for learning common symbols, terminology, and abbreviations, as well as for recognizing normal and abnormal extraoral and intraoral conditions.

▶ The dental assistant will be responsible for obtaining accurate diagnostic impressions. Later, these impressions will become diagnostic models that are made of plaster for use in diagnosis and case presentations.

BIBLIOGRAPHY

Coleman GC, Nelson JF: *Principles of oral diagnosis,* St Louis, 1992, Mosby.

Kerr DA, Ash MM, Millard HD: *Oral diagnosis,* ed 6, St Louis, 1983, Mosby.

Thibodeau G, Patton K: *Anatomy and physiology,* ed 2, St Louis, 1993, Mosby.

Woodall IR: *Comprehensive dental hygiene care,* ed 4, St Louis, 1993, Mosby.

25 Managing Emergency Needs of Patients

LEARNING OBJECTIVES

You will have mastered the material in this chapter when you can:
▶ Define the key terms
▶ Identify medical conditions or health changes that may affect a patient's dental treatment
▶ Explain the management of common dental emergencies
▶ Explain the management of common medical emergencies
▶ Describe the appropriate emergency equipment for a dental office
▶ Identify the ABC's of emergency care
▶ Describe the chain of command in a dental emergency
▶ Explain the procedure for CPR
▶ Describe the Heimlich maneuver

KEY TERMS

ABC's of emergency care
Abscess
Advanced cardiac life support (ACLS)
Anaphylactic shock
Avulsed tooth
Cardiopulmonary resuscitation (CPR)
Emergency medical service (EMS)
Epilepsy
Grand mal seizure
Heimlich maneuver
Hyperglycemia
Hypoglycemia
Jacksonian epilepsy
Petit mal seizure
Psychomotor seizure
Stoma
Syncope

Each patient who visits the dental office for treatment brings a unique set of needs—needs that may be compounded by systemic diseases, recent changes in general health, prescribed medications, allergies, a disability, emotional stresses, or an unknown health problem that can trigger an emergency.

In the previous chapter, emphasis was placed on the need to collect the most current and thorough knowledge about a patient's health history when dental treatment is provided. This chapter concentrates on understanding the relationship between a patient's medical health and dental care, on learning to recognize symptoms that are common to dental and medical emergencies, and on understanding the role of the dental assistant in managing life-threatening situations.

Effect of Medical Health on Dental Care

Common situations that confront dental assistants every day involve questions that patients pose about inquiries on health questionnaires. A patient may not understand the relationship between his or her general health and dental care. Consequently, it is vital for the dental assistant to have a complete understanding of how specific medical conditions affect a patient's dental treatment. Several situations may present themselves each day in the dental office, ranging from a patient who is being treated for a malignant cancer and is to receive dental care to a patient who has had a sudden weight loss and is to have an oral prophylaxis. Each situation poses special problems and each patient requires special care.

Many categories of medical disorders pose potential complications in dental treatment, including cardiovascular disease, diabetes, a fractured limb, renal failure, or various infectious diseases. Several of these categories are described in the following discussion. Table 25-1 lists common diseases and changes in general health that may directly affect the patient's dental care. A review of this table will aid the dental assistant in understanding the effect certain diseases or physical changes have on dental care. Alternatives in dental treatment may warrant consultation with the patient's physician, adjustment in a patient's medication, modification of the dental treatment plan, or simply an adjustment made in the position of the dental chair.

Systemic Diseases

A positive response on a health questionnaire about rheumatic fever, mitral valve prolapse, or any placement of prosthetic replacement parts should initiate the dentist's questioning the patient to determine the extent of damage, to ascertain whether the patient is presently under a physician's care, and to determine the preoperative precautions that must be taken during routine dental care. History of a heart murmur may increase the risk of subacute bacterial endocarditis (SBE) and may require the use of antibiotic therapy before an oral prophylaxis or extractions. The dental team must be aware of current drug treatment guidelines for treatment against SBE during dental care.

Cardiovascular disease, such as arteriosclerosis or myocardial infarction, may indicate a patient is on some form of blood-thinning medication, such as Coumadin.

TABLE 25-1 COMMON DISEASES AFFECTING DENTAL CARE

Condition	Oral manifestation	Relation to dental tx.
Epilepsy	Gingival hyperplasia as a result of drug therapy	Seizures that are not controlled by drug therapy may occur during dental treatment
Pregnancy	Poor nutrition may result in increased carious activity or in a periodontal condition	Potential harm to fetus from radiation (x-ray examination) or drugs
Sexually transmitted disease	Soft tissue lesions, chancre, stomatitis, periodontal disease, hairy leukoplakia, lymphadenopathy, Kaposi's sarcoma, squamous cell carcinoma, xerostomia	Transmission of infectious disease during dental treatment may increase risk of infections and potential for bleeding
Joint/artificial prosthesis	None	Dental treatment may introduce bacterium into body systems causing secondary infections; bleeding might be excessive if anticoagulants have been taken
Diabetes mellitus	Oral ulcerations, possible periodontal disease, and abscesses	Potential increase for infection; wound healing may be compromised in uncontrolled diabetic patient
Murmur	Usually none	If functional, treatment is normal; if organic, premedication may be necessary to avoid infection or SBE
Tuberculosis	Ulcerations, lymph node involvement	Infection may be transmitted from patient to dental team member or from dental team member to patient
Cardiac arrhythmia	Medical treatment may result in ulcerations, petechiae, xerostomia	Use of epinephrine or increase in stress may cause arrhythmias; cardiac pacemaker patient may be at risk if interference occurs in the function from electric pulp testers or dental chairs

For this reason, further inquiry must be made to determine the treatment the patient is currently receiving. Diseases such as tuberculosis, hepatitis, and AIDS were all discussed earlier in Chapter 8, *Infection Control.* However, such questions must be included on the health questionnaire and follow-up queries, regarding the status of the disease, are necessary.

Patients with pulmonary disease, such as emphysema, require special attention, since the use of an inhalation type of sedation may pose a serious risk. Certain chair positions, such as the supine position, may cause the patient to have difficulty with breathing.

Gastrointestinal disease, such as hiatal hernia or peptic ulcer, present special dental needs. A diet and the frequency of feedings for a patient with peptic ulcer may present a situation that causes a high cariogenic level. This condition may require special home care instructions.

A patient with any of the endocrinopathies, such as diabetes mellitus, hyperthyroidism, Addison's disease, or a patient who is taking steroids presents special problems in dental treatment. When a patient with diabetes is treated, the dentist must know how to control the disease if the patient depends on insulin and must be knowledgeable about the type of insulin that is being taken. Infection and healing are primary concerns for a patient with this disease. Treatment for a patient with hyperthyroidism may need to be postponed until the patient is in a controlled state. Excess stress and the potential of infection must be avoided with patients who have this disease. A patient who has Addison's disease must avoid dental treatment during stressful times because the patient may be weak or may display hypotension or dizziness. If a patient is taking steroids, the type of steroid, the dosage, and the expected length of therapy must be known.

▶ Cancer Patients

A thorough head and neck examination must be performed as part of routine patient examination. Early detection of cancerous or precancerous lesions could result. Prompt diagnosis and treatment of cancerous lesions have a direct correlation to the patient's survival rate. The clinician must be cognizant of abnormalities in the oral tissues and surrounding areas. If necessary, the patient should be referred for biopsy and further treatment.

When a patient has received a diagnosis of cancer, pretreatment dental care may become an important part of the overall approach to the cancer. Pretreatment care for a cancer patient requires that the oral cavity be free of any active caries or sources of infection before any palliative therapy. Treatment can be planned for the patient with a cancerous lesion that is removed with local excision just as it can be planned for any other patient; the timeliness of the care may be important. The patient is monitored regularly for any recurrence of the disease after treatment.

The patient who receives radiation therapy, which includes penetration of the radiation beam through the dental arches and salivary glands, may anticipate radiation caries. Teeth that are nonrestorable or those that have support structures which involve advanced periodontal disease are usually removed through extraction before therapy, allowing adequate time for healing before radiation therapy begins.

Radiation caries can quickly involve pulpal tissues, with subsequent involvement of surrounding structure. Secondary oral infections, such as candidiasis, as well as other bacterial and viral infections, are often found in the oral cavity following radiation therapy. With a decrease in salivary secretions, teeth may become hypersensitive; some relief is found when topical fluoride is applied. Radiation therapy may cause a loss of appetite for the patient. The appetite will often return in 3 to 4 months after treatment is completed. During the interim, however, the lack of stimulation and the patient's diet may complicate the health of the oral tissues. Other complications of radiation therapy may be mucositis, xerostomia, osteoradionecrosis, and muscular dysfunction.

Dental treatment for chemotherapy patients must include relief of all sources of oral infections. Good oral hygiene habits must be encouraged. For children who receive chemotherapy, all primary teeth that are slightly mobile should be extracted before treatment begins. Teeth that are being orthodontically treated must be free of bands. If a prosthesis is needed because of the removal of cancerous tissue, impressions should be taken before radiation therapy begins.

If emergency dental care is needed during the regimen of chemotherapy treatment or radiation therapy, the dentist should seek medical consultation. If treatment is needed, antibiotic therapy may be recommended, particularly if surgery or other invasive care is provided.

Managing Dental Emergencies

The dental assistant may encounter calls from patients who are experiencing emergency needs. It is the responsibility of the dental assistant to screen these calls to determine the nature of the emergency and to obtain as much information as possible about the patient's needs. Several important concepts about emergency care should be considered at this time.

▶ Displaying a Caring Attitude

When a patient experiences pain it is often a crisis for him or her and the assistant must display a caring and concerned attitude. The patient, regardless of whether he or she is a patient of record or a new patient, has called your office and expects service. To delay the patient's emergency needs for several days or weeks will cause the patient to seek treatment elsewhere.

The patient is often anxious and frightened when he or she experiences pain or trauma. Therefore, a calm voice and a display of a caring attitude may sound like this: "Mrs. Brown, I'm sorry to hear you are having such discomfort. Could you tell me a little more about the problem?"

▶ Obtaining Pertinent Emergency Information

When a patient calls the dental office during an emergency, it is important to obtain as much pertinent information about the emergency situation as possible. Ask the questions carefully and concisely, and avoid repeating the same question; however, be certain to ask the questions that will provide complete and accurate information (Box 25-1).

▶ Determining an Office Policy for Emergencies

The dentist and staff need to determine a policy for handling medical or dental emergencies. Factors to be considered in establishing this policy should include the following:

1. Who determines if the situation is life threatening?
2. What is the chain of command when the person who usually makes this decision is absent from the office?
3. What procedures are implemented to transfer a patient to another dental office or facility?

Certainly one factor that will generally make scheduling easier is to set aside some buffer time—approximately 15 minutes—each morning and afternoon that can be used for emergencies. Many dentists like to reserve late morning or afternoon for emergencies or to catch up on other unfinished work. The later time is often more convenient for patients also because they may not contact the office first thing in the day. When a buffer time is set aside, the patient can be told that he or she can be seen at a specific time.

▶ Respecting Other Patients' Time

Be considerate of other patients when an unexpected emergency arises. If a patient who has an emergency is seen during midmorning or afternoon, causing a significant delay in the day's appointment schedule, look ahead and determine whether future appointments can

---

BOX 25-1

GATHERING COMPLETE AND ACCURATE INFORMATION WHEN HANDLING EMERGENCY SITUATIONS ON THE TELEPHONE

1. Obtain the patient's correct and complete name. If a patient says, "This is Mrs. Brown, and I am having a lot of pain in one of my teeth," you need to inquire, "Mrs. Brown, may I have your first name and the correct spelling of your last name?" Accurate identification of a patient will help locate the proper clinical record.
2. Ask the patient to describe the discomfort, and as he or she responds, determine the following:

   ▶ Type of pain: sharp or dull, continuous or periodic, increasing or subsiding in intensity
   ▶ Length of time the pain has been experienced: days, hours, weeks
   ▶ Sensitivity to temperature: hot or cold
   ▶ Discomfort on biting or chewing
   ▶ Swelling or redness in a specific area; if yes, where?
   ▶ Specific tooth that can be identified as causing the discomfort

3. If the call relates to an accident, determine if the tooth is fractured, if the tooth is avulsed, if soft tissues are cut, or if bleeding has occurred.
4. Determine if this emergency can be handled in the office.
5. If the doctor is not available, follow a predetermined plan for referring the patient to another doctor.
6. If the patient is to be treated in the office, survey the appointment book and schedule a time to treat the patient. If the patient has been in an accident, he or she needs to be seen as soon as possible in the office.
7. Reassure the patient that the staff will attempt to do everything possible to provide comfort. Be personable, display empathy, and let the patient know that he or she is important and that his or her dental care is of primary concern.

---

be rescheduled. Patients appreciate courtesy and respect for their time and may be willing to reschedule the appointment, rather than to come to the office and wait for an hour.

Handling Specific Dental Emergencies

Specific dental emergencies occur frequently. In the following discussion some of the most common dental emergencies have been described with suggestions for obtaining information, common symptoms, and some recommendations for these problems.

▶ Abscess

Two types of abscesses may occur in the oral cavity: periapical or periodontal; each can present significant discomfort to the patient. The periapical abscess is described in Chapters 6 and 33. The periodontal abscess is discussed in detail in Chapters 7 and 37. Symptoms frequently identified with the periapical abscess may include the following: sensations of pressure, severe pain, severe reaction to hot temperatures but relief with cold temperatures, edema, redness, a fistula on the oral mucosa near the apical end of the tooth, or discomfort on biting. The symptoms of the periapical abscess may also be identified by pain; however, these symptoms may be accompanied by bleeding, redness, edema, and blunted gingival tissues.

In each of these situations the patient must be seen by the dentist as soon as possible. It may not be possible for the dentist to complete a treatment procedure for the patient during one appointment. Endodontic treatment may be necessary for the periapically involved tooth, and a series of appointments may be needed for the periodontally involved tooth. The patient needs to be informed that the doctor will be able to see him or her at a certain time to determine the nature of the problem and perhaps to render some treatment; however, future appointments may need to be rescheduled.

▶ Avulsed Tooth

An avulsed or dislodged tooth presents a real emergency to the dental office staff. Replanting permanent teeth into the alveolus enjoys a relative success. This type of accident occurs frequently in young children, and success is predicated on quick action on the part of the parent or caregiver and the dental staff. The child must be seen immediately. Studies have shown that the success rate of replants is correlated with the time that has elapsed between the dislodging and the replant. Replants done within 20 minutes have greater retention success than those that are performed after an hour.

The caregiver should be instructed to wrap the tooth in a clean moistened gauze or fabric (even immersing the tooth in milk is acceptable) and bring it and the patient to the dental office immediately. Also, instruct the caregiver to place a gauze or small piece of fabric over the tooth socket, and direct the child to bite on the gauze. The pressure on the socket will help to control the bleeding. The procedure for replanting the avulsed tooth is described in detail in Chapter 36, *Pediatric Dentistry;* a child in contact sports is most susceptible to this injury.

▶ Fractured Tooth / Restoration of Loosened Crown

When a patient calls and states that he or she has broken a tooth or has lost a crown or other type of restoration, the primary concerns will include the following:
  ▶ Whether the patient has the crown
  ▶ If there is discomfort
  ▶ If sharp areas on the tooth are irritating the tongue or cheek

If a crown or fixed prosthesis has loosened (and if the crown is available) an appointment can be scheduled to determine if the restoration can be recemented. If so, the crown is recemented. If not, the crown may be used as a temporary, and new appointments need to be made to prepare the tooth for the new restoration. If the restoration is an intracoronal, the fractured material has no value.

A fractured tooth or a fractured restoration is not unlike the situation just described. The difficult task is to determine on the telephone the type of restoration that is needed for patient comfort and whether this requires replacing the restoration or whether a more extensive restoration is needed. Whichever the case, it is wise to inform the patient that the initial appointment will be made to determine the nature of the problem and that if time permits, the doctor will also attempt to place the restoration. However, if some other type of restoration is needed, additional appointments will be scheduled.

▶ Lost Temporary Restoration or Interim Dressing

A temporary restoration is often placed, while a permanent restoration (often a casting of some type) is constructed in the laboratory. Since the temporary restoration is used initially to protect the tooth from discomfort, fracture, hypereruption, or potential drifting, it is important that the temporary be replaced. If the patient is not experiencing discomfort and if an appointment can be scheduled within a day, the doctor may suggest that the patient wait until the originally scheduled appointment. If not, the patient should be seen as soon as possible.

A similar situation may occur when a patient has had an interim periodontal dressing placed; this dressing might fracture away and not remain intact. The same approach just discussed for the fractured temporary restoration may be taken. If it will be several days before the patient's scheduled appointment, consult the doctor to determine if the dressing warrants replacement. In this situation the dressing needs to be replaced, since the tissue healing is enhanced by retaining the dressing; therefore, the patient can be scheduled for an appointment to replace the dressing. If the dressing is not to be replaced, the patient should be cautioned to avoid hot and spicy foods and trauma that could be caused by toothbrushing.

▶ Broken Prosthesis

When the patient calls about a broken denture or partial denture, he or she is usually concerned about esthetics. If the fracture can be treated in the office, the patient can wait while the repair is being made. In some circumstances it may not be possible to repair the denture quickly, and the patient may return later that day or the next day. For such a procedure, check with the dental laboratory to determine the repair schedule for the patient.

▶ Displaced Orthodontic Band

This type of emergency is not unlike the lost restoration, yet it may require less time to replace. If the patient has the band, it should be brought with him or her to the office and an appointment scheduled for cementing it.

Managing Medical Emergencies

When the dental team finds itself in the middle of a medical emergency, individuals must work as a *team*. The informed response and teamwork of the dental professionals may be synonymous with the patient's survival.

▶ Establish a Chain of Command

At the time of any medical emergency in a dental office, all personnel must be aware of their own responsibilities during the emergency. Prior delegation of responsibilities to ensure a swift and competent response to an emergency situation is mandatory for an efficient functional team to meet the patient's needs.

Normally, more than one team member is present at all times when patients receive dental treatment, furnishing a team approach to managing medical emergencies. All vital signs should be monitored for patients on a regular basis—every 6 months, or more often if necessary. Usually, the dentist determines the individual responsibilities of the team and is also the team leader, directing others in their duties. Without a clear delineation of responsibilities and leadership, an incident could result in confusion and possibly lead to a more involved medical emergency.

All members of the team should be aware of the location of emergency equipment and be familiar with its maintenance and use. The assistant is usually responsible for organizing the emergency kit as directed by the dentist. All drugs in the kit must be replaced before the expiration date. Oxygen cylinders are kept full and are maintained; all equipment should be easily accessible.

Emergency telephone numbers must be current and posted at all telephone locations.

Certification in a clinical course of basic life support and additional training of all office personnel in management of medical emergencies are recommended. Some states require current certification of dental personnel in cardiopulmonary resuscitation techniques for renewal of their individual dental licenses. Basic life support knowledge and application are probably the most important preparation in management of medical emergencies.

Fortunately, the incidence of medical emergencies in dental offices does not occur frequently. Even though emergency skills may not be tested regularly, the dental team must always be ready to shift into the emergency mode with automatic responses. Emergency practice sessions, simulating different medical situations, should be conducted periodically to test the team's ability to meet the anticipated needs. Practice in medical emergencies is the only insurance the team has of efficient performance in an actual emergency.

▶ Emergency Equipment

Every dental office should have complete and current emergency equipment. The emergency equipment should include an emergency drug kit with injectable and noninjectable drugs, as well as other items, including an oxygen delivery system, suction and suction devices, syringes, tourniquets, cricothyrotomy needle or scalpel, variously sized artificial airways and airway adjuncts (shown in Chapter 10).

All emergency drugs in the kit are available in *unit doses* or in preloaded syringes. But the use of drugs is not a recommended course of action until the ABC's of basic life support techniques have been tried without success. Often the use of oxygen or basic life support would be the common course of care in most situations in dental offices.

INJECTABLE DRUGS

Injectable drugs are usually divided into three groups: essential, nonessential, and the **advanced cardiac life support (ACLS)** drugs. The ACLS drugs are usually kept separate from the basic emergency kit. ACLS drugs are kept in dental offices that have personnel with advanced training in ACLS.

Essential drugs are those that are deemed necessary to manage emergency situations and include the following:

Epinephrine—selected to manage immediate allergic reactions

Antihistamine (chlorpheniramine)—used to treat allergic reactions that have a longer period (1 hour) of onset

Anticonvulsant (diazepam)—used to manage seizure disorders

Narcotic antagonist (naloxone)—used to act against narcotic and respiratory depression

Nonessential drugs are not always considered part of an emergency kit because clinical application requires additional clinician background in their use. These drugs include the following:

Analgesics (morphine)—for use with pain, anxiety, and congestive heart failure

Vasopressors (Vasoxyl)—to raise blood pressure in unknown cardiac situations

Corticosteroid (Solu-Cortef)—to deal with acute allergic reactions after use of epinephrine and antihistamines

Antihypoglycemics (50% dextrose solution)—to control seizures and unconsciousness from an unknown source

ACLS drugs are administered by those individuals with ACLS training for care of patients with emergency cardiac care situations. ACLS drugs include the following:

Sodium bicarbonate—used during cardiopulmonary arrest

Atropine sulfate—applied in severe sinus bradycardia with hypotension

Lidocaine—for use in tachycardia and fibrillation

Calcium chloride—used during cardiac arrest

NONINJECTABLE DRUGS

The category of noninjectable drugs is probably more familiar to the dental assistant, since contact with these drugs may be more common in the dental office. This category includes the most important drug in the emergency kit: oxygen. The noninjectable drugs include the following:

Oxygen—used at times in emergency situations where respirations are difficult or do not exist

Vasodilator (nitroglycerin)—particularly used with chest pain, often angina pectoris and acute myocardial infarction

Respiratory stimulant (aromatic ammonia)—an aromatic ammonia vaporole to stimulate respiratory centers

Antihypoglycemic oral (carbohydrate)—particularly used with diabetes mellitus or nondiabetic patients with hypoglycemia

Bronchodilating agent (metaproterenol)—used for respiratory difficulty from asthma or allergic reactions

The emergency drug kit and equipment in your dental office could be the only barrier between life and death for a patient. The regular maintenance and refurbishing of all emergency apparatus are the responsibility of all dental personnel. A record of this routine care should be maintained. One individual may be responsible for maintaining current inventory. Various substances in the

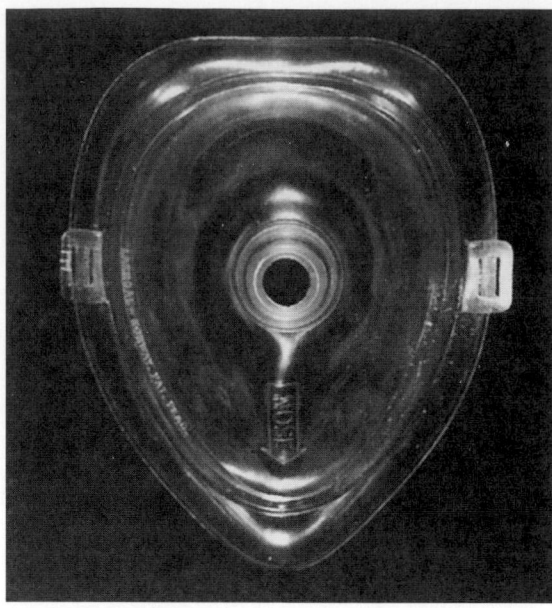

FIG. 25-1   Protective face shields and masks are important parts to an emergency kit.

emergency drug kit have a limited shelf life and must be replaced regularly. Universal barriers should be maintained with the emergency equipment. Protective gloves, masks, and glasses are included in this equipment, as well as face shields and masks that are placed between the mouth of the rescuer and the victim (Fig. 25-1).

Emergency Action and Cardiopulmonary Resuscitation

Emergency action principles and **cardiopulmonary resuscitation (CPR)** techniques are lifesaving skills that all individuals—especially health professionals—should be capable of performing when an emergency situation arises. CPR skills are needed to assist individuals who have respiratory and cardiac emergencies. An emergency could involve an infant, a child, or an adult; consequently training should involve first aid for patients of all ages. Lifesaving skill levels are designed to help individuals in particular age groups: infants, children who are 1 to 8 years, children who are 9 years of age and above, and adults.

An important factor in the successful outcome of any emergency situation requires consistent repetition of steps. The repetition of steps ensures remembering the steps in an emergency situation.

▶ Emergency Action Principles

When a health professional faces an emergency situation in a dental office, the principles advocated by the

American Red Cross and American Heart Association apply. The patient should be comforted if he or she is conscious and should be assured that the professional is trained in first aid. The patient should be assessed for responsiveness by positioning yourself near the patient, touching the patient, and shouting "Are you OK?"

If the patient does not respond, shout for help to draw attention if you are alone, so that they will alert the EMS system. At this point the patient must be placed on his or her back. The rescuer should place personal protective barriers and then survey the patient's condition to determine the patient's ABC's: airway, breathing, and circulation levels.

▶ Rescue Breathing

The next step in administering emergency aid to the patient is the *A* of the ABC's: opening the patient's *airway*. This is accomplished by a technique called the head-tilt/chin-lift. Place your hand closest to the patient's head on the forehead and apply force backward, tilting the head back. The patient's chin is brought forward until the teeth almost contact. With this step the tongue is lifted away from the back of the throat and the airway is opened. After the airway is opened, move on to *B:* check for maintenance by looking, listening, and feeling for any activity of *breathing* for 3 to 5 seconds. If you see chest movement and can hear and feel air passage, the patient is breathing; however, if there is only chest movement, the patient may not be breathing.

If the patient is not breathing, place the patient's head in the head-tilt/chin-lift position and close the nose opening by pinching the nostrils closed. Open your mouth, take a deep breath, and immediately seal your lips tightly over the patient's mouth. Force 2 full breaths at 1 to 1½ seconds per breath into the mouth, with pauses between to replenish your air supply and to watch for the patient's chest to fall after you have removed your mouth. At this point repeat the techniques for listening and feeling the air releasing from the patient's chest.

If any resistance is met when breath is released into the patient's lungs, the tongue may be blocking the airway and the head position may need to be adjusted. The *C,* or checking of *circulation* as you check the carotid pulse, follows to determine if the patient's heart is beating. If **EMS**, an **emergency medical service**, was not called before these steps were performed, they should be called at this point and informed if the patient is conscious, is breathing, and has a pulse.

If the patient has a pulse but is not breathing, rescue breathing is begun by maintaining the airway and administering a breath every 5 seconds and by checking the rise and fall of the chest and the pulse. This procedure must be maintained until EMS personnel arrive and relieve you of your responsibilities. During rescue breathing the rescuer may force air into the patient's

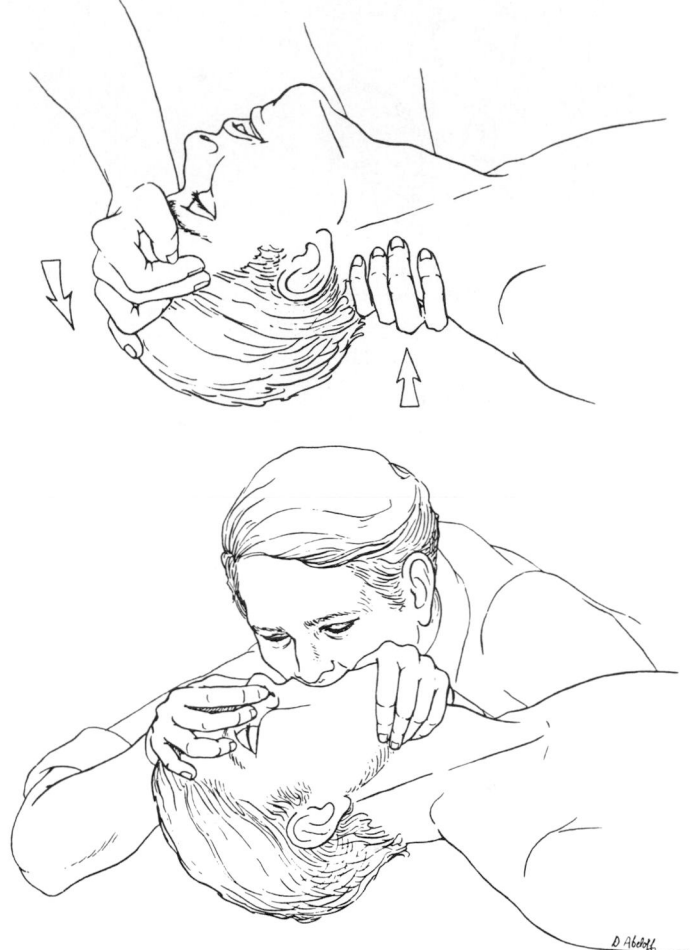

FIG. 25-2 Rescue breathing series.

stomach, which can cause vomiting; the stomach contents can be aspirated into the lungs, which could lead to death. Make sure the patient's head is tilted properly, do not breathe too fast into the lungs, and do not breathe into the lungs after the chest has risen to prevent the patient vomiting (Fig. 25-2, *A* and *B*).

Certain situations require other techniques to access air to the patient's lungs. If the airway is not clear, it may be necessary to perform mouth-to-nose breathing, or if the patient has a **stoma** (a surgically prepared opening in the throat because of medical complications), mouth-to-stoma breathing may be required. If a patient who wears dentures requires rescue breathing, the dentures should be left in place, giving support to the mouth and cheeks; however, if the dentures are loose to the point of blocking the airway, they should be removed.

▶ Airway Obstruction

It is possible for a patient to aspirate a dental object during treatment when a rubber dam is not used for

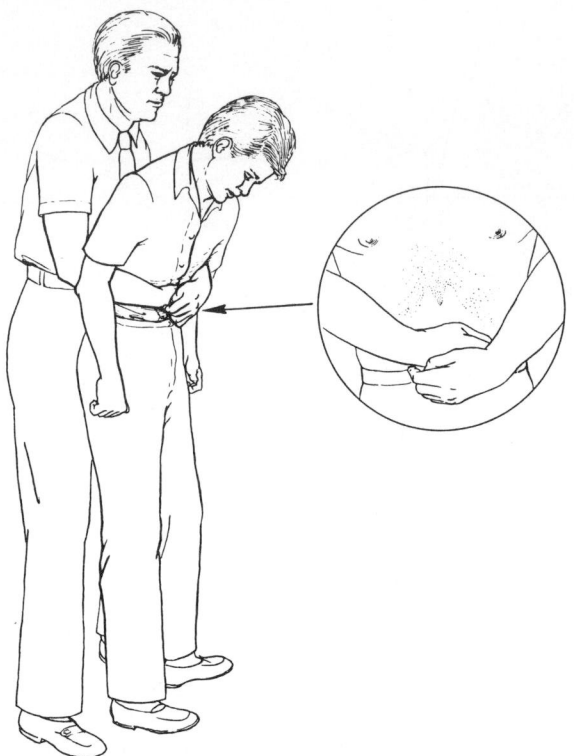

FIG. 25-3   Heimlich abdominal thrusts series.

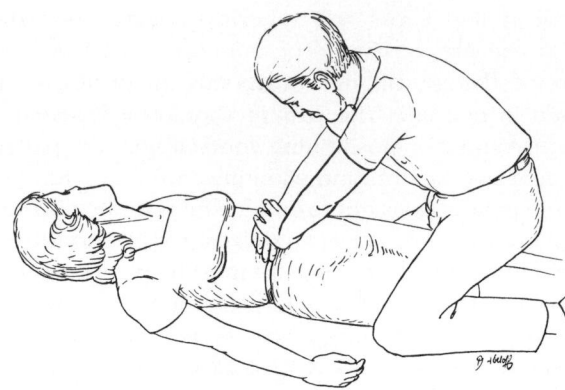

FIG. 25-4   Abdominal thrusts series.

isolation. Everyone has heard of people whose airway becomes obstructed in a restaurant or in the home and who need emergency first aid to assist in breathing.

When you are faced with this situation as a rescuer, you must first question the person by asking "Are you choking?" If the person has a partially obstructed airway with good air exchange, the person can cough or wheeze. In this circumstance you should stay with the person but do nothing else; allow the patient to cough up the object to clear the airway. If the patient has a poor air exchange (indicated by a weak cough and a high-pitched noise), provide assistance as if there were a complete airway obstruction that would not allow the person to breathe, cough, or speak.

After a determination of choking is confirmed, EMS should be called and informed of the situation. The **Heimlich maneuver**, or abdominal thrust technique, requires the patient to be in a standing or sitting position; the rescuer stands behind the patient, wrapping both arms around the patient's waist. A fist is made with one hand, and the thumb of the fist is placed against the middle of the patient's abdomen, above the navel and below the lowest edge of the breastbone (Fig. 25-3). The opposite hand grasps the fist and with both elbows positioned out from the patient's sides, the fist is pressed into the abdomen on the midline with a quick upward thrust.

The thrusts are repeated until the obstruction to the airway is released or until the person becomes unconsciousness. If the person becomes unconscious, he or she should be lowered to the floor, a finger sweep should be done to open the airway, and two breaths should be administered. If the air does not fill the lungs, six to ten abdominal thrusts should be given. This action is repeated until the obstruction is freed or until EMS arrives and assumes responsibility.

When the administration of abdominal thrusts is difficult (e.g., with someone who is nearing term in pregnancy or who is obese), chest thrusts are performed in place of the abdominal thrusts (Fig. 25-4).

After assistance has been provided for a patient in an emergency the patient should then be taken to the nearest hospital for evaluation. When abdominal or chest thrusts are administered, internal injuries may result, and the patient must be seen by a physician to ensure that no injuries or complications exist.

COMPLETE AIRWAY OBSTRUCTION IN AN UNCONSCIOUS ADULT

In this situation repeat the steps just described. If you are unable to breathe air into the patient, the patient's head must be retilted and you must provide two additional breaths. At this point and with the patient lying down, administer six to ten abdominal thrusts as you straddle the patient's thighs. The heel of one hand is placed in the middle of the patient's abdomen in a similar position for the thrusts administered in the earlier description; the second hand is positioned directly on top of the first, with the fingers of the second pointed upward. The abdomen is pressed quickly, with an upward thrust, six to ten times. After the thrusts are accomplished, a finger sweep of the mouth should be performed. If nothing is removed from the airway, these steps are repeated until the airway is cleared or until EMS personnel take over.

▶ Cardiopulmonary Resuscitation (CPR)

Many of the same steps mentioned in previously described emergency situations are repeated for the adult patient whose heart has stopped beating. The primary survey is performed by checking the ABC's, followed by a study to affirm the patient's level of responsiveness. If the patient is not responsive, shout for help, and position the patient on his or her back. The airway is opened; look, listen, and feel for breathing; then administer two full breaths in the patient if he or she is not breathing. At this time the carotid pulse is checked and someone else should be contacting EMS for assistance.

If the patient has no pulse after checking the carotid for 5 to 10 seconds, CPR is begun. This is accomplished by kneeling beside the patient and over the chest positioning the hands on top of each other with the fingers interlaced and over the breastbone. The chest is compressed pushing the breastbone down approximately 1½ to 2 inches in smooth, even strokes. Fifteen administered compressions followed by two full breaths complete a cycle. The rate of compressions should be 80 to 100 per minute (Fig. 25-5, *A* through *E*).

Recheck the patient's carotid pulse after completing 4 cycles of CPR. If no pulse is felt, two breaths are given, and CPR is continued. CPR should be continued until the heart starts beating, until another CPR-trained rescuer arrives, until EMS takes over, or until you physically cannot continue CPR. If you find a pulse, check for breathing; if the patient is breathing, maintain the open airway and observe the breathing and pulse closely.

If no one responds to your shouts for help, CPR should be administered for 1 minute, shouting for help as you are able. If no one has answered the shouts for help after this length of time, the patient must be left for the minimal time that is necessary to phone EMS; then return and continue CPR. See Fig. 25-3 for a review of the step-by-step rescue breathing procedures.

If a second trained rescuer is available during CPR, this person should notify EMS and then relieve you when you become exhausted. You then observe the rise and fall of the patient's chest and check the carotid for a pulse during compressions. The second rescuer can also provide compressions as the first rescuer administers ventilation. The first rescuer gives directions so that the team can work efficiently. As one rescuer becomes fatigued, positions can be exchanged.

When you are faced with a medical emergency, the dental professional's initial response is to satisfy the immediate needs of the patient. Concern must be taken, however, not to abandon infection control procedures or to overlook the potential for transmission of disease. Mouth pieces are available (shown in Fig. 25-2) to avoid mouth-to-mouth or mouth-to-stoma contact.

NOTE: this segment of the chapter is not intended to

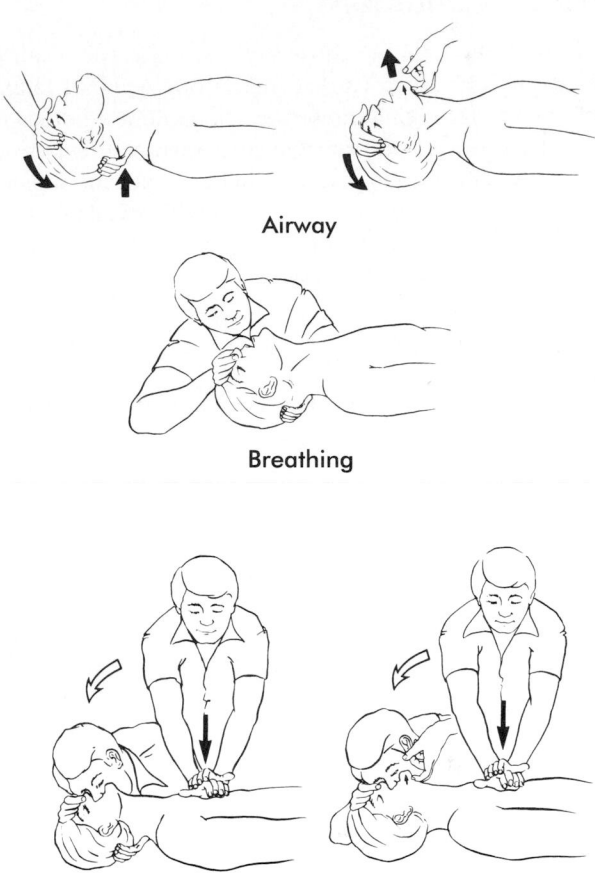

Airway

Breathing

Circulation

FIG. 25-5 The ABCs of CPR. The airway is opened, preferably by head tilt-chin lift maneuver (*Airway*), after which mouth-to-mouth ventilation is performed (*Breathing*). External chest compression (*Circulation*) is then combined with breathing to become cardiopulmonary resuscitation. The previously used head tilt-neck lift method is also illustrated here, though the chin lift is easier to learn and may be more effective. Therefore, it is being recommended as the preferred technique.

replace the need for emergency training and CPR classes; it is an overview of the skills that will be necessary for you to use in an emergency situation. Additional procedures and techniques for assisting children and infants are similar but vary to some extent.

Medical Conditions

Certain systemic or physical conditions require the dental professional to put into practice the skills that have been discussed in this chapter. A patient's medical status may create an unexpected emergency situation which will warrant the emergency actions of the dental professional.

▶ Heart Conditions

Obviously, the patient whose heart stops as the result of a heart attack, a myocardial infarction, or heart failure will need to have CPR; however, the patient who has an angina pectoris condition will not warrant this type of treatment. The angina patient will have extreme substernal pain that can radiate to the arm, with swelling in the extremities. The patient may also experience shortness of breath and increased anxiety.

TREATMENT

The most comfortable position for this patient is to lie at a 45 degree angle. The angina patient usually carries nitroglycerin tablets that are placed under the tongue and are absorbed through the mucous membranes. A second tablet can be administered in approximately 20 minutes. If a patient wears a transdermal patch the second tablet is not always recommended. The attack of angina usually subsides in 2 to 4 minutes after nitroglycerin is taken. The use of oxygen aids in relieving the attack. Oxygen usage during dental treatment may act as a preventive step for the angina patient.

▶ Syncope

The patient who is experiencing **syncope**, or a temporary loss of consciousness, may not always provide the dental professional with an advance warning. Potential problems may be found when vital signs are obtained. A patient who displays symptoms that include a change in pallor and possible excess perspiration provides insight to potential medical needs.

TREATMENT

The patient is placed in the dental chair, or, if necessary, on the floor, in a supine position. The patient's feet are positioned higher than the head, allowing the blood to flow away from the stomach and to the brain. An ammonia inhalant is broken and passed by the nostrils, forcing the patient to inhale quickly, which in turn forces extra oxygen to into the system. A record of this incident is made in the patient's file with the pulse and blood pressure.

▶ Anaphylactic Shock

Anaphylactic shock results from an extreme allergic reaction to an allergen, such as food, an insect bite, or a specific drug. The allergen causes a release of histamines, which in turn cause edema and a decrease in vascular movement. The swelling of the larynx and bronchi forms a blockage of the airway, resulting in cyanosis.

TREATMENT

Treatment, similar to that used for syncope, is administered immediately to ensure patient recovery; an antihistamine is also used to reduce edema. Epinephrine is usually the drug of choice in a dose of 1:1000 of 0.5 ml, followed by contact made with the patient's physician. The use of oxygen may make the patient more comfortable as long as breathing continues. An entry of the patient's allergen is made in the record.

▶ Diabetes Mellitus

Diabetes mellitus is a disease found in millions of individuals throughout the world. Hyperglycemia and hypoglycemia are two clinical complications that may be encountered with the diabetic patient. The patient that is diabetic is also susceptible to other complications, such as large blood vessel disease, small blood vessel disease, greater risk of infection, and poor healing process.

Patients may have insulin-dependent diabetes mellitus (IDDM, or Type I) or noninsulin-dependent diabetes mellitus (NIDDM, or Type II). Each diabetes mellitus patient is unique and must be able to monitor his or her own disease. This is accomplished by the self-monitoring of the blood glucose levels and by management of the disease by making the appropriate changes in food intake, insulin dose, or even exercise.

▶ Hyperglycemia

Hyperglycemia may result in hyperglycemic coma, also known as diabetic acidosis. This might occur when the patient has an increased blood sugar level, possibly caused by eating too much sugar, has an infection, or has not taken the appropriate dosage of insulin. Symptoms of hyperglycemia are a rapid or weak pulse; rapid breathing; and dry mouth, with an acetone breath. The patient becomes less responsive or nonresponsive and may lose consciousness.

TREATMENT

The patient who is hyperglycemic needs insulin or other medications that are normally taken immediately. Contact with the physician of record should follow. This emergency may require the care of an EMS team, followed by physician direction for care.

▶ Hypoglycemia

The **hypoglycemic** patient may be diabetic or nondiabetic. This patient has blood glucose levels that have dropped below 50 mg/100 ml from a high level of insulin. The onset of symptoms may lead to the loss of consciousness or insulin shock. The symptoms of hypoglycemia include disorientation, fatigue, hunger, and/or pallor, and during stressful situations, may result in temperature changes, convulsions, tachycardia, and possibly syncope. Factors that cause hypoglycemia are not eating meals, excessive exercise before meals, or an overdose of insulin.

TREATMENT

If the patient is conscious, the ingestion of sugar increases the blood sugar level and results in the loss of symptoms. A cup of orange, apple, cranberry, or pineapple juice could be administered to increase the blood sugar level. Ten lifesavers or several pieces of hard candy might also increase the blood sugar. If the patient is unconscious, it may be necessary to administer an injection of glucose.

▶ Seizure Disorders

Convulsive episodes are usually a result of transient alterations in brain function. The onset of a convulsive episode in a patient is not normally life threatening, and action on the part of someone witnessing a seizure is usually not necessary. If multiple seizures occur (or status epilepticus) a medical emergency may result. The seizure causes changes in the state of consciousness, motor activity, or sensory phenomena and is often short in length. **Epilepsy** is a recurrent convulsion that is caused by various cerebral and noncerebral disorders; it is seen through a tonic state, with constant muscular contraction, and produces an appearance of stiffness or rigidity. Other seizure reactions appear as intermittent muscle contractions and then relaxation periods, producing a convulsive seizure or stertorous:snoring. Seizures may be symptomatic epilepsy, in which the cause of the epilepsy is known, or they may be idiopathic epilepsy, in which the cause is not known.

GRAND MAL

Grand mal seizure is a form of epilepsy that finds the patient in a tonic-clonic form of seizure and usually lasts 2 to 5 minutes. Tonic-clonic seizures involve spasms of muscles and are followed by loss of consciousness, muscle rigidity, and uncoordinated movement of limbs. The majority of people with epilepsy have grand mal seizures. This form of epilepsy is found in all age groups.

PETIT MAL

Petit mal seizure may be the only seizure disorder the patient has, or it may be combined with other forms of seizures. A lapse of consciousness of approximately 5 to 10 seconds is normal; a 30-second lapse may occur in some situations. The patient does not normally move, other than a possible blinking of the eyelids or dropping of the head; this absence of movement is sometimes combined with a blank staring. This form of epilepsy usually develops in childhood and may decrease as the person ages; it is often not found past the age of 30.

JACKSONIAN EPILEPSY

Jacksonian epilepsy is also referred to as a simple partial seizure, since the patient does not always lose consciousness. The seizure usually begins in a limb or a part of the face as a spasm and then spreads.

PSYCHOMOTOR SEIZURES

Psychomotor seizures are usually combined with another form of seizure and are considered minor by comparison. The patient has a loss of contact with the environment for 1 to 2 minutes. A few symptoms of this seizure are smacking of the lips, movement of the eyes, incoherent speech, turning the head, and amnesia.

The course of treatment for epileptic seizures usually involves phenytoin (Dilantin), resulting in a side effect of hyperplasia of the gingival tissues; therefore, proper oral hygiene is important. In some extreme cases where the hyperplastic tissue covers large portions of the teeth, surgical excision may be necessary to maintain good oral health.

TREATMENT

In most circumstances, treatment is not necessary in the majority of epileptic seizures. The patient should be allowed to let the seizure run its normal course. To avoid injuries, care should be taken to remove any objects the patient may hit or that might fall on him or her during the seizure.

▶ Cerebral Palsy

A cerebral palsy patient has a neural disorder that results in brain damage, which was caused at the time of birth or during the postnatal period before the complete development of the central nervous system. Motor centers of these patients are affected by the disease, with muscle weakness, paralysis, and other possible disorders. The disease can manifest itself in two forms: spasticity, or muscle tension, and athetosis, or uncontrolled body movements.

The cerebral palsy patient often has poor oral hygiene techniques caused by lack of motor control. Consequently the patient may need to be premedicated to relax him or her and to reduce unexpected movements during treatment.

▶ Older Adults

Though the aging process is not a medical condition, older adult patients often present a variety of treatment complications during dental care. This is becoming more apparent as the number of aging patients continues to increase in the United States. Many of the medical complications are not dissimilar to those previously discussed. The older adult patient is discussed in other areas of the text; however, several factors should be considered when the elderly patient receives treatment.

▶ **Drug interaction.** A thorough and accurate review of the health questionnaire must be completed before treatment. The patient may not be aware of all of the medication that he or she is taking, and it may be necessary to consult with a caregiver or a physician before treating the patient.

▶ **Physical mobility.** Aging patients may have impaired physical mobility or sensory perception; the breathing patterns may be irregular; or they may not be able to tolerate a great amount of activity. Consequently, some older adult patients find it difficult to sit for long periods of time in a dental chair or they may reject being placed in a supine position.

▶ **Oral conditions.** As a person ages the teeth become more brittle and fracture more easily and oral tissues tend to change rapidly. Xerostomia: dry mouth, is more apparent in the older adult patient.

KEY POINTS

▶ The medically compromised patient may present complications to dental treatment. These complications may include cardiovascular disease, diabetes, fractured limbs, bodily function failures, and infectious diseases.

▶ Certain patients such as those diagnosed with cancer may require interceptive dental treatment before the treatment for the disease.

▶ Dental emergencies require a caring attitude and an ability to quickly assess the situation.

▶ Treatment of the dental patient who presents with an emergency requires gathering information, assessing patient needs, and treatment scheduling.

▶ Medical emergencies in a dental office require the need for current certification in emergency techniques, implementation of the established chain of command, maintenance of emergency equipment, and the dental staff working as a team.

▶ Emergency kits should include injectable and noninjectable drugs, suction equipment, syringes, tourniquets, airways, various other devices, and universal barriers.

▶ Determining emergency needs of a patient requires implementing emergency action principles, evaluating patient alertness, providing rescue breathing, clearing an airway obstruction, and CPR techniques.

▶ Medical emergencies commonly faced by the dental team may require changes in care and include heart conditions, syncope, anaphylactic shock, diabetes mellitus, hyperglycemia, hypoglycemia, seizure disorders, and the physically challenged.

BIBLIOGRAPHY

American Red Cross Community CPR, St Louis, 1993, Mosby Lifeline, Mosby.

Hooley JR, Daun G: *Hospital dental practice*, St Louis, 1980, Mosby.

Little JW, Falace DA: *Dental management of the medically compromised patient*, ed 4, St Louis, 1993, Mosby.

Malamed SF: *Medical emergencies in the dental office*, ed 4, St Louis, 1993, Mosby.

Oral management of the cancer patient: a guide for the health care professional, Kansas City, 1981, The Curators of the University of Missouri.

Silverman S Jr, Borsky M, Losada F: Oral leukaplakia and malignant transformation: a follow-up study of 257 patients, *Cancer* 53:563-568, 1984.

26 Preventive Dentistry

LEARNING OBJECTIVES

You will have mastered the material in this chapter when you can:

▶ Define the key terms
▶ Describe the factors relating to prevention in dentistry
▶ List common preventive procedures
▶ Describe motivation skills needed in patient education
▶ Define diet analysis
▶ Explain home care instructions for a variety of oral conditions
▶ Describe the techniques for the use of various oral hygiene devices
▶ Select appropriate toothbrush, floss, and auxiliary aids for patients with various needs
▶ Explain how an oral prophylaxis is a preventive procedure
▶ Describe the armamentarium and procedure for an oral prophylaxis
▶ Explain the function of fluoride and pit and fissure sealants as preventive agents
▶ List three types of topical fluoride, and explain how they are applied in an office setting
▶ List common types of self-administered topical and systemic fluorides
▶ Describe the armamentarium and procedure for applying topical fluorides and pit and fissure sealants

KEY TERMS

Bass technique
Charters technique
Dentrifice
Diet analysis
Disclosing agent
Flossing
Fluoride
Fones technique
Interdental aids
Modified Stillman's technique

Motivation
Oral hygiene aids
Oral hygiene score
Oral prophylaxis
Patient education
Pit and fissure sealants
Press-roll technique
Preventive dentistry
Scaler

According to the American Dental Association, (ADA) *preventive dentistry* involves the "procedures in the practice of dentistry and community health programs which prevent the occurrence of oral diseases and abnormalities." The ADA also stated that "optimum oral health is within the reach of every individual, but achievement requires the combined efforts of the practitioner, the patient, and the community."

Prevention in Dentistry

The prevention of oral disease involves the creation and implementation of a preventive program. A preventive program in a dental office must consider the following:

1. Patient education
2. Brushing and flossing the teeth to prevent periodontal disease and dental decay
3. Routine dental care, including examinations, prophylaxis, radiographs, and other preventive and restorative procedures
4. Provision of mouthguards

Other factors that influence a preventive program are as follows:

1. The relationship of a patient's dental needs to his or her oral hygiene habits, eating habits, and socioeconomic conditions
2. The need to motivate the patient to make changes in food selections and eating habits
3. Educating the patient in the correct oral hygiene techniques
4. How the dental staff works as a team to provide optimal patient education programs

Preventive dentistry places responsibility on the patient and the dental team. The patient assumes responsibility for proper home care, and the dental professionals provide routine preventive procedures in the dental office. These procedures include a personalized patient education program, an oral prophylaxis, topical fluoride treatments, the application of pit and fissure sealants, and the provision of mouthguards. Each of these procedures will be described in this chapter.

Motivation

Motivation is the incentive that arouses a particular behavior. A part of motivation is education. Motivating a patient requires an understanding of the patient's needs, a positive attitude, encouragement, and good follow-up. Examples of motivational approaches include the following:

▶ Explaining to a patient how the development of good oral hygiene habits can enable him or her to keep his or her own teeth for a lifetime
▶ Telling a patient that tooth loss is not a part of the aging process

▶ Pointing out how a healthy smile is one of the first things that people notice
▶ Explaining that the patient possesses the power and ability to have a healthy clean smile
▶ Reinforcing the rewards of conscientious dental care and a healthy smile for a lifetime

If the patient does not respond to the positive approach and motivational suggestions, it may be necessary to use a different approach. Other approaches may include the following: remind the patient that bacteria and food debris left in the mouth tend to become malodorous and can lead to dental decay, gingival infection and disease, eventual tooth loss, and extensive dental treatment. Stress to the patient that he or she has a choice to actively pursue a program of prevention, to maintain good home care, and to visit the dental office regularly for routine preventive treatment. The alternative is to neglect the teeth, with the potential for pain, discomfort, and eventual tooth loss. The patient needs to understand that the dental health professionals are there as resource persons to offer further direction and encouragement, but that the patient is ultimately responsible for his or her own dental health.

Patient Education

Patient education is the process of using a variety of teaching aids to inform the patient of dental needs; it becomes the first step in a successful prevention program. In many offices the primary responsibilities for preventive education may be delegated to the dental hygienist, but every member of the dental health team must be skilled in patient education. Regardless of who provides the education, each team member should be aware of available preventive dental products and must assist the patient in making the best choice based on personalized needs. The dental assistant should be able to educate the patient in wise food choices to maintain a healthy mouth and a healthy body.

Patient education requires that the dental professional not only be a teacher, but also be a good listener and role model. Every patient is an individual who has priorities, ideas, needs, skills, and a lifestyle. For teaching to be effective, these variables must be considered before making a final recommendation to the patient. For example, the dental professional must be aware of the patient's oral hygiene history, lifestyle, and economic background before an individual patient education program can be designed. The choice of a toothbrush and auxiliary aids will depend on this information.

To begin a patient education program, the patient must first be given information about healthy oral tissues. This could be done with the use of visual aids, brochures, and patient education packets. Many of these materials are available through dental manufacturing companies and the ADA. A hands-on approach can be accomplished by providing the patient with a hand mirror and by identifying examples of healthy and unhealthy tissue in his or her own mouth. Unless a patient can identify healthy tissue, that is tissue that is unblunted, void of inflammation, firm, or does not bleed when brushed, he or she will not be able to recognize unhealthy tissue. The patient observes the oral tissues every day and should be encouraged to recognize abnormalities in his or her own mouth.

When teaching oral hygiene procedures it is necessary to initiate the following:

▶ Provide the patient with a toothbrush and mirror
▶ Have the patient demonstrate his or her toothbrushing technique and evaluate the patient's skills
▶ Give directions for improvement
▶ Demonstrate the technique to the patient
▶ Provide encouragement throughout

This same procedure can be followed when teaching a patient to use any **oral hygiene aid**: a device used to clean, stimulate, maintain, or modify healthy oral tissues.

This procedure ensures that the patient will understand directions and allows the dental assistant to evaluate the patient's skills. During the teaching process the assistant should encourage questions, maintain eye contact, and provide an enthusiastic, positive attitude. To reinforce instructions, provide the patient with written information about the technique. If the patient has difficulty brushing a certain area in the mouth, helpful hints may be written on a professional note pad. A personalized preventive program takes extra time, but it is worth the effort. This personalized attention can contribute to establishing a positive bond of trust between the patient and dental team.

Since a multitude of products are available, recommendations for specific brand names of dental products is helpful to the patient. Patients look to the dental professional for expert advice, so it is necessary for each dental staff member to maintain a current knowledge of products on the market. When it is possible, give the patient a sample product that is recommended. In this way the patient can take the product home and begin using it immediately. When the scheduled appointment is concluded, data should be recorded in the patient's record that include the type of toothbrushing method that was recommended and the hygiene aids that were provided to the patient.

Diet Analysis

Another aspect of patient education in preventive dentistry is diet analysis. **Diet analysis** is the evaluation of a diet on the basis of caloric intake and dietary components. In dentistry an analysis is concerned with the sugar intake, the consumption pattern, and the types of foods that are consumed. The relationship of diet and dental disease is discussed in Chapter 5, *Nutrition*. The following list of suggestions will help the patient to develop good dietary patterns:

▶ Ask the patient to complete a food anaylsis form/questionnaire (a history of food habits)
▶ Educate the patient about the relationship of diet to the development of dental caries and periodontal disease
▶ Guide the patient in identifying adequate and inadequate nutritional patterns in the diet, such as the following:
    Physical form of sugar items
    Frequency of intake of sugar items
    Consumption pattern
▶ Provide guidance in developing a nutritional diet

Food habits are usually behavioral patterns that may not be recognized and are often difficult to change. To identify eating patterns, ask the patient to maintain a 5-day diet diary. Use a blank chart form that is supplied by the dental office and filled out by the patient, or the patient can simply record all food and beverage items on a sheet of paper. Advise the patient to include all nonfood items, such as cough drops, breath mints, chewing gum, or condiments on the list. The amount of each item and the time of day the food was consumed is essential for an accurate diary. Fig. 26-1 is an example of a completed diet analysis form.

At a subsequent appointment a dialogue with the patient regarding the diet diary is needed to:

▶ Review and identify nutritional adequacy and offer positive reinforcement on good food choices
▶ Identify food groups that may contribute to dental disease
▶ Describe various foods and critical nutrients of the food pyramids
▶ Analyze eating patterns and offer alternative suggestions for change
▶ Review the effect of systemic nutrition and local food factors on dental disease

If the dental professional and the patient have agreed that dental caries is a major concern, circling (or underlining) any potentially cariogenic items on the diary can provide a good point of reference for the patient. Alternative foods and beverages should be suggested and written down to replace those that are circled. Explain to the patient the difference in retentive qualities and consistencies of various foods, and how these qualities affect the cariogenic potential. Use Fig. 26-1 as an example; the following recommendations can be made:

▶ A sugar substitute can be used in coffee, instead of granulated sugar
▶ A toasted English muffin or bagel can be eaten, instead of the blueberry muffin or cinnamon roll

Patient's Daily Diet Diary

Breakfast

1 Blueberry muffin
1 Glass orange juice
Coffee, with 1 spoon sugar

Midmorning snack

1 Cinnamon roll
Coffee, with 1 spoon sugar

Lunch

Salad (lettuce, carrots, tomatoes,
celery, bean sprouts, and 1000 Island dressing)
1 Small bag potato chips
12 oz Diet cola
1 Cup cherry gelatin

Afternoon snack

12 oz Diet cola
1 Chocolate candy bar

Supper

1 Fried chicken breast
1 Baked potato, with butter and sour cream
1/2 Cup green beans, with butter
1 Slice white bread, with butter
Coffee, with 1 spoon sugar
1 Brownie

Evening snack

12 oz Diet cola
2 Cups caramel corn

FIG. 26-1   Completed diet analysis form.

▶ Sugar-free gelatin can replace gelatin containing sugar
▶ Cheese cubes and soda crackers, instead of a chocolate candy bar
▶ Fresh fruit or fresh fruit salad as an alternative to a brownie
▶ Plain popcorn can replace caramel corn

These few suggestions can reduce simple sugars in the patient's diet. A pamphlet with additional recommendations for a low sugar diet that is produced in the office or obtained from the ADA can be given to the patient. A pamphlet that is designed by a dental office staff is an excellent reinforcement tool and can enhance public relations for the office. Similar patient education materials can be provided to the patient with special needs, such as the periodontal patient.

Dr. Washington Wentworth Sheffield developed the squeezable toothpaste tube in 1892. From 1892 to 1900 the sales record of Dr. Wheffield's Creme Dentrifice was extraordinary, and both an industry and a cultural icon were born. Also, it was the beginning of conflict among family members over whether to squeeze the toothpaste tube in the middle or to neatly roll up the ends. (From Curtis EK, Inscriptions, *J Arizona State Dent Assoc,* Nov 1992.

Home Care

Home care is the primary responsibility of the patient in an effective preventive program. Home care begins with patient education in the dental office, followed by a regimen of brushing and flossing and by eating a proper diet at home. If the patient has not been motivated to preventive education, home care may not be successful. The needs of a patient may dictate a specialized plan of home care. For instance, if a patient does not have the manual dexterity to use the traditional toothbrush, it may be necessary to alter the toothbrush handle or to recommend a mechanical device. Home care includes instructions in the use of the toothbrush, flossing techniques, choice of dentrifices, and the use of other auxiliary aids.

Toothbrushing

The ultimate goal of brushing is mechanical removal of bacterial plaque and debris and the stimulation of soft tissues. Since plaque accumulates in significant amounts within 24 to 48 hours, daily removal of these deposits is necessary. It is recommended that a patient brush at least twice a day or brush as the dentist directs for the patient's specific needs. The patient must be advised that it is the quality and not the quantity of brushing that helps to ensure healthy tissues. Excess brushing done incorrectly can lead to toothbrush abrasion, which results in tooth sensitivity and potential loss of tooth structure.

The toothbrush is composed of the handle, the shank, and the head, which holds the bristles (Fig. 26-2, *A*). Individual bristles that are bound together in groups are called tufts. The two primary tuft designs of the past are referred to as the tufted brush, and the multitufted brush. The tufted brush contains five or six spaced tufts that are two or three rows wide. The multitufted version has ten to twelve closely spaced tufts that are three to four rows wide.

A recent design in toothbrushes employs the use of rippled bristles, which are designed to gain greater

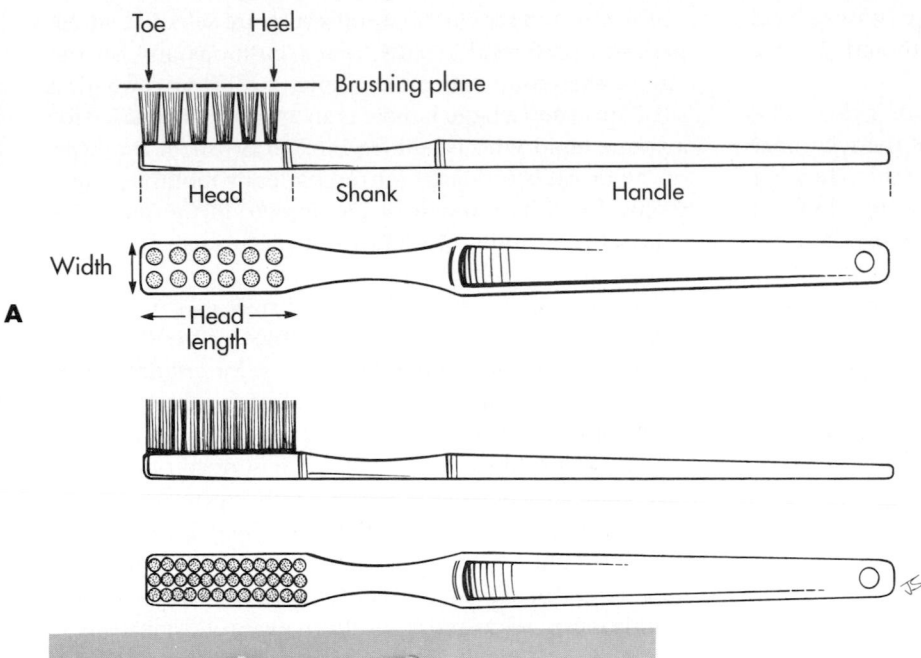

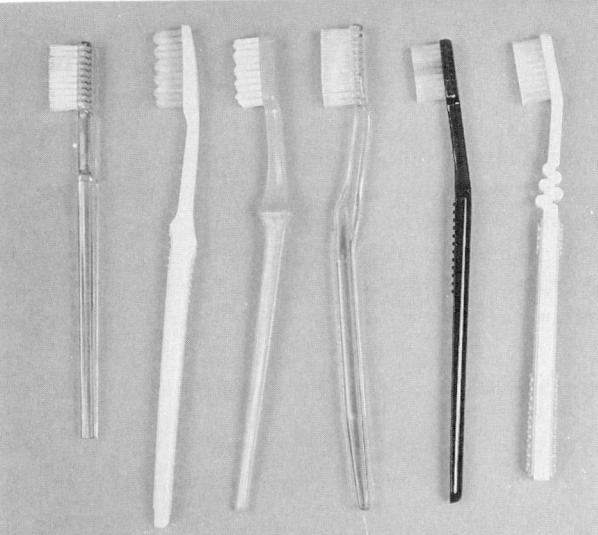

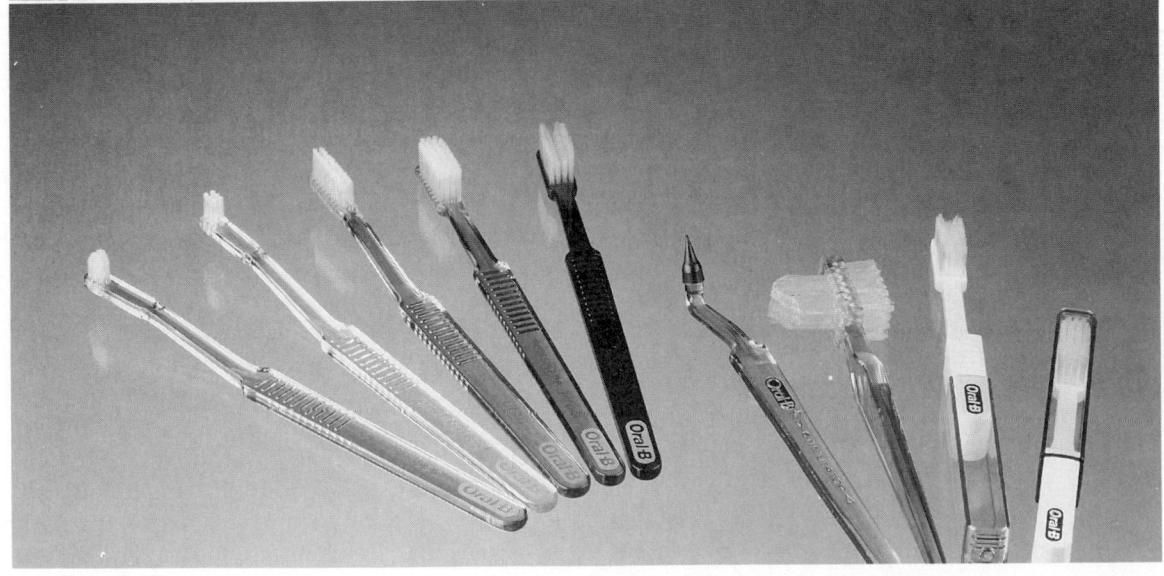

FIG. 26-2   *A,* Parts of a toothbrush. *B,* Variations of toothbrush styles seen in a lateral view. *C,* Additional variations in toothbrush design, including on the right a rubber stimulator, denture brush, orthodontic brush, and travel brush.

(*C,* Courtesy of Oral B Laboratories, Redwood, California.)

access to proximal surfaces of teeth. These brushes have end-rounded bristles, which are often mounted on a tapered head and neck.

Toothbrush bristles are either natural or nylon. The natural bristle is obtained from the hair of the wild boar or hog; these bristles are not uniform in size. They are stiffer, are hollow, can split, can absorb water, and can stay soggy longer. The wild boar or hog bristles may harbor microorganisms that can cause soft tissue damage. The nylon bristle, on the other hand, is manufactured to specific instructions. These bristles are uniform in size (0.006 to 0.008 inch in diameter for soft bristles); rinse clean, and dry quickly; hold their shape longer; and can be polished or end-rounded.

The round and polished ends of bristles prevent damage to tooth structure. Soft-, medium-, and hard-bristled toothbrushes are available. Soft bristles are recommended most often because they are more flexible in adapting to tooth contours and less damaging to soft tissue than are the hard and medium versions.

It is recommended that patients replace their toothbrushes at least every 3 months or as soon as the bristles appear bent. Bent or splayed toothbrush bristles will not clean effectively and may injure soft tissues. The toothbrush should also be replaced after an illness because bacteria and viruses may harbor within the bristles, with the potential to reinfect the patient. Some patients prefer to have more than one toothbrush; they can be used alternately, allowing each to dry thoroughly between uses.

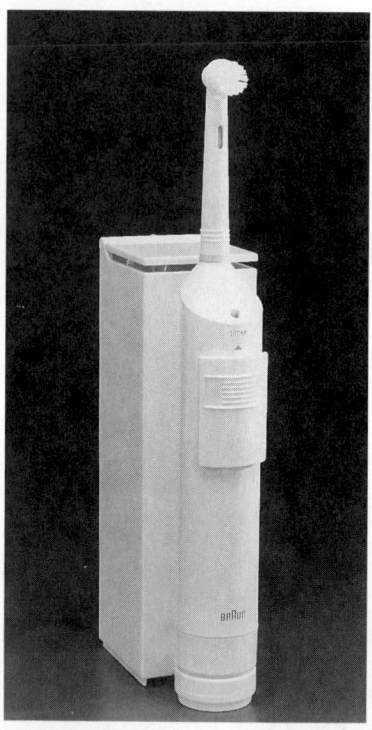

FIG. 26-3   Automatic toothbrush.

(Courtesy of Braun Company.)

The size and style of the toothbrush are selected on the patient's preference, skills, oral conditions and on the size of the mouth. As an example, a toothbrush with a small head and a large handle is an appropriate choice for a young child who is still learning to brush. If the head of the brush is too large for the patient's mouth, plaque removal will be difficult or incomplete in the posterior areas of the mouth. Variations in toothbrush styles are shown in Fig. 26-2, *B* and *C*.

The automatic or electric toothbrush can be recommended for the patient who is disabled or bedridden or has a low level of manual dexterity or for children (Fig. 26-3). A variety of designs are available to meet special needs of the patient. The bristle motion is built into the automatic toothbrush; thus, the patient need only direct the handle and head of the brush to the appropriate area in the mouth and turn on the brush. Since little skill and time are required, the poorly motivated patient may also find the automatic toothbrush convenient. The aspirating toothbrush is discussed as an alternative style of brushing in the *Special Needs* section of this chapter.

▶ Brushing Methods

The brushing method chosen for a patient should be based on the patient's age, his or her manual dexterity or skill, and preexisting oral conditions. Many types of brushing methods are recommended today. In this chapter the Bass, Fones, press-roll, modified Stillman's, and Charters will be discussed. In the descriptions that follow, the term *area* refers to approximately three teeth, depending on the size of the teeth. The entire procedure is repeated five or six times in each area before moving on to the next site.

BASS OR SULCULAR TECHNIQUE

The **Bass technique** is based on the concept that the bristles of the brush are positioned in the gingival sulcus and a vibrating motion is used. This technique is recommended for patients with periodontal disease, loss of gingival contour, or heavy cervical plaque.

A soft-tufted brush is suggested for use in this method (Fig. 26-4). To perform this technique refer to Box 26-1.

PRESS-ROLL TECHNIQUE

The **press-roll technique** is easily taught to children and adults who exhibit healthy gingiva and normal oral tissue contour. This technique is designed to press the bristles against the gingival tissue and roll the toothbrush toward the crown. A soft or medium toothbrush is recommended for this method. To perform this technique refer to Box 26-2.

For the lingual surfaces, the same technique is used.

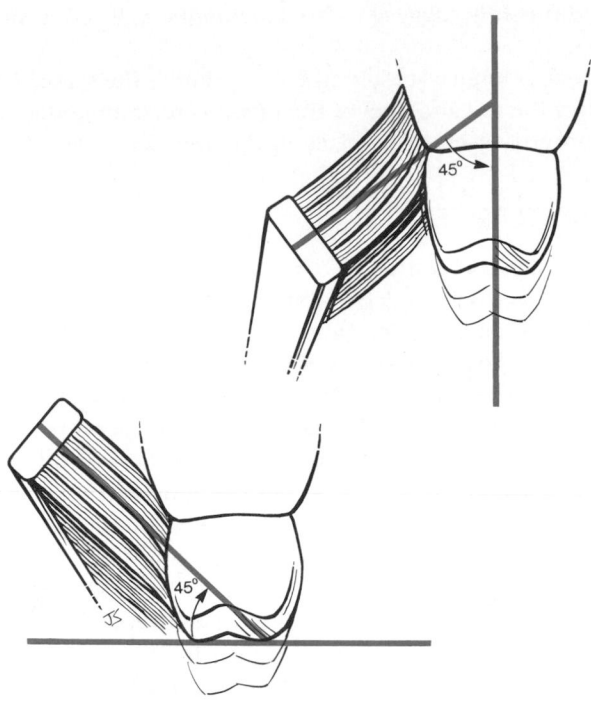

FIG. 26-4 Bass brushing technique.

However the heel and toe of the brush may be used for easier access, especially on anterior teeth.

Dr. Alfred C. Fones, 1869 to 1938, is credited with the evolution of dental hygienists. He trained the first dental hygienist and organized the first school of dental hygiene. Many graduates of the first class were hired by the Bridgeport Connecticut School System, and they performed prophylaxis and patient education for children. The result was a 75% reduction in dental caries rates of participating children.

FONES OR MULTITUFTED TECHNIQUE

The **Fones technique** uses gentle pressure on the bristles and rotates the brush in small circles. This technique is sometimes referred to as the *circular scrub* method and is useful for children and adults with healthy gingiva and normal tooth position. A soft multitufted toothbrush is recommended to perform this technique, which is outlined in Box 26-3.

MODIFIED STILLMAN'S TECHNIQUE

Originally, this technique was developed to simply massage the gingiva. The ***modified* Stillman's technique** now includes cleaning the entire tooth. It is recommended for those patients with gingival recession and/or puffy gingival tissue. A soft or medium tufted

---

BOX 26-1

BASS TECHNIQUE

1. Place the bristles at a 45 degree angle to the long axis of the tooth.
2. Position the bristles in the sulcus and come into contact with the gingiva and tooth simultaneously.
3. Gently vibrate the brush in short, back-and-forth strokes while the bristles remain in the sulcus.
4. Vibrate the brush in each area for a count of five to ten.
5. Clean the lingual areas in a similar manner, with the toe of the brush used on the anterior teeth.

BOX 26-2

PRESS-ROLL TECHNIQUE

1. Place the side of the toothbrush bristles on the gingiva, with the tips of the bristles pointing apically.
2. Press the bristles against the tissues until they slightly blanch.
3. Roll the brush so that the bristles slowly point towards the facial surface of the tooth and then continue to move the brush toward the crown.
4. Replace the bristles to the apical position and repeat the entire procedure.

BOX 26-3

FONES TECHNIQUE

1. Close the teeth, and place the bristles at a 90 degree angle to the teeth in the maxillary molar area.
2. Use gentle pressure, and rotate the brush in small circles, covering the teeth from the maxillary gingiva to the mandibular gingiva.
3. Count to five as you brush in each area.
4. To brush the anterior teeth, bring the teeth together in an end-to-end position, and continue brushing in small circles.
5. To brush the lingual surfaces, follow the same technique, but use the toe of the brush for the anterior areas.

MODIFIED STILLMAN TECHNIQUE

1. Place the toothbrush bristles at a 45 degree angle to the long axis of the tooth, pointing it apically. The bristles should contact the gingiva and the cervical area of the tooth. Do not position the bristles into the sulcus itself.
2. Press the bristles until the tissue blanches slightly.
3. Vibrate the brush in approximately 20 short back and forth strokes, while gradually moving the toothbrush coronally.
4. Replace the bristles to the original position and repeat this procedure for each area in the mouth.

CHARTERS TECHNIQUE

1. Direct the bristles toward the occlusal/incisal surface at a 45 degree angle to the long axis of the tooth. The bristle tips should contact both the gingiva and the cervical area of the tooth.
2. Press the brush to flex the bristles between the teeth.
3. Move the brush to a count of 10 in short vibrating strokes, keeping the bristles in place.
4. Repeat this procedure for each subsequent area, taking care to see that the bristles reach each interproximal area.

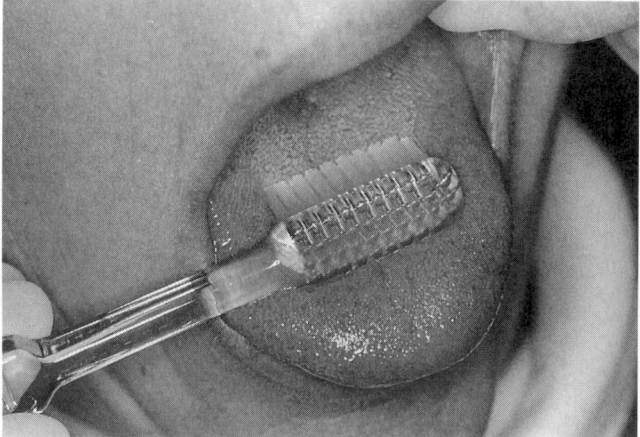

FIG. 26-5　Brushing the tongue.

toothbrush is suggested. This technique is listed in Box 26-4.

For the lingual surfaces the procedure is the same. The use of the toe and heel of the brush is recommended for improved access, especially in the anterior areas.

CHARTERS TECHNIQUE

The **Charters technique** directs the bristles toward the incisal/occlusal surface and uses a vibrating action. It is also recommended for gingival massage. Patients with a loss of gingival contour, with single or abutment teeth, or postperiodontal surgery are good candidates for this brushing technique. The method requires good manual dexterity and sufficient motivation to be successful. For these reasons, patient selection is important. A soft- or medium-tufted design is the toothbrush of choice. The performance of this technique is listed in Box 26-5.

The lingual surfaces are cleaned, using the same technique. Once again, the anterior areas may be better reached by using the toe of the brush.

All five methods conclude with occlusal brushing and brushing of the tongue (Fig. 26-5). The posterior chewing surfaces are scrubbed in a back and forth motion, placing the bristles so that the occlusal pits and fissures are cleaned effectively.

To brush the tongue the bristles of the brush are placed on the dorsal surface of the tongue and as posterior as patient comfort will allow. The brush is pulled forward to the anterior tip of the tongue, and the step is repeated until the tongue is cleansed. Toothbrushing should last for 2 minutes or more to do a thorough job.

Flossing

The primary function of **flossing** is to remove bacterial plaque from interdental surfaces of each tooth. The goal of flossing is to mechanically remove plaque and debris from between the teeth, where a brush cannot reach. Dental floss has been shown to be the most effective auxiliary aid for plaque removal. Daily plaque removal is a responsibility of the patient during home care. A patient is directed to floss once a day for the cleansing of the teeth and for stimulation of the interproximal tissues.

▶ Types of Floss

Floss is available in several forms today (Fig. 26-6, *A* and *B*), including waxed versus unwaxed, extra-fine to flat tape or tufted, white versus colors, plain versus flavored (including bubble gum flavored for children). Recommendation of a particular floss product should be based on the patient's dentition, age, and manual skills.

Waxed and unwaxed floss each present advantages and disadvantages. Many dental professionals believe that the

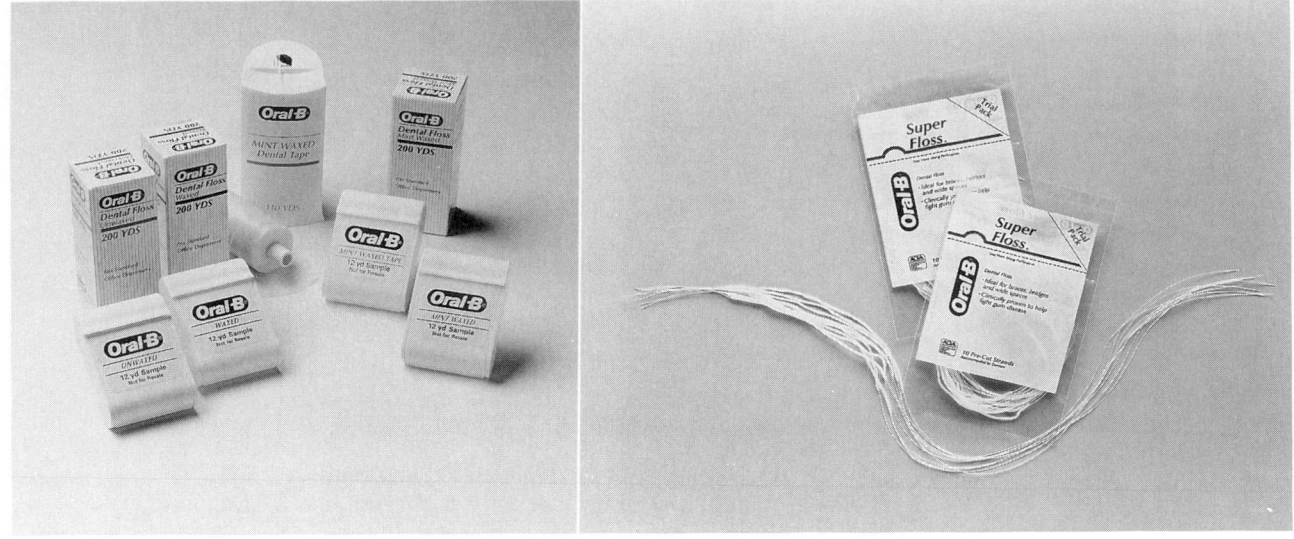

FIG. 26-6   *A*, Types of dental floss. *B*, Superfloss.

(Courtesy of Oral B Laboratories, Redwood, California.)

unwaxed floss offers some clinical advantages. Since the floss filaments are not impregnated with wax, they tend to fan out over the tooth and break up the microcoshs as they cut through and dislodge the plaque deposits. Some clinicians also believe the unwaxed floss aids in carrying away the plaque debris from the teeth and sulcus. The waxed floss provides a distinct advantage in tight contacts and roughened surfaces, while an unwaxed floss might fray in these areas. Because of this the waxed version can be suggested for beginners or for patients with many proximal restorations.

Waxed dental tape is a thicker version of waxed floss. It is used for broad surface cleaning, such as under the pontic of a fixed bridge. The flavored flosses are not easier to use, but they offer another alternative to motivate the patient to floss more often.

▶ Flossing Technique

The technique for flossing (Fig. 26-7, *A* and *B*) is as follows:

1. Begin with a 12- to 18-inch piece of dental floss.
2. Wrap the floss around the middle fingers of both hands, leaving a short span (1 to 2 inches) between the hands, with no slack.
3. The ends of the floss are either kept wound on the fingers or are held in the palm of the hand.
4. The thumb and forefingers guide the floss into the interdental space.
5. A gentle sawing motion of the floss inserts it between the teeth and into the sulcus. Caution is taken to avoid snapping the floss into the interproximal area.

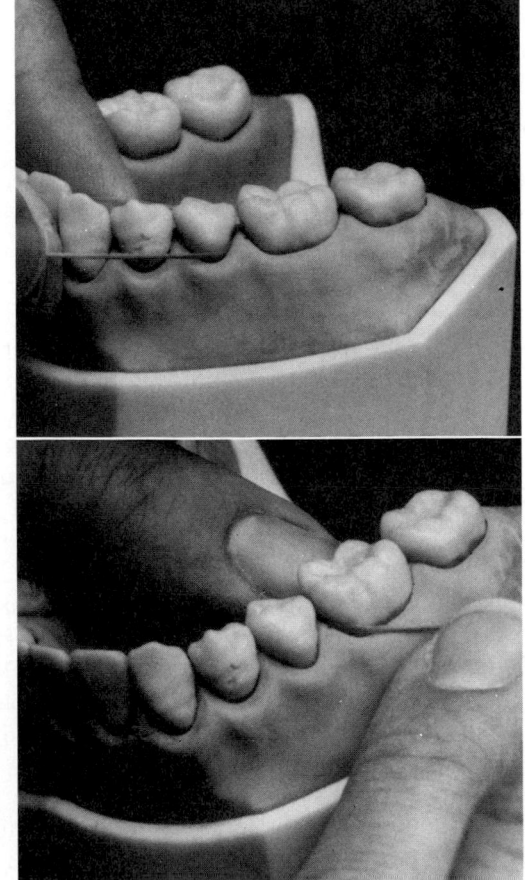

FIG. 26-7   Floss placement around distal and interproximal areas and sublingually.

(From Genco RJ, Goldman HM, Cohen DW: *Contemporary periodontics*, St Louis, 1990, Mosby.)

6. The floss is wrapped around the tooth in a C shape so that it can slide up and down the proximal surface of the tooth to remove the plaque.

7. The floss is advanced on the fingers to a new area after each tooth is cleaned.

8. The mesial and distal surfaces of all teeth are flossed. The patient is instructed not to neglect those areas without adjacent teeth, such as third molars.

If the patient finds this technique difficult to follow, an alternative one can be suggested that uses a circle of floss. A circle of floss can be made by using approximately 12 inches of floss tied at the ends. This technique of flossing may be easier for the patient who has trouble holding and maneuvering the floss. The floss is placed between the teeth and moved in the same manner described in the wrapped finger method.

Auxiliary Oral Hygiene Aids

In addition to the toothbrush and dental floss, various auxiliary aids are available to the patient; these aids include dentrifices, interdental aids, disclosing agents, and anticariogenic substances.

▶ Dentrifices

A **dentrifice** is no longer just ordinary toothpaste. A dentrifice is a compound used in conjunction with a toothbrush to clean the teeth. Most dentrifices contain mild abrasive, detergent, flavoring agent, coloring, optimal deodorants, and/or various medicaments, such as fluoride, that are designed to prevent dental caries. Some dentrifices are designed to prevent tartar accumulation or to desensitize teeth. When the use of a toothpaste or any product is suggested to the patient, make certain that it has earned the American Dental Association, or ADA, approval; this will ensure that the product has been tested extensively and is proven to do what the manufacturer claims.

Currently, most ADA-approved fluoride toothpastes contain 1000 to 1100 ppm fluoride in one average application of paste. This fact is important when discussing toothbrushing with the caregiver of a young child. Many children tend to swallow toothpaste instead of expectorating it. Some children are not able to effectively *spit*, or they like the toothpaste's taste. In either case the dental professional must stress to the parent or caregiver that large amounts of fluoride can be ingested each time the child swallows the paste. Explain to the patient that excess fluoride could cause mottled tooth enamel. To prevent this, instruct the care giver to use only a small amount of paste on the child's brush and closely supervise the brushing. Fluoride toothpastes

tested by the ADA over the years have been proven to reduce dental decay by 15% to 25%.

Patients who suffer from toothbrush abrasion or tissue resorption may experience mild or severe discomfort during brushing and may benefit from one of the ADA toothpastes designed to be used with sensitive teeth. These toothpastes, when they are used on a regular basis, are shown to be effective in decreasing the sensitivity of teeth.

Tartar control toothpastes contain ingredients that help inhibit the growth of supragingival calculus. Remind the patient that this dentrifice will not prevent calculus below the gingiva and that it is not a replacement for flossing.

▶ Disclosing Agents

A **disclosing agent** is a color substance that is applied to the teeth on which bacterial plaque is not ordinarily visible to the patient. Liquid disclosing agents can be used in the office setting, or a tablet form is available for home use (Fig. 26-8). The main ingredient of this agent is a harmless dye, usually red; it stains any plaque or debris that remain on the teeth—a technique that is useful in illustrating to the patient that plaque exists on the teeth, even though it wasn't visible. The disclosing agent shows where the patient needs to brush and floss better.

While the patient is in the dental office, use a disclosing agent in conjunction with a plaque control chart (Fig. 26-9) as a visual aid that illustrates to the patient the areas in the mouth where debris remains after flossing and brushing. These areas can then be marked on the plaque control chart. An **oral hygiene score** brings to light the percentage of teeth on which plaque is present. This percentage can be determined by using a simple formula: the total number of disclosed tooth

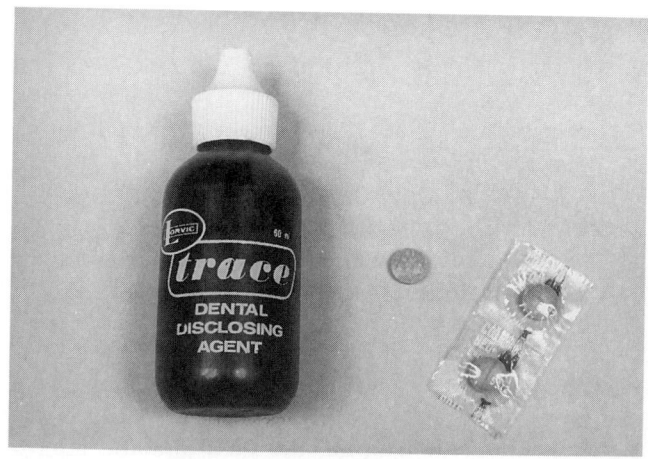

FIG. 26-8   Disclosing agents.

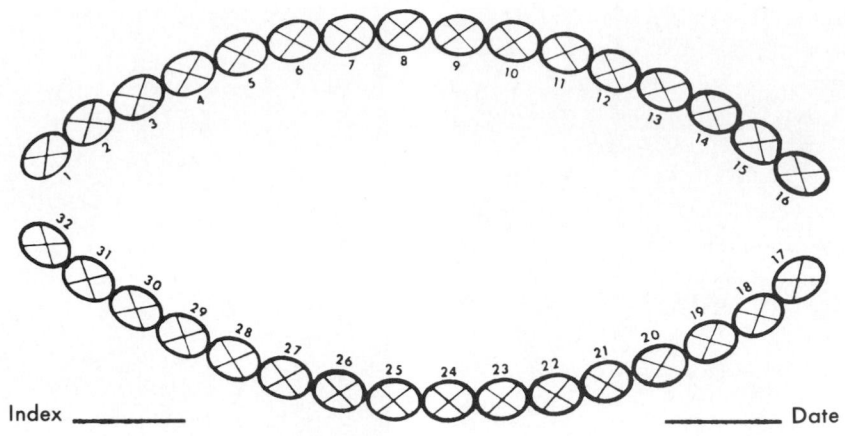

FIG. 26-9   Plaque control chart.

(From Woodall IR: *Comprehensive dental hygiene care,* ed 3, St Louis, 1993, Mosby.)

surfaces divided by the total number of tooth surfaces × 100% = oral hygiene score %; or it can be presented in the following formula:

$$\frac{\text{Sum of disclosed surfaces affected by plaque}}{\text{Total tooth surfaces}} \times 100 = \% \text{ index}$$

For instance, if a patient has 28 teeth and the plaque is detected on 12 of the teeth, the patient's oral hygiene score would be approximately 43%. The patient should strive for a lower percentage each office visit. The initial score can serve as a baseline, and as the patient improves his or her skills, a lower score—15% or 10%,—would show improvement. Each score should be documented in the patient record at the time of the appointment.

Obtain the oral hygiene score in the following manner:
1. Instruct the patient to brush thoroughly.
2. Apply lubricant to the lips of the patient to avoid staining.
3. Use a cotton-tipped applicator, and paint the solution onto the teeth. If the tablet form is used, instruct the patient to chew one tablet thoroughly and to swish the dye around the mouth completely.
4. Rinse the area thoroughly.
5. Use a mouth and hand mirror to illustrate the areas that are disclosed.

 In 1788 William Bartram, a Quaker botanist, discovered that Cherokee Indians used plant roots that were dried into small, clear amber pieces and chewed on to clean the teeth and to sweeten the breath.

Interdental Aids

Interdental aids are devices that stimulate the tissue between the proximal surfaces of adjacent teeth or aid in cleaning the interproximal surface of the teeth. Common aids include floss holders, rubber or wooden stimulators, floss threaders, interproximal brushes, water irrigators, mouthrinses, and chewing gum.

▶ Floss Holder

A **floss holder** is a device that is designed to assist the patient in flossing (Fig. 26-10). A Y-shaped plastic device holds the floss in a short, taut span. The patient directs the floss gently through the contact area with the handle. The handle is moved forward and back and up and down to clean the proximal areas. The floss is moved forward on the holder as it is used.

▶ Rubber or Wooden Stimulator

A **rubber tip stimulator** is a small cone-shaped rubber device that is found on the end of the toothbrush handle

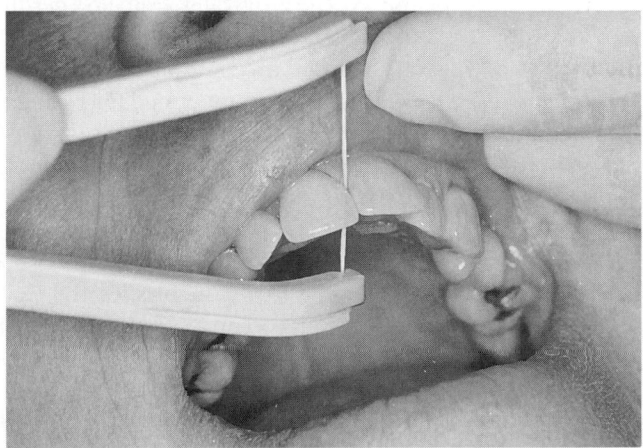

FIG. 26-10   Floss holder.

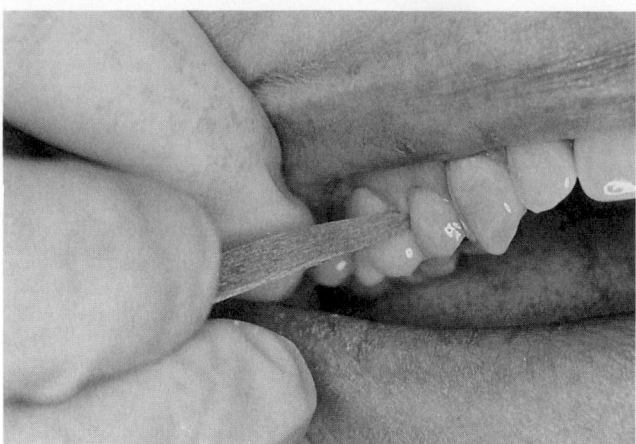

FIG. 26-11   Wooden stimulator placed at the interproximal space.

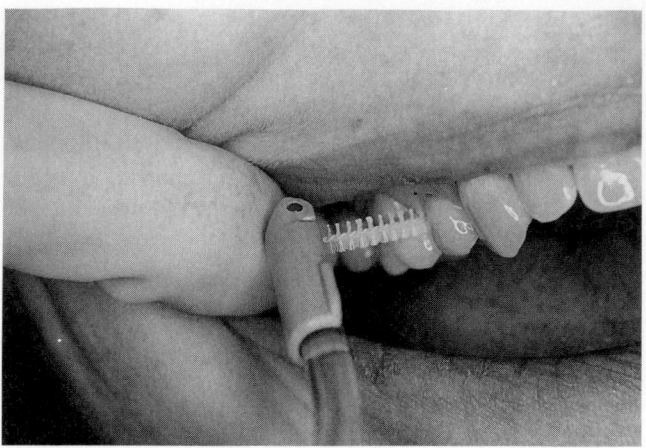

FIG. 26-12   Interproximal brush placed at the interproximal space.

or on a separate handle (see Fig. 26-2, *C*). This device is indicated when a large interproximal space exists and/or when loss of papillae occurs. The patient places the rubber tip in the interdental space, angles it towards the occlusal surfaces, and uses a gentle rotary motion. The gingiva is massaged and stimulated and some plaque is removed.

A **wooden stimulator** (Fig. 26-11) is an interdental aid that is made of a soft wood, usually balsam, and is designed in an elongated wedge shape. As with the rubber tip stimulator this wooden aid is indicated when there is a loss of papillae or when a large interdental space is present. Before the wood stimulator is used, it is softened with water or saliva and then placed between the teeth, angling it toward the occlusal. Use an in and out motion, rubbing the wood against the tooth surface. This action removes plaque and stimulates the tissue.

An additional aid that is similar to the stimulators is the Perio Aid trademark. This device consists of a plastic handle with holes at either end. A moistened toothpick or wooden point is placed in each hole. The point is carefully placed just below the gingival margin and gently moved from a distal to mesial direction. This motion removes subgingival plaque and stimulates the soft tissue. Normally, this device is recommended for patients that are highly motivated and who have some form of recession, periodontal disease, or furcation involvement.

Interproximal Brush

Interproximal brushes are soft nylon bristles that are usually cone shaped and are placed on a plastic or twisted wire handle (Fig. 26-12). This device can be recommended for the following:

- Cleaning in and around orthodontic wires and brackets
- Cleaning an open bifurcation or trifurcation

- Stimulating and cleaning an open contact area or site where there is a loss of papillae

For proper use, place the brush in the desired area, apply light pressure, and use a rotary motion.

Water Irrigation Devices

Water irrigation uses a steady or pulsating stream of water to help remove nonadherent debris and food, especially for those patients with fixed bridges or fixed orthodontic appliances (Fig. 26-13). It is not, however, a replacement for proper brushing and flossing because it does not eliminate adherent plaque. Instruct the patient in careful placement of this device. These devices can be used with a self-administered prevention solutions.

In the correct position the water stream is pointed in a horizontal direction that is perpendicular to the tooth and gingiva. Never aim the water into the gingival sulcus, as this could cause damage to the gingiva and periodontium by forcing debris further into the sulcus. This device is not recommended for patients who have subacute bacterial endocarditis (SBE).

Floss Threader

Floss threaders can be found in numerous sizes and shapes (Fig. 26-14) that are commonly made of a stiff plastic that is designed like a small needle with an eye through which the floss is threaded. These help to remove plaque and debris from under fixed bridges and retainers, and between orthodontic wires. Instruct the patient to thread the floss or tape (or a piece of synthetic yarn if the opening is large) through the *eye* of the device. The patient can direct the stiff end of the threader with the floss under or through the contact and then remove the threader, leaving the floss. The floss is now in posi-

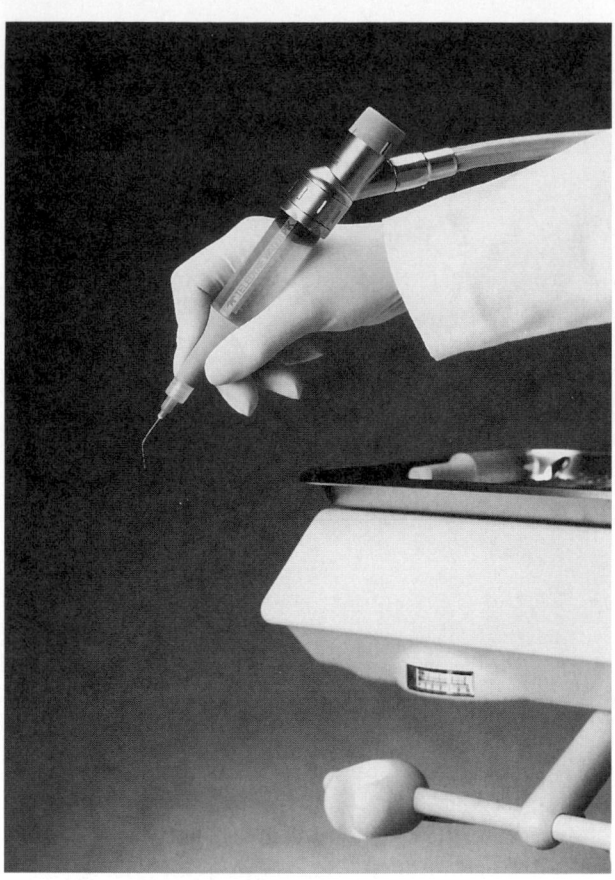

FIG. 26-13   Water irrigation device.

(Courtesy of Teledyne, Fort Collins, Colorado.)

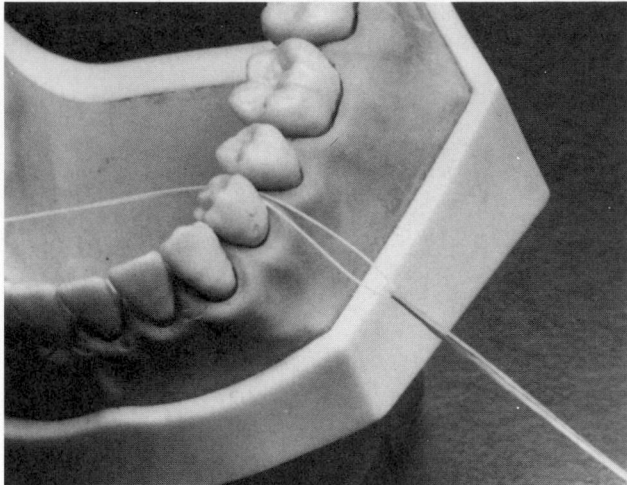

FIG. 26-14   Floss threaders.

(From Genco RJ, Goldman HM, Cohen DW: *Contemporary periodontics*, St Louis, 1990, Mosby.)

tion in the hard-to-reach area, and effective cleaning can take place.

▶ Oral Rinses

Originally **oral rinses** were mouth rinses that were intended to freshen the breath. Today the ADA has given approval to oral rinses that contain fluoride and help to reduce dental decay, supragingival plaque, and gingivitis. A cautious recommendation should be given when using these rinses. The composition of the rinse may include substances that could cause harm if they are ingested. An oral rinse is intended (as it states) to be placed in the mouth, swished about, and removed from the oral cavity. For this reason the rinse is not recommended for use by young children or by those who are unable to effectively expectorate.

▶ Chewing Gum

Recently some antibacterial chewing gums have been researched and found to show some caries inhibiting properties when chewed after eating a fermentable carbohydrate. The concept is that when the gum is chewed, the body secretes more saliva. The increase of saliva in the mouth produces a buffering action that helps neutralize the plaque acids. This, in turn, decreases some caries production, and the mechanical action of the oral tissues on the teeth helps in the removal of food particles.

Care of Prosthetic Devices

Not all patient education and oral hygiene instructions relate to maintaining the health of natural teeth. The dental professional must also be concerned with caring for prosthetic devices, replacements for missing teeth and tissues, and orthodontic bands and appliances. Often the dental assistant is responsible for demonstrating the care and maintenance of prosthetic devices to the patient during oral hygiene instructions. The assistant may also be responsible for cleaning the devices in the dental laboratory when the patient receives treatment.

▶ Fixed Bridge

The patient with a fixed bridge needs to be reminded that extra care is required in this situation to maintain optimal oral health. Cleaning under the pontic (the artificial tooth) of the fixed bridge is essential and can be accomplished by using one of the auxiliary aids previously discussed for this purpose (Fig. 26-15, *A* through *C*).

▶ Orthodontic Bands and Appliances

In the case of the orthodontic patient with fixed appliances, a special orthodontic toothbrush can be

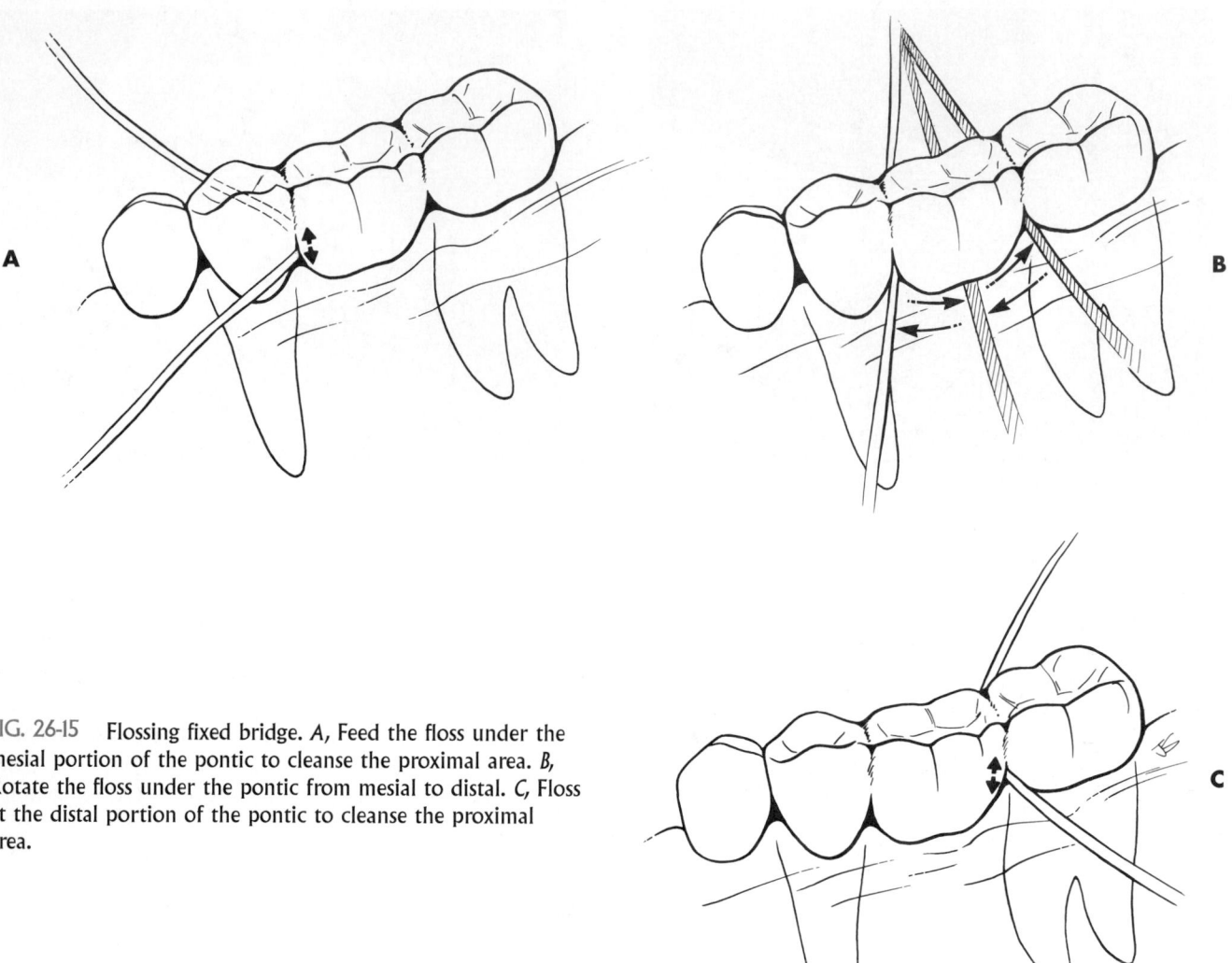

FIG. 26-15   Flossing fixed bridge. *A,* Feed the floss under the mesial portion of the pontic to cleanse the proximal area. *B,* Rotate the floss under the pontic from mesial to distal. *C,* Floss at the distal portion of the pontic to cleanse the proximal area.

suggested (Fig. 26-16). This brush is designed with a center row of shorter bristles to fit over the orthodontic brackets and aid in their cleaning. Instruct the patient to use short vibrating strokes with the brush to clean and stimulate the gingiva. Caution the patient that if proper care is not taken during active orthodontic treatment, carious lesions can occur around and under the brackets and bands. Regular fluoride treatments are often prescribed for the patient during the course of orthodontic treatment to reduce the risk of carious activity.

Removable Prostheses

All removable dentures and appliances should be taken out of the mouth and cleaned at least once a day; also at the least they should be rinsed following a meal. Cleaning of the removable prostheses can be accomplished by various methods:

▶ Rinse under water only when other methods are not available
▶ Brush with a denture brush (Fig. 26-17) and a mild soap or toothpaste; avoid coarse abrasives; they may be damaging to the appliance or soft tissue
▶ Immerse in commercial chemical soaking solutions or in a solution that is made at home of the following ingredients:
    1 tsp. bleach
    2 tsp. Calgon (anticorrosive agent)
    1 cup warm water

If calculus is observed, the appliance can be soaked in the following dilute vinegar solution:
    1 to 2 tsp. white vinegar
    1 cup warm water

These solutions should only be used occasionally—not used on a daily basis. Caring for the removable appliance is only half the oral hygiene process. The soft tissue

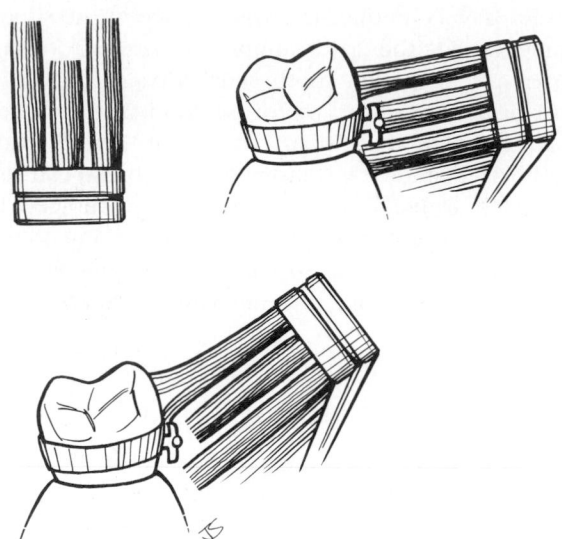

FIG. 26-16   *A,* End view of orthodontic brush. *B* and *C,* Brush placement.

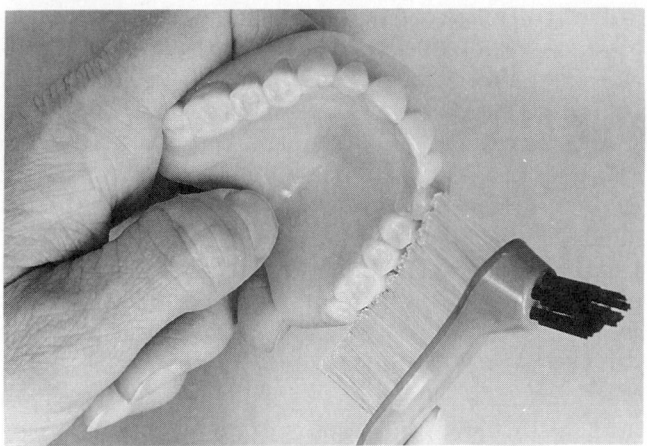

FIG. 26-17   Denture brushing.

underneath the appliance needs attention also. At least once a day the tissue should be cleansed with a soft bristle brush. The purpose of cleaning the tissue is to maintain circulation and to aid in fighting against tissue trauma.

Denture patients are advised to remove and clean their full and partial dentures daily. When using a manual denture or clasp brush, the procedure should take place over a sink. Place a paper towel or washcloth in the bottom of the sink, and fill the sink with approximately an inch of water. This will prevent possible breakage of the denture if it is dropped. Hold the denture or partial denture securely to facilitate removal of plaque and debris. A commercial or home-prepared chemical immersion may also be used on a daily basis. In addition, brushing any remaining teeth, soft tissue, and palate should be performed every day.

Oral Hygiene for Patients with Special Needs

Customized oral hygiene instructions must be created for patients with special needs, including the disabled, those with cancer, the older adult and the pregnant patient.

▶ Physically Challenged Patients

The instruction and home care of the physically challenged patient will depend on the type and the severity of the disability. The patient who has a mild physical or mental disability can be taught a simple brushing method, such as the Fones or press-roll method. Supervision by the parent or caregiver may be required at one

of the daily brushings, preferably the evening one. The more seriously impaired patient may be instructed in the use of an electric toothbrush. The patient should also be encouraged to brush the teeth by himself or herself during the day. This will serve the following two purposes:

1. To reinforce the concept that the teeth should be cleaned at least twice daily
2. To give the patient a sense of responsibility for his or her own care

Toothbrushes can be personalized according to the patient's needs. Examples of such individualized care might be by fashioning a wooden tongue blade to add length to the toothbrush handle or by bending the toothbrush handle, changing the angle to compensate for the disability. Hot water often will soften the plastic handle to allow bending. A bicycle handle grip or rubber ball attached to the toothbrush handle can also make the brush easier for the patient to hold and maneuver. If the patient has the necessary skills and interest, flossing can be taught. A floss holder is a useful device if the patient's manual dexterity is limited. The *circle of floss* method is also an acceptable alternative.

Severely disabled and some bedridden patients may require that the caregiver provide all of the oral hygiene needs for that patient. In some cases the patient who is still capable of mobility may resist receiving care. Assistance in the delivery of oral hygiene care may be necessary in these circumstances. The assistance might be in the form of another person restraining the patient or simply holding the patient's hands. This prevents injury to the patient and caregiver and allows for easier access to the mouth. The patient who is uncooperative or unable to hold the mouth open for any period of time may necessitate the use of a mouth prop. One can be made by using four or five tongue blades secured together, or a commercial mouth prop may be obtained.

When a manual or an automatic toothbrush is used, toothpaste should be applied sparingly. Wipe the teeth and soft tissues after brushing with a moist gauze or cloth to remove excess toothpaste and debris.

An *aspirating toothbrush* might be considered in the situation just described. This toothbrush consists of a flexible tube that is connected at one end to a suction device. The opposite end connects to the back of the head of a manual toothbrush. The suction unit is turned on, and brushing can begin. This type of system allows for simultaneous brushing and removal of oral fluids and debris for a clear working field. Rinsing and suctioning with water and wiping the teeth and soft tissues with a moist gauze will complete the cleaning procedure. Many situations call for the caregiver to also inspect the mouth for any noticeable changes or abnormalities. These observations should be brought to the attention of the dentist to avoid major problems. Complete cleaning and inspection of the mouths of these patients need to be accomplished daily.

▶ Cancer Patients

Cancer patients may exhibit a variety of oral manifestations as a result of cancer treatment. Rampant or root caries, xerostomia, gingival bleeding, or loss of facial and masticatory muscle function may create complications to oral hygiene. The immune system of the patient is often compromised during cancer therapy. Effective plaque removal is imperative to avoid additional infection in the mouth because of poor oral hygiene. Unusually sensitive gingiva that bleeds easily may require an extrasoft toothbrush or a foam toothbrush. One similar to those given postperiodontal surgery patients may be suggested. The frequent use of home topical fluoride with custom-fitted trays helps to reduce the incidence of decay. The critically ill patient may be difficult to motivate. Therefore, great effort must be made to be empathetic, caring, and encouraging.

▶ Older Adult Patients

The older adult patient has many years of experience and skill; however, he or she may also have limitations. The responsibility of the dental professional is to select and teach home care methods that are based on observations. Because of the many advances in dentistry, patients are now able to retain their natural teeth longer. Some patients may have considered dentures and *old age* as synonymous, but with preventive dental care this no longer is true. However, gingival fragility, recession, and cervical abrasion are often problems that face the older adult patient. Recommend a soft toothbrush to avoid aggravating existing conditions. A brush-

ing method that concentrates on the cervical area, such as the Bass technique, is a wise choice in the situation. Home fluoride therapy is important to deter root surface caries and to lessen tooth sensitivity.

Arthritis or reduced motor function that is caused by a stroke may necessitate the need for a modified toothbrush handle. An automatic toothbrush can also be suggested. Dental flossing needs to be encouraged, but it may be difficult for these patients. Recommend a floss holder or the *circle of floss* method as possible alternatives. The importance of home care cannot be overemphasized.

▶ Pregnant Patients

Pregnancy gingivitis is commonly seen in the pregnant patient. In discussing home oral hygiene care, the patient must first understand why this type of gingivitis is occurring. Thorough daily brushing and flossing are essential to avoid serious gingival problems that are complicated by hormonal changes. During pregnancy the patient may be easily nauseated and consequently toothpaste odors and flavorings may be difficult for her to tolerate. Suggest to the patient that she might switch to a milder tasting brand or that she might not use *any* toothpaste during this time. Frequent *morning sickness* or vomiting will create an acidic environment in the mouth; this may cause tooth erosion or increased dental caries. Encourage the pregnant patient to brush or rinse frequently to lessen the chance of this happening. During the home care instruction an excellent opportunity exists to offer suggestions about the new baby's teeth and their care. It may be suggested that the patient consult with her physician about the possibility of a prescription for vitamins with fluoride to be taken prenatally.

Explain to the mother that she must brush the baby's teeth or wipe them with a moist gauze daily as soon as they erupt. Caution her to eliminate the possibility of *nursing bottle decay* by never putting the baby to bed with a bottle filled with anything but water. The ADA provides a variety of educational materials for distribution to patients in the dental office. For instance, brochures such as *Nursing Bottle Mouth, For the Pregnant Mother, Your Child's Teeth, Smokeless Tobacco*, are only a few samples of educational materials that are available for specific needs of your patients.

Oral Prophylaxis

The term *prophylaxis* is familiar in our society today because it refers to the prevention of disease. An **oral prophylaxis** is the prevention of dental disease and consequently it is more than just having the teeth *cleaned*. The patient must understand that an oral or dental prophylaxis is the removal of calculus—subgingival and supragingival—from all surfaces of the teeth, the removal of stains, the polishing of the teeth, and the thorough examination of all intraoral soft and hard tissues, as well as an examination of the extraoral tissue. To call this procedure a *cleaning* is to understate its purpose. Prophylaxis is a preventive procedure intended to prevent periodontal disease and to examine oral tissue for early signs of oral diseases, lesions, and other anomalies. A professional oral prophylaxis should be done on a regular basis. A Record is made on the patient's chart of any changes in the oral tissues. Commonly this procedure is recommended at 6-month intervals, but it may extend to 12 months or be as frequent as 3 or 4 months, depending on the patient's needs.

The basic steps in an oral prophylaxis procedure include an initial oral examination; a disclosing procedure; patient education; scaling, polishing, and flossing the teeth; and a final examination and charting of oral conditions.

▶ Basic Prophylaxis Instruments

Before the actual prophylaxis is begun, an understanding of the instruments that are used in this procedure is appropriate. Various specialized instruments are used during an oral prophylaxis. As with the hand cutting instruments described in Chapter 18, each dentist may use instruments of personal preference. Many of the instruments used in a prophylaxis will require frequent sharpening. These instruments must remain sharp to remove the calculus from the teeth. The basic technique for this procedure is described in Chapter 18, also.

As with all procedures the explorer, mirror, and cotton pliers are used on a prophylaxis setup. Other instruments include a periodontal probe, scalers, polishing paste and holder, polishing cups and brushes, and articulating paper, as well as auxiliary items common to most preset trays.

PERIODONTAL PROBE

The **periodontal probe** is the primary instrument used in a periodontal examination. It is used to examine the gingiva for bleeding and to determine the depth of the gingival sulcus. Detailed information on this instrument is given in Chapter 18.

SCALER

A **scaler** is the workhorse of an oral prophylaxis procedure. The primary function of this instrument is to remove supragingival and subgingival calculus from the tooth. Scalers are available in manual or mechanical forms. The manual scalers are the most widely used; perhaps this is because of the tactile ability with these instruments. The mechanical scalers are more often used for specialized situations. The basic shapes are available in both forms. The most common shapes of scalers are the curet and sickle, with the chisel and hoe scalers also available for use in specific areas.

Curet Scalers

The **curet scaler** is the most effective instrument for removal of calculus and for smoothing root surfaces. Curets are supplied as SE or DE instruments. Two types of curets are available: universal and Gracey, or area specific. The physical characteristics of a curet scaler are distinguished by two cutting edges (one on each lateral surface) that converge into a rounded flat end. The slender curved blade of a curet scaler resembles a spoon excavator, and the cross section of the blade is half-moon shaped (Fig. 26-18, *A* and *B*). The universal curet scaler can be used on all surfaces of the teeth (Fig. 26-18, *C*) and is especially effective when subgingival calculus or fine supragingival calculus is removed. Heavy or rigid curets are well suited for supragingival calculus, while the fine curets are used for subgingival application.

The **Gracey scalers** are designed with additional angles and variations in their shanks (see Fig. 26-18, *A* and *B*). These angles adapt to specific areas on tooth surfaces, such as furcations or deep root surfaces. These modifications aid the operator in removing subgingival calculus and in smoothing rough cementum or root surfaces.

Sickle Scalers

The **sickle scaler** is distinguished by two straight cutting edges that terminate in a sharp point. The cross section of this instrument blade is triangular (Fig. 26-19, *A*). The sickle scaler is designed for removal of supragingival calculus or to remove deposits that extend only slightly below the free gingival margin. Two basic types of sickle scalers are used in a prophylaxis: the straight or anterior, and the modified—contra-angle or universal. The basic difference in these two instruments is found in the angle of the blade. The blade of the modified or universal sickle scaler sits at a right angle to its shank. This angle allows for the instrument to be used in any area of the mouth, whereas the straight sickle is limited primarily to the anterior segment of the mouth. Three common sickle blades are shown in Fig. 24-19, *B*. Anterior sickle scalers as shown may be supplied with a straight or a curved blade, and the modified or posterior scaler has the blade at a 90 degree angle.

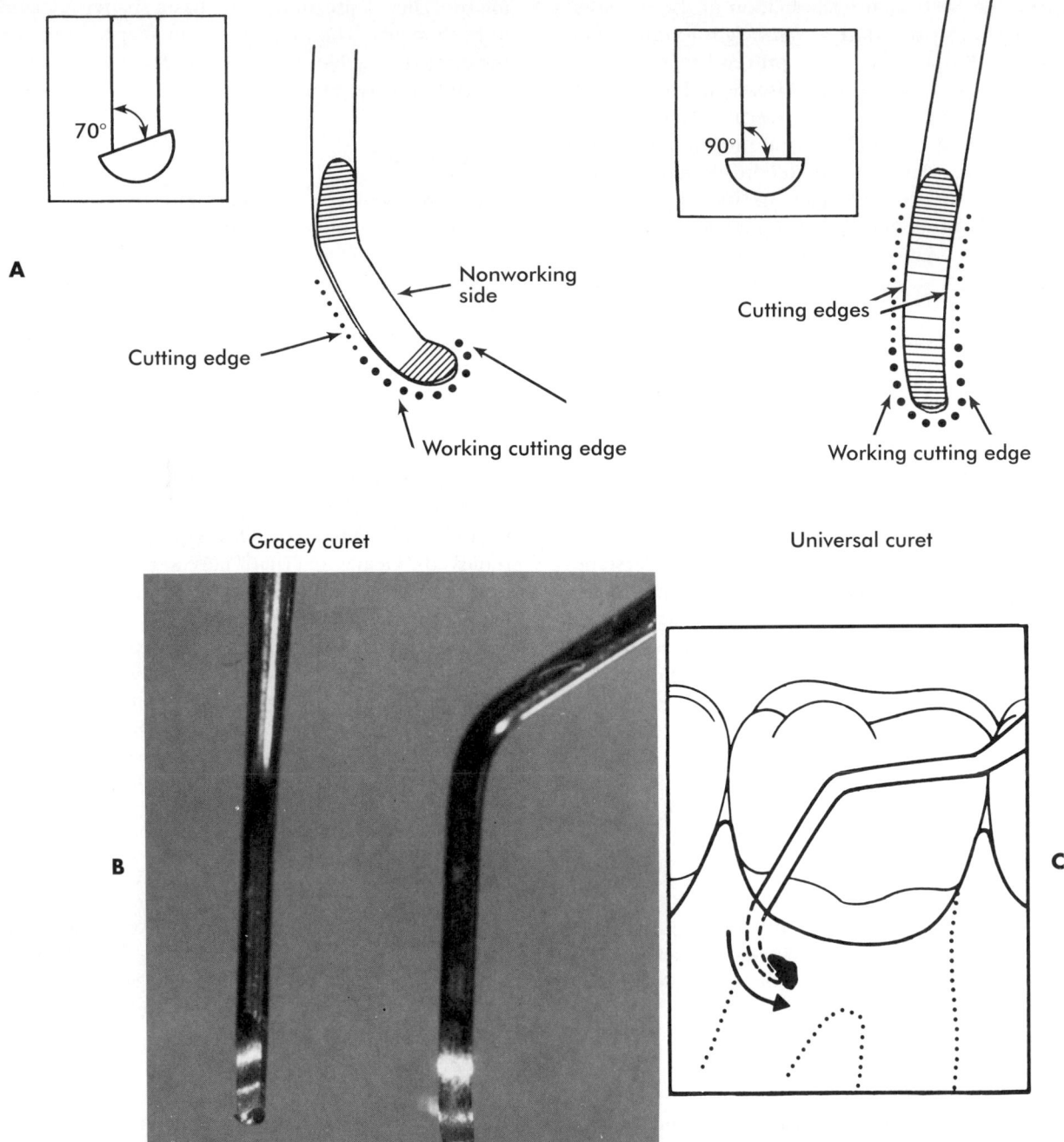

FIG. 26-18   *A* and *B,* Curet scalers, universal, and Gracey. *C,* Curet scaler being used on one of many areas.

(From Genco RJ, Goldman HM, Cohen DW: *Contemporary periodontics,* St Louis, 1990, Mosby.)

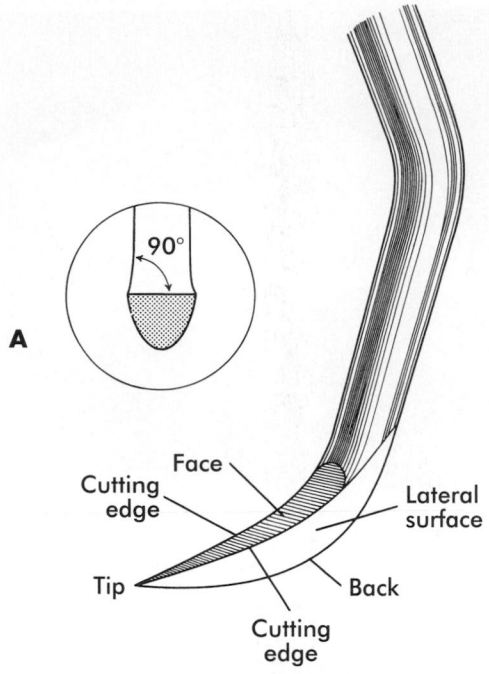

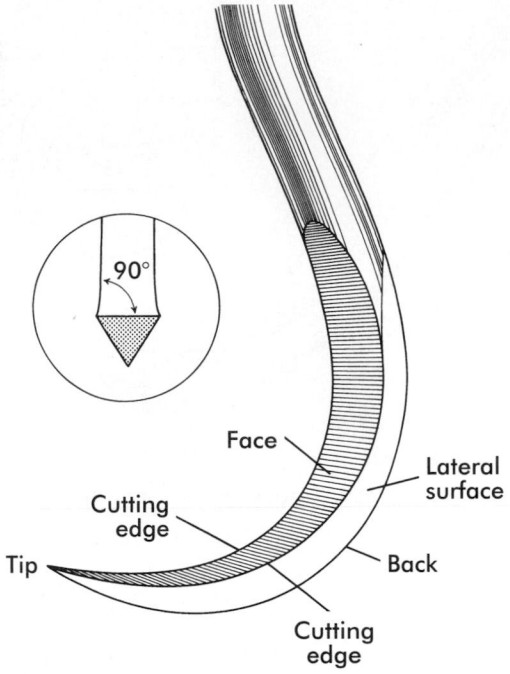

FIG. 26-19 *A,* Sickle scalers. *B,* Three common sickle scalers.

(*A* from Genco RJ, Goldman HM, Cohen DW: *Contemporary periodontics,* St Louis, 1990, Mosby.)

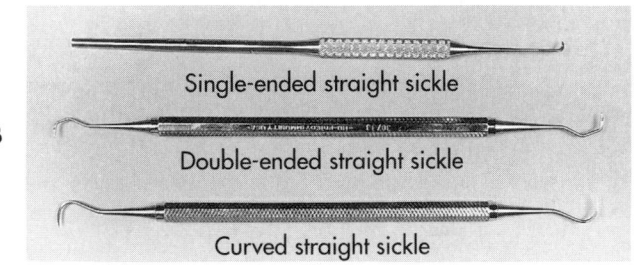

Single-ended straight sickle

Double-ended straight sickle

Curved straight sickle

Hoe Scaler

The **hoe scaler** is designed for removing or dislodging heavy supragingival and subgingival calculus in easily accessible areas.

The cutting edge is at a near right angle to the blade (Fig. 26-20) and resembles a garden hoe. It is a bulky instrument used with a pull action, and its use should be limited to the buccal or lingual surfaces or proximal surfaces adjacent to edentulous areas. This instrument is not likely to be part of a routine prophylaxis, but it is available for use in a special situation.

CHISEL SCALER

Like the hoe scaler, this is not a routine instrument for a prophylaxis tray setup. It is designed with a single

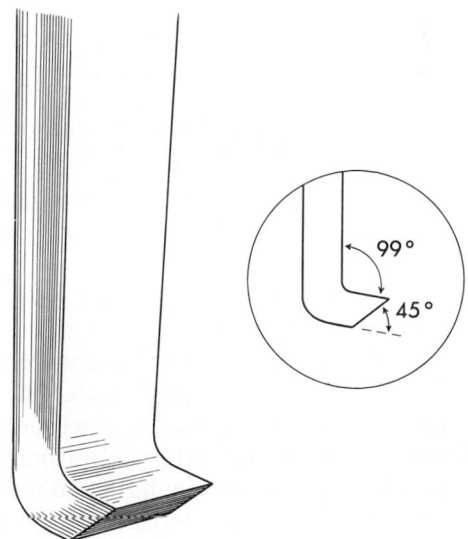

FIG. 26-20 Hoe scaler.

(From Genco RJ, Goldman HM, Cohen DW: *Contemporary periodontics,* St Louis, 1990, Mosby.)

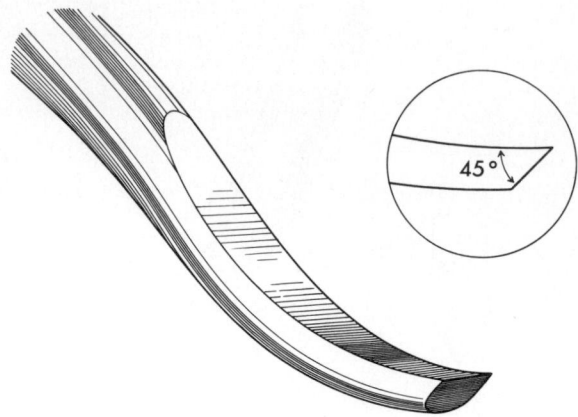

FIG. 26-21   Chisel scaler.

(From Genco RJ, Goldman HM, Cohen DW: *Contemporary periodontics,* St Louis, 1990, Mosby.)

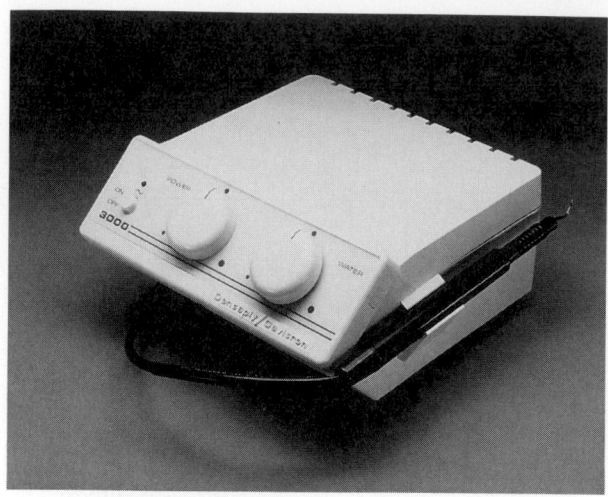

FIG. 26-22   Mechanical scaler.

(Courtesy of Teledyne, Fort Collins, Colorado.)

straight cutting edge (Fig. 26-21) and is used primarily for the removal of heavy supragingival calculus in anterior areas. This instrument is primarily used in a carefully managed push motion to dislodge and loosen the calculus.

ULTRASONIC/MECHANICAL SCALER

A **mechanical or ultrasonic scaler** can be a useful device in gross calculus removal in specific situations. This unit, shown in Fig. 26-22, is electrically powered or is air driven. It removes calculus with a high-frequency vibrating, scaler-shaped tip. Because this system generates heat, it is supplied with a built in water coolant. When this device is used, the assistant must use the HVE to remove excess water and aerosol sprays in the patient's mouth. A variety of tips are available for the ultrasonic scaler; each one resembles a manual scaler. When this device is used, the operator activates the tip of the ultrasonic scaler with a foot control. As with any clinical procedure, universal barrier techniques are used.

The mechanical scaler has been shown to be effective when it is used for the following:

▶ Removal of heavy, tenacious supragingival calculus
▶ Removal of heavy staining, which is difficult to remove with conventional hand instruments
▶ Use with patients who have acute necrotizing ulcerative gingivitis (trench mouth) because manual scaling may cause discomfort to the inflamed tissues

The ultrasonic scaler is contraindicated in the subgingival area because of its bulk and the need for water irrigation. Water irrigation is needed to reduce the heat that is generated by the device. In general, the tips of the ultrasonic scaler are more bulky than those of a fine curet.

Polishing Devices

An array of devices are available for polishing the teeth. Polishing is achieved with the use of manual or power driven polishing devices and dental floss. Polishing the teeth during an oral prophylaxis is done to accomplish the following:

▶ Remove extrinsic stains for improved esthetics
▶ Create a smooth finish on existing restorations to enhance their longevity
▶ Remove plaque from the tooth surface to create a less adherent surface and a fresh clean mouth

A disadvantage to polishing if care is not used in the polishing process is the removal of fluoride-rich enamel layer and the trauma to the gingival tissue.

▶ Manual Polishing Devices

Once the most common manual polishing device, the porte polisher (Fig. 26-23, *A* and *B*) is still available but is rarely used in practice today. This manual device is designed to hold small orangewood sticks or wooden pegs at the working ends. These wooden pegs are available in various shapes and are adapted to the tooth shapes. This instrument is used by hand to polish each surface of every tooth individually.

▶ Rotary Polishing Devices

A more common procedure is to use a rotary device, such as a prophylaxis angle or contra-angle (Fig. 26-24). These angles are supplied in a metal sterilizable version or in a disposable style. Attached to the angle is either a rubber cup or a polishing brush. Polishing cups are provided in

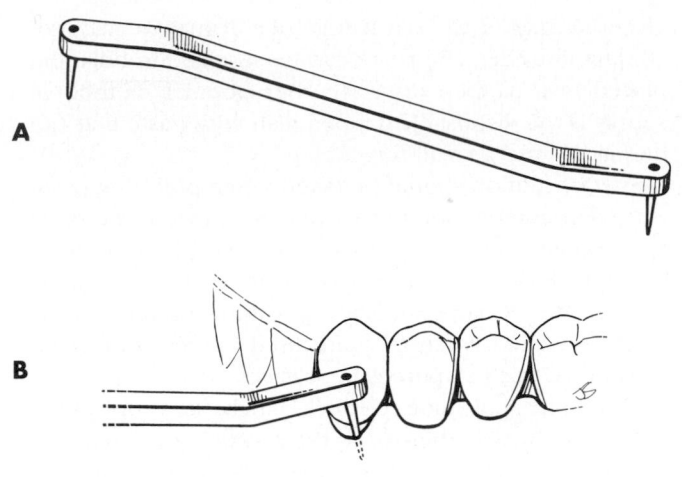

FIG. 26-23 *A*, Porte polisher. *B*, Porte polisher in position.

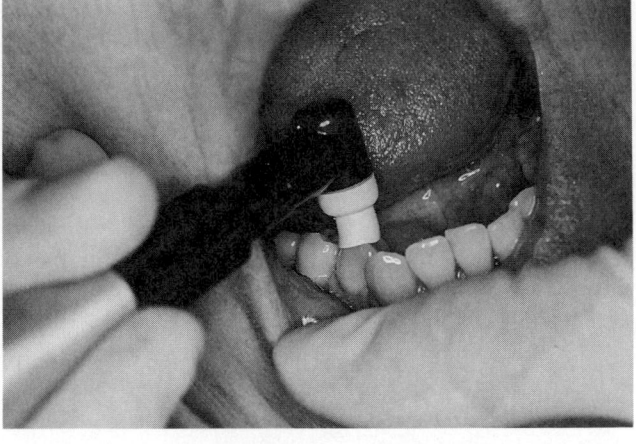

FIG. 26-24 Prophylaxis angle and cup polishing a tooth.

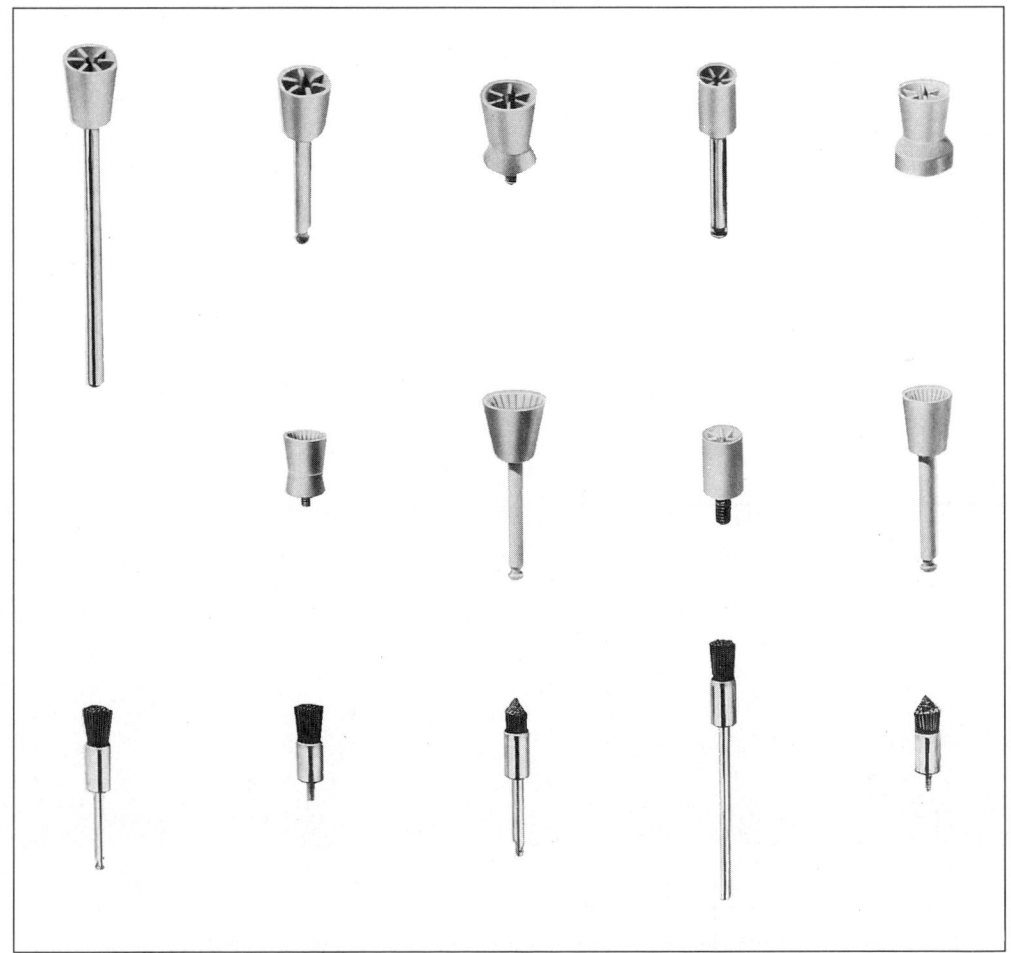

FIG. 26-25 Various prophylaxis cups and brushes.

several forms (Fig. 26-25): webbed or unwebbed, ribbed or plain, flexible or rigid, and pointed or assorted shanks for attachment to the appropriate angle or the alternative shapes. The rubber cup is used to polish the smooth surfaces—buccal, labial, and lingual—and may be used for the occlusal. Brushes are supplied in various shanks, shapes, and flexibility. The brush is used for the occlusal, pit, and fissure surfaces and is helpful in removing stains in these areas. The brush, used with care, can also be applied on the lingual of the anterior teeth where stain often occurs.

▶ Polishing Paste

Each of the devices just described requires the use of some form of abrasive to polish the teeth. Polishing paste is basically flour of pumice, with flavoring, coloring, and glycerine matrix to hold it together. It may or may not contain fluoride. The paste can be supplied in bulk and placed in a dappen dish. Another popular method of supply is the disposable dappen dish with paste that can be placed into a small finger ring.

Special caution should be taken when polishing paste is used in conjunction with other treatment at the same appointment. For instance, a nonfluoridated paste may be used during coronal polishing if sealants are to be placed later. Coarse abrasive polishing pastes can be contraindicated when they are used in areas of a fixed prosthesis, such as porcelain surfaces.

Automatic polishing devices, such as prophy-jets, which can be less abrasive to the enamel in the removal of debris, are available. These devices also provide a jet of water simultaneously to rinse the area.

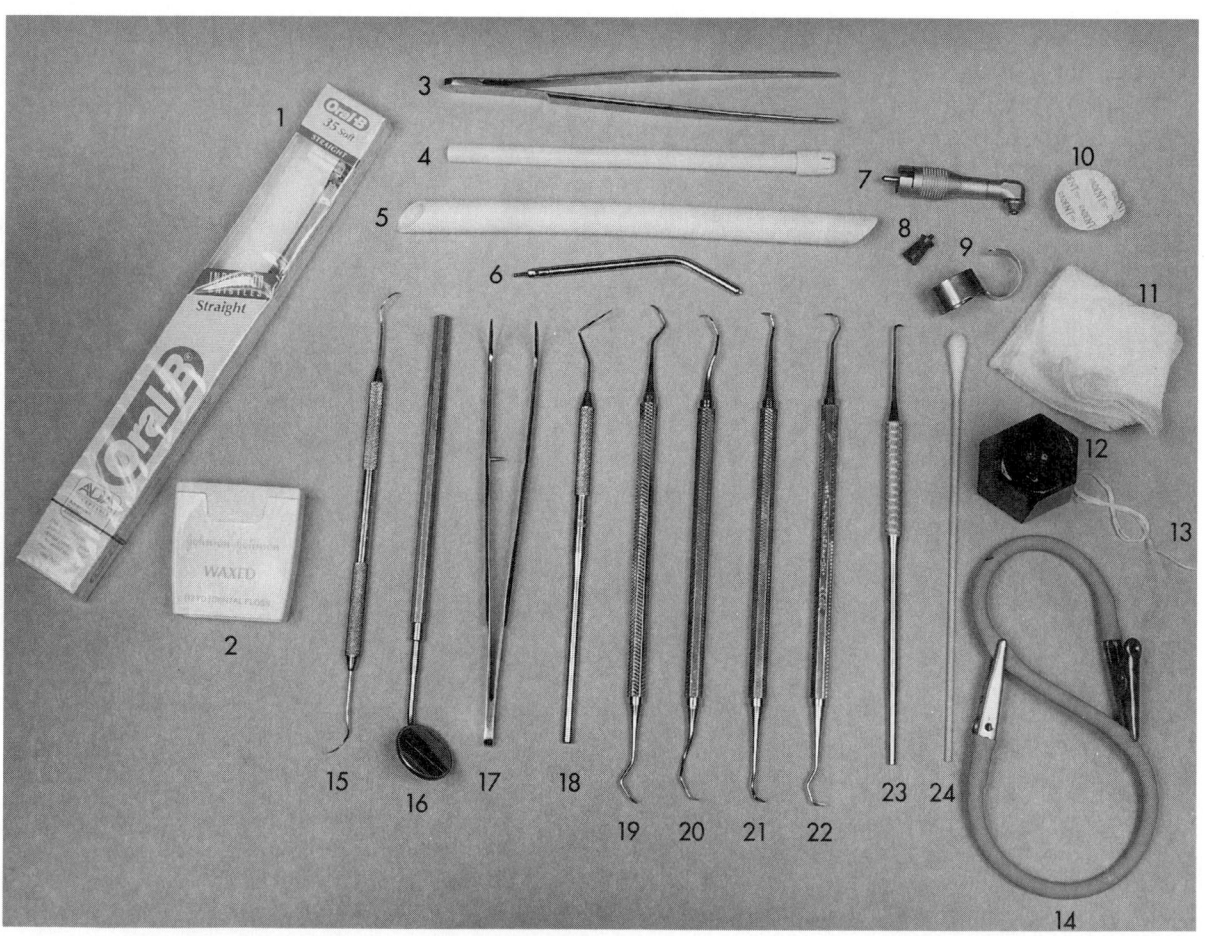

FIG. 26-26   Armamentarium for a prophylaxis. *1,* Patient toothbrush. *2,* Patient dental floss. *3,* Thumb forceps. *4,* Saliva ejector. *5,* HVE tip. *6,* A/w tip. *7,* Prophylaxis angle. *8,* Prophylaxis cup. *9,* Prophylaxis paste ring. *10,* Prophylaxis paste. *11,* 2 × 2 gauze. *12,* Dappen dish. *13,* Dental floss. *14,* Napkin chain. *15,* Siphon. *16,* Mirror. *17,* Cotton pliers. *18,* Periodontal probe. *19,* Curet scaler. *20,* Gracey scaler. *21,* Modified sickle scaler. *22,* D/E straight sickle scaler. *23,* SE straight sickle scaler. *24,* Cotton-tipped applicator.

▶ Dental Floss

Many practitioners like to use dental floss for polishing the interproximal surfaces of the teeth before a final rinsing of the patient's mouth is completed. Since some of the abrasive polishing paste may still be in the mouth, it allows for the floss to carry some of the abrasive through the interproximal and to aid in polishing each of the smooth proximal surfaces. Waxed or unwaxed floss can be used during this step.

Oral Prophylaxis Procedure

Whether the oral prophylaxis is performed by the dentist or the hygienist, the utilization of a chairside assistant increases the efficiency of the procedure. The following provides a list of supplies and an efficient step-by-step procedure for a manual oral prophylaxis:

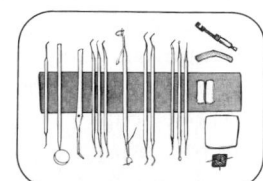

Armamentarium (Fig. 26-26)

Protective glasses for patient
Disclosing solution

ORAL PROPHYLAXIS

▶ Are all universal barrier techniques being used?
▶ Is all the armamentarium available and prepared for use?
▶ Are the instruments arranged in sequence of use?
▶ Am I prepared for alternative treatment plans?
▶ Is the necessary equipment turned on and ready to operate?

The role of the dental assistant during manual scaling and polishing includes the following:

1. Seat and drape the patient with a patient napkin or apron, and offer safety glasses
2. Pass the mirror and explorer for the initial oral examination
3. Exchange the explorer for a periodontal probe. Then exchange the probe for an applicator with lubricant that is placed on the lips before the disclosing solution is applied; the assistant holds the disclosing solution while the operator applies it to the teeth
4. Return these instruments to the mobile cart, and rinse the patient's mouth
5. Pass the hand mirror to the patient for the operator to illustrate the disclosed area to the patient
6. Pass the scalers in sequence of operator's choice
7. Keep the mirror clear of debris, and evacuate the mouth as necessary
8. Be prepared to rinse the site as bleeding occurs, to evacuate the area, or to spray air on a specific site as the operator needs a clear field
9. Keep instruments free of debris by wiping the instruments during use in the transfer area; by using the HVE tip close to the instrument, debris will not accumulate on the instrument end; HINT: if the instrument is wiped manually, care should be taken to grasp the instrument on the sides of the blade with the 2 × 2 gauze instead of the tip end, and wipe in a direction away from the shaft of the instrument; this avoids accidental puncture of the gloves
10. Rinse and evacuate as necessary; constantly observe the patient's mouth as bleeding occurs or as saliva accumulates in the mouth
11. When scaling is completed, pass the handpiece with the prophylaxis angle and cup attached; position the handpiece for the appropriate arch (a specific coronal polishing procedure in the box on p. 666)
12. Hold polishing paste in the transfer zone so that it is always available for operator to use
13. Evacuate saliva and polishing paste; NOTE: some polishing pastes and viscous saliva cause splatter, and it is helpful to place the HVE tip as close to the polishing cup as possible, and yet not draw the paste from the cup before it is used
14. Change from the polishing cup to a brush as needed
15. Pass the dental floss
16. Perform a complete mouth rinse (see Chapter 21, *Oral Evacuation*)
17. Pass mirror and explorer for the final oral examination; some operators may opt to redisclose the patient's mouth at this time
18. Pass 2 × 2 gauze for soft tissue examination of the tongue and the floor of the mouth
19. Chart oral conditions as dictated; this may be done before scaling and at the option of the operator
20. Offer the patient a cup of water for rinsing; pass the saliva ejector or evacuate with HVE
21. Check the patient's face for debris, and wipe with a damp tissue; dry the face thoroughly; if the procedure has been done by a hygienist, the dentist may complete an oral examination at this time, according to the state board of dentistry licensure regulations
22. Reposition the patient and direct them to the rest room if they wish to freshen up before leaving the office
23. Follow the suggested disinfection and sterilization procedures

---

▶ Are the appropriate universal barrier techniques removed?
▶ Have all of the appropriate surfaces been cleaned and disinfected?
▶ Has all armamentarium been removed?
▶ Has all equipment been repositioned?
▶ Has all the equipment been disinfected/sterilized according to OSHA guidelines?

Explorer
Mouth mirror
Cotton pliers
Periodontal probe
Curet scaler
Straight sickle scaler
Modified sickle scaler
Cotton tip applicators
Lubricant
Prophylaxis angle or contra-angle or the appropriate
Handpiece
Rubber cup
Bristle brush
Polishing paste
Dappen dish or prophy ring
2 × 2 gauze
Oral evacuation tip
Saliva ejector
Dental floss or tape, approximately 18 inches
HVE tip
Disposable drinking cup
Mouthwash
Disclosing solution
Hand mirror
Patient's chart, radiographs, and exam sheet
Sterile writing devices

[AF]

CORONAL POLISHING PROCEDURE

1. Place the polishing paste onto the cup by lightly rotating the cup in the paste.
2. Develop a sequence for polishing; for instance, polish all of the buccal surfaces of an arch and then the lingual and occlusal surfaces. Follow this same pattern in the next arch.
3. Avoid damaging gingival and tooth tissues during polishing by the following methods:
   a. Use a moist polishing paste
   b. Begin the rotation of the cup before placement on the tooth surface
   c. Rotate the polishing cup only at a low speed
   d. Avoid using excessive pressure of the cup on the tooth
   e. Tilt the polishing cup toward the occlusal rather than the gingival surface of the teeth
   f. Avoid forcing the cup edge too far gingivally

Fluoride

As early as 1874 fluorine was thought to have a preventive effect on dental caries. In 1908 a dentist in Colorado Springs, Colorado, Fredrick McKay, suggested that brown mottling that is found on the teeth of children in that area could be attributed to excess fluorides found in the water supply. Without having confirmed data, McKay began to work with G.V. Black and a publication arose that suggested fluorine was the responsible agent of the mottled teeth; however, the publication did not suggest that fluorine lowered the incidence of caries.

The cities of Grand Rapids and Muskegon, Michigan, as well as Newburgh and Kingston, New York, were the test cities for fluoride-containing and fluoride-deficient water in studies conducted during the 1940s.

In 1925 Dr. McKay was consulted in a case from Oakley, Idaho, about children who had mottled teeth. Dr. McKay recommended finding a source of surface water rather than using deep-well water, and no new cases of enamel mottling resulted in subsequent years. This correlation gave rise to Dr. McKay's announcment that "caries was inhibited by the same water which produced mottled enamel." After much research a definite inverse relationship between the fluoride content of the water and dental caries was discovered.

Fluoride is found naturally in some water supplies and today is considered an important substance in the prevention of dental disease. An optimum level of one part per million was found to give positive caries reduction without creating mottling effects. The city of Grand Rapids, Michigan, was the first to have sodium fluoride added to the public water supply in 1945. A control group in Muskegon, Michigan, had no additional fluoride added to their water. The study was scheduled to last 15 years. After 6 ½ years, however, the results of decreased dental decay were so impressive that other cities joined in by adding fluoride to their public water reservoirs. From that time to the present, fluoride has been proven over and over again to provide substantial protection against dental caries. Two forms of fluoride are useful in controling dental caries: systemic or topical application.

▶ Systemic Fluoride

Systemic fluoride is ingested into the body and incorporated into the developing teeth. In the presence of this fluoride, fluorapatite and hydroxyapatite crystals are formed as a component of the tooth structure; this provides the tooth enamel with increased caries protection even before tooth eruption and can be accomplished by adding fluoride to the water supply. If this option is not available, fluoride can be obtained by prescription in chewable or liquid drop supplements.

The patient's water supply must be evaluated to determine its natural fluoride content before a prescription for fluoride supplements is dispensed. Most local health departments make such testing available. Systemic fluoride supplements, if needed, should be given from birth to age 12 or 13 or when the second permanent molars erupt. Up to 60% reduction in dental caries has been shown with systemic fluoride. Excessive amounts of ingested fluoride should be avoided because this could cause *endemic dental fluorosis* or mottled enamel, as Dr. McKay noted nearly 100 years ago.

▶ Topical Fluoride

Once the tooth has erupted, fluoride can be topically applied in many ways, each providing various degrees of caries reduction. This form of fluoride is most effective on the smooth surfaces of the teeth. Topical fluoride protects the tooth in two ways: it is taken up by the exposed tooth surface and makes the tooth more resistant to plaque acid demineralization, or it is deposited on decalcified areas and assists in their remineralization. Topical fluoride has also been shown to be effective in desensitizing teeth. With all three types of the topical fluoride, uptake of fluoride by the tooth is at its peak during the first years following tooth eruption.

Topical fluoride is available in many forms: through the use of fluoridated toothpastes, mouth rinses or topical application.

One of the most common forms of topical fluoride is fluoridated dentifrice. This formulation of toothpaste usually contains between 1000 to 1100 parts per million of fluoride per dose, and has offered 15% to 30% reduction in dental caries. Supervision of young children is essential to avoid excessive fluoride consumption during brushing.

Fluoride mouth rinses, both those that are sold over the counter and those that are prescribed, are another means of topical fluoride application. These are known to reduce the caries experience by 20% to 50%. Nonprescription ADA-approved fluoride rinses can be recommended and readily purchased by patients with a high caries rate. Adults with gingival recession and exposed root surfaces also benefit from this product, as root surface decay can be a major concern. Fluoride rinses should not be suggested for the very young children or for those who are unable to effectively expectorate the product from their mouths.

Professionally applied and home topical fluoride treatments offer between 40% and 50% caries reduction. This type of topical fluoride is commonly found in three forms: sodium fluoride, stannous fluoride, and acidulated phosphate fluoride. With each of these types of fluoride the professional application of the fluoride treatment is done in the dental office. Variations in the fluoride gels have allowed for home use through patient administration. The home gel fluoride treatments contain a lesser degree of fluoride concentration, thus the uptake percentage is reduced in each application.

The armamentarium used during the professionally applied fluoride treatment includes the following (Fig. 26-27).

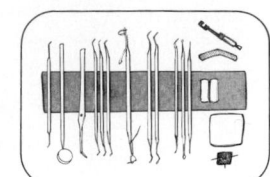

Fluoride gel
Saliva ejector
Upper and lower
  arch foam trays
Cotton rolls and holders
  (optional)
Cotton-tipped applicator
Timing device

ACIDULATED PHOSPHATE FLUORIDE APPLICATION

Acidulated phosphate fluoride (APF) in gel form is currently the most widely used topical agent. Acidulated phosphate fluoride is available in a 1.23% gel in both 1- and 4-minute formulas. A 4-minute, single professional application of this gel twice a year will give valuable caries protection. APF is a stable solution with a long shelf life. It is available in many agreeable flavors. Uptake of fluoride by the tooth is good because of the low pH of the gel. APF is contraindicated because of the low pH for use on inflamed tissues or esthetic restorations; etching could occur. APF can also be suggested for home use with custom-fitted trays, using a 0.5% gel solution. If the APF is the preferred choice and the above-mentioned contraindications exist, then an APF with a neutralizer must be used.

APPLYING ACIDULATED PHOSPHATE FLUORIDE (APF)

1. Seat patient in an upright position
2. Try in the trays
3. Fill trays ⅓ full with APF gel
4. Place cotton rolls in vestibule areas if necessary
5. Dry the teeth thoroughly with compressed air
6. Insert foam trays—one at a time, or as a set—into the patient's mouth (Fig. 26-28)
7. Insert a saliva ejector and cotton rolls at the corner of the patient's mouth, and instruct the patient to gently chew for 1 minute
8. Four minutes after the saliva ejector has been inserted, remove it and discard the cotton rolls; remove the foam trays
9. Remove excess fluoride from the mouth with the saliva ejector; direct the patient to empty excess gel from his or her mouth before swallowing
10. A dry gauze may be used to further wipe off the teeth and tongue if necessary
11. Instruct the patient not to eat, chew, drink, smoke, or rinse for 30 minutes following this treatment

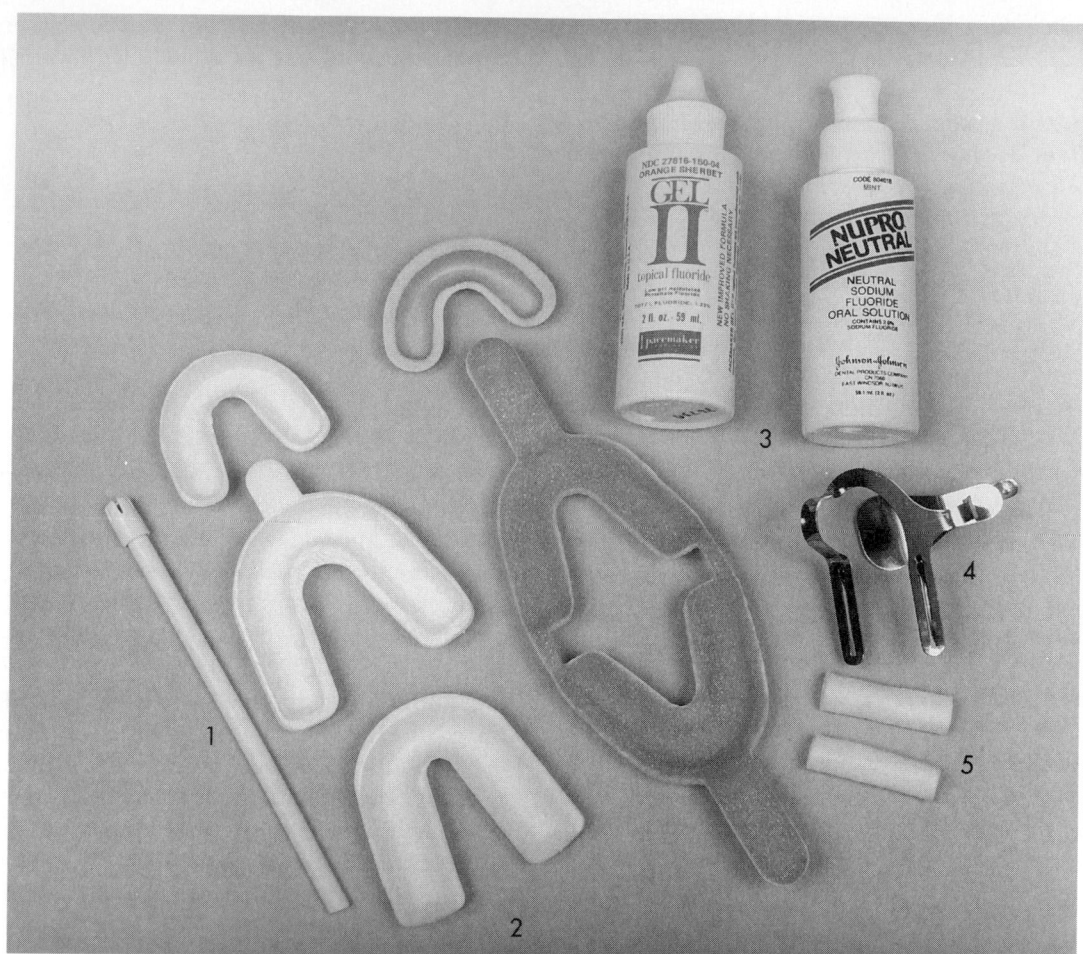

FIG. 26-27   Armamentarium for a fluoride treatment. *1,* Saliva ejector. *2,* Assorted fluoride treatment trays. *3,* Fluoride gels. *4,* Cotton roll holder. *5,* Cotton rolls.

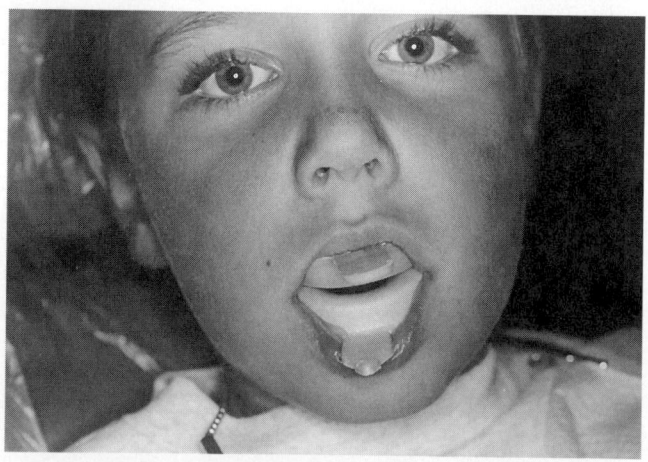

FIG. 26-28   Fluoride trays in place.

STANNOUS FLUORIDE APPLICATION

Stannous fluoride is an unstable solution and must be mixed fresh for each patient. A single four-minute application of an 8% or 10% liquid mixture is recommended at 6-month intervals for caries protection. This solution possesses a metallic taste and cannot be flavored. Brown staining of the teeth, especially decalcified areas, and anterior restorations is a noticeable disadvantage to the fluoride agent. Irritation to soft tissues has also been noted. Stannous fluoride in a 0.4% gel may be recommended for home use. This gel is applied with a toothbrush, with cotton-tipped applicators, or with the solution in custom-fitted trays. Stannous fluoride in this form is more stable and can be pleasantly flavored.

SODIUM FLUORIDE APPLICATION

The success of sodium fluoride depends on a sequence of four, 3-minute applications that are spaced 2 to 7 days apart. These professional treatments are scheduled when the child is approximately 3, 7, 10, and 13 years old to coincide with the eruption of new teeth. A single dose of sodium fluoride may be recommended at 6-month intervals for additional caries reduction. As with all three of the topical fluoride agents, uptake of fluoride by the tooth is at its peak during the first years following eruption. Sodium fluoride has an agreeable flavor, and will not cause tooth discoloration. Irritation of soft tissue has not been an issue. A concentration of 1.1% sodium fluoride is used for home application in custom-fitted trays.

This entire treatment must be applied in a series of four consecutive appointments that are approximately a week apart.

Pit and Fissure/Enamel Sealants

As teeth develop in the bone, deep grooves and pits may form on the tooth surface. When these teeth erupt into the mouth they become susceptible to dental decay. **Pit and fissure sealants** are a clear or shaded resin material placed on the pits and fissures of premolars and molars. It is virtually impossible for the patient to completely clean these *pit and fissure* areas. Material that is referred to as pit and fissure sealants or enamel sealants offers a barrier between these vulnerable tooth surfaces and bacterial plaque. For optimal protection the material should be placed soon after the tooth erupts. When the material is properly applied, sealants provide excellent caries protection.

Many brands of pit and fissure sealant materials are available, including those that are self-curing and light-cured, tinted, or opaque and clear. The manufacturer's directions should be carefully followed. When selecting teeth for sealant placement avoid those teeth that exhibit the following characteristics:

▶ Hypoplastic enamel
▶ Amalgam restorations
▶ Gold inlays or foils
▶ Deep carious lesions
▶ Synthetic porcelain restorations

The ideal teeth for successful sealant placement are the occlusal surfaces of premolars and molars. Studies have shown that the retention rate (the period of time that the sealant maintains margin integrity) on premolars is higher than on molars. As treatment progresses towards the posterior in the oral cavity, the retention rate tends to lessen, usually caused by the increased difficulty of access in placement.

It is also thought that the retention rate in mandibular teeth is higher than maxillary teeth. Again the reason suggested for this factor is that access to the mandibular teeth is more convenient than it is to the maxillary arch.

▶ Rationale for Sealant Placement

Sealants reduce the risk of dental decay on primary and permanent teeth. Sealants have also been shown to contain no toxic or carcinogenic agents that could have an adverse effect on the body. The cost of placing sealants compared with the cost of placing a restoration that may have a life of 15 to 20 years is much less. Although sealants may not last as long as a restoration, the amount of tooth structure removed during the pit and fissure procedure is microscopic in size, while tooth structure that is lost during the placement of a restoration is

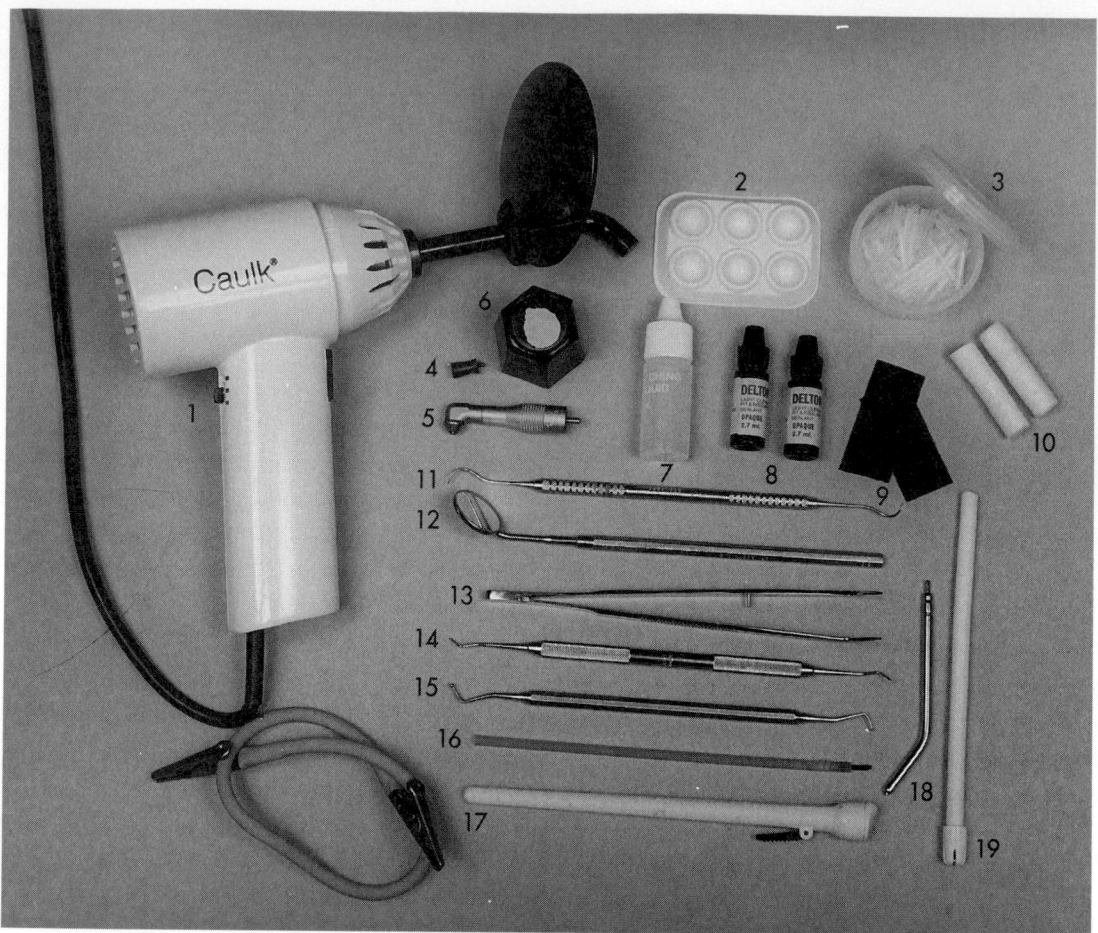

FIG. 26-29 Armamentarium for pit and fissure sealants. *1,* Light-curing device. *2,*
Welled-solution devices. *3,* Tubes for P & F application. *4,* Prophylaxis cup. *5,* Prophylaxis
angle. *6,* Dappen dish, with nonfluoridated paste. *7,* Acid etch solution. *8,* Sealant. *9,* Articulating paper. *10,* Cotton rolls. *11,* Explorer. *12,* Mirror. *13,* Cotton pliers. *14,* Spoon excavator. *15,*
Ball burnisher. *16,* Brush. *17,* Sealant applicating device. *18,* A/w tip. *19,* Saliva ejector.

considerable. An even greater amount of tooth structure
is usually lost during the removal and replacement of a
restoration. If a sealant is lost or is defective, unlike a
restoration, there appears to be no increase in caries
incidence of these surfaces over teeth where no sealants
have been placed.

In certain circumstances studies have shown that
where decay is minimal on the occlusal surface, placement of pit and fissure sealants has arrested the dental
decay. The residual bacteria is sealed off from its nutrient
supply and thus prevents acid accumulation. The cessation of acid accumulation arrests the decay progress.

▶ Sealant Procedure

The technique and instruments that are used during the
procedure vary with each clinician. However, some basic
instruments and steps are common to all. The steps

involved in applying pit and fissure sealants are listed
below.

▶ Armamentarium (Fig. 26-29)

Many of the following instruments and devices have been
discussed at length in this or other chapters in text, so the
level of explanation of instrument description and use is
limited in this procedure.

    Rubber cup or bristle brush
    Pumice or *nonfluoridated* prophylaxis paste
    Isolation materials
    Explorer
    Mouth mirror
    Cotton pliers
    Articulating paper
    Etchant
    Sealant

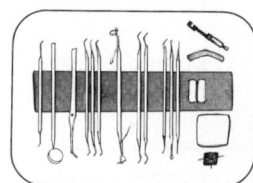

BASIC STEPS IN APPLYING PIT AND FISSURE SEALANT

1. Prepare armamentarium
2. Update medical history
3. Examine and determine absence of caries in teeth that will receive pit and fissure sealants
4. Pumice tooth with nonfluoridated pumice
5. Rinse and evacuate
6. Check occlusal relationship
7. Isolate
8. Dispense and place acid etchant
9. Rinse thoroughly, evacuate, and dry the teeth
10. Isolate again with dry cotton rolls
11. Dispense and apply pit and fissure sealant
12. Check occlusal relationship and correct if necessary

Disposable sable brush tips, skubes, or cotton pledgets
Brush tip holder
Plastic dispensing well
Sealant applicator and tube
Curing light
Rotary instruments, including handpiece

The application of a sealant is usually limited to one or two quadrants at a time. The teeth may be isolated before or after the pumicing step, depending on the operator's preference. To effectively isolate all quadrants at once and to place the sealant is sometimes difficult, particularly if it is kept in mind that the greatest reason for sealant failure is due to inadequate isolation techniques that occur during the application. Rubber dam or cotton rolls are used for isolation. If rubber dam is used, a single quadrant is isolated and dried; however, if the cotton roll technique is preferred, one side of the mouth could be isolated. The cotton rolls are placed in the maxillary arch near the parotid gland; four are placed in the mandible, two are placed sublingually, and two are placed in the vestibule area.

Polish the Teeth

1. The teeth are cleaned of any debris and fluoride remnants by using a rubber cup or bristle brush to apply a nonfluoridated pumice to the occlusal surfaces. The operator must cover all occlusal surfaces during this preparation step to ensure adequate etching. 2. Once they are polished with pumice, the teeth are rinsed and dried thoroughly. 3. If cotton rolls were placed, they may need to be removed and replaced to ensure complete isolation for the next step.

Assess Occlusion

1. Articulating paper is positioned over the teeth that are to have sealants placed to determine the contact points during articulation. This step aids the operator in determining the extent of sealant placement on the occlusal surface. If the articulation is not determined, the sealant may be placed over a contact point, which could cause interference in the patient's bite. 2. Remove any interference that could lead to an open margin and subsequent failure of the sealant. NOTE: If rubber dam isolation was selected, checking the articulation is impossible, unless the isolation is placed after the polishing of the teeth is completed.

ACID ETCHING

1. The acid etchant, either a gel or a liquid, is dispensed into the dispensing well and passed to the operator with the application device of choice. 2. The brush, skube, or pledget with cotton pliers is immersed in the etchant and applied to the tooth surface for 60 seconds for a permanent tooth or 90 seconds for a primary tooth. 3. The liquid etchant is lightly bathed over the tooth surface with a single application, not rubbing it on the enamel. 4. The gel etchant is constantly applied to the enamel for the whole time. 5. As the etchant is passed to the operator, care is taken to avoid any spillage as the acid could slightly burn tissues.

6. After the prescribed period of time has elapsed, the tooth surface is rinsed completely with an aerated spray for 30 seconds. 7. The occlusal surface is dried completely, disclosing a white, chalky enamel surface. If the enamel does not appear chalky, the procedure must be repeated to ensure proper bonding of the resin to the enamel. 8. The moist cotton rolls are carefully removed and replaced with dry ones if they are being used for isolation. 9. If any moisture touches the etched surfaces, the etching step must be repeated.

RESIN APPLICATION

1. The resin material is placed in the dispensing well and the application device is selected for placement. 2. If the resin is of a chemically cured design, equal amounts of the resin are dispensed and mixed until the two are homogeneous. 3. If the kit provides an applicator, the tube is placed in the applicator. 4. The lever of the applicator is forced down and the tip of the tube is placed in the resin (Fig. 26-30, *A*). 5. The lever is released, and through capillary action the resin is drawn into the tube. 6. The applicator is passed to the operator, who places the tube tip on the most distal surface of the tooth. The operator presses the lever lightly as the applicator is pulled toward the mesial of the tooth, laying a thin layer of resin over the etched tooth surface. 7. The procedure is repeated on the next tooth if more than one is receiving the sealant.

If a skube, pledget, or brush is used to apply the sealant, the device is immersed in the sealant, placed on

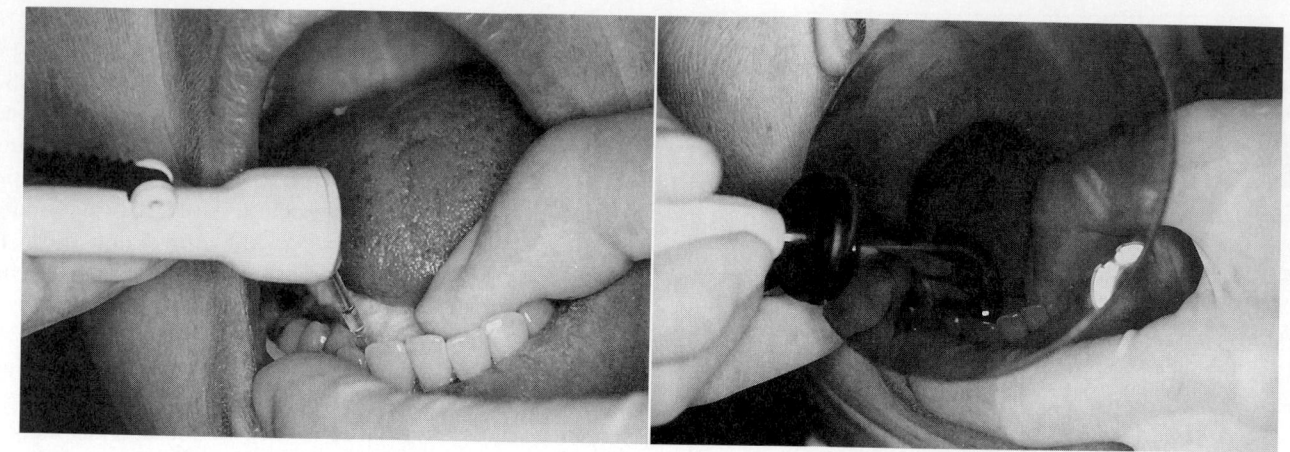

FIG. 26-30   *A*, Application of pit and fissure sealant. *B*, Curing the pit and fissure sealant.

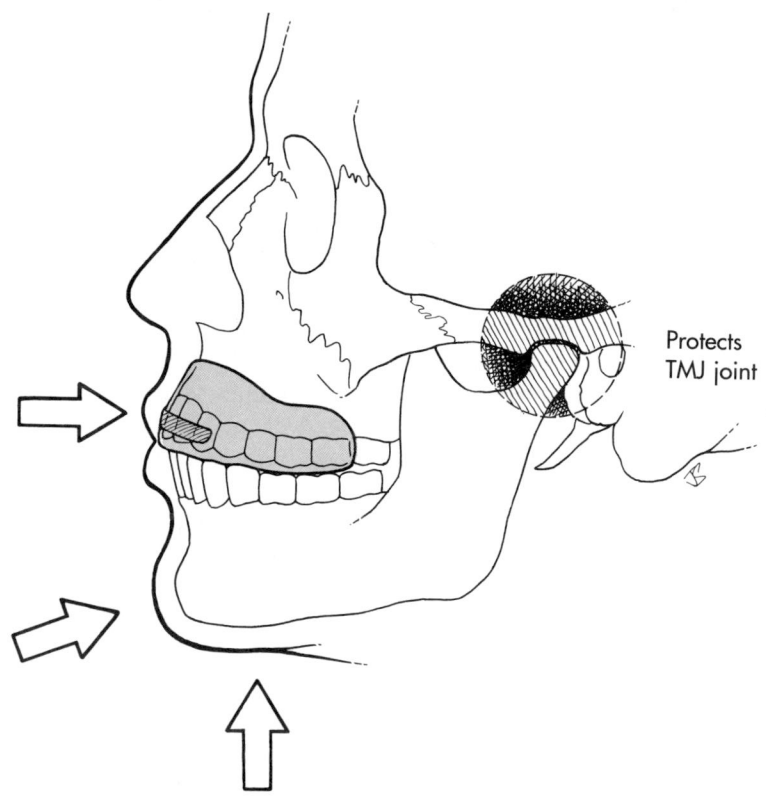

Protects
TMJ joint

FIG. 26-31   Sites of impact where trauma can be prevented through the use of a mouthguard. Arrows represent points of impact. A mouth guard may prevent oral lacerations, tooth injury, jaw fractures, TMJ trauma.

the distal surface, and drawn toward the mesial covering with a layer of resin. The device is immersed in the resin as often as is necessary to cover the etched surface.

8. The applicator is passed back to the assistant, and the curing light is positioned over the resin. 9. The patient is directed to close his or her eyes, and the operator and assistant do not look directly at the light during operation; or a curing shield may be used. The curing light is activated for approximately 20 seconds as the tip is held close to the tooth surface (Fig. 26-30, *B*). 10. At the end of curing time the explorer is exchanged to test an outer margin for hardness. The operator must be careful not to dislodge a margin at this time, since this could lead to sealant failure. 11. If the sealant is of a chemically cured design, the assistant can determine the hardness of the resin by checking any excess material in the dispensing well with an explorer.

Isolation Removal and Articulation Check

1. The isolation is removed. 2. The articulating paper is placed over the sealed teeth, and the patient is directed to bite up and down and from side to side. 3. If any areas that are covered with the sealant are marked by the articulating paper, it may be necessary to use a rotary device to correct; this is not the ideal, since the margins of the sealant can be opened with the use of a rotary instrument.

The properly placed sealant can provide many years of service for a caries protection. When sealants become defective, they can be replaced with a new sealant.

Mouthguards

Mouthguards as described in Chapter 11 are protective devices used in contact sports or physical activities. Various devices are available for patients, and the construction of a custom-made mouthguard is described in Chapter 40. Mouthguards are usually made of polyvinylacetate-polyethylene and absorb impact to the oral structures during physical activities. Fig. 26-31 illustrates the potential areas of trauma which can be prevented or reduced by the use of a mouthguard.

KEY POINTS

▶ Preventive dentistry not only involves the private practice of dentistry, but also goes beyond it to include community health programs that prevent the occurrence of oral diseases and abnormalities. Prevention is a process that requires an understanding of patient needs, a willingness to listen, good motivating skills, and an ability to use positive reinforcement. Prevention is the foundation for a successful dental practice.

▶ A prevention program in the dental office includes patient education, an oral prophylaxis, the application of topical fluoride, and the use of pit and fissure sealants. To be totally successful, however, any prevention program requires that the patient be motivated to achieve optimal dental health.

▶ Each dental professional in the office must take an active role in prevention; this requires a thorough understanding of the relationship of diet and nutrition to dental health, as well as knowledge and skill to teach common oral hygiene techniques that are appropriate to a patient's individual need. The dental professional also assumes responsibility for evaluation of oral products that confront the consumer on the market today, including the following: dentifrices, flosses, toothbrush styles, oral rinses, fluoride, and a myriad of interdental aids.

▶ Dependent on the individual state dental practice act, the qualified dental assistant will be responsible for various treatment as part of preventive dentistry. This treatment will include fluoride application, placement of pit and fissure sealants, coronal polishing, and diet analysis, as well as assisting with the oral prophylaxis procedure.

BIBLIOGRAPHY

Hoag PM, Pawlak EA: *Essentials of periodontics,* ed 4, St Louis, 1990, Mosby.

Mosley DC, Megginson LC, Pietri PH: *Supervisory management: the art of working with and through people,* ed 2, Cincinnati, 1989, South-Western.

Weiss RL, Swearingen RV: *Chairside psychology in patient education: a self-instruction course,* U.S. Department of Health, Education, and Welfare, 1969, The Department.

Woodall IR: *Comprehensive dental hygiene care,* ed 4, St Louis, 1993, Mosby.

UNIT VI RESTORATIVE PROCEDURES

27 Amalgam Restoration

LEARNING OBJECTIVES

You will have mastered the material in this chapter when you can:

▶ Define the key terms
▶ Describe the use of amalgam as a restorative material
▶ Review the G.V. Black cavity forms
▶ Describe the steps of a cavity preparation
▶ Identify and explain the phases of an amalgam procedure
▶ Identify the armamentarium and materials used in the amalgam restorative procedure
▶ Identify the parts and describe the assembly of a circumferential matrix band and retainer
▶ Describe the function of basic instruments used in the amalgam restorative procedure
▶ Explain procedural modifications in different amalgam procedures
▶ Explain the indications for a pin-retained amalgam and identify the associated armamentarium

KEY TERMS

Anatomic carving	Outline form
Caries removal	Resistance form
Convenience form	Retention form
Extension for prevention	Smooth surface carving
Opening phase	

An amalgam procedure is considered a restorative procedure: one in which tooth structure is restored with a man-made substance. The substance is used to recreate anatomy that no longer exists on a tooth. The placement of an amalgam restoration involves a single appointment, step-by-step procedure that includes the following:

▶ Examination of the treatment site
▶ Preparation of the area
▶ Medication of the preparation
▶ Placement and finishing of the amalgam material

This procedure allows the operator to replace lost tooth structure with a metallic material that is an amalgamation of several substances, such as mercury, silver, tin, and copper.

The amalgam restoration is a dental procedure performed on teeth to restore surfaces that have been lost to trauma, to defects, or to carious lesions. Amalgam restorations are placed in cavity preparations that are predominantly on posterior tooth surfaces of the primary and permanent dentition, including Class I, II, V, and VI carious lesions.

Amalgam is not a particularly esthetic material, and its use in the anterior segment of a patient's mouth would be prohibitive. An exception could be the use of amalgam in a Class III preparation on the distolingual surface of a cuspid, or Class I pit on the lingual of an anterior tooth.

As discussed in Chapter 6, the original G.V. Black cavity classification included Class I through Class V preparations of teeth. A Class II classification identifies cavities on one or both proximal surfaces of premolars and molars. A modification of Black's classification has been made to differentiate the Class II classification, which includes only one proximal surface, from that of a modified Class II, which includes both proximal surfaces. This latter classification has been designated as a Class VI by many dentists. For the sake of clarity a Class II cavity is referred to as a cavity that includes one proximal surface and a Class VI is sometimes referred to as a modified Class II, which includes both proximal surfaces.

The cavity classifications noted above are all intracoronal restorations since they are contained in the crown of the tooth. Amalgam does not possess adequate compressive strength to be used when the crown of a posterior tooth needs to be completely restored. However, amalgam may be used as a core material to rebuild tooth structure that has been extensively lost due to fracture or decay. The core of amalgam placed on the tooth usually serves as a base for a cast metal restoration.

Dental Amalgam

Dental amalgam: a combination of mercury and alloy that consists primarily of silver particles, is still a commonly used restorative material in dentistry. Because of its mercury content, amalgam has always been the subject of controversy; however, in 1983 the ADA Council on Dental Materials, Instruments, and Equipment and the Council on Dental Therapeutics declared amalgam safe for all dental patients, except those who are allergic to it. In July, 1989, the same Councils confirmed their positions with publications supporting the original reports. Mercury exists in our environment, and it is harmful to human existence when we are exposed to unsafe amounts. The proper safety guidelines as described in Chapter 11 can reduce or eliminate mercury contamination in a dental office.

Cavity Forms

G.V. Black, who is sometimes referred to as the father of scientific dentistry, developed standardized rules for cavity form during the preparation of all teeth that are to receive different restorative materials. Cavity form is the actual shaping of the cavity walls and floors as the tooth is prepared to receive various types of restorative

---

BOX 27-1

CAVITY FORMS

OUTLINE FORM

The form of the cavity preparation as it meets the tooth surface when it has been expanded to include all carious areas

RESISTANCE FORM

A shape that is given to a cavity that enables a restoration to withstand the stress that occurs during mastication

RETENTION FORM

Shaping the cavity preparation to prevent the restoration from being displaced; a large part of this is provided by the resistance form; in most cavities the retention form is made by shaping certain of the opposing walls so that they will be parallel or slightly undercut

CONVENIENCE FORM

The changes that are made in the basic outline form to facilitate visibility and placement of the restorative material

REMOVAL OF CARIES

The actual removal of carious or decalcified tissue from the tooth

FINISHING ENAMEL WALLS AND MARGINS

The placement of angles and bevels in the cavity preparation, and the final smoothing of the cavity walls

EXTENSION FOR PREVENTION

The extension of the original cavity preparation includes pits and fissures that could become carious at a later time.

---

materials. Cavity form phases include the **opening, outline, resistance, caries removal,** and **retention** phases. Additional phases to cavity form may also be used when necessary to create a certain preparation. These phases include **convenience, finishing walls and margins, and extension for prevention.** Each of these phases requires different designs and various instruments depending on the type of restorative material that is to be placed. All members of the operative team must understand the principles of cavity form before they participate in the operative procedure. The cavity forms that provide guidelines for a cavity preparation (shown in Box 27-1) lead to a successfully retained restoration.

 Greene Vardiman (G.V.) Black, who first became a licensed physician in 1878 and later served as Dean of Northwestern University Dental School in Chicago, was also an educator, researcher, biologist, and author. He made two major contributions to dentistry: the principle of *extension for prevention,* which allows for the extension of margins of cavity preparations to a point where a patient can easily reach with a toothbrush, and the standardized rules of cavity preparation. Before his death in 1915 he claimed that "the day would come in the not too distant future when emphasis in a dental practice would be on prevention rather than reparative dentistry."

Common Armamentarium for an Amalgam Restoration

Before the steps of the restorative procedure are addressed, a review of the instruments is necessary. Each clinician has favorite instruments and devices to use in a given restorative procedure. The summary of armamentarium that follows offers some traditional options for the amalgam restorative procedure. Often, as a dental assistant begins to study a new area, it is helpful to group or categorize materials and instruments. The armamentarium is grouped in phases for treatment. The descriptions and basic use of each instrument are discussed in Chapter 18, *Basic Dental Instruments.*

The function of the instruments as they apply to the amalgam procedure are addressed in this chapter.

BOX 27-2

COMMON STEPS OF AN AMALGAM RESTORATION

1. Prepare the armamentarium
2. Update medical history
3. Examine treatment site
4. Determine occlusal relationship
5. Administer anesthesia
6. Isolate with rubber dam
7. Open cavity preparation
8. Outline/resistance form of cavity preparation
9. Remove caries
10. Place retention form
11. Isolate with cotton rolls (alternative isolation)
12. Place cavity medication
13. Place matrix band, retainer, and wedge(s)
14. Insert and condense amalgam
15. Perform initial carving
16. Remove matrix retainer, wedge, and band
17. Perform interproximal carving
18. Complete final carving
19. Remove isolation
20. Check the articulation
21. Burnish the margins
22. Give postoperative instructions
23. Finish, and polish (Optional)

The techniques of the amalgam procedure followed by each operator may vary, but certain fundamental phases are common to all. Box 27-2 lists common steps in a Class II amalgam procedure. The manipulation of amalgam as a restorative material is explained in Chapter 11, *Dental Materials.*

▶ Examination Phase

The instruments in the examination phase: the explorer, mirror, and cotton plier, are used to check the tooth for anomalies, retraction, visibility, and illumination and to pass small items to and from the mouth. Even though the instruments are categorized in the examination phase, some are used throughout the procedure for other purposes, such as removing excess amalgam.

EXPLORER

The explorer is used to detect anomalies in tooth structure, to remove excess amalgam between the matrix band and restorative material at the marginal ridge, and to check margins. An additional function of the explorer is to check for flash or excess at the cavosurface margins.

MIRROR

The mirror is used to reflect light or to provide indirect vision to a tooth or into a cavity preparation. It also aids in the retraction of tissue.

COTTON PLIERS

This instrument transfers items, such as varnish-soaked cotton pledgets, to the preparation; it also transfers wedges, cotton rolls, and articulating paper to check articulation.

▶ Preparation Phase

The instruments in the preparation phase are used to remove carious debris, to plane and cleave walls, to remove unsupported enamel, to place cervical and pulpal floor bevels, to remove tooth structure or restorative material during cavity opening, to outline, for caries removal, and for retention phases in a procedure.

SPOON EXCAVATOR

The spoon excavator is usually used to remove carious tissue from the preparation. A large spoon excavator, such as the #26, may also be used to carve excess amalgam and to refine the occlusal surface of the restoration.

ENAMEL HATCHET

The enamel hatchet is used to plane and cleave unsupported enamel, as well as to smooth the vertical walls of the preparation.

MESIAL AND DISTAL GINGIVAL MARGIN TRIMMERS

The gingival margin trimmers (GMT) place bevels on the cervical margin and the pulpal floors. The mesial GMT is used on the mesial proximal box, and the distal GMT is used on the distal proximal box.

BURS

Certain burs, such as the amalgam removal diamond, are designed for specific purposes. A #34 FG inverted cone or a #1 or 2 FG round bur are often used to open a preparation. A straight fissure plain cut bur (a #55-57 FG), may be used for the outline/resistance form. Round burs, such as #2, #4, #6, or #8 FG or RA can be used for caries removal, while a #¼ or #½ round bur is used to place retentive grooves on the floors of the preparation.

▶ Placement Instruments and Devices

The instruments and devices of this phase of the procedure are used to place, condense, and retain the amalgam in the cavity preparation.

AMALGAM CARRIER/SYRINGE/GUN

This instrument can be single or double ended and made of metal or plastic. The design varies according to the specific type of amalgam placement device that is used; however, a hollowed end to carry the amalgam to the preparation is common to all.

#1 and #2 Amalgam Condensers/Pluggers

The design of the amalgam condensers/pluggers can be manual or mechanical. A common denominator is a flat working end with various shapes and sizes.

#1 Amalgam Condenser/Plugger

This smaller instrument condenses the first amalgam increments in the cavity preparation.

#2 Amalgam Condenser/Plugger

This larger instrument condenses additional amalgam increments as the preparation is filled.

Automatic Condenser

The automatic condenser condenses amalgam by a mechanical instrument.

MATRIX RETAINERS, BANDS AND WEDGES

Tofflemire/Ivory matrix retainer aids in restoring lost proximal walls by holding the matrix band around the tooth to provide support for the amalgam during condensation.

Matrix bands (universal, contoured, Ivory, T-band) are bands that are made of different gauges of metal and provide a partial circumferential or total circumferential surrounding of the tooth to retain amalgam that is placed primarily in the proximal box area.

A contoured band is designed so that the metal extends cervically in the areas of the proximal box to provide support at a greater depth than does a universal band.

An Ivory band is used when a single proximal wall is removed in the preparation.

A T-Band is often used in pediatric dentistry to provide support on a tooth without using a retainer to hold the band in place.

Each type of band may need to be contoured with the rounded handle of an instrument or with contouring pliers to adapt it to the individual shape of a tooth.

Class V contoured matrices are those that are designed specifically for contouring amalgam in Class V preparations.

Wedges hold the matrix band against the tooth when a proximal wall is being restored (to maintain the proximal opening) to avoid overhangs of amalgam and to maintain proximal contact.

In a Class II preparation, a single wedge is used; in a Class VI preparation, two wedges are needed. Each wedge may have to be contoured to fit the proximal space in which it is being placed (Fig. 27-1, *A* and *B*).

▶ Carving Instruments

After the amalgam is placed in the cavity preparation, it must be carved to restore the original anatomy of the tooth. Carving includes **anatomical** and **smooth-surface carving**. Anatomical carving involves placement of occlusal fissure, grooves, and cusp positions in the tooth's surface. Smooth-surface carving occurs on the less anatomically pronounced areas of the tooth, such as the buccal, lingual, and proximal surfaces. The first step in carving is referred to as gross or initial carving, which requires the removal of large portions of excess amalgam from the pits and fissures of a tooth. Final carving is accomplished with instruments that are similar to those that are used in initial carving but are usually smaller in size. Smooth-surface carving requires using instruments

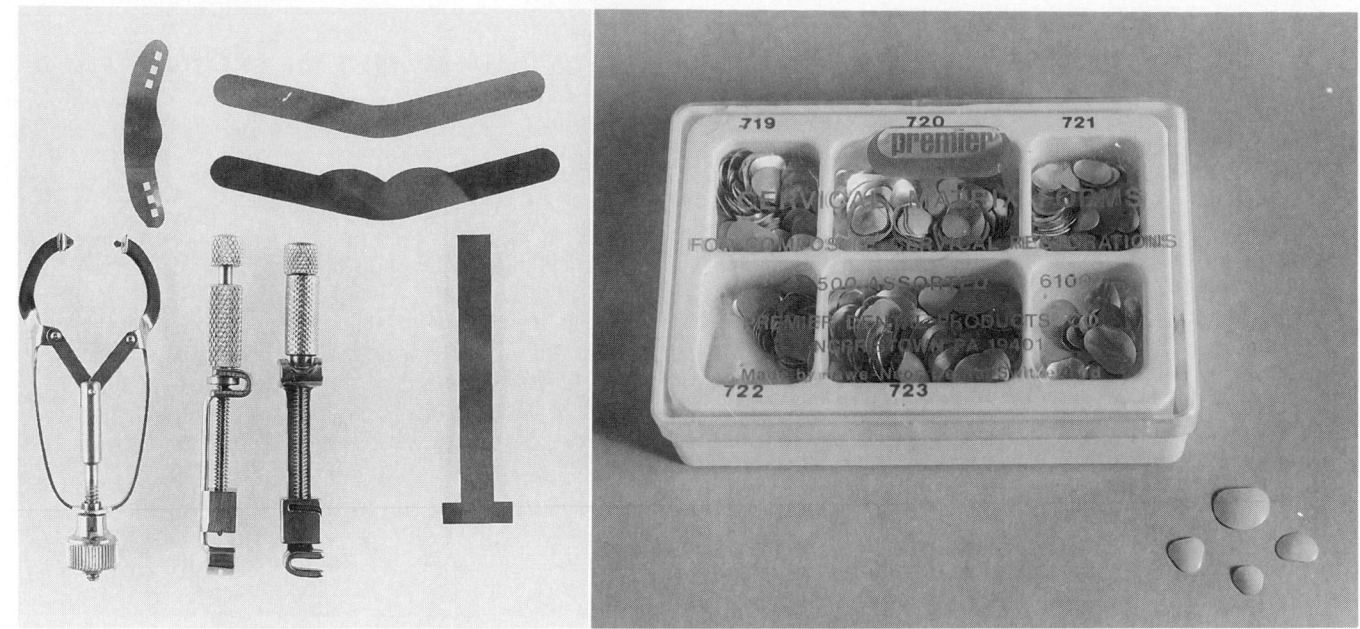

FIG. 27-1 *A,* Ivory band; universal and contoured Tofflemire band; Ivory retainer; Tofflemire retainers and T-band. *B,* Contoured Class V matrices.

(Courtesy of Whaledent International, New York, New York.)

that are adapted to the smooth surfaces of the tooth. The following instruments aid in achieving this step.

ANATOMIC CARVING INSTRUMENTS

#7 C Cleoid-discoid carver — removes initial or gross amalgam on the occlusal surface of the amalgam restoration

#5 C Cleoid-discoid carver — carves the final anatomical areas of the occlusal surface

#26 Spoon excavator — removes initial or gross amalgam on the occlusal surface of the amalgam restoration

Anatomical/lateral burnisher — may be used in initial carving or later in burnishing

SMOOTH SURFACE CARVING INSTRUMENTS

Ward's or **Hollenback carver** — carves interproximal amalgam or smooth surfaces

An explorer is often used to refine the carving and to check the margins of a restoration.

▶ Finishing Instruments

After the amalgam is carved, the margins and surfaces are refined and finished to a smooth surface with the following instruments:

Ball burnisher — burnishes and refines the amalgam surface and cavosurface margins

Anatomical burnisher #21B — initially carves amalgam or burnishes anatomy

T-ball/beavertail burnisher — burnishes and refines amalgam surface and cavosurface margins

▶ Additional Armamentarium

The following armamentarium is necessary in an amalgam procedure to achieve the ideal restoration:

Dappen dish/amalgam well — holds amalgam before placement in the cavity preparation

Articulating paper — determines proper occlusal relationship through marking of tooth surfaces before and after the restorative procedure

Cotton rolls — isolates structures

Cotton pellets — used to place medication, isolate, and dry

Cotton gauze — cleanses instruments and other surfaces

Articulating paper holder — holds articulating paper while occlusal relationship is determined

Rubber dam armamentarium

Anesthesia armamentarium

Finishing and polishing armamentarium
    Rubber cup/soft bristle brush
    Finishing strip
    Dental floss/tape
    Polishing agents
    Finishing and polishing burs, points, and knives

Dental materials armamentarium

PARTS OF THE TOFFLEMIRE RETAINER

Outer knob — A knob that is used to adjust the tightness of the spindle on the band inside of the vise

Inner knob — A knob used to move the vise to increase or decrease the size of the band to accommodate the size of the tooth

Frame — The part of the retainer that connects the outer and inner knobs, vise, and spindle

Spindle — A threaded rod that holds the end of the matrix band in the vise

Vise — The device that clamps tight to hold the ends of the matrix band in the retainer

Guide slots — Slots at the end of the retainer and in the area of the vise that allow the band to be directed to certain areas as selected (Fig. 27-2)

MATRIX BAND AND RETAINER PREPARATION

1. Adjust the outer knob so that the spindle is short of entering the vise slot.
2. Turn the inner knob clockwise so that the vise is $\frac{3}{16}$ inch from the end of the retainer.
3. Hold the matrix band with the gingival aspect above the occlusal aspect. (The band position simulates a smile.)
4. Pull the free ends of the band toward you, with the occlusal aspect below the gingival aspect.
5. Place the occlusal, larger part of the circle into the slots of the retainer first. (The size of the circle that extends from the retainer should correlate to the size of the tooth on which it will be placed.)
6. Look at the gingival aspect of the retainer and band and place the loop out the right side of the retainer for the mandibular left quadrant or the maxillary right quadrant. If the loop is out the left side of the retainer, it is assembled for the mandibular right and the maxillary left quadrants.
7. Tighten the outer knob, securing the spindle against the band.
8. Smooth the loop of the band with a mirror handle if it is crimped.

THE TOFFLEMIRE RETAINER

Of the instruments that were just listed, some require assembly before use. For instance, if the preparation requires using a matrix band and retainer, the assistant should assemble the band and retainer as a unit before the first step of the amalgam procedure. The matrix band and retainer are usually assembled during treatment room preparation to maintain efficiency and reduce time and motion during the actual procedure. A circumferential matrix band and retainer, such as the Tofflemire band and retainer, are commonly used in Class II or Class VI amalgam procedures (Box 27-3). A complete understanding of the assembly of this procedure is necessary (Box 27-4).

Preparation of the Tofflemire Retainer

When the retainer is assembled, two orientations of it should be considered: the gingival aspect and the occlusal aspect.

Gingival aspect: from the side of the retainer that is to be placed near the gingival openings, the guide slots and the diagonal slots are visible (Fig. 27-2).

Occlusal aspect: from the side of the retainer that will be placed near the occlusal surface, openings of the guide slots and the diagonal slots are not visible.

It is necessary to understand these orientations when the assembly and placement of the matrix band into the retainer are discussed.

The retainer should be prepared first in the following stages of assembly:

1. Hold the retainer with the gingival aspect facing upward.
2. Adjust the outer knob by turning it clockwise; stop

turning the knob before the spindle enters the vise slot.

3. If the knob is turned too far, entry to the diagonal vise slot is blocked, and the matrix band will not slide into place.
4. Turn the inner knob clockwise to move the vise $\frac{3}{16}$ inch from the end of the retainer.
5. If the outer knob needs to be adjusted, move the spindle to the end of the diagonal vise slots (Fig. 27-2).

Placing the Universal Matrix Band in the Retainer

The following steps are provided as guidelines for the assembly of the matrix band and retainer:

1. The universal matrix band, like the contoured and Ivory band, have a gingival and occlusal edge. (Because the T-band has equal surface area on both sides of the band, it can be placed toward the gingiva or the occlusal surface.)
2. Hold the band with the gingival aspect above the occlusal aspect.
3. The band position is that of a ***smile*** toward the operator (Fig. 27-3).
4. Pull the two ends of the band toward you (Fig. 27-4).
5. The larger part of the circle, the occlusal edge, is

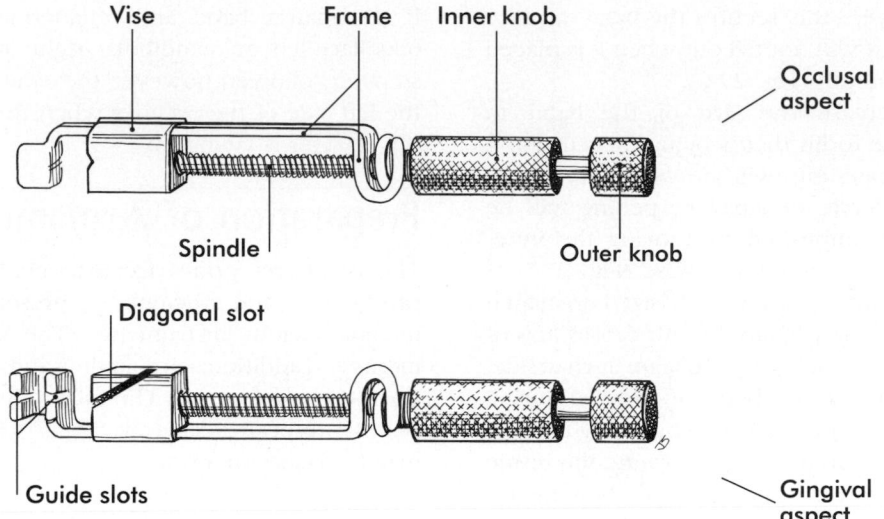

Vise   Frame   Inner knob

Occlusal aspect

Spindle

Outer knob

Diagonal slot

Guide slots

Gingival aspect

FIG. 27-2   Gingival and occlusal aspect of Tofflemire retainer.

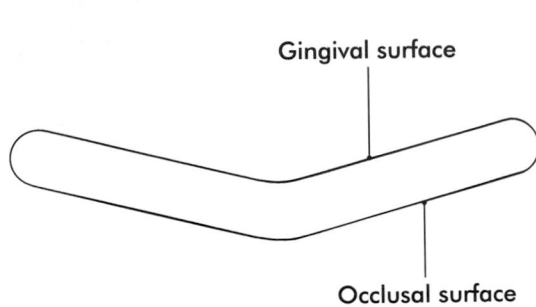

Gingival surface

Occlusal surface

FIG. 27-3   Tofflemire matrix band, positioned with gingival aspect on top, and the occlusal aspect on the bottom of the loop.

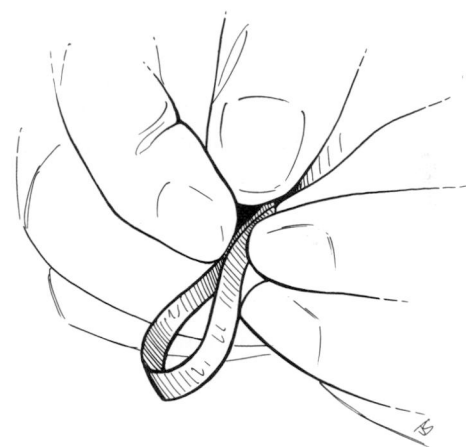

FIG. 27-4   The matrix band ends are pulled together to form a loop.

down; the smaller part of the circle, the gingival edge, is up.

NOTE: This size correlates with the shape of the tooth; it is narrow at the gingiva and wide at the occlusal

6. Place the occlusal edge of the band into the diagonal slot first, with the loop extending toward the end of the retainer

7. With the gingival aspect of the retainer and the band facing up, place the thumb over the slots to stabilize the band. The opening of the loop should be as close as possible to the size of the tooth on which it is to be placed. For instance, if a premolar is being prepared, the loop, when it is first placed into the retainer, should be smaller than it is for a molar.

8. Force the loop of the band up, lifting it through the right side opening of the retainer and sliding it firmly into place (Fig. 27-5).

9. Tighten the outer knob into the ends of the band by

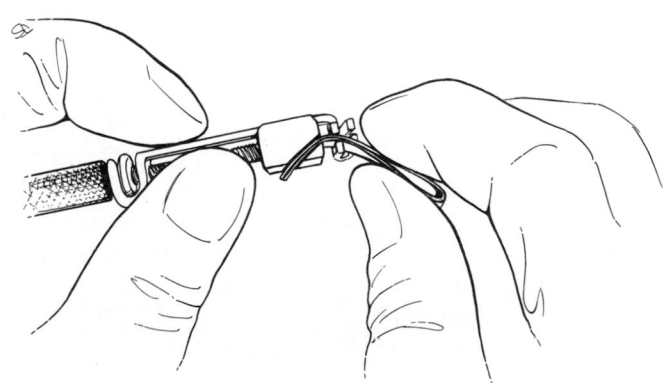

FIG. 27-5   The band ends are placed in the diagonal slots of the retainer, and the loop is fed through the slot.

turning it clockwise; this secures the band in place and ensures that it will not fall out when it is placed in the patient's mouth (Fig. 27-6).

10. Increase or decrease the size of the band to accommodate the tooth that is being treated. For a molar, a large opening will be necessary; for a premolar, a moderate or smaller opening will be used. This is accomplished by moving the inner knob clockwise or counterclockwise (Fig. 27-7, *A* and *B*). A band that is not correctly sized or shaped to the contour of the prepared tooth causes loss of time and motion for the operating team at chairside.

11. The loop of the band may become crimped during preparation; this can be smoothed by taking the end of a mirror handle and running it around the inside of the loop, while it is tightly held by the retainer. The thumb is used to create a controlled pressure on the mirror handle against the band. This establishes again the round shape of the band that is needed to obtain a good contour around the tooth. Since bands are sterilizable, they can be distorted through repeated use.

12. The band and retainer are now prepared for the maxillary right or the mandibular left quadrant (Fig. 27-8, *A* and *B*).

If the matrix band and retainer are needed for the maxillary left or mandibular right quadrants, the same steps are followed; however, the band loop is directed out the left side of the retainer when the gingival aspect of the retainer is facing up.

Preparation of Armamentarium

The use of preset trays decreases chairtime and increases productivity and efficiency. A preset amalgam tray will include various instruments. The selection of instruments and additional armamentarium will depend on the operator's preference. The following is an example of a typical preset amalgam tray. Fig. 27-9 illustrates items that may be found on a tray.

Armamentarium

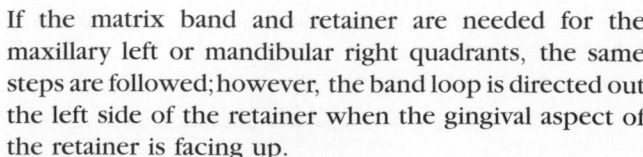

Explorer
Mirror
Cotton pliers
Spoon excavator
Enamel hatchet
Mesial gingival marginal trimmer
Distal gingival marginal trimmer
Amalgam carrier
#1 Condenser
#2 Condenser

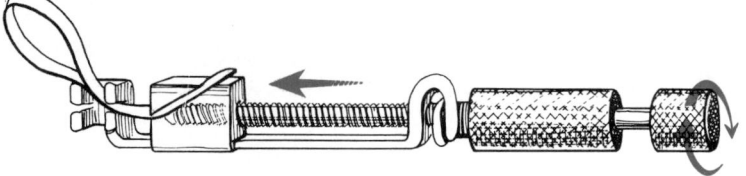

FIG. 27-6 The outer knob of the retainer is turned clockwise, tightening the spindle against the ends of the matrix band.

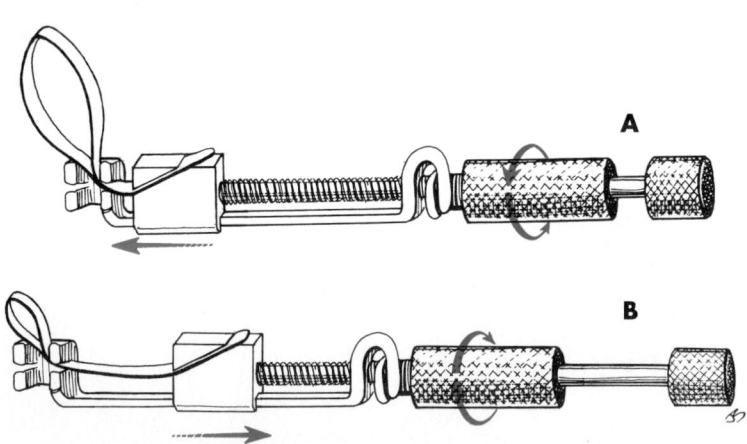

FIG. 27-7 *A* and *B*, The band size loop can be increased and decreased in size by turning the inner knob of the retainer.

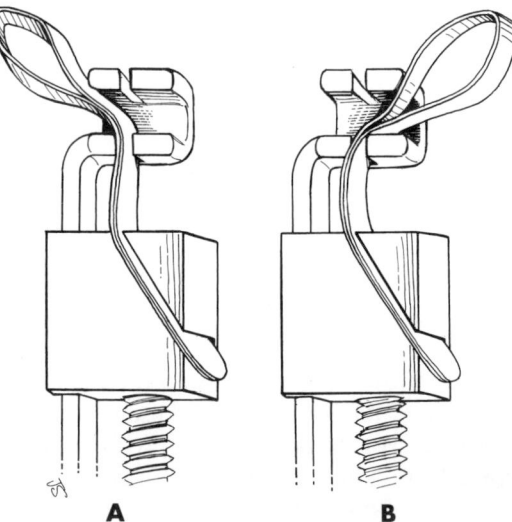

FIG. 27-8 *A*, Retainer and band, prepared for the maxillary left and the mandibular right. *B*, Retainer and band, prepared for the maxillary right and the mandibular left.

#7 Cleoid-Discoid carver
Ward's carver
#5 Cleoid-Discoid carver
Anatomical burnisher
Ball burnisher
Articulating paper holder
Thumb forceps
HVE tip
Articulating paper
2 × 2 gauze

Patient napkin chain
Tofflemire matrix retainer and band
Wedges
a/w Tip
a/w Tip cover
Plastic pad
Cotton pellets
Dappen dish
Bur block and burs
Cotton rolls

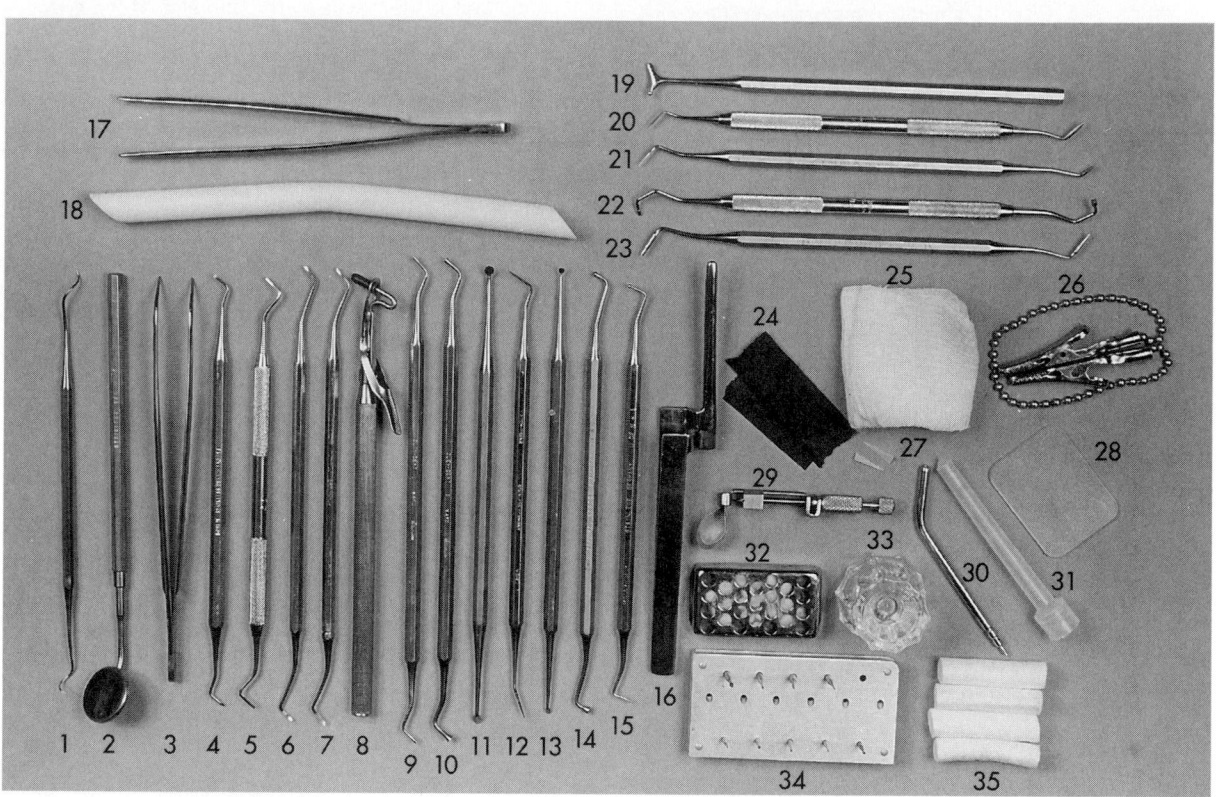

1. Explorer
2. Mirror
3. Cotton pliers
4. Spoon excavator
5. Enamel hatchet
6. Mesial gingival marginal trimmer
7. Distal gingival marginal trimmer
8. Amalgon carrier
9. #1 Condenser
10. #2 Condenser
11. #7 Cleoid-discoid carver
12. Ward's carver
13. #5 Cleoid-discoid carver
14. #21B Anatomical burnisher
15. Ball burnisher
16. Articulating paper holder
17. Thumb forceps
18. HVE tip

19. Beavertail burnisher
20. Hollenback carver
21. Smooth and anatomical carver
22. Back-action condenser
23. Wesco 25
24. Articulating paper
25. 2 × 2 Gauze
26. Patient napkin chain
27. Wedges
28. Plastic film divider to mix liners
29. Tofflemire matrix band and retainer
30. A/W syringe tip
31. A/W syringe tip cover
32. Cotton pellets
33. Dappen dish
34. Assorted burs
35. Cotton rolls

FIG. 27-9   Example of armamentarium for an amalgam procedure.

AMALGAM PROCEDURE

- Are all universal barrier techniques being used?
- Is all of the armamentarium available and prepared for use?
- Are the instruments arranged in sequence of use?
- Am I prepared for alternative treatment plans?
- Is the necessary equipment turned on and ready to operate?

A common procedure that is frequently accomplished in a dental office is a Class II amalgam restoration. Since this particular cavity classification encompasses most of the basic concepts of an amalgam procedure, this section will describe a step-by-step procedure for placing a Class II amalgam restoration on a posterior tooth. Later in this chapter examples of simple and more complex procedures are described to aid in identifying the differences in the procedure for various cavity classifications, teeth, and other special situations. Box 27-2 is a brief overview of the amalgam procedure. The following discussion provides a chronologic description of each of these steps.

Update Medical History

A **current health history** is obtained from the patient who is being seen for restorative treatment. In this situation no health contraindications warrant any special care. As discussed earlier in the text, current health history is important to alert the dental team of any problems that might complicate the procedure and require additional steps.

Examine the Treatment Site

The **site of treatment is examined** by the operator as the assistant passes the explorer and mirror. The operator confirms the area and the extent of treatment to be rendered.

Determine Occlusal Relationship

The first step that is completed before any restorative procedure is begun **determines the occlusal relationship** and any interference. The assistant dries the surfaces of the teeth with a 2×2 gauze sponge and holds articulating paper between the arches with articulating paper forceps or cotton pliers. The patient is directed to bite firmly up and down and then to grind the teeth side to side.

The identification of centric stops and the excursive contacts will aid the operator as the restorative material is placed and carved into the prepared tooth surfaces. It is necessary to obtain this information to avoid fracturing the restorative material by extreme occlusal contact.

Anesthesia Administration

After the occlusion has been established, the next step is to **administer the anesthesia.** A detailed explanation of this procedure is found in Chapter 23. The following steps provide a review:

Assembly (Complete prior to seating the patient.)

Remove the syringe and additional items from sterilized packaging.

Select a 1 ⅝ inch needle and an anesthesia carpule with a vasoconstrictor based upon the treatment plan and the patient's health history.

Remove the protective shield from the hub end of the needle and attach the needle to the hub end of the syringe.

Pull back on the plunger of the syringe, increasing the opening of the breech.

Drop the anesthetic carpule into the syringe, with the hub end of the carpule facing the hub end of the syringe.

Release the plunger, which forces the hub end of the needle to engage the diaphragm of the carpule.

Engage the harpoon into the plunger of the anesthetic carpule.

Test the harpoon for engagement into the plunger of the carpule.

Any air drawn into the carpule is expressed.

Loosen, *but do not remove, the needle sheath/cover.*

Place the prepared syringe that is ready to use near the treatment area.

Administering Anesthesia

The operator palpates the site of the injection.

Pass the 2×2 gauze sponge to dry the site.

Exchange the gauze with a cotton-tipped applicator with topical anesthesia.

Retrieve the applicator, and slightly raise the operating light.

Pass the syringe, using the hidden syringe technique.

Retrieve the syringe and recap, using OSHA accepted techniques, and pass a 2×2 gauze to dry the site.

Rubber Dam Isolation

During the few minutes it takes for complete anesthesia to occur, the **rubber dam isolation** procedure may begin. The rubber dam has been prepared in anticipation of use. The rubber dam may be punched in a number of ways, as described in Chapter 22. One of these techniques has been selected for use in this procedure. The holes are punched for four teeth: one posterior to the tooth to be prepared, the tooth that is to be treated, and the two teeth anterior to the tooth that is being prepared. The assistant flosses the interproximal spaces of the teeth to determine that the contacts are not too tight, allowing for easier placement of the rubber dam material.

The rubber dam assembly, including dam material, frame, molar clamp that is in position with floss attached, and rubber dam forceps, is passed to the operator. The operator places the clamp on the second molar as the assistant stabilizes the assembly. The operator positions the holes over the first molar, second premolar, and first premolar as the assistant

AMALGAM PROCEDURE—cont'd

flosses the dam down in the interproximal spaces. The assistant passes the floss from the lingual to the buccal to force the dam interproximally. Pulling the floss up through the occlusal surfaces is likely to carry the dam with it. Once all the dam is through the contacts, the assistant places an anterior ligature in the mesial contact of the first premolar stabilizing the rubber dam assembly.

The rubber dam napkin or gauze is placed under the assembly to protect the patient's facial surfaces. The assistant passes the spoon excavator, beavertail burnisher, or plastic instrument to the operator to begin the cuffing or inverting procedure. As the operator inverts the dam into the gingival sulcus, the assistant dries the tooth surfaces with air to facilitate the inversion. The assistant receives the spoon excavator and places a saliva ejector under the rubber dam on the right side of the patient's mouth to aid in saliva control.

Cavity Preparation
Opening Phase

At this point, the cavity preparation begins with the **opening phase.** The opening phase is the process of using a dental bur to make an opening through the enamel and into the dentin tissues of the tooth. The operator uses a high-speed handpiece with either a #34 FG inverted cone or a #1 or #2 FG round bur to open the enamel on the occlusal surface. The assistant obtains position, within the oral cavity, with the high-velocity evacuator tip on the surface of the tooth that is closest to the assistant and slightly towards the distal of the tooth. Keeping the HVE tip in this position will reduce the accumula-

tion of oral fluids. As the operator removes the handpiece from the oral cavity, the assistant should immediately rinse and dry the cavity preparation. This is done by placing the a/w syringe over the opening of the tooth and using an aerated spray. The tooth is dried thoroughly, and any additional fluids should be evacuated (Fig. 27-10, *A*).

Outline or Resistance Form Phase

The operator continues the opening, and, when that is completed, begins the **outline phase,** which is an extension of the preparation that includes shaping and designing the wall and floor shapes of the preparation. This may be accomplished with a #55, #56, or #57 FG on the high-speed handpiece that the assistant delivers during a handpiece exchange. The process of the outline phase could also result in development of the **resistance form.** The resistance form is created when the operator positions walls in the internal portion of the preparation. The relationship of the walls is similar to the outer walls of a pyramid. The walls are closer together near the occlusal surface and further apart toward the floor of the preparation. This allows the restorative material to be placed when it is malleable and as it hardens it is locked in place through the shape of the preparation.

The assistant maintains the position of the HVE. As the operator signals, the assistant again rinses and dries the preparation and exchanges the explorer as the operator determines areas of additional decay. When the opening of the preparation is adequately expanded from the occlusal

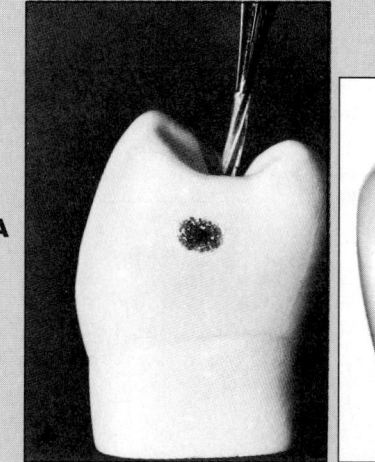
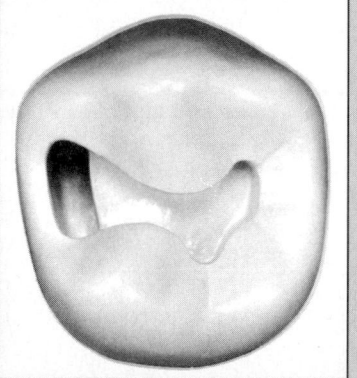

FIG. 27-10   *A,* Opening phase of the cavity preparation. *B,* The occlusal view of a step in the outline phase of the preparation.

(From Sturdevant CM et al: *The art and science of operative dentistry,* ed 2, St Louis, 1985, Mosby, pp. 21 5 and 216.)

Continued.

AMALGAM PROCEDURE—cont'd

surface across to the distal proximal wall, the operator may use hand cutting instruments to continue the preparation procedure (Fig. 27-10, *B*). The enamel hatchet is exchanged for the handpiece so the operator can remove the final thin layer of enamel in the distal proximal box area. The use of the enamel hatchet rather than a rotary instrument provides the operator with a controlled removal, which is not easily provided with a handpiece (Fig. 27-11, *A* through *C*). The integrity of the mesial surface of the second molar can be ensured with the enamel hatchet. When all unsupported enamel has been removed by the planing and cleaving process, the operator uses the distal

gingival margin trimmer. Either end, the right or left, of the distal gingival margin trimmer may be passed first, since both will be used to place bevels on the line angles of the cervical and pulpal floors. These bevels will provide strength to avoid fracture of the restoration (Fig. 27-12). If the cavity preparation had been a Class II or a Class VI preparation (mesial-occlusal-distal), the mesial and distal margin trimmers would both be used. After the hand cutting instruments are used, the assistant rinses and dries the site in preparation for the caries removal step.

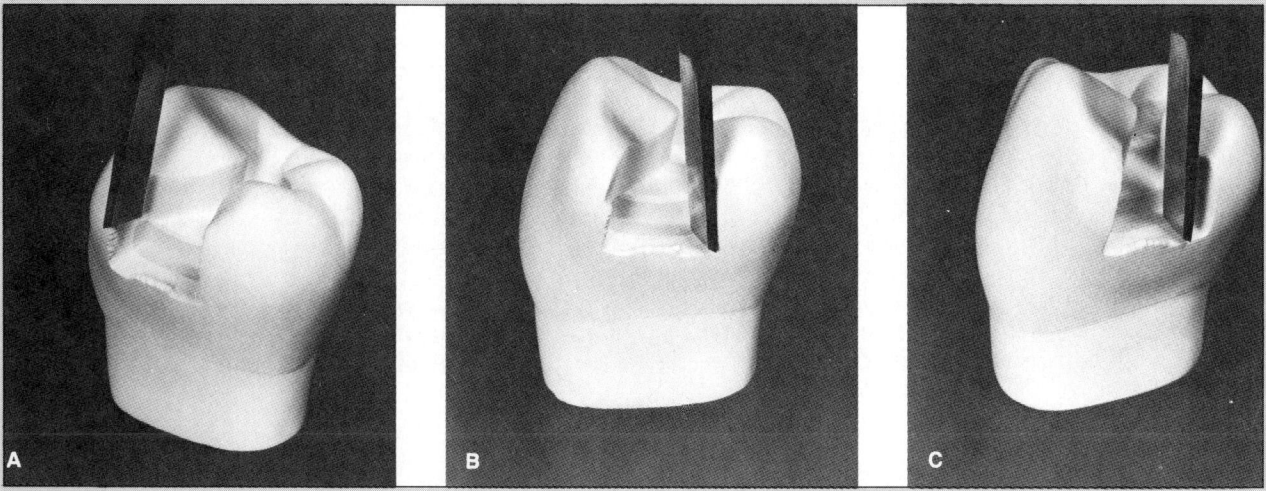

FIG. 27-11   *A* through *C,* Enamel hatchet used on the wall of the preparation.

(From Sturdevant CM et al: *The art and science of operative dentistry,* ed 2, St Louis, 1985, Mosby, p. 219.)

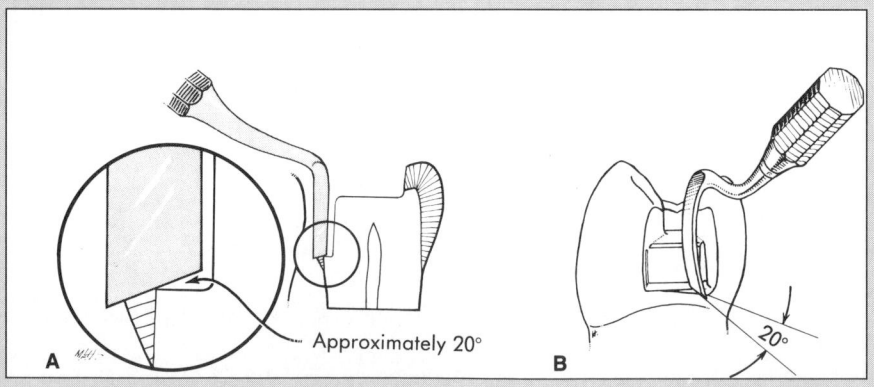

FIG. 27-12   Placement of bevels with GMT.

(From Sturdevant CM et al: *The art and science of operative dentistry,* ed 2, St Louis, 1985, Mosby, p. 222.)

AMALGAM PROCEDURE—cont'd

Caries Removal

Caries removal involves the removal of any carious tissues through mechanical or manual means. By manual means, a spoon excavator is used to remove carious tissue. Mechanically, caries is removed through the use of the slow-speed handpiece with a round bur. Choice of caries removal is determined by the depth of the carious tissue and by operator preference. If the carious tissue is near the pulp chamber, the operator may opt to use manual removal to avoid a pulp exposure. Under less than optimal circumstances, most caries removal is completed mechanically.

In this situation the operator exchanges the hand cutting instrument for the low-speed handpiece with either a #2, #4, or #6 FG or RA bur for **caries removal.** The size of the bur is determined by the size of the tooth and the extent of the carious lesion. Occasionally caries may be removed by instrumentation with the spoon excavator (Fig. 27-13, *A* and *B*). As the carious tissue is removed mechanically with the handpiece, tooth debris will accumulate within the preparation. A slight spurt of air directed into the preparation will force the debris away. Air rather than aerated spray is used at this time to maintain a dry field. The operator often exchanges the handpiece for the explorer during this phase to determine all areas of remaining decay. When the decay is completely removed, the assistant returns the handpiece to the dental unit and rinses and dries the cavity preparation.

Retention Phase

The retention form is a step to assist in the retention of the restoration in the preparation. Sometimes this is considered to be part of the resistance phase. Usually the retention phase involves the placement of small grooves on the pulpal and cervical floors of the preparation to assist in mechanically locking the amalgam in place.

This phase is begun when all decay is removed, so that the final phase of the cavity preparation, the **retention phase,** can proceed. The assistant passes the operator the low-speed handpiece, which has been prepared with a retention bur. Retentive grooves are usually placed with a ¼ or ½ FG or RA round bur. The grooves are placed on the pulpal and cervical floors to aid in the retention of the restorative material (Fig. 27-14). The assistant again provides an occasional spurt of air to clear the site. The explorer is exchanged with the handpiece again to inspect the grooves. When the retentive grooves are adequate, the assistant receives the explorer and rinses and dries the cavity preparation.

Cotton Roll Isolation

At this point the cavity preparation is completed, having provided recommended outline, resistance, and retentive forms to ensure a quality prepared tooth structure. If cotton roll isolation is used instead of rubber dam isolation, the cotton rolls are placed at this point.

FIG. 27-13   *A,* Caries removal with a small bur. *B,* Caries removal with a spoon excavator.

(From Sturdevant CM et al: *The art and science of operative dentistry,* ed 2, St Louis, 1985, Mosby, p. 195.)

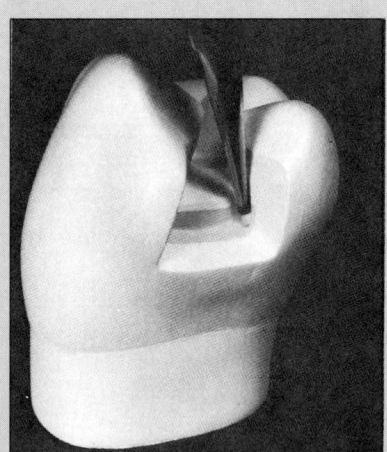

FIG. 27-14   Retentive grooves placed with a ¼ to ½ round bur.

(From Sturdevant CM et al: *The art and science of operative dentistry,* ed 2, St Louis, 1985, Mosby, p. 223.)

Continued.

AMALGAM PROCEDURE—cont'd

 STOP

Cavity Medication Placement

The **cavity medication phase** may proceed as indicated by the depth of the prepared tooth and the closeness of the pulpal tissues. Cavity depth determines the type of medication necessary to seal the dentinal tubules, provide insulation, act as an obtundant, stimulate the pulp and create an ideal depth in the preparation. Table 27-1 illustrates various cavity depths and medications that are needed to provide patient comfort (Fig. 27-15).

Medicating the cavity preparation is necessary to maintain the health of the pulpal tissues and to ensure that the restorative material is placed at ideal depth. In this procedure the depth of the first molar is beyond the ideal, as discussed in Chapters 6 and 11, because of the extent of decay. The assistant rinses and dries the preparation and then dips previously prepared cotton pledgets (that are held in the cotton pliers) into the cavity varnish. The assistant passes the pledget (a piece of tightly rolled cotton) to the operator who places the varnish over the cut dentin tubules. If a second application of varnish is needed, the assistant prepares a second pledget in a new pliers and exchanges these for the first set. The use of a second set of cotton pliers prevents contamination of the varnish container. If a light-cured varnish is used, follow manufacturer's directions for manipulation of the material (Fig. 27-16).

Once the varnish has set and a dry field has been maintained, the cement base of choice is prepared by the assistant. If zinc phosphate is selected, the assistant prepares

TABLE 27-1   COMMON MEDICATIONS UNDER AMALGAM RESTORATIONS

Cavity depth	Type and sequence of medication
Ideal or minimal cavity	Cavity varnish
Extended beyond ideal; extensive, but no invasion of the pulp	Cavity varnish, zinc phosphate, or glass ionomer bases
Near exposure; thin layer of dentin remains	Zinc oxide–eugenol, cavity varnish, zinc phosphate, or glass ionomer base
Small exposure; minimal in size	Calcium hydroxide, zinc oxide–eugenol, cavity varnish, zinc phosphate, or glass ionomer base

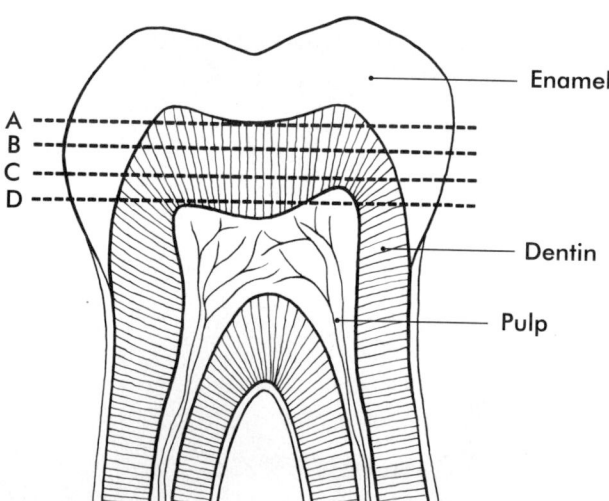

FIG. 27-15   Cavity depths. *A,* Ideal. *B,* Beyond ideal. *C,* Extensive. *D,* Near exposure. *E,* Pulp exposure.

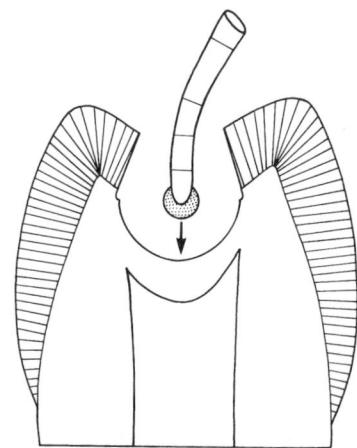

FIG. 27-16   Cavity varnish applied to provide seal for the dentinal tubules.

(From Sturdevant CM et al: *The art and science of operative dentistry,* ed 2, St Louis, 1985, Mosby, p. 196.)

AMALGAM PROCEDURE—cont'd

 STOP

the base as the manufacturer directs for the secondary consistency, placing a small amount of primary consistency in the upper left corner of the glass slab as described in Chapter 11.

The assistant passes the operator the instrument of choice, FP1, condenser or other placement instrument for the cement insertion (Fig. 27-17). An FP 1 plastic instrument is used to place a small amount of primary consistency into the preparation to aid in retention of the secondary consistency. The assistant holds the slab just beneath the patient's chin with one hand and a 2 × 2 gauze sponge to wipe the instrument with the other hand. The operator may then use another instrument, such as a Wesco 25 or a #1 amalgam condenser, to place the secondary consistency. It is important for the assistant to have additional cement powder on the slab into which the operator may place the end of the instrument. Placing the cement increment into the preparation and the instrument into the powder, while condensing the base, avoids having the cement stick to the instrument, pulling out of the preparation. The cement base is placed and condensed in all areas to replace removed dentin. At this point the operator may use an explorer to refine the cement.

Matrix Band, Retainer, and Wedge Placement

The next step in the procedure is the placement of the previously prepared **matrix band and retainer.** By examining the treatment plan, the assistant can determine whether the band and retainer should be prepared for the first molar before the start of the procedure.

It may be necessary to place a wedge first for a few minutes between #19 and #18 to force the teeth apart and to allow for easier placement and adaptability of the matrix band and retainer. If this step is not needed, the band and retainer are placed on the first molar. Once the band is adapted to the cervical and completely surrounds the tooth, the retainer is tightened and the band circumference is reduced to a snug fit.

The interdental space and a wedge are shaped like a triangle with two equal sides and one unequal side that is the base. The base of the wedge is placed in cotton pliers so that it can be placed against the base of the interdental space or the cervical. Fig. 27-18 illustrates the position of the wedge as it is directed from the lingual into the proximal space of the four quadrants in the mouth. The wedge is directed into this space from the lingual surface of the tooth. The wedge against the band is like a wooden form used when concrete is poured, to retain the required shape. The operator uses the explorer to examine the band around the proximal box. Occasionally, the band is not contoured properly and must be removed. A contouring pliers is used to adjust the shape of the band and it is placed again. A deep interproximal preparation might call for a contoured matrix band rather than the commonly used universal band (Fig. 27-19).

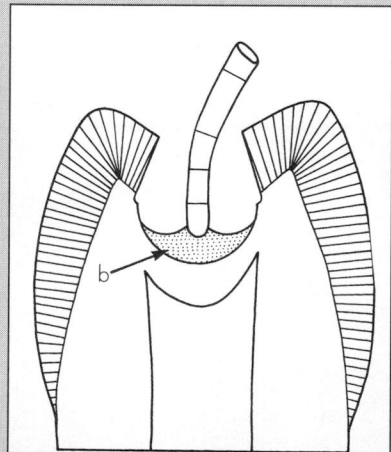

FIG. 27-17   Cavity depth may require the placement of a cement base to provide patient comfort.

(From Sturdevant CM et al: *The art and science of operative dentistry,* ed 2, St Louis, 1985, Mosby, p. 196.)

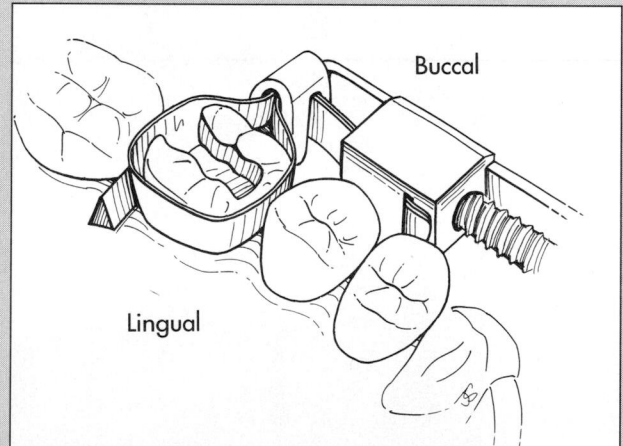

FIG. 27-18   The matrix band, retainer, and wedge are properly placed before insertion of the amalgam.

Continued.

Amalgam Insertion

After the matrix band, retainer, and wedge are placed, the **insertion phase** begins with the assistant rinsing and drying the treatment site. To avoid contamination of the capsule activator and the amalgamator, overgloves may be placed over treatment gloves. Through use of these gloves during preparation and mixing of the amalgam, disinfection of the capsule activator and amalgamator can be eliminated. This reduces time and motion between teardown and preparation of the treatment room for the next patient treatment.

In China around A.D. 659 the Materia Medica of Su Kung mentions silver paste, a combination of 100 parts of mercury, 45 parts of silver, and 900 parts of tine that was triturated to form a paste.

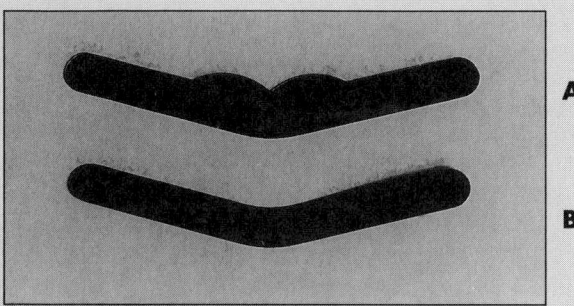

A

B

FIG. 27-19   *A,* A contoured matrix band may be needed for deep proximal preparation instead of *B,* a universal matrix band.

For this particular procedure the assistant would select a double spill and activate the preproportioned amalgam capsule. The capsule is placed in the amalgamator and is mixed for the proper length of time, as directed by the manufacturer. The assistant prepares the dappen dish or amalgam well and the amalgam insertion instrument of choice: an amalgam carrier, gun, or syringe. When the amalgam is mixed and placed in the dappen dish, the assistant fills the amalgam carrier completely and passes it to the operator. The operator places the first increment in the least accessible area, the proximal box, and the assistant exchanges the carrier with the #1 amalgam condenser or plugger (Fig. 27-20, *A* and *B*). The assistant may sometimes place the increments into the cavity preparation under the direction of the operator if it is allowed by state dental practice law. The assistant continues the process of filling the carrier as it is emptied and exchanges it with the condenser. As the preparation becomes full, a larger condenser may be used. When the carrier is filled and only enough amalgam remains to fill one more carrier, the assistant should apprise the operator of the situation. The operator may then determine if another spill of amalgam is needed. If so, the assistant mixes an additional spill, as time is of the essence.

Initial Carving

When the preparation is completely overfilled, the **initial carving phase** commences. The assistant passes the operator the instrument of choice, a #7 cleoid-discoid carver, a #26 spoon, or even a #21B anatomical burnisher to remove the gross amount of amalgam and surface mercury. The contouring of the amalgam begins with this step. It is important for the

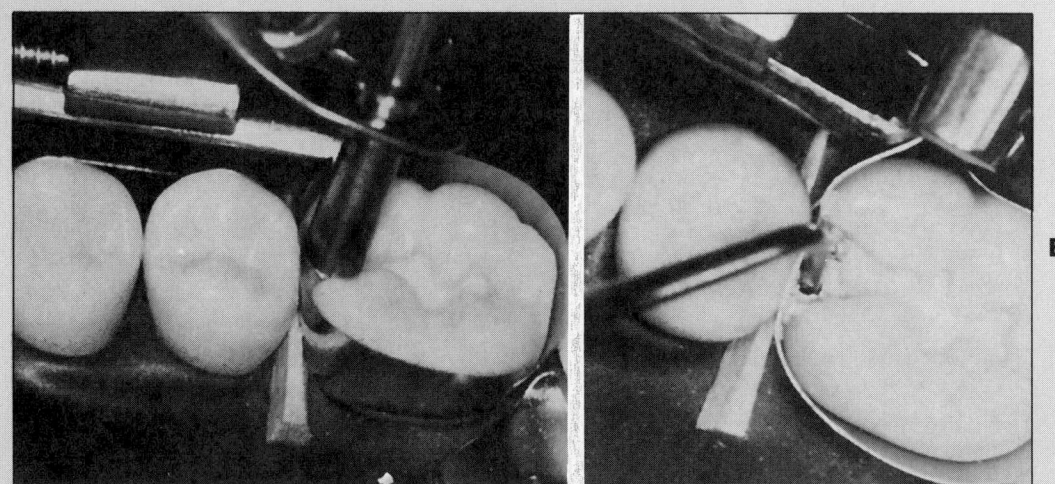

A

B

FIG. 27-20   *A* and *B,* The first increment of amalgam is placed in the proximal box of the preparation and is condensed in the preparation.

(From Spohn EE, Halowski WA, Berry TG: *Operative dentistry procedures for dental auxiliaries,* St Louis, 1981, Mosby, pp. 153, 154.)

assistant to position the HVE, as before, near the site, to remove the excess amalgam as it is carved away. The carver should be placed on the cavosurface margin, partially on the tooth, as well as on the restorative material. This position functions as a fulcrum to prevent the tendency to overcarve the amalgam and create an underfilled area at the cavosurface margins. Underfilled areas could result in an increased possibility of microleakage.

An overcontoured surface results in an undercarved restoration. By the same token, an undercontoured surface results in an overcarved restoration (Fig. 27-21, *A*). An overcontoured restoration may result in fractures of the material that extend beyond the cavosurface margin or in an occlusal relationship that is uncomfortable for the patient. The overcontoured restoration can be finished later with a handpiece. An undercontoured restoration can be corrected only by removing the restoration and placing a new one (Fig. 27-21, *B*). Next the #7 carver is exchanged for the explorer or Ward's C carver, which is used to remove amalgam from the contact at the marginal ridge and the band (Fig. 27-22). The contact is not opened but is contoured as the natural tooth would be as it contacts the abutment tooth. Care must be taken during this step to avoid any fractures of the amalgam. Additional amalgam that was forced down around the band in other areas, such as the buccal or lingual, is removed by slightly rotating the instrument through these areas. The operator returns the instrument to the assistant who rinses and dries the site.

Matrix Retainer, Wedge, and Band Removal

The assistant passes the cotton pliers for the first step of the **removal of the matrix band and retainer.** The wedge is removed first by using the cotton pliers; then the retainer is loosened

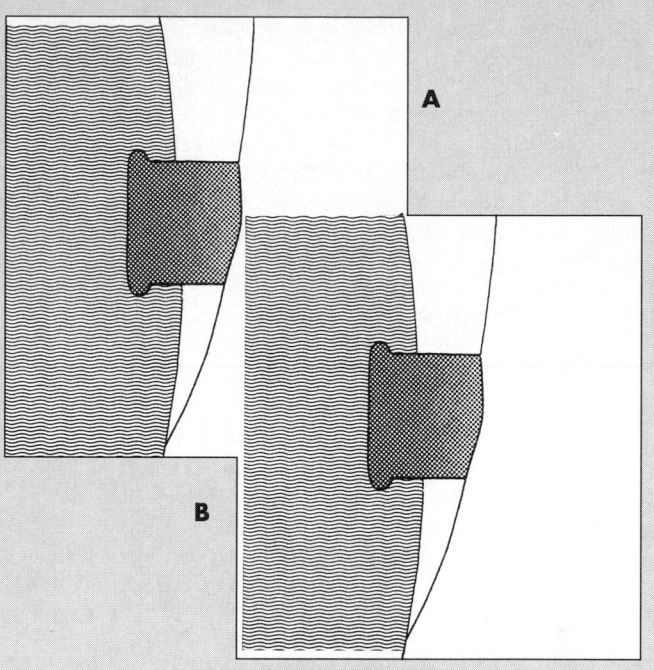

FIG. 27-21   *A,* The overcontoured surface of the amalgam restoration. *B,* The undercontoured surface of the amalgam.

(From Spohn EE, Halowski WA, Berry TG: *Operative dentistry procedures for dental auxiliaries,* St. Louis, 1981, Mosby, A, p. 111; B, p. 112.)

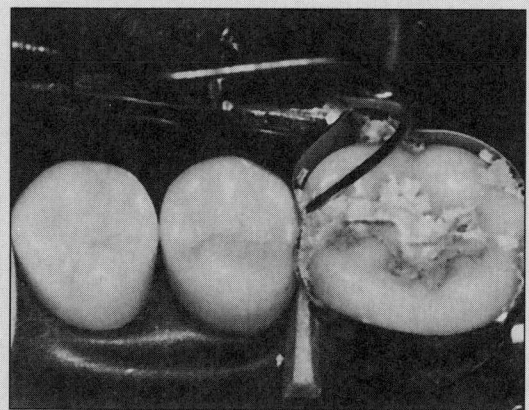

FIG. 27-22   The marginal ridge area is rounded with the explorer tip.

(From Spohn EE, Halowski WA, Berry TG: *Operative dentistry procedures for dental auxiliaries,* St Louis, 1981, Mosby, p. 157.)

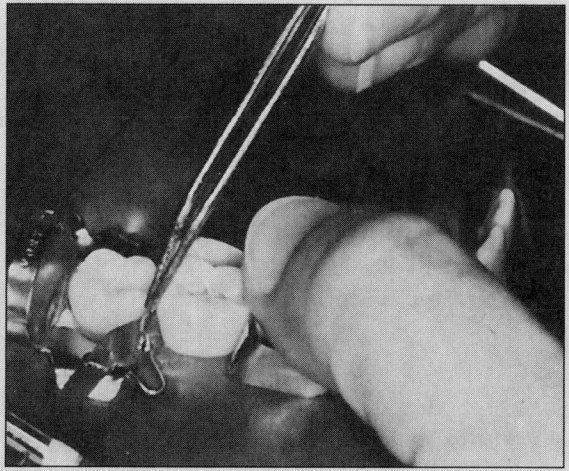

FIG. 27-23   The cotton forceps are used to remove the matrix band.

(From Spohn EE, Halowski WA, Berry TG: *Operative dentistry procedures for dental auxiliaries,* St Louis, 1981, Mosby, p. 158.)

Continued.

AMALGAM PROCEDURE—cont'd

and removed. The assistant receives both, and loads a cotton pellet in the cotton pliers, positioning it lightly over the marginal ridge as the operator removes the matrix band (Fig. 27-23). This step is done to avoid fracturing the marginal ridge, but it may not always be included. Cotton pliers may be used to remove the matrix band, or it may be removed by hand. The steps for removal of the wedge, retainer, and band may vary, according to the operator's preference and the treatment situation.

Interproximal Carving

The assistant receives the band by exchanging the Ward's C carver or the explorer for the **interproximal carving** to contour the least accessible area: the distal proximal surface. It is important to gain access early to avoid being unable to remove excess amalgam that may cause problems for the patient later such as overhangs (Fig. 27-24).

The blade of the carver is positioned interproximally and is raised towards the occlusal until resistance is met. The carver is then pulled cervically against the amalgam surface, carving the excess away. The operator uses the explorer next to check the area carved with the Ward's C carver, ensuring that no overhangs exist. The explorer provides the ability to feel the finer surfaces that are not always visible to the operator and to determine the existence of any excess amalgam that may have to be removed with the Ward's C carver. The assistant will rinse and dry the field, removing any fluids and debris from the carving phase.

Final Carving

The operator exchanges the explorer for the #5 cleoid-discoid carver for the **final carving** of the occlusal surface. The majority of the occlusal contour is developed at this point, and it is a meticulous stage. The original tooth anatomy is reestablished in the amalgam with a #5 cleoid-discoid carver, deepening and accentuating the grooves and fissures that were placed with the #7 cleoid-discoid carver (Fig. 27-25). The same techniques used with the #7 cleoid-discoid carver are followed, taking care not to overcontour the amalgam. The cleoid end of the instrument develops the grooves, and the discoid end creates natural slopes of the cusps. The operator will often use the explorer to check the margins after carving with the #5C. The assistant receives the explorer from the operator and rinses and dries the site.

Isolation Removal

The rubber dam removal is the next step in the process. The assistant cuts the interproximal areas of the rubber dam as the operator pulls it away from the teeth. The anterior ligature is also removed, and the assistant then passes the rubber dam forceps to the operator, who carefully lifts the clamp off the tooth. At times the clamp will be free of the dam; at other times the assembly lifts off as one unit. The assistant takes the rubber dam from the operator and checks it to ensure that no pieces are left in the gingival sulcus areas. If pieces are missing, the assistant removes them by passing floss in the areas to pull the pieces through the interproximals. The assistant completes a full mouth rinse to remove any particles from the patient's mouth and to remove any fluids. For a review of rubber dam removal refer to Chapter 22.

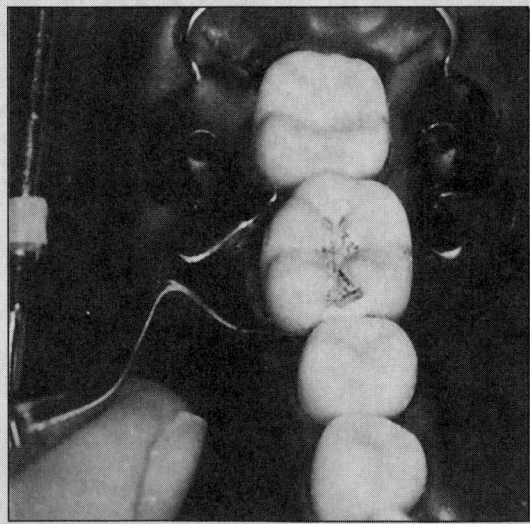

FIG. 27-24   Interproximal carving may begin with the use of the amalgam knife or with a smooth surface carver on the proximal surface.

(From Spohn EE, Halowski WA, Berry TG: *Operative dentistry procedures for dental auxiliaries*, St Louis, 1981, Mosby, p. 160.)

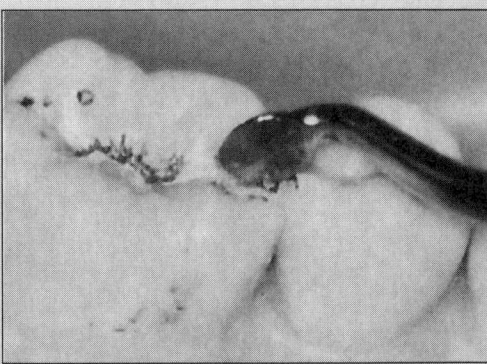

FIG. 27-25   The final occlusal carving is accomplished with a smaller anatomical carver.

(From Spohn EE, Halowski WA, Berry TG: *Operative dentistry procedures for dental auxiliaries*, St Louis, 1981, Mosby, p. 162.)

AMALGAM PROCEDURE—cont'd

Checking the Articulation

The assistant passes the operator the **articulating paper to check the occlusion** of the newly restored surfaces. The patient is directed to bite gently up and down on the paper. The assistant readies the anatomical carver for use. If the paper marks the amalgam surface, the operator is passed the #5 cleoid-discoid carver to remove the excess amalgam where the patient is occluding too heavily (Fig. 27-26). The articulation may be checked and the occlusal surface may be carved several times before the occlusal contact is correct and comfortable for the patient. The patient may not be able to determine if heavy contact is made during occlusion because the anesthesia is still effective; this may cause an inability to assess the contact accurately. The patient may find after the effect of anesthesia subsides that it feels as if contact is heavy on the recently restored tooth; the patient may need to return to the office to have the occlusal contact adjusted.

Burnishing

The articulation is checked again by the operator or the assistant. If the amalgam is not marked, the operator receives the ball burnisher (or burnisher of choice) and smooths the cavosurface margins and all other areas. Special care is given to the area of the marginal ridge, which can still fracture easily. Additional anatomy can be placed on the occlusal surfaces during the burnishing (Fig. 27-27, *A* and *B*).

Occasionally, the operator needs to exchange the burnisher for the explorer to remove any flash of amalgam. Flash, an overextension of the amalgam on the tooth surface, must be removed or it may fracture away, leaving an open margin that could eventually decay. The operator will exchange the explorer for the burnisher to burnish the surface again, removing any scratches and providing a smooth finish. The assistant receives the burnisher and provides the patient with a thorough mouth rinse, making sure to remove all small pieces of amalgam that have become trapped under the tongue or in the posterior pillar area. Criteria for a clinically acceptable amalgam restoration is listed in Box 27-6.

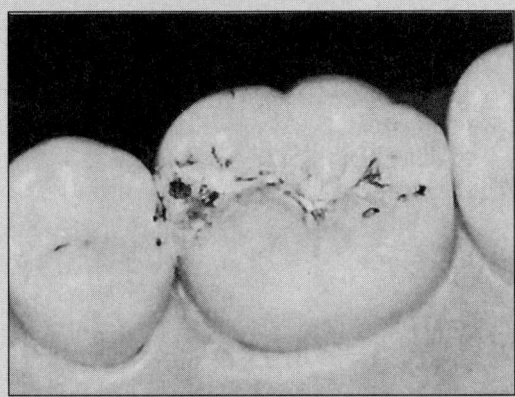

FIG. 27-26 The articulation paper marks heavy in areas that must be removed on the restored surfaces, and excess material is removed.

(From Spohn EE, Halowski WA, Berry TG: *Operative dentistry procedures for dental auxiliaries,* St Louis, 1981, Mosby, p. 162.)

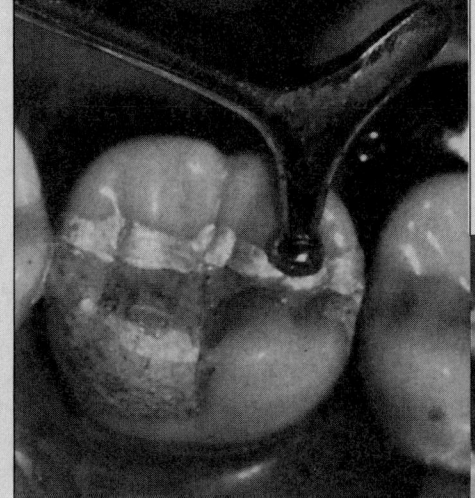

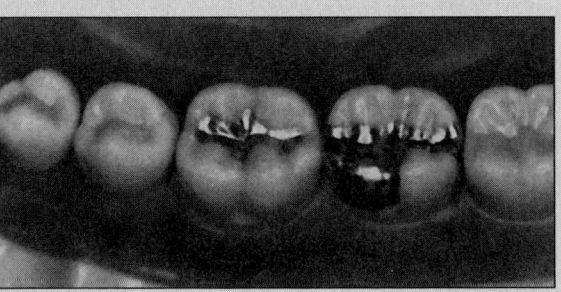

FIG. 27-27 *A* and *B,* Burnished restoration.

(From Spohn EE, Halowski WA, Berry TG: *Operative dentistry procedures for dental auxiliaries,* St Louis, 1981, Mosby, p. 188.)

Continued.

AMALGAM PROCEDURE—cont'd

Finishing and Polishing

With certain types of amalgam, finishing and polishing can be accomplished at this appointment. With the use of other types of amalgam a longer setting time may be required, necessitating another appointment. The assistant passes a slow-speed handpiece using a series of plug finishing burs on the occlusal surfaces. The larger burs are used first, followed by a succession of smaller burs to refine the contour of the amalgam surfaces across the occlusal and the margins of the restoration. Occlusal margins can also be contoured with flame- or carrot-shaped stones. When all adjustments are made on the anatomical surfaces (Fig. 27-28), the cervical areas may be finished with the use of narrow water-resistant finishing strips. The assistant cuts a point at one end of the strip and passes it to the operator, who threads it into the interproximal surface. The strip is pulled back and forth, contacting the amalgam surface. The strip is exchanged for the explorer, and the surface is checked for smoothness. An unwebbed rubber cup with a slurry of polishing agent (silex, as an example) is prepared on the slow-speed handpiece and exchanged for the explorer. This is used to finish the surfaces accessible with the rubber cup. With the slurry still in place, the handpiece is exchanged for dental floss or tape, which is used on the proximal surfaces to refine the polishing procedure. A second slurry of tin oxide, used with a cup or soft polishing brush, is rotated over all areas, completing the finishing and polishing the restoration. The assistant receives the handpiece and provides the patient with a complete mouth rinse.

Postoperative Instructions

The patient is given postoperative instructions by the assistant or the operator, regarding the length of time that the anesthesia may remain in effect. If this were a child patient, the parent or caregiver would be given these instructions. The patient is also advised when and what he or she may eat for

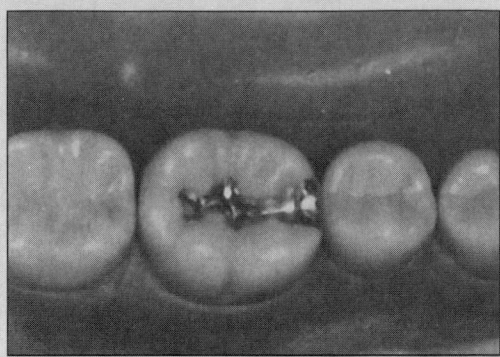

FIG. 27-28   **Polished amalgam restoration.**

the rest of the day; then the patient is dismissed. If finishing and polishing will be done at a later date, as directed by manufacturer's instructions, the patient is advised to schedule another appointment before leaving.

▶ Are the appropriate universal barrier techniques removed?
▶ Have all of the appropriate surfaces been cleaned and disinfected?
▶ Has all armamentarium been removed?
▶ Has all equipment been repositioned?
▶ Has all of the equipment been disinfected/sterilized according to OSHA guidelines?

Additional instruments that are seen in Fig. 27-9 and that may be used in an amalgam procedure are as follows:

T-ball or beavertail burnisher
Hollenback carver
Combination smooth and anatomical carver
Back-action condenser
#25 Wesco condenser

Before the amalgam procedure is begun, the assistant must determine whether all equipment and armamentarium are prepared for the procedure. A consistent pattern of preparation and a few simple ideas that are repeated before the procedure can assist in enhancing the efficiency of patient treatment.

The amalgam procedure is the most common restorative procedure in dentistry and requires that the dental assistant have a thorough understanding of each of its phases. The procedures described in this chapter are common to most amalgam procedures. The assistant, however, must be prepared to adapt to special situations as they arise during the treatment procedure. The assistant must anticipate the needs of the operator by closely observing changes that take place in the procedure, as well as in the patient's needs. Be prepared to adapt instruments and medications to accommodate the situation that might be used with different cavity classifications. Occasionally, problems that can occur during a procedure require changes as noted in Table 27-2.

TABLE 27-2 COMMON PROBLEMS SEEN DURING AMALGAM PROCEDURE

Problem	Solution
1. Fracture of the marginal ridge during removal of the matrix band and retainer	Place a cotton pellet over the marginal ridge during removal of the band
2. Fracture of the marginal ridge during carving sequence	Place less pressure on the amalgam by resting the instrument on tooth structure and the restoration during carving to diffuse any pressure
3. Matrix does not extend to cover the complete proximal box area	Select and use a contoured band that provides coverage of the box; it may be necessary to cut the side opposite the preparation; contour and crimp into original shape through the use of contouring pliers
4. Crumbly amalgam	Increase the mixing time of the amalgam capsule
5. Soupy amalgam	Decrease the mixing time of the amalgam capsule
6. Overhang	Recarve proximal surface if amalgam is still soft enough; use amalgam knife or rotary instrument if hardened.
7. More amalgam is needed to fill the prepared tooth	Always discuss the treatment plan with the operator to determine the number of spills necessary to fill the preparation; if more spills are needed than was expected, the amalgam must be mixed quickly to afford a cohesive surface between the spills of amalgam

Modifications of the Procedure

The example just used was for a conventional Class II preparation and restoration. Other situations and unique circumstances require modifications. It is important to understand which steps can be modified. The first six steps described in the common phases of an amalgam procedure, the updated medical history, examination of the treatment site, checked occlusion, administration of anesthesia, isolation of the area, and the opening of the preparation are basically the same for all cavity classifications and would follow similar step-by-step procedures. Other aspects of the procedure would vary with every cavity preparation. In the cavity medication phase, for example, cavity depth may range from ideal to a pulp exposure and would be treated with medications according to the specific depth as discussed in Chapter 11.

▶ Example of Procedural Modifications
Class I — Caries on #3 Lingual Surface

Variations in procedures are necessary when different cavity classifications are involved in a procedure. In a Class I carious lesion on #3 the outline form may be established with different burs rather than straight fissure burs and the caries removal could possibly be performed with a smaller round bur. The use of a single spill of amalgam would be likely and gingival margin trimmers, matrix bands, retainers, wedges, occlusal anatomical carvers, or anatomical burnishers would not be needed. Smooth surface carvers, such as a Ward's C or Hollenback carver, would be needed more often.

Class I — Caries on #18 Occlusal Surface

In this situation caries removal would likely be performed with a smaller round bur because the cavity preparation may be smaller. A single or double spill of amalgam may be needed, depending on the size of the preparation. The matrix band, retainer and wedges, gingival margin trimmers, Ward's C carver or any other smooth surface carvers would not be needed. However, occlusal anatomical carvers, such as the cleoid-discoid carvers would be needed more often.

Class III — Caries on #11 Distal Surface

Occasionally, Class III carious lesions on canines are restored with amalgam, and when amalgam is used, the outline form may be completed with different burs rather than with straight fissure burs. The caries removal would likely be performed with a smaller, round bur, since the cavity preparation may be smaller. A single spill of amalgam would likely be used, and a matrix band, retainer, and one wedge could be needed. A single gingival marginal trimmer may be needed, depending on which proximal surface is involved.

Class V — Caries on #30 Buccal Surface

The outline form in this situation may be completed with different burs rather than with straight fissure burs, and caries removal would likely be performed with a smaller, round bur, since the cavity preparation may be smaller. A matrix band, retainer and wedges, gingival margin trimmers, occlusal anatomical carvers, and anatomical

TABLE 27-3   AMALGAM TRAY USAGE

	2[B]	12[O]	14[6]	19[MO]	21[DO]	30[MOD]	32[L]
Anesthesia							
Long				X	X	X	X
Short	X	X	X				
Rubber dam							
Teeth isolated	*1,2,3,4	10,11,12,13	12,13,14,15	18,19,20,21	20,21,22,23	28,29,30,31	30,31,32
Clamp on	1	13	15	18	20	31	32
Explorer	X	X	X	X	X	X	X
Mirror	X	X	X	X	X	X	X
Cotton pliers	X	X	X	X	X	X	X
Spoon excavator	X	X	X	X	X	X	X
Hatchet/chisel	X	X	X	X	X	X	X
Mesial margin trimmer				X		X	
Distal margin trimmer					X	X	
Amalgam carrier	X	X	X	X	X	X	X
#1 condensor	X	X	X	X	X	X	X
#2 condensor	X	X	X	X	X	X	X
Ward's C carver	X			X	X	X	X
7C		X	X	X	X	X	
5C		X	X	X	X	X	
Ball burnisher	X	X	X	X	X	X	X
Anatomic burnisher		X	X	X	X	X	
Matrix band				X	X	X	
Matrix retainer				X	X	X	
Wedges							
1.				X	X		
2.						X	
Dappen dish/amalgam well	X	X	X	X	X	X	X
Cotton pellets	X	X	X	X	X	X	X
Articulating paper		X	X	X	X	X	

*Rubber dam optional; additional teeth may be isolated at operator's preference.

burnishers would not be needed. However, smooth surface carvers, such as Ward's C or Hollenback carvers, would be needed more often.

Modified Class VI — Caries on #2 Mesial, Occlusal and Distal Surfaces

The matrix band, retainer, and two wedges would be needed in this situation, and a double spill of amalgam if not more would also be needed. The carving must occur on both proximal surfaces, since both boxes are being restored. Additional caution must be taken when removing the matrix band, retainer, and wedges, as well as when carving the marginal ridges.

Modified Class VI - Caries on #19 Mesial, Occlusal, Distal and Buccal Surfaces

The matrix band, retainer, and two wedges would be needed, as well as a double spill of amalgam, if not more. There must be carving on both proximal surfaces, since both boxes are being restored. Additional caution must be taken when removing the matrix band, retainer, and wedges, as well as when carving the marginal ridges and buccal cusp area.

Table 27-3 provides a chart of various common treatment situations and the types of instruments and armamentarium that are necessary to complete the procedure.

Pin-retained Amalgam Restoration

Occasionally, a patient might have a more extensive restorative situation that requires additional steps to assist in the retention of the restorative material. One such situation would be the pin-retained amalgam restoration which uses a threaded-pin system. Normally, amalgam is retained within the confines of the structure of the tooth.

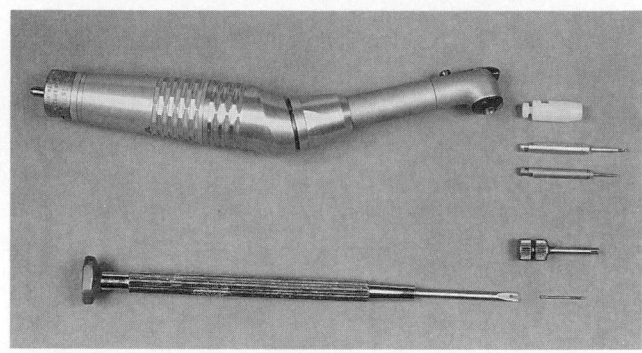

FIG. 27-29   Example of pin placement devices and pins.
(Courtesy of Whaledent International, New York, New York.)

When tooth structure is lost from decay or trauma, the tooth may not be structurally capable of retaining the restorative material—be it amalgam or composite. Pin techniques are used to assist in these situations with amalgam or composite restorative procedures.

▶ Procedure

The operator makes a starter hole with a ¼ or ½ round bur and then expands the hole with a spirec drill on the slow-speed handpiece. Each type of pin system provides or recommends the use of a particular spirec drill for the pin technique (Fig. 27-29). The pin is placed in the hole with a pin wrench or an autoclutch, a mechanical means of pin placement. If an autoclutch is used, it is placed on the slow-speed handpiece with a plastic latch-type, shanked pin, allowing the pin to be twisted in automatically. Since the pin is a self-shearing device, it will shear off as the pin reaches the correct pinhole depth. Placing more than one pin requires a multipin threaded system. Two pins attached to a plastic latch-type shank device, piggy back pins, allow placement of the pins without removing the device from the autoclutch (Fig. 27-30, *A* and *B*).

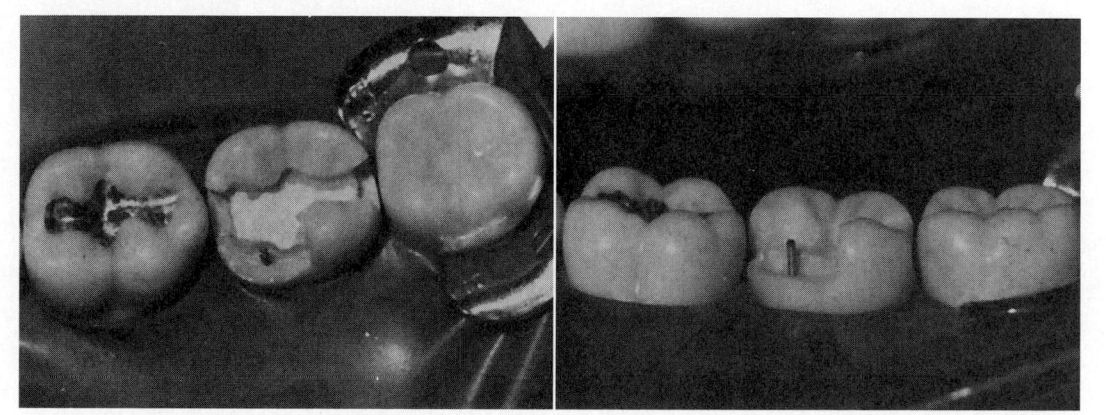

FIG. 27-30   *A* and *B*, Pin placed in prepared tooth to assist in retention of restorative material.
(From Spohn EE, Halowski WA, Berry TG: *Operative dentistry procedures for dental auxiliaries*, St Louis, 1981, Mosby, p. 166.)

TEAM APPROACH

Amalgam Procedure

OPERATOR	ASSISTANT
	Select and prepare all armamentaria
	Prepare the treatment room and escort the patient in to be seated
	Assist in administration of anesthesia and placement of isolation
	Pass mirror and explorer
Examine treatment site	Exchange instruments for opening bur in high-speed handpiece
Open the preparation	Place HVE and a/w syringe to maintain clear field of operation
	Prepare explorer to pass
	Exchange explorer for handpiece
Examine site with explorer	Insert outline and resistance form bur in handpiece and exchange handpiece for explorer
Create outline resistance form	Maintain clear field of operation
	Exchange hand cutting instruments for handpiece
Receive and use hand cutting instruments to place bevels and remove unsupported tooth structure	Exchange slow-speed handpiece with caries removal bur for hand cutting instruments
Remove caries	Maintain clear field of operation
	Exchange explorer for handpiece
Check preparation for complete caries removal of explorer	Exchange retentive bur in handpiece for explorer
Place retentive grooves	Maintain clear field of operation
	Exchange explorer for handpiece
Place cavity medication	Prepare cavity medication and exchange placement instrument for explorer
	Keep 2 × 2 gauze and medication in transfer zone operator access
	Exchange instrument for explorer
Use the explorer to remove excess cement	Maintain clear field of operation
	Exchange prepared matrix retainer and band for explorer
Place matrix retainer and band	Pass cotton pliers and wedge
Place wedge interproximally	Exchange explorer for cotton pliers
Evaluate placement of retainer, band, and wedge	Mix amalgam and receive explorer
	Fill amalgam carrier and pass

TEAM APPROACH
Amalgam Procedure-cont'd.

OPERATOR	ASSISTANT
Place amalgam preparation	Exchange carrier for condenser and fill carrier The exchange of the amalgam carrier and condenser continues until the preparation is overfilled with the HVE in the area to remove excess pieces of amalgam Exchange anatomical carver for condenser
Initially carve restoration removing gross amounts of excess	Maintain clear field of operation Exchange carver and for explorer
Remove excess from marginal ridge area	Exchange explorer for cotton pliers
Remove wedge	Receive wedge
Remove retainer	Receive retainer
Remove band	Exchange smooth surface carver for band and cotton pliers
Carve smooth surface	Exchange carver for explorer
Check smooth surfaces with explorer	Prepare anatomical carver Exchange explorer for anatomical carver
Refine anatomical carving	Maintain clear field of operation Exchange carver for burnisher
Burnish the restored surfaces	Exchange burnisher for explorer
Remove flash	Remove carved flash with HVE
Remove isolation	Assist in removal of isolation Exchange articulating paper and paper holder for explorer
Check articulation	Exchange holder for carver
Remove excess with carver	Exchange carver for articulating paper
Check articulation	Exchange articulating paper for carver or burnisher
Carve or burnish as necessary	Receive instruments Remove debris, and provide full mouth rinse Provide postoperative instructions, and dismiss patient Record treatment on the patient's chart Follow OSHA guidelines for cleanup

After all the pins are placed in the preparation, the procedure would continue as any other Class II or Class VI procedure. The matrix band, retainer, and wedge/s would be placed, and the amalgam would be inserted over the pins. The pins work like pilings on a highway bridge: they provide strength to the structure to avoid fractures and further damage to the tooth. If the pin height is excessive it may need to be reduced in height through the use of a bur to cut the pin. A different style of pin may be needed to allow coverage of the restorative material.

KEY POINTS

▶ The amalgam restorative procedure, using concepts of four-handed dentistry with the operator and the chairside assistant working as a team, increases productivity and efficiency. The use of four hands provides the patient with a more comfortable and expeditious experience.

▶ The steps in the amalgam procedure include examination, preparation, medication, placement of the amalgam, and carving and finishing. Modifications in this procedure are common, and the dental team must be prepared at all times to meet the patient's needs.

▶ Dental amalgam is used as a restorative material for intracoronal preparations where adequate tooth structure remains to retain the amalgam.

▶ Amalgam restorations are most often placed in Class I, II, V, and VI cavity preparations. Since it is not an esthetically pleasing restorative material, it is not usually placed in areas of the mouth that would be visible.

▶ Cavity forms include steps of opening, outlining, resistance, caries removal, retention, convenience, and extension for prevention. The phases or forms are necessary to sustain the health of the tooth and the retention of the restoration.

▶ Modifications in an amalgam procedure involve preparation of different surfaces of the tooth, variables in use of instruments and materials, and the need for placement of pins to aid in the retention of the restorative material.

BIBLIOGRAPHY

Council on Dental Materials, Instruments and Equipment, and Council on Dental Therapeutics: Safety of dental amalgam, *Am Dent Assoc J* 106:519, 1983.

Ring ME: *Dentistry, an illustrated history,* St Louis, 1985, Mosby.

Spohn EE, Halowski WA, Berry TG: *Operative dentistry procedures for dental auxiliaries,* St Louis, 1981, Mosby.

Sturdevant CK, Heymann H, Robertson TM, Sturdevant JR: *The art and science of operative dentistry,* St Louis, 1994, Mosby.

28 Composite Restorations

LEARNING OBJECTIVES

You will have mastered the material in this chapter when you can:
▷ Define the key terms
▷ Describe the use of composite resin as a restorative material
▷ List the types of cavity preparations that are common with the use of composite resin as a restorative procedure
▷ Identify the steps of the composite resin restorative procedure
▷ Identify the armamentarium and materials used in the composite resin restorative procedure
▷ Describe the function of each instrument during the procedure

KEY TERMS

Bonding
Centrix syringe
Compules
Polymerize
Shade selection

The composite restorative procedure, like the amalgam procedure, allows for the replacement of lost tooth structure, while retaining healthy tissue. The steps in the procedure are similar to the amalgam procedure, examination, preparation, medication, placement and finishing, but also include acid etching and bonding. This procedure is used to restore various cavity classifications and also is used in the bonding procedure of cosmetic dentistry. The bonding procedure involves the layering of esthetic material on the facial or lingual surfaces of teeth to improve esthetic value.

One of the most important concerns to a dental patient, aside from relief of pain, is to receive a restoration that is esthetically pleasing. An esthetic restoration is a restoration in the oral cavity of which a patient may be consciously and visually aware. A patient does not want an amalgam restoration placed in an anterior tooth, nor does a patient want to have a restoration placed that will stain or corrode. In the 1880s porcelain inlays were fabricated for placement in cavity preparations. Present day esthetic filling materials change regularly to meet patients' and practitioners' needs.

The composite resin procedure is becoming increasingly more popular as the materials supplied by the manufacturers meet more of dentistry's needs. As new materials and technologies are developed, the dental assistant must become familiar with their use. The assistant needs to be curious and to perpetuate an interest in current product information by reading dental literature. Restorative dentistry is ever changing, and introducing new concepts and materials to the practice is part of that change.

Today, it is estimated that the average dental practitioner spends 10% to 15% of treatment time on procedures that are related to a patient's appearance. It is projected that by the end of this decade the percentage of time allocated to esthetic dentistry will triple. In our society great emphasis is placed on esthetics. With the development of various new techniques and materials, esthetic dentistry can be done faster and can be less expensive, more attractive, and longer lasting.

In 1972 approximately 2.7 billion teeth in the United States were in need of dental treatment. It is estimated that by the year 2030 the number will increase to 5 billion teeth, and of those, many will require a course of treatment that improves a patient's appearance and restores function.

Esthetic Dentistry

The types of treatment that enhance a patient's appearance through esthetic dentistry include bonding and contouring, bleaching discolored teeth, porcelain laminates, direct bonded resin veneers, porcelain and resin crowns, inlays, onlays, direct posterior composites, and fixed bridges that are made of combinations of porcelain, composite, and metal. Some of these procedures can be accomplished in a single appointment; others take multiple appointments. As dentistry uses computers, new techniques are being explored. An example of this new technology is CAD-CAM, a computer-generated system that provides the operator with the ability to fabricate and place partial crowns and veneers for a patient in a single appointment. A video of the tooth is taken after the tooth has been prepared to receive the restoration. The information is input to a computer immediately, and a shaping device that is attached to the computer fabricates a restoration within minutes. It is hoped this system can be used in the fabrication of full crowns in the near future. See Chapter 40 for more details of this technology. This chapter will emphasize the conventional procedure of providing the patient with an esthetically pleasing composite resin restoration.

Composite Materials and Uses

Esthetic filling materials usually are placed in areas of the oral cavity that are readily visible when the patient smiles or talks. To obtain the best esthetic restorative material has been a goal of the dental profession. Materials that are used include veneers, glass ionomers, and chemically and light-cured composite resins. A material that comes the closest to providing the best esthetic restoration in a single appointment procedure is the microfilled composite restorative material. Placement of the composite materials in anterior teeth is as common as placement of amalgam in the posterior teeth. Positive aspects of the material would be the ability to obtain the correct color and translucency match. The microfilled composites are one of the most commonly used composite materials because the surfaces can be finished to an extreme level of smoothness. Macrofilled and minifilled composite materials are also available. Each has certain aspects that warrant use and are discussed in Chapter 11, *Dental Materials.*

Microfilled composite resin materials are usually bonded in place on a tooth. **Bonding** is a common procedure to attach the restorative material to the tooth surface. Previous to the development of the bonding technique, restorative materials were held in place through a system of mechanical lock. The mechanical lock was established with the use of burs and stones used to create undercuts to aid in the retention of the restorative material. It is common to use a combination of mechanical retention and the bonding technique in a preparation to ensure retention of a restoration. The bonding technique involves the placement of an acid etchant on the enamel surface of the tooth. The etched enamel provides a slightly porous surface for the bonding material to adhere. The composite resin material then adheres to the bonded resin. With the use of a bonding material less tooth surface has to be removed to retain a restorative material. In some circumstances, burs are not even used to create a preparation before the placement of the restorative material, the surface is simply acid etched and bonded.

In the past most composite restorations were placed in the anterior segment of the mouth and on buccal surfaces of all other teeth, since these areas are often visible. As technology has improved, posterior composite restorative materials are used more frequently in other cavity classifications. The high compressive strength of the microfilled materials has provided an avenue for practitioners to place esthetic restorative materials in nontraditional cavity preparations (i.e., Class II and Class VI).

The common classifications of cavities usually restored with composite material include the following:

- ▶ **Class I** — buccal pit lesions of posterior teeth, lingual pit lesions of incisors, defects of the incisal two thirds of anterior teeth
- ▶ **Class III** — lesions on proximal surfaces with no involvement of the incisal angle of anterior teeth
- ▶ **Class IV** — lesions on proximal surfaces with involvement of the incisal angle of anterior teeth
- ▶ **Class V** — lesions on the cervical one third of all teeth

Composite filling material is also used on a regular basis as a core material to reconstruct major tooth structures before a crown preparation. If a composite resin restoration fails, it is usually attributed to color change and excess washing or to wear in the contour of the material.

The steps for cavity preparation outlined for the amalgam procedure are followed for the composite procedure (i.e., retention form, caries removal). Generally, the procedure is less extensive for a composite restoration than it is for an amalgam. That is particularly true with resin composite that is used in conjunction with acid etching and bonding. Less tooth structure is removed during this procedure when it is compared with placement of amalgam or a cast alloy restoration. To review the procedure for the preparation steps, refer to Chapter 27.

Common Armamentarium for a Composite Restorative Procedure

As stated in Chapter 27, the clinician will have favorite instruments and devices to use in a given procedure. The following summary of armamentarium and instruments includes examples of traditional selections.

The techniques of the composite restorative procedure that are followed by each operator may vary; however, certain fundamental steps are common. Box 28-1 lists the common steps in a Class III composite procedure. The manipulation of composite resin as a restorative material is explained in Chapter 11, *Dental Materials.*

▶ Examination Phase

The instruments in the examination phase are used to check the tooth for anomalies, retraction, visibility, and illumination and to pass small items to and from the mouth. Although the instruments are categorized in the examination phase, some are used throughout the procedure for other purposes. The instruments and devices of the examination phase are the explorer, the mirror, cotton pliers, and shade guides.

Explorer — checks the tooth for anomalies, and inspects for flash or defects in restorations

Mirror — provides retraction, visibility, and illumination

Cotton pliers — places and removes wedge(s), places articulating paper and cavity medication, and aids in placement of acid etch and bonding agent

Shade guides — used to obtain an accurate composite shade for tooth structure that is to be replaced

Rubber cup and pumice — polish teeth before shade selection to remove stain and fluoride remnants

▶ Preparation Phase

The instruments in the preparation phase are used to remove carious debris, plane and cleave walls, remove unsupported enamel, place cervical and pulpal floor bevels, remove tooth structure or restorative material during cavity opening, outline, to remove caries, and to establish retention phases in a procedure.

Spoon excavator — removes carious debris, inverts rubber dam, places cement bases

Wedelstaedt chisel — planes and cleaves walls, removes unsupported enamel

Triple-angle chisel — planes and cleaves walls, using pull action

Burs — #½, #1, #2 Round FG — opens the cavity preparation

  #55, #56 Straight Fissure FG — places the outline form of the cavity preparation

  #2 Round RA or FG — removes caries

  #¼, #½ Round RA or FG — places retentive grooves

  #7901 flame finishing — places bevel to aid in finishing the restorative material

▶ Placement Instruments and Devices

The instruments and devices of this phase of the procedure are used to prepare tooth surfaces for placement of the material and to place, retain, and cure the filling material.

Rubber cup — used with pumice on tooth surface to remove debris

Acid etch — prepares the enamel surface for good bond strength

Bonding agent — polymer liquid that leaves polymer tags on enamel surface

Light-activating device — polymerizes the resins (restorative and bonding material)

Teflon/plastic instrument — places restorative material

BOX 28-I

STEPS OF COMPOSITE RESTORATION

1. Update medical history
2. Examine treatment site
3. Determine occlusal relationship
4. Administer anesthesia
5. Polish the tooth with pumice
6. Select shade
7. Isolate with rubber dam/cotton roll(s)
8. Open cavity preparation
9. Place outline and resistance form
10. Remove caries
11. Place retention
12. Place cavity medications (base)
13. Place matrix strip and wedge(s)
14. Acid etch (reisolate if necessary)
15. Apply bonding material
16. Insert filling material
17. Remove matrix and wedge
18. Finish and polish
19. Remove rubber dam/cotton roll(s)
20. Check articulation
21. Give postoperative instructions

Composite syringe, tip and, plunger — places restorative material in areas difficult to reach

Mylar/celluloid matrix strip — aids in the retention of the restorative material in the preparation during insertion

Wedge(s) — holds celluloid matrix strip against the tooth, and provides adequate interdental space during insertion of material

Matrix strip holder — holds strip, while it surrounds restorative material in preparation

Skubes/disposable brushes/cotton pledgets — used in placement of acid etch and bonding material

▶ Finishing Instruments

After the composite filling material is placed and cured, excess material is removed and the surfaces are finished and polished to a fine smoothness, restoring the anatomic shape.

12B scalpel blade and handle — removes excess composite material

Finishing strip — used to shape and contour restorations on proximal surfaces

Articulating paper — determines proper occlusal relationship before and after the restorative procedure

Articulating paper holder — holds articulating paper while occlusal relationship is determined

Finishing and Polishing Armamentarium

Round green stone	Round white stone
Carrot-shaped green stone	Carrot-shaped white stone
Mandrel	Composite finishing disks
Composite finishing points	7900 Finishing burs

▶ Additional Armamentarium

The following armamentarium is needed for the composite restorative procedure:

Rubber dam armamentarium or cotton rolls — used for isolation

Cotton pellets — used to place medication, to isolate, to place acid etch and bonding agent, and for drying

Cotton gauze — cleans instruments and other surfaces

Rubber dam armamentarium

Anesthesia armamentarium

Composite Resin armamentarium

Dental Materials armamentarium

Preparation of Armamentarium

The use of preset trays is common for operative procedures. A preset composite tray includes a variety of instruments. The selection of instruments and additional armamentarium depends on the operator's preference. The following is an example of a typical preset composite tray. The devices are listed as seen in Fig. 28-1.

ARMAMENTARIUM FOR THE COMPOSITE PROCEDURE

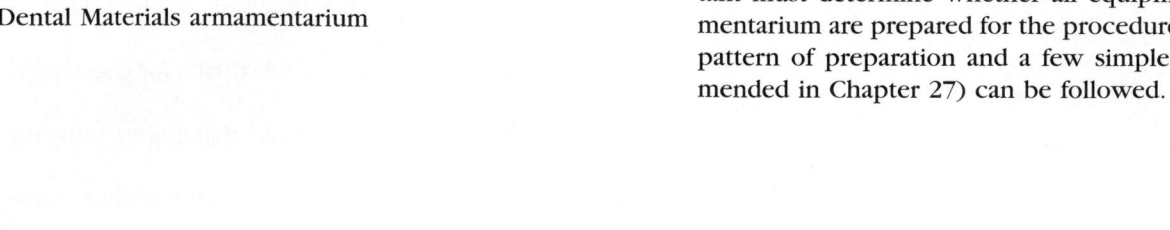

Explorer
Mirror
Cotton pliers
Spoon excavator
Binangle or triple angle chisel
Wedelstaedt chisel
Teflon plastic instrument
12B scalpel blade and handle
Articulating paper holder
Thumb forceps
HVE tip
Articulating paper
Mylar matrix strip
Matrix strip holder
Wedge(s)
Skubes/disposable brushes
Shade guides
Finishing strips
a/w Tip
a/w Tip cover
Plastic pad
Cotton pellets
2 × 2 gauze
Rubber cup and pumice
Patient napkin chain
Dappen dish
Bur block and burs
Finishing and polishing devices
Cotton rolls
Composite materials including acid etch and bonding
Curing light
Composite syringe (if necessary)

Before beginning the composite procedure the assistant must determine whether all equipment and armamentarium are prepared for the procedure. A consistent pattern of preparation and a few simple ideas (recommended in Chapter 27) can be followed.

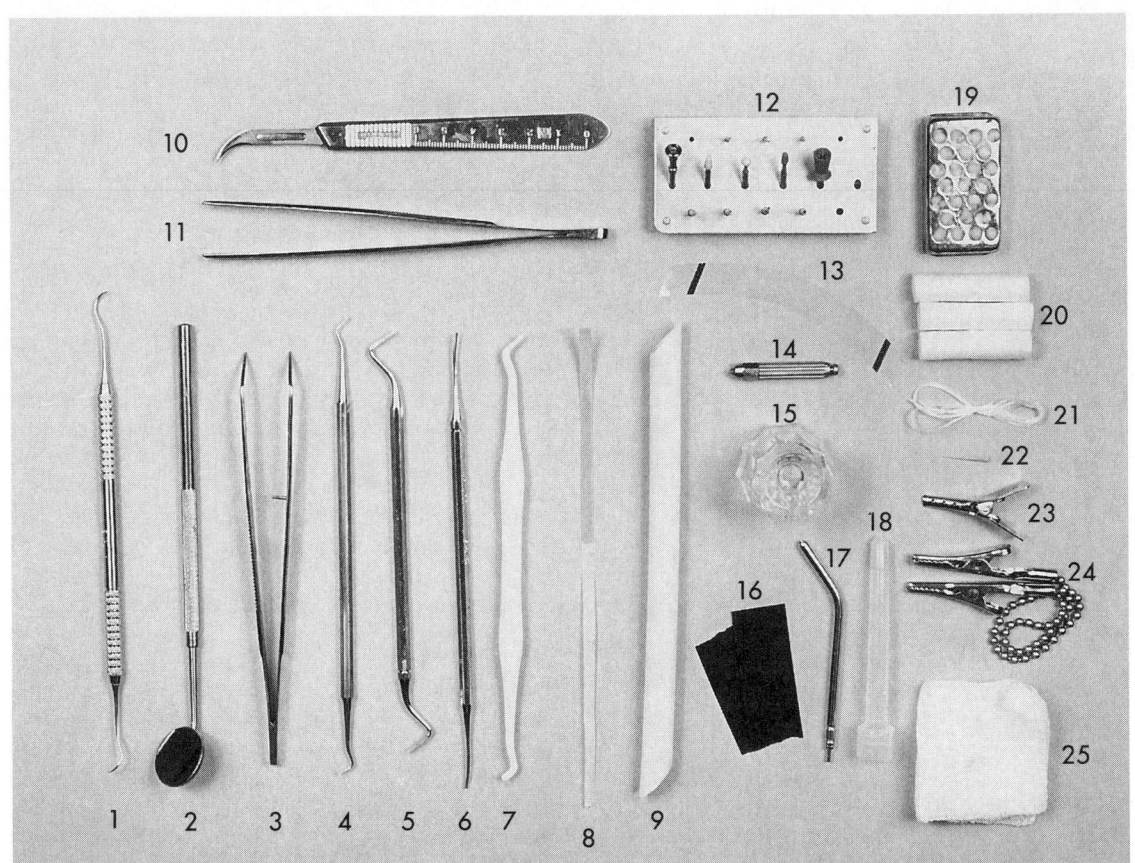

FIG. 28-1   Example of a composite tray set-up. *1,* Explorer. *2,* Mirror. *3,* Cotton pliers. *4,* Spoon excavator. *5,* Binangle chisel. *6,* Wedelstaedt chisel. *7,* Plastic Teflon instrument. *8,* Linen strip. *9,* HVE tip. *10,* #12B scalpel blade and handle. *11,* Thumb forceps. *12,* Bur block, with assorted burs and stones. *13,* Mylar/celluloid matrix strip. *14,* Bur tool. *15,* Dappen dish. *16,* Articulating paper. *17,* a/w tip. *18,* a/w tip cover. *19,* Cotton pellets. *20,* Cotton rolls. *21,* Floss. *22,* Wedge. *23,* Matrix strip holder. *24,* Napkin chain. *25,* 2 × 2 gauze.

CLASS III COMPOSITE PROCEDURE

One of many forms of composite procedures performed daily in a general dentistry practice is a Class III restoration. The following sections describe a step-by-step procedure for placing an acid-etched and bonded composite resin, using light-cured composite resin.

▶ Are all universal barrier techniques being used?
▶ Is all of the armamentarium available and prepared for use?
▶ Are the instruments arranged in sequence of use?
▶ Am I prepared for alternative treatment plans?
▶ Is the necessary equipment turned on and ready to operate?

Update Medical History

A **current health history** is obtained from the patient who is being seen for treatment on the distal surface of an anterior tooth. In this situation the patient has a medical history of rheumatic heart fever at the age of 5 years. Since the patient was scheduled 2 weeks in advance for this appointment, the dentist prescribed an antibiotic regimen before treatment.

Examination of Treatment Site

The **site of treatment is examined** by the operator as the assistant passes the explorer and the mirror. During the examination the operator confirms the area and the extent of treatment to be rendered.

Determine Occlusal Relationship

The first step that is completed before any restorative procedure is to determine the **occlusal relationship** and to identify any interferences that may exist. The assistant dries the surfaces of the teeth with a 2 × 2 gauze sponge and holds articulating paper between the arches, with articulating paper forceps or cotton pliers. The patient is directed to bite firmly down and then to grind side-to-side, as well as to slide forward and back.

The identification of centric stops and the excursive contacts will aid the operator as the restorative material is placed in the preparation. If the operator extends the filling material beyond the margins or into an area that occludes heavily with an opposing tooth or teeth, it will complicate the finishing step. It is necessary to obtain this information to avoid spending excess time to remove the hardened restorative material during the finishing and polishing steps.

Anesthesia Administration

After the occlusion has been established, the **administration of anesthesia** begins. The anesthesia syringe is prepared by selecting an anesthetic with vasoconstrictor, when no contraindications are noted in the patient's health history. A 1-inch needle is selected, since access to the area is rather simple during infiltration, to achieve innervation. The assembly and passing of the syringe is described in Chapter 23.

When the syringe is passed by the assistant, using the hidden syringe technique, it may be necessary to place the HVE tip near the injection site during or immediately after the injection. The tissue into which the solution is placed is taut, and some of the solution may leak from the site. The anesthesia solution is extremely bitter, and the HVE is used for the patient's comfort. After the anesthesia has been administered, the assistant completes a full mouth rinse on the patient.

Polishing the Tooth With Pumice

If a routine preparation is being completed, this step may not be performed. If bonding is being done on an unprepared tooth, the following procedure needs to be completed. The area of the tooth that is to be restored must be cleansed of all debris and any fluoride remnants before the acid etched composite procedure is performed. This step ensures a successful bond of tooth and material. It is accomplished as the operator uses a rubber cup that is placed on the low-speed handpiece with a nonfluoridated flour of pumice slurry or prophylaxis paste. The surfaces of the tooth are polished and then rinsed and dried thoroughly. (Steps in coronal polishing were identified in Chapter 26, during the prophylaxis procedure.)

Shade Selection

After the tooth has been polished, the **shade selection,** which determines a hue of tooth color, is easier to match with the resin. A shade guide with lettered or numbered buttons that correspond to the restorative material is provided with each kit of resins. It is important to ensure that the correct shade is selected under natural conditions. The shade is selected without the rubber dam in place, with saliva moistening the shade button, and in natural light. If natural light is not available, the operating light should be turned away from the oral cavity as the operator/team decides the correct shade. Shade selection consists of not only determining the correct shade, but also determining the level of translucency (Fig. 28-2). Usually, a separate translucency paste is provided with each composite kit.

Often, the operator will ask the patient for input in the shade selection, since the patient must be pleased with the color of the restorative material. Shades can be combined or layered during placement to obtain the shade that correctly compliments the tooth that is being restored. This could occur when natural tooth color is different in one area than it is in another, such as on the incisal edge as opposed to on the cervical area. A comparison of the same tooth in the opposite quadrant is made, since coloring is often similar.

CLASS III COMPOSITE PROCEDURE—cont'd

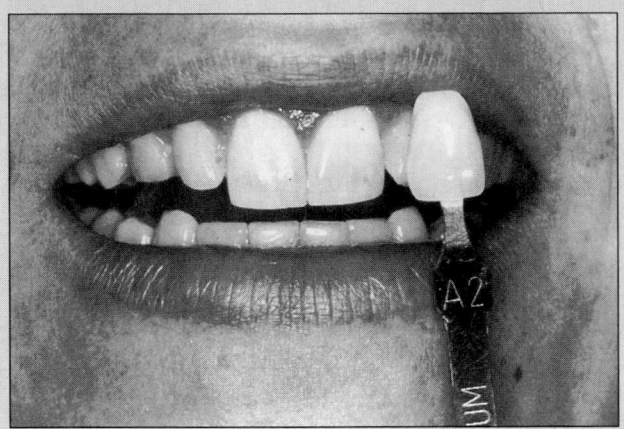

FIG. 28-2 Shade selection involves selection of the hue from a shade tab or a guide.

(From Sturdevant C: *Art and science of operative dentistry,* St Louis, 1985, Mosby.)

The assistant retrieves the material that corresponds to the selected shade of restorative material from the available selections with either overgloves or noncontaminated thumb forceps. If the assistant uses gloved hands that have been involved in the procedure, contamination of the kit of material could occur. At all times during any restorative procedure the dental team must be aware of cross-contamination of instruments and materials.

Isolation with Rubber Dam

A composite restorative procedure is an excellent example for the ideal use of rubber dam isolation, since total isolation must be maintained during various phases of the procedure. The step-by-step procedure is described in Chapter 22. The use of clamps is optional because the rubber dam can be anchored with ligatures of rubber dam material, floss, or other devices. These options provide better access to the tooth that is being restored and reduce potential of contaminated aerosols.

Cavity Preparation

Cavity preparation in a composite restorative procedure may not be necessary in some circumstances. If the patient has a fractured incisal edge, the extent of treatment may be pumicing, etching, bonding and placement, curing and finishing of the restorative material. Other situations warrant the removal of tooth structure as in this example.

Opening Phase

Extension of a cavity preparation to prevent future decay is not a great concern during the composite preparation procedure because anterior teeth have less defined anatomi-

cal structure: grooves and fissures. The removal of the existing carious tissue, while developing conventional preparation and retentive forms, is more important; this is usually attempted as the operator preserves all possible tooth structure. If the carious lesion begins on the lingual of the distal proximal surface, all attempts are made to preserve the facial surface of the distal; or if the decay occurs on the facial surface, an effort is made to maintain the lingual area.

In this treatment situation the decay has begun on the facial surface and penetrated to the lingual, forcing the removal of the proximal area completely. The assistant prepares a #½ or 1 round FG bur on the high-speed handpiece and passes it to the operator. The preparation is started with the penetration of the bur from the lingual surface on the tooth as the assistant places the HVE tip on the facial surface (Fig. 28-3). The assistant retracts the lip with the HVE and also evacuates the handpiece spray simultaneously. A constant stream of air is placed on the mirror by the assistant with the a/w syringe. This helps to maintain visual contact with the preparation for the operator. The HVE tip may be placed posterior to the surface to pick up excess water; however, if this is done, the assistant will still have to retract the maxillary lip with a finger and keep the mirror clean.

When the operator stops the preparation procedure, the assistant rinses and dries the preparation site thoroughly and exchanges the handpiece with the explorer, so that the site can be checked for additional decay. The operator may exchange the explorer for the handpiece again to continue the convenience form and to extend the preparation through the facial surface. All attempts must be made to maintain the integrity of the incisal edge, to prevent the preparation from being extended into a Class IV classification.

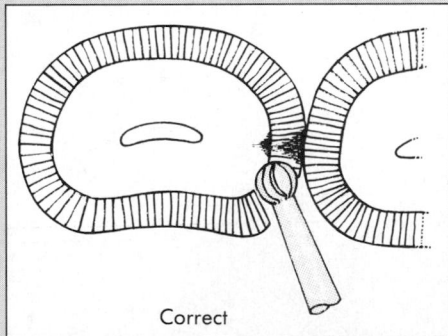

FIG. 28-3 Opening phase of the preparation.

(From Sturdevant C: *Art and science of operative dentistry,* ed 3, St Louis, 1994, Mosby.)

Continued.

CLASS III COMPOSITE PROCEDURE—cont'd

Outline and Resistance Phase

The assistant passes the operator the second high-speed handpiece, with the #55 straight fissure FG bur, to extend the preparation in the outline form and then repositions the HVE and triplex syringe. The operator uses the bur at a right angle on the enamel surfaces to preserve all the tooth structure possible by keeping within the parameters that were established during the opening phase. The handpiece is exchanged for a wedelstaedt, binangle chisel, triple-angle chisel or even an enamel hatchet. The instrument is used to

cleave the unsupported enamel and to finish the walls (Fig. 28-4).

The operator has the assistant place a #7901 finishing bur or diamond bur on the high-speed handpiece for an optional step. This bur is used on the cavosurface margins to place bevels on the enamel surface (Fig. 28-5). This step aids later in the finishing phase of the procedure.

Caries Removal

If all the carious tissue was not removed during the previous steps the assistant exchanges the hand instrument for the low-speed handpiece with a #1 or #2 RA round bur. The conventional-speed handpiece is the device commonly used to preserve as much tooth structure as possible. Tooth structure can be removed quickly with the use of a high-speed handpiece and natural tooth surfaces are preferred over resin surfaces. An optional instrument for caries removal is a spoon excavator.

The assistant occasionally positions the a/w syringe over the preparation and forces a spurt of air into it. Any debris from the site is forced out and a dry field is maintained for the operator. When the operator signals, the assistant exchanges the handpiece for the explorer, so that the operator can confirm complete removal of all carious tissue.

Placement of Retentive Grooves

The assistant places the #¼ or ½ RA round bur in the conventional-speed handpiece, while the operator uses the explorer. The exchange occurs, and the operator places retentive grooves in the dentin along all existing walls. This step will help to retain the restorative material in the preparation (Fig. 28-6). The assistant retrieves the handpiece and completely rinses and dries the preparation.

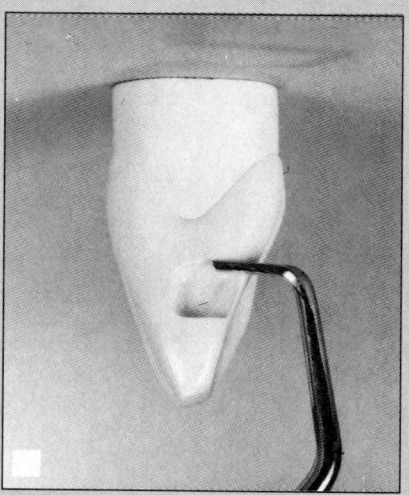

FIG. 28-4   Resistance phase of the preparation.

(From Sturdevant C: *Art and science of operative dentistry,* ed 3, St Louis, 1994, Mosby.)

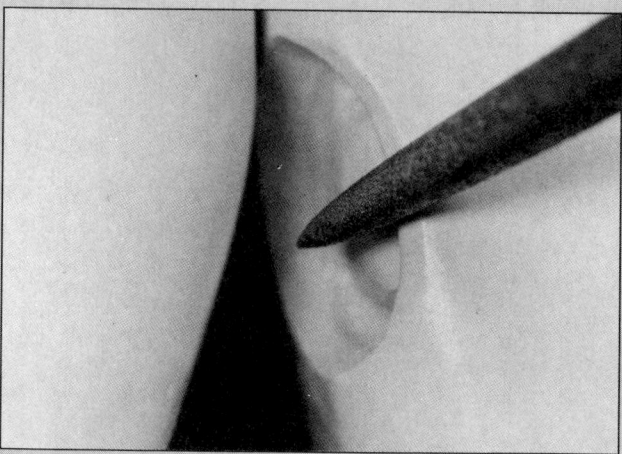

FIG. 28-5   Placement of cavosurface bevels.

(From Sturdevant C: *Art and science of operative dentistry,* ed 3, St Louis, 1994, Mosby.)

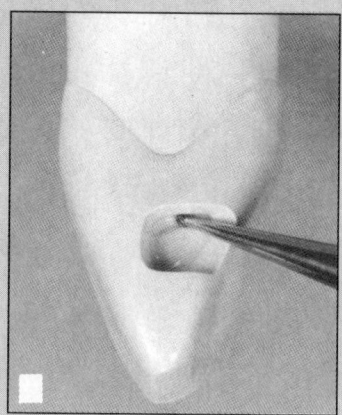

FIG. 28-6   Placement of retentive grooves.

(From Sturdevant C: *Art and science of operative dentistry,* ed 3, St Louis, 1994, Mosby.)

CLASS III COMPOSITE PROCEDURE—cont'd

Placement of Cavity Medication

The selection of cavity medication is predicated on several factors: the thickness of the remaining dentin, pulpal protection, and the type of restorative material that is to be placed. To use conventional cavity varnish or zinc–oxide eugenol cements beneath a resin restorative material is not recommended. These materials will create an undesirable or incomplete set of the resin. Currently glass ionomer or light-cured calcium hydroxide are considered selections in a cavity preparation of minimal depth, such as in this case.

The assistant mixes a thin paste consistency of glass ionomer on the slab, places a small amount on a ball-type applicator, and passes it to the operator for placement in the site. A 2 × 2 gauze sponge is kept in the transfer zone by the assistant to wipe excess material off of the instrument.

Placement of Matrix Strip and Wedge

After the ionomer has hardened, the assistant passes a curved or a straight celluloid matrix strip to the operator, and it is placed interproximally. The strip is placed approximately 1 mm below the cervical wall; then a test determines whether the strip is contoured properly to the tooth surface (Fig. 28-7). The wedge is selected and passed to the operator with cotton forceps or in the assistant's palm. The placement of the wedge may be done from the lingual or facial aspect because the purpose is to secure the position of the matrix strip during the insertion of the restorative material (Fig. 28-8). The wedge also forces the teeth apart, assisting and assuring the operator of the proper interproximal contact.

Acid Etching

The acid etching procedure is a step that is taken to obtain an ideal bond of the surfaces when composite resin materials are used. The assistant dispenses the acid etch material—usually phosphoric acid—on a plastic slab or a welled device that is provided by the manufacturer. The placement device of choice is prepared: a ball-tipped applicator, a spoon excavator, a bristle brush, disposable applicator or a **skube** (a small piece of sponge or a piece of endodontic paper point that is held in cotton forceps). If a paper pad is provided by the operator, contamination of the pad might occur during the placement of the etching material. The applicator is passed, and the acid is held in the transfer zone for the operator to dip the instrument into the etchant and apply it to the *thoroughly* dried tooth surface. This step roughens the enamel surface and removes debris. The etchant can be liquid or of a gel consistency. The application technique varies, depending on the type of etchant. If the etchant is in a liquid form, it should be applied to the surface and then reapplied every 20 seconds, for a total of 1 minute. If the etchant is gel form, a single application that is left on the surface for 1 minute is adequate. It is necessary to have the matrix strip in place during this step to avoid etching adjacent tooth surfaces. After 1 minute the operator passes the instrument back to the assistant, and the tooth is thoroughly rinsed from the etched enamel surface for at least 30 seconds and is then dried. The etched enamel will appear white and chalky; however, if the surfaces do not appear white and chalky, they may have to be etched again. During the re-etching procedure, the same steps are

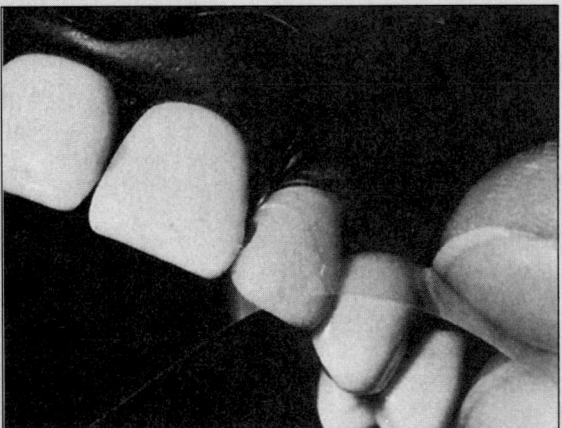

FIG. 28-7 **Matrix strip in position.**

(From Spohn EE et al: *Operative dentistry procedures for dental auxiliaries,* St Louis, 1981, Mosby.)

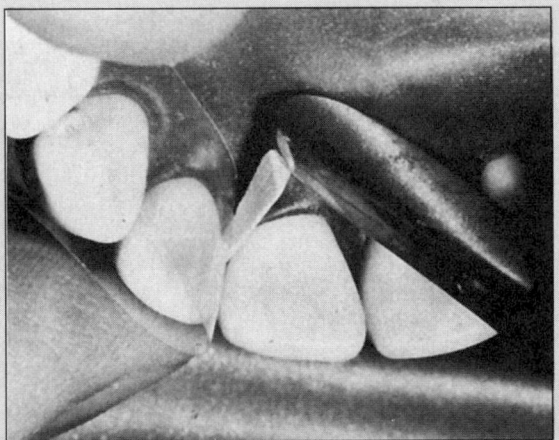

FIG. 28-8 **The wedge is positioned to secure the position of the matrix.**

(From Spohn EE et al: *Operative dentistry procedures for dental auxiliaries,* St Louis, 1981, Mosby.)

Continued.

followed. If the same matrix strip is used, it must be completely dried, or, if necessary, it may be removed and replaced. If rubber dam is not used for isolation, cotton rolls are removed and replaced at this time.

Placement of Bonding Material

The bonding material is supplied as a single, self-curing resin, as a two-paste system, or as a light-cured type. The selection is based on the operator's preference and on the type of composite restorative material that is being placed. The two-paste system is used in this situation. The assistant places equal portions of catalyst and base on a work surface and mixes the material with a ball-tipped applicator, until it is homogeneous. The placement instrument may be any of those discussed in the acid-etching step of the procedure. The operator maintains complete isolation during the preparation of the bonding material, since it is vital to the success of the bond. The materials are passed to the operator, who places the bonding material on the etched surfaces and prepares for the curing of the material, whether the material self cures is chemically cured, or is light cured.

Insertion of Filling Material

Composite filling materials are available as chemically cured, two-paste systems or as light-cured, single-paste systems (Fig. 28-9, *A* and *B*). This specific procedure will be completed with a light-cured material. The preselected light-cured filling material is dispensed by the assistant. The material is sensitive to light and may begin to cure from artificial light sources, so it should be dispensed for immediate use. The syringes of material that are provided in the composite kits are usually made of an opaque material that does not allow

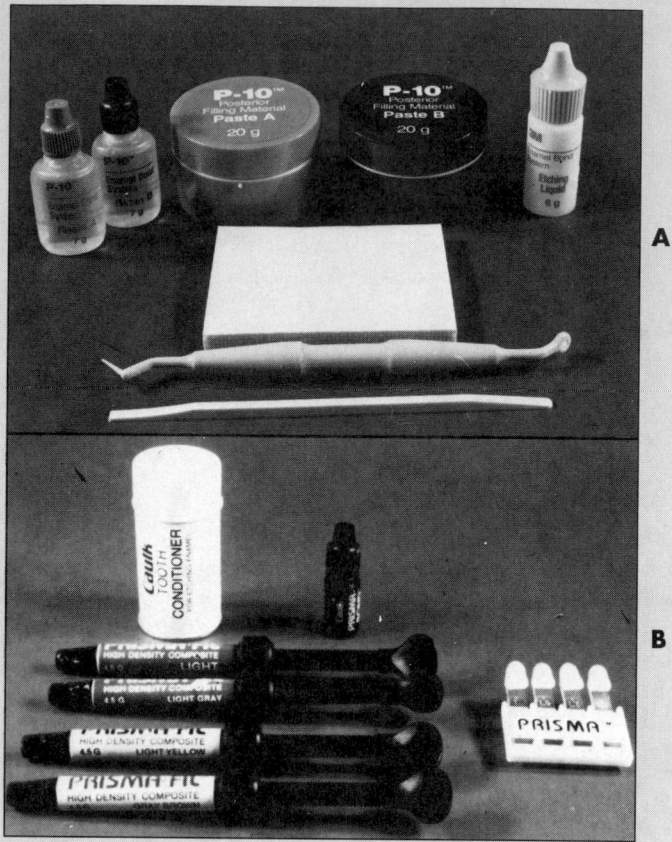

FIG. 28-9   *A* and *B,* Chemically and light-cured composite restorative systems.

(From Craig RG, O'Brien WJ, Powers JH: *Dental materials: properties and manipulation,* ed 5, St Louis, 1992, Mosby.)

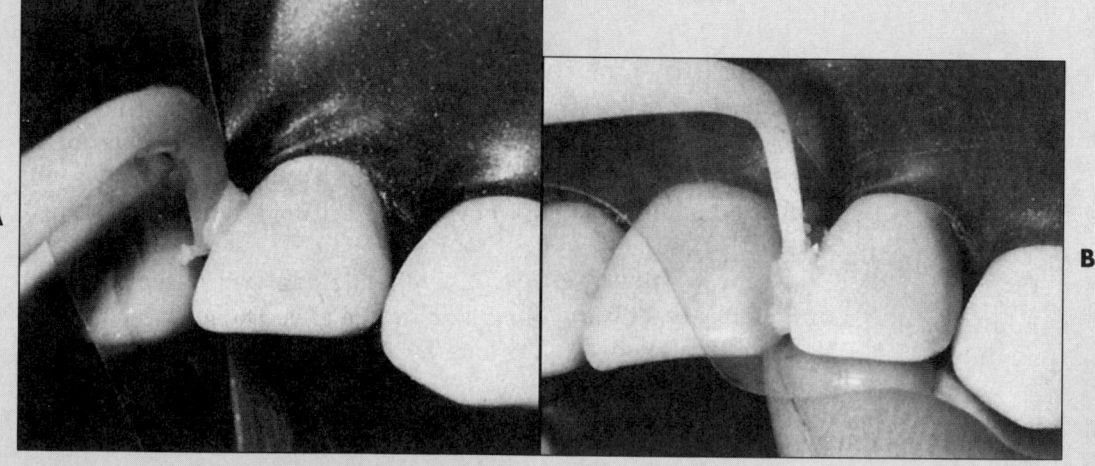

FIG. 28-10   *A* and *B,* Placement of the restorative material.

(From Spohn EE et al: *Operative dentistry procedures for dental auxiliaries,* St Louis, 1981, Mosby.)

CLASS III COMPOSITE PROCEDURE—cont'd

light to penetrate the composite material. While the over-gloves are worn, the necessary amount of material is dispensed onto a paper pad or a plastic slab by turning the key of the syringe in a clockwise direction. Once the appropriate amount of material has been dispensed, the assistant reverses the direction of the key to pull the material into the syringe. The syringe is recapped. This type of material is relatively expensive, and it is important to conserve costs for the operator and the patient by dispensing only the amount needed. At no time should the composite placement instrument contact the source of the composite material, thus contaminating the remaining material.

The resin material may also be provided in preproportioned **compules** that are used in conjunction with a **centrix syringe.** Once they are used, the compules should be discarded. When the compules are placed in a patient's oral cavity, they become contaminated.

The assistant passes the disposable or sterilizable work surface and a placement instrument to the operator, who places the material into the preparation in increments [Fig. 28-10, *A* and *B*]. Time is not as significant a factor with the light-cured material as it is with the chemically cured material. The increment amounts placed in the preparation normally should not exceed 2.0 mm in thickness before the material is cured or **polymerized,** which involves the process of setting. The ability of the curing light to penetrate the inner surfaces may be questionable. If more than 2.0 mm of material is needed, it is recommended that the first thickness be cured and the second layer of material be placed and cured. After the material is placed, the matrix strip is contoured around the resin as the operator pulls the ends tautly towards the midline and holds the strip. The ends may also be held in place by a matrix strip holder, freeing the operator's hands for other activities.

The light-curing wand (on which a protective barrier cover may be placed), with an attached, protective shield, is passed to the operator. The patient is directed to close his or her eyes during this step to avoid any damage to the retina.

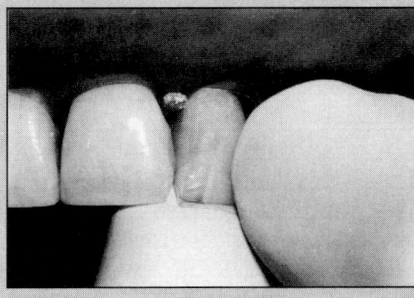

FIG. 28-11 **Curing the light-activated restorative material.**

(From Sturdevant C: *Art and science of operative dentistry,* ed 3, 1994, Mosby.)

Protective eyewear may be worn by the operator and assistant, or vision is directed from the light source. The curing wand is placed approximately 1 mm from the restorative material, and the timer is set for 20 to 30 seconds [Fig. 28-11]; this amount of time will allow the light source from the unit to polymerize the restorative material. If a second layer of material is added, the procedure is repeated.

Removing Matrix Strip and Wedge

After curing is completed, the assistant passes the operator the explorer and receives the light wand. Any flash of the material that extends from the preparation is tested for hardness. The wedge, matrix holder (if used), and matrix strip are removed. The wedge may be removed by hand or with the cotton pliers that are passed by the assistant. The matrix holder is unclamped, the strip is pulled through the proximal area, and both are returned to the assistant. If any voids in the material are observed, additional amounts can be easily added when the light-cured material is used. If a chemically-cured material was used, the restorative material would have to be removed and the procedure, repeated.

Finishing and Polishing

The finishing and polishing procedure is extremely important. Obviously, esthetics is important to the patient, but a finely finished surface also reduces the potential for accumulation of debris and subsequent staining. Finishing begins with the removal of excess material, and this can be accomplished by hand or mechanically. The #12B Bard-Parker scalpel is passed to the operator to remove flash from the tooth surfaces. The instrument is held almost parallel to the surface and is drawn over the restoration to remove gross amounts of excess. Slivers of material dislodge, and the assistant uses the HVE to retrieve these pieces from the oral cavity or from the instrument surface. It is *not* recommended to remove the material from the instrument's surface with a 2 × 2 gauze because the 12B scalpel is extremely sharp and can puncture protective gloves easily.

Other devices may be used for gross removal of excess restorative material. Coarse disks that are placed on mandrels in the low-speed handpiece remove excess amounts of material, more quickly than do finer disks. The assistant replaces each disk, descending in a sequence from coarse to fine, to allow refinement of the surfaces as they are contoured. The labial surface and portions of the lingual surface can be contoured with these disks; however, the cingulum of a tooth may need the use of finishing stones that vary in size and grit. The stones have shapes that match the areas that are to be contoured: round, carrot, or biscuit, for example. When finishing devices are used, the operator may like the restored surfaces to be moist; this can be accomplished by placing a lubricant that is supplied by the

Continued.

CLASS III COMPOSITE PROCEDURE—cont'd

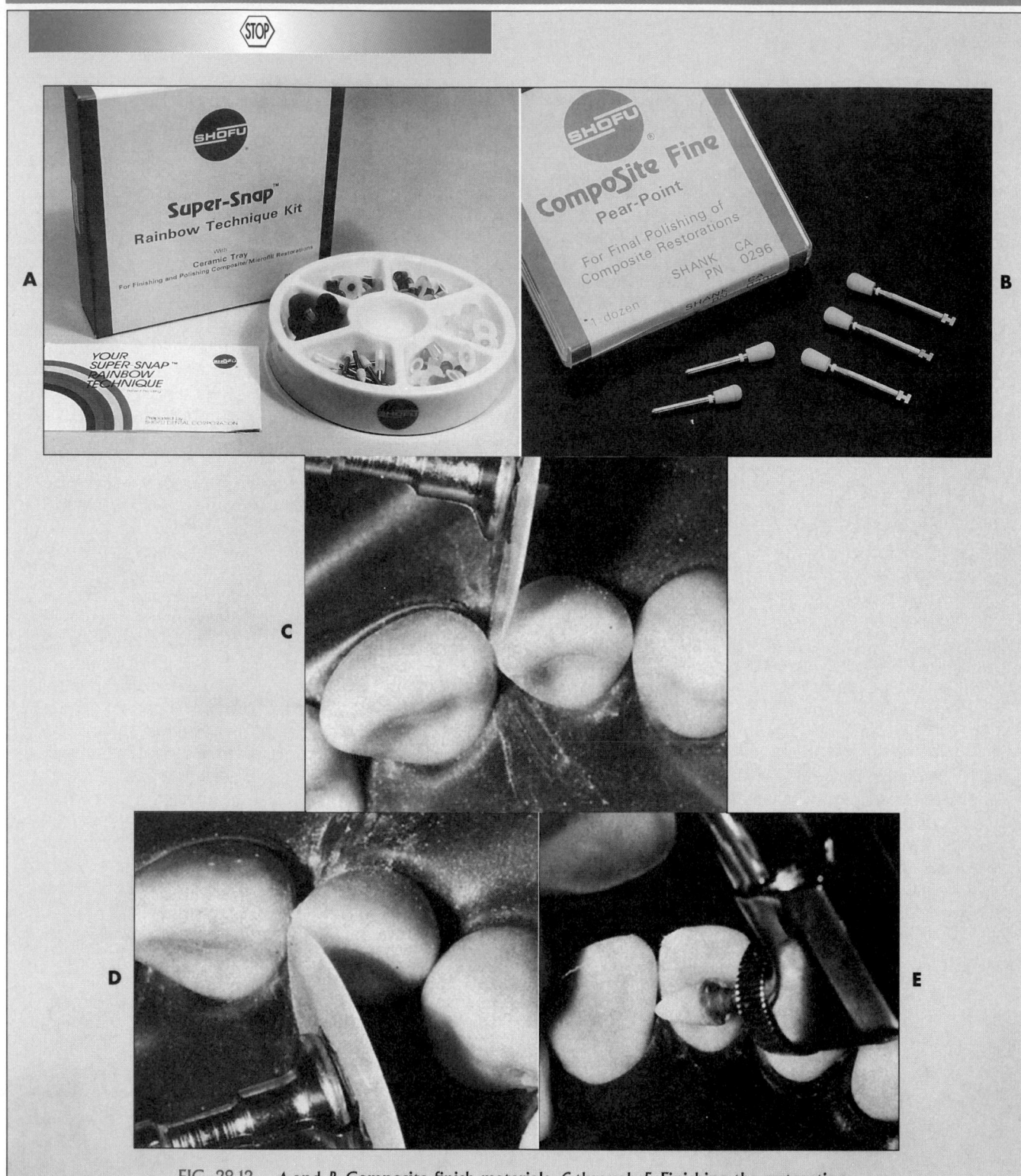

FIG. 28-12   *A* and *B,* Composite finish materials. *C* through *E,* Finishing the restoration.

(From Spohn EE et al: *Operative dentistry procedures for dental auxiliaries,* St Louis, 1981, Mosby.)

CLASS III COMPOSITE PROCEDURE—cont'd

manufacturer or by the assistant spraying water intermittently on the surface. Other rotary devices that may be used are the #7901 finishing bur series or diamonds. These devices provide a smooth surface when they are used with the high-speed handpiece.

Various composite finishing and polishing points, disks, and stones are available in kits that are specific to certain resins. These kits provide various rotary devices that perform well during the finishing and polishing procedure (Fig. 28-12 *A* through *E*).

A finishing strip is trimmed to a point on one end and is passed to the operator, who threads the surface with grit into the interproximal area to finish the distal area. The strip may also have a surface in the middle without grit that can be placed like floss. The strip is worked carefully back and forth on the interproximal surface to provide a smooth distal area. The operator exchanges the strip for the explorer to examine the restoration for smoothness. Dental floss may also be used interproximally, moving from the cervical to incisal area and examining the material for any surface roughness. However, when finishing and polishing is complete, the objective is to provide the patient with a well-contoured and smooth-finished restoration.

Removal of Rubber Dam

The rubber dam is removed as described in Chapter 22. Caution in removal is not as important to the restored surfaces of a composite as it is in the amalgam procedure, since the material has already reached final set. If a rubber dam has been used for isolation, dehydration of the tooth can occur, resulting in a temporary change in color of the tooth surface.

Check Articulation

After the rubber dam is removed, the patient should receive a complete mouth rinse. The site is thoroughly dried and the assistant places the articulating paper at the restored site, either by hand or with an articulating paper holder. The patient is directed to bite down and side-to-side and to slide the teeth forward and back. If any abnormally marked areas are noted, the excess composite material is removed by the operator with a finishing device that is passed by the assistant. The articulation is checked again by the same procedure. If the restored surface is not excessively marked (indicating proper articulation), the operator will likely want to smooth the surface again. The tongue is extremely sensitive to that which the eye cannot see. The patient should be directed to test the surface with his or her tongue. If any roughness is indicated by the patient, the operative team continues to make adjustments.

Postoperative Instructions

The tissue in the area may still be anesthetized, and the patient should be informed of the expected duration of the anesthesia. The material has reached final set, so directions to avoid certain foods is not necessary. Occasionally, after the rubber dam is used, the color of the teeth that have been isolated may not match because the tooth may have dehydrated. The patient should be apprised of the situation and shown the difference. The tooth will hydrate naturally in a short period of time from the normal fluids in the oral cavity.

- ▶ Are the appropriate universal barrier techniques removed?
- ▶ Have all of the appropriate surfaces been cleaned and disinfected?
- ▶ Has all armamentarium been removed?
- ▶ Has all equipment been repositioned?
- ▶ Has all the equipment been disinfected/sterilized according to OSHA guidelines?

▶ Modifications of the Procedure

The example just used was for a conventional Class III preparation and restoration with resin. Additional situations and unique circumstances require modifications to the procedure. The basic steps may be similar, but the armamentarium may vary.

EXAMPLES OF PROCEDURAL MODIFICATIONS
Class I — Caries on #24 Lingual Surface

Variations in the restorative procedure are necessary when different cavity classifications are involved. In a Class I carious lesion on #24 the shade selection may not be as critical, since the restoration will not be visible when the patient smiles or talks.

Determination of the occlusal contact is not as necessary, since there are no contact areas with an opposing tooth. The matrix strip is not to be used during the insertion phase, since a proximal surface is not involved in the preparation. The restorative material could be placed, contoured, and then cured without the use of the matrix strip and also without a proximal surface involved. The finishing and polishing may not be completed with disks, since the lingual surface would

TEAM APPROACH
Composite Procedure

OPERATOR	ASSISTANT
	Select and prepare all armamentarium
	Prepare the treatment room, and escort the patient in to be seated
	Assist in administration of anesthesia
Examine treatment site	Pass mirror and explorer
Select composite shade	Receive instruments, and pass shade guide
	Assist in shade selection
Place isolation	Pass isolation setup, and assist in placement
	Pass opening bur in high-speed handpiece and mirror
	Place HVE and a/w syringe to maintain clear field of operation
Open the preparation	Evacuate and dry the site
	Exchange explorer for handpiece
Examine site with explorer	Insert outline/resistance form bur in handpiece, and exchange for explorer
Create outline/resistance form	Maintain clear field of operation
	Exchange hand cutting instrument for handpiece
Place bevels and remove unsupported tooth structure	Exchange low-speed handpiece with caries removal bur for hand cutting instrument
Remove caries	Maintain clear field of operation
	Exchange explorer for handpiece
Check preparation for complete caries removal with explorer	Exchange retentive bur in handpiece for explorer
Place retentive grooves	Maintain clear field of operation
	Exchange finishing bur in high-speed handpiece for explorer
Feather preparation cavosurface margin	Maintain clear field of operation
	Pass matrix strip
Place matrix strip	Prepare and pass etching agent
Etch tooth structure	Thoroughly rinse, dry, and evacuate field
Remove matrix strip	Exchange used matrix strip for new strip
	Prepare and pass bonding agent
Place bonding agent	Maintain clear field of operation
	Pass composite resin material and placement instrument
Place composite material	Exchange curing device for placement instrument
Cure the composite material	Exchange explorer for curing device
Check for set of composite	

TEAM APPROACH
Composite Procedure—cont'd

OPERATOR	ASSISTANT
Remove matrix strip	Exchange strip for 12B scapel Maintain clear field of operation
Remove flash composite material	Exchange scalpel for finishing device in handpiece
Smooth and finish composite surfaces	Maintain clear field of operation Exchange handpiece for explorer
Check restoration for smoothness	Exchange explorer for articulating paper and holder
Check occlusion	Exchange holder for handpiece if additional finishing is necessary Exchange finishing strip
Finish interproximal surfaces	Receive finishing strip and provide patient with full mouth rinse Provide postoperative instructions Perform cleanup according to OSHA Record treatment on patient record

be difficult to reach, but stones and points would be possible choices.

Class IV — Caries on #8 Mesial Surface

In this example the occlusal relationship can be difficult to establish again in a restorative procedure when an incisal edge is involved. A greater understanding of the occlusal relationship might be achieved during the finishing and polishing procedure after the restorative material is placed. Extensive removal of excess material might be necessary, since the occlusal determination is difficult.

During tooth preparation it is important to have a defined labial bevel to establish adequate retention and color match. A matrix strip or a preformed celluloid crown form can be used to provide a mold for the lost tooth structure. The crown forms are stock that are formed for each tooth. A hole is usually placed in the mesial-incisal corner to allow excess material to extrude from the form. The incisal and mesial surfaces of the crown form may be cut away from the rest of the form and used as a matrix to hold the material on the tooth during the placement and curing. The form is removed by lifting the edge and cutting the form off with a scalpel after the restorative material has hardened. The necessary finishing and polishing is then completed.

If it is necessary in this situation, a threaded pin can be placed to provide support for the restorative material. This step may not be as necessary as it was in the past, because of the newer and stronger resins that are available and the bonding steps that are performed. The threaded pin technique is discussed in Chapter 27.

Class V — Caries on #11 Labial Surface

The matrix strip may not be used in a Class V restorative procedure. In its place a preformed Class V matrix may be used. The matrix is sized for the various designs of cavity preparations. It will allow penetration of the blue/white light during the curing stage.

KEY POINTS

▶ The composite resin procedure uses concepts of four-handed dentistry, with the operator and chairside assistant working as a team to increase productivity and efficiency. The steps in this procedure involve the assistant's being active in isolation and maintenance of the oral fluids. Without these important steps the likelihood that the restorative procedure will succeed is reduced.

▶ Composite restorative material is selected for use because of the esthetic value it offers the patient. The patient is consulted in the selection of the material shade that is used in this procedure.

▶ The steps in this procedure are similar to those of the amalgam restorative procedure but are often somewhat less involved; possibly influenced by the amount of tooth structure that has been lost or that has to be replaced by the process.

BIBLIOGRAPHY

Charbeneau GT: *Principles and practice of operative dentistry,* ed 3, Philadelphia, 1988, Lea & Febiger.

Craig RG: *Restorative dental materials,* ed 7, St Louis, 1985, Mosby.

Landman P: Cosmetic dentistry in the nineties, *J Am Dent Assist Assoc* 60:6, 1991.

Spohn EE, Halowski WA, Berry TG: *Operative dental procedure of dental auxiliaries,* St Louis, 1981, Mosby.

Sturdevant CM, Barton RE, Sockwell CL, Strickland WD: *Art and science of operative dentistry,* St Louis, 1985, Mosby.

29 Introduction to Prosthodontics

LEARNING OBJECTIVES

You will have mastered the material in this chapter when you can:

▶ Define the key terms
▶ Describe the scope and objectives of prosthodontics
▶ Differentiate between the various types of fixed and removable dental prostheses
▶ Describe the function of various types of dental prostheses
▶ Describe the advantages and disadvantages of various types of fixed and removable prosthetic restorations
▶ Describe the preliminary steps to prosthodontic treatment
▶ Explain the factors to be considered by the dentist when various prostheses are recommended to a patient
▶ Explain factors that are involved in becoming a successful prosthetic patient
▶ Explain the dental assistant's role in prosthodontics

KEY TERMS

Abutment
Bilateral
Bridge
Cantilever bridge
Cosmetic imaging
Denture
Edentulous
Fixed prosthodontics
Full-coverage crown
Implant
Inlay
Laminate
Maryland bridge
Obturator
Onlay
Overdenture
Pontic
Porcelain crown
Post and core
Prosthesis
Prosthodontics
Removable prosthodontics
Retainer
Surveying
Three-quarter crown
Tissue conditioning
Unilateral

In the previous chapters that relate to restorative dentistry, a dental material, such as amalgam or composite, is used to restore a diseased or injured tooth to its normal function by placing the material directly into a cavity preparation that is designed to retain the material as an intracoronal restoration. When the intracoronal restoration is inserted, the dental material is in a malleable or moldable state, which allows the material to be placed into the tooth. As the restorative material hardens it is carved or trimmed to normal anatomic structure.

This chapter will describe a dental **prosthesis** (plural is prostheses), which is the device that is used to replace missing teeth and tissues. A prosthesis is constructed outside the oral cavity after a series of appointments and will require various methods of insertion, depending on the type of prosthesis. The materials used in dental prosthetics include various precious and nonprecious metals, plastic, and porcelain.

The dental assistant will be introduced to an overview of prosthodontics, both **fixed** (not able to be removed from the oral cavity) and **removable** (capable of being removed from the mouth by the patient). Through a series of descriptions and illustrations, the dental assistant should understand the reasons a dentist will prescribe a specific type of prosthesis for a patient with certain oral conditions.

In the two ensuing chapters fixed and removable prosthodontics will be presented in detail, with emphasis on the role of the dental assistant during the procedural steps that prepare the mouth to receive one of the common dental prostheses.

Objectives of Prosthodontics

Prosthodontics is the art and science of designing and fitting artificial substitutes to replace lost or missing tissues. When it is properly designed, a fixed or removable prosthesis can meet the objectives of prosthodontic service that are identified in Box 29-1.

When a patient loses a significant number of teeth, it can be difficult to carry on normal oral functions. Teeth serve to:

1. Aid the tongue and lips to form sound in speech
2. Give support to the facial musculature which aids the lips and cheeks in performing the function of manipulating food and expressing emotion
3. Divide food finely into a larger surface area for the natural action of digestive juices

The loss of just a single tooth can be the beginning of the collapse of a dental arch (Fig. 29-1) by creating movement of individual teeth, which can cause the loss of interproximal contacts and, ultimately, gingival deterioration. Teeth are needed to provide function that is necessary to minimize the risk of caries caused by food impaction; preserve the health of soft tissues through the massaging action of the food; and to prevent drifting, rotation, or hypereruption of other teeth. Further, when a patient loses all of his or her teeth, becoming **edentulous**, he or she is faced with the following:

1. Limitations in the daily diet; hard and fibrous foods must be finely chopped or potential digestive problems can occur
2. Difficulty with speech; the tongue cannot come to proper rests on the teeth to form certain consonant sounds

3. The appearance of premature aging; musculature support is lost, causing the cheeks and lips to sag, the soft tissues to bunch up around the mouth, and the chin and nose to become abnormally close

Consequently, a fixed or removable partial or full denture prosthesis for a patient can literally add years to his or her life by the following:

- Improving dietary consumption
- Providing mastication
- Assisting in normal speech
- Preserving the health of the soft oral tissues
- Eliminating the potential for future dental diseases
- Improving esthetics, which not only creates an improved appearance but can result in an improved self-image

Regardless of whether teeth are lost because of caries, periodontal disease, or trauma, the teeth should be replaced as soon as possible to maintain optimal oral health. Although a fixed prosthesis might be desired over a removable prosthesis, it may not be feasible because of the anatomic structure of a patient's mouth or the ability to maintain good oral hygiene, or because the cost may be prohibitive. A fixed prosthesis is secured in the mouth without attachments and avoids movement on tooth surfaces. The removable prosthesis offers an alternative that provides function and esthetics to the patient.

BOX 29-1

OBJECTIVES OF PROSTHODONTICS

Replace lost tissues with like tissues
Replace missing teeth and tissues with biologically acceptable restorations
Improve phonetics and esthetics
Provide restorations that are comfortable to the patient
Improve masticatory function
Preserve teeth and tissues that will enhance either a fixed or removable prosthesis design
Prevent future dental disease or loss of oral structures
Promote good oral health
Improve the general health and well-being of the patient

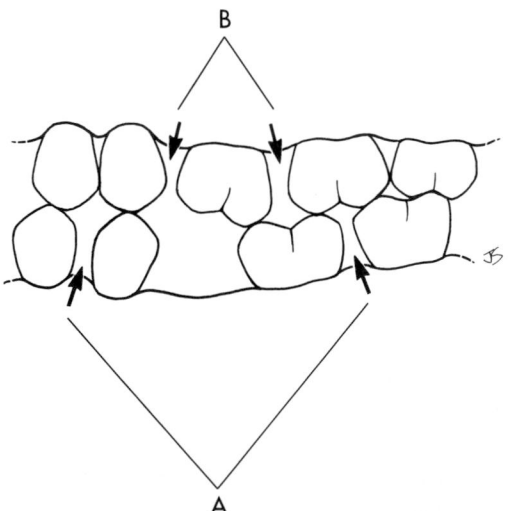

FIG. 29-1 The result of the loss of a single tooth in an arch creates possible open contacts resulting in a potential for tooth drifting, hypereruption, periodontal trauma, ridge distortion, food impaction, loss of esthetics, difficulty in mastication, and change in phonetics.

Types of Prosthodontics

Many times the damage to a tooth is so extensive that the tooth must be removed or the amount of tooth structure that remains is inadequate to support an intracoronal restoration without further trauma to the tooth. Trauma and disease can also cause damage to maxillofacial structures, requiring an extraoral prosthesis to be designed. Treatment at this point then involves the creation of a dental prosthesis: an artificial device that is designed to restore or replace one or more missing teeth and associated structures. Prosthodontics has three main branches: *fixed prosthodontics, removable prosthodontics, and maxillofacial prosthetics.*

Fixed Prosthodontics

This branch of prosthodontics is responsible for creating a fixed dental prosthesis. A **fixed prosthesis** is an artificial replacement for missing teeth and associated structures that is secured to the supporting teeth in the mouth. This type of restoration cannot be removed to clean or inspect.

▶ Types of Fixed Prosthodontics

Several types of fixed prostheses are commonly used in dentistry today. These include a variety of extracoronal restorations, such as **bridges**, **implants**, and **fixed partial dentures**. Table 29-1 provides a list and illustrations of various types of fixed prostheses (Fig. 29-2).

TABLE 29-1 COMMON TYPES OF FIXED AND REMOVABLE PROSTHESES

Restoration/Drawing	Definition
Inlay	A cast restoration involving the occlusal surface and one or more proximal surfaces FIG. 29-2, A
Onlay	A cast restoration that includes the complete occlusal table, both proximal surfaces and some or all of the cusp surfaces to avoid future fracture FIG. 29-2, B
¾ Crown	A cast restoration that covers ¾ of the tooth, with the buccal or lingual surface remaining intact FIG. 29-2, C
Full cast crown	A restoration that completely circumscribes the tooth and may be made of cast alloy or a combination of alloy FIG. 29-2, D

*From Dentsply International, York Division, York, Pennsylvania.
†From McGivney GP, Castelburg DJ: *McCracken's removable partial prosthodontics,* St Louis, 1987, Mosby.

Continued.

TABLE 29-1   COMMON TYPES OF FIXED AND REMOVABLE PROSTHESES

Restoration / Drawing	Definition
Porcelain fused to metal crown	Cast crown with porcelain that is fired to one or more surfaces

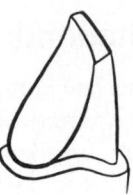 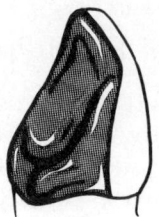

FIG. 29-2, E

| Full porcelain crown | A restoration that completely circumscribes the tooth and is made entirely of porcelain |

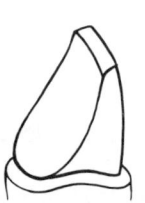 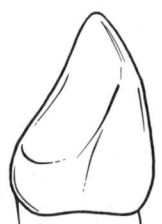

FIG. 29-2, F

| Fixed bridge | A restoration that replaces missing teeth and is supported by abutment teeth, with the replacement tooth or teeth referred to as pontics |

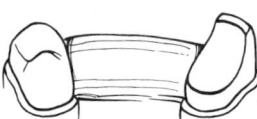 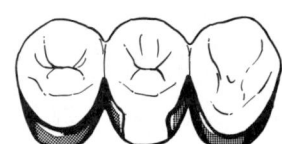

FIG. 29-2, G

| Cantilever bridge / cantilever partial denture[†] | A prosthesis in which only one side of the device is attached to a retainer / abutment |

Occlusal load

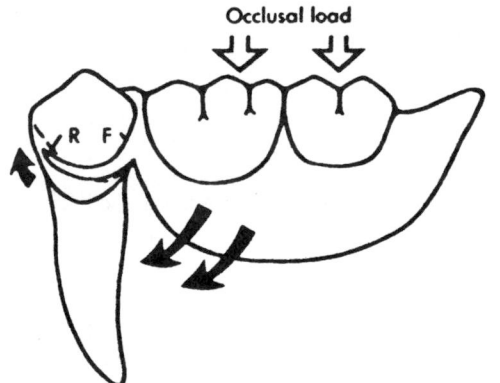

FIG. 29-2, H

| Maryland bridge | A conservatively prepared resin-retained bridge that requires a bonding procedure |

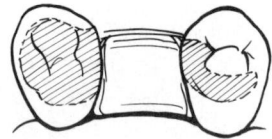 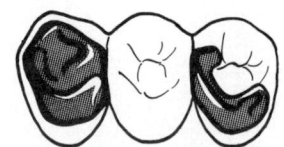

FIG. 29-2, I

---

*From Dentsply International, York Division, York, Pennsylvania.
†From McGivney GP, Castelburg DJ: *McCracken's removable partial prosthodontics,* St Louis, 1987, Mosby.

TABLE 29-1   COMMON TYPES OF FIXED AND REMOVABLE PROSTHESES—cont'd

Restoration / Drawing	Definition
Laminate 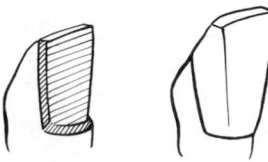	A veneer restoration made of a thin layer of porcelain or resin commonly used on anterior teeth FIG. 29-2, J
Post and core* 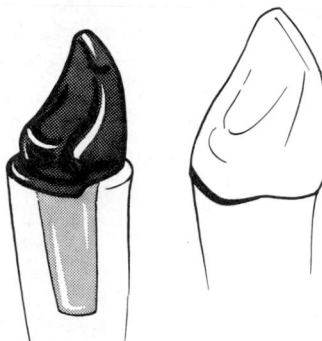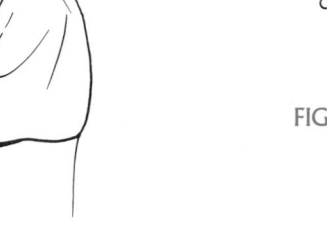	Used on endodontically treated teeth that have lost a significant amount of tooth structure; the post fits in the pulp chamber and canal, and the core resembles a tooth that is prepared for a full-coverage crown FIG. 29-2, K
Complete denture* 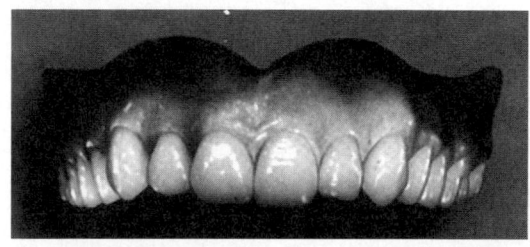	A dental prosthesis that replaces all of the natural teeth and associated structures of the maxilla or mandible FIG. 29-2, L
Partial denture* 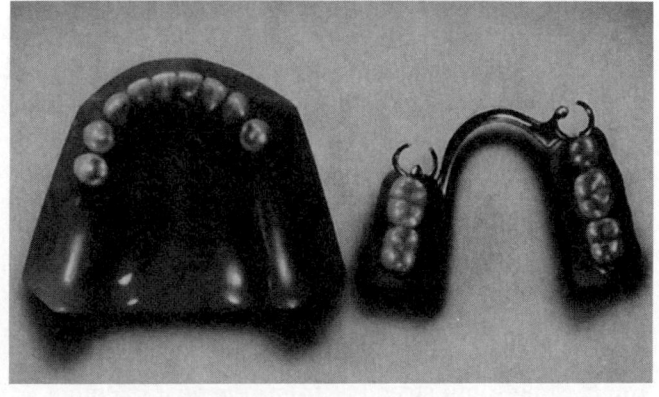	A dental prosthesis that replaces one or more, but not all, of the natural teeth and associated structures; *bilateral partial* replaces teeth and structures on both sides of an arch and a *unilateral partial* replaces teeth and structure on only one side FIG. 29-2, M

Continued.

TABLE 29-I COMMON TYPES OF FIXED AND REMOVABLE PROSTHESES—cont'd

Restoration / Drawing	Definition
Precision attachment† 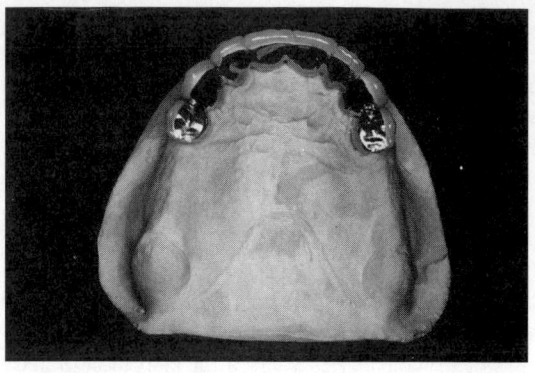 FIG. 29-2, N	A direct type of retainer used in a fixed removable partial denture; a female portion is placed within the coronal portion of the abutment crown, and the male portion is an attachment that is fitted to the denture
Implant† (See Chapter 31 for illustration)	Placement of an artificial tooth or teeth into the alveolar process or frame that is attached to the alveolar process; referred to as endosseous, subperiosteal, or mucosal implant

Extracoronal restorations, referred to as fixed restorations, are designed to replace missing tooth structures and may provide partial or complete coverage of a tooth. This type of restoration includes *inlays, onlays, three-quarter and full-coverage crowns, bridges, laminates, implants,* and *post and cores.* An extracoronal restoration may be fabricated from several materials, including precious and nonprecious metals, plastic, and porcelain. The selection is often dictated by the location of the restoration in the oral cavity. The design of an extracoronal restoration or prosthesis that replaces missing tooth tissue will circumscribe (encircle) all or a portion of a tooth, unlike an intracoronal restoration that is predominantly encircled by the tooth. Each of these restorations will be discussed in detail in the chapter on fixed prosthodontics.

An extracoronal restoration in the anterior segment of the mouth may be made completely of porcelain or porcelain ceramic that is fused to alloy to provide more pleasing esthetics. In less obtrusive areas, such as the posterior segment of the mouth—particularly second molars, a restoration of precious metal alloy may be selected because of its strength and durability.

A fixed prosthesis accurately replicates the natural tooth and is designed to transmit function to the teeth in a relatively stress-free manner. A fixed prosthesis, such as a crown, inlay, or bridge, may be constructed of precious or nonprecious metal. For esthetics, porcelain or ceramic may be fused to the metal alloy on the buccal or facial surfaces or on any other surface that would enhance

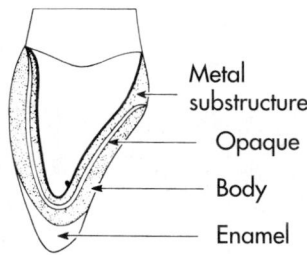

FIG. 29-3 Layers of material in a porcelain, fused-to-metal restoration.

esthetic value to the patient. Additionally, the use of an opaque liner (a substance placed on the restoration or natural tooth), as illustrated in Fig. 29-3, can enhance the appearance of the restoration by eliminating the darkness of the metal beneath the porcelain or ceramic material.

An **inlay** (see Table 29-1) is possibly the most conservative approach to restoring a tooth, by using a cast or porcelain restoration. An inlay is placed as an intracoronal restoration and involves the occlusal surface, with one or both of the proximal surfaces included. In addition, the operator may extend the coverage to include a portion of the cusps by extending the preparation beyond the cusp tip. This extension protects the existing tooth structure from potential fracture.

When an inlay design cannot adequately restore complete function to a tooth, an **onlay** (see Table 29-1) may provide the necessary coverage. An onlay is a cast or porcelain restoration that includes the complete occlusal surface and both proximal surfaces. Unlike the inlay, it extends to cover the entire cuspal surface. Coverage of the cusps is intended to avoid future fracture. This type of restoration also preserves the integrity of most of the gingival surfaces. This is true except when it is necessary to involve the proximal gingival surfaces to reduce the possibility of recurrent decay.

A **three-quarter coverage crown** (see Table 29-1) is a less conservative approach in restoring a tooth to normal function. Typically, this restoration covers three quarters of the tooth, with the buccal surface remaining intact. This type of preparation is an extension of the onlay. The preparation is extended beyond the occlusal surface to the margin of the lingual or buccal surface, with a finish line or a margin near the cervical margin of the tooth.

A **full-coverage crown** (see Table 29-1) is prepared when no other options are available in the restoration design. This type of coverage is used when a significant amount of tooth structure has been lost to decay or fracture. It may be necessary to remove additional tooth structure during preparation to prevent future fracture or to create retention. A full crown completely covers the tooth with the metal restoration, providing strength and protection to the remaining tooth structure.

A full coverage crown may be constructed entirely of metal alloy or porcelain that is fused to metal (sometimes referred to as a porcelain veneer crown). The latter is preferred for anterior teeth or posterior teeth where esthetics is a major factor. Two approaches to this concept include making the base of metal for strength and covering it completely with porcelain on all coronal surfaces for esthetics or making the crown of metal and baking porcelain only to the facial aspect of the crown for esthetics. Both of these approaches would provide strength and esthetics and would likely involve an opaque liner beneath the facial porcelain to enhance the esthetics.

A second option to the full coverage crown, where esthetics is a factor, is the **porcelain crown** or **jacket**, which is made entirely of porcelain. This type of crown presents more risks of fracture for the patient than the porcelain veneer crown.

A **fixed bridge** (see Table 29-1) is also an extracoronal restoration, which not only restores missing tooth structure but also replaces one or more missing teeth. Sometimes, this restoration is referred to as a fixed partial denture—a misnomer, since the fixed bridge is not removable. The teeth which support this type of restoration are referred to as **abutment teeth** and the replacements for the missing teeth are referred to as **pontics**.

Although less traditional than the fixed bridge, the **cantilever bridge** (supported by only one abutment tooth) is an option for a more conservative preparation. Like the traditional bridge the cantilever-type bridge is used to replace a missing tooth. The cantilever bridge, however, is designed with the retainer placed on a single abutment tooth, which is attached to the pontic. The retainer in this situation is the restoration that is placed on the abutment tooth to provide retention for the bridge. The assurance of healthy periodontium of the tissues involved in the placement of a cantilever bridge is vitally important. The use of a cantilever bridge may be considered in situations where there is no traumatic occlusion and the opposite abutment is a virgin tooth.

Like the cantilever bridge, the **Maryland bridge** (see Table 29-1) is an example of a more conservative approach to replacing missing teeth. The Maryland bridge is relatively new to dentistry and is fabricated to restore function and esthetics for teeth. This restoration includes a pontic that is connected to thin metal retainers placed on the lingual (anterior) or occlusal (posterior) surfaces of abutment teeth. Preparation for this type of bridge involves little or no reduction of tooth structure and is cemented in place by using composite resins to assist in retention.

A **dental laminate** presents a similar concept to the Maryland bridge in that limited, if any, reduction of tooth structure is necessary. This veneer restoration of the facial surface of an anterior tooth is fabricated as a laminate, thin layer, or sheet of porcelain or resin. The laminate is bonded to etched enamel surfaces. Laminates may be used in conjunction with an opaque liner to reduce the translucency and appearance of stain underneath the restoration.

A **fixed partial denture** is a tooth-supported partial denture that is designed to be permanently attached to the teeth or roots that furnish support to the restoration. A portion of this device can be removed for cleaning and inspection. An **implant** (see Table 29-1) is a device that is surgically placed into or onto the alveolar process and is designed to be used as a prosthetic abutment or support. Typically, one portion of the implant fits into the alveolar process, and then a fastening screw is attached to the implant over which is placed a precision plastic or precious alloy sleeve onto which a crown or partial denture is attached. The importance of an implant is the additional stability that is provided for the final restoration.

The placement of a **post** and **core** (see Table 29-1) is used in restoring endodontically involved teeth. When an endodontically treated tooth is restored, the operator is not only confronted with the endodontic condition but may encounter extensive loss of tooth structure through caries or existing restorations. The post portion of this type of restoration fills the opened pulp chamber and a portion of the canal, lending strength to the final restoration. The metal core resembles a tooth that is prepared for a full-coverage crown. The post and core are cast as one restoration and are cemented in place as a single unit. After this procedure a full-coverage crown is designed and cemented on the core. It is possible to make the crown and post and core as a single unit, replacing the two-step procedure. The dentist will make

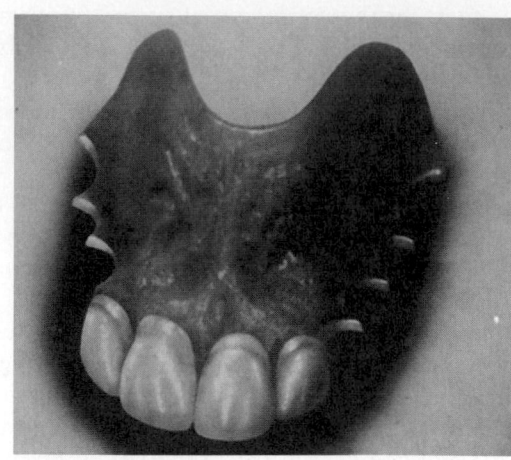

FIG. 29-4 An interim partial denture; flipper; used for a short period of time.

(From Dentsply International.)

the decision involving which option is best for the situation. In the past a core buildup for a nonendodontically involved tooth was made of amalgam or even a pin-retained casting. Today, this type of core will generally be made of a composite or glass ionomer material as opposed to amalgam, allowing for reduced thermal conductivity and cost to the patient.

Each type of dental prosthesis presents unique advantages and disadvantages. In general, full coverage provides greater retention than a more conservative approach. A fixed prosthesis can provide stability to the tooth, improve esthetics, and be less irritating to abutment teeth and adjacent tissues than can a removable prosthesis. The disadvantages of a fixed prosthesis include extensive loss of tooth structure for some types of preparations, possible gingival irritation that is caused by an unnatural material being placed at the gingival margin, possible fracture of some ceramic materials, and using an alloy that may create the potential for galvanism (Box 29-2).

Removable Prosthodontics

A removable dental prosthesis is, by definition, an artificial substitute for missing teeth and supporting tissues that can be removed by the patient to be cleaned and inspected.

▶ Types of Removable Prosthodontics

Removable prosthodontics can be classified into the following categories: complete, partial, overdenture, fixed removable, or interim denture. When a patient has lost all of the teeth in an arch because of advanced decay or periodontal disease, a *complete denture* may be made to replace all of the teeth.

A **partial denture** is a prosthesis which replaces one or more teeth but replaces less than all of the natural teeth in an arch. A partial denture may be bilateral, replacing teeth on both sides of an arch, or unilateral, replacing teeth only on one side of the arch.

An **overdenture** (sometimes referred to as a *fixed removable partial denture*) is a complete or partial denture that is supported by retained roots that provide improved support, stability, and tactile sensation and reduce alveolar ridge resorption. An **interim partial** or **full denture** is a denture that is used for only a short period of time. Such a denture might be a *flipper* type partial denture that is used after an accident in the anterior region of the mouth, while waiting for healing to take place before the placement of a fixed prosthesis (Fig. 29-4).

Precision attachment is a term frequently associated with a special type of retainer that is used in the construction of a removable partial denture. The retainer is constructed with a female portion that is placed in the coronal portion of the abutment crown; the male portion is attached to the denture.

Similar to the purpose of fixed prostheses, the purpose of dentures, complete or partial, is twofold: function and esthetics. Although some patients may be

ADVANTAGES AND DISADVANTAGES OF REMOVABLE PROSTHESIS

ADVANTAGE OF A REMOVABLE PROSTHESIS

▶ Improves mastication
▶ Eliminates aging appearance
▶ Prevents drifting
▶ Improves speech
▶ Improves self-image

DISADVANTAGES OF A REMOVABLE PROSTHESIS

▶ Clasp-type attachments of partial dentures can cause trauma to abutment teeth
▶ Can create gingivostomatitis
▶ The use of clasps can create poor esthetics
▶ If it is not cleaned regularly, the prosthesis can create tissue trauma or decay to the abutment teeth
▶ If it is not worn routinely, drifting and hypereruption can occur
▶ Could be lost or damaged if left out of the mouth

concerned more about esthetics, function is an important reason for replacing teeth for the overall general systemic health of the patient. The overall advantages and disadvantages of removable prosthesis are listed in Box 29-3.

Maxillofacial Prosthodontics

This branch of prosthodontics is involved with replacing missing parts of the stomatognathic (mouth and jaws) system. This includes structures responsible for speech, mastication, and deglutition of food. It is not uncommon in this phase of prosthodontics to see patients who have cleft palate, who have lost portions of the head and neck tissues because of cancer or other diseases, or who are trauma victims. For these patients specialized prostheses are designed, including obturators and other devices that are used to replace missing tissues in the maxillofacial region. An **obturator** is a prosthesis that is used to close a congenital or acquired opening in the palate.

Factors to Consider When Selecting a Prosthesis

The type of extracoronal restoration or prosthesis that is planned for a patient is based on many factors that have been described previously, including esthet-

ics, oral hygiene practices, level of function that is needed to correct the condition that requires the prosthesis, patient's attitude toward his or her oral health, patient's financial ability to make the investment, skill of the dentist, and technical laboratory support services.

Although the dental assistant is not responsible for the diagnosis and treatment plan, he or she must understand why the recommendations are made for specific treatment plans in various situations. A patient may often seek the advice of the dental assistant or ask why it is necessary to have a specific type of prosthesis versus an alternative.

It is vital for the dental assistant who works in a dental office where prosthetic dentistry is practiced to have a commitment to the philosophy of that practice. As discussed earlier two basic objectives of the dental profession are to save teeth and to aid patients in retaining their teeth for a lifetime; these should be continuing goals of all dental professionals. At times, however, teeth are lost because of neglect and disease; the other objectives of dentistry then must be recognized: to relieve patients of pain, to prevent disease, to aid patients in being able to chew, and to maintain pleasing esthetics. Consequently, the specialty of prosthodontics is confronted not only with the need to retain and restore existing teeth to a healthy status, but also to replace missing teeth in the oral cavity to restore normal function and esthetics.

Preliminary Treatment

Just as it is with any other dental treatment, it is necessary to complete several preliminary steps before a thorough diagnosis can be made or before any form of prosthodontic treatment can begin. These steps include the following:

▶ Complete medical and dental history
▶ Intraoral and extraoral examination
▶ Radiographic examination
▶ Diagnostic models
▶ Case presentation
▶ Oral cavity preparation, including periodontal, endodontic, orthodontic, occlusal equilibration, or surgical treatment

Since many of these steps have been reviewed in Chapter 24, emphasis will be placed on the impact of these procedures as they relate to preparing for prosthodontic treatment.

▶ Patient History

The patient's medical and dental history is obtained in advance of treatment as it is with all dental care and is kept current with periodic updates. Some special interest questions, however, are more specific to prosthodontics than some of the other specialty areas. Since a prosthodontic procedure often requires the use of invasive materials that may not always be used during routine care, it is important to be aware of patient sensitivity to chemicals and to medication that is currently being taken by the patient.

In addition, the dental assistant must understand the reasons that certain conditions exist in a patient's mouth. The dentist needs to know if the loss of a tooth or teeth was caused by a congenital condition, trauma, dental disease, or neglect. It is also wise to gain an understanding of the patient's attitude toward dental care, his or her interest in maintaining any remaining teeth, and his or her willingness to participate in decisions about the dental care. A patient's occupation may also be important in making decisions about placing a dental prosthesis in the patient's mouth. For instance, a wind instrument player may require special attention if changes are to be made in the anterior teeth. Likewise, patients who are intimately involved in public appearances may have a major interest in esthetics and speech.

Intraoral and Extraoral Examination

The intraoral and extraoral examinations are not unlike examinations that were done previously in oral diagnosis. During the intraoral examination, evidence of missing or drifting teeth and irritated tissues may exist. Likewise, loss of musculature because of loss of teeth may be evident. Recording all data is important in preparing for the future treatment plan. Clinical charts for prosthodontics often include profile drawings that enable the assistant to indicate tooth mobility or musculature changes.

Radiographic procedures in prosthodontics usually include the typical periapical exposures. However, in edentulous arches a panograph may enhance the dentist's perspective not only of the teeth but also of the adjacent structures.

Diagnostic Impressions

The initial alginate impressions will have been procured for diagnostic models during the initial examination procedure. These same models can be used for the construction of custom-made trays to be used during the final impression phase.

Diagnostic models are used not only to discuss the case with the patient, but also are the initial casts which the dentist uses to determine the design of a fixed or removable prosthesis. It is important that the models be accurate (review the section on alginate impressions in

Chapter 24), since the dentist must determine answers to many of the following questions from these models:

1. Are the proposed abutment teeth favorable for clasping or for use as abutment tooth?
2. Are there any interferences, such as undercuts, tori, or malposed teeth?
3. Will restorative treatment be necessary to achieve the required retention or articulation?
4. What are the best types of connectors or retainers to use in this case?
5. Is clearance adequate for the proposed prosthesis? Will the vertical dimensions have to be opened, or will the teeth need to be reduced?
6. Will the ridge, as it exists, provide stability for the prosthesis?
7. Is the occlusion adequate, or will it be necessary to adjust the occlusion?

Answers to these questions combined with the results of the clinical examination will aid the dentist in designing the proposed prosthesis on the diagnostic models.

Model Surveying

Before proceeding with treatment a dentist will generally have the models surveyed by the dental laboratory that is going to construct the prosthesis. **Surveying** is the procedure of studying the parallelism or lack of parallelism of the teeth and associated structures to select a path

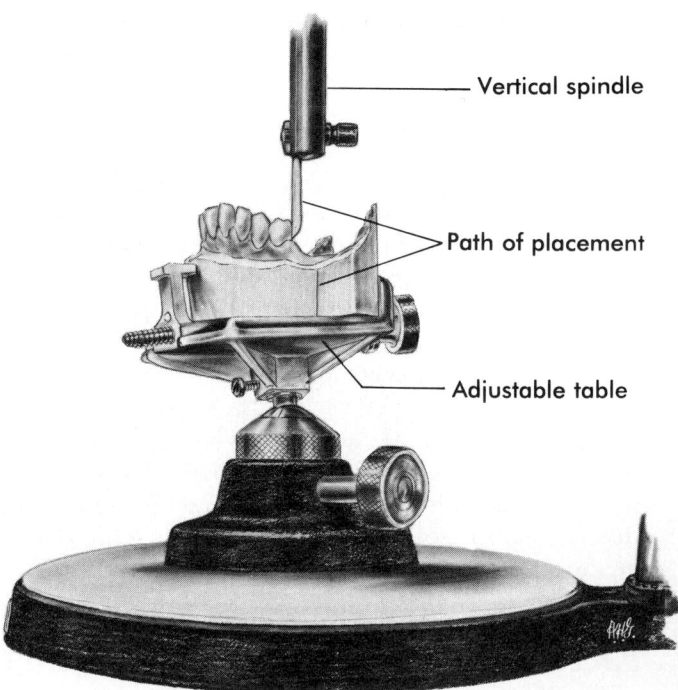

FIG. 29-5   Model being surveyed.

(From McGivney GP, Castleberry D]: *McCracken's removable partial prosthodontics*, St Louis, 1994, Mosby.)

for placement of the components of the prosthesis. In anticipation of having a case surveyed the models should have been poured in stone rather than plaster to provide a more rigid surface for surveying. This process ensures that the clasps, rests, retainers, and connectors (devices used to retain the prosthesis in the mouth) are placed in positions that will provide adequate and balanced retention, without causing stress or interference to the teeth and soft tissues, and yet will provide a prosthesis that is esthetically acceptable. An example of a model that has been surveyed by the laboratory is shown in Fig. 29-5.

Once the surveying is complete and the design is determined, the next step in the use of the diagnostic models is the construction of custom-made trays. Trays that are used for the final impression must fit adequately and compensate for any undercuts that are created by tori or malposed teeth. The construction of custom-made trays is discussed in Chapter 40.

▶ Case Presentation

During the case presentation it is essential that the patient understand in simple terms what the treatment involves and what his or her responsibility is to maintain the prosthesis and oral tissues. As mentioned previously it is important that the patient have a good mental attitude about the prosthesis that is to be constructed and a willingness to maintain this device. Without the compliance of the patient you will not gain his or her acceptance and the dentist may be faced with a patient who may constantly find fault with the prosthesis. A dissatisfied patient is often a patient who did not thoroughly understand the process or one who did not accept the treatment plan in the beginning.

The patient must be involved in the treatment selection and have a thorough understanding of the processes, the advantages and disadvantages of proposed treatment, the consequences of neglect, and the alternative options that are available. For effective treatment planning and case presentation the use of visual aids becomes an invaluable tool.

Various visual aids, including the patient's diagnostic models, comparative models, radiographs, and examples of various types of dental prostheses that include models with crowns, bridges, inlays, implants, full or partial dentures, and photos of completed cases can enhance any presentation. Pamphlets or video materials can also serve to increase the patient's understanding during the case presentation. Pamphlets can also be taken home to share with family or friends during decision making. Many excellent materials are available through the ADA, prosthodontic societies, and dental manufacturing companies.

Diagnostic models can demonstrate to the patient the need for prosthodontic treatment. A patient may not completely understand the consequences of loss of tooth structure caused by decay and trauma, until he or she visualizes this through illustrated models. An excellent way to visually demonstrate the need for a fixed bridge is by showing the mesial drift that occurs to a tooth and by describing the consequences of continued drift, using comparative models at different stages of development.

Not only are diagnostic models important for patient education, but also they can be used for the fabrication of custom acrylic trays and the interim temporary restoration that are placed until the permanent restoration is cemented. Diagnostic models aid the dentist in performing diagnostic tooth preparation. The models allow the operator to simulate the restoration on the model teeth. This step is extremely helpful, particularly when several preparations are to be completed for a multiple unit bridge. When the models are surveyed, the dentist is able to determine the draw or parallelism on the individual preparations and to see how each unit relates to the other. A wax simulation of the restoration can be made, and if the wax-up is able to be removed from the model, without fracture, then the dentist can be assured that replication of the preparation in the mouth will be successful. The wax simulation can also serve to give the patient an opportunity to see what the completed

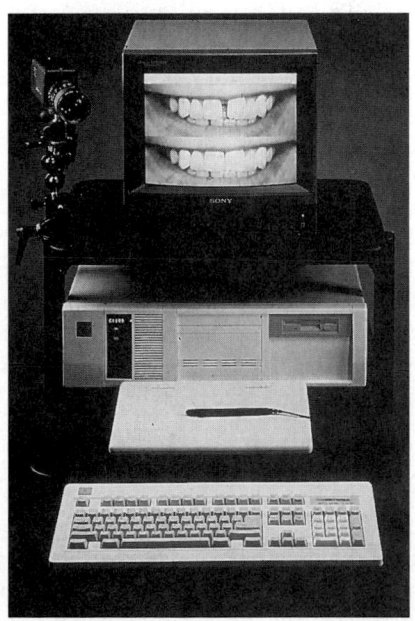

FIG. 29-6 Cosmetic imager; computer equipment with monitor, showing projection of before and after image of maxillary diastema.

(Courtesy of Dental Vision Plus.)

restoration will look like when it is cemented in place in the oral cavity.

Cosmetic imaging is also a valuable adjunct to a case presentation. Unlike the intraoral imager that is described in Chapter 24, the cosmetic imager allows the dentist to generate an image of the proposed treatment and provide a pictorial copy of this image. The patient, who may be apprehensive about a specific type of treatment, is able to see how he or she will look with the prosthesis in place (Fig. 29-6). The image substitutes for the patient's imagination. A cosmetic imager can be a successful marketing tool and is used in many other areas of dentistry, such as orthodontics.

▶ Mouth Preparation

The importance of preparing the mouth before inserting a dental prosthesis cannot be overlooked. Two goals of mouth preparation in planning for prosthodontic treatment are to obtain optimal health of the foundation tissues and to provide adequate mouth preparation for the insertion of a fixed prosthesis or a full or partial denture. Specialized mouth preparation for either the fixed or removable prosthesis will be covered in the following chapters.

OBTAINING OPTIMAL HEALTH

It is a well accepted concept that to build a house on a faulty foundation is unwise. To insert a dental prosthesis into a mouth that is not free of periodontal disease; one that has active dental caries; or one that is in need of endodontic, orthodontic, or occlusal equilibration treatment is to destine prosthesis failure.

Each type of prosthesis requires that various preparatory treatment stages be completed before the actual prosthesis is constructed. Different treatment approaches are used for patients who are to have a fixed prosthesis as opposed to those who need a partial or a full denture; some cases involve a combination of these restorations. Each of these situations incorporates similarities; however, in general, many of the following stages will be completed for most patients.

PREPARATORY SURGERY

This phase of treatment should be accomplished as soon as possible to provide for adequate healing, while other treatment is in progress. In removable prosthetics preparatory surgery will be completed first to provide the patient with relief from pain. Beyond this, any teeth that cannot be retained because they are nonusable and nonvital, severely malpositioned, unerupted, or nonrestorable because of extreme caries or periodontal disease

will be extracted. Any root remnants, cysts, or tumors need to be removed. In fixed prosthetics it may be necessary to perform electrosurgery (method of removing soft tissue by using a surgical instrument that uses electricity) around abutment teeth to remove excess soft tissues that may impinge on cervical marginal areas.

In addition, it may be necessary to recontour hard tissues, including knife edged ridges, tori, bone nodules, undercuts, and prominent tuberosities, or soft tissues, such as prominent frena, hyperplasia from previous dentures, or flabby, fibrous ridges. It is likely that most of these surgical procedures will be done by a maxillofacial oral surgeon.

ORAL PROPHYLAXIS AND PERIODONTAL TREATMENT

For the patient who is retaining teeth in the oral cavity and who will be receiving a fixed bridge or partial denture, a thorough oral prophylaxis must be performed. The prophylaxis and any necessary periodontal treatment should be completed as soon as possible. The patient must learn early in the treatment sequence how to adequately care for his or her mouth. As treatment progresses, home care should be evaluated routinely and the patient should be informed of his or her progress or need for improvement. How a patient takes care of his or her mouth during this initial periodontal phase will give an indication as to how the patient will likely care for the future proposed prosthesis.

ENDODONTIC TREATMENT

If any teeth require endodontic treatment, this procedure should be completed before prosthetic treatment. It would not be wise to place a fixed prosthesis or a removable prosthesis and then complete endodontic treatment.

RESTORATIVE PROCEDURES

Restorative treatment of all nonabutment teeth should be done before beginning the prosthodontic procedures; this would include the placement of amalgam and composite restorations, implants, and recontouring of any natural teeth. When a partial denture is placed in conjunction with fixed bridgework, the fixed prosthesis is completed before the removable prosthesis.

ORTHODONTIC TREATMENT

As prosthodontic treatment is considered for a patient, other factors must be considered in the treatment planning, such as adjunctive orthodontic treatment.

Unless orthodontic factors, such as malocclusion, oral habits, or jaw formation, are considered, the prosthetic restoration may result in additional problems.

The acceptance of teeth in their present position in the mouth may not be the most progressive means of providing a patient with effective treatment. The position of the teeth in the oral cavity result in dynamics that should be addressed during treatment planning. Often the general practitioner works cooperatively with the orthodontist to provide treatment to teeth that are malpositioned. To provide the patient with maximum benefit from prosthodontic treatment, it may be necessary to postpone prosthetic treatment until orthodontic treatment is completed.

OCCLUSAL EQUILIBRATION

Another consideration before prosthodontic treatment occurs when a patient presents with temporomandibular joint dysfunction. The patient who complains of *pain in the TMJ area* or that *the teeth no longer fit together as before* may require intervention treatment before prosthodontic treatment is started. The elimination of occlusal interference through occlusal equilibration techniques or through the use of an intraoral occlusal appliance may be suggested before additional care.

TISSUE CONDITIONING

In achieving optimal oral health it may be necessary to condition irritated tissues, especially in situations where a patient has had an ill fitting prosthesis or where an irritation is present at the future site of a prosthesis. **Tissue conditioning** is the process of removing irritants and treating the soft tissues so that they can return to a healthy state. There are three approaches to tissue conditioning: complete tissue rest, surgical intervention, or the use of a tissue treatment agent.

When complete tissue rest is recommended, a patient is advised to remove the present prosthesis, a partial, or the full denture from the mouth and leave it out of the mouth until the irritation is removed or healed. Although this would appear to be the most efficient and cost-effective method for many patients, it is often not a feasible solution, since the patient cannot maintain normal esthetics and carry on activities that might require contact with other people.

Similar to the method that was just described, surgical removal of unhealthy tissue is not always the preferred choice. Surgery subjects the patient to discomfort and may require the removal of tissue that is vital to retain the prosthesis. If a prosthesis is being worn at the time of the surgery, it may be necessary for the patient to refrain from wearing the prosthesis until healing has taken place.

The most favored choice for tissue conditioning is the use of a material that can line the inside of the partial or full denture for several days, acting as a soft cushion between the prosthesis and the irritated soft tissues. A tissue conditioner is commonly a powder/liquid system. The powder is a polyethyl-methacrylate to which plasticizers and retarders have been added to control the polymerization and to prevent the material from hardening. The mixed material is placed inside the prosthesis and allowed to remain for 3 or 4 days to adapt to the ridge. The material may be replaced several times, until the irritation has subsided. The use of this tissue conditioner may require removal of some denture base material in order to obtain an adequate fit.

Criteria for a Successful Prosthetic Patient

The success of any dental prosthesis is predicated on the condition of the mouth, the patient's attitude toward wearing the prosthesis, the skill of the dentist, and the technical laboratory support services, as well as on adequate patient education.

▶ The Condition of the Mouth

Earlier discussion about the condition of the mouth relates directly to a fixed prosthesis. However, one of the primary concerns in the success of a denture is the potential retention ability. Retention is the process of holding the prosthesis in place; it is directly affected by the shape of the alveolar ridge and sulci and by the formation of the palate. A patient with a well-developed ridge that is not abnormally thick and who has a moderate palatal vault has favorable conditions for a successful denture. However, a patient, who has a flat palate with small ridges and shallow sulci or tori interference presents a less-than-favorable condition for a removable or partial denture. Various ridges and palatal conditions are shown in Fig. 29-7.

An edentulous alveolar ridge is not a natural condition. The shape and size of the ridge are the result of the individual's inherited bone and tooth size, the amount of bone lost because of extraction of teeth and periodontal disease, and the amount of resorption. Patients who have had ill-fitting dentures may also experience changes in the shape of the alveolar ridge because of resorption.

The tongue also plays an important role in the function of a fixed or removable prosthesis. The tongue controls food during mastication and swallowing and aids in forming the sounds of speech. Care must be taken in placing teeth and other components of a dental prosthe-

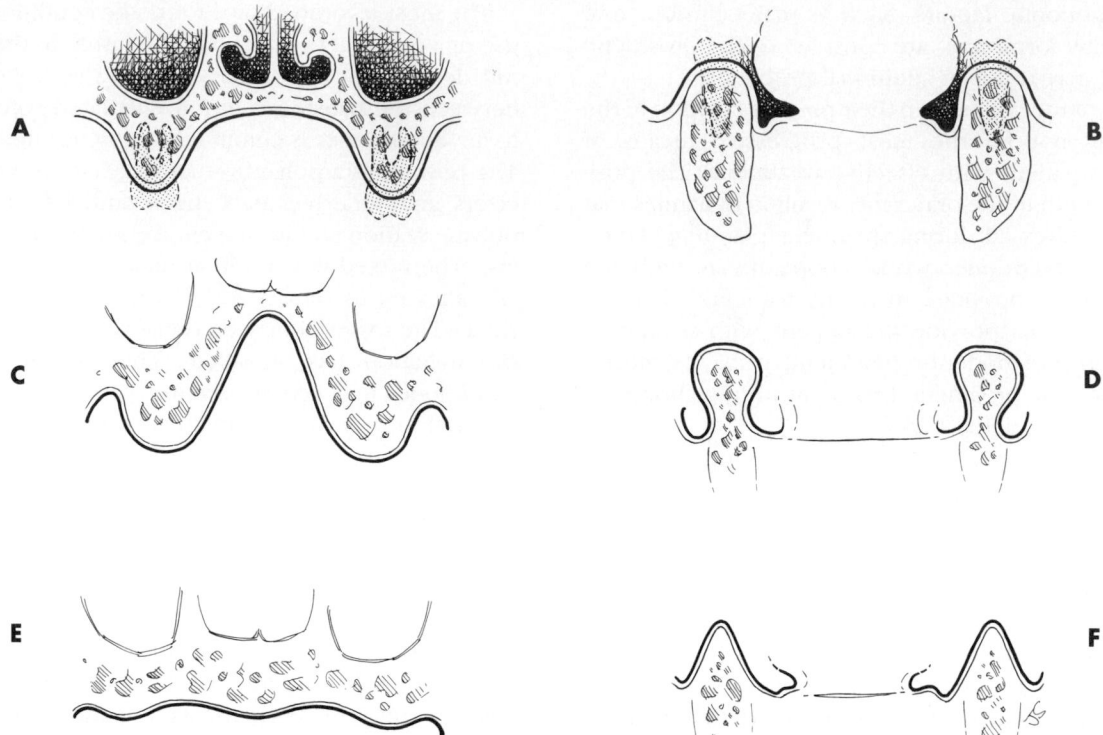

FIG. 29-7   Various conditions of ridges in a partially or completely edentulous patient. *A,* Normal maxillary ridge. *B,* Normal mandibular ridge. *C,* Vaulted maxillary ridge. *D,* Rolled ridge creating undercuts and tissue. *E,* Flat palate. *F,* Sharp pointed ridges.

sis to avoid interference with the tongue, which could result in the patient's inability to eat or articulate.

The patient needs to be made aware that regardless of what type of prosthesis is being inserted in the mouth, it will be different from his or her own teeth and tissues and that a period of adjustment will be necessary. The patient also needs to know that the prosthesis may feel bulky and that the feelings he or she is having are normal during the adjustment to the new appliance.

▌ Musculature Adjustment

For the patient who is to have a removable or full denture prosthesis, there will probably be more musculature adjustment than with the fixed bridge prosthesis. The patient who has a removable prosthetic device may find it necessary to retrain the muscles, using the tongue and cheek muscles differently to aid in retention of the prosthesis. The patient needs to understand the limitations of the prosthesis and to realize that a period of time will be necessary to adjust to this new device. As with any new activity some discomfort can be expected in the facial muscles, which have not been used for a while.

▌ Patient Attitude

Success or failure is determined significantly by a person's attitude. Often a patient's attitude is dictated by his or her own previous experiences or by the experiences of friends and family. When a dental prosthesis is recommended to a patient, it is possible that he or she has no awareness of the function of the prosthesis. Sometimes a lack of knowledge is more beneficial because the dental practitioner can present a positive case for the prosthesis. However, the risk of the patient having a negative attitude may exist because a member of the family or a friend may have had an unfavorable experience. For instance a patient may need a full cast crown and his or her only knowledge of such a restoration comes from a brother who had a full cast crown and later had to have the tooth removed. The suggestion for a full crown may cause the patient to relate to this situation. The patient needs to be reminded that first, no restoration is going to last for a lifetime but that the loss of the brother's tooth may have been related to other conditions, such as the lack of proper oral hygiene or because the tooth became devital because of trauma or other disease and not because of the cast crown.

A similar situation might arise with a removable prosthesis. If, for instance, before being completely edentulous a patient had a favorable experience with a partial denture, it is likely that he or she will have a more positive attitude about a complete denture. The patient, however, needs to realize that the full denture will present a different set of adjustment processes than did the partial denture. For instance, there are no longer other teeth to provide support or stability, and if it is a maxillary prosthesis, the palate will be covered with a denture base. Similarly, if a patient has previously worn a denture with relative comfort and efficiency and then a new denture is constructed, a successful experience with the new denture may be anticipated.

On the other hand, if a patient has had no previous prosthetic experience and has heard negative responses from family or friends, it poses a challenge to the dentist and staff to create a positive attitude and to teach the patient good habits in developing muscle control to use the prosthesis. Such education cannot be taught in a few minutes, but it is a gradual process that must be ongoing at each appointment. The patient must be told what to expect, must be provided with suggestions to overcome potential problems, and must be encouraged to develop a positive attitude.

▶ Patient Education

Patient education becomes an important factor in ensuring the success of the restored area. If the oral health of the tissues is not maintained, periodontal involvement may result in premature loss of the restoration or tooth.

It is not wise to wait until the prosthesis is inserted to discuss oral hygiene with the patient. Patient education must be periodically reinforced. For instance, oral hygiene instructions may be given at the onset of treatment, but as treatment progresses the oral care is reviewed and reemphasized as needed. If a patient neglects to floss adequately this should be noted, and the patient should be informed of the consequences of such neglect when the prosthesis is inserted. At the appointment for prosthesis insertion, instructions for home care of the prosthesis are given to the patient. Specific care of various types of prostheses will be covered in the following chapters.

Dental Assistant's Role in Prosthodontics

It is important for the dental assistant to have an understanding of the various types of fixed and removable restorations that can be placed in different situations, the purpose for selecting a particular restoration for a given situation, the steps necessary to accomplish the procedure, care and cost of the prosthesis, advantages and disadvantages of each type of restoration, home care, and the consequences of neglect. The assistant must also be capable of describing the procedure and purpose of the restoration to the patient and have the ability to anticipate the operator's needs during a given procedure. The current health history alerts the dental team to any problems that could complicate the procedure and require special action on the part of the team.

The dental assistant is vital to all phases of prosthodontics but becomes a valuable asset in fixed prosthodontics. Without an assistant during cavity preparation, impression taking, temporization, cementation, and home care instructions the procedure can become lengthy, stressful for the operator and patient, and not cost effective.

Removable prosthetic dentistry may be perceived as a specialty area where four-handed dentistry is not applicable. Although the preparatory phases of denture and partial denture construction may require more concentrated time on the part of the dentist, this should not be interpreted as an ineffective application for dental assistant utilization.

Many advanced functions are being delegated in prosthodontics to the qualified dental assistant. These duties include fabricating temporary crowns, bridges, and inlays; obtaining opposing models; placing gingival retraction cord; and fabricating custom-made trays.

Four-handed dentistry can be used during all phases of prosthetic dentistry, including impression taking, mouth preparation, shade and mould selection, try in, and insertion of the prosthesis. The dental assistant will also play a vital role in scheduling appointments, performing basic laboratory procedures, coordinating surgical and laboratory schedules, providing patient education and support, and preparing appropriate claim forms for third party payments.

KEY POINTS

▶ Prosthodontics is the specialty that is involved with designing and fitting artificial replacements for lost or missing tissues. Dental prosthodontics can be categorized into the three following phases: fixed, removable, and maxillofacial prosthodontics.

▶ The dental assistant is an integral part of the prosthodontic team from the initial examination for diagnosis through the actual preparation and delivery appointments.

▶ Types of dental prostheses that can be designed for patients include inlays, onlays, ¾ and full crowns, bridges, obturators, precision attachments, and full and partial dentures.

▶ Before the placement of a dental prosthesis designed to replace missing teeth and oral tissues, it is necessary to complete an oral prophylaxis and periodontal treatment, endodontic and orthodontic, occlusal equilibration, and tissue conditioning.

▶ Several factors are involved in creating a successful experience for the prosthodontic patient; these include the condition of the mouth, musculature, patient attitude, and patient education.

BIBLIOGRAPHY

Dyer MRY, Roberts BJ: *Notes on prosthetic dentistry,* London, 1989, Wright.

Grazzo JE, Miller EL: *Removable partial prosthodontics,* St Louis, ed 3, 1991, Mosby.

Halperin AR, Grasser GN, Rogoff GS, Plekavich EJ: *Mastering the art of complete dentures,* Chicago, 1988, Quintessence.

McGivney GP, Castleberry DJ: *McCracken's removable partial prosthodontics,* ed 9, St Louis, 1994, Mosby.

Neill DJ, Nairn RI: *Complete denture prosthetics,* ed 3, London, 1990, Wright.

Renner RP, BLJ: *Removable partial dentures,* Chicago, 1987, Quintessence.

Zarb GA, Bolender CL, Hickey JC, Carsson GE: *Boucher's prosthodontic treatment for edentulous patients,* ed 10, St Louis, 1990, Mosby.

30 Fixed Prosthodontics

LEARNING OBJECTIVES

You will have mastered the material in this chapter when you can:
- Define the key terms
- Define the principles of tooth preparation for fixed prosthodontics
- Describe the basic procedural sequence for the preparation, fabrication, and cementation of a fixed restoration
- Explain the role of the dental assistant in a fixed prosthodontic procedure
- Describe common dental materials used in a fixed prosthetic procedure

KEY TERMS

Biologic principle	Luxating
Bite registration	Mechanical principle
Burnishing	Occlusal clearance
Cast	Opposing model
Cementation	Shade
Coping	Shimstock
Crucible former	Sprue
Draw	Surfactant
Esthetic principle	Tachycardia
Film thickness	Tissue retraction
Investing procedure	Undercut
Ischemia	Wax elimination
Laboratory prescription / requisition	

In the previous chapter an overview of prosthodontics and the purpose of this specialty of dentistry was discussed. Fixed prosthodontics involves the preparation or shaping of a tooth or teeth for a prosthesis that will be cemented into the mouth as a permanent restoration. As described previously this type of restoration may be an intracoronal or extracoronal restoration and usually requires a minimum of two appointments: one for tooth preparation and a later appointment for **cementation** or final insertion of the restoration. In some instances interim appointments are necessary to try in the restorations or components of the prosthesis. The steps in the preparation and insertion of a fixed prosthesis will be discussed in detail in this chapter.

Principles of Tooth Preparation

Several factors in cavity preparation for a fixed prosthesis differ from the previously described intracoronal restorations, such as amalgam and composite. A dentist must first decide which type of coverage is necessary to restore a tooth or area to function. These options include the following: (1) inlay; (2) onlay; (3) ¾ crown; (4) full crown; (5) esthetic coverage; and (6) bridges, were discussed in detail in Chapter 29. Once the type of restoration has been selected the technical components of the preparation must be considered. Although tooth preparation is the responsibility of the dentist, the dental assistant must have an understanding of the basic concepts to anticipate the needs of the dentist.

 The first articulator that created movement of jaws in three dimensions was designed in 1840 and patented by an American dentist, Dr. Daniel Evans.

Preparing a tooth to receive a fixed restoration requires (1) reducing the tooth shape to remove a portion of the occlusal surface from contact with the opposing tooth; (2) decreasing the circumference of the tooth; (3) creating a margin that allows for smooth transition from the tooth to the restoration; and (4) removing any carious lesion.

Several design factors must be considered when a fixed prosthesis is constructed. These include the biologic, mechanical, and esthetic principles of cavity preparation. Each of these principles has an interrelationship with the other and may affect the integrity of the restoration, which can result in success or failure. A balance of these three principles is critical and must be achieved with careful planning and preparation. A thorough understanding of the complexities of cavity design requires a broad background in scientific principles. It seems appropriate, however, that a basic overview of the factors involved in cavity design be presented for the assistant.

▶ Biologic Principles

The **biologic principle** of tooth preparation refers to creating a balance between tooth conservation and retention of the restoration. In reality, the dentist needs to design a preparation that maintains as much tooth structure as possible and yet create a restoration that can be held in place through retention. Care must be taken not to extend the preparation to a point that causes a fracture of the tooth. The preparation must also allow for the creation of occlusal harmony and for protection of the oral tissues. If an excess of tooth structure is removed during the preparation, pulpal damage may occur as a result of temperature change, chemical irritation or

bacterial attack. The operator will also take care to ensure that the restoration has been properly adapted to the gingival margin to prevent plaque build up and to avoid the irritation of gingival tissue.

▶ Mechanical Principles

Mechanical principle refers to the components in the preparation design that will aid in the retention of the restoration. Here the dentist is concerned with the physical design of the preparation, the type of cement used in final placement, and the physical properties of the restorative material, such as deformation.

▶ Esthetic Principles

Esthetics refers to the theory of beauty and fine arts. In fixed prosthodontics the concern for esthetics refers to the creation of a pleasant smile and good appearance, while still maintaining a functional dentition. The responsibility for esthetics involves the patient and dental team. The operator must assess the patient's appearance when he or she is smiling or speaking to determine the appropriate dental material for a restoration. For instance, if the patient has a broad smile that exposes the maxillary first molar, then the use of a ceramic fused to alloy restoration may be the appropriate choice as a restoration in the posterior of the mouth. If, however, the tooth is not exposed as the patient smiles and speaks, the use of a gold alloy may be more appropriate to regain function of the tooth. In either case the patient must be informed about the treatment that is planned and become a partner in the decision making. Likewise, when a **shade** (color of the tooth) is chosen, it is vital to have the patient involved in this selection to ensure patient satisfaction.

Design Factors Applied to Fixed Restorative Procedure

During the fixed prosthetic procedure the dentist must keep in mind several factors that relate to the biologic, mechanical, and esthetic principles to ensure success in the final restoration. These factors are often directly related to the use of specific instruments or materials which the dental assistant must prepare and have ready for use.

▶ Retention and Resistance Form

Retention and resistance form in fixed prosthodontics differs from an amalgam and composite preparation. Fixed prosthodontics include the use of grooves and pinholes to ensure retention instead of undercuts. For instance, an **undercut** (cut made under a cavity wall that will lock in a restoration) used in an amalgam or

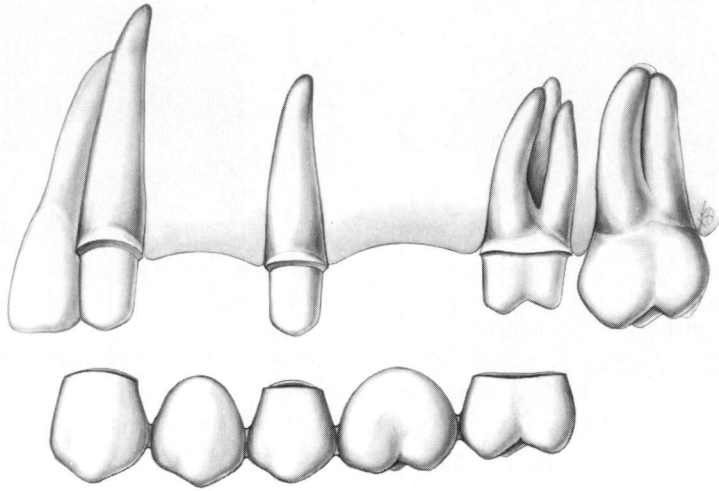

FIG. 30-I   Prepared teeth demonstrate draw.

(From Rosenstiel SF, Land MF, Fujimoto J: *Contemporary fixed prosthodontics*, ed 3, St Louis, 1995, Mosby.)

composite preparation cannot be present in a cast restoration, since it is necessary to place the restoration on and off of the tooth before final cementation.

Draw

Draw: a taper or divergence of the intracoronal or extracoronal walls of a preparation must be present to allow for the insertion of the cemented restoration (Fig. 30-1). Improper draw results in the inability to seat a cast restoration in the preparation because the walls are not aligned properly. Walls must be tapered to allow the withdrawal of the cast restoration in an occlusal direction.

Use of Pins

When pins are used as part of a cast restoration, it is necessary for them to be parallel to each other in order to place and remove the casting. Pins provide greater retention of the restoration. The assistant can often aid the dentist visually in establishing parallelism from the assistant's side of the mouth.

Occlusal Forces

Concern for natural occlusal forces must be noted. The operator considers the patient's normal masticatory and bruxing processes during the cavity design. If these forces are not considered, the new restoration may interfere with the patient's normal chewing patterns and could result in damage to the teeth and associated structures.

Occlusal Clearance

The amount of **occlusal clearance**: space between the prepared and opposing tooth/teeth, must be adequate. The removal of a sufficient amount of tooth tissue will provide for an adequate thickness of metal in the cast restoration to resist stress and to allow for reproduction of natural tooth morphology, yet it will not interfere with occlusal harmony.

If the occlusal clearance is not reduced sufficiently, attrition will occur on the new restoration. A similar situation can occur when insufficient tooth structure is removed from the facial surface of an anterior tooth that is to receive a ceramic fused to metal crown. If inadequate space is left for the porcelain to be baked onto the metal, the strength of the porcelain to withstand the forces in the oral cavity is reduced. Consequently, through normal masticatory processes a fracture of the porcelain could occur.

Margin Design

Ideally, the margin of a preparation is placed supragingival, since periodontal disease has been related to subgingival margin placement. The preparation of supragingival margins provides easier access for the operator during the preparation and seating appointment, and it makes it easier for the patient to maintain good oral hygiene. Other factors for placement of the margin supragingival include greater ease in obtaining the final impression and better access in finishing the margins during placement. Situations that prohibit the operator from placing supragingival margins are the extent of

BOX 30-I

VARIATIONS OF MARGIN DESIGNS
(Fig. 30-2, *A* through *E*)

Chisel edge — used for the margins of teeth that are rotated or tilted from normal position

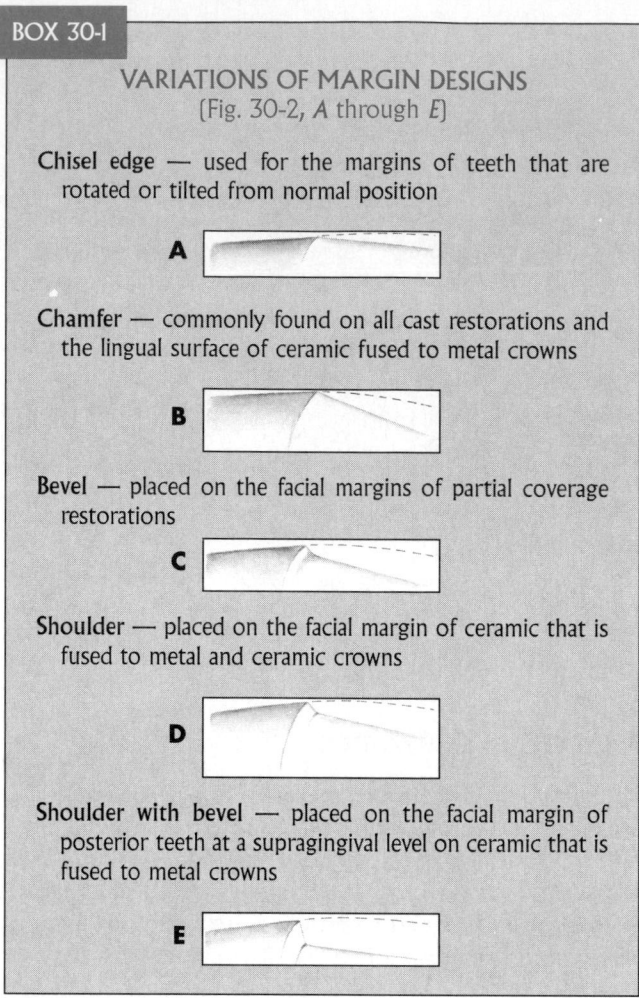

Chamfer — commonly found on all cast restorations and the lingual surface of ceramic fused to metal crowns

Bevel — placed on the facial margins of partial coverage restorations

Shoulder — placed on the facial margin of ceramic that is fused to metal and ceramic crowns

Shoulder with bevel — placed on the facial margin of posterior teeth at a supragingival level on ceramic that is fused to metal crowns

FIG. 30-2   Variations of margin designs.

(From Rosenstiel SF, Land MF, Fujimoto J: *Contemporary fixed prosthodontics,* ed 3, St Louis, 1995, Mosby.)

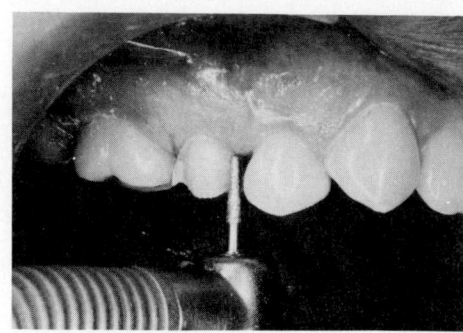

FIG. 30-3   Diamond is used in tooth reduction and in placing margins.

(From Rosenstiel SF, Land MF, Fujimoto J: *Contemporary fixed prosthodontics,* ed 3, St Louis, 1995, Mosby.)

caries below the ideal, root sensitivity that may warrant extension of the restoration to include coverage, and the need for greater retention forcing the need to extend the restoration. Esthetics may also play a role in the extension to subgingival length if the patient does not want the margin of a ceramic fused to metal crown visible.

Commonly, five categories of margin designs are placed on teeth in fixed prosthodontics, as shown in Box 30-1, Fig. 30-2.

The selection of the margin design is determined by the operator to remove the least amount of tooth possible to accommodate the preparation design, to allow for adequate bulk of the restorative material and wax pattern, and to be easily seen in the final impression. The dental assistant should become familiar with these terms and the instruments that the dentist uses for placing these margins. Differently shaped burs and diamonds are used for many of these margins and will likely depend on the operator's preference (Fig. 30-3).

▶ Type of Dental Material

The appropriate dental material must be chosen to withstand the patient's occlusal forces. For instance, in Chapter 11 the various types of gold alloys, Type I, II, or III, were described. To choose a gold alloy that is inadequate for the natural forces generated by the patient's occlusion would cause deformation of the metal, ultimately causing distortion of the restoration and possibly interfering with the opposing tooth or teeth.

▶ Internal Surface Roughness

It is necessary to have surface roughness on the inside of the cast restoration to achieve an interface with the luting cement. Little or no surface roughness on the interior of a restoration will result in the cement not interfacing with the casting and may result in failure of the restoration to be retained on the tooth.

▶ Use of Dental Cement

It is not intended that the dental cement retain the restoration, but rather that the mechanical design of the preparation be such that the restoration can be retained by itself.

The type of cement used and its luting consistency is important to retention. A thin layer of cement, referred to as **film thickness**, is placed on the inner surface of the restoration. The assistant must prepare the dental cement according to specific manufacturer's instructions to ensure maximum strength. A cement mixed to a thickness greater than film thickness does not allow for correct seating of the restoration. Likewise, a cement of less viscosity than film thickness does not assist in the retention of the restoration.

Procedure Sequence for a Fixed Prosthesis

The procedure to create a fixed prosthesis includes three major phases:

1. *Preparation* includes reducing the tooth structure, creating retention, taking the bite registration, taking the impression and opposing impression, and temporization.
2. *Laboratory processing* includes creating casts and dies; fabricating the wax pattern; investing the pattern; and creating, finishing, and polishing the casting.
3. *Cementation* includes removal of the temporary restoration, trying the cast restoration, checking margins and occlusion, and cementing the cast.

Commonly, this procedure is done in multiple appointments. Typically, the preparation is done at the first appointment, and the patient is dismissed, wearing some form of temporary restoration on the prepared tooth. During the interim, laboratory procedures take place to create the restoration. In some situations additional appointments are necessary for trying in the castings before soldering the units together to determine appropriate fit or before porcelain is fired to the casting. The final appointment is the cementation or seating appointment when the temporary restoration is removed and the fixed prosthesis is tried in and cemented in place.

In each phase of fixed prosthodontics several basic steps must be completed before the next phase can begin. Box 30-2 lists the procedures necessary to complete each of the phases of fixed prosthodontics for a full cast restoration.

The dental assistant plays a vital role in fixed prosthodontics, preparing the armamentarium for each phase of the preparation and cementation, performing basic laboratory procedures, communicating with the laboratory, and scheduling patient appointments, as well as providing patient education. This prosthetic procedure is

---

BOX 30-2

PROCEDURAL STEPS IN FIXED PROSTHODONTICS

PREPARATION PROCEDURE

1. Prepare the armamentarium
2. Update patient's medical history
3. Examine treatment site
4. Determine occlusal relationship
5. Administer anesthesia
6. Prepare tooth
   Remove caries and place core material to build up tooth as necessary
   Reduce occlusal surface
   Place occlusal grooves
   Check occlusal clearance
   Reduce axial walls
   Place axial grooves
   Remove caries as necessary
   Refine and finish margins
7. Dry and isolate site
8. Place cavity medication if needed*
9. Retract gingiva
10. Obtain final and opposing impressions
11. Obtain bite registration
12. Fabricate and place temporary restoration
13. Postoperative instructions
14. Prepare case according to OSHA guidelines and prescription for laboratory

LABORATORY PROCEDURE

1. Disinfect impression according to OSHA guidelines
2. Produce die and cast from impression
3. Articulate the casts
4. Fabricate wax pattern on die

5. Invest wax pattern
6. Eliminate wax
7. Cast the alloy
8. Recover the cast
9. Remove sprue
10. Remove imperfections
11. Finish the cast restoration

CEMENTATION PROCEDURE

1. Disinfect cast and restoration
2. Administer anesthesia if necessary
3. Remove temporary restoration and excess cement
4. Try in cast restoration
   Assess stability
   Check contacts
   Check occlusion
   Determine margin integrity
   Make necessary adjustments
5. Finish margins
6. Complete final laboratory finish and polish
7. Disinfect cast restoration
8. Isolate tooth
9. Prepare final cement
10. Place thin film of cement on inner surface of casting
11. Cement cast restoration on tooth
12. Remove excess cement
13. Reevaluate occlusal contact and margins
14. Make final adjustments if necessary
15. Postoperative instructions

---

* This step may be eliminated if it is completed in core build up.

one of many that exercises all of the clinical chairside skills of the qualified assistant. Depending on the particular state dental practice act the dental assistant may be permitted to take the opposing impressions, place tissue pack for gingival retraction, fabricate, and place and remove temporary restorations in addition to the traditional chairside duties. Many assistants who display the interest and skill may also assume responsibility for fabricating the wax pattern, investing, and casting and finishing the final restoration.

The following discussion presents an overview of the step-by-step procedure for each of these phases. A description of variations for different types of fixed restorations follows this discussion.

Procedure for a Full-Coverage Crown

This type of preparation usually requires the removal of a thin layer of tissue from all surfaces of the tooth. The removal of tissue is necessary to (1) provide an adequate thickness of metal in the cast restoration to resist stress and to reproduce tooth morphology; (2) to ensure equal removal of tooth tissue from all areas of the tooth; and (3) to eliminate axial undercuts, while obtaining draw and retention.

The techniques that are used to prepare the tooth, obtain an impression and casts, wax the pattern, cast the restoration, and seat a fixed prosthesis vary with the tooth that is being restored and with the individual operator's technique. The full-coverage cast crown is probably one of the most common prosthetic restorative procedures that is performed, particularly on posterior teeth. Therefore, we have opted to present in this chapter a step-by-step procedure for the preparation and final seating of a full-coverage cast alloy crown.

The basic format for this type of procedure includes common steps that are followed for most fixed prosthetic restorations. There are, however, variations in the process, and several of these are noted in Table 30-1.

The patient is involved in the selection of the fixed restoration and provides informed consent for the procedure. A complete and thorough health history and patient record is produced. The diagnostic models that were taken at a previous appointment are used by the dental assistant to fabricate a custom acrylic impression tray. A **coping**, a thin plastic reproduction of existing structure, is used as a mold to create an acrylic temporary (if this type of temporary restoration is selected); this reproduction can be made in advance from the models and used until the final restoration is seated.

▶ Armamentarium Preparation

As with previous clinical procedures all armamentarium is prepared and universal precautions are implemented. The armamentarium for this procedure is more extensive than the typical intracoronal restoration. It will be necessary, in most cases, to assemble the armamentarium in sequence of use. For instance, the anesthesia and preset preparation tray can be placed on the mobile cabinet, and the impression and temporization materials can be placed on the fixed cabinetry nearby. Then with

TABLE 30-I   PROCEDURAL MODIFICATIONS AS COMPARED TO FULL CAST CROWN

Type of restoration	Preparation	Laboratory	Cementation
Inlay/onlay	More conservative	Same as cast crown; no lab needed if CAD/CAM design	Same
¾ Crown	Less tooth preparation	Same	Same
Porcelain jacket	Modified margin design; shade selection	Not a cast procedure; porcelain is baked	Same; dependent on type of cement
Porcelain veneer	Modified margin design; shade selection	May need an opaque liner	Same
Fixed bridge	Multiple tooth preparation; possible shade selection	Possible try in appointment; opaque liner when needed	Same
Cantilever bridge	Conservative preparation	Same	Same
Resin-retained bridge	Minimal tooth reduction	Wax and cast framework and create and bake porcelain pontic	Rubber dam preferred; use of resin cement
Post and core	Canal preparation first appointment; second appointment for impression of cemented post and core	Create two working casts and dies; possible opaque liner	Cement post with core; cement crown over post and core

a Class IV or V movement the assistant can transfer the preassembled setups into the static zone as they are needed.

The armamentarium for the preparation procedure will vary according to the specific tooth that is being prepared and to the operator's individual choice of instruments or materials (Fig. 30-4). Box 30-3 is a generic list of instruments and materials that are used by many operators.

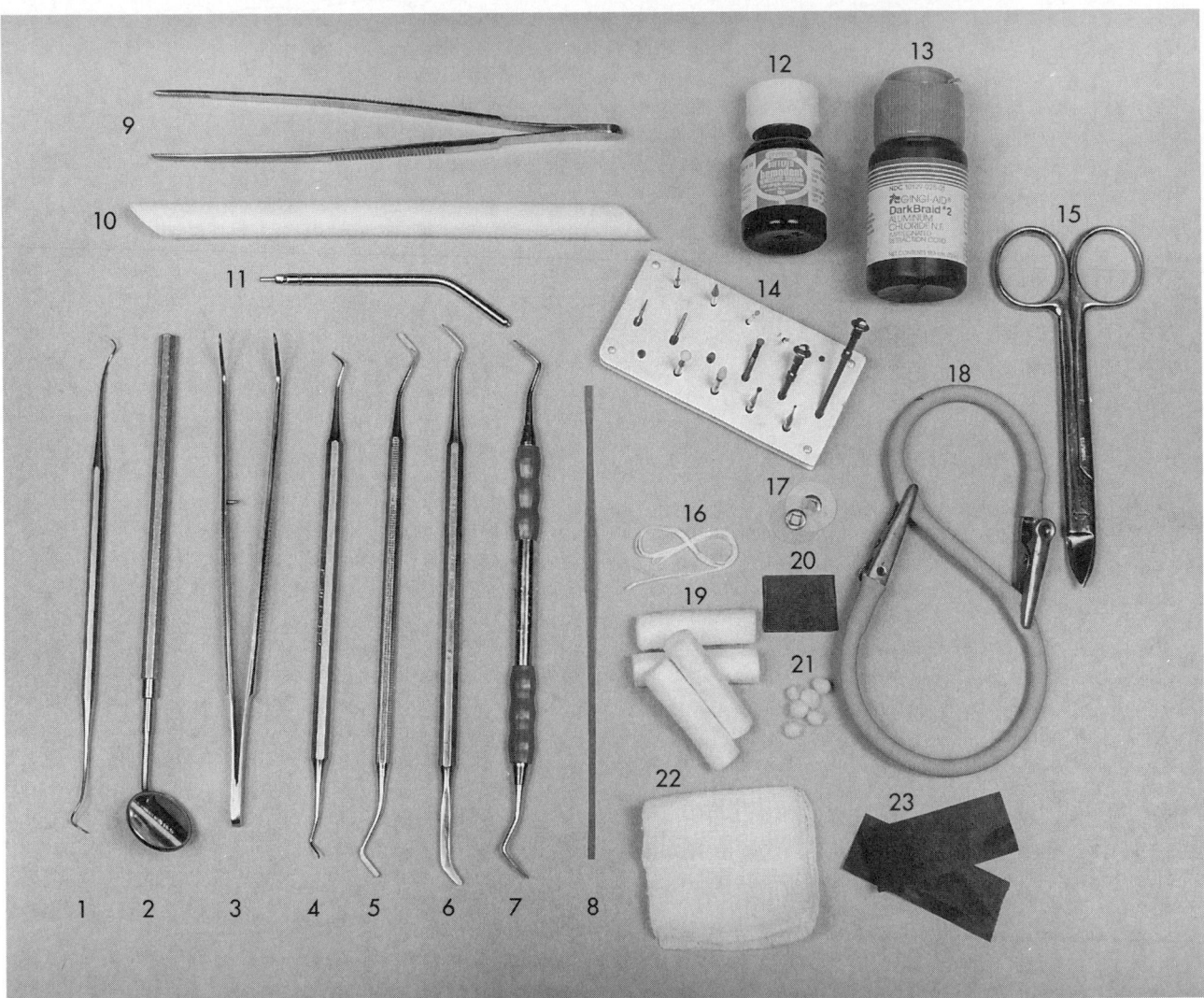

1. Explorer
2. Mirror
3. Cotton pliers
4. Spoon excavator
5. Enamel hatchet
6. Plastic instrument
7. Retraction cord placement instrument
8. Lightening strip
9. Thumb forceps
10. HVE tip
11. A/W tip
12. Hemostatic agent
13. Retraction cord

14. Assorted burs, stones and mandrels
15. Crown and collar scissors
16. Dental floss
17. Abrasive disks
18. Patient napkin
19. Cotton rolls
20. 28q Green wax
21. Cotton pellets
22. 2 × 2 gauze
23. Articulating paper

Not pictured: impression-taking armamentarium and temporization armamentarium

FIG. 30-4 Preparation tray set-up.

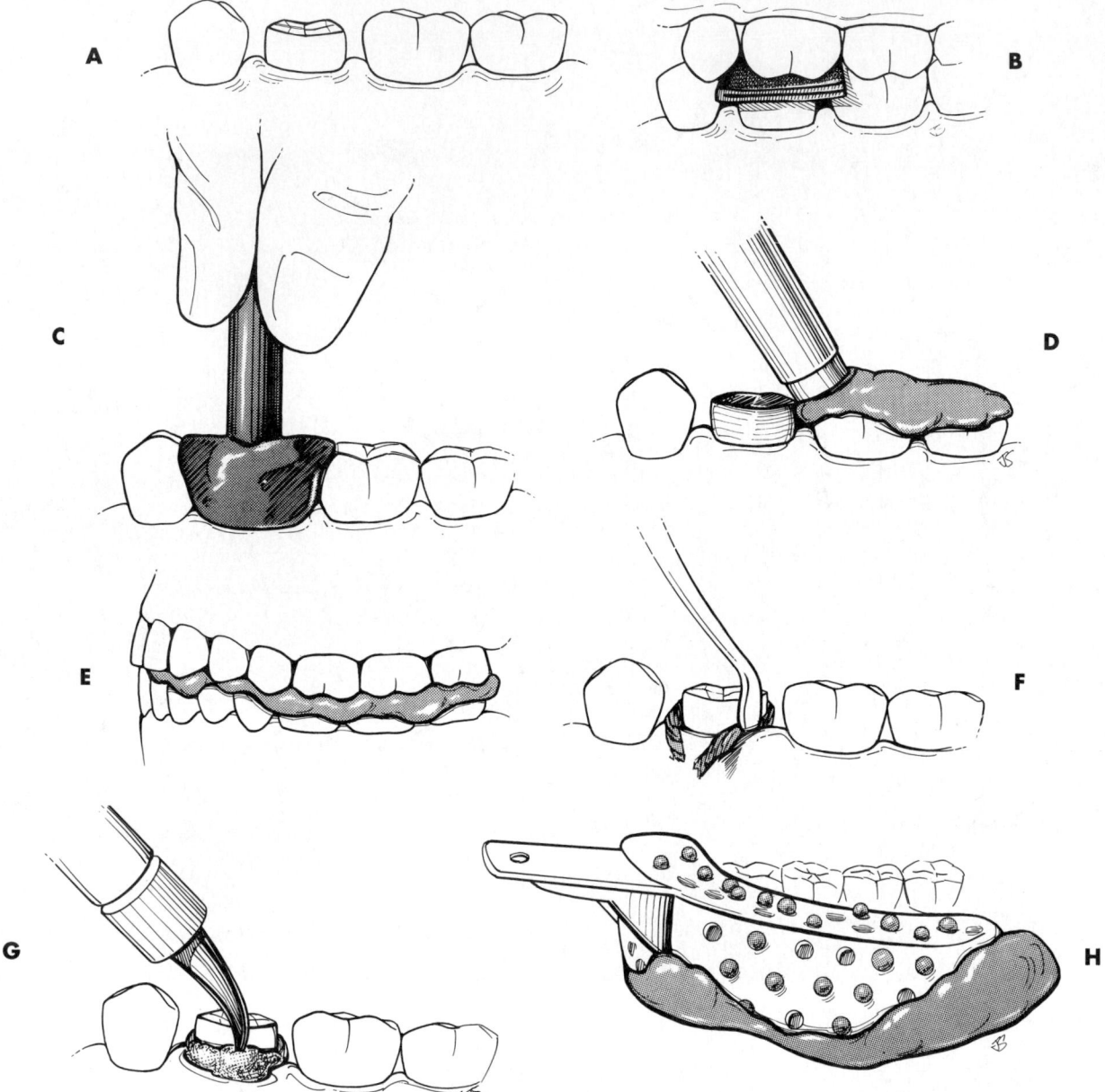

FIG. 30-5   *A,* The tooth is prepared. *B,* Occlusal clearance is evaluated. *C,* Snap impression determines draw and accuracy of preparation. *D* and *E,* Bite registration is obtained. *F,* Placement of retraction cord. *G* and *H,* Final impression is taken.

PROCEDURE FOR A FULL-COVERAGE CROWN

- ▶ Are all universal barrier techniques being used?
- ▶ Is all of the armamentarium available and prepared for use?
- ▶ Are the instruments arranged in sequence of use?
- ▶ Am I prepared for alternative treatment plans?
- ▶ Is the necessary equipment turned on and ready to operate?

Preparation Procedure

The following discussion presents a step-by-step procedure for the preparation appointment outlined in Box 30-2. An overview of these steps is illustrated in Fig. 30-5, *A* through *G.*

Examination of the Treatment Site

Before the actual treatment occurs, the updated medical and dental history is reviewed to alert the dental team to any health contraindications that could complicate the procedure and require intervention.

The dental assistant passes the operator a mirror and explorer and the site is examined. At this point the operator may determine the expected level of margin placement, furcation involvement, relation of opposing and hypererupted teeth, and any other factors to be considered in the preparation design.

Determine Occlusal Relationship

The occlusal relationship of the arches before the preparation is an important factor for the operator to consider. The relationship that exists between the opposing arches must be replicated to restore proper function for the patient. To determine the occlusal relationship, articulating paper is placed in the mouth to mark the occlusal contacts. These contacts are then examined. The dental assistant may pass the articulating paper to the operator or place it directly on the site.

Anesthesia Administration

Anesthesia is administered to achieve patient comfort for the dental procedure. A review of the medical history will dictate the type of anesthesia to be administered. The assistant will follow the procedure that is outlined earlier in this text for the preparation, transfer, and administration of local anesthetic.

Placement of Occlusal Grooves and Surface Reduction

The reduction of the tooth is completed with various rotary instruments. Most commonly, a wheel-shaped diamond is used to reduce the occlusal cusps, and tapered diamonds and carbide burs are used to form walls of the preparation.

Initially, the operator may place depth grooves or holes in the central, mesial, and distal fossae. The operator can then connect the depth markers creating a line through the central groove of the tooth and into the mesial and distal marginal ridge areas. Guiding grooves are placed on the buccal and lingual grooves and on each of the triangular ridges to connect to the central

groove. It is necessary to reduce the functional cusp depth to 1.5 mm while nonfunctional cusp depth is reduced to 1 mm. These guiding grooves provide the operator with a reference point for tissue removal, thereby minimizing the amount of structure that is removed in the preparation. If the grooves are not placed accurately and equal in depth, more tooth structure may be removed than is necessary. It is helpful for the operator and the assistant to know the diameter of rotary instruments to assist in ensuring the adequate placement of these grooves. Fig. 30-6, *A* through *C,* illustrates the placement of guiding grooves with a diamond bur.

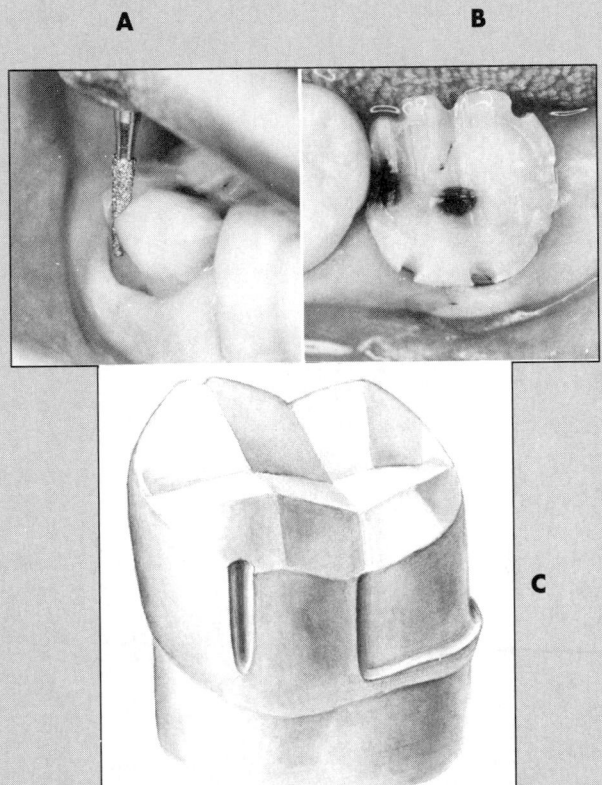

FIG. 30-6   *A,* The diamond is aligned parallel to the long axis of the tooth, as the buccal guiding grooves for axial alignment are placed. *B,* After all six grooves have been placed, note that they are quite deep occlusally but are shallower toward the cervical margin. *C,* If axial reduction is completed first on either the distal or the mesial half of the tooth, evaluation is simplified because the remaining intact tooth can serve as a reference.

(From Rosenstiel SF, Land MF, Fujimoto J: *Contemporary fixed prosthodontics,* ed 3, St Louis, 1995, Mosby.)

Continued.

PROCEDURE FOR A FULL COVERAGE CROWN—cont'd

The occlusal reduction can be completed in two steps. The tooth structure is removed on either the mesial or the distal half of the tooth, while the other half remains intact, providing the operator with a reference point because one half of the tooth is maintained intact with original tooth structure and the other half is reduced for occlusal clearance. The other half of the occlusal reduction is completed the same as the first half. The role of the dental assistant during the procedure involves performing constant oral evacuation and retraction of the soft tissues. Once the handpiece is removed, the site is rinsed and dried so that the operator can examine the progress of the preparation.

During this phase of the procedure the assistant evacuates the oral cavity, dries the preparation site as necessary, and observes the patient to determine the level of comfort. Periodic bur changes may be necessary.

Check Occlusal Clearance

The occlusal clearance of the prepared tooth can be verified after occlusal reduction is completed or the operator may opt to perform this task after the preparation is completely finished. Occlusal clearance may be determined by using a piece of 28-gauge casting wax that is folded into three thicknesses that is slightly larger than the occlusal surface of the tooth. The wax is placed on the reduced occlusal surface, and the patient is directed to close the arches firmly (Fig. 30-7, *A*). The wax is removed from the mouth and is evaluated for thin areas in which the teeth are occluded (Fig. 30-7, *B*). If it is desired, the thickness of the wax can be measured with a dial caliper.

If the thickness is adequate, new wax is placed in the patient's mouth and the patient is directed to move the mandible in protrusive and excursive directions. The wax is removed again and reevaluated for thickness during the intercuspal movements. If at any point a less-than-adequate thickness of wax, 1.5mm to 1 mm, is not maintained, the tooth structure in the area of penetration of the wax is removed and the occlusal clearance is checked with another piece of wax.

For the assistant this step will require preparation of multiple pieces of wax and handpiece exchange as necessary, until the appropriate clearance is obtained.

Placement of Axial Grooves and Reduction

Alignment grooves for axial reduction are placed on the buccal and lingual surfaces, parallel to the long axis of the tooth. These grooves are approximately 1 mm deep. The thickness will vary to allow for taper to the cervical finish of the tooth. The axial reduction is done with the removal of tooth surface and by placing a minimum of 5 degrees of taper on the axial walls from

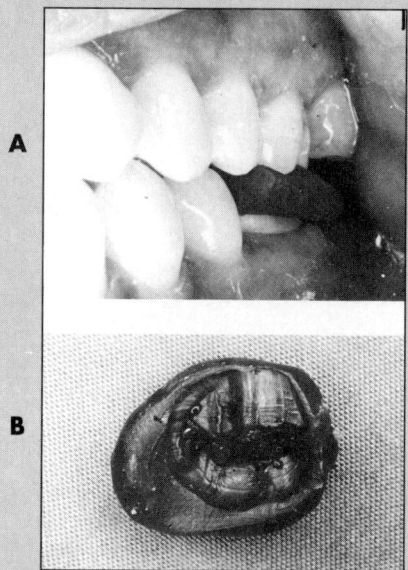

FIG. 30-7 Evaluation of the adequacy of occlusal clearance. *A,* The patient is asked to close into softened wax. *B,* The thickness of the wax can be assessed visually and is measured with a wax caliper after it has been removed from the mouth.

(From Rosenstiel SF, Land MF, Fujimoto J: *Contemporary fixed prosthodontics,* ed 3, St Louis, 1995, Mosby.)

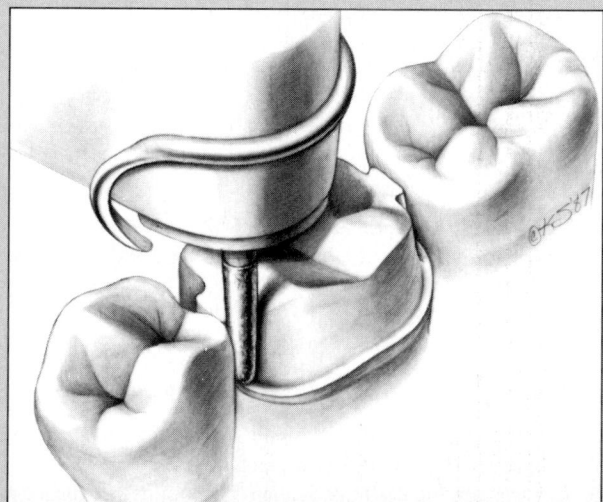

FIG. 30-8 If large contact areas exist, axial reduction can be completed except for the proximal contact, broken with a narrower diamond rotary instrument.

(From Rosenstiel SF, Land MF, Fujimoto J: *Contemporary fixed prosthodontics,* ed 3, St Louis, 1995, Mosby.)

PROCEDURE FOR A FULL COVERAGE CROWN—cont'd

the occlusal to the cervical (Fig. 30-8). The operator may use a diamond with a taper of 5 to 6 degrees, allowing for the shank of the diamond to be placed parallel to the path of withdrawal of the restoration. This technique allows the operator to produce a taper to the axial walls that is identical to the taper of the diamond. The cervical area of reduction will be approximately half the width of the tip of the diamond. This amount of taper will accommodate impression taking and placement of the cast restoration to ensure retention to the preparation. An increase in taper of the axial walls will reduce the retentive qualities of the preparation.

During reduction of the axial surfaces of the tooth the operator must take caution to avoid damaging the abutment tooth or teeth with the diamond or bur. A metal matrix band can be placed around the adjacent tooth to protect it from damage. If the proximal surface of an adjacent tooth is damaged, it must be polished and even given a fluoride treatment to avoid demineralization of the surface. If this option is chosen, the assistant can play a role in observing contact on adjacent teeth and can aid in holding the matrix strip. As in the occlusal preparation the primary responsibility of the assistant is to maintain oral evacuation and retraction.

Refine Margin and Finish

Placement of the cervical margin is often completed as the operator is performing the axial reduction. Regardless of the design of the cervical margin the width of the margin should be uniform throughout the tooth and should be a smooth continuous line completely around the tooth. The operator will check this margin with an explorer. If there is a distinct displacement of an explorer as it is drawn vertically from below the margin or as the explorer is forced cervically from prepared

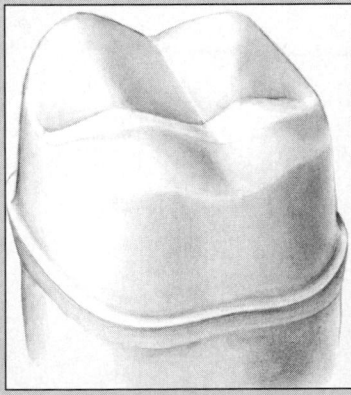

FIG. 30-9 **The completed preparation is characterized by a smooth, even chamfer, a 6-degree taper and gradual transitions between all prepared surfaces.**

(From Rosenstiel SF, Land MF, Fujimoto J: *Contemporary fixed prosthodontics,* ed 3, St Louis, 1995, Mosby.)

tooth surface to nonprepared areas of the tooth the margin must be refined.

The finish of the preparation should allow for a smooth transition from one surface to another. A fine grit, round-tipped diamond that is used on a lower speed can assist in completing the finish. This area of transition (as with all others) should be slightly rounded to allow for ease of impression taking, waxing the pattern, investing and casting the restoration. Sharp corners that are sometimes found when axial walls meet cervical bevels and floors of a preparation must be slightly rounded to avoid fracture (Fig. 30-9). If additional retentive features are desired, they can be placed at this time. This refinement phase requires the assistant to maintain a clear dry field at all times and to be prepared to exchange the explorer and various diamonds and stones until the margins have been finished completely.

Determine Draw and Accuracy

At this point the preparation can be evaluated for accuracy through the use of a snap impression technique. A small amount of impression compound is heated and softened with lubricated gloves and then gently forced over the entire preparation. The impression compound is immediately cooled with water from an a/w syringe to reduce the heat and to decrease the setting time. The assistant cools the area and evacuates the residual water with the HVE. After it has hardened, the impression compound is removed from the preparation and inspected for taper or draw, margin definition, and fracturing. If the margin is not accurate in the snap impression, the operator may elect to refine it at this point. If the impression should fracture on removal, it may have been caused by the design of the preparation, which may need to be altered. It is possible that undercuts are not immediately visible in the oral cavity, which stressed the impression compound on removal and caused the fracture. Again, the preparation must be modified to correct this problem before the final impression is taken.

At this point the assistant rinses and dries the site. During the repeated checks of the preparation it is wise to let the patient rest his or her mouth. During the long periods of preparation the mouth remains in an open position, which can be tiring to the patient's jaw.

Bite Registration

To recreate the correct occlusion of the patient on the models that are being obtained requires a bite registration. Although it may be possible to accomplish the articulation by looking at previous study models, a bite registration can make this task easier, especially if opposing teeth have been altered during tooth preparation. One means of obtaining a bite registration is through the use of specially prepared waxes (some have metal between the two layers of wax to increase strength) that are produced in the shape of the arch. Other waxes, such as

Continued.

PROCEDURE FOR A FULL COVERAGE CROWN—cont'd

baseplate wax, can be folded twice to increase the thickness and rigidity and then are placed in the mouth to register the patient's bite. The wax is placed on either arch, allowing the patient to bite into the mass, thereby obtaining bite registration (Fig. 30-10). If necessary the wax may be preheated to make it more pliable to obtain a more accurate registration of the occlusal surfaces. The patient then is directed to bite firmly into the wax and to hold the position until the warmed wax has cooled. To cool the wax more quickly, the assistant applies water from the syringe over the surface of wax and removes the water with the oral evacuation system.

Bite registrations may also be produced through the use of a rigid impression material; this bite registration paste is dispensed in equal portions, mixed, and placed on a frame for the quadrant. The mesh material on which the paste is placed holds the mixture in place until it hardens. Before the impression material is placed in the mouth, it is necessary to lubricate the teeth that will contact the mixture or the mixture may adhere to the tooth surface. The bite registration material is placed in the mouth, and the patient is directed to close and to hold the arches together. Cool water from the a/w syringe may again be sprayed on the material to decrease the setting time. Care must be taken when using this form of bite registration material because a degree of flow might result in the material being locked in undercuts; this in turn will result in difficulty in removing the bite registration—if not in fracture of the registration—at the time of removal from the oral cavity.

A third form of bite registration is produced through the use of a Triple Tray (brandname). This particular tray allows the operator to secure in one step a bite registration, an opposing bite, and the final impression. The dental material is placed on both sides of the tray and positioned in the mouth when the final impression is taken, allowing the operator to obtain all the desired information in one impression.

A newer form of elastic bite registration material can be injected onto the occlusal surfaces with a syringe-type device. Once the registration material is placed, the patient is directed to occlude onto the material, and it is allowed to set. After the material hardens to a rubberized state, it can be removed and disinfected as directed.

The dental assistant's role during the bite registration procedure is to assemble the armamentarium, to prepare the material, to dispense and evacuate water from the oral cavity, and to properly disinfect the final bite registration. Regardless of the type of bite registration that is used, each one will be checked for accuracy and then disinfected according to OSHA guidelines.

Tissue Management and Retraction

A **cast,** the replica of the prepared structures, is fabricated from the impression, and the fixed prosthesis is made from the cast and die. Thus, an impression or a negative production of the area must be obtained. The **die** is a replica of a single tooth or several teeth. A **wax pattern,** a pattern of the actual shape of the future restoration, is fabricated indirectly on a die outside

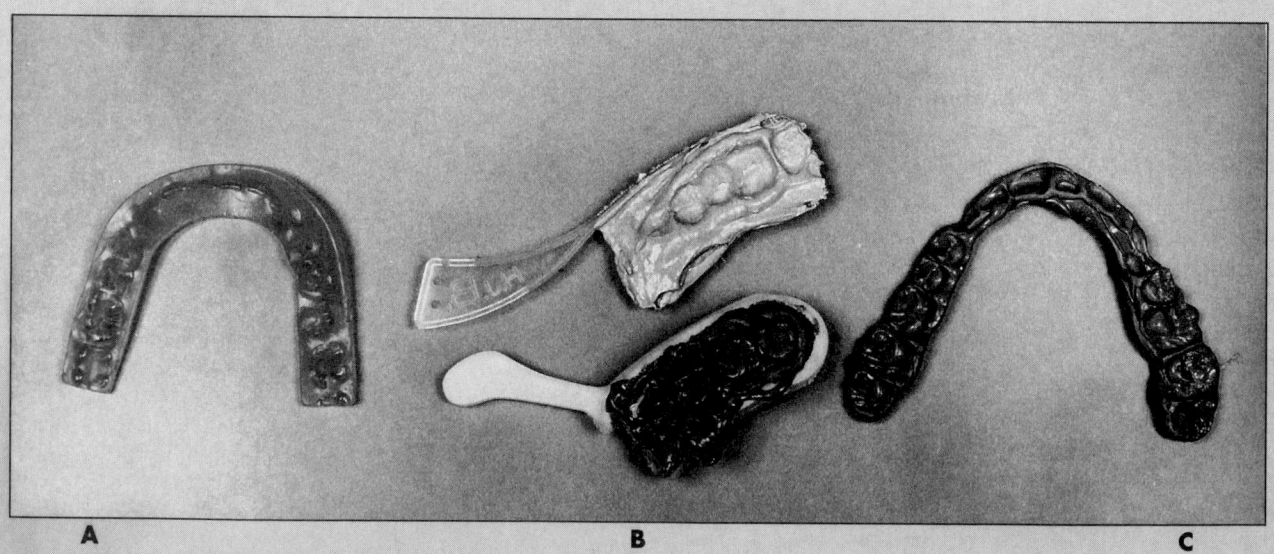

A   B   C

FIG. 30-10   Wax bite. Rigid bite registration. Triple tray. Flexible bite registration.

PROCEDURE FOR A FULL COVERAGE CROWN—cont'd

the patient's mouth. A wax pattern is constructed on the replica of the teeth that becomes the pattern for the cast restoration. To arrive at an acceptable finished restoration an accurate impression must replicate the prepared tooth or teeth, adjacent tissues surrounding the preparation must be free of voids. Before an accurate impression can be obtained, three factors must be considered: tissue health, isolation of the site, and gingival retraction.

Tissue Health

Before the impression is taken, the health of the soft tissue surrounding the prepared tooth is accessed. If the gingiva is inflamed or overly extended, it may interfere with the accuracy of the impression. Measures that are implemented to remove the excess tissue or to reduce the inflammation before impression taking can minimize time and motion later. A dentist may opt to perform an electrosurgery procedure. An **electrosurgery unit**, illustrated in Fig. 30-11, *A* through *C*, can be used for minor tissue removal before taking an impression or to eliminate interference of the tissue at the margin to enlarge the sulcus area.

An electrosurgery unit passes high-frequency current through the tissue from a large to a small electrode, which results in tissue removal. The unit actually cauterizes the tissue, resulting in tissue being removed without bleeding occurring; this is especially important, since bleeding could interfere with obtaining an accurate impression. Several factors that should be considered before using an electrosurgery unit include the following:

1. Use of this machine is contraindicated on or near a patient who has a cardiac pacemaker or a debilitating disease that delays healing or on a patient who is receiving radiotherapy.
2. Metal HVE tips or other metal instruments can not be used with this machine.
3. Soft tissue anesthesia must be maintained.
4. Reduction of odors from the cauterized tissue can be accomplished through the use of the HVE at the surgery site.
5. The sulcus should be cleansed with hydrogen peroxide after the treatment.
6. An impression can be taken immediately following the procedure.

Moisture Control

To maintain the patient's comfort and to ensure an accurate impression, a dry field must be maintained in the preparation during the impression procedure. Many techniques discussed in Chapter 22 can be implemented here. The most common method of maintaining a dry field during this procedure is to use cotton rolls. A svedopter with a tongue flange can be used in the mandibular arch to retract the tongue and to aid in removing saliva. The assistant has primary responsibility for moisture control during the procedure.

If local anesthesia is used, it may reduce saliva flow because of the action the anesthesia has on the periodontal ligament through the nerve impulses. A medication, such as atropine and dicyclomine or anticholinergics, may be prescribed to reduce salivary action from the parasympathetic nerves. However, caution must be taken when prescribing these drugs to patients who are older adults, who have heart disease, or who have glaucoma.

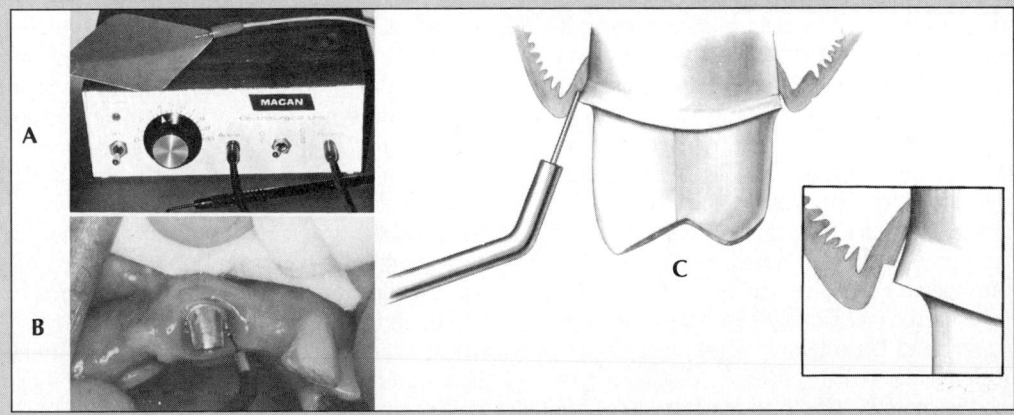

FIG. 30-11 *A,* An electrosurgery unit. *B* and *C,* Unit in use to enlarge the gingival sulcus.
(From Rosenstiel SF, Land MF, Fujimoto J: *Contemporary fixed prosthodontics,* ed 3, St Louis, 1995, Mosby.)

Continued.

PROCEDURE FOR A FULL COVERAGE CROWN—cont'd

Tissue Retraction

To obtain an accurate impression of the prepared area, the soft tissue surrounding the gingival margins must be displaced. Not only is access to the margins increased, but also the space for placement of the impression material is increased to ensure adequate thickness of the impression material.

Tissue retraction or displacement of the gingival tissue is accomplished with the placement of retraction cord in the sulcus. Gingival retraction cord may be impregnated with an astringent of aluminum salts or aluminum chloride to create a transient **ischemia,** also known as a shrinking of the tissues. The cord also assists in controlling seepage of gingival fluids. A previously popular retraction cord was impregnated with a vasoconstrictor, epinephrine, which aids in controlling bleeding. This is not recommended for use since it may cause **tachycardia,** abnormal, rapid heartbeat. Nonimpregnated cord can also be used but is usually left in place for a longer period of time.

The placement of the retraction cord involves cutting a piece of cord of sufficient length to encircle the prepared tooth. If the cord is a nonbraided type, a slight twist in the cord is recommended before placing it around the tooth. The cord is looped and positioned around the crown of the tooth (Fig. 30-12, *A*). The operator gently forces the cord into the sulcus area with an instrument, such as a Geyer 7 or a FP1 plastic instrument. The cord should be placed apical to the cervical margin of the preparation (Fig. 30-12, *B*).

Retraction cord is usually left in place for 5 to 10 minutes to achieve adequate access to the sulcus area. If retraction is not accomplished or if bleeding exists upon removal of the cord, a second attempt may be required. If either of these factors exist at the time a second cord is removed, it may be necessary to place the temporary restoration and have the patient return at a later time for the impression when the tissue is healthier.

Final Impression/Opposing Impression

The final impression is necessary to obtain an accurate recording of the tissues. The technique that is used to obtain a final impression was discussed in detail in Chapter 11. The impression is usually obtained through two steps in the procedure: by using the syringe-tray technique or the putty/wash system. The impression materials of choice include any of the polyether, polysulfide, silicone rubber, or agar hydrocolloid material.

The tray impression material is placed into a custom acrylic or stock impression tray—either a quadrant or full arch tray, depending on the operator's choice and the extent of the preparation. Using a custom acrylic tray ensures that the tray will fit the configuration of the patient's mouth, reducing the amount of impression material that is needed. Whichever type of tray is selected, the impression material must be retained in the tray when it is removed from the mouth after reaching a final set. To retain the material in the tray may require the use

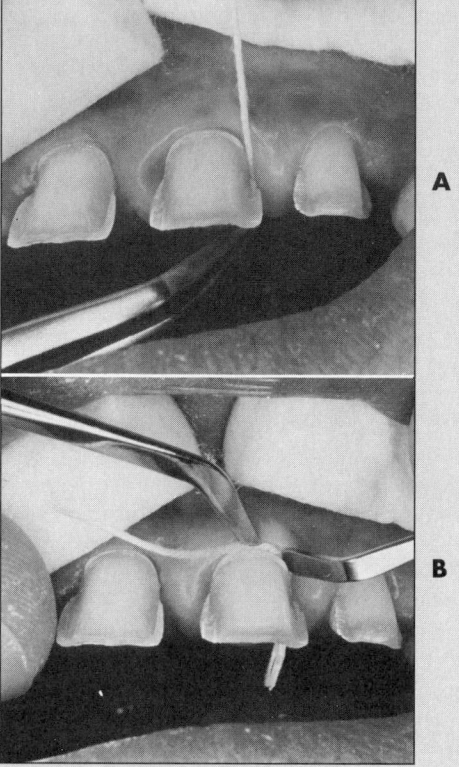

FIG. 30-12   *A,* Retraction cord is positioned at the cervical area. *B,* Second instrument is used to place cord in sulcus area.

(From Rosenstiel SF, Land MF, Fujimoto J: *Contemporary fixed prosthodontics,* ed 3, St Louis, 1995, Mosby.)

of a manufacturer's prepared adhesive and/or the placement of holes in the tray. The impression materials are transferred to the mobile cabinetry for easy access for the assistant.

During the syringe-tray technique of impression taking, both materials are dispensed, and the syringe material is mixed first and loaded into the syringe as described in Chapter 11. The operator observes the assistant mixing the material and, as it nears completion, removes the retraction cord with a cotton forceps, and passes the cord to be discarded (Fig. 30-13). The assistant should be able to pause long enough to transfer the forceps and continue mixing the tray material. The operator evaluates the condition of the sulcus for fluid and retraction; if there is no fluid, the operator receives the loaded syringe from the assistant and begins injecting the material into the sulcus around the preparation and onto the adjacent teeth (Fig. 30-14, *A*). If moisture exists just before the syringe material is injected,

PROCEDURE FOR A FULL COVERAGE CROWN—cont'd

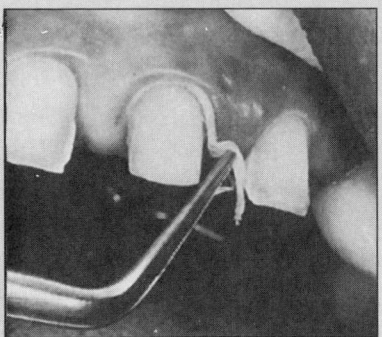

FIG. 30-13 Cord is removed with cotton pliers after approximately 5 minutes.

(From Rosenstiel SF, Land MF, Fujimoto J: *Contemporary fixed prosthodontics,* ed 3, St Louis, 1995, Mosby.)

cotton pellets must be transferred quickly to absorb the moisture. To ignore the moisture can only result in potential voids, requiring a retake of the impression. This is a critical time in the procedure, and the assistant may need to be attentive to multiple areas of responsibility at the same time.

As the operator injects the syringe material, the assistant mixes and places the tray material in the impression tray. Trapping air in the tray must be avoided because this may create voids in the impression, causing a situation that will require taking another impression. To avoid trapping air in the impression, scoop all the tray material onto the mixing spatula and place it in the tray with one continuous movement. As the tray material is prepared and loaded into the tray, the operator or the assistant removes any remaining cotton rolls and excess saliva and the operator immediately places the tray in position

over the prepared area (Fig. 30-14, *B*). After the first few minutes the patient may be placed in a semivertical position for comfort. A saliva ejector should be available to remove any excess saliva.

The assistant continues to monitor the patient during this entire procedure. The operator may leave the patient at this time to perform treatment in another room; if so, the assistant remains with the patient and must monitor the patient's eye movement, facial coloring, ability to breathe, and overall comfort. It may be necessary to remove saliva with the HVE, taking care not to displace the impression tray or material. It is also comforting to the patient to have someone speak to him or her while the impression is reaching the final set. Avoid discussion that would warrant a response from the patient, since he or she is unable to respond.

Once the impression reaches the final set, it is removed from the mouth, rinsed thoroughly under water, dried, and evaluated for accuracy (Fig. 30-14, *C*). If voids or tears are present or if definition of the margins is inadequate, it may be necessary to repeat the previous steps and to retake the impression. The assistant's attention should then turn to the patient, while the operator examines the impression. The patient's mouth can be rinsed, and any debris from the impression can be removed; thank the patient for being so cooperative during the procedure.

An impression of the opposing arch may need to be taken at this time if this has not been done at a previous appointment or if treatment has been provided after the diagnostic models were constructed. If changes in the oral cavity have occurred since the diagnostic models were made, discrepancies in occlusal and proximal contacts may exist. This necessitates a new alginate impression to ensure accuracy for the future laboratory procedures. A quadrant or full-arch impression is taken following the procedures outlined in Chapter 24. When all of the impressions have been taken and are

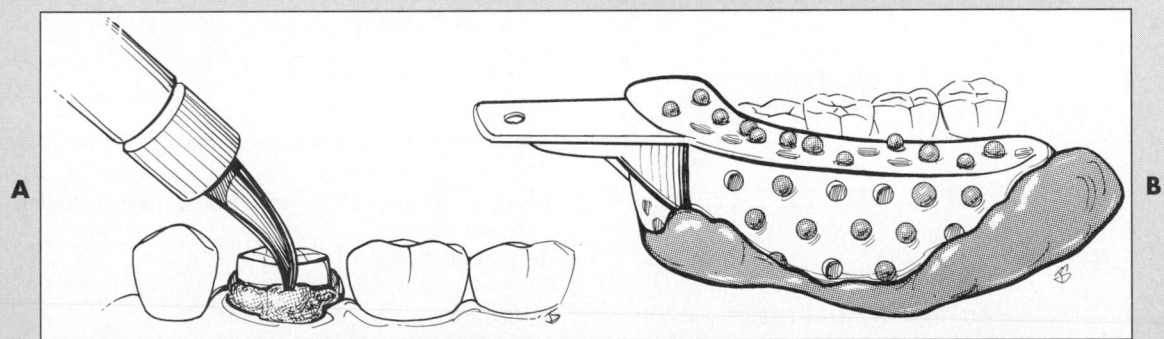

FIG. 30-14 *A,* Injection of syringe material around prepared and adjacent teeth. *B,* Placement of tray material over syringe material.

Continued.

PROCEDURE FOR A FULL COVERAGE CROWN—cont'd

 (STOP)

acceptable, they are disinfected as required by OSHA guidelines.

Temporization

Temporary coverage of the prepared tooth or teeth is made to (1) protect the pulp; (2) maintain periodontal health; (3) prevent the drifting of teeth; (4) prevent fracture of the preparation; and (5) maintain the occlusal relationship. A temporary restoration also restores masticatory and phonetic function of the tooth while it provides esthetics.

The technique for the construction of various temporary restorations is discussed in Chapter 32, *Temporary Restorations.* The choice of a temporary restoration is determined by the operator's preference, the period of time the temporary restoration must remain in the mouth, and the location of the preparation.

Postoperative Instructions

The treatment just described is a relatively invasive procedure that may involve trauma. At the end of the treatment, anesthesia may still be effective, creating a false sense of comfort. Potential discomfort may occur later to the surrounding tissues, with possible sensitivity to the prepared structures and of the temporary restoration.

It is important for the patient to have an understanding of the conditions in the mouth before he or she leaves the treatment room. Not all patients experience discomfort with this treatment; however, it is possible that they may experience some tissue discomfort for a couple of days.

The temporary restoration may also be more sensitive to temperature changes than is tooth tissue. The patient must also be informed of the importance of maintaining the temporary restoration in the mouth. If it should become displaced, the patient is directed to call the dental office to obtain an appointment to replace the temporary restoration. The patient should also be told to avoid eating or chewing sticky or extremely hard foods in the area of the temporary restoration because each may contribute in displacing the restoration.

 (STOP)

- Are the appropriate universal barrier techniques removed?
- Have all of the appropriate surfaces been cleaned and disinfected?
- Has all armamentarium been removed?
- Has all equipment been repositioned?
- Has all of the equipment been disinfected/sterilized according to OSHA guidelines?

BOX 30-3

ARMAMENTARIUM FOR PREPARATION APPOINTMENT

Explorer
Mirror
Cotton pliers
Cotton rolls
2 × 2 gauze
Anesthesia setup
Spoon excavator
Gingival retraction packing
    instrument (Geyer 7, FPI)
Retraction cord
Astringent agent
Scissors
Rotary instruments for high- and low-speed usage
    Diamond burs or stones
    Fissure burs, tapered and straight
    Diamond disks
    Mandrels and assorted finishing disks

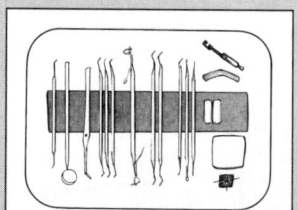

28 gauge casting wax
Maxillary and mandibular impression trays, quadrant or full
    arch as needed
Impression material for
    Opposing model
    Final impression
Mixing pads/bowls, spatulas, and syringe for impressions
Bite registration material and armamentarium
Means of temporization: acrylic, preformed aluminum
    crown, coping
Temporary cement
Floss
Articulating paper
Articulating paper forceps
Thumb forceps
Cement placement instrument

LABORATORY PRESCRIPTION/REQUISITION

It is common for the dentist to use the services of a commercial laboratory for the construction of the fixed restoration. A **laboratory prescription**, specific directions from the dentist to the laboratory technician, must be sent to a commercial laboratory with each case. The impression, casts, bite registration, and other materials, such as a shade button are sent with the prescription. Included on the prescription is a description of the type of prosthesis that is to be constructed, the type of alloy or other dental material that is to be used, shade selection, a diagram of the device, possibly a diagram that indicates areas in which different shades may be requested. Other vital information includes the dentist's name, address, and phone number, as well as the patient's name and case number. If a try in is desired, a date is designated and the date for the final restoration is requested.

Laboratory Procedure

The laboratory phase (Box 30-2) actually begins the minute the impression is complete. The impression is disinfected, wrapped in toweling, and placed in a plastic bag before sending it to the laboratory technician. Some dentists or other team members actually perform some of the laboratory procedures in the office. It is possible to make the die and cast in the office and articulate the models before the case is transferred to a commercial laboratory. Continuation of the laboratory procedures in the dental office is possible to the point of actually fabricating the cast.

It is wise for the assistant to have an understanding of the laboratory process to comprehend the many steps in a fixed prosthodontic procedure, which will enable the assistant to understand the value of the investment in this type of restoration. This comprehension and understanding will enable the assistant to articulate the procedure and its value to the patient.

▶ Armamentarium for the Laboratory Procedure

The following list includes instruments and materials that are used to fabricate the full cast crown. The armamentarium is divided into four phases:
Phase I — Creating casts and dies
Impression of prepared areas of the mouth
Opposing impression or model
Die material
High strength stone
Mixing bowls and spatulas
Dowel pin
Separating agent
Die space
Articulator
Sticking wax and sticks
Bite registration
Phase II — Fabricating the wax pattern
Casting wax for patterns
Waxing instruments including #7 spatula
Bunsen burner
Phase III — Investing the wax pattern
Crucible former
Sprue material
Ring liner
Casting ring
Surfactant
Sable brush
Investment material and armamentarium
Phase IV — Making the casting
Furnace
Centrifuge and crucible
Air/gas torch
Flux
Alloy
Tongs
Pickling solution
Finishing and polishing devices

Creating Casts and Dies

The most common procedure used in dentistry to create a metal casting is referred to as the **indirect technique**: the wax pattern for the metal casting is produced indirectly on a replica of the actual tooth. The laboratory procedure begins with the construction of working casts and dies, since this method of fabrication of a restoration is efficient, less time consuming, more convenient, and less susceptible to fracture than a **direct** procedure, which creates the wax pattern on the actual tooth in the oral cavity. Before the wax pattern is made, a **working cast** and opposing model must be made. A cast is a working replica of the prepared tooth or teeth, the supporting tissues, and all relevant soft tissues and their contours. An **opposing model** is a replica of the opposite arch, including the teeth in occlusion with the preparation. These models are articulated together to recreate the existing conditions of the patient's oral cavity, which can then be used to create the fixed prosthesis in the laboratory. Within the arch of the cast the prepared tooth or teeth are separated from the cast to create a **die**. The die is a portion of the cast, the prepared tooth, or the area in which the fixed prosthesis is to be fabricated. The die can be taken out of the cast to enable the technician to work on the individual tooth or teeth. The accuracy of the cast and die depend on the accuracy of tissue registration and impression.

▶ Types of Dies

The gypsum products used to construct models, casts, and dies were discussed extensively in Chapter 11. While study models are usually produced from model plaster, an arch is used as an opposing model for articulation of both arches and is made from dental stone for greater strength. A die, if constructed of gypsum, is usually done so with high-strength stone (Fig. 30-15, *A* and *B*). If model plaster or even dental stone is used for a die, the gypsum would succumb to abrasion during instrumentation of the wax and the cast restoration. Thus, a material must be used that can withstand these forces.

A die can also be fabricated from epoxy or through electroplating techniques. An **epoxy die** is composed of epoxy resin that is used to fabricate a precision die.

Electroplated dies are an alternative to gypsum dies, which require a coating of pure silver or copper on the impression, particularly in the area of the prepared tooth and the abutment teeth. Various cast and die systems may be employed during this procedure. Two commonly accepted systems are the removable die system and the solid cast with the individual die system. Alternative die systems, such as the Di-Lok (brandname) and the Divestment (brandname) techniques, require the use of different materials and procedures. The following text addresses the fabrication of a die and cast through the use of the removable die technique.

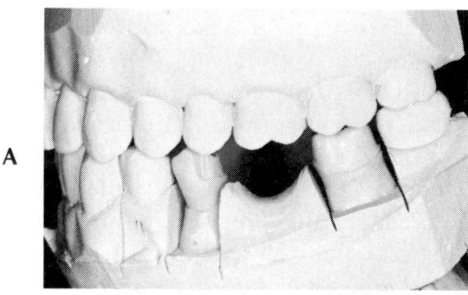
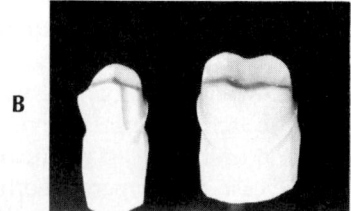

FIG. 30-15 Removable die system. *A,* Working cast. *B,* Individual dies.

(From Rosenstiel SF, Land MF, Fujimoto J: *Contemporary fixed prosthodontics,* ed 3, St Louis, 1995, Mosby.)

▶ Die Techniques

The **removable gypsum die technique** requires a two-pour system of creating a cast and die. Type IV stone, possibly of two different colors, is used to pour the die first and then the remaining cast. Strips of stainless steel can be positioned between the teeth in the impression to create an area of separation. The area of the prepared tooth and abutment teeth is poured with stone. Before the stone is completely set, a dowel pin, with one flattened side, or a brass pin is placed directly over the prepared tooth and secured in position (Fig. 30-16, *A*). A separating medium is placed over the dowel pin and stone for ease in separation from the rest of the cast later. The remainder of the impression is poured as seen in Fig. 30-16, *B*.

The cast is separated from the impression and inspected for any voids after the stone has hardened (Fig. 30-16, *C*). The doweled areas are tapped to remove the die from the cast. The separating strips are also removed. The buccal and lingual sulcal areas are trimmed in the area of the removable section of the cast. If the metal separators were not used, a hand saw is used to carefully place cuts between the preparation and the abutment teeth, leaving the margins and the proximal contact of the preparation intact (Fig. 30-16, *D*). The proximal cuts must be completely through the first pour of stone to release the die from the rest of the cast. A slight tap on the end of the dowel pin should dislodge the die from the cast.

The die is trimmed, removing excess stone that surrounds the preparation through the use of an arbor band, carbide burs, or a scalpel. The die is replaced in the cast in the correct position (Fig. 30-16, *E*).

 F Y I Teeth with inlays of jade and turquoise can be traced back to the Mayan skulls in the ninth century, A.D.

ARTICULATING THE CASTS

It is critical for working casts to be accurately mounted to an articulator. A less-than-accurate articulation of the casts may produce a cast restoration that does not fit the prepared tooth or teeth, resulting in increased chairside time during cementation.

An **articulator** is a device that simulates a patient's jaw relationships and movement. Since articulators are mechanical devices, the ability to reproduce all movement of the mandible is limited; the articulator can only be expected to provide a minimal level of clinical acceptance. Articulators are available with a variety of features. Each patient's case will dictate the type of articulator that is needed for each process (Fig. 30-17).

The bite registration that is taken during the prepara-

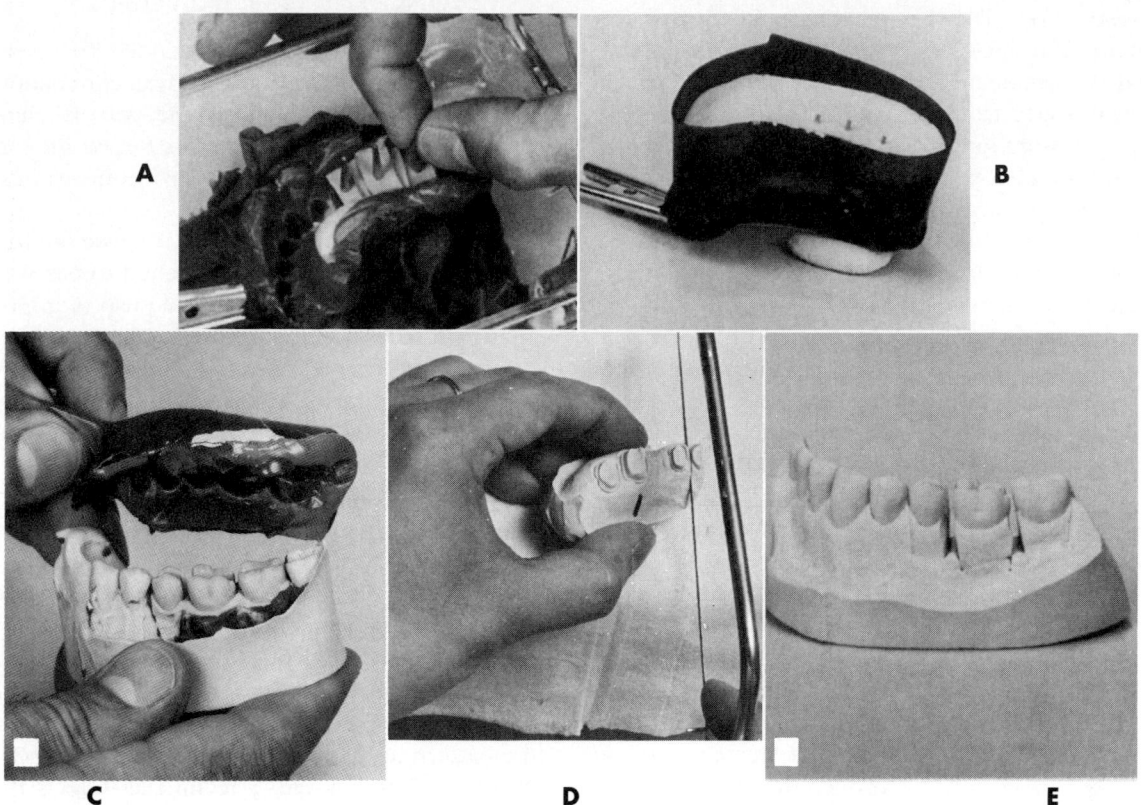

FIG. 30-16   *A,* The dowel pin is positioned in the stone before it is set. *B,* Boxed and poured impression. *C,* Withdrawing cast from impression. *D,* Hand saw used to section dies. *E,* The trimmed die is positioned in the cast.

(*A, B, C,* and *E* from Sturdevant CM et al: *The art and science of operative dentistry,* ed 3, St Louis, 1994, Mosby; *D* from Rosenstiel SF, Land MF, Fujimoto J: *Contemporary fixed prosthodontics,* St Louis, 1995, Mosby.)

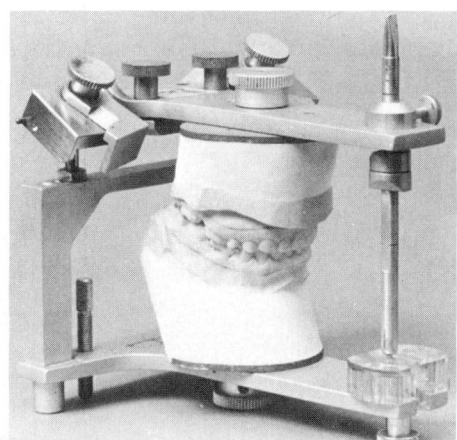

FIG. 30-17   Working cast and opposing model are articulated on the articulator.

(From Rosenstiel SF, Land MF, Fujimoto J: *Contemporary fixed prosthodontics,* ed 3, St Louis, 1995, Mosby.)

tion appointment provides a guide to the centric relationship and the working and balancing relationship of the arches. Assembling the casts with dies, bite registration, and articulator as one working unit may be necessary to replicate the patient's articulation.

FABRICATING THE WAX PATTERN

To create a wax pattern on a die requires the armamentarium shown in Phase II of the laboratory armamentarium list.

The **wax pattern** is the reproduction of tooth structure that will become the cast restoration. The pattern must be accurate, with limited or no distortion, and must fit correctly on the prepared tooth. The steps in the fabrication of the wax pattern include placing the die spacer, flowing the wax on the die, and carving the wax pattern to the desired tooth morphology.

A die spacer is placed on a die to accommodate the space necessary for the cement during cementation of the cast restoration. The die spacer is painted over the surface in an even thickness. After the spacer is dry, the margins of the preparation are marked with a pencil to distinguish this area from the rest of the die.

Waxing a restoration requires knowledge of tooth anatomy and the ability to reproduce three-dimensional structures. The person waxing the pattern can use the abutment teeth, the opposing teeth, and the same tooth in the opposite quadrant as anatomic references during the carving procedure.

One of the pattern waxes described in Chapter 11, *Dental Materials,* is used to create the wax pattern. Each of these waxes has different characteristics, and the laboratory technician makes the decision based on the physical properties of the material and how it is to be used.

The removable die provides ease in handling the prepared tooth, allowing for visual access to all areas of the die. The first step in creating the wax pattern is the application of a die lubricant. Before any wax is placed, the lubricant must be completely dry. The waxing instrument is heated on the shank in a Bunsen burner to allow the wax to flow off the tip of the instrument. The wax is flowed onto the die from a heated waxing instrument. The wax must be applied in small portions, since wax has a memory, which can cause distortion. This *memory* means that unless the wax is completely liquified it maintains some elasticity that can cause distortion. By placing the wax in small molten drops on the pattern this memory is removed.

The laboratory technician uses a #7 wax spatula, Ward's carver waxing instruments, and other carving instruments and creates a wax pattern that simulates natural anatomy, with properly trimmed margins. The wax is built up on the die, establishing margins, proximal and occlusal or incisal contacts, cusp height and location, and axial contour. Each addition of wax to the die is allowed to cool before more wax is applied. The wax is removed from the die periodically to evaluate the developing pattern (Fig. 30-18). Once this procedure has been completed, the pattern is invested.

INVESTING THE WAX PATTERN

The wax pattern must be surrounded by a heat-resistant investment material to allow for wax elimination through heat. The area from which the wax is eliminated is replaced by molten alloy that is forced into the investment. The technique for this procedure varies, but the final result is similar.

After the wax pattern is made, a sprue pin that is made of wax, plastic, or metal is attached to the wax pattern at the bulkiest and least involved cusp (Fig. 30-19). The **sprue** provides a tunnel through which the molten alloy flows from a crucible to the area in which the wax has been eliminated. Hot wax is added at the point where the sprue is attached to the pattern. The pattern and sprue are removed from the die and placed in the hole of the sprue former. This assembly is secured in place with hot wax at the base of the sprue and the former (Fig. 30-20).

A wax pattern cleaner, or **surfactant**, is carefully painted over the pattern to increase the wetting of the pattern during investing. A casting ring is lined with a moist ring liner and positioned evenly inside the ring. The ring is positioned over the crucible former and the sprued pattern to ensure adequate space from the tip of the pattern to the top of the investment ring (Fig. 30-21, *A* and *B*). The laboratory technician selects the type of investment material that is to be used, according to the casting procedure and type of alloy to be cast.

The two methods of investing a wax pattern are manual and mechanical. Following the manufacturer's directions the investment material is mixed with the appropriate amount of water and is mixed by hand or is attached to a vacuum investment hose. Using a brush the pattern is painted with the investment material and is gently vibrated over all surfaces. The casting ring is attached to the sprue former, and the investment material is poured into the ring, using either a vibrator for the hand technique or the vacuum machine for a mechanical process (Fig. 30-22). Care should be taken to avoid air

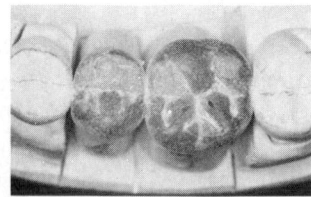

FIG. 30-18   **Wax pattern on die.**

(From Rosenstiel SF, Land MF, Fujimoto]: *Contemporary fixed prosthodontics,* ed 3, St Louis, 1995, Mosby.)

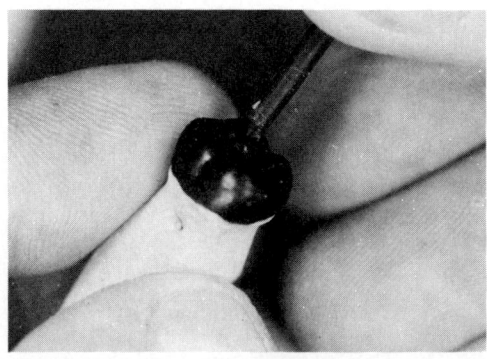

FIG. 30-19   **A wax sprue is attached to the wax pattern.**

(From Rosenstiel SF, Land MF, Fujimoto]: *Contemporary fixed prosthodontics,* ed 3, St Louis, 1995, Mosby.)

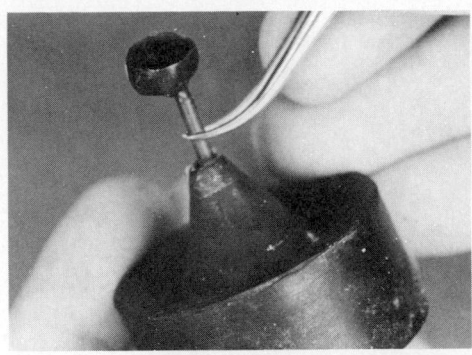

FIG. 30-20   The wax pattern and sprue are attached to the former.

(From Rosenstiel SF, Land MF, Fujimoto J: *Contemporary fixed prosthodontics,* ed 3, St Louis, 1995, Mosby.)

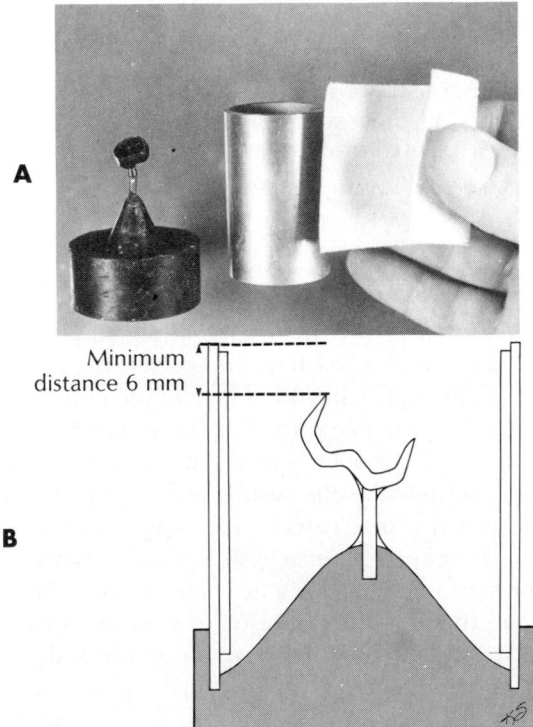

Minimum distance 6 mm

FIG. 30-21   *A,* A ring liner is placed in the investment ring that is positioned over the wax pattern and crucible former. *B,* The pattern must be positioned ⅛ to ¼ of an inch from the end of the investment ring.

(From Rosenstiel SF, Land MF, Fujimoto J: *Contemporary fixed prosthodontics,* ed 3, St Louis, 1995, Mosby.)

being trapped during the process and to ensure that the thickness of the investment material is uniform between the pattern and casting ring. The investment material is allowed to harden for approximately 1 hour; this hardening process may take place on the counter or in a hygroscopic water bath.

ELIMINATING WAX

The lost wax technique used in dentistry today has changed little from its earlier days in the eighteenth century. Today, this same casting process is used for the creation of rings, brooches, tie pins, and fine jewelry.

The **lost wax technique** is based on the principle that a pattern is made in wax, placed into a container that is surrounded by an investment plaster that hardens in the mold, and when the mold is heated, the wax pattern melts away or is *lost.* Metal is then cast into the cavity that is left by the *lost wax* and duplicates the original wax pattern. The mold is then destroyed to recover the casting.

To create the cast crown from the previously invested wax pattern, the crucible former is removed from the investment ring; if a metal sprue has been used, it is removed at this time. If a wax or plastic sprue has been used, it can remain to melt away. The ring is placed in a furnace at a temperature and for a length of time that is determined by the type of investment material. During this time the casting ring may need to be repositioned. After the appropriate burnout time, the investment is ready to be cast.

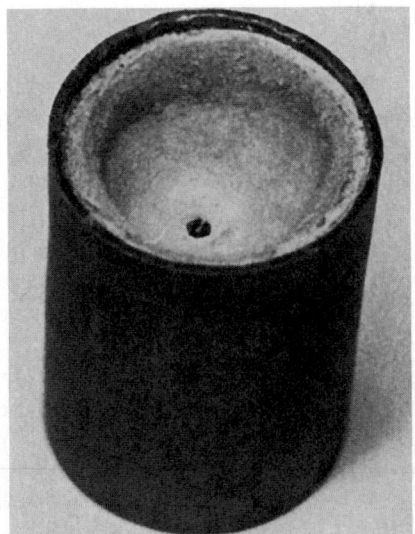

FIG. 30-22   Investment mixing machine.

(From Craig RG, Powers JM, O'Brien WJ: *Dental materials,* ed 5, St Louis, 1992, Mosby.)

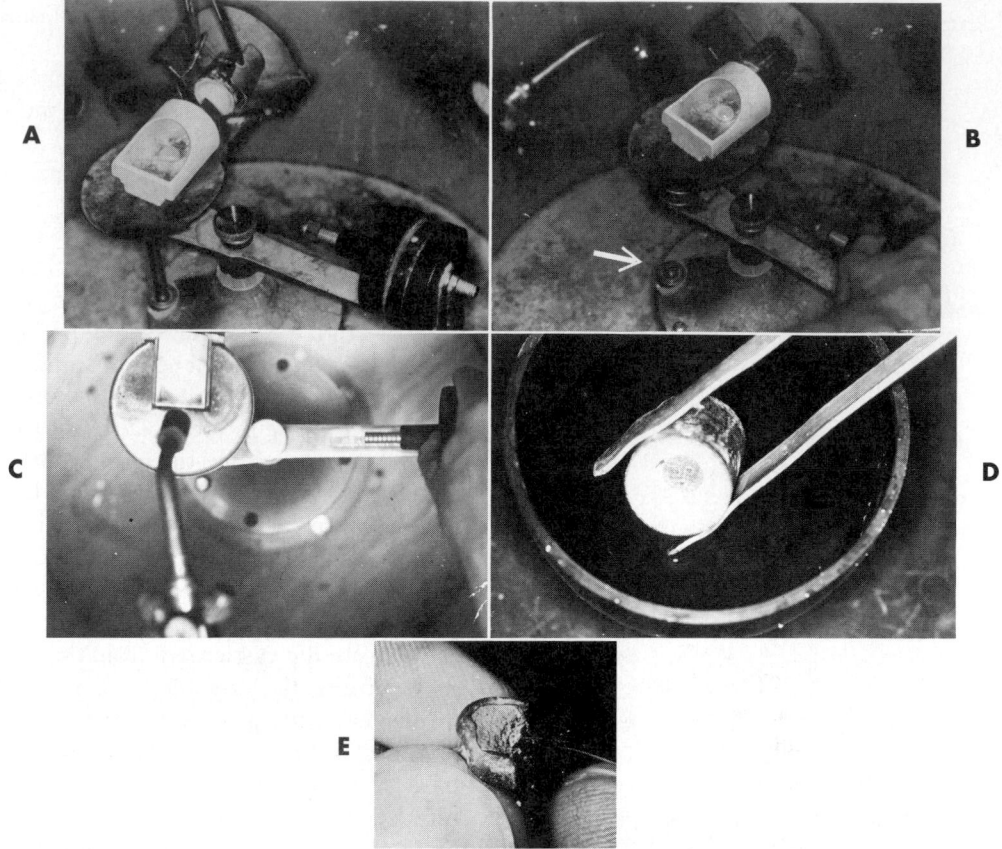

FIG. 30-23   *A,* The alloy is heated in the crucible. *B,* The investment casting ring is removed from the oven and placed on the crucible platform. *C,* The alloy is heated until it becomes molten. *D,* The ring is quenched in cold water. *E,* The casting is removed from the investment.

(From Rosenstiel SF, Land MF, Fujimoto J: *Contemporary fixed prosthodontics,* ed 3, St Louis, 1995, Mosby.)

CASTING THE ALLOY

Several steps occur simultaneously in the wax elimination process, and the casting of the alloy occurs simultaneously. The casting step in the laboratory procedure involves the use of a broken-arm centrifugal casting machine and an air/gas casting torch. The casting machine is turned clockwise three times and is secured in place with a pin. A crucible with a liner is placed in the cradle of the machine. The operator must have protective eyewear in place.

The air/gas torch is lit and adjusted for maximum effectiveness, and the armature, cradle, and crucible are all preheated. The alloy is placed in the crucible and melted in the reducing portion of the flame. Once the alloy is molten, **flux** (a powder that is sprinkled over the alloy to remove impurities) is placed on the molten alloy (Fig. 30-23, *A*). The alloy looks different when it is molten, depending on its content. Gold alloy becomes red, balls up, is shiny and moves freely.

Tongs are used to remove the casting ring from the furnace and quickly place it on the crucible platform with the sprue opening facing the orifice of the crucible (Fig. 30-23, *B*). The crucible platform is moved to contact the sprue opening. The alloy is heated until it is molten, and the pin is dropped as the casting arm is pulled forward and the armature is released to spin (Fig. 30-23, *C*). The centrifugal force of the machine forces the molten alloy into the sprue opening. The machine begins to slow the spin, and the tongs can be used to stop the turning. A commercial laboratory may use an automated casting machine for this process.

RECOVERING THE CAST

Once the bright red glow of the molten alloy subsides, the casting ring is removed from the crucible platform and placed in a bowl of water (Fig. 30-23, *D*). The investment material begins disintegrating as it is submerged in the water. Once it is cool to the touch, any remaining investment material can be removed with a brush (Fig. 30-23, *E*). The internal surface integrity must be maintained because any scratches or margin damage can result in damage to the die when the casting is fitted in place.

FINISHING THE CAST RESTORATION

The first step in finishing is to pickle the casting to remove tarnish and oxides. This process is accomplished by placing the casting in a heat-resistant container that is filled with pickling solution. The container is placed over an open flame; however, it is not allowed to boil, but it is heated thoroughly to enable the solution to work on the surfaces of the casting. Any instrument used to retrieve the casting from the pickling solution must be protected with a plastic coating; otherwise the surface of the instrument will become etched. The casting and instrument are rinsed thoroughly under running water to remove all residue.

The cast restoration is then cut free of the sprue and the **sprue button**, excess alloy that is needed to maintain flow during the casting procedure; these are cut from the casting with a disk (Fig. 30-24). The casting is then recontoured, finished, and polished before it is returned from the laboratory for placement in the patient's mouth.

The internal surface of a casting does not require any finishing or polishing because it has been constructed to fit the tooth with adequate space for the cement, yet still maintaining retentive qualities. Disks and stones are used to adjust the contour of the casting. Various stones and burs, such as green stones and finishing burs, can be used to place a satin finish on the alloy, while the refining occlusal morphology of the restoration is placed.

The restoration is placed on the die of the working cast and is evaluated for proximal and occlusal contact, margin definition, and overall contour. Adjustments to any of these areas are made, and the restoration is reevaluated.

Assorted abrasives, disks, points, and polishing wheels are used to finish the cast restoration. The finishing and polishing process begins with the use of the most coarse material or device and continues to the least abrasive, going from a finishing level to a polishing level. Common polishing materials include Tripoli, rouge, and other buffing compounds that are often used on rag wheels to obtain a high gloss on the surface of the restoration (Fig. 30-25).

Cementation Procedure

The cast restoration that is returned from the laboratory needs to be disinfected as described by OSHA regulations before it is placed in the patient's mouth; this process includes rinsing the casting thoroughly under running water and placing it in a disinfectant for approximately 10 minutes. The casting then is removed and rinsed again to flush any disinfectant residue from the casting. The patient may not need to be anesthetized for this procedure; it is often helpful if the patient is not anesthetized. The patient who is anesthetized may not be as sensitive to occlusal contact or proximal pressure during try in and cementation. Therefore, if the tooth is not uncomfortable, the dentist may opt to seat the casting without anesthesia.

As noted in Box 30-2 the cementation appointment involves removing the temporary restoration, cleaning and drying the preparation, anesthesia (if necessary), isolation, trying in the casting to determine contact and occlusion, adjusting the casting to proper contact and occlusion, seating the casting, and burnishing and finishing the margins.

▶ Armamentarium for Cementation Procedure

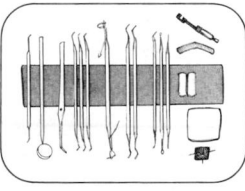

The armamentarium needed in the cementation procedure includes the following:
Cast restoration and working cast

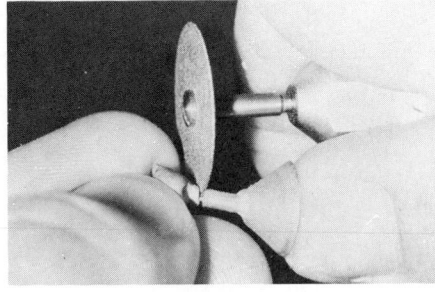

FIG. 30-24   The sprue button is removed from the cast restoration.

(From Rosenstiel SF, Land MF, Fujimoto J: *Contemporary fixed prosthodontics*, ed 3, St Louis, 1995, Mosby.)

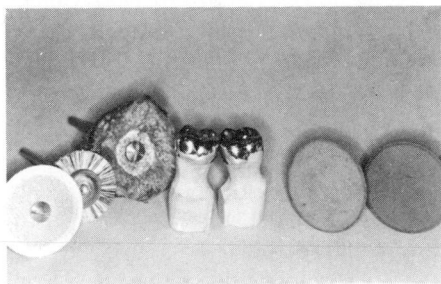

FIG. 30-25   The cast restoration is polished to a high gloss with buffing compounds and rag wheels.

(From Rosenstiel SF, Land MF, Fujimoto J: *Contemporary fixed prosthodontics*, ed 3, St Louis, 1995, Mosby.)

Explorer

Mirror

Cotton pliers

Cotton rolls and gauze

Rubber dam setup (optional procedure)

Spoon excavator

Instruments for removing the temporary restoration and the final restoration before cementation: modified sickle scaler, curet scaler, large spoon excavator, crown remover

Finishing and polishing devices, such as rubber wheels, finishing burs and stones, mandrels, and disks

Articulating paper and holder

Shimstock

Floss

Burnishers, ball/2 to 3S

Tripoli and rag wheel

Cement and necessary armamentarium

Cooley peg

Orangewood stick

Lubricant

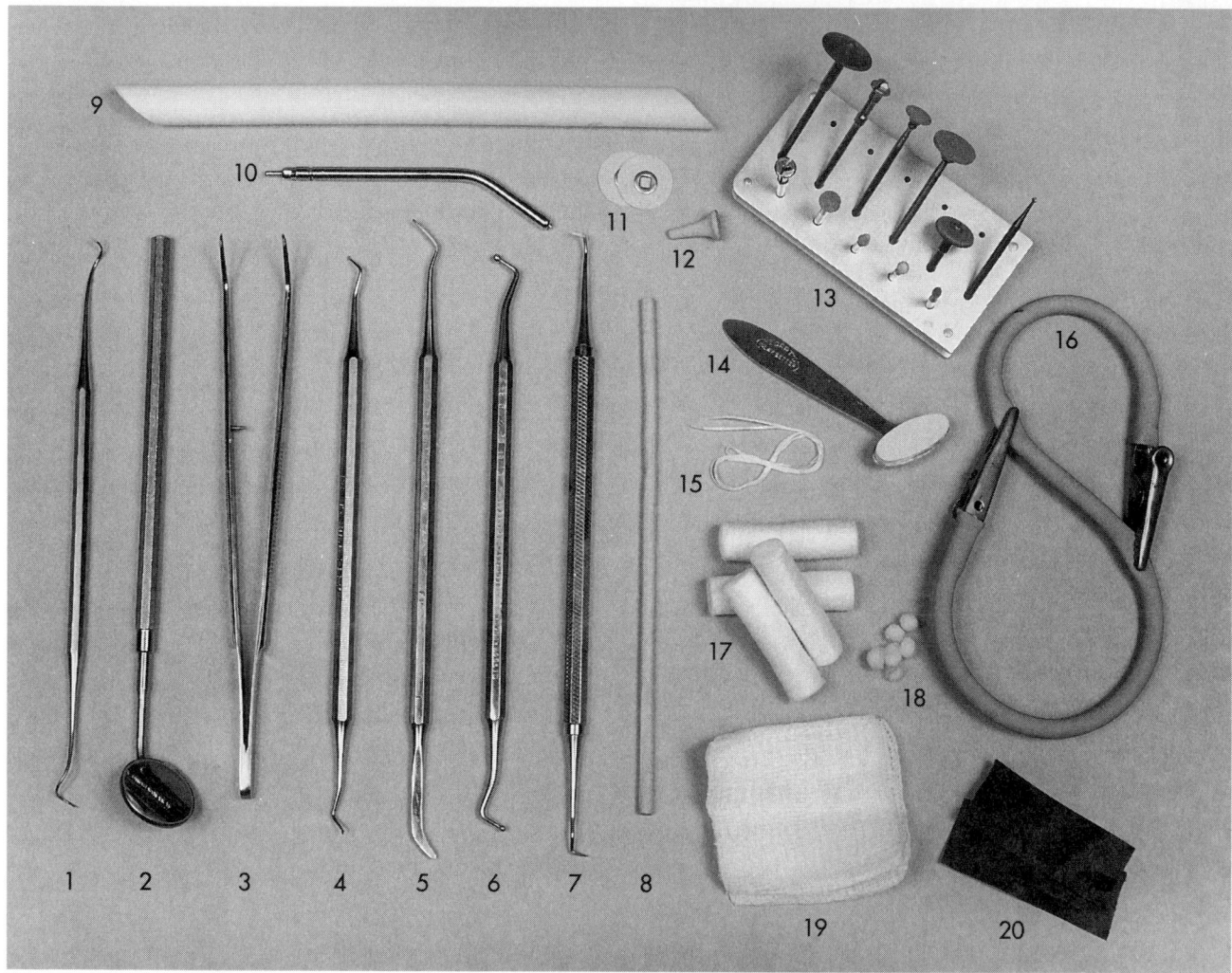

1. Explorer
2. Mirror
3. Cotton pliers
4. Spoon excavator
5. Plastic instrument
6. Ball burnisher
7. Modified sickle scaler
8. Orangewood stick
9. HVE tip
10. A/W tip
11. Abrasive disks

12. Cooley peg
13. Assorted stones and disks
14. Inlay seater
15. Dental floss
16. Napkin chain
17. Cotton rolls
18. Cotton pellets
19. 2 × 2 gauze
20. Articulating paper

Not pictured: final restoration and cementation armamentarium

FIG. 30-26   Example of a cementation tray set-up.

SEATING THE CAST RESTORATION

Removing the Temporary Restoration

To remove the temporary restoration, the assistant passes an instrument, such as a modified sickle scaler or a crown remover. The dentist places the device at the most accessible margin and luxates (twists, dislocates) or loosens the temporary restoration from the tooth. The temporary restoration may be resistant to this action; it may require numerous attempts to dislodge the temporary restoration.

The temporary restoration and any remaining cement are removed from the prepared tooth. Excess cement left in place interferes during the try in of the cast restoration. The tooth may be lightly polished with a polishing paste and cup to remove any residual cement. If the preparation is an intracoronal restoration, the procedure is not significantly different. Again, a scaler may be used to loosen the cement, followed by removal of any remaining cement. The primary task is to loosen the temporary cement and to lift it out. It is helpful to allow a temporary restoration, such as a full coverage crown, to remain intact during removal if possible. If the temporary restoration must be replaced because the cast restoration fits inaccurately, time and motion can be saved by using the same temporary again.

Trying in the Cast Restoration

The initial try in of the casting involves checking the contact relationship, checking the occlusion, and determining the margin integrity.

Checking the Contact

The casting is passed to the operator to insert. At first, the operator uses hand pressure to seat the crown; some resistance may be met. If the crown does not go into place, the first area of adjustment is usually the proximal contact. The contact may be heavy, which results in the incomplete seating of the casting and the inability to pass floss through the contact, and in pressure at the contact points. If the contact is light, the restoration will fall into place without any resistance. A contact that is ideal will allow for a snapping action of the floss as it is passed through the contact.

The area of excessive contact can be determined by placing a matte finish with a rubber wheel on the surface of the restoration. The restoration is placed on the tooth and a shiny scratch mark will appear at the point of contact. Reduction of the area and the replacement of the matte finish before a subsequent try in will allow for the testing of the contact again. The patient will be able to indicate if pressure is felt when the restoration is placed and may have the feeling that teeth are being forced apart. A slight amount of tightness should be present before the final polish of the restoration. Polishing the cast will remove a slight amount of material. The assistant will be involved in a continuous exchange of materials, such as stones, disks, and burs on the handpiece, explorer, and other instruments, as well as floss, while the restoration is adjusted.

During this time the assistant must also maintain a clear, dry site that is free of debris.

If the contact is too light, it will be necessary to add solder to establish a contact. This process is described during modifications of the procedure later in the chapter.

The consequence of an improper contact can result in damage to the tissues later. If a contact is left open or is light, the patient can trap food, causing trauma to the interdental papilla. If it remains tight, the patient will be unable to pass floss through the contact area to maintain healthy oral tissues.

Checking Margin Integrity

Once the proximal contact is established and the restoration is seated on the tooth, the margin integrity is assessed. An explorer is passed to the operator, and it is moved from the restoration to the tooth and from the tooth to the restoration. During this probing procedure, no evidence of resistance should be apparent. If resistance is found in both directions, there is an opening in the area, which can result in an ill-fitting casting, with the potential for bacterial invasion, eventually resulting in loss of the restoration. If the casting has inadequate margins, a new impression must be obtained, and the laboratory procedure must be repeated to create a new casting. If the resistance is in a single direction, the situation is corrected by finishing the margin areas. The assistant exchanges various burnishers, fine point stones, and rubber points on the slow-speed handpiece, until the margins do not offer any resistance during probing. Only when the margins have been deemed adequate does the operator proceed to the next step.

Checking Occlusion

The occlusal contact of the maxillary and mandibular teeth is evaluated to ensure that distribution of contact exists throughout the mouth; the operator can determine this by having the patient close on the restoration and by visually assessing the areas. Shimstock, a narrow strip of silver Mylar, is placed throughout the mouth at contact areas (Fig. 30-27). If resistance is met when an attempt is made to pull the Mylar strip from the closed mouth, contact is confirmed in this area. This technique can be used to confirm contact throughout the mouth. If contact is not confirmed, the operator may test the same area without the new restoration in place. The open contact may be a normal situation in the patient's mouth, or the new restoration may need adjustment on the occlusal to allow greater closure of the arches.

Articulating paper is used to mark any interference in the relationship of the arches. The paper is held in place, and the patient is directed to close in the centric position and to shift from working to balancing relationships; this information will alert the operator to the need for additional adjustments in the restoration. If it appears that too much adjustment has occurred because the occlusal plane of the cast restoration is thinning or if excessive relief of the opposing tooth to the

Continued.

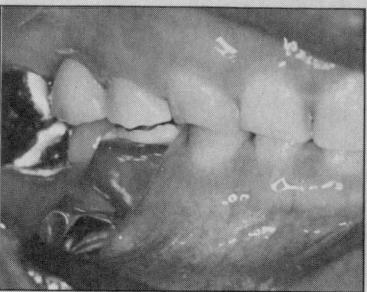

FIG. 30-27   Shimstock used to check centric tooth contact.

(From Rosenstiel SF, Land MF, Fujimoto J: *Contemporary fixed prosthodontics,* ed 3, St Louis, 1995, Mosby.)

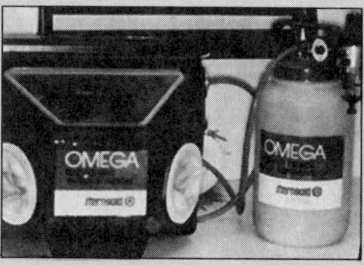

FIG. 30-28   Occlusal prematurities can be identified by giving the casting a matte finish with an air abrasion unit. The prematurities will appear as shiny areas.

(From Rosenstiel SF, Land MF, Fujimoto J: *Contemporary fixed prosthodontics,* ed 3, St Louis, 1995, Mosby.)

restoration is necessary, the operator must decide whether to take a new impression and make a new casting.

Occlusal contacts can be evaluated with a technique that is similar to the proximal contact: a matte finish is placed on the surface through the use of rotary instruments or a sandblast unit (Fig. 30-28). The patient is directed to occlude, and heavy contact areas will appear scratched giving the operator guidance for relief of the area. Occlusal indicator pastes and other such systems are also available for use in this step.

During this procedure the dental assistant will be responsible for numerous exchanges of instruments and devices, as well as for placement of articulating paper as needed. Markings and residue may be removed from the articulating paper and the indicator pastes with gauze sponges that are wiped over the occlusal surfaces.

When all the adjustments for seating have been made, the final finish and polish of the restoration is complete. The

dentist may likely move from the treatment room to the laboratory equipment in the office to perform these tasks. When this is done, the operator must be concerned about cross-contamination. If contamination occurs, the laboratory equipment must be properly disinfected and sterilized. The restoration is brought to a high polish to reduce the possibility of food and plaque adhering to the surface. The cast restoration is disinfected after polishing to remove any contaminants before cementation.

Cementing the Cast Restoration

In certain situations the operator may elect to temporarily cement a restoration. If the tooth becomes symptomatic during the procedure, the operator may suspect future endodontic involvement with the tooth. Rather than diminish the integrity of the new restoration by opening the tooth for endodontic access later, the operator may opt to cement the restoration temporarily. In this situation a temporary ZOE cement that allows easy removal of the restoration at a later time is ideal.

The permanent cementation of the restoration involves the selection of a luting agent that has a relatively long working time, adheres well to the tooth and the restoration, establishes a good seal, has compressive strength, is nonirritating to the pulp, and has low viscosity and solubility characteristics. Currently, no cement can supply all of these characteristics to the operator. However, many cements provide most of these factors, including the most commonly used luting agents, such as zinc phosphate, glass ionomer and zinc polycarboxylate cements. Each has specific characteristics as described in *Dental Materials;* Chapter 11, the operator chooses the materials to use in a given situation.

Cementation

The restoration and the tooth are inspected for any debris or contaminants. The field must be isolated, the tooth is dried and the patient is directed to remain with the mouth open. The dental assistant prepares the cavity varnish, if needed, to limit any pulpal irritation that might occur from the luting agent.

The dental assistant prepares the luting agent. In this case, a zinc phosphate cement is prepared for a primary consistency. A thin layer of lubricant can be applied to the exterior of the crown for ease in removing cement that exudes during placement of the restoration. Care must be taken not to place any lubricant on the interior of the crown because this would interfere with the function of the luting agent and the integrity of the margin seal. A thin coat of cement is placed to cover all internal surfaces of the restoration completely. The tooth is dried again.

The assistant places the crown in the palm of a hand, with the internal surface facing into the palm. This allows the crown to be passed easily to the operator for cementation. The restoration is seated on the tooth, and the patient is directed to bite on an orangewood stick that is rocked back and forth across the occlusal surface of the restoration. The margins are checked with an explorer to ensure that the crown is seated completely. The patient may continue to bite with a constant pressure on the orangewood stick. Other devices that could be used for biting include a Cooley peg, a cotton roll, or a similar seating device.

The operator may opt to use a hand burnisher, such as a ball burnisher or 2 to 3S burnisher, at this time to burnish the margin. A burnisher that is mounted on a slow-speed handpiece can also be used for this purpose. The burnishing activity is known to spin the gold to create a desirable surface to the alloy. As the cement becomes elastic, its removal can begin. Dental floss is forced through the proximal contact and pulled to the side. The floss is not brought up through the contacts from the cervical because this may dislodge the restoration. It is possible

to tie a small knot on the end of the floss and to pull the knot through the proximal space to remove excess cement. An explorer, curet, spoon excavator, or other instrument of choice is used to remove cement from the exterior of the crown. All cement must be removed from the crown, especially the gingival sulcus. The restoration is checked again for proper occlusal contact. Once the crown is cemented and cleaned of cement, the patient is given postoperative instructions.

During this time the assistant will aid in transfer of instruments, in mixing of cement, and in oral evacuation. A 2×2 gauze sponge that is held nearby will aid in removing cement from the operator's instrument.

▶ Modifications in Procedure

The previously described procedure for the preparation, laboratory procedure and cementation of a single unit crown is common to everyday general dentistry. However, several modifications of treatment depend on the type of restoration that is to be placed for various functions. The dental assistant must develop an understanding of the various changes that may occur as the choice of restorative material, dental cement, or restoration design are altered. The descriptive chart in Table 30-1 includes some of the common changes or techniques that may be encountered as the various changes occur. This chart identifies the changes that are made, either in preparation, laboratory, or cementation procedures, as they compare to the previously described full-cast coverage crown procedure.

The following steps may be necessary in specific situations as discussed in the narrative. They have not been included in the previous chart because they may be generic to several procedures.

SOLDERING

Sometimes solder must be placed on the proximal surface of a metal crown. This step is required when the proximal contact is light or nonexistent. Contact must be created to maintain the position of the tooth on the arch and to retain healthy gingival tissue. Soldering is accom-

plished through the use of an intermediate metal, with a melting point that is less than the metal in the restoration. The solder that is selected for use with a particular parent metal is specifically formulated for use with that metal. The surface that is to be soldered must be free of any oxides and must be smooth to allow for a free flow of the solder on the surface. This is accomplished through the use of flux on the area that is to be soldered. Antiflux stops any flow of the molten metal and is placed where the solder is not to go. In place of the antiflux the surface of gold that is to be soldered is ground to remove any shiny surface.

A piece of solder is held in place with a petroleum jelly–based flux and the casting is heated in the flame of a Bunsen burner. The solder slumps, and the casting is quickly removed from the burner to cool. The solder is added to provide adequate contact and form and to allow the material to be blended with the casting. Once the solder has cooled, the surface of the restoration is finished and polished before try in is attempted.

Soldering is also necessary when a multiple unit prosthetic device, such as a fixed bridge, is treatment planned. The pontics and abutments can be fabricated separately and soldered together as a single restorative device before try in. Another alternative to soldering the units before placement in the mouth is to try in each unit individually. The assembly can be connected as one with the use of sticky wax or another adhesive substance. The assembly, with each component relationship determined, is removed and fused as one with a soldering technique.

TRY IN PROCEDURE

Try in of a metal substructure for a metal-ceramic restoration is common practice to ensure accurate fit of the restoration before the porcelain is placed. Try in is also helpful to determine the areas in which the veneer should extend. The short time that is taken by the operator for a try in appointment to discover and correct small discrepancies is considered minimal compared with the amount of time that might be required later to correct these discrepancies. Certainly other techniques and materials used in prosthodontic treatment are available and used daily. To cover all the variables that are practiced would require a text that addresses only prosthodontics. For additional information on these procedures, it is wise to become involved in any of the prosthodontic organizations that offer a wide range of educational seminars for its members.

KEY POINTS

▶ Fixed prosthodontics is the preparation of a tooth or teeth to receive inlays; onlays; full or partial coverage crowns; post and cores; bridges; and resin-retained, veneer restorations that are permanently affixed in the mouth.

▶ A fixed prosthesis requires a minimum of two appointments to complete. The procedure requires a tooth or teeth to be prepared, an impression to be taken, and a temporary restoration to be placed. The cementation procedure involves removing the temporary restoration, try in and adjusting the cast restoration, and seating the final restoration.

▶ During the laboratory procedure for a fixed prosthesis the cast and die are fabricated and mounted with the opposing arch to an articulator; and the wax pattern is formed on the die and is invested, cast, and recovered for finishing and polishing. These procedures are commonly performed in a commercial laboratory but, with the appropriate skills, can be performed by a dentist or auxiliaries in the dental office.

▶ The dental assistant plays an important role in fixed prosthodontics and must develop a thorough understanding of each phase of the procedure to anticipate the needs of the operator and also to communicate the value of the procedure to the patient.

BIBLIOGRAPHY

Craig RG, O'Brien WJ, Powers JM: *Dental materials: properties and manipulation,* ed 5, St Louis, 1992, Mosby.

Myers GE, Lorey RE, Clayton JA, McPhee ER: *An outline of fixed prosthodontics,* ed 3, Ann Arbor, Mich, 1983, School of Dentistry, University of Michigan.

Naylor WP, Beatty MW: *Materials and techniques in fixed prosthodontics,* vol 36, no. 3, Saunders, Pa, 1992, Dental Clinics of North America.

Padilla MT, Bailey JH, *Margin configuration, die spacers, fitting of retainers/crowns and soldering,* vol 36, no. 3, Saunders, Pa, 1992, Dental Clinics of North America.

Rosenstiel SF, Land MF, Fujimoto J: *Contemporary fixed prosthodontics,* St Louis, 1988, Mosby.

31 Removable Prosthodontics

LEARNING OBJECTIVES

You will have mastered the material in this chapter when you can:
- Identify the key terms
- Briefly describe the Kennedy classifications of removable prostheses
- Differentiate between the various types of removable prostheses
- Outline the typical appointment schedule for common removable prostheses
- Define the components of a removable prosthesis
- Describe the basic procedural steps necessary to create a removable prosthesis
- Describe home care for a removable prosthesis
- Define the various types of implants
- Describe the implant process

KEY TERMS

Adjustment	Immediate denture
Alveolar ridge	Mortise
Bar	Mould
Baseplate	Muscle trimming
Border molding	Occlusal rim
Centric relationship	Osseointegration
Clasp	Partial denture
Complete denture	Precision attachment
Connector	Rebase
Conventional denture	Reline
Denture base	Rest
Diatoric hole	Retentive area
Duplicate denture	Ridge
Endosteal	Saddle
Face-bow	Stippling
Facing	Subperiosteal
Flask	Tenon
Framework	Vertical dimension
Free way space	

Removable prosthodontics as described in Chapter 29 refers to the replacement of missing teeth and tissues with a prosthetic device that can be removed from the mouth to clean and examine. When it is properly designed, a removable prosthesis can meet the objectives of prosthodontic service by replacing lost tissues with prostheses that simulate missing tissues, by improving phonetics and esthetics, and by providing restorations that are comfortable to the patient. The purpose of these prostheses is the improvement of masticatory function, preservation of teeth and tissues, which will enhance and promote oral health, as well as improve the health and general well being of the patient. Although a patient may prefer to have a fixed prosthesis, it may not be feasible because of the anatomic structure of the mouth, the ability to maintain good oral hygiene, or prohibitive cost.

Consequently, some form of removable prosthesis offers an alternative that provides function and esthetics to the patient.

Types of Removable Prosthodontic Restorations

The most common removable prostheses are complete dentures and removable partial dentures. Each of these devices will be described in detail in this chapter.

▶ Complete Dentures

A **complete denture**, a prosthesis that replaces all of the natural teeth and associated structures of the maxillae and mandible can be prepared for insertion by two different methods: immediate or conventional. The **immediate denture** is delivered immediately at the time the natural teeth are extracted. It is common to remove some of the posterior teeth in advance of taking impressions for this type of denture. This process generally involves removing the posterior teeth, allowing

these tissues to heal, taking impressions, and designing the denture. A try in of the denture set-up is done with the anterior teeth still intact. Then on the day that the denture is delivered, the remaining teeth are extracted, and the denture is inserted immediately. The patient is encouraged to leave the denture in place for the next 24 hours. The denture serves to restrict edema, promote healing, and aid the patient in maintaining esthetics during this time.

A **conventional denture** requires that all of the natural teeth be removed in advance of denture construction. The tissues are allowed to heal for 6 to 8 weeks; then the patient returns for the denture construction process. This method may be an option for the patient who has a severely diseased mouth and is not gravely concerned about esthetics for a few weeks or for the patient who has had a previous denture. If the patient has had a previous denture and if it is not injurious to the tissues, it can be worn during the construction of the new denture.

A **duplicate denture** is a second denture constructed to be a copy of the first denture. This denture acts as a spare or backup denture for the patient. Although such an investment may seem an unnecessary one for some

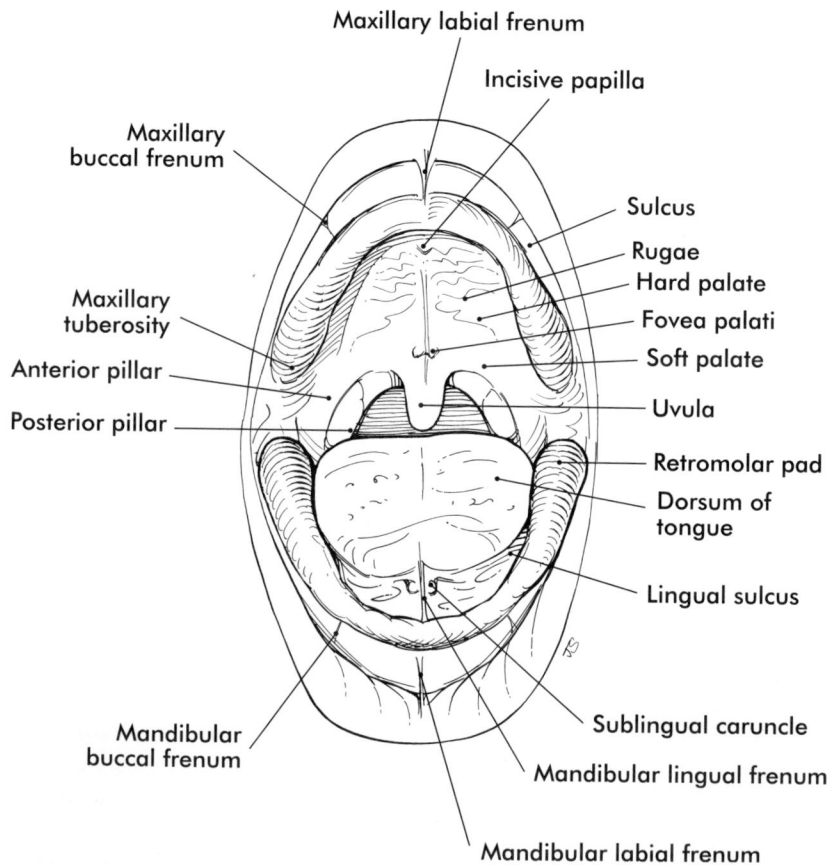

FIG. 31-1   Open edentulous mouth, with landmarks identified. The tongue is retracted to improve identification.

patients, it may be a distinct advantage for those individuals who make public appearances daily. Since this denture is constructed primarily as a backup, the teeth are commonly made of autopolymerizing acrylic rather than premanufactured denture teeth. The teeth are made directly in an alginate impression which has been imbedded into a **flask**, a holding device for processing a denture. When it is set, the denture base resin is poured into the flask. The denture is cured and finished in a manner similar to that of the original denture.

Emphasis is placed on the anatomic structures of a dentulous mouth. However, since fewer edentulous patients are encountered in most general practices today, many dental assistants will not be as familiar with the anatomic structures of an edentulous patient. When all of the teeth are missing from the mouth, it may be difficult to orient oneself to the oral anatomy. In Chapter 9 emphasis is placed on exposing dental radiographs for completely or partially edentulous patients, and a dental assistant working in a prosthodontic office should become familiar with the edentulous landmarks. Fig. 31-1 illustrates an open edentulous mouth with its visible structures. The tongue is retracted to improve visibility.

▶ Partial Dentures

Partial dentures, which replace one or more missing teeth, can be prepared in many styles; the most typical style is the extracoronal clasp retainer style. The intracoronal **semiprecision attachment** or the **precision attachment** partial (which has no visible external components) provides a more esthetic approach but involves a greater initial investment for the patient. In addition, a removable partial overdenture can be designed like a full overdenture except that the denture base overlies one or more natural tooth roots that have been endodontically treated; these tooth roots are used for support in retention.

As with other situations in a patient's mouth, the edentulous conditions can be classified into several categories. The Kennedy classification system is a well accepted classification that is used in partially edentulous mouths to identify the status of the remaining teeth. Table 31-1 identifies most of the common edentulous conditions according to the number of teeth that remain in the arch, to the position of the teeth, and to their relationship with one another. These conditions are illustrated in the table in Fig. 31-2, *A* through *F.*

TABLE 31-1   KENNEDY CLASSIFICATION SYSTEM FOR PARTIALLY EDENTULOUS CONDITIONS IN THE ORAL CAVITY

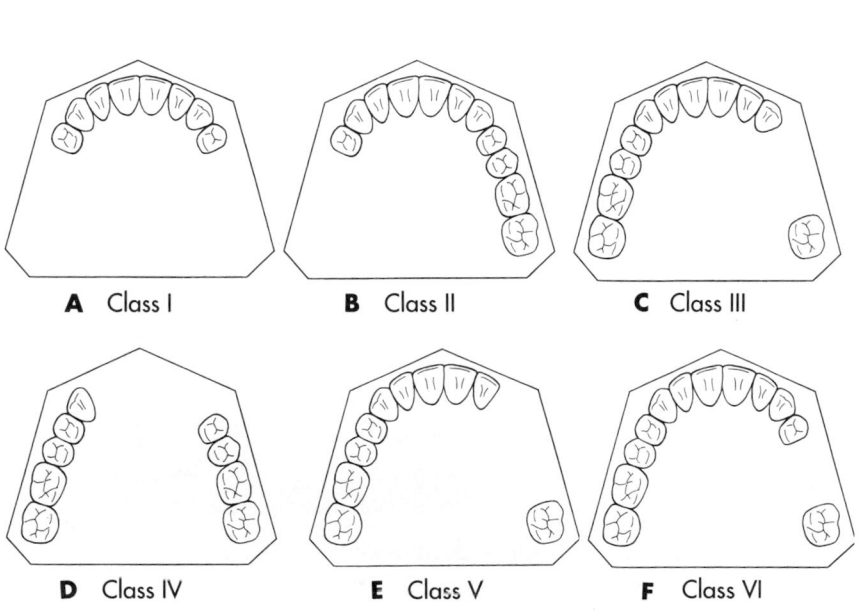

A Class I   **B** Class II   **C** Class III

D Class IV   **E** Class V   **F** Class VI

FIG. 31-2   Kennedy classification of edentulous mouth.

An edentulous situation in which all remaining teeth are anterior to the bilateral edentulous areas (Fig. 31-2, **A**).

An edentulous situation in which the remaining teeth of either the right or left side are anterior to the unilateral edentulous area (Fig. 31-2, **B**).

An edentulous situation in which the edentulous area is bounded by teeth that are *unable* to assume total support of the prosthesis. These abutments require the aid of teeth that are remotely located, so that the principles of cross-arch splinting and counter leverage can be used to resist lateral tilting forces (Fig. 31-2, **C**).

An edentulous situation in which the remaining teeth bound the edentulous area posteriorly on both sides of the median line (Fig. 31-2, **D**).

An edentulous situation in which teeth bound the edentulous area anteriorly and posteriorly but where the anterior abutment tooth is *not* suitable for normal abutment service (Fig. 31-2, **E**).

An edentulous situation in which the boundary teeth are capable of total support of the required prosthesis (Fig. 31-2, **F**).

Many combinations of treatment plans can be made for the partially edentulous patient. It is not uncommon to see treatment plans that call for combinations of prostheses, including fixed bridgework in combination with a removable prosthesis; a full maxillary denture opposing a removable clasp or a semiprecision attachment partial denture on the mandible; precision or semiprecision attachment partial on both arches; or any of these prosthesis on one arch with natural teeth on the opposite arch.

▶ Components of a Partial Denture

The dental assistant needs to be familiar with the components of a partial denture. Whether a clasp or a precision type partial denture is to be designed, the assistant must understand the function of each of the components to communicate with other professionals, as well as to describe the functions and care to a patient.

COMPONENTS OF A CLASP PARTIAL DENTURE

The components of a typical clasp partial denture are described in Box 31-1. These components are illustrated in Fig. 31-3.

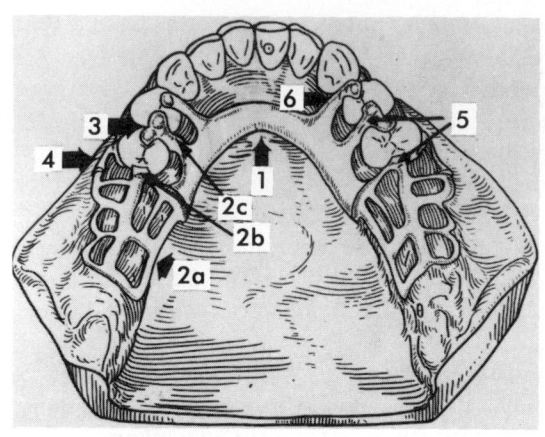

FIG. 31-3   Components of a partial denture. *(1)* Lingual bar major connector; *(2)* minor connector to which acrylic resin denture base will be attached; *(3)* occlusal rests; *(4)* direct retainer arm, part of total clasp assembly; *(5)* stabilizing components of clasp assembly, two minor connectors and two rests, and *(6)* an indirect retainer, consisting of a minor connector and an occlusal rest.

(From McGivney GP, Castleberry D]: *McCracken's removable partial prosthodontics*, ed 8, St Louis, 1989, Mosby.)

COMPONENTS OF A CLASP PARTIAL DENTURE

1. **Direct retainer**—a clasp or an attachment on the removable prosthesis that is applied to an abutment tooth to provide retention to the removable prosthesis; these may be extracoronal in the clasp-style partial denture (Fig. 31-4) or internal attachments (Fig. 31-5) in an intracoronal precision or semiprecision partial; extracoronal clasps can be classified according to type of construction—cast, wrought-wire, or combination; or the clasp can be categorized according to the design—circumferential or bar type as shown in Fig. 31-6 *A* and *B*
   a. **Circumferential type** clasp is one that encircles more than 180 degrees of the tooth and one terminal end is placed in the infrabulge area or in the undercut of the crown of the tooth (Fig. 31-6, *A*)
   b. **Bar type** clasp originates from the denture base or from a major connector and approaches the undercut from a cervical direction (Fig. 31-6, *B*)
2. **Major connector**—this part of the device that is generally a plate, strap, or bar that connects the sides or bases of a partial denture; on the maxillary arch this connector may be in the form of a horseshoe, a palatal strap, a palatal bar, or a complete palatal plate (Fig. 31-7); on the mandible this connector may take the

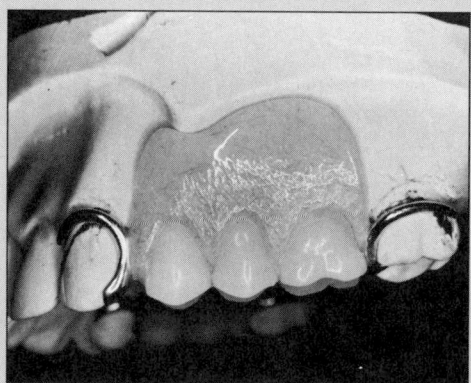

FIG. 31-4   Partial denture with cast circumferential retentive clasps.

(From McGivney GP, Castleberry D]: *McCracken's removable partial prosthodontics*, ed 9, St Louis, 1995, Mosby.)

COMPONENTS OF A CLASP PARTIAL DENTURE—cont'd

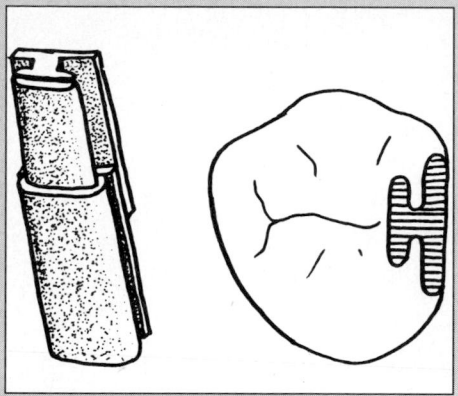

FIG. 31-5 Intracoronal retainer consists of a male (tenon) and female (mortise) portion.

(From McGivney GP, Castleberry D: *McCracken's removable partial prosthodontics*, ed 8, St Louis, 1989, Mosby.)

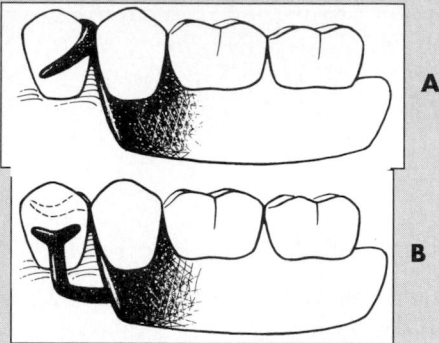

FIG. 31-6 Extracoronal clasps. *A*, Cast circumferential clasp arm. *B*, Bar clasp—T-bar style.

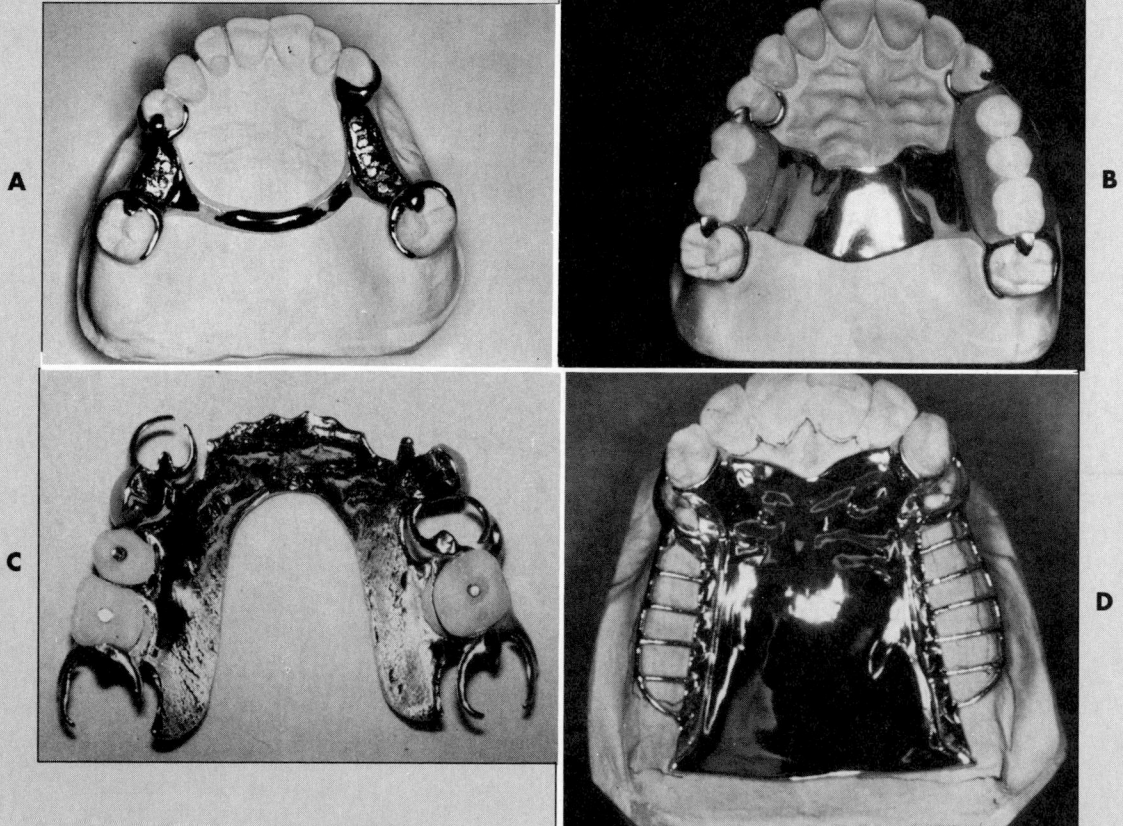

FIG. 31-7 Major connectors on maxillary partial dentures.
A, Single palatal strap. *B*, U-shaped. *C*, Anteroposterior palatal strap. *D*, Palatal plate.

(From McGivney GP, Castleberry D: *McCracken's removable partial prosthodontics*, ed 9, St Louis, 1995, Mosby.)

BOX 31-1

COMPONENTS OF A CLASP PARTIAL DENTURE—cont'd

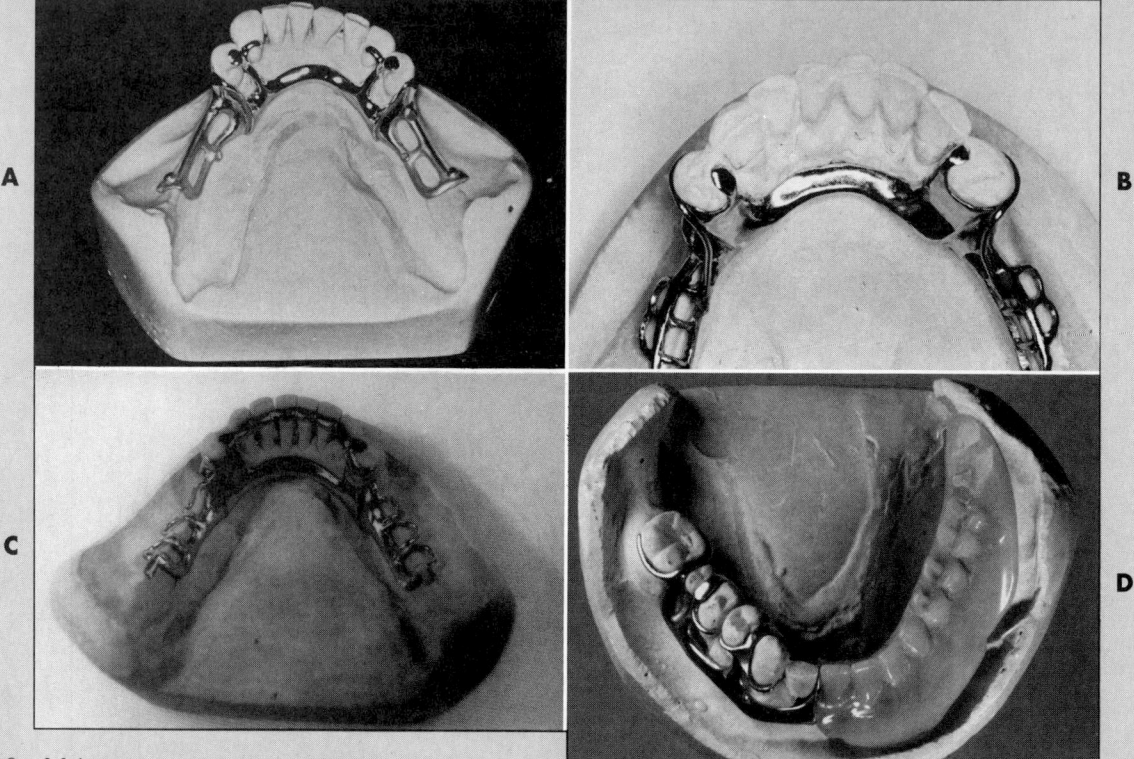

FIG. 31-8   Major connectors on mandibular partial dentures. *A*, Lingual bar. *B*, Lingual bar with continuous bar retainer. *C*, Linguoplate. *D*, Labial bar.

(From McGivney GP, Castleberry D]: *McCracken's removable partial prosthodontics*, ed 8, St Louis, 1989, Mosby.)

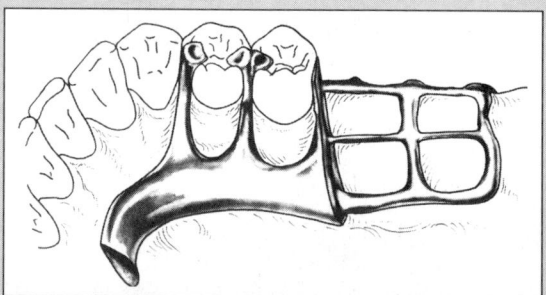

FIG. 31-9   Minor connectors extend from the lingual bar to the occlusal rests and distal connector on the second premolar.

(From McGivney GP, Castleberry D]: *McCracken's removable partial prosthodontics*, ed 9, St Louis, 1995, Mosby.)

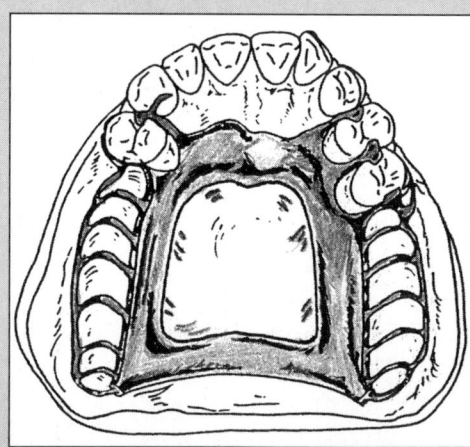

FIG. 31-10   Plastic retention area is a mesh-like area that is designed to retain acrylic denture base.

(From McGivney GP, Castleberry D]: *McCracken's removable partial prosthodontics*, ed 8, St Louis, 1989, Mosby.)

shape of a lingual bar, a lingual plate, a double lingual bar, or even a labial bar (Fig. 31-8)

3. **Minor connector**—this is a connecting link between the major connector or base and the other parts of the prosthesis, such as the clasps and rests (Fig. 31-9)

4. **Rest**—this is a rigid extension of the partial denture that contacts a tooth to dissipate vertical and horizontal forces; an incisal, occlusal, cingulum, or ball type rest may be placed (see Fig. 31-3)

5. **Indirect retainer**—this is a part of the partial denture that functions as a lever to prevent displacement of the partial denture, thereby eliminating rotation between the rest and the support areas; an indirect retainer may be a rest, an extension, a secondary lingual bar, or a lingual plate (see Fig. 31-3)

6. **Plastic retention area**—this is a loop or mesh-like area that is designed to retain the acrylic base material (see Fig. 31-10)

7. **Base**—this is the portion of the partial denture that rests on the oral mucosa to which teeth are attached; the term *saddle* is often used to describe this portion of the appliance, since it fits over the alveolar ridge in a saddle-like style; the base may be made of metal or plastic resins (Fig. 31-11)

8. **Teeth**—Teeth placed on a partial denture may be resin, porcelain, or even metal; they may be denture teeth, tube teeth, facings, or metal teeth (Fig. 31-11)

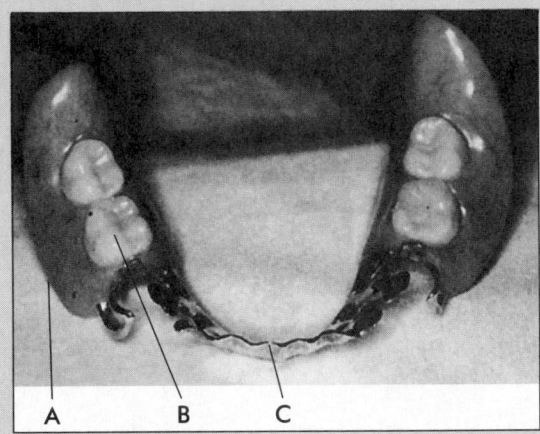

FIG. 31-11 **Partial denture with base,** *A;* **denture teeth,** *B;* **and saddle area,** *C.*

(From McGivney GP, Castleberry D]: *McCracken's removable partial prosthodontics,* ed 8, St Louis, 1989, Mosby.)

COMPONENTS OF AN INTRACORONAL PARTIAL DENTURE

Intracoronal components of a partial denture provide retention by internal frictional resistance. The terms *precision, semiprecision,* and *spring lock attachment* refer to some type of prefabricated interlocking mechanism with two matched parts. Typically, a crown covers the abutment tooth into which is imbedded one part (i.e., the **mortise** [female] portion) of the attachment. The removable partial denture houses the **tenon** (male) portion of the attachment instead of a clasp as shown in Fig. 31-5. Advantages of the precision attachments include the following:

▶ Improved esthetics
▶ Reduction of food impaction, plaque, and caries
▶ Resistance to rotational forces to displace the partial denture
▶ Improved patient comfort
▶ Improvement in the support of the forces of mastication

The precision attachment requires more clinical and laboratory time; more abutment tooth considerations and an increased investment on the part of the patient.

Components of a Denture

The two basic parts of a denture are the base and the teeth (Fig. 31-12, *A* through *E*). A **denture base** is the part of the denture which simulates the gingival mucosa, alveolar mucosa, and hard palate and is available in a variety of tissue colors that reflect the patient's complexion and that can be characterized to create a natural appearance. The **denture teeth** provide the functional portion of the denture and are supplied in various shades or colors, in different shapes or moulds, in various sizes, and in an assortment of arrangements that enable the operator to recreate the patient's natural look.

▶ Denture Base

Placing special characteristics in the denture base can be as important in personalizing the denture as it is in selecting the correct type of teeth to create a natural appearance. The complexion of the patient dictates the type of denture base material to use. Various shades of acrylic are available to match the patient's tissue tone. **Stippling**, the orange-peel, pebble-like appearance that exists in the natural attached gingiva, can be recreated in the denture base by contouring the finished denture. Small, colored fiberglass fibers are added to some acrylic bases to simulate capillaries.

Though acrylic resin is most often used as a denture base, metal may be chosen as an alternative base. Bases are made of different materials, such as gold, platinum, cobalt chromium alloys, and stainless steel and provide greater thermal conductivity, as well as increased tissue tolerance. The increased weight of a metal base can be a disadvantage to a maxillary denture but may be the choice for the mandible denture because it can increase retentive qualities.

For esthetics and function, root indication areas are made on the buccal and labial portions of the denture base to point out the various natural alveolar prominences.

▶ Denture Teeth

The selection of denture teeth, whether for a full or a partial denture, is an important aspect of prosthesis construction. The types of teeth used in removable prosthetics include facings, tube teeth, and denture teeth. These teeth are made of either porcelain, plastic, or metal.

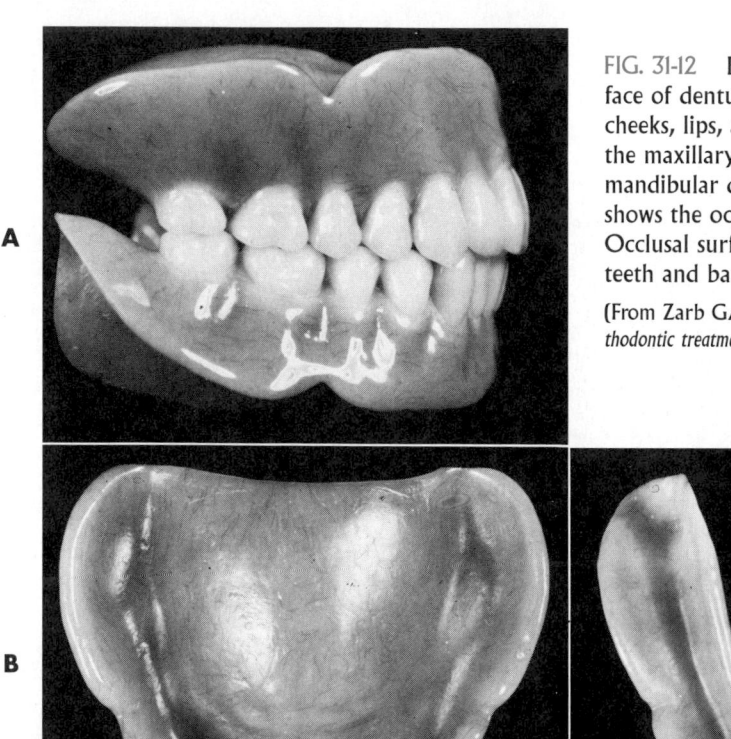

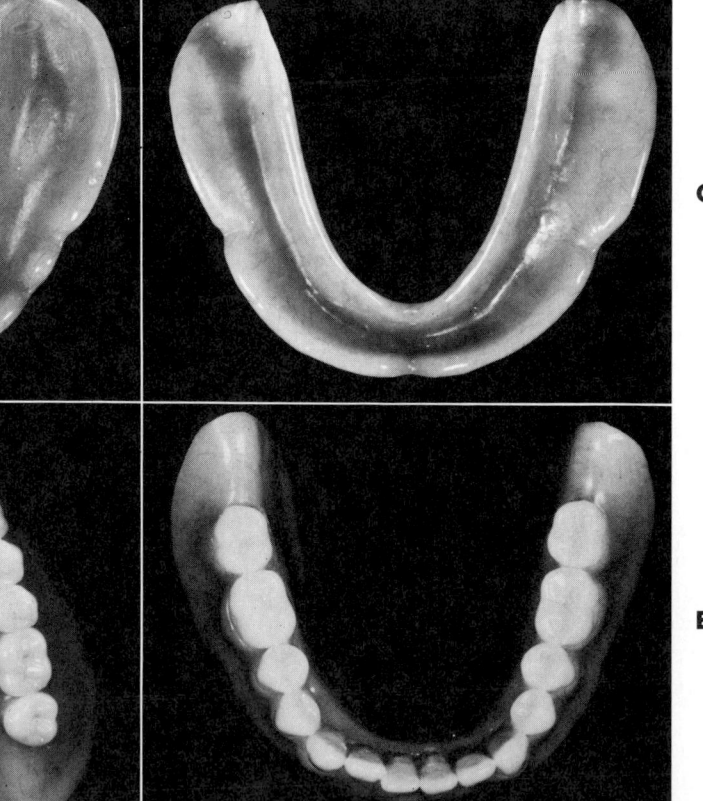

FIG. 31-12 Basic parts of a denture. *A,* Labial and buccal surface of denture base is polished to support and contact the cheeks, lips, and tongue. *B,* Internal base (mucosal surface) of the maxillary denture. *C,* Internal base (mucosal surface) of the mandibular denture. *D,* Occlusal surface of maxillary denture shows the occlusal of teeth and palatal surface of base. *E,* Occlusal surface of mandibular denture shows the occlusal of teeth and base of denture.

(From Zarb GA, Bolender CL, Hickey JC, Carlsson GE: *Boucher's prosthodontic treatment for edentulous patients,* ed 10, St Louis, 1990, Mosby.)

Generally dental assistants have little contact with denture teeth unless they are working in a prosthodontic practice. Typically, most general dental practices rely on commercial laboratories to set denture teeth. However, it will be necessary to order these teeth sometimes for replacements if a denture repair is done in the office.

Facings are most commonly used for anterior teeth in partial dentures. The facing attaches to a metal slot on a metal backed prosthesis; they are often used for a single tooth replacement or where minimal space is available. Facings present the disadvantage of poor esthetics because of their opacity when backed with metal.

Tube teeth are designed by altering a resin or porcelain denture tooth to fit onto a metal partial base. A hole is ground in the denture tooth that fits over a projection in the cast partial framework. Tube teeth can be attached to the partial denture with autopolymerizing resin or traditional crown and bridge cement.

DENTURE TEETH

Denture teeth are carded in full sets of maxillary or mandibular anteriors (1×6s) (Fig. 31-13, *A*) and maxillary and mandibular posteriors (1×8s) (Fig. 31-13, *B*). The arch can be distinguished on the card as noted in Fig. 31-13, *B*, since the teeth are set in the same position as they are in the mouth. To order denture teeth for a complete set of dentures, it would be necessary to order four different sets of teeth: one maxillary 1×6, one mandibular 1×6, one maxillary 1×8, and one mandibular 1×8.

PORCELAIN VERSUS PLASTIC TEETH

The type of denture teeth used in a prosthesis is determined by the dentist. Plastic teeth are easily adjusted, they will not wear opposing natural tooth structure or gold, and they are more commonly used in

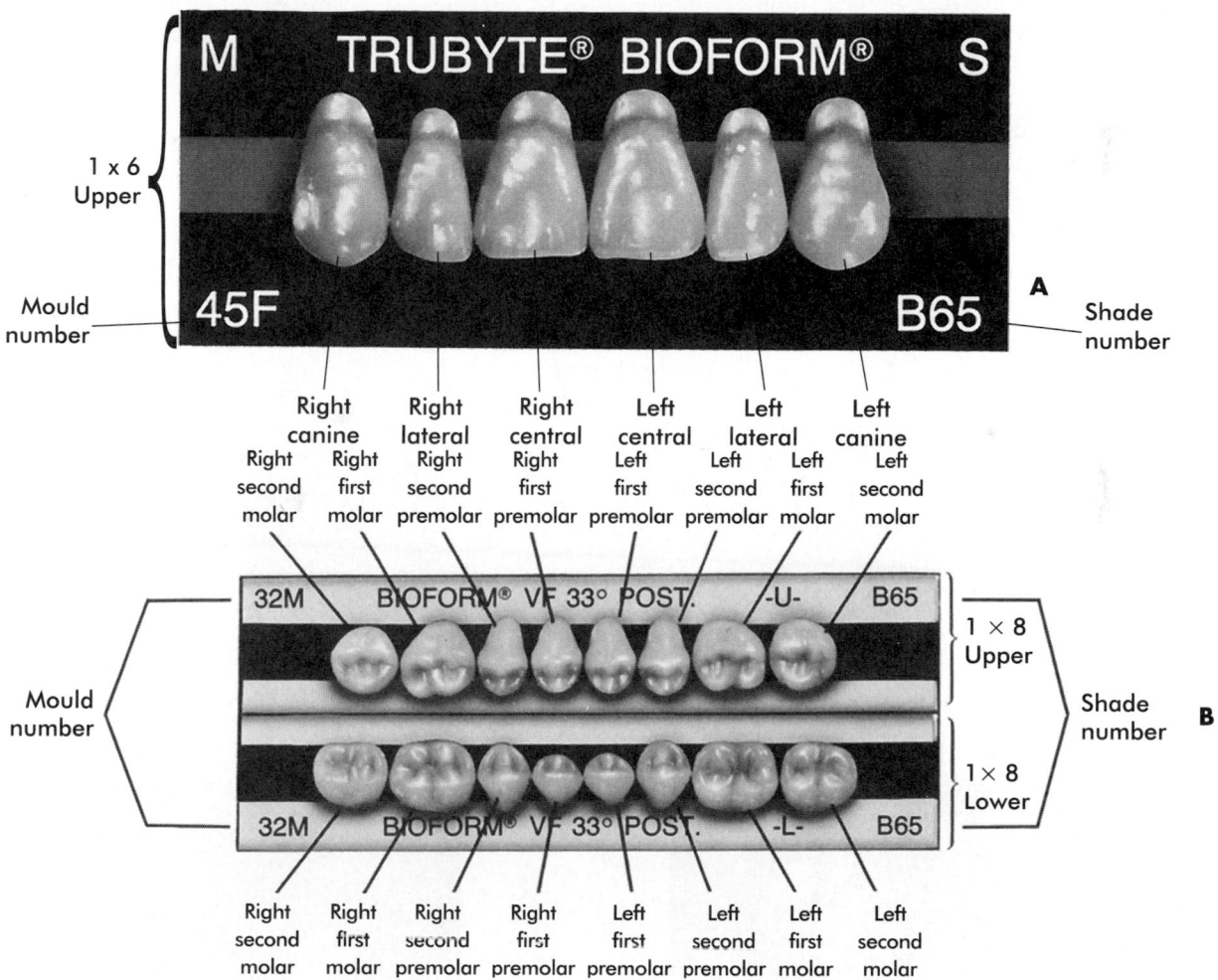

FIG. 31-13 *A,* Carded set of maxillary anterior denture teeth. *B,* Carded sets of mandibular and maxillary posterior denture teeth.

(Courtesy of Dentsply International.)

a removable prosthesis, since they can withstand considerable grinding and adjusting. Porcelain teeth, on the other hand, are more difficult to grind and adjust; such grinding leaves an unglazed surface on the porcelain, which is difficult to polish. Porcelain teeth do not wear but cause wear to natural tooth structure including gold and resin teeth in the opposing arch.

Anterior porcelain denture teeth are distinguished from plastic anterior teeth by small pins that project from the lingual surface. These pins provide a mechanical lock for retentive purposes in the acrylic denture base. Plastic anterior denture teeth do not have these pins, since they are held in the base by a chemical bond with the plastic denture base.

Porcelain posterior denture teeth have no pins, but rather a **diatoric hole** which is molded into the center back of the tooth. The fluid denture base material flows into the hole, and when it hardens, it provides a lock with the denture base. Small vent holes are provided in porcelain teeth that allow air to escape as the denture base material flows into the diatoric hole. Posterior plastic teeth, like anteriors, have no additional locking mechanism, since the chemical bond is adequate here too. On both styles of posterior teeth a separate dot appears on the tissue base of the tooth to aid in identification of first and second molars and premolars.

One dot is for first premolars and first molars, and 2 dots are for second premolars and second molars. In addition, each tooth is identified with a mould number (see Fig. 31-14).

METAL OCCLUSALS

Metal occlusals on teeth can be constructed for partial or full dentures. Metal occlusals are waxed and cast in the same manner as any other metal casting, except that all of the occlusal surfaces are attached together as one unit. Metal occlusals provide strength and can be designed to occlude with the patient's existing teeth. The application of metal occlusals is often indicated in situations where the occlusion in the removable prosthesis opposes cast gold restorations (Fig. 31-15).

SHADE AND MOULD SELECTION

Of major importance is the selection of denture teeth for the anterior region of the mouth. The two basic factors that need to be considered when selecting anterior teeth are shade and mould. **Shade** is the color of the teeth and **mould** is the shape of the teeth.

The selection of teeth, especially when a full denture is being constructed, is important to a patient, since this

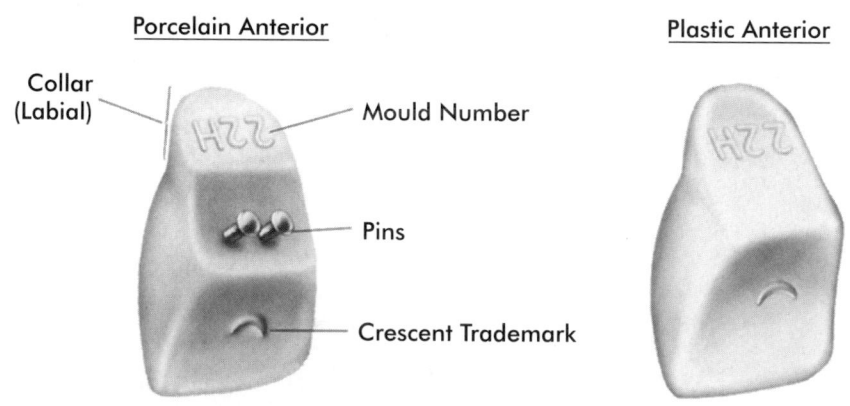

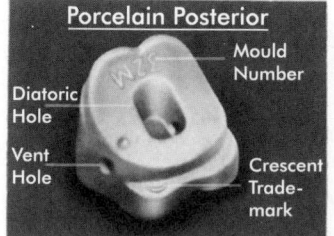
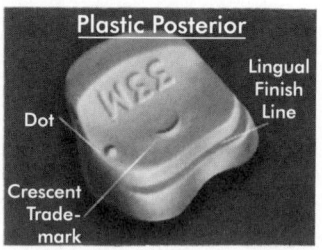

FIG. 31-14   Denture teeth, with appropriate nomenclature.
(Courtesy of Dentsply International.)

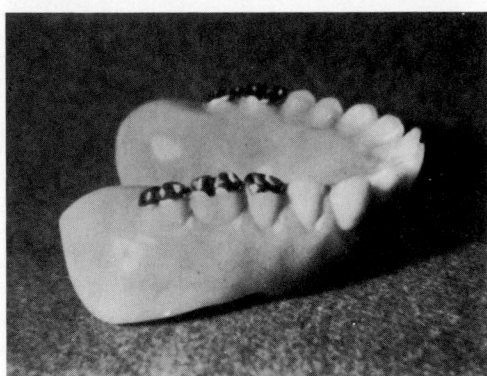

FIG. 31-15   Metal (gold) occlusal surfaces on a denture.

(From Zarb GA, Bolender CL, Hickey JC, Carlsson GE: *Boucher's pros-thodontic treatment for edentulous patients*, ed 10, St Louis, 1990, Mosby.)

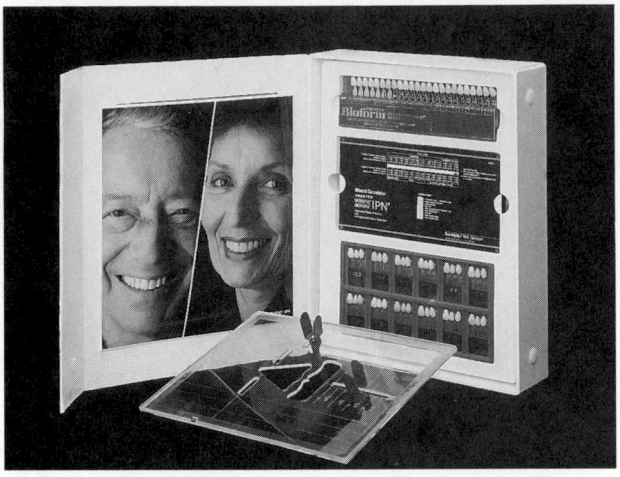

FIG. 31-16   Esthetic Denture System (trademark) provides trubyte tooth indicator to aid in determining appropriate tooth size for a denture.

(Courtesy of Dentsply International.)

will have a direct effect on his or her acceptance of the denture. The patient needs to be directly involved in this decision. Many companies who manufacture denture teeth provide the dentist with various selection systems that aid in choosing the correct mould and tooth shade. For instance the Dentsply Company provides an entire Esthetic Denture System (trademark), including a Trubyte Tooth Indicator, which aids in translating the vertical and horizontal measurements into appropriate tooth sizes.

MOULD SELECTION

The Trubyte Tooth Indicator can be used to select the mould by placing this transparent device over the patient's face, allowing the nose to come through the center triangle (Fig. 31-16). The pupils of the eyes are centered in the eye holes and the indicator is held in position, with the center line coinciding with the median line of the face. The form of the face is noted in comparison to the vertical lines of the Tooth Indicator. It is also possible to obtain an approximate size of the maxillary central incisors by using this indicator in the same position and moving the vertical arm up to touch the chin and moving the horizontal arm in, just until it touches the face. The width of the upper central incisor can then be read from the chart in millimeters.

The tooth mould is determined by the shape of the patient's face. The four basic face forms, square, square tapering, tapering, and ovoid, are illustrated in Table 31-2. Since teeth are not naturally arranged perfectly, it is wise to consider individualized anterior arrangements for teeth. For instance, the patient's natural teeth may have been crowded, asymmetric, or spaced, and the patient may wish to maintain this same natural look. Such an arrangement can be chosen so that the teeth are set in the

TABLE 31-2   FACE FORM USED IN SELECTING NATURAL ANTERIOR TOOTH ARRANGEMENT

	Facial descriptions
A	Square face—the sides of the face from the hairline to levels of the condyles to the angles of the jaw are straight and parallel
B	Square tapering face—the sides of the head are parallel from the condyles upward; from the condyles downward along the sides of the face, the outline tapers in to the angles of the jaw
C	Tapering face—this face is widest at the hairline and narrowest at the angles of the jaw; the lines converge in toward the jaw
D	Ovoid face—the ovoid face is widest through the center at the level of the condyles; it curves upward and downward to form an oval outline

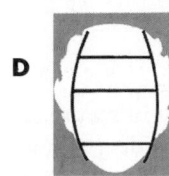

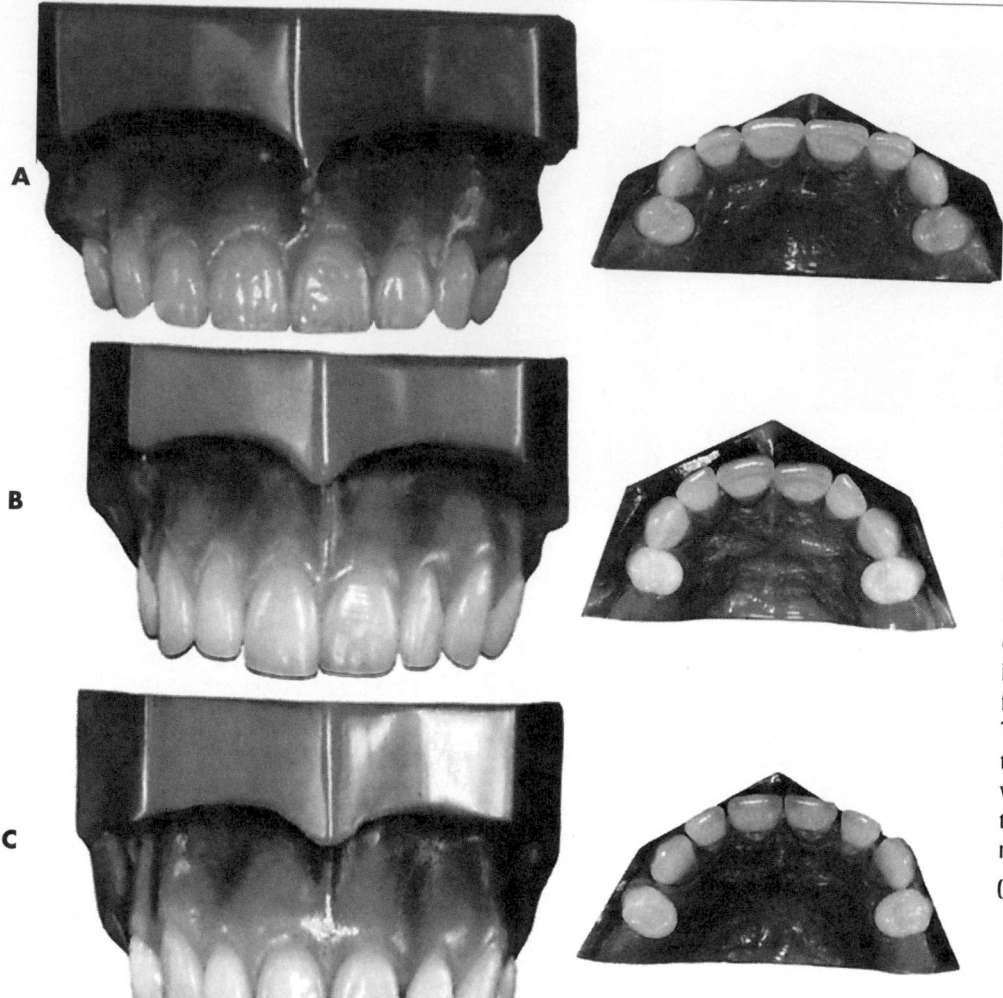

FIG. 31-17   (*A,* A medium-sized typal Square tooth set in a typal arch form. Note that the centrals are set practically straight across, with the laterals also having a full labial aspect. *B,* Normally, a crowded condition is not usually found in the Square arch because of its broadness and resulting adequate room for the eruption of all teeth. However, in some instances, particularly where the natural teeth may be slightly larger than normal, this does result in a crowded condition. In this arrangement the centrals and laterals are lapped and rotated to produce the effect of crowding. *C,* In the Square arch form, spacing is more likely to be found than the crowded condition. The spacing condition in the Square arch obviously results from the opposite cause of crowding. The natural tooth form is smaller than normal, and variable spaces develop between practically all of the teeth. In this arrangement there is mild spacing between all teeth.

(Courtesy of Dentsply International)

denture to meet the personal needs of the patient (Fig. 31-17, *A* and *B*). Other individual characteristics can be added to retain the natural look: e.g., even a gold crown or inlay, which may have been characteristic of the patient's natural appearance, may be added. Often a dentist may ask a patient to provide a photo that was taken at an earlier time, showing the patient's natural teeth; this will aid the dentist in recreating a natural appearance in the new prosthesis.

A mould number is placed on each individual tooth and on the carded set of teeth (see Fig. 31-14). The manufacturer will correlate the anterior mould shapes to the opposite arch, as well as to the appropriate shape of posterior teeth.

SHADE SELECTION

A shade guide is provided to aid in determining the color of the teeth (Fig. 31-18). This shade guide provides a complete range of natural tooth colors to aid in selecting

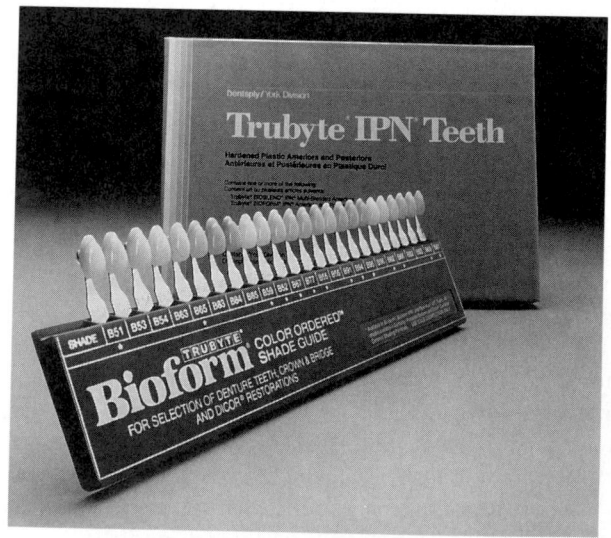

FIG. 31-18   Shade guide.

(Courtesy of Dentsply International.)

the appropriate tooth shade that will harmonize with the patient's hair, eyes, and complexion. The shade is selected under the same conditions as shades for any other esthetic restorations. The shade button is wetted with saliva and placed behind the lip, near the location of the tooth or teeth to be replaced; the shade is selected under natural light and with the input of the patient. Once a shade is selected, its number and the mould number are entered on the patient's clinical chart and is placed on a laboratory requisition when the case is sent to the dental laboratory. It is possible to characterize the shade of individual denture teeth by adding stain to recreate natural staining. This may be used in a patient who has a dark cervical line on certain teeth or perhaps a darker yellow on the cervical of the cuspids.

ANATOMIC VERSUS NONANATOMIC POSTERIOR TEETH

No one specific type of posterior teeth can satisfy the needs of all patients. Posterior teeth are manufactured with anatomic, semianatomic, and nonanatomic characteristics. Generally, as a patient ages, he or she is more likely to have worn down the occlusal surfaces of the teeth. While anatomic teeth with high cusps tend to improve a person's chewing ability, the shape of the edentulous **ridge**: that portion of the alveolar process where teeth formerly existed, may not be able to support the high cusp teeth; for this reason a less anatomic type tooth must be used. Box 31-2 describes the application of anatomic versus nonanatomic denture teeth.

▶ Factors to Consider in Creating Esthetics

When a denture is being constructed the patient may refer to the new prosthesis as *false teeth*. Many people have replacement teeth that do not look natural. The teeth may appear monotone in color, may be placed too evenly, and may be too small or too large for the size of the patient's mouth. During denture construction the objective for the dentist, staff, and technician should be to choose teeth that look natural, have color variations, and reflect a natural and attractive look. Factors affecting esthetics are described in Box 31-3.

Typical Appointment Sequence for Removable Prosthesis

Although the procedural sequence for the construction and insertion of a removable prosthesis varies from type to type, some common procedures are followed for each prosthesis. In the following discussion each phase that is involved in the production of various types of prostheses—partial dentures, immediate full dentures, and conventional full dentures—is discussed. Boxes 31-4 through 31-7 list typical appointment schedules for each type of prosthesis. Even though the technique may vary with the type of prosthesis, the type of dental material that is used, or the variations in procedures that occur, these steps represent the basic processes that must be completed before an appliance can be delivered to a patient.

At this point of discussion it is assumed that all diagnostic procedures have been completed, that the patient has provided informed consent, and that the mouth has been restored and prepared to a point of optimal health, so that the only remaining treatment is the construction of the prosthesis.

▶ Preliminary Impressions

These impressions are taken at the patient's initial appointment and are used during oral diagnosis. During

BOX 31-4

APPOINTMENT SCHEDULE FOR A PARTIAL DENTURE

The following appointments are scheduled for a patient who is to receive a partial denture after the complete oral examination, the surveying of the models, the consultation, and the acceptance of the treatment plan:

- Mouth preparation, including surgical, endodontic, periodontal, and restorative
- Tooth preparation for partial denture retention
- Preliminary impressions
- Final impressions of prepared teeth, remaining teeth, and edentulous ridges
- Try in framework, and adjust as necessary
- Final impression of edentulous ridge may be taken if required
- Bite relationships
- Shade and mould selection as needed
- Insert partial denture
- Adjustment appointments as necessary

BOX 31-5

APPOINTMENT SCHEDULE FOR AN IMMEDIATE DENTURE

The following appointments are scheduled for a patient who is to receive an immediate denture after the complete oral examination, the consultation, and the acceptance of the treatment plan:

- Extraction of posterior teeth on one side of the mouth
- Extraction of posterior teeth on opposite side of the mouth
- Four to six weeks later, initial impressions are taken of arches with remaining teeth and edentulous ridges
- Final impressions of remaining teeth and edentulous ridges
- Jaw relationships; shade and mould selection
- Try-in and set-up approval
- Extraction of remaining teeth and insertion of denture; surgery may be done by maxillofacial oral surgeon
- Day after surgery; follow up visit to examine denture and tissues
- Adjustment appointments as necessary
- Six to eight months later; recall visit to examine denture fit and need for reline

BOX 31-6

APPOINTMENT SCHEDULE FOR A CONVENTIONAL DENTURE

The following appointments will be scheduled for a patient for a nonimmediate denture after the complete oral examination, the consultation, and the acceptance of the treatment plan:

- Tissue conditioning as needed
- Initial impressions of arches and edentulous ridges
- Final impressions of arches and edentulous ridges
- Jaw relationships; shade and mould selection
- Try-in and set-up approval
- Denture insertion
- Adjustment appointments as necessary

BOX 31-7

INTERIM LABORATORY PROCEDURES

The following activities are completed at various times during a typical prosthetic procedure:

- Survey casts
- Custom tray construction
- Master cast construction
- Cast framework, if partial denture
- Construct baseplates and occlusal rims
- Set-up trial, full, or partial denture
- Process final, full, or partial denture
- Process reline for full or partial denture

removable prosthetics these models are used to survey the case for proper placement of components or to determine any surgical procedures that need to be performed. If restorative treatment has been completed after the diagnosis, new preliminary impressions must be taken before the next step is initiated. Refer to Chapter 24 to review the proper diagnostic impressions procedures.

If a patient is to have a complete denture, the dentist

may wish to relieve the peripheral borders of the preliminary impression or the custom tray to allow for border molding at a later appointment. **Border molding** is a process of recording the denture border by manipulating the tissues adjacent to the borders. Therefore, before an impression is poured or a custom tray is constructed, the dentist should be consulted on the appropriate technique to follow to allow space in the peripheral region for border molding. This is done by placing warmed dental compound on the periphery of the tray, placing the tray into the patient's mouth and asking the patient to move the cheeks, tongue, and lips in various positions.

Custom Tray Construction

The trays that are used for the final impression must adequately fit the arch, whether it is narrow or wide, and must compensate for any undercuts that are created by tori or malposed teeth. The construction of custom-made trays is discussed in Chapter 40.

Before the tray is used for an impression, the dentist will try it in to ensure that the fit is adequate and that it compensates for all of the soft tissues in the mouth. The tray should not impinge on the labial frenum, and adequate room must be available to place dental compound during the border molding process.

When the custom tray is constructed for use in removable prosthodontics, two options are available: (1) construct the tray as a solid piece with or without a

handle, and use some form of adhesive to retain the impression material in the tray (Fig. 31-19, *A* and *B*); or (2) construct the tray with or without a handle and make holes all over the tray with a fissure bur to create mechanical retention of the impression material (Fig. 31-19, *C* and *D*).

Final Impressions for Master Casts

The objective of this appointment is to obtain an accurate impression from which to construct a denture. To achieve a retentive denture, the denture base must be well adapted to the mucous membrane, must cover the maximum available area, and must establish an effective seal with the tissues at the border. To accomplish all of these criteria, it is necessary to have an accurate final impression. The criteria for an accurate final impression are noted in Box 31-8.

The final impression appointment includes two phases: (1) the border molding of the periphery of the tray; and (2) the impression of the soft and hard tissues of the arch.

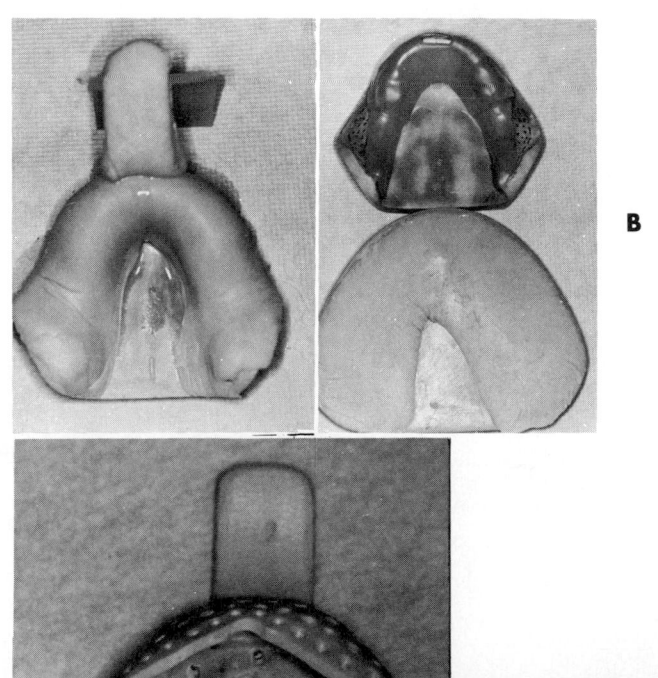

A

B

C

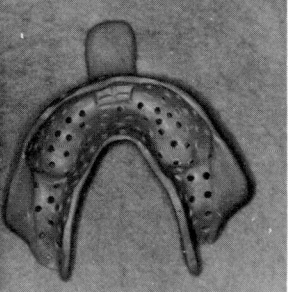

D

BOX 31-8

CRITERIA FOR ACCURATE FINAL IMPRESSIONS IN DENTURE CONSTRUCTION

- Close contact with the surface of the mucous membrane on which the denture will rest
- Include a complete registration of the mucolabial fold
- Extend the impression distally to include all tissues that will be involved in the design of the denture to obtain an adequate seal
- Include detailed reproduction of all soft and hard tissues
- Be free of voids

FIG. 31-19 Custom-made acrylic trays for final impression and border molding. *A,* Solid, with handle. *B,* Solid, without handle. *C,* Maxillary, with holes. *D,* Mandibular, with holes.

(From McGivney GP, Castleberry D]: *McCracken's removable partial prosthodontics,* ed 9, St Louis, 1995, Mosby.)

This appointment requires that all of the armamentarium be assembled in advance on the mobile and fixed cabinetry. Although this procedure includes many areas that are conducive to four-handed procedures, some operators may prefer a set-up that provides easy access to the materials during the border molding process. This requires that the bunsen burner and water bath be placed near the operator for easy access. The materials that the assistant mixes should be placed on the mobile cabinetry in the normal position for easy access during transfer.

Armamentarium

The armamentarium necessary for this procedure includes the following (Fig. 31-20):

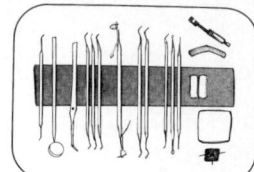

Prepared custom-made trays
Low-fusing compound
Heating bath
Laboratory knife
#7 wax spatula
Bunsen burner
Matches
Cold cream or petroleum jelly
Impression materials: zinc oxide–eugenol impression paste or elastomer-type impression material, such as polyvinylsiloxane, polysulfide rubber base, or polyether materials
Mixing pads and spatulas for impression materials

FIG. 31-20   Armamentarium for border molding and final impressions appointment.

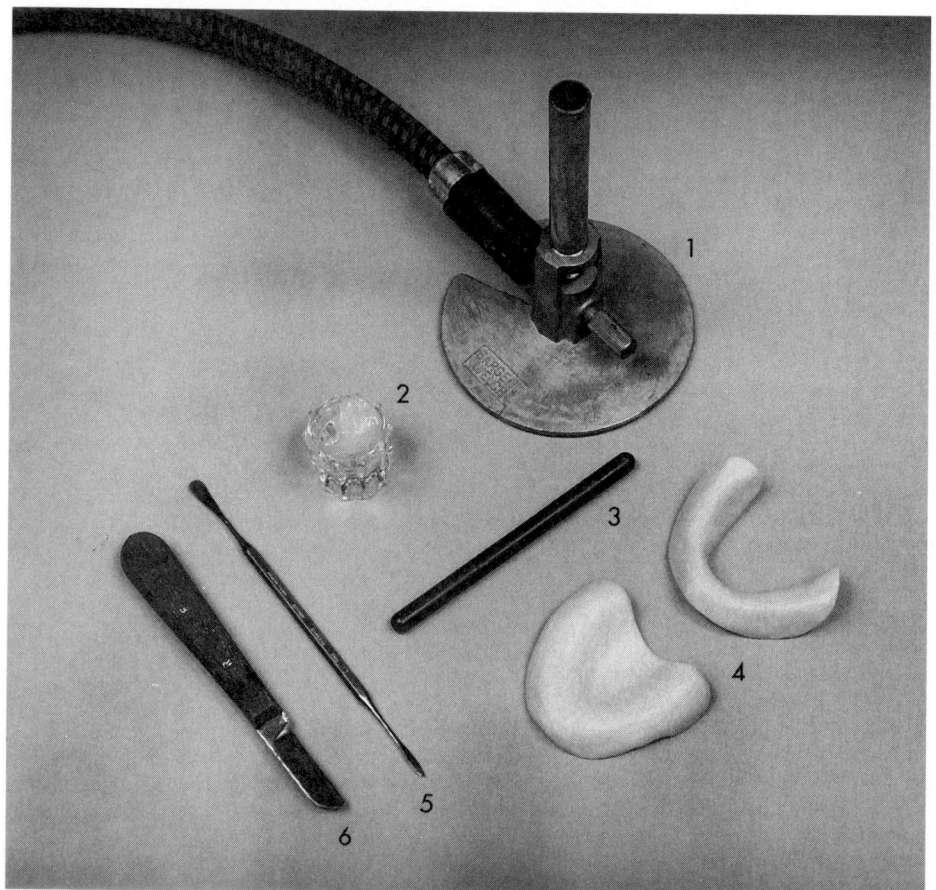

1. Bunsen burner
2. Vaseline
3. Compound stick
4. Custom made acrylic trays
5. #7 Wax spatula
6. Laboratory knife

Not pictured: water bath and impression material armamentarium

BORDER MOLDING

- Are all universal barrier techniques being used?
- Is all of the armamentarium available and prepared for use?
- Are the instruments arranged in sequence of use?
- Am I prepared for alternative treatment plans?
- Is the necessary equipment turned on and ready to operate?

Border molding, or **muscle trimming,** is a common procedure for complete dentures. It is also a process that is completed on the tissue areas of partial dentures, such as the saddle or tuberosity areas. No appreciable difference in technique exists in the border molding procedure for the maxillary or the mandibular arch. In each case the primary objective of border molding is to obtain an impression that replicates the border of the denture, while the tissues are being manipulated or are actively moving. In the mandibular impression, however, it will be necessary for the patient to activate the tongue in many different positions to create action that might cause denture movement to occur.

To achieve border molding the dentist will perform the following procedures:

1. Coat the periphery of the custom-made tray with warmed dental compound
2. Place the tray into the patient's mouth
3. Manipulate the soft tissues
4. Ask the patient to move the lips, cheeks, or tongue in various directions to recreate the common masticatory and speech actions that are a normal part of the patient's oral activity

The custom-made tray with relieved peripheral borders is used during the border molding. The tray is trimmed about 2 to 3 mm short of the planned denture border. This relief of the tray allows for the extension of the borders in dental compound. The steps in Box 31-8 are typically followed to achieve border molding on a custom tray. Various steps in this procedure may lend themselves to four-handed procedures, depending on the arrangement of the treatment room. The assistant needs to arrange the equipment as close to the site of treatment as possible, but he or she may have to adapt the environment to compensate for the Bunsen burner or the heating bath. Much of this procedure requires the dentist to work intraorally and does not require frequent instrument exchanges. The preparation of the materials and mixing of impression material becomes the primary responsibility of the assistant.

Steps in the Border Molding Procedure

1. Warm the compound in a flame from a Bunsen burner until it is softened.
2. Fill the relieved areas on the peripheral border of the tray with dental compound.
3. Use a flame from an alcohol torch to soften the compound on the tray.
4. Dip the tray into a water bath at the working temperature of the dental compound to temper and soften the material so that it will be comfortable when it is placed in the patient's mouth.
5. Place the tray slowly into the patient's mouth and seat it firmly in place. This will allow the compound to flow.

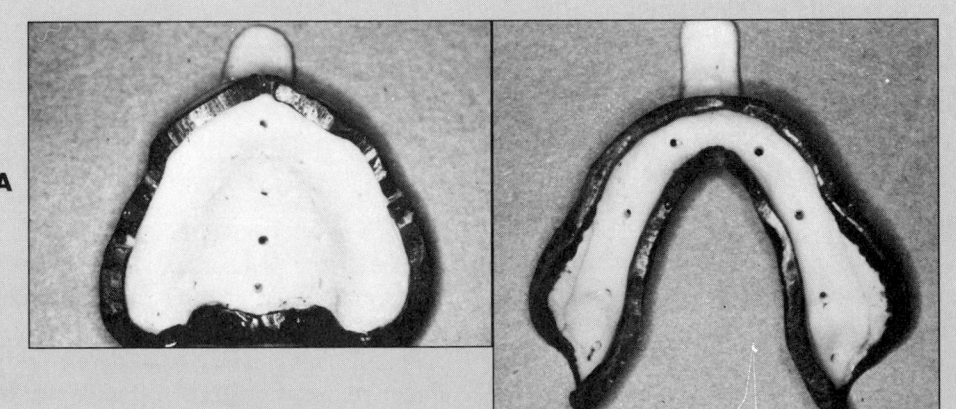

FIG. 31-21 Border molding completed on maxillary, *A,* and mandibular, *B,* trays.

(From Zarb GA, Bolender CL, Hickey JC, Carlsson GE: *Boucher's prosthodontic treatment for edentulous patients,* ed 10, St Louis, 1990, Mosby.)

Continued.

BORDER MOLDING—cont'd

6. Remove the tray from the mouth and chill in cold water to harden the compound.
7. Remove the excess compound from the peripheral border with a laboratory knife or a wax spatula.
8. Rewarm the compound in the water bath, and reinsert the tray in the patient's mouth.
9. Instruct the patient to activate various muscle groups by asking the patient to perform such actions as extending the tongue, opening the mouth widely, swallowing, everting the lips, or biting down.
10. In addition, the dentist will massage various groups of muscles, feel and observe the cheeks, frena, and various flange areas to ensure that no overextensions of the tray will create poor denture design. Adequate extensions promote the creation of an adequate seal in the finished denture.
11. This process is continued until the dentist has ensured that all border extensions are adequate to provide the necessary support and retention in the denture (Fig. 31-21, *A* and *B*). During this procedure the normal actions of opening and closing, swallowing, yawning, talking, and puckering the lips to whistle must be duplicated because the denture must be retained during each of these actions.

12. Once the border molding is completed, a *wash*-type impression of zinc oxide–eugenol, rubber base, or silicone can be taken of the ridges and supporting structures. Because this custom-made tray is closely adapted to the tissues, a minimal amount of impression material will be needed to obtain the wash. The impression procedure for all of these materials is described in Chapter 11.
13. The impression is disinfected (follow OSHA guidelines) before sending it to the laboratory for the master cast to be poured.

▶ Are the appropriate universal barrier techniques removed?
▶ Have all of the appropriate surfaces been cleaned and disinfected?
▶ Has all armamentarium been removed?
▶ Has all equipment been repositioned?
▶ Has all of the equipment been disinfected/sterilized according to OSHA guidelines?

NOTE: Be certain to follow the laboratory as well as the clinical OSHA guidelines when working with prosthetics.

▶ Interim Laboratory Procedures

A laboratory requisition is sent with the final impression, indicating that the case is ready to have a master cast poured and a record base or baseplate designed. Commonly the impression is boxed (as illustrated in Chapter 11) before pouring to preserve the extension of the impression and the thickness of the border. The interim laboratory procedure includes boxing the impression and constructing baseplates and occlusal rims.

Boxing the Impression

1. The impression is thoroughly dried.
2. The mandibular impression tongue area is blocked out with wax and sealed to the lingual border of the impression.
3. A wax rope, approximately 4 mm wide, is adapted around the periphery of the impression approximately 3 to 4 mm beneath the border of the impression.
4. The wax is sealed carefully with a warmed spatula.
5. A strip of boxing wax is warmed and adapted around the wax rope to form the base of the cast.

6. This boxing wax strip is sealed with a hot spatula, and the finished boxed impression is ready to be poured with a high strength stone (Fig. 31-22, *A* and *B*).
7. When the models are separated, they are prepared by the laboratory technician and mounted on an articulator. From these models a baseplate is constructed for each arch (31-22, *C* and *D*).

CONSTRUCTING BASEPLATES AND OCCLUSAL RIMS

A record base or **baseplate** is an acrylic resin or shellac substance that is used as the denture base in making maxillomandibular jaw relationship records. An occlusal rim or bite rim, which is built from wax, is secured on the baseplate. This rim is used to determine the maxillomandibular jaw relationships and will later be used as a base into which the teeth will be set for the prosthesis. Some dentists may opt to perform this procedure in the office, while others work closely with a commercial laboratory during construction of the prosthetic device. Fig. 31-23, *A* and *B*, illustrates the relationship of the baseplate, occlusal rims, and master casts.

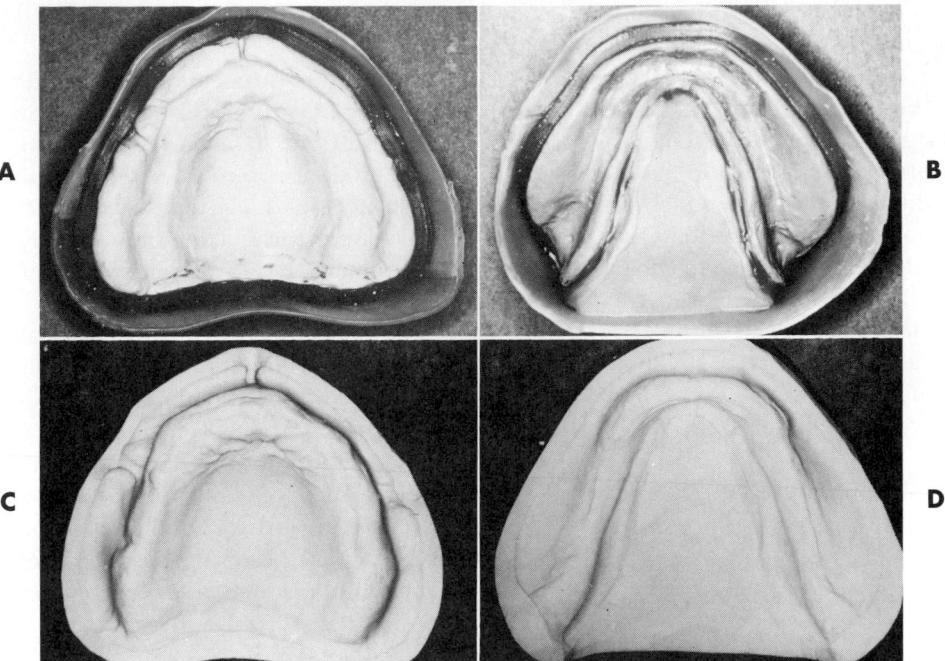

FIG. 31-22   Boxed maxillary and mandibular final impressions. *A,* The vertical wall of the boxing is securely attached to the boxing strip. The height of the wall allows the base of the cast to be about ⅜ to ⅝ inches thick. *B,* The wall of the boxing wax is securely attached to a strip of boxing wax and to the posterior extent of the tongue space filler. *C,* The final maxillary cast provides an accurate record of all of the oral tissues. *D,* The final mandibular casts are formed so that the posterior ends of the residual ridges are well supported.

(From Zarb GA, Bolender CL, Hickey JC, Carlsson GE: *Boucher's prosthodontic treatment for edentulous patients,* ed 10, St Louis, 1990, Mosby.)

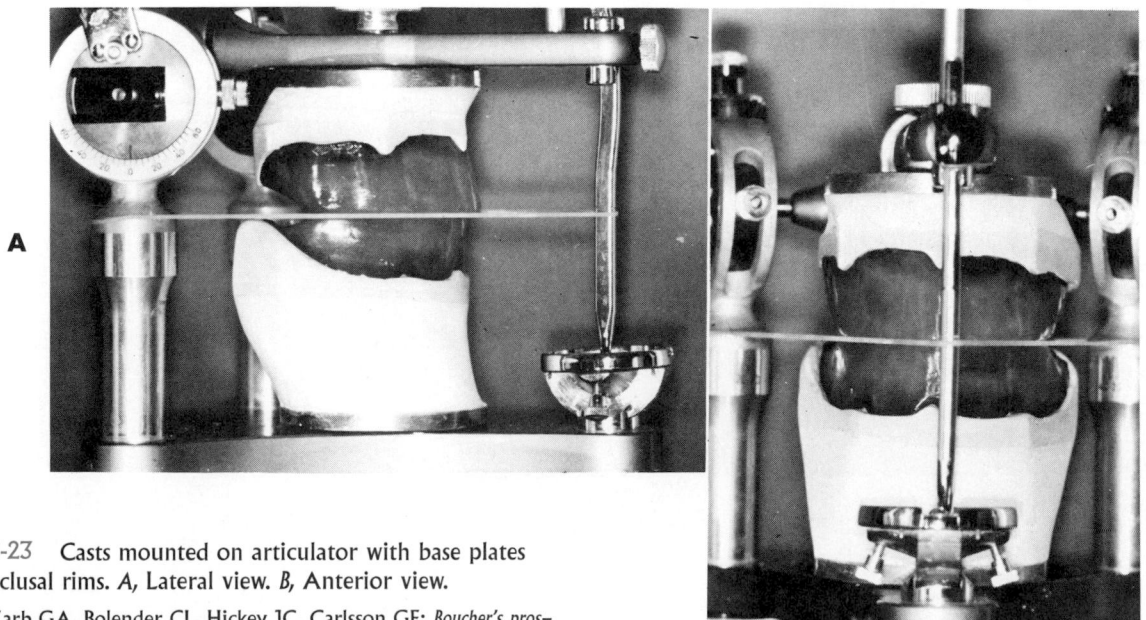

FIG. 31-23   Casts mounted on articulator with base plates and occlusal rims. *A,* Lateral view. *B,* Anterior view.

(From Zarb GA, Bolender CL, Hickey JC, Carlsson GE: *Boucher's prosthodontic treatment for edentulous patients,* ed 10, St Louis, 1990, Mosby.)

Before the set-up is returned to the dental office, the laboratory technician will have also stabilized the baseplate. Warpage may have occurred during the processing of the baseplate. The baseplate must be adapted closely to the master cast to ensure proper retention. Typically, the laboratory technician performs the following:

- Block out all undercuts on the model with wax
- Place aluminum foil over the master cast
- Place a thin layer of zinc oxide–eugenol impression paste into the tissue side of the baseplate
- Seat the tray on the foil covered model
- When set, remove the baseplate
- Peel off the aluminum foil
- Remove all excess material from the peripheral borders
- Store the baseplate back on the master cast
- Return the case to the dental office

FIG. 31-24 Armamentarium for jaw relationship appointment.

▶ Jaw Relationships

During this procedure the dentist must select the appropriate articulator for the specific case. Articulators are available in a variety of designs. Commonly, in prosthodontics a more complex articulator will be used that includes some type of *condyle* design. The Hanau (trademark) articulator shown in Fig. 31-23 is a popular instrument that is used in many complex prosthodontic procedures.

Several different activities will take place during the jaw relationship appointment, including making a face-bow record; determining vertical, centric, protrusive, and excursive jaw relationships; and completing the shade and mould selections. Before any of these procedures can be completed, the dental assistant must prepare the armamentarium and the dentist determines whether the baseplates fit adequately, then the occlusal rims can be attached to the baseplates.

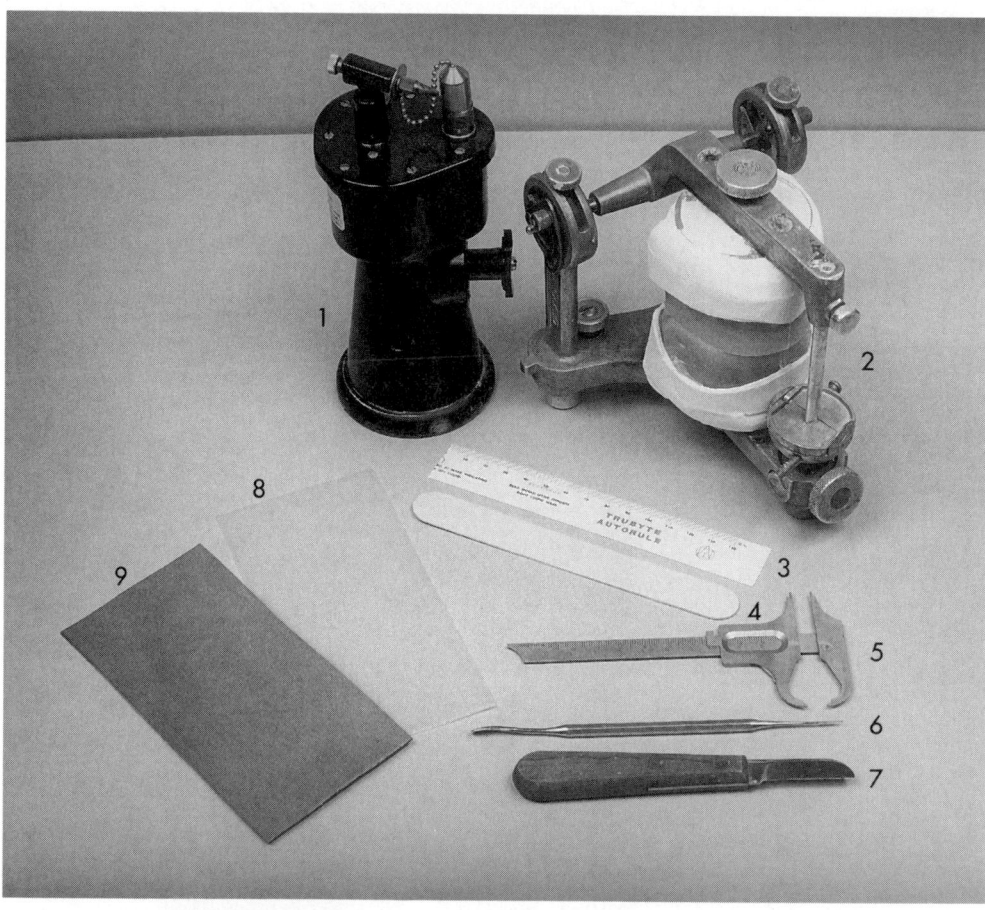

1. Alcohol lamp
2. Baseplate/biterim set-up
3. Millimeter ruler
4. Tongue blade
5. Boley gauge
6. Wax spatula #7
7. Laboratory knife
8. Baseplate wax
9. Aluwax

Not shown: water bath

JAW RELATIONSHIPS

Checking the Fit of the Baseplates

The dentist places the baseplates into the patient's mouth to ensure that they are stable and comfortable. If the bases are not stable to finger pressure, it may be necessary to correct the baseplate or even to begin with a new final impression. To determine tissue comfort, some pressure indicator paste is placed on the inner surface of the baseplate with a small brush. Any pressure areas should be relieved before continuing with jaw relationships.

Attaching the Occlusal Rims

Once the baseplates have been deemed stable, the dentist proceeds to attach the occlusal rims by using either a sheet of baseplate wax, which has been rolled into a tight rope, or by using a preshaped wax occlusal rim. The occlusal rim is attached to the ridge of the baseplate (Fig. 31-22).

Making a Facebow Record

A **facebow** is a caliper-like, adjustable device that is used to establish the relationship between the mandibular condyle of the temporomandibular joint and the maxillary dental arch. This dimensional relationship is transferred to the articulator to simulate jaw movement during the construction of the dental prosthesis. Making the face-bow record includes the following steps:

1. Place ear rod of the face-bow into the external auditory meatus.
2. Place the maxillary baseplate, to which the bite fork has been attached, in the patient's mouth (Fig. 31-25, *A*).
3. Position the face-bow apparatus to fit into the bite fork arm, and adjust the side axis arms, so that they are an equal distance from the axis points that have been marked on the face. The arms should just touch the marked points.
4. Readjust the arms, until they lightly touch the face, and take a reading on the numbered index scale. This number is recorded on the patient record.
5. Remove the face-bow and baseplate from the patient's mouth, and attach it to the articular condyle rods of the articulator.
6. Adjust the anterior height of the maxillary occlusal rim by moving the face-bow up and down, so that the incisal edge of the maxillary occlusal rim is level with the line on the incisal guide pin.
7. Mount the ring of the articulator to the prepared maxillary cast with stone.
8. Remove the bite fork from the set-up by warming the handle of the fork in a direct flame. The heat is transferred to the bite portion of the fork and allows for easy removal. A wax spatula can aid in smoothing any voids in the occlusal rim (Fig. 31-25, *B*).

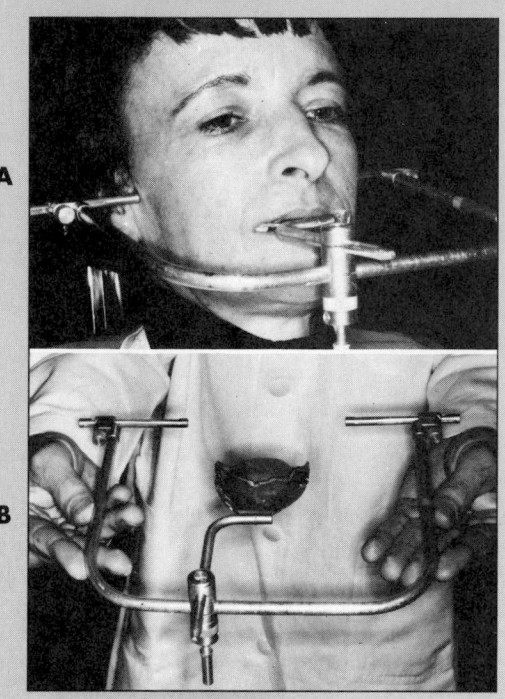

FIG. 31-25   *A,* Hanau facebow fork attached to the maxillary occlusal rim properly locates the facebow on the patient's face. *B,* Completed facebow record.

(From Zarb GA, Bolender CL, Hickey JC, Carlsson GE: *Boucher's prosthodontic treatment for edentulous patients,* ed 10, St Louis, 1990, Mosby.)

The next step in the procedure is to obtain **vertical dimension** relationships. Vertical dimension refers to the distance between two arbitrary fixed points: one on the maxilla, and one on the mandible when the jaws are at rest. This measurement is used to establish the height of the occlusal tables and the **freeway space** in denture construction. The freeway space is the amount of space between the maxillary and mandibular teeth when the jaws of an individual are at rest. The **vertical dimension of occlusion** refers to the face height that exists when the teeth are in occlusion. The vertical dimension of rest is defined as the habitual postural position of the mandible when the patient is resting comfortably in an upright position and the condyles are in a neutral unstrained position. Obtaining vertical dimension requires the dentist to:

1. Select two points to determine facial height: one on the mandible, and the other on the maxilla (Fig. 31-26).

Continued.

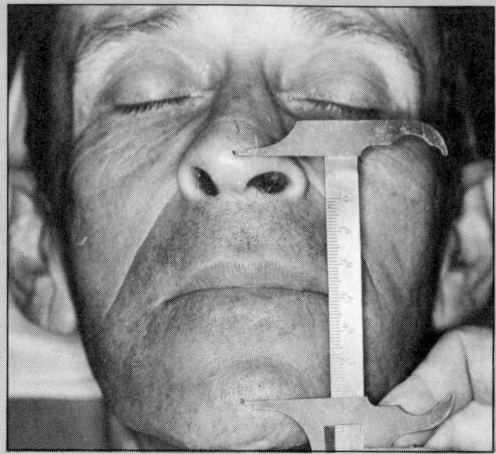

FIG. 31-26   A measurement is made between two points on the face when the jaws are at the vertical relation of a physiologic rest position.

(From Zarb GA, Bolender CL, Hickey JC, Carlsson GE: *Boucher's pros-thodontic treatment for edentulous patients,* ed 10, St Louis, 1990, Mosby.)

2. Take a measurement of the patient's vertical dimension while at rest and in occlusion, using a millimeter ruler and tongue blade. Several methods can be used to determine an accurate measurement. These include asking the patient to speak, swallow, bite forcefully, or swallow.
3. The dental assistant records these measurements; however, this dimension will be checked later because it is possible for these measurements to vary with different patient activities.

Often, accurate measurements are difficult to obtain with baseplates, and the dentist may need to make a tentative decision until the teeth are set up in the trial denture.

Once the vertical dimension has been obtained, the dentist obtains centric relationships. Two factors are considered in this relationship: centric occlusion, and centric jaw relation. **Centric occlusion** is the relation of opposing occlusal surfaces that provides the maximum contact or intercuspation. **Centric jaw**

relation is more complex and includes the relation of the mandible to the maxilla when the condyles are in their most posterosuperior, unstrained positions in the glenoid fossae, from which lateral movements can be made at the occluding vertical relation normal for the patient. Centric relation is a relation that exists at any degree of jaw separation.

To determine centric relation the dentist will perform the following:

1. Make a V-shaped notch approximately 1 to 3 mm in the mandibular occlusal rim.
2. Rub the surface with petroleum jelly, and insert the mandibular occlusal rim into the patient's mouth.
3. Prepare the maxillary occlusal rim by relieving the wax occlusal rim vertically, approximately 4 mm in the posterior area that opposes the mandibular occlusal rim.
4. Add warmed, softened Aluwax (trademark) to the relieved area on the maxillary rim, and guide the patient to bite into the wax. The dentist will ask the patient to remain in this position until the wax is hardened.
5. Remove the occlusal rims, and cool to set the wax.

The dentist will return the baseplates and bite rims to the articulator frequently, until all vertical, centric, excursive (side-to-side), and protrusive (anterior-to-posterior) recordings have been completed. Each time a relationship is recorded on the articulator, the dentist will adjust various settings on the condylar element to simulate the patient's various jaw relationships.

In addition, at this appointment, it will be necessary to make available the following materials for shade and mould selection:

▶ Appropriate shade guides
▶ Trubyte Tooth Indicator (trademark), optional

Use the suggestions made earlier in this chapter to select a shade and mould for the denture teeth. The assistant records the selections on the patient's record and transfers this information to the laboratory requisition.

Armamentarium

The armamentarium necessary for this procedure includes the following (Fig. 31-24):

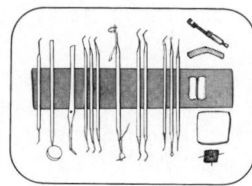

Articulated set up with the baseplates and occlusal rims
Sharp lab knife
Hanau torch (trademark)
Wax spatula
Face-bow assembly
Baseplate wax
Millimeter ruler
Caliper or Boley gauge
Bite wax, such as Aluwax
Tongue blade

The case is disinfected according to OSHA guidelines and transferred to the dental laboratory with the appropriate instructions on the laboratory requisition.

▶ Interim Laboratory Procedures

Arranging and articulating artificial teeth on the occlusal rims are critical tasks of the dental laboratory technician at this point of the treatment procedure. Data provided by the dentist are used to select the appropriate teeth and to set them into the bite rim. The trial denture also involves contouring the wax on the gingival mucosa areas to reproduce the contours of the original tissues in the dentulous mouth. When this task is done carefully, it will be easier for the dentist and the patient to evaluate the appearance, comfort, and speech during the try in appointment.

When the trial denture has been completed, it is returned to the dental office for a try in appointment.

▶ Denture Try-In

This is an important appointment for the dentist and the patient. It is the time to check the tooth arrangement and to ensure that the denture provides for adequate speech and mastication and that a pleasing appearance has been achieved. This is the final appointment before the completion of the denture; if any changes are to be made, they must be done at this appointment. During the appointment the denture is evaluated to ensure the following:

1. Adequate tongue space for proper speech
2. Correct fullness in the cheek and lip areas
3. Proper vertical and centric dimension
4. Correct shade and mould
5. Adequate buccal and labial tooth position to avoid biting the cheeks and lips

DENTURE TRY-IN

The denture is disinfected before trying it in the patient's mouth. The denture is then passed to the dentist for insertion and the following steps are followed. Check the

1. Occlusal vertical dimension, using the caliper and millimeter ruler. The patient is asked to perform the same type of verbal activities as done during the initial appointment.
2. Centric occlusion.
3. Tooth position. Ask the patient to speak to verify the lingual position is adequate.
4. Appearance. Observe the lip and cheek fullness to ensure that adequate bulk is present. If the cheeks are too full, the teeth may need to be repositioned or some of the wax, removed. If the cheeks are too shallow or if a sunken appearance is evident, the teeth may need to be repositioned or may need to be added.
5. Orientation of the occlusal plane to ensure that it is even with the lip line and that an adequate amount of tooth length is showing.
6. Shade and mould of the teeth for a blend with the patient's complexion and face shape.
7. Arrangement of the teeth to verify that they provide a pleasing appearance.

If any of these check points are not satisfactory, it may be necessary to heat a wax spatula or knife, remove the teeth, reset the teeth, or recontour the mucosa wax. When the trial denture is accepted by the dentist and the patient, it is disinfected and returned to the laboratory for final processing. Again, a laboratory requisition accompanies the case, with details for the final insertion.

Armamentarium

Armamentarium that may be used at this appointment include the following (Fig. 31-27):

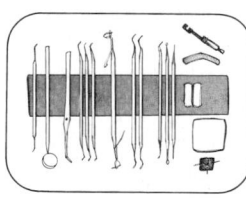

Waxed dentures on the articulator
Millimeter ruler
Bunsen burner
Wax spatula
Wax knife
Baseplate wax
Bowl of cold water
Boley gauge
Hand mirror, or access to wall mirror

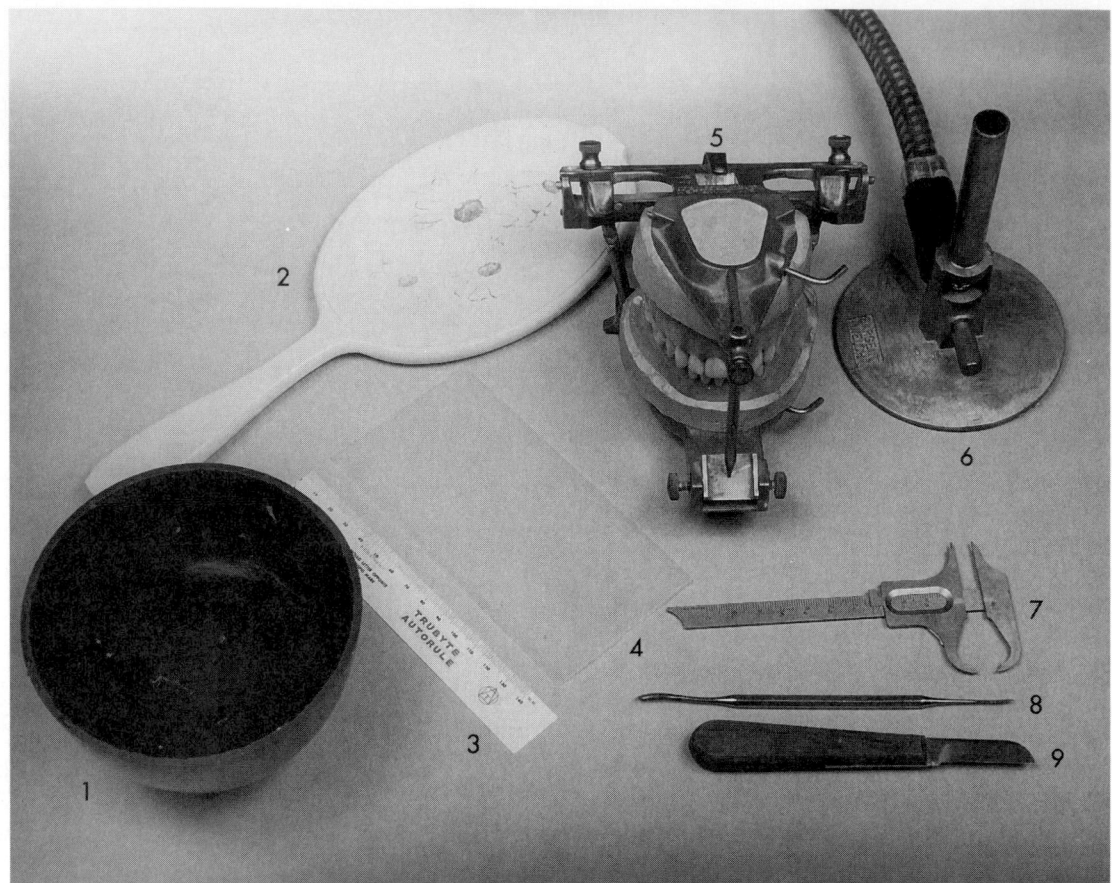

1. Rubber bowl with cold water
2. Patient face mirror
3. Millimeter ruler
4. Baseplate wax
5. Hanau articulator with waxed denture set-up
6. Bunsen burner
7. Boley gauge
8. #7 Wax spatula
9. Laboratory knife

FIG. 31-27   Armamentarium for try-in appointment.

Final Laboratory Procedures

Denture processing is the process of converting the wax pattern of a denture or a trial denture into a denture with a base that is made of another material, such as acrylic resin. To accomplish this task the denture goes through a flasking process, where the cast and wax denture are placed into a flask to prepare for molding the denture base material into the form of the denture (Fig. 31-28, *A* through *C*).

Prosthesis Insertion

The type of insertion appointment depends on the type of prosthesis that is to be delivered to the patient. For instance, if complete immediate dentures are to be inserted, it is likely that the dentures will be delivered to a maxillofacial oral surgeon, who will perform the surgery and insert the dentures initially. This procedure is described in Chapter 37. If the prosthesis is a nonimmediate denture or a partial denture, the prosthesis is sent directly to the dentist who has been preparing the prosthesis. At this appointment the assistant must perform the following tasks:

1. Check the retention of the denture
2. Ensure the accuracy of the jaw relations
3. Determine tissue comfort
4. Instruct the patient in the correct insertion and use of the dentures
5. Provide instructions for proper home care, and explain the limitations of the prosthesis
6. Where necessary, adjust the denture, using a variety of stones and burs

The procedural description for inserting full nonimmediate dentures follows.

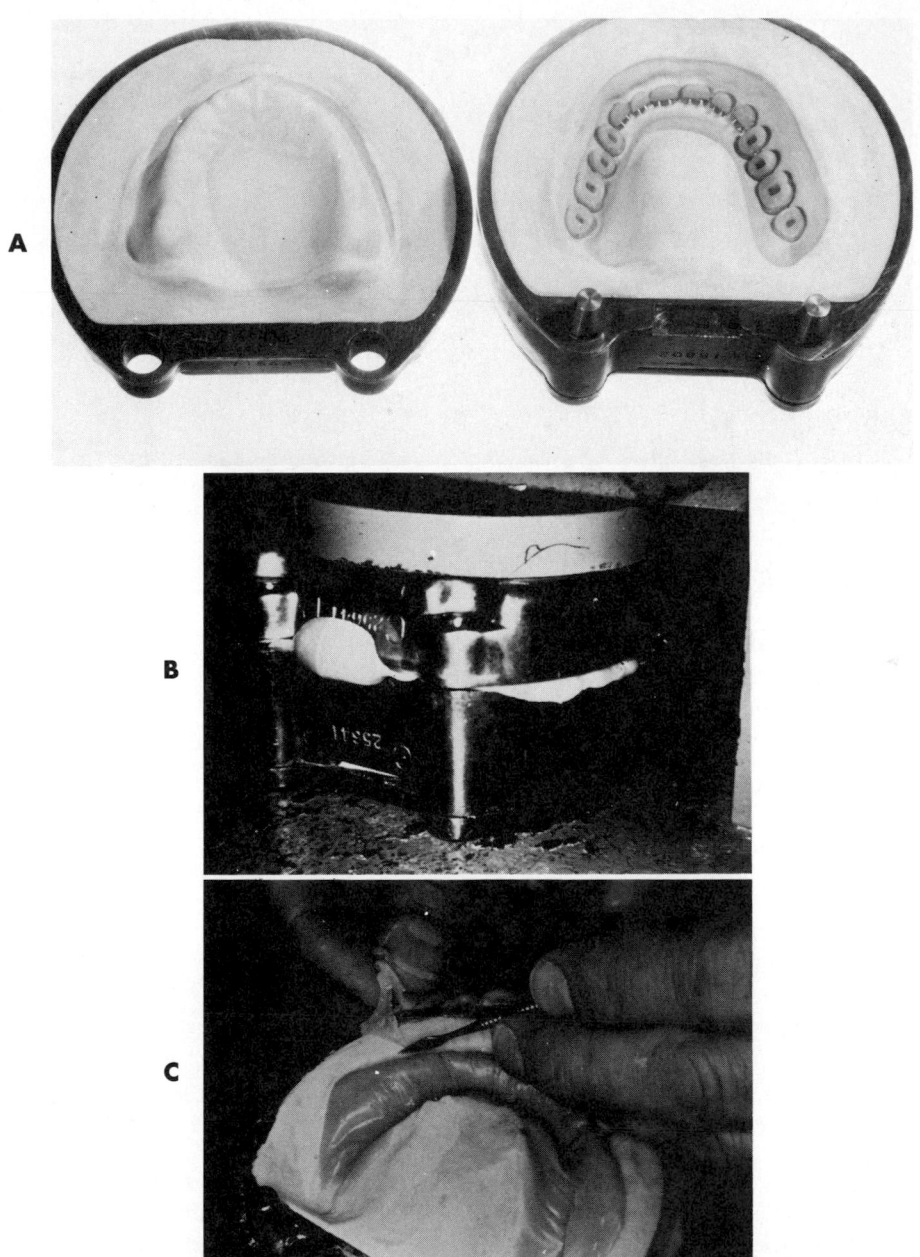

FIG. 3I-28   Denture flask. *A,* Two parts of the denture flask; just before packing the acrylic dough. *B,* Excess dough is forced out of the flask under pressure. *C,* Excess, or flash, is trimmed away.

(From Craig RG, Powers JM, O'Brien W]: *Dental materials,* ed 5, St Louis, 1992, Mosby.)

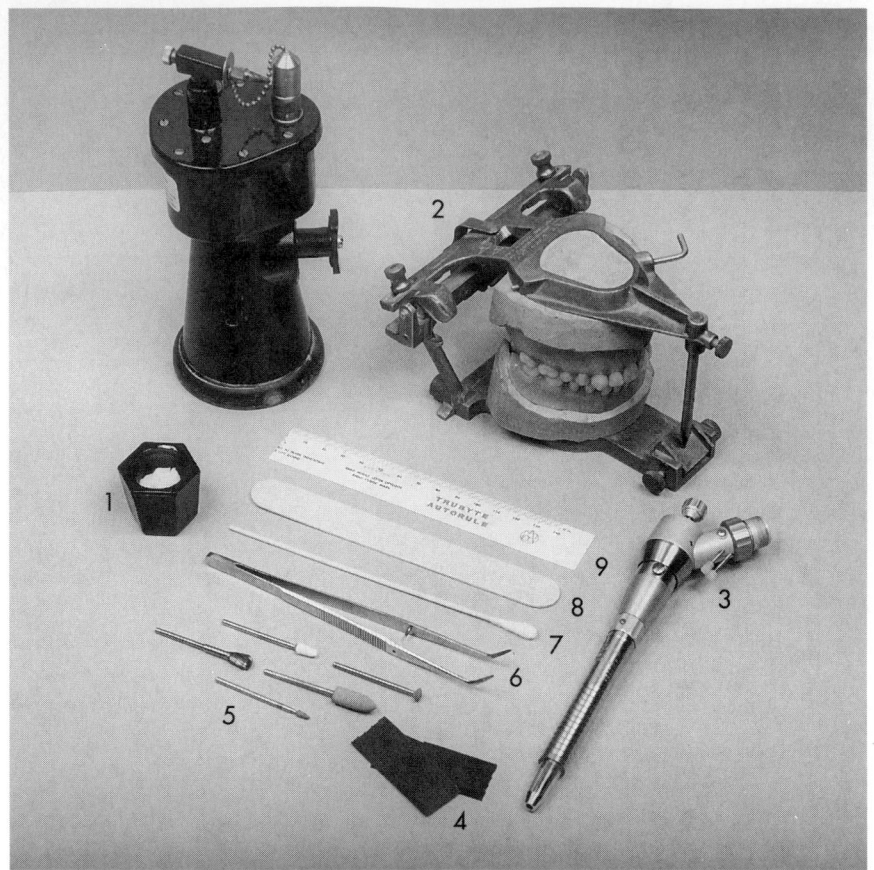

FIG. 31-29   **Armamentarium for denture insertion appointment.**

1. Dappen dish with pressure indicating paste
2. Hanau articulator with denture set-up
3. Slow-speed handpiece
4. Articulating paper
5. Assorted stones and burs
6. Cotton pliers
7. Cotton-tipped applicator
8. Millimeter ruler
Not shown: face mirror

PROSTHESIS INSERTION

Before inserting the denture, it is disinfected. The following procedures are followed during denture insertion:

1. The denture is examined to ensure that no nodules or sharp edges are present that could injure the soft tissues.
2. The maxillary denture is inserted with a firm upward and backward motion. With a finger in the palatal area, the dentist seats the denture firmly.
3. The denture is removed to verify retention by grasping at the buccal surfaces of the denture with thumb and forefinger, and pressure is applied in a downward, pulling motion.
4. The maxillary denture is reinserted, and the mandibular denture is then inserted.
5. The retention of the lower denture is tested by placing force in an upward direction.

6. Internal tissues are checked by brushing pressure indicator paste inside the denture. Where evidence of extreme pressure is apparent, the acrylic is removed with a small bur or stone.
7. The occlusion is checked with the use of articulating paper. High contact points are adjusted with stones or burs.
8. The markings are removed with a tissue or with 2×2 gauze. If the marks cannot be removed manually, it may be necessary to transfer the denture to the polishing wheel in the office laboratory.

The patient is shown a mirror and allowed to practice taking the dentures in and out to ensure proper placement and comfort.

Armamentarium necessary for this procedure includes the following (Fig. 31-29):

Completed dentures
Burs and stones
Slow-speed handpiece
Millimeter ruler
Articulating paper and forceps
Pressure indicating paste set-up

Home Care Instructions

Several points need to be reviewed with the patient about home care instructions, including initial and future soreness and discomfort, coping with the prosthesis, and maintaining the oral tissues and the prosthesis.

▶ Soreness and Discomfort

The patient needs to know that some initial soreness may occur in the soft tissues for a few days after insertion of the prosthesis. If the prosthesis is a partial denture discomfort may be present in some of the natural teeth. The oral tissues are sensitive, and it may take some time for these tissues to adjust to the new pressures that are being placed on them. The patient needs to know also that the dentist is available to adjust the new prosthesis during this time and that he or she is expected to contact the office if the discomfort does not subside in a few days.

The patient must also be informed that if discomfort occurs after several weeks or months the cause may be tissue changes, and the patient must be seen by the dentist to determine what changes have occurred. The patient should be informed that he or she should not use home remedies to avoid an office visit. Remedies such as using a wood file or an emery board on a prosthesis may result in creating rough surfaces or may improperly alter the denture, resulting in further discomfort.

▶ Potential Damage from Denture Neglect

If a patient does not observe changes taking place in the mouth or continues to neglect symptoms, damage may occur to the surrounding tissues and existing teeth and gingiva. These conditions may be acute, causing severe pain a short time after the denture is inserted, or the conditions may be chronic, developing over a longer time period, and they may not be painful.

Acute conditions are often evidenced by pain, redness of tissues, and the presence of ulcerated tissue. These conditions are frequently the result of discrepancies in the fit of the prostheses: an overextension of the denture base; a vertical dimension that is too great; teeth that are set in the wrong position; clasps on a partial denture that gouge into undercut areas, causing periodontal involve-

ment; connectors damaging the mucosa; an allergy to a constituent in the denture base; improperly polished surfaces, or improperly cleaned prosthesis. Each of these conditions can generally be corrected at chairside, with the exception of the allergy, which may require the construction of a new denture.

Chronic conditions are generally the result of a lack of attention to home care and as a result may cause chronic damage to the oral tissues. Evidence of this neglect results in increased resorption of alveolar ridges, production of bony or soft tissue abnormalities, hyperplasia of the oral mucosa, denture stomatitis, or hyperkeratosis. Partial dentures may cause chronic damage to restorations or abutment teeth, leading to fracture or loss or to potential TMJ symptoms caused by poor occlusion.

Edentulous patients often feel that regular visits to the dentist are no longer necessary except for major problems, such as fracture or a lost denture tooth. A recall system for denture patients is encouraged and can become part of the education program. Denture wearers should realize that the insertion of complete dentures is not final dental treatment. They need to understand the value of follow-up appointments for tissue examination, future reline and rebasing, and new dentures that are made at periodic times. The need for such treatment is evidenced by the benefit coverage by most major insurance carriers. Most carriers make some provision for replacement dentures in 5 to 8 years. Thus, a denture is not a lifetime replacement.

Coping with the Prosthesis

In Chapter 29 emphasis is placed on patient education and the need to lay a foundation for positive acceptance of the new prosthesis. The new prosthesis wearer will need to learn new coping techniques in specific areas, including how to speak distinctly, how to eat, and how to manage an increased salivary flow and excessive bulk in the mouth.

For the new wearer speaking may seem difficult if the device covers a major portion of the palate. Sometimes the bulk and placement of the palatal coverage may make it difficult at first to place the tongue in the normal position. The assistant may suggest that the patient try reading and speaking aloud in private or with family members at home to overcome the fear of speaking and to develop confidence.

▶ Managing Bulk and Salivary Flow

When a new prosthesis is placed in a patient's mouth, he or she often has a feeling of fullness and crowding of the tongue. Sensory receptors in the tongue are stimulated, causing the patient to be aware of the new prosthesis. For a short period of time the sensory receptors in the mouth may also induce increased salivary flow. Fortunately after a period of time these reactions will generally subside. The patient must understand that these reactions are normal, and that they will subside after the prosthesis has been worn for a time.

Maintaining Oral Tissues

Whether the new prosthesis is a full or a partial denture, the patient needs to receive instructions in maintaining the oral tissues beneath the prosthesis and in how to care for the prosthesis. The patient who wears the partial denture must learn how to care for the natural teeth, as well.

▶ Caring for the Natural Teeth

A patient who has a partial denture has obviously lost teeth because of disease or trauma. If the loss has been caused by disease, the patient is already aware of the results of neglect. Having a partial denture requires that the patient spend more time in oral hygiene to maintain the remaining teeth. Chapter 26 provides the recommended oral hygiene techniques for a prosthesis wearer. Emphasis, however, must be placed on the need to rinse the mouth after eating and to give special attention to the care of the abutment teeth.

▶ Caring for the Soft Tissues

The underlying tissues beneath the prosthesis must be well maintained. It is unnatural to have the oral mucosa covered 24 hours a day. To promote healthy capillary action, the tissues need to be exposed for several hours at a time. The easiest and most convenient method of cleaning and massaging the soft tissues is to use a soft tooth brush. Another method of cleaning and massaging these tissues is to use a moist washcloth. The washcloth is moistened and is placed over the forefinger, and the gingival and supporting tissues are scrubbed thoroughly.

▶ Caring for the Prosthesis

Be certain to point out to the patient that food debris and calculus can adhere to a partial or full denture and offer advice on care of the prothesis.

These suggestions might include the following:
1. Use a soft brush to clean the prosthesis. Avoid using a hard brush or any abrasive substance, especially for acrylic bases because they can be scratched easily.
2. Clean the prosthesis over a bowl of cold water, so that if the device slips and falls, the fall will be broken by the water.
3. If calculus forms on the prosthesis, use a cleaning

agent that will dissolve the calculus. To be helpful, provide the patient with a sample of such a material.
4. Avoid wearing the prosthesis all night. The underlying tissues need time to rest.
5. When the prosthesis is inserted, it should be placed by hand to avoid trauma to the denture; it should not be bitten into place.
6. When the prosthesis is not worn, it should always be stored in water to avoid dimensional changes caused by a loss of absorbed water.

Since this is a busy appointment for the patient, it is helpful to provide written instructions on the care of the prosthesis. Instructions, such as those as shown in Box 31-9, can be taken home for later review.

Initial Adjustment

A **denture adjustment** is the process of removing excess denture base to relieve an area where soft tissue is being irritated or to alter the occlusion. The follow-up appointment is generally scheduled within 24 to 48 hours following insertion of the prosthesis. For an immediate denture the appointment is scheduled 24 hours after insertion, whereas for a nonimmediate denture or a partial denture the follow-up appointment may be scheduled after a longer period of time. For the immediate denture patient, this will be the first time the denture has been removed. It will also be the first time the patient will have experienced the feeling of oral tissues without the presence of teeth.

After the patient has been seated, the dentist will observe the extraoral tissues to note any asymmetry caused by edema. Some bruising from the trauma of the surgery may be evident. The patient should be informed that these conditions are normal and that they will subside in a few days.

Armamentarium

Armamentarium for this appointment may include the following:

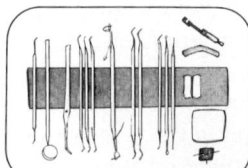

Mouth mirror	Articulating paper
Mouthwash	Articulaalting paper forceps
Pressure-indicating paste	Assorted burs and stones

Rebasing and Relining

Relining is the process of adding denture base material to the tissue side of the removable prosthesis to improve its adaptation to the tissues. Relining of a complete denture is done to improve retention and stability; this is especially important in an immediate denture because the tissues of the posterior area will resorb as they heal following surgery. **Rebasing** is the replacement of all of the acrylic resin base material without changing the occlusal relationships. Indications for a reline or rebase include noticeable movement in a partial denture that causes the retainer rests to be raised or even unseated; instability in a denture over which a patient has no control; or irritation of the soft tissues, caused by the unstable denture.

To complete a relining or rebasing the patient needs to be informed of the length of time it will take to complete this process. Unless the patient has a duplicate denture, he or she will be without the prosthesis for a period of time while it is processed. Commonly, a patient may come to the office early in the day and be able to have the prosthesis returned later in the day.

Armamentarium

Armamentarium may include the following:
Prosthesis to be relined
Acrylic bur or flange
Petroleum jelly or cold cream
2 × 2 gauze sponges

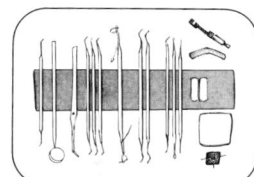

The following steps are used in the initial denture adjustment appointment:

1. The denture is gently removed.
2. The patient is allowed to rinse the mouth gently, without forcefully swishing the mouthwash about to avoid dislocation of any blood clots. The mouthwash is removed gently with the HVE tip avoiding contact with the soft tissues.
3. The denture is rinsed by the assistant.
4. The dentist examines the oral tissues to identify any areas that may be irritated by the denture.
5. The denture can be dried and pressure-indicating paste inserted in the tissue portion of the denture. The denture is reinserted and removed to identify pressure points. These pressure points can be relieved with a bur or stone.
6. The denture is reinserted, and the occlusion is adjusted. Minor adjustments may be made at this initial appointment, since discomfort from the surgery or other sore spots may impede a realistic occlusal registration.
7. The patient is then shown how to take the denture in and out of the mouth and is allowed to practice this procedure.
8. A review of the home care procedure and the need to observe the changes in oral tissues is provided the patient.

At this point the patient is informed of the need for future follow-up appointments and is encouraged to contact the office in case of discomfort.

To reline a denture the following steps are used:

1. Clean the tissue surface of the denture manually or in the ultrasonic.
2. Remove all undercuts from the denture to ensure that the denture can be removed from the stone casts after the reline has been cast.
3. Remove flanges of the denture with an acrylic bur or stone to avoid overextension.
4. Correct minor defects or base extension with low heat stick compound.
5. Take an impression by placing the impression material in the tissue side of the denture and inserting it into the patient's mouth. If a zinc oxide–eugenol paste is used, lubricate the patient's extraoral tissues before insertion.
6. Remove the denture from the patient's mouth.
7. Disinfect the denture and transfer to the laboratory, with instructions for the reline and the delivery time included.

Impression material: Zinc oxide–eugenol, polyvinyl siloxane, or polysulfide

The dental laboratory will cast impressions in stone and process the dentures in a manner similar to that of flasking the new denture. After the flasking procedure the laboratory technician polishes and finishes the denture and returns it to the office. The reinsertion of the denture follows the steps that are used for the initial delivery. The patient should be informed that, like the original insertion, he or she can anticipate some soreness or discomfort because the tissue surface of the denture has been readapted to the oral tissues.

Osseointegration

Osseointegration, the growth of the alveolar process around the mortise of a dental implant, is an integral aspect of prosthetic dentistry. Implanting single tooth restorations or multiple teeth in combination with bridges, partial or full denture is an alternative for some patients. Certain oral conditions must exist for successful implants, including an alveolar process that is of adequate height, width, and density and gingival tissues that are healthy.

Several dental implants are available, but the two most common are the **endosteal** and **subperiosteal** implants. The endosteal implant involves the use of screws, cylinders, or blades that are implanted in the alveolar process (Fig. 31-30). Each implant is capable of holding a single restoration or a combination of prosthetic teeth. A subperiosteal implant is positioned over the alveolar process, and a framework of metal posts extends from the gingival tissue after implantation to assist in retaining a prosthesis.

▶ Implant Process

The implant process may take 3 to 9 months from the beginning to completion. The steps in the plantation process include placing the anchor or the fixture

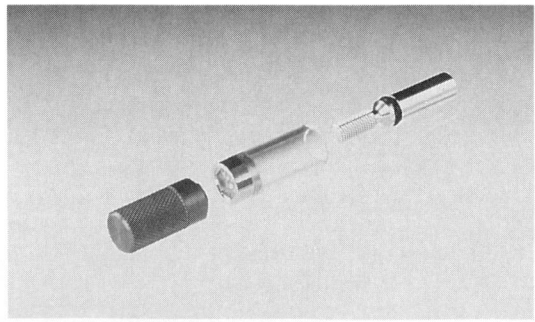

FIG. 31-30   Universal combo abutment, hexed with long screw; Branemark analog.

(Courtesy of IMPAC.)

installation; attaching the abutments; and creating and placing the restoration(s). The first phase may be completed under local or general anesthesia. The following appointments may require the use of local anesthesia alone.

ANCHOR PLACEMENT

The first step in the implant process is the surgical placement of the anchors for the restoration/prosthesis (Fig. 31-31). This process may occur in a dental office or in a hospital setting. Often, before the surgical procedure the patient is requested to take an oral antibiotic to prevent infections. To reduce potential infection just before the surgical procedure, the patient may be asked to brush the teeth thoroughly and to rinse with an antiseptic mouthwash.

The placement of the implant anchors involves making a surgical opening in the gingival tissues to expose the bone. Initially, the alveolar bone is surgically prepared by creating a small hole opening with a round bur. Spiral drills of increasingly larger sizes are then used to enlarge the hole. The anchor or fixture is positioned in the hole opening, often through a process of countersinking the fixture. Throughout the process to place the anchor, the area must be irrigated with room-temperature saline solution and evacuated to reduce friction and mechanical trauma.

Once the anchor is securely positioned, a cover or cover screw is positioned in the mortise or anchor. The coverage of the opening prevents bone growth over the anchor head during the healing process. The gingival tissues are sutured over or around the anchor. Suture removal occurs after 1 week; however, the process of healing extends to approximately 4 to 6 months.

POSTSURGICAL CARE: FIRST APPOINTMENT

Throughout the healing process, maintenance of healthy tissue is extremely important to the success of the procedure. Postsurgery instructions must be given to prevent infection and to aid in the healing process. The patient may begin a soft diet and also begin the oral hygiene procedure, using a small soft brush. Beyond normal hygiene care the patient must continue dental visits to evaluate the healing and osseointegration process. The patient is directed to avoid pressure on the alveolar process and may be directed not to wear prosthetic devices.

ABUTMENT CONNECTION

The second appointment (a surgical setting) requires the same pretreatment preparation as the first appointment (Fig. 31-32). The operator will determine the site of the implantation area(s), with the use of an explorer to find the cover screws.

At this point a surgical opening is made through the oral mucosa to expose the anchors. All soft and hard tissue remnants are removed from the surgical site, and the area is thoroughly rinsed and evacuated.

Once the anchor is exposed, an abutment is placed in the opening at the top of the anchor. The abutment may be permanent, or it may be a temporary connector. After this procedure, trauma is significantly less apparent than it was after the first surgical procedure.

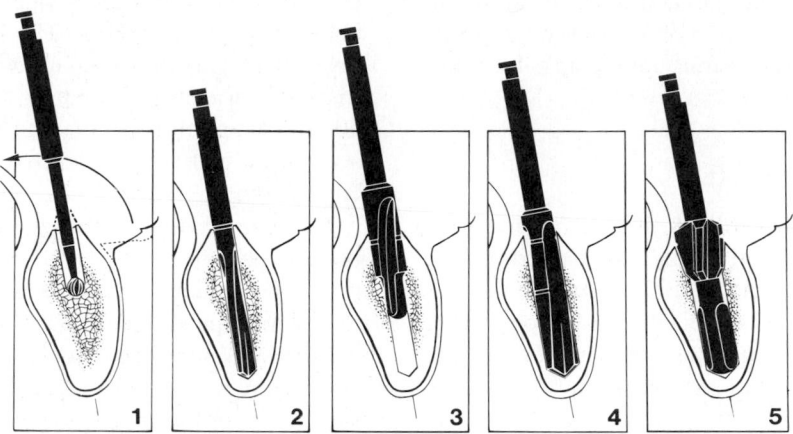

FIG. 31-31 Surgical procedure for osseointegration, first surgical appointment. *1 to 4,* Steps in preparing the site for a titanium root analogue; *5,* flap preparation and gradual widening of the fixture site; countersinking for access to the fixture site; installation of the fixture, and placement of a cover screw under the mucoperiosteal flap.

(From Zarb GA, Bolender CL, Hickey JC, Carlsson GE: *Boucher's prosthodontic treatment for edentulous patients,* ed 10, St Louis, 1990, Mosby.)

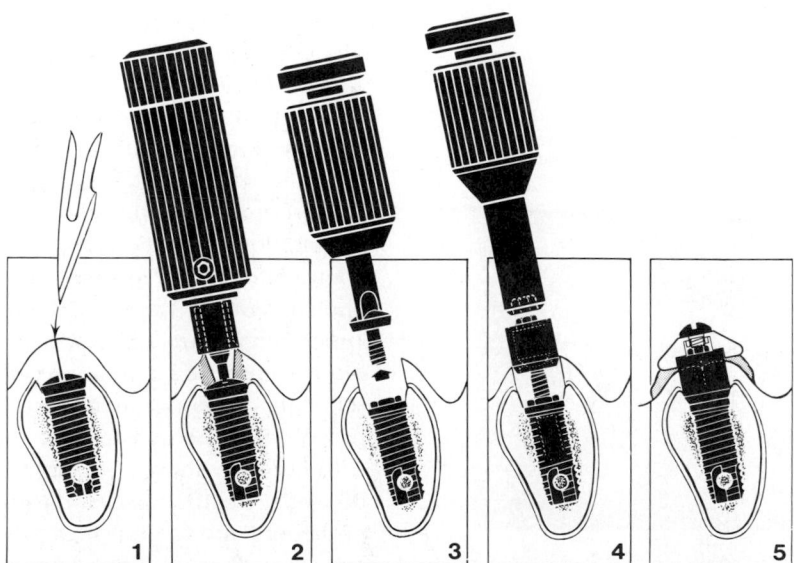

FIG. 31-32 Second surgical appointment, *1* and *2.* Location of the cover screw and surgical excision of the overlying mucosa, *3* and *4.* Removal of the screw and connection of the abutment, *5.* Abutment in place with a surgical pack retained by means of a disposable healing cap.

(From Zarb GA, Bolender CL, Hickey JC, Carlsson GE: *Boucher's prosthodontic treatment for edentulous patients,* ed 10, St Louis, 1990, Mosby.)

POSTSURGICAL CARE: SECOND APPOINTMENT

As it is with the initial surgery, home care is integral to preventing infection, and it aids in the healing process. A few days after the surgical procedure the patient may begin to clean the abutments with a small, soft toothbrush. Initially, the diet should be soft, but as healing progresses the patient is encouraged to alter the diet to his or her level of comfort. Fig. 31-33, *A*, shows implants in place on a model. A panoramic radiograph illustrates a completed implant case in Fig. 31-33, *B*.

RESTORATIVE PROCEDURE

The restorative procedure in this process is similar to those discussed in this chapter if the patient is to receive a partial or a complete denture and those discussed in Chapter 30 if the patient is to receive a fixed prosthetic restoration. This process may include impression, bite registrations, try ins and patient education.

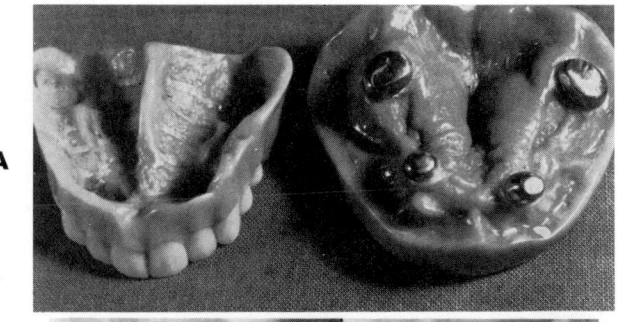

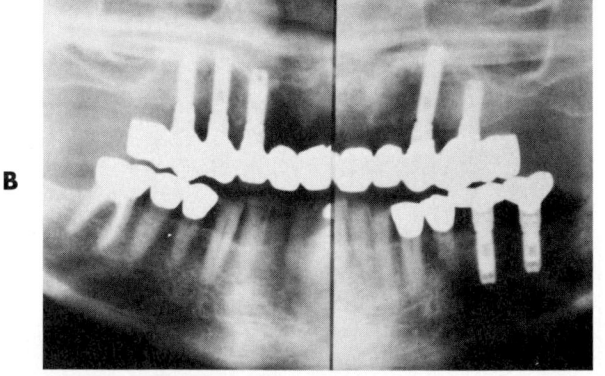

FIG. 31-33   *A,* Implants in place for an overdenture. *B,* Panoramic radiograph of a completed implant.

(From McGivney GP, Castleberry DJ: *McCracken's removable partial prosthodontics, ed 8, St Louis, 1989, Mosby.*)

Modifications in Prosthesis Construction

The procedure just described covers many facets of a typical prosthetic procedure. However, in other types of prosthetic construction, such as in removable partial dentures or in implantology, additional stages or modifications in appointment sequences may be required to achieve the final results. The dental assistant plays an important role in these modifications since, in most instances, the changes require that the assistant schedule additional appointments with the patient and coordinate schedules with other dentists or with the prosthetic laboratory.

Immediate dentures often require the coordination of patient appointments with the maxillofacial oral surgeon. The laboratory needs to know the delivery date and where the final denture is to be delivered. Since the denture will be inserted by the oral surgeon, follow-up appointments for denture checks need to be scheduled for the patient in the office, either following surgery or a day later, to examine the denture.

Partial dentures may require additional appointments with the patient to check cast framework before jaw relationships are completed. If intracoronal attachments are used in the removable partial, additional preparatory appointments are necessary to prepare the abutment teeth, to take the necessary impressions, and to seat any castings that are used. Many variations exist in this type of partial denture, and it is the assistant's responsibility to develop a thorough understanding of the common procedures that are used in the office.

Interim dentures that have been placed temporarily need follow-up appointments with the patient to determine healing of tissues and to schedule future appointments to complete the final prosthesis.

Implants, like specialized partial dentures, require preparation time. For instance, it will be necessary to coordinate patient appointments with the maxillofacial oral surgeon for the insertion of the implant. Follow-up appointments are scheduled to determine readiness for future impression appointments. After this time the basic schedule of appointments can be arranged for the final prosthesis to be constructed.

In any of these situations the flow of treatment depends on the assistant's ability to understand the procedure and to coordinate the prosthetic, laboratory, and surgical procedures. Important, too, is the ability to follow up on the activities that are taking place outside the office and to always inform the patient of the next step in the procedure.

KEY POINTS

▶ The most common types of removable prostheses are complete or partial dentures. A complete denture replaces all of the teeth in an arch, and a partial denture replaces one or more teeth.

▶ Complete dentures are inserted by two different methods: conventional or immediate. Conventional dentures are constructed after all of the teeth have been removed, or they may be a replacement denture. An immediate denture is designed for the patient who first has the posterior teeth removed and then, on the day of denture insertion, has the anterior teeth removed. A denture has two basic parts: the denture base and the teeth.

▶ Partial dentures can be prepared with extracoronal clasp retainers or with intracoronal semiprecision or precision attachments. Partial dentures are designed by using a variety of components that relate to the retention of the prosthesis.

▶ The edentulous conditions of a patient's mouth can be categorized according to the status of the remaining teeth in a system that is referred to as the Kennedy Classification System.

▶ The construction of any removable prosthesis requires several appointments, including preliminary impressions; border molding and final impressions; selection of mould and shade; try-in of the set-up; insertion; and adjustment. Each of these appointments requires the dental assistant to coordinate schedules between the dental office, the patient, and the dental laboratory or other professionals, such as the maxillofacial oral surgeon.

▶ Each appointment in a removable prosthetic practice may not require four-handed dental procedures. However, each phase of the procedure demands complex set-ups, various laboratory tasks, jaw relationship records, and coordination of activities that require the skills of a qualified dental assistant with outside laboratories and individuals who are responsible for various phases of treatment.

BIBLIOGRAPHY

Dyer RY, Roberts J: *Notes on prosthetic dentistry,* London, 1989, Wright.

Grasso JE, Miller L: *Removable partial prosthodontics,* ed 3, St Louis, 1991, Mosby.

Halperin R, Grasser N, Rogoff S, Plekavich J: *Mastering The art of complete dentures,* Berlin, Germany, 1988, Quintessence.

McGivney GP, Castleberry DJ: *McCracken's removable partial prosthodontics,* ed 8, St Louis, 1989, Mosby.

Zarb GA, Bolender CL, Hickey JC, Carlsson GE: *Boucher's prosthodontic treatment for edentulous patients,* ed 10, St Louis, 1990, Mosby.

32 Temporary Restorations

LEARNING OBJECTIVES

You will have mastered the material in this chapter when you can:

▶ Define the key terms

▶ Identify the difference between intracoronal and extracoronal temporary restorations

▶ Explain the functions of a temporary restoration

▶ Describe the procedure for the construction of temporary restorations

▶ Describe the procedure for the placement of all temporary restorations

▶ Identify the criteria for a clinically acceptable temporary restoration

KEY TERMS

Acrylic crown
Aluminum crown
Coping
Extracoronal dressing
Festoon
Interim dressing
Intracoronal dressing
Stainless steel crown
Temporary restoration

A primary responsibility of a dental professional is to provide relief, comfort, and a stable environment in the oral cavity. A temporary restoration placed in or on a tooth will often fulfill this need. In some states the dental assistant who is educated in advanced functions is delegated the responsibility for providing a temporary restoration for the patient. The different types of temporary restorations, uses, and step-by-step procedures that are involved with each restoration are discussed in this chapter.

In many states the task of placing temporary restorations is delegated to the credentialed dental assistant or hygienist. The delegation usually occurs with a patient of record and is assigned to the team member under direct or general supervision of the dentist. The operator in procedural examples in this chapter could be the assistant, the hygienist, or the dentist. This delegated responsibility can increase productivity and efficiency in the dental practice and can relieve the dentist of these duties.

Types and Uses

Temporary restorations are interim dressings: fillings that are placed for a short period of time to protect the tooth until a permanent restoration can be placed; these restorations are designed in two basic forms. A temporary restoration may be an **intracoronal dressing**: a dental material that is placed directly into the crown or a cavity preparation. For example, this type of temporary restoration may be used when a tooth is prepared for the placement of an inlay. Another reason to use an intracoronal restoration may be when a patient has a deep carious lesion on a tooth. The operator may select a temporary dressing, often a zinc oxide–eugenol (ZOE) cement, and wait to place the amalgam at a later appointment. An **extracoronal** temporary restoration, one that surrounds a large portion or all of the crown of a tooth, is used when teeth have been prepared for crown or bridge procedures. This type of temporary is usually a full-coverage temporary that is constructed from self-curing acrylic or is designed from preformed plastic or metal crowns.

The functions of temporary restorations are wide ranging. These types of restorations can accomplish the following: (1) aid in mastication; (2) prevent hypereruption of the prepared and the opposing tooth until a permanent restoration is placed; (3) avoid further trauma to the tooth; (4) avoid mesial drift of an abutment tooth and thus (5) maintain space for the permanent tooth eruption; (6) provide an esthetic appearance; (7) relieve discomfort by creating an anodyne effect; and (8) deter the decay process.

PATIENT EDUCATION

A patient must be advised that a temporary restoration is not to be considered final treatment for the specific tooth. The patient may have a chief complaint—a tooth ache or a fractured tooth—and want relief. Once relief is provided, sometimes in the form of a temporary restoration, the patient must be educated about the need for further treatment. Eventually, a temporary restoration will fail; the cementing agents that have been used will begin to wash away or crumble, and teeth will drift mesially; the patient will be left with the same, or an even more complicated, dental need.

If the temporary restoration has been placed as an interim dressing until a permanent crown or bridge can be completed by the dental laboratory, it is even more important that the patient returns for the cementation appointment. If the patient is comfortable with the temporary restoration, it may not seem necessary to return for the permanent restoration, and if the patient fails to return, the dental practice is faced with a laboratory case that is not seated and with the expense of the preparation procedure and the laboratory costs. Mesial drift and/or hypereruption make it impossible for the operator to seat the permanent restoration after delays.

Patient education is extremely important to successful dental treatment, and the need for temporary restorations to be temporary is a major part of any patient education program. This responsibility may fall to the operator alone or it may be delegated to any or all members of the dental team (see *Patient Education for Temporary Restorations*).

Patient Education Tips for Temporary Restorations

▶ Brush the temporary restoration as any other tooth.
▶ Floss the teeth, but pull the floss through the contact toward the buccal, or cheek side, to avoid disturbing the temporary restoration.
▶ Temporary cement is weak, and the temporary restoration can easily be lost.
▶ If the temporary is dislodged, immediately call the dental office to arrange to have it recemented to avoid mesial drift and hypereruption.

▶ Mesial drift and hypereruption may result in the permanent restoration not fitting properly.
▶ The temporary may be sensitive to temperature.

Intracoronal Temporary Restorations

Intracoronal temporary restorations are usually constructed of plastic or of a temporary cement. The acrylic or plastic temporary restoration is designed, contoured, and often cemented with a temporary zinc oxide-eugenol cement that can be easily removed. The cement intracoronal temporary is fabricated of a zinc oxide-eugenol cement to provide an anodyne effect and for ease in the removal of cement at a later appointment. Occasionally, a permanent cement of greater strength, zinc phosphate, could be placed if the temporary restoration remains in place for more than 3 to 4 weeks.

BOX 32-1

CRITERIA FOR A PROPERLY CONTOURED INTRACORONAL TEMPORARY

Temporary cement is adapted to the margins
Interproximal contact is established
Marginal ridge is contoured to the same height as abutment tooth/teeth
Interproximal contour is the same as natural tooth structure
Occlusion is adjusted to allow proper articulation
Excess cement is removed from all areas, especially the gingival sulcus

---

▶ Cement Temporary

A patient who has a fracture of the mesiobuccal cusp of the mandibular left first molar may require treatment with a cement intracoronal temporary. The tooth is symptomatic and sensitive to heat, and the operator decides to place a cement temporary until a later appointment. The procedure that follows is an example of the type of treatment provided for this patient.

Armamentarium

Armamentarium that is used for a cement temporary includes the following: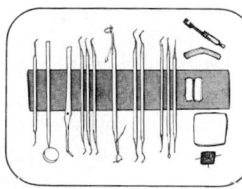

▶ Dental cement (one of the following)

(Short term cement)	(Longer term cement)
ZOE	Zinc phosphate
Cavit	Polycarboxylate

CEMENT TEMPORARY

▶ Are all universal barrier techniques being used?
▶ Is all of the armamentarium available and prepared for use?
▶ Are the instruments arranged in sequence of use?
▶ Am I prepared for alternative treatment plans?
▶ Is the necessary equipment turned on and ready to operate?

Update Medical History

When any patient is treated it is important to obtain a current health history. The medical history is especially important if the dentist considers providing the patient with medication to relieve the pain caused by treatment. All medications that are currently being taken by the patient and his or her overall physical well-being need to be considered to correctly prescribe any medication.

Examination of the Treatment Site

The site of treatment is examined by the operator with the mirror and explorer. If the operator is unsure about the integrity of the pulpal tissues, one option that demonstrates a conservative approach to treatment is to provide a temporary restoration, allowing time for the tooth to become asymptomatic or for evidence to appear that suggests the pulpal tissues are dying and that endodontic treatment is necessary. As the operator examines the tooth, any carious debris is removed and the site is rinsed and dried completely.

Determine Occlusal Relationship

As it is with the placement of a permanent restoration, the occlusal relationship also must be determined before placement to aid in proper positioning and to avoid occlusal disharmony in the temporary restoration. The operator directs the patient to bite down and to grind side-to-side and forward and back on articulating paper that is held between the dental arches.

Placement of Isolation

Cotton rolls are placed in the buccal vestibule, in the sublingual area, and in the maxillary arch near the parotid gland.

Matrix Band, Retainer, and Wedge Placement

The matrix band, retainer, and wedge are prepared, passed, and placed as described in Chapter 27.

Placement of the Cement

A temporary cement is mixed to base consistency (described in Chapter 11), cut into small increments, and passed to the operator, along with a small condenser or other instrument of choice for placement. The operator places an increment of cement in the preparation, working it firmly into the opening (Fig. 32-1). Each increment is added; the cement is condensed and formed against the tooth structure and the matrix band, if it is used. Because no cavity preparation has been performed no margins are defined.

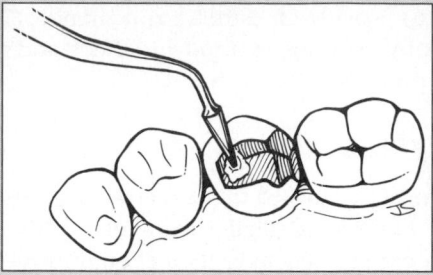

FIG. 32-1   Cement is placed in small increments in the preparation.

A larger condenser may be used to complete the condensation. As the cement is placed, the operator occasionally places the end of the condensing instrument into extra cement powder on the pad. The cement powder on the instrument tip helps avoid the increments that stick to the instrument during condensation and eliminates the material from being pulled out while increments are added. The cement placement is similar to the amalgam placement: each increment is placed and compressed in the tooth with the condenser.

Initial Carving

The fractured area is overfilled with cement, and the operator begins to carve the material to the correct shape of its original anatomy. In this procedure the material may be carved with various instruments; one example is a 7C cleoid-discoid carver (Fig. 32-2). The carver rests on the existing tooth structure, across the cavosurface margin and onto the cement. The cement is refined with small carving movements.

The excess cement is carved from the occlusal surface, and the normal anatomy of the tooth is restored in the cement. The carver is exchanged for the explorer to remove excess cement from the marginal ridge and matrix band.

Removal of Matrix Retainer, Wedge, and Band

The same technique as described for the amalgam procedure (see Chapter 27) is used to remove the wedge, retainer, and band. Removal of the band may need to be delayed until the cement becomes hardened to avoid fractures.

Final Carving

The least accessible area, the interproximal space, must be carved as soon as the matrix band is removed. The operator may use a Ward's C carver or other smooth surface carvers to remove the smooth surface excess, contouring the cement to the tooth structure. It is easy to force cement into the sulcus area, which may cause gingival irritation. The cement is a mechanical irritant, and if it is not removed, the sulcus area becomes inflamed and tender; therefore, the carver should be used in an upward stroke, towards the occlusal, rather than up and down. Objectives of this step are the recreation of the

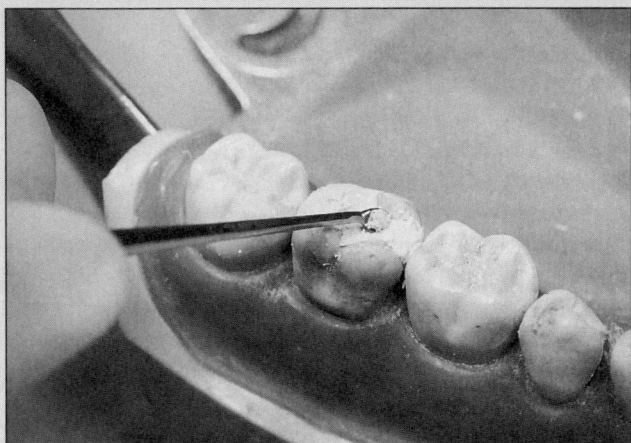

FIG. 32-2 An anatomic carver is used to simulate the patient's anatomy in the cement.

interdental space and the marginal ridge contact. The carver is exchanged for the explorer as the operator examines the carved surface for smoothness and for removal of any cement from the sulcus.

An anatomic carver, such as the #5 C carver, is exchanged with the explorer to place more refined occlusal anatomy in the cement. The operator takes care to remove excess cement that has extended beyond the fractured surfaces. Placement of anatomic grooves and fissures and refinement of the marginal ridge is just as important in a temporary restoration as it is in the amalgam restorative procedure. Box 32-2 lists criteria for a properly placed intracoronal temporary restoration.

The cement temporary is burnished and finished for patient comfort and smoothness to the tongue. Burnishing and finishing can create a high level of shine and smoothness in dental cement. A burnisher is used to accentuate grooves and fissures, highlighting the anatomy that is normally found on the occlusal surface. The smoothness can also be increased by rubbing the cement surface with a cotton pellet that has been saturated with water and placed in cotton pliers.

Removal of Cotton Roll Isolation

The assistant removes the cotton rolls with the cotton pliers. If the cotton is dry, it should be completely saturated with water so that it does not adhere to the oral tissues and cause abrasion.

Check Articulation

A complete mouth rinse is performed to remove all debris and to refresh the patient's mouth. Articulation paper that is attached to an articulating paper holder is positioned over the tooth that has been temporized with cement. The patient is directed to bite up and down and side-to-side and to slide back and forth on the articulation paper. As heavy blue markings appear on the cement, the assistant prepares and passes a carving instrument to the operator. After carving the instrument is exchanged for a burnisher to smooth the cement once again. The occlusion is checked by the operator, and if necessary the carving and burnishing are repeated until the occlusal contact is correct.

Postoperative Instructions

The temporary restoration is not as strong as a permanent restorative material. Fractures can occur easily from biting pressure and from everyday hygiene procedures. The patient is given this information and is asked to return for the future appointment to replace the temporary restoration with a permanent restoration.

- Are the appropriate universal barrier techniques removed?
- Have all of the appropriate surfaces been cleaned and disinfected?
- Has all armamentarium been removed?
- Has all equipment been repositioned?
- Has all of the equipment been disinfected/sterilized according to OSHA guidelines?

- Instruments/armamentarium

Explorer	Ward's C carver	#1 Amalgam condenser	#26 Spoon excavator
Mirror	Ball burnisher	#2 Amalgam condenser	Anatomic burnisher
Cotton pliers	Articulating paper	Tofflemire matrix band and retainer	Cotton rolls
Spoon excavator	2 × 2 gauze		Cotton pellets
FP1 plastic instrument	Cement spatula	Wedge	Mixing pad
5C cleoid-discoid carver		7C cleoid-discoid carver	

CRITERIA FOR A PROPERLY TRIMMED ACRYLIC TEMPORARY

▶ Acrylic is adapted to the preparation margins
▶ Interproximal contact is established
▶ Marginal ridge is contoured to the same height as the abutment tooth/teeth
▶ Interproximal contour is same as natural tooth structure
▶ Occlusion is adjusted to allow proper articulation
▶ Excess cement is removed from all areas, especially the gingival sulcus

▶ Acrylic Temporary

If a patient has a fracture of the mesiobuccal cusp of the mandibular left first molar, another form of temporary restoration is possible. The dentist can treatment plan the tooth for a final restorative procedure by preparing the tooth for a Class II or Class VI cast alloy inlay restoration. The cast alloy procedures are described in Chapter 30, so specific details regarding the procedure are not included in this chapter. The operator completes the preparation, and a member of the team is directed to place an acrylic temporary restoration.

Armamentarium

Armamentarium for an intracoronal acrylic temporary include the following:

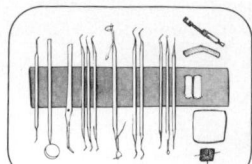

Temporary dental cement
Acrylic material
Explorer
Mirror
Cotton pliers
Spoon excavator
FP1 plastic instrument
2×2 gauze
Cement spatula
Dappen dish
Flour of pumice
Modified sickle/curet scaler
Lubricant
Articulating paper
Cotton rolls
Cotton pellets
Mixing pad
Floss
Finishing/polishing burs and disks
Polishing wheel

The temporization procedure begins with the mixing of the acrylic, since the preparation steps have been completed. The preparation includes placement of defined walls and floors, which allows positioning of an acrylic temporary that will not be locked in undercuts and grooves. Acrylic cannot be used as easily in the same way as a cement temporary because acrylic hardens to a pattern of the inside of the preparation and is then cemented in place. A preparation that does not allow placement and removal of the temporary due to lack of wall and floor taper would lock the acrylic in place.

PREPARATION AND PLACEMENT OF THE ACRYLIC TEMPORARY

Most acrylics are provided by the manufacturer as a liquid and powder, with various shades of color from which to select. The color selection is not as critical for an acrylic temporary that is to be placed in a posterior tooth as it is for the material that is to be placed in an anterior tooth. The use of acrylic and the chemical and physical properties that are associated with its use are discussed in Chapter 11.

Cotton rolls are placed to provide isolation. The assistant dispenses acrylic powder in a dappen dish or similar deep-welled device. Acrylic liquid is added until the powder does not absorb the liquid any longer. The material may be mixed with a spatula or an FP1 instrument until it is homogeneous. The consistency of the acrylic should be doughy. The material loses its gloss as it begins to reach a workable stage. The operator places

lubricant on the abutment tooth to avoid adherence of the acrylic to that tooth. A small amount of lubricant can also be applied to the preparation to assist in the removal of the acrylic temporary after the material has set. Too much lubrication can result in some distortion of the acrylic.

A ball of mixed acrylic is passed to the operator and is pressed into the prepared tooth. Care is taken to ensure that the placement of the acrylic extends to all cavosurface margins. The acrylic can be molded by hand or with an instrument to form it in the preparation. If the acrylic extends beyond the cavosurface margins it may be cut away with a hand instrument before it hardens. However, if the acrylic extends beyond the cavosurface margin and is allowed to harden, it can be trimmed away with rotary instruments later. The majority of carving and refining of the anatomy is made after the material has set; however, excess material can be removed by carving it away with an instrument before it has set.

A small amount of acrylic can be kept in reserve by the assistant. It is usually held between the assistant's fingers to simulate the temperature in the patient's mouth. Once this sample piece has hardened, the material in the patient's mouth has also become hard.

Some operators may like to remove the acrylic temporary before it reaches a final set, ensuring the operator that the temporary is not trapped in undercuts. The operator may ask the patient to bite down on the acrylic before it has reached the final set. This provides guides as to how the opposing tooth/teeth occlude on the temporary and will aid in the finishing and trimming steps.

If the temporary is difficult to remove, a modified sickle scaler, curet scaler, or spoon excavator can be used against an edge of the acrylic to lift it out of the preparation (Fig. 32-3). Once it is removed, the final set can be accelerated by placing the acrylic temporary in a bowl of warm water. If the acrylic temporary is removed from the preparation too soon, a distortion may occur that will not allow the acrylic temporary to reseat. If this occurs, the completion of the procedure is delayed so that another temporary can be fabricated.

Trimming the Acrylic Temporary

If the auxiliary is delegated to construct the temporary, the use of rotary instruments must be outside the patient's mouth or in a laboratory setting. The temporary will most likely need to be trimmed extensively to fit in the tooth. The trimming can be accomplished by the use of finishing stones, burs, and disks that vary in grit (from coarse to fine) and in size.

As the rotary instrument is used it is important to establish a fulcrum to maintain complete control of the handpiece during the trimming of the acrylic (Fig. 32-4). If a fulcrum is not maintained, the rotary instrument can wander from the desired position and may remove acrylic from an incorrect area (Box 32-4).

The rotary instrument is pointed in the direction from the occlusal to the cervical (Fig. 32-5). This position allows the operator to use the rotary instrument to feather or thin the cervical margin, removing bulk acrylic that causes gingival irritation that acts as a mechanical irritant. The feathering continues around the circumference of the tooth, reducing thickness throughout.

As the trimming continues toward the proximal surface, the operator does not remove acrylic from the marginal ridge contact area unless the contact is tight when it is evaluated, using floss. If the contact is light (meaning that it does not touch the adjacent tooth at the marginal ridge), the temporary may have to be reconstructed. Occasionally, extra acrylic can be added to the surface in a second mix, but the two mixes may not always adhere successfully.

The occlusal guides are established by the patient's occluding on the soft acrylic. The excess acrylic that is observed after this movement is removed with a carving instrument before the material hardens. The remainder of the trimming is completed

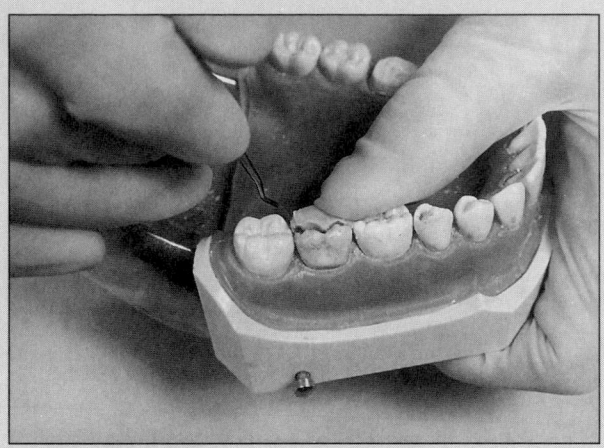

FIG. 32-3 **During fabrication of the acrylic temporary restoration it may be necessary to remove it with an instrument.**

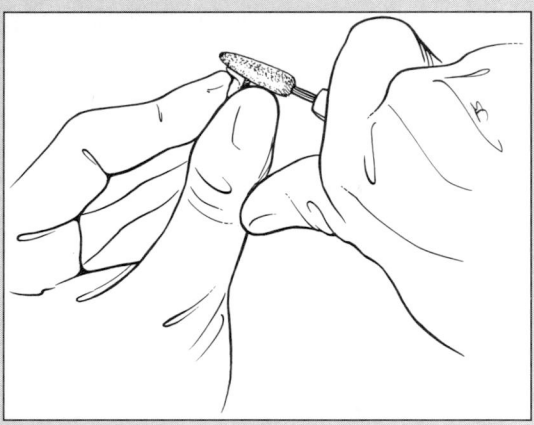

FIG. 32-4 **Fulcrum position of the right hand on the left to stabilize the rotary instrument.**

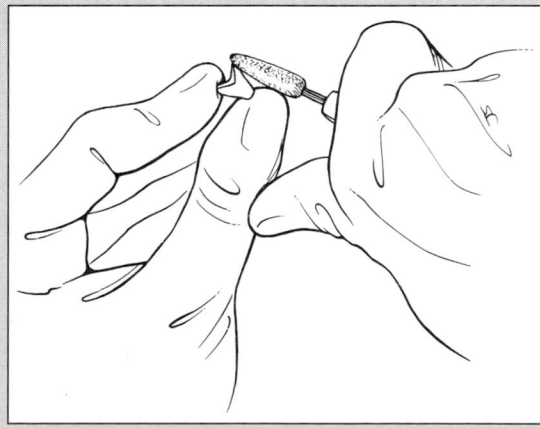

FIG. 32-5 **The rotary instrument is directed from the occlusal toward the cervical to reduce the thickness of the temporary at the cervical margin.**

Continued.

PREPARATION AND PLACEMENT OF THE ACRYLIC TEMPORARY—cont'd

with stones or acrylic burs, placing grooves and developing occlusal anatomy. The operator must be well acquainted with tooth anatomy to recreate the anatomy in restorations. The temporary is tried in the preparation many times during this adjustment phase of the procedure.

The temporary is placed in the preparation, and the occlusion is checked with the articulating paper. If marked heavily, the temporary is removed and adjusted as described. The temporary is placed again, and the operator runs floss through the proximal contact. The floss should slide through the contact without interruption. If the floss can not be pulled through the contact, the temporary restoration is removed and the contact is adjusted by removing a slight amount of acrylic with a rotary instrument.

Even though the temporary is in place for a short period of time, concern is shown for the health of the gingival tissues. The temporary restoration should not impinge on gingival tissue, possibly causing irritation. The temporary is polished with a slurry of pumice on a wetted polishing wheel that is placed on a lathe. A high luster on the acrylic can be achieved during this step. The temporary is rinsed and thoroughly dried. The laboratory equipment is disinfected or sterilized according to OSHA guidelines following this procedure.

Cementing the Acrylic Temporary

The preparation is dried, and isolation is continued with the use of newly placed cotton rolls. It is beneficial to place lubricant on the exterior surfaces of the temporary before cementation. The layer of lubricant eliminates the cement adhering to the external surface of the acrylic temporary, thus making cement removal easier.

The assistant dispenses a temporary cement, such as ZOE—in this case, a two-paste system—on a plastic pad and mixes it with a spatula until it is homogeneous. An even thickness of cement is placed on the interior surfaces of the temporary with an FPI plastic instrument or with any instrument of choice. The temporary is passed to the operator with

the cement-covered surfaces facing down into the assistant's palm. This allows the operator to easily pick up the temporary and slide it into the preparation. The patient is directed to bite firmly on a cotton roll that is placed on the occlusal of the temporary. While the cement is hardening, the assistant passes an explorer to the operator, who then checks the margins to ensure proper placement in the preparation. The cement takes approximately 3 to 5 minutes to set; the excess cement exudes beyond the margins and can be removed with an instrument. Cement along the margins, in the gingival sulcus, and in all other areas must be removed. The cement removal instrument, a spoon excavator, a scaler, or an explorer, is exchanged for floss that is passed through the interproximal and pulled to the buccal side of the mouth carrying cement through the contacts, rather than leaving it or forcing it into the sulcus further. The assistant completely rinses and dries the area removing all loosened cement.

The patient is directed to bite on the articulating paper; however, no excessive articulation markings should show on the temporary, since articulation was checked earlier. If the temporary appears high or if the patient occludes on the temporary more than on the other teeth, it can be adjusted in the oral cavity with a rotary instrument.

Postoperative Instructions

The instructions are similar to any temporary restoration, but good oral hygiene must be maintained during this time.

The previous example centered around the use of the acrylic without any prefabricated form. Many devices can be used to provide the operator with a positive reproduction of the tooth that is to be temporized. A discussion of these options will be included after the acrylic crown example which follows.

Extracoronal Temporary Restoration

When excess amounts of tooth structure have been lost to decay, to trauma, or to the preparation procedure, the temporary restoration becomes extracoronal, or it covers the clinical crown that exists. Extracoronal temporary restorations might include a pontic in the configuration of the temporary restoration. The pontic helps to maintain the integrity of space that once was occupied by a tooth and will be replaced by a portion of the permanent restoration. Examples of extracoronal temporary restorations that are prefabricated full coverage protection include the **stainless steel**, **aluminum, and acrylic crowns**, while other temporary restorations are made of acrylic to fabricate customized crowns and bridges. The extracoronal temporary is fabricated from aluminum, stainless steel, or acrylic crown materials.

▶ Acrylic Temporary Crown

The following discussion examines the preparation and placement of an acrylic temporary crown on an anterior tooth. For reasons of esthetics an aluminum crown would not be acceptable in the anterior segment of a patient's mouth, so an acrylic temporary crown must be fabricated according to the criteria listed in Box 32-3.

The operator may select a preformed acrylic crown or construct a crown from a coping.

Before treatment commences, the dental assistant is responsible for fabricating a coping for this procedure. A **coping**—a piece of plastic that is formed over a model of the tooth/teeth before the beginning of the preparation—is created. The first step in this procedure is to recreate the anatomy of the tooth that was lost because of fracture. The incisal edge and segments of the mesial and distal are fractured. These fractured surfaces are replaced with wax that is heated and formed on the replica of the tooth in the study casts that were made from alginate impressions. This build-up and carving away of the wax create a tooth on the study cast that is similar to the natural tooth before the fracture occurred.

CONSTRUCTION OF A COPING

A coping starts as a sheet of cloudy plastic that is approximately 5 inches × 5 inches. The plastic is placed and secured in the hinged frame of the Omnivac machine (brandname). The Omnivac is a device that provides heat (through a heating element in the top of the machine) and a vacuum effect (in the base). The frame that is holding the plastic sheet is positioned at a stop near the heating element. The study cast, with wax in place on #8, is placed on the vacuum plate base, which has many small holes. The heating element switch is placed in the *ON* position, and the plastic begins to warm. As the plastic sheet is heated, it begins to lose its cloudiness and to droop. The edges of the plastic are not warmed, allowing the plastic to continue to be held in the frame. The plastic sheet droops within 1 inch of the occlusals of the study cast to ensure accurate adaptation of the plastic over the cast.

The vacuum motor is turned on, and the assistant pulls the frame that holds the melted plastic sheet down on top of the study cast. The vacuum pulls all the air from the area allowing the plastic to adapt closely over the form. The heat button is turned off, the vacuum is turned off, and the heating coil is positioned to the side of the Omnivac. The plastic sheet that tightly surrounds the cast is removed from the frame.

The plastic coping begins to cool immediately, but care is taken not to burn fingers when touching it. The study cast is removed from the coping. Three teeth, the tooth to be restored, #8, and the abutment teeth, #7 and #9, are cut from the square of plastic with scissors or a scalpel (Fig. 32-6). The cut extends approximately 1 to 2 mm below the cervical tissue line.

> **BOX 32-3**
>
> ### CRITERIA FOR A PROPERLY CONTOURED ACRYLIC CROWN
>
> ▶ Acrylic is adapted and trimmed to the margins
> ▶ Interproximal contact is established
> ▶ Interproximal contour is the same as natural tooth structure
> ▶ Incisal length is adjusted to match adjacent teeth
> ▶ Occlusion is adjusted to allow proper articulation
> ▶ Excess cement is removed from all areas, especially the gingival sulcus

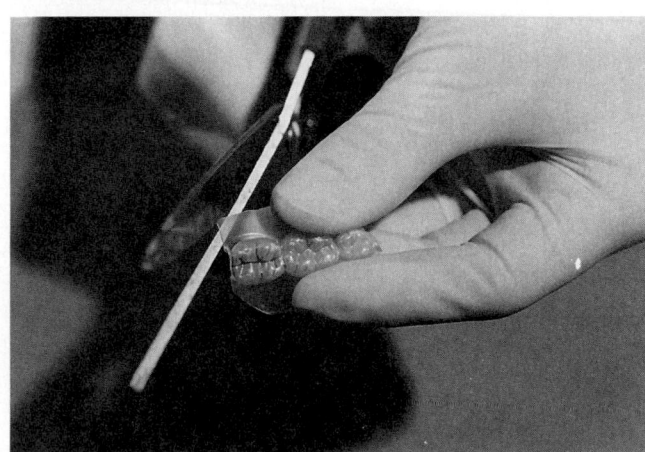

FIG. 32-6 A coping is used in conjunction with the fabrication of an acrylic temporary restoration.

Armamentarium

Armamentarium for an acrylic temporary crown, using a coping, includes the following:

Explorer
Mirror
Spoon excavator
Scaler
FP1 plastic instrument
Scissors
Temporary coping material

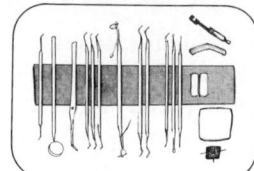

Omnivac
Cotton rolls
Acrylic
Temporary cement
Acrylic burs
Lubricant
Polishing wheels
Flour of pumice
Floss
2 × 2 cotton gauze

THE ACRYLIC COPING TEMPORARY

The patient returns for the preparation appointment, and the step-by-step procedure for the temporization phase continues. The coping is tested on the teeth for fit before the tooth is prepared. The coping should cover the tooth and fit closely, forming itself around all anatomic structures.

Fabrication of the Acrylic Temporary

The selection of the acrylic powder color is important because the temporary will be seen in the oral cavity. The patient will want an esthetic restoration, even though it is a temporary restoration. A variety of shades are available and can be mixed to provide the patient with an esthetically pleasing temporary crown. A light covering of lubricant is placed over #7 and #9 with a cotton roll or a cotton pellet that is held in cotton pliers. The acrylic is mixed as described in the intracoronal temporary example, or the acrylic powder can be placed in the coping at the site of #8 and liquid can be added to it until it is completely wetted. An FPl plastic instrument is used to reposition any acrylic that flows onto the adjacent teeth of the coping. The coping, with acrylic in it, is placed on the lubricated teeth in the mouth and allowed to set. Often, excess acrylic will exude from the coping and is removed with an instrument, avoiding any injury to the gingiva.

Trimming and Polishing the Temporary

When the acrylic has set, the coping and acrylic form are removed from the mouth, and the acrylic is removed from the coping. Excess material is trimmed away with rotary instruments, and the criteria for the temporary are as described with the previous acrylic temporary. The cervical margins must be feathered to a correct thickness, so that excess bulk is not left at the tissue line to cause irritation. This feathering process is accomplished with acrylic burs and disks, reducing the thickness, contouring the contacts, correcting the length, and adjusting for excess contact when articulation is checked. The acrylic crown must have proximal contact to avoid mesial drift, not be excessive in length to ensure that the temporary is not displaced during mastication, and not hit excessively on the lingual contact. The cervical margin of the crown should meet that of the tooth, providing a smooth transition from acrylic to tooth when examined with an explorer.

Cementation of the Temporary Crown

The temporary crown form is cemented like the other temporaries previously described. As the cement sets, the explorer is used to examine the margins for correct placement. All excess cement is completely removed from all surfaces of the crown and in the sulcus area.

Checking Articulation

Articulating paper is placed between the arches, and the patient is directed to bite down. If the patient occludes heavily on the temporary crown, the marked area is removed with a rotary instrument.

Postoperative Instructions

The postoperative instructions are the same as the other temporaries, except the patient should *definitely* not bite directly on the temporary, since it could fracture or be displaced.

Metal Temporary Crown

The less esthetic metal temporary crown is placed in the posterior segment of the mouth.

The three available types of prefabricated metal crown forms that are placed in posterior crown preparations are aluminum crown, stainless steel crown, and tin crown forms (Fig. 32-7). The aluminum and stainless steel crown forms are more anatomically correct than the tin crown forms and are used more often to provide the patient with anatomy that is normal to the mouth. The most common application for stainless steel crowns is in pediatric dentistry.

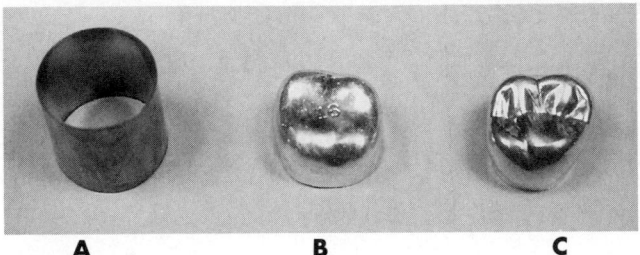

FIG. 32-7   Examples of metal crown forms. *A,* Copper band. *B,* Metal crown form. *C,* Anatomic crown form.

BOX 32-4

CRITERIA FOR A PROPERLY CONTOURED ALUMINUM CROWN FORM

▶ Adapted to margins of prepared tooth
▶ Interproximal contact is established
▶ Crown is in the plane of occlusion
▶ Marginal ridge is contoured to the same height as abutment tooth/teeth
▶ Interproximal contour is the same as natural tooth structure
▶ Occlusion is adjusted to allow proper articulation
▶ All areas of the crown are smooth, avoiding accumulation of debris
▶ Excess cement is removed from all areas, especially the gingival sulcus

Armamentarium

Armamentarium for a metal temporary crown includes the following:

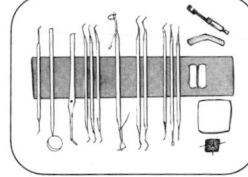

Explorer
Mirror
Cotton pliers
Spoon excavator
FP1 plastic instrument   Temporary cement
Ball burnisher   Lubricant
Contouring pliers   Floss
Crown and collar scissors   Cotton rolls
Aluminum crown kit   2 × 2 gauze

TEMPORARY ALUMINUM CROWN

 STOP

The patient is scheduled to have tooth #4 prepared for a full-coverage cast alloy crown. The step-by-step procedure for tooth preparation will not be reviewed here but can be found in Chapter 31. The preparation and impression have been completed and temporization is the next step to be performed.

The operator is passed a temporary sizing device. Most aluminum crown form kits provide a sizing device for measuring. The distance between the abutment teeth is measured by placing the device over the prepared occlusal surface of #4 and measuring from distal to mesial (Fig. 32-8). A number found on each end of the measuring device correlates to the different sizes of prefabricated crowns. If the exact size is not available, select a crown form that is slightly larger to establish proximal contacts, rather than selecting one that is smaller,

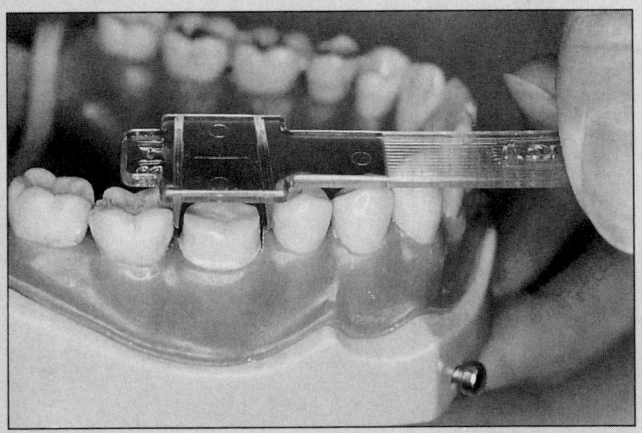

FIG. 32-8   The mesial and distal relationship, or distance between the adjacent teeth, is measured to assist in selection of the prefabricated crown form.

Continued.

TEMPORARY ALUMINUM CROWN—cont'd

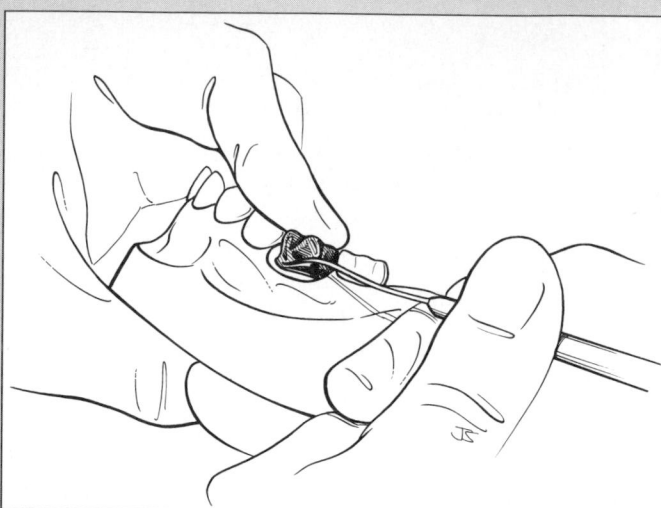

FIG. 32-9   The margins of the aluminum crown form are scored with an explorer to determine the area to cut for the temporary.

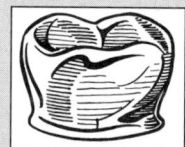

FIG. 32-10   The flair of the cervical margins provides a guide to the amount of excess that is to be removed.

with possibly light or no contacts. In this case the distance measured is 11.5 mm between the distal of #5 and the mesial of #3. Since tooth #4 is found in the maxillary right quadrant, the assistant selects the crown from the maxillary right quadrant section of the kit. The crown form selected is number U66.

The assistant passes the crown form to the operator, who tries it on the prepared tooth structure. Usually, if the initial placement of the crown form does not fit correctly, the goal is to determine if the form will provide contact with the abutment teeth after it is trimmed. The form *should not* be placed back in the kit if it does not fit; it can be sterilized and replaced in the kit later if it has not been distorted.

The appropriate length of the crown is determined when the tooth is placed. An explorer is held at the cervical margin, marking the exact location of the margin on the crown of the tooth. When the crown form is placed on the tooth and extends beyond this marked length, it is scored; this is accomplished by the tip of the explorer etching a line around the circumference of the crown form at the location of the margin. The scoring/etching provides a guide to trim the length of the crown form. The criterion for the length of the crown form is at or within 1 mm of the margin but not beyond the margin (Fig. 32-9).

Another method can be used to determine the correct length of an aluminum crown form. When the crown is placed on a prepared tooth, the excess length on the form flairs out; this flair of aluminum occurs at the site of the cervical margin, providing another guide to indicate the proper length to which the form should be trimmed (Fig. 32-10). If the temporary crown is too long, the gingival tissues become irritated and inflamed, creating difficulties for the operator, who attempts to seat the permanent cast alloy restoration at a later appointment.

The operator uses the crown and collar scissors to trim the excess metal from the cervical area. The scissors are held parallel to the edge of the metal, and long, smooth strokes are used to cut around the circumference of the crown form (Fig. 32-11). If

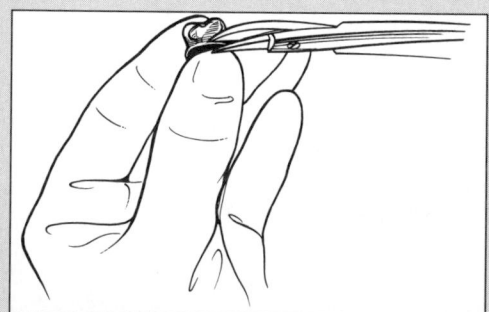

FIG. 32-11   The scissor blades are paralleled with the edge of the crown form.

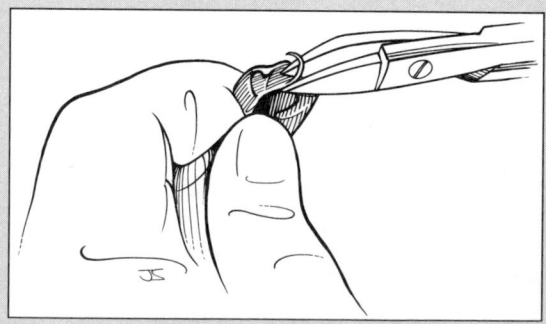

FIG. 32-12   The metal flairs out from the blades of the scissors as it is cut.

the cuts are short and jerky, tags of aluminum are left or the form may be distorted. As the cuts are made the metal flairs out and the natural contour of the original form is not retained (Fig. 32-12). Contouring pliers are used; the ball segment of the pliers is placed inside the crown to contour the cervical of the form (Fig. 32-13). The crown form is placed back on the tooth, and the contouring is checked.

Cutting, contouring, and trying in the form may be done several times to ensure a correct fit. If at some point the proximal contact is open, it must be reestablished by placing the crown form occlusal side down on several 2 × 2 gauze sponges. A ball burnisher is positioned on the inside of the form at the marginal ridge area (Fig. 32-14). Force is placed against the aluminum to press it out at the marginal ridge; this expands the aluminum crown and provides a marginal ridge contact for the form when it is placed on the tooth. The form is tried back on the tooth, and if necessary the step can be repeated until the ridge contact is reestablished.

Once the cervical margins and marginal ridge contact are correct, the occlusal contacts must be rechecked. If the contacts are high, the cervical margins must be recontoured to enable the form to be pushed down further on the tooth. The crown form is checked again, and once the objectives have been met, it is polished with a cratex wheel, a burlew wheel, or another rotary instrument. Smoothing the metal surfaces eliminates areas of possible plaque accumulation on the crown form.

Cementation of the Aluminum Temporary Crown

Like the acrylic intracoronal temporary, the lubricant is placed on the external surface of the crown form. The temporary cement is mixed, and a thin layer is placed inside the crown form, with some excess near the occlusal. The form is passed to the operator, with the occlusal resting in the palm of the assistant's hand. The form is positioned, and a cotton roll is set on the occlusal surface; the patient is directed to close firmly, holding the cotton roll in place.

The operator checks the margins with an explorer to ensure proper placement of the form. If the form is short of the margins the patient is directed to bite harder on the cotton roll, forcing the form to the cut length. Once the cement has set, the excess is removed with the instrument of choice, possibly a scaler, spoon excavator, or explorer. The cement is removed from all areas, especially the interproximal area. If the cement is not removed until the subsequent dental appointment, the oral tissues will have become inflamed and irritated. When the operator attempts to seat the permanent restoration, the patient will experience excessive bleeding and discomfort.

Floss is passed through both contacts and pulled to the lingual or buccal to avoid forcing any cement into the gingival sulcus or popping the temporary off the tooth. The articulation is checked again because the cementation may have left the crown form high. If this has happened, the operator can remove the high spot with a rotary instrument.

Postoperative Instructions

After refinement of the temporary restoration is completed the patient is given the following directions:

▶ Do not chew on that side of the mouth
▶ Avoid sticky food as much as possible
▶ Call the office if the crown becomes loose, so that it can be recemented immediately, again avoiding mesial drift and hypereruption and possible discomfort

Occasionally, the stock aluminum crown forms do not fit the prepared tooth structure as well as the operator would prefer. An acrylic wash can be placed inside the crown form after the metal is trimmed and contoured but before the

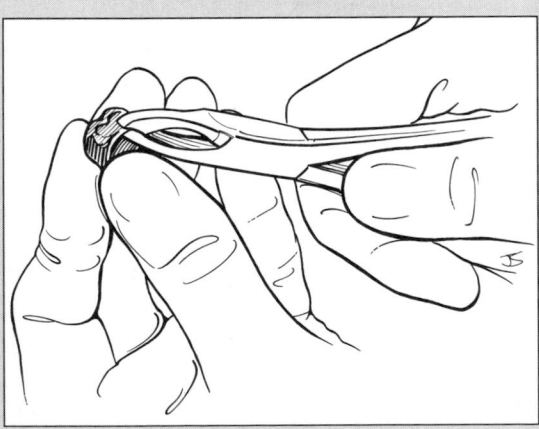

FIG. 32-13 Contouring pliers are used to contour the margins of the crown form to fit the prepared tooth.

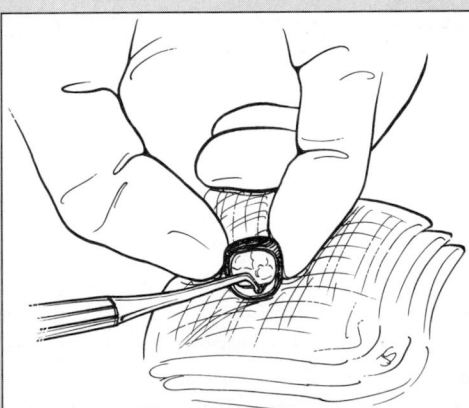

FIG. 32-14 The marginal ridge area can be extended inside the crown form by applying pressure with a ball burnisher.

Continued.

TEMPORARY ALUMINUM CROWN—cont'd

cement is placed inside the crown form. The prepared tooth is isolated and lubricated. The acrylic powder is placed directly into the crown, followed by the liquid and until the liquid is completely absorbed by the powder. The form with the acrylic is placed on the prepared tooth and allowed to set. If excess acrylic extrudes from the cervical margins, it must be trimmed away to provide the patient with a temporary that will not cause irritation to the gingival tissues. Once the acrylic is trimmed away, the same cementation steps are followed as discussed previously. This step provides the patient with a temporary that can be more stable and resilient to normal everyday mastication.

Alternative Temporary Procedures

Additional methods of fabricating temporary crowns are alternatives to the examples previously described. Each of the following procedures affords the operator with a selection of different temporization techniques. Surely, other techniques for making temporary restorations are practiced; the previous examples are just a few that might be encountered in dentistry.

▶ Polycarbonate Crown Forms

Instead of using a coping to provide a form for placing acrylic, prefabricated stock acrylic crown form kits (also known as polycarbonate crown forms) are available for use. A crown form is selected from a kit. The kits are similar in style to those of aluminum crown forms, with a variety of each type of tooth available in a shell of acrylic that fits over a prepared tooth structure.

The polycarbonate crown forms are anatomically correct, but the length and width may need to be adjusted for any particular tooth. The forms are shells that can be customized to fit a tooth by using an acrylic wash inside the form and then positioning it over the prepared tooth (as with the wash technique described for the aluminum crown temporary). Any excess material is removed with rotary instruments and contoured as previously described. The adaptation of the crown form with an acrylic wash provides a stronger and better adjusted temporary that fits more accurately.

▶ Temporary Restorations from Study Model Impressions

Another technique to develop a temporary crown is accomplished with the study model impression that is taken before the preparation of a tooth. If the tooth is somewhat intact, not fractured or decayed substantially, the alginate impression is used to make a form for a temporary. The acrylic is placed in the impression over the prepared tooth, and the impression with the acrylic is positioned back in the patient's mouth. The acrylic is allowed to set and both impression and acrylic are removed. The acrylic is separated from the impression and is trimmed, contoured, and cemented in place.

▶ Temporary Bridges

Yet another form of temporary restoration is that of a temporary bridge. When a patient is treatment planned for a bridge to replace a missing tooth or teeth, a temporary bridge must be placed in the interim period from preparation of the abutment teeth to the placement of the permanent bridge. Many of the described techniques can be used, but the need for the temporary restoration is similar to any other: provision for covering the teeth temporarily, maintaining space, aid in mastication, and providing comfort and esthetics.

KEY POINTS

▶ Temporary restorations are interim dressings that are categorized as intracoronal or extracoronal restorations.

▶ Temporary restorations aid in mastication, prevent hypereruption, avoid addition trauma, maintain oral space, relieve discomfort, and deter the decay process.

▶ Intracoronal temporary restorations are usually fabricated from cement and acrylic, while extracoronal temporary restoration are formed from acrylic, aluminum, and stainless steel.

▶ A clinically acceptable intracoronal or extracoronal restoration should reduce pain or trauma, reduce inflammation, and maintain space.

BIBLIOGRAPHY

Craig RG, O'Brien WJ, Powers JM: *Dental materials: properties and manipulation,* ed 5, St Louis, 1992, Mosby.

Project Accorde: *Restoration of cavity preparations with amalgam and tooth-colored materials,* U.S. Department of Health, Education, and Welfare, 1974.

Rosenthiel ST, Land MF, Fujimoto J: *Contemporary fixed prosthodontics,* ed 2, St. Louis, 1994, Mosby.

Sturdevant CM, Heymann H, Robertson TM, Sturdevant JR: *The art and science of operative dentistry,* ed 2, St Louis, 1985, Mosby.

UNIT VII   SPECIALIZED PROCEDURES

33 Endodontics

LEARNING OBJECTIVES

You will have mastered the material in this chapter when you can:
- Define the key terms
- Describe the scope of endodontics
- Describe the symptoms and etiology of an endodontically involved tooth
- Identify diagnostic tests used in endodontics
- Explain the importance of radiography in endodontics
- Identify and explain the function of specialized endodontic armamentarium
- Describe the physical characteristics and function of common intracanal instruments
- Identify the use of common intracanal medications
- Describe the basic procedures common to an endodontic practice
- Describe surgical procedures commonly found in endodontics
- Explain the function and process of vital and nonvital bleaching
- Identify the role of the dental assistant in various phases of endodontic treatment

KEY TERMS

Abscess
Actinomycosis
Apexification
Apexogenesis

Apical periodontitis
Apicoectomy
Bacteremia
Bicuspidization

Biomechanical cleansing
Bleaching
Broach
Buccal object rule
Cellulitis
Endodontic file
Extirpation
Fistula
Hemisection
Hyperemia
Master cone
Necrosis
Obturation

Osteomyelitis
Periapical abscess
Periodontal involvement
Pulpectomy
Pulpitis
Pulpotomy
Pulp stone
Reamer
Replant
Splinting
Transillumination
Trial point radiograph

To a patient a referral or a visit to an endodontic practice indicates the need for root canal treatment. An endodontist provides many services beyond a root canal or pulpectomy. Although the **pulpectomy**, a complete removal of pulpal tissues, is one of the most common forms of treatment performed by this specialist, other procedures performed by the endodontist include a pulpotomy, an apicoectomy, root resections, replants, and the bleaching of vital and nonvital teeth.

The endodontist must be concerned about the pulpal and periodontal tissues of the tooth. There is a symbiotic relationship between the pulp and periodontal ligament because of the existence of the apical foramen, dentinal tubules, lateral canals, and other accessory canals. It is possible to have a tooth with a primary endodontic lesion with secondary periodontal involvement (Fig. 33-1, *A* through *F*), and likewise a peridontally involved tooth may have secondary endodontic involvement. During a clinical examination a tooth may indicate mobility, furcation or bone loss, sensitivity to percussion, or may display a draining **sinus tract**, canal, or passage that leads to an abscess in the gingival sulcus. Initially, the dentist may consider these symptoms an indication of periodontal disease, but to make a final diagnosis, the dentist must conduct a battery of tests to determine whether the tooth discomfort is attributed to an endodontic or a periodontic problem (Fig. 33-2, *A*). The relationship between these tissues also relates to the potential success or failure of endodontic treatment. For instance, a tooth that is in need of endodontic treatment but is supported by unhealthy periodontal tissues is not a good candidate for treatment unless the periodontal prognosis is good (Fig. 33-2, *A* through *C*).

 In 1570 to 1085 B.C. in Saqqara of the New Kingdom a skull with a severely carious lesion on the mandibular first molar also had two cylindrical holes drilled at the area of the apices. It is suggested that these holes were placed to relieve pressure from exudate that had accumulated in this area.

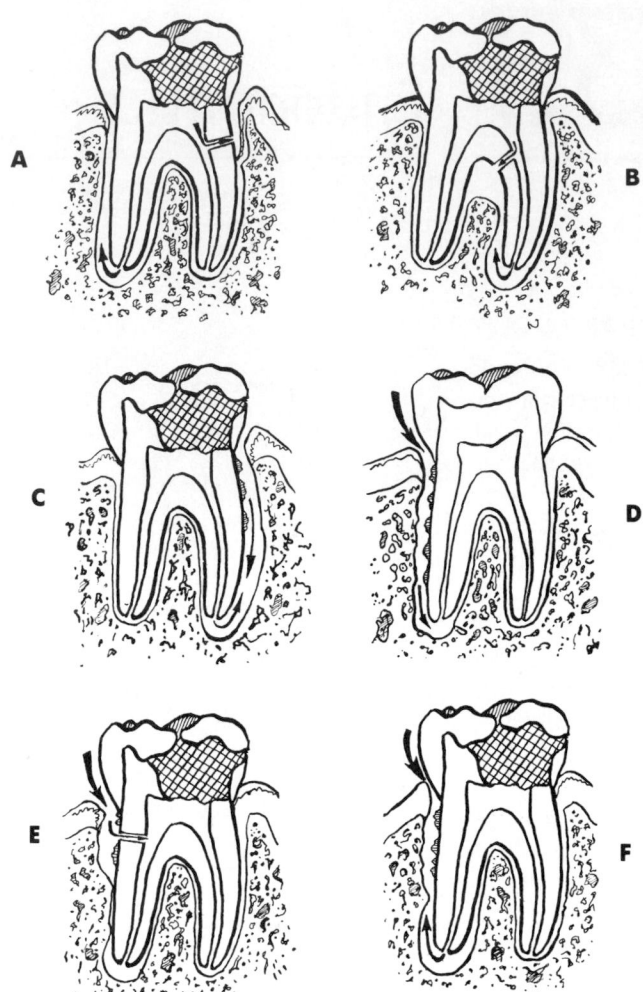

FIG. 33-1   Endodontic lesions: *A,* A fistula is evident through the periodontal ligament from the apex or from a lateral canal. *B,* Fistulation through the apex or a lateral canal, causing bifurcation involvement *C,* Secondary periodontal involvement. With the passage of time the pathway through *A* will encounter plaque and calculus formation from the cervical line. Periodontal lesions. *D,* Progression of periodontitis to apical involvement, with vital pulp. *E,* Secondary endodontic involvement. The primary periodontal involvement at the cervical margin and the resultant pulpal necrosis, once the lateral canal is exposed to the oral environment, produce this condition. *F,* Combined lesions, coalescence.

(From Cohen S, Burns RC: *Pathways of the pulp,* ed 6, St Louis, 1994, Mosby.)

One of the objectives of dentistry is to help a person maintain his or her teeth for a lifetime. Endodontics provides the patient with the opportunity to prevent the loss of a tooth through specialized treatment. Premature loss of teeth in a child because of pulpal damage from traumatic injury or because of extensive dental caries can result in mesial drift of permanent teeth and can ultimately lead to malocclusion. An adult who loses a tooth is faced with similar mesial drift, loss of esthetics, impaired speech, and, unless this space is restored, may

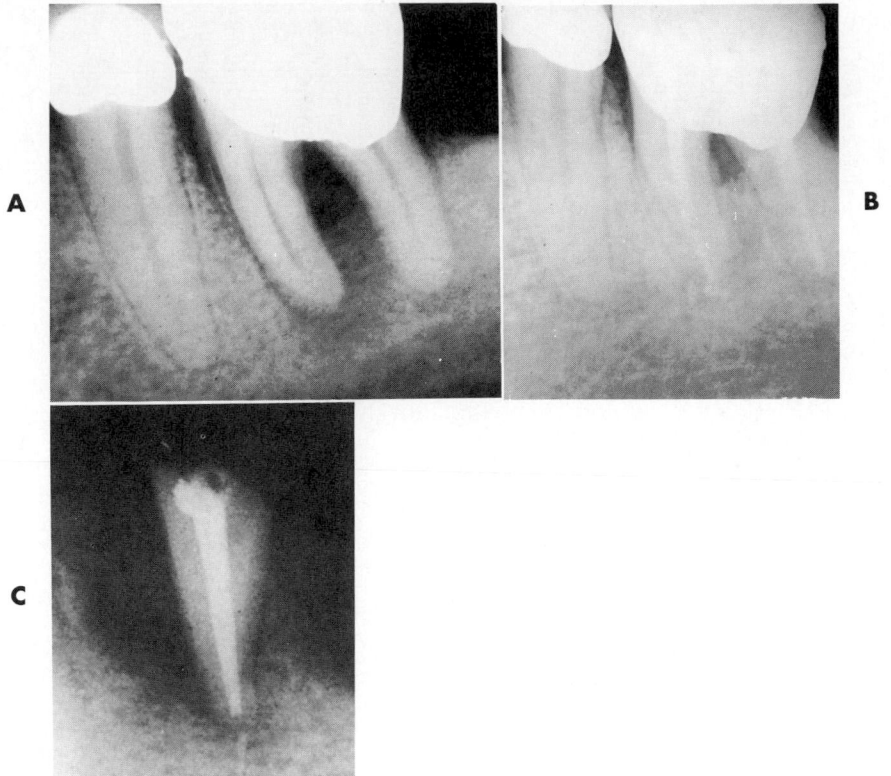

FIG. 33-2 *A,* Tooth with bone demineralization in the furcal and apical areas; root canals are necrotic but periodontal involvement is evident. *B,* Two-year recall after endodontic therapy shows nearly complete healing, with some furcation involvement, possibly as a secondary condition to the endodontic status. *C,* Periodontal disease. Endodontically treated tooth to have been used for an overdenture has periodontal disease that prohibits the tooth from being a support.

(From Cohen S, Burns RC: *Pathways of the pulp,* ed 6, St Louis, 1994, Mosby.)

face periodontal complications or a multitude of other dental problems.

Pulpal Pathoses

Various diseases and injuries can cause the dental pulp to degenerate, resulting in the need for endodontic therapy. The following is an overview of pulpal pathoses most commonly encountered in endodontics today. Table 33-1 represents a condensation of these pulpal pathoses, the symptoms, the reactions to common diagnostic tests, and the prognosis and treatment.

▶ Hyperemia

Pulpal hyperemia is not a disease in itself but is the first stage of inflammation and is indicated by an increased or excessive amount of blood in the pulpal tissue. Pulp tissue that has received an injury from chemical or mechanical irritation, dental caries, or a traumatic blow may become hyperemic, or engorged with blood. The pressure of the increased blood enclosed within the tooth and having no place to escape can sensitize the nerve fibers, which in turn creates severe discomfort for the patient.

▶ Reversible Pulpitis

Pulpitis is an inflammation of the pulpal tissue, and like an inflammation in any other body tissues, it is the response to an irritant that has injured the cells. The pulpal cells can be injured in the same manner as described previously in the hyperemic condition. Pulpitis can also be a secondary inflammation from a periodontal inflammation or may result from **bacteremia**: bacteria in the blood. If pulpitis is treated in its early stages by removing the irritating factor and placing a sedative dressing before performing a permanent restoration, the prognosis is often good, and no further treatment may be needed. If it is left untreated, the sequelae of pulpitis will include the following:

TABLE 33-1   REACTIONS TO COMMON ENDODONTIC DIAGNOSTIC PROCEDURES

Symptoms	EPT/DPT	Heat	Cold	Percussion	Radiograph	Prognosis	Treatment
REVERSIBLE PULPITIS Acute pain, short duration, or clinically observed in dental radiograph	Positive	Normal, indicating vitality	Normal, indicating vitality	Negative	Caries invades dentin near pulp	Good—can return to normal, develop secondary dentin	Protection with sedative dressing, e.g., ZOE cement
IRREVERSIBLE ACUTE PULPITIS Severe pain, increasing in duration and intensity Analgesics often provide limited relief	Positive	Positive, may react more severely, or may be more prolonged than normal	Positive, may provide relief	Negative, unless inflammation spreads to periapical tissue	Negative for bone change	Pulp is degenerating to potential for recovery	Pulp extirpation/endodontic treatment
CHRONIC PULPITIS May be asymptomatic, often occurs in older patients in teeth that have been restored	Positive, may require more electric current to react	Excess amount needed to elicit reaction	Excess amount needed to elicit reaction	Negative	May note a resorption in canal; evidence of bone change	No recovery	Pulp extirpation/endodontic treatment; endodontic treatment or asymptomatic teeth as a prophylactic measure
ACUTE APICAL ABSCESS Severe pain; no relief from analgesics Intraoral or extraoral swelling present Possible draining sinus/fistula	Negative	No response	No response	Positive, often severe, reactions	If early stage, no bone change; latent stage thickening of periodontal membrane is evident	No recovery	(1) Establish drainage through occlusal/lingual opening apex of tooth with file or incision of soft tissue (2) Prescribe antibiotic (3) Hot salt oral rinses (4) Medication for pain; narcotic optional (5) Treat endodontically at later date

NECROSIS May be asymptomatic or previous pain	Negative	No response	No response	Negative	No change evident	No recovery	Pulpectomy and endodontic treatment
CHRONIC APICAL PERIODONTITIS Mild degree of pain; sensitivity less than pulpitis Tooth may feel *high* and discomfort is evident on biting or clenching teeth	Negative	No response	No response	Negative	Bone resorption evident; radiolucent lesion at apex	No recovery	Pulpal extirpation and endodontic treatment
ROOT FRACTURE May be asymptomatic; paresthesia may occur after traumatic blow; dull feeling	Negative	No response	No response	Painful	May indicate fracture, if extensive; hairline fractures may be blocked	No recovery	Extirpation and endodontic treatment; root removal or removal of tooth
CHRONIC APICAL SUPPURATIVE Draining sinus or gingival abscess is present; may be mild degree of pain	Negative	Negative	Negative	Negative	Radiolucent lesion at apex	No recovery	Pulpal extirpation and endodontic treatment

1. **Irreversible pulpitis** — Inflammation of pulpal tissues to an extent that no recovery is imminent
2. **Granuloma** — Pulpal inflammation progresses into the periapical tissues
3. **Periodontal involvement** — Pulpal disease can progress beyond the apical foramen and involve the periodontal ligament with the inflammation
4. **Periapical abscess** — The inflammation process extends past the tooth apex and becomes a localized collection of exudate (pus); all tissue in the local area is destroyed in this highly acidic environment
5. **Extraoral fistula** — Result of the body turning the abscess into a chronic lesion and creating a drainage to an outer or external surface
6. **Cellulitis** — When the abscess spreads along facial planes, it can become a serious infection
7. **Osteomyelitis** — A latent stage of the progression of a periapical infection, which results in the infection spreading into the bone
8. **Actinomycosis** — Bacterial infection that spreads to the mouth, throat, and neck

▸ Irreversible Pulpitis

This form of pulpitis has progressed to a stage that may not allow the pulpal tissue to recover and thus is referred to as **irreversible pulpitis**. The pain for a patient is severe and of longer duration; pulp degeneration is inevitable. The only treatment for this tooth is pulpal **extirpation** (removal).

▸ Necrosis

Necrosis is the death of cells or group of cells. Pulpal necrosis is the death of pulp cells and is generally attributed to irreversible pulpitis. It is possible for exudate that is created from pulpitis to drain through a carious lesion or other channel in the oral cavity, which results in delaying pulpal necrosis. However, if the tooth is intact and if the exudate has no drainage site, the death of the pulpal tissue occurs more rapidly.

▸ Acute Apical Periodontitis (AAP)

Acute apical periodontitis is an extension of pulpal inflammation into periapical tissues. This condition is often the result of irritants from bacteria and toxins (by-products of the necrotic pulp), or it may be the result of a tooth in hyperocclusion. The irritation also may be caused by overextension of instrumentation or by chemicals that are used while cleaning and shaping the root canal during endodontic therapy. Generally, once the irritant is removed or the occlusion is adjusted, the apical periodontitis will subside.

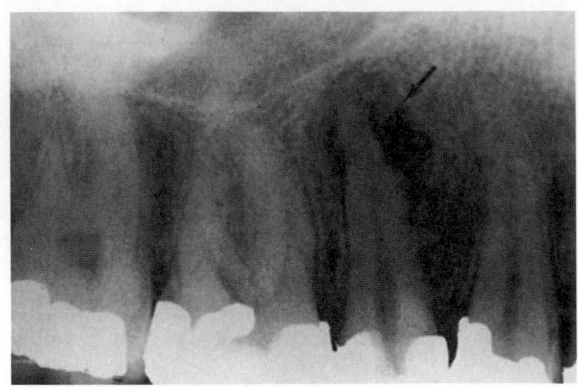

FIG. 33-3   Periapical granuloma.

(From Chasteen JE: *Essentials of clinical dental assisting,* ed 4, St Louis, 1989, Mosby.)

▸ Chronic Apical Periodontitis (CAP)

When the irritant in the acute stage of apical periodontitis is not removed, a chronic state typically follows. In a radiograph this is noted by an interruption in the lamina dura or evidence of more extensive tissue destruction in the periapical region. Few other symptoms are evident.

▸ Periapical Granuloma

A **periapical granuloma** is the result of pulpal inflammation emanating into the periapical tissues. A periapical granuloma (Fig. 33-3) is a lesion that is caused by trauma or irritants from the pulp that may include microorganisms, bacterially produced toxins, or by-products of protein degradation. In this illustration of the apex of a premolar tooth a large area of bone is replaced by granulation tissue, which contains numerous inflammatory cells. If the irritating factor is removed, the exudate will subside and cell repair can take place, resulting in healing of the tissue. If a periapical granuloma is not treated, the potential exists for the formation of cysts.

▸ Apical Periodontal Cyst

Fig. 33-4 is an illustration of an apical cyst, which is a closed epithelium-lined space that contains fluid or semifluid. This cyst forms when a mass of epithelial cells in a granuloma proliferates extensively; the central cells outgrow their vascular supply, become necrotic, and liquefy, creating a cavity that is filled with fluid and semisolid material and is partially lined with stratified squamous epithelium. The epithelium is surrounded by connective tissue that contains all of the cells identified in the granuloma. Once a cyst has formed, periapical curettage and proper pulp canal therapy are needed to enable the periapical tissues to regenerate. If a cyst remains after the inflammatory irritant has been eliminated, it may continue to accumulate fluid and enlarge, thereby destroying the surrounding tissue with its pressure.

▶ Periapical Abscess

An abscess is a localized accumulation of exudate in a cavity that is formed by tissue degeneration. A **periapical abscess** at the periapical region of a premolar tooth is shown in Fig. 33-5. This abscess is partially filled with liquefied necrotic tissue that forms a semiliquid material or exudate. An abscess can create great pressure, resulting in the fluid's being forced through the buccal cortical plate to emerge into the gingival mucosa, creating periodontal involvement as shown in Fig. 33-1.

A cutaneous abscess can develop (Fig. 33-6); this periapical abscess was forced through the bone into a

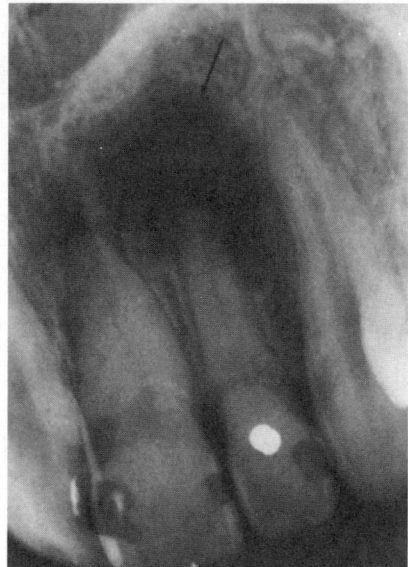

FIG. 33-4   Periapical cyst.

(From Chasteen JE: *Essentials of clinical dental assisting,* ed 4, St Louis, 1989, Mosby.)

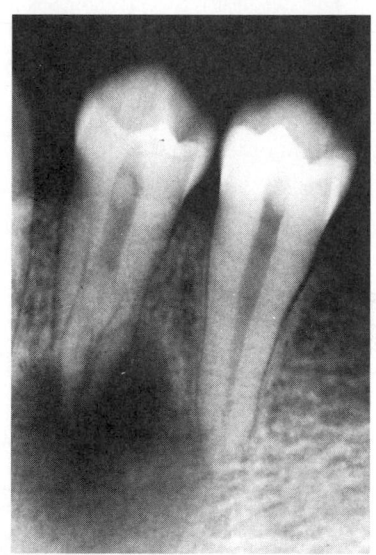

FIG. 33-5   Periapical abscess.

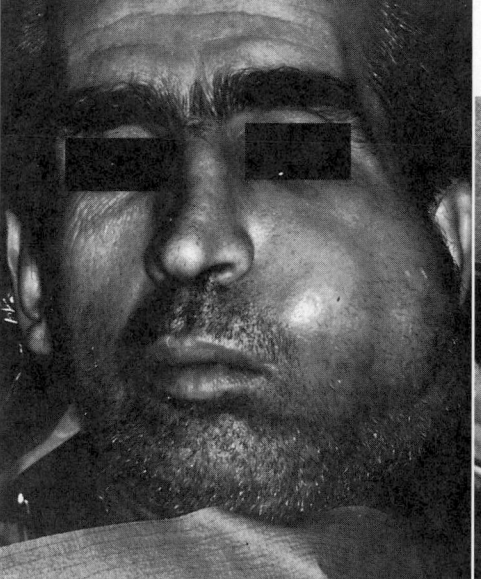

A

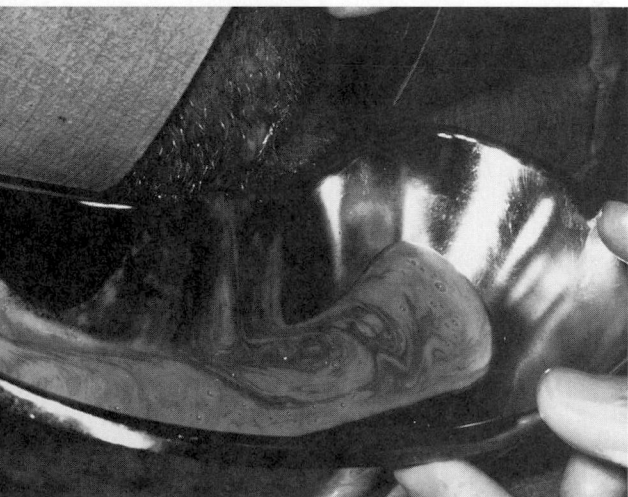

B

FIG. 33-6   *A,* Clinical photograph of an acute periapical abscess. *B,* Pus and blood draining externally into a basin from the incised abscess.

(From Cohen S, Burns RC: *Pathways of the pulp,* ed 6, St Louis, 1994, Mosby.)

region that led to the masticatory space. The exudate buried itself in the subcutaneous tissue as a cutaneous abscess and eventually would have erupted through the skin to expel its purulent contents.

Cellulitis

Cellulitis is an extension of a periapical inflammatory process. The inflammation spreads along fascial planes into fibrous connective tissue that envelops organs and structures within the body, and through tissue spaces creating marked edema (Fig. 33-7).

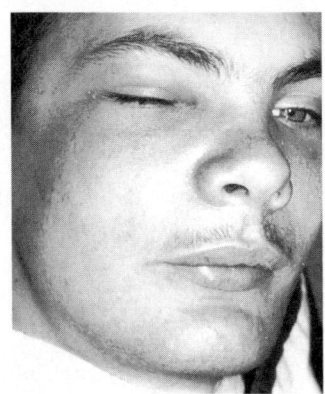

FIG. 33-7   Cellulitis has created edema around the right mandibular region.

(From Cohen S, Burns RC: *Pathways of the pulp*, ed 6, St Louis, 1994, Mosby.)

Pulpal Stone

A **pulp stone** is a calcification that occurs in the coronal region of the pulp (Fig. 33-8). A diffuse or linear calcification in the form of a spicule may occur in the pulp canal and is usually aligned near a vessel or nerve. Typically, pulp stones have no clinical significance; however, they may increase in frequency and size with age or with irritation. Large pulp stones can complicate gaining access to a canal during root canal therapy.

Injuries

Each day in a person's life can present a myriad of opportunities for traumatic injury to the teeth. Injuries can result from contact sports, automobile or household accidents, dental procedures, or domestic violence. Trauma to the teeth can generally be categorized as luxation injuries, avulsion injuries, alveolar fractures, or mechanical injuries to the pulp.

LUXATION INJURIES

Luxation injuries occur when a blow or hit to the mouth results in trauma to the supporting tissues. A tooth with luxation injury is generally sensitive to percussion and may have mobility. A **luxated tooth** is one that has been moved from its normal physiologic position. It is common with this type of injury for the tooth to become

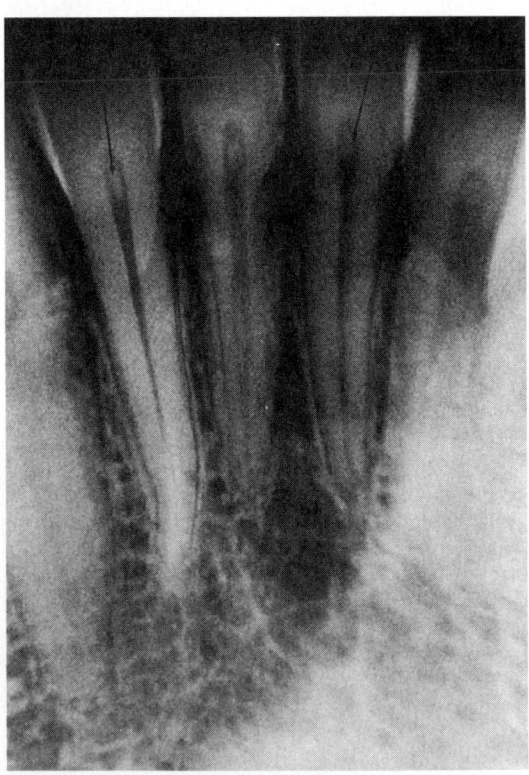

FIG. 33-8   Pulp stones are found as isolated calcifications.

(1) extruded, displaced out of the socket, along its long axis; (2) intruded, forced into its socket in an axial or apical direction; or (3) laterally luxated, rotated out of normal position from its long axis in a buccal, lingual, mesial, or distal direction.

Depending on the extent of the injury it may be necessary to reposition the teeth, splint the luxated teeth, or perform root canal treatment if evidence of irreversible pulpitis is apparent. Various types of injuries are shown in Fig. 33-9, *A* through *C*. Such injuries may require consultation with other specialists, including an orthodontist or oral maxillofacial surgeon.

A patient with this type of injury must be monitored to verify the pulp status through various tests, radiographs, and visual observation of color changes.

AVULSION

An **avulsed tooth** is a tooth that has been knocked completely out of its socket. The tooth can be replanted; however, time is a most important factor in the success of such treatment (Fig. 33-9, *D*). In this situation the dental assistant plays an important role in providing first aid instruction to the patient, parent, athletic teacher, or other responsible person. For immediate replantation the following instructions can be given:

▶ Rinse the tooth gently in tap water.
▶ Do not scrub the tooth.
▶ Gently place the tooth into the socket in as close to normal position as possible; the patient may bite down on a piece of soft fabric or handkerchief to help maintain the position.
▶ See a dentist immediately.

If the tooth cannot be reinserted in the socket, the following directions should be given to the patient or transport person:

▶ Place a clean cloth over the site of the injury, and ask the patient to bite on it.
▶ Transport the patient and the tooth to the office immediately.
▶ Transport the tooth in a liquid medium, such as saline, saliva, or milk. Water is not considered a good medium for transport because it does not maintain the vitality of the periodontal ligament cells.

Time is the primary factor in the success of replantation. Therefore, the patient should be brought to the office promptly and seen immediately upon arrival.

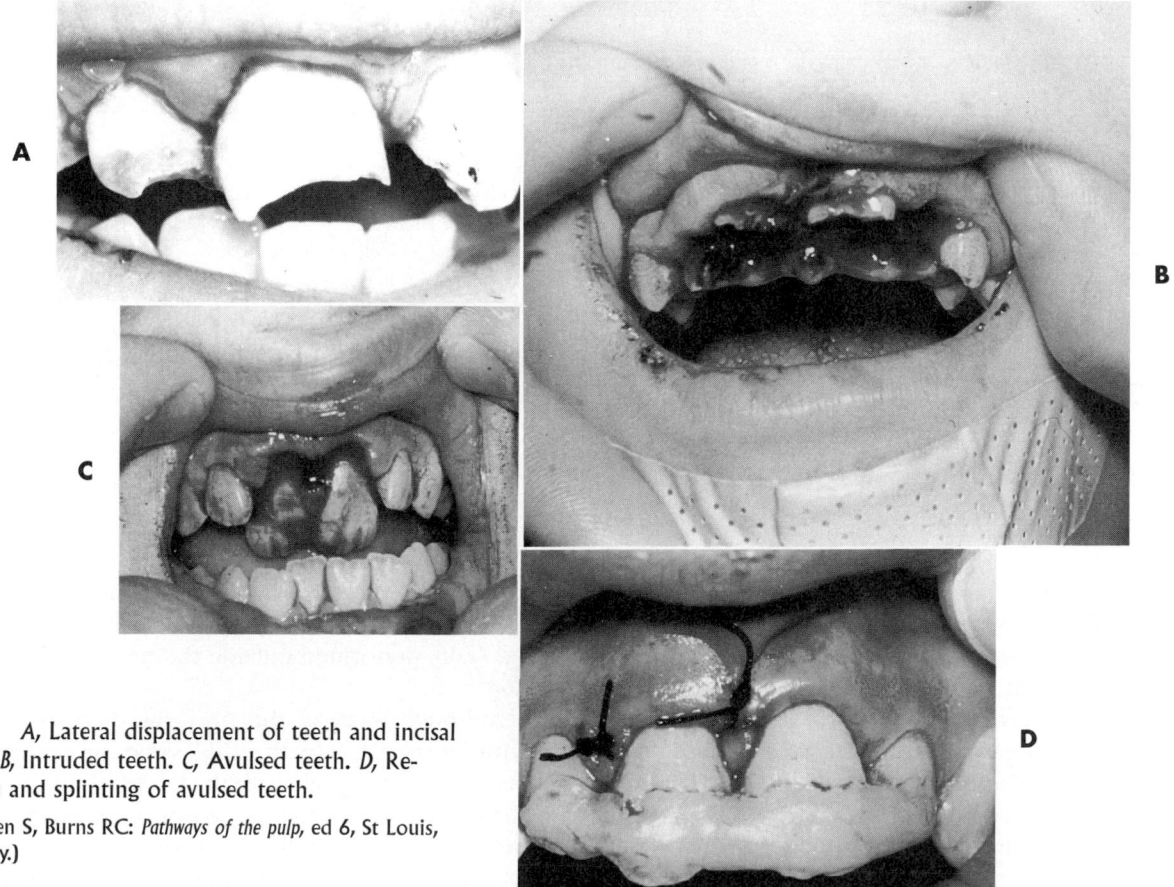

FIG. 33-9   *A,* Lateral displacement of teeth and incisal fractures. *B,* Intruded teeth. *C,* Avulsed teeth. *D,* Replantation and splinting of avulsed teeth.

(From Cohen S, Burns RC: *Pathways of the pulp,* ed 6, St Louis, 1994, Mosby.)

REPLANTATION OF TEETH WITH LESS THAN 2 HOURS EXTRAALVEOLAR TIME

- ▶ Are all universal barrier techniques being used?
- ▶ Is all of the armamentarium available and prepared for use?
- ▶ Are the instruments arranged in sequence of use?
- ▶ Am I prepared for alternative treatment plans?
- ▶ Is the necessary equipment turned on and ready to operate?

The following procedure is followed once the patient has arrived in the office with the avulsed tooth.

1. Place the tooth in a cup of saline.
2. Radiograph the area of injury; look for evidence of alveolar fracture.
3. Examine the avulsion site carefully for any loose bone fragments that can be removed.
4. Gently irrigate the socket with saline; it is not necessary to remove blood clots.
5. Grasp the tooth from the cup of saline with extraction forceps to avoid handling the root surface.
6. Examine the tooth for debris, which, if present, can be removed with cotton pliers.
7. Reinsert the tooth into the socket; after partial insertion, using the forceps, the remainder of the procedure can be accomplished by gentle finger pressure or by letting the patient bite on a 2 × 2 gauze until the tooth is seated.
8. Check the tooth for proper alignment; avoid hyperocclusion.
9. Stabilize the tooth for 1 to 2 weeks with a nonrigid splint.
10. Prescribe antibiotics as necessary for mild to moderate oral infections. A tetanus booster injection is recommended if the last one was administered more than 5 years previously.
11. Supportive care includes a soft diet and mild analgesics as needed.

REPLANTATION OF TEETH WITH MORE THAN 2 HOURS EXTRAALVEOLAR TIME

The following procedure illustrates replantation with more than 2 hours having elapsed after tooth avulsion.

The following procedure is followed once the patient has arrived in the office and provided the avulsed tooth.

1. Examine the patient and the area of tooth avulsion; examine the radiographs for evidence of alveolar fractures.
2. Examine the tooth, and remove debris and any pieces of soft tissue that may be adhering to the root surface.
3. Soak the tooth in a fluoride solution for at least 5 minutes.
4. Extirpate the pulp and fill the root canal, while holding the tooth in a fluoride-soaked piece of gauze. Often, the root canal procedure can be accomplished from an apical direction if the tooth is less than fully mature.
5. Carefully suction the alveolar socket; for this type of replantation, it will be beneficial to remove blood clots. Irrigate the socket with saline. Anesthetic may be necessary first.
6. Gently replant the tooth into the socket; check for proper alignment and occlusal contact.
7. Stabilize the tooth for 1 to 2 weeks.

- ▶ Are the appropriate universal barrier techniques removed?
- ▶ Have all of the appropriate surfaces been cleaned and disinfected?
- ▶ Has all armamentarium been removed?
- ▶ Has all equipment been repositioned?
- ▶ Has all of the equipment been disinfected/sterilized according to OSHA guidelines?

Once the patient is in the office and seated, the sequence of the procedure for replantation within 2 hours may be followed.

Commonly, when a tooth has been replanted within 2 hours, it will be necessary to perform root canal therapy on the tooth within 2 to 3 weeks after replantation. In immature teeth where the apex has not completely developed and is open, the root canal is generally not performed immediately but is evaluated over the next year at regular intervals. However, in teeth which have not been replanted in this short period of time or have not been kept moist and the periodontal ligament and fibers have not survived, the root canal therapy is generally performed outside the mouth before replantation.

Although most of the previous discussion has dealt with permanent teeth, this same procedure can be performed for primary teeth. Often, the replantation of an avulsed deciduous tooth is not considered as a primary treatment choice. If, however, the tooth is to be retained for 1 to 2 years before natural exfoliation, the procedure may be an effective method of space maintenance. This procedure involves young children and may be difficult to complete so obviously the dentist must weigh several factors before such treatment is begun.

ALVEOLAR FRACTURE

During a traumatic blow an alveolar fracture may occur and pulpal necrosis may develop. Typically, an oral maxillofacial surgeon sees the patient when such a traumatic injury occurs, but the follow-up visit with the general practitioner or endodontist should include periodic radiographs and vitality tests to determine when and if future root canal treatment is necessary.

Diagnosis

The components of most endodontic procedures include a complete dental and medical history, clinical evaluation, diagnosis, presentation of a treatment plan, the treatment procedure, and a recall appointment for the follow-up visit.

In Chapter 24, emphasis is placed on the important role the dental assistant has in obtaining vital data to ensure an accurate diagnosis for a patient. Endodontics is no exception. Here, too, the dental assistant often is the first person with whom the patient comes in contact when he or she is having severe discomfort that later may be diagnosed as an endodontically involved tooth.

Initial Complaint

Commonly, the patient will contact the dental office by telephone and identify that he or she is having a problem. As discussed in Chapter 24 the dental assistant needs to ask specific questions to determine the nature of the complaint. Obviously, questions to the patient may vary in an endodontic specialty office, since much of the information may have be obtained from the referring dentist. However, to determine whether a tooth has potential endodontic involvement, several of the following questions are beneficial.

1. *"Which tooth is causing the pain?"* In a telephone conversation the patient may describe whether the tooth is an upper or lower one and where it is located. If the patient is in the office, the patient may point to the tooth. The assistant needs to record the specific location of the discomfort on the health questionnaire.
2. *"Describe the pain. When does it bother you? Does anything trigger the pain; i.e., such as hot or cold temperatures?"* The patient may describe the pain as "constant" or that the pain is worse when he or she has a hot cup of coffee or after he or she eats. Again, information specific to the type of pain is recorded on the patient's record.
3. *"How long does the pain last?"* The pain may only occur when the site is stimulated, such as when eating or drinking liquids of different temperatures.
4. *"Do you ever get any relief? If so, how?"* The seriousness of the problem often can be narrowed with this question. If the patient gets relief from taking an over-the-counter medication such as aspirin, the condition may be less serious than it is with the patient who gets little relief from a stronger medication, such as Darvocet. Caution should be taken, however, in making this decision, since the pain threshold of patients varies greatly.
5. *"Does the pain keep you awake at night?"* If the patient states that the pain is constant and that he or she cannot sleep, obviously the patient needs to be seen immediately. To ignore the patient at this point means that his or her general health may deteriorate and problems may arise, such as changes in blood sugar or blood pressure levels, or other systemic infections may occur.

▶ Diagnostic Tests

As in any diagnosis a variety of tests are used. In endodontics these tests include a complete medical and dental history; clinical examination; radiographs; percussion; palpation; thermal, electronic (EPT), or digital pulp test (DPT); bite test; periodontal probe; transillumination; or a test cavity. One test alone may not conclusively prove that the tooth is devital and warrants endodontic treatment. Consequently, the dentist frequently relies on results of several of these tests to verify the final diagnosis.

MEDICAL/DENTAL HISTORY

The need for a thorough medical history on an endodontic patient does not differ from other phases of dentistry. The dental history portion of the questionnaire for a patient with a suspected endodontic condition addresses different concerns, however. Special attention is given to previous accidents or traumatic injuries that may now be the cause of a devital tooth. The patient may indicate that he or she was in an auto accident several years previously or that he or she was hit in the mouth once while participating in a contact sport. Complaints about a specific tooth over a period of time may also aid in diagnosing the tooth in question.

ENDODONTIC CHARTING

As with other dental specialties most endodontists use a specially designed chart to record pertinent data about their findings. Standardized charts for general dentistry do not include appropriate space to record the results of specific endodontic tests.

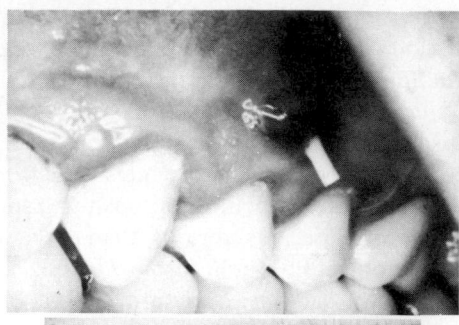

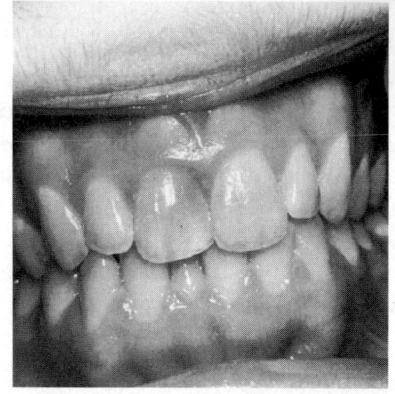

FIG. 33-10   *A,* External fistula. *B,* Discolored tooth.
(From Cohen S, Burns RC: *Pathways of the pulp,* ed 6, St Louis, 1994, Mosby.)

CLINICAL EXAMINATION

As they are in a routine clinical examination, the external tissues are first observed. When the patient arrives in the office, attention should be given to facial asymmetry to determine if any edema exists that may be caused by dental pathology or trauma. An external fistula, as shown in Fig. 33-10, *A,* may indicate a draining sinus from intraoral tissues.

During the intraoral examination attention should be given to the following:

Discolored teeth — Teeth with necrotic pulp are often darker in color or less translucent than healthy teeth (Fig. 33-10, *B*).

Soft tissue lesions — Periapical or periodontal abscesses may be identified by areas of bony or soft tissue swelling. Draining sinuses in the vestibular or palatal area may be traced to a chronic abscess.

Fractured teeth — Hair-line fractures of the enamel may go undetected and may extend to the dentin, resulting in pulpal damage.

Deep caries or extensive restoration — Caries that has extended to the pulp generally will do irreparable damage to the pulpal tissue. Likewise, pulpal damage may have occurred to the tooth during the preparation for an extensive restoration that is within close proximity of the pulp. The dentist may have taken all of the necessary precautions, but the extent of damage to the pulp may have been irreparable. Such damage can also be the result of an uncooperative patient who was unable to restrain movement, thereby causing the handpiece to enter the pulpal tissue.

Malocclusion — Constant traumatic occlusion may result in damage to the periapical and pulpal tissues.

▶ Radiographs

Radiographs are important for several reasons in endodontics. Later in this chapter, radiographs are discussed as they relate to treatment procedures. However, periapical, Panorex, and bite-wing radiographs are valuable diagnostic tools in endodontics when they are used in conjunction with other diagnostic tests. The use of radiographs in the endodontic diagnosis has several limitations and should not alone be considered a conclusive diagnostic tool. First, radiographs are only two-dimensional, and a variety of angles may be needed to create a three-dimensional perspective. Further, pathologic changes in the early stages of pulpitis or periapical disease may not be visible on radiographs. Periapical lesions are only noted in radiographs as the inflammatory process spreads into its latent stages where a break in the lamina dura or the presence of a granuloma is evident (see Fig. 33-3).

BUCCAL OBJECT RULE

One of the disadvantages of dental radiographs in endodontics is the lack of a third dimension, which causes difficulty in distinguishing between two structures that appear superimposed. The use of the *buccal object rule* is used to define the buccolingual relationship between two superimposed structures. To apply this rule, two radiographs are taken. The first is taken using standard periapical technique. The second exposure is made in the same way, except that the tube is shifted about 20 degrees in either the vertical or the horizontal angulation. When the two radiographs are compared, the buccal object will appear to have moved in the opposite direction from the tube shift (Fig. 33-11, *A* through *F*). For instance, if the tube is shifted mesially by changing the horizontal angulation, the buccal object will appear to have moved distally. The basic concept is *buccal opposite* when this rule is applied. Thus, if a radiograph were taken of a mandibular molar and the vertical angulation is increased by moving the beam down, the buccal object will appear to have moved superiorly on the film.

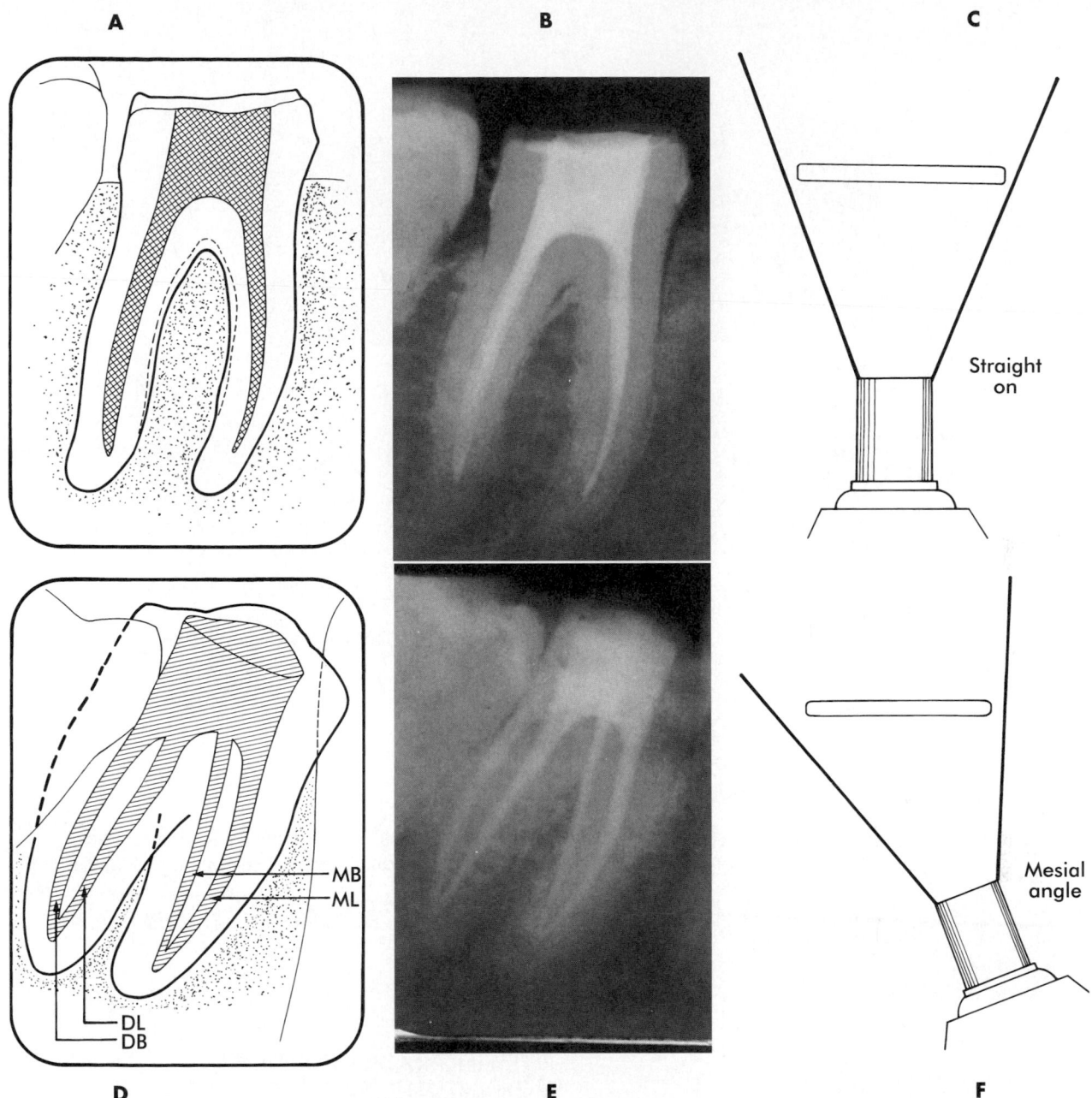

FIG. 33-11 Comparison of straight-on and mesial-angled views of an endodontically treated mandibular molar with four canals. *A,* through *C,* Straight-on view of the mandibular molar shows superimposition of the root canal fillings. *D,* through *F,* Mesial-to-distal angulation produces separation of the canals. The mesolingual and distolingual root-filled canals move mesially (toward the cone), and the mesiobuccal and distobuccal root-filled canals move distally (away from the cone) on the radiograph.

(From Cohen S, Burns RC: *Pathways of the pulp,* ed 6, St Louis, 1994, Mosby.)

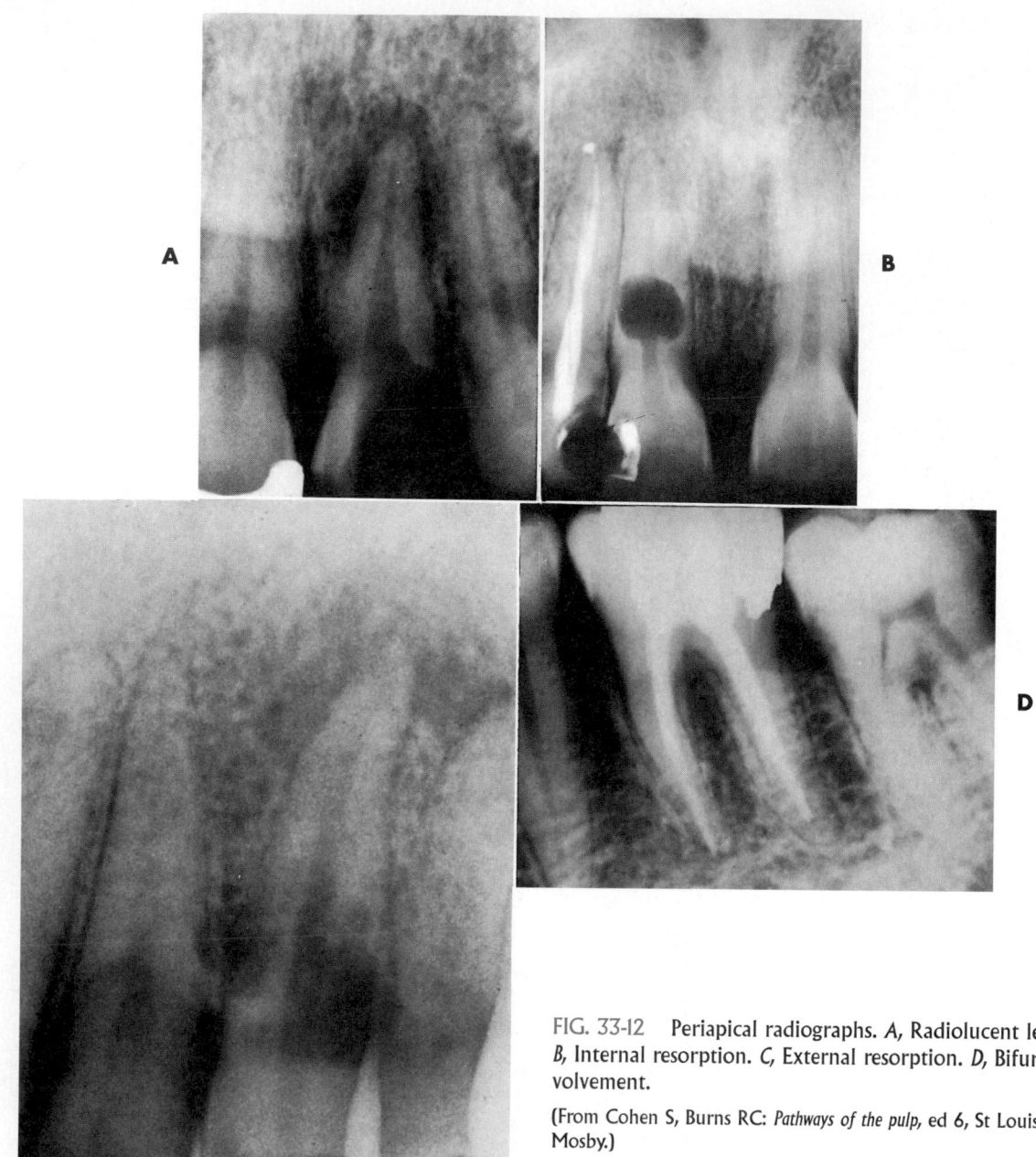

FIG. 33-12   Periapical radiographs. *A*, Radiolucent lesion. *B*, Internal resorption. *C*, External resorption. *D*, Bifurcation involvement.

(From Cohen S, Burns RC: *Pathways of the pulp*, ed 6, St Louis, 1994, Mosby.)

PERIAPICAL RADIOGRAPHS IN ENDODONTIC DIAGNOSIS

When it is used in endodontics, a periapical radiograph will indicate the following:

1. Presence of radiolucent areas (Fig. 33-12, *A*)
2. Internal or external resorption or calcification of the pulp chamber or root canal (Fig. 33-12, *B* and *C*)
3. Involvement of disease into the periapical or periodontal tissues
4. Presence of pulpal stones (see Fig. 33-8)
5. Bone loss and furcation involvement (Fig. 33-12, *D*)

BITEWING RADIOGRAPHS IN ENDODONTIC DIAGNOSIS

From a bite-wing radiograph the dentist can determine the following:

1. Extent of dental caries
2. Level of bone loss

PANORAMIC RADIOGRAPHY IN ENDODONTIC DIAGNOSIS

From a Panorex radiograph the dentist can determine the conditions evident in a periapical radiograph and can also

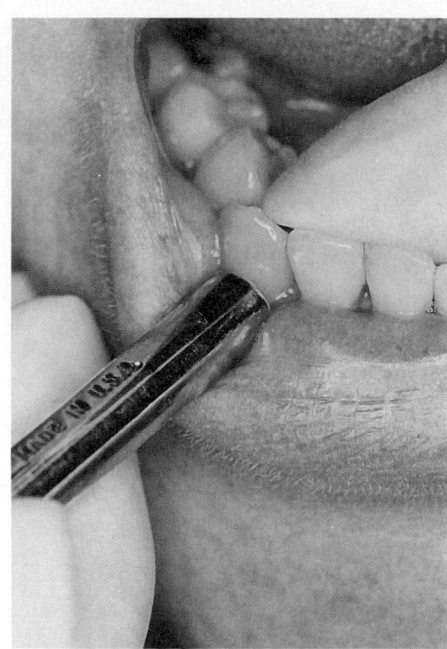

FIG. 33-13   Percussion test, with mirror handle.

gain a broader perspective of the entire oral cavity, as well as a better comparison of adjacent and opposing structures.

▶ Percussion Test

This test is frequently done by tapping the handle of a mirror on the symptomatic tooth (Fig. 33-13). Indicate to the patient the expected reaction when a healthy tooth is tapped, and then perform the test on the suspected tooth. When percussion is used on a tooth with a periapical lesion, the patient will likely experience a sharp pain or severe discomfort. A devital tooth or a fracture may result in a dull thud-like sound or in no response at all.

▶ Bite Test

A bite test is not unlike a percussion test. This test may be done by asking the patient to bite normally or by placing a cotton roll or a tongue blade wrapped with gauze over the suspected tooth and asking the patient to bite. If the patient indicates discomfort while biting on a specific tooth, additional tests can be conducted to verify the findings.

▶ Palpation

Similar to the percussion and bite tests the palpation tests help to determine the extent of inflammation in the periapical tissues. The dentist will apply pressure with a gloved finger over the apical region of the suspected

tooth. If the patient reacts to this pressure by indicating that pain is present, the inflammation evidently has invaded the periapical tissues and is present in the bone and mucosa of the apical region.

During the palpation test, mobility of the tooth can also be determined. By using two gloved fingers the dentist is able to create lateral pressure on the tooth. The ball of one finger can be placed on the lingual aspect, and pressure with the mirror handle can be applied to the tooth from the opposing surface. If the mobility exceeds a Class III level, the tooth likely has little periodontal support and may not be a candidate for successful endodontic treatment.

Gutta percha, used today in endodontic treatment, had its origin in 1850; then it was made from exudate of the trees of the sapodilla family and was mixed with lime, quartz, and feldspar. It was first marketed under the name of Hill's Stopping and was used as a temporary filling.

▶ Thermal Test

Two types of thermal tests are used to elicit response from the patient to determine the presence of an inflammation in the tooth. Like many of the other tests, thermal tests alone cannot be reliable. A *cold test* uses dry ice (CO_2), refrigerant (ethyl chloride) (Fig. 33-14, *A*), or regular ice that is made into an ice stick by freezing water in the noninjection end of a protective needle cover or in prefabricated ice stick forms (Fig. 33-14, *B*). The latter method—the ice stick—is a simple and popular technique. A *heat test* is performed by placing a heated instrument, such as a ball burnisher, directly on the tooth (Fig. 33-14, *C*); by heating gutta percha in a bunsen burner and applying it to the tooth; or by rotating a dry rubber prophy cup on the tooth to create frictional heat (Fig. 33-14, *D*). Care should be taken when administering a heat test to avoid injury to adjacent tissues, especially if a heated instrument is used.

To administer any of these tests, the suspected tooth and comparison teeth are isolated and dried with cotton pellets. Thermal tests are less reliable on posterior teeth than anterior teeth because of the bulk of a posterior tooth. To apply the ice, the stick is held between the gloved fingers and placed on the labial or buccal surface. On a vital tooth this test will elicit a sharp pain that quickly disappears when the ice is removed. If the sharp pain increases in intensity and persists even after the ice is removed, an irreversible pulpitis probably exists in the tooth. In necrotic teeth no response occurs with cold stimulation.

When heat is applied to the isolated tooth the temperature gradually increases until pain is elicited. As in the cold test, a sharp, nonlingering pain indicates a

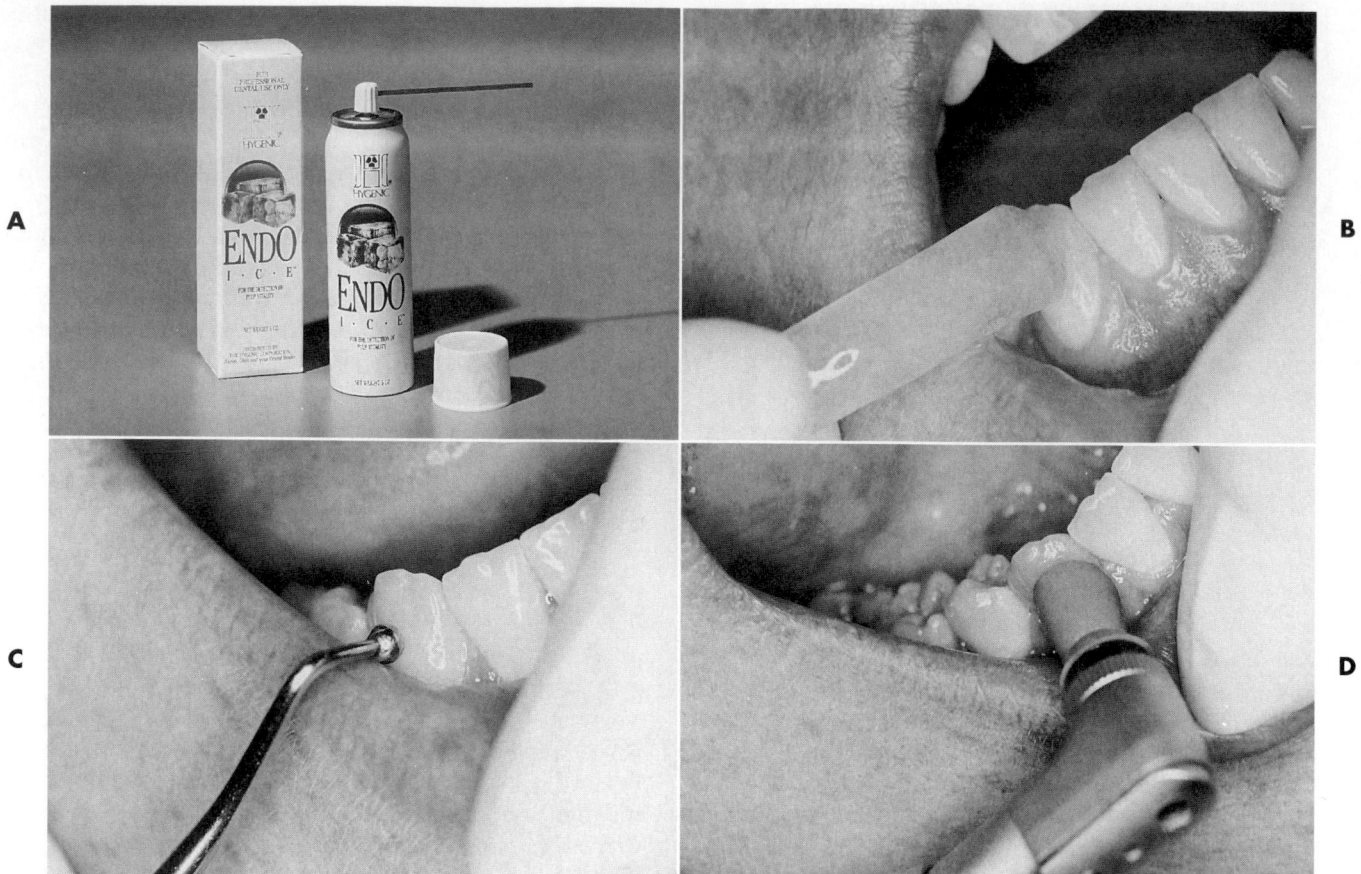

FIG. 33-14   Thermal test. *A,* Ethyl chloride spray. *B,* Prefabricated ice stick. *C,* Heated ball burnisher. *D,* Rotating a dry rubber prophy cup on a tooth.

(*A* from Hygenic Corporation. *B* and *C* from Chasteen JE: *Essentials of clinical dental assisting,* ed 4, St Louis, 1989, Mosby.)

vital tooth and a sharp nonsubsiding response generally indicates an irreversible pulpitis. Likewise, a lack of response will indicate a necrotic pulp. A combination test that uses heat and cold can also verify irreversible necrosis. Heat can be applied, and if the reaction is severe it can be followed by a cold application. If relief occurs when cold is applied to the tooth, it is likely that an irreversible pulpitis exists.

▶ Electronic Pulp Test (EPT)/Digital Pulp Test (DPT)

Electronic pulp testers are powered by direct electric current or batteries, providing a high-frequency current that creates an electrical stimulus to generate a reaction in the tooth. The amount of current can be varied; however, it should be noted that the variance in the current level does not indicate the level of vitality or degeneration of the tooth.

The difference between an EPT and a DPT is the

method of providing the readout (Fig. 33-15). The DPT provides a digital readout, and many dentists feel it is easier to use.

Both testers operate similarly. The tooth is isolated and dried and a saliva ejector is placed. A small amount of toothpaste or similar medium is placed on the tip of the electrode and the tip is then placed on the labial or buccal surface of the tooth (Fig. 33-16). Care should be taken to place the tip on the natural tooth surface and not on a restored surface or on gingival tissue. Many types of pulp testers require adjunct connectors to come into patient contact at two points to complete the circuit. As the test begins, the rheostat on the tester is slowly advanced to increase the amount of current. The patient is instructed to raise a finger when sensation is noted. Often the patient will indicate a tingling or *hot* feeling, identifying the presence of vital tissue. The absence of such a response generally indicates pulpal necrosis. It is important to make comparison tests with adjacent *normal* teeth to validate the results of the test. The typical recording on most pulp testers is between 0 to 10. The

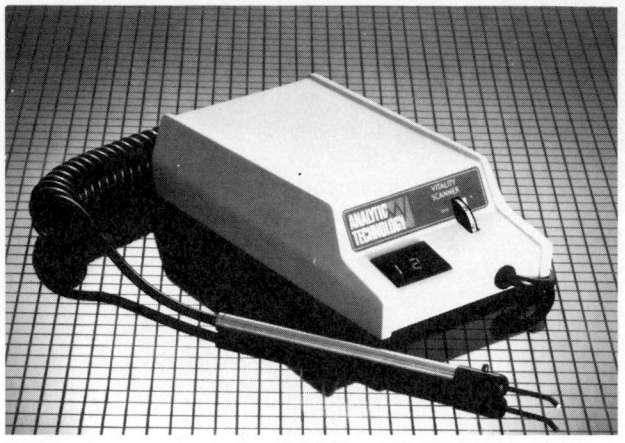

FIG. 33-15   Digital pulp tester.

(From Cohen S, Burns RC: *Pathways of the pulp,* ed 6, St Louis, 1994, Mosby.)

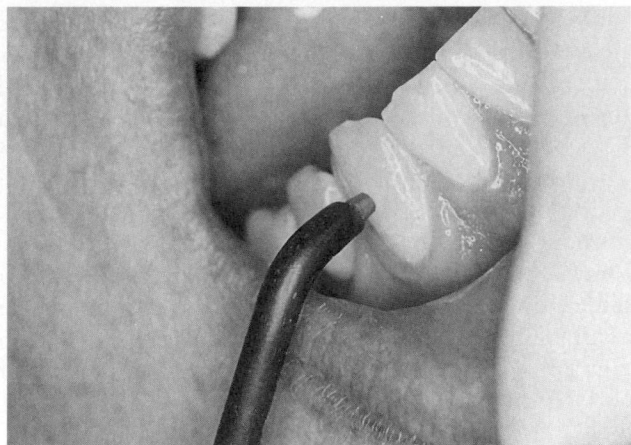

FIG. 33-16   Toothpaste or similar medium placed on tip of pulp tester, which is placed on isolated tooth to determine vitality.

higher the reading, the greater the amount of current needed to create the stimulus, indicating the tooth is probably devital.

▶ Periodontal Probing

This test is vital to determine the status of periodontal health and lends credence to the prognosis for endodontic treatment. For instance, when the dentist probes the periodontal tissues and determines that the periodontal attachment is in relatively good health, the potential for success of root canal therapy is greater. However, the tooth with a vital pulp that warrants endodontic therapy but has severe periodontal disease with furcation involvement can be a potential for failure.

If the patient experiences discomfort during this probing activity, a local anesthetic may be needed. As the dentist probes all of the root and furcal surfaces, the dental assistant carefully records the periodontal findings to be used later in combination with the other endodontic tests to determine the final diagnosis.

▶ Transillumination

With the advent of fiberoptics this particular test has increased in use. A **transillumination** test allows for a concentrated amount of intense light to pass through a tooth from the lingual to the labial surface (Fig. 33-17). In a tooth with a necrotic pulp the outline of the pulp chamber is visible as a dark outline. In a normal tooth, no color differentiation is visible between the pulp chamber and adjacent tooth structure. This test is most effective in the anterior region of the mouth.

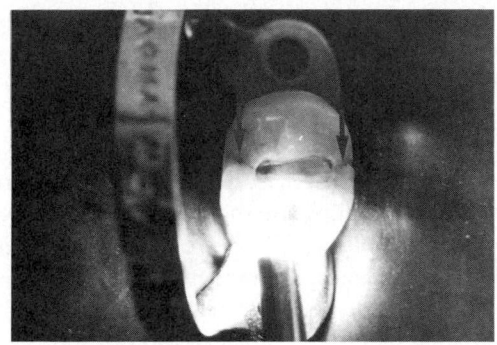

FIG. 33-17   Transillumination. All restorations are removed, the tooth is isolated with a rubber dam, and dentin is dried with cotton pellets. A strong fiberoptic light is directed in through the buccal or lingual wall. A vertical fracture in the dentin may appear as a dark line.

(From Cohen S, Burns RC: *Pathways of the pulp,* ed 6, St Louis, 1994, Mosby.)

▶ Test Cavity

When a degree of uncertainty exists in a diagnosis, the dentist may select to perform a test cavity. This perhaps is the least common test; however, when no definitive diagnosis can be made, an opening is made (without anesthesia) in the occlusal or lingual surface of the tooth through the enamel or through an existing restoration. If during this opening procedure the patient indicates pain from the heat of the handpiece as the bur reaches the dentin, it can be determined that the tooth has vitality and can render a previously made devital diagnosis negative. The test can be terminated at this point, and a permanent restoration can then be placed.

Once a tooth has been diagnosed as needing endodontic treatment, a consent form must be reviewed with the patient and signed by the patient or responsible party if the patient is a minor (see Fig. 14-16). Appointments can be scheduled for the patient, and treatment can begin. The assistant must be familiar with the procedure for each phase of treatment. This chapter includes a basic introduction to the pulpotomy, pulpectomy, apicoectomy, and bleaching of vital and nonvital teeth. Before an understanding of any procedure can develop, the dental assistant needs a working knowledge of several basic concepts and of the instrumentation that is used in endodontics.

ANESTHESIA

Anesthesia is an important component of endodontics. Even though it seems unnecessary to anesthetize a tooth that is necrotic and that has a periapical lesion, frequently vital tissue exists in the apical region of the root canals. The obvious goal of the dentist is to make the patient comfortable during all phases of treatment. Consequently, anesthesia is frequently used in the initial appointments, although it may not be used in the obturation appointment.

The traditional anesthetic techniques can be used in endodontics, including the maxillary division block, the inferior alveolar block, and intraligamentary injections. An infiltration may also be used as the dentist attempts to block any accessory nerves that lead to the tooth. An intrapulpal injection that is placed directly into a vital and sensitive pulp may be needed. Although this type of injection can be extremely painful, it is of short duration and may be needed to achieve a profound effect in a patient who experiences severe discomfort.

Difficulty in achieving profound anesthesia often occurs in a patient who has a highly inflammatory condition. In this situation the doctor may try alternative methods of local anesthesia, including inhalation or intravenous anesthesia. For an infection, the dentist may prescribe an antibiotic, open the tooth and place a cotton pellet to promote drainage, and wait until the inflammatory state subsides.

Isolation

The isolation method of choice in root canal therapy is the rubber dam. This method of isolation offers the benefits identified in Box 33-1.

Rubber dam armamentarium used in endodontics is not unlike the materials described in Chapter 22. However, several suggestions are made for use of equipment in endodontics that can expedite the treatment procedure.

Rubber dam selection itself varies in color and weight,

BOX 33-1
RUBBER DAM ISOLATION FOR ENDODONTIC TREATMENT
▶ Improves visibility
▶ Reduces salivary leakage to promote a dry field
▶ Decreases exposure to cross-contamination
▶ Confines intracanal irrigants and medicaments to eliminate distaste to the patient
▶ Decreases interference of soft tissues
▶ Increases patient comfort
▶ Increases efficiency
▶ Improves standard of care; all dental schools in the United States require the use of rubber dam during endodontic procedures; its use obviously decreases potential negligence

as discussed in Chapter 22. For endodontics the light-colored material is often chosen, since it allows for greater illumination and, since it is somewhat transparent, the lighter color aids in film placement when radiographs are taken. The heavyweight dam material is not required, since gingival retraction is unnecessary in this procedure. The lightweight dam material may promote leakage, which could cause contamination. Therefore, a medium weight is often chosen because it is relatively easy to apply and can eliminate salivary leakage.

The choice of frames is a concern in endodontics. A metal frame, such as the Young's frame, is radiopaque and must be removed when the radiograph is taken. The Nygaard-Ostby and the Star Visi frames are radiolucent and need not be removed during the radiographic exposure.

Clamps used in endodontics are the choice of each dentist. Among the popular choices are the Ivory #0, #1, #9, #14A, and #26 that are shown in Chapter 22. Each is a winged clamp that provides good rubber dam retention, and the #14A adds additional retention because of its gingival retraction capability.

The last major difference in rubber dam usage from operative dentistry is the need to punch only one hole. The adjacent teeth need not be exposed for contact access; therefore, only the tooth being treated is exposed, and the clamp is placed directly on this tooth.

Endodontic Radiography

Earlier in this chapter the importance of radiographs in diagnosis is discussed. Radiographs play a major role in various stages of endodontic treatment and several concerns should be considered to provide the most accurate radiograph possible.

▶ Avoid Distortion of the Film

For diagnosis and treatment the film must not be bent and the image must not be distorted. Special film holders, including the Endo Ray, Easy Grip IIE, and the Snap-a-Ray (see Fig. 9-11), all aid in positioning the film and in preventing movement or bending of the film. When the rubber dam is in place, a hemostat is used and the patient is asked to hold the film in place. Care must be taken when the hemostat is placed on the film (Fig. 33-18) to avoid the interference of the beaks in the film.

▶ Position the Film

The film must be positioned to provide a clear and complete view of the apex of the tooth. In Fig. 33-19, *A*, the film was improperly positioned and the apices of the teeth are not visible. Correct positioning ensures that the complete apical region is visible and is near the center of the film, while all of the occlusal surfaces and the surrounding alveolar tissues are completely visible.

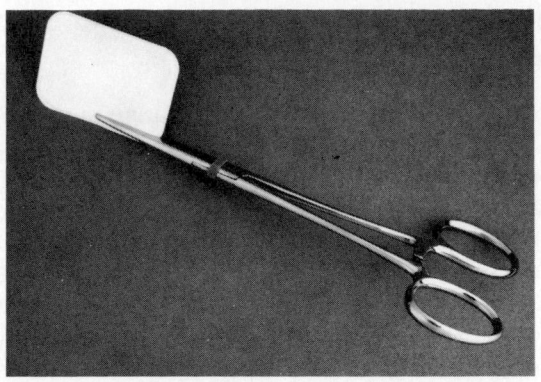

FIG. 33-18   Hemostat aids in film placement and in cone alignment.

(From Cohen S, Burns RC: *Pathways of the pulp*, ed 6, St Louis, 1994, Mosby.)

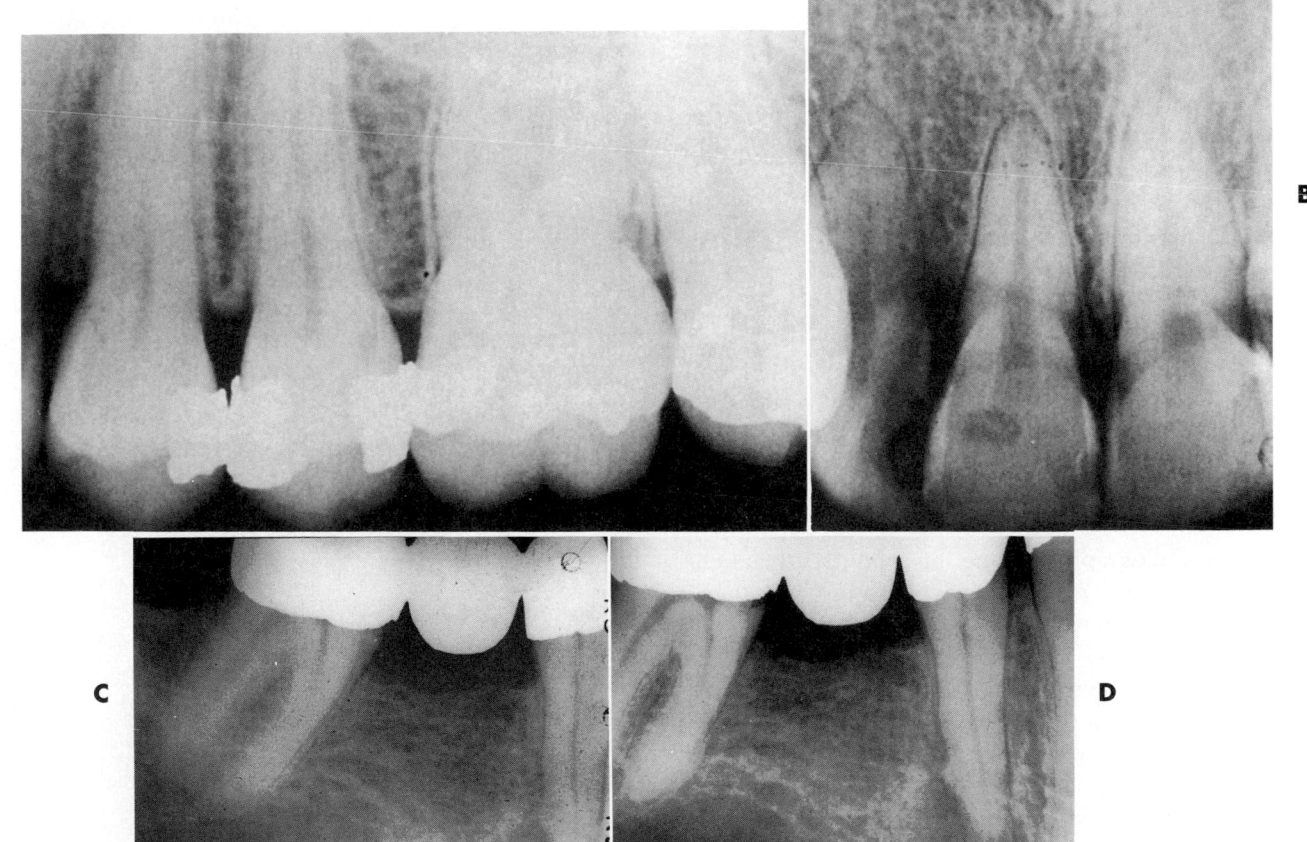

FIG. 33-19   *A*, Elongated and distorted radiograph, caused by poor PID placement. *B*, Foreshortened image. *C*, Improperly exposed or poorly processed radiographs such as this will make diagnoses difficult. *D*, Crown, roots, and surrounding tissues of teeth can only be seen with properly prepared radiographs.

(*A* and *B* from Frommer HH: *Radiology for dental auxiliaries*, ed 5, St Louis, 1992, Mosby. *C* and *D* from Cohen S, Burns RC: *Pathways of the pulp*, ed 6, St Louis, 1994, Mosby.)

◗ Eliminate Elongation and Foreshortening

The importance of obtaining an accurate image of the tooth cannot be overemphasized. Bent films can cause distortion; likewise, improper cone placement can create elongation (previously shown) or foreshortening (Fig. 33-19, *B*). Such errors can give a misleading length for the dentist during biomechanical preparation. It is suggested that the paralleling technique be used to avoid distortion and to provide greater clarity in the film. If the patient has a low palatal vault or tori or is uncooperative, alternative methods may need to be considered. Whichever film technique is used during endodontic radiography, it should be repeated at subsequent appointments to ensure the same anatomic reproduction. Film processing, like film exposure, is important to endodontics. Improperly processed film can make a diagnosis difficult (Fig. 33-19, *C* and *D*).

◗ Working Radiographs

Radiographic films will need to be exposed during various stages of treatment. Commonly, radiographs can be used during treatment to:
1. Determine the shape, number, location, and direction of the root canals
2. Determine the length of the canal before biomechanical preparation
3. Verify working or trial length of files during biomechanical preparation
4. Verify malpositioned or broken files
5. Confirm location of master cone
6. Examine final root canal filling
7. Observe and evaluate surgical treatment site
8. Evaluate tissue changes at recall appointment

◗ Processing the Film

Processing radiographs during endodontic treatment needs to be done more quickly than do traditional developing procedures. Typically, it takes 10 to 20 minutes to process a radiograph, even in an automatic processor. During actual root canal therapy and endodontic surgical procedures this time is prohibitive. Having a radiograph processed in less than a minute is often necessary in endodontics. The processing time can be decreased by increasing the strength of the developer and fixer, and in some instances the temperature of the solutions must be accelerated. Success can be attained by immersing the film in the developer for about 5 to 10 seconds, rinsing, and then placing the film in the fixer for about 15 to 20 seconds, until the film is clear.

Traditional developing tanks do not meet these criteria, so those dentists who practice endodontics exten-sively or the endodontist may create their own version of such a developing tank or they may purchase a commercial tank, such as the Chairside Darkroom.

Sterilization

Sterilization of endodontic instruments is not significantly different from other dental instruments. However, two factors can pose potential complications to successful treatment. The first is the evidence of stress, fatigue, or damage to the fine delicate intracanal instruments. Small instruments, such as #8, #10, or #15, are disposable and are discarded after only one use. These fine instruments can seldom withstand the stress of high-heat sterilization, and to risk reuse presents the potential for instrument fracture within the canal. Although larger instruments can be reused for one or more cases after sterilization, they lose their cutting efficiency with reuse. Each instrument must be examined at the time of sterilization and again before it is inserted into a canal to ensure a sound instrument that is free of stress or damage.

Steam and dry heat sterilization may be used for sterilization of endodontic instruments, according to manufacturers' recommendations. If steam is used, the instruments must be protected with a protective emulsion to avoid damage to the instrument. However, some dentists prefer to avoid the emulsion and to use dry heat. This method, however, poses potential damage to delicate instruments that is caused by the high heat over a longer period of time.

At chairside, a small, rapid method of sterilization is often needed, which can be accomplished by using a salt sterilizer (Fig. 33-20). A file may need to be curved with

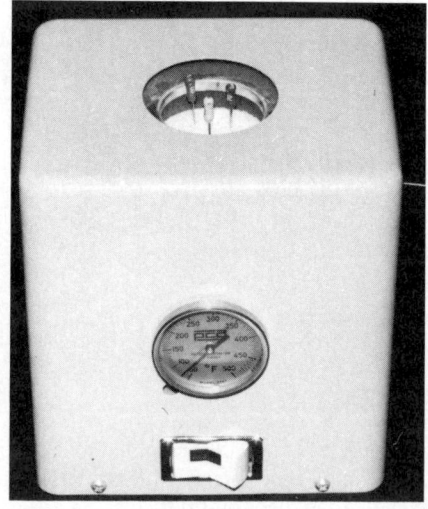

FIG. 33-20 High temperature endodontic sterilizer.

(From Cohen S, Burns RC: *Pathways of the pulp*, ed 6, St Louis, 1994, Mosby.)

the gloved fingers or with a nonsterile forceps. Before the file is inserted into the canal, the instrument is submerged into the salt sterilizer for 5 to 10 seconds at 450° F to sterilize it.

Specialized Endodontic Instruments

A plethora of specialized instruments are used in the practice of endodontics, and for the most part they are dissimilar from other operative instruments. Since many of these instruments are used within the canal, common instruments, such as spoon excavators and explorers, frequently have longer shanks, or the instruments may be smaller devices, such as intracanal files and reamers. Table 33-2 describes and illustrates instruments that are common to most endodontic procedures. Endodontic instruments can be divided into several basic categories: examination, intracanal, cleansing, medicating, obturation, and rotary instruments.

Examination and preparation instruments include the longer shank explorer and the spoon excavator, which enable the operator to gain access to the pulp chamber and to identify the location of the canals more easily. The endodontic locking forceps enable materials such as small cotton pellets and paper points to be put into and taken out of the tooth without the fear of dropping the items.

Before the actual canal can be filed or prepared, access must be gained to the canals. Several types of rotary instruments can be used to widen or to open the canals. These instruments can be easily attached to an angle on the slow-speed handpiece and come in an assortment of sizes. Typically, the occlusal or lingual of the tooth is opened with a high-speed handpiece, using a #34 or #2 bur. After this, a Gates Glidden drill, an orifice bur, or a Peeso reamer can aid in widening the coronal opening of the root canal, removing curvatures of the orifice or preparing the tooth for a post.

Intracanal instruments include the small endodontic file, the reamer, the broach, the canal finder, and the apex locators. Although several of these are available in rotary form, most are used as manual instruments that are held in the fingers to remove pulpal tissue from the canals. Files are the most common form of instruments that are used during the preparation of the canal and are available as K-style files and Hedstrom files. Through research the ADA has established specific standards for the manufacture of endodontic files. ADA specifications #28 and #58 identify the sizing, fracture resistance, stiffness, and corrosion resistance of files. From these specifications have come the standardized measurements and handle colors of intracanal instruments. The importance of this standard for the assistant is the ease of identification of files by size and color. Table 33-3 lists the common files and sizes.

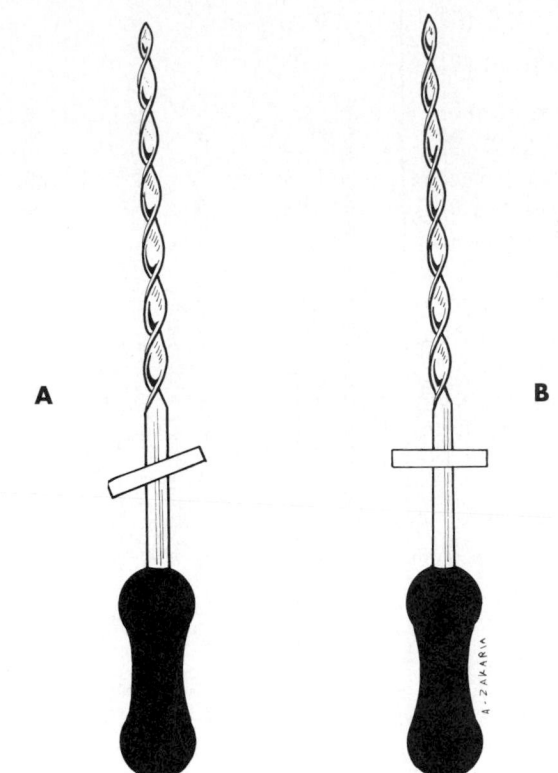

FIG. 33-21   *A,* Incorrect placement of stop. *B,* Correct placement of stop.

(From Bence R: *Handbook of clinical endodontics,* ed 2, St Louis, 1980, Mosby.)

During the biomechanical preparation of the canal a *stop* is placed on the file to indicate its working length. Small silicone rubber stops are available for such use and are placed on the file perpendicular to the handle (Fig. 33-21) for accurate measurement. To aid in accurate placement of the stops, several items can help: a ruler, a stop gauge, or an automatic stop dispenser gauge, which places the stop on the file automatically. A holding device for files must be at chairside during the biomechanical preparation. Some operators may choose to use a finger-holding device, while others opt for a small endodontic instrument stand, which will hold a dozen or more small finger instruments.

▶ Cleansing Instruments

During biomechanical cleansing of the canal an irrigating syringe with a large gauge needle must be used to flush the canal with sodium hypochlorite and absorbent paper points to dry the canal. Paper points are supplied in various sizes, from extra fine to extra coarse. The use of two locking pliers makes it easy to transfer the points to

TABLE 33-2 COMMON ENDODONTIC INSTRUMENTS

Instrument/device	Purpose	Distinguishing characteristics
GATES GLIDDEN DRILL	▶ Facilitates preparation of the canal ▶ Aids in opening access to canal ▶ Removes curvature of the orifice ▶ Prepares tooth for a post	▶ Long-shanked rotary device ▶ Elliptically shaped with cutting end resembling a football ▶ Used with latch-type, slow-speed handpiece ▶ Rotates in clockwise direction ▶ Available in six sizes ▶ #1 Size = to #50 K-style file ▶ Scribed mark on side of shank indicates size, single indentation = #1, double = #2 and so forth ▶ Designed as a safe tip instrument, requiring a prior hole be made for this instrument to be used
PEESO REAMER	▶ Widens coronal access quickly ▶ Opens the orifice ▶ Aids in removing curvatures of the orifice ▶ Used in canal in conjunction with enlarging instruments ▶ Used intermittently with moderate rotation	▶ Long shanked rotary instrument with sharp parallel flutes ▶ Tungsten carbide ▶ Available in six sizes ▶ #1 Size = to a #70 K-style file ▶ Scribed mark on side of shank indicates size, single indentation = #1, double = #2 and so forth
ORIFICE BUR	▶ Used to roughly enlarge root canal after instrumentation is complete ▶ Excavation of root caries ▶ Opens orifice or difficult bicuspid and molar root canal ▶ Opens tooth to drain canal	▶ Flame-shaped rotary device resembling Gates Glidden ▶ Used on latch-type contraangle ▶ Available in only one or two sizes, commonly 1.6 diameter
ENDODONTIC EXPLORER	▶ Probes the chamber and canals ▶ Identifies location of canals	▶ Long-shanked ▶ Generally doubled ended ▶ Common #s are 2, 16, 17 (right angle at one end), and shepherd's hook
ENDODONTIC SPOON	▶ Aids in removing debris and other materials from chamber ▶ Aids in placing temporary in canal	▶ Long shank ▶ Spoon-like shape ▶ Generally double ended
ENDODONTIC PLIERS	▶ Grasp instruments and points for transport to canals ▶ Locking style permits transport without loss of material	▶ Central groove along axis ▶ Available in locking or nonlocking ▶ Commonly about 6 inches long ▶ Many styles available
PLASTIC INSTRUMENT	▶ Used to place and pack temporary filling material into chamber area	▶ Common styles include nib, paddle, ball or condenser-like working end

Continued.

K-STYLE FILE

- Scrape against side of canal wall
- Remove necrotic tissue until clean dentin is reached
- Widen the preparation

- Varying sizes from 8 to 140
- Number of size on handle
- Greater number and more angular flutes than a reamer

HEDSTROM FILE

- Quickly plane walls of canal
- Useful on canals with irregular walls
- Aids in removing instruments

- Varying sizes from 10 to 140
- Number of size on handle
- Flutes are ground to form successively larger cones
- Resembles a pine tree shape
- Sharp blades
- Cuts more aggressively than a K-style file or reamer
- Must never be rotated in the canal, or will bind in the dentin

REAMER

- Used in a reaming or revolving action in canal
- May be used to remove old gutta percha fillings
- Aids in placing paste fillers near apex
- Not as frequently used as files

- Varying sizes from 6 to 140
- Number of size on handle
- Less flutes than a file

BARBED BROACH

- Remove soft tissue from canal
- Remove intracanal dressings

- Sizing from coarse, medium, fine to xxxx fine
- Notched to form sharp barbs on instrument
- Never rotate a broach in a canal
- Not recommended for use until the canal can accommodate a #35 file

Gates Glidden drill

K-style file

Hedstrom file

Reamer

Barbed broach

Continued.

TABLE 33-2 COMMON ENDODONTIC INSTRUMENTS—cont'd.

Instrument/device	Purpose	Distinguishing characteristics
LENTULO SPIRAL	▶ Carries and places root canal cement apically in clockwise rotation	▶ Delicate, flexible, strong, spring type ▶ Used on latch-type contra angle ▶ Reverse spiral shape ▶ Available in four to six sizes ▶ Size range 0.25 mm to 0.44 mm, smaller than most K-style files
FINGER PLUGGER	▶ Used with finger pressure for apical condensation of gutta percha	▶ Smooth, tapered with dull-tipped instrument that is shaped like a file with no flutes ▶ Sizes from 15 to 40 consistent with standard file sizes
FINGER SPREADERS	▶ Used with finger pressure for lateral condensation of gutta percha	▶ Smooth, tapered, sharp-pointed instrument, shaped like a file with no flutes ▶ Sizes range from extra fine to medium
ENDODONTIC SPREADER	▶ Used manually for lateral condensation of gutta percha	▶ Long shank with pointed tips ▶ Available in sizes equivalent to #25 to #40 K-style file ▶ Single ended
ENDODONTIC PLUGGER	▶ Vertical condensation of gutta percha	▶ Long shank with dull tip ▶ Single or double ended ▶ Size ranges equal to #25 to #85 K-type file
ROOT CANAL PLIERS	▶ Used to retrieve points, file, or other materials from canal ▶ Transport and grasp materials for canals	▶ Grooved and serrated ▶ May resemble hemostat or plier handle
ENDODONTIC UTILITY SCISSORS	▶ Used to cut gutta percha and paper points	▶ Typical scissor style ▶ Delicate sharp beaks
RETRO MIRROR	▶ Used to observe retrograde filling at apex of tooth	▶ Small face ▶ Angled shank to aid access
RETRO FILLING AMALGAM PLUGGERS	▶ Aid in placement of apical amalgam	▶ Resembles back action amalgam condenser ▶ One end multiple angled and opposite and commonly at right angle ▶ Small diameter of tip
RETRO AMALGAM CARRIER	▶ Transport small amount of amalgam to small retro fill preparations	▶ Carrier and diameter small: 3/64 inch to 5/64 inch ▶ Delicate tip end ▶ Resembles thumb forceps
MICRO-CONTRAANGLE	▶ Used for retrograde amalgam preparation	▶ Small head ▶ Adjustable head
ENDO-HEAD CONTRAANGLE	▶ Aid in using specialized rotary devices	▶ Generally latch type ▶ Oscillating, quarter turn movement ▶ Operates at speeds up to 3000 rpm ▶ Reduction style contra angles rotate at speeds between 500 and 1000 rpm ▶ Maintain high torque at low speeds

ENDODONTIC AMALGAM GUN

- To place apical amalgam

- Resembles anesthetic syringe
- Nozzles available, straight or angled
- Diameter of nozzle tips 1 mm to 1.5 mm

GUTTA PERCHA POINTS

- Used to obturate the canal

- Thermoplastic
- Compressible to adapt to shape of canal
- Radiopaque
- Dense, stiff, and unbreakable
- Soluble in chloroform
- Dimensionally stable when hardened
- Sizes correspond to K-file from #15 to #140

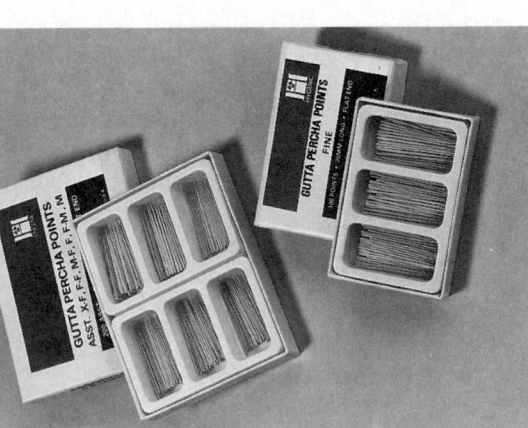

SILVER POINTS

- Used for obturation of canals
- Not frequently used today

- Rigid silver point
- Made of bactericidal silver
- Matched to sizes of standard K-style file #8 to #140
- Retains shape
- May be configured to fit curved canal

ABSORBENT PAPER POINTS

- Used to dry canals
- Introduce medication and sealers
- Culture canals

- Absorbent
- Made of high-quality bibulous paper
- Sterilized and nonsterilized available
- Can be sterilized
- Sizes correspond to K-style file from #15 to #140

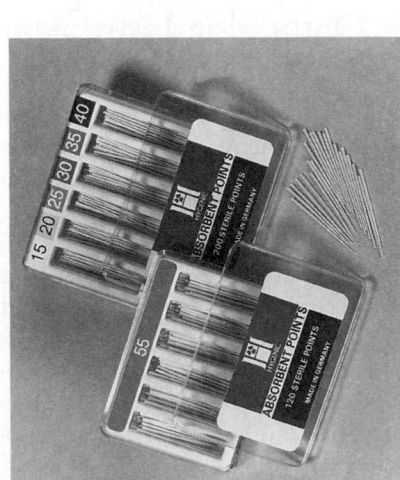

TABLE 33-3 STANDARDIZED SIZE AND HANDLE COLORS OF INTRACANAL INSTRUMENTS

Size	Handle color code
08	Gray
10	Purple
15	White
20	Yellow
25	Red
30	Blue
35	Green
40	Black
45	White
50	Yellow
55	Red
60	Blue
70	Green
80	Black
90	White
100	Yellow
110	Red
120	Blue
130	Green
140	Black

the operator because many points are used during each appointment to adequately dry the canal.

Medicating Instruments

When medications are used, they are typically applied to a cotton pellet, which is placed into the pulp chamber, followed by a temporary restoration that includes gutta percha, Cavit (trademark), or a ZOE cement. The pellet is inserted with a sterile cotton forceps; to place the interim dressing, a plastic instrument is used.

Obturation Instruments

A great variety of obturation instruments are available, and the choice of these instruments is the dentist's. The standard gutta percha points used for master cones are supplied in sizes coordinating with the file sizes as described earlier. These master cones are disinfected before insertion in a small liquid sterilizer at chairside. Root canal sealer is used to secure the master cone and accessory cones; this may be pumped into the canal manually with a small file or carried to the canal with a rotary instrument, such as the lentulo spiral. Endodontic pluggers are used for vertical condensation of gutta percha, and spreaders are used to aid in lateral condensation.

Surgical Instruments

When a surgical process such as an apicoectomy is done, it may include placing an amalgam restoration at the apex of the tooth. Small angled instruments are needed to perform this procedure. These instruments include a micro contra angle, a retro filling amalgam carrier, a retro filling amalgam plugger, and a Messing root canal gun with a delicate angled tip. A retro mirror that has a small 4 to 8 mm face with a specially angled shank will improve visibility.

Miscellaneous Instruments

Several instruments are used in all phases of the treatment. These include an instrument tray or organizer in which instruments are stored and sterilized. These trays (Fig. 33-22, *A* through *D*) provide space for most intracanal instruments to be stored in sequence of use. Files that are to be used can be removed with a sterile forceps and placed on a sterile towel or holding device for easy transfer to the dentist. Contaminated instruments are not returned to this tray, but are placed on another sterile towel or holding device.

A special endo-head contra angle is available for all of the rotary instruments just described. This specialized contra angle has an oscillating, quarter-turn movement and operates at speeds up to 3000 rpm, thus providing a safety factor for intracanal use. A reduction style contra angle is also available, which operates at an even lower speed of only 500 to 1000 rpm.

Intracanal Medications or Solutions

Substances used in pulp canal therapy can be categorized into irrigants, dentin softeners, lubricants, and medicaments. Each of these has a specific purpose but not all substances are used in every case. Typically, the irrigants and medications are used more routinely, but special situations may require the use of either of the other substances.

Irrigation Solution

An irrigating solution is used primarily as a biomechanical cleaning agent to flush the canal free of debris. This solution should be nontoxic, allow the instruments to slide freely into the canal, act as a disinfectant, be a tissue solvent when possible, and be relatively inexpensive. Sodium hypochlorite (NaOCl), or household bleach, is the most common biomechanical cleaner. At one time hydrogen peroxide was used because its effervescent quality was thought to be beneficial in debriding the canal. This has not proved true, and sodium hypochlorite continues to be the more widely used solution.

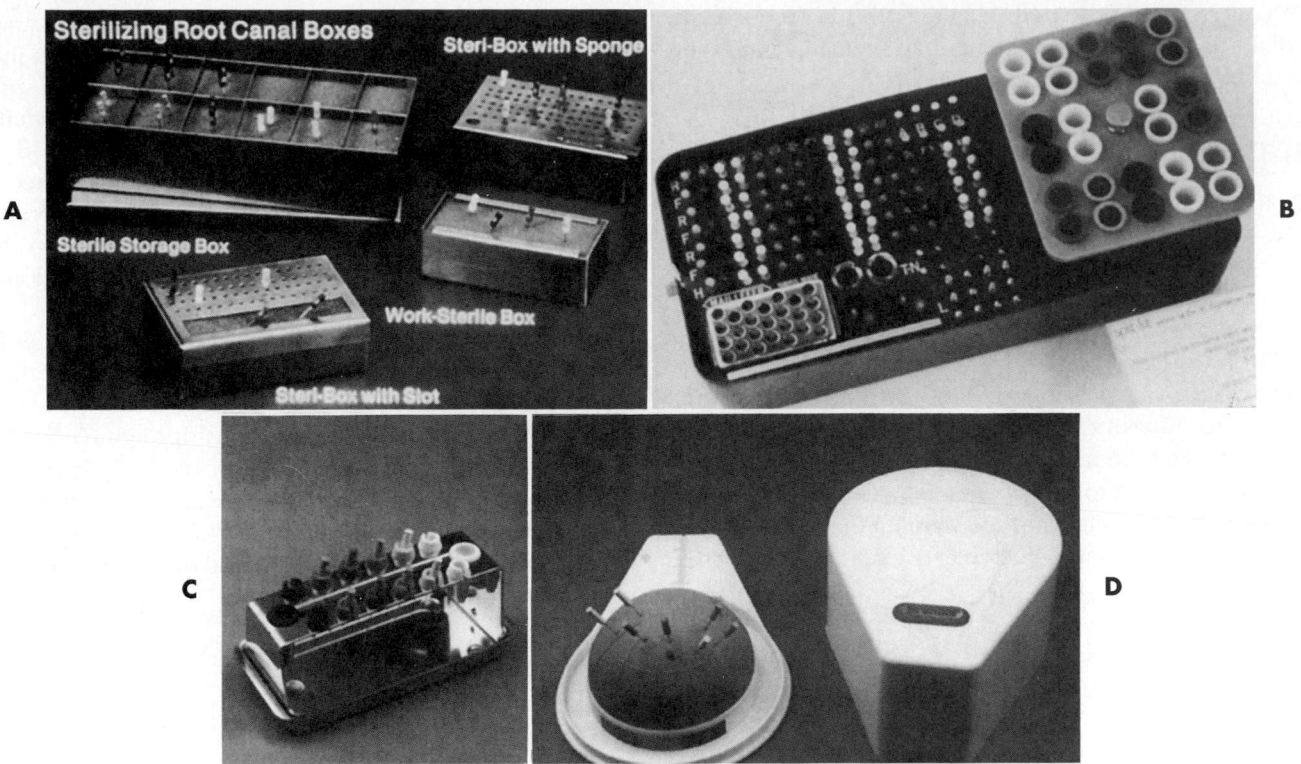

FIG. 33-22 File storage, sterilization, and delivery. *A,* Sterilizing boxes. *B,* Split kit. *C,* File stand. *D,* File sponge.

(From Cohen S, Burns RC: *Pathways of the pulp,* ed 5, St Louis, 1991, Mosby.)

▶ Dentin Softeners

The primary function of a dentin softener is to remove mineral deposits, such as calcium, from the dentin. These products known as chelators remove metallic ions, such as calcium and decalcifiers, which are chemicals that remove mineral salts in solution. Two common chelators are EDTA (ethylenediaminetetraacetic acid) and dilute citric acid. The ability to increase the removal of tissue does not appear significantly greater than the use of a file to cut away the tissue and debris. The application of these substances may be more significant in canals with restrictions, which a file is unable to navigate.

▶ Lubricants

These substances aid the dentist in gaining access to the full length of the canal during filing. A lubricant can also aid in negotiating small constricted canals. These substances do not dissolve tissue, thus they are not an aid when a file comes to a stop in the canal. Glycerin is a sterile, inexpensive, and nontoxic substance that works effectively as a lubricant. It is water soluble and can be removed from the canal easily after its use.

▶ Canal Medication

Over the years the use of and reasons for intracanal medication have undergone change. At one time success of the root canal was thought to be based on the medication that was used during the interim appointments. Later, it appeared that some of the medications that were used might even be toxic, rather than therapeutic. Today, greater emphasis is placed on the mechanical preparation of the root canal rather than on the use of medicaments. The few medications that are used today are considered significant in providing comfort and preventing pain after biomechanical preparation, providing antimicrobial action in the pulp and periapical tissues, and neutralizing the canal remnants to make them inert.

Three medications appear to be used currently in endodontics. They are formocresol (FC), camphorated monochlorophenol (CMCP), and calcium hydroxide (CaOH), with the first, FC, being the most widely used.

The typical method for application of the medicaments is the use of a small cotton pellet, the size of the access opening, that is saturated in the substance. The pellet is tapped dry on a sterile gauze and then placed into the coronal portion of the pulp chamber; this is then sealed in place with a temporary cement and remains until the next appointment within 3 to 10 days.

Pulpotomy

When trauma occurs to the pulp of a tooth in a young child—either by accident or because of extensive dental caries—it is likely that the apical constriction is not complete and that the root may have an open apex. Two treatment alternatives are available to the dentist: apexification or apexogenesis.

Apexification, chosen for a tooth with necrotic pulp, is the procedure of creating an environment within the root canal and periapical tissues to allow a calcified barrier to form across the open apex. Typically, this procedure involves cleaning and shaping the root canal to remove toxic agents and bacteria, drying the canal with absorbent paper points that are inserted into the canal, and placing a radiopaque calcium hydroxide paste into the canal. The access opening is closed with a zinc oxide–eugenol cement followed by a permanent cement. The patient is recalled at a later date, and the tooth is examined clinically and radiographically. If evidence is apparent of a calcified stop at the apex, routine root canal therapy can be completed, and the canal can be obturated to this new apical stop. If the stop has not develop, apexification may be reattempted.

Apexogenesis is the treatment of a vital pulp by a **pulp capping** or **pulpotomy** (removal of the coronal portion of the pulp) to permit continued closure of the open apex and growth of the root (Fig. 33-23, *A* through *E*). This is the procedure of choice when possible. A formocresol pulpotomy is a surgical procedure that is commonly performed on the pulpal tissues of young children. This process not only removes the coronal portion of the pulp

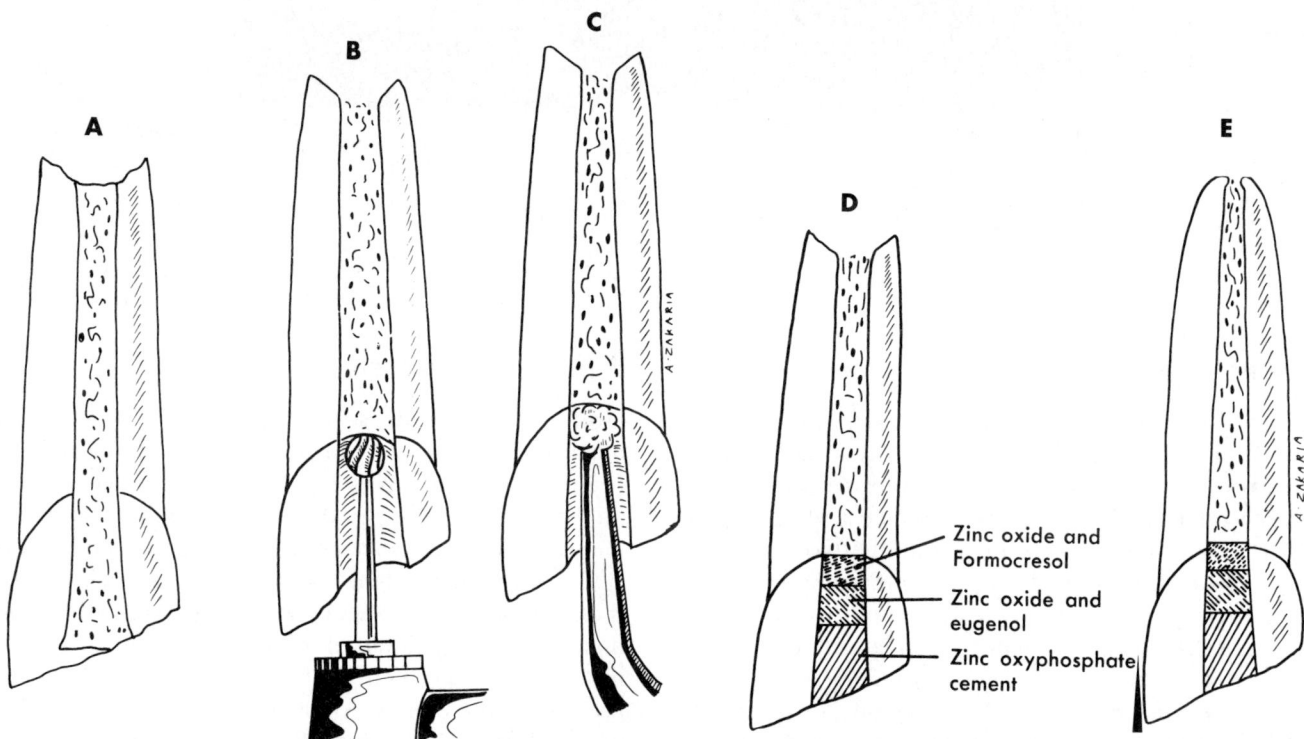

FIG. 33-23   Traumatic pulp exposure in a tooth, with incomplete root formation. *A,* Not an indication for a pulpectomy because of the wide apical opening; it would be impossible to condense a filling material into the canal that would seal the apex. *B,* A formocresol pulpotomy is performed by removing the injured pulp tissue with a sterile round bur. *C,* Placing a pellet moistened with formocresol over the pulp stump for 3 minutes. *D,* A paste of zinc oxide and formocresol is placed over the mummified tissue, and the opening is sealed with zinc oxide and eugenol, followed by zinc phosphate cement. *E,* The pulp in the apical portion of the root canal is not disturbed, and root development will continue. When the apical portion of the root develops, the remaining pulp tissue is removed and the canal is debrided and filled as described in a pulpectomy procedure.

(From Bence R: *Handbook of clinical endodontics,* ed 2, St Louis, 1980, Mosby.)

PULPOTOMY (FIG. 33-23)

1. The tooth is anesthetized, and the segment is isolated with a rubber dam.
2. The tooth is opened with a #34 bur on a high-speed handpiece, and the basic outline form is completed with a #57 bur. The cavity walls are extended to provide adequate access to the pulp chamber. The burs may need to be modified, depending on the amount of tooth structure previously lost to decay or on the specific tooth involved.
3. A #4 or #6 round bur is used on the slow-speed handpiece to slowly remove the large carious lesion. A large spoon excavator may be used to aid in caries removal.
4. A sterile round bur #4, #6, or #8 is then used in the low speed to remove the remaining dentin and to expose the occlusal portion of the pulp chamber. The occlusal portion of the pulp chamber is extirpated to the level of the pulp canals.
5. With a sterile cotton pellet, pulpal debris is removed. Hemorrhaging is likely to occur, and the cotton pellets aid in controlling the bleeding. Do not use air because this will desiccate the pulpal tissue and contaminate the site.
6. Dip a sterile cotton pellet into formocresol (FC), and pass it to the dentist. The cotton pellet is placed in the pulp chamber for about 5 minutes.
7. At the end of 5 minutes the cotton pellet is removed. The FC will have fixed or mummified the pulpal tissue that remains in the pulp canals. The pulpal stumps will have a dark brown appearance.
8. A ZOE cement is mixed, and a drop of FC is incorporated as part of the liquid. The cement is mixed to a secondary consistency and passed to the dentist with a cement plugger; the mix is placed over the pulpal stumps to a thickness of about 2 to 3 mm.
9. A permanent cement, perhaps a zinc phosphate or a polycarboxalate, could be inserted before the tooth is prepared for the stainless steel crown.
10. The final restoration may be placed at the dentist's discretion. If not, a temporary restoration is placed until it is determined that no postoperative complications exist.
11. The isolation is removed, and the patient is dismissed.
12. The parent or caregiver for the child should be instructed to contact the office immediately if evidence of severe discomfort arises at a later time. Before the patient leaves the office, the dentist provides instruction for pain medication, if necessary, and explain any postoperative complications that might arise.

chamber but mummifies the occlusal tips of the pulp canals. In the following procedure the tooth involved is a maxillary right central incisor that has been traumatically injured in a bicycle accident. The tooth has no other indication of pathology, tooth mobility, or sensitivity to percussion, and no evidence of radiolucency exists in the radiographs. It appears that the tooth is not undergoing any pulpal degeneration and thus is a good candidate for a pulpotomy.

Following the pulpotomy a restoration is placed on the tooth, and in this case, since it is an anterior tooth, a polycarbonate crown is likely to be the restoration of choice. This procedure is described in Chapter 32, *Temporary Restorations*. As long as the tooth remains asymptomatic following this procedure, the treatment should provide for the retention of the tooth until the apex is closed and additional endodontic treatment is done when the patient is older.

▶ Armamentarium

Explorer
Mirror
Cotton pliers
Spoon excavator
Rubber dam set-up
Sterile cotton pellets
Burs
  Opening #34, #57, or other choice
  Removing dentin and coronal pulp #4 or #6, sterile
Formocresol (FC)
Zinc oxide–eugenol cement (ZOE)
Permanent cement
Temporary crown set-up

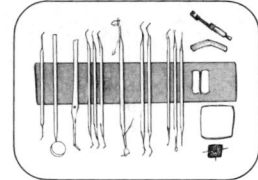

Pulpectomy

A **pulpectomy**, commonly called a root canal by most patients, is the complete removal of the pulp tissue from the pulp chamber to the dentinocemental junction at the apex of the root. This procedure can be done in a single appointment but commonly is done in a sequence of two or three appointments (see Box 33-2 for the basic steps of the multiple appointment procedure).

▶ Single Visit Versus Multiple Visits

Two approaches to appointment scheduling exist when performing a pulpectomy for a patient. In the single appointment approach the tooth is opened; canals are identified, debrided, and shaped; and the canal is obturated or filled. Advantages to this approach include the following:

1. Eliminates multiple patient appointments, while maintaining success of treatment

BOX 33-2

TYPICAL APPOINTMENT SEQUENCE FOR A PULPOTOMY

INITIAL APPOINTMENT FOR PULPECTOMY

1. Anesthetize tooth if necessary
2. Place rubber dam isolation
3. Disinfect treatment field
4. Make occlusal opening for access
5. Locate the root canals
6. Determine tooth length, and set rubber stops for reference points
7. Determine working length
8. Complete biomechanical preparation of the canals
9. Take trial point radiograph
10. Flush canals with sodium hypochlorite
11. Dry canals with sterile paper points
12. Place intracanal medication
13. Place interim dressing in the occlusal opening, and adjust occlusion
14. Remove rubber dam

INTERIM APPOINTMENT FOR PULPECTOMY

1. Anesthetize tooth if necessary
2. Place rubber dam isolation
3. Disinfect treatment field
4. Remove the interim dressing
5. Check for dryness of canals by placing a dry absorbent point in each canal
6. Irrigate canals with sodium hypochlorite
7. Complete the biomechanical preparation
8. Verify the length of the canal with a radiograph of the final size file in place

9. Flush the canal with sodium hypochlorite
10. Dry the canal with absorbent paper points
11. Place intracanal medication
12. Place interim dressing and adjust occlusion
13. Remove rubber dam

The dentist may need to provide the patient with a prescription for an antibiotic or analgesic at this appointment or at the first appointment depending on the inflammatory state or amount of discomfort the patient is experiencing.

OBTURATION (FINAL) APPOINTMENT FOR PULPECTOMY

1. Anesthetize tooth if necessary
2. Place rubber dam isolation
3. Disinfect treatment field
4. Remove the interim dressing
5. Check for dryness of canals by placing a dry absorbent point in each canal
6. Irrigate canals with sodium hypochlorite
7. Place the final file to length to verify the canal length
8. Dry the canal with sterile absorbent points
9. Select the master cone, and adjust to final length
10. Take a trial point radiograph with the master cone in place
11. Obturate the root canals
12. Expose a final radiograph
13. Place final or temporary restoration
14. Remove rubber dam

2. Eliminates interappointment contamination and potential flareup because of loss of the temporary seal in severely broken down teeth
3. Eliminates the need for the dentist to become familiar with the anatomic structure of the canal at subsequent visits
4. In fractured teeth the completed canal can be used immediately for retention of a post to construct a temporary restoration, which is a distinct advantage in anterior teeth where the crown has been fractured at the gingival margin and an esthetic temporary restoration is needed for the patient

Of course, several situations in which the one patient visit would be contraindicated include the following:

1. Presence of periapical symptoms, which might include edema, periapical tenderness, or the presence of exudate in the oral cavity
2. Anatomic structure, which makes the identification of the pulp canals difficult, including receded pulp chambers, calcified canals, or severely curved or bifurcated canals

3. Multirooted teeth; although this situation can be treated in one visit, many dentists believe that it is too difficult and time consuming to complete such a procedure in one visit

When the multivisit approach is used, the patient may be seen for two or three appointments. The first appointment involves opening the occlusal access, locating the canals, and if time permits biomechanical preparation of the canals is begun. At the end of the appointment an interim dressing is placed and the patient dismissed. At the second appointment the temporary is removed, the final biomechanical preparation is completed, and a trial point radiograph is taken to determine if the canal has been filed to the apical stop. Again, the patient is sent home with an interim dressing. At the final appointment the canal(s) is obturated or sealed and a final radiograph is taken. Subsequent recall appointments are necessary to follow up the healing process of the periapical tissues and to examine the tooth for color and mobility.

The controversy continues about which approach to

take for a pulpectomy treatment. In general, it should be realized that in skilled hands on single-rooted, asymptomatic teeth, the single visit appointment can be an effective, cost-saving approach to treatment. However, many dentists opt to use the multiple visit sequence for various reasons.

▶ Stages of Treatment

Regardless of the appointment concept that is used, basic stages of treatment must be followed to complete a pulpectomy. These stages include the opening, biomechanical preparation, biomechanical cleansing, trial point, and final cone radiographs, canal medication, temporization, and obturation (Fig. 33-24, *A* through *R*). Only the medication is bypassed if the single appointment is used. Although it is possible to place a final restoration on the day of obturation, it is likely that a temporary may still be placed.

OPENING

Before the tooth is opened, it is anesthetized and isolated with a rubber dam. The treatment field is disinfected with a cotton applicator or cotton pellet that is placed in a forceps and dipped in a disinfectant; this can be done by the assistant alone or as a four-handed procedure. As in an amalgam preparation an occlusal opening is made for access to the canals; this may be done with a #34 or #2 bur in the high-speed handpiece. The assistant will use the HVE to evacuate fluid and debris from the treatment site as it accumulates on the rubber dam. The assistant should keep the HVE tip near the tooth because it is possible for exudate to extrude from the canal. If the exudate has been under pressure and an opening appears in the occlusal, the exudate may exit with some force. With the HVE nearby the exudate can be picked up rapidly, reducing odors. The dentist may exchange the #34 bur for a #57 or another bur to complete an outline form of the access opening.

At this point the dentist removes any carious material, debris, or necrotic material that is in the pulp chamber before proceeding with the canal preparation. To do this, a low-speed handpiece with a #2 bur may be used. The use of a spoon excavator may aid in manual debridement of the chamber.

Once the opening is made in the tooth and the chamber area is completely clean, the dentist will use an endodontic explorer to locate the root canals. **DO NOT** blow air or water spray into the tooth after the pulp chamber is opened. The dentist may wish to irrigate the site with NaOCl at this point. If so, the syringe is passed, and the assistant places the HVE tip close to the opening to remove excess NaOCl.

BIOMECHANICAL PREPARATION

The primary objective of this stage of endodontic treatment is to remove all debris from the pulp chamber and root canals and to shape the canals to receive a filling material.

Working Length Radiograph

Once the opening has been made and the dentist is able to place a file into the canal, the working length of the canal must be determined. To do this, a small file, generally a #10 or a #15 is passed to the dentist and the file is placed into the canal to determine the length. A radiograph is taken with the file in place. A hemostat or film holder is used to position the film. The patient is instructed to hold the handle of the hemostat to secure the film in place. A knowledge of accurate tooth length is an important part of this treatment. Tooth length is determined when the file reaches the apical constriction which is at the dentinocemental junction (Fig. 33-25). The dentist files to this constriction and later places the filling material at this point. If the preparation is filed short of the apical constriction, it is possible to leave infected or necrotic material in the canal that can develop into a site for inflammation. If, on the other hand, the canal is filed and filled beyond the apical constriction, an irritation of the periapical tissues can result in discomfort during treatment and may result in failure of the root canal.

The dentist studies the radiograph, compares it with the original diagnostic radiograph, and confirms the working length of the file; this working length is recorded on the patient's clinical chart. Silicone stops are then placed to this length on all future files to aid the dentist in placing the file. The stops must be perpendicular to the handle (Fig. 33-23). The assistant may need to pass the forceps periodically if the stop position needs to be adjusted.

Filing

Filing is one of the primary tasks in biomechanical preparation of the canals. It is accomplished by using a series of endodontic files in numeric sequence, from the smallest to largest. Since most canals have some form of curvature, the dentist may need to curve the files to prevent gouging or ledging the walls within the canal.

To shape the root canal, the dentist generally begins with a file that is significantly smaller than the diameter of the canal to avoid packing pulpal tissue or debris into the apical portion of the canal. When the canal is being filed the dentist seats the file completely, carefully presses laterally against the wall of the canal, turns the file only a quarter of a turn and then places pressure on the withdrawal of the file. The dentist takes care to work

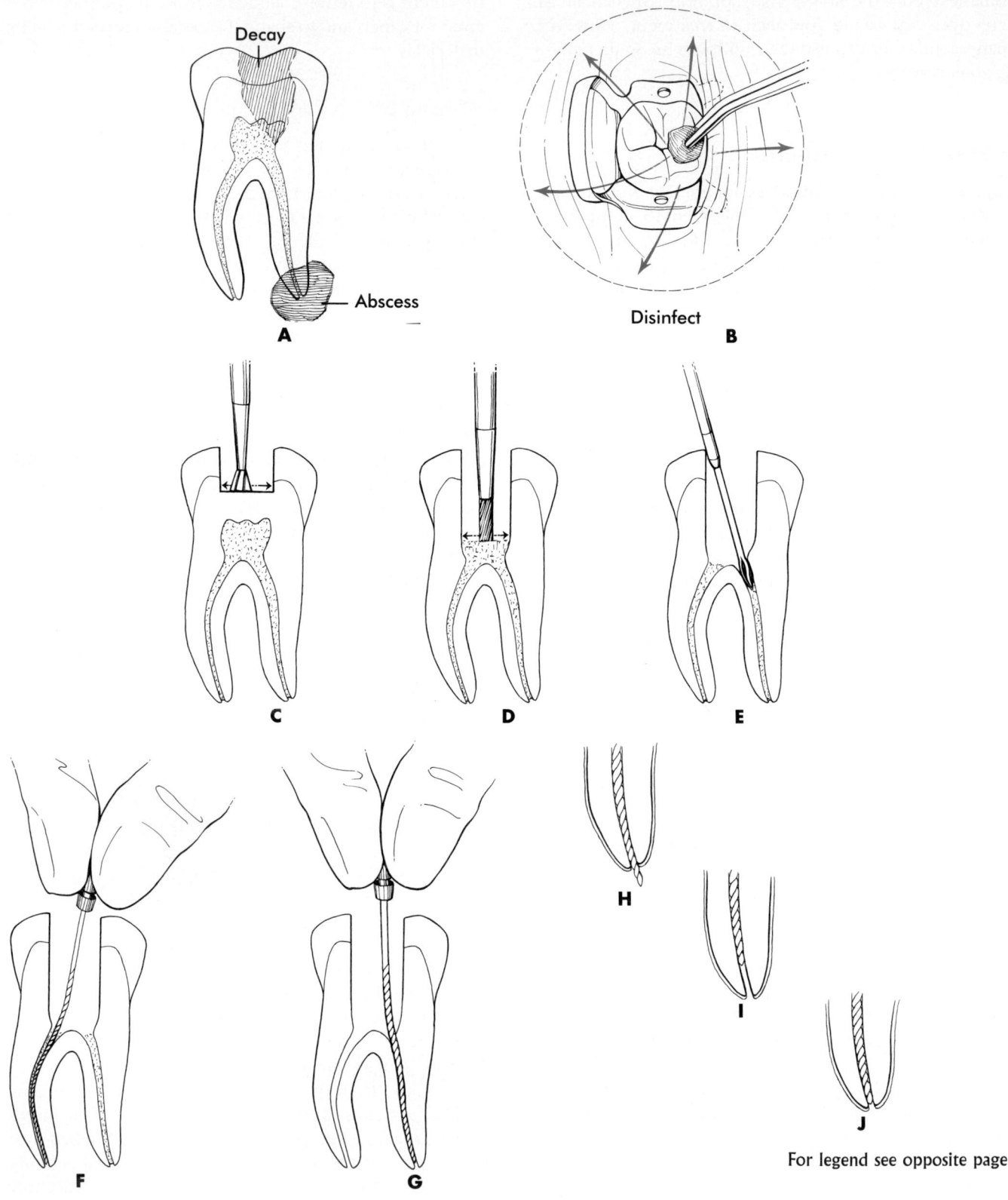

Decay

Abscess

A

Disinfect

B

C

D

E

F

G

H

I

J

For legend see opposite page.

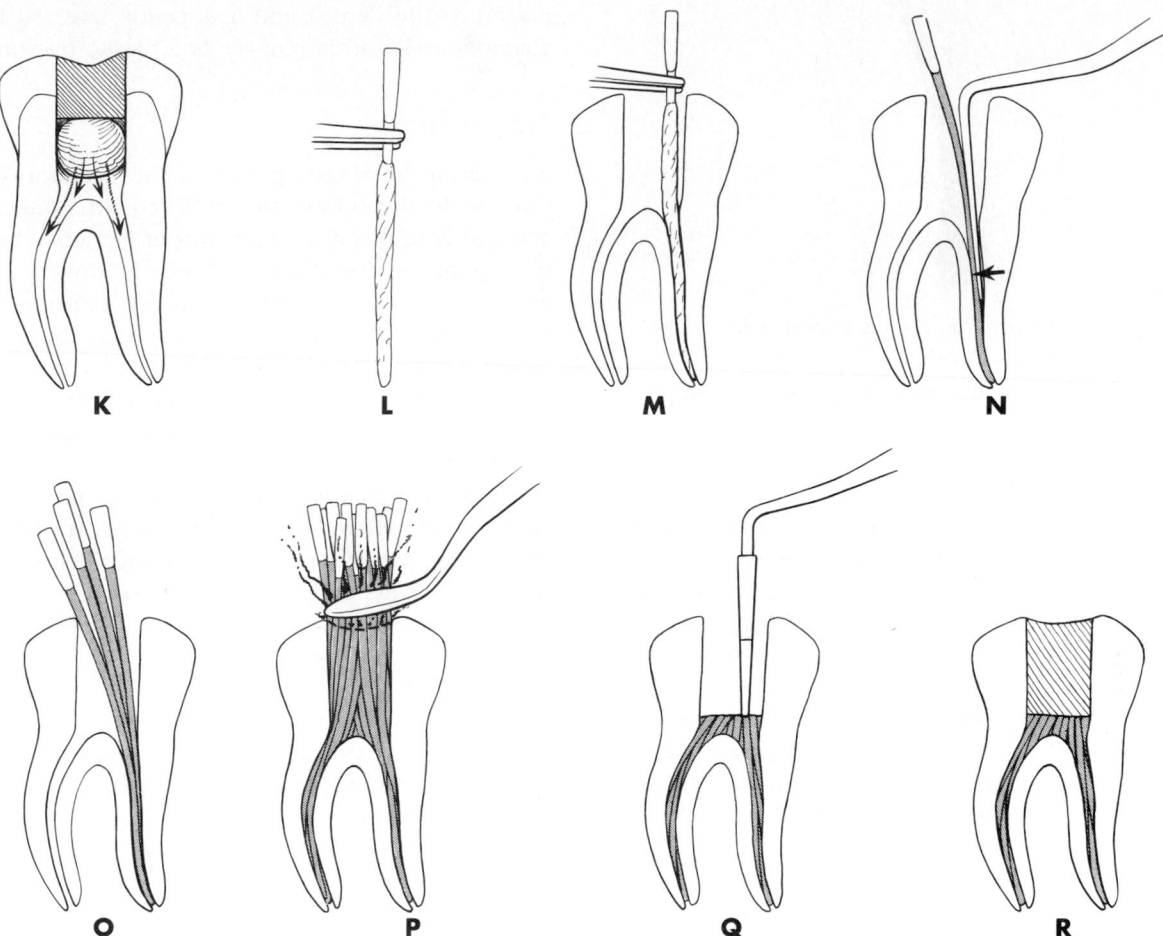

FIG. 33-24   Pulpectomy procedure. *A,* Carious lesion extends into the pulp chamber, with periapical involvement. *B,* Molar is isolated with rubber dam, and site is disinfected. *C,* Access to pulp chamber is accomplished with a round or inverted cone bur on high-speed handpiece. *D,* Enlargement and flaring of preparation are done with a fissure bur. *E,* Peeso reamer is used to gain access to canals. *F,* Intracanal instruments are angled to gain access to canals. *G,* Bio-mechanical preparation continues. During this phase the pulp chamber is flushed with sodium hypochlorite and the canals are shaped and cleaned. *H,* Radiographs are obtained to determine that the length of the files are not too long, *H,* are not too short, *I,* or are approximately 1 mm from the apical opening *J. K,* After the canals are flushed with sodium hypochlorite and dried with paper points, the tooth can be medicated with a cotton pellet that is saturated with formocresol or chlorbutanol, and a small amount of Cavit or ZOE cement can be placed over the pellet. *L,* Obturation will take place at a later appointment, with a gutta percha point that has been coated with a sealer. *M,* The master cone is placed into the canal, and laterally condensed, *N. O,* Auxiliary gutta percha cones are placed into the canal and laterally condensed. *P,* Both canals are filled, and the excess gutta percha is removed with a heated spatula. *Q,* A plastic instrument is used to condense the gutta percha in the coronal portion of the tooth. *R,* Temporary restoration is placed, and the patient is referred to the general dentist for a final restoration.

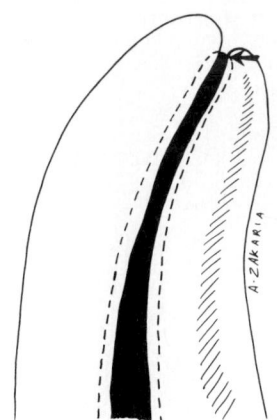

FIG. 33-25   Canal preparation creates a constriction at the dentinocemental junction (*arrow*).

(From Bence R: *Handbook of clinical endodontics*, ed 2, St Louis, 1980, Mosby.)

the file slowly and never screws the file within the canal. As the procedure progresses the dental assistant continues to transfer the files to the dentist in numeric sequence, from smallest to largest, never skipping a file. This process continues until clean white dentinal filings appear on the file.

Files need to be cleaned often and may be wiped on a cotton roll that is saturated with sodium hypochlorite. Used files are returned to the tray or other holder. During the biomechanical preparation procedure the canal must always be kept moist with NaOCl.

Record the final file sizes to which the canal was filed. Other information of importance, such as unfound canals, files that are short of length, or perforations, should be recorded on the patient record.

Biomechanical Cleansing

The canal is flushed with sodium hypochlorite, and the assistant removes any excess with the HVE. When the syringe is passed to the dentist for flushing, be cautious that no solution is on the tip of the needle and that it is not passed over the patient's eyes or clothing.

Pass sterile paper points to the dentist to dry the canal. The size of the points will depend upon the size of the last file that was used. The use of two cotton forceps to pass the paper points expedites this process.

Medication

During the multiple visit appointment approach, most dentists place some type of medication in the canal, as described earlier in this chapter. Either formocresol or chlorobutanol may be placed on a sterile cotton pellet that is appropriate to the size of the occlusal access

opening. The pellet is held in the forceps, and excess medication is removed from the pellet by tapping it on a sterile gauze. Excess medication can be an irritant if it is allowed to permeate the periapical tissues. The pellet is passed to the dentist and it is gently inserted into the chamber area with a plugger or a plastic instrument.

Temporization

An interim dressing is placed in the occlusal opening. Commonly, this is Cavit or a ZOE cement. Some dentists may prefer to place an extra layer of gutta percha before placement of the Cavit. If this is done, a plastic instrument is warmed and a small amount of material is removed from a gutta percha stick. After the cement or Cavit is in place, a small wet cotton pellet can be passed to the dentist to smooth the occlusal surface of the material and to secure the seal; this will also accelerate the material's setting time.

Before the occlusion can be checked, the rubber dam must be removed and the patient's mouth must be rinsed. Articulating paper is used to check the occlusion, and if adjustment is needed, a spoon excavator, condenser or, occlusal carver may be used.

Obturation

Obturation is the procedure for filling and sealing the root canal and is the final step in the pulpectomy procedure; it is accomplished only after the canals have been completely debrided and shaped appropriately to receive a filling material and after the tooth is asymptomatic and the canals are completely dry.

Successful obturation of the canal requires the use of a solid material, the master cone, in combination with some form of paste. In past years silver cones were used as the master cone in conjunction with a sealing paste. Silver cones do not fit the canal as precisely as gutta percha, and they present more difficulty in canal preparation for a post-type restoration. Today, gutta percha points are used more often with a pulp canal sealer. These points may be seated manually or automatically and are available in several forms. A master gutta percha cone can be inserted into the canal with auxiliary cones that are condensed laterally adjacent to the master cone, until the entire canal is obturated.

Another form of obturation is a Thermafil (trademark) method, which is an endodontic obturator that consists of a flexible central carrier—metal or plastic—that is sized and tapered to match standard endodontic files and that is uniformly coated with a layer of refined and tested gutta percha. The Thermafil cone (Fig. 33-26) is commonly heated in an oven and sealed into place with a sealer.

An injectable form of gutta percha is also available and

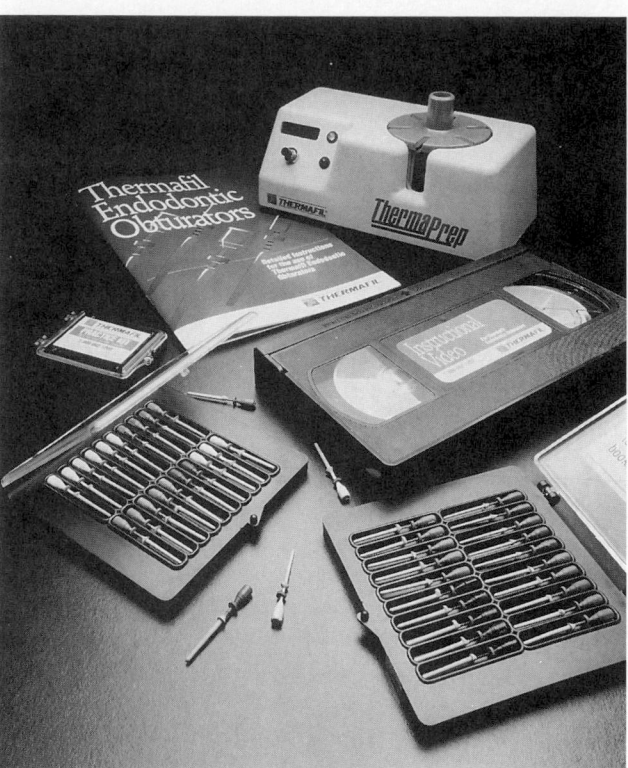

FIG. 33-26   Thermofil System.
(Courtesy of Thermafil Corporation.)

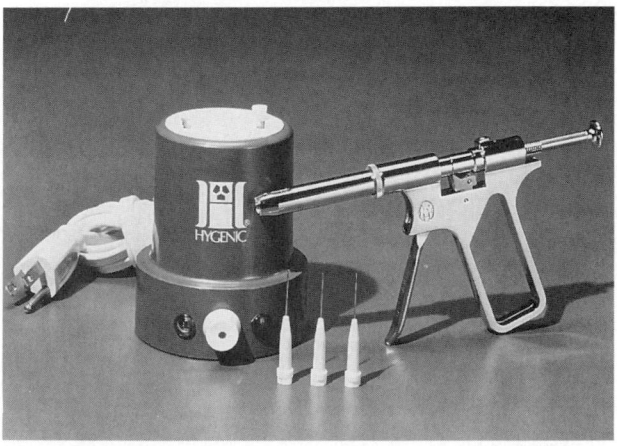

FIG. 33-27   Injectible gutta percha system.
(From Hygenic Corporation.)

is provided in a gun-like device (Fig. 33-27). A specially formulated gutta percha is placed into the gun, which heats and softens the material; it is then injected directly into the canals. The heating device provides a temperature that enables the material to become viscous enough to flow but that does not liquefy the material to a state that would cause the material to flow from the canal.

With the exception of the last technique, some form of sealer must be used to secure the points in place. Dr. Louis Grossman, the *father of modern endodontics,* identified the characteristics of a sealer. These characteristics are listed in Box 33-3.

Until recently and with the advent of the heated gutta percha systems the most common sealers were a powder/liquid or two-paste systems. Most products are formulated by using a zinc oxide–eugenol cement. Silver and barium compounds are added to the powder to create a radiopacity; iodine is included for an antiseptic property, and rosins are used to accelerate the setting time and to modify the film thickness. The paste is mixed on a sterile slab with a sterile spatula and may be spun into the canal with a lentulo spiral or placed onto the master cone and gently pumped into place.

Postoperative Instructions

The patient should be informed about what to expect after each phase of the procedure. After the initial biomechanical preparation some discomfort may arise, and the dentist may recommend an analgesic or prepare a prescription, depending on the nature of the problem and the patient's pain threshold.

Record final instructions and/or medications that are prescribed for the patient on the record. Observe the patient's face to make certain that it is clean and free of debris before dismissal from the chair.

▶ Pulpectomy Procedure

The following pulpectomy sequence describes the step-by-step procedure for multivisit appointments. This sequence was outlined in Fig. 33-24, *A* through *R,* as a single appointment. Note that since each appointment

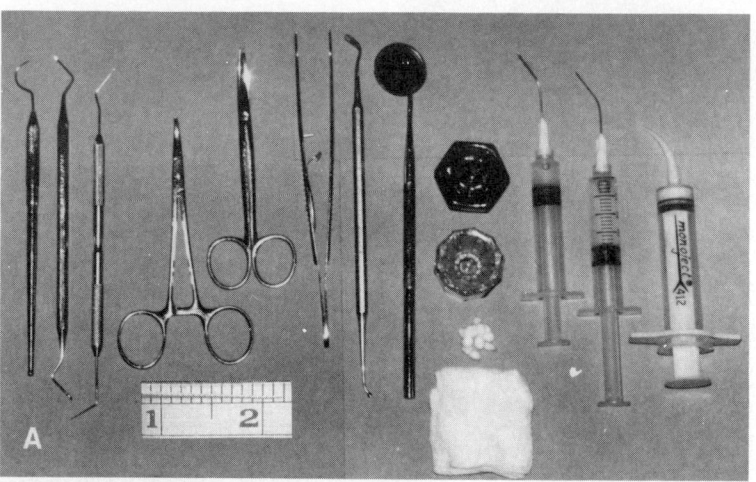

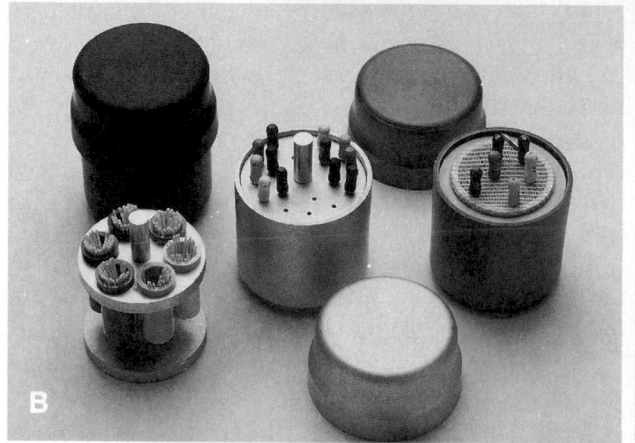

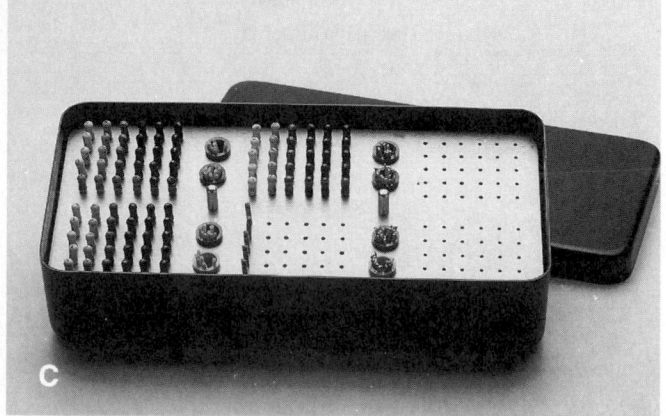

FIG. 33-28   Armamentarium for first appointment for pulpectomy. *A*, Basic endodontic tray setup. From left to right: endodontic explorer; spoon excavater; DG-16 explorer; mosquito hemostat; iris scissors; endodontic cotton pliers; plastic instrument; mirror; Dappen dish (two); cotton pellets; 2 × 2 gauze sponges; assorted irrigation syringes; ruler. *B* and *C,* Instrument boxes to store and autoclave intracanal instruments and paper points.

(From Bessner E, Michanowicz AE, Michanowicz JP: *Practical endodontics: a clinical atlas,* St Louis, 1994, Mosby.)

requires you to **STOP AND THINK** beforehand and afterward, the logo is used only in the beginning and end of the entire procedure, but it is highlighted where applicable in the appointment sequence.

FIRST APPOINTMENT

If time permits, the dentist may accomplish some of the treatment, such as the opening and the canal location, on the day the patient is first seen for diagnosis. If not, the patient is rescheduled for the entire appointment series. The primary objective at this first appointment is to relieve pain if it exists and to begin biomechanical preparation, which includes the complete debridement of the canals and the reshaping of the canal for the intended filling material.

Armamentarium (Fig. 33-28)

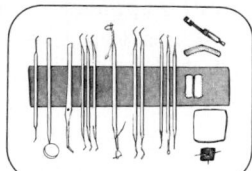

Anesthesia set-up
Rubber dam set-up, with clamp for the appropriate tooth
Endodontic explorer
Mirror
Endodontic locking pliers
Endodontic excavator
Plastic instrument

PULPECTOMY: MULTIVISIT (FIRST VISIT)

1. The tooth is anesthetized if necessary.
2. Place rubber dam isolation (Fig. 33-24, *A*).
3. Disinfect the treatment field with a cotton applicator or cotton pellet that is dipped in disinfectant (Fig. 33-24, *B*).
4. Make an occlusal opening for access to the canals. The assistant passes a high-speed handpiece with a #34 bur to the dentist and uses the HVE to evacuate fluid from the treatment site as it accumulates on the rubber dam. The dentist may exchange the #34 bur for a #57 or other bur to complete an outline form of the access opening (Fig. 33-24, *C*).
5. Exchange the handpiece for an endodontic explorer, so that the root canals can be located. **DO NOT** blow air or water spray into the pulp chamber. The dentist may wish to irrigate the site with NaOCl at this point. If so, pass the syringe; the assistant uses the HVE tip.
6. Pass a small file, generally a #10 or #15, to the dentist, who places the file into the canal to determine the length (Fig. 33-24, *F*).
7. Tooth length is determined, and the silicone stops are placed on all future files to be used. Pass the forceps periodically if the stop position needs to be adjusted (Fig. 33-24, *G*).
8. A radiograph is taken with the file in place, using the hemostat or film holder to position the film. After the length is determined, record it on the patient's record.
9. Biomechanical preparation of the canals is completed by passing files in numeric sequence, from smallest to largest, to the dentist (Fig. 33-24, *H* through *J*). The dentist returns the used file; it is positioned on the tray or other holder, while the dentist receives a new file. During the biomechanical preparation procedure the canal must always be kept moist with NaOCl.

10. Record the final file sizes to which the canal was filed. Other important information, such as unfound canals, file short of length, or perforations, should be recorded on the patient's record.
11. The canal is flushed with sodium hypochlorite (NaOCl), and the assistant removes any excess with the HVE (Fig. 33-24, *K*).
12. Pass sterile paper points to the dentist to dry the canal. Two cotton forceps expedites this process.
13. At this point the operator places the intracanal medication, either formocresol or chlorobutanol. Saturate the pellet with the medication, using a sterile forceps to enter the bottle. Tap the pellet dry on a sterile 2 × 2 gauze, and pass it to the operator. Transfer a plugger or a plastic instrument to push the pellet into place.
14. The plastic instrument can be used to insert the temporary cement. A small amount of Cavit or ZOE cement is prepared on the mixing pad and inserted into the occlusal opening. A small wet cotton pellet is used to smooth the occlusal surface of the material and to secure the seal. This moist pellet also accelerates the material's setting time.
15. Remove the rubber dam, and rinse the patient's mouth. Observe the patient's face to make certain it is clean and free of debris. The occlusion is checked with articulating paper. If adjustment is needed, a spoon excavator, condenser, or occlusal carver may be used.
16. Provide postoperative instructions.
17. Record any final instructions to the patient on the record, and dismiss the patient from the chair.

Endodontic ruler
Irrigating syringe, with sodium hypochlorite (NaOCl)
Gauze sponges
Cotton pellets
Disinfectant
Cotton applicator (optional)
Endodontic tray, with files, reamers, and broaches
File holder (optional)
Appropriate handpieces and contra-angles
HVE tips, standard and surgical
Radiographic film
Film holder or hemostat
Temporary filling material

SECOND OR INTERIM APPOINTMENTS

The first part of this appointment preparation is repeated from the first appointment. This appointment may vary in its routine, depending on how much was accomplished at the first appointment. For instance, in multirooted teeth all of the biomechanical preparation may be incomplete, and the second appointment commences where the first one ended. Also if all the preparation was completed at the first appointment and

---

PULPECTOMY: MULTIVISIT (SECOND VISIT)

 STOP

1. Tooth is anesthesized if necessary.
2. Place rubber dam isolation.
3. Disinfect treatment field with a cotton applicator or a cotton pellet in forceps that is dipped in disinfectant.
4. Pass a spoon excavator to remove the interim dressing.
5. Pass a sterile paper point to the operator to be inserted into each canal to check for dryness of canals or for the presence of a purulent odor.
6. Pass the irrigating syringe to irrigate the canals.
7. Complete the biomechanical preparation.
8. Verify the length of the canal with a radiograph of the final size file in place.
9. Flush the canal with sodium hypochlorite.
10. Dry the canal with absorbent paper points.
11. Place intracanal medication.
12. Place interim dressing, and adjust occlusion.

The dentist may need to provide the patient with a prescription at this appointment for an antibiotic or an analgesic, depending on the inflammatory state or on the amount of discomfort that the patient is experiencing. If a prescription was given at the first appointment, instructions for completion of the prescription should be clarified.

 STOP

---

if the tooth is asymptomatic, the second appointment could be eliminated, going directly to the obturation or the final appointment. Further, an additional interim appointment may be added if the patient is experiencing discomfort or if the canals cannot be accessed in a second appointment. The following description of this appointment is in an abbreviated form since it includes steps repeated from the first appointment.

Armamentarium

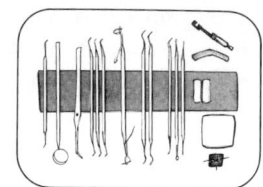

The tray set-up for this appointment is the same as it was for the first appointment. Some dentists may select a master cone at this appointment if the treatment progresses satisfactorily. This armamentarium is noted in the obturation appointment.

OBTURATION OR FINAL APPOINTMENT

At this appointment the root canal will be sealed or obturated. As described earlier, this phase of the treatment is done only after the canal has been filed completely and after the tooth is asymptomatic. At the conclusion of this appointment a final restoration must be placed. If the obturation is done by an endodontist, the patient is referred to the primary dentist for this restoration and an interim dressing is placed after the obturation procedure.

Armamentarium (Fig. 33-29)

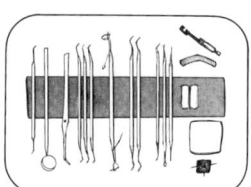

Rubber dam set-up with clamp
   for the appropriate tooth
Endodontic explorer
Mirror
Endodontic locking pliers
Endodontic excavator
Plastic instrument
Endodontic spreader
Absorbent paper points
Heat source
Root canal pluggers
Master cone or filling material
Auxiliary cones as needed
Root canal sealer

RECALL APPOINTMENT

Follow-up on the patient who has had a pulpectomy is important. Depending on the dentist's philosophy, the follow-up appointment may be scheduled in 6 weeks and again in 3 to 6 months. The patient is seen at least every

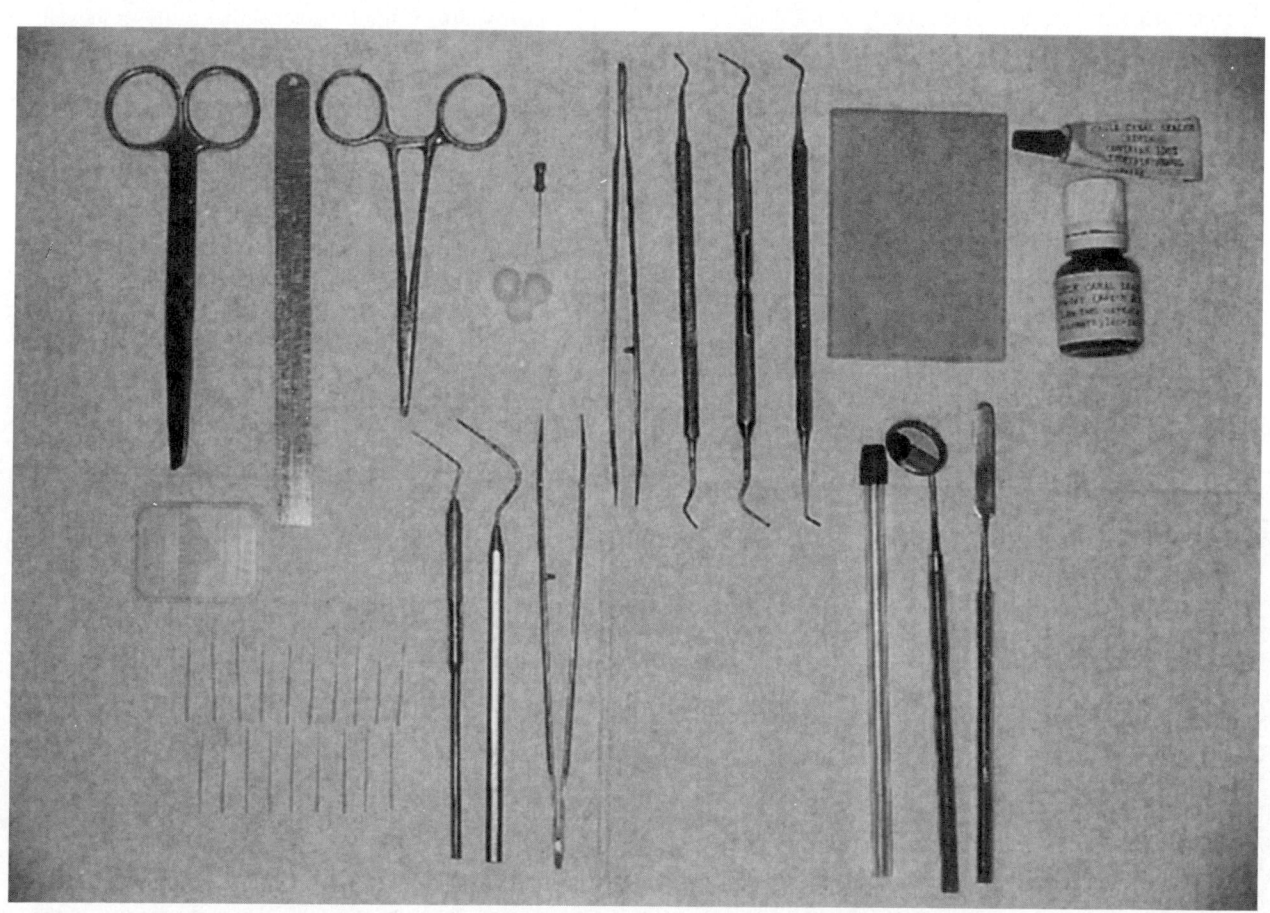

FIG. 33-29   **Armamentarium for obturation appointment.**

PULPECTOMY: MULTIVISIT (FINAL VISIT)

1. Anesthetize tooth if necessary.
2. Place the rubber dam isolation.
3. Disinfect the treatment field.
4. Pass the excavator to remove the interim dressing. Exchange the spoon for an explorer, if necessary, to remove the cotton pellet. Use the HVE to remove the debris from the opening. **DO NOT IRRIGATE THE CANALS.**
5. The canals are checked for dryness. Pass a dry absorbent point to the dentist to place in each canal.
6. Pass the irrigating syringe to the dentist and place the HVE near the tooth that is to receive irrigating fluids.
7. Pass the final files on which silicone stops have been set to final working length. The files are placed into the canals to reorient the dentist and to verify that the length is correct and that the canals have been filed to completion. A radiograph may be taken at this point.
8. Final irrigation is done by passing the irrigating syringe, followed by a series of paper points to dry the canal. Use two cotton forceps to expedite this procedure.
9. The dentist will select the master cone and adjust it to final length; the assistant can then place the cone in a chairside sterilizer or petri dish filled with full strength NaOCl. Allow the points to remain for at least 1 minute. Remove the master cone from the disinfectant, and blot it dry on a sterile gauze or towel.
10. Pass the master cone to the dentist who will insert it into the appropriate canals. If the cone needs to be adjusted, pass a pair of curved crown and collar scissors, and the dentist will cut off the excess.
11. Once the master cone is adjusted and seated in place, the dentist will want to check for snugness of fit. Pass a cotton forceps to test the cone seating. A trial point radiograph with the master cone in place is taken at this time. Develop the film, and pass it to the dentist to verify the correct length. If the points are correct, proceed to the obturation step. However, steps 9 and 10 may need to be repeated if the master cone is not the correct length, or it may even be necessary to return to the filing procedure. Be prepared to repeat any of the necessary steps.
12. The dentist removes the cone from the canal and passes it to you. Place the point on a sterile towel or gauze. If multiple canals are being filled, place the points in a specific order that can be identified for each canal.
13. Place the final point and auxiliary points in the disinfectant solution. After a minute, remove them from the dish and dry them thoroughly on a dry towel.
14. Mix the root canal sealer on a sterile slab, according to the manufacturer's directions. Select a file that is one or two sizes smaller than the final file size. Pass the file to the dentist, and hold the mixing slab with the sealer in the passing zone. The dentist will saturate the file with the sealer and place it into the canal, rotating the file counter clockwise and using a pumping action. The objective is to coat the walls but not to fill the canal with sealer.
15. Pass the master cone to the dentist, using the cotton forceps (Fig. 33-24, *L*). Some dentists prefer to dip the master cone tip in some of the sealer, so position the sealer near by if this procedure is followed. The dentist then seats the master cone (Fig. 33-24, *M*).
16. Pass the spreader to the dentist (Fig. 33-24, *N*). Prepare to pass the auxiliary cones in the cotton forceps. Pass the spreader. Continue to exchange the spreader and the cotton forceps filled with auxiliary cones until the canal is filled (Fig. 33-24, *O*). After each use, wipe the excess sealer off the spreader with a gauze sponge. If multiple canals are to be filled, this process is repeated for each canal.
17. Heat a plastic instrument or plugger in a flame until it is warm enough to melt the gutta percha inside the crown of the tooth. Pass it to the dentist who places the instrument into the crown of the tooth to remove the excess gutta percha (Fig. 33-24, *P*). Use the HVE tip near the tooth to pick up any smoke that may be created. Wipe the end of the plugger with a gauze. Repeat this procedure if necessary. The dentist may want to return to the plugger to pack the remaining gutta percha into the occlusal access opening. Often, a cold instrument is preferred (Fig. 33-24, *Q*).
18. Mix a temporary cement to cover the gutta percha filling. If this procedure is being done in a general practice office, some dentists may place the final restoration at this time, but often, a temporary restoration is still placed to verify the comfort of the tooth (Fig. 33-24, *R*).
19. Remove the rubber dam.
20. A final radiograph is taken. This radiograph is important, since it will be a reference radiograph for follow-up appointments in future years.
21. Inform the patient about recall appointments every 6 months over the next 2 years.
22. Make certain the patient's face is clean and free of debris. Dismiss the patient from the chair.

NOTE: If a heat-softened gutta percha obturation technique is used, the manufacturer's directions for use of the material will be followed.

6 months for the next 2 years. If the treatment is performed in a general practice, the follow-up is often done at the patient's routine prophylaxis visit. At this recall appointment the intraoral tissues, the tooth mobility, and the tooth color are examined. Follow-up radiographs are also taken to observe the periapical tissues.

Surgical Endodontics

The most common types of surgical endodontic procedures may include incisions for drainage of an apical abscess; an apicoectomy (the surgical removal of the apical portion of the root); or root amputation, hemisection, or bicuspidization. Each of these procedures is described in the following discussion.

▶ Drainage of an Apical Abscess

When a patient arrives for treatment with severe edema that results from pulpal necrosis, it is typically treated by drainage. The choice of treatment is to open the tooth through the occlusal to provide drainage. However, if adequate drainage is not accomplished through this route, it may be necessary to establish apical drainage. If a fluctuant swelling is obvious (a fluid-containing mass), an incision can be made to release the purulent (pus-like) substance; providing the patient with immediate relief. The procedure is accomplished in the following steps illustrated in Fig. 33-30, *A* through *F*.

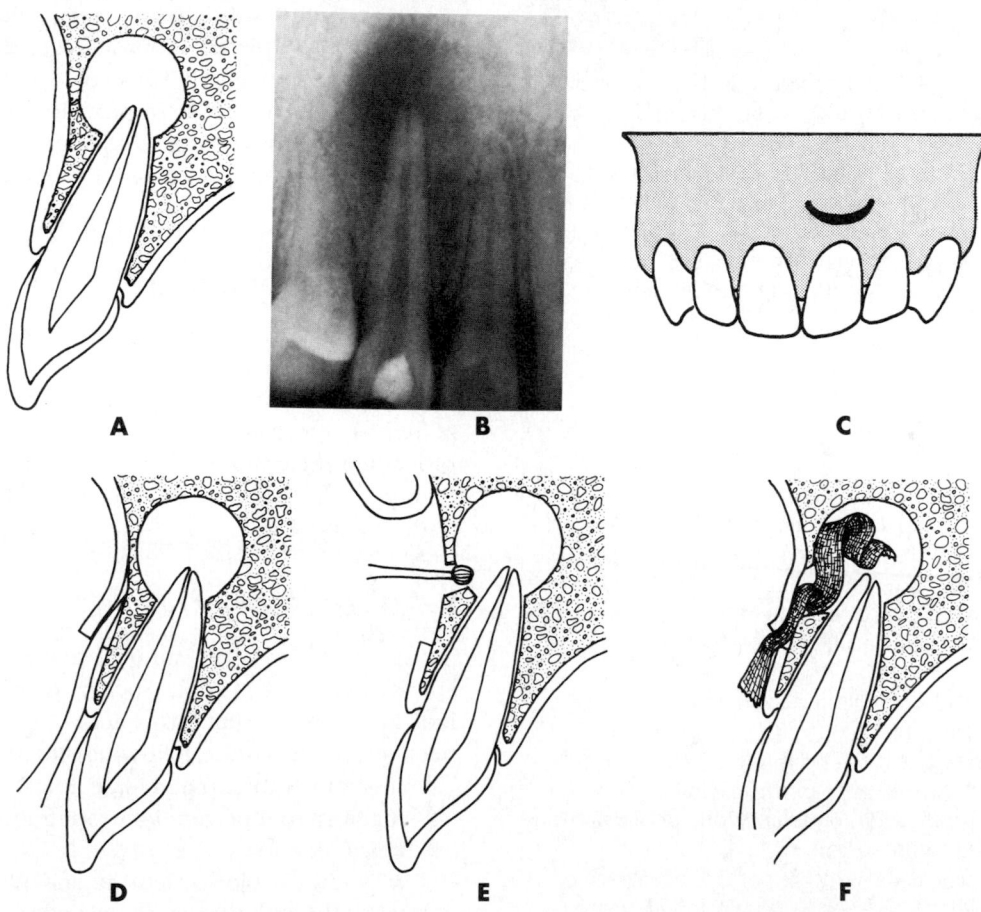

FIG. 33-30   Drainage of an apical abscess. *A*, Graphic location of an apical abscess. *B*, Radiographic illustration of apical abscess. *C*, Incision is made on labial surface. *D*, Tissue is elevated to gain exposure. *E*, Round bur prepares an opening through the cortical plate. *F*, The incisional site is kept open by a gauze drain that is inserted into the lesion and extends out the path of entry.

(From Cohen S, Burns RC: *Pathways of the pulp,* ed 5, St Louis, 1991, Mosby.)

Armamentarium

Anesthetic set-up
Explorer
Mirror
Cotton forceps
2 × 2 gauze sponges
HVE tip
Periosteal elevator
#11 or #15 scalpel
Drain, rubber or iodoform
Hemostat
Irrigating syringe
Sterile saline solution

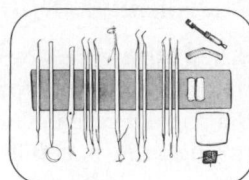

DRAINAGE OF AN APICAL ABSCESS

1. The patient is anesthetized, using a field or mandibular block. Infiltration anesthesia may prove painful and ineffective.
2. Once anesthesia is obtained pass a #11 or #15 scalpel blade to be used to make an incision directly into the edematous mass. Exudate will generally flow out immediately, followed by some hemorrhaging. The dental assistant should keep the HVE tip near the site to remove all fluids.
3. Pass a closed small hemostat or needle holder to the operator to enlarge the opening, allowing additional drainage.
4. Pass a 2 × 2 gauze to wipe the site free of hemorrhage or exudate.
5. If the site is to be irrigated, transfer sterile saline solution to the operator in an irrigating syringe. The assistant should hold the HVE tip nearby to collect fluids that drain from the site.
6. If a drain is to be placed, pass the drain in the forceps for insertion. This drain will be kept in place for 3 to 5 days.
7. Wipe the patient's face clean of any debris before dismissal from the chair.
8. Indicate to the patient the need to retain the drain in place. Record the treatment on the clinical chart, and indicate if a prescription for an antibiotic or analgesic is provided to the patient.
9. Provide the patient with written postoperative instructions as shown in Box 33-4. Be certain to indicate to the patient to notify the office if he or she experiences severe discomfort or excessive drainage.

Hemisection

A hemisection is the process of surgically removing a single root from a multirooted tooth, while the remaining root or roots are left intact. High-speed handpieces, surgical chisels, elevators, and forceps are used to separate the tooth buccolingually through the furcation region. The diseased root and its portion of the crown are removed. This procedure removes the periodontally involved root and allows for retention of the remaining roots, which can be treated with traditional endodontic procedures (Fig. 33-31, *A* and *B*).

Bicuspidization

This surgical procedure is used when severe bone loss is confined to the furcation area. The process actually creates two premolars (bicuspids) from a mandibular molar. In Fig. 33-31, *C,* the severe bone loss in the furcal region requires that a pulpectomy be performed on both roots, and the tooth is then cut in half with a bur in a high-speed handpiece. A thorough curettage of the furcal area is completed, and full crown coverage is placed over the two premolar teeth. To provide added support, the crowns are splinted, with adequate opening provided at the furcal region to enable the patient to perform thorough oral hygiene.

Root Amputation

This surgical procedure is not significantly different from a hemisection. It is more commonly done on maxillary teeth than mandibular and involves the surgical removal of one or more roots on a multirooted tooth. In this procedure the entire crown is left intact and endodontic therapy is performed on the remaining root(s) (Fig. 33-32, *A* and *B*).

Apicoectomy

An apicoectomy is the surgical removal of the apex or apical portion of a root. Such a surgical procedure is indicated when traditional endodontic therapy has not been successful in the following situations:

▶ It is impossible to eliminate apical pathology resulting from root perforation, root fracture, or recurring apical disease
▶ It is impossible to debride and fill the entire root using the traditional coronal approach, such as teeth with severe root curvatures or with calcified canals
▶ Treatment has failed because of broken instruments, apical perforation, or incomplete canal obturation

The components of an apicoectomy procedure include an apical curettage—the debridement of the apical lesion; a reverse or retrofilling—the sealing of the canal at the

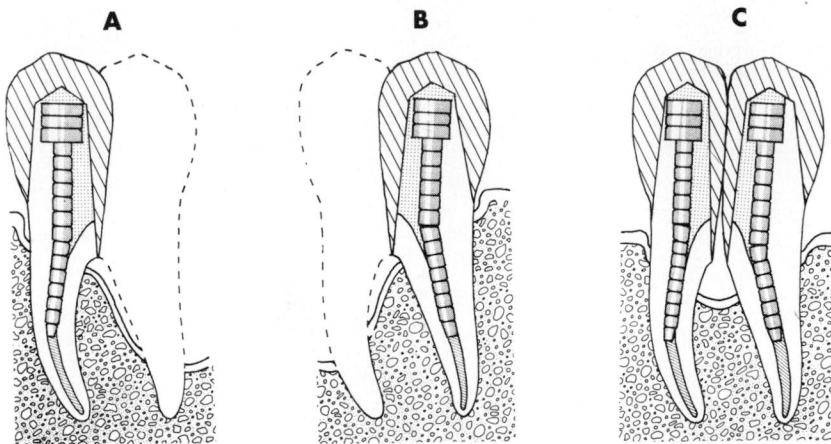

FIG. 33-31 Hemisected mandibular molar and bicuspidization. *A,* Amputation of the distal root. Note the dowel reinforcement. *B,* Amputation of the mesial root. Note the dowel reinforcement. *C,* Bicuspidization. Each remaining root should be dowel reinforced. Note that dowel is shaped with three-pronged clasp bending pliers.

(From Cohen S, Burns RC: *Pathways of the pulp,* ed 5, St Louis, 1991, Mosby.)

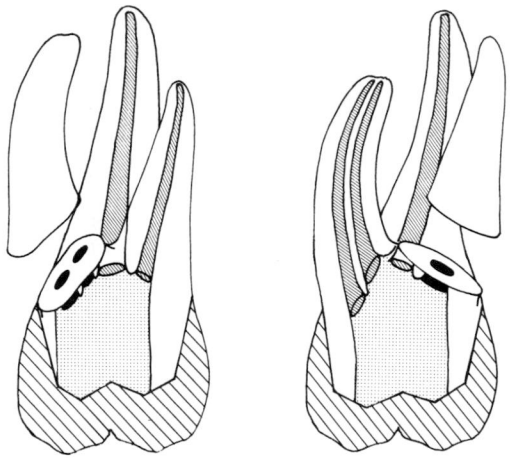

FIG. 33-32 Mesiobuccal and distobuccal root amputation of a maxillary molar.

(From Cohen S, Burns RC: *Pathways of the pulp,* ed 5, St Louis, 1991, Mosby.)

BOX 33-4

PROCEDURE FOR APICAL SURGERY

▶ Anesthetize
▶ Make a flap incision
▶ Retract tissue flap
▶ Gain access to the apex
▶ Perform apical curettage
▶ Perform apicoectomy
▶ Complete retrograde preparation and restoration
▶ Replace flap and suture
▶ Give postoperative instructions

FIG. 33-33 A large round bur is used to remove cortical and cancellous bone. The initial approach is, *A,* to identify the correct root and then, *B,* enlarge the window to expose the lesion and the apex, facilitating curettage. *C,* When the lesion is completely exposed, the concave surface of a sharp curette will strip the tissue from bone; and once the tissue is free, it can be spooned from the bone cavity. The specimen should not be pulled from the crypt.

(From Cohen S, Burns RC: *Pathways of the pulp,* ed 5, St Louis, 1991, Mosby.)

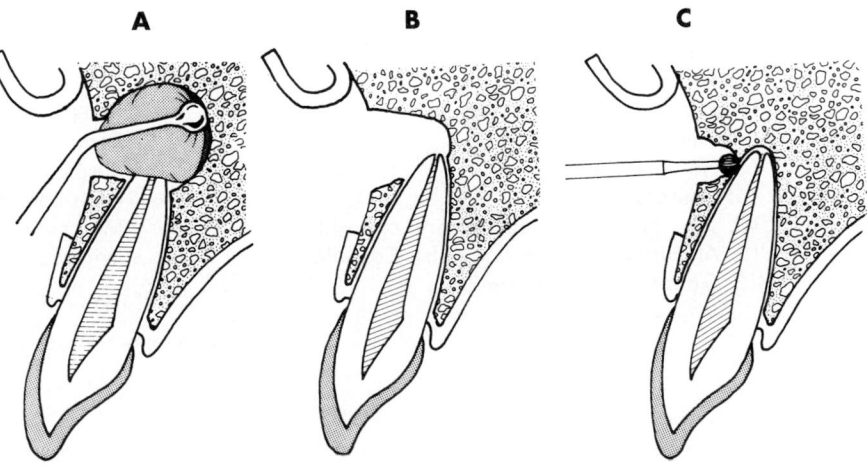

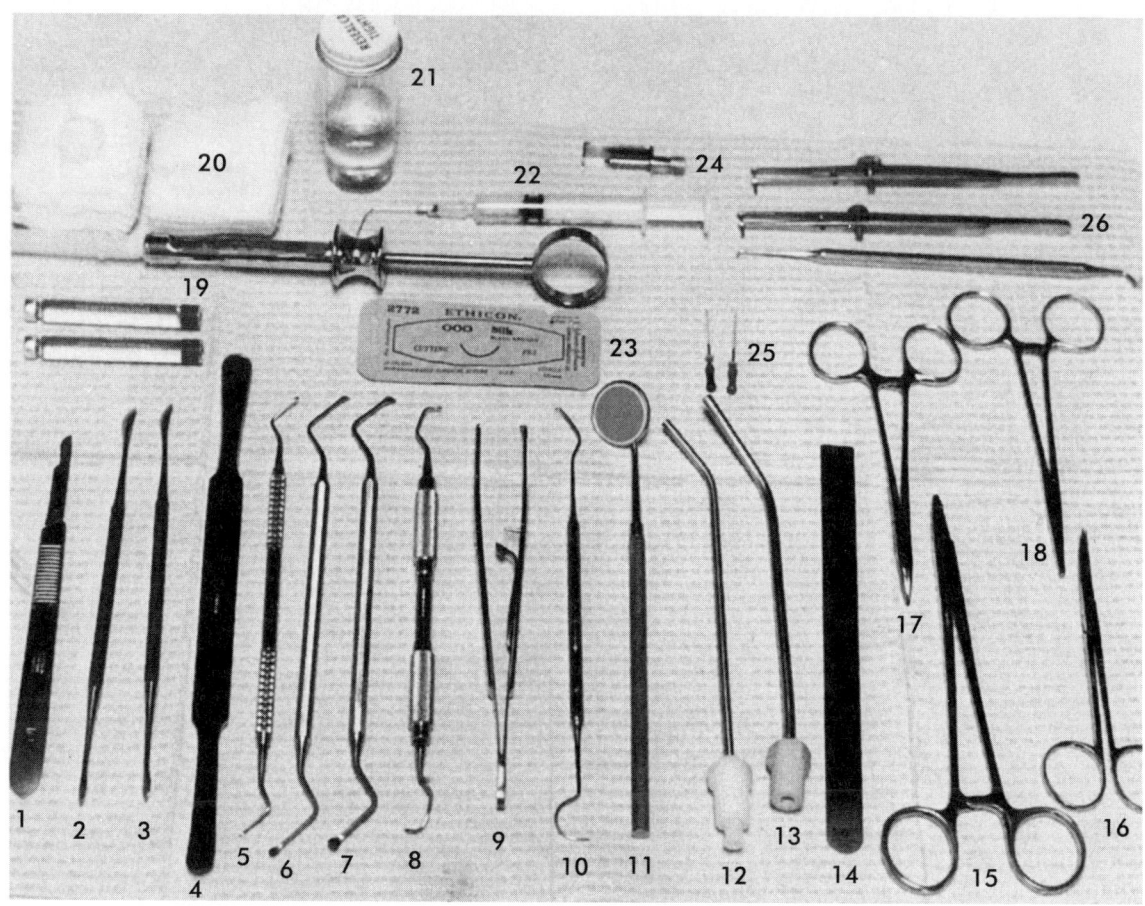

1. Scalpel
2. Periosteal elevator
3. No. 7 wax spatula
4. Retractor
5-8.   Curettes (three surgical and one periodontal)
9. Locking pliers
10. Explorer
11. Mirror
12, 13.   Aspirator tips (two sizes)
14. Millimeter ruler
15. Hemostat-scissors
16. Scissors
17, 18.   Hemostats (curved and straight)
19. Anesthetic syringe and extra Carpules
20. Gauze and cotton pellets

21. Biopsy bottle
22. Irrigating syringe
23. Suture material
24. Bur changer
25. Files (to aid in locating apex)
26. Amalgam carriers and condenser

Other items, not shown in photograph:
Regular-length burs (Nos. 700, ½)
Surgical-length burs (Nos. 700, ½, 4, 6)
High-speed handpiece
Mini contra-angle with No. 1 bur
Irrigating solution (sterile distilled saline water)

FIG. 33-34   Apicoectomy tray set-up.

apical region; and the actual apicoectomy—cutting away of an apical portion of the tooth. The steps for this procedure are listed in Box 33-4.

The procedure includes anesthetizing the patient, making a flap type incision, retracting the flap, locating the apex, removing bone that overlies the apex of the tooth, and curetting the lesion (Fig. 33-33, *A* through *C*). A typical preset tray for this procedure is shown in Fig. 33-34.

To perform the apicoectomy, a beveled cut is made on the root tip at a distance that is predetermined by the dentist. The amount of root that is removed is determined from the radiograph and is dictated by the reason for the apicoectomy. Once it has been determined that the apical seal is adequate and that fractures or other complications are not apparent, the canal can be sealed at the apex. A preparation that is similar to the amalgam preparation is made. A retrograde filling material, such as amalgam, composite, gutta percha, or even Cavit (trademark), is placed in the apical preparation (Fig. 33-35, *A* through *C*). Miniature instruments, such as the micro-contra angle, the small amalgam carrier, and the small amalgam condenser, can be used in the preparation for and insertion of the amalgam into the preparation.

At the conclusion of the apicoectomy the tissue flap is repositioned and the surgical site is sutured. The patient's face is cleaned of any debris before dismissal, and postoperative instructions are given to the patient in printed form as shown in Box 33-5.

BOX 33-5

CARE AND INSTRUCTIONS FOLLOWING APICAL SURGERY

1. To minimize swelling, apply an ice bag with minimal pressure to the area, alternating 10 minutes on and 10 minutes off for the remainder of the day.
2. Brush the teeth in the normal manner, but be cautious at the site of the surgery.
3. Some oozing of blood may occur. If so, place a sterile moistened gauze over the site with finger pressure for 15 minutes. If the bleeding does not subside, call the office.
4. Avoid chewing hard foods. Eat a soft diet, but be sure to eat. Drink plenty of fluids.
5. Rinse the mouth with warm salt water tomorrow; this can be done every 3 hours. Avoid forceful rinsing.
6. Refrain from smoking or consuming alcoholic beverages for 24 hours.
7. Avoid lifting the lip to look at the area. The stitches may tear.
8. Some discomfort may occur. This is normal. If a prescription is given for a pain medication, take it according to the prescribed directions. If no prescription is given and discomfort occurs, take a nonprescription medication that you would normally take for pain.
9. If severe pain or excessive swelling or bleeding occurs, contact the office.
10. Sutures need to be removed in 7 to 10 days. If a drain has been placed, it will be removed in 3 to 5 days.

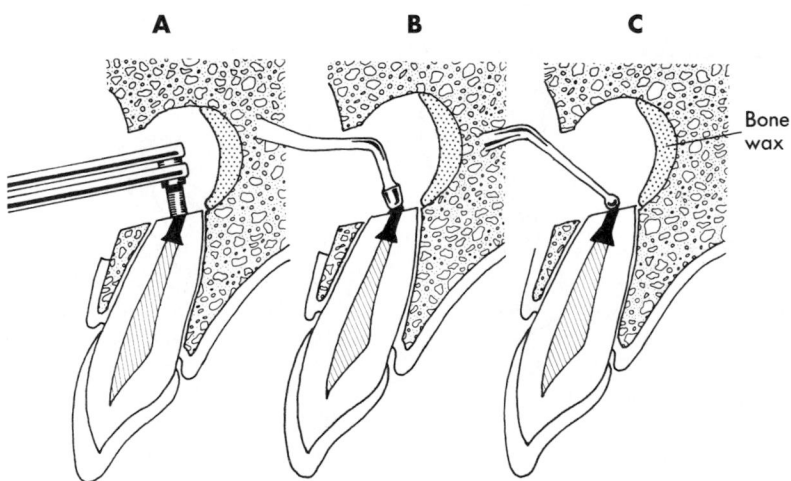

FIG. 33-35   When the preparation is complete, *A*, carry the amalgam to the opening, *B*, condense it with a miniplugger, and then, *C*, curette.

(From Cohen S, Burns RC: *Pathways of the pulp*, ed 5, St Louis, 1991, Mosby.)

Bleaching

Teeth may become discolored for various reasons. Natural or acquired stains are caused from pulpal necrosis; and developmental defects in the enamel are caused by fluorosis, systemic drugs, such as tetracycline, or other systemic diseases. *Iatrogenic* or inflicted stains are often caused by chemicals or materials that are used in dentistry. Most commonly, this type of discoloration comes from metallic restorations, such as amalgam, which, over a period of time, may turn the dentinal tissues gray. Pulpal fragments left in the tooth during endodontic therapy can gradually discolor. Finally, the use of some obturating materials, such as root canal sealers that contain silver particles, are left in the coronal portion of the tooth and may come in contact with oral fluids through percolation, causing a darkening of the tooth.

If a patient is bothered by the discolored tooth, he or she may opt to bleach the tooth or to have porcelain veneer, laminate, or full-coverage restorations placed on these teeth. The patient must be presented with all of these options and should be told of the fee and potential success of each technique. The restorative methods are described in Chapter 29, and an overview of the bleaching technique follows.

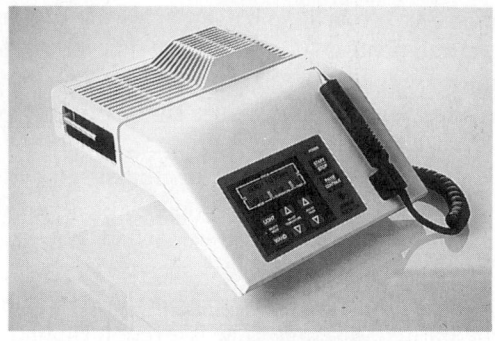

FIG. 33-36   A combined bleaching light and heat wand with LED sensor has been incorporated into the state-of-the-art *Illuminator*.

(Courtesy Thermafil Corporation.)

Various bleaching techniques are available: internal, external, and even home bleaching. Various oxidizing agents have been used for internal bleaching, including sodium hypochlorite, hydrogen peroxide, and sodium perborate. Methods of application for internal bleaching include the following:

▸ Thermocatalytic technique, which involves the placement of the chemical in the pulp chamber and

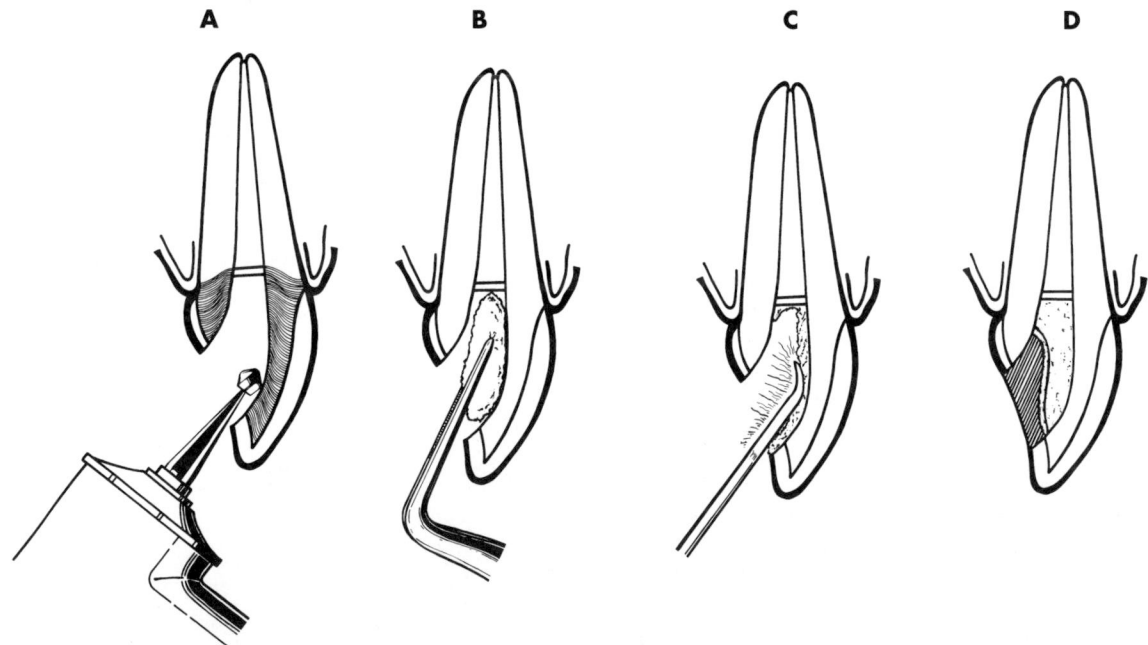

FIG. 33-37   *A,* Gutta percha is removed from coronal portion of tooth and canal is sealed with zinc phosphate cement 1 mm coronal to the cementoenamel junction (*A*). *B,* All debris and surface stains are removed. *C,* Cotton pellet saturated with 35% hydrogen peroxide is placed into pulp chamber. *D,* Heated tip from bleaching instrument is inserted into chamber.

(Courtesy Dr. A.C. Goerig.)

then the application of heat; this method of application has been controversial because of the potential damage of heat to the cervical periodontium

- Walking bleach technique, which requires the affected teeth to be isolated with a rubber dam and existing restorations and cement bases removed; the pulpal chamber may be cleaned with a solvent; a paste of sodium perborate and water or anesthetic solution is mixed to the consistency of wet putty; the paste is placed into the chamber, and a temporary cement can then be placed; the patient is rescheduled for two or three similar appointments; this technique is a gradual process, and the bleaching is not quickly evident
- Light activated technique, which uses an ultraviolet beam; the light is applied to the tooth after a cotton pellet that is saturated with a 30% to 35% hydrogen peroxide solution has been inserted into the chamber (Fig. 33-36)

External or vital bleaching is not dissimilar in its technique to vital or internal bleaching. Using the hydrogen peroxide technique the teeth are isolated and a solution of 30% hydrogen peroxide is applied to the enamel with a heat application. The benefits of this bleaching method are not definitive, and the effect of the solution on the enamel and the potential damage of the heat on the pulp raise significant questions about this technique. An alternative method of vital bleaching is to mix a paste of 35% hydrochloric acid with an equal volume of water to which flour of pumice is added. This mixture is applied to the enamel surface and rubbed for 5 seconds, followed by rinsing for 10 seconds. Although this latter method has proven effective, concern for safety because of enamel decalcification and potential chemical burns to the soft tissue often outweigh the benefits. A bleaching technique is illustrated in Fig. 33-37, *A* through *D*.

KEY POINTS

- The practice of endodontics is primarily concerned with the diseases of the pulp. This specialized area offers the chairside dental assistant challenging opportunities, including comforting the patient, assisting with diagnostic tests, providing accurate radiographs, and preparing and assisting during a variety of endodontic procedures, from a basic pulpotomy to a complex periapical surgical procedure.

- Pulpal pathoses that can cause the dental pulp to degenerate include hyperemia, reversible and irreversible pulpitis, acute or chronic apical periodontitis, periapical abscess, pulp stone, or traumatic injuries.

- Traumatic injuries occur when a blow to the mouth occurs, resulting in trauma to supporting tissues. Trauma can result in various injuries to the teeth, including luxation, avulsion, intrusion, and fractures, and requires endodontic therapy—in some situations even replantation.

- Diagnostic tests to determine the health of a tooth include clinical examination; radiographs; thermal, electronic, or digital pulp tests; percussion; palpation; transillumination; or a test cavity.

- Endodontic treatment can include various procedures, such as a pulpotomy, pulpectomy, and bleaching and surgical procedures, including an apicoectomy, hemisection, and root amputation.

BIBLIOGRAPHY

Bence Richard: *Handbook of clinical endodontics,* ed 2, St Louis, Mosby, 1980.

Cohen S, Burns R: *Pathways of the pulp,* ed 5, St Louis, 1991, Mosby.

Corcoran JF et al: *Endodontics I,* ed 3, Ann Arbor, Mich, 1992, University of Michigan Dental Publications.

Greene HA, Wong M, Ingram III TA: Comparison of the sealing ability of four obturation techniques, *J Endodont* 9:423-428 1990.

Walton R: Current concepts of canal preparation, *Dent Clin No Am* 36(2): April 1992.

34 Oral and Maxillofacial Surgery

LEARNING OBJECTIVES

You will have mastered the material in this chapter when you can:

▶ Define the key terms
▶ Describe the role of the oral surgery assistant
▶ List differences in design between an oral surgery and a general dental office
▶ Identify common medical conditions that can affect dental treatment
▶ Identify various types of antianxiety techniques, and describe the advantages and disadvantages of each
▶ Name and describe the function of the types of instruments that are normally found on an oral surgery tray
▶ Describe the steps in tooth extraction
▶ Describe other common oral surgical procedures
▶ Explain common postoperative instructions for an oral surgery patient
▶ Discuss the role of the hospital in operative dentistry and maxillofacial surgery procedures

KEY TERMS

Anesthesiologist	Nitrous oxide
Biopsy	Orthognathic surgery
Chisel	Periosteal elevator
Conscious sedation	Pulse oximeter
Electrocardiogram (ECG)	Rongeur forceps
Elevator	Stent
Endotracheal tube	Surgical curette
Exfoliative cytology	Surgical dressing
Exodontia	Surgical forceps
Extraction	Surgical HVE or aspirator tip
Frenectomy	Suture
Intravenous (IV) administration	Titration
Maxillofacial	Trendelenburg

Oral and maxillofacial surgery is the dental specialty that deals with the diagnosis and surgical treatment of diseases, injuries, and deformities of the face and jaws. The term **maxillofacial** refers to the portion of the face that includes the maxilla and mandible.

In this chapter the dental assistant will be introduced to specialized armamentarium and basic surgical procedures that are performed in a maxillofacial oral surgery practice. This chapter will also focus on the importance of patient management. Since this specialty often involves invasive procedures that create anxiety, this chapter will also address designing an office for patient comfort and creating an atmosphere of caring.

In addition to extracting teeth (**exodontia**) the oral surgeon treats oral pathology (diseases of the mouth and jaws) or facial injuries and trauma such as broken bones, practices preprosthetic surgery to prepare the mouth to receive prosthetic devices such as dentures or implants, and performs **orthognathic surgery**, that is, surgery of the jaws to correct deformities, making the jaws more functional. Orthognathic surgery is always performed in a hospital; the patient receives general anesthesia that is administered by an **anesthesiologist**, a physician who specializes in anesthesiology, which is the specialty of administering medication that causes a loss of sensation with or without a loss in consciousness. Oral surgery that is performed in the dental office also can involve either general anesthesia or conscious sedation. In the office, however, the oral surgeon usually administers the anesthesia and performs the surgery.

 Ambroise Pare, often referred to as the father of surgery, made significant contributions to dentistry by designing the first oral obturator and numerous surgical instruments and by replacing extracted anterior teeth with bridges that were made of ivory teeth set in gold bases and then attached to adjacent teeth with gold wire.

An individual who wishes to specialize in oral surgery must first complete dental school and then generally spends an additional 4 years in a hospital residency program. During this residency the oral surgeon receives extra training in internal medicine, general surgery, anesthesia, and oral and maxillofacial surgery. Some individuals spend 2 additional years to earn the Medical Doctor (MD) degree. After the residency is completed, a state, regional, or national specialty board examination must be passed and practice is restricted to oral surgery. Oral surgery is also practiced by general dentists, but they usually restrict themselves to less involved cases and usually do not practice in the hospital setting.

Role of the Dental Assistant

In the oral surgery office, more than in any other dental specialty, the dentist and the assistant must work together as a team for safety reasons and for convenience. Oral surgery assistants may be registered or certified dental assistants who have received additional experience in an oral surgery office. A specialty exam for assistants who are in oral maxillofacial surgery assisting is available through the Dental Assistants' National Board (see Chapter 2). Some assistants also take a home study course that is sponsored by the American Association of Oral and Maxillofacial Surgeons, which allows them to sit for an examination for certification as an oral surgery anesthesia assistant. The assistant must also be well trained in cardiopulmonary resuscitation and first aid because many patients that are referred to the oral surgery specialty practice may be either in poor health or victims of trauma.

▶ Intraoral Responsibilities

The assistant is responsible for preparing all of the armamentarium medications that will be used in administering the anesthesia and in performing the surgical procedure. During oral surgery procedures the assistant must maintain a clear surgical field for the surgeon by efficient use of evacuation and retraction. Oral surgery patients are often heavily sedated or anesthetized for these procedures. The assistant observes the patient's vital signs and monitors the patient's blood pressure, pulse, and respiration rate to ensure that the patient is responding safely to the surgery and anesthesia. In some states, advanced functions, such as suture removal, may be delegated to qualified assistants in this specialty.

▶ Patient Management

Oral surgery challenges the surgery assistant's patient management skills. The assistant plays a major role in reassuring the patient and helping him or her to relax, while the surgeon performs the procedure. A friendly smile, a comforting hand on the shoulder or even holding a patient's hand during the administration of anesthesia can make a patient feel better during this stressful time, especially if the patient is a child. Most oral surgeons prefer that a child's parent not be present in the room during surgery, since patient management is often easier without the parent present. Young children can be frightened being in a strange environment without the parent. The oral surgery assistant can help the child to feel at ease and less frightened in this setting.

▶ Teaching

At times, the assistant's role involves a significant amount of teaching by providing pre- and postoperative instructions for a patient. After a surgical procedure the patient may experience hemorrhaging and can expect postoperative pain. The assistant must inform the patient about what to expect, how to stop the bleeding, and how and when to take pain medication. The assistant can also make a follow-up call to the patient later in the day to make sure that he or she understands the instructions, answering any questions or discussing any complications that may have arisen. This follow-up call may avoid patient panic and after-hour emergency calls.

▶ Maintaining Infection Control Standards

As in any dental office the oral surgery office practices universal precautions, so instrument preparation and sterilization and management of medical waste are vital. Because oral surgery involves invasion of tissues, proper sterilization becomes vitally important. For a review of infection control refer to Chapter 8.

Office Design

With a few modifications the oral surgery office can be similar in design to a general dental office. Because of the increased anxiety that patients feel when they are about to have surgery, it is important that the environment be as soothing as possible. Soft music, subdued colors, rounded edges of counters and door frames, etc. can lend a subtle calming effect that rock music, bright colors, and hard edges cannot achieve.

▶ Reception Room and Hallways

Patient seating in the reception area must be comfortable and well lighted. Unlike most general dental offices, oral surgery patients are accompanied to the office by a driver, who must wait in the reception area until the

patient's procedure is completed. Hallways in the oral surgery office should be wider than in the general dental office. Not only does this give an effect of spaciousness, which can be calming, but since many oral surgery patients are sedated for the procedures, they must be supported while exiting the office, so that they don't stumble. The hallways must be wide enough for two individuals to walk comfortably abreast.

▶ Oral Surgery Treatment Rooms

Similarly, the oral surgery treatment room must also be wider than the general dental treatment room. Often times, during oral surgery procedures, two assistants participate in the procedure. Both assistants and the dentist must have plenty of room to stand or sit comfortably to allow the surgical procedure to proceed as smoothly as possible and to decrease the operator's stress. The ideal width of an oral surgery treatment room is at least 10 feet, which allows the second assistant to easily walk around the operator to get to an area where extra assistance may be needed. Ideally, there should be two entrances into the treatment room (Fig. 34-1) so that neither the operator or the assistant is trapped in a corner. There should also be room at the foot of the chair for an assistant to walk around if necessary. Adequate counter space is necessary in the treatment room to accommodate the various instruments that are used to monitor patient functions, such as blood pressure, pulse, and respirations. At least one sink, preferably two, must be included in the treatment room to allow for hand washing before and after gloving. Oxygen, nitrous oxide, and other gases, such as nitrogen (used for some oral surgery handpieces), should be plumbed into the wall directly behind the patient's head, so that the cords do

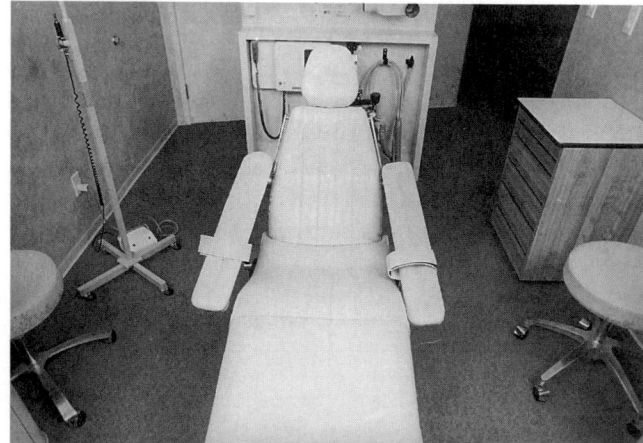

FIG. 34-1 Typical surgery treatment room with two entrances, and surgical chair with IV arm.

(Courtesy of Helen Zylman, D.D.S., Ann Arbor, Michigan.)

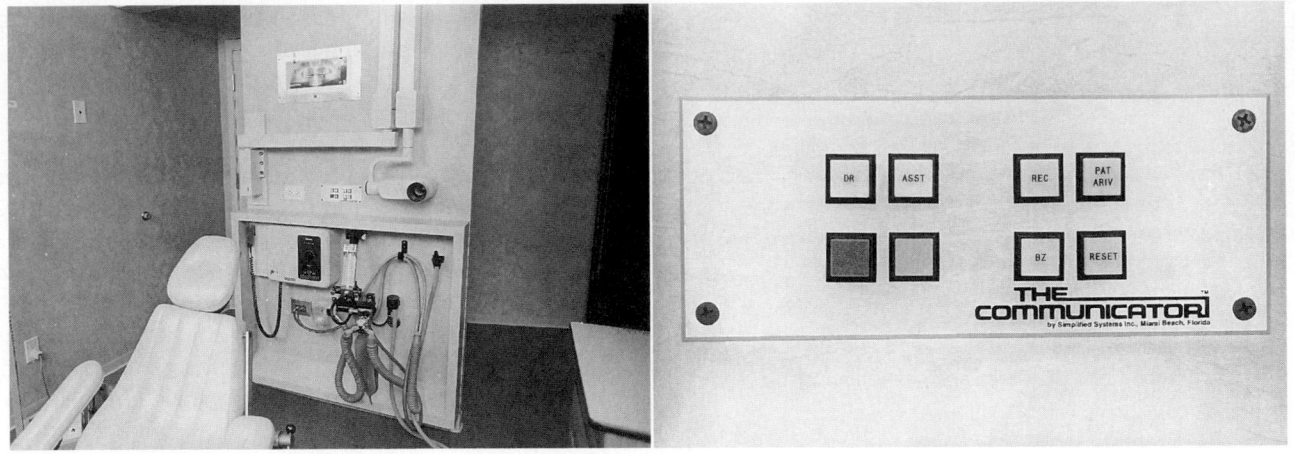

FIG. 34-2   *A,* Nitrous oxide and other gases are plumbed into the wall behind the patient's chair. *B,* Communication system in wall behind patient's chair.

(*A* courtesy of Helen Zylman, D.D.S., Ann Arbor, Michigan; *B* courtesy of Simplified Systems Inc., Miami Beach, Florida.)

not interfere with the operator's view (Fig. 34-2, *A*). In this same area a communication system (Fig. 34-2, *B*) and suction must be available. Whether the surgical tray is positioned behind the patient's head or directly over the patient's chest, the instrument tray should not be present in the room when the patient is initially seated to allay potential patient fears.

The dental chair is slightly different in oral surgery than it is in the general dental office. Many oral surgeons work standing up rather than sitting down, so it must be possible to elevate the chair high enough so that the surgeon does not have to stoop. Because many oral surgery patients are sedated for the procedures, the chair must have a flat arm that can easily support a sedated patient's arm with an IV in place (see Fig. 34-1). The oral surgery chair must be equipped to function in emergencies. It must be strong enough to withstand CPR compression and must be able to be placed in the **Trendelenburg** position—a position in which the patient's head is below the level of the feet.

▶ Adjunct Rooms

As in a general practice the sterilization area must be central to the treatment rooms to allow easy access during cleanup and to provide adequate storage.

The oral surgery office, just as the general dental office, must have an area that is set aside for radiography. Whereas most general dentists rely primarily on intraoral radiographs, oral surgeons typically work from extraoral radiographs, such as panoramic films or cephalograms. The panoramic radiograph machine is rather large and

cumbersome and is usually placed in its own separate area.

Many oral surgery offices have separate recovery rooms where patients who have had conscious sedation or general anesthesia can wake up; these are often small rooms with a bed or cot. A small sink, suction, and oxygen must be easily available to aid the patient as the need arises.

The restroom and business office in this specialty are not unlike most general dental offices. Special attention should be given to making the restroom handicapped accessible and provide adequate room for a patient who needs assistance. This assistance is usually provided by the patient's family member, not by the dental assistant. Usually in the oral surgery business office the *checkout* area is slightly more private than in the general dental office. A separate private exit is advised for patients who have just had surgery, so that patients who are sitting in the reception area cannot see sedated patients, or those with gauze in their mouths, leaving the office.

Medical Evaluation

A detailed history and careful examination are essential to safe and effective patient treatment. Many oral surgeons schedule a separate patient appointment to review the health questionnaire, to expose and evaluate radiographs, and to examine the patient. At this appointment the informed consent can be discussed, providing the patient an opportunity to ask questions. Box 34-1 is an example of an informed consent for oral surgery. Also, other tests, such as blood studies, may need to be

BOX 34-1

INFORMED CONSENT FOR ORAL AND MAXILLOFACIAL SURGERY

Procedure: Extraction (removal) of teeth _____
Alternatives to surgery
I understand that if this tooth/teeth are not removed my condition may worsen, resulting in complications that include, but are not limited to, the following
1. Infection
2. Loss of additional teeth
3. Pain
Possible complications that have been explained to me are:
1. Dry socket
2. Infection
3. Swelling
4. Bleeding and bruising
5. Injury to adjacent teeth or fillings
6. Decision to leave a small piece of root in the jaw when its removal would require extensive surgery and increased risk of complications
7. _____
I have had the opportunity to discuss my surgery with Dr. _____ and to ask questions. I consent to surgery as described.

_____   _____
Patient, parent or guardian   Date

_____   _____
Doctor   Witness

ordered, and the oral surgeon may possibly want to confer with the patient's physician regarding the patient's health before he or she returns for surgery. The oral surgeon must try to achieve an optimal state of health in the patient, especially with elective surgery. In an emergency situation, the oral surgeon does not have the advantage of this separate appointment with the patient; however, the oral surgeon must still evaluate the patient carefully.

▶ Health Questionnaire

Usually, the first step in evaluating the patient is to have him or her fill out a health questionnaire (see Fig. 14-11). Information on this form allows the oral surgeon to quickly assess the patient's general state of health. The form is generally designed so that a healthy individual would answer "no" to each question, allowing the surgeon to rapidly skip to the areas that need greater attention. The form should provide space for the patient to write down his or her reason for the visit and to list any medical or dental problems not otherwise covered.

▶ Evaluating Heart and Lungs

The areas that are probably most important to evaluate are the patient's heart and lungs. Physician consultation is always recommended in situations where a patient has significant medical problems. Special considerations for patients with these conditions include the following:

1. A patient who has had a heart attack within the past 6 months is not a candidate for elective surgery, since the risk of further heart damage from secondary infections is significant.
2. Patients with heart disease of any sort are best handled in a low-stress environment, possibly with either oral or intravenous sedation. These appointments should be relatively short and are best scheduled in the morning. It is important to make sure that the patient takes all regularly scheduled medications on the morning of his or her appointment.
3. A patient with lung disease, such as asthma or tuberculosis, might best be treated with some nasal oxygen during the procedure.
4. Preventive medication, such as nitroglycerine for individuals who have angina or inhalers for those who have asthma, should be readily available during the procedure and in many cases should be given before the procedure for safety reasons.

Find out if the patient has a heart murmur. Even if it is a relatively mild murmur, it can put the patient at risk for subacute bacterial endocarditis (SBE) if it goes unrecognized and untreated. A heart murmur can indicate an underlying abnormality in the heart that can cause an irregular flow of blood through the heart. Any bacteria that invades the bloodstream during the oral surgery procedure will tend to lodge in the wall of the heart in the area of irregular blood flow, causing an infection that is difficult to treat and can even be life threatening. Bacterial endocarditis can in most cases be prevented by treatment with antibiotics, both before and after any procedure that could cause the invasion of bacteria into the bloodstream. The current recommendation of the American Heart Association for antibiotic prophylaxis (or preventive pretreatment) is to have the patient take 3 g of amoxicillin 1 hour before the dental procedure, and then follow up with 1½ g of amoxicillin 6 hours later. This antibiotic regimen should be followed any time an invasive procedure is scheduled. The dental assistant must ask the patient whether he or she took the premedication and at what hour. The antibiotic must have time to get into the bloodstream before the procedure is started. Ideally, this information should be written in the patient's chart to document that appropriate premedication was administered.

Hypertension

Patients with hypertension can be difficult to assess in the oral surgery office. Both anxiety and pain can increase a patient's blood pressure, and both are often present in patients who need oral surgery. Many patients only have an elevated blood pressure in situations of stress. To review blood pressure refer to Chapter 24.

Systemic Diseases

The history of kidney or liver diseases is important to dental treatment (see Chapter 24, *Oral Diagnosis*). In oral maxillofacial surgery these diseases can affect the way various drugs, including local anesthetics and antibiotics, are metabolized. Patients with these problems should be evaluated carefully before surgery. Medical consultation is often recommended. A patient who is undergoing kidney dialysis needs special protocols to schedule antibiotic doses and surgery at the most opportune time relative to his or her dialysis treatment.

Patients with kidney and liver diseases often have bleeding problems that must be taken into account when surgery is scheduled. Often, cardiac patients are taking medications, such as coumadin, that will thin the blood. Patients who have a history of bleeding problems or who are taking blood-thinning medication will need several blood tests before surgery to ensure that the blood will clot after surgery. Some medications may need to be discontinued 1 or 2 days before surgery. The drug that is probably the most likely to cause bleeding problems in the general dental population is aspirin. Many individuals fail to realize that even one aspirin that is taken 2 weeks before surgery can thin the blood enough to increase bleeding. Many individuals now take aspirin daily to reduce the risk of heart attacks or inflammation. Patients must be questioned specifically about aspirin use, since often they do not consider it a drug and do not list it as a daily medication on the health questionnaire.

Pregnancy

Pregnancy can be another relative contraindication to oral surgery. If it is at all possible, oral surgery should be postponed until the second trimester of the woman's pregnancy. During the first trimester the risk of spontaneous abortion and birth defects is increased. During the third trimester the stress of the procedure can bring about early labor. Obviously, in an emergency situation, such as a severe infection or a fractured jaw, these guidelines cannot be followed. The oral surgeon must work with the obstetrician to make the procedure as safe as possible for the woman and the fetus.

Diabetes

Diabetes is another systemic disease that can have an impact on oral surgical care. Diabetics who receive daily insulin injections are particularly important to evaluate before surgery. The amount of insulin a person takes depends on the number of ingested calories, which presents a problem, since the individual who needs oral surgery is often asked to fast before the procedure and often doesn't eat normally afterwards. In this unique situation the patient is scheduled early in the morning and is asked to take one half of the normal morning dose of insulin and to eat a light breakfast. In this way the blood sugar is unlikely to drop too low, since only half of the dose of insulin was given, and the patient may be able to eat soft food by lunch time. Insulin doses for the remainder of the day are determined by checking the blood glucose levels with finger sticks. Since those with diabetes are more susceptible to infections than other patients, many surgeons prefer to premedicate them with antibiotics. It is always imperative to consult with the patient's physician when a change is made in a drug regimen.

Other Drugs

As mentioned in Chapter 10, an important part of the health questionnaire deals with drugs that the patient takes routinely, particularly prescription and nonprescription drugs and alcohol. The surgeon must carefully evaluate the list of medications and decide whether the drugs might interact with those medications that will be used in surgery or in anesthesia. The patient must be warned about any possible interactions. For example, it has recently been shown that antibiotics can partially inactivate oral contraceptives; this should be made known to all women who are taking oral contraceptives and are also on an antibiotic regimen. Another example of this would be a patient who is taking a monoamine oxidase inhibitor—a drug that is used to treat depression; this drug causes individuals to be extremely sensitive to epinephrine and requires a change in local anesthetic.

Both alcohol and drug abuse can alter a patient's reaction to medications such as sedatives or even local anesthetics. Also, patients who are *recovering alcoholics,* or *chemical dependents* who are currently free of drugs may prefer to avoid using any narcotic medications, either during or after surgery. Often, these patients might choose to have a long-lasting local anesthetic injected, so that they need not take such strong analgesics after surgery.

▶ Allergies

Drug allergies are also noted on the health questionnaire. Some patients are overly cautious and say that they are allergic to a drug when it gives them an upset stomach. Other individuals may actually have an allergy to a medication that could be life threatening. The surgeon must carefully question each patient about his or her allergies to discover which ones are true allergies and which ones cause sensitivities to the patient, such as an upset stomach.

▶ Infectious Patient

Questions included on many surgeons' health questionnaires relate to infectious disease, such as HIV; this issue is a sensitive one. Since universal precautions should be practiced in all dental offices, the answer to this question should not cause a change in office procedure, other than possibly premedicating the patient with antibiotics to reduce the increased risk of infection. Since many HIV-positive patients experience discrimination, it is not unheard of for an HIV-positive person to state that he or she is negative, while others who have never been tested may not know their status. This is exactly why universal precautions are practiced. As with any patient's medical history, confidentiality must be maintained.

Radiographic Evaluation

At the preoperative appointment the oral surgeon usually directs the assistant to expose appropriate radiographs to evaluate the area that requires surgery. In most cases a panoramic radiograph is the most effective, since it covers a wide area (see Fig. 9-40). In addition to showing the teeth, the sinuses, the condyles of the mandible, and the inferior alveolar nerve are all revealed. It is often difficult to expose excellent periapical films of the third molar areas, since these teeth are often out of the line of occlusion. The panoramic radiograph clearly demonstrates these teeth, even when they are in extreme positions. When a single tooth or small area is to be visualized, a periapical film can be used. Occasionally, occlusal films, cephalograms, or other extraoral radiographs can also be used. For a review of dental radiographic techniques refer to Chapter 9.

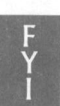

John M. Riggs is credited with extracting the first tooth under anesthesia; the tooth belonged to Horace Wells.

Anesthesia / Premedication / Sedation

Most patients who present themselves for oral surgery are anxious. For some individuals the only reason that they have come to the oral surgery office is because they are in pain. They may have neglected their teeth for years and avoided dental treatment. For these patients, try to make the procedure as easy as possible for them so that they may want to try some preventive treatment next time. Other individuals desire preventive treatment but are still frightened. Pain control and treatment of anxiety are therefore an important aspect of the oral surgeon's practice.

Patient anxiety is a factor that must be dealt with in a surgery practice, and this anxiety can sometimes be allayed by establishing rapport with the patient. The oral surgery assistant can play a significant role in this process by providing information and by maintaining a professional and caring manner in all patient interaction. The child patient may need to meet the surgeon and the staff at a time other than the surgery appointment to create a sense of trust and comfort as discussed in Chapter 36, *Pediatric Dentistry.*

Patient anxiety can be relieved through personal interaction; however, conventional anesthesia, premedication, and sedation techniques are also used to reduce anxiety. These techniques can be divided into the three following general classes: oral medications, inhaled gases, and intravenous medications. If a patient is to receive sedation, instructions need to be given at the consultation appointment before treatment (Box 34-2).

BOX 34-2

INSTRUCTIONS TO PATIENTS WHO DESIRE SEDATION

1. You may eat a light breakfast or lunch the day of your appointment, but please do not eat or drink anything 6 hours before your scheduled appointment time.
2. You may take prescription medication on the morning of your surgery appointment, unless otherwise instructed.
3. Please wear loose, comfortable clothing, with short sleeves. Do not wear high-heeled shoes.
4. You must have a responsible adult accompany you to the office to drive you home. You will not be able to drive for 24 hours. You may not leave the office alone, even in a taxi cab.
5. If you wear contact lenses, please remove them before you are seated for your surgery.

[Courtesy of Helen Zylman, D.D.S., Ann Arbor, Mich.]

Oral Medications

The oral premedications most commonly used can be classified as chloral derivatives, such as chloral hydrate; antihistamines, such as Atarax and Vistaril; or antianxiety agents, such as Valium. Oral medications are most often used with small children, although occasionally adults can benefit from them as well. These premedications can be administered by the parent at home before the appointment. Some surgeons prefer to have the parent administer the premedication when he or she arrives for the surgery appointment. The advantage of this method is that there is more supervision and help in case of an unusual reaction to the medication.

The advantage in using oral premedications is that they are easy to administer, even to a small child, and needles or syringes are not needed. Another advantage is that oral medication is less expensive than intravenous or inhaled medications. Fortunately, these medications are safe, and it is unusual for a patient to have a significant reaction to them. A disadvantage of oral medication is that the effects may be unpredictable. Unlike injectable premedication, oral medications are absorbed through the lining of the stomach. The rate of this absorption can be affected by the presence or the absence of food in the stomach and can even be affected by the patient's state of anxiety. At best, the medications take 45 minutes to 1 hour to take effect. If the medication affects the patient either too well or not well enough, it is difficult to remedy that problem in a timely fashion.

Inhaled Gases

This form of anesthesia for **conscious sedation**, an anesthetic procedure in which anesthesia and analgesia are accomplished without loss of consciousness, has a rapid onset and the patient recovers quickly. Different drugs are used in the administration of conscious sedation, and the choice is predicated on the patient's health history, physical examination, and the projected level of apprehension.

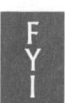 Horace Wells is credited as the first to use nitrous oxide as an anesthetic during surgery in 1844.

NITROUS OXIDE

A form of inhaled gas that is used in the anesthetic process is that of **nitrous oxide** or N_2O. Nitrous oxide is the most common anesthetic gas used in the dental office, and it was one of the first anesthetics used to provide comfort to the patient. Another substance that was used as an inhaled gas at the time nitrous oxide was developed is ether. Before the use of nitrous oxide or

ether, alcohol and opium were used as a means of anesthesia.

Nitrous oxide can be used as an analgesic gas alone, or it can be used in conjunction with other inhaled or injected agents. Nitrous oxide is a sweet-smelling gas that affects patients within 2 to 5 minutes after breathing it, rather than the hour or more required by oral premedication. It results in a pleasant, somewhat disoriented, feeling that is often accompanied by a sensation of numbness.

Nitrous oxide is sometimes referred to as *laughing gas* by the lay person, since some patients start to giggle within a few minutes after breathing the gas, although a small number of individuals paradoxically start to cry after inhaling it.

In addition to having a much more rapid onset of symptoms than are seen with oral sedatives, nitrous oxide can also be titrated to a desired effect. **Titration** refers to the ability of the surgeon to administer small amounts of medication periodically, until the patient is nicely relaxed. The oral surgeon or the delegated team member administers the gas until the patient reaches the desired state of relaxation and reduced anxiety, usually within 3 to 5 minutes. The dosage is then adjusted to maintain that same level for the patient. Unlike oral sedatives the depth of sedation can rapidly be adjusted upward or downward to achieve the required result. When the dental procedure is over, the patient inhales 100% oxygen for approximately 5 minutes and quickly recovers. Once the patient is feeling normal again, he or she is allowed to leave the office unescorted. With oral medication the patient might be sedated for hours after the procedure has been completed and must always be accompanied by another adult driver. Box 34-3 examines the levels of nitrous oxide that can be administered and the patient's response.

BOX 34-3

LEVELS OF NITROUS OXIDE VERSUS PATIENT REACTION

10% to 15% Nitrous oxide — produces limited numbness in extremities, sedation, and tingling

35% to 40% Nitrous oxide — sedative effects are increased; analgesic effect is that of 15 mg of administered morphine; sensation of heaviness or of floating; room noises sound distant

50% Nitrous oxide — intensified analgesic symptoms; patient becomes increasingly sleepy and may become unconscious; this is a dangerous state of general anesthesia

One disadvantage of nitrous oxide is that the patient must be able to breathe through the nose for the gas to be effective, since it is administered by a nasal mask; it doesn't work well with individuals who have a cold or who are mouth breathers. In addition, certain individuals may become nauseated by the gas, especially if it is administered at a high level or for a long period of time.

The administration of nitrous oxide is primarily the responsibility of the dentist, but in some states this duty is delegated to the hygienist. In certain states the dental assistant is delegated the responsibility of monitoring the administration of nitrous oxide to the patient.

Nitrous oxide is always administered with oxygen. Normal room air contains about 20% oxygen. Any anesthetic gas that is administered must have at least as much oxygen as room air; because of this, many nitrous oxide machines are made to be *fail safe*. The system is manufactured so that it is impossible to administer any more than 70% nitrous oxide and, therefore, also impossible to administer any less than 30% oxygen. If for some reason the oxygen tank becomes empty and this circumstance is not recognized, the nitrous oxide machine turns itself off rather than deliver 100% nitrous oxide. In this way the patient always receives at least as much oxygen as he or she needs, and the risk to the patient is greatly reduced. Nitrous oxide is administered to the patient through a disposable or sterilizable mask that covers the nose only (Fig. 34-3). Since the patient sometimes continues to breath through the mouth (especially if he or she is talking), most nitrous oxide machines are equipped with scavenging equipment that suctions the exhaled gases from around the patient's mouth and evacuates these gases into the central suction for the office; thus

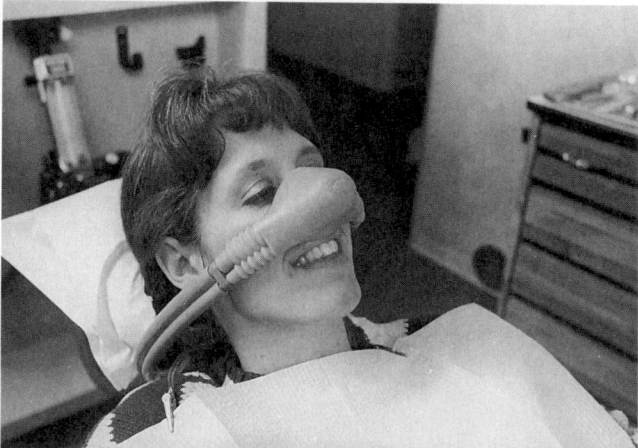

FIG. 34-3   Disposable or sterilizable mask is placed securely over patient's nose to administer nitrous oxide.

(Courtesy of Helen Zylman, D.D.S., Ann Arbor, Michigan.)

the administration of the nitrous oxide gases is a bit safer, not for the patient, but for the staff, since recent reports suggests a relationship between nitrous oxide and spontaneous miscarriage.

Nitrous oxide must be used only under the direct supervision of the oral surgeon. The assistant may help to place the mask before the procedure and may remove it after the procedure has been completed and after the patient has been breathing 100% oxygen for 5 to 10 minutes. In some states the law requires that the assistant should not be left alone with a patient who is breathing the gas and is not allowed to adjust the dose. The assistant is also responsible for turning on the tanks of oxygen and nitrous oxide in the morning and turning them off again in the evening, checking the level of the gases in the tanks. A backup oxygen tank always should be available. Many offices have an alarm system that sounds when the level of the gases is too low, indicating that the tanks need to be switched. In addition, the assistant is responsible to ensure that the scavenging system is always functional.

Nitrous oxide can be classified as an *analgesic* rather than an anesthetic gas. It helps to relieve mild pain sensations, but administration of local anesthesia is required to ensure that the procedure is totally painless. Some oral surgeons use other anesthetic gases that render the patient unconscious; this procedure is usually performed in a hospital setting. These agents are actually supplied to the oral surgeon in liquid form; however, when the liquid is introduced into the anesthesia machine, it is converted into a gas inside of a vaporizer and is then mixed with oxygen and possibly nitrous oxide. This mixture of gases is then delivered to the patient through a flow meter, which carefully controls the ratio of gases and the rate of delivery. Some of the general anesthetic gases are halothane (Fluothane), enflurane (Ethrane), and isoflurane (Forane). These agents are usually administered in a slightly different modality than the nitrous oxide. Usually, with a general anesthetic gas an endotracheal tube is placed through the patient's nose or mouth and into the windpipe or trachea. **Endotracheal** means inside the trachea. The anesthetic gases are administered through this tube in a controlled fashion.

Sometimes, the anesthesia is light enough that the patient is still breathing on his or her own; but sometimes, the oral surgeon actually has to help the patient breathe by squeezing a breathing bag. This type of system holds less risk of exposure to exhaled gases for the dental team, since the gases go directly from the patient's lungs into the anesthesia machine and are disposed of without being discharged into the treatment room. Because the patient is unconscious and is using artificial respiration, the risk is significantly greater for the patient than it is when nitrous oxide is used and the patient is conscious and breathing on his or her own. Because this system is so complex and because the risk is greater, a second individual, usually the anesthesiologist (other than the treating surgeon), administers the anesthesia.

▶ Intravenous (IV) Administration

The final technique that is discussed here to provide patient comfort and to relieve anxiety is the technique of **intravenous administration**, that is, injecting anesthetic drugs into a vein. The most common types of drugs used for this purpose today are narcotics, such as Demerol; sedative-hypnotics, such as Versed; or ultra short-acting barbiturates, such as Brevital. These medications can be used in various ways to result in either conscious sedation, where the patient has a rational response to commands with unassisted breathing, or in general anesthesia, where the patient is actually unconscious during the procedure. The latter technique is usually warranted when a patient is extremely anxious or when the ailment is difficult to treat because of the patient's physical or mental condition. This form of anesthesia depresses the central nervous system and alters the level of consciousness. Depressed levels of consciousness can result in depression of vital functions or can trigger cardiac arrhythmias. Arthur E. Guedel, an American anesthesiologist, developed a system that describes the accepted stages of anesthesia. The stages of anesthesia that are described in Box 34-4 can assist the operator in observing signs that the patient may exhibit during treatment.

Usually, local anesthetic is administered in conjunction with conscious sedation or general anesthesia; this is mandatory with conscious sedation, since the patient would still be able to feel pain without the local anesthesia. Local anesthesia is often administered in conjunction with general anesthesia, since it reduces the depth of general anesthesia that is necessary to make the patient comfortable. The epinephrine in local anesthesia helps to control bleeding, and as the patient recovers from the procedure, there is no sudden burst of pain.

The techniques of intravenous conscious sedation and general anesthesia can also be combined. Some surgeons prefer to have the patient unconscious through difficult times, such as when local anesthesia is administered, and then the level of anesthesia is lowered, so that the patient is merely sedated for the rest of the procedure.

One significant advantage of using intravenous anesthesia over oral medication is the rapid onset of action of most intravenous medications. Most often, a patient reacts within 20 to 30 seconds as the medication reaches the central nervous system, as opposed to the 45 minutes to 1 hour that it takes for the oral medication to become effective. This time lapse allows the surgeon to titrate the amount of anesthesia to a certain result. This technique is different from the technique that uses oral medication,

---

BOX 34-4

GUEDEL'S SIGNS

Stage 1 — (amnesia and analgesia) begins with the administration of an anesthetic and continues until the patient has lost consciousness; respiration is quiet, sometimes irregular; reflexes are still present

Stage 2 — (delirium or excitement) begins when the patient has lost consciousness and with the onset of total anesthesia; the patient may move the limbs, chatter incoherently, hold the breath, or become violent; vomiting, with possible danger of aspiration, may occur

Stage 3 — (surgical anesthesia) begins with stable breathing patterns and total loss of consciousness; first signs of respiratory or cardiovascular failure appears

    Plane 1 — all movement ceases, and respiration is regular; eyeball movements are marked

    Plane 2 — eyeballs are fixed centrally; respiration remains regular

    Plane 3 — pupils no longer react to light; total muscle relaxation occurs; intercostal paralysis, or paralysis between the ribs is present

    Plane 4 — deep anesthesia occurs; no spontaneous respiration; sensation is absent

Stage 4 — (premortem) signals danger; pupils are dilated to a maximum, and the skin is cold and ashen; blood pressure is extremely low; brachial pulse is feeble or absent; cardiac arrest is imminent

---

where the doctor must approximate the amount of medication to prescribe for the desired result.

Probably the greatest advantage of intravenous medication using either a sedative-hypnotic, such as Versed, or general anesthesia is that the patient has amnesia and has no recollection of the procedure. Even if the patient is carrying on a conversation during the procedure, he or she won't remember any part of it when it is over.

One disadvantage of intravenous techniques is that the patient must be monitored much more carefully, since the patient cannot communicate his or her state of health. The patient cannot protect his own airway and extra precautions must be taken to make sure that the patient does not choke. Also, the more medications that are given, the greater is the likelihood that a patient will have a reaction to one of the medications.

▶ Monitoring Vital Signs

To make the procedure as safe as possible, the patient's vital signs must be monitored regularly. The blood pressure must be assessed frequently throughout the procedure with an automatic blood pressure monitor, so that the assistant does not break the chain of asepsis; this eliminates the need to change gloves every time the blood pressure is taken. Since the patient's level of breathing may be depressed, the amount of oxygen in the patient's bloodstream and his or her respirations must also be evaluated throughout the procedure with a **pulse oximeter**, a photoelectric apparatus that determines the amount of oxygen in the blood. It is also helpful for the surgeon to have an **electrocardiogram (ECG)** strip that runs throughout the procedure to warn of unusual heart action. The ECG is a record of electrical activity of the heart.

In addition to the use of just conscious sedation or of intravenous general anesthesia, some surgeons add some nitrous oxide and oxygen along with the sedation, which is administered before the IV is started, helping the patient to relax for that procedure. This is helpful for the following reasons: (1) the combination of the two methods helps to keep the patient sleepier during the procedure; (2) because the effect of the nitrous oxide can be eliminated in less than 5 minutes with the introduction of oxygen, it helps the patient to awaken faster after the procedure is completed; and (3) it also gives the dentist more control over the anesthesia during the procedure; if the patient becomes too sedated, the nitrous oxide is turned down or off and the patient will begin to *lighten up* or awaken slightly. This technique is preferable to reversing the medication by giving another drug intravenously to provide a countereffect to the first drug. The patient breathing nitrous oxide and oxygen and is always breathing a minimum level of oxygen (as in room air or more pure air); this method helps to ensure that enough oxygen is getting to the brain in cases where the patient's breathing might be slightly decreased from normal.

The assistant aids in the administration of intravenous general anesthesia and conscious sedation. After the patient is escorted into the treatment room, the assistant connects the monitors to the patient. Fig. 34-4 shows a patient who is attached to a pulse oximeter and an ECG machine with an automatic blood pressure monitor. The

pulse oximeter is the easiest monitor to apply. The patient places one finger in the finger clip that is attached by cord to the machine. A small red light within the finger clip can read the amount of oxygen in the bloodstream of the patient through the thin skin at the finger tip. Fingernail polish is not a contraindication to use of the pulse oximeter and does not affect the readings from the machine.

BLOOD PRESSURE MONITORING

The automatic blood pressure cuff is applied as a manual blood pressure cuff. The assistant needs to judge the size of the patient's arm (a variety of cuff sizes are available) and then must make sure that the blood pressure cuff is tight around the patient's arm. The wrist clips—plastic clips that fit snugly over the patient's wrist—are applied. Small metal plates in the clips pick up an electrical signal from the patient's pulse and transmit it through the wires to the EKG machine, where this electrical activity is displayed on a screen. In a hospital setting the patient must undress and have adhesive patches applied to the chest rather than the wrist. The newer machines for outpatient surgery now use wrist clips, which are much more convenient for staff and patients. To ensure that a clear electrical signal is received, a conductive spray must be used to moisten the patient's wrists before the clips are placed. Reassure the patient that some of the movement that is seen on the ECG screen is caused by artifact, or movement, and does not indicate that the heart is malfunctioning. Describe the extra marks as being similar to static on the radio—an image that most people can understand.

PREPARATION OF THE IV

The assistant must also prepare the IV bag and draw up the medications. IV bags come in several sizes: most commonly 250 ml, 500 ml, and 1000 ml. The IV bag is sealed and stored in a plastic overwrap. The steps in setting up the IV include:

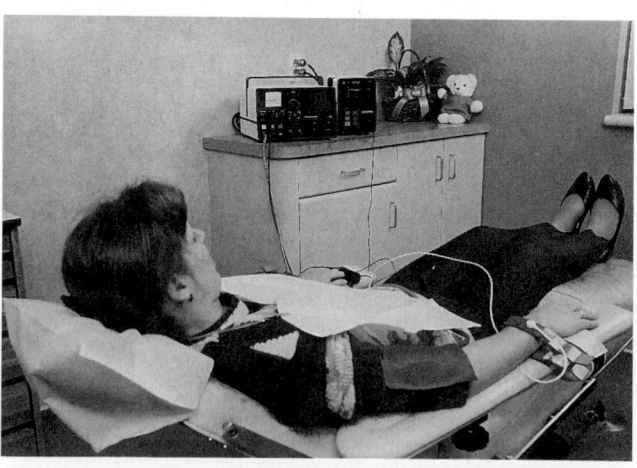

FIG. 34-4   Patient is attached to monitors.

(Courtesy of Helen Zylman, D.D.S., Ann Arbor, Michigan.)

PREPARING THE IV BAG

1. Open the overwrap and remove the sterile IV bag. With the port end of the bag held upside down so that the fluid cannot leak out, pull the seal from the neck of the bag.
2. Remove the protective cover from the pointed end of the drip chamber of the IV tubing set, and with a twisting motion insert it into the port of the IV bag (Fig. 34-5).

3. Turn the bag so that the port and the IV tubing are at the bottom. Place the bag on the stand. Gently squeeze the drip chamber of the IV tubing, filling it about half full (Fig. 34-6).
4. Remove the protective cover of the opposite end of the IV tubing, and allow the fluid to flow through the tube. When the fluid reaches the end, tighten the adjustable clamp to stop the flow. Then replace the protective cover over the end, until the tubing is attached to the IV needle that is placed in the patient's arm.

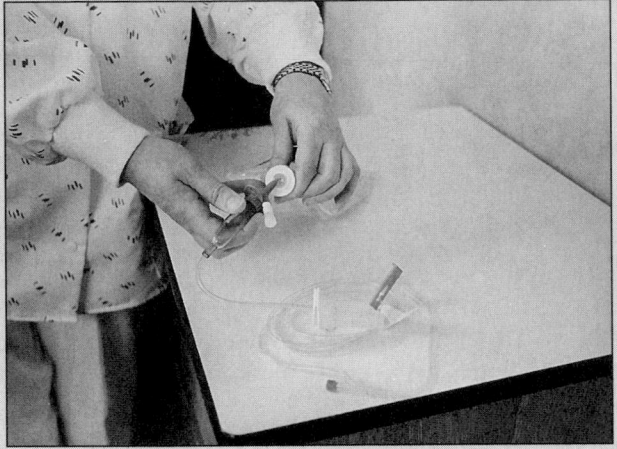

FIG. 34-5   After the IV bag is opened the IV tubing is inserted into the bag.

(Courtesy of Helen Zylman, D.D.S., Ann Arbor, Michigan.)

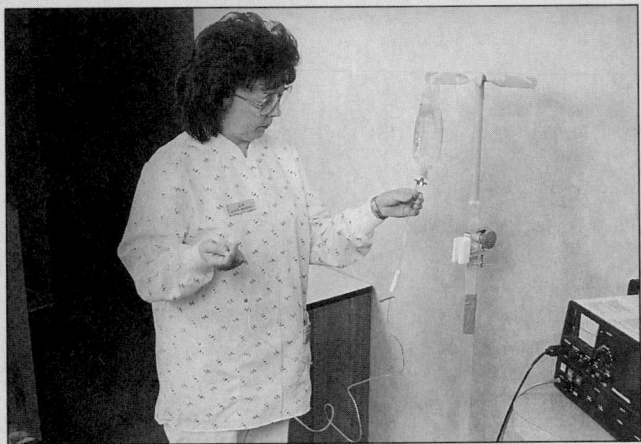

FIG. 34-6   IV is placed on stand, and drip chamber is checked.

(Courtesy of Helen Zylman, D.D.S., Ann Arbor, Michigan.)

MEDICATION PREPARATION

The assistant also prepares the medication syringes. Some oral surgeons use manufacturers' prefilled syringes, but most use multidose vials and draw up set amounts of medications into each syringe. It is important that each syringe be labeled so that the medications are not mistakenly administered (Fig. 34-7). The syringes and medications should be kept in a locked cupboard for protection and when it is specified by law. When a medication syringe is prepared, the assistant should first check the expiration date of the medication, read the label before filling the syringe, and recheck the label again after filling the syringe to ensure that the proper medication has been prepared. To prepare medications from a multidose vial, observe the following suggested steps:

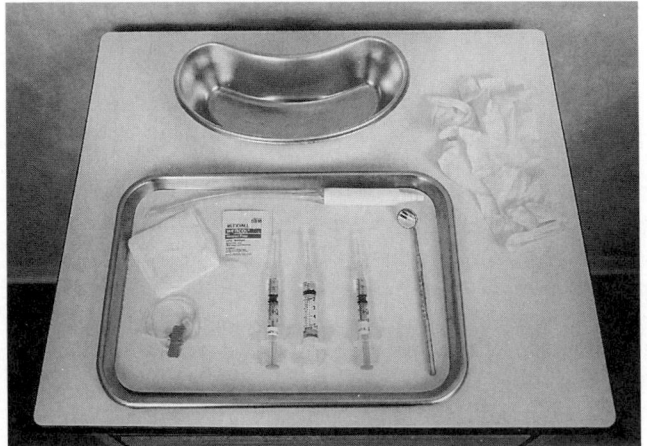

FIG. 34-7   Drug syringes are assembled with labels.

(Courtesy of Helen Zylman, D.D.S., Ann Arbor, Michigan.)

PREPARING MEDICATION FROM A MULTIDOSE VIAL

1. Wipe the rubber diaphragm on the top of the vial with an alcohol sponge, and dry it with a sterile sponge.
2. To withdraw liquid from the vial, which is under a vacuum, inject air into the vial; to accomplish this, pull back the plunger of the syringe until it reaches the specific gradation mark that indicates the proper amount of medication to be used. In other words, if the syringe is to be filled with 3 cc of medication, withdraw the plunger to the 3 cc mark.
3. Hold the vial with the diaphragm facing the floor, and remove the needle cap. Do not touch the sterile end of the needle. Pierce the rubber diaphragm.
4. After the top of the vial is pierced with the needle and with the vial still in an inverted position, push down on the plunger, thus injecting 3 cc of air into the vial.
5. Pull back on the plunger again, withdraw the desired amount of medication to fill the syringe.
6. If bubbles enter the chamber, remove them by gently tapping the syringe, with the needle end of the syringe pointing upward, sending the bubbles to the top of the medication. Then expel the bubbles by slightly pressing the plunger forward.
7. After the syringe is filled, withdraw the needle from the vial, and place the cap back over the needle again.
8. To avoid accidental needle sticks, a recapping device or the one-handed scoop technique should be used to assist in this process.
9. If additional medication is needed, the process is repeated, filling a sterile syringe each time.

Surgical Instruments

The oral surgeon uses a number of instruments that are also used in general practice, such as mouth mirrors and cotton pliers. A vast majority of instruments are unique to surgery. Most surgical instruments have polished working ends of stainless steel. The handle of the instrument is textured, so that the oral surgeon will be able to maintain a firm grasp on the instrument during the procedure.

This portion of the chapter describes a number of commonly used surgical instruments. A comprehensive list of all surgical instruments is virtually impossible. Oral surgeons usually have a few instruments that are commonly used. The oral surgery assistant must become familiar with the instruments used in the practice. Look carefully at each instrument as it is being cleaned and

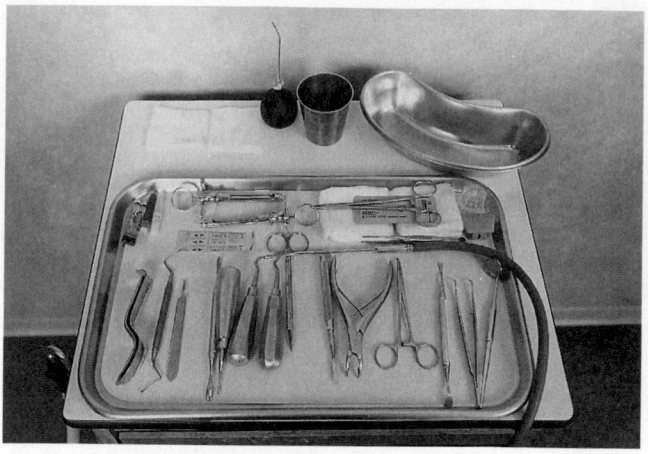

FIG. 34-8 Typical surgical tray set-up.
(Courtesy of Helen Zylman, D.D.S., Ann Arbor, Michigan.)

sterilized. One other way of becoming familiar with the surgical instruments is to look through an instrument catalog. The pictures of the instruments are usually shown at half size, and it is easy to see the similarities and the differences between the different styles.

Surgical Tray Set-up

Fig. 34-8 shows a typical tray set-up for the surgical extraction of a tooth. Some surgeons have a smaller tray that is used just for simple extractions. Simple extractions with complications, such as root fracture, may turn into a complex or a surgical extraction, thus making it easier to have one basic tray set-up for dental extractions of all types. The description of the instruments basically follows the order in which they are used. Just as in general dentistry, it is helpful to have the instruments arranged in a sequential order. An instrument can be found on an organized tray more easily than it can on a tray where the instruments are in disarray. The following instruments and descriptions are those that are common to a basic surgical tray set-up.

Anesthetic Syringes

The first instrument is the anesthetic syringe. Almost all dentists today use aspirating syringes to prevent injection of anesthetic into the blood vessels as described in Chapter 23. If both long and short injection needles are used, it is helpful to have two syringes set up, one with each length of needle. Enough anesthetic carpules should be set out for the planned procedure, with additional carpules available nearby for patients who require extra anesthesia.

▶ HVE Hosing and Tips

HVE tubing and the aspirator tip are vital devices that are used in the surgical procedure. The typical HVE hose used in general dentistry does not work well in the oral surgery practice. The hose itself is too heavy and inflexible to be used easily for surgical procedures. Surgical HVE tubing can be sterilized, unlike the typical HVE hose in the general dental office. The **surgical HVE** or **aspirator tip** is also different than the standard HVE tip. The orifice or opening at the end of most surgical HVE tips is smaller, only a few millimeters in diameter. The surgical tip may be fabricated from metal or disposable plastic. A variety of sizes and shapes are available. One particular type of HVE tip that should always be available is the Yankauer or tonsil suction tip; this has a larger diameter at the tip, but it is rounded so that it will not lacerate the fragile tissue of the throat. The Yankauer suction tip is used to clean out the throat if a patient is choking, or if he or she has vomited and it is necessary to prevent choking (Fig. 34-9).

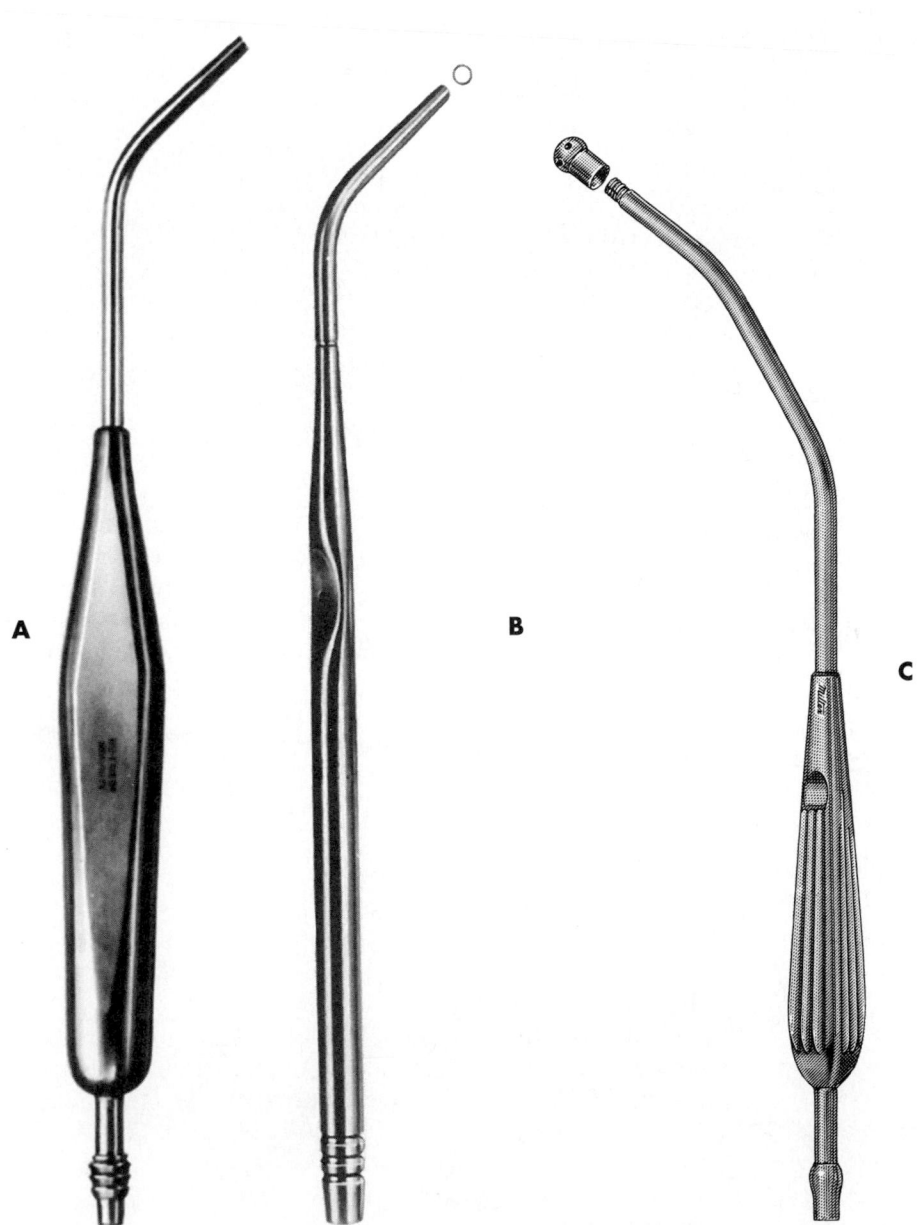

FIG. 34-9 Variety of surgical aspirators. *A,* Coupland. *B,* Cogswell. *C,* Yankauer.

(*A* and *B* courtesy of Hu Friedy; *C* courtesy of Miltex.)

▶ Retractors

Lip and cheek retractors provide clear vision for the oral surgeon. Some oral surgeons prefer to use the mouth mirror for retraction of the cheek. Unfortunately, the thin handle of the mouth mirror can pull on a patient's lip, sometimes resulting in a cut or bruised lip. Some oral surgeons use the periosteal elevator (to be described later) for retraction of the tissues. Because this instrument has a thin handle and a small working surface,

trauma to the tissues may result; it does not protect the tissue as well. One retractor with a broad base and handle that seems to work well is the University of Minnesota retractor. The right angle bend in the handle keeps the retractor out of the line of vision. Various lip, cheek, tongue, and tissue retractors are available (see Fig. 34-10, *A* and *B*), and each surgeon probably has one or two favorites. A mouth prop may be needed when a patient is unable to cooperate, especially if the patient is sedated. Examples of two types of props are shown in Fig. 34-11.

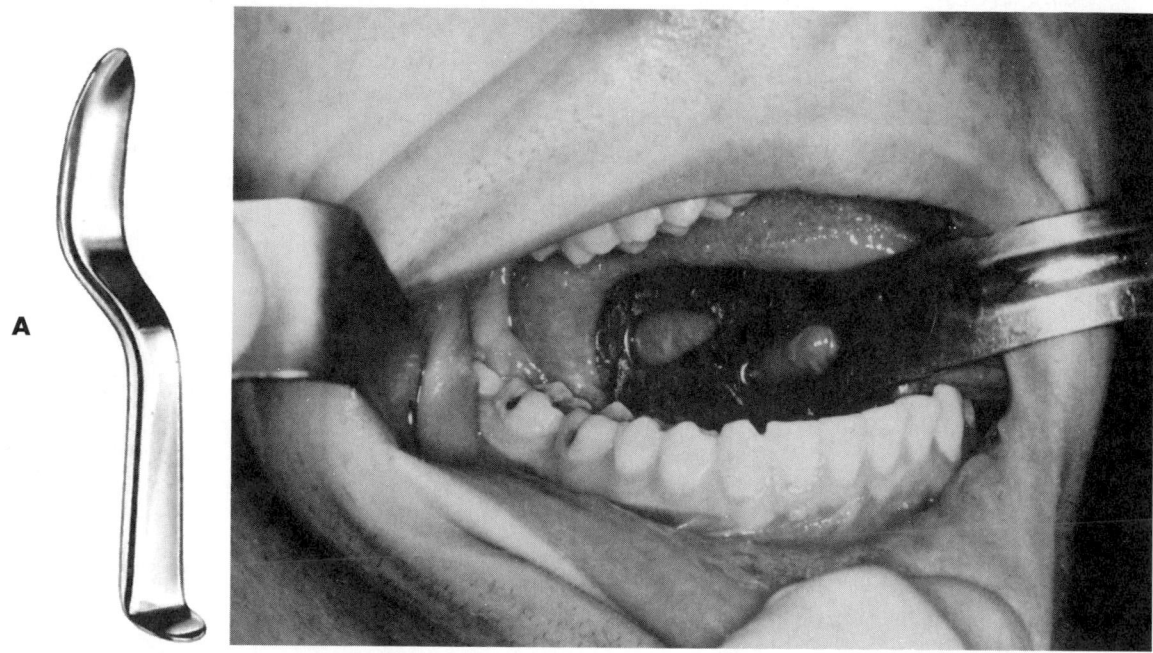

FIG. 34-10 *A*, Tongue and cheek retractor. *B*, Retractor in place.

(*A* courtesy of Hu Friedy; *B* from Peterson LJ, Hupp J, Ellis III E, Tucker M: *Contemporary oral and maxillofacial surgery*, ed 2, St Louis, 1992, Mosby.)

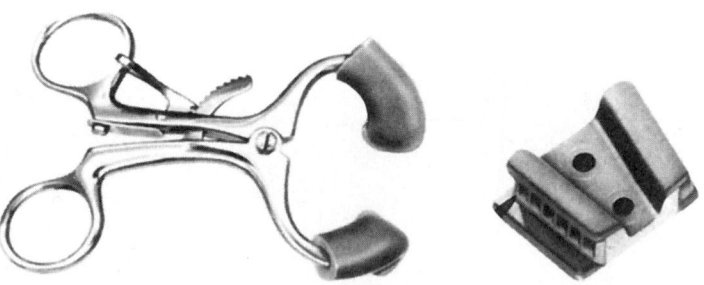

FIG. 34-11 Mouth props.

(Courtesy of Hu Friedy.)

▶ Scalpels

A **scalpel**, a thin sharp blade that is used to make a cut or incision, is common to most surgical tray set-ups. Most surgeons today use reusable and sterilizable scalpel handles, with disposable sterile scalpel blades. To remove a scalpel blade safely, a scalpel blade remover is used. A wide variety of blades and handles are available, depending on the needs and desires of the surgeon.

Blades can be short, long, curved, or straight. Four common blade sizes and shapes are #11, #12, #12B, and #15. The letter *B* beside the number denotes that both edges of the blade have a cutting surface. Some surgeons prefer a round handle, while others prefer a flat handle. The type of blade and handle that are used may vary from case to case, depending on accessibility and preference. Variations of these devices are shown in Fig. 34-12.

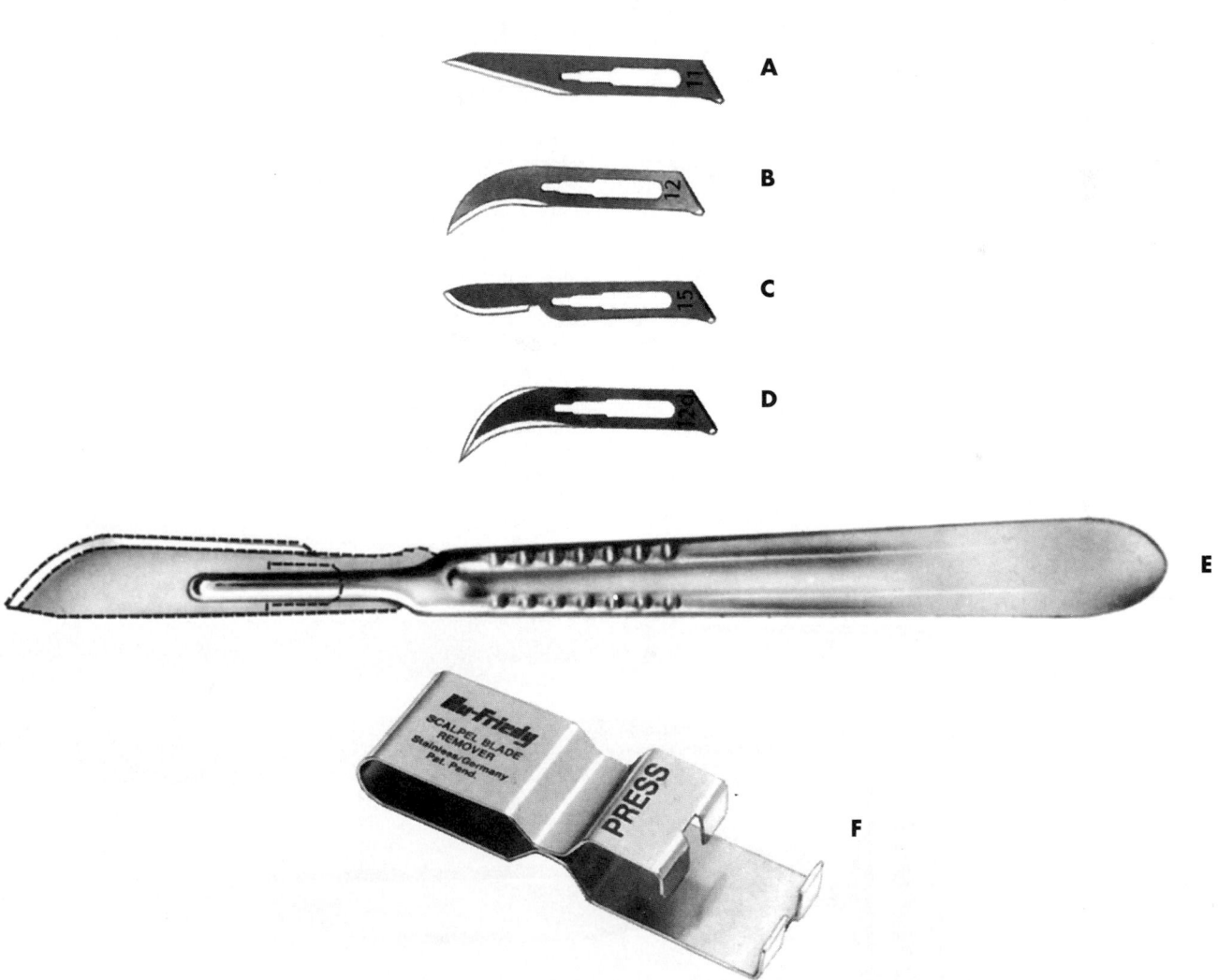

FIG. 34-12 Surgical blades and handles. *A,* #11 blade. *B,* #12 blade. *C,* #15 blade. *D,* 12 B blade (double-sided). *E,* Sterilizable scalpel handle (removable scalpel blade). *F,* Scalpel blade remover.

(Courtesy of Hu Friedy.)

▶ Periosteal Elevator

Once an incision has been made, a **periosteal elevator** is used to reflect, pull away, or detach and lift the tissue (including the periosteum) from the bone. There are several types of periosteal elevators. Most have one sharp and one rounded end (Fig. 34-13). The sharp ends are used to scrape the tissue away from the bone. Some oral surgeons also use the periosteal elevator to retract tissue. The surgeon will place the periosteal elevator between the soft tissue to protect the tissue from injury.

▶ Chisels

Chisels are instruments that are often used to remove bone from around an impacted tooth. If the bone is soft, as it is over an impacted maxillary third molar that is close to the surface, the chisel can be used along with finger pressure. Where the bone is more calcified, such as around mandibular third molars, a **mallet** may be used to tap the end of the chisel to remove the bone. Chisels and mallets are also used to split teeth. Chisels can either be single beveled, with one flat side and one sharp angled side, or bi-beveled, with two sharp angled sides. Chisels and a mallet are shown in Fig. 34-14, *A* through *C*.

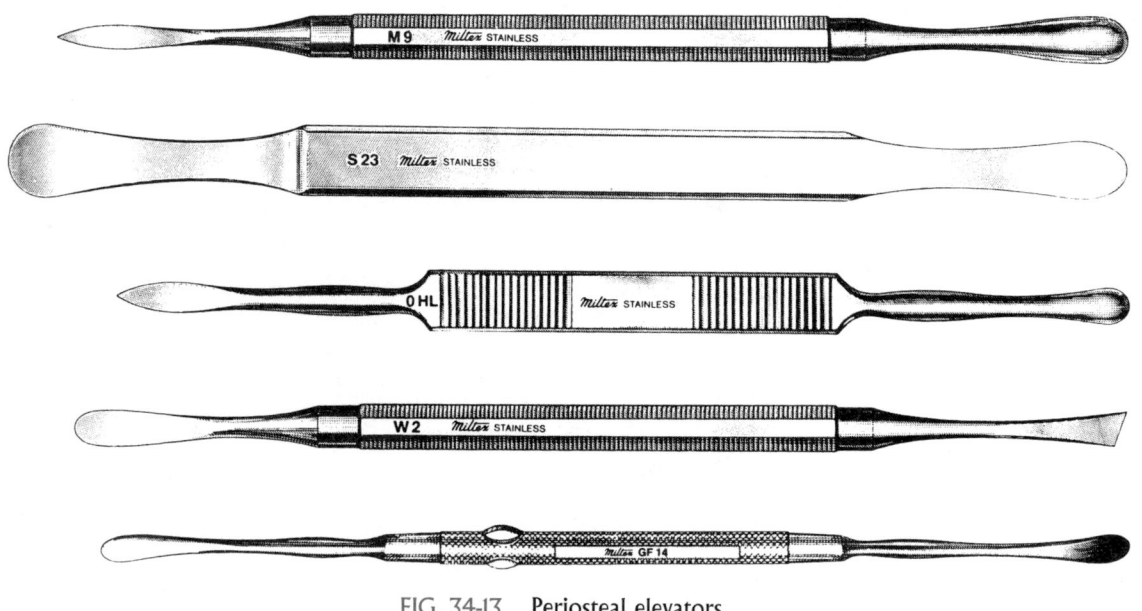

FIG. 34-13   Periosteal elevators.
(Courtesy of Miltex.)

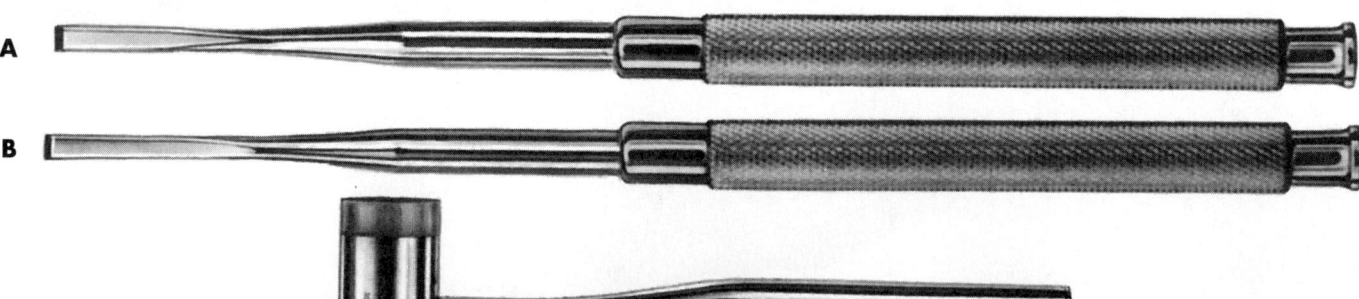

FIG. 34-14   Chisels. *A,* Single. *B,* Bi-beveled. *C,* Mallet.
(Courtesy of Hu Friedy.)

▶ Elevators

Dental elevators are the workhorses of the surgical extraction tray. Although forceps are used routinely to **luxate** (loosen) erupted teeth, most of the time they cannot be used for removal of impacted teeth or fractured roots. Even when teeth are fully erupted, elevators are often used to help loosen the structural attachment around the tooth. The elevator is wedged between the tooth to be extracted and the adjacent bone. It is then rotated, using the bone as a fulcrum, without pushing on the adjacent teeth, to compress the space between the

tooth and the bone. The elevator is also often used, rather than the mallet and chisel, to split teeth. In this situation a groove is made part of the way through the tooth, using a handpiece and a bur. The elevator is then put into that groove and rotated, thus completing the fracture of the tooth.

Elevators can be divided into two major classes, straight and angled. The angled elevators are usually used as a pair, a right and a left. The surgeon may alternate between right and left to remove the tooth. Fig. 34-15 illustrates a number of different types of elevators, both single and paired. As it is with many other types of

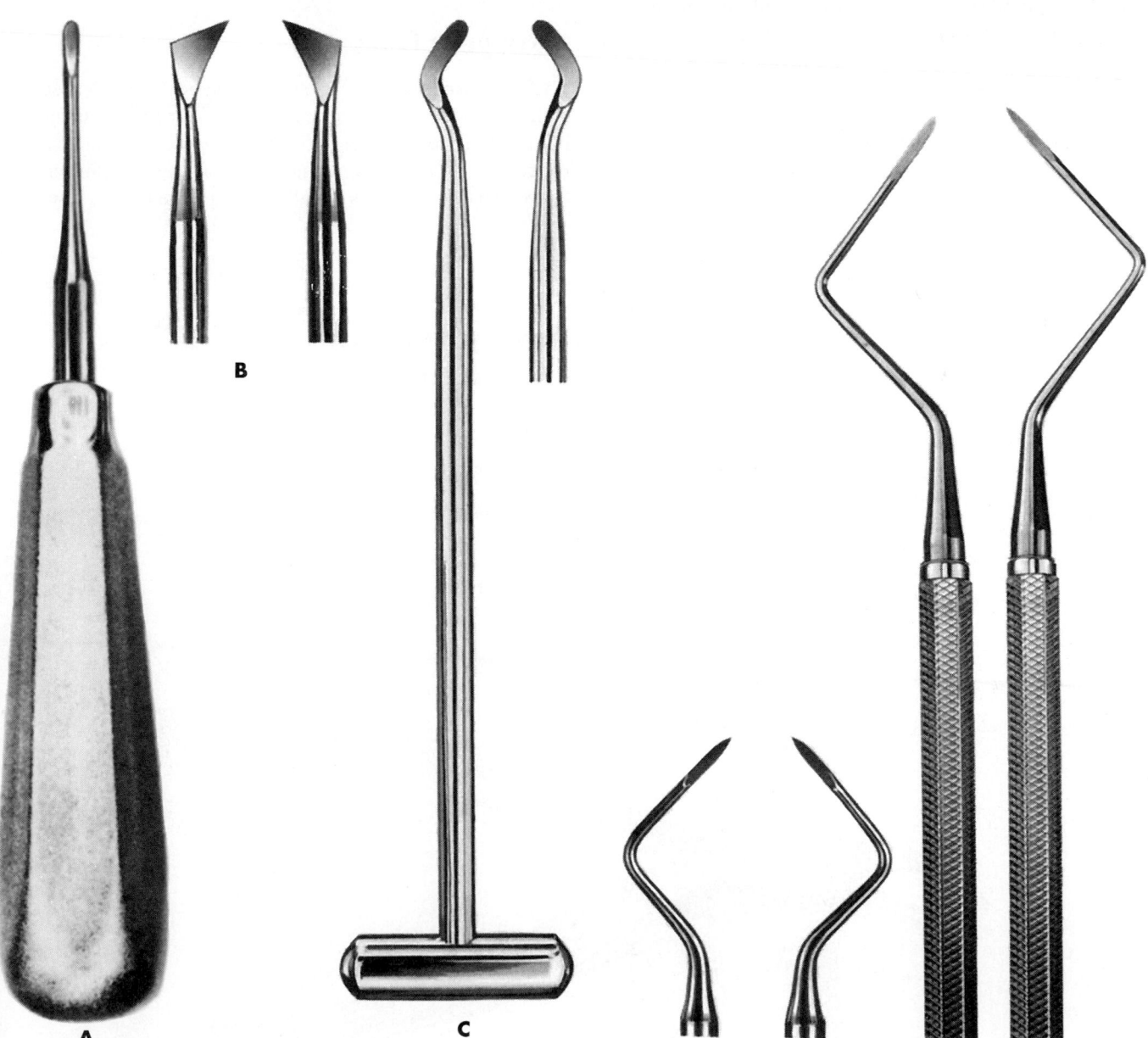

FIG. 34-15   Variety of dental elevators. *A,* Straight. *B,* Cryer, paired. *C,* Potts, paired.

(*A* through *C* courtesy of Hu Friedy).

FIG. 34-16   Two styles of root tip elevators or picks.

(Courtesy of Hu Friedy.)

surgical instruments, a large variety is available, and each assistant needs to be familiar with the types of elevators that are used in the practice. Some oral surgeons refer to an elevator by manufacturer's number, while others refer to it by the name of the individual who designed it. For example, Potts elevators are also known as #6 and #7, while Cryer elevators have three sets of numbers, depending on the size of the tip. Examples of the numbers are #30 and #31, #39 and #40, #34 and #34 S.

Root tip elevators or root tip picks are similar to dental elevators but usually are much thinner and finer (Fig. 34-16) and are available in right and left pairs. The angulation of these paired root picks allows easier access to root tips in confined areas. They can range in size from substantial for large fractured roots to extremely fine for smaller root fragments. It should be noted that these instruments are designed to tease fractured root tips out of sockets and not to expand the bone as do the elevators. The root tip picks are much less substantial, can be bent, and may break if too much pressure is used.

▶ Surgical Curette

After a tooth has been removed from a socket, the socket must be cleared of tissue fragments and infected material, such as abscesses. A **surgical** or **bone curette** is used for this purpose. Surgical curettes are similar to periodontal curettes because the blade of the instrument is sharp; however, the shape of the blade is much different. Surgical curettes are usually double ended, like the periodontal curette; they usually have a round tip that is used to scoop material out of dental sockets. The ends are polished steel and range from rather small to rather large. Surgical curettes are shown in Fig. 34-17.

▶ Rongeur Forceps

The **rongeur forceps** is also used to remove excess tissue from around the site of an extracted tooth; but it can also be used to remove or to contour excess bone. The rongeur is an instrument that looks similar to a forceps; however, the handle is usually spring loaded. The edges

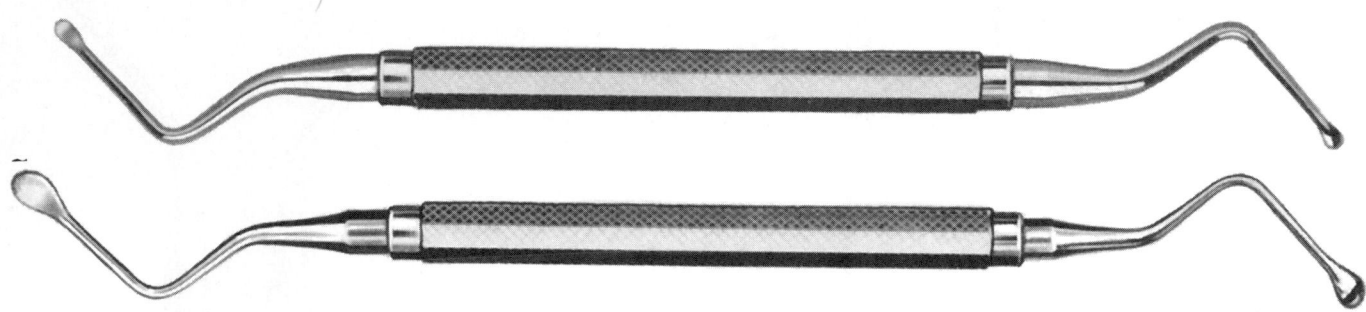

FIG. 34-17   Two styles of surgical curettes.
(Courtesy of Hu Friedy.)

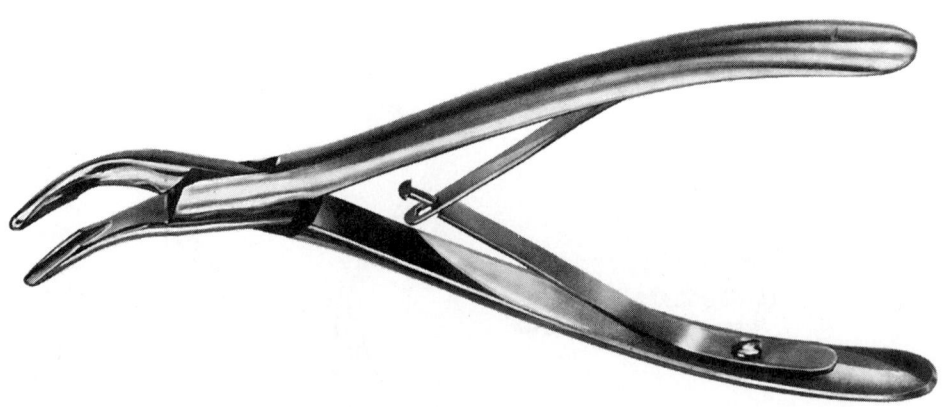

FIG. 34-18   Rongeur forceps.
(Courtesy of Hu Friedy.)

of the beaks are sharp and are used to tug tissue away from bone and to nip sharp edges of the bone to smooth it. The rongeur is particularly useful in preparing an alveolar ridge for dentures after extractions. Fig. 34-18 shows a rongeur forceps.

▶ Bone Files

A **bone file** is used after the rongeur to smooth the sharp edges of the alveolar ridge. This process helps to seat future dentures and to prevent sharp fragments of bone from working through the tissue at a later time. Most bone files are double ended and usually have files of differing sizes on each end. A bone file can be seen in Fig. 34-19.

▶ Surgical Scissors

Scissors are used routinely in oral surgery. The most common use for the scissors is to cut sutures. In addition, scissors are used to undermine tissue or to spread it away from other tissue; they are also used to trim tissue, rather than using a scalpel blade. Surgical scissors are available in sizes ranging from 4 inches to 7 inches long. The scissors tips can be blunt, sharp, curved, or straight or many combinations of the above. Sometimes more than one set of scissors are needed: perhaps a small, sharp, curved scissors for undermining tissue or a larger scissors for trimming tissue or snipping sutures. Several varieties of scissors are shown in Fig. 34-20.

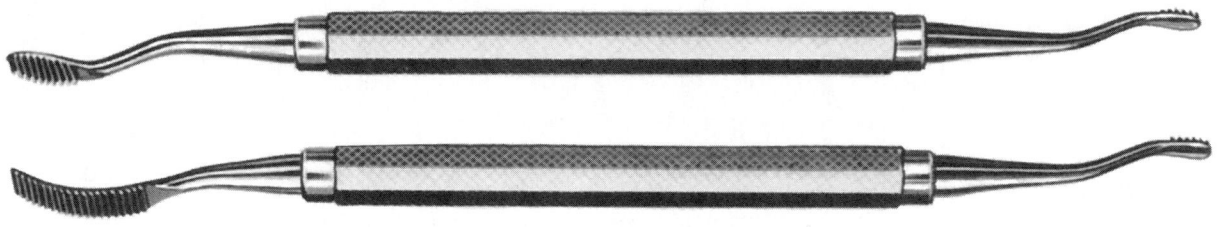

FIG. 34-19   Two styles of bone files.
(Courtesy of Hu Friedy.)

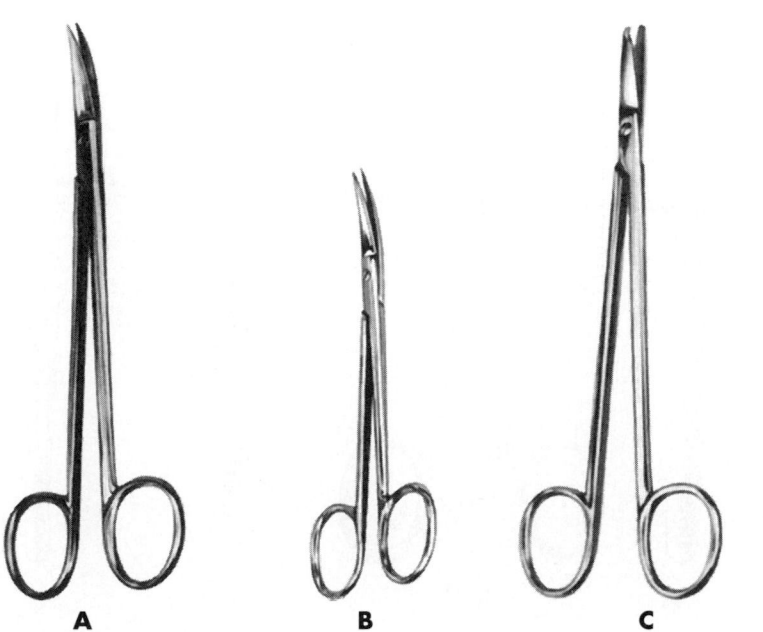

A   **B**   **C**

FIG. 34-20   Variations in surgical scissors. *A* and *B*, Two styles of tissue scissors. *C*, Suture scissors.
(Courtesy of Hu Friedy.)

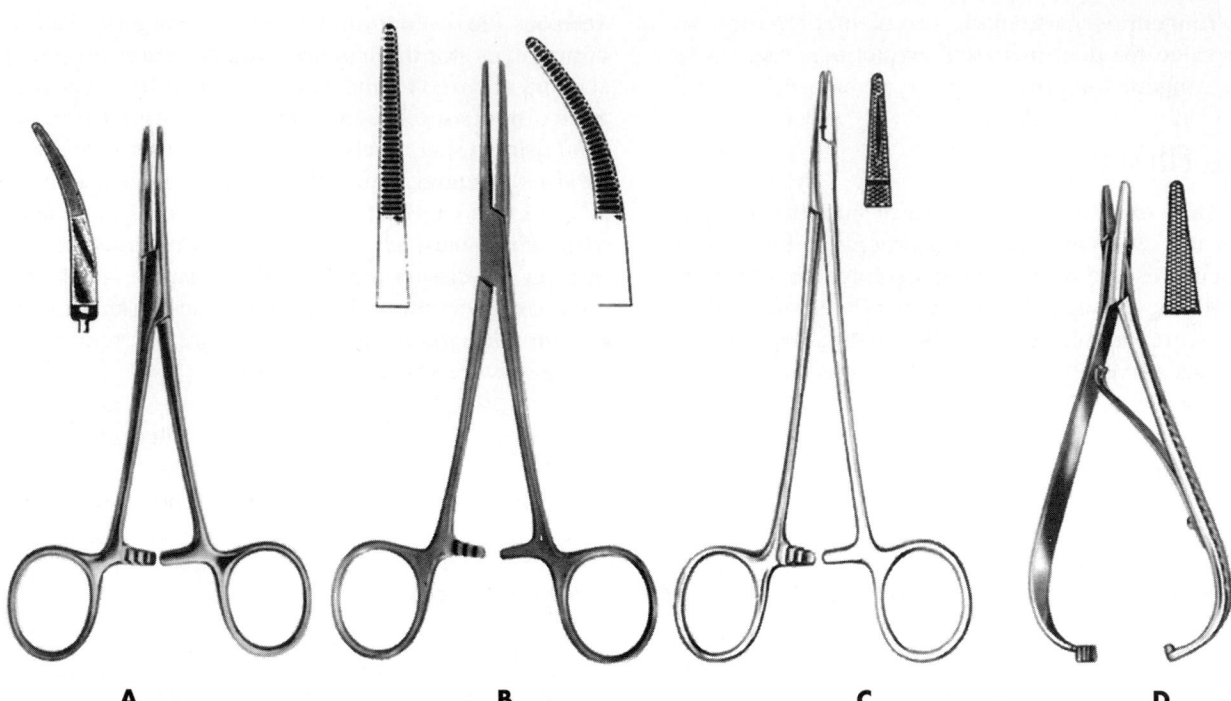

FIG. 34-21   Curved hemostats and needle holders. *A* and *B,* Hemostats. *C* and *D,* Needle holders.

(Courtesy of Hu Friedy.)

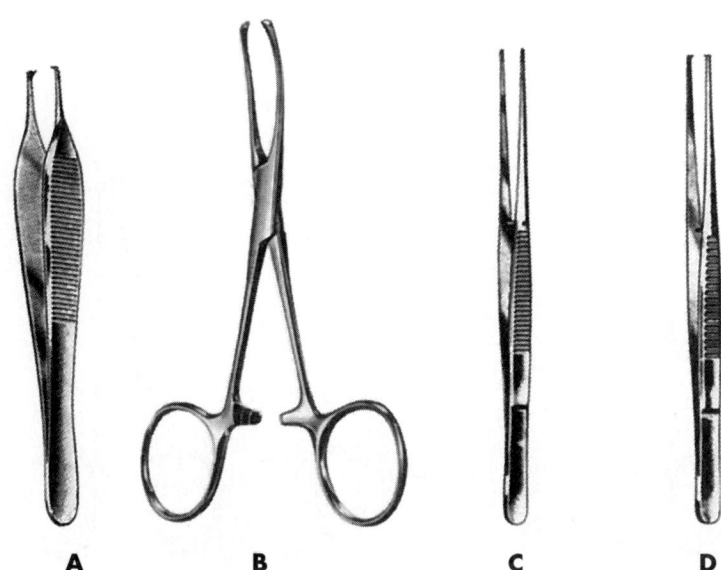

FIG. 34-22   Variations in tissue forceps and tissue pliers. *A,* Allison baby tissue forceps. *B,* Adson 1 × 2 tissue pliers. *C,* Straight Semkin-Taylor tissue pliers. *D,* Straight Semkin-Taylor 1 × 2 tissue pliers.

(Courtesy of Hu Friedy.)

▶ Hemostats and Needle Holders

Hemostats and needle holders are instruments that are often confused with each other. **Hemostats** are primarily used to grasp tissue and to clamp off blood vessels, while **needle holders** are used to hold suture needles. Hemostats can be curved or straight, while needle holders are generally straight. Hemostats are usually narrower than the more blunted and heavier needle holders. The serrated portion of the beaks of the hemostat is also longer than the same area on a needle holder. Often, a needle holder has a criss-cross pattern on the internal portion of the beaks or a slotted groove down the midline of the beak. Fig. 34-21 demonstrates several variations of hemostats and needle holders.

▶ Tissue Pliers

Tissue pliers and forceps are instruments that are used to hold tissue during surgery and during suturing. **Tissue pliers** are similar to cotton pliers. They are usually very fine instruments. Usually the ends of the tissue pliers have small teeth to aid in holding the tissue. Tissue forceps are fashioned similarly to a hemostat and are designed to hold larger portions of tissue, such as a fragment for a biopsy. Fig. 34-22 shows tissue forceps and pliers.

▶ Surgical Forceps

A **surgical forceps** is a dental instrument that permits the surgeon to grasp the crown of the tooth beyond the cementoenamel junction and luxate the tooth for removal. Forceps are not always needed for extractions, and when impacted teeth are removed, forceps are almost never used. Many surgical trays (especially if they are intended for removing third molars) are set up without any forceps, although usually at least one pair of forceps is kept handy in a sterile package and ready for use if needed. Routine or simple extractions are usually accomplished with forceps.

The two major divisions of surgical forceps are **maxillary** and **mandibular** forceps. Usually, with maxillary forceps the direction of the beaks parallels the direction of the handle. With mandibular forceps the direction of the beaks is usually at a right angle to the direction of the handle. Fig. 34-23 shows a #150, a maxillary universal forceps, and a #151, a mandibular universal forceps. These forceps are called *universal,* since they can be used for incisors, cuspids, premolars, and roots; they are not often used for molars, however. After careful examination of the illustration the difference in the position of the beaks of the forceps can be seen and compared with the handle.

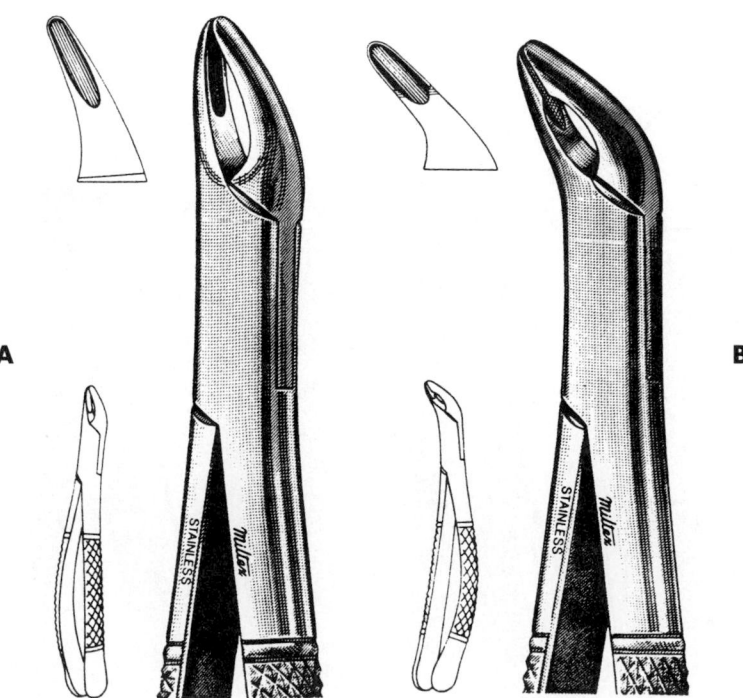

A   **B**

FIG. 34-23   *A,* #150 maxillary forceps. *B,* #151 mandibular forceps. (Courtesy of Miltex.)

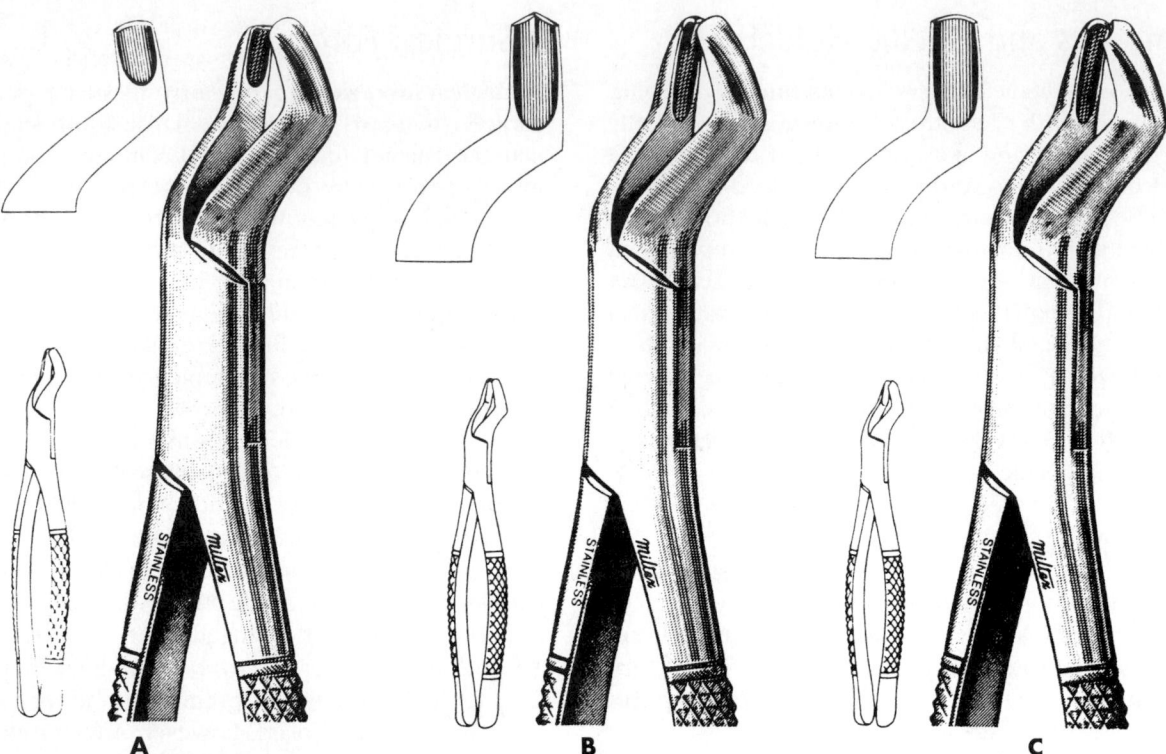

FIG. 34-24   *A,* #210 S maxillary third molar forceps. *B* and *C,* #53 R and 53 L maxillary right and left molar forceps.

(Courtesy of Miltex.)

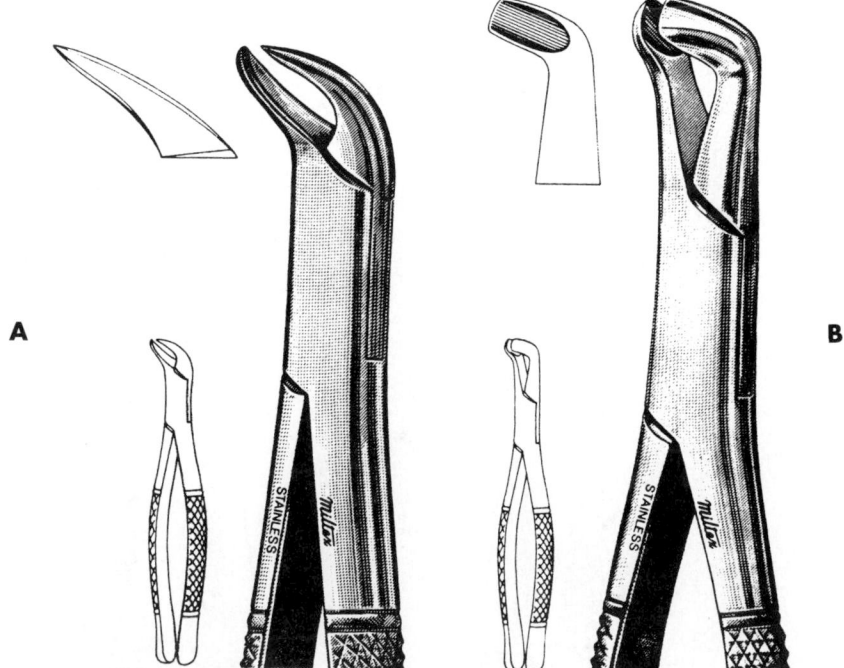

FIG. 34-25   *A,* #16 mandibular molar cowhorn forceps. *B,* #222 mandibular molar and third molar forceps.

(Courtesy of Miltex.)

Another type of forceps that differs in shape from the universal forceps is the *bayonet forceps.* These are maxillary forceps that are used for removing molar teeth. Because the molar teeth are more posterior in the arch, access is slightly more limited. As a result the shape of the beak is somewhat different to compensate for these differences. Although the beaks come close to being parallel to the handles, they are offset slightly to allow greater access to the posterior of the mouth. Bayonet forceps are available in two different types: (1) the universal type (#210 S), in which both jaws are identical; and (2) right and left pairs (#53 R and #53 L), in which one beak is pointed. The point of the beak is placed between the bifurcation of the two buccal roots. Usually the #210 S is used with maxillary third molars, which may not have well defined bifurcations, while the #53 R and L are used with maxillary first and second molars. Fig. 34-24 shows these three forceps.

The *cowhorn forceps* have somewhat rounded, pointed beaks that resemble a cow's horns. These forceps are usually used for the removal of mandibular molar teeth. The two beaks grasp the tooth in the furcation between the roots and below the level of the crown. If the crown of the tooth is slightly broken down or partially decayed, a firm grasp can allow the operator to remove the tooth. The #16 forceps is a typical cowhorn forceps. A slightly different type of forceps is #222, which is used primarily for removal of mandibular third molars. The beaks on this forceps are much shorter, again because of the relative lack of space in the posterior part of the arch. Fig. 34-25 illustrates both of these forceps. Surgical forceps that are used for the removal of primary teeth are similar to those that are used for permanent teeth, although they are smaller. Fig. 34-26 shows a photograph of #150 S for maxillary primary teeth, and #151 S and #16 S for mandibular primary teeth. The #150 S and #151 S can also be used for permanent premolars and roots, especially in situations where crowding exists and access is difficult.

Many other forceps are available for use in special situations. It is impossible to describe them all in this textbook. Each assistant needs to become acquainted with the forceps that are used in the office. Table 34-1 illustrates the use of some of the basic instruments that are routinely used in oral surgery.

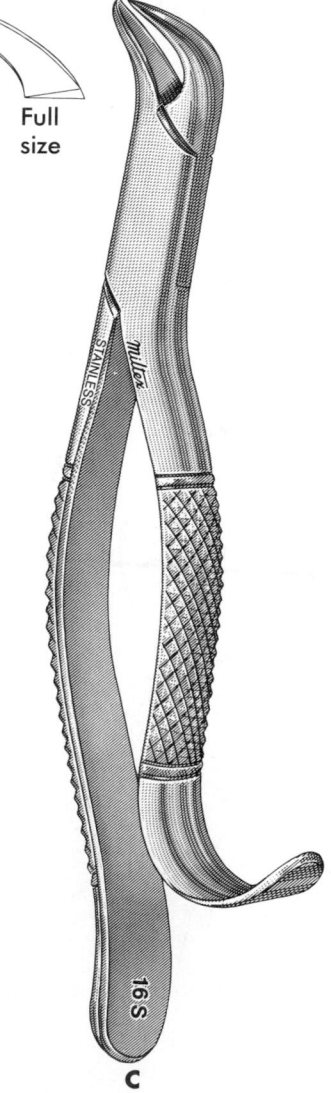

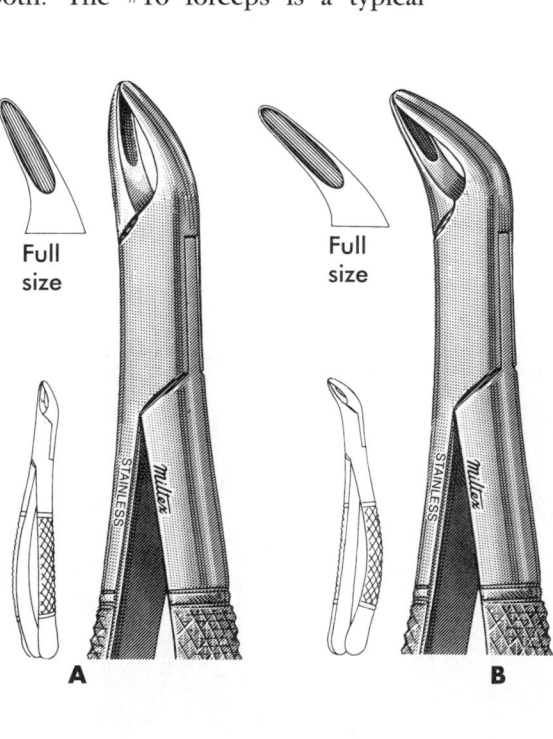

FIG. 34-26 Pediatric forceps. *A,* #150 S maxillary primary universal forceps. *B,* #151 S mandibular primary anterior forceps. *C,* #16 S mandibular primary molar forceps.

(Courtesy of Miltex.)

TABLE 34-1   FUNCTION OF BASIC SURGICAL INSTRUMENTS

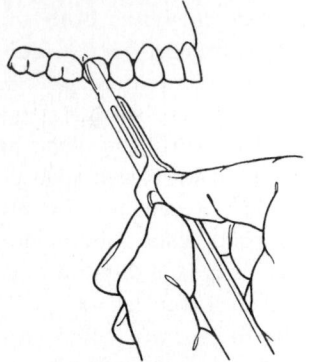

A. Scalpel is used to incise gingival sulcus

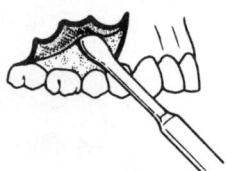

B. Periosteal elevator is used to reflect tissue

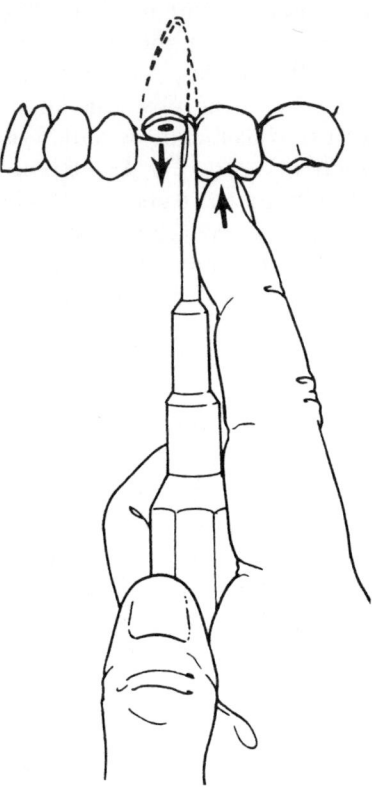

E. Small, straight elevator is used to luxate tooth root from its socket

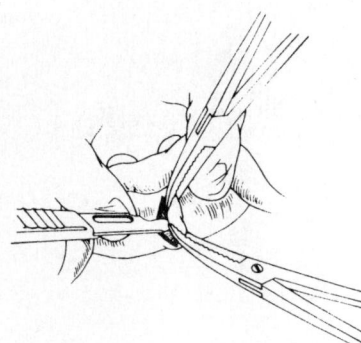

C. Hemostat is used to grasp tissue

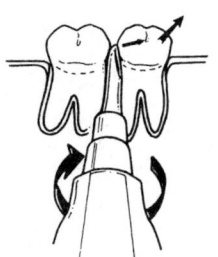

D. Straight elevator is placed on the tooth and turned toward the tooth to luxate before removal

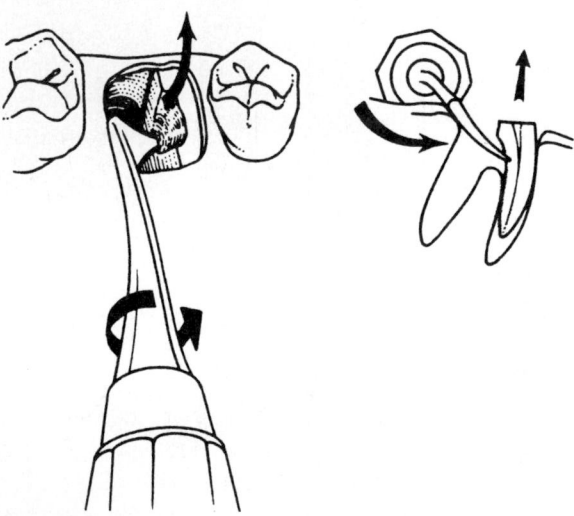

F. Triangular cryer elevator is used to retrieve roots from the socket

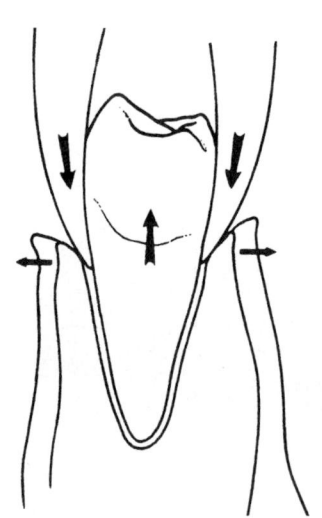

G. Jaws of forceps act as wedge to expand alveolar bone and to remove tooth in occlusal direction

From Peterson LJ, Hupp J, Ellis III E, Tucker M: *Contemporary oral and maxillofacial surgery,* St Louis, 1990, Mosby.

Additional Armamentarium

Other items are used in conjunction with the surgical instruments to perform oral surgery. The armamentarium in cludes dressing materials, lubricant, and suture materials.

▶ Surgical Dressings

Some oral surgeons have a medicated **surgical dressing**, such as tetracycline, on the surgical tray to place in the socket of extracted teeth to aid in healing and to control hemorrhaging. Tetracycline is placed on the tray in a small dappen dish and made into a paste with a drop or two of sterile saline solution. The Gelfoam, a surgical packing medium, is cut into small pieces and dipped into the tetracycline paste. A cotton pliers is used to transport the tetracycline on the gel foam to the socket where it is placed to promote healing.

▶ Surgical Suture Material

Suture material is used to close the surgical site to promote the healing process and to reduce the possibility of debris lodging in the socket and causing trauma. Exodontia sutures are supplied most commonly, attached to a sterile needle (Fig. 34-27). The suture material, generally about 18 inches in length, may be made of silk, gut, or Dacron. The material is supplied either plain or braided. The half-circle–shaped needle is available in an assortment of sizes, generally from 1 to 20, with the smaller number correlating with the larger needle. Sutures are in many different configurations. Variations of the single, multiple, and continuous sutures are shown in Fig. 34-28, *A* through *D*. The step-by-step procedure for placing sutures is illustrated in Fig. 34-29, *A* through *G*.

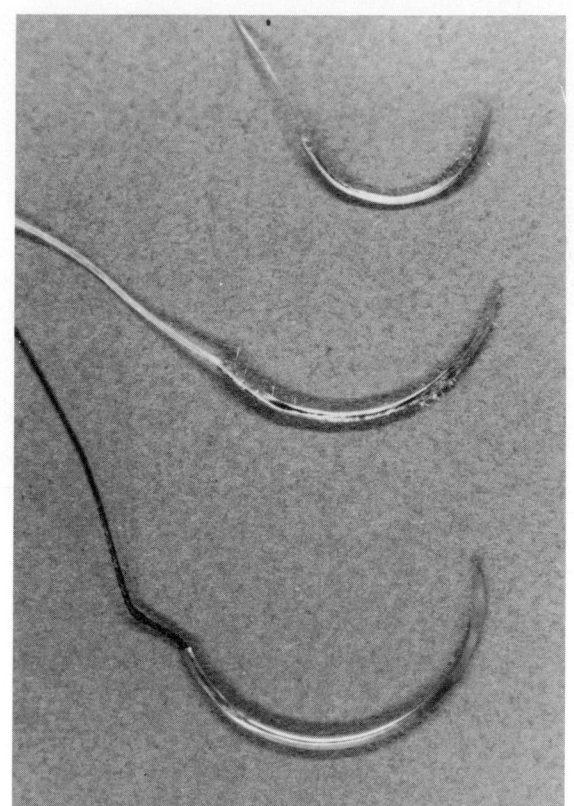

FIG. 34-27   Suture needles used in oral surgery are ⅜ circle cutting needles. Middle needle is #F 5-2, and lower needle is X-I.

(From Peterson LJ, Hupp J, Ellis III E, Tucker M: *Contemporary oral and maxillofacial surgery,* ed 2, St Louis, 1992, Mosby.)

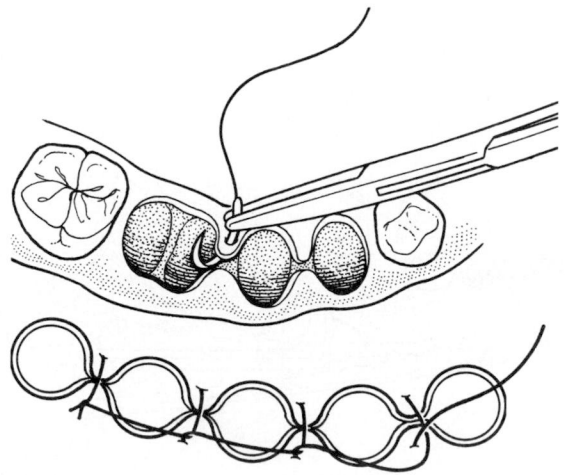

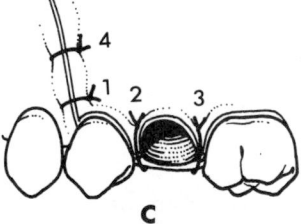

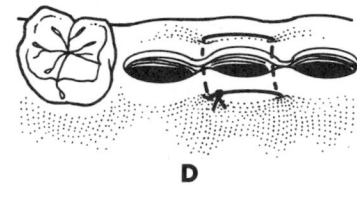

FIG. 34-28   Different styles of sutures. *A,* Single interproximal suture. *B,* Continuous suture. *C,* Flap suture, with four individual stitches. *D,* Single horizontal mattress.

(From Peterson LJ, Hupp J, Ellis III E, Tucker M: *Contemporary oral and maxillofacial surgery,* ed 2, St Louis, 1992, Mosby.)

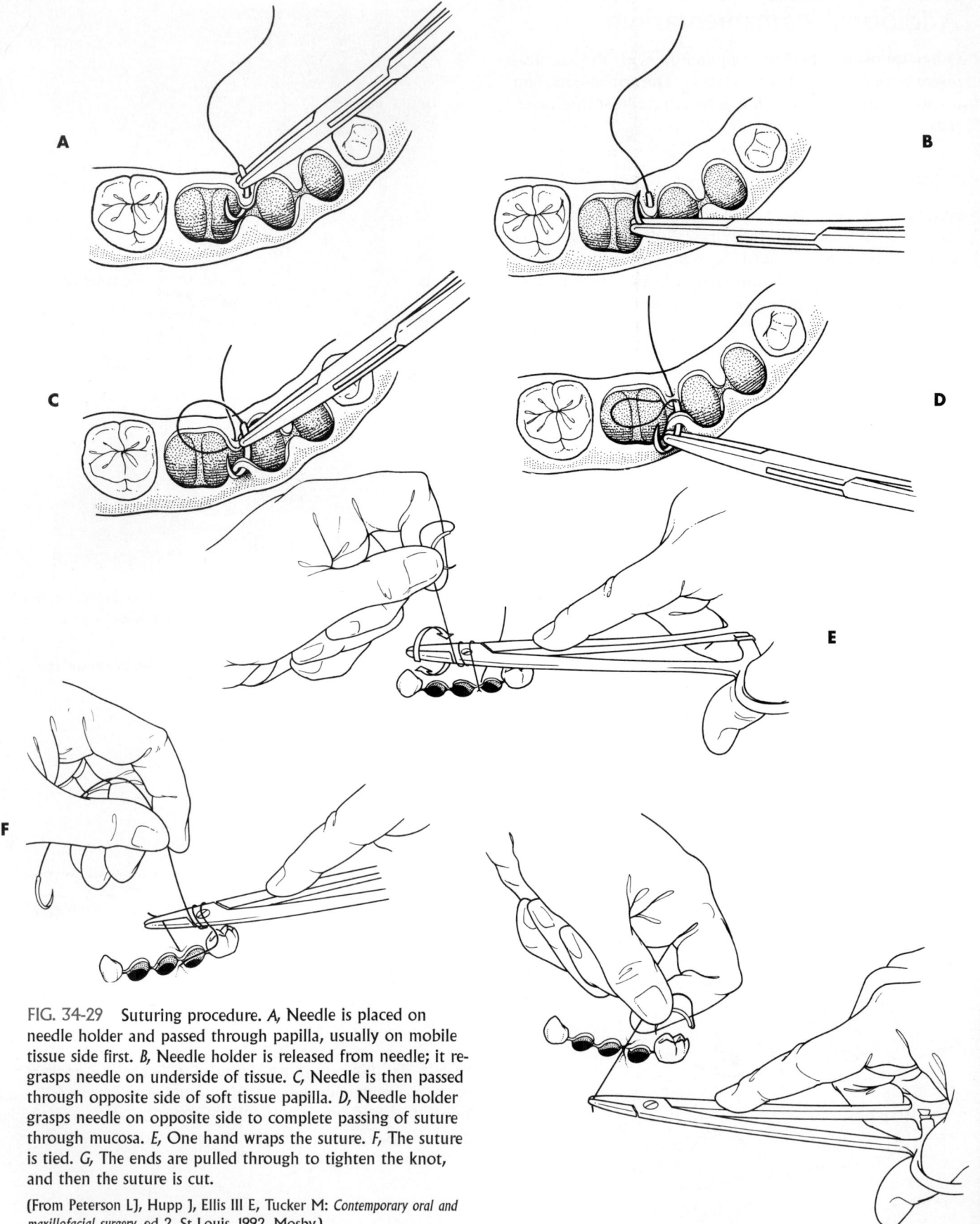

FIG. 34-29   Suturing procedure. *A,* Needle is placed on
needle holder and passed through papilla, usually on mobile
tissue side first. *B,* Needle holder is released from needle; it re-
grasps needle on underside of tissue. *C,* Needle is then passed
through opposite side of soft tissue papilla. *D,* Needle holder
grasps needle on opposite side to complete passing of suture
through mucosa. *E,* One hand wraps the suture. *F,* The suture
is tied. *G,* The ends are pulled through to tighten the knot,
and then the suture is cut.

(From Peterson LJ, Hupp J, Ellis III E, Tucker M: *Contemporary oral and
maxillofacial surgery,* ed 2, St Louis, 1992, Mosby.)

Lubricant

One last item that is helpful to have on the tray is a cotton applicator that is dipped in a lubricant. The patient's lips become quite dry during oral surgery, and a lubricant helps to keep the lips from cracking. Also, a lubricated lip does not adhere to the retractor as much and is less likely to become bruised. One way to avoid placing lubricant on the tray with the instruments is to take the clear hub end of an anesthetic needle and fill it with lubricant. This can then be used as a carrier; the cotton tip applicator is dipped into the lubricant, and it is applied to the patient's lips.

Preparation for Surgical Procedures

This portion of the chapter will attempt to specifically describe the assistant's role in a number of commonly performed procedures in the oral surgery specialty office. Many different techniques are used by oral surgeons throughout the country. Obviously, each one of these techniques cannot be discussed here because space is limited. The information that is contained here is intended to give the assistant a general background in the specialty.

Preparation

Just as it is in restorative dentistry, preparation is one of the most important functions of the dental assistant in oral surgery. The middle of a surgical procedure is no time to realize that a particular instrument is needed and is missing. Much of the preparation time can be eliminated by having preset trays; however, before the patient is seated, the assistant must stop and think whether any additional items are needed for this particular situation. It is often helpful to have less frequently used items, such as forceps, bagged separately, so that they are not needlessly contaminated. These items can be stored on a back counter or in a nearby drawer; if they are needed, they are easily accessible. The tray set-up should be arranged in an orderly sequence for easy access during the surgical procedure. In addition to preparing the surgical tray, the surgical assistant must draw up any medications that may be needed for sedation or general anesthesia. Often, it is helpful to have a separate smaller tray with all the items necessary for the anesthesia, so that a particular procedure can be accomplished without contaminating the entire surgical tray. The additional instruments that are added to each tray are usually bagged separately and are opened only when needed. This process also reduces the necessity of purchasing large numbers of instruments.

It is important to have enough instruments and sterile tray set-ups, so that the surgeon and patient never have to wait for instruments to be sterilized. Extra supplies, such as anesthetic carpules and 3×3 gauze, should also be easily accessible.

Barrier Techniques

Universal barrier techniques are essential in the surgery practice. Since blood and saliva are present in the surgery office during every procedure, every possible precaution must be taken to protect both the staff and the patients and to prevent contamination of the equipment. Sterility is vital in an oral surgery office. For example, sterile surgical gloves are required for each case rather than nonsterile gloves, which can be used in other procedures. The assistant is responsible for setting out masks and gloves and for ensuring that all members of the surgical team wear masks, gloves and eye protection. Additional protective coverings, such as hospital gowns, are used as directed by OSHA regulations.

Managing Medical Wastes

The oral surgery office presents many opportunities for producing regulated wastes and hazardous materials: extracted teeth, diseased tissues, needles, and scalpel blades. The policies for management of these wastes are regulated by OSHA Rule 29 CFR and by individual state regulations. The staff in an oral surgery office must maintain a constant update of these regulations. To review the management of these wastes, refer to Chapter 8, *Infection Control,* which provides information regarding the application of this OSHA rule in the daily activities in a dental office.

Patient Preparation and Monitors

Once the assistant is certain that the room is completely prepared, the patient can be seated. Some surgeons ask the patient to prepare the oral cavity by either brushing the teeth or by using an antibiotic mouth rinse or both. Following this the assistant verifies that no changes have occurred in the patient's health since the initial office visit. If changes have occurred, the surgeon is alerted, so that a determination can be made regarding changes in the treatment plan. If the patient has experienced no health changes, the assistant uses a standard set of questions for the patient to make certain that the patient is ready for the procedure. The checklist in Box 34-5 indicates several questions and steps that must be considered before progressing with the procedure.

After the assistant has documented all the answers to these questions, the next step is to assess the patient's vital signs. Electronic monitoring is popular in oral surgery offices today, since it greatly increases both the safety of the procedures and the ease of evaluating the

PREPARATORY STEPS BEFORE SURGERY

▶ Verify patient consent form is signed and accurate
▶ Confirm a driver is present for sedated patients
▶ Request patient remove contact lenses if he or she is to be sedated or to receive general anesthetic
▶ Verify that any prescribed premedication has been taken
▶ Confirm patient's height and weight to determine anesthetic dosage
▶ Review and confirm information on health history form
▶ Determine if a female patient is pregnant or is taking contraceptives
▶ Determine time of last meal for patients to be sedated or to receive general anesthesia
▶ Provide antimicrobial rinse
▶ Check vital signs and record status of vital signs in record before and after the surgical procedure
▶ Connect monitors; blood pressure, ECG, and pulse oximeter
▶ Provide antimicrobial rinse before seating patient
▶ Use universal precautions
▶ Assist with the administration of all forms of anesthesia

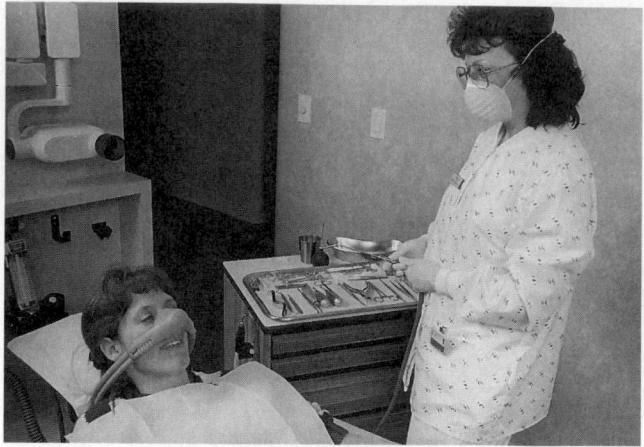

FIG. 34-30   Patient is prepared for surgery, with nitrous mask in place, and set-up is prepared on mobile cart.

(Courtesy of Helen Zylman, D.D.S., Ann Arbor, Michigan.)

necessary parameters. In patients who are having local anesthesia only, only the blood pressure needs to be taken. In some offices this is done manually, but in other offices this is checked electronically. The use of the automatic blood pressure monitor, the EKG machine, and the pulse oximeter have been described earlier in this chapter. After the patient is hooked up to the monitors, both machines are started. Most EKG machines with automatic blood pressure monitors and some pulse oximeters include a printout and a recording device. Periodically, they print out a record of the blood pressure, an EKG reading, and a percentage of oxygen in the bloodstream. This information can be attached to the patient's chart, although the initial and final readings are usually written down on the surgical record. The pulse oximeter continuously monitors the oxygen level throughout the procedure. The automatic blood pressure machine continuously monitors the EKG but reads the blood pressure only periodically. Most machines can be set to record once each minute and up to once every 30 minutes. As long as a patient is stable, it is usually sufficient to monitor every 10 or 15 minutes.

▶ General Anesthesia / Sedation

The surgeon has many types of sedation or general anesthesia available, and each surgeon chooses the type to be used based on patient need and operator preference. This section describes a combined technique that uses nitrous oxide analgesia, as well as conscious sedation. The procedures that have been described would be similar if only one of these types of sedation were being used. If intravenous general anesthesia were used without an endotracheal tube, it would also be similar. Once the monitors have been applied and vital signs have been recorded in the chart, it is time for the surgeon to begin. The surgeon usually converses with the patient to ensure that the patient has no further questions about either the procedure or the consent form that has already been signed. At this point, the surgeon places the patient into a reclining position, applies the nitrous oxide rubber mask to the patient's nose (Fig. 34-30), and tightens the cord, so that the mask does not slip off. The patient is then allowed to breathe a fairly high rate of nitrous oxide/oxygen (i.e., 60%/40%) for a few minutes. This helps to reduce anxiety, reduces the discomfort of the venipuncture, and gives the surgeon a chance to evaluate the patient's reaction to an easily reversible analgesic. The patient is told that in a few minutes he or she will notice a sweet smell from the nitrous oxide and will start to feel more relaxed. The patient may also feel a sensation of numbness or tingling in the extremities. The patient must never be left alone once the nitrous oxide is introduced. Although it is a safe anesthetic technique to use, occasionally patients have an unusual reaction to the gas or become frightened by it. Some patients, who have a tendency towards claustrophobia, object to the mask on their faces. Usually, they get used to it after a short time. It is not wise to insist that a patient use a particular technique if it obviously is not working for him or her.

STARTING THE IV

▶ Are all universal barrier techniques being used?
▶ Is all of the armamentarium available and prepared for use?
▶ Are the instruments arranged in sequence of use?
▶ Am I prepared for alternative treatment plans?
▶ Is the necessary equipment turned on and ready to operate?

1. Pass the tourniquet to the surgeon, who places the tourniquet tightly above the patient's elbow. The patient is instructed to make a fist, or is given an object to squeeze to make the veins protrude at the elbow or on the back of the hand.
2. Open the alcohol wipe packet. Hold the outside of the paper packet, while the surgeon takes the alcohol wipe from inside the packet. Wipe the patient's arm with the alcohol to clean it before placing the IV (Fig. 34-31, *A*).

3. Retrieve the used alcohol wipe, and pass the surgeon a dry gauze to dry the area (Fig. 34-31, *B*). It is more uncomfortable for the patient if the intravenous puncture is done while the arm is still wet with alcohol.
4. Take the butterfly needle (some surgeons use other types of needles, with a slightly different technique), slightly loosening the plastic shield over the needle without touching the needle. Bend up the wings of the needle, so that the surgeon can take the needle in the proper position for use (Fig. 34-31, *C*). Hold the plastic shield as the surgeon slides the needle out.
5. As the surgeon inserts the needle into the patient's vein (Fig. 34-31, *D*), take a piece of tape (which has already been laid out) and hand it to the surgeon to fasten the needle in place as soon as the needle is in the vein and

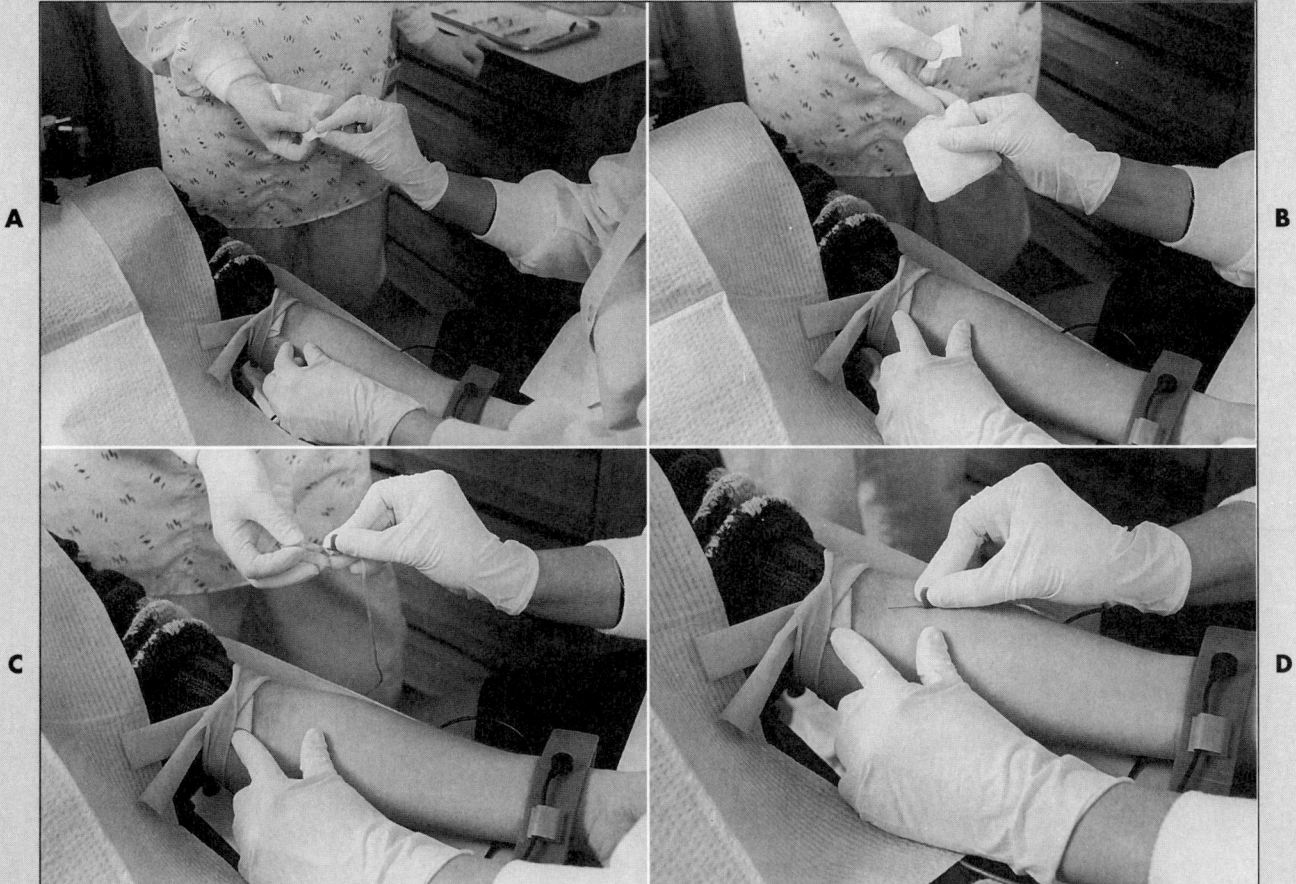

FIG. 34-31   IV is started. *A,* The tourniquet is applied, and the assistant passes a disinfectant sponge to clean injection site. *B,* The alcohol sponge is exchanged for a dry gauze, and the site is dried. *C,* The assistant grasps the protective cover over the needle, and transfers it to the surgeon. Surgeon grasps the needle. *D,* Surgeon inserts needle in vein.

Continued.

blood can be seen in the small plastic tube that is attached to the needle.

6. The surgeon then takes the cap off the end of the butterfly tubing, allowing blood to flow to the end of the tubing, and releases the tourniquet. Meanwhile, move to the IV stand, remove the cap from the end of the intravenous line, and hand the end to the surgeon to attach to the butterfly tubing (Fig. 34-31, E).

7. Once the IV line is attached to the tubing, open the clamp on the IV line, allowing the contents to start flowing into the vein. A final piece of tape is then applied to the needle and tubing to hold everything in place during the procedure, and the patient's arm is secured to the chair to reduce the chance of dislodging the intravenous catheter (Fig. 34-31, F).

8. If a high dose of nitrous oxide and oxygen has been used to provide anxiety control or mild analgesia during this portion of the procedure, the level of nitrous oxide is turned down to a maintenance dose, approximately 30% nitrous oxide and 70% oxygen.

▶ Are the appropriate universal barrier techniques removed?
▶ Have all of the appropriate surfaces been cleaned and disinfected?
▶ Has all armamentarium been removed?
▶ Has all equipment been repositioned?
▶ Has all of the equipment been disinfected/sterilized according to OSHA guidelines?

FIG. 34-31, cont'd   E, Surgeon takes cap off the end of butterfly tubing, and it is connected to the IV line. F, The tubing is taped in place. G, The assistant passes the anesthetic syringe to the surgeon, who then administers anesthesia.

(Courtesy of Helen Zylman, D.D.S., Ann Arbor, Michigan.)

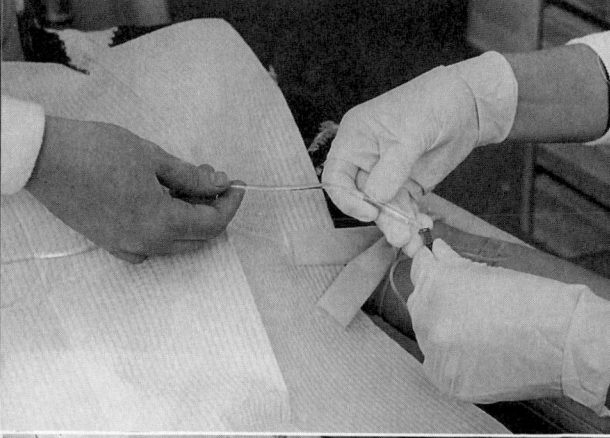

E

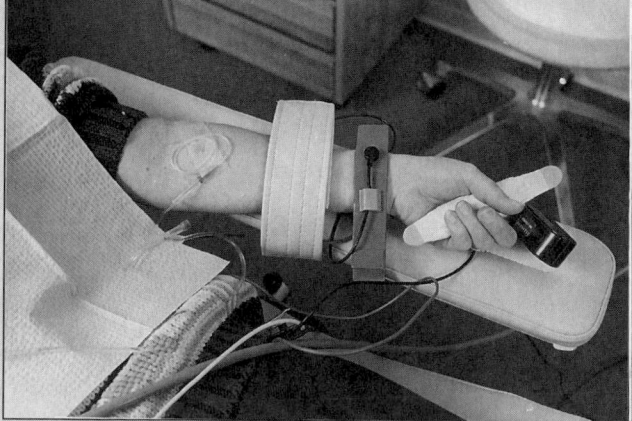

F

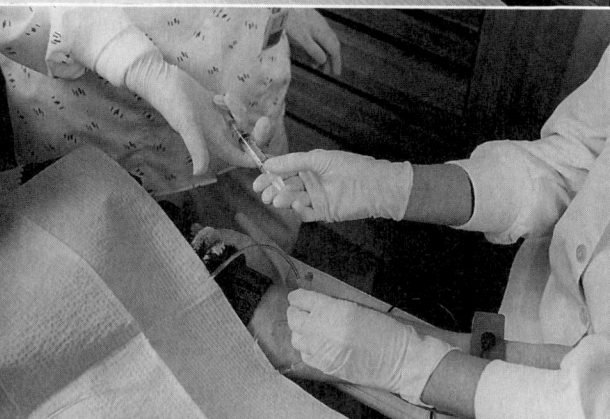

G

Once the nitrous oxide has had an effect, it is time to start the IV. If intravenous sedation is not being used, the next step is to use a local anesthesia. On the other hand, some surgeons do not use any nitrous oxide at all and begin with an IV. While the patient is breathing the nitrous oxide, the assistant should finish preparing the anesthesia tray.

The next steps in the anesthesia/sedation procedure are the same whether or not nitrous oxide is used in a combination technique and are similar for both conscious sedation and for intravenous general anesthesia. The assistant secures the first of the prefilled syringes and passes it to the surgeon (Fig. 34-31, *G*). Depending on the technique this may be a narcotic, such as Demerol or fentanyl; an ultra-short–acting barbiturate, such as Brevital; or a sedative-hypnotic, such as Valium or Versed. Each syringe on the tray should be labeled, so that the wrong medication is not given to the patient by mistake. According to the techniques practiced by the surgeon, one or more anesthetic agents are titrated for the patient to reach the desired end point of anesthesia. During the time the anesthesia is administered the surgeon usually tells the patient that he or she will become drowsy, may see the lights move, and probably will not remember anything from that point onward. At this point the surgeon tries to achieve the desired level of anesthesia; noise in the treatment room must be kept at a minimum. The assistant should also remain alert for any problems that might develop, such as the patient becoming severely nauseated and starting to vomit. A tonsil suction tip and emesis basin must be kept close by. Once the patient is sedated and the IV lines are secured, the surgeon and the assistant can wash their hands, put on their masks, eye protection, and surgical gloves. The next step is administration of local anesthesia.

▶ Local Anesthesia

Regardless of the method of anxiety control, whether it is intravenous sedation, nitrous oxide, or oral premedication, every oral surgical procedure must include profound local anesthesia. Even patients who are receiving general anesthesia usually receive local anesthesia, both for control of bleeding during surgery and for pain control immediately after the patient wakes up.

The technique for administration of local anesthesia for oral surgery is similar to the technique that is used in general dentistry. One difference is the amount of anesthesia that is administered. Usually, oral surgery requires the use of more local anesthesia, since the procedure involves a greater part of the mouth than a restorative dentistry procedure. For example, it is common for an oral surgeon to remove third molars in all four quadrants of the mouth in one procedure. Instead of needing one injection to achieve anesthesia for this procedure, the surgeon may need to administer as many as eight injections. As a result, some surgeons choose to use two local anesthetic syringes. The assistant removes the empty carpule from the one syringe while the surgeon is using the second syringe. Then the syringes are exchanged in the typical syringe exchange technique, and the surgeon immediately moves to the next quadrant without waiting for the syringe to be refilled.

Local anesthesia for oral surgery must also be more profound than that which is used for restorative dentistry. In oral surgery not only the teeth, but also the soft tissue and bone around the teeth, must be anesthetized; to do this, extra injections must be administered. In the maxilla and in addition to infiltration of the buccal mucosa next to the tooth, the palatal tissue must also be anesthetized with a second injection. In the mandible and in addition to the mandibular block injection, a second *long buccal* infiltration is required to anesthetize the soft tissue that lies above the third molars. Usually the lingual nerve is anesthetized at the same time as the mandibular block. If sensation remains in the lingual tissue, then that nerve must be anesthetized again.

Another difference in techniques involves sedated patients. The medications used in conscious sedation render a patient relaxed and sleepy but still able to feel pain. As a result, administration of local anesthetic can be quite uncomfortable for the patient, especially if they have a low pain tolerance. Since the sedation reduces patient inhibitions, often, the patient reacts to the stimulus of the needle by either moving his or her head or by reaching up a hand to try to move the painful stimulus out of the way; this is especially common with palatal injections, since they tend to be particularly uncomfortable. As a result, the assistant must always be ready to help hold the patient still or to prevent the patient's hands from bumping the surgeon and possibly causing breakage of a needle or inadvertent laceration with the needle. If the patient is uncooperative, a second assistant may be brought in exclusively to restrain the patient. Often, Velcro arm straps are used, especially in sedated patients. The patient who is awake may like to have the assistant hold his or her hand during this time; this works well with small children. They are told that the second dental assistant "likes to hold hands with the patients." Most children do not mind holding hands with an adult, especially if their caregivers aren't present. The assistant can then comfort and restrain the child simultaneously.

The dental assistant must keep track of the amount of anesthetic that has been administered. Since oral surgery involves the use of more local anesthetic, it is more likely that the maximum dosage of anesthetic will be reached. When the amount of anesthetic starts getting close to the recommended maximum amount, the assistant must remind the surgeon of the number of carpules already administered.

Surgical Procedures

The following descriptions of surgical procedures are presented as actual cases. Since a patient's history often dictates changes in surgical procedures, these cases are representative of situations that would commonly confront the oral surgery team. The actual case is described in narrative form followed by a step-by-step procedure. During each surgical procedure the assistant performs several tasks at one time. Many of these tasks are identified in Box 34-6.

▶ Routine Extractions (Case Scenario #1)

The patient is a 65-year-old female in good health, who has some mild hypertension that is well controlled with routine blood pressure medication. The patient is to have a periodontally involved maxillary right first premolar removed (Fig. 34-32). The tooth has been abscessed several times in the past, but the periodontist now believes that the prognosis is hopeless and has advised that the tooth be removed to avoid further involvement of adjacent oral tissues and before a severe infection endangers the health of the patient. The patient does not present any apprehension over the surgery and prefers a local anesthetic. The choice of anesthetic is approved by the surgeon.

Armamentarium Preparation

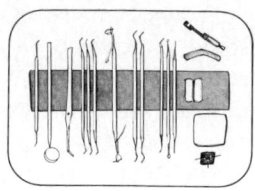

Before the patient is seated, the assistant follows the preparatory steps, preparing the anesthesia and the set-up. The basic armamentarium for this procedure includes the following:

    Local anesthetic set-up
    Nitrous oxide set-up (optional)
    Oximeter
    Automatic blood pressure cuff

    The armamentarium just listed is repeated in each of the surgical scenarios. The symbol is used to indicate this repeated set-up for the procedures.

Routine Extraction Set-Up

Mirror
Periosteal elevator
Surgical curette
Retractor
Straight elevator
Maxillary universal forceps
Ronguers
Surgical HVE tip
3 × 3 Gauze sponges
Irrigating syringe or set-up, with sterile saline solution
Cup with sterile water for clearing the suction tip
Surgicel (placed nearby)
Lubricant

BOX 34-6

RESPONSIBILITIES OF A DENTAL ASSISTANT DURING SURGERY

Transfer instruments in sequence of use
Observe changes in treatment site
Monitor patient's vital signs
Observe patient's nonverbal cues
Monitor patient's movements
Inform surgeon of changes in patient's status
Observe and retract tissues to avoid injury
Maintain a clear working field, free of blood and oral fluids
Keep instruments clean and free of debris
Clear HVE line frequently
Aid in irrigation
Keep track of amount of local anesthesia being used
Keep track of number of sutures placed
Dispose of medical wastes according to OSHA guidelines
Clean blood from patient's face
Accurately and thoroughly record treatment

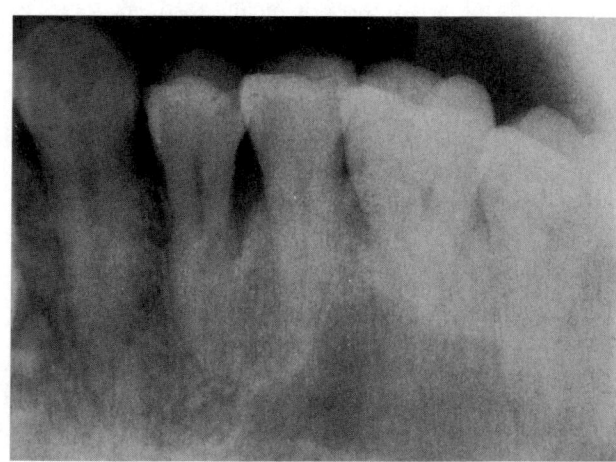

FIG. 34-32 **Radiograph of periodontally involved tooth #5.**
(Courtesy of Helen Zylman, D.D.S., Ann Arbor, Michigan.)

ROUTINE EXTRACTIONS

Anesthesia Administration

A topical anesthetic is applied to the mucosa, and local anesthetic is injected on the buccal side of tooth #5 and on the palatal side. The assistant rinses and evacuates the area to remove any bitter taste from the patient's mouth and then remains with the patient.

After sufficient time has elapsed for the anesthesia to take effect, the assistant hands the surgeon a double-ended curette. This relatively sharp instrument is used to assess the tissue on either side of the tooth to ensure that it is anesthetized. The surgeon may use a finger from the left hand to retract the tissue or may choose to use a mirror or a retractor, such as a Minnesota retractor. If the surgeon prefers to use an instrument, it is passed with the curette, one instrument for each hand. If the patient still feels a sharp sensation when the curette is touched to the tissue, more local anesthesia would be administered to achieve the level of anesthesia needed; this is not uncommon when a tooth is abscessed, since the infection in the area tends to inactivate the local anesthetic.

Extraction Procedure

The extraction procedure may vary with each surgeon. The following step-by-step procedure, however, includes the common steps that are performed by most operators.

Routine Extraction (case scenarios #1 and #2)

1. Pass the surgeon a surgical curette or a periosteal elevator to detach the periodontal ligament from around the tooth.
2. Exchange this instrument for a straight (#77) elevator.
3. The surgeon places the elevator on the mesial side of the tooth and applies pressure in a distal direction. Since the tooth is already slightly mobile, a great deal of pressure is not needed.
4. The surgeon exchanges the elevator for a maxillary universal forceps (#150). This can be done with either a one- or two-handed transfer, whichever works best for the surgical team. The advantage of using the one-handed transfer is that the other hand is still available for evacuating and retracting tissue.
5. Observe the surgical site and remove excess blood with the HVE tip as it accumulates, maintaining a clear field of operation for the surgeon.
6. The surgeon then luxates the tooth with the forceps.
7. Watch closely and keep the HVE tip nearby. The tip can be used for tissue retraction and also for evacuation of debris, such as a fragments of tooth or amalgam that fractures when the forceps is placed firmly on the tooth. Periodically, clear the suction line with sterile water to prevent clogging.
8. When the tooth is sufficiently mobile, the surgeon lifts the tooth out of the socket. (Oral surgeons never really *pull* teeth. They spread the bone around the neck of the tooth, making room to lift the tooth out of the socket. A tooth that is *pulled* may break.) Refer to Table 35-2, *A* and *B*.

9. Have your left hand prepared to receive the forceps from the surgeon. The surgeon holds the forceps by the handle. Take the working end of the forceps and the extracted tooth in the palm of the hand, while transferring a surgical curette to the surgeon. The apex of the tooth must be observed to ensure that the root has not fractured. If the tooth is not intact, obtain root tip elevators to retrieve the remainder of the root.
10. The surgeon uses the curette to remove granulation tissue and dental abscesses from the socket. Once the curette is exchanged to the surgeon, be ready to evacuate the surgical site.
11. Hold the rongeur in readiness for transfer to the surgeon as soon as the socket has been curetted. The ronguer is used to remove the tissue which was loosened from the base of the socket.
12. While the rongeur is being used, the surgeon periodically brings the instrument out of the patient's mouth, since it holds tissue debris. Use a 3×3 gauze to efficiently remove the tissue from the rongeurs, without ever taking the instrument from the surgeon. Ideally, the surgeon's eyes should never leave the operating field.
13. When the surgeon has finished with the rongeurs, make the curette available to exchange in case it is needed again.
14. Regularly pass the HVE tip over the surgical site during this procedure, so that vision of the site is not impaired by bleeding.
15. Once the surgeon is satisfied that the socket is sufficiently clean, transfer an irrigating syringe to the surgeon to use at the site. Usually, a sterile saline (salt water) solution is used rather than tap water, since the sterile saline is less damaging to the tissue.
16. While the area is being irrigated, ask the patient to turn to one side or the other, so that all the irrigation solution does not fill the back of the throat and cause choking. Since this is a relatively simple extraction, sutures are not needed to close the tissue.
17. Finally, fold a 3×3 gauze into a small pillow and either give it to the surgeon to place or place it directly over the surgical site.
18. Instruct the patient to apply a firm biting pressure to the area to control the bleeding and to aid in clot formation.
19. In this case, there was not an exceptional amount of bleeding during the procedure, so the surgical dressing mentioned earlier was not used.
20. Take a moistened gauze and use it to wipe any blood from the patient's lips and cheeks.
21. The surgeon decides what type of pain medication to give the patient, signs the prescriptions, and then moves on to the next patient.
22. Be certain that data which includes a description of the surgery, the type and amount of anesthetic, and the pain prescription are entered on the patient record.
23. Dispose of medical wastes and barrier covers, according to infection control policies.

BOX 34-7

GENERAL INSTRUCTIONS*

1. Keep the pressure gauze firmly over the surgery site for 30 to 45 minutes, unless instructed otherwise. After this it may be discarded.
2. Do not rinse your mouth or spit forcefully the day of surgery. Starting the next evening it may be beneficial to use a warm salt water rinse (⅓ teaspoon salt to a full glass of warm water) gently twice a day, or use the Peridex rinse if it has been prescribed.
3. Do not brush your teeth in the area of surgery the day your teeth are removed. After that, gentle brushing is recommended, until the area is healed.
4. If it is more comfortable, or if you are instructed to do so, eat soft or liquid foods but **DO NOT STOP TAKING NOURISHMENT.** Do not drink through a straw. Change to a regular diet as soon as possible, but do not miss a single meal.
5. Do not smoke for at least 24 hours.
6. The **PRESCRIPTION SCHEDULE** follows.

YOU MAY HAVE THE FOLLOWING:

1. **PAIN** Start taking the pain medication that is prescribed for you before the anesthetic wears off. Follow the instructions written on the medicine bottle—do not take more medication than you are instructed to take. If the medication does not give you sufficient relief, please call the office. All pain medication should be taken with milk, yogurt, or food to prevent nausea.
2. **BLEEDING** You may experience slight oozing of blood the first day and night after surgery. If this seems excessive, place a pad of gauze folded so that it is at least an inch thick directly over the surgery site and close your teeth together firmly. (Do not use absorbent cotton or paper tissues.) If no gauze is available, a small clean handkerchief or a tea bag will do. Do not become excited. Sit quietly, putting pressure on the gauze for 30 minutes. If bleeding persists, repeat the pressure with a fresh gauze pad for 30 minutes more. If you are still concerned about the bleeding, call the office.
3. **SWELLING** It is common to experience a temporary swelling of your cheeks after surgery. An ice pack placed over your cheek for 30 minutes out of each hour for the first 12 to 24 hours after surgery will help keep the swelling to a minimum. Any swelling which does occur will subside in 4 to 6 days.

4. **JAW STIFFNESS** This, like the swelling, is a natural reaction of your body to surgery and should disappear completely within 4 to 6 days. Starting 72 hours after the surgery you may use warm, moist towels, a hot water bottle, or an electric heating pad to help reduce the swelling or stiffness. Make sure that the heat is not excessive, though, since extreme heat can cause painful skin burns.
5. **FACIAL DISCOLORATION** A day or so after the surgery you may notice a yellow, blue, or brown color appearing on the skin of the face adjacent to the surgery area. This, too, is temporary and will disappear after a few days.
6. **SUTURES** You may have sutures (stitches) placed at the time of surgery. These will dissolve within 4 to 6 days. You do not need to return to have these removed.
7. **OTHER** If you have any questions or concerns, please call the office. Please try to call during office hours, unless it is an emergency.

HELEN ZYLMAN, DDS (313) _ _ _-_ _ _ _ or _ _ _-_ _ _ _
3250 PLYMOUTH ROAD   TELEPHONE ANSWERED
ANN ARBOR, MI 48105   24 HOURS

Note:
   On the day of surgery please follow the schedule below. On the day after, try taking the Motrin only. If you need the Tylox/Zydone, go ahead and use it, but it is a narcotic, so we would like you to stop taking it as soon as it is no longer necessary.
Today:
   Tylox/Zydone: __   __   __   __   __
   Motrin: __   __   __   __
   Other: __   __   __
Tomorrow:
   Try taking Motrin only.
   If an antibiotic has been prescribed, continue taking it as prescribed, until all the tablets are gone.
Tomorrow Evening:
   Start Peridex Rinses/salt water rinses and continue as prescribed for 1 to 2 weeks.

*(Courtesy of Helen Zylman, DDS, Ann Arbor, Michigan.)

Postoperative Instructions

The assistant is now responsible to give the patient instructions about what to do and what to expect over the next few days. The patient is given a sheet of written instructions (Box 34-7) for later reference. The assistant also explains the prescriptions and the time schedule for taking the medication. If the patient is older and possibly forgetful, is a child, or has been sedated, the assistant invites the person who has accompanied the patient into the treatment room to listen to the instructions. Before this patient is discharged, the assistant also demonstrates how to change the gauze and provides some extra gauze to take home. If the procedure is difficult, the assistant gives the patient an ice pack. After the assistant is certain that the patient has no more questions, he or she walks with the patient to the business desk. The patient may feel lightheaded or faint after a procedure such as this, and the assistant must continue to monitor the patient and assist if necessary.

▶ Multiple Routine Extractions (Case Scenario #2)

This patient is a healthy 11-year-old female with mild crowding of the dentition (Fig. 34-33). The orthodontist has completed a thorough examination before starting full orthodontic treatment and has indicated that because of the amount of crowding, the shape of her arch, and the fact that there is insufficient room for the cuspids, the four first premolars must be removed.

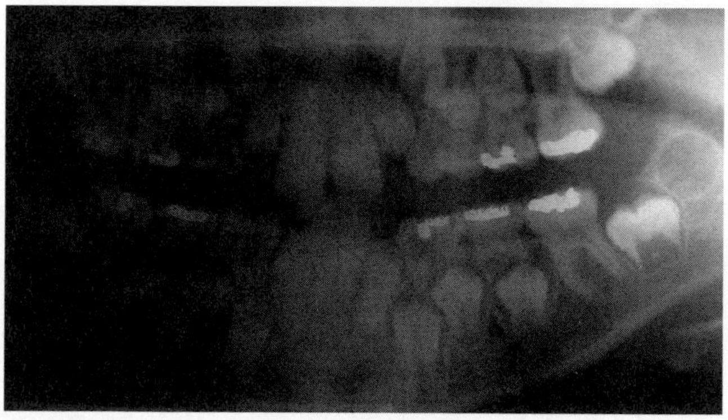

Armamentarium Preparation

Anesthesia/Patient Monitor Set-Up
Multiple Routine Extraction Set-Up

The set-up for the routine extraction is used, with the addition of a mandibular anterior forceps, #151.

Postoperative Instructions

In this case the parent/caregiver is called into the treatment room and the assistant goes through the instructions with her. Usually, children like to take the teeth home with them after the extraction; so the teeth must be cleaned and placed in an envelope for the tooth fairy.

▶ Surgical Extractions (Case Scenario #3)

This procedure involves the extraction of a badly broken-down tooth that may not come out in one piece. This patient is a 70-year-old male who has spent many hours in the dental chair over the years. The maxillary right first molar has had periodontal therapy, endodontic treatment, and a crown. Now, however, decay is in the trifurcation area of the crown of the tooth and the dentist has decided that the tooth is nonrestorable (Fig. 34-34). The dentist refers the patient for extraction, and the tooth will be replaced with a bridge. The patient had rheumatic heart disease as a child, and in preparation for his surgery he took 3 g of amoxicillin 1 hour before his appointment.

Teeth that have had endodontic therapy are often brittle, making it difficult to remove them without fracture. The amount of decay in the trifurcation area suggests that the crown will fracture from the roots when the tooth is removed. For this reason it is best to plan on a surgical extraction of this tooth.

FIG. 34-33 Radiograph of orthodontic patient with crowding. Four first premolars are to be removed.

(Courtesy of Helen Zylman, D.D.S., Ann Arbor, Michigan.)

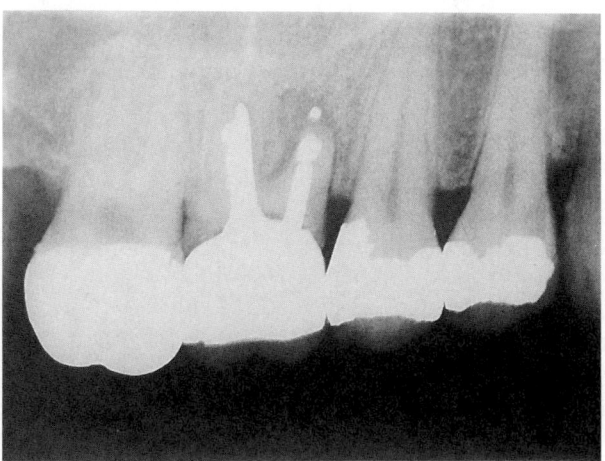

FIG. 34-34 Radiograph of nonrestorable tooth #3

(Courtesy of Helen Zylman, D.D.S. Ann Arbor, Michigan.)

MULTIPLE ROUTINE EXTRACTIONS

Anesthesia Administration

The procedure for removing these teeth is similar to that used with the patient in case #1. When the young patient is seated the parent/caregiver remains in the reception room, since most children behave better without this person present in the treatment room. The patient takes no premedication, the vital signs are normal, but the patient is a bit anxious about the procedure. In this procedure, nitrous oxide is used. Local anesthetic is administered; this is a difficult time for many children, and the assistant must anticipate any undesired reactions with the child. Usually, with verbal reassurance or possibly a hand to hold, most children pull through without too much difficulty.

Each oral surgeon has a preferred way of removing multiple teeth. A common procedure is to start in the maxillary left quadrant, with the patient in a reclining position, move to the maxillary right, then raise the back of the chair slightly, and proceed to first the mandibular left quadrant and then the mandibular right. This routine is used for local anesthesia, as well as the extractions. The order of extracting teeth does not really matter; however, a set pattern helps both members of the surgical team to know what to expect next.

With multiple extractions such as this, the two-syringe technique is used, since many injections are needed. The procedure is identical to that described for the single extraction. The patient is told that her lips will start to feel *fat*. Many children today have no caries and have not experienced local anesthesia before having some orthodontic extractions. It is helpful to warn the children about how they will feel and also to caution them not to bite the lips while they are numb.

Extraction Procedure

The procedure is essentially the same as for the single extraction (see Routine Extraction steps) with the following changes:

1. When the patient is a child, it is particularly important to let them know what to expect next, such as pressure or noise, etc.; demonstrate whenever possible. For example, the HVE tip can be applied to the assistant's gloved hand to demonstrate the action (placing it on the child's hand could contaminate the tip). The patient can be told that it is like a "little vacuum cleaner."
2. With extraction of healthy teeth, such as in orthodontic extraction, usually it is not necessary to use the surgical curette after extraction.
3. The tooth is luxated with the elevator (some operators skip this step in orthodontic extractions); then the forceps is used and the tooth is removed from the mouth.
4. After each extraction a gauze pad is placed to help control bleeding. The patient should be allowed to bite on the gauze briefly; this gives the patient a chance to rest slightly after each extraction.
5. After all the extractions are complete, the patient's mouth is rinsed and one piece of folded gauze is placed on each side.

Armamentarium Preparation

Anesthesia/Patient Monitor Set-Up

SURGICAL EXTRACTION SET-UP

Mirror
Retractor
Cotton pliers
Surgical curette
Scalpel handle, with blade, #11, #12, or #15
Periosteal Elevator
Straight elevator #77
Root tip elevators

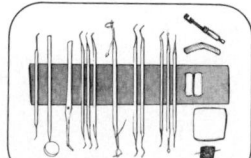

Bayonet forceps #210-S
Rongeurs
Bone file
Surgical HVE tip
Surgical burs with handpiece
Irrigating syringe, with sterile saline
Cup, with sterile water
Suture, placed in sterile water to soften
Needle holder
3 × 3 gauze sponges
Lubricant

SURGICAL EXTRACTIONS

Extraction Procedure

1. Simultaneously, pass the retractor and the curette to the surgeon for the purpose of assessing the level of anesthesia. Since the patient feels only pressure and no sharp sensation when the area is checked, the surgeon hands the curette back to the assistant and the procedure begins.

2. Exchange the curette for the #77 elevator. The surgeon attempts to luxate the tooth, but as expected, it doesn't move easily. Rather than placing the forceps on the tooth, with the high probability of fracture, the surgeon decides to remove the tooth surgically.

3. The surgeon returns the elevator to the assistant in exchange for a scalpel with a #15 blade. Safety is important and care must be taken anytime sharp instruments such as this are exchanged; it might be easy to cut oneself through a glove if careless.

4. The surgeon makes an incision along the margin of the gingiva and down to the bone. The incision usually extends the width of one tooth on either side of the tooth to be extracted. If the incision is less than or equal to the width of the tooth, vision will not be clear and the tissue may be torn. A sharp, clean incision heals more quickly than a jagged tear. When maxillary teeth are removed, a vertical releasing incision is usually added to one end or the other of the incision to add visibility (Fig. 34-35).

5. At this point the surgeon uses a retractor in the left hand to keep the cheek out of the way, while using the scalpel in the right hand. The assistant uses the HVE tip in the right hand to keep the surgical site clear, while keeping the left hand free to exchange instruments. If this were an extraction in the mandibular right quadrant instead of the maxillary arch, the HVE tip might also

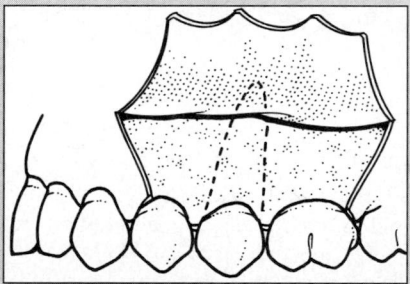

FIG. 34-35   **Diagram of envelope flap, with vertical release.**

(From Peterson LJ, Hupp J, Ellis III E, Tucker M: *Contemporary oral and maxillofacial surgery*, ed 2, St Louis, 1992, Mosby.)

be used as a retractor for the tongue. The surgical HVE tip does not need to be in the mouth at all times, but the assistant must keep a close watch on the surgical field to make sure that the area is as clean and dry as possible.

6. Once the incision has been made, exchange the surgeon's scalpel for a periosteal elevator. Usually the pointed end of this instrument is used to start reflecting the mucoperiosteal flap (the full thickness soft tissue flap, including the top or mucosal layer and the inner layer, which covers the bone—the periosteum). Once the flap is partially reflected, the instrument can be turned and the flatter end can be used to complete the reflection. During this process, the surgeon places the Minnesota retractor between the reflected tissue and the bone to see the site of operation.

7. The surgeon returns the periosteal elevator to the assistant. Some surgeons use this elevator as a retractor, rather than one of the specific retractors; therefore, it is helpful to have two periosteal elevators on the tray, one for reflection and one for retraction. The surgeon receives the surgical handpiece with a round bur from the assistant.

8. Pick up the irrigating syringe. Some handpieces have a device that provides automatic irrigation during use, so that the irrigating syringe is not needed. The surgeon uses the handpiece and the retractor, while the assistant uses the irrigating syringe and the HVE tip. Whenever a handpiece is used to remove bone, the area must be irrigated simultaneously; this helps to keep debris from the flutes of the bur, it keeps the bone from desiccating (overheating and burning), and it helps to keep the area clean, so that the surgeon has good visibility. A slight stream of water must be kept on the end of the bur.

9. Place the HVE nearby, so that the mouth does not fill with water, but do not keep it so near that the liquid from the irrigating syringe goes directly into the HVE tip without ever touching the bur.

10. As the surgeon moves the handpiece and bur, follow closely, making sure that the water always stays on the end of the bur.

11. Occasionally, when bone relief or sectioning is done, the assistant will have to stop and refill the syringe. If the surgeon asks, it is helpful occasionally to irrigate and clean the entire surgical site and to evacuate the patient's mouth. During this point in the procedure, the surgeon's goal is to remove enough bone (usually a small amount) to be able to visualize the roots of the tooth and to divide them.

Continued.

SURGICAL EXTRACTIONS—cont'd

STOP

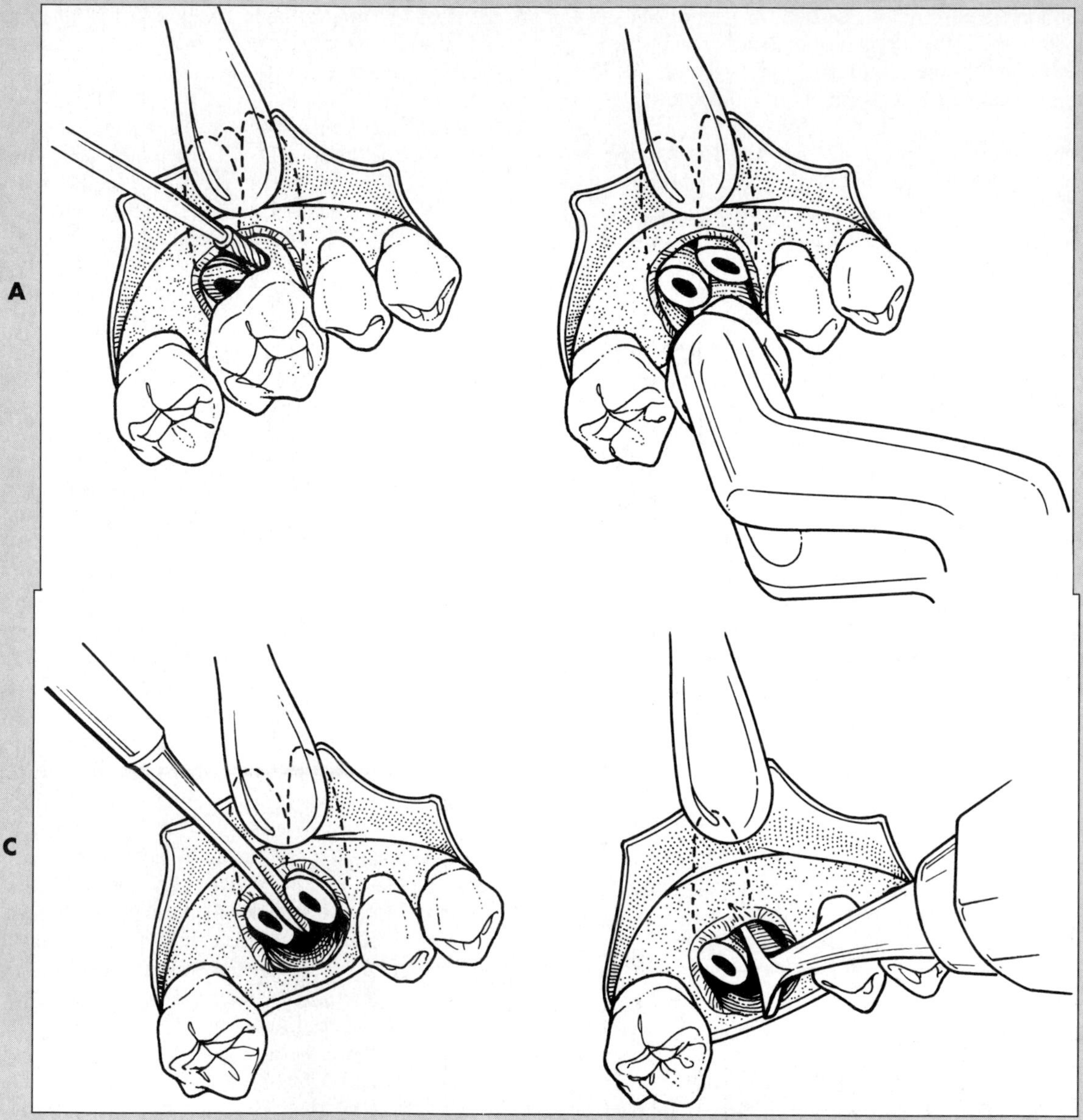

FIG. 34-36 Sectioning a maxillary molar. *A,* Small envelope incision is made, and small amount of bone is removed with a bur. *B,* Molar forceps is used to remove crown portion of tooth along with palatal root. *C,* Straight elevator is used to mobilize buccal roots and may deliver the roots. *D,* Cryer elevator can be used to rotate and deliver remaining root.

(From Peterson LJ, Hupp J, Ellis III E, Tucker M: *Contemporary oral and maxillofacial surgery,* ed 2, St Louis, 1992, Mosby.)

12. In this situation the roots are exposed and the two buccal roots are divided from the rest of the tooth. To accomplish this, a groove is made part of the way through the roots of the tooth. Some surgeons prefer to switch to a different bur, such as a straight fissure bur, at this point.

13. Pass the surgeon a straight elevator to complete the split from the rest of the tooth.

14. Sometimes the roots easily come out at this point; at other times a root tip elevator (#2 or #3) will be needed to lift the roots from the socket. The common sequence is to remove the buccal root tips and the rest of the tooth; the palatal root can be luxated and removed as a single-rooted tooth.

15. Pass the root tip or cryer elevators individually to the surgeon, who will use these instruments to loosen the root tips.

16. Transfer forceps, such as the rongeurs, to the surgeon for removal of the root tips. Occasionally, the tips may be removed by the assistant with the surgical HVE tip. Care should be taken to clear the HVE tip.

17. After these root tips are removed, the rest of the tooth and the palatal root can be luxated and removed almost as a single-rooted tooth (Fig. 34-36).

18. The surgeon then takes the bayonet forceps (#210 S) and removes the rest of the tooth. The assistant takes the tooth and the forceps together in the palm of the left hand. The surgeon is simultaneously handed a curette to check for abscess formation (described with the routine extraction).

19. When a tooth is removed surgically, sharp bony edges must often be smoothed. After the surgeon has finished with the curette, the instrument is exchanged for a double-ended bone file. If only one tooth has been removed, the smaller end of the bone file usually is used; but if multiple teeth have been removed, the larger end is often used. The sharp edges of the instrument are passed along the edge of the bone to smooth it.

20. When either the curette or the bone file is handed back to the assistant, the HVE tip or a gauze sponge should be used to clean the end of the instrument to make it ready for use again; this also helps cut down on the instrument cleaning later, since blood and bone fragments can be much more difficult to remove once they have dried than they were initially.

21. When the surgeon decides that the bone is sufficiently smooth and that the socket is clean, the bone file is exchanged for an irrigation syringe and the entire area is irrigated. All bone fragments and tooth debris must be removed from the area; otherwise they may cause an infection. The assistant may find it easier to have the patient turn to one side to gain access to the fluid in the mouth.

Suture Placement

1. Next, hand the surgeon the needle holder with the needle attached, having placed the needle into the holder so that the needle points in the proper direction to pass through the tissue. The position of the needle should enable it to pass through the tissue from the most mobile tissue (the reflected flap) to the least mobile tissue (the unreflected soft tissue), with the tip of the holder just grasping the needle at right angles and approximately two thirds of the way from the tip (Fig. 34-37). One surgical knot is placed in each interproximal area. At least one additional knot is placed in the vertical extension.

2. When the surgeon has passed the suture through both sides of the tissue, the suture is tied. The surgeon needs both hands to tie the knot, so the assistant must retract the tissue. This may be done with the HVE tip, with a mirror, with a retractor or by hand. The assistant needs to reach around the back of the patient's head to retract the cheek on the right side of the mouth because the surgeon's view would be impaired if the assistant's arm were across the face of the patient. At times the assistant may need to retract both cheek and tongue, such as in the lower right quadrant.

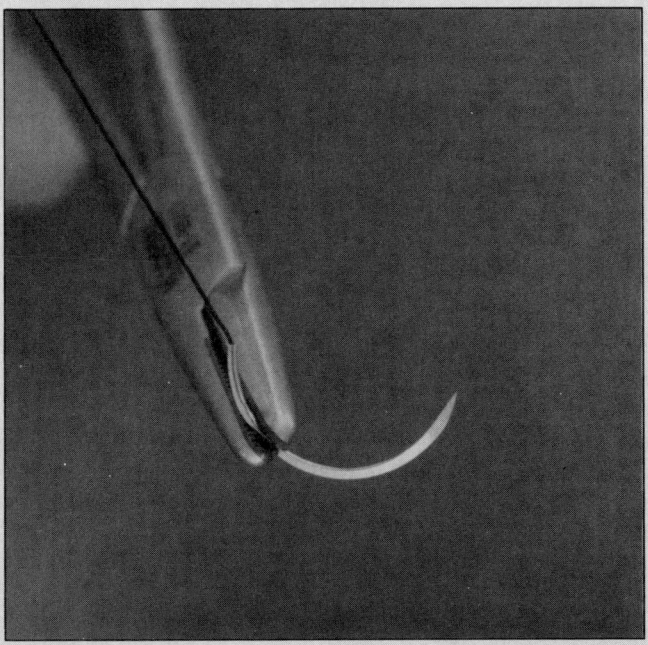

FIG. 34-37   Needle holder grasps curved needle two thirds of the distance from the tip of needle.

(From Peterson LJ, Hupp J, Ellis III E, Tucker M: *Contemporary oral and maxillofacial surgery*, ed 2, St Louis, 1992, Mosby.)

Continued.

SURGICAL EXTRACTIONS—cont'd

3. After the knot is tied, the suture must be cut, usually by the assistant, although some dentists like to cut the suture themselves.

4. Hold the scissors with the thumb and the fourth (ring) finger. This technique gives much more stability than when the scissors are held with the thumb and the third finger. Most surgeons use suture scissors that are slightly curved. The assistant brings the scissors into the oral cavity with the beaks closed and the tips pointing away from the alveolar ridge. This affords a measure of safety because the assistant may inadvertently cut the patient this way.

5. The suture should be cut with the tips of the scissors, and the assistant must watch carefully when cutting to protect the patient. The length of the suture ends should be approximately 2 mm, although again, this de-

pends on the preference of the surgeon. Silk sutures that must be removed usually are left with longer tails than resorbable sutures, which dissolve and come out on their own.

During the course of the extraction the assistant must keep the tray neat and orderly, returning used instruments to their original position on the surgical tray. A basin or bag should be available for trash, such as empty suture packets and used gauze. Used sharps must be kept separately. Trash must not cover the tray, impeding easy access to the instruments. Some surgeons may request that the used anesthetic carpules be kept separately from the rest of the trash, so that an easy accounting of the carpules can be made.

Postoperative Instructions

After the suturing is complete, a gauze square is placed directly over the surgical site and the patient is instructed to bite firmly. The assistant wipes the patient's mouth, and the chairback is elevated slightly, allowing the patient to relax for a few minutes before the assistant goes over the postoperative instructions and the postoperative pain medications. The patient has taken amoxicillin for SBE prophylaxis and needs to be reminded to take a second dose 6 hours after taking the first one. After the remainder of the instructions have been covered, the patient can be scheduled for a suture removal appointment in 5 to 7 days and then discharged.

In this case the patient was sitting up and was almost ready for discharge when he mentioned feeling lightheaded and nauseated. The assistant immediately reclined the chair again, so that the patient was lying almost flat. It is almost impossible for a patient to faint in the supine position. In this type of situation the assistant should give the patient an emesis basin to hold (these should be easily accessible at all times). A cool damp cloth should be placed on the patient's forehead, since patients often feel hot when they are about to faint. At this point the assistant should notify the surgeon, who may order some oxygen for the patient, or if the patient is having chest pain, the surgeon might order a nitroglycerine tablet. If there is a call box in the treatment room, the assistant can call for help immediately. The assistant should not leave the patient alone when going for help. A calm demeanor must be maintained because

patients can become frightened by the assistant's sudden changes in motion and urgency. The patient should be reassured that he or she will be feeling better soon.

Assuming that the patient starts to feel better, he or she should slowly be raised to an upright position; this should not be hurried, or a relapse may occur. The patient should not be allowed to leave the office until he or she is feeling normal. It may even be necessary to arrange for transportation because the patient should definitely not drive even if the lightheadedness has abated.

▶ Multiple Extractions with Immediate Denture Placement (Case Scenario #4)

The techniques used in this next case study will involve all those already learned. The patient is a 55-year-old male and has been struggling with periodontal disease and decay during his adult life. He has now decided to have the remaining mandibular teeth removed and a denture fabricated.

The patient's prosthodontist has already made the denture and it is to be inserted immediately after the teeth have been removed, so that the patient will not be without teeth. The disadvantage to this technique is that the prosthodontist needs to make a denture based on a *projected* ridge and not the actual ridge after the teeth have been removed. Also, the oral tissues will shrink considerably after the denture has been placed, requiring the denture to be relined in a year. An alternative to an immediate denture would be to have the patient wait for

MULTIPLE EXTRACTIONS WITH IMMEDIATE DENTURE PLACEMENT

Anesthesia Administration

This is a prolonged procedure, and the patient has never been comfortable in the dental chair, so the surgeon has elected to use intravenous sedation. Intravenous sedation is given and local anesthetic is administered. Since multiple injections are needed to anesthetize the mandibular arch, two syringes are used. The patient will not remember any of this, so topical anesthetic is not used; however, a second dental assistant is brought in to restrain the patient's hands, because the anesthetic makes the patient drowsy; the injections are uncomfortable, so the patient wants to push the doctor's hand away.

If general anesthesia or deep sedation is used, a second assistant may be needed to monitor the patient's airway during surgery. A deeply sedated patient may be so relaxed that he or she cannot keep the airway open. The anesthesia assistant may need to place his or her hands behind the angles of the patient's mandible, using forward traction to lift the mandible slightly and keep the airway open. If a patient is snoring, the airway may be partially obstructed, and the patient must either be stimulated to open the airway or the assistant must do it.

Extraction Procedure

1. Hand the curette and retractor to the surgeon. This time, when the areas are evaluated for adequate anesthesia, the patient's response indicates that several spots are painful.

2. Return the curette and retractor to the tray, and pass the syringe to the surgeon for more anesthesia.

3. Once the level of anesthesia is adequate, hand the scalpel to the surgeon, who makes an incision through the soft tissue in the mandibular right quadrant (again, this is a totally arbitrary place to begin surgery; each surgeon has his or her own preferred area to initiate the procedure).

4. Exchange the scalpel for a periosteal elevator; the surgeon reflects a small mucoperiosteal flap to allow access to the teeth.

5. Retrieve the periosteal elevator, and pass a straight elevator, which is used to luxate teeth, to the surgeon.

6. The surgeon removes the remaining teeth with forceps as described earlier in the previous extraction procedures.

7. After all of the teeth in this quadrant have been removed, hand the curette to the surgeon for removal of any pathology in the alveolus. Throughout this procedure use the HVE to maintain a clear field of operation for the surgeon. Extractions of periodontally involved teeth can be quite bloody, and the need for the HVE tip needs to be anticipated.

8. Exchange curette for a ronguer to be used in removing any tenacious bits of tissue that are clinging to the bone. At this point the surgeon looks at the overall shape of the arch. The arch must be free of sharp edges, and undercuts should be kept to a mini-

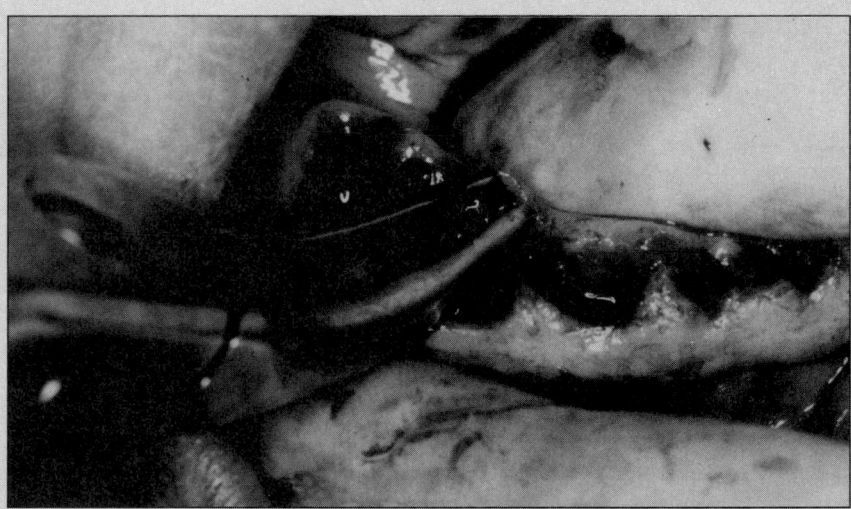

FIG. 34-38   Use of rongeur forceps to reduce prominent bone.

(From Peterson LJ, Hupp J, Ellis III E, Tucker M: *Contemporary oral and maxillofacial surgery*, ed 2, St Louis, 1992, Mosby.)

Continued.

MULTIPLE EXTRACTIONS WITH IMMEDIATE DENTURE PLACEMENT—cont'd

mum. The patient has one area of especially prominent bone over the edge of the mandibular right first premolar (Fig. 34-38).

9. The surgeon now uses the rongeur to remove most of this excessive bone. Each time the surgeon removes a piece of bone with the rongeur, hold out a gauze square and wipe the beaks of the instrument free of debris.

10. After the surgeon is satisfied with the shape of the bone, exchange the rongeur for a bone file. In this case the large end of the bone file is used, since there is a lot of bone to smooth.

11. After the ridge is smooth, exchange the file for the irrigating syringe. The surgeon irrigates the site, while the assistant evacuates. Suturing, which would ordinarily be done now, is delayed until after completion of the entire procedure.

Attention now is turned to the mandibular left quadrant. The procedure here is identical to the one performed on the

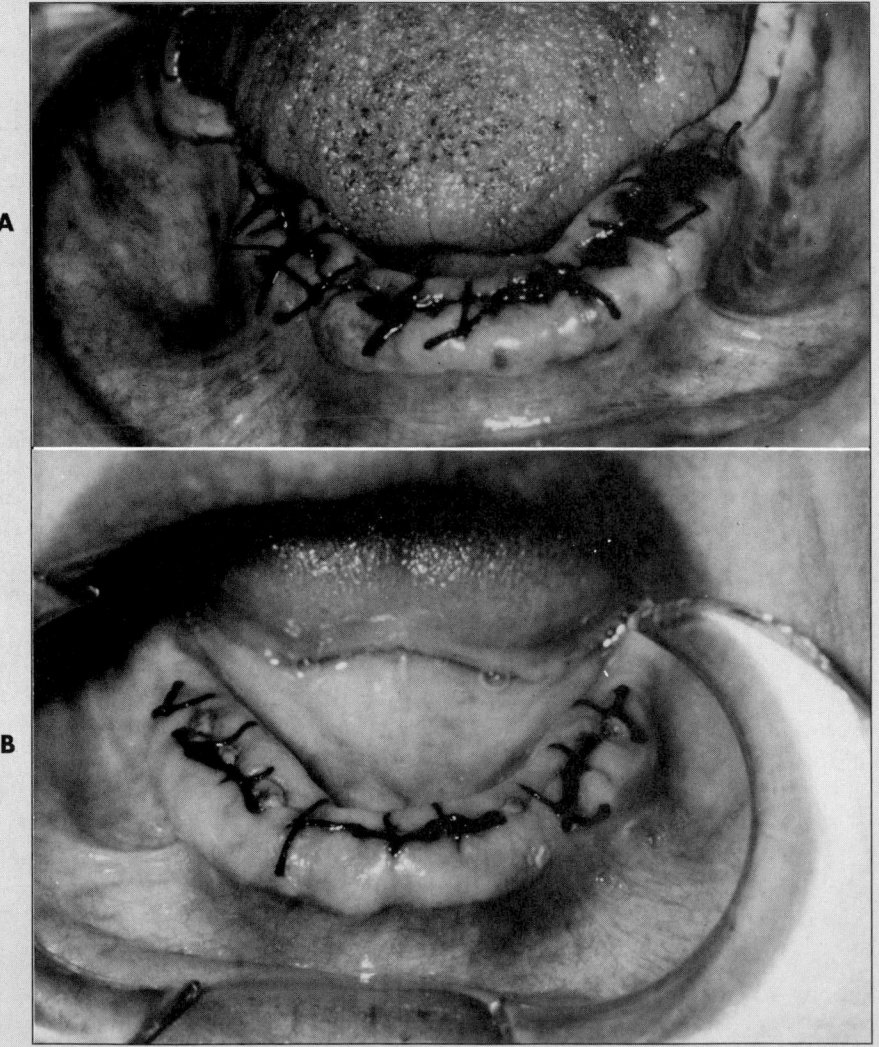

FIG. 34-39   *A,* Tissue is closed. *B,* Patient returns 1 week later for suture removal.

[From Peterson LJ, Hupp J, Ellis III E, Tucker M: *Contemporary oral and maxillofacial surgery,* ed 2, St Louis, 1992, Mosby.

MULTIPLE EXTRACTIONS WITH IMMEDIATE DENTURE PLACEMENT—cont'd

mandibular right quadrant. The difference that arises in this quadrant is that during the extraction of tooth #19, the mesial root fractures. Since a flap has already been reflected, it is a relatively easy procedure to remove the root tip.

12. The surgeon can handle a fractured mesial root in the following manner:
    a. Forceps are used on the root tip if it is accessible
    b. Since roots usually aren't accessible enough, bone is removed to make the roots accessible; a medium-sized root pick (#2 or #3) is used to lift the root out of the socket, using the palatal portion of the socket as a fulcrum; in this case the root tip is located towards the buccal
13. The surgeon makes a small perforation through the bone at the apex of the root tip with the handpiece and uses the root elevator to ease the root tip out.
14. The remainder of this procedure, including the extraction of the six anterior teeth, proceeds as described in Case #2. Often, extraction of the cuspids is a surgical procedure because the cuspids usually are strong teeth with excellent bone support, making them difficult to remove. The surgical site is shown complete with sutures in Fig. 34-39, *A* and *B*.

Stent Try In / Denture Insertion

When all of the teeth are removed, the ridge is prepared, and before suturing begins, the plastic stent is tried in. A stent is a clear plastic denture base, which is made on the same model as the denture; the surgeon can see through the stent to the arch beneath to identify areas that impinge on the stent.

1. Hand the stent to the surgeon to try in. The stent does not seat correctly; the surgeon can see that the area already trimmed is the problem area.
2. The surgeon hands the stent back and removes more bone from this area, using the handpiece with a bone trimming bur.
3. After the area is irrigated, the denture is tried in again. This time it fits. If a stent had not been used, it probably would have been more difficult to determine interferences that were causing the denture not to seat properly.

Suture Placement

Now that the denture fits, the soft tissue is sutured. It is the surgeon's choice whether to use individual knots or to use a continuous suture. With a continuous suture, a traditional knot is tied at one end of the arch. Only the short end of the knot is trimmed, and the long end is used to sew the tissue closed. Usually a knot is tied in the midline and a second suture is started from the other end. When it is time to tie the second knot, the needle is passed through the tissue; however, the last loop of suture is not pulled tight. Instead it is used to make a knot with the remainder of the suture which is attached to the needle. Refer to Fig. 34-28, *B,* for suture placement.

---

about 6 weeks for healing of the gingiva and alveolar process before inserting the denture. (See Chapter 31 for further discussion of this process.)

Armamentarium Preparation

Anesthesia / Patient Monitor Set-up

SURGICAL EXTRACTION SET-UP

Mirror
Retractor
Cotton pliers
Surgical curette
Scalpel handle, with blade, 11, 12, or 15
Periosteal elevator
Straight elevator #77
Assorted forceps (optional)

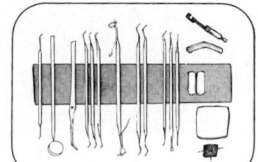

Mandibular universal forceps #151
Mandibular molar forceps #23
Maxillary right and left molar forceps #53 R and L
Rongeurs
Bone file
Surgical HVE tip
Surgical burs with handpiece
Irrigating syringe with sterile saline
Cup with sterile water
Suture, placed in sterile water to soften
Needle holder
3 × 3 gauze sponges
Lubricant
Surgicel (placed nearby)
Root tip elevators (optional)
Stent
Denture

Postoperative Instructions

After the suturing has been completed, and the denture is inserted, the patient is informed that the procedure has been completed, is cautioned that the denture may need adjustment (usually an adjustment appointment is scheduled soon after the immediate denture placement), and is advised that it will take some time to get used to talking and eating with the new denture. The assistant removes the monitor leads and the IV, and the patient's companion is brought back to listen to the instructions. The patient was sedated and may not remember all the instructions; so it is helpful if a companion listens as well and is given written instructions. Once recovery from the anesthesia has occurred, the patient can be discharged and is directed to visit the prosthodontist as previously arranged. The patient should return in a week for a follow-up visit, at which time the sutures are removed and the tissue is evaluated.

▶ Third Molar Extractions
(Case Scenario #5)

In the modern dental office (caries being greatly reduced), third molar removal is probably the most common reason patients are referred to an oral surgeon. This procedure combines most of the techniques already discussed in this chapter. The patient is an 18-year-old female and, except for having insulin-dependent diabetes, is healthy. She has recently been feeling some pressure in her mouth. Her family dentist saw from her bitewing radiographs that the patient's third molars were impacted, so she was referred to the oral surgeon, where a panoramic film was exposed (Fig. 34-40). It is obvious from this film that there is insufficient room in the patient's mouth for these teeth, and the surgeon recommends that all of the third molars be removed before they cause problems, such as crowding, infection, or cyst formation. The surgeon also tells the patient that removal of teeth becomes much more difficult as a patient gets older and that removal before the age of 20 is highly recommended.

Armamentarium Preparation

Anesthesia/Patient Monitor Set-up
SURGICAL EXTRACTION SET-UP
Mirror
Retractor
Cotton pliers
Surgical curette
Scalpel handle, with blade, 11, 12, or 15
Periosteal elevator
Straight elevator #77
Assorted forceps (optional)
  Maxillary universal forceps #150
  Maxillary posterior bayonet forceps #210S
  Maxillary right and left molar forceps #53R and L
Rongeurs

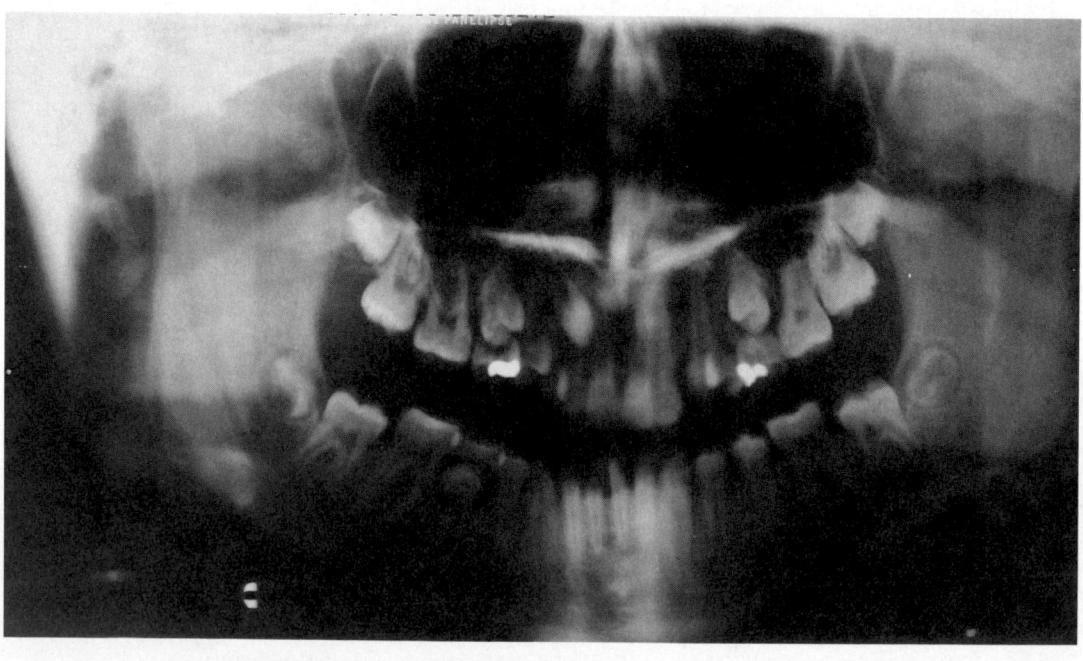

FIG. 34-40   Panorex of crowded third molars.

(Courtesy of Helen Zylman, D.D.S., Ann Arbor, Michigan.)

THIRD MOLAR EXTRACTIONS ·

Anesthesia Administration

Since this patient is diabetic, the assistant asks her about her last meal. The patient tells the assistant that she ate a light breakfast approximately 1 hour before coming into the office; she also took half of her normal morning dose of insulin. The primary care physician and the surgeon also had recommended that the patient be premedicated with an antibiotic to lessen the possibility of postoperative infection.

The patient is to have a combination of nitrous oxide and intravenous sedation. The surgeon then comes in and reclines the chair and places the nitrous oxide mask on the patient's nose. The level is set at 60% nitrous oxide and 40% oxygen. The patient is advised that soon she will begin to feel some tingling in her hands and feet. As the nitrous oxide begins to take effect, the surgeon and the assistant place the IV as described in earlier procedures in this chapter. In this case, Versed and Demerol will be used. First, Demerol is administered, and the patient is warned that occasionally patients experience some stinging in the area where the IV has been placed but that this will go away quickly. Then the Versed is titrated in slowly. The patient is told that she will start to feel as if she is floating and will notice that the lights appear to be moving, that it will become difficult for her to talk and that she will not remember anything of the procedure. The patient must be informed of the effect of the sedative.

To use the nitrous oxide in addition to the intravenous sedation gives the surgeon more control over the anesthesia than if only the sedation were used. The nitrous oxide potentiates the effect of the sedation, making sedation more effective at lower doses. Therefore, the patient is relaxed and comfortable throughout the procedure and has a quick recovery after the surgery. The extra oxygen that is supplied to the patient is helpful in cases of sedation; it eases breathing and reduces anxiety during recovery.

Local anesthetic is administered. Approximately 1¼ carpules are used for each third molar; one is used to infiltrate the mucosa next to the upper third or to block half of the mandible and approximately ¼ carpule is used to infiltrate the palatal and the long buccal nerves; the technique for this is identical to that described earlier in this chapter.

Extraction Procedure
Maxillary Left Third Molar

1. Pass the retractor and the curette to the surgeon. Assess the soft tissue posterior to tooth #15 for patient reaction. When the patient indicates there is no pain when the curette is used, the procedure continues.
2. Exchange the curette for a scalpel; the surgeon makes an incision through the tissue in the posterior left maxilla. Using the HVE tip on the tissue before the first incision is made keeps saliva to a minimum, and optimum vision is maintained. The incision parallels the ridge that is posterior to the second molar tooth, follows the gingival crevice around the second molar to the papilla, and is extended vertically up into the vestibule.
3. Exchange the scalpel for the periosteal elevator; pass this to the surgeon with the pointed end available for immediate use. The surgeon uses the retractor in the left hand to hold the patient's cheek out of the way and elevates the mucoperiosteal flap with the periosteal elevator in the right hand. Once some of the tissue is reflected, the surgeon places the retractor between the tissue and bone to continue to facilitate vision.
4. When the flap is completely reflected, the surgeon returns the periosteal elevator and receives a chisel or a bone bur in a surgical handpiece. Surgeons vary the technique, based on the amount and density of the bone to be removed.
5. When a surgical handpiece is used, follow the technique for removing an erupted tooth. Hold the HVE tip in the right hand, and hold the irrigation syringe in the left hand. Drip a slow steady stream of sterile water or saline solution onto the bur to prevent heat generation. Use the HVE tip to keep the surgical site clear.
6. When this procedure is used for maxillary teeth, the mandibular arch and posterior pillar region must be evacuated occasionally. Remember to be alert to the patient's needs because the patient has diminished gag reflex when he or she is sedated.
7. Once an adequate amount of bone has been removed from the buccal surface of the tooth, the surgeon exchanges the handpiece for a #77 elevator (or other preferred elevator).
8. The surgeon positions the elevator between the tooth and the edge of the bone and pushes the impacted third molar distally out of the socket, using the bone as the fulcrum. Support the patient's head as needed during this step, since a sedated patient has lost muscle strength and will move along with the pressure of the elevator. When the head is supported, the pressure from the elevator is more effective.
9. If the tooth does not move easily, the elevator is exchanged for the handpiece to remove more bone.
10. Once the tooth has been elevated from the socket, the surgeon exchanges the elevator for a bayonet-type forceps. The angle on the end of the forceps allows the instrument to be placed in a small area.
11. If the elevator dislodges the tooth, the surgeon may ask for a rongeur or a forceps to remove the loosened tooth from the mouth. Sometimes, it can be brought out with the elevator, or it can be removed from the oral cavity with the HVE tip.

Continued.

12. Keep the HVE tip in place until the tooth is removed from the mouth. Teeth can be quite slippery, and occasionally a tooth may pop out of the socket and into the patient's mouth, where it could be swallowed or aspirated, so position the HVE tip between the tooth and the throat as a precautionary measure.

13. Once the tooth has been removed, assess the roots of the tooth for fractures.

14. If one or more of the root tips is sharp or appears to be fractured, notify the surgeon. Many surgeons examine extracted teeth themselves. In case scenario #5, all of the root tips came out intact.

15. The surgeon receives the curette from the assistant and uses it to remove the dental follicle—a sac of slightly thickened membrane—from the socket; this is something that occurs routinely when third molars are removed from young individuals. The follicle is part of the developing tooth. As an individual gets older, the follicle shrinks and eventually disappears. It is important to remove the follicle, however; if it remains, it might develop into a cyst.

16. Exchange the curette for the rongeur, and while the surgeon is removing tissue from the socket, prepare a gauze sponge to remove any tissue from the ends of the rongeur.

17. When the surgeon is finished with the rongeur, the instrument is returned.

18. Once the socket has been cleaned, pass the bone file to the surgeon, who smoothes the edge of the socket. Occasionally, the surgeon might extend the bone file toward you, so that the end of it can be cleaned with the HVE.

19. The surgeon exchanges the file for the irrigating syringe. Evacuate the entire surgical site as it is irrigated with sterile saline or water. The surgeon returns the syringe.

20. Pass the needle holder with the suture needle placed so that the surgeon can suture from posterior to anterior.

21. When the surgeon is ready to tie the suture, retract the oral tissues so that the surgeon can use both hands to tie the suture.

22. In the maxillary and mandibular left quadrants and with a right-handed surgeon, you can cut the suture, but often it will be difficult for the assistant to see well enough to do this on the right side of the patient's mouth. If this is the situation, the surgeon cuts the suture. Usually, three sutures are needed to close the third molar incision: one interproximally; one posteriorly; and one in the vertical extension of the incision.

23. If a removable suture is used, record the number of sutures used in each area on the patient chart.

24. After this extraction has been completed, put a folded gauze sponge over the extraction site.

Maxillary Right Third Molar

1. Turn the patient's head to the left, and adjust the light to shine over the maxillary right quadrant.

2. The surgeon receives the retractor and the curette and begins the procedure again. Tooth #1 is removed in the same fashion as #16.

3. Once the extraction of #1 has been completed, raise the patient to a semisitting position. Readjust the patient's head to the right, and adjust the light.

Between each of these procedures, the assistant should take the opportunity to reorganize the tray. Any used sponges are discarded appropriately, and the instruments are repositioned. The assistant checks the length of the remaining suture to make sure that there is enough to continue (this may be a problem when suturing after the last tooth has been extracted). Some surgeons may want the scalpel blade to be changed at this point. The surgeon also assesses the patient's state of relaxation. In this particular case the patient had started to awaken so more of the sedative drug Versed is administered. Refill the irrigation syringe and prepare more gauze sponges for later use. Once the procedure begins, it is vital to keep the chair time to a minimum.

Mandibular Right Third Molar

The procedure for removing the mandibular third molars is similar to that for removing the maxillary third molars, with several important differences.

1. Ask the patient to open the mouth widely. Remove any gauze sponges that are present.

2. Because the patient is drowsy and it is difficult to keep the mouth open, place a rubber bite block on the right side of the mouth. This helps to stabilize the jaw and protects against closing down on the bur or scalpel and possibly causing pain.

3. The surgeon assesses the anesthesia with the curette as before. In this particular case the patient did not react to the curette, but she did react slightly when the incision was extended to the interproximal space between teeth #18 and #19. This indicated that the anesthesia from the long buccal injection, which covered the area directly over the third molar area, was adequate but the mandibular block was not completely successful; this block controls anesthesia of the tooth, bone, and soft tissue from the interproximal area forward.

4. Exchange the scalpel for the anesthetic syringe. The surgeon administers another mandibular block to provide complete anesthesia.

THIRD MOLAR EXTRACTIONS—cont'd

5. Once the anesthesia is adequate, pass the scalpel to the surgeon, who makes an incision.

6. Exchange the scalpel for a periosteal elevator, and the surgeon begins the reflection of the flap. The design of the flap is diagrammed in Fig. 34-41, *A* and *B*. The surgeon makes an angled incision over the soft tissue that lies immediately over the third molar and extends this incision forward along the gingival margin and through the interproximal papilla. In this particular flap design a vertical extension is not used, although some surgeons do use a vertical extension routinely.

7. Often, during reflection of this flap, the situation requires the surgeon and the assistant to alternate the scalpel and the periosteal elevator several times. Keep the scalpel ready for reuse until the surgeon indicates that it is no longer needed. On the patient's left side, help retract the patient's cheek with the HVE tip. On the patient's right side, help retract the patient's tongue with the HVE tip. In the mandibular arch, gravity tends to direct the saliva, irrigation, and blood into and over the surgical site, so be efficient with the HVE tip.

8. The surgeon finishes with the periosteal elevator and returns it. In this particular case, however, the surgeon is not satisfied with the exposure that has been achieved with the periosteal elevator alone.

9. Transfer the scissors to the surgeon, who places them in the posterior portion of the incision, between the bone and periosteum and with the beaks closed and the tip curved toward the bone and away from the tissue. The surgeon then opens the beaks of the scissors, stretching the tissue and improving visibility.

10. This opening and closing may need to be done several times before the surgeon is ready to return the scissors and exchange it for the periosteal elevator to make the final reflection of the flap.

11. The surgeon receives the rongeur and removes some fibrous material from over the tooth.

12. After the surgeon removes this bone he or she can opt to use a handpiece with a bur or a mallet and chisel. Most surgeons today use the handpiece.

13. The surgeon holds the retractor in the left hand and the handpiece in the right. Hold the HVE in the right hand, both for evacuating and for retracting, and hold the irrigation syringe in the left hand. Use the single-handed instrument transfer to retract in the mandibular arch. That way, one hand is always free.

14. The surgeon removes bone from the surgical site until the tooth is exposed and follows the outline of the tooth with the bur to expose as much of the crown of the tooth as possible. Always warn the surgeon when the end of the water supply is near. Another assistant

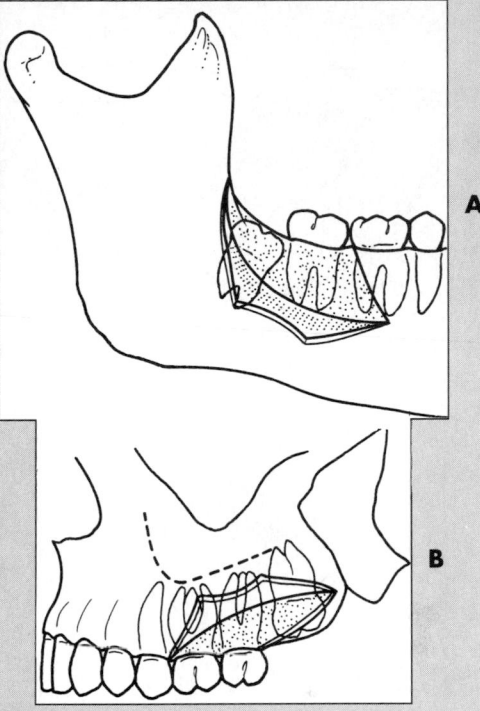

FIG. 34-41 Diagrams of reflected flaps on *A,* mandibular third molar and, *B,* maxillary third molar.

(From Peterson LJ, Hupp J, Ellis III E, Tucker M: *Contemporary oral and maxillofacial surgery,* ed 2, St Louis, 1992, Mosby.)

may need to fill the sterile water supply. Do not leave chairside to obtain more solution.

15. Once the tooth is exposed, the surgeon might ask for an elevator to luxate the tooth. In this particular case, however, the tooth cannot be lifted out in one piece, so the surgeon asks the assistant to refill the irrigation syringe. The next task will be to divide the roots of the tooth.

16. The surgeon makes a vertical groove along the central groove of the buccal surface of the tooth. A straight fissure bur may be used to extend the groove about half way through the tooth. Then exchange the handpiece for a #77 elevator. Various techniques for this procedure are illustrated in Fig. 34-42, *A* through *I.*

17. The surgeon places the elevator into the groove in the tooth and rotates it distally. This completes the crack through the crown of the tooth. Now that the fragments are loosened, the elevator can be used to remove them.

Continued.

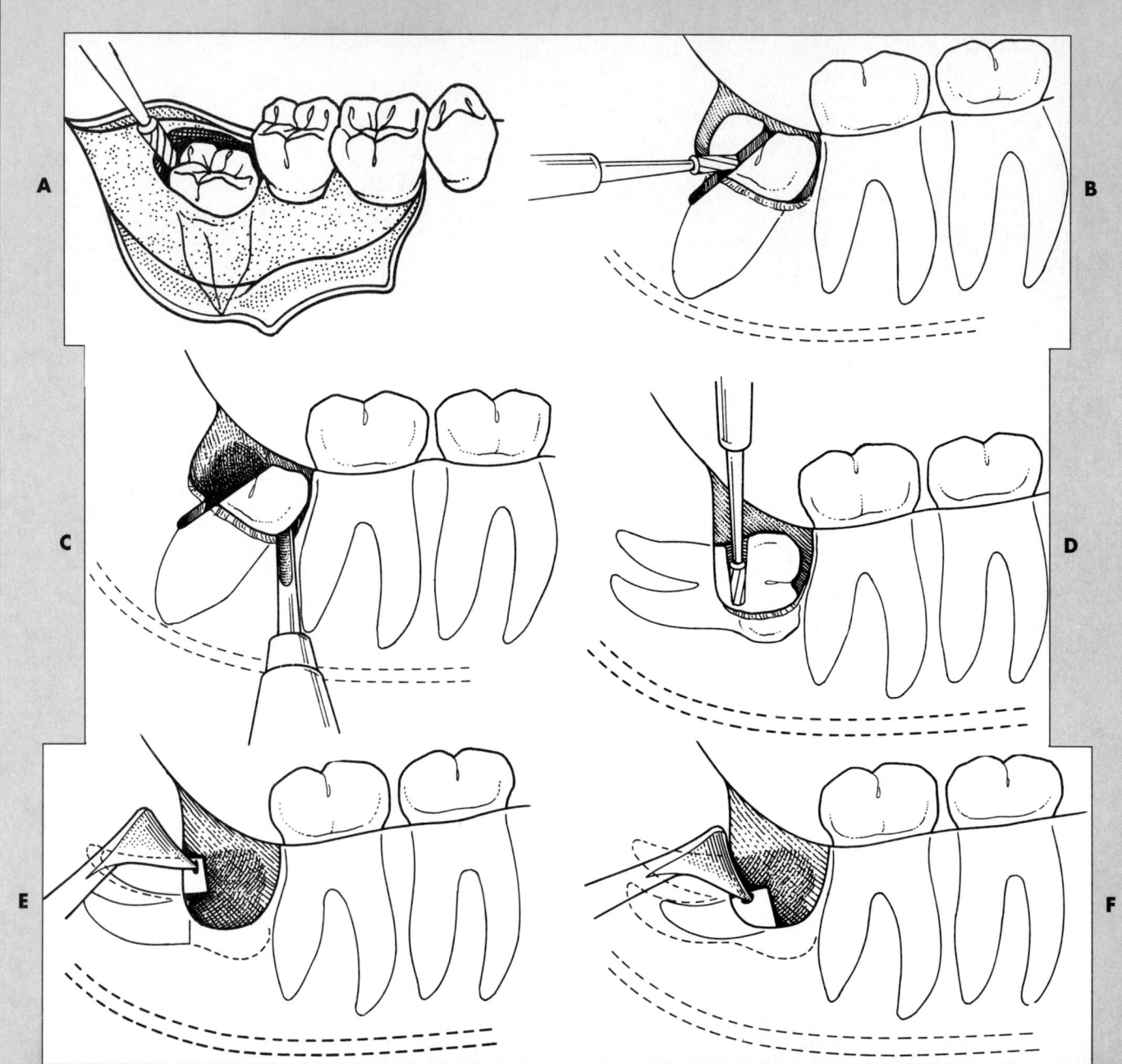

FIG. 34-42   Diagram of sectioning of mandibular third molar. *A,* Soft tissue flap is made, and bone on buccal and distal aspect of impacted tooth is removed with a bur. *B,* Buccal and distal bone is removed to expose crown of mesioangular impaction, and distal aspect of crown is sectioned. *C,* A small straight elevator is used to rotate and elevate remainder of tooth. *D,* A horizontal impaction requires that overlying bone be removed with a bur. *E* and *F,* The crown is sectioned with a cryer elevator, and the roots are lifted out in two separate parts.

THIRD MOLAR EXTRACTIONS—cont'd

18. Completion of this extraction is almost identical to that of the extraction of the maxillary third molar. The only difference is that the surgeon may decide to place a medicated dressing made of Gelfoam and tetracycline in the socket.
19. In earlier preparations a dappen dish with tetracycline powder was placed on the tray. Mix this with sterile saline to make a slurry paste.
20. Dip a piece of Gelfoam into the solution with a cotton forceps.
21. Transfer this to the surgeon after the suture has been placed for the last stitch but before the knot is tied.
22. The surgeon places the Gelfoam into the socket, returns the cotton pliers, and finishes tying the suture knot.
23. Remove the bite block, evacuate the patient's mouth, and allow the patient to close the mouth and rest for a moment before the last tooth is removed.
24. Inspect and reorganize the tray and refill the irrigating syringe.

Mandibular Left Third Molar

1. The surgeon asks the patient to turn to the right and open wide.
2. Place the bite block and adjust the light before the procedure begins again.
3. Everything proceeds identically to the previous extraction, with one exception. On this side, after the crown of the tooth is sectioned, both halves of the crown are removed, but the root tips fracture. Slightly more bone is removed to expose the root tips, and then they are edged out with a fine root tip pick. The remainder of the procedure is identical to that in case scenario #4.

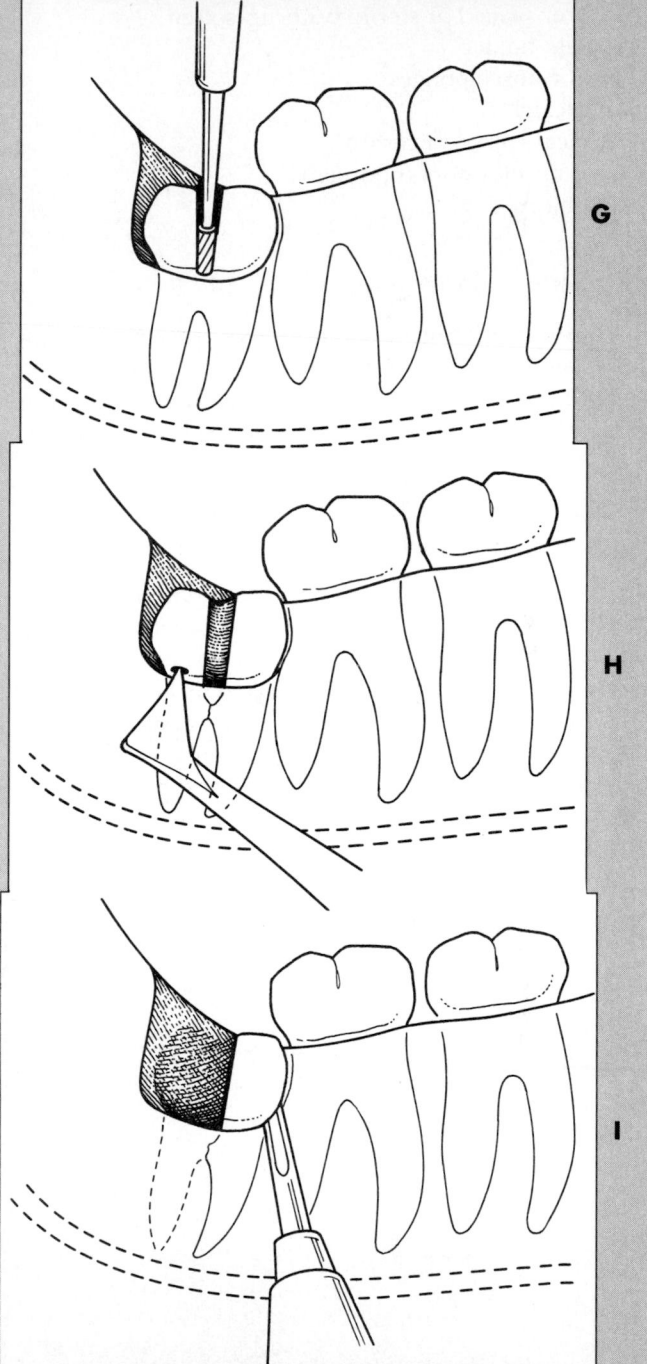

FIG. 34-42, cont'd *G,* A vertical impaction requires removing bone on the occlusal, buccal, and distal; the tooth is then sectioned into mesial and distal parts. *H,* The use of a cryer removes the distal root. *I,* the straight elevator can be used to elevate the mesial root.

(From Peterson LJ, Hupp J, Ellis III E, Tucker M: *Contemporary oral and maxillofacial surgery,* ed 2, St Louis, 1992, Mosby.)

Bone file
Surgical HVE tip
Surgical burs, with handpiece
Irrigating syringe, with sterile saline
Cup, with sterile water
Suture, placed in sterile water to soften
Needle holder
3 × 3 Gauze sponges
Lubricant
Surgicel (placed nearby)
Root tip elevators (optional)
Bite block

Postoperative Instructions

The postoperative instructions for this procedure are not significantly different from those in the previous cases. The primary concern is that the patient be reminded to eat a proper diet as described earlier in the chapter.

▶ Exposure of Impacted Cuspid (Case Scenario #6)

This procedure will be slightly different from those already discussed. To this point the procedures have involved the removal of teeth. This case concerns a female patient, age 11, who is referred by her orthodontist for exposure of her impacted right maxillary cuspid (Fig. 34-43). The orthodontist has been observing this tooth for the last 2 years and now believes that this tooth has moved as far as possible on its own. The orthodontist is concerned that by leaving the tooth in place, the root of the lateral incisor may be compromised.

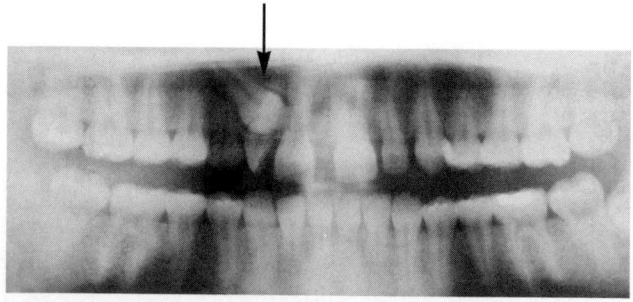

FIG. 34-43   Radiograph of impacted cuspid.

(Courtesy of Helen Zylman, D.D.S., Ann Arbor, Michigan.)

Armamentarium Preparation

Anesthesia / Patient Monitor Set-up

SURGICAL EXTRACTION SET-UP
Mirror
Cotton pliers
Surgical curette
Scalpel handle, with blade, #11, #12, or #15
Periosteal elevator
Bone chisel
Rongeurs
Surgical HVE tip
Surgical burs, with handpiece
Irrigating syringe, with sterile saline
Cup with sterile water
Suture, placed in sterile water to soften
Needle holder
3 × 3 gauze sponges
Lubricant
Periodontal dressing
Root tip elevators (optional)

Postoperative Instructions

After the surgeon is satisfied with the dressing, tip the patient upright and begin to remove monitor leads and the IV. Gauze pressure packs are not needed for this patient because the periodontal dressing covers the area completely. Usually, after this dressing is placed, there is little bleeding. The patient's mother is brought to the treatment room. Review the instructions with the mother and child. Although the patient has done well all through the procedure, once she sees her mother in the room, she starts to cry. Reassure the mother that this is not unusual at all, especially with young children. Try to distract the young patient with a treat that is given only to *good patients.* An appointment to return in 1 week for the removal of dressing is scheduled. The patient will see the orthodontist that same day and may possibly have an orthodontic bracket bonded to the tooth. In some instances this procedure can be done during the surgical procedure as illustrated in Fig. 34-44, *A* through *D.*

▶ Frenectomy (Case Scenario #7)

Occasionally patients present with a thick, fibrous frenum, either in the maxillary or the mandibular arch; this can occasionally contribute to a diastema (space between the teeth) or to difficulty with speech, or it may interfere with prosthesis placement. To close the

Text continued p. 912.

EXPOSURE OF IMPACTED CUSPID

Anesthesia Administration

The patient is quite anxious about having this procedure done because she has never had local anesthetic. As a result her mother has given permission for her to be sedated. The procedure is much the same as the ones previously described, except now the surgical team has the responsibility of managing child behavior, by encouraging the child to trust them. In this particular case, all of the equipment was demonstrated at the preoperative visit to reduce the patient's anxiety. At this appointment the patient is still a little nervous, so some nitrous oxide and oxygen are used to help her relax before insertion of the IV needle. Once the IV is placed and flowing, the patient is sedated. Patient positioning is important for this procedure. Most of the work will be done on the patient's palate, and she is placed in a complete supine position or even slightly beyond supine position, so that the surgeon's vision is as unobstructed as possible. The light is adjusted so that it shines on the palate without being blocked by the surgeon's or the assistant's head. The local anesthetic is administered, and the nitrous oxide is discontinued. After 5 minutes on 100% oxygen, the mask is removed; the position of the mask would press on the lip and thus interfere with the surgeon's view. In this case, local anesthetic is infiltrated on both buccal and palatal sides of the arch from just posterior to tooth #6 to the midline.

Exposure Procedure

1. As usual, hand the surgeon a curette to assess anesthesia.
2. If the anesthesia is adequate, exchange the curette for a scalpel; the surgeon makes an incision on the palatal side of the involved area.
3. The surgeon alternates the scalpel with the periosteal elevator, while reflecting the flap because palatal tissue is fibrous and can be difficult to reflect.
4. The surgeon then removes a thin layer of bone that overlies the impacted tooth. The surgeon must be careful during this procedure because the tooth must not be scarred by the bur. Often, when the bone gets to be quite thin, the surgeon completes the remainder of the bone relief by using a bone chisel. Use caution during irrigation to avoid water entering the posterior of the mouth.
5. Once the surgeon exposes the crown of the tooth, there is usually a fairly good-sized follicle that must be removed. Exchange either the handpiece or the chisel for a curette. Often the surgeon uses a periodontal curette, which is more useful in removing a follicle.
6. Be ready with the rongeur because once the follicle is loosened, the surgeon will want to use the rongeur to remove any loose tissue.
7. After the follicle is removed and the tooth is clearly exposed, the surgeon returns the curette and the rongeur to the assistant and prepares to irrigate the site.
8. Receive the irrigating syringe and any retractors that the surgeon has used. Transfer a tissue pliers and either a scalpel or a tissue scissors to the surgeon. These are used to trim the tissue so that the tooth can be clearly seen.
9. The surgeon hands the excised tissue to the assistant. Transfer the suture set-up and the needle holder; the surgeon places one suture in each interproximal area.
10. Once the flaps are repositioned and sutured, place some gauze sponges in the patient's mouth to keep the area as dry as possible.

Dressing Placement

1. Mix a periodontal dressing to be used to cover and protect the area while it is healing.
2. Give the surgeon some lubricant to prevent the gloves from sticking to the dressing.
3. When the dressing begins to stiffen, pass the material to the surgeon.
4. The surgeon receives a plastic instrument to place the dressing around the surgical site, while you retract the tissues.
5. Remove debris from the plastic instrument when necessary.
6. The surgeon asks the patient to tap the teeth together a few times to make sure that the dressing does not interfere with occlusion. If the dressing is marked by tooth marks, it must be adjusted so that the dressing will not be dislodged by chewing.
7. Tell the patient to eat only soft foods for the next week and not to chew gum until the dressing is removed 1 week later at the follow-up appointment.

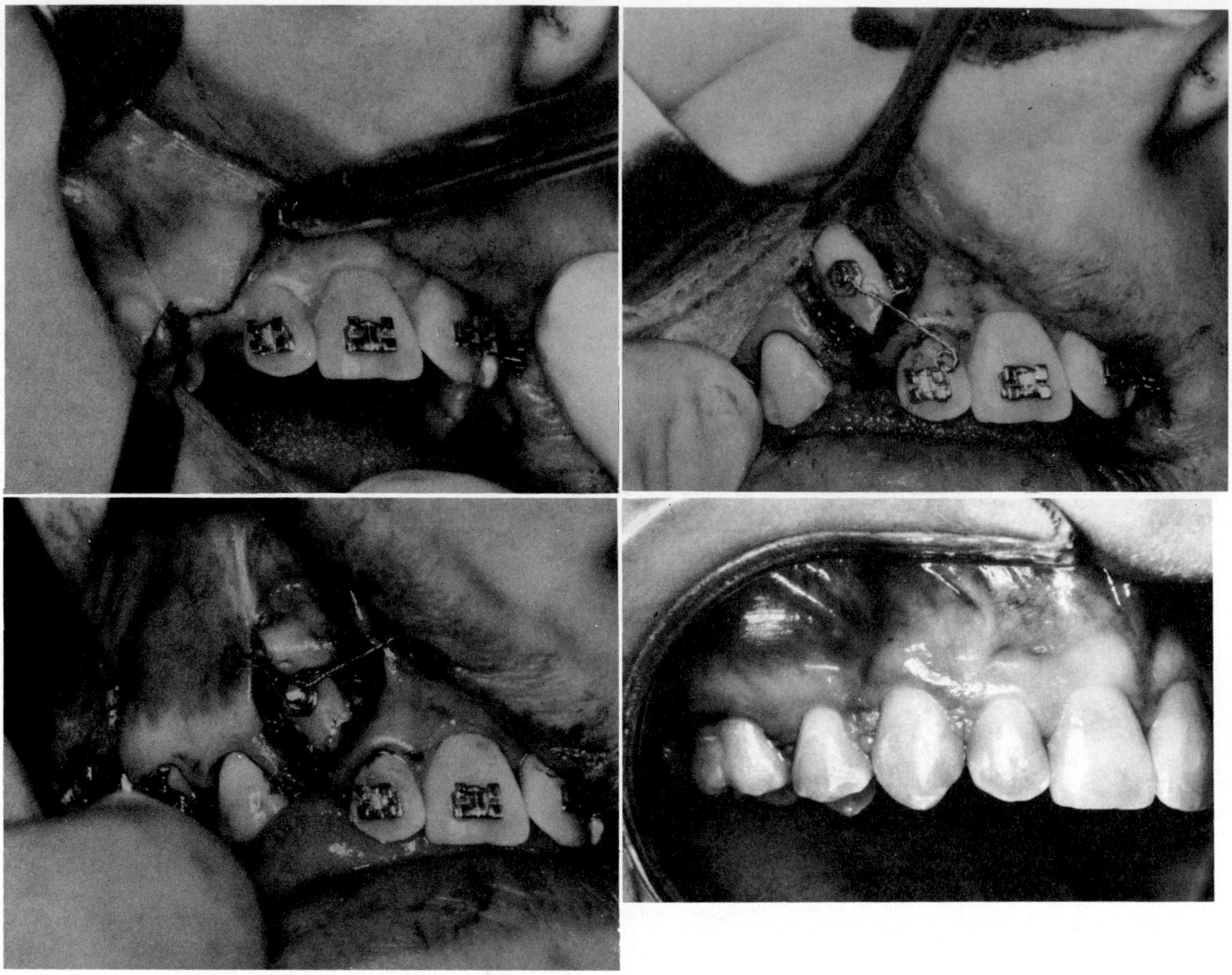

FIG. 34-44   **Removal of impacted cuspid.** *A,* Mucoperiosteal flap is made with scalpel. *B,* Tissue is retracted, and bracket is bonded to tooth. *C,* Flap is sutured apically to tooth. *D,* After 6 months, the exposed tooth is in the desired position.

(From Peterson LJ, Hupp J, Ellis III E, Tucker M: *Contemporary oral and maxillofacial surgery,* ed 2, St Louis, 1992, Mosby.)

FRENECTOMY

Anesthesia Administration

The patient is prepared and anesthetized in the usual fashion.

Frenectomy Procedure

1. The surgeon assesses for adequate local anesthesia by pinching tissue with a tissue pliers. The patient agrees that this does not feel sharp.
2. The surgeon everts and exposes the frenal attachment area (Fig. 34-45, *A*). Exchange a straight hemostat for the tissue pliers. The hemostat is used to grasp the tissue of the frenum. The surgeon locks the hemostat closed and uses it as a handle for the tissue.

3. Pass the surgeon a scalpel, and retract the lip. During this time, the surgeon runs the scalpel down either side of the hemostat, removing a thin section of tissue along with the hemostat (Fig. 34-45, *B*). When the lip is relaxed, this leaves a diamond-shaped incision (Fig. 34-45, *C*).
4. The surgeon then takes the sharp tissue scissors, undermines the tissue, and irrigates the area.
5. The surgeon now closes the incision with three or four sutures, leaving a vertical incision (Fig. 34-45, *D*).
6. Follow-up 3 months later reveals a healing of the area and a diastema that is closing.

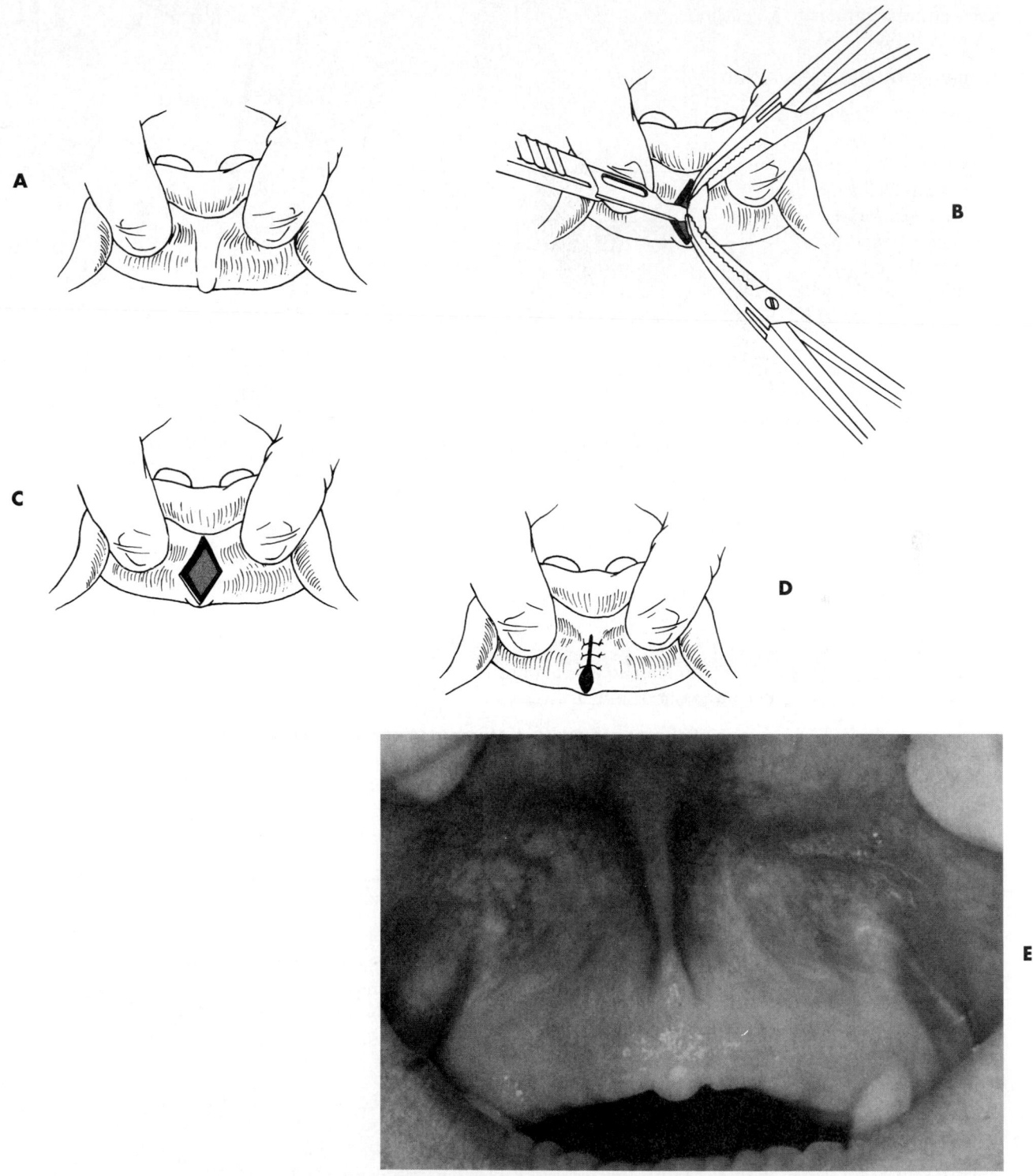

FIG. 34-45   Frenectomy procedure. *A,* The tip is retracted and the surgical site is identified. Frenum is grasped in a curved hemostat and is released by an incision on either side of its base. *B,* Eversion and exposure of frenal attachment area. *C,* Excised tissue is removed and a diamond-shaped defect is left. *D,* Sutures are placed. *E,* Follow-up 3 months later; healing is completed.

diastema, the frenum must be cut and some of the muscle fibers must be removed.

In an edentulous situation a frenum may need to be released to accomodate a denture.

Armamentarium Preparation

Anesthesia/Patient Monitor Set-up

FRENECTOMY SET-UP

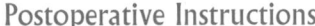

Mirror
Tissue pliers
Tissue scissors
Straight hemostat
Surgical curette
Scalpel handle with blade,
    #11, #12, or #15
Surgical HVE tip
Irrigating syringe with sterile saline
Cup with sterile water
Suture, placed in sterile water to soften
Needle holder
3 × 3 gauze sponges
Lubricant

Postoperative Instructions

When the procedure is over, prepare the patient for discharge the same way as in the preceding procedures. Assess vital signs, remove the monitors and IV, and turn off the machines. Review the postoperative instructions with the patient, as in other procedures, and answer all of the patient's questions.

▶ Biopsy/Cytology Smear
(Case Scenario #8)

The last procedure to be described in this chapter is biopsy of a suspicious lesion. A biopsy is the removal of a small piece of living tissue from an organ or part of the body for microscopic examination to confirm a diagnosis, a prognosis, or a follow-up on the disease. In the following case an **incisional biopsy** (Fig. 34-46, *A*) will be done. This means that only a small section of the lesion is removed, along with some normal tissue. The other type would be an **excisional biopsy** (Fig. 34-46, *B*), which involves the removal of the entire lesion plus some normal tissue around the edge, necessitating removal of quite a bit of tissue; this procedure is reserved for small lesions, usually those under a centimeter in size. Occasionally, a nonsurgical procedure that includes scraping or wiping the lesion is done. This process is called **exfoliative cytology** and may be used as an adjunct to the surgical procedure.

The patient is a 64-year-old male who has been a smoker during his adult life; he admits smoking at least

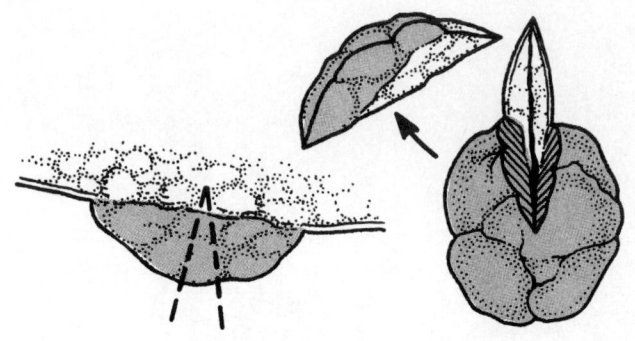

A

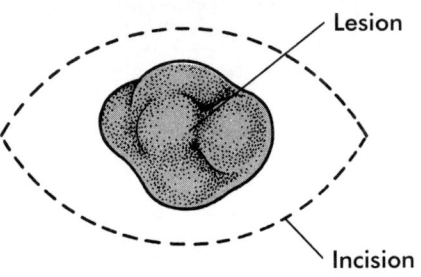

Lesion

B

Incision

FIG. 34-46   *A,* Incisional biopsy. *B,* Excisional biopsy.

(From Peterson LJ, Hupp J, Ellis III E, Tucker M: *Contemporary oral and maxillofacial surgery,* ed 2, St Louis, 1992, Mosby.)

1½ packs of cigarettes each day. He also drinks approximately ½ pint of whiskey every day. One month ago the patient noticed an ulcer on the inside of his lower lip that would not heal. The patient's physician recommended that the ulcer be biopsied.

The ulcer is about 2 cm in diameter, and the surgeon plans an incisional biopsy. Further treatment is planned after the pathologist gives a diagnosis.

Armamentarium Preparation

Before the patient is seated, the assistant follows the preparatory steps for the anesthesia and the set-up. The basic armamentarium for this procedure includes the following:

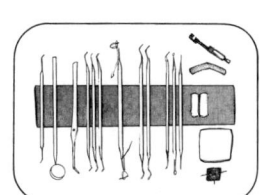

Anesthesia/Patient Monitor Set-up

BIOPSY SET-UP

Mirror
Tissue pliers
Tissue scissors
Straight hemostat
Surgical curette
Scalpel handle, with blade, #11, #12, or #15
Surgical HVE tip

BIOPSY PROCEDURE

The area is anesthetized by infiltrating local anesthetic around the lesion.

1. Transfer the scalpel to the surgeon who then makes a wedge-shaped incision through the edge of the lesion.
2. Pass the surgeon a tissue forceps to hold the biopsy specimen while it is released from the underlying tissue. Two dental assistants are needed for procedures such as these. Retract the lip, holding it out with fingers on either side of the lesion. The lip is pinched tightly to help control the bleeding. The second assistant passes instruments and evacuates in the usual fashion; during the actual biopsy procedure, it usually works better to simply blot the surgical site frequently with gauze rather than to use suction on the soft tissue.
3. After the surgeon has removed the wedge of tissue, provide a small bottle of 10% Formalin into which the specimen is dropped. Tightly close the lid, and then irrigate the surgical site. The surgeon closes the incision.
4. Prepare the specimen with the necessary data, including the patient's name, the date, the site of the biopsy, a history of the lesion, and a tentative diagnosis. Send the biopsy to the laboratory for analysis.
5. Give the patient an appointment to return in 1 week to get the results of the biopsy.

SUTURE REMOVAL

▶ If any of the procedures just described require suture removal, this task is delegated to a qualified assistant in some states. Typically, removable sutures are left in place 5 to 7 days. If the sutures remain longer, they may increase the contamination of the underlying tissues. Suture removal includes the following steps:

1. Examine the patient's record to determine the type and number of sutures that were previously placed.
2. Clean surface debris from the site with a cotton-tipped applicator that has been soaked in peroxide, iodophor, or other antiseptic solution.
3. Cut the suture with a sharp, pointed, or specially designed suture scissors. If the suture was a continuous-style suture, a single suture is cut at a time.
4. With a cotton pliers, remove the suture by pulling it toward the incision line—not away from the suture line. However, if the suture knot is positioned on the incisional side, the suture is removed from the knot side.
5. Wipe the area with a cotton gauze.
6. Record the appearance of the tissue and the number of sutures that are removed on the patient's record.

Irrigating syringe, with sterile saline
Cup with sterile water
Suture, placed in sterile water to soften
Needle holder
3 × 3 gauze sponges
Lubricant
Small bottle, with 10% formalin
Since this biopsy is a short procedure, local anesthesia is selected.

Postoperative Care

When the procedure is over, prepare the patient for discharge as in the preceding procedures. Assess the vital signs, remove the monitors and IV, and turn off the machines. Review the postoperative instructions and answer all of the patient's questions.

Hospital Dentistry

It seems appropriate that hospital dentistry be reviewed in this chapter, since many of the procedures that are described in this chapter, especially the anesthesia technique, may be performed in a hospital setting. Many hospitals include operating suites that are completely equipped to perform clinical dentistry—restorative and surgical. A dentist who frequently practices hospital dentistry may use the services of his or her own dental assistant during these procedures. The protocol of the individual hospital is followed to meet the appropriate credentials, staffing, scheduling, and facility use.

Although many hospitalized patients require dental treatment because of illness or traumatic injury, the major portion of hospital dental patients are admitted specifically for dental treatment. These patients include the following:

▶ Medically compromised patients who, because of systemic diseases, present a greater-than-normal risk for treatment in the general practice office; these

TEAM APPROACH

Routine Extraction of Maxillary Right First Pre-Molar

Before this procedure, monitors will be connected and anesthesia will be administered. When the patient is sufficiently anesthetized the procedure begins.

OPERATOR	ASSISTANT
	Pass curette or periosteal elevator
Grasp instrument and detach periodontal ligament; return curette or periodontal elevator	Exchange instrument for straight elevator
Grasp elevator; place elevator on tooth; apply pressure and luxate tooth; return elevator	Exchange elevator for universal maxillary forceps
Receive forceps; grasp tooth; luxate	Observe site; evacuate blood; keep HVE tip near site to pick up debris and tooth fragments; retract tissue as necessary
Lift out tooth; examine apex of tooth; transfer forceps with tooth	Grasp forceps with left hand; if root was not intact, root tip elevator is passed; transfer curette
Grasp curette, and remove granulation tissue or any abscess from socket	Place HVE near site to withdraw debris and blood
Return curette	Exchange curette for rongeur forceps
Grasp rongeur and use to remove tissue that has been loosened from bony socket	Wipe off tips of rongeur forceps as needed; pass HVE over site to clean area
Return rongeur	Exchange for curette
Grasp curette and clean socket	Use HVE to clean site
Return curette	Receive curette, transfer irrigating syringe with sterile saline
Grasp irrigating syringe; ask patient to turn on side; irrigate the area	Use HVE to collect fluids; fold 3 × 3 gauze into small pillow
Return irrigating syringe	Exchange syringe for folded gauze
Place gauze over extraction site; ask patient to close on gauze	Use moistened gauze to wipe blood from patient's lips and cheeks
Remove gloves and other surgical attire as necessary	
Sign prescriptions	Provide postoperative instructions; enter clinical data on chart; dispose of medical waste following OSHA standards

patients may warrant close observation during treatment, such as patients with diabetes or coronary disease or those who are under special therapy

▶ Disabled patients, who, because of their physical or emotional disability are unable to tolerate care in the private dental office; patients with Down's syndrome, severe arthritis, or Parkinson's disease may be unable to control motions and may present potential safety complications during treatment

▶ Trauma patients with jaw fractures or head and neck injuries, who may not be able to be transferred to a dental chair

▶ Extensive oral procedures, such as multiple extractions, alveoloplasty, or other full mouth construction

▶ Individuals who have been hospitalized for cancer treatment and who are to receive radiation treatment before hospital release

▶ Patients who seek hospital dental care for convenience, out of irrational fear, or because the dental care is in conjunction with other head and neck surgical procedures

The actual practice of dentistry in a hospital is no different than in a private practice. The environment and number of team members may change, but the ideas expressed in this chapter regarding surgical teamwork, thorough medical evaluation, constant monitoring of the patient, the use of sterile techniques, and the safe management of medical wastes are all principles that must remain the same in a hospital setting.

KEY POINTS

▶ The specialty of maxillofacial oral surgery presents the qualified dental assistant with challenging opportunities to work directly with patients in obtaining vital data, assist during simple to complex surgical procedures, provide patient management during stressful experiences and be a source of patient education. The procedures vary greatly from those used in chairside assisting in most general dental offices.

▶ The office design in this specialty must consider an environment that is comfortable, provides a calming effect, and provides adequate space for increased personnel, adjunct equipment, and maneuverability of patients when they are assisted by staff or a family member.

▶ Treatment in this specialty may require the use of oral medications, inhaled gases, and local anesthetic and will involve many types of invasive procedures. Consequently, medical evaluation must be completed with a thorough review of health history, an evaluation of heart and lungs, a medication and drug history, and a review of systemic diseases. In addition, dental radiographs and laboratory studies must be made available.

▶ The assistant is responsible for assembling the armamentarium for the anesthesia and surgical procedure, for applying the monitoring devices, and for observing these devices for the patient's vital signs during the entire procedure. At the end of a procedure the assistant removes these monitoring devices, reviews postoperative procedures with the patient and the person who has accompanied the patient, and dismisses the patient.

▶ Assorted surgical materials and instruments are available for this specialty. The assistant should be familiar with the basic instruments, their styles, and their uses.

▶ In the dental office, basic surgical procedures often will include single, multiple, or third molar extractions; preprosthetic surgery; frenectomy; exposure of unexposed teeth for orthodontic purposes; or biopsies. Hospital oral maxillofacial surgery is performed for special needs situations, facial injuries and trauma, implants, or other orthognathic surgery.

BIBLIOGRAPHY

Davis K: *The training manual for anesthesia assisting in the oral and maxillofacial surgery office*, ed 2, 1988, Training Manual Publishing Company.

Malamed F: *Sedation: a guide to patient management*, St Louis, 1985, Mosby.

Pollack BR: Legal considerations in sports dentistry, *Dent Clin North Am* 35(4):809-829, 1991.

35 Orthodontics

LEARNING OBJECTIVES

You will have mastered the material in this chapter when you can:
- Define the key terms
- Identify and classify the different types of malocclusion
- Describe the dental discrepancies that may be present in a malocclusion
- Identify the possible causes of malocclusion
- Differentiate between interceptive and corrective phases of orthodontic treatment
- Describe the types of diagnostic records used in orthodontic treatment planning
- Differentiate between removable and fixed appliances
- Identify the components of the fixed appliance system
- Describe the biologic mechanism of tooth movement
- Identify the basic orthodontic instruments and their use in placement of the appliances

KEY TERMS

Angle's classification of malocclusion	Headgear
Archwire	Interceptive treatment
Bracket	Ligature tie
Class I	Malocclusion
Class II	Orthodontic band
Class III	Overbite
Corrective treatment	Overjet
Crossbite	Prognathic
Elastics	Removable appliance
Fixed appliance	Retrognathic
	Separator

Orthodontics is the specialty of dentistry that involves the diagnosis, prevention, and treatment of dental and facial irregularities. An orthodontist must receive at least 2 additional years of formal education in an accredited university after attaining a dental degree. To become certified or licensed as an orthodontic specialist, a specialty examination is administered by a state or regional board of dentistry. Membership in the American Association of Orthodontists denotes that the individual has met these standards of education and experience.

 Norman W. Kingsley, who is considered the father of orthodontics, published *Treatise on Oral Deformities as a Branch of Mechanical Surgery* in 1880.

While the orthodontic specialist provides the majority of orthodontic treatment these days, a number of family dentists or pediatric dentists perform orthodontic treatment of an interceptive or a corrective nature in less involved cases.

The dental assistant is invaluable in a modern orthodontic practice. Most state laws allow the assistant to perform many of the tasks described in this chapter, such as sizing and placing bands and placing ligature ties and separators. These procedures may be carried out independently with the patient, so that assisting in orthodontics involves more one-to-one patient interaction and less four-handed dentistry than in other dental disciplines. The dental assistant may not only perform tasks that are related to the placement of the appliances, but also may be responsible for the education and motivation of patients in the use and care of their appliances. Working directly with the orthodontic patient can be challenging from the standpoint of patient management and from the standpoint of employing procedures that are unique to this specialty. With a basic knowledge of orthodontic diagnostic and treatment procedures and with practice, these skills may soon be mastered.

In this chapter the dental assistant is introduced to the diagnosis and etiology of malocclusion, the different types of orthodontic appliances, and the basic orthodontic instruments and their functions.

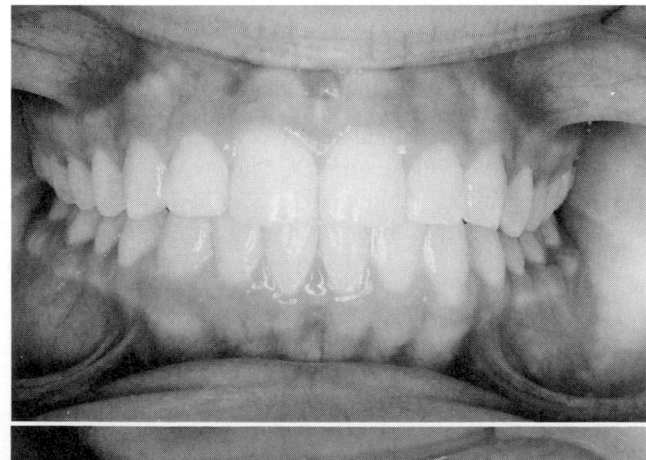
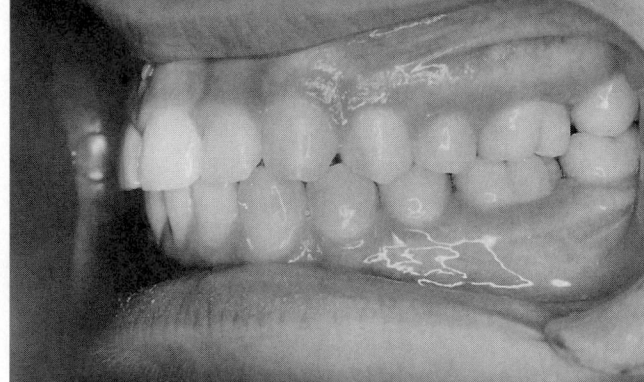

FIG. 35-1　Ideal occlusal relationship. *A,* Frontal view. *B,* Lateral view.

(Courtesy of Daniel R. Balbach, D.D.S., M.S., and John G. Clinthorne, D.D.S., M.S., Ann Arbor, Michigan.)

Malocclusion

The orthodontists's primary role is the correction of malocclusion. The word **malocclusion** literally means *bad closure* and refers to irregularities in the positions of teeth and the bite relationships. Most malocclusions result from irregularities, not only in the positions of teeth, but also in the facial bones and the oral musculature. To understand malocclusion more thoroughly, the dental assistant must first understand what constitutes a normal occlusion.

In the ideal occlusal relationship (Fig. 35-1, *A* and *B*) note that the cusps of the maxillary posterior teeth fit neatly into the embrasures or grooves of the mandibular posterior teeth. The mesiobuccal cusp of the maxillary first permanent molar coincides with the buccal groove of the mandibular first permanent molar. The maxillary cuspid fits neatly into the embrasure between the mandibular cuspid and first premolar. Also note that the maxillary teeth overlap the mandibular teeth slightly in both a horizontal and a vertical direction in the anterior and posterior segments of the dentition. The horizontal overlap of the incisor teeth is referred to as **overjet** (Fig. 35-2). The overjet is most commonly measured as the distance from the labial surface of the mandibular central incisors to the labial surface of the maxillary central incisors and is in the range of 2 to 3 mm in the ideal

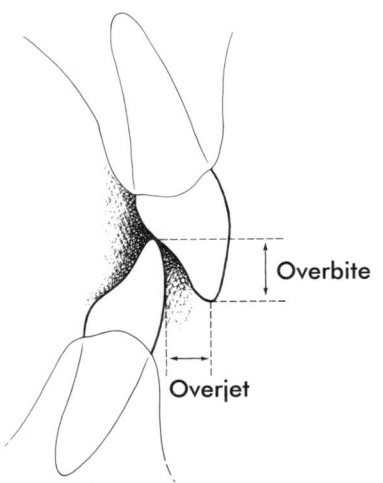

FIG. 35-2　Measurement of overbite and overjet.

occlusion. The extent to which the maxillary incisors overlap the mandibular incisors in a vertical direction is referred to as the **overbite** (Fig. 35-2). This measurement may also be 2 to 3 mm in the ideal situation.

Classifications of Malocclusion

Rarely do we find dentitions that naturally conform to these ideal relationships. To separate and categorize the different types of occlusal irregularities, Dr. Edward Angle in 1899 introduced a classification of malocclusion based on the relationship of the maxillary and mandibular first permanent molars. These are now referred to as the **Angle Classifications of Occlusion** (Fig. 35-3).

CLASS I

A **Class I relationship** exists when the mesiobuccal cusp of the maxillary first molar occludes in the buccal groove of the mandibular first molar (Fig. 35-4). The occlusal relationships of the cuspids and premolars may also be taken into account to determine the classification of occlusion.

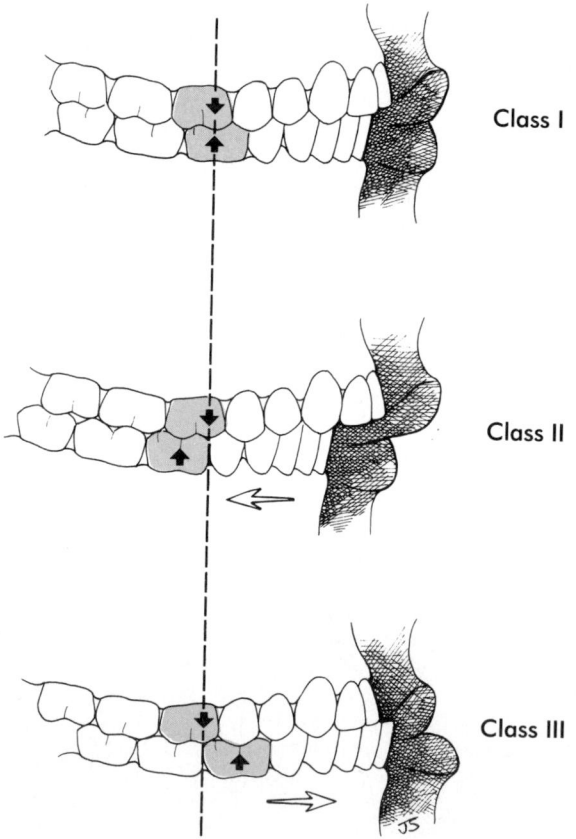

FIG. 35-3   Angle's classifications of occlusion.
(Line drawing by J. Schlesinger.)

CLASS II

A **Class II relationship** denotes that the mesiobuccal cusp of the maxillary first molar occludes anteriorly to the buccal groove of the mandibular first molar (Fig. 35-5). The mandible is retruded, thus **retrognathic**; the mandible has a distal relationship with the maxilla. This classification is then further divided into two types, division 1 and division 2, based upon the positions of the incisor teeth. In the Class II, division 1 malocclusion the maxillary incisors are all inclined and protruding anteriorly resulting in a large overjet. The Class II, division 2 malocclusion is found when the maxillary central incisors are inclined posteriorly, while the maxillary lateral incisors are frequently tipped labially (Fig. 35-6).

CLASS III

A **Class III malocclusion** occurs when the mesiobuccal cusp of the maxillary first molar occludes posteriorly to the buccal groove of the mandibular first molar. In this type of malocclusion, note that the maxillary incisors are actually occluding lingually to the mandibular incisors, resulting in negative overjet (Fig. 35-7). The mandible is protruded, thus **prognathic.** The mandible has a mesial relationship with the maxilla.

▶ Dental Irregularities in Malocclusion

Each type of malocclusion may exhibit a variety of associated dental discrepancies. These irregularities may be found within the dental arch (e.g., crowding) or may describe a variation from the normal relationship between the maxillary and mandibular dental arches upon closure.

CROWDING

Crowding occurs when the teeth are too large for the perimeter of the dental arch (Fig. 35-8); this results in rotation, tipping, and displacement in the positions of individual teeth within the dental arch.

SPACING

Spacing may result when the teeth are too small in comparison to the dental arch (Fig. 35-9). Both crowding and spacing problems are caused primarily by hereditary factors.

DEEP OVERBITE

A **deep overbite** refers to excessive vertical overlap of the incisors upon closure (Fig. 35-10). This type of relationship may be functionally unhealthy for the dentition. In the extreme case, the mandibular incisors may occlude

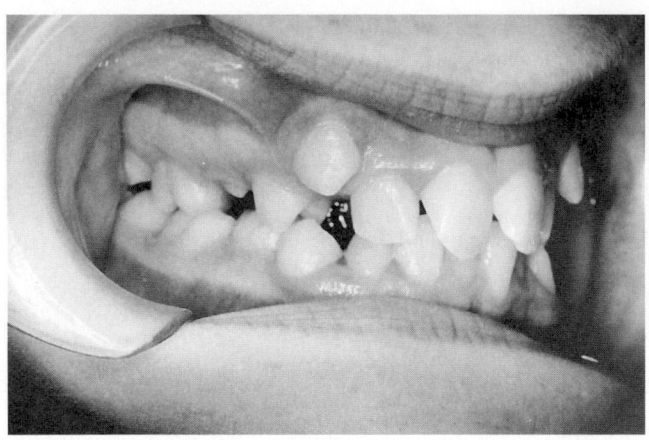

FIG. 35-4   Class I malocclusion.

(Courtesy of Daniel R. Balbach, D.D.S., M.S., and John G. Clinthorne, D.D.S., M.S., Ann Arbor, Michigan.)

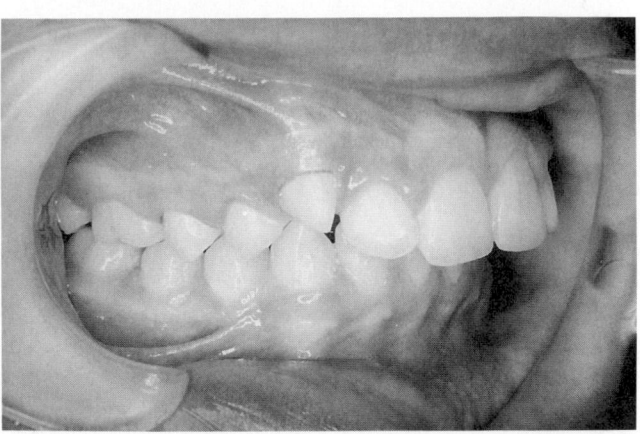

FIG. 35-5   Class II, division I, malocclusion.

(Courtesy of Daniel R. Balbach, D.D.S., M.S., and John G. Clinthorne, D.D.S., M.S., Ann Arbor, Michigan.)

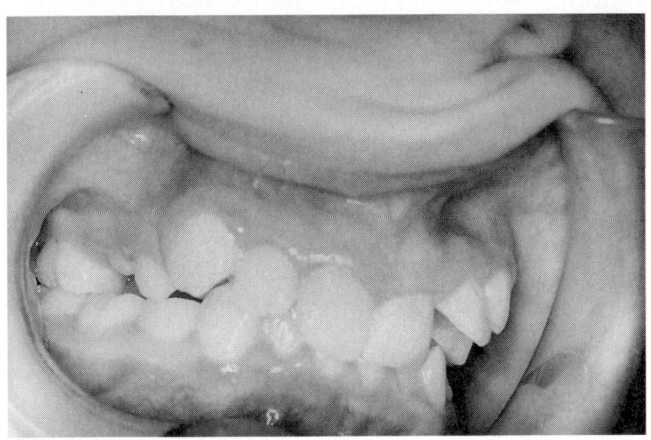

FIG. 35-6   Class II, division 2, malocclusion.

(Courtesy of Daniel R. Balbach, D.D.S., M.S., and John G. Clinthorne, D.D.S., M.S., Ann Arbor, Michigan.)

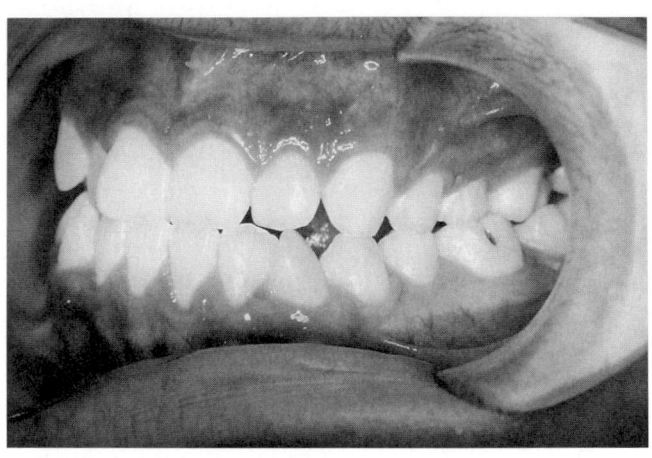

FIG. 35-7   Class III malocclusion.

(Courtesy of Daniel R. Balbach, D.D.S., M.S., and John G. Clinthorne, D.D.S., M.S., Ann Arbor, Michigan.)

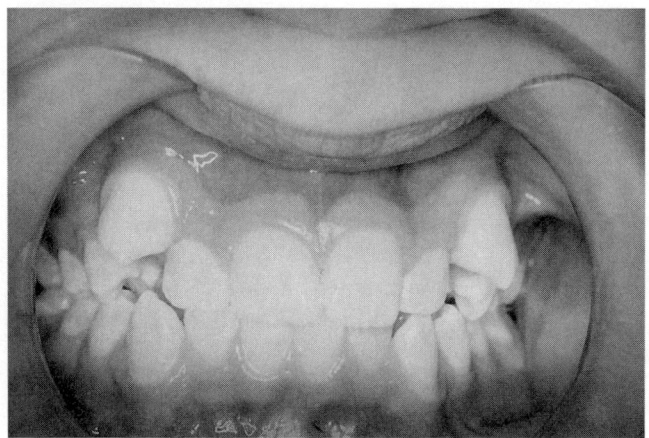

FIG. 35-8   Crowding. The maxillary cuspids have coupled labially because of lack of space.

(Courtesy of Daniel R. Balbach, D.D.S., M.S., and John G. Clinthorne, D.D.S., M.S., Ann Arbor, Michigan.)

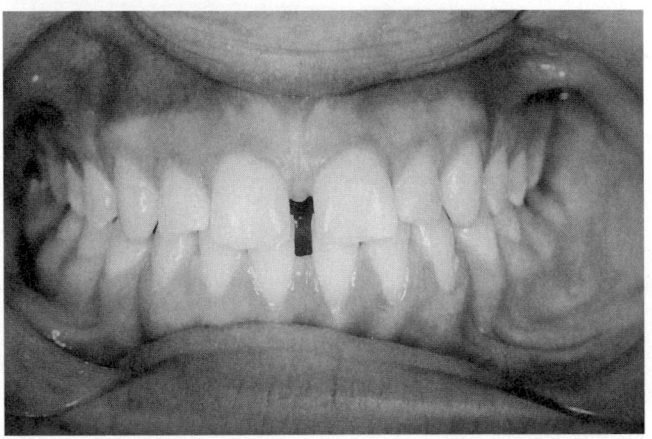

FIG. 35-9   Spacing.

(Courtesy of Daniel R. Balbach, D.D.S., M.S., and John G. Clinthorne, D.D.S., M.S., Ann Arbor, Michigan.)

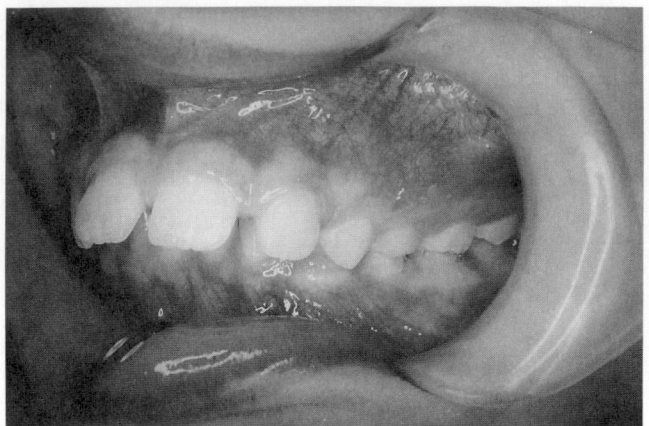

FIG. 35-10   A deep, impinging overbite.

(Courtesy of Daniel R. Balbach, D.D.S., M.S., and John G. Clinthorne, D.D.S., M.S., Ann Arbor, Michigan.)

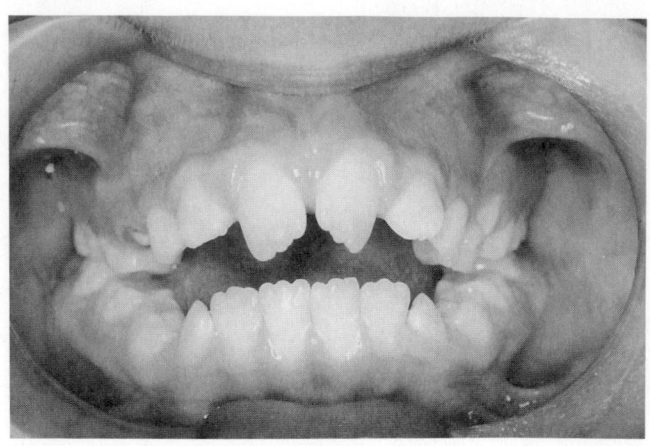

FIG. 35-11   An open bite.

(Courtesy of Daniel R. Balbach, D.D.S., M.S., and John G. Clinthorne, D.D.S., M.S., Ann Arbor, Michigan.)

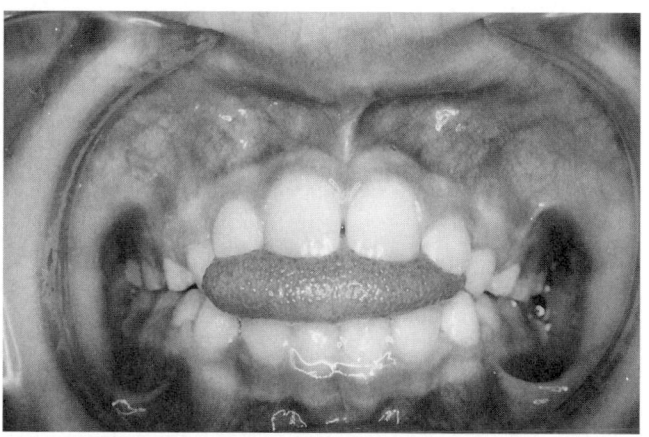

FIG. 35-12   Open bite with anterior tongue thrust.

(Courtesy of Daniel R. Balbach, D.D.S., M.S., and John G. Clinthorne, D.D.S., M.S., Ann Arbor, Michigan.)

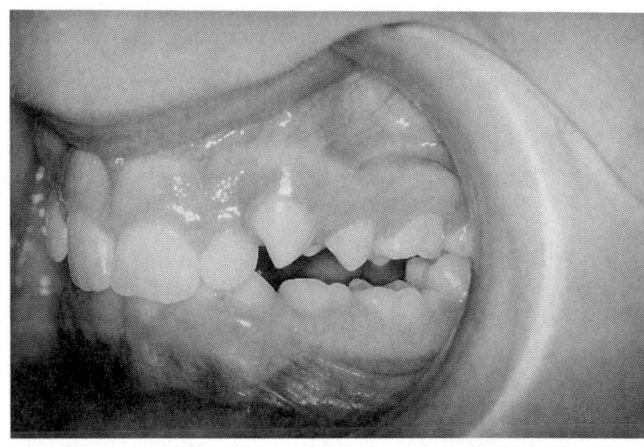

FIG. 35-13   Posterior open bite with ankylosis of primary molars.

(Courtesy of Daniel R. Balbach, D.D.S., M.S., and John G. Clinthorne, D.D.S., M.S., Ann Arbor, Michigan.)

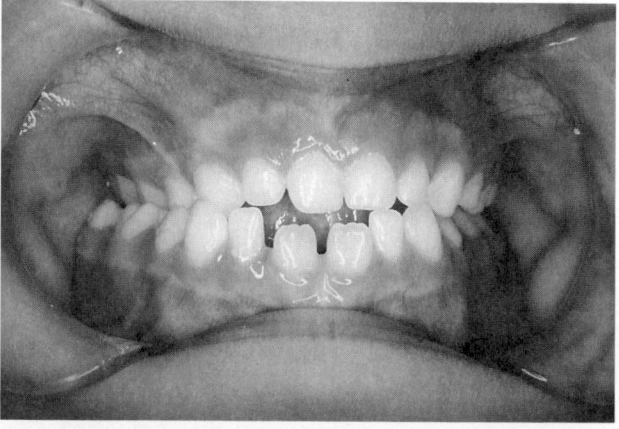

FIG. 35-14   Posterior unilateral crossbite. The buccal cusp of the maxillary molars occlude lingual to the buccal cusps of the mandibular molars on the right side.

(Courtesy of Daniel R. Balbach, D.D.S., M.S., and John G. Clinthorne, D.D.S., M.S., Ann Arbor, Michigan.)

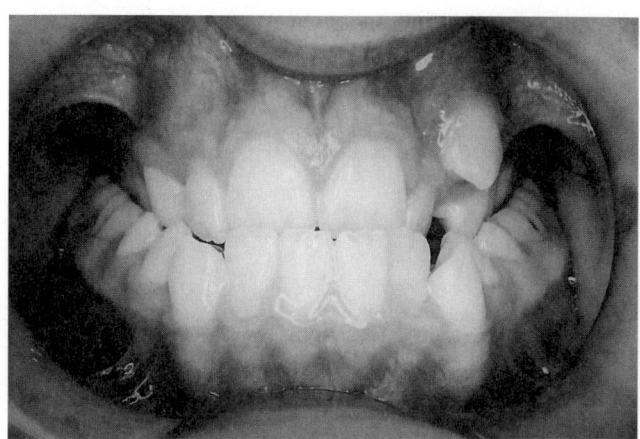

FIG. 35-15   Anterior and bilateral posterior crossbites associated with Class III malocclusion.

(Courtesy of Daniel R. Balbach, D.D.S., M.S., and John G. Clinthorne, D.D.S., M.S., Ann Arbor, Michigan.)

on the palatal gingiva, resulting in an **impinging overbite.** If it is left untreated, this type of discrepancy may result in periodontal problems and eventual loss of the anterior teeth.

OPEN BITE

The opposite of a deep overbite is the **open bite** (Fig. 35-11), which occurs when, upon closure, there is no vertical overlap and no contact between certain maxillary and mandibular teeth. Open bites occur most frequently in the anterior region and are commonly associated with an oral habit, such as thumb sucking or tongue thrusting (Fig. 35-12). Posterior open bites are also possible, although they are much less common and may be associated with lateral tongue thrusting or ankylosis of primary molars (Fig. 35-13).

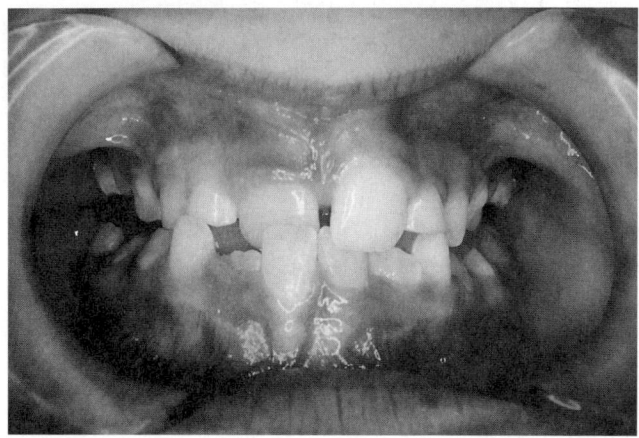

FIG. 35-16 Anterior crossbite involving one incisor.

(Courtesy of Daniel R. Balbach, D.D.S., M.S., and John G. Clinthorne, D.D.S., M.S., Ann Arbor, Michigan.)

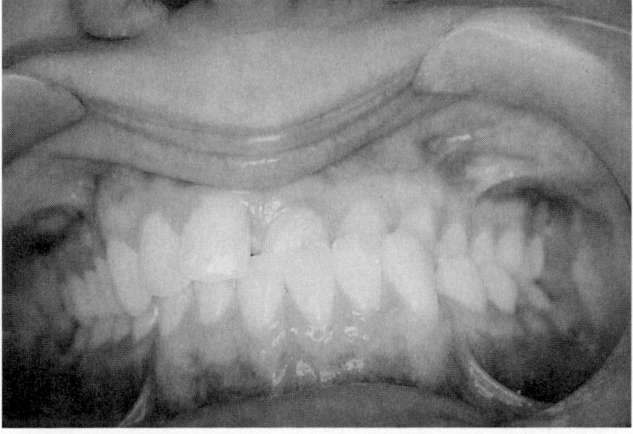

FIG. 35-17 Anterior and unilateral posterior crossbite.

(Courtesy of Daniel R. Balbach, D.D.S., M.S., and John G. Clinthorne, D.D.S., M.S., Ann Arbor, Michigan.)

CROSSBITE

A **crossbite** refers to an abnormal buccolingual relationship of the teeth. A **posterior crossbite** (Fig. 35-14) may exist when the buccal cusps of the maxillary molars or premolars occlude lingually to the buccal cusps of the mandibular posterior teeth. This problem may occur on just one side (unilateral posterior crossbite) or on both sides (bilateral posterior crossbite) and may involve one or several teeth (Figs. 35-15 and 35-16). In an **anterior crossbite** the maxillary incisors may occlude lingually to the mandibular anteriors. This situation is frequently associated with a Class III malocclusion when it involves several teeth, or it may be just an isolated problem when it involves the displacement of a single tooth (Fig. 35-17).

Etiology of Malocclusion

The two major causes of malocclusion are genetic and environmental factors.

▶ Genetic Factors

By far the most common cause of malocclusion is heredity. Genetic factors may result in an imbalance in the size of the teeth compared with the size of the jaws, as in crowding. Disharmony in the size and relationship of the maxilla and mandible may also be passed on from generation to generation, resulting in hereditary Class II or Class III malocclusions.

▶ Environmental Factors

Environmental factors may also produce significant irregularities of the teeth. Premature or delayed loss of primary teeth may cause displacement or impaction of the permanent successors (Fig. 35-18). The presence of supernumerary teeth (Fig. 35-19) or congenital absence of teeth (Fig. 35-20) may also result in malocclusion. Oral habits, such as thumb sucking, can distort the dental arches, affecting the positions of the teeth and the occlusion (Fig. 35-21; Box 35-1).

BOX 35-1

DENTAL DISCREPANCIES ASSOCIATED WITH A LONG-TERM THUMB-SUCKING HABIT

Protrusion of the maxillary incisors
Excessive overjet
Open bite
Posterior crossbite

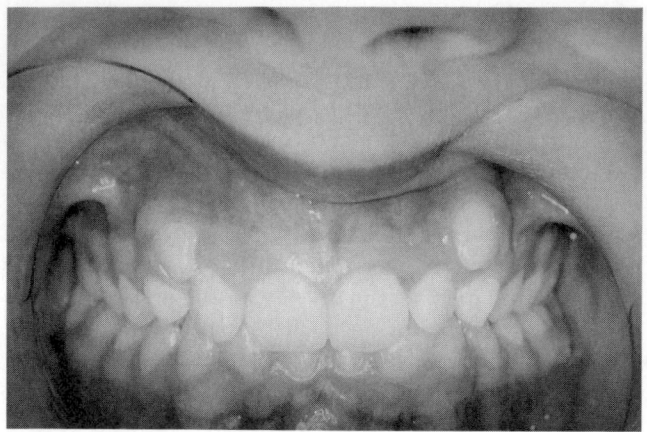

FIG. 35-18   Example of delayed loss of primary cuspids and ectopic eruption of permanent cuspids.

(Courtesy of Daniel R. Balbach, D.D.S., M.S., and John G. Clinthorne, D.D.S., M.S., Ann Arbor, Michigan.)

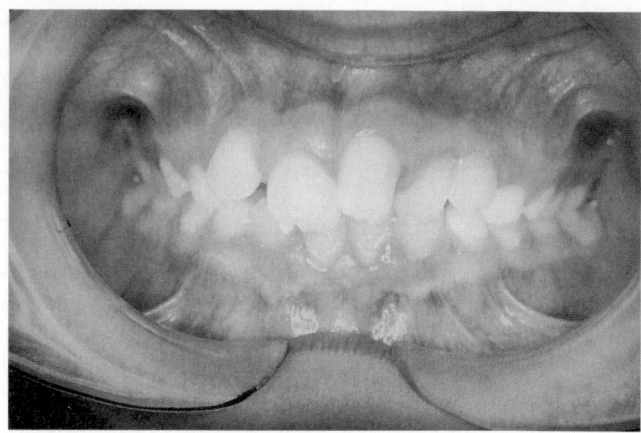

FIG. 35-19   A maxillary supernumerary incisor has erupted in the midline.

(Courtesy of Daniel R. Balbach, D.D.S., M.S., and John G. Clinthorne, D.D.S., M.S., Ann Arbor, Michigan.)

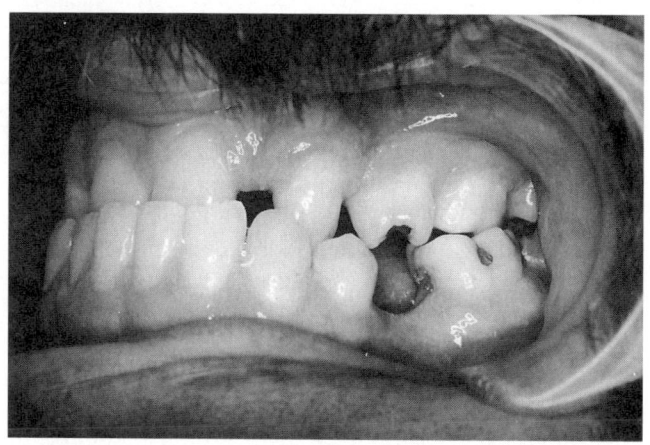

FIG. 35-20   Congenital absence of several teeth has resulted in this malocclusion.

(Courtesy of Daniel R. Balbach, D.D.S., M.S., and John G. Clinthorne, D.D.S., M.S., Ann Arbor, Michigan.)

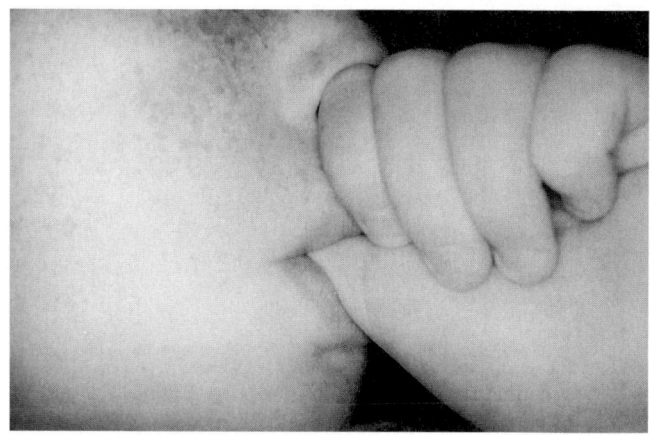

FIG. 35-21   Discrepancies are caused by thumb-sucking habit.

(Courtesy of Daniel R. Balbach, D.D.S., M.S., and John G. Clinthorne, D.D.S., M.S., Ann Arbor, Michigan.)

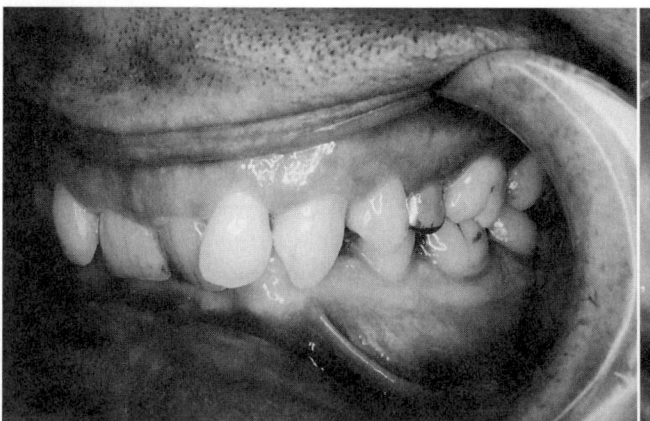
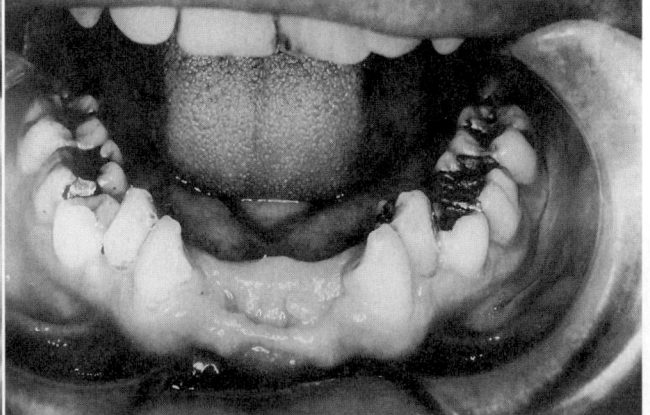

FIG. 35-22   Untreated Class II, division 2, malocclusion, resulting in loss of the lower incisor teeth because of periodontal problems.

(Courtesy of Daniel R. Balbach, D.D.S., M.S., and John G. Clinthorne, D.D.S., M.S., Ann Arbor, Michigan.)

Tongue thrusting is a deviation from the normal pattern of swallowing; the tongue is pushed anteriorly between or against the maxillary and mandibular anterior teeth upon swallowing. This action inhibits the alveolar bone growth and development in the arc of the thrust and usually results in an open bite. A tongue thrust may also be secondary to the open bite that is created by thumb sucking and may be retained even after elimination of the thumb habit, resulting in a permanent deformity. Mouth breathing is another oral habit which may affect the growth of the entire dentofacial complex. Thus the underlying factors in the etiology of a malocclusion may be either genetic or environment but are frequently an interaction of both.

The discrepancies that are present in a malocclusion can often affect the long-term health of the dentition and the surrounding oral structures. If problems are left untreated, many tend to gradually get worse (Fig. 35-22, *A* and *B*). Teeth that are crowded may have a greater risk of tooth decay and periodontal disease and possible subsequent tooth loss. Malocclusion may also result in excessive and uneven wear on the enamel surfaces of the dentition. Incorrect bites may cause stress on the jaw muscles and joints and become a contributing factor in temporomandibular joint dysfunction. Several of these dysfunctions are described in Chapter 24. Orthodontics is an important factor in the maintenance of oral health and masticatory function, as well as in the patient's self-esteem when facial esthetics are affected.

Timing of Orthodontic Treatment

Suspected skeletal or dental problems should be evaluated as soon as possible by an orthodontist, so that the appropriate timing for the correction can be determined. The American Association of Orthodontists has recommended that the proper age for a child's first visit to the orthodontist is at 7 years. This age frequently corresponds with the eruption of the permanent incisors and first molars—a time when many orthodontic problems are first noted. The child's general dentist or pediatric dentist is instrumental in the diagnosis of these early signs of malocclusion, and he or she refers the patient to the orthodontist if appropriate.

While many malocclusions are amenable to treatment at any age, there is usually a certain optimal age at which to achieve the correction. This decision is based upon the level of dental development, the timing of skeletal growth, and the nature of the problem.

The goal of early orthodontic treatment, during the mixed dentition, is to improve the environment for dental development to reduce or minimize the orthodontic needs in the future. Early treatment may be divided into two categories; interceptive treatment and corrective treatment.

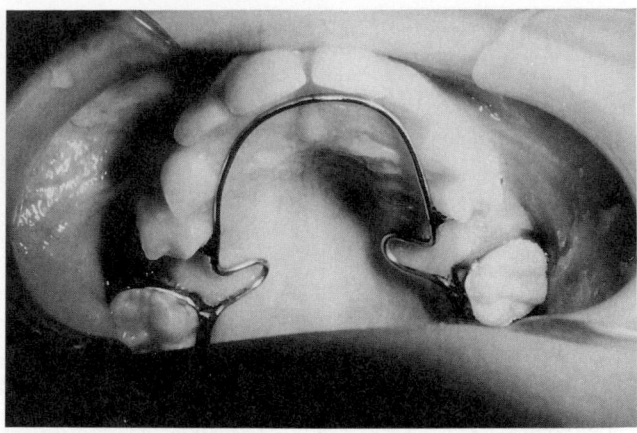

FIG. 35-23   Space maintainer in maxillary arch.

(Courtesy of Daniel R. Balbach, D.D.S., M.S., and John G. Clinthorne, D.D.S., M.S., Ann Arbor, Michigan.)

▶ Interceptive Treatment

Interceptive treatment proposes to head off certain problems before they can have a negative effect on the developing dentition. One example of interceptive orthodontic treatment may be the placement of a space maintainer when a primary tooth has been lost prematurely (Fig. 35-23); this prevents drifting of the adjacent teeth into the edentulous area, which would subsequently result in impaction or displacement of the permanent successor. Control of deleterious oral habits, such as thumb sucking and tongue thrusting, is also an important interceptive measure.

▶ Corrective Treatment

The goal of corrective treatment during the early to midmixed dentition is the improvement of existing problems. Correction of anterior and posterior crossbites may be undertaken at this stage of development and are examples of early corrective intervention (Fig. 35-24). In cases of severe skeletal imbalances, as in Class II and Class III malocclusions, early treatment may be initiated to improve the relationships of the jaws and to reduce the amount of orthodontic treatment that may be needed in the future. Removable devices called functional appliances are frequently used at this stage and for this purpose.

Most orthodontic treatment is initiated in the late mixed dentition or the early permanent dentition. At this stage, since most of the permanent teeth are present, the orthodontist now has control over the development of the final occlusion. In addition, most patients in this age group are undergoing a pubertal growth spurt, and this represents an excellent time for the correction of most

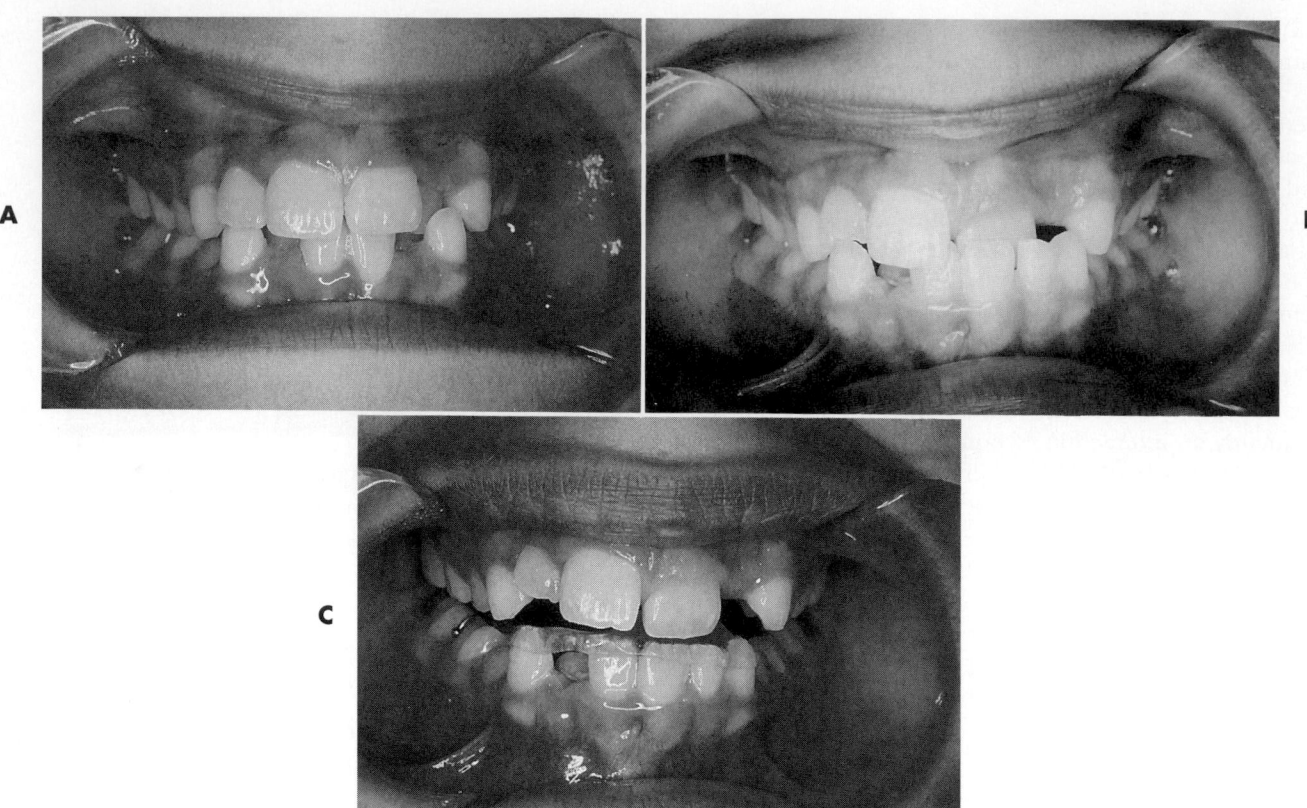

FIG. 35-24   Maxillary central incisor crossbite corrected with a removable appliance. *A,* Crossbite before treatment. *B,* Treatment phase. *C,* Maxillary central crossbite corrected.

(Courtesy of Daniel R. Balbach, D.D.S., M.S., and John G. Clinthorne, D.D.S., M.S., Ann Arbor, Michigan.)

dental and skeletal discrepancies. Comprehensive fixed appliance therapy, commonly known as *braces,* is the most common treatment modality in this age group.

▶ Adult Treatment

Since orthodontic tooth movement is possible at any age, increasing numbers of adults are seeking treatment. Currently, adults make up approximately 25% of all of the active orthodontic patients in the United States. Many adult patients seek treatment for esthetic reasons when orthodontic correction was not available to them as adolescents. Others require orthodontics for corrective reasons, such as for the enhancement of restorative dentistry, periodontics, or TMJ therapy. Because of the lack of growth in the adult patient, there may be some limitations and compromises in the treatment goals. For this reason a combination of orthodontics and orthognathic surgery (described in Chapter 34) is often necessary to resolve severe skeletal imbalances in adult patients.

Orthodontic Records

Diagnosis and treatment planning in orthodontics include many of the techniques described in Chapter 24, *Oral Diagnosis.* The following list indicates the diagnostic aids that are used in orthodontics to define the problem and to arrive at a treatment plan.

1. Medical history
2. Dental history
3. Clinical examination
4. Panoramic radiographs
5. Cephalometric radiograph and tracing
6. Intraoral and extraoral photographs
7. Study models
8. Additional radiographs as necessary (TMJ radiographs, periapicals, occlusal radiographs, etc.)

To effectively evaluate a patient's problem and to determine the appropriate treatment, a thorough diagnostic procedure must be employed.

Medical History

A complete medical history is essential in evaluating a patient before orthodontic treatment is begun. A variety of medical conditions and medications may affect the movement of the teeth, the growth of the jaws, or the patient's ability to cope with the treatment. Children with a history of heart murmur or of rheumatic fever may be at risk for life-threatening infections and are treated by SBE prophylaxis. Severe infections and rapid periodontal breakdown may also occur with routine orthodontic care during the active phases of leukemia, sickle cell anemia, or uncontrolled diabetes. Juvenile onset of rheumatoid arthritis may affect the growth sites of the lower jaw, resulting in deficient bone growth and malocclusion. Medications that are used to control seizures may result in gingival hyperplasia, interfering with tooth movement. Since orthodontic treatment may extend over several years and the patient's medical status may change rapidly, the medical history must be updated periodically.

Dental History

The dental history may give some insight into the nature and cause of the orthodontic problem. Family traits, such as crowding or congenital absence of teeth, may be explored, past caries incidence can be determined, and the presence of deleterious oral habits may be confirmed. The patient's attitude toward dental treatment is also an important aspect of the dental history.

Clinical Examination

During the clinical examination the patient's teeth and jaw relationships are evaluated, as well as the surround-

ing oral and facial soft tissues. The stage of dental development may be recorded by charting the primary and permanent teeth that are present at the time. Any abnormalities in the shape, size, color, and position of the teeth are noted. The Angle classifications of occlusion is determined on both the right and left sides and any deviation in the occlusion, such as a crossbite, may be recorded. Overjet, overbite and the amount of crowding or spacing may be measured precisely. Abnormal, functional, and neuromuscular patterns (e.g., tongue thrusting, mouth breathing, bruxism) may also be noted at this time.

Radiographs

Panoramic and full mouth series of radiographs (see Fig. 9-40) are commonly used to determine the positions of the teeth and the health of the dentition and supporting structures.

A cephalometric radiograph, or lateral head radiograph, allows the orthodontist to more accurately determine the specific areas of imbalance, measure the degree of discrepancy, and project the future growth of the bones of the face (Fig. 35-25). This radiograph is taken on a device called a cephalostat, which is designed

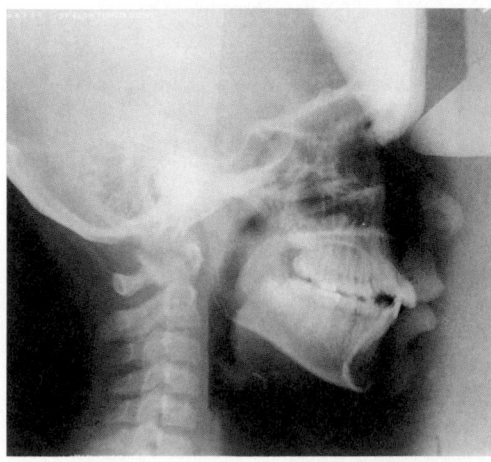

FIG. 35-25 Cephalometric radiograph.

(Courtesy of Daniel R. Balbach, D.D.S., M.S., and John G. Clinthorne, D.D.S., M.S., Ann Arbor, Michigan.)

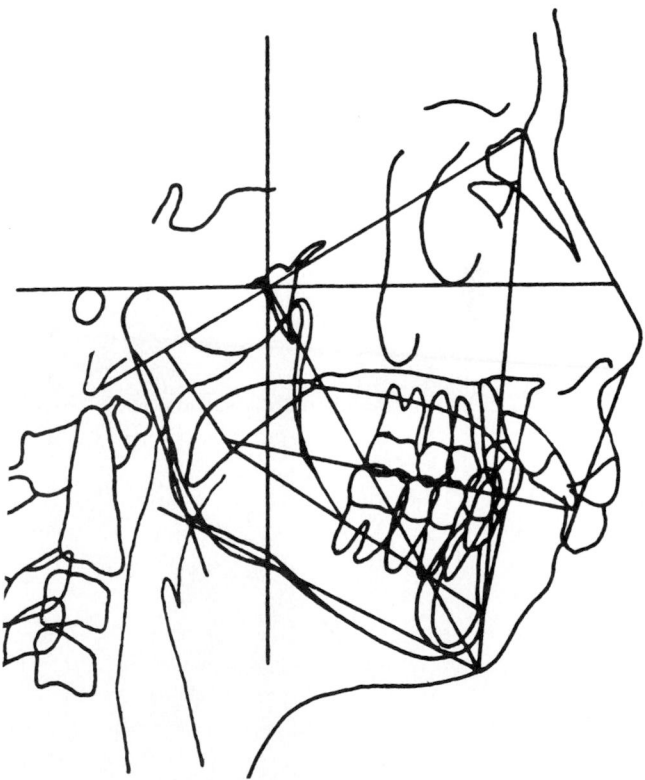

FIG. 35-26 Cephalometric tracing.

(Courtesy of Daniel R. Balbach, D.D.S., M.S., and John G. Clinthorne, D.D.S., M.S., Ann Arbor, Michigan.)

to hold the head in a specific position. The head position can then be accurately reproduced for future cephalograms that can be superimposed and compared with the original; this allows the orthodontist to observe the growth that has occurred, as well as the effects of the treatment upon the skeletal and dental development. Tracing the cephalogram on acetate tracing paper (Fig. 35-26) will facilitate the measurements of the positions of the teeth and jaws. These measurements may be compared to various cephalometric standards, which are based upon good dentoskeletal balance.

Most orthodontic practices use panoramic and cephalometric radiographs routinely, but occasionally, additional radiographs are indicated for a more complete diagnosis. Periapical and occlusal radiographs may give a closeup view of any irregularity that is noted on the panoramic radiograph. TMJ x-rays or tomograms may be indicated if a more accurate view of the temporomandibular joint is required.

▶ Diagnostic Photographs

Diagnostic photographs are also a vital part of orthodontic records. Intraoral photographs (Fig. 35-27, *A* through

C) are taken of the teeth in frontal, left and right lateral, and maxillary and mandibular occlusal views. Extraoral photographs (Fig. 35-28, *A* and *B*) are taken of the patient's head in frontal and lateral views. Both sets of photographs may be exposed by a 35 mm camera that is fitted with a special lens and flash attachment that is designed for this purpose. These photographs serve as a visual record of the dentition before orthodontics and as a record of the progress of treatment.

▶ Study Models

Study models that accurately reproduce the teeth and occlusion are an invaluable aid in the diagnostic procedure (Fig. 35-29). Meticulous impression technique is imperative, so that not only are the teeth recorded accurately, but also the alveolar mucosa is recorded to the depth of the buccal and lingual vestibule. Orthodontic impression trays (Fig. 35-30) have been designed specifically for this purpose; the extended buccal and lingual flanges can be noted. The edges of the impression trays may also be extended with rope-wax (Fig. 35-31) as necessary to attain a more accurate impression of these areas. After pouring the impressions, the study models

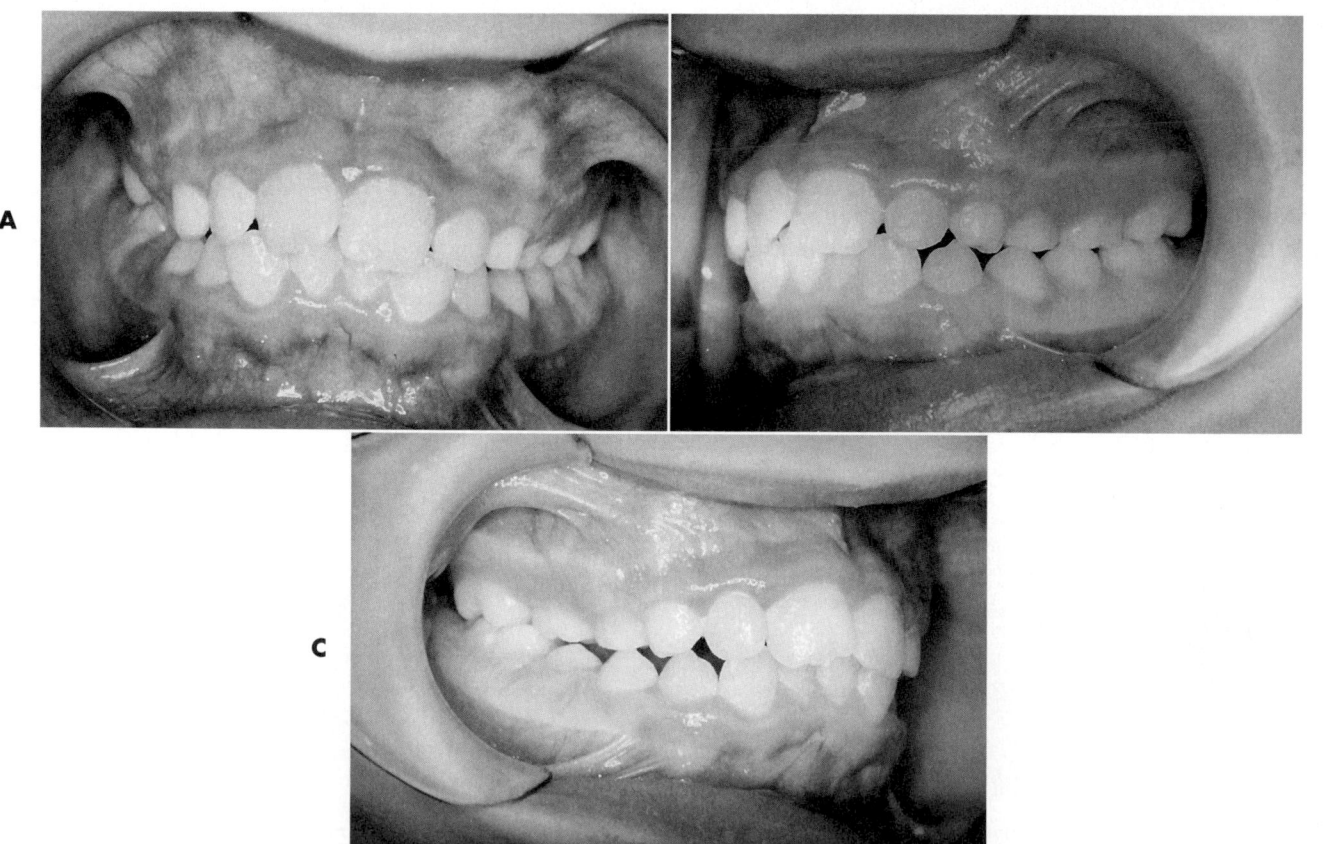

FIG. 35-27   Series of intraoral photos. *A,* Frontal view. *B,* Left side. *C,* Right side.

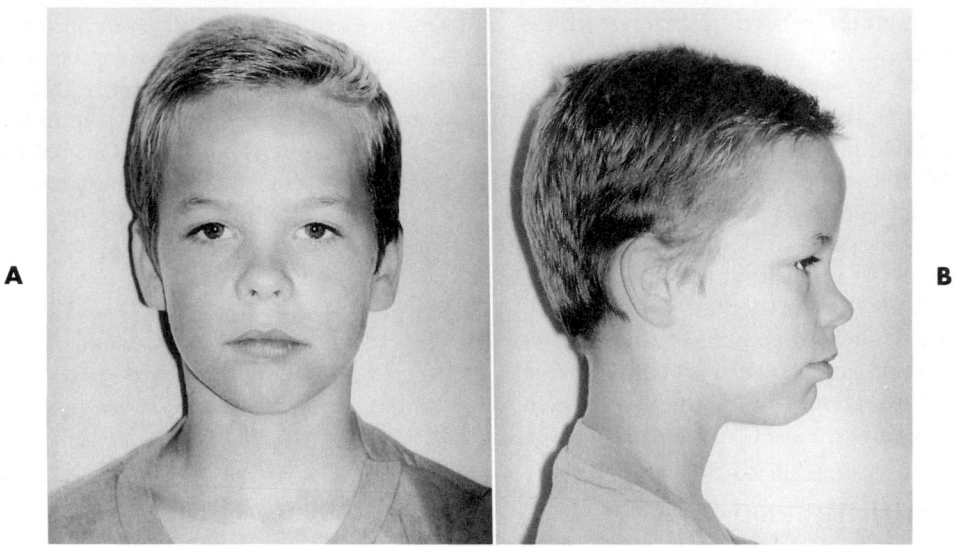

FIG. 35-28   Extraoral photos. *A,* Frontal view. *B,* Lateral view.

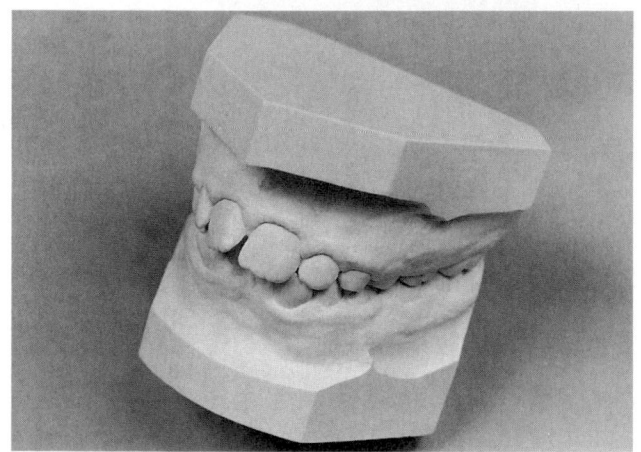

FIG. 35-29   Orthodontic study models.

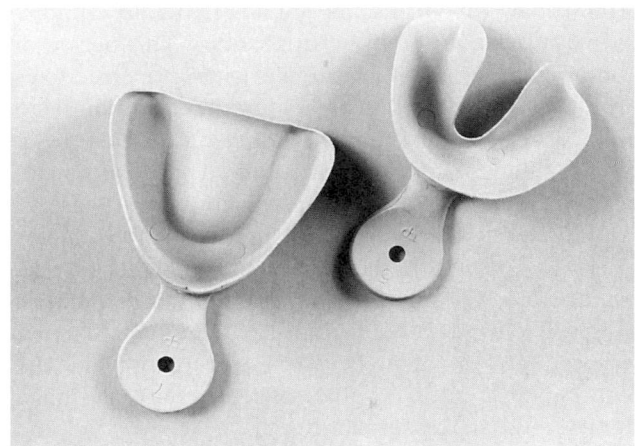

FIG. 35-30   Orthodontic impression trays.

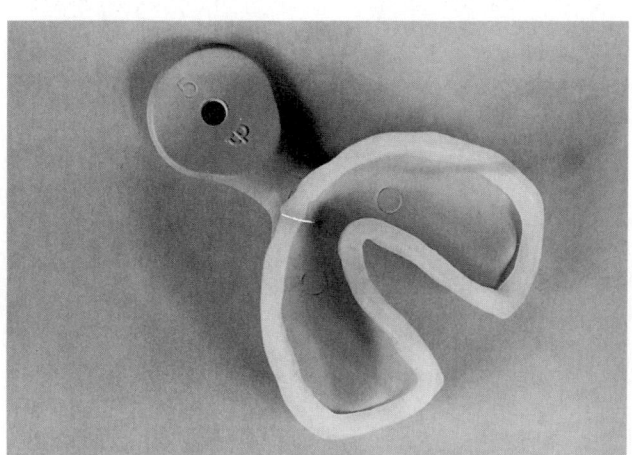

FIG. 35-31   Edges of the tray extended with rope-wax.

are trimmed according to the procedure that is outlined in Chapter 40. It is important to have the backs of the casts trimmed in such a manner that when they are placed on a flat surface, the maxillary and mandibular teeth occlude in exactly the same position as they do in the patient's mouth. The models are usually finished by soaking them in a special solution, model gloss or soap, that gives them a smooth surface, resistant to the staining, which may occur upon frequent handling.

Using these materials the orthodontist is able to determine the nature of the problem and the treatment that will be necessary to correct it. The records also serve as a reference point throughout the treatment by which the patient's progress can be closely monitored.

Treatment Planning

Once the nature of the malocclusion has been clarified, the orthodontist must determine the appropriate timing and implement the treatment. In severe skeletal imbalances or dental discrepancies, early interceptive or corrective treatment may be initiated, before comprehensive treatment with fixed appliances. This period of treatment in the mixed dentition is usually referred to as Phase 1 treatment, and it may last from a few months to several years, depending on the nature and severity of the problem. When comprehensive fixed appliances are placed in the permanent dentition, known as Phase 2, the patient is usually seen at monthly intervals for adjustments in the appliance. Most malocclusions require about 24 months of active treatment, although this can vary widely, depending on the patient's age, the rate of growth, and the complexity of the problem. Once the functional and aesthetic goals of treatment have been achieved, the fixed appliances are removed and the retention phase of treatment begins. During this phase of treatment, removable appliances called retainers are used to allow further stabilization of the teeth, bones, and oral musculature. The patient is frequently monitored for several years during the retention phase, although appointments are much less frequent than during the active stage of treatment.

Mechanism of Tooth Movement

When a continuous gentle pressure is applied to a tooth, changes will occur in the alveolar bone that surrounds the root, allowing the tooth to move. A force applied to a tooth results in an area of compression of the periodontal ligament on one side of the root and an area of tension in the periodontal ligament on the opposite side. The body reacts by sending specialized bone cells called **osteoclasts** to the area under compression, which dissolve or resorb the alveolar bone, creating freedom for tooth movement in that direction. On the tension side,

bone cells called **osteoblasts** deposit new bone into the area from which the tooth has moved. The efficiency of tooth movement may depend on three factors: (1) the magnitude of the force; (2) the duration of the force; and (3) the direction of the force. This remodeling process of bone that allows tooth movement may occur at any age, although the rate of movement is often slower in adults than in children.

Orthodontic Appliances

An orthodontic appliance is a device that is used to produce changes in the relationships of the teeth and the skeletal structures.

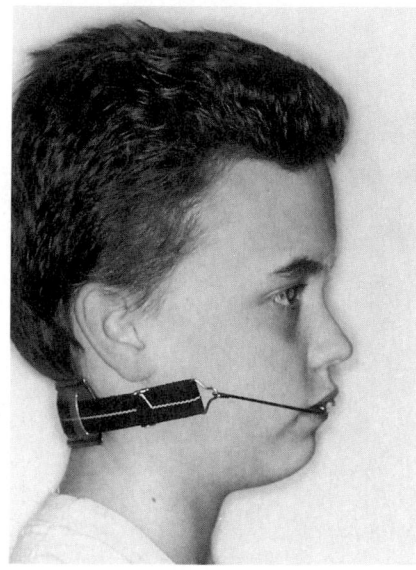

FIG. 35-32   Headgear in place.

(Courtesy of Daniel R. Balbach, D.D.S., M.S., and John G. Clinthorne, D.D.S., M.S., Ann Arbor, Michigan.)

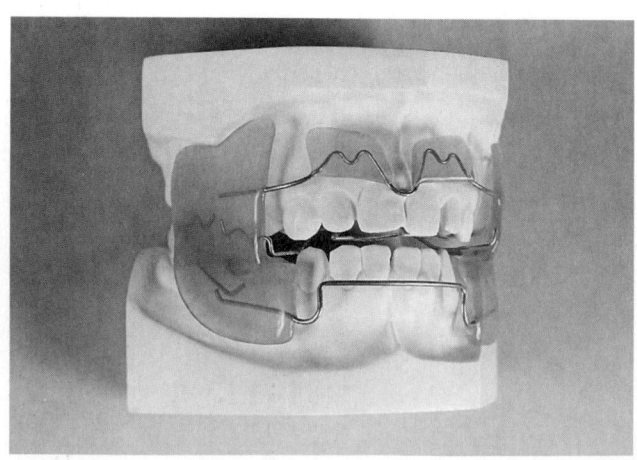

FIG. 35-33   The Fränkel appliance.

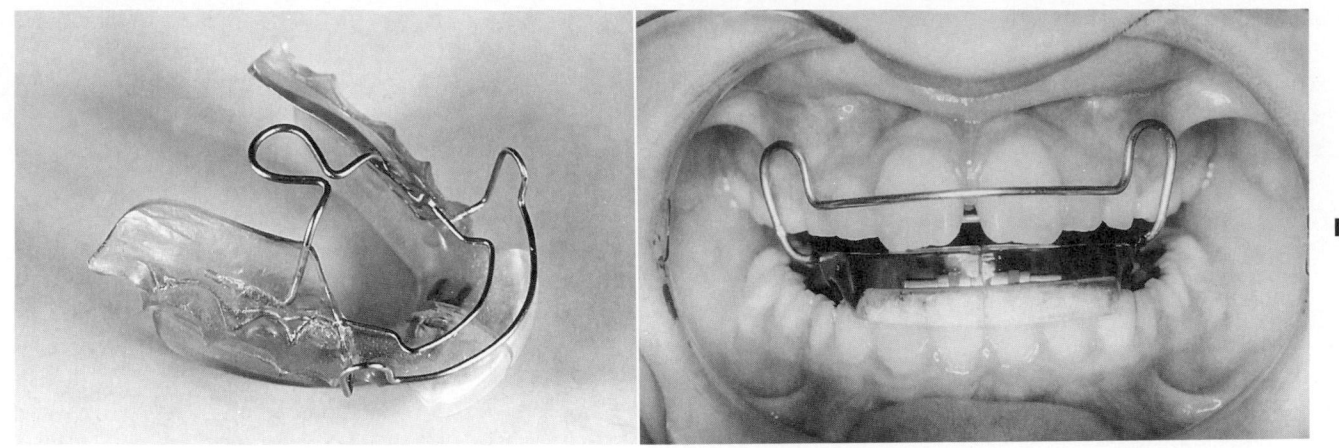

FIG. 35-34   *A*, The bionator. *B*, Bionator in place.

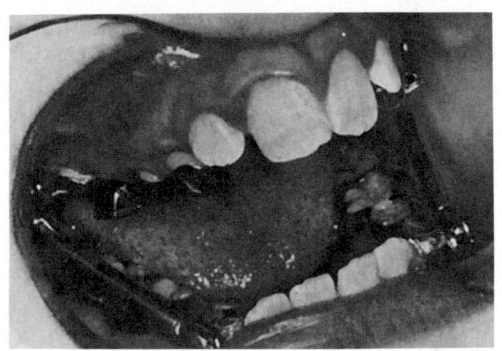

FIG. 35-35   The Herbst appliance in place.

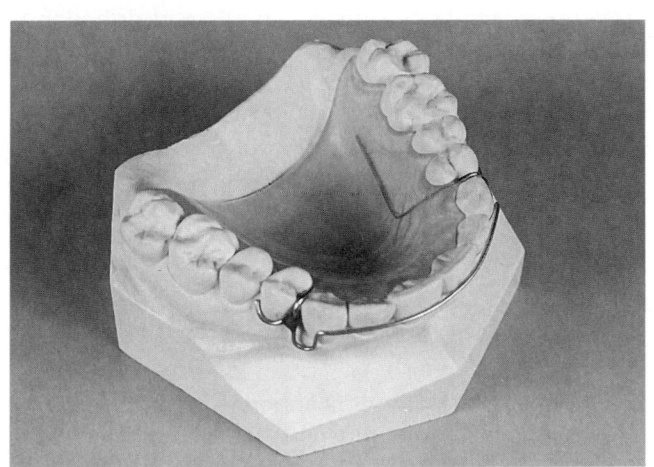

FIG. 35-36   Maxillary Hawley retainer.

▶ Removable Appliances

A **removable appliance** can be inserted into the mouth and removed by the patient. A **headgear** (Fig. 35-32) is an example of a removable appliance that can be used in conjunction with fixed appliances. Functional appliances are removable devices that are frequently used in Phase 1 or early corrective treatment before the placement of fixed appliances. Functional appliances are used to effect changes in the differential growth rate of the jaws when a skeletal imbalance is present. Common examples of functional appliances are the Fränkel appliance (Fig. 35-33), the Bionator (Fig. 35-34, *A* and *B*), and the Herbst appliance (Fig. 35-35). Retainers (Fig. 35-36) are removable appliances that are used to hold or *retain* the alignment of the teeth after fixed appliance therapy. A

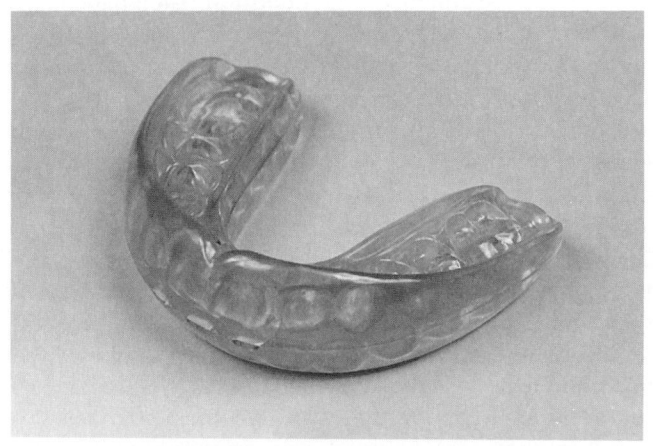

FIG. 35-37   Positioner appliance.

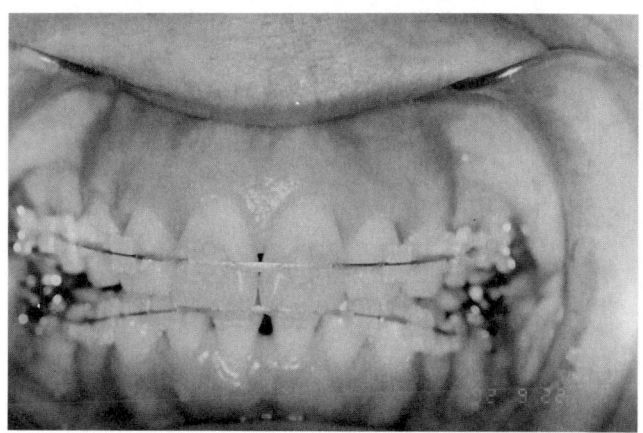

A

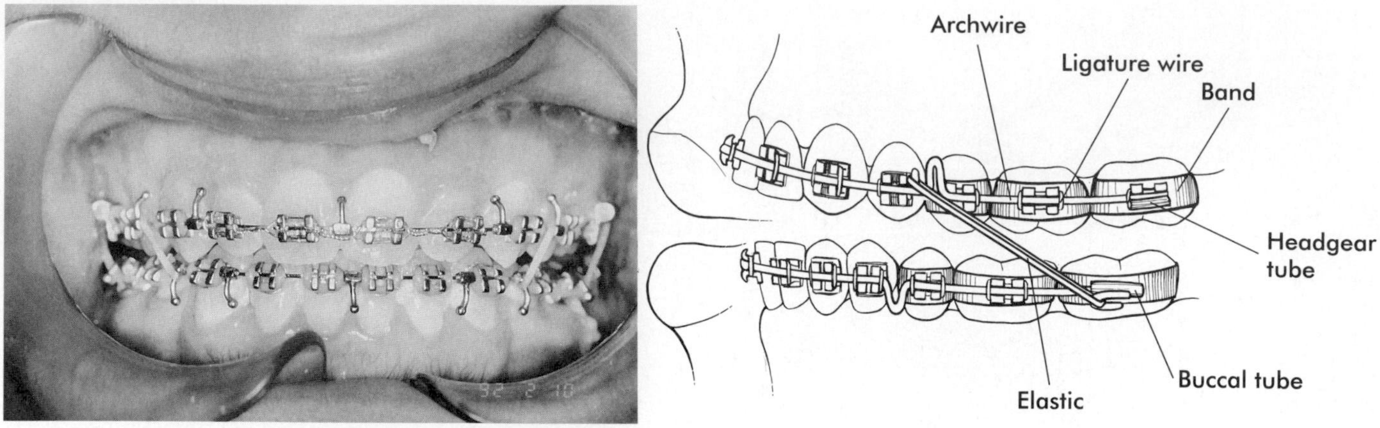

B

Archwire

Ligature wire

Band

Headgear tube

Buccal tube

Elastic

FIG. 35-38   *A,* Fixed orthodontic appliances. *B,* Components of fixed orthodontic appliances.

(Courtesy of Daniel R. Balbach, D.D.S., M.S., and John G. Clinthorne, D.D.S., M.S., Ann Arbor, Michigan.)

removable appliance called a positioner may also be used to retain the teeth after the active phase of orthodontic treatment. This appliance is fabricated from a soft, resilient plastic and is made to fit over the maxillary and mandibular teeth simultaneously (Fig. 35-37). Generally, removable appliances are worn from 12 to 24 hours a day to produce the desired effects.

▶ Fixed Appliances

Fixed appliances are cemented to the teeth and cannot be removed by the patient; these are commonly referred to as *braces* and consist of several important parts (Fig. 35-38, *A* and *B*). **Orthodontic bands** are stainless steel rings that encircle the tooth and are cemented with zinc phosphate or glass ionomer cement; these come in a variety of sizes. Each tooth must be individually sized and fitted before cementation. Bands are most commonly used on molar and premolar teeth because they are strong enough to withstand the heavy occlusal forces in the posterior segments of the dentition. Each band has a **bracket** or tube that is welded to the facial surface, which serves as a means of attachment for the archwires. Orthodontic brackets are usually bonded directly on the enamel surface of the anterior teeth, using an acid etch technique and acrylic bonding resin. Orthodontic brackets are made of stainless steel translucent ceramic or acrylic (Fig. 35-39). In certain cases, specially designed brackets may be placed on the lingual surfaces of the teeth, making the fixed appliances barely visible when the patient is smiling or talking. The band and brackets would have little value by themselves without the **archwire,** the means by which forces are applied to the dentition. The archwires fit into the horizontal slot in the brackets or slide into the buccal tubes on the molar teeth. Archwires come in a variety of diameters and com-

FIG. 35-39   Ceramic brackets are a less visible alternative to stainless steel brackets.

(Courtesy of Daniel R. Balbach, D.D.S., M.S., and John G. Clinthorne, D.D.S., M.S., Ann Arbor, Michigan.)

positions, which affect the magnitude of the force that is applied to the teeth. To secure the archwires into the brackets, **ligature ties** are used. These ligatures may be made of thin wire or tiny elastic bands. Removable auxiliary attachments, such as headgears or **orthodontic elastics,** may be attached to the fixed appliances to provide additional support for the desired tooth movements.

Instruments and Procedures

The dental assistant must be familiar with orthodontic procedures because many state laws permit the assistant to perform certain tasks. The procedures and instru-

PLACEMENT AND REMOVAL OF SEPARATORS

- Are all universal barrier techniques being used?
- Is all of the armamentarium available and prepared for use?
- Are the instruments arranged in sequence of use?
- Am I prepared for alternative treatment plans?
- Is the necessary equipment turned on and ready to operate?

Placement of Separators, Using Separating Pliers (Fig. 35–40, A)

1. Engage a separator on the tips of the separating pliers, and squeeze the handles gently to slightly stretch the elastic band (Fig. 40, *B*).
2. Place the separator on the embrasure area between the teeth where separation is desired (Fig. 35-40, *C*).
3. Using a back-and-forth *sawing* motion that is similar to inserting dental floss, work down one side of the separator through the interproximal contact, until it

rests completely beneath the contact. The occlusal portion of the separator should remain in the embrasure between the teeth, resting above the proximal contact (Fig. 35-40, *D*).

3. Once the separator is properly positioned, release the tension on the plier handles and remove the separating plier. This procedure is repeated at each interproximal contact where future orthodontic band placement is anticipated.

Placement of Separators, Using Dental Floss

1. First, insert two strands of dental floss through the lumen of the separator (Fig. 35-41, *A*)
2. Then, double over the ends of the floss, wrapping it around the middle finger of each hand. Stretch the separator slightly.

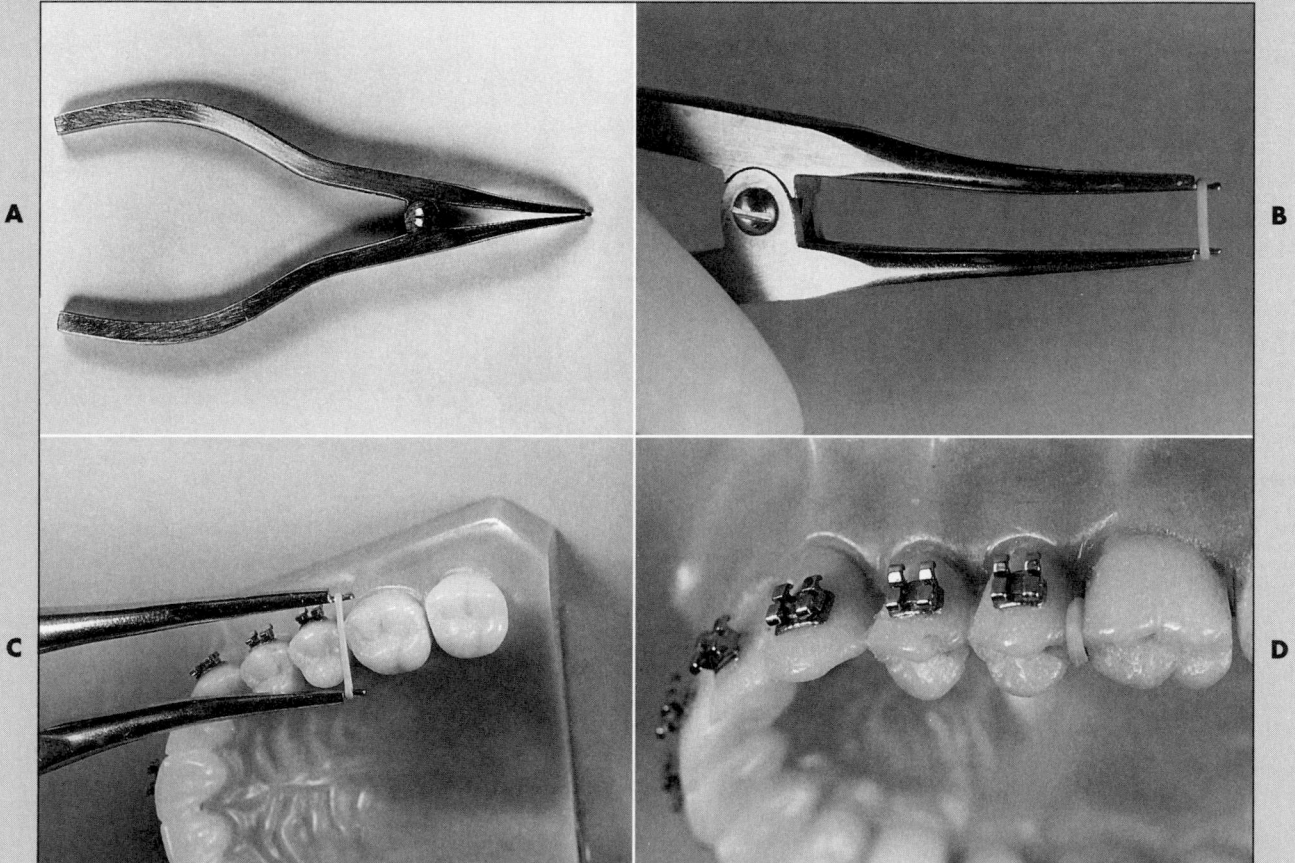

FIG. 35-40   *A,* Separating pliers. *B,* Pliers with separator engaged. *C,* Placement of separator. *D,* Properly positioned separator.

PLACEMENT AND REMOVAL OF SEPARATORS—cont'd

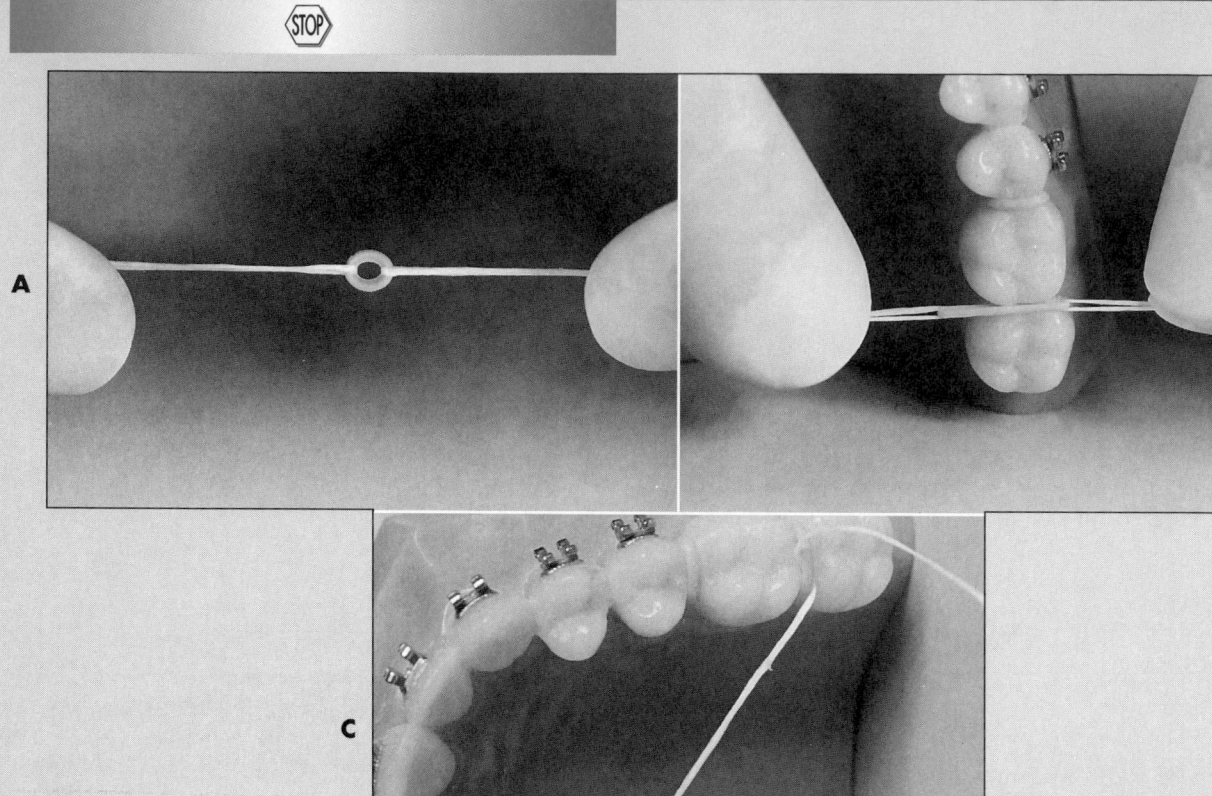

FIG. 35-41   *A,* Placement of dental floss through the separator. *B,* Insertion of separator. *C,* Removal of floss.

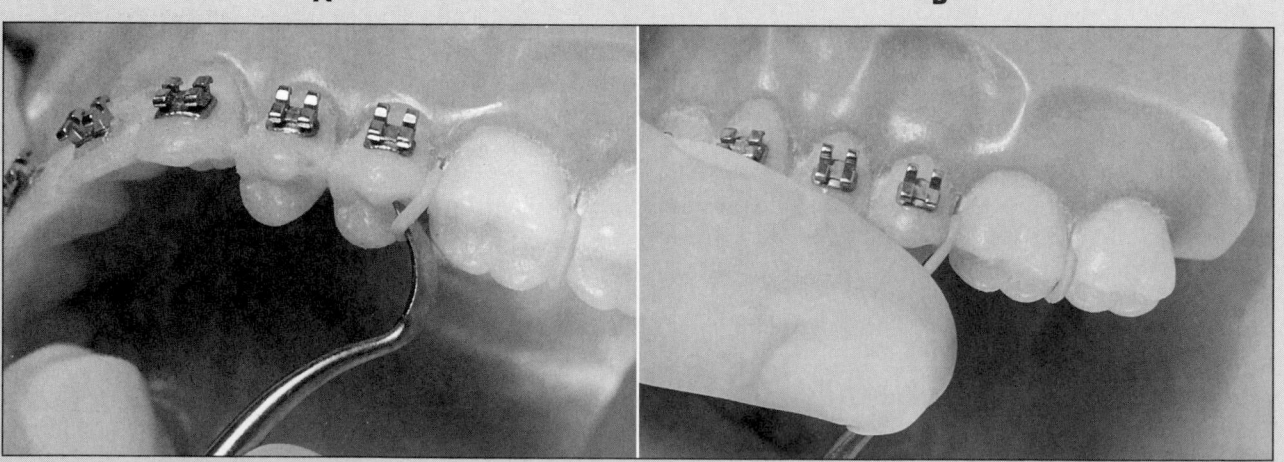

FIG. 35-42   *A,* Placement of scaler to remove separator. *B,* Removal of separator.

3. Insert the separator in a manner that is similar to flossing; one side of the separator is passed through the proximal contact area between the teeth (Fig. 35-41, *B*).
4. Once the separator is properly positioned, with one side of the elastic ring below the contact area and the other side above the contact, remove the strands of floss by pulling one end of each piece (Fig. 35-41, *C*).

Removal of Separators

1. Before the orthodontic bands are placed, the separators must be removed. For removal, hook one end of a scaler or explorer beneath the occlusal aspect of the separator (Fig. 35-42, *A*).
2. Place the index finger of the opposite hand over the top of the separator to prevent injury to the patient if the elastic band should snap (Fig. 35-42, *B*).

3. Pull gently on the instrument in an occlusal direction to disengage the separator.

▶ Are the appropriate universal barrier techniques removed?
▶ Have all of the appropriate surfaces been cleaned and disinfected?
▶ Has all armamentarium been removed?
▶ Has all equipment been repositioned?
▶ Has all of the equipment been disinfected / sterilized according to OSHA guidelines?

ments may vary slightly from one practice to another, but the techniques outlined here provide a good basic knowledge on which to build.

▶ Placement of Separators

For patient comfort and ease of placement a slight amount of space must exist between the teeth to fit the orthodontic bands. This is accomplished through the use of orthodontic **separators**, which are usually placed 1 week before the banding appointment. Although separators are supplied in metal, the most commonly used type of separator today is an elastic band, which is placed between the teeth. The separator encircles the proximal contact and provides a gentle force, which, over a period of days, moves the teeth apart. Separators may be placed with a special plier that is designed for this purpose or with dental floss. The following step-by-step procedure explains the placement of separators, using both placement methods, as well as removal of the separators.

Sometimes the separators are lost before the patient's next appointment because as the contact between the teeth opens, the separator becomes loose. When a patient returns to the office and it appears that a separator has been lost, examine the area carefully to make certain that the separator has not been displaced completely beneath the interproximal contact into the gingival tissue. An impacted separator can result in acute periodontal problems.

▶ Sizing and Fitting of Orthodontic Bands (Instruments shown in Fig. 35-43)

Orthodontic bands come in a large range of sizes and may be precontoured to fit specific teeth. Thus, maxillary molar bands are different from mandibular molar bands,

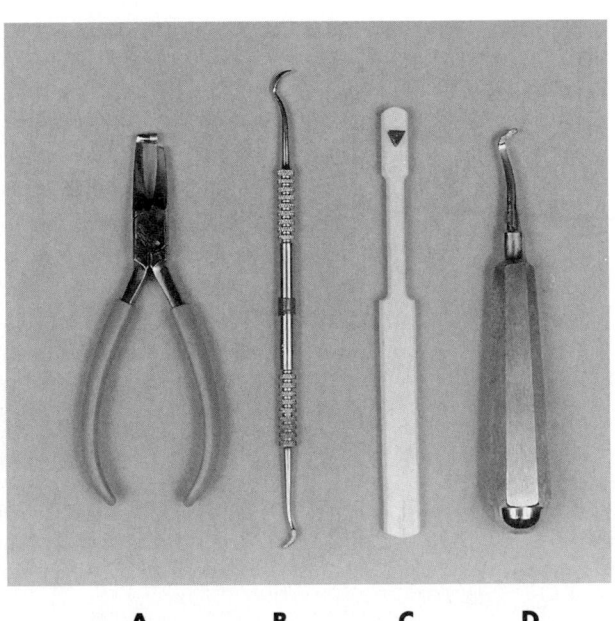

A B C D

FIG. 35-43 Instruments used to adapt orthodontic bands. *A,* Band-removing pliers. *B,* Schure #349 scaler. *C,* Band biter. *D,* Band seater / adapter.

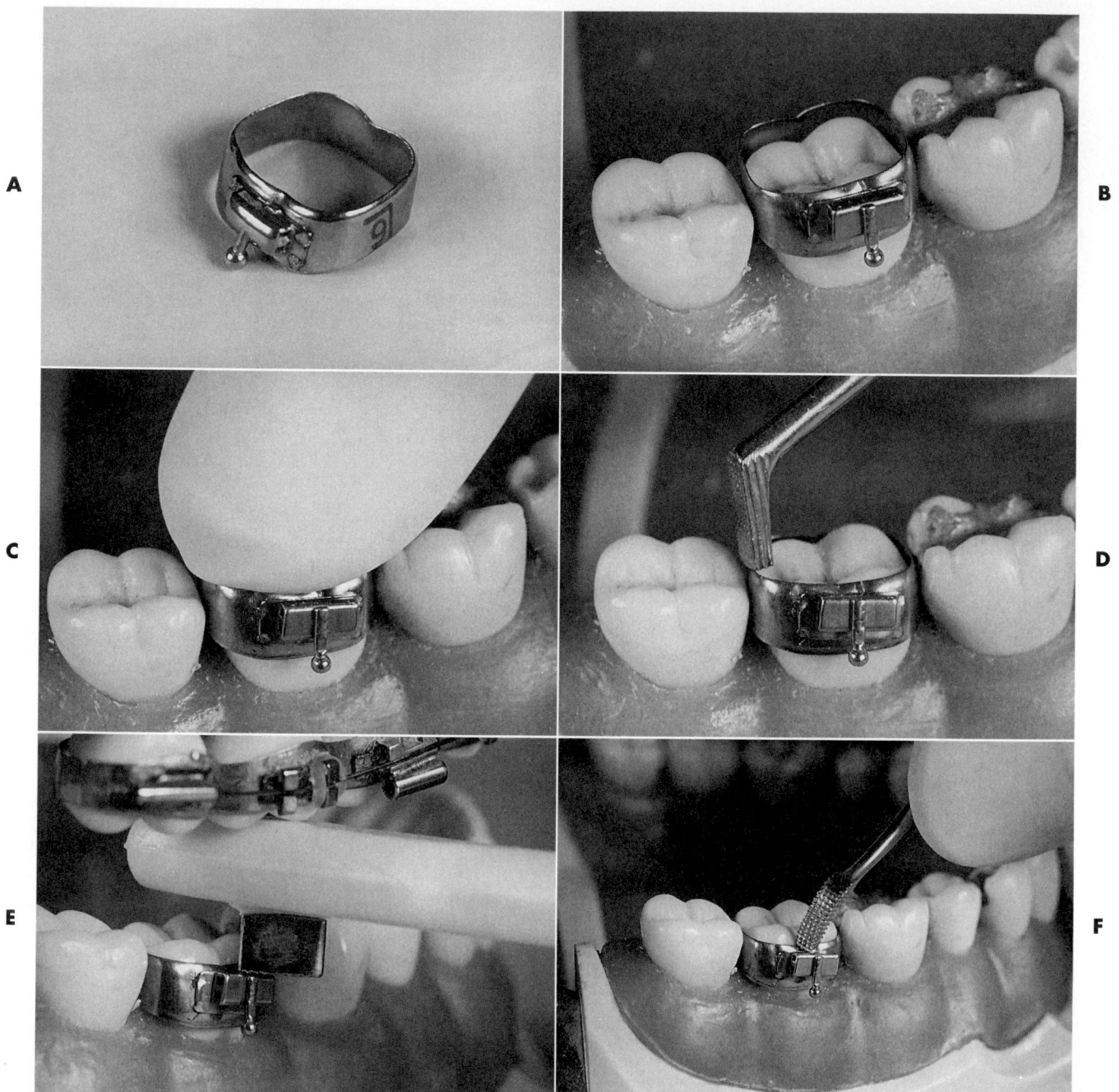

FIG. 35-44 *A,* Orthodontic band, showing size designation. *B,* Estimating size from study model. *C,* Using finger pressure to seat the band. *D,* Further seating with band adaptor. *E,* Placement of the band biter. *F,* Adaptation of the band, using the Schure instrument.

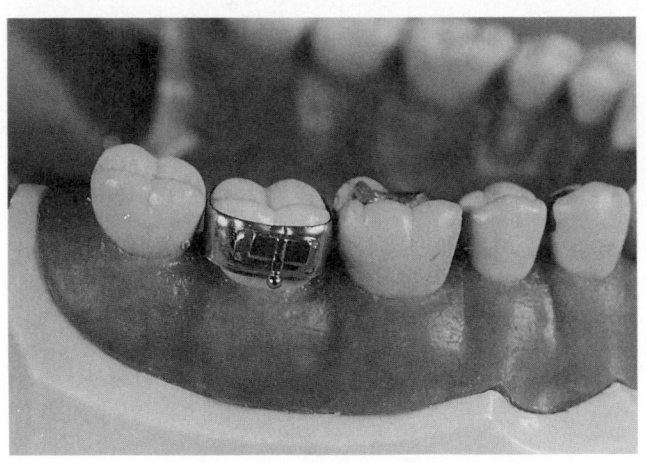

FIG. 35-45   Properly fitted band.

and even the right and left sides are contoured differently to best conform to the shape of a particular tooth. The size, arch, and right or left designation are imprinted on each band for ease of identification (Fig. 35-44, *A*). The following step-by-step procedure is the common method for trial sizing and fitting the bands.

A properly adapted band should fit tightly around the tooth, with no space visible between the edges of the band and the tooth (Fig. 35-45). The occlusal edges of the band should be positioned approximately 1 mm cervical to the marginal ridges of the tooth, and the band should not rock back and forth when buccal or lingual pressure is applied. The bands that were previously tried on but were not selected, are autoclaved, sorted, and returned to the box for future use.

SIZING AND FITTING ORTHODONTIC BANDS

1. First, estimate size of the band by placing it on the tooth on the patient's study model (Fig. 35-44, *B*).
2. Use finger pressure in the patient's mouth and push down the preselected band over the tooth (Fig. 35-44, *C*). If the band slides down too easily, it is probably too large, and a smaller size is selected. If the band cannot be pushed down at all, then it is too small, and a larger size is then chosen.
3. Place the serrated end of the Schure instrument or band adaptor on the edges of the band at the mesial and distal marginal ridges. Apply pressure in an attempt to push the band further in a cervical direction (Fig. 35-44, *D*).
4. Use the band biter for the final seating of the band onto the tooth. Place the serrated metal tip of the instrument on the edges of the band, and then ask the patient to bite down on the plastic handle to produce the desired force. Pressure will frequently need to be applied alternately at several areas on the band to ensure complete seating (Fig. 35-44, *E*). The best area for the application of biting pressure to seat a maxillary band is on the lingual surface, whereas the best area to seat a mandibular band is on the buccal surface (Fig. 35-44, *F*).
5. Then use the Schure instrument or band adaptor to contour the band into the grooves and around the marginal ridges by pressing the band material toward the tooth for a close fit. Since substantial pressure is applied, use extreme care to avoid patient injury.

CEMENTATION OF ORTHODONTIC BANDS

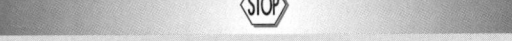

1. Place the plastic tip of the band-removing pliers on the occlusal surface of the tooth, while the opposing metal tip grasps the cervical edge of the band. Gentle pressure on the plier handles lifts the band from the tooth. As it is in band seating, mandibular bands are most easily removed by placing the tip of the pliers on the buccal surface, while removal of the maxillary bands is most easily approached from the lingual surface (Fig. 35-46).
2. Prepare the bands for cementation by rinsing and drying, and fill the brackets and tubes with soft beeswax to prevent them from getting filled with cement.
3. Polish the teeth with pumice; then rinse, dry, and isolate with cotton rolls.
4. Slowly mix zinc phosphate cement on a refrigerated slab to increase the working time. The proper consistency of the cement should be slightly thicker than the primary consistency used to cement inlays and crowns.
5. Place the cement inside the band and seat the band onto the tooth, using finger pressure, the band adaptor, and the band biter in the same sequence as used previously.
6. Once the cement has completely set, carefully remove the excess by using the scaler end of the Schure instrument (Fig. 35-47).

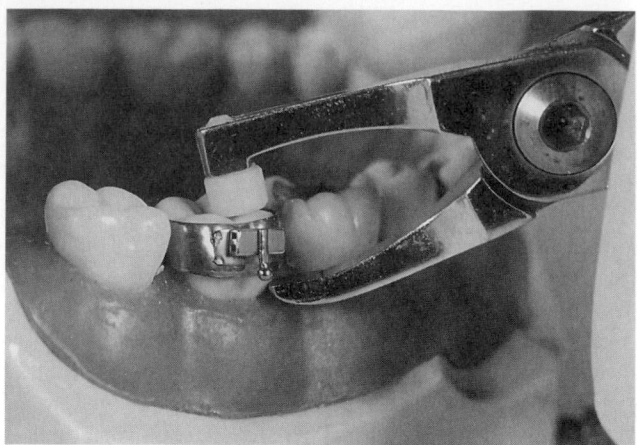

FIG. 35-46   Placement of the band-removing pliers.

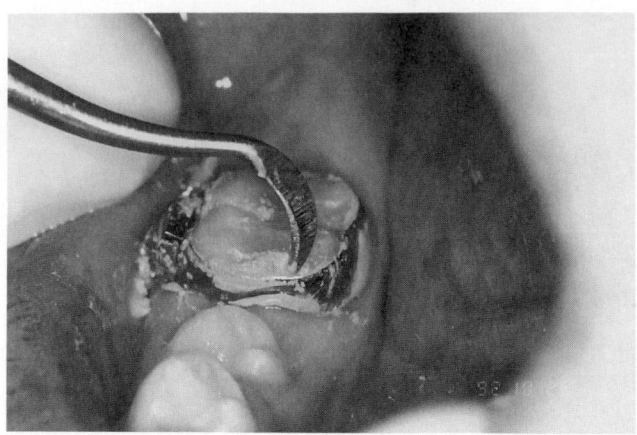

FIG. 35-47   Removal of excess cement with Schure instrument.

DIRECT BONDING OF ORTHODONTIC BRACKETS

1. Arrange the brackets on an adhesive pad next to the tooth number corresponding to the specific bracket. The brackets are color coded for each quadrant by a small dot on the distogingival corner of the bracket face (Fig. 35-48, *B*).
2. First, polish the teeth to be bonded with pumice, and then rinse and dry. Prophylaxis paste should not be used because some of the additives interfere with the bonding (Fig. 35-48, *C*).
3. Isolate the areas to be bonded with cheek retractors, saliva ejector, and cotton rolls to retain a dry field (Fig. 35-48, *D*).
4. Apply phosphoric acid etching gel to the enamel surfaces where the brackets will be attached. Allow the etching gel to remain on the teeth for 30 to 60 seconds (Fig. 35-48, *E*).
5. Thoroughly rinse and dry the teeth. This is one of the most critical steps. An inadequate rinse or moisture contamination may cause the bonding agent not to adhere properly. (Fig. 35-48, *F*).
6. Apply the bonding agent to the enamel surface. Mix and apply the bonding agent to the back of the bracket, according to the manufacturer's specifications (Fig. 35-48, *G*).
7. Use special forceps to place the bracket on the tooth. The cement reaches its initial set within approximately 30 seconds. Repeat the last two steps for each of the brackets to be bonded (Fig. 35-48, *H*).
8. Remove excess cement with a scaler before the resin has polymerized. Allow the cement to set for at least 5 minutes before the isolation is removed.

▶ Cementation of Orthodontic Bands

Once the bands have been sized and fitted, they must be removed and cemented in place. A permanent cement, such as a zinc phosphate or glass ionomer, is used to cement the bands. The following step-by-step procedure is used when orthodontic bands are placed.

▶ Direct Bonding of Orthodontic Brackets

The bonding of orthodontic brackets directly to the enamel surfaces allows for improved patient comfort and oral hygiene. While the brackets do not usually have to be sized and fitted before cementation, the individual brackets, like orthodontic bands, are specific for each tooth in the arch. The procedure for bonding requires careful preparation of the tooth surface, which is critical to the adhesion of the bracket. The armamentarium is assembled as shown in (Fig. 35-48, *A*). The step-by-step procedure is outlined as follows:

Cementation of the appliances is done by the orthodontist; however, the assistant may perform many of the sizing, fitting, and tooth preparation tasks.

▶ Placement of Archwires and Ligature Ties

Instruments used to place archwires and ligature ties are shown in Fig. 35-49. Insertion of the archwires is the next step in the placement of the orthodontic appliance.

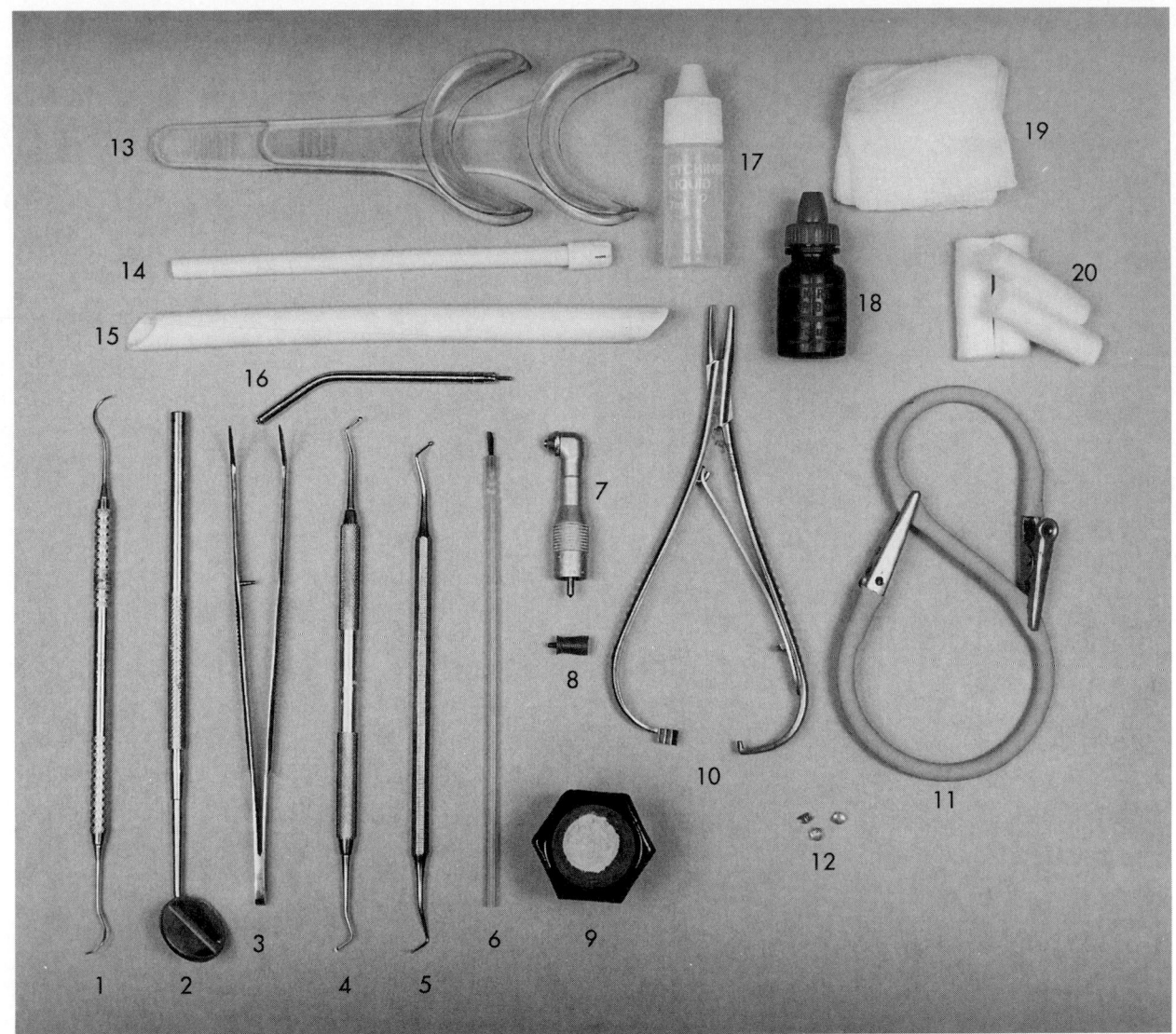

1. Explorer
2. Mirror
3. Cotton pliers
4. Spoon excavator
5. Ball burnisher
6. Disposable brush
7. Prophylaxis angle
8. Prophylaxis cup
9. Dappen dish with flow of pumice
10. Hemostat
11. Napkin chain
12. Brackets
13. Mouth props
14. Saliva ejector
15. HVE tip
16. a/w Tip
17. Etching liquid
18. Bonding material
19. 2 × 2 gauge
20. Cotton rolls

FIG. 35-48 *A,* Armamentarium for bonding orthodontic brackets. *Continued.*

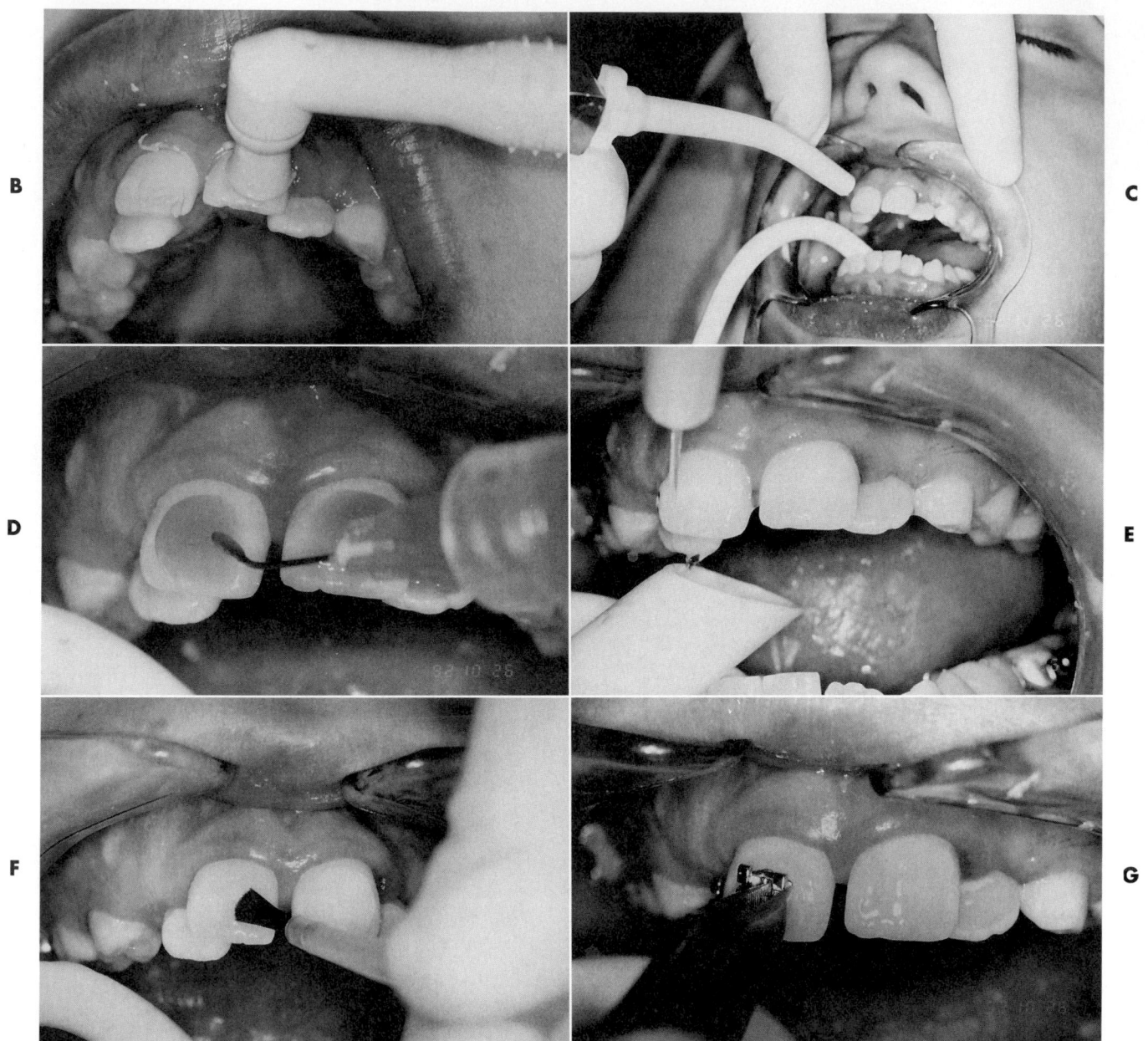

FIG. 35-48, cont'd.   *B,* Polish the teeth with pumice. *C,* Dry and isolate the site. *D,* Apply etching gel to surface where brackets are to be attached. *E,* Rinse and dry the teeth thoroughly. *F,* Mix and apply the bonding agent. Place on enamel surface and back of bracket. *G,* Place the bracket.

(Courtesy of Daniel R. Balbach, D.D.S., M.S., and John G. Clinthorne, D.D.S., M.S., Ann Arbor, Michigan.)

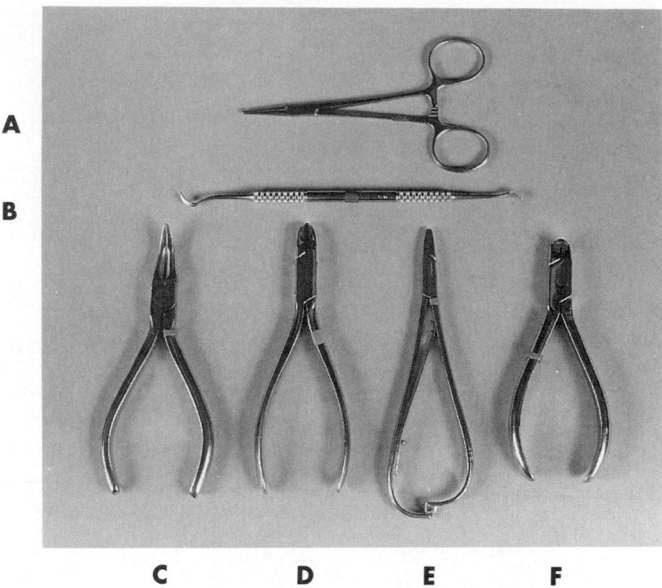

FIG. 35-49   Instruments used to place wires and ligatures. *A,* Weingart utility plier. *B,* Ligature cutter. *C,* Ligature tying plier. *D,* Distal end cutting plier. *E,* Schure #349 scaler. *F,* Hemostat.

PLACEMENT AND REMOVAL OF ARCHWIRES AND LIGATURES

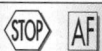

1. Select the appropriate wire.
2. Estimate the length of the wire on the study models, and cut off the excess with the wire cutters.
3. Use the Weingart pliers to insert the wire into the buccal tubes of the molar bands (Fig. 35-50). Care must be taken not to injure the soft tissues with the sharp wire ends during insertion and removal. The Weingart pliers may also be used to fit the wire into the horizontal slots in the brackets.

4. If excess wire still remains distal to the ends of the buccal tubes on the molar bands, remove it or cut it with the distal end cutting pliers (Fig. 35-51).

The archwires must now be secured by the placement of ligature ties. Two types of ligatures may be used, wire ties and elastic ties.

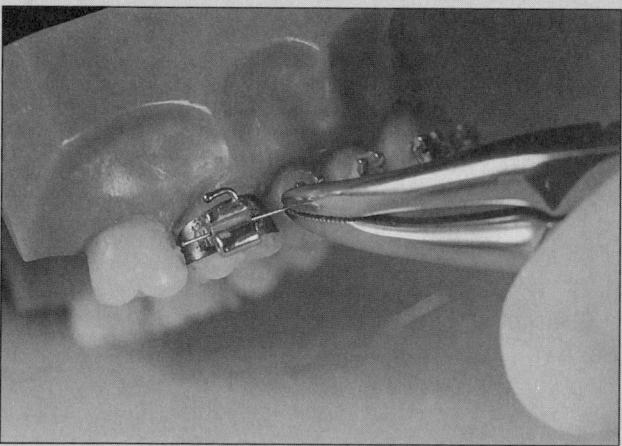

FIG. 35-50   Placement of wire into tube with Weingart plier.

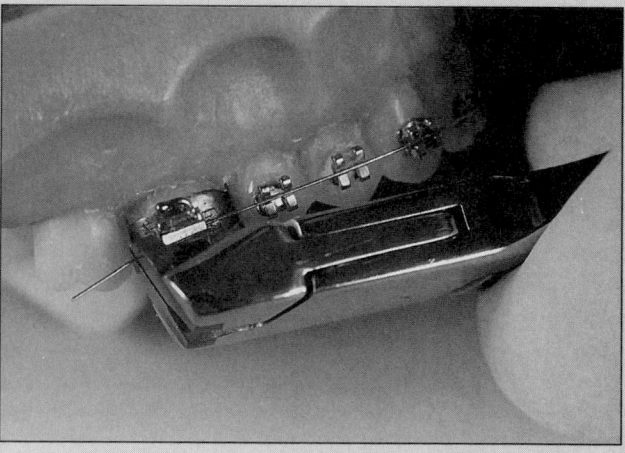

FIG. 35-51   Cutting distal end with distal end cutter.

Continued.

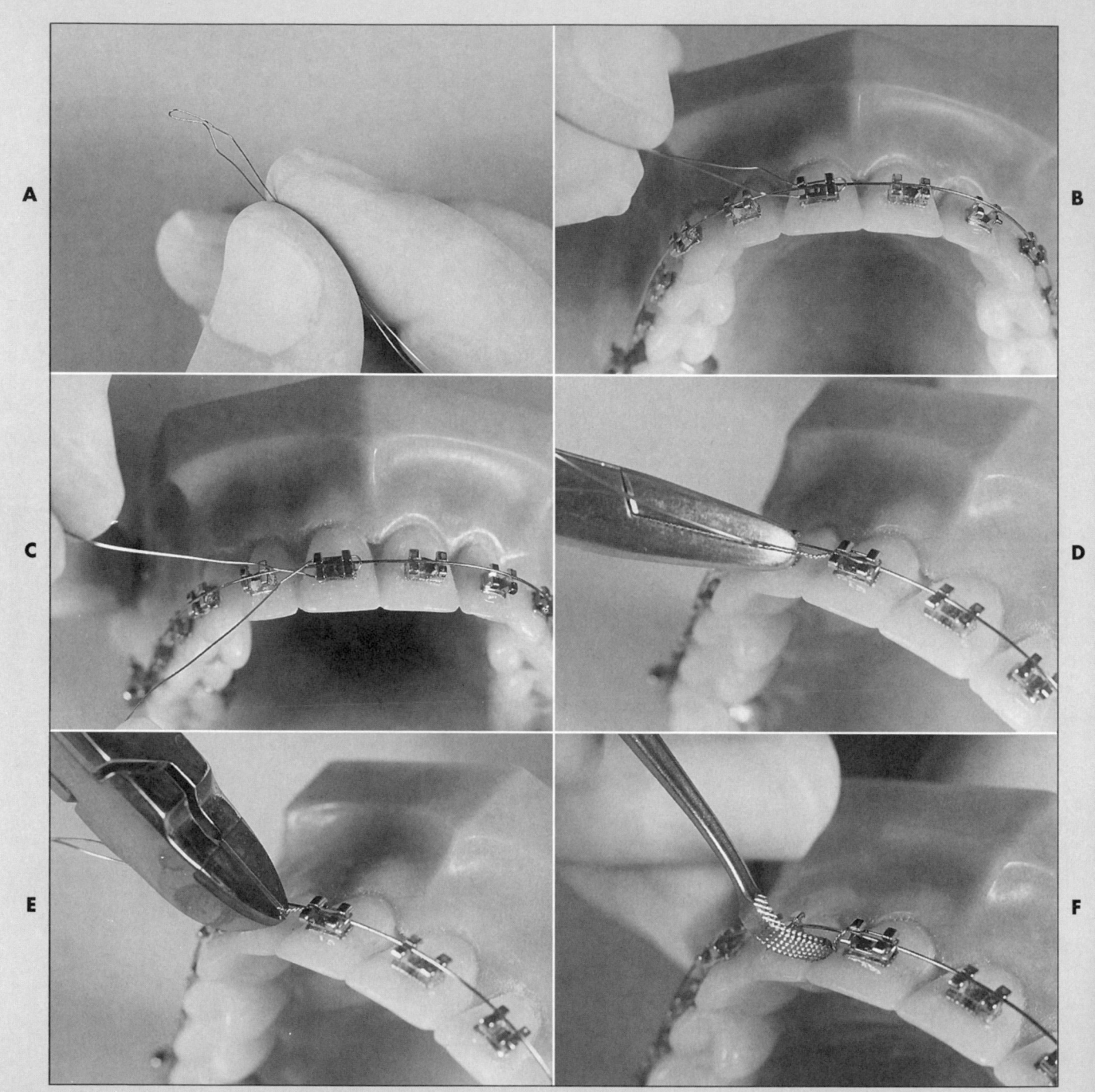

FIG. 35-52 Ligature wire placement sequence. *A,* Bend the loop at a slight angle before placement. *B,* Slide the loops around the wings of the bracket. *C,* Cross the ends of the ligature wire over the top of the archwire at the side of the bracket. *D,* Place the ligature tying pliers about 4 to 6 mm from the bracket, and rotate the pliers several times to twist the wires tightly together. *E,* Cut the excess ligature wire leaving a 3 mm *pigtail. F,* Tuck the sharp twisted end of the tie under the archwire.

Placement of Wire Ligatures

1. It may help to bend the loop at a slight angle before placement (Fig. 35-52, *A*). Slide the preformed wire loops horizontally around the bracket, so that one side of the loop rests under the gingival tie wings on the bracket and the other side rests under the occlusal tie wings (Fig. 35-52, *B*).
2. Cross the ends of the ligature wire over the top of the archwire at the side of the bracket (Fig. 35-52, *C*).
3. Place the ligature tying pliers on the tie wire crossing 4 to 6 mm from the bracket. The handles of the pliers are squeezed to engage the wire and to lock the pliers.
4. Rotate the pliers several times so that the wires are twisted tightly together (Fig. 35-52, *D*).
5. Squeeze the pliers handles to disengage the wires.
6. Use the ligature cutting pliers to cut the excess ligature wire, leaving a 3 mm *pigtail* of twisted wire next to the bracket (Fig. 35-52, *E*).
7. The serrated tip of the Schure instrument may be used to tuck the sharp twisted end of the tie underneath the archwire where it will not irritate the lips or buccal mucosa (Fig. 35-52, *F*).

Removal of Wire Ligatures

The ligature ties are removed at each appointment where the archwire is changed.

1. Place the ligature cutter at the mesial or the distal side of the bracket on the ligature wire. The cutting edges may be nearly parallel to the archwire (Fig. 35-53).

2. Grasp the cut ligature with the ligature cutters and gently release it from the tie wings of the bracket.
3. Take care when handling the cut ligature wires because the sharp ends can easily penetrate oral mucosa, as well as latex treatment gloves and fingers.

Placement of Elastic Ligatures

Elastic ligature ties may be used as an alternative to wire ties.

1. Use the hemostat to grasp elastic ligatures and remove them from the holder (Fig. 35-54, *A*).
2. Carefully stretch the ligature around the gingival tie wings of the bracket, over the archwire, and around the occlusal tie wings (Fig. 35-54, *B*).
3. Release the hemostat, leaving the ligature securely encircling the bracket. The procedure is repeated until all brackets have been ligated to the archwire (Fig. 35-54, *C*).
4. The elastic ligature ties may be removed by inserting the tip of the scaler beneath the tie and between the occlusal tie wings, gently releasing it from the bracket (Fig. 35-54, *D*).

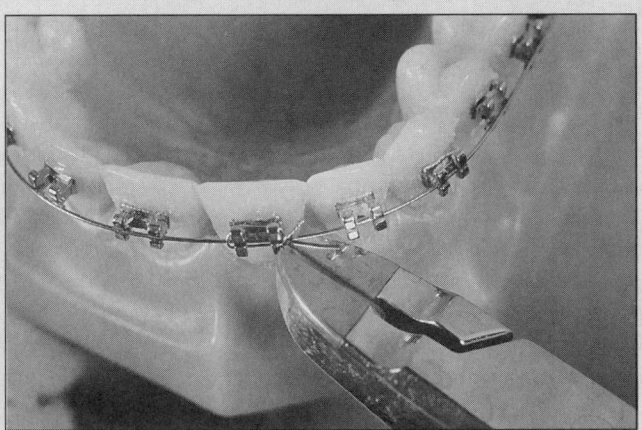

FIG. 35-53 **Cutting ligature wire.**

Continued.

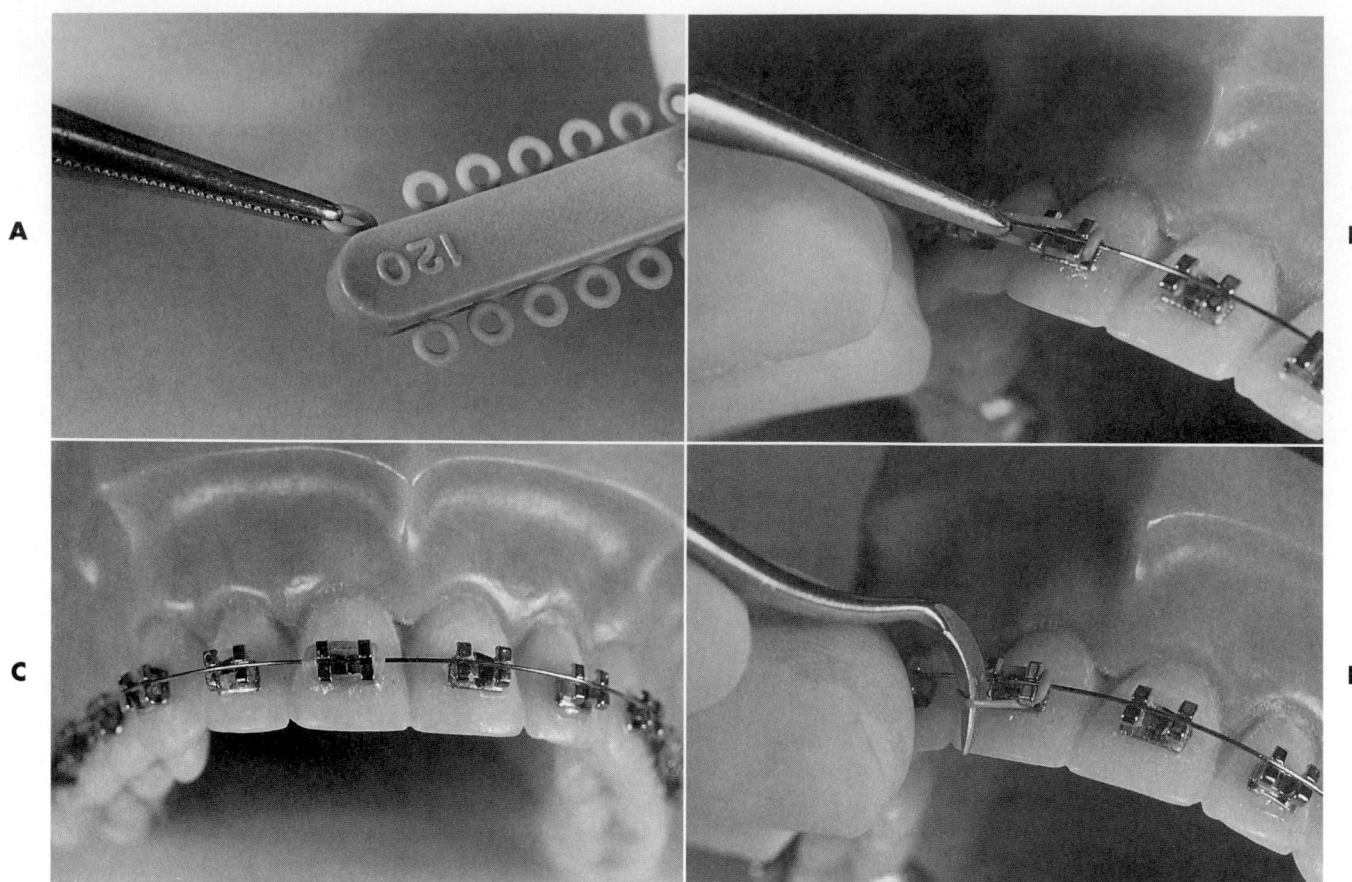

FIG. 35-54   Placing plastic ligatures. *A,* Attach hemostat to plastic ligature. *B,* Stretch ligature over bracket tie wings and archwire. *C,* Attached plastic ligature. *D,* Place scaler beneath tie to release plastic ligature from bracket.

Oral Hygiene

People who wear orthodontic appliances are more susceptible to dental decay around the bands and brackets because food trapped in these areas can lead to the build-up of plaque. Plaque accumulation tends to occur along the gingival border of the brackets and in the interproximal areas beneath the archwire. If the plaque is not removed frequently, it may dissolve the enamel of the teeth underneath the surrounding brackets, resulting in permanent decalcification or decay.

The dental assistant is the prime motivator for and educator about oral hygiene for the orthodontic patient. The assistant evaluates the patient's toothbrushing at every appointment and demonstrates the proper techniques for reaching the troublesome areas.

The orthodontic patient must spend additional time brushing and using special techniques to thoroughly remove plaque from around the fixed appliances. An orthodontic toothbrush is frequently recommended be-cause it has rows of bristles that are specially contoured to fit around the brackets more easily. (See Chapter 26 for examples of this brush style.) One of the most critical areas to brush is the facial aspect of the teeth between the bracket and the gingival margin. The toothbrush is placed in this area with the bristles at about a 45-degree angle, with the ends pointing towards the brackets. A small circular motion is used, starting at one side of the arch and continuing around to the other side. The complete arch should be brushed in this manner, rather than skipping from one spot to another. The facial surfaces of the teeth are then cleaned by brushing the area between the brackets and the incisal edges, rotating the brush at a slight angle, with the bristles pointing toward the brackets. With each pass, the bristles should be worked underneath the archwire to remove plaque from the interproximal areas. A special interdental brush may also be used in these areas to ensure complete plaque removal. The lingual and occlusal surfaces of the teeth may be brushed as usual, unless appliances are present on these surfaces.

Flossing is also an important part of oral hygiene for orthodontic patients. The floss must be inserted beneath the archwire at each interproximal area, and a floss threader may be used to facilitate its placement. The floss is then gently worked between the interproximal contact, and the opposing surfaces of the adjacent teeth are flossed separately. The dental floss is then carefully pulled from beneath the archwire and the process is repeated for the next interproximal contact.

The orthodontic patient should brush after every meal and perform one session of complete flossing and brushing once a day. One of the most important habits to develop is to examine the teeth for complete plaque removal after brushing. Disclosing tablets are sometimes used to highlight areas that the patient missed.

Oral irrigation devices may also be used as an adjunct to oral hygiene for the orthodontic patient. The jet stream of water helps loosen particles of food and plaque from around the brackets, but this is no substitute for thorough brushing.

KEY POINTS

▶ The specialty of orthodontics offers the dental assistant an exciting challenge with varied duties, including the opportunity to work independently with the patient in performing a variety of tasks that are delegated as advanced functions in different states, assist in collection of data for diagnostic aids, expose radiographs, and aid in patient management.

▶ The patient in this practice will generally be under treatment for nearly 2 years. During this time the dental assistant will face the challenge of understanding the patient's treatment plan, the progression of treatment, the motivational needs of the patient, and the patient's many physical and systemic changes that transpire during this period of treatment.

▶ Malocclusion can be categorized in many different ways. One of the most common methods is the Angle's Classifications of Occlusion, based on a relationship of the maxillary and mandibular first permanent molars. Classifications are identified in this system as Class I, Class II, or Class III.

▶ Malocclusion can result in a variety of dental discrepancies, including crowding, spacing, overbite, open bite, or crossbite.

▶ Interceptive treatment is a concept that proposes to supersede certain problems before they have a negative effect on the developing dentition.

▶ Orthodontics, like other phases of dentistry, relies on a collection of data in making a thorough diagnosis and treatment plan. These diagnostic aids include a medical and dental history; clinical examination; panoramic, cephalometric, and intraoral radiographs; study models; and intraoral and extraoral photographs.

▶ Orthodontic appliances are categorized as removable or fixed. Examples of removable appliances include a headgear, functional appliances, and retainers. Fixed appliances are cemented to the teeth and include various components, such as bands, brackets, archwires, ligature ties, and orthodontic elastics.

BIBLIOGRAPHY

Gottlieb GL, Nelson A, Vogels DS: 1990 JCO study of orthodontic diagnosis and treatment procedures, *J Clin Orthodont* pp. 145-156, March 1991.

Graber TM, Vanarsdall RL: *Orthodontics: current principles and techniques,* ed 2, St Louis, 1994, Mosby.

Profitt WR: *Contemporary orthodontics,* ed 2, St Louis, 1993, Mosby.

36 Pediatric Dentistry

LEARNING OBJECTIVES

You will have mastered the material in this chapter when you can:
▶ Define the key terms
▶ Define the specialty of pediatric dentistry
▶ Describe the scope of pediatric dentistry
▶ Explain the role of the dental assistant in pediatric dentistry
▶ Describe common behavior patterns or stages in children
▶ Describe behavior management of children in the dental office
▶ Identify common treatment procedures in pediatric dentistry
▶ Identify urgent care treatment in pediatric dentistry
▶ List the signs and symptoms of child abuse
▶ Identify materials and equipment unique to pediatric dentistry

KEY TERMS

Behavior management techniques
Behavior patterns
Flooding
Hand-over-mouth (HOM)
Modeling
Papoose board
Pediatric dentistry
Show-and-tell
Validation

Pediatric dentistry is one of the eight recognized specialties of dentistry and involves the delivery of dental treatment to children from birth through the age of mixed dentition. The focus of pediatric dentistry has changed to meet the needs of today's children. The National Institute of Dental Research (NIDR) produced the National Caries Prevalence Study in 1981, which indicated a visible decline in dental caries in children of school age. This study confirmed that 17 million children were caries free, equivalent to an 11% decrease in decay. Further information gathered showed a decline in the occurrence of multiple surface lesions, pulpal therapy in primary teeth, and the number of applied stainless steel crowns. This same study confirmed an increase in the application of fluoride and sealants and in the use of a more conservative approach during the placement of restorations.

The American Society for the Promotion of Children's Dentistry was founded in 1927; later, in 1940, it became the American Society of Dentistry for Children.

These statistics were used to change the delivery of care in pediatric dentistry from a restorative to a preventive approach. The scope of pediatric dentistry today allows the practitioner to devote more time to new concepts that meet the needs of the patient, which include greater emphasis on diagnosis and prevention and on increased involvement in the correction of malocclusion. But often, the foremost need in the delivery of dental treatment to children is the ability to manage the patient's needs, fears, and individual emotional variations.

Behavior Management

It is important to understand that a child is not just a small adult. Each year brings changes and new experiences to a child's mental and physical development, and the dental assistant must be able to communicate at their level, without being demeaning. The appropriate application of **behavior management** techniques (used to modify a response from a patient) is relative to the success of the dental procedure.

Probably one of the more difficult situations confronting a dental staff in the treatment of children is the potential for behavior management problems. Children seen in a pediatric dental office vary in physical age, emotional age, and level of maturity. The dental team is challenged with delivery of care to patients ranging from a child of 2 or less, who might not be able to identify pain, to a young teenager, who feels grown up and prefers to be seen by a general practitioner, as well as physically and emotionally disabled children, who have multiple physical and behavior problems. A range of skills is necessary to address all of these needs, but underlying this demand is a basic need to understand developmental growth patterns and the emotional and physical development of children.

Childhood Development

Although development varies with each child, certain levels of emotional, chronologic, and intellectual growth can be expected at particular ages. Knowledge of these levels of development assists the dental team in evaluating the child and providing treatment. The following describes common levels of development for each age group.

▶ Birth to Two Years

From birth to age 2 a child begins to develop trust in surroundings as nurturing needs are met through food, sucking, and general care. A child that is brought to a dental office at this age is not able to respond rationally to questions that relate to dental needs. The caregiver must be informed of the treatment and any postoperative instructions.

▶ Two Years

A child of 2 is rapidly developing physically, emotionally, and intellectually. Normally a child becomes toilet trained during this year, instilling a sense of pride in achievement and independence from the caregiver. The vocabulary increases, both in usage and comprehension.

The 2-year-old child relies on feelings for understanding and depends on tone of voice and facial expression to completely understand certain situations. Since sudden movements and sounds will sometimes frighten this child, the dental experience must be handled with great care. Each change in chair position, sound, and activity must be explained so that the child is less fearful of the experience. The pediatric dentist may feel more comfortable or find it necessary to have a caregiver in the treatment room with the child.

▶ Three Years

A 3-year-old child is developing socially, with increased vocabulary skills and greater outside experiences through separation from parents. In modern society many children of this age have had the opportunity to experience preschool and outside authoritative figures and consequently are more willing to be left alone in a treatment room with another person.

▶ Four Years

The 4-year-old child may be less cooperative and he or she may be assertive, aggressive, and even resistant to any direction. The child fears the unknown but is less fearful of strangers because of increased social experiences. Although both direction and understanding used by the dental team can produce a patient who is cooperative, this child may respond negatively to minor pain that is induced in dental treatment. Therefore, the dental staff should take every precaution possible to avoid or eliminate any discomfort for the patient.

▶ Five Years

As early childhood comes to an end the 5-year-old accepts separation from caregivers. The child is capable of interacting socially through verbal and physical activity and is usually quite interested in discussions of accomplishments, possessions, and themselves.

▶ Six Years

The 6-year-old child is embarking on a major change in experiences as school begins. The pressure and involvement of peer groups greatly influence a child at this age. The type of interaction that involves evaluation by peers and authority figures helps in developing self-esteem. With the introduction of another authority figure, the teacher, a child is more responsive to directions from other adults; this allows the dental team to direct the child toward a positive response to dental treatment.

▶ Seven to Twelve Years

From 7 to 12 years the child is physically and intellectually more capable of dealing with situations that might create anxiety. The level of maturity of this age child reflects a knowledge of the reality of having to deal with unpleasant situations, which is how the dental visit may be viewed.

These descriptions are only generalizations, and therefore the dental team must be prepared to deal with the child patient whose behavior might differ. It is possible to have a child in the dental chair who, chronologically, is 10 years old, intellectually, 7 years old, and emotionally, 5 years old. The needs and conditions of dealing with this child may necessitate careful instruction, demonstration, caring, and a great deal of patience to provide a dental experience that will not result in a negative memory.

Behavior Patterns

The dental team must be able to recognize and respond appropriately to any **behavior pattern**, a repeated response or reaction to a stimulus, demonstrated by a child before or during dental treatment. Once a child has been successful in having his or her own way in a dental office through the use of a particular behavior pattern, the behavior will be repeated at a later date to accomplish the same goal. The following categories describe behavior that is often encountered when treating children in a pediatric or a general dental practice.

The *cooperative* child is seen most often in a dental office. This child is willing to accept well-defined explanations and respond positively to directions. The child who *lacks cooperative ability* is unable to understand explanations of procedures or to communicate this inability. This type of child is usually one who is very young or who is mentally or physically disabled, with restricted communication levels and skills.

Potentially uncooperative behavior can be exhibited by any child seen in an office. Usually fear is the stimulus for the uncooperative behavior. This fear may manifest from past negative dental experiences or from discussions of negative dental experiences with parents, peers, or siblings. This child might demonstrate uncontrolled, defiant, timid, tense-cooperative, whining, or stoic behavior. It is possible that each behavior pattern

requires a different response from the dental team. Techniques used to manage these patients are discussed later in this chapter.

Parent/Caregiver Attitude

Many, if not all, of the previously mentioned behavior patterns may depend on the interaction a child has with the primary caregiver. Dental professionals not only are providing a service to patients, but also need to be detectives in the day-to-day interaction with patients. The power of observation plays an integral part in determining a potential behavior problem with a child. Talking with and observing a caregiver's interaction with the child provides information regarding parental attitudes. These attitudes may be adopted by the child and may lead to unacceptable behavior patterns in their children.

If a caregiver is overprotective, the child does not have the opportunity to experience different lessons of life. The child of a caregiver who exhibits this attitude is often shy, afraid of new experiences, and may lack self-confidence and self-esteem. The caregiver may have had a negative dental experience and has imparted these fears and anxieties to the child.

An overindulgent attitude of the caregiver toward the child creates in the child a sense of being able to demand and expect reactions to his wishes. When the child is faced with a situation in a dental office where his or her demands are not met, the result can be disruptive. For example, the child might request the caregiver to stay in the treatment room during a procedure. If the child does not receive compliance with demands, a temper tantrum may result. The dental team may have to disrupt a pattern of care to address this problem. Children of overauthoritative caregivers are expected to act an age other than their own. These children are overly criticized and may resent people with authority giving direction, including the dentist.

Underaffectionate caregivers can display a range of attitudes toward their children. The caregiver may show the child a lack of interest or an obvious rejection or may be physically abusive. The child in this situation exhibits low self-esteem, is stoic, and may even be nonresponsive; but often, in an attempt to seek attention, the child may be loud and aggressive.

Behavior Management Techniques

Before employing any behavior management technique, the behavior must be identified correctly to provide the proper response. *Communication* is the primary means of response to a behavior management situation.

Once the lines of communication are open, the ability to continue with treatment is much easier. Children are individuals and have specific interests, needs, desires, and personality characteristics. They have needs that are similar to those of adults and desire to be treated with respect, whether it is a cognizant feeling or not. A child should be met with a friendly greeting, and every attempt should be made to make eye contact with the child. The dentist questions the child about interests and establishes a line of communication. This interaction usually relaxes the child and allows the dentist to continue with an explanation of the treatment that will be rendered.

An *atmosphere* that relaxes a child is conducive to achieving a positive relationship. At times this can be accomplished by creating a setting that makes the child comfortable and trusting. Pediatric dental offices should be designed for the comfort of the child but still be functional for the dental team.

The reception area of a pediatric office is designed to entertain and educate the children as they wait for dental treatment. Sometimes a patient's caregiver will bring other children to wait for the patient. As one sibling waits for another, boredom and antagonistic behavior can develop. A reception area that is colorful and full of activities for various age levels can keep the children occupied. A specific theme can be woven into all the areas of the office for the children's enjoyment.

Books, dental educational tools, puzzles, small jungle gyms, toys, and videocassette or audiocassette players all entertain children. A bulletin board that contains pictures of children in the practice and articles about their achievements, which are visible to all the children, acts as a positive public relations tool and allows the children to see themselves or their friends given special attention.

The uniforms worn by the pediatric dental staff should be more colorful and attractive to relieve the anxiety that may be associated with white coats but should still maintain OSHA uniform guidelines. Identification tags can be worn so that the child can attach a name with a face and feel more at ease and among friends.

▶ Dental Semantics

The treatment must be explained at a level that the patient can understand. Dental terminology that is used with an adult must be replaced with words the child can comprehend. This does not mean the dentist should use *baby talk* but should change the terminology to meet the child's level. The words and the actions associated with them must not frighten the child. An example of word exchanges follows:

Anesthesia — Makes a sleepy tooth that will feel fat
Rubber dam — Looks like a raincoat and is placed on the tooth to keep it dry
HVE — A vacuum cleaner for the mouth
Explorer — A tooth feeler

Allowing the child to feel things such as the HVE and the rubber cup for polishing helps to allay the fears of the procedure.

▶ Authoritative Figure

The dentist usually takes the lead in providing the child with directions and instructions. This allows the child to focus on what one person is saying and to not become confused over directions given by two people. The ability to distinguish between the directions given by two people may become difficult as the fear of the unknown overrides the child's abilities.

Before treatment begins the child must understand the rules involving any dental procedure. A complete and thorough explanation of the rules prevents problems later. The child is told to keep the hands in the lap, to remain still, and to not make any loud noises that might upset other children in the office.

▶ Validation

Many children become fearful of unfamiliar situations, and their behavior may become uncooperative. When this happens, the child's fear must not be denied, but through **validation** the child's feelings should be acknowledged and confirmed by the dentist, who indicates that being afraid is all right and who explains the treatment to the child again. Denying the child's fear creates a feeling of distrust for the dentist because the child believes the dentist is being untruthful.

▶ Voice Control

Children will attempt to use excuses to delay treatment if they are uncomfortable. Tactics that a child might take to delay treatment include being overly talkative and wanting to tell the dentist everything about himself or herself, having the need to visit the bathroom several times, or claiming to be ill. Occasionally it may be necessary to use *voice control* to regain a child's attention. The dramatic change in the dentist's tone of voice directing the child to "be quiet and open your mouth" gains the child's attention. This technique reminds the child that the dentist is an authority figure and demands cooperation and respect. Once the child complies with the instructions, the dentist reinforces the good behavior by thanking the child for the cooperation.

Certain individuals do not feel comfortable commanding a child to obey. They believe they should ask for the child's approval. But the response from the child might be negative. Children should have the opportunity to make decisions when it is appropriate, such as in selecting a flavor of fluoride. This gives the child some sense of ownership in the activity and makes for a more cooperative patient.

Modeling

Other forms of behavior modification include **modeling**, desensitization, and flooding techniques. In **modeling** a child who exhibits good behavior in a dental office is the model for a child who may be a potential problem or for a child who has already exhibited inappropriate behavior. The dentist may use an open bay concept for treatment room design to allow children to see another child during treatment. This is often effective when treating siblings. This concept promotes an opportunity to use peer pressure to help the child respond in a positive manner.

Show-and-Tell

The child who visits a dental office with preconceived or established fears may have to be desensitized through a **show-and-tell** technique. For example, the sound and feeling that are associated with the HVE frighten some children. The dentist should turn the HVE on and explain its use. The child is allowed to feel it on a hand before it is placed in the mouth, allowing the child to experience its use. The child then has reduced fears and a base of knowledge regarding the use of the HVE without associating it with pain.

Flooding

Flooding techniques are steps that are taken in behavior therapy to reduce anxiety that is associated with phobias. The techniques usually provoke anxiety desensitization. These behavior modification techniques need to be discussed with the primary caregiver before implementation, since these actions are more drastic than the ones previously described.

The first technique is known as the **hand-over-mouth (HOM) technique**. HOM is normally used on children who are 3 years and older and who are not physically disabled or mentally compromised. A child who is uncooperative—screaming, biting, or kicking—must be dealt with immediately. The child must be told that this is unacceptable behavior, that it prolongs treatment time, and that it will not be tolerated. The child is held in the chair and the dental assistant holds the arms and legs as the dentist firmly places a hand over the mouth and whispers in the child's ear, "I want to talk with you. I will take my hand away when you are quiet and are holding still. Do you understand?" As the dentist makes eye contact and the child agrees to the dentist's request, the child is thanked for his or her cooperation. If the technique must be repeated, the child must not see anger

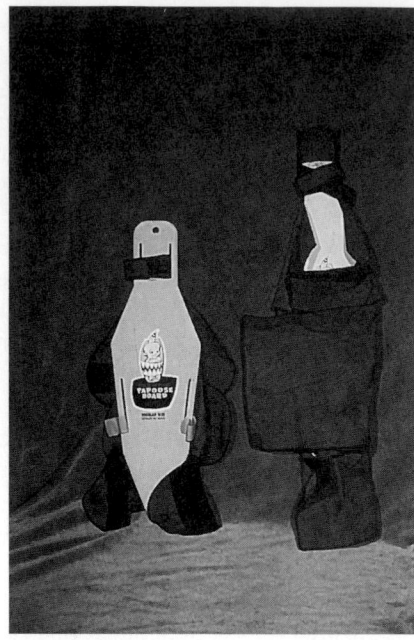

FIG. 36-1   Restraint of a child can be achieved through the use of a papoose board.

on the part of the dental team. This attempt by the child to avoid treatment will end once the child is able to deal with the fears and anxieties.

The HOM technique is not the choice of technique in all situations. The child may need only to be physically restrained with a **papoose board** to gain cooperation. The use of the least amount of restraint is preferred and ranges from holding a child's hands to completely immobilizing the child through the use of a body restraint or a papoose board (Fig. 36-1). As the child's resistance wanes, the restraints can be removed. In severe behavior problems, where the aforementioned behavior management techniques do not gain the child's cooperation, the use of pharmacologic substances may be necessary.

Medication

Certain patient situations warrant the use of medication before dental procedures are performed. Premedication is used for some patients to restrict anxiety and pain that is related to dental procedures. Various types and dosages of medication are given, and each is based on the weight and height of the child. Barbiturates and tranquilizers are two of the most common categories of medication to relieve anxiety. Each of these would be used in conjunction with local anesthesia, nitrous oxide, and general anesthesia. The use of medication is discussed in Chapter 34.

If the patient is under the age of 3 years, the ability to comprehend and deal with fear is seldom possible. Often the caregiver must accompany the child into the treatment room. If this is the case, ideally, the caregiver sits quietly within the child's view. If the child will not sit quietly in the dental chair, it may be necessary to have the caregiver and the dentist hold the child. The two face each other, touching knees, with the child's head in the dentist's lap. The caregiver gently restrains the arms and legs.

At times, the parent/caregiver being in the treatment room causes anxiety, and the child begins to cry. The dental team is not only providing treatment for the pediatric patient, but must also educate the parent before any treatment begins. It is helpful to provide the caregiver with information before treatment to forestall any problems. An anxious caregiver can create greater distress in the patient. The child is capable of reading facial expressions and recognizing changes in the tone of voice, which can increase fear and anxiety. The caregiver who has a complete and thorough understanding of the treatment and techniques to be used is an asset to the dental team in creating a positive dental experience for the child.

Information on office policy regarding the caregiver's presence in the treatment room and the recommended responses for the caregiver during treatment is helpful. An office policy may offer suggestions to the caregiver about not speaking to the child during treatment and not ridiculing or threatening the child with punishment to exact proper behavior. Communication is a common thread in creating a positive experience for treatment. Communication with caregivers and with the child reduces and may eliminate potential problems during dental treatment.

Common Treatment Procedures in Pediatric Dentistry

Several specific procedures are performed predominantly for the pediatric patient (Box 36-1).

Certain treatment is provided for children in different

BOX 36-1

COMMON PEDIATRIC PROCEDURES

Placement of stainless steel crowns
Placement of space maintainers
Treatment of fractured teeth
Pulp therapy
Manufacture of mouthguards

BOX 36-2

PREVENTIVE PEDIATRIC PROCEDURES

Oral examination
Prophylaxis
Pit and fissure sealants
Fluoride treatments
Restorative and surgical procedures as needed

---

age groups, including preventive oral hygiene procedures (Box 36-2).

Preventive Procedures

The preventive procedures performed on children are similar to those used for adults. It is vital to educate and encourage caregivers and children to adopt the concept of *keeping their teeth for a lifetime.* A caregiver who does not understand the need for a child to retain the primary teeth until the natural exfoliation develops sets a pattern and instills a lack of concern for oral hygiene habits in the child. The primary teeth aid in mastication, speaking, and appearance; affect the health and development of the permanent dentition; and act as a guide for the permanent dentition.

One of the first free dental clinics for schoolchildren, founded in the United States, emerged from the Rochester Dental Society and was founded in 1909 by George Eastman.

▶ Initial Visit

A child's initial visit to the dental office can set the tone for subsequent dental visits. A primary responsibility of the dental team is to create a sense of comfort and relaxation when a child is first exposed to the dental office; this can be accomplished by having the caregiver bring the child to the office for a nontreatment appointment.

This appointment may be a responsibility delegated to the dental assistant alone, or it may be handled with a team approach. Initially the child is greeted and called by name. A tour is provided of the dental office, with introductions to staff and explanations of each area, so that the child can begin to feel comfortable with the surroundings. In the treatment room the dental assistant describes the movement of the chair and helps the child into it. The chair is placed in a supine position, and the child is allowed to adjust to the change. Often, it is helpful to suggest that the chair is similar to a rocket ship or an airplane, so that the child can relate it to something of interest.

The assistant turns the treatment light on and explains that this helps the dentist to see the inside of the mouth more easily. The dentist shows the child the dental mirror and has the child look at himself or herself in the mirror to become familiar with the mirror before it is placed in the mouth. The dentist may even use the explorer to *feel* the teeth. After the child is released from the treatment chair and escorted to the reception area, a reward for good behavior, followed by praise, allows the child to leave the dental office with positive feelings.

If the child reacts negatively to any of these activities, additional explanation may be necessary to make the child more comfortable with the situation. If the child resists and shows signs of fear, it may be necessary to provide additional explanation. Foremost in this visit is to make the child feel important and comfortable with dental treatment and the office surroundings. To force the child excessively at this point may create a negative impression of dentistry, which makes future appointments less productive.

▶ Oral Diagnosis

As it does with treatment for an adult, oral diagnosis plays an important role in pediatric dentistry. As described in Chapter 24, the patient examination includes not only the examination of the oral cavity, but also considers the health of the whole person. The task of determining whether other physical factors are affecting the health of the patient is a major responsibility of the dentist during the dental examination.

▶ Medical/Dental History

A child's first treatment appointment can be extremely uncomfortable if one of the previously described behavior patterns has been established or if the child is in need of dental treatment as a result of trauma. Normal first appointments usually are similar to those for adult patients (Box 36-3).

A complete and comprehensive health history may require follow-up questions to obtain adequate information that is necessary for diagnosis. These questions may include more in-depth queries of the patient or the caregiver. For example: *"Has the child received fluoride treatments? If so, has the fluoride been provided through drinking water, fluoride tablets, or other supplements?"* If the caregiver indicates that the child is being given fluoride supplements through vitamins and has no knowledge of the amount of fluoride in the drinking water from a well, then some concern about the amount of fluoride the child is receiving may be realistic.

BOX 36-3
FIRST APPOINTMENTS
Complete and thorough medical and dental history is completed by the caregiver
Radiographs
Intraoral and extraoral examination
Study casts
Prophylaxis
Possibly fluoride treatment, and/or placement of pit and fissure sealants

---

This information forewarns the operator about the possibility of a problem from over- or underfluoridation. As described in Chapter 6, underfluoridation of the developing teeth may produce an oral cavity that is more susceptible to carious lesions. Overfluoridation causes enamel mottling. After the examination of the child and with the knowledge from the question, it can be determined whether the child is receiving enough fluoride. Obtaining a sample of the water and having it tested for fluoride can ensure the level of fluoride that is being received by the child. If the fluoride level is not adequate, the operator could prescribe additional fluoride through fluoride treatments, oral tablets, fluoride rinses, and toothpastes or by any combination of the fluoride forms.

Likewise, if evidence arises during the examination that indicates an excess of fluoride, the source of the fluoride and the amount must be determined. Recommendations can be made to reduce the amount of fluoride that the child is receiving. The reduction may preclude the use of the orally ingested fluoride or it may necessitate an analysis of the family water supply and subsequently the need to use water from an outside source if it is found to be beyond the recommended fluoride levels for human consumption. (The recommended fluoride levels are addressed in Chapter 26, *Preventive Dentistry.*)

Another question that is asked on the health questionnaire is: *"Does the child still receive a bottle; if so, what liquids does the child ingest? When does the child receive a bottle and does it include bedtime?"* When an infant or young child is fussy and uninterested in sleeping, a caregiver may respond by giving the child a baby bottle that contains milk or juice. The sugar contained in the liquids is allowed to bathe the child's teeth during sleep, since some liquid is usually left in the mouth after sucking. The sugar combines with the oral bacteria and plaque and develops into acid that attacks the structures of the teeth. Eventually the resistance of the enamel is depleted, allowing the decay to establish a foothold on the teeth. This condition is known as *nursing bottle syndrome.*

Parents may be completely unaware of the damage this activity causes. Once the damage has occurred, a caregiver may think the teeth need not remain in the mouth and request that the affected teeth be extracted. Premature removal of primary teeth results in the need to maintain the space that results from the extraction. If the space is not maintained through the use of an orthodontic appliance, such as a fixed or removable space maintainer, the teeth posterior to the space will drift mesial. The primary teeth are the guide for the succedaneous permanent teeth. Excess spacing may result in an arrangement of permanent teeth on the dental arches that requires orthodontic treatment. (The use and placement of space maintainers and other orthodontic appliances are discussed in detail in Chapter 35.)

The caregiver should be directed in techniques to avoid this syndrome. These techniques include the following:

Provide only water in the child's bottle

Wipe the alveolar ridge and erupted teeth with a small towel to remove debris

Do not allow the child to have a bottle

Finally, another health question is: *"Has the child ever been treated with or exposed to medication; when did this occur?"* This will indicate whether drugs have been ingested at an early age. Medication given to infants and young children and to expectant mothers may affect the development of the primary and permanent tooth buds before eruption. A complete medication history informs the dentist of the occurrence of a disease and the type of medication that was prescribed for the individual.

It may also be advantageous to determine any medication the child's mother took while pregnant, such as the antibiotic tetracycline. Tetracycline prescribed for a mother in the second trimester or to a child through the age of 8 may cause permanent staining of teeth (Fig. 36-2). The stain can be slight, appearing gray or yellow without banding over all teeth; moderate, as a darker discoloration and again without banding; or severe, with even darker discoloration of a gray and blue with possible banding at the cervical area of the teeth. Many individuals with this type of disfigurement of the dentition become extremely self-conscious about their appearance and seek cosmetic treatment. Advanced techniques in bonding and bleaching procedures or possibly cast prosthetic procedures as the child matures into adulthood may be needed to cover the staining, since these stains are intrinsic and cannot be removed by polishing.

Various oral conditions or abnormalities may be discovered during the initial visit of a pediatric patient. Some of these conditions, such as intruded or fractured teeth and pulp polyps, may warrant immediate treat-

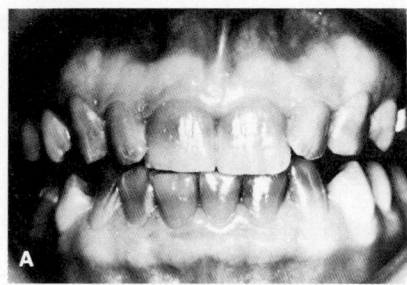

FIG. 36-2   Tetracycline stain in a pediatric patient.

(From Sturdevant CM et al: *The art and science of operative dentistry*, ed 3, St Louis, 1994, Mosby.)

ment. Other situations, such as the staining of teeth from a systemic agent, will likely become part of the treatment plan for the patient.

Oral Examination

The examination of the oral cavity that is performed for a child is no different from that for an adult. Similar conditions, such as gingivitis, abnormal growths, and carious activity, found in the oral cavity of an adult may be discovered in a child. What may be different are the approach the dentist takes and the clinical examination chart that is used. Examination charts that are commonly used in pediatric dental offices are designed to be able to chart primary and secondary dentition (Fig. 36-3). Any of the common tooth numbering systems discussed in the oral anatomy chapter are practiced in a pediatric examination.

Dental Radiographs

Dental radiography is an extremely important factor for diagnosis of dental health in any patient, including children. The use of dental radiographs enables the dentist to determine the position of the unerupted permanent teeth in relation to the primary teeth, discover any anomalies in the dental arches and surrounding structures, and assess the health of the existing teeth in the oral structures. The type of radiographic series for a child is determined by the age and the ability of the child to tolerate the experience. Commonly, panoramic radiographs are used as diagnostic tools, since they indicate information such as missing teeth and the position of teeth in the arch. Occlusal radiographs are used in pediatric dentistry for diagnosis and to provide information on tooth positioning and abnormal growth. (These radiographs and others are discussed at length in Chapter 9.)

The justification for dental radiographs may be questioned by the caregiver. The public is barraged with

PEDO EXAM RECORD

Last name	First name	Recommended by	Name of physician
Address		Address	Address or telephone
City	State Zip	Referred by Dr.	Date of examination Age

X-RAY EXAMINATION	ORAL EXAMINATION
Date	Date
Full mouth	Bite:
Bite wings	Occlusion
Anterior	Eruption
Periapical	Alignment
Remarks:	Serial extractions indicated: Yes No
	Remarks:
	Orthodontics required: Yes No Date
Birthdate	Discussed with parents: Yes No Date
School	Consultation with Dr. Date
Skeletal frame: Small Large Average	Remarks:
Under the care of physician now	
For what reason	
Any allergies	
Novocaine Penicillin	Study Model Yes No Date
Others	
Childhood diseases (list)	Fluoride in water supply: Yes No Tablets: Yes No
	Reaction to dentistry
	Attitude of parent
	Remarks:

Prophylaxis indicated: Yes   No

Inflammation present: Yes   No

Remarks:

Condition of saliva:

Habits—thumb or finger sucking

Item 92 © 1952, 1960, Rev. 6/89 • SYCOM® Madison, WI Printed in U.S.A.

various information regarding health issues through the media, but the whole story is not always explained to the extent that is appropriate. The caregiver may say "I don't want Tommy to have x-rays because I have read radiation will cause cancer." An educated response to the caregiver is necessary to provide the patient the most current and valid information regarding safety. The patient and caregiver need to understand that the dental professional cannot see everything about the child's development without the use of radiographs. Here is an opportunity to illustrate, with the use of radiographs and models, everything that can be seen with a radiograph. Dental radiographs do cause a risk, but the benefit of the diagnostic information received outweighs the possible harm from the radiation. The National Bureau of Standards, which provides standards for exposure limits, maintains that the dose to the body for 1 year should not exceed 5 rad of radiation. For a full series of radiographs the dose is approximately 0.0003 R. Areas of the body that are more sensitive to radiation, such as the thyroid and the reproductive organs, are protected from exposure with the use of a lead apron. Quality assurance techniques are used as well. Given an educated response to their concerns, most people will allow the procedure to continue for the benefit of the patient. Several informational pamphlets are available through the ADA to assist in this educational process.

RE-EXAM RECORD

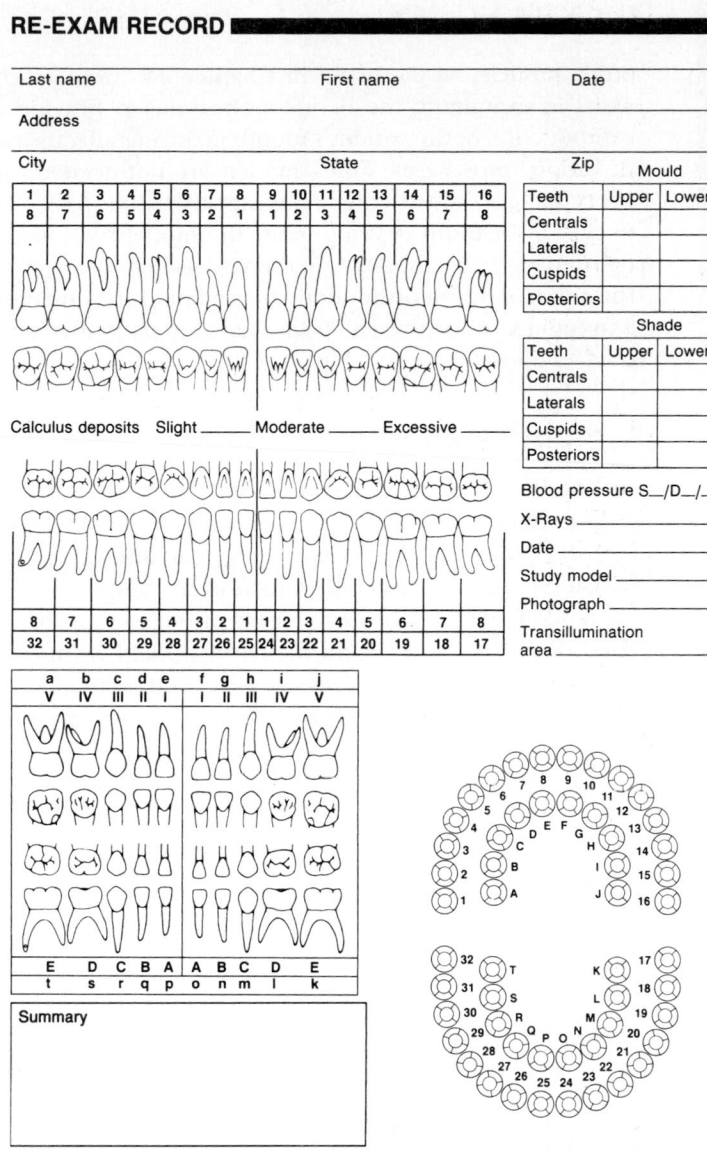

Last name

First name

Date

Address

City   State   Zip

Calculus deposits   Slight _____ Moderate _____ Excessive _____

Mould		
Teeth	Upper	Lower
Centrals		
Laterals		
Cuspids		
Posteriors		

Shade		
Teeth	Upper	Lower
Centrals		
Laterals		
Cuspids		
Posteriors		

Blood pressure S__/D__/__

X-Rays _____

Date _____

Study model _____

Photograph _____

Transillumination area _____

Summary

Item 4057 © 1960, 6/89 SYCOM® Madison, WI Printed in U.S.A.

FIG. 36-3   Pediatric clinical charts.

(Courtesy of Sycon Corporation.)

▶ Oral Hygiene Instructions

Children mimic caregivers' actions and habits. A positive role model, who encourages good oral hygiene habits, is desirable. Consequently, a caregiver who does not practice recommended oral hygiene procedures is not a good model for a child. To ask a child to perform a task that a caregiver does not perform may be unrealistic. If educating the caregiver is not successful, then educating the child is necessary.

Educating a child in correct oral hygiene techniques must be coordinated with the child's ability to comprehend and his or her physical capability to accomplish the task. Children up to 2 years are not able to comprehend or perform toothbrushing or flossing at an acceptable level. The caregiver should start this routine of brushing early, before the primary teeth have erupted, by placing a toothbrush in the child's mouth and gently moving it over the oral mucosa daily. Also, a finger wrapped with gauze or cloth is acceptable. This begins to set a pattern in the child's daily routine that becomes an accepted habit.

As the child reaches 2 to 5 years, he or she can accept the responsibility for brushing the teeth. The caregiver assumes the role of an observer and provides guidance as it is warranted.

When a child is given toothbrushing instructions, position the child in front of a mirror and hold the

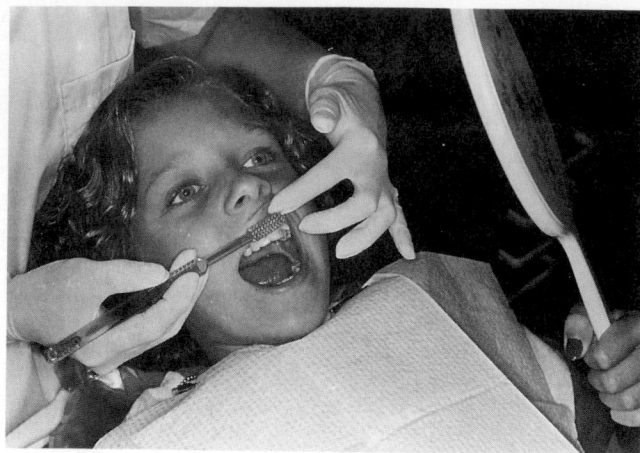

FIG. 36-4 Provide toothbrushing instruction to a child, and then ask the child to demonstrate the technique.

toothbrush to demonstrate the technique (Fig. 36-4). With the maxillary and mandibular arches closed, the brush is angled toward the facial surfaces of the posterior teeth. The brush is moved in a circular motion over the facial surface of the teeth, including two or three teeth in each placement. The brush is moved forward or, when toothbrushing is complete on one side, the brush is moved to the opposite side of the mouth, and the brushing is repeated. The child is then directed to open the mouth and is shown the circular brush motion on the lingual surfaces of the teeth. After the lingual surfaces are cleansed, the occlusal surfaces of the teeth are brushed in a back-and-forth action. A child should also be shown how to brush the tongue by placing the brush as far back on the tongue as is tolerated, and then the brush is pulled forward to the tip of the tongue. This action can be repeated 3 or 4 times to completely cleanse the tongue.

The toothbrushing may be done with a dry brush or with a brush that has a small amount of toothpaste applied. A small amount of toothpaste can be an incentive to some children, since the flavor may be desirable. Many toothpastes and brushes are designed specifically for children. Manufacturers have developed flavors of toothpaste that appeal to the young child, such as bubble gum and grape. Toothbrushes also are available with a picture of a currently favorite cartoon character or environmental concern, another motivational factor for brushing.

Flossing a child's teeth is a task that the caregiver must perform until the child has developed the manual dexterity to avoid any injury to the soft tissue. The child should watch the caregiver during flossing to understand the technique before being allowed to try it alone; then the child can demonstrate the flossing technique to the caregiver. Again, flavored floss is available to pique a child's interest to floss on a regular basis.

Study Models

Study models, as discussed in Chapter 24, are used to assist in examining the dental arches and to provide a reproduction of the patient's mouth in the manufacturing of various prostheses. Study models are not needed for every patient, but if concern exists about the patient's occlusion or tooth development, the models will likely be prepared. The models can then be used to determine the need for future orthodontic treatment or to construct a mouthguard for the child who actively participates in contact sports.

Mouthguards

As stated earlier, the concept of *keeping their teeth for a lifetime* becomes a critical issue with the child who is a sports enthusiast. As a child develops an interest in any contact sport, the idea of protection from injury must become integral to the mechanisms of the sport itself. A child does not go to bat on the baseball field without a protective helmet in place; likewise, a child participating in a contact sport should have protection for the mouth. The use of protective mouthguards for children is extremely important to avoid traumatic injury.

The dental professional who gathers as much information as possible about the patient, whether he or she plays sports or prefers to read books, is helping the child keep the teeth for a lifetime. Questioning the child about his or her activities can determined whether the child needs a mouthguard. The mouthguard can then be produced on the study models that have been created. (The fabrication of a mouthguard is discussed in Chapter 40.)

Urgent Care Needs

Beyond the normal realm of everyday dental care exists the potential dental emergency. These dental needs require immediate attention by the dental team to stabilize or provide treatment for the patient.

Trauma

Statistics support the fact that most trauma to the head and mouth occurs to children, with the possible exception of automobile injuries. The daily activity of a child usually involves situations that could lead to an accident, such as bicycling, baseball, football, and skating. So, it is not uncommon for children to be seen in the dental office with intruded, avulsed, or fractured teeth and lacerated lips, tongue, or mucosa.

Fractured Teeth

Tooth fracture usually results from a traumatic blow that often affects the crown of the tooth. The anterior segment of the oral cavity is usually affected in tooth fracture accidents. The vitality of an injured tooth must be determined to develop a course of treatment for each situation. Testing involves the sensitivity of the tooth to hot, cold, air, and pressure. (The devices used to determine vitality are discussed in Chapter 33.)

The fracture of the crown may occur in primary or permanent teeth. The Ellis classification system qualifies the extent of tooth structure lost in each situation. A Class I fracture involves the loss of enamel and can be treated by smoothing the fractured surfaces for the patient's comfort. A Class II fracture is more extensive in that the dentin is also involved in the traumatized area. This type of fracture is treated by placement of a bonding agent and a composite resin layer to restore the tooth to normal. Ellis Class III fractures include not only the enamel and dentin, but the fracture also encroaches on the pulpal tissues. The extent of the pulpal exposure may be minimal—a pinpoint exposure requiring a direct pulp cap—or extensive, necessitating a pulpotomy or pulpectomy. (Each of these procedures is discussed at length in Chapter 33.)

Partially Developed Teeth

Teeth may not be fully developed at the time they are traumatized, which can result in additional problems. Apexogenesis and apexification, discussed in Chapter 33, are two treatments that involve the status of the root development. When apexogenesis, the development of the root of the tooth as it narrows to the apex, has not been completed before the traumatic injury, further complications occur. If treatment of the vital pulp through direct pulp capping or pulpotomy is not provided, the root and apex will not form properly. Either of these treatments allows maintenance of pulp vitality in the root and the continued formation of the root and apex.

If the tooth is no longer vital and the root and apex are not completely developed, apexification is necessary to close the apex. This procedure involves the complete eradication of the pulp, similar to that of endodontic treatment but short of filling the canals with the appropriate material. Instead, calcium hydroxide is placed at the apex of the incompletely formed tooth and a sterile cotton pellet is placed between it and an interim restoration. The calcium hydroxide stimulates the cementum to close the apex, after which endodontic treatment continues and a final restoration is placed.

Pediatric Surgery

Trauma to the oral cavity may result in the need for pediatric oral surgery. An extensively fractured tooth, where only a minor portion of the root is left in the socket, requires removal through a surgical procedure.

(The steps involving root retrieval and other oral surgery procedures are discussed in Chapter 37.)

Luxation

Injuries to the oral cavity also involve teeth that are luxated. The tooth may be intruded (pushed into the socket or bone) or extruded, with a degree of movement out of the socket. The course of treatment for teeth that are luxated is determined by whether it is a primary or a permanent tooth. (An in-depth discussion of luxated teeth is found in Chapter 33.)

A primary tooth that is luxated is usually extracted to protect the developing permanent tooth. A radiograph may be taken to predict the eruption time of the permanent tooth that is still unerupted. If it is determined that eruption will not be soon, a space maintainer can be positioned in the space that is vacated by the lost primary tooth, thereby allowing the permanent tooth to erupt in the proper position. The caregiver may not realize the importance of the maintenance of this space and question the need for this treatment. It may be the responsibility of the dental assistant to instruct the caregiver on the importance of this appliance and on the necessity of maintaining the abutment teeth in their positions so that the permanent tooth can erupt correctly.

A repositioned primary tooth is susceptible to periodontal infection, which could damage a developing permanent tooth. A permanent tooth that is luxated is usually returned to the normal position in the arch and

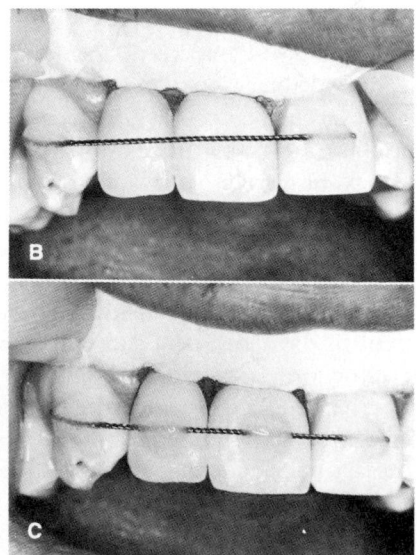

FIG. 36-5   Stabilization of traumatized teeth.

(From Sturdevant CM: *The art and science of operative dentistry*, ed 3, St Louis, 1994, Mosby.)

stabilized for approximately 7 to 10 days. The stabilization may be done with the use of orthodontic wire that is bonded in place on the facial surfaces of the luxated tooth and the surrounding teeth, which act as the anchor for the injured tooth (Fig. 36-5, *A* and *B*). A more extensive technique may be required through the use of a temporary splint to maintain the position of the tooth in the dental arch. (The fabrication of a splint is discussed in more detail in Chapter 37.)

▶ Avulsed Tooth

A tooth that is avulsed has been completely removed from the mouth as a result of a traumatic injury. An avulsed primary tooth normally is not replaced within the alveolus because of the possibility of periodontal infection. A permanent tooth that is avulsed must be replanted immediately, followed by stabilization until the tooth is secure in approximately 7 to 10 days.

Educating a patient and the caregiver to the potential problems involving avulsed teeth has resulted in the successful replantation of teeth. The factor that is of most importance in replantation is time. A tooth that is outside of the socket for an excess of 30 minutes is less likely to survive this procedure. The avulsed tooth should be immediately rinsed off with water and replaced in the socket if possible. If the tooth cannot be replanted, it should be kept in oral fluids inside the cheek, only if the patient is conscious and aware of this action. If the patient is not conscious or willing to have the tooth immediately replanted, it should be stored in milk or cold water until the dental visit. Successful reimplantation may require subsequent dental care: endodontic treatment to maintain the tooth in the mouth or splinting. (A detailed description of endodontic treatment procedures is discussed in Chapter 33.)

Urgent care may also come in the form of a child who has a loosened primary tooth. Caregivers may find themselves in circumstances where the child has a loosened primary tooth that needs to be removed. The child may not want to remove it alone or will not allow the caregiver to remove the tooth. This may necessitate a trip to the dental office. Primary teeth with resorbed roots may be attached only through soft tissue. The tissue attachments can be extremely sensitive and painful, and any movement of the tooth may cause discomfort.

Another factor to be considered is that the child may not have experienced dental pain in the past and may be frightened with the impending treatment. It will probably be necessary to comfort the child and to explain the procedure to reduce fear and anxiety. The dental assistant must explain that this is a common procedure and that sometimes the primary teeth need additional assistance in exfoliation.

Child Abuse

The previously described categories each represent the traditional types of preventive treatment in a dental office. Child abuse, however, is a less traditional but a serious problem that all health professionals confront each day, since abuse continues to increase at a rapid pace. The National Commission for the Prevention of Child Abuse in 1991 reported 1033 deaths caused annually as a result of abuse. Each year, more than 2.7 million children are abused or neglected. These statistics reflect only reported incidences, and a much larger number of actual cases might occur. Statistics indicate alarming increases in suspected and reported cases of child abuse. A dental visit provides an opportunity to observe conditions that might be indicators of child abuse. It is the dental assistant's responsibility with other team members to be aware of techniques to recognize abuse and to know the protocol for reporting suspected abuse to the appropriate authorities. Unfortunately, no two cases of child abuse are the same, and thus it is often difficult to recognize. Several types of child abuse can be evident, including shaking, slapping, choking, and squeezing, lacerations, genital trauma, bone fractures, burns and scalds, as well as life-threatening injuries to the intraabdominal area, eyes, and cranium.

▶ Bite Marks

Bruising in various stages of healing caused by the dentition is a form of child abuse that is being studied with greater depth by forensic odontologists. Bite marks provide specific evidence that all health professionals should be aware of and be able to identify when faced with a possible child abuse situation. Although bite marks go undetected as common bruises, each is a replica of the tooth that made the bite mark.

Usually bite marks are oval or elliptical imprints of the maxillary and mandibular arches as seen in Chapter 38. The bruise that results from a bite varies, depending on the level of force that is applied during the bite. Discoloration of the surrounding tissue may be apparent, but usually the skin is left intact from the trauma. The greater the force that is applied during the bite, the more the damage to the area and to the deeper layers of the muscle tissue.

Proof of child abuse may be evident or not. If a child arrives for dental appointments with bruises and cuts in various places the dentist may question the child as to the origin of the injuries. The child may be reluctant, afraid, or unable to answer the questions or may provide excuses for the injuries, such as falling down the stairs. If the child is unwilling to answer the question or if the answer is suspicious, the same question can be asked of the caregiver to see if the answers support each other.

Further questioning may be necessary to provide enough information to determine whether abuse may have occurred.

Typically, when a child falls, he or she falls face forward. If a child falls off a swing, trampoline, or other recreational device, the knees, elbow, face, and frontal surfaces are scratched, bruised, or skinned. If, however, the injuries are in locations such as the shoulders or the back, it may be an indication of abuse. Another clue is the child who wears long sleeves and pants all year long to disguise evidence of bruises or cuts.

If suspicion of child abuse exists, it is more than the health care professional's *responsibility* to notify the appropriate authorities—it is a *legal mandate*. Responsible agencies, such as social service departments, child care institutions, and law enforcement agencies in every state are able to respond to suspected incidences of abuse or neglect. For efficient management of such cases the dental assistant must have readily available the telephone number of the appropriate agency to contact if child abuse is encountered. Some states also have provided *good faith* protection clauses to conceal the identity and protect the individual who has submitted the abuse case to the authorities. Once the case is submitted, the social service department notifies law enforcement agencies. (Further information regarding the liability of health care professionals aware of child abuse situations is discussed in Chapter 38, *Forensic Dentistry.*)

Restorative Procedures for Children

Restorative procedures for children are similar to those performed on adult patients. Variations in the procedures usually involve the size of the instruments and the approach that is taken. Examples of these instrument variations are the dental handpiece and burs, matrices, and rubber dam clamps.

The use of rubber dam isolation is common in pediatric dentistry. Preparation and placement of the rubber dam are similar to the procedure discussed in Chapter 22, *Isolation.* Variations in the size of rubber dam clamps, rubber dam material, and the number of teeth that are isolated may vary, but the technique is the same. Remember to explain the procedure and the materials that are to be used to the pediatric patient.

Rubber dam clamps are designed to fit certain teeth. Clamps are available that approximate the contour of primary teeth, allowing for greater stability of the rubber dam assembly. Clamps that are too large may cause damage to the gingival tissues, as well as provide a less-than-desirable isolated area.

Pediatric dental handpieces have a more compact head to allow greater access into the oral cavity of a child. To assist in gaining access, a pediatric bur (Fig. 36-6) that has

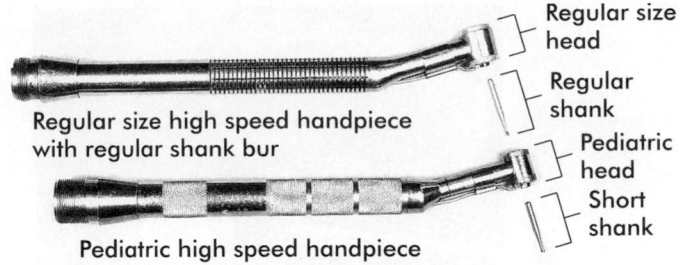

FIG. 36-6 Pediatric handpiece that has a smaller head and a short shank bur.

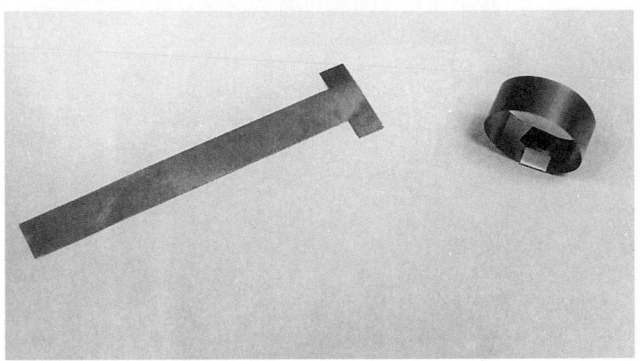

FIG. 36-7 T-band style matrix that is used in pediatric preparations involving proximal surfaces.

a shorter shank is also available. When these two instruments are used together, they provide the operator with greater access in a much smaller mouth.

Dental matrices vary tremendously to meet the needs that are created by the size and shape of the teeth and by the dimensions of the cavity preparation. The assembly and use of the Tofflemire matrix band and retainer are discussed in Chapter 27. In pediatric treatment it is not uncommon to create customized matrices for each situation. One such matrix is the T-band (Fig. 36-7), which is used predominantly in pediatric dentistry on primary teeth. The loop of the band is shaped to approximate the circumference of the tooth, and the T ends are folded around the circle with the free end of the excess of the band through the T. The band is placed into the interproximal spaces gingivally to cover the extent of the preparation, with the free end on the buccal surface of the tooth. As the band is positioned, the free end is pulled to tighten the fit of the band around the cervical portion of the tooth. The end of the band is bent back toward the T or the distal surface of the tooth to allow the band to be secured. Excess band material is removed with scissors. The band is wedged and burnished as it is with the Tofflemire band.

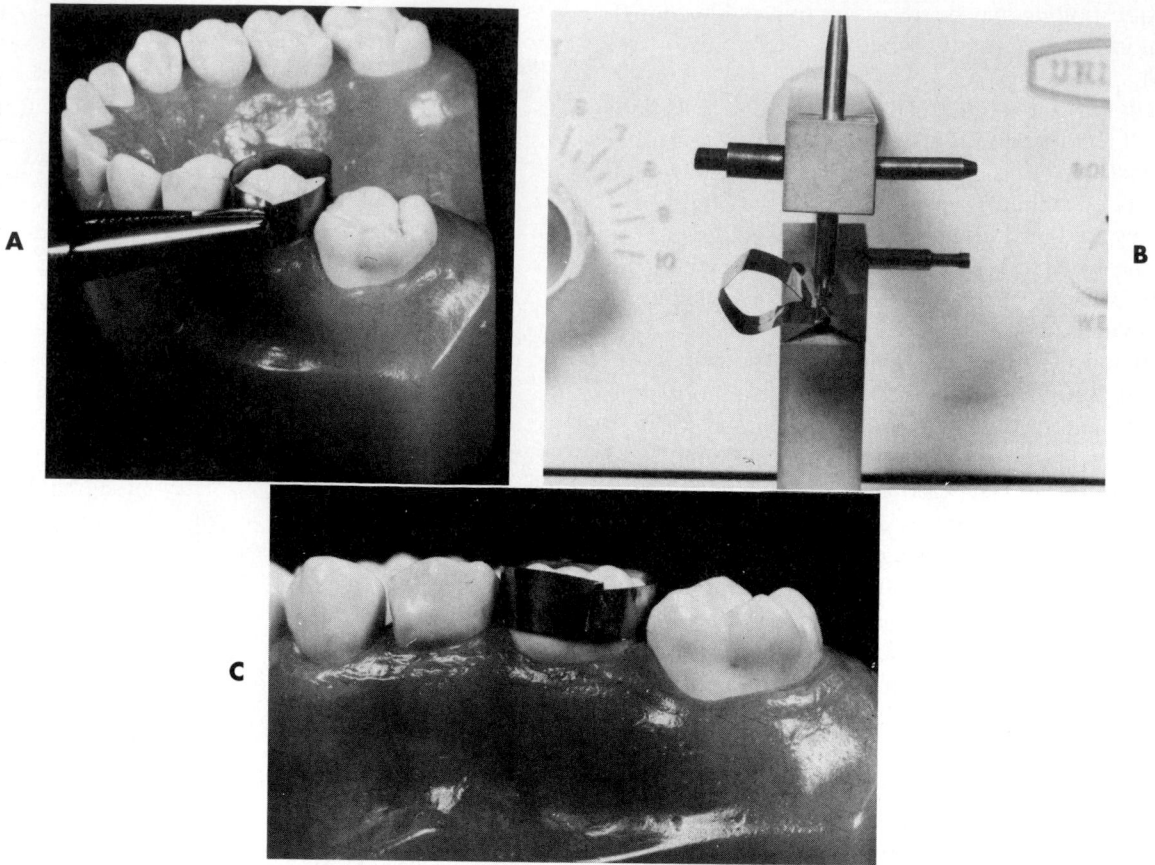

FIG. 36-8   Fabrication of spot-welded matrix band. *A,* Pinching band with hemostat. *B,* Welding band. *C,* Finished band in place.

(From Chasteen JE: *Essentials of clinical dental assisting,* ed 4, St Louis, 1989, Mosby.)

Another form of customized matrix band is the spot-welded matrix for primary teeth. The matrix material is fabricated in rolls of ¼- to ³⁄₁₆-inch width and 0.002-inch thickness and can be cut to the approximate length that is needed to fit an individual tooth. The matrix is placed through the interproximal space, and the free ends are brought to the buccal surface to lap over. An explorer is used to mark the overlap area, and the band is removed. An electric welding unit (Fig. 36-8) is used to fuse the metal ends together at the cervical and the occlusal areas of the band. The excess band is trimmed from the spot-welded matrix band, and the band is repositioned on the tooth and secured in place.

Amalgam and composite resin restorations are placed on primary and permanent teeth; the procedures are the same as in adult dentistry. An exception is the placement of permanent cast restorations on primary teeth and partially erupted permanent teeth. Sometimes a permanent tooth that is completely erupted may not be prepared for a permanent cast restoration until the child reaches a stage when all permanent or adjacent permanent teeth have fully developed and erupted.

Stainless steel crowns are usually selected for placement on posterior teeth. As a result of trauma or decay, coverage might be necessary to protect a tooth from sensitivity or further damage. This type of protection can be gained through the use of temporary crowns.

Temporary Crowns

The need for temporary crowns in pediatric dentistry is an interim measure to retain primary teeth before the natural exfoliation process: until the permanent teeth erupt. Temporary crowns are placed on a pediatric patient for various reasons (Box 36-4).

The type of temporary crown is determined by the location of the tooth in the oral cavity. A custom composite resin crown or polycarbonate crown is placed in areas visible under normal circumstances, and a stainless steel or aluminum crown is selected for the posterior areas of the mouth. (The fabrication of temporary crowns, with the exception of the stainless steel crown, is discussed in Chapter 32.) The physical characteristics of stainless steel crowns make them the crown of choice in pediatric treatment. Stainless steel crowns are capable of enduring the forces of mastication in the oral cavity for a greater period of time than is an aluminum shell crown, making the use of a stainless steel crown more common when a primary tooth that is decayed or fractured needs protection. This crown may need to remain in place for several years, until the permanent tooth erupts, or the crown may be placed on a permanent tooth until a permanent cast restoration is planned. The fabrication of a stainless steel crown is similar to the fabrication of an aluminum shell crown. A recap of the criteria of the step-by-step procedure is found in Box 36-5.

KEY POINTS

▶ Pediatric dentistry, one of eight areas of specialty in dentistry, involves the provisions of dental care to children.

▶ The knowledge of the physical, emotional, and intellectual level at which a child is expected to be functioning will assist in managing situations and in providing dental treatment.

▶ Behavior patterns seen in the pediatric patient can be categorized as cooperative, lacking cooperative ability because of the inability to comprehend, and potentially uncooperative because of past negative situations.

▶ To effectively manage the behavior of a child, the dental team must be able to communicate with the patient and to provide an atmosphere that is comfortable.

▶ Techniques that are employed in management of pediatric patients include validation, voice control, modeling, show-and-tell, flooding, and medication.

▶ Dental procedures completed on pediatric patients may be different from those for adult patients.

▶ The signs and symptoms of child abuse must be known and used by the dental team to assist any possible abuse victim.

BIBLIOGRAPHY

Rock WP, Grundy MC, Shaw L: *Diagnostic picture tests in paediatric dentistry,* Ipswich, England, 1988, Wolfe Medical Publications.

Goran K: *Pedodontics: a clinical approach,* ed 2, St Louis, 1992, Mosby.

Wright GZ: *Behavior management in dentistry for children,* Philadelphia, 1975, WB Saunders.

Shaw L: *Self-assessment picture tests in dentistry: pedodontics,* St Louis, 1993, Mosby.

Wolff JM: Bite marks: recognizing child abuse and identifying abusers, *Fam Soc J Contemp Human Serv,* October 1990.

American Humane Association: *Highlights of official child neglect and abuse reporting, 1986,* Denver, 1988, The Association.

37 Periodontics

LEARNING OBJECTIVES

You will have mastered the material in this chapter when you can:

▶ Define the key terms

▶ Describe the role of the dental assistant in periodontics

▶ Describe types and signs of periodontal disease

▶ Record periodontal conditions, and state why each is important

▶ Identify and describe instruments and procedures used in periodontics

▶ Explain human relations practices that contribute to the success of periodontal treatment

KEY TERMS

Attachment width (AW)
Bone swaging
Coronaplasty
Crevicular fluid
Curettage
Debridement
Digitized radiography
Donor tissue
Excise
False pocket
Festoon
Flap surgery
Furcation involvement
Gingivectomy
Gingivectomy knife
Gingivoplasty
Graft
Granulation tissue
Incise
Index
Infrabony pocket

Irrigation
Keyes technique
Mucogingival surgery
Mucoperiosteal flap
Mucosal flap
Occlusal equilibration
Osseous surgery
Oxygenating agent
Periodontal dressing
Periodontal surgery
Physiologic contour
Recession
Recipient tissue
Reflect
Resection
Root planing
Splint
Sulcular fluid
Sulcus temperature gauge
Suprabony pocket

This chapter examines periodontal disease: what it is and how it is described and treated. Additionally, it concerns the role and responsibilities of the dental assistant in periodontics and describes periodontal examinations, instruments, and procedures. It concludes with specific directions for the technical procedures that dental assistants commonly perform. Demographics indicate that in the coming decades there will be an increased need for periodontal care and a corresponding need for qualified dental assistants.

Periodontal Disease

Periodontics refers to procedures for prevention and treatment of periodontal disease. Periodontal disease is an episodic, site-specific infection of the dental supporting tissues. The American Academy of Periodontology estimates that 3 out of every 4 adults will acquire some form of this disease during their lifetime; adults are also more likely to lose teeth as a result of periodontal disease rather than as a result of caries. Children do not develop periodontal disease at the same rate as adults, but they do contract it, and some juvenile forms are severe and progress rapidly.

Gingivitis and periodontitis are two basic types of periodontal disease. Gingivitis is confined to the gingiva; periodontitis extends into the periodontal ligament, cementum, and/or alveolar bone. A variety of forms of the two types appear, and disease in a specific patient is described on the basis of extent, severity, resistance to treatment, age of onset, duration, speed of progression, and etiologic agent, if known. Table 37-1 lists the forms of periodontal disease and the terms (and their meanings) most commonly used to characterize each form. Only the characteristics important to the disease in a specific patient are described and recorded, such as chronic generalized mild periodontitis or gingivitis associated with diabetes.

Infected periodontal tissues can mar the patient's appearance, bleed, swell, produce an odor and exudate, taste bad, loosen teeth, make chewing difficult, and export pathogenic microorganisms to other parts of the body. When disease is far advanced, otherwise healthy teeth can be lost for lack of support. A healthy periodontium looks, feels, smells, and tastes fine. It contributes greatly to the patient's sense of attractiveness, comfort, and social acceptance. The periodontics assistant works as part of a team to help patients achieve and maintain comfortable, healthy tooth support structures as an important ingredient in physical and mental well-being.

 Investigation of the ancient Lebanese city of Sidon has produced evidence of a mandible showing periodontal disease, with recession of the gingiva and the bone. Treatment involved the use of gold wire to splint the incisors together.

The Periodontics Team

The periodontics team consists of the patient and selected dentists, dental assistants and dental hygienists, who work as a group to help the patient achieve periodontal health. Each member has a specific role and responsibilities that contribute to treatment success.

▶ Importance of Human Relations

Good human relations are vital to the success of periodontal therapy. The patient generally sees at least two dentists, the primary care dentist and a periodontist, as well as the various assistants and hygienists in each of these offices. In a given treatment facility each of these people must in turn relate to the patient and to each other. The duties performed by the various team members may overlap. The dentists and their staff members must coordinate the therapy between the two practices to provide comprehensive care to the patient. Periodontal treatment may extend over several months, and the goal of therapy must be maintained indefinitely. The responsibility of each dental professional must be clearly defined. To avoid error and misunderstanding, everyone must maintain the three *C*s: consultation, communication, and coordination.

▶ The Patient

The patient is the most important member of the treatment team. The patient must realize the importance of his or her role before any treatment is rendered. The patient's appearance, comfort, and senses of smell and taste are of major concern. The patient provides consent for treatments that are provided, pays the bills for treatment received, and is responsible for maintaining

TABLE 37-1   FORMS OF PERIODONTAL DISEASE

Characteristic	Forms described	Meaning
Extent	Localized	In small area
	Generalized	Over large area
Severity	Mild	Gingivitis
	Moderate	Progressing to periodontitis
	Severe	Significant tissue loss
Resistance to treatment	Refractory	Resistant
Age of onset	Prepubertal	Preteen years
	Juvenile	Childhood
	Adult	After teenage years
Duration	Acute	Short, rapid
	Chronic	Long, slow
Speed of progression	Rapid	Swiftly moves to periodontitis
	Slow	Varying progression
Etiologic agent	Infection	Microorganisms; often complicated by poor tissue contour, functional trauma, improper diet, systemic disorder, or genetics

tissue health once it is achieved. Patient attitudes about periodontal care and a willingness and ability to perform oral hygiene procedures are major factors in the success or failure of therapy. Consequently, as with all dental care, the patient continues to be the primary concern for every member of the team.

▶ Dentists

At least two dentists are on the periodontal team: the patient's general dentist and the periodontist. Periodontal patients may, however, have many types of problems that affect their periodontal health. Conditions such as caries, malocclusion, missing or nonvital teeth, infection, and improper contour of bone or soft tissue may prevent periodontal disease control. Appropriate restorative, endodontic, orthodontic, surgical, and prosthodontic care must then be coordinated with periodontic care to create total oral health. Accordingly, comprehensive periodontal treatment is considered to have four phases: initial, surgical, reconstructive, and continuing. The patient undergoes only those phases that are required.

Team leadership shifts from one dentist to the other as the patient progresses through the phases of treatment. Periodontists direct the initial phase, provide periodontal surgical care, and coordinate any associated specialty care. General dentists provide restorative care and may direct the reconstructive phase. Specialists direct their particular portion of surgical or reconstructive care. Either the periodontist or general dentist may supervise continuing care; often the responsibility is shared.

▶ Dental Assistants

Assistants in a periodontic office begin by performing all of the duties common to any assisting position in their state. In addition, they serve as surgical assistants to the dentist, periodontic educators, operators in technical periodontic procedures, and assistants to dental hygienists. During periodontal surgery the assistant may prepare patients, treatment rooms, anesthetics, instruments and materials for surgery, assist with surgical procedures, supervise patient recovery, provide postoperative instructions, apply and remove periodontal dressings, remove sutures, and dispose of surgical wastes in accordance with local, state, and federal regulations. As educators, assistants provide information about office policies and procedures, surgery, oral hygiene, and the nature and control of periodontal disease. As operators, assistants take impressions, prepare models, apply fluorides and sealants, polish teeth, expose intraoral radiographs and photographs, run videocameras, and operate computerized

systems for radiography, tissue visualization, and data recording. The assistant is also responsible for helping the dental hygienist during treatment, performing the traditional business office and laboratory procedures, and maintaining infection control.

▶ Dental Hygienists

Usually two hygienists are on the team, one each from the general and periodontics practices. Hygienists provide initial and continuing care, with duties that include screening examinations, exposure of radiographs, preparation of models, performance of diagnostic tests, scaling, root planing, polishing, fluoride treatments, placement of sealants, and application of medications to relieve root sensitivity or alter the microbial flora.

The Periodontal Therapy Process

Periodontal therapy has the following six basic steps:
1. Development of rapport
2. History and examination
3. Evaluation
4. Case presentation
5. Treatment
6. Continuing care

Coordination of periodontal care with restorative, surgical and reconstructive care occurs at the treatment stage.

▶ Developing Rapport

Psychologically, patients and dental personnel are in two different worlds. Dental professionals talk about health, but patients are concerned with comfort, an attractive smile, odor-free breath, and affordability. Patients understand that health is a basic goal, but for most, healthy tissues just do not have the same emotional impact as attractiveness or social acceptability.

Each patient has a self-image. Part of the image is a set of expectations for how the mouth should look, feel, and taste, and feelings about how much value the patient places in the dental care in terms of time, effort, money, inconvenience, and pain. These feelings and expectations are not always readily apparent, but they have much to do with whether the patient develops enough trust and confidence in the periodontic team to become an enthusiastic member.

Trust and confidence develop over time. The first seed is planted with rapport, a feeling that the patient and team members understand and can talk to each other. The assistant in a periodontic office responds not only to what the patient is doing and saying but also to the deeper level of what it means to open the door to rapport.

Caring attitudes, professionalism, efficient methods, taking time to explain with a friendly smile or touch, all speed the treatment process. The periodontic team really must sell itself, its concepts, and its services. When the patient decides to become part of the team, acceptance of its values results. Values motivate learning and behavior change. Over time, achieving and maintaining periodontal health require both.

Periodontal Examination

An examination of existing conditions is made to collect information on which diagnosis and treatment decisions are based. As treatment proceeds, subsequent data are collected and compared to evaluate progress.

Periodontists provide complete examinations for their patients just as any other dentist would. The process begins with a thorough history, then moves to clinical examination of the head and neck, temporomandibular joint, lips, oral mucosa, gingiva, teeth, and occlusion. Radiographs, photographs, impressions for study models, diagnostic tests, and diet counseling are included as indicated to meet the needs of specific patients. Emphasis is placed on observation and recording of periodontal conditions. Either the dentist or hygienist may perform the examination. Dental assistants perform parts of the examination—which parts depend on the dental practice act of the state in which you are employed.

SEQUENCE

Similar to the procedure described in Chapter 24, periodontal clinicians follow a standard routine to ensure that all aspects of the examination are completed. The sequence of the routine varies with the operator's preference. Most operators begin with the extraoral area, then move into the oral cavity to complete the procedure. General aspects of the head and neck—the eyes, ears, skin, and hair—are observed first. Next the action of the temporomandibular joint is assessed, and the masseter muscle, accessible salivary glands, and lymph nodes surrounding the ear and extending along the side of the neck are palpated. The operator then completes the external portion of the examination by palpating the lips and perioral area.

The internal portion of the examination begins with an assessment of the status of the vestibule, buccal mucosa, and central and lateral frena. The palatal and pharyngeal mucosa is then observed, followed by all surfaces of the tongue, the lingual frenum, and the floor of the mouth.

Next the teeth are examined. Missing teeth, caries, restorations, malpositions, occlusion, and jaw relationships are noted.

The dental supporting structures are examined last. The gingiva is observed for its height, color, contour, consistency and texture. Periodontal probing is done to measure the depth of the sulcus and check for the presence of bleeding. The width of the attached gingiva is measured. Each tooth is moved in its socket to determine whether it is excessively mobile. The presence of debris, plaque, and calculus is noted. Finally, radiographs are taken to observe the condition of the bone, and impressions are made for study models.

Nimazi females, members of an indigenous forest tribe, continue an ancient tradition of purposely developing periodontal inflammation as part of their initiation into a special society of women.

INDICATIONS OF PERIODONTAL DISEASE

The clinician is looking for evidence, or signs, of past or current periodontal disease, as well as existing factors that contribute to periodontal disease development. Table 37-2 lists periodontal disease signs and what they mean; Table 37-3 lists the major contributing factors and how they assist disease development. Signs and contributing factors considered together give the clinician a picture of the disease process in a given patient. Treatment is then planned to eliminate or control present disease and contributing factors.

PROCEDURE

The operator observes, measures, evaluates, and announces the conditions present. The dental assistant transfers or operates the instrumentation, maintains excellent visibility of and access to the examination site, accurately records the conditions observed, monitors the patient's reactions, and assists the patient with physical needs or psychologic comfort as indicated. As always, accuracy in recording is essential. If you do not hear or understand the conditions that are dictated, ask for clarification. Treatment will be based on what you record.

EXAMINATION INSTRUMENTATION

Manual examination instruments include a mirror, an explorer, a periodontal probe, an air syringe, and dental floss. Many of these instruments have previously been

TABLE 37-2   SIGNS OF PERIODONTAL DISEASE

Sign	Appearance	Significance
Inflammation	Red, swollen	Indicates current infection
Bleeding on probing	Blood present	Early sign of inflammation
Changes in gingiva		
Color	Red	Inflammation is acute
	Purple	Circulation is stagnant
	White	Tissue is fibrotic
Contour	Swollen	Edema is present
	Papillae rounded, flattened, or rolled	Impairs self-cleaning
	Cleft	Traps food, debris, microorganisms
Consistency	Soft	Extra fluid present (blood, tissue fluid and/or pus)
	Hard	Infection is chronic
		Reparative fibers have grown into connective tissue
Texture	Smooth surface	Fibers are losing their elasticity
	Shiny surface	Epithelium is thin
Pocketing	Gingival	Sulcus enlarged
		Traps plaque, debris, toxins
	Suprabony	Loss of attachment
	Infrabony	Difficult to debride
Decrease in attachment width	May appear normal	Loss of fiber attachment
	Root may be exposed	
Bone loss	Ragged or cupped alveolar crest	Beginning of bone loss
	Localized	Loss of tooth support
	Generalized	
Mobility	Tooth moves too much	Anchoring ligament fibers weakened
		Inadequate bone support remaining
		May be infection at root end

TABLE 37-3   FACTORS CONTRIBUTING TO PERIODONTAL DISEASE

Contributing factor	Mechanism of action	Result
Plaque	Harbors microorganisms	Produces toxins, enzymes
Calculus	Surface rough, irregular	Harbors debris, toxins
	Hard composition	Cannot be removed by brushing
	Securely attached	Difficult to debride
	Forms along tooth roots, furcations	Interferes with oral hygiene procedures
Malocclusion	Poor distribution of occlusal forces	Bone may resorb
		Mobility may develop
Missing teeth	Ligament fibers not present to exercise tendon on bone	Bone loss, hypereruption; adjacent tooth drifting
Frenum pull	Tension on soft tissue	Gingival recession
Improper diet		
Too soft	Food sticks between and around teeth	Gingival irritation
Too hard	Gingival trauma	Laceration
Deficient in essential nutrients	Unknown	Tissue integrity impaired
Systemic disease		
Diabetes	Impaired immune response	Poor healing
AIDS	Unknown	Severe, rapidly progressing periodontal disease
Heredity		
Poor host response	Unknown	Difficulty in controlling periodontal disease
Gene structure	Unknown	Development of juvenile forms

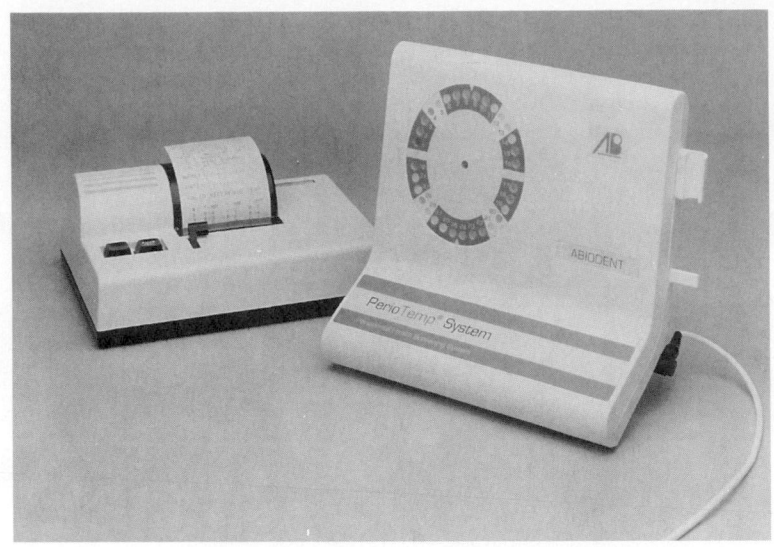

FIG. 37-I   Automated sulcus temperature gauge. Machine with data printout.

introduced but may have functions that are specific to periodontics.

AUTOMATED INSTRUMENTS

Automated instruments that were described in Chapter 24, such as the Perioprobe and the dental imager, have particular application in this specialty. The operator may use automated instruments to collect, record, and analyze examination data. Such machines save time, increase accuracy, and standardize results. For periodontal patients, the use of automated instrumentation can serve as a motivation tool.

SULCUS TEMPERATURE GAUGE

A Perio-Temp is a gingival **sulcus temperature gauge** and recorder (Fig. 37-1). Sulcus temperature is of interest because the inflammatory process creates heat. Inflammation occurs, and the temperature of the sulcus fluid rises when periodontal disease is present. To measure the temperature of **crevicular fluid**, an altered serum fluid in the sulcus, a handpiece sensor tip is first placed under the tongue to obtain a baseline oral temperature for the patient. Each sulcus is then probed, by positioning the sensor in the sulcus and activating a foot switch. The machine records a temperature for the sulcus and compares it to the established baseline. Temperatures exceeding upper limits of a range around the baseline activate a red light, indicating inflammatory *hot spots.* Those within normal limits activate a cool green light, and those nearing an upper limit activate a cautionary yellow. A hard copy printout of temperatures is made as probing proceeds.

AUTOMATED BITE RECORDER

Bite force can be measured by computer. The operator keyboards the patient's name and other identifying data into the machine, inserts a preformed bite sheet with disposable cover into the patient's mouth, and asks the patient to bite slowly but firmly and carefully, then hold this position for a short time. Sensors relay occlusal loads of the various teeth to the computer, which creates a three-dimensional image of bite forces throughout the dentition. This graphic is relayed to a monitor and may be printed as well.

PERI-OPTIK PROBE

A Peri-Optik probe (Fig. 37-2) may be used to improve field visualization at the examination site. This instru-

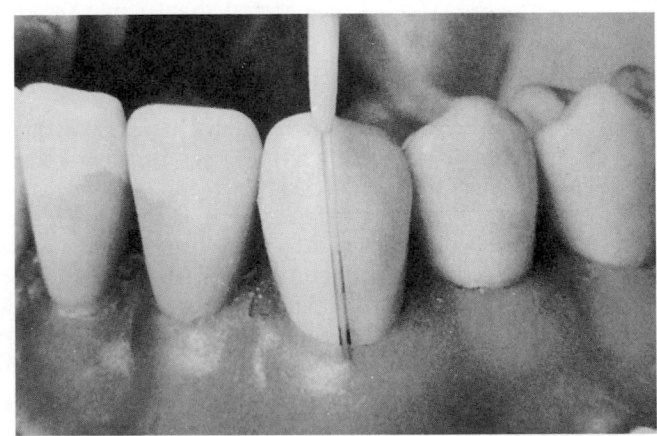

FIG. 37-2   Peri-Optik probe and close-up of wand with controla showing.

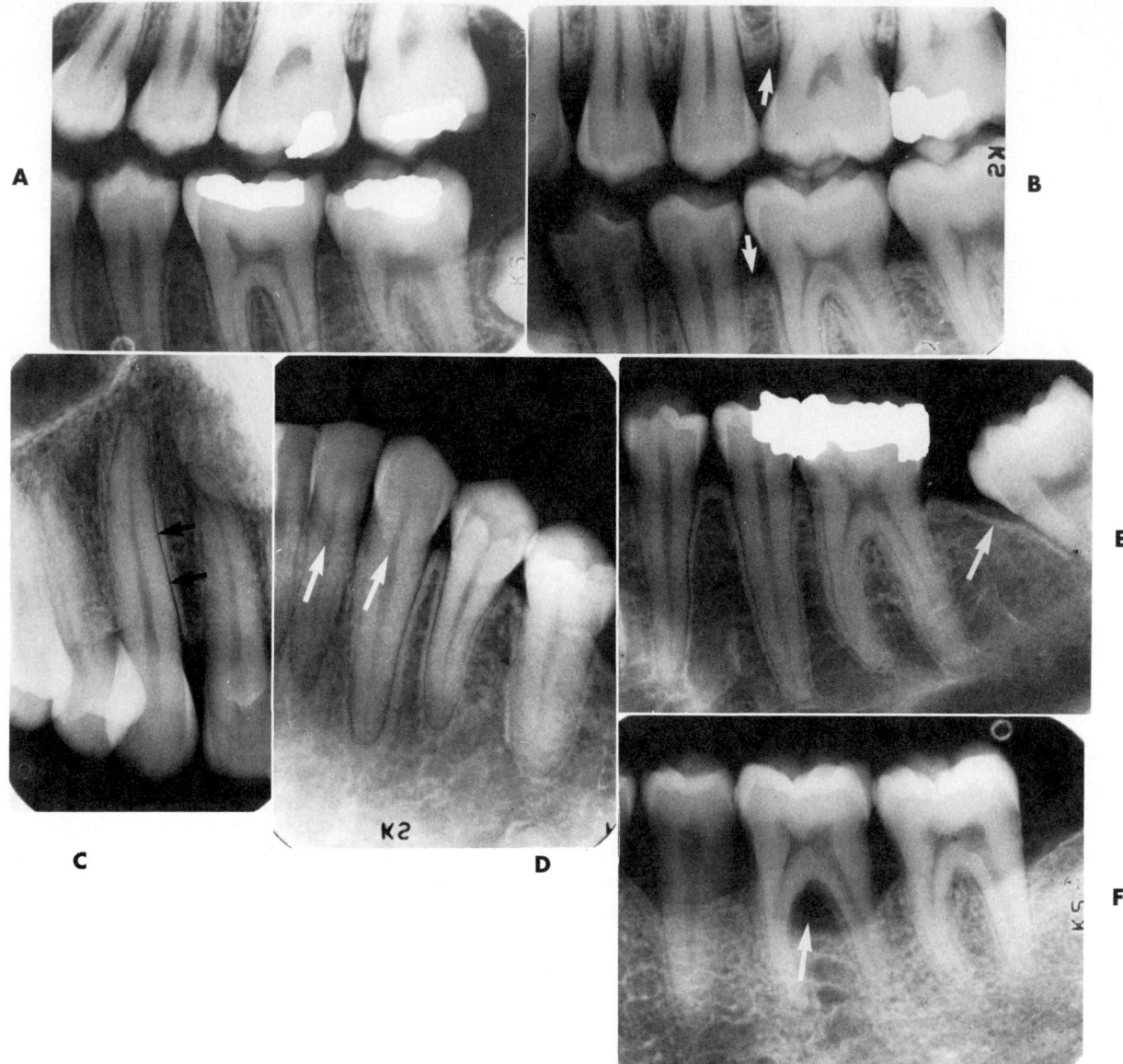

FIG. 37-3   A, The normal alveolar crest lies 1 to 1.5 mm below the adjacent cementoenamel junctions and forms a sharp angle with the lamina dura of the adjacent tooth. B, Initial periodontal disease is seen as a loss of cortical density (*arrows*) and a rounding of the junction between the alveolar crest and lamina dura. C, The periodontal ligament space appears wide on the mesial surface of this canine (*arrows*) and thin on the distal surface. D, Inconsistent bony margins are seen as irregular coronal edges of the buccal or lingual cortical plates superimposed over an image of the tooth roots (*arrows*). E, An intrabony defect demonstrates vertical loss of interdental bone adjacent to the tooth surface (*arrow*), with preservation of the buccal and lingual cortical plates. F, Advanced destruction of the periodontal bone has led to destruction of both cortical plates and interradicular bone in the furcation region of the first molar (*arrow*). G, Periodontal cyst between mandibular premolars. Radiograph shows a well-defined oval lesion subcrestally. Sulcus did not communicate with osseous defect. Diagnosis was confirmed following a periosteal flap and biopsy.

(*A through F from Goaz PW, White SC: Oral Radiology, ed 2, St Louis, 1987, Mosby; G, from Genco RJ, Goldman HM, Cohen DW: Contemporary periodontics, St Louis, 1990, Mosby and courtesy of Wilford Hall, USAF Medical Center.*)

ment consists of a fiberoptic wand of sufficient size to use as a tissue retractor. Light shines out the ends of the fibers, and air and water sprays can be activated. Enhanced vision, retraction, flushing, and drying of an area can thus be accomplished as needed, using only one hand.

VOICE-ACTIVATED DATA RECORDING SYSTEM

A device is available to record electronically any data observed on examination. Before using it on a patient, the operator records a series of words that will be used to describe conditions seen. For example, the operator might say normal, the numbers from 1 to 32, millimeters, and red. During the examination the operator wears a headset and speaks into its microphone. The examination is completed in a standard order. As the operator speaks, the machine recognizes the words that were recorded earlier and converts them to data records. For example, saying "Number 1; 3, 4, 4" would indicate pocket depths of 3, 4, and 4 mm for the distobuccal, buccal, and mesiobuccal surfaces of tooth no. 1. Data are stored electronically and may also be printed in chart form. Operator, assistant, and patient are able to see at a glance the pictorial record of all conditions and to compare the printed charts to see changes over time.

RADIOGRAPHY

Paralleled bite-wings and periapicals are the radiographs of choice for routine applications in periodontics. (Chapter 9 discusses these radiographic techniques.) The periodontist is looking primarily at the condition of the alveolar bone and the width and shape of the periodontal ligament space but also notes factors contributing to periodontal disease, such as restoration contours, overhangs, calculus, and caries. Parallel vertical bite-wings and periapicals provide the most accurate and complete view of the ligament space and interdental bone.

CRITERIA FOR RADIOGRAPH ASSESSMENT

Alveolar bone should follow the contour of the cementoenamel junction and be slightly apical to it; the alveolar crest and lamina dura should be clearly defined lines. A widened periodontal ligament space indicates inflammation has extended into bone. An indistinct lamina dura or a ragged or cupped out alveolar crest indicates early bone loss. Apically angled bone adjacent to the tooth indicates bone resorption in a particular area; it is often associated with tooth malposition and resulting traumatic occlusion. Decrease in the height of bone around several teeth or an entire arch indicates a more generalized loss and is likely to be associated with generalized inflammation. **Furcation involvement**, which concerns the area where the root divides, indicates advanced disease. A radiolucent area next to the tooth may indicate a periodontal abscess or cyst. Fig. 37-3, *A* through *G,* illustrates these radiographic conditions.

The periodontist will diagnose radiographic conditions, but you should understand their significance and recognize them on radiographs once the periodontist has made decisions. This will enable you to use radiographs as an aid to patient education.

RADIOGRAPHY TECHNIQUES

Periodontists may use conventional, digitized, or subtraction radiography. (Conventional technique is discussed in Chapter 9.)

DIGITIZED RADIOGRAPHY

Digitized radiography is similar to conventional radiography except no film is used and the image may be manipulated to suit operator preferences before it is finalized (Fig. 37-4). A small camera is covered with a disposable plastic sheath and placed lingual to the teeth of interest just as a film would be. A lead apron is not

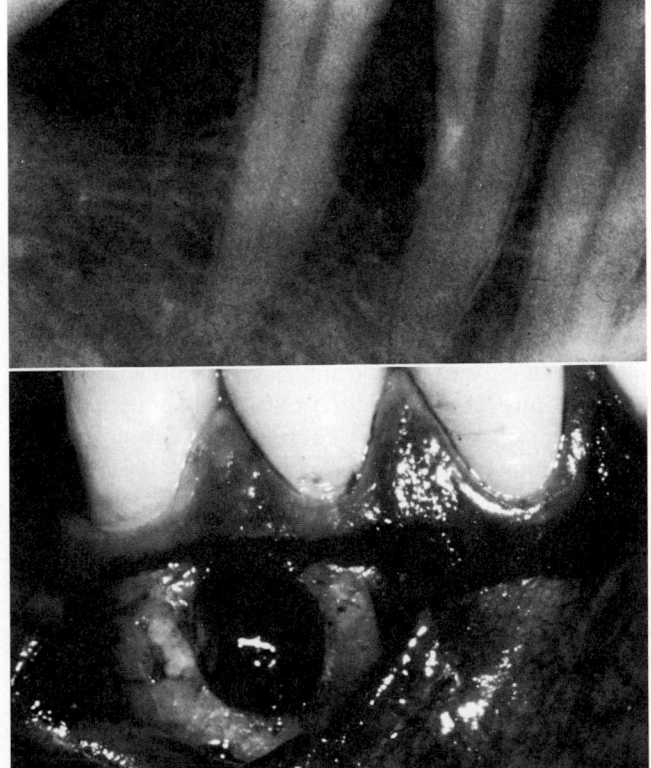

G

FIG. 37-3, cont'd.   For legend see opposite page.

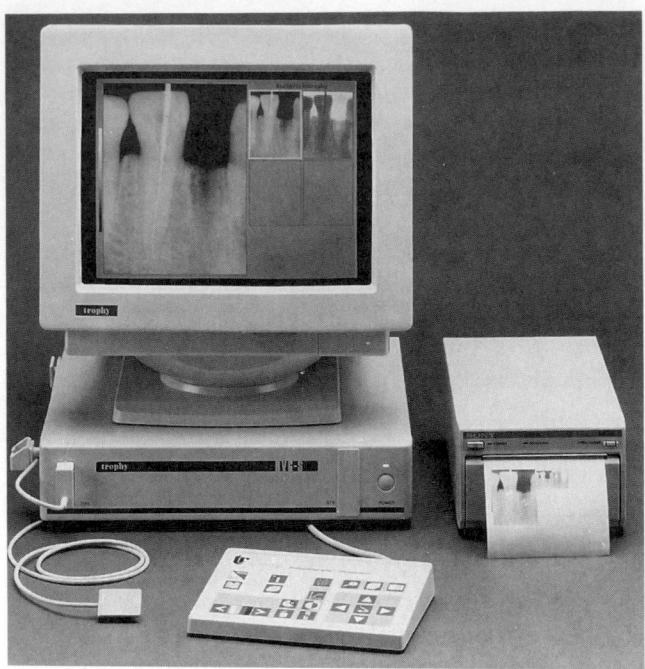

FIG. 37-4   Digital radiography technique. Machine showing a close-up of control console and digitized image of apical area of tooth in socket.

used. The image is recorded electronically and projected on a small screen at the control console. The operator can then alter the density or contrast or zoom in on a close-up view of a specific area of interest, if desired. When an optimal image is achieved, a button is pressed to obtain a hard paper copy. Only the image on the viewscreen can be printed; once printed, an image is not retained in digital form.

SUBTRACTION RADIOGRAPHY

Subtraction radiography uses a series of radiographs taken over time to visualize areas of bone loss. Either a conventional or digitized system may be used. Exposure technique must be parallel because consistent film or camera placement is necessary. The finished films or paper prints are placed in an image digitizer and compared electronically. Unchanged areas are subtracted from the image, so that only the changed areas remain. The final view, composed only of areas of loss, is then printed as a positive image. Conventional radiographs are negative images in which light gray areas indicating bone, and clear areas where bone should be indicate loss. Subtraction radiograph images are just the opposite: dark areas indicate loss and clear areas indicate bone.

Charting

Most periodontists use charting forms that differ slightly from those used by general dentists. There are many variations of periodontal charts, but most include lines across and small boxes above and below the tooth roots. The lines are used as guides for drawing in the height of the gingival margin and the alveolar bone. The boxes are used to record measurements made of the sulcus depth and width of attached gingiva. Additionally, many periodontal forms have an area where oral hygiene conditions are recorded. Refer to Figs. 14-11 and 14-16 for illustration of periodontal chart and informed consent to periodontal surgery. A detailed explanation of the abbreviations such as PD, AW, M, and OH is found in Box 37-1. These abbreviations refer to pocket depth, attachment width, mobility, and oral hygiene. Since these are important terms in periodontics, the assistant should know their meanings. You may want to refer to other symbols and abbreviations from Chapter 24. Individual periodontic office use of symbols can vary according to geographic area. Some may opt to use symbols, and other offices may use color coding to differentiate various conditions.

Evaluation

When all the examination data have been collected, the dentist must analyze and evaluate them to arrive at a diagnosis and treatment plan. The periodontist considers the oral presentation conditions, any medical factors of importance, and various alternative diagnoses that might appropriately describe the disease before making a diagnosis. The prognosis for the diagnosed condition, the patient's medical factors, available treatments, and the dentist's personal beliefs about the efficacy of each are then factored into a decision regarding a treatment plan.

The treatment plan should include a definite sequence in which the treatment tasks are to be performed, the time allocated for each task, interim appointment times, and procedure fees. The dental assistant assumes responsibility for scheduling and coordinating appointments and arranging payment plans.

Case Presentation

The case presentation follows the guidelines that are described in Chapter 24. Full information regarding examination findings, diagnosis, goals of treatment, recommended treatment procedures, available alternatives, the time and discomfort involved, fees, insurance coverage, and available payment options is provided to the patient. Discussion should be clear, specific, and succinct. Open communication allows the patient to

COMMON PERIODONTAL SYMBOLS

PD = POCKET DEPTH: DISTANCE IN MILLIMETERS FROM GINGIVAL MARGIN TO BASE OF POCKET

Important facts about pocket depth
  Normal sulcus depth is 0.5 to 3 mm
  Epithelial attachment migrates apically in periodontal disease
  Resulting deepened sulcus is termed a pocket
  Pockets may be false, suprabony, or infrabony
    False pocket is gingival swelling without apical migration of attachment
    Suprabony pocket has apical migration of attachment and base above the alveolar crest
    Infrabony pocket has apical migration of attachment and base below the alveolar crest
  PD measurement indicates how deep the pocket has become
  Six measurements are taken: mesiofacial, facial, distofacial; mesiolingual, lingual, and distolingual
  Measurements are entered in order in boxes above facial and below lingual of each maxillary tooth; below facial and above lingual of each mandibular tooth

AW = ATTACHMENT WIDTH: DISTANCE IN MILLIMETERS FROM THE BASE OF THE POCKET TO THE MUCOGINGIVAL LINE

Important facts about attachment width
  Indicates the amount of attached gingiva remaining
  AW measurement = total gingiva minus pocket depth
  Measurements made at same points and placed in boxes in same manner as pocket depth

M = MOBILITY: HOW FAR BEYOND NORMAL THE TOOTH MOVES IN ITS SOCKET

Important facts about mobility
  Tooth is rocked between clinician's index fingers or one finger and instrument handle
  Resulting motion is assigned a class
    N = Normal
    Class 1 = <1 mm
    Class 2 = 1 to 2 mm
    Class 3 = >2 mm
  If class is normal, mobility is **not** considered to be present

OH = ORAL HYGIENE: NUMBER DESCRIBING THE ORAL HYGIENE CONDITION OF A SINGLE TOOTH OR ALL TEETH IN THE MOUTH

Important facts about an oral hygiene score
  Indicates the average amount of debris on a tooth
  Each tooth assigned a single score;
    the larger the score, the more debris
  Scoring system is termed an **index**
  Many scoring systems and **indices** are available;
    assistant should learn index preferred in periodontics practice in which employed

---

speak freely, ask any questions, and voice any concerns. Some practices use automated equipment to enhance their presentations. The two types commonly used are an intraoral video camera and an esthetic imager (discussed in Chapter 24).

▶ Decision

Ideally, a decision to accept the treatment plan should be made at the end of the presentation. During the case presentation it is desirable for the patient to bring a friend or family member along for consultation or support in decision making. However, if this is not possible and the patient needs to consider the case presentation for a short period, a staff member should follow up the consultation with a phone call within 1 or 2 days. Many patients want to think about what they have heard before they make a final decision. Some patients also may think of questions that were not addressed during consultation. Therefore, the follow-up call can often clarify any uncertainties.

Whenever the decision is made to proceed with treatment, a series of appointments can be made to ensure the necessary time is available in the practice and is convenient for the patient.

Treatment

Periodontal therapy is individualized to meet the patient's needs; generally, it follows a predictable pattern. Initial **debridement**, the removal of plaque and calculus, is done first to eliminate periodontal infection and to promote formation of healthy tissue. Dental infections are then eliminated with endodontic therapy. Oral and maxillofacial surgery follows to eliminate bone and soft tissue infection and to prepare for implants. Carious teeth are then restored. Next, orthodontic treatment is provided to establish physiologic jaw and tooth alignment and the major outlines of bone and soft tissue. Periodontal surgery follows to complete calculus debridement, as well as to establish fine bone and soft tissue contour. Prosthetic procedures are completed last to ensure that crowns, bridges, implants, and removable appliances are precisely fitted to the newly established fine tissue contours and to promote ease of oral cleaning. At this point treatment is essentially complete, but in periodontics the patient is never *done*. Continuing care is always provided to help maintain the gains achieved. A review of these phases is shown in Box 37-2.

▶ Initial Periodontal Treatment

The initial periodontal treatment extends over a series of appointments and cannot be accomplished at one sitting. Initial treatment is conservative and nonsurgical. The

A TYPICAL SEQUENCE OF PERIODONTAL THERAPY

Initial debridement of plaque and calculus, to eliminate periodontal infection and promote healthy tissue

Endodontic treatment, to eliminate dental infection

Oral and maxillofacial surgery, to eliminate hard and soft tissue infection and to prepare for implants if necessary

Restoration of carious teeth, to eliminate dental infection

Orthodontic treatment, to establish physiologic jaw and tooth alignment and establish major outline of bone and soft tissue

Periodontal surgery, to complete calculus debridement and establish fine bone and soft tissue contour

Prosthetic procedures completed to newly established tissue contours, to promote ease of oral hygiene

least intrusive procedure that can accomplish the desired result is selected. Procedures that are used include scaling, root planing, irrigation, Keyes technique, splinting, occlusal equilibration, and patient education and home care.

Periodontal treatment has been performed for thousands of years. Albucasis, the great physician of ancient Persia, cradled his patients' heads in his lap when scaling their teeth.

▶ Scaling

The scaling procedure done in this phase of periodontal treatment is similar to the procedure that is described under routine prophylaxis in Chapter 26.

Scaling involves debridement of plaque and calculus deposits from tooth surfaces. Calculus is hardened plaque. Brushing and flossing will not remove it. Its surface is rough and pitted, like a cement sidewalk. This roughness collects debris, more plaque, and microorganisms. A layer of plaque is always present on the calculus surface. Microorganisms in the plaque release tissue toxins into the sulcus and sometimes enter and infect the tissue itself. Additionally, calculus interferes with oral hygiene procedures; it is simply in the way. Removal of calculus on root surfaces is essential to disease control. It helps to shrink pockets, permit thorough oral hygiene procedures, and smooth the root surface for attachment of soft tissue fibers.

Scalers are the instruments that are used to remove plaque and calculus. These instruments are described in detail in Chapter 26. As in a prophylaxis and during hand scaling the assistant uses the standard or surgical HVE tip placed adjacent to the area where the operator is working

to control bleeding and to remove pieces of calculus that have been dislodged. Periodically, of course, the HVE is placed in the posterior pillar area to evacuate saliva. Tissues obstructing the operator's view are retracted, and a 2×2 gauze square is available to wipe clean any instrument ends that become clogged with blood, tissue, or bits of calculus. With a skilled chairside assistant the instrument can be carefully cleaned to provide an instrument free from debris.

ROOT PLANING

Root planing is removal of rough and diseased cementum and smoothing of the root surface until it feels as smooth as glass. Studies have shown that sulcus epithelium will reattach easier to a smooth, disease-free surface. Curets are used for root planing. Repeated small scaling strokes are made in several directions on the root surface. This removes small bits of calculus, embedded or calcified periodontal ligament fiber ends, and a thin layer of the cementum itself to expose healthy cementum and to produce the desired smoothness. As one area is finished, another is completed, until all rough areas and diseased cementum have been removed and the underlying healthy tissue is completely smooth. Root planing takes a considerable amount of time and can be painful; local anesthesia is typically used (Fig. 37-5, *A* through *E*).

Table 37-4 is an overview of instruments and devices commonly used during periodontal therapy. These devices may be used for surgery, smoothing and polishing tooth surfaces, and aiding in contouring rough surfaces.

IRRIGATION

Irrigation is the use of a syringe or nozzle to flush a pocket clean of debris or place medication within it. **Sulcular fluid** is fluid that has flowed from the sulcula epithelium; its precise mechanism of formation is not completely known, but the selective barrier concept is believed to apply. This means that some components of the tissue fluid enter the crevice and some enter at a higher-than-expected rate. Accordingly, it often works better to place the medication directly into the sulcus to ensure that it actually reaches the pathogenic microorganisms that live there. Various medications are used, depending on the specific needs of the patient. The sulcular fluid is cultured to see what types of microorganisms are infecting the area. An antibiotic, an **oxygenating agent** (a chemical containing oxygen), or another drug can then be prescribed to target those organisms.

Both manual and automated irrigating devices are available. Manual syringes include a root canal irrigating syringe, with the tip removed; a surgical irrigating syringe; and a bulb irrigator. Automated systems include a small electric system with a single fluid reservoir, a delivery

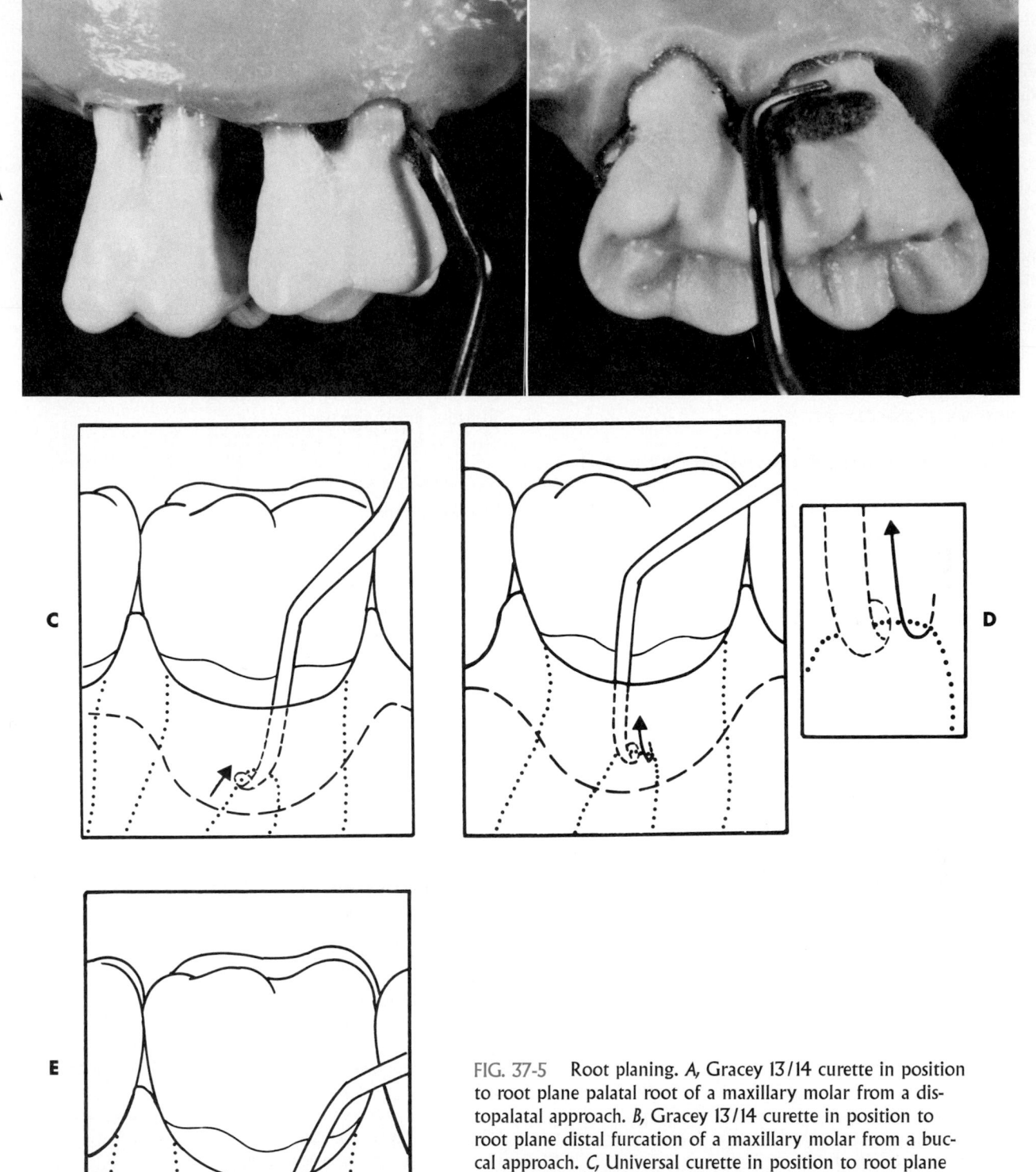

FIG. 37-5 Root planing. *A,* Gracey 13/14 curette in position to root plane palatal root of a maxillary molar from a distopalatal approach. *B,* Gracey 13/14 curette in position to root plane distal furcation of a maxillary molar from a buccal approach. *C,* Universal curette in position to root plane mesial aspect of distal root. *D,* Curette in position to root plane trunk of furcation. *E,* Curette in position to root plane distal aspect of mesial root.

(From Genco RJ, Goldman HM, Cohen DW: *Contemporary periodontics,* St Louis, 1990, Mosby.)

TABLE 37-4   PERIODONTAL INSTRUMENTATION

Instrument/use	Design characteristics
HAND EXAMINATION INSTRUMENTS	

Mirror
  Vision
  Retraction
	Reflecting surface

Explorer Detect hard deposits, caries, roughness	Small, thin, flexible tip

Periodontal probe
  Locate pockets
  Measure pocket depth, attachment width, size of lesions
	Thin, may be round or flat, tip blunt, often tapered, usually marked in millimeters

Air/water syringe Increase visibility	3-way: air, water, spray

Dental floss
  Detect overhangs, tight contacts
  Remove debris
	Operator's preference for waxed or unwaxed, floss or tape

SCALERS	

Sickle
  Remove supragingival deposits
  3 types:
    Curved (universal); straight (for anterior surfaces); modified (for posterior proximals)
	2 cutting edges converge to pointed tip
	Triangular in cross section

Curet
  Remove subgingival deposits
  2 types:
    Universal (all surfaces)
    Area-specific (specified surfaces)
	Spoon-shaped blade with rounded tip
	
	2 cutting edges of same length; both edges used
	2 cutting edges, 1 longer; only longer edge used

Hoe Remove heavy supragingival deposits	Similar to small garden hoe Blade may be straight or curved
Chisel Remove deposits from exposed proximal surfaces of anteriors	Blade flat, beveled at 45-degree angle with shank Cutting edge slightly curved

File
  Crush calculus deposits
  Smooth restoration margins
	Multiple cutting edges
	Blades appear as series of small cutting edges on oval or round base

Sonic scaler Remove stain, hard deposits and restoration overhangs	Air-powered Rapid tip oscillation Several interchangeable tips

Ultrasonic scaler
  Remove stain, hard deposits and restoration overhangs
  Flush sulcus
	Electric powered
	Uses water spray
	Very rapid tip oscillation
	Several interchangeable tips

Diamond file	Wedge-shaped rotary instrument Gingival side smooth Working side diamond or aluminum dust
POLISHING/SMOOTHING	

Prophylaxis angle
  Remove stain
  Polish surfaces
	Small, right/contra-angle, slow speed; sterilizable or disposable

Porte polisher
  Remove stain
  Polish surfaces
  Massage gingiva
  Apply medication
	Manual instrument handle
	Uses disposable orangewood points

Air polisher Remove heavy stain	Air powered Spurts water/sodium bicarbonate slurry through nozzle

TABLE 37-4   PERIODONTAL INSTRUMENTATION—cont'd.

Instrument/use	Design characteristics
Polishing cup	Rubber rotary instrument round with flexible edges
Remove light stain	
Polish surfaces	
Cleaning brushes	Rotary instrument
Remove moderate stain	Hard black or soft white bristles
Amalgam knife	Straight sickle-shaped blade
Contour amalgam restorations	
Enamel file	Coarse, medium or fine file on straight or oval base
Smooth enamel/restoration margins	Rounded end

HAND SURGICAL INSTRUMENTS

Pocket marker	Similar to cotton pliers except has sharp triangular projection on
Mark level of pocket base	one arm
Scalpel	Single, sharp, beveled edge
Incise soft tissue	Several blade shapes
Periodontal knife	Kidney-shaped blade
Incise gingiva	
Interdental knife	Triangular with 2 beveled blades
Incise interdental gingiva	
Electrosurgery	Powered by high-frequency current
Cut soft tissue and seal circulatory vessels	Wand with interchangeable tips
Soft-tissue scissors	Pointed ends, curved blades
Cut and contour soft tissue	
Nippers	Small spring-loaded clippers
Clip tissue tags	
Remove bone spicules	
Surgical scalers and curets	Similar to regular scalers except larger and with longer shanks
Remove hard deposits	
Burs	Many shapes
Cut, contour, and smooth bone	Often large and low speed
Surgical chisel	Similar to chisel scaler
Remove exostoses	May have slightly curved blade
Surgical curet	Similar to curet scaler but larger
Remove necrotic bone	
File	Round or oval base with multiple blades
Contour and smooth bone	
Periosteal elevator	Paddle or claw ends
Reflect incised soft tissue	
Suture needle/thread	Small, curved, usually prethreaded, disposable
Sew wound edges in position	
Needle holder	Similar to scissors except has blunt nose, ratchet handle
Position needle for use	
Suture scissors	Blunt nose
Cut suture thread	One arm has half-moon cut-out

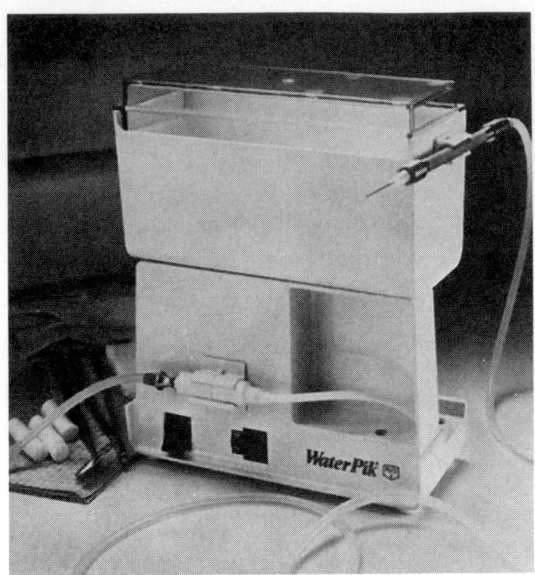

FIG. 37-6   Professional irrigating machine. (From Woodall IR: *Comprehensive dental hygiene care*, ed 4, St Louis, 1993, Mosby.)

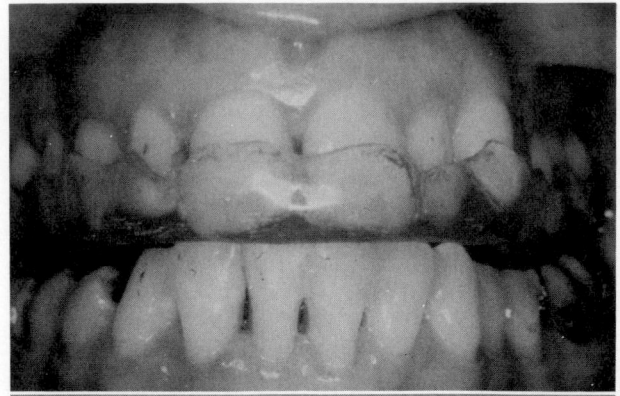

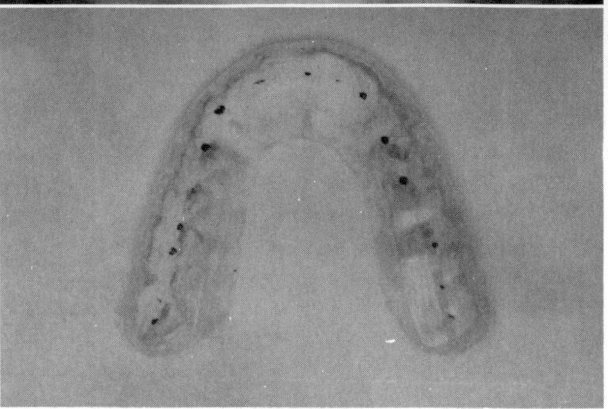

FIG. 37-7   *A,* Maxillary full occlusal splint. Occluding surface is flat, with as little guidance as can be tolerated. *B,* Each opposing tooth touches occluding surface of night guard with at least one contacting point.

(From Genco RJ, Goldman HM, Cohen DW: *Contemporary periodontics,* St Louis, 1990, Mosby.)

tube and several interchangeable nozzles; and a larger system that permits tube and nozzle delivery of a choice of several premixed solutions by activating a footswitch (Fig. 37-6).

KEYES TECHNIQUE

Patients using the **Keyes technique** clean their teeth with sulcus brushing and a paste of baking soda, salt, and hydrogen peroxide. Chemically speaking, baking soda is a very basic substance, salt is hypertonic, and hydrogen peroxide liberates oxygen. The chemical ingredients of the paste are thus antimicrobial, and some studies have found using it regularly significantly reduces the bacterial population of the sulcus. Patients often find the taste of the paste objectionable and may not use it regularly. Adding a drop or two of peppermint or wintergreen oil will improve the flavor greatly and increase most patients' willingness to adhere to the regimen.

SPLINTING

A **splint** is a device that fits over or is bonded to teeth to broaden the area over which biting forces are distributed. They may cover the occlusal or incisal surfaces of a few teeth or a whole arch or connect adjacent portions of lingual tooth surfaces of single teeth (Fig. 37-7, *A* and *B*). Full-arch splints are made of acrylic and are used to relieve the pain and mobility associated with temporomandibular joint dysfunction. Small-area splints are used to control mobility from trauma or periodontal disease long enough to permit strong fiber reattachment in the

area. They are made by etching the lingual surfaces of the recipient teeth and bonding plastic material to them. There are two basic methods by which a splint can be fabricated—full-arch acrylic (processed extraorally) or a small-area composite splint (processed intraorally). The extraoral full-arch splint is removable; the intraoral small-area composite splint is retained in the mouth.

PREPARATION OF SPLINTS

Full arch, acrylic type (extraoral):

Armamentarium

Alginate impression tray, impression material and powder measure
Rubber bowl and alginate spatula
Water and alginate water measure

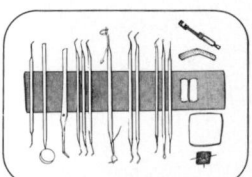

PROCEDURE FOR FABRICATION OF EXTRAORAL SPLINT*

1. Obtain and disinfect alginate impression
2. Pour impression in class II stone, and allow to harden
3. Trim excess stone from model to gain access to the anatomy
4. Block out undercuts on model with wax, and coat with a thin layer of petroleum jelly
5. Bend and cut wire to fit lingual curve of arch
6. Mix acrylic powder and liquid according to manufacturer's directions
7. Adapt thin layer of soft acrylic to model, and place wire cervical to occlusal surface on lingual portion of acrylic layer
8. Adapt second layer of acrylic over wire, blend with first layer and allow to set
9. Remove splint from model; trim rough edges with quartz wheel
10. Smooth splint with rag wheel and polishing compound; buff splint with chamois wheel

*Follow OSHA guidelines as they apply.

PROCEDURE FOR FABRICATION OF SMALL-AREA COMPOSITE SPLINT

1. Cut short piece of wire to act as ligature
2. Isolate teeth, and paint with acid etch according to manufacturer's directions
3. Flush, dry, and check for chalky appearance
4. Reisolate tooth, and dry thoroughly
5. Paint with bonding agent, and cure
6. Place composite to form small bridge between adjacent tooth surfaces, and embed ends of wire in uncured composite
7. Smooth composite to desired shape and cure
8. Polish composite with disks, abrasive paste, and cup
9. Pass dental floss through interproximal area to be sure the area can be satisfactorily cleaned

Dental stone, graduated cylinder, and water
Plaster spatula
Separator (petroleum jelly)
Acrylic powder and liquid
Disposable paper cup
Cement spatula
Reinforcing wire, bending pliers, and cutting pliers
Quartz, rag, and chamois wheels for lathe
Acrylic polishing compound
Small area composite type splint

Armamentarium

Cotton rolls
Acid etch and application brush
Timing device
Light-cured bonding agent and application brush
Light-cured composite and plastic instrument
Curing light
Reinforcing wire and cutting pliers
Small wax spatula
Composite finishing disks
Abrasive polishing paste
Contra-angle and rubber cup
Dental floss

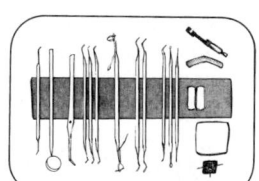

ORAL HYGIENE AIDS

The use of oral hygiene aids, such as floss, interdental brushes, interdental tips, implant cleaners, therapeutic mouthwashes, and preventive toothpastes is an integral part of patient education in a periodontal practice. The application of each of these materials or devices was described in Chapter 26. The dental assistant should be familiar with all of these materials and be able to describe their functions during periodontal therapy.

OCCLUSAL EQUILIBRATION

Occlusal equilibration, also termed **coronaplasty**, involves reshaping the occlusal or incisal surfaces of selected teeth to improve the bite. Carbide burs and occlusal registration paper are used for equilibration. The periodontist uses the handpiece like a paintbrush to *draw* the new shape of the cusp or incisal surface, then checks for result with bite registration paper. When blue paper is used, a high spot appears as a blue dot. When red paper is used, a red halo appears around the high spot. During the shaping process a thin stream of air or water coolant is blown on the tooth surface to prevent tissue damage from the heat that is generated by the rapidly rotating bur. On completion, either the dental assistant or the dentist may make a more accurate bite registration with zinc oxide and eugenol paste, wax, or vinyl polysiloxane bite impression material. Before dismissing the patient, the dentist makes a final check of this registration for accuracy of equilibration and then completes any remaining minor adjustments.

PATIENT EDUCATION

Patient education is the backbone of successful periodontal treatment. No amount of scaling, root planing, or other treatment is effective for long if the patient does not appreciate and maintain the gains achieved through treatment. The patient must understand what has been done, why it was done, and what needs to be done to keep the supporting structures healthy. The dental professional must be alert for opportunities to educate the patient and use these opportunities wisely. Education works best when it is related to conditions in the patient's own mouth, is couched in language the patient understands, and is delivered as an ongoing part of the treatment process.

The dental professional must understand that education is vital; if it is unsuccessful, everything else is a waste of time. All team members educate patients in a periodontal practice. Education is part of total care and cannot be charged as a direct service to the patient. Education is an integral part of successful periodontal practice. Although it is time consuming, the economics of this time investment are offset by the positive patient response and potential success of treatment.

Some concepts, such as oral hygiene techniques, work best when the patient is focused on learning. Others, such as surgical procedures, work best when education is part of everyday conversation. Educating as you work saves time for yourself, lets the patient learn easily in a bit-by-bit manner and still gets the job done well. Observe the patient as the education is presented. If it appears that the patient does not understand or accept the material, stop and focus on teaching. Observing patients' reactions in various situations improves your ability to educate different patients in various types of treatment.

During patient education each patient should learn the following:

1. The definition of periodontal disease
2. The status and appearance of his or her periodontal disease
3. What normal healthy periodontal conditions are, and how they appear
4. How to achieve and maintain the healthiest conditions possible in the patient's mouth

The patient needs not only to learn about periodontal disease and mouth care, but also needs to put knowledge into action by faithfully following recommended home care procedures. Conscientious home care flows from education. The dental assistant needs to teach the patient what to do, when and how to do it, the pitfalls and success signs to look for to evaluate daily progress, and how to make corrections in technique when the pitfalls appear. Home care techniques that are used include brushing, flossing, oral hygiene aids, irrigation, therapeutic mouthwashes, preventive toothpastes, and wise food choices. Nutritional counseling techniques and oral hygiene procedures are presented in Chapters 5 and 26.

Surgical Treatment

When initial therapy is not adequate to overcome either ongoing periodontal disease or conditions that are left from prior episodes, surgery may be indicated. The need for surgery is usually determined after initial therapy has been completed. Thorough reexamination and reevaluation of the patient's periodontal status are made. Conditions such as deep or inaccessible pockets, irregular bone contour, furcation involvement, mucogingival defects, and persistent inflammation might not be successfully treated without the quality of deposit removal, tissue debridement, and recontour afforded by surgical therapy.

Even when indications for surgery exist, not every patient is a candidate. Some patients are medically compromised, mentally or physically unable or unwilling to cooperate in the surgical process, do not have enough bone remaining to justify periodontal treatment, or decide not to make the necessary financial investment. The dentist considers the *whole patient*—periodontal condition, local and systemic contributing factors, and patient cooperation—before recommending surgery. The patient makes the final decision.

The overall objective of periodontal surgery is to eliminate the conditions that predispose to periodontal disease: poor tissue contour, pockets, and plaque accumulation. When diseased tissue is removed and **physiologic contour** (tissue that best promotes tissue health) is reestablished, oral hygiene procedures are more easily performed, plaque accumulation decreases, and the host's defenses can more easily eliminate infective agents. The result is better tissue health.

▶ Types of Procedures

Periodontal surgery is performed on both hard and soft tissues (Table 37-5). Common soft tissue procedures are curettage, gingivectomy, gingivoplasty, gingival graft, and flap surgery. Hard tissue procedures are osseous surgery and root resection. The gingivectomy surgery may include many of these procedures, such as the gingivoplasty, flap surgery, curettage, and bone augmentation.

TABLE 37-5   PERIODONTAL SURGERY PROCEDURES

Procedure	Definition	Indications
Curettage	Removal of diseased soft tissue lining the pocket wall	Inflammation and edema of suprabony pockets
Gingivectomy	Removal of marginal and interdental gingiva	Suprapockets
		Periodontal abscesses
		Gingival enlargements
Gingivoplasty	Reshaping of gingiva	Gingival defects
Free gingival graft	Transfer of small piece of mucosal tissue from one site to another	Gingival recession
		Exposed roots
Flap surgery	Surgical separation of all or part of soft tissue in an area from underlying tissues, completion of other procedures, then return of soft tissue to same or adjacent area	Inaccessible root deposits
		Diseased hard and soft tissue
		Infrabony pockets
Osseous surgery	Sculpting of alveolar bone height and contour by addition or removal of bone or bone substitute	Bone roughness
		Bone defects or loss
		Infrabony pockets
		Exostoses
Root resection	Amputation of one root of a multirooted tooth	Extensive furcation involvement

CURETTAGE

Curettage is the surgical removal of diseased soft tissue that lines the sulcus. It is preceded by scaling and root planing and aims to eliminate inflamed epithelial and **granulation tissue**, highly vascular tissue that is formed in response to inflammation, edema, and **suprabony pockets**—a pocket with a base above the level of the alveolar crest. When these local factors are removed, swelling subsides, pocket depth is reduced, and physiologic contour is reestablished. If the curettage has been extended subgingivally, new fiber attachment occurs at a more apical level on the root. The two types of curettage are closed and open.

CLOSED CURETTAGE

Closed curettage takes place in a closed field: the gingival tissue remains in position around the tooth. In this instance a curet is turned around so that the blade faces the soft tissue rather than the root surface. Careful horizontal strokes are used to remove the sulcus wall and to detach the junctional epithelium. Curettage may also be extended subgingivally and may be referred to as subgingival curettage. The area is flushed with water and the tissue is readapted to the tooth surface. Healing usually occurs within 2 weeks.

OPEN CURETTAGE

Open curettage is done in an open field: after a flap (a section of soft tissue) has been incised and pushed back to expose underlying tissues. **Reflecting** the flap (displacing the flap from the surgical site) improves visibility and access to the site. The remaining calculus is then removed, root planing is done, diseased soft tissue is cut away, the flap is sutured back into position, and a periodontal dressing is placed. Healing requires approximately 6 weeks.

GINGIVOPLASTY

Gingivoplasty involves shaping the gingival tissue to physiologic contour. Gingival aberrations, such as hyperplasia, clefts, craters, **festoons**, poor contour, and bulbous or misshapen papillae, are sculpted into correct forms by the use of soft tissue cutting instruments, then repositioned and sutured as indicated. Healing time depends on the type and extent of the wound.

FLAP SURGERY

Flap surgery consists of lifting a section of gingiva and/or mucosa from the underlying tissue, completing other procedures in conditions of good visibility and access while the flap is elevated, then repositioning and suturing the flap. Some flaps are repositioned in the same area and some are displaced laterally, apically, or coronally. The various types fit into two basic classes: **mucoperiosteal flap**, full-thickness, and **mucosal flap**, split-thickness. All soft tissues in an area, epithelium, connective tissue, and periosteum, are incised and elevated for a split-thickness flap; this gives excellent access and visibility for work on the bone. Only epithelium and part of the underlying connective tissue are elevated for a full-thickness flap; this leaves the bone covered with periosteum and a layer of connective tissue and is the flap of choice when apical repositioning occurs. Apical repositioning is a widely used technique in pocket elimination surgery because it helps to increase the width of the gingiva. Healing requires 4 to 8 weeks.

MUCOGINGIVAL SURGERY

Mucogingival surgery is plastic surgery of the gingiva and/or mucosa. It seeks to correct mucogingival defects that help to maintain or exacerbate periodontal disease. A variety of procedures is available to increase the width of the attached gingiva, cover exposed tooth roots, reduce frenum or muscle attachment pull of soft tissue away from the tooth, and widen or deepen the vestibule. The dental assistant is most likely to encounter gingival grafting and the use of displaced flaps.

LATERAL FLAP DISPLACEMENT

A laterally displaced flap is used to cover isolated areas of exposed root, such as those created by deep clefts, **recession,** retraction of tissues, or frenum pull. Gingiva in the recipient (affected) site is excised and resected down to the periosteum. The root surface is scaled and planed. Donor tissue is obtained by creating a partial-thickness flap in the laterally adjacent soft tissue. The open end of the flap is then moved sideways, adapted to cover the exposed area, and sutured into position. The area is covered with a periodontal dressing. Complete healing requires 2 to 3 weeks.

GINGIVECTOMY

Gingivectomy is the cutting away of gingiva. It is done to provide visibility and access for scaling and root planing, to **excise** (cut away or remove) enlargements and eliminate suprabony pockets or periodontal abscesses. Cutting may be done with periodontal knives, electrosurgery, or chemicals. Most commonly, knives are used. The depth of the pocket is measured and the measurement is transposed to the gingival surface. The base of each pocket is marked on the outside of the gingiva with a pocket marker (Fig. 37-8, *A* through *C*). The resulting line of dots is then connected with incisions (Fig. 37-9, *A* and *B*). A flap is reflected with an elevator (Fig. 37-9, *C*). A surgical hoe or curet scaler is used to remove the incised marginal and interdental gingiva, the area is washed with water, granulation tissue and remaining root surface deposits are removed, and rough areas on the root surface are planed (Fig. 37-9, *D*). The area is thoroughly flushed, then blotted with a gauze sponge, until hemorrhage is controlled and a clot has formed. The flap is repositioned over the wound area. The wound may be protected with sutures and a periodontal dressing (Fig. 37-9, *E* and *F*). Complete healing requires nearly 2

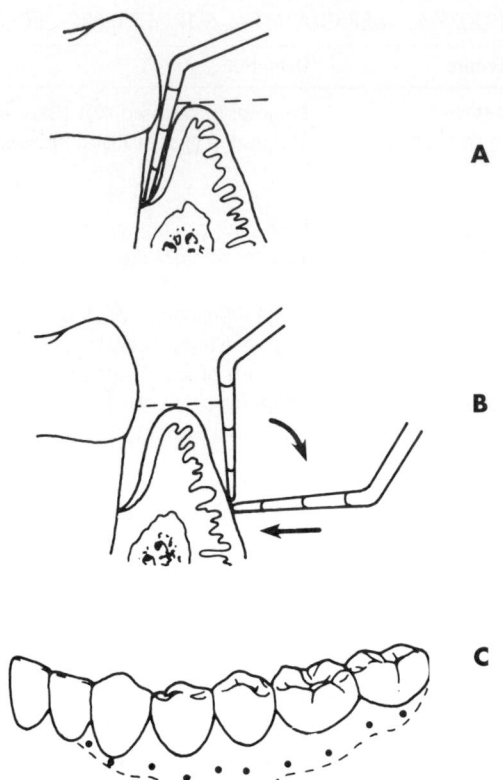

FIG. 37-8   Marking periodontal pockets for gingivectomy procedure. *A,* Measuring depth of pocket. *B,* Transposing measured depth to gingival surface. *C,* Gingiva is marked by puncturing mucosa at level of pocket depth. Incising just apical to puncture marks.

(From Chasteen JE: *Essentials of clinical dental assisting,* ed 4, St Louis, 1989, Mosby.)

months. Fig. 37-10, *A* through *U,* photographically depicts the gingivectomy procedure.

GINGIVAL GRAFTING

A **graft** is the moving of tissue from one area to another. A gingival graft is done to increase attached gingiva. Pocket walls in the area are cut away and root surfaces are scaled and planed. The **recipient tissue,** the area where the graft is placed, is prepared by surgically creating a connective tissue bed in which to place the graft. **Donor tissue,** the tissue to be placed in the site, may be either gingiva or thick mucosa. A template of the prepared bed is made and used as a pattern for excising the graft. The graft is placed in the recipient bed, sutured into position,

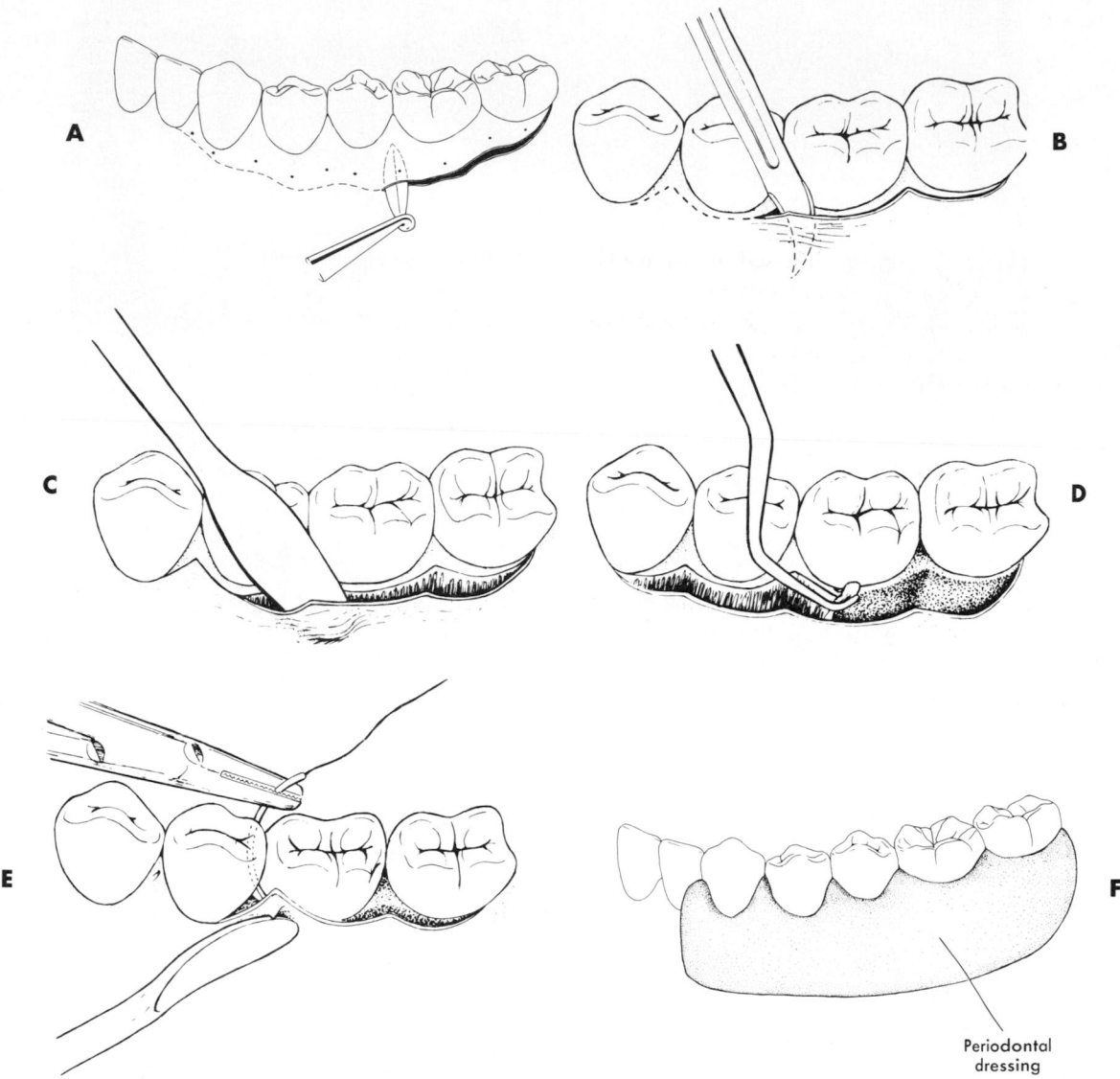

FIG. 37-9 *A,* An incision is made along the marked *dots* for resecting the gingiva. *B,* A surgical blade is used to incise the remainder of gingival tissue. *C,* The flap is reflected with a periosteal elevator. *D,* The curet is used to remove granulomatous tissue. *E,* The suture material is placed. *F,* The periodontal dressing is placed.

(From Chasteen JE: *Essentials of clinical dental assisting,* ed 4, St Louis, 1989, Mosby.)

and protected with a periodontal dressing (Fig. 37-11, *A* through *E*). Healing requires about 2½ weeks.

▶ Osseous Surgery

Osseous surgery, or bone surgery, can be either augmentive or resective. Augmentive surgery is the addition of bone or bone substitute to fill bony defects.

Resective surgery may be either bone or root resection, involving removal of hard tissue.

BONE AUGMENTATION

Augmentive procedures add bone or bone substitute to fill in bony defects. Added bone may come in the form of a bone graft from a different site in the same patient or

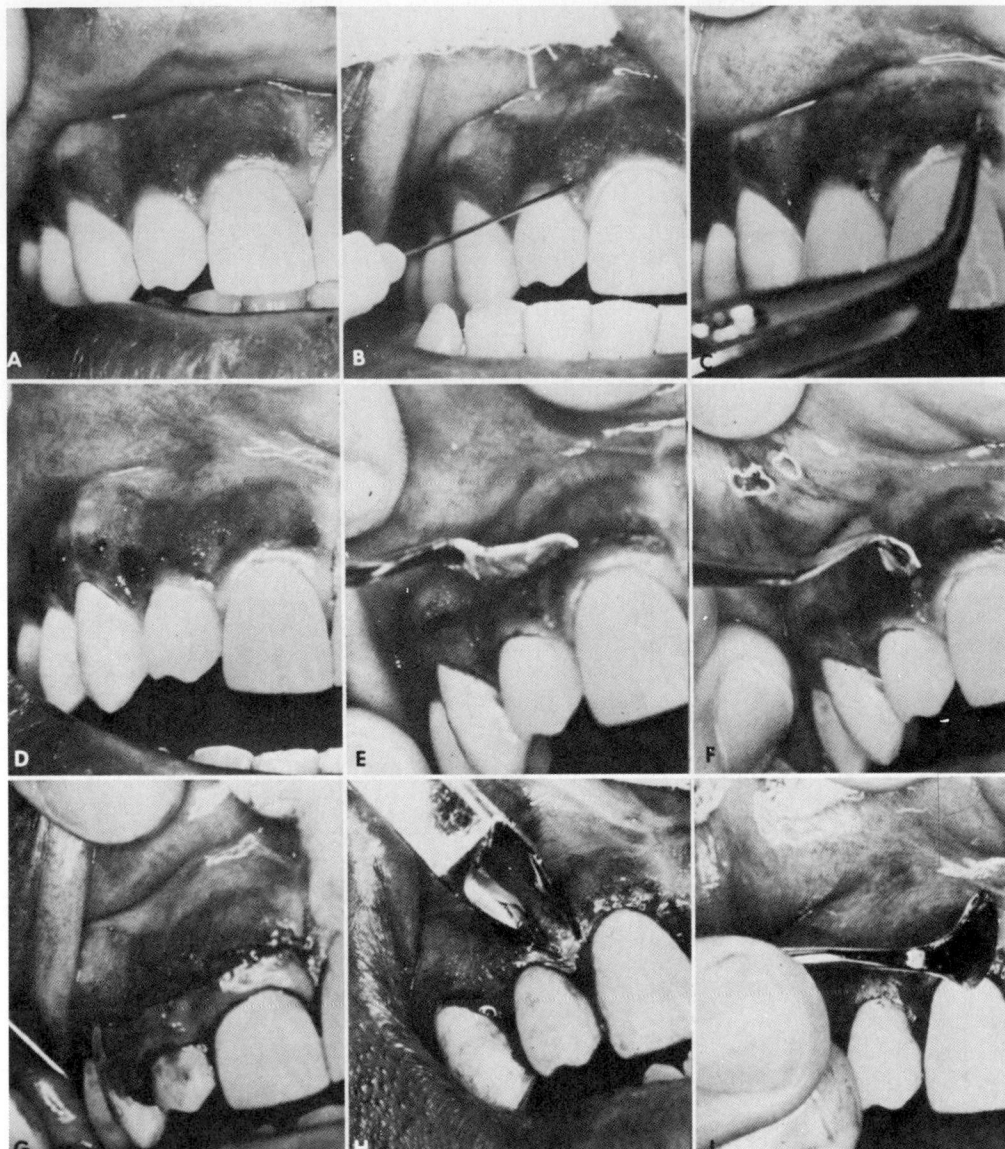

FIG. 37-10   Step-by-step procedure for gingivectomy. A local anesthetic has been injected
into mucogingival area, resulting in anesthesia of area. Anesthetic fluid is also injected into
palatal area corresponding to mucogingival site. *A,* Appearance before anesthetic. *B,* Injection
of anesthetic into buccal peaks; this is also done in palatal peaks. By doing so, tissue becomes
firmer and thus easier to contour. *C,* Pocket marking is then performed. Beaks of pocket
marker must be parallel to root surface. Markings are made on mesial, central marginal, and
distal aspects. *D,* Markings are then surveyed to ascertain relative levels of resultant gingival
margins after resection on a continuous line guided by markings. *E* and *F,* Interdental cut
is then made. Knife is inserted into primary incision and extended interdentally as far as possible. *G,* Surgical surface is then inspected carefully. Teeth are dried to see if any calculus is
present and scaled if necessary. Gingival topography usually needs further correction, and tissue tabs must be removed. For this, nippers, *H,* scraping with knife, *I,* and a curette, *J,* are
useful. Resultant surface should be smooth and clean, *K* and *M.* Use of dental tape will release
any loosened tissue. Operator must probe each margin to ascertain that all detached tissue
has been removed. Same procedure is performed on palatal aspect. *T,* Interdental tissue must
be left smooth. *N* through *S,* Step-by-step procedures for palatal aspect. Use of a diamond
stone to shape gingival tissue is seen in *Q,* Interdental sluiceways are easily produced by this
method. *L* and *U,* Gingival area is then covered with a periodontal dressing.

(From Genco RJ, Goldman HM, Cohen DW: *Contemporary periodontics,* St Louis, 1990, Mosby.)

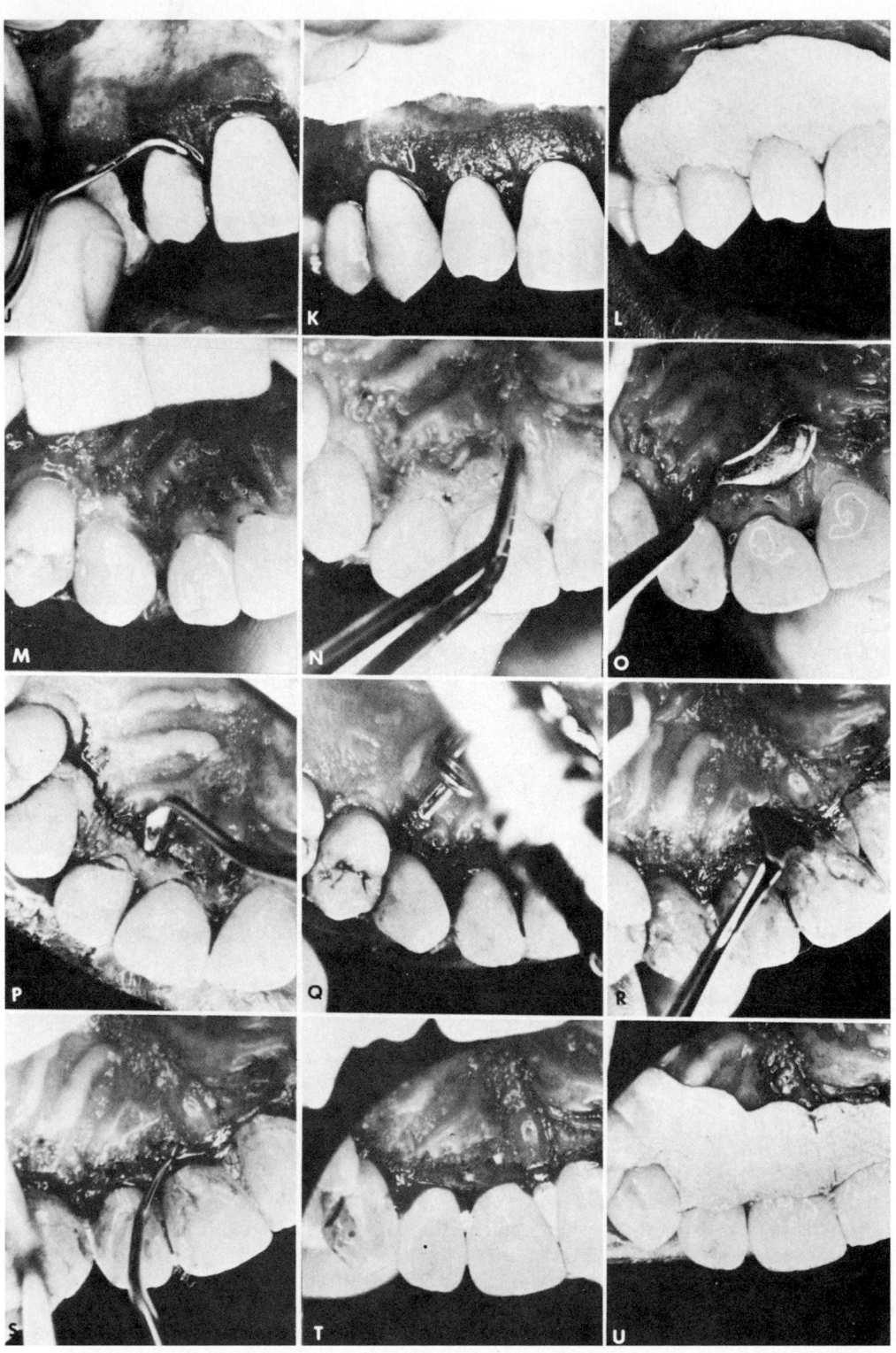

FIG. 37-10, cont'd.   For legend see opposite page.

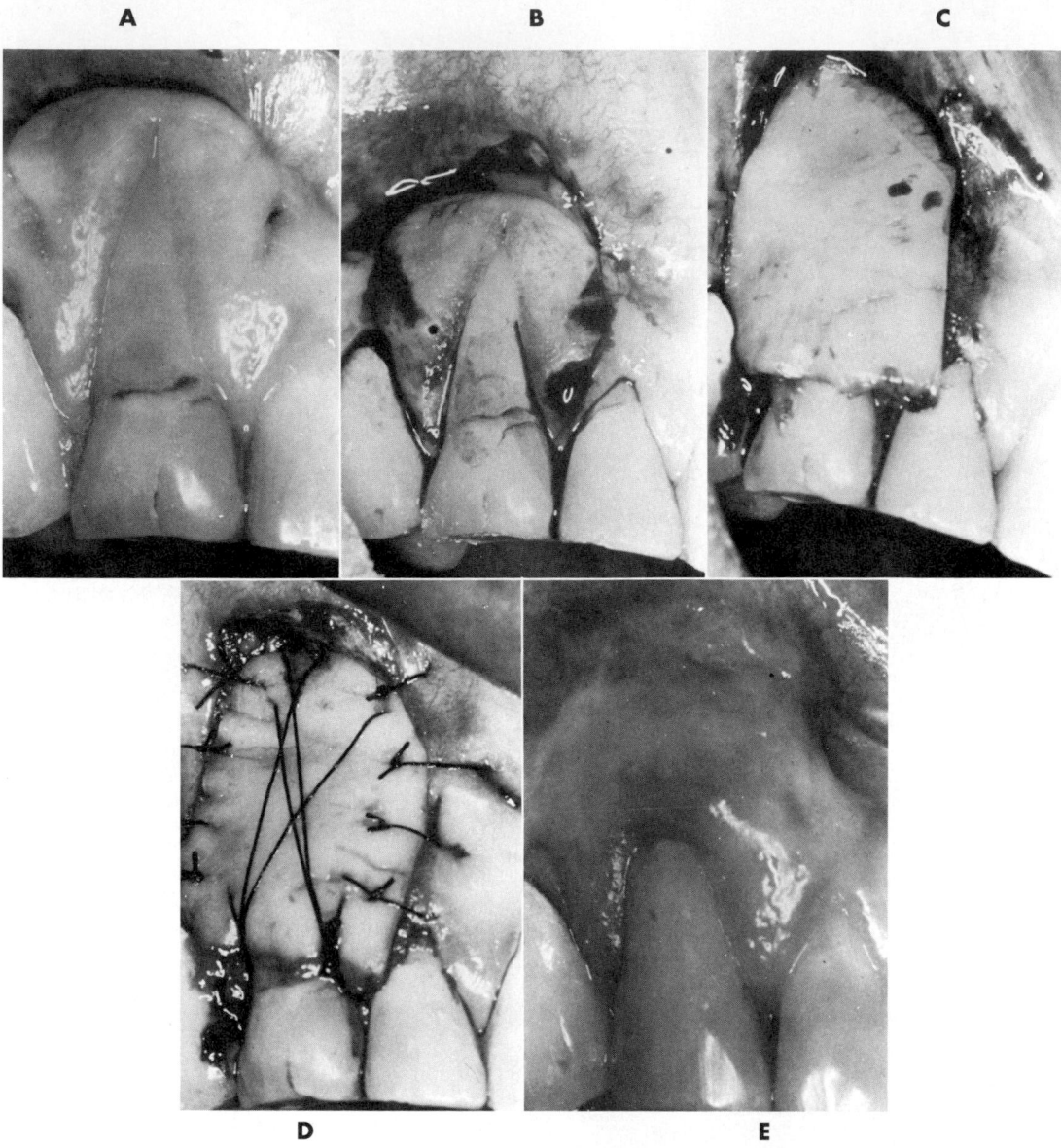

FIG. 37-11 Illustration of a free gingival graft to cover recession over a maxillary canine. Deep area of recession exists over maxillary canine, which is broad coronally and narrow apically and extends within 1 mm of mucogingival junction. *A,* Preoperative photograph. *B,* Initial incision before removing gingiva in interproximal areas mesial and distal to area of recession to prepare recipient bed. *C,* Graft (from palatal donor site of patient) is approximately one fourth to one third larger than area taken from gingival epithelium. *D,* Free gingival graft sutured into place over recipient bed and area of recession. *E,* Two-year postoperative view showing large band of attached gingiva covering approximately one half of original area of recession, resulting in an esthetic scallop matching that of adjacent teeth.

(From Genco RJ, Goldman HM, Cohen DW: *Contemporary periodontics,* St Louis, 1990, Mosby.)

from a different patient altogether. Bone from the same patient is well tolerated but involves creating two wounds in the same patient. Two surgical procedures separated by days or weeks are required. Bone from a different person raises questions of tissue compatibility and possible rejection of the graft. Sometimes these problems can be avoided by using a **bone swaging** technique. Swaging is similar to lateral flap displacement; it displaces bone laterally to fill in a vertical defect. The alveolar bone adjacent to the bony defect is freed at the top and sides (but not at the base) to a predetermined depth, then adapted laterally to fill in the defect. Bone to be moved is freed by cutting away an undermining wedge of bone on the side farthest from the defect. The area from which bone was cut away fills in with the beginnings of new bone in 6 weeks, and complete healing requires approximately 6 months.

BONE RESECTION

Resection is the process of removing tissue. Bone resective procedures remove bone. They involve chiseling, clipping, filing, cutting, and smoothing to create the most physiologic bone contour possible for a given patient. Each periodontist has specific preferences, but in general, steps proceed from gross to fine removal, followed by contouring and smoothing.

Following any type of bone surgery, covering soft tissue is contoured and sutured into place. The area is gently irrigated and blotted with 2 × 2 gauze squares to ensure that the sutures are well placed and a clot is beginning to form. A periodontal pack is used to protect small areas or those with poor soft tissue coverage. Large sutured areas with adequate soft tissue coverage may not be dressed.

ROOT RESECTION

When periodontal disease of a multirooted tooth has caused extensive bone loss around one root but adequate bone remains around the other(s), the seriously involved root may be amputated. Such resection aims to eliminate furcation involvement and bony defects and to promote ease of cleaning. A full-thickness flap is elevated, and a bur is used to amputate the root. The root stump is smoothed and contoured with diamond points, remaining roots are scaled and planed, the area is washed, the flap is repositioned and sutured, and the wound is covered with a periodontal pack. Soft tissue repair is completed in about 2 months; bone fill-in occurs in approximately 6 months.

Surgical Instrumentation

Surgical armamentaria are of five types: soft tissue cutting instruments, hard tissue cutting instruments, surgical scalers, miscellaneous instruments, and suturing items.

▶ Soft Tissue Cutting Instruments

Soft tissue cutting instruments are used to **incise** (cut away or contour) gingiva and underlying connective tissue (see Table 37-4). Pocket markers are inserted in pockets and used to cut minute holes on the outside of the gingiva to mark pocket base locations. Scalpels slice soft tissue; electrosurgery units cut and cauterize it (seal it off by burning). Periodontal and interdental knives incise and cut away gingival tissue; rotating stones used with a light touch contour and smooth it. Scissors cut and contour gingiva, and nippers clip off tissue tags.

When the periodontist is cutting soft tissue, the assistant must carefully use a surgical high-volume evacuator tip to control bleeding, permit visibility, and pick up small pieces of excised tissue. A disposable cup and 2 × 2 gauze squares are kept nearby to receive larger bits of tissue and wipe soiled instrument tips. Periodic evacuation of saliva from the retromolar area and retraction of tissue to avoid obstructed vision are necessary. The anticipation and preparation of the appropriate instrument or supply to be used next increase the efficient progression in the treatment. When an electrocautery device is used, the assistant must position the end of a *plastic* HVE tip immediately adjacent to the area of surgery to remove the odor that results from burning of soft tissue. As always, monitor the patient's physical and psychologic condition, and notify the dentist if any untoward effects are observed.

▶ Hard Tissue Cutting Instruments

Hard tissue cutting instruments are used to cut and contour bone and teeth (see Table 37-4). Burs are used to cut windows in bone, to gain access to tooth roots, and to resect them. Curets are used to spoon out necrotic bone, chisels and mallets to cut away exostoses, rongeurs to clip small bone spicules, files and burs to finely contour and smooth. When burs are used on bone, the assistant irrigates the area with sterile saline solution. In addition to the usual tasks of field maintenance and patient monitoring just described, during bone surgery the assistant must keep 2 × 2 gauze squares and a disposable cup nearby to wipe bone bits from instrument tips, unclog bur's, file blades that fill with bone debris, and receive pieces of bone.

SCALERS

Scalers used in surgery are often the Gracey style. The principal difference is that these scalers have longer, more angled shanks and sometimes longer, finer blades to access and remove deposits in root furcations and deep bony defects. Even though scaling is done before surgery, studies indicate that tenacious calculus deposits are still present when the tissue is flapped and reflected.

MISCELLANEOUS INSTRUMENTS

A periosteal elevator looks like a double-ended paddle or hockey stick. A true periosteal elevator is a larger surgical instrument than an often preferred #7 spatula, which resembles the periosteal elevator but is more delicate. Both are used to reflect soft tissue at the surgical site. Diamond files are wedge-shaped rotary instruments that are placed in a handpiece and used to remove calculus deposits. Periodontal files are delicate instruments used to smooth or plane rough tooth surfaces. An amalgam knife looks like a large straight or modified sickle scaler; it is used to contour amalgam overhangs. An air-water syringe is used to flush away blood, toxins, and tissue bits and to dry selected areas to increase visibility. See Table 37-4 for illustrations of miscellaneous periodontal surgery instruments.

SUTURING ITEMS

Periodontal suturing is the process of reapproximating soft tissues to ideal position to promote healing. Several types of suturing are used in periodontal surgery, including interrupted, continuous ligation, and periosteal suturing.

Periodontal suturing is much more delicate than many other types of surgical suturing, since the needles and suture material are quite fine. The sutures are supplied on sterile curved, prethreaded disposable needles and are used with soft tissue scissors, mirrors for retraction, and several 2×2 gauze sponges. The periodontist cleanses the area, then carefully positions and sutures the soft tissue.

PERIODONTAL DRESSINGS

Periodontal dressings are used to protect surgical sites by covering the areas to avoid additional trauma during healing. These protective surfaces also provide a guide to contour regenerating gingival tissue, support for mobile teeth, and protection from hot and spicy foods. Many state laws provide for the placement and removal of these dressings by the dental assistant.

There are two types of dressings, eugenol and noneugenol. Eugenol types may be prepared in advance and stored in the refrigerator for several days. Dressings are mixed, placed, and contoured to physiologic form while soft, then allowed to harden and left in place for a week to 10 days. The patient returns to have the dressing removed, and the healing is assessed. Occasionally, dressings are removed earlier than a week after surgery, left in position longer than 10 days, or removed and replaced one or more times. The dentist determines when the dressings are to be removed, based on the healing assessment.

The noneugenol type of dressings are more widely

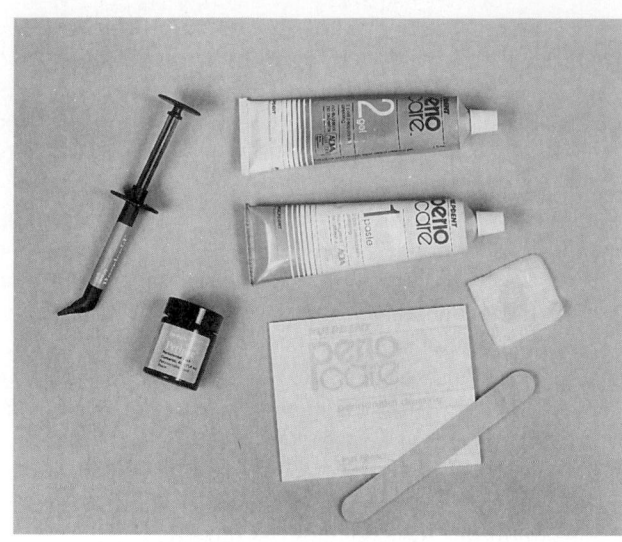

FIG. 37-12   Periodontal dressings. Two paste and light-cured systems.

used because they are less irritating to the tissue, cause fewer allergic reactions, and take less time to prepare. This type of dressing is provided in a two-paste or a light cured system (Fig. 37-12).

SURGERY TRAY

Each periodontist has a preferred surgery tray. There are similarities, however, and it is necessary for the assistant to quickly learn the dentist's preference. The tray set-up illustrated in Fig. 37-13 is representative of most periodontal surgery trays. Optional items that are used less frequently might include a chisel and mallet, antibiotic ointment, prepared bone allograft and packing instrument, and gore-Tex periodontal membrane material for removal of bone exostoses, addition of bone, or guidance and control of soft tissue regeneration. A suture setup would be added as indicated.

Surgery

A basic sequence of steps in periodontal surgery is used, with slight variation for most procedures. As with other dental procedures, it is necessary for the dental assistant to anticipate the operator's needs and to be able to adapt to the procedure when a variation in steps occurs.

The sequence in periodontal treatment should include the following appointments:

1. Prescaling of the teeth
2. Gingival surgery, including pocket elimination, root planing, residual calculus removal, suturing and

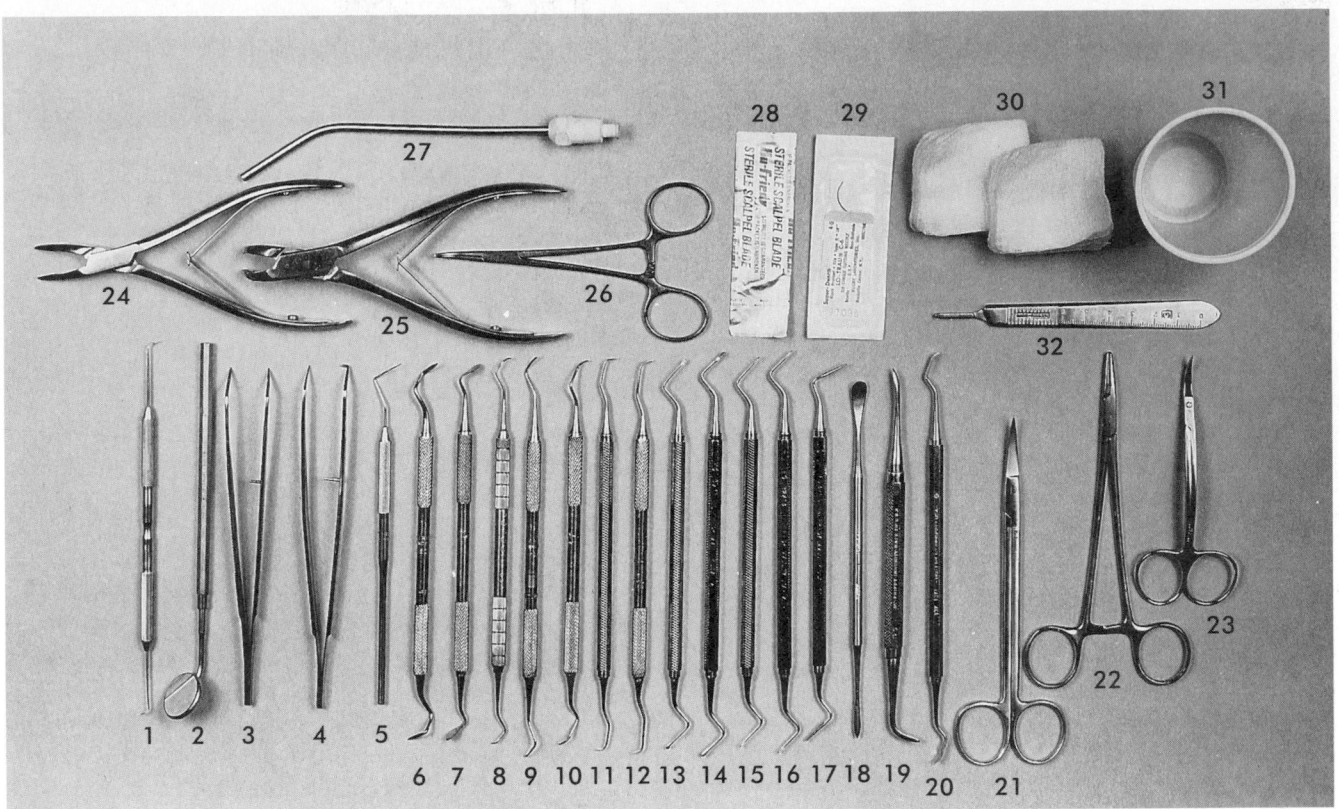

FIG. 37-13 Surgery tray. *1,* Explorer. *2,* Mirror. *3,* Cotton forceps. *4,* Pocket marker. *5,* Periodontal probe. *6,* Orban instrument. *7,* Kirkland gingivectomy knife. *8* through *12,* Various scalers. *13* and *14,* Various surgical curets. *15* and *16,* Hoes. *17,* Sugarman file. *18,* Small periosteal elevator; #7 spatula. *19,* Periosteal elevator. *20,* File. *21,* Surgical scissors. *22,* Hemostat. *23,* Tissue scissors. *24,* Ronquer. *25,* Tissue nipper. *26,* Needle holder. *27,* Surgical suction tip. *28,* Scalpel blade. *29,* Suturing items. *30,* 2 × 2 gauze. *31,* Sterile cup. *32,* Scalpel handle.

placement of a dressing, and providing home care instructions

3. Removing the dressing and sutures, rinsing the area and gently polishing the teeth, and placing a second dressing if necessary

4. Optional appointment to change dressing, rinse and polish teeth, and provide home care instructions

5. Recall to evaluate healing and home care

BOX 37-3

PERIODONTAL SURGERY SEQUENCE

Anesthetize site
Examine and mark pockets
Incise and reflect soft tissue
Scale and root plane
Debride site of diseased bone and tissue
Smooth and contour hard and soft tissue
Flush site
Place sutures to close wound
Place protective dressing
Record procedure
Give postoperative instructions

During each of these phases, records management is an integral part of patient care and is particularly important in protecting the operating team. Box 37-3 lists the sequence of the periodontal surgical procedure.

▶ Surgery Procedure

In the following discussion each of these phases is described in a step-by-step procedure, with emphasis on the techniques and the dental assistant's responsibilities. The armamentarium for a surgical procedure is as follows:

Armamentarium

Anesthesia setup
Knives
Mirrors
Cotton forceps
Pocket marker
Periodontal probe

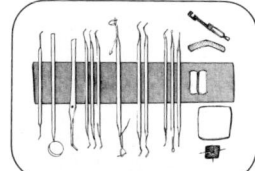

Explorers
Scalpel with handle and blades
Specialized scalpels
Periosteal elevators
Specialized curets
Sharpening stones
Chisels/scalers
Burs and stones
Interproximal files
Rongeurs
Surgical curet
Tissue nippers
Surgical scissors
Hemostat
Needle holder
2 × 2 gauze
Dressing material and armamentarium
Suture setup
Surgical HVE tip
Sterile saline solution

PERIODONTAL SURGERY PROCEDURE

▶ Are all universal barrier techniques being used?
▶ Is all of the armamentarium available and prepared for use?
▶ Are the instruments arranged in sequence of use?
▶ Am I prepared for alternative treatment plans?
▶ Is the necessary equipment turned on and ready to operate?

1. Anesthetize the patient.
2. Pass the explorer to the dentist to examine the site. Exchange the explorer for a periodontal probe for examination of the periodontium.
3. Pass the pocket marker for the dentist to mark the base of the pocket.
4. After this is done, exchange the instrument for a periodontal knife. Some dentists may prefer to use a standard scalpel, such as a 12 B to detach the periodontal ligament before the periodontal knife is used.
5. Use the surgical HVE tip close to the surgical site to remove oral fluids and blood. Hold a 2 × 2 gauze sponge in the passing zone for the operator to pass cut tissue and for the assistant to clear the instrument tip.
6. Exchange the scalpel intermittently for surgical scissors to cut the tissue. Use a forceps or hemostat to grasp tissue, making it easier for the dentist to cut the tissue. Grasping the tissue permits it to be easily removed, thus avoiding the removal of tissue by the HVE tip. Such tissue removal could clog the tip.

7. The operator may use a surgical bur to cut a window in the bone when necessary, to gain access to the surgical site.
8. After the soft tissue is removed, exchange a variety of scalers and periodontal files. During this debridement and root planing procedure, flush the site with sterile water, using an irrigating syringe. Constant use of HVE and 2 × 2 sponges is necessary to clear instruments and the site.
9. If a suture is to be placed, pass it at this time and prepare to cut the suture as the operator indicates.
10. Place either a eugenol or a noneugenol dressing, according to the manufacturer's directions.
11. Place the dressing to meet the criteria in Box 37-4.
12. Provide postoperative instructions (see Box 37-5 and 37-6).
13. Make entries on the patient record, including the type of anesthesia, surgery, number and type of sutures placed, type of dressing, patient reactions, and additional notations.

▶ Are the appropriate universal barrier techniques removed?
▶ Have all of the appropriate surfaces been cleaned and disinfected?
▶ Has all armamentarium been removed?
▶ Has all equipment been repositioned?
▶ Has all of the equipment been disinfected/sterilized according to OSHA guidelines?

Irrigation syringes and cups

Antibiotic ointment

Lubricant

Before the surgical procedure the patient's health form will have been reviewed and updated. In addition, the patient's allergies must be reviewed to ensure that there will be no reaction to any drugs, medications, or dressings that are to be used.

PLACING SUTURES

The purpose for placing sutures is to reapproximate the position of tissue to promote ideal healing. After the site has been cleansed and profuse bleeding has been minimized to the greatest extent, suture placement proceeds.

The assistant prepares the suture by placing the needle holder securely on the heel of the suture needle. The needle, suture material, and needle holder are passed to the operator as the assistant ensures that no tangling of the suture material has occurred. The assistant may lightly grasp the end of the suture material apical to the surgical site and allow passage of the material through the fingers and off the patient's face.

The assistant gently retracts obstructing tissue, transfers and receives instruments and materials, and cuts the finished sutures at the length the dentist indicates. When suturing is complete, the operator will want a gauze sponge to examine for optimal stitch placement and beginning clot formation. The assistant provides the patient with directions for postoperative care if periodontal dressing is not placed at this time. In some states the assistant is legally delegated the duty of suture removal, described in Chapter 34.

PLACING PERIODONTAL DRESSINGS

Periodontal wounds or surgical sites are dressed to protect them from injury during healing, guide the contour of regenerating gingival tissue, and support mobile teeth. Dressings may be thought of as soft tissue bandages. Many state laws permit them to be applied and removed by the dental assistant.

The mixing and placement of eugenol and noneugenol periodontal dressings are similar. Variations in the steps and technique for mixing depend on the type of material selected. Two types of dressings are described in the following discussion. The first material is a eugenol or noneugenol paste type dressing and the second is a light-cured material.

MIXING AND PLACING EUGENOL AND NONEUGENOL DRESSINGS

1. Coat the patient's lips with a thin layer of lubricant.
2. Dispense proper proportions of the dressing as directed by the manufacturer.
3. Incorporate catalyst into the base using the tip of the tongue depressor with circular strokes, until the mass is streaked in color.
4. Switch to the side of the depressor, and complete the mix with figure-eight motions; the mix is complete when the color is homogeneous.
5. Gather the mix on the tongue depressor, and place it in cold water, until it may be easily handled.
6. Once the material becomes tacky, coat your gloves with a thin layer of lubricant.
7. Roll the mass into a thin rope that is the length of the wound and approximately 3 mm in diameter.
8. Pinch the rope into two halves, and shape one half to fit the lingual side of the surgical site.
9. Isolate the surgical site with cotton rolls or gauze sponges; dry and maintain the area by blotting gently with sterile gauze.
10. Adapt the lingual half of dressing, using gentle finger pressure, to fit the material into the interdental spaces.
11. Adapt the other half to the facial area in the same manner.
12. Gently press the two halves into interproximal areas until they meet, and lock the two pieces together.
13. Remove excess material with a plastic instrument or scaler.
14. Use the back of the beaks of the cotton pliers to adapt the material into the interdental space more accurately.
15. Muscle trim the material through the manipulation of the lips and cheek to ensure that the material does not impinge on movement; remove any excess with the scaler.
16. Smooth the cut edges, and contour the material around the teeth, using a spoon excavator.
17. Contour the material on the tooth surface not to exceed ⅓ the length of the tooth and to avoid any interference with occlusion.
18. Create a smooth and even thickness of material.
19. Wet a gauze sponge, and gently massage the dressing material to increase the smoothness. (See Box 37-4).

PLACEMENT OF LIGHT-CURED MATERIAL

1. Prepare all necessary armamentaria.
2. Isolate and dry the surgical site.
3. Lubricate gloves.
4. Dispense material on a mixing pad, and with a lightly lubricated finger, roll the ribbon of dispensed material off the pad and onto the surgical site.
5. Muscle trim the material through manipulation of the lips and cheeks.
6. Contour the material as described in the previous technique.
7. Expose each area of the dressing, four teeth at a time, for at least 40 seconds under the curing light.
8. Curing must be done on the lingual, as well as the buccal or facial, surfaces.
9. If the dressing interferes with the occlusion or is uncomfortable to the patient, after hardening it can be contoured with a finishing bur on a slow-speed handpiece. [See Box 37-4.]

STOP

Armamentarium for Paste Dressing Placement

Lubricant
Dressing base and catalyst
Paper pad and tongue depressor
Disposable cup of cold water
Mirror
Cotton pliers
Spoon excavator
Curet scaler
Plastic instrument
Crown and collar scissors
2 × 2 gauze sponges

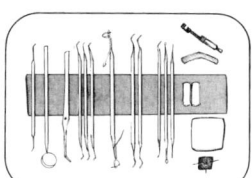

Provision of Postoperative Directions for Care of Surgical Sites

Both oral and written directions for postoperative care should be provided to every patient who has had surgery. The patient must be able to understand them, therefore they should be given in the patient's native language if that is possible and to an interpreter if it is not. They must be provided at a vocabulary level the patient can comprehend.

The three types of directions that are given are (1) care of a site with a periodontal dressing (Box 37-5); (2) care

BOX 37-4

CLINICAL CRITERIA FOR EVALUATING THE PLACEMENT OF A PERIODONTAL DRESSING

Dressing material should:
Be firm but not tacky
Have smooth edges and surfaces
Extend 3 mm beyond the margins of cut soft tissue
Cover the cervical third of any teeth adjacent to the wound
Follow the contours of the teeth and interdental gingiva
Attach securely
Avoid excessive thickness or shelflike projections
Ensure that it feels comfortable to the patient

BOX 37-5

POSTOPERATIVE INSTRUCTIONS FOR PERIODONTAL DRESSINGS

Dressing should remain in place for 7 to 10 days or as directed by the operator.
Brushing should be done as usual.
Avoid hot, spicy, and hard foods.
Small pieces of the dressing may crumble and fall off; do not be alarmed.
If large pieces or the entire dressing is lost, call the practice to arrange for replacement or removal as indicated.
Make an appointment for observation and probable dressing removal in 7 to 10 days.

of a site without sutures (Box 37-6); and (3) care of a site with sutures. Any site with a dressing is considered to fall into the first example, regardless of whether it has sutures.

PERIODONTAL DRESSING REMOVAL

The removal of the periodontal dressing is usually done 7 to 10 days after the surgical procedure. The removal of the dressing allows the operator to inspect and assess the surgical site for healing. This duty may be delegated to the dental assistant as directed by each state's dental practice act.

Armamentarium for Dressing Removal

Mirror
Explorer
Cotton pliers
Spoon excavator
Curet scaler or plastic instrument

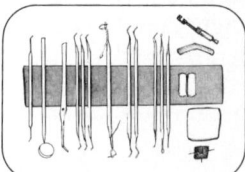

BOX 37-6

CARE OF A SURGICAL SITE WITHOUT SUTURES

Bite on a folded gauze square for the next 30 minutes.

Slight bleeding may occur for the next 24 hours.

Do not eat or drink for 2 hours.

Avoid rinsing or brushing the area for 24 hours. After that time you should brush as usual.

Avoid hot, spicy, and hard foods for the next few days.

Take the medication(s) prescribed by the dentist according to the directions on the package.

Call the office if you experience heavy bleeding, severe pain, or any unexpected symptom. (Office or clinic phone number should be provided.)

Make an appointment to return for the dentist to observe the area in ____. (Fill in the blank with the appropriate number of days or weeks for the patient.)

PATIENTS WITH SUTURES

These patients receive the same directions as above with the following additions:

They are informed of the type of sutures they received (resorbable or nonresorbable) and what this means in terms of whether they must return for suture removal.

Patients who must return are told the time interval for their return, and an appointment is made.

Suture patients are also told that some of the sutures may loosen and be lost. They should not be concerned unless bleeding returns after the loss.

REMOVAL OF THE PERIODONTAL DRESSING

1. Irrigate the area with warm water.
2. Remove facial portion first by **working gently and carefully** to place the instrument under the distoapical margin of the dressing and working forward.
3. Pry the dressing loose.
4. If the sutures are embedded in the dressing, cut the dressing into sections with an instrument blade, work loose one section at a time, and cut the sutures that prevent a section from loosening easily.
5. Remove interproximal debris with an explorer **or** with floss that has a single knot tied in it.
6. Irrigate the site with antiseptic solution.
7. Grasp the free end of each remaining suture above and close to the knot with cotton pliers.
8. **Gently** elevate the knot.
9. Slip one blade of the scissors under the suture, and cut the thread near the tissue.
10. Pull the cut thread (**never the knot**) through the tissue; save removed sutures on a gauze square; **count to verify all have been removed.**
11. Irrigate the area with sterile water.
12. Verify that all dressing fragments, debris, and suture ends have been removed.
13. Have the patient rinse with mouthwash.
14. **Record removal on the patient's record; include the suture count.**
15. Have the dentist examine the healing area.
16. Transfer the mirror and gauze sponge for healing examination.

Delicate suture scissors

Irrigating syringe with tip removed

Antiseptic irrigating solution (commercial or hydrogen peroxide in water)

HVE tip

Floss

2 × 2 gauze sponges

Cup and diluted mouthwash

Continuing Care after Periodontal Therapy

Patients who have received periodontal therapy must receive continuing care. Studies consistently show that patients who practice thorough, daily oral hygiene procedures and who return to the dentist at prescribed intervals are most likely to maintain the status of periodontal health that is achieved in treatment. Without such care, deterioration is more likely and may be more rapid and severe.

Continuing care actually begins during treatment. As each phase is completed, the patient is taught about the new conditions in the mouth and is helped to master necessary cleaning techniques. Treated periodontal tissues tend to be positioned more apically than previously. Roots or furcation areas may be exposed and interdental areas enlarged. Teeth may be mobile. Extensive restorations or prosthetic devices may be present. The patient may need to be taught to prevent root caries and to use interproximal oral hygiene aids or to care for splints, bridges, fixed or removable partial dentures, and implants or dressings. The assistant provides much of this education as a part of ongoing duties during the treatment phase.

When therapy is complete, the patient is entered into a maintenance program. Maintenance appointments are a monitoring and early warning system; they consist of a standard series that can be readily varied to adapt to the

TEAM APPROACH
Periodontal Surgery Procedure

OPERATOR	ASSISTANT
Anesthetize patient	Assist with anesthesia
	Pass the explorer
Grasp explorer; examine site	
Return explorer; receive periodontal probe, and examine periodontium	Exchange the explorer for a periodontal probe
Return periodontal probe	Receive periodontal probe, and pass the pocket marker
Receive marker, and mark the base of the pocket	
Return pocket marker	Exchange marker for periodontal knife or scalpel
Receive scalpel, and make a flap/incision at marked site	Place surgical HVE tip close to the surgical site to remove oral fluid and blood
	Hold a 2 × 2 gauze sponge in the passing zone for the operator to pass cut tissue and to clear the instrument tip
Return scalpel Scale and plane exposed areas	Receive scalpel; pass surgical scissors or burs if needed to cut gingival tissues or bone; retract tissues as needed; transfer and exchange a variety of scalers and periodontal files; wipe tips of instruments with gauze sponge; keep HVE tip near surgical site; flush site with sterile saline solution as needed
Return scalers and files	Receive scalers and files; prepare suture needle, and pass if needed
Receive needle, and place sutures	Retract tissues; evacuate site
Return suture needle	Receive suture needle; prepare dressing; pass lubricant to operator; pass dressing
Receive dressing; place dressing; adapt dressing to site	Pass placement instrument and dressing material; wipe instrument as needed
Return placement instrument	Receive instrument
	Clean patient's face; provide postoperative instructions; dismiss patient; record treatment

needs of the individual patient. At each maintenance appointment the periodontal condition is reexamined and reevaluated; the patient is made aware of the results and is educated and motivated to perform any indicated home care procedures; routine scaling and root planing are done; and arrangements are made to treat any recurrent disease while it is still manageable.

The importance of education and motivation at maintenance appointments cannot be overstated. Periodontal health maintenance procedures must continue indefinitely. It is easy to forget or to tire of educating and motivating. One of the most effective and important services that is performed as a dental assistant in a periodontic practice is to stimulate and motivate patients' interest in tissue maintenance. It is periodic professional care plus good daily home care that makes a difference, and faithful home care most likely happens when meticulous, caring attention is paid to patient education, reeducation, and motivation at maintenance appointments.

Maintenance appointments are scheduled similarly to recall patients in a general practice. The patient may make another appointment before leaving or elect to be notified later of the need to do so. In either case a recall system is established, usually by the office manager. The patient's name, address, telephone number, date for return, and time that is required for the next appointment are entered in a computer or a card file and indexed by name or number under the planned month and week of return. At a predetermined interval before the return, usually 2 to 4 weeks, a card is sent to remind the patient of the appointment or of the need for rescheduling. Patients with definite appointments are called the day before to confirm the appointment. These calls are made as part of the regular office appointment reminder system. In many practices, maintenance patients are scheduled with the hygienist, and the dentist consults as necessary.

The prognosis for patients in continuing care depends primarily on the type and severity of the periodontal disease that has been treated and on the thoroughness of home hygiene procedures. Other considerations include age, degree of inflammation, amount of remaining bone support, occlusion, and quality of host response to disease episodes. Patients with a greater degree of inflammation from local factors tend to have a better prognosis. Extensive bone loss, malocclusion, and some systemic disorders mitigate against successful maintenance. The role of host factors, such as immunity and genetic inheritance, is not yet completely understood. With few exceptions, the patient who maintains excellent oral hygiene and receives prompt professional treatment of any site where disease recurs is likely to be able to maintain the periodontal health he or she, you, and the other team members have worked to achieve.

KEY POINTS

▶ Periodontal disease is site specific and episodic. The two major types are gingivitis (inflammation of the gingiva) and periodontitis, which extends into the periodontal ligament, cementum, and/or bone. Initially, both diseases are treated with scaling and root planing, elimination of factors contributing to the disease, and excellent home care. Extensive cases may require surgery as well.

▶ Dental assistants in a periodontic office work as part of a team to develop rapport, examine, present findings, treat, and provide continuing care to patients with periodontal disease. The responsibilities of the assistant in periodontics are vital to successful treatment and smooth team functioning.

▶ Assistants in periodontics care for periodontal instruments, prepare tray setups, prepare occlusal registrations, assist in surgery, maintain infection control procedures, provide postoperative directions, remove sutures, and place and remove periodontal dressings.

BIBLIOGRAPHY

American Academy of Periodontology: *Current procedural terminology for periodontics,* ed 5, Chicago, 1987, The Academy.
Genco RK, Goldman HM, Cohen DW: *Contemporary periodontics,* St Louis, 1990, Mosby.
Hoag PM, Pawiak EA: *Essentials of periodontics,* ed 4, St Louis, 1990, Mosby.
Grant DA, Stern IB, Listgarten MA, editors: *Periodontics in the tradition of Gottlieb and Orban,* ed 6, St Louis, 1988, Mosby.
Ishikawa J et al, editors: *Recent advances in clinical periodontology,* New York, 1988, Excerpta Medica.
Lindhe J: *Textbook of clinical periodontology,* ed 2, Copenhagen, 1988, Munksgaard.
Wilkins M: *Clinical practice of the dental hygienist,* ed 6, Philadelphia, 1989, Lea & Febiger.

38 Forensic Dentistry

LEARNING OBJECTIVES

You will have mastered the material in this chapter when you can:

- Define the key terms
- Explain the importance of accurate patient records and radiographs to the identification of human remains
- Explain the process of dental identification of human remains
- Describe the role of the dental assistant in forensic odontology
- Explain the organization and duties of a forensic dental identification team
- Identify the armamentarium used in the identification of human remains
- Explain the rationale for marking of dental prostheses and appliances
- List situations when bite marks might occur
- List the protocol for bite mark case management
- List the components of child abuse and the likely subject of abuse
- List the signs of child abuse
- Explain the responsibilities for reporting suspected child abuse by health care professionals
- Explain the significance of forensic odontology to public service

KEY TERMS

Adjudication	Identification
Antemortem	Litigation
Assailant	Mass disaster
Coroner	Medical examiner
Forensic anthropologist	Perpetrator
Forensic odontology	Postmortem

Forensic Odontology

Forensic odontology, or forensic dentistry, is the art and science of dentistry as it relates to civil and criminal law. Forensic dentistry as practiced in the 1990s can be divided into the following five major areas:

  Identification of human remains
  Mass disasters
  Bite and tooth mark recognition and case management
  Child abuse and battered adult recognition

Dentists who practice forensics are often required to testify as expert witnesses regarding dental evidence in civil and criminal **litigation**, which is a legal contest by judicial process.

Although forensic odontology is not a recognized dental specialty, it requires training and expertise beyond that of the general dental practitioner or the dental specialties. The American Board of Forensic Odontology certifies dentists who have demonstrated expertise in forensic odontology by examination as diplomates.

▶ Role of the Dental Assistant

Forensic dentistry is not practiced in the traditional office setting, and the role of the dental assistant may be limited. **Identification** is providing a proof of identity for human remains and is usually done in morgues, in the offices of medical examiners or coroners, or in funeral homes. Bite mark evidence may be collected in hospitals or law enforcement facilities. The traditional role of the chairside assistant is not necessary, although auxiliaries may assist the dentist in recording data, making radiographs, and taking impressions. In mass disasters, dental teams are often composed almost exclusively of dentists; however, auxiliary personnel can assist with charting, record keeping, and radiographs.

Every dental assistant can play a significant role in two areas. First, every patient record in a practice should be legible, accurate, and as complete as possible. Mass disasters are natural or human-created events that can result in the death of a large number of people in a localized area. When individuals die in a mass disaster, such as floods, hurricanes, tornadoes, plane crashes, or hotel fires or under circumstances in which their identities are questioned, requests for records, including radiographs and casts, if available, are conveyed to the dentist. The accuracy of charting and the quality and proper mounting and labeling of the radiographs may make a difference in the ability of the forensic team to positively identify the deceased individual.

Second, dental assistants may observe evidence of child abuse in patients seen in the dental office. Suspected abuse should be called to the attention of the dentist, who is mandated by law to report these incidents to the appropriate authorities.

▶ Identification of Human Remains

No two individuals, including identical twins, have exactly the same dentition. Since teeth withstand both fire and decomposition, they can be used in identifying unknown persons if accurate antemortem (before death) dental records are available for comparison. Bodies that are burned beyond visual recognition usually have much of the dentition intact. Although the unprotected anterior teeth are often charred, the posterior dentition is protected by the cheeks and usually remains intact. Victims of drowning are frequently distorted, preventing positive visual identification. Decomposed and even skeletal remains can be positively identified by comparing postmortem (after death) and antemortem dental data.

> **F Y I** In 1776 the body of General Joseph Warren was identified by Paul Revere on the basis of a dental prosthesis that Revere had made for him. This was the first recorded identification by dental means in U.S. history.

If the dentition is not intact because of decomposition, dismemberment, or fire, the area where the body was found should be carefully searched for teeth and other dental evidence. The age, race, and sex of decomposed bodies or skeletal remains can be determined in conjunction with a forensic anthropologist, who studies the science of human beings in application to the legal system and law (Fig. 38-1).

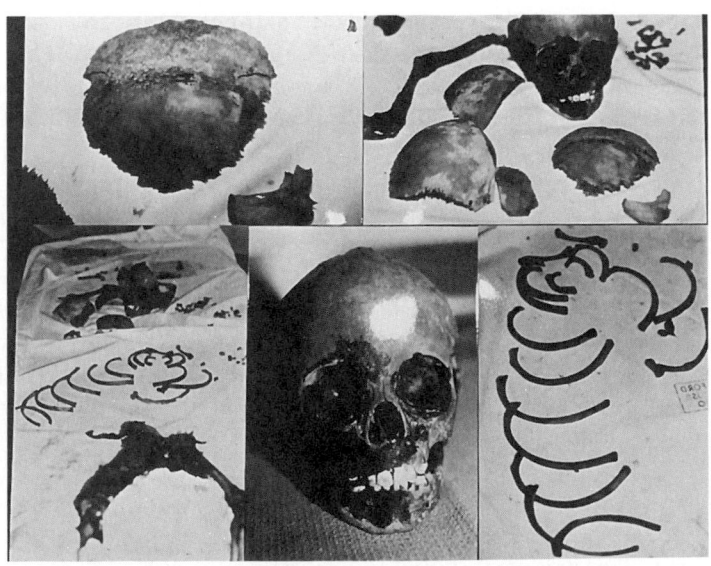

FIG. 38-1   All available human remains are gathered for examination and identification purposes.

(Courtesy of Allan J. Warnick, D.D.S., Wayne County Medical Examiner's Office, Detroit, Michigan.)

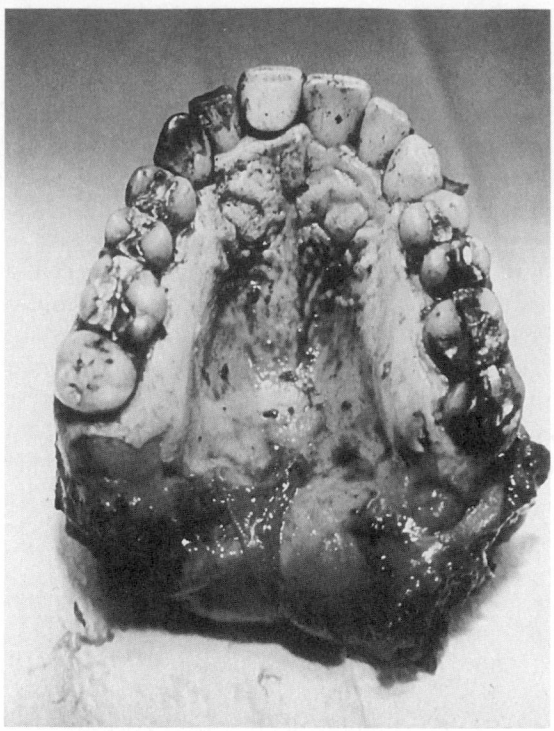

FIG. 38-2   Maxillary arch from the remains of a body that has been charted tooth-by-tooth for comparison to antemortem records.

(Courtesy of Allan J. Warnick, D.D.S., Wayne County Medical Examiner's Office, Detroit, Michigan.)

POSTMORTEM DATA COLLECTION

Unless the body is to be prepared for viewing, the jaws are usually resected to allow better access for charting and radiographs (Fig. 38-2). The dentition of the postmortem remains is visually charted tooth by tooth, noting all dental restorations and their types, apparent caries, anomalies, abrasions, erosion, implants, prostheses, and missing teeth. (Teeth that are missing post mortem that were apparently present before death are noted as *missing post mortem* to distinguish them from those teeth that are missing ante mortem. Other information, such as the victim's periodontal condition and occlusal relationships (including single malpositioned teeth), is also recorded when possible. Periapical and bitewing radiographs are made for comparison with antemortem films. Photographs of the oral structures may also be helpful.

In addition to collecting data for identification, forensic odontologists examine victims of homicide for evidence of bite and tooth marks. This evidence should also be documented as discussed below because since it may be needed to identify the assailant, the aggressor in a confrontation between two individuals, or the perpe-

trator, the individual who committed the crime in question.

ANTEMORTEM DATA COLLECTION

An antemortem charting is compiled from the dental records and the supporting information that is obtained from the dentist of record for the individual in question. A form similar to that used for the postmortem charting is employed to allow ease in comparison (Fig. 38-3).

COMPARISON

If the remains are suspected to be a particular individual, the postmortem and antemortem data are compared for similarities. Restorations, crown and root morphologies, pulp chamber morphology, sinuses, and trabecular bone patterns can all be used for comparison. If sufficient consistencies are present without any discrepancies, a positive identification can be made. If the remains are of an unknown individual, then comparisons can be made with available records of missing persons for a possible identification. Records of missing persons may be supplied by the National Crime Information Center. If the available evidence is not sufficient to allow the dentist to form a conclusion, no identification can be made.

Mass Disasters

Large numbers of people may die as the result of natural or human-created disasters. Identification of the remains requires a team effort and is coordinated through the Office of the Medical Examiner or Coroner within whose jurisdiction the disaster occurs. The **medical examiner** is an appointed public official who makes postmortem examinations of bodies to determine the cause and manner of death. This position is held by a physician, usually a forensic pathologist. The coroner is an elected official who inquires by inquest into the cause of any death in which there is reason to suspect that death is not due to natural causes. Forensic odontologists work together with forensic pathologists and anthropologists, the FBI, and supporting personnel to identify the victims of the disaster. Dental hygienists and assistants may work with dentists in recording antemortem and postmortem data and in the exposure of postmortem radiographs.

 The Jonestown, Guyana, massacre/suicide in 1979 was the largest mass disaster to date in which forensic dentistry was used to identify the 913 victims.

▶ Forensic Dental Identification Team

Forensic dental identification teams have been organized in a number of states through district dental societies for

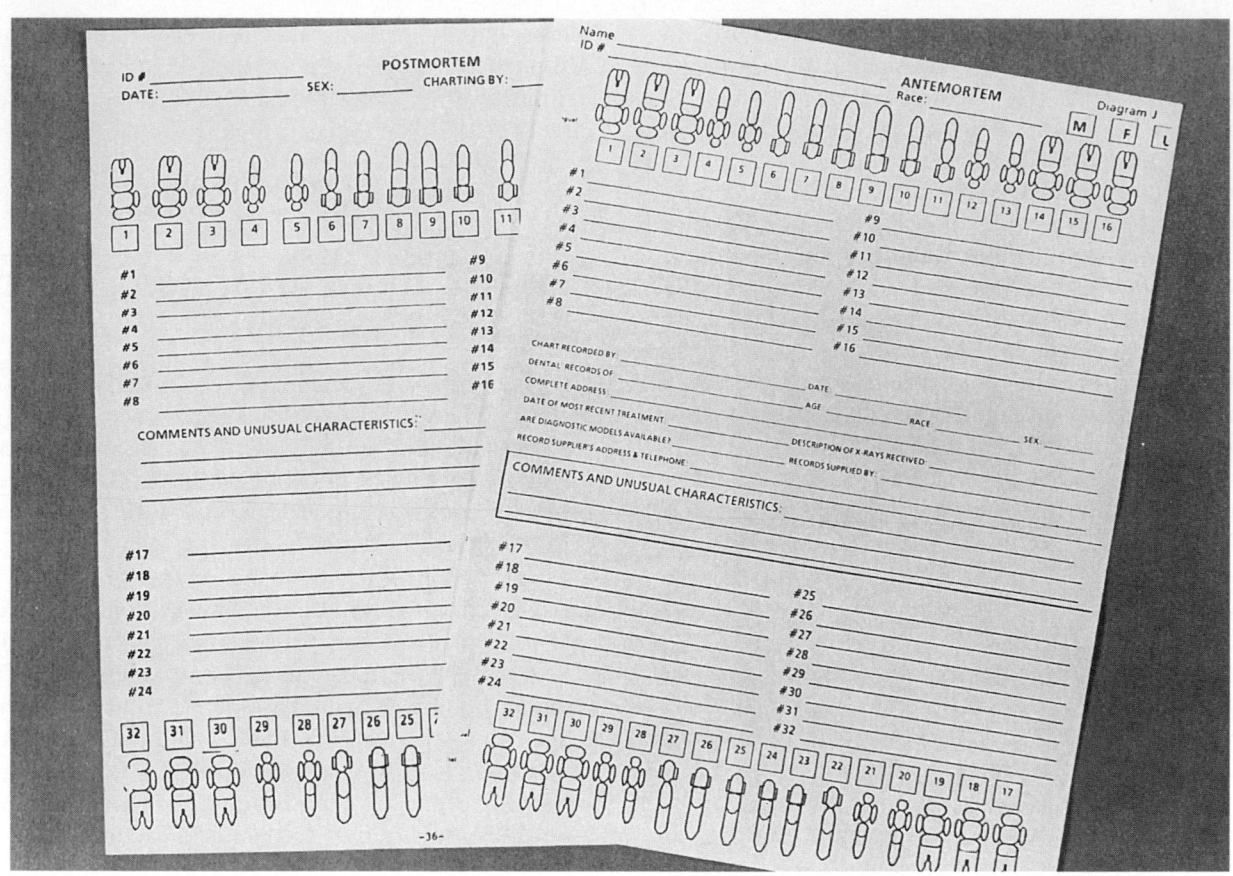

FIG. 38-3   Comparison of antemortem and postmortem clinical records.
(Courtesy of Allan J. Warnick, D.D.S., Wayne County Medical Examiner's Office, Detroit, Michigan.)

the purpose of responding in the event of a disaster in the area. Preparedness cannot be overemphasized. The team should have a team leader who is certified in forensic odontology to coordinate the team's efforts and act as the liaison between the team and the Office of the Medical Examiner or other agency in charge. Forensic dental teams are typically divided into four sections: postmortem, photography and radiography, antemortem, and comparison. Each section should have a leader or supervisor who is responsible for coordinating the section's efforts and for conveying the section's results to the team leader.

POSTMORTEM AND THE PHOTOGRAPHY AND RADIOGRAPHY SECTIONS

The remains are transported to a designated location. In airline disasters such a location has often been an available hangar. Refrigerated trucks can also be used as holding facilities. Personal effects, fingerprints, identifying markings (tattoos, scars), and pertinent anthropologic data are documented by the appropriate individuals (medical examiner, FBI) as belonging to the corpse, which is assigned an identifying number.

Dental data are collected as described above. Postmortem dental section members work in teams of three. The three individuals may be three dentists or two dentists and one auxiliary. One dentist examines the remains, another dentist or the auxiliary records, and the third dentist confirms the data. There is no room for error in identifying the victims of a mass disaster. Additional team members from the photography and radiography section work in pairs to photograph the dentition and to expose periapical and bitewing radiographs. Forms such as those presented in Fig. 38-3 are employed for recording the data. Standard designations are employed to represent the various restorations and other findings. Ideally both an anatomic charting and a written description are employed.

ANTEMORTEM SECTION

Dental and medical records of those individuals who were likely to be involved in the disaster are requested in writing from the dentist on record, either by the responsible agency or by their designee. Upon receipt, these must be cataloged. Medical records may also be cataloged in the antemortem dental section and made available to the medical examiner.

Dental data are recorded on a standardized form similar to that used in recording postmortem data to afford ease in comparison. Again, standard designations are used in recording data. Teams of three dentists or two dentists and one auxiliary work together to interpret the submitted records. Inaccurate, illegible records frequently make this task difficult to impossible. The section leader or his or her designee may telephone the office, supplying the records to aid in the interpretation. Occasionally, records that indicate contradictory information are obtained from multiple dentists for the same individual. The necessity for accurate, legible records cannot be overemphasized.

COMPARISON SECTION

After all postmortem records are recorded and the antemortem data have been compiled, the process of comparison can begin. In disasters involving large numbers of victims, computer systems have become a valuable, time-saving asset. By entering postmortem and antemortem data into a data base, possible matches can be obtained by comparing each postmortem record with each antemortem record. Those records that are a possible match can then be directly compared by section leaders. If no inconsistencies are found, a positive identification based on dental information can be made.

Armamentarium for Identifications

Identification kits typically include a wide variety of supplies, including staplers, marking pens, zip-lock plastic bags, modeling clay, plastic buckets, dental x-ray film, cotton rolls, and toothbrushes. Identification kits include traditional dental instruments, such as mirrors, explorers, scalers, and scalpels but also include mallets, chisels, and long-handled pruning shears. Scissors, tissue forceps, portable x-ray units, automatic developers, x-ray view boxes, and personal protective equipment are a few of the other items needed for mass identifications.

Marking of Dental Prostheses

A number of states now require that all newly fabricated removable dental prostheses and appliances contain identifying markings, such as the name and social security number of the individual for whom the device is made. In addition to its obvious usefulness in identifying unknown persons, this information is particularly useful in nursing homes or in other extended care facilities where elderly patients may misplace their dentures. Although it has happened, individuals rarely wear a denture or other dental appliance fabricated for someone else.

Bite and Tooth Mark Recognition and Case Management

Bite and tooth mark evidence is recognized by the courts and may be important in criminal and civil litigation that result in adjudication, a judicial decision or sentence. Initial recognition of bite and tooth marks, followed by proper recording and documentation of the lesion, is critical as trace evidence.

It is possible for bite marks to be present in any situation that involves direct, violent contact between two individuals. Tooth pattern injuries can be seen in sexual assaults (heterosexual or homosexual), nonsexual assaults, homicides, and child abuse and battered adult cases. Any victim of an assault may have been bitten. Conscious victims should be questioned regarding the possibility of having been bitten or of having bitten the assailant. Unconscious or deceased victims should be examined thoroughly, since any part of the body may show evidence of bite and tooth marks. Bite and tooth mark injuries can show brush/rub or bruiselike patterns, laceration, avulsion of tissue, or a combination of all of these (Fig. 38-4).

Individuals who seek treatment for human or animal bites may present to the emergency room or the dental office. The primary concern of the health care professional must be the care of the victim/patient; the collection of bitemark evidence must never interfere with timely patient treatment. Whenever possible, authorization for collecting evidence should be received before any procedures. The collection of evidence should follow a routine procedure once the bite mark has been recognized and described in the medical/dental record.

▶ Bite Mark Protocol

Photographs are noninvasive and need not interfere with prompt patient treatment. Photographs should include both orientation and closeup views (see Fig. 38-4). These should be made before the area is sutured, whenever possible. Collection of trace salivary evidence should also be undertaken by swabbing of the wounds. Approximately 80% of the population secretes blood type proteins in their saliva. This laboratory data can be used as evidence in implicating the perpetrator.

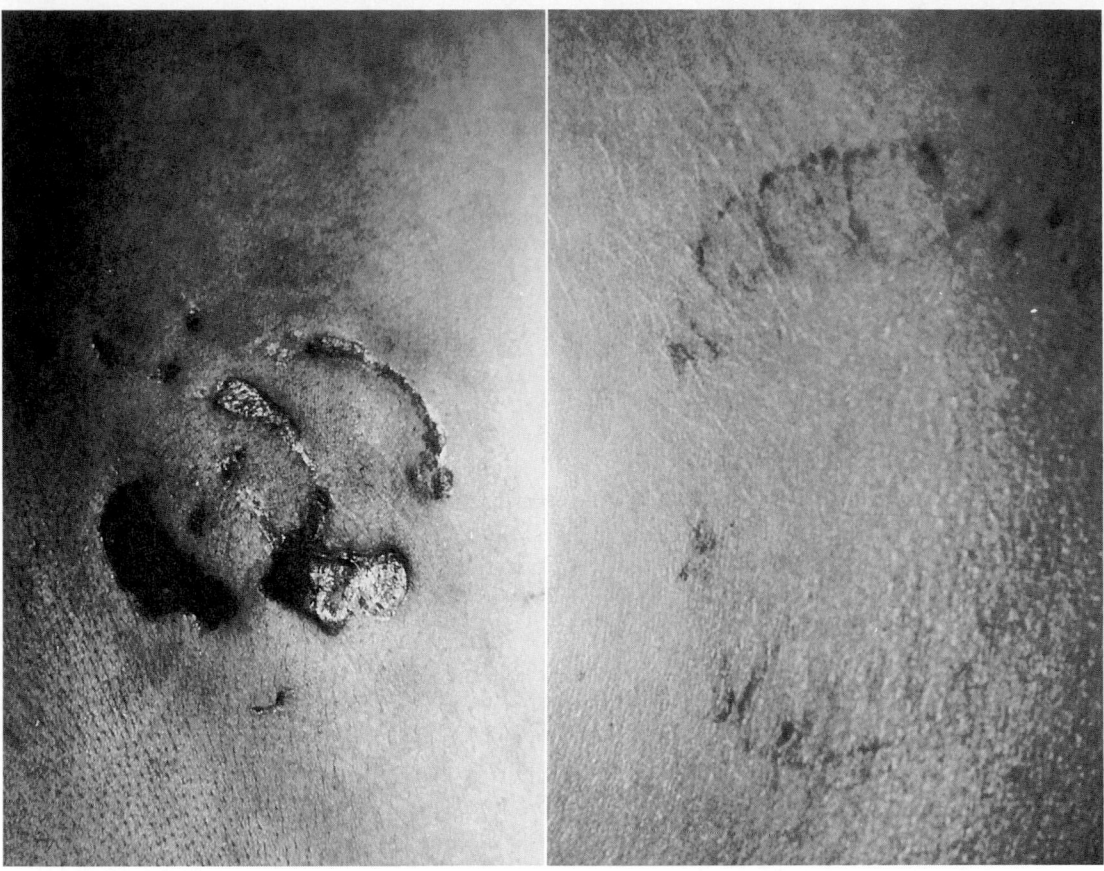

FIG. 38-4   Teeth marks on a victim's body can identify the assailant.

(Courtesy of Allan J. Warnick, D.D.S., Wayne County Medical Examiner's Office, Detroit, Michigan.)

 In 1906 tooth imprints left on a piece of cheese at the scene of a burglary in England were used to convict one of two suspects. This was the first use of bite mark evidence in a court case.

Impressions of the wound pattern are useful if there are dimensional changes in the area after it has been bitten. Wound pattern impressions can be obtained from victims who are living or deceased. The impression should be made with a resilient dental impression material, such as a vinyl polysiloxane, which is routinely used by the dentist in his or her practice. Various methods are used for making a nondistortable backing for the impression. The resultant impression is poured in commercial die stone first for a master model and poured again for a duplicate working model. Both the impressions and the models are retained as evidence.

Follow-up photography may be used to elicit wound patterns at a later date. Infrared and ultraviolet photog-raphy can be used to visualize old wound patterns that cannot be seen by routine procedures; these are especially helpful in detecting old wounds in abuse cases.

▶ Forensic Dental Workup of the Suspect

Dental data must be collected from the suspected assailant when the victim presents with a bite or a tooth mark. A search warrant that describes all procedures necessary for documentation must be obtained. Saliva and blood samples are taken for comparison with the salivary evidence. A complete oral examination, intraoral and extraoral photographs, dental impressions, and bite registrations are obtained by the forensic dentist. In addition, the dentist photographs and makes impressions of any marks on the suspect that might be relevant to the case.

▶ Armamentarium for Bite and Tooth Mark Evaluation

Instruments that are used to examine and to make impressions are necessary; these are usually transported in a portable case. When dental evidence is collected from living suspects, sterile instrument packs and impression trays must be available. In the documentation of bite and tooth marks, a quality 35-mm camera with a macrolens is a necessity.

▶ Evaluation of Bite and Tooth Mark Evidence

The evaluation of bite and tooth mark evidence should be undertaken only by a trained forensic odontologist. Methods for comparing evidence include overlays, video superimposition, scanning electron microscopy, transillumination, and alternative light photography.

Clear plastic overlays can be used to trace tooth patterns from 1:1 ratio photographs of the bite or tooth mark and the dentition of the suspect. These can then be superimposed. Videos can now be used for the same purpose. Scanning electron microscopy is sometimes used to magnify unique patterns found in the wound and on the dentition of the suspect, thus making them more apparent.

Transillumination involves the visualization of underlying patterns from tissue samples of the bite mark obtained from a dead victim. Alternative light photography is the use of infrared and ultraviolet photography to visualize old wound pattern injuries that can no longer be seen by the naked eye.

Child Abuse

Each year more than 2.7 million children are abused or neglected by caregivers, relatives, or strangers. Over a thousand children die annually as a result of this abuse; 1033 deaths that are caused by abuse were reported to the National Commission for the Prevention of Child Abuse in 1991. Child abuse may be classified as physical, sexual, emotional, or overall neglect.

Abuse occurs at all educational, economic, and social levels. Any child can be the subject of abuse. Health professionals are mandated by law to report suspected abuse in all states, and in most states they are given immunity from civil or criminal liability when the report is made in good faith. Furthermore, reporting suspected abuse may prevent the additional suffering and possible death of an innocent child.

Dentists are faced with child abuse in two ways. The forensic dentist may be presented with a postmortem case of a child who has bite or tooth marks. Second,

patients in the dental practice may be victims of child abuse.

▶ Suspicion of Child Abuse

Children who show signs of overall poor care and neglect, who are unduly aggressive or withdrawn, or who bear signs of previous injuries should be suspected as being victims of child abuse. The victim's behavior is particularly relevant. Abused children may exhibit atypical fear of the dental visit or withdraw and become silent or otherwise inhibited in the presence of the parents (the possible perpetrators). Abused children may also manifest various neuroses, encephalopathies, autism, or childhood schizophrenia. Psychotic withdrawal in abused children is characterized by a shuffling gait with eyes focused on the floor and unresponsiveness to the environment.

Abusive parents are frequently distrustful of others and reluctant to give information regarding the child's injuries. They may be overly critical of the child or totally ignore the child. They may refuse to cooperate with the suggested treatment and fail to keep follow-up appointments.

▶ Examination of the Child

The child should be interviewed without the parents present. The extraoral and intraoral examination should include both visual and palpable examination of the head, neck, and all oral structures. Exposed body parts should be viewed for obvious scars, keloids, lacerations, bruises, possible bite and tooth marks, and other signs of injury. The intraoral examination may reveal suspicious findings, such as untreated fractures of teeth, discolored or devital teeth, fistulous tracts, oral burns, and lacera-

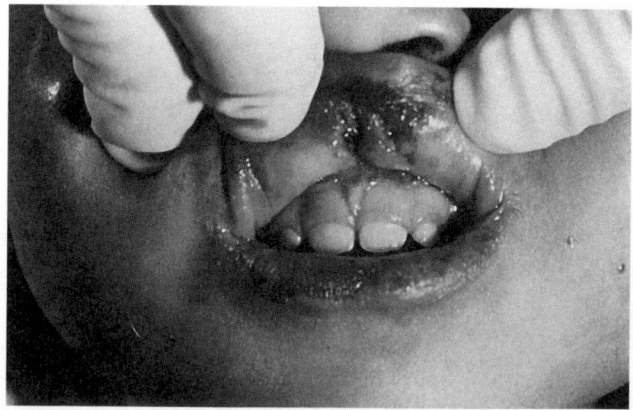

FIG. 38-5   Labial laceration can be a sign of child abuse, depending on the child's age and mobility.

(Courtesy of Allan J. Warnick, D.D.S., Wayne County Medical Examiner's Office, Detroit, Michigan.)

tions of the lip, frenum, or uvula. A torn labial frenum is common in children learning to walk but should prompt suspicion when it is observed in infants or children who are freely ambulatory (Fig. 38-5).

▶ Bite and Tooth Marks

Bite and tooth marks may be found on any area of the body. They are most commonly seen on the cheek, shoulders, chest, abdomen, arms, legs, and buttocks. Bite marks may be single or multiple. Single tooth marks may also be observed. Bite marks may appear as bruising, *suck-like* marks; incised marks, with bruising lacerations; and even avulsion of tissue. If the dental assistant is suspicious, he or she should ask the child about being bitten. Siblings may sometimes be the aggressors in situations where other signs of abuse are not apparent. Markings made by belts, belt buckles, cords, wires, and other tools may also be seen in child abuse.

▶ Documentation and Reporting

Injuries should be documented in the medical and dental records. Photographs with a reference scale should be made. Parental consent is usually not necessary for photographs of visible areas or radiographs that are taken to document suspected abuse.

Reports of suspected abuse should be made to the state or county Social Services Office, the Bureau of Child Welfare, the Department of Family Services, or the local police department. In most states, failure to report suspected abuse is a misdemeanor.

Battered Adults

Adults, particularly those who are dependent on others, may be victims of abuse. The dental team should be aware of the possibility of abuse in adults who present with traumatic injuries, especially when the stated cause is inconsistent with the injury, when dental injuries are repeated, or when evidence of bruising or bites exists. Women and older adults are most often victims. If the perpetrator brings the patient to the dental office, he or she may be reluctant to allow the patient to be alone with dental office personnel.

If abuse of a competent adult is suspected, the dentist should make the patient aware of the phone numbers of possible social services agencies that might be of assistance. Documentation should be placed in the patient record. If the patient is mentally challenged or otherwise incompetent, the dentist should notify appropriate authorities of suspected abuse.

Public Service

Forensic odontology is frequently undertaken as a public service to the community. Although most dentists who are regularly involved in forensics are paid for their expertise, the satisfaction of providing a service to the community by identifying a deceased individual or by assisting a child or other victim in need is frequently the major reward for such a service. The families of individuals who have died in a mass disaster or as the victim of a brutal homicide or suicide need the certainty of knowing that the body is indeed that of their loved one. An identification of a nonrecognizable body by dental means allows the family to begin the process of accepting their loss.

KEY POINTS

▶ Forensic odontology involves dentistry in relation to civil and criminal law. Dentists who are trained and have expertise in this area can become involved in identifying human remains, in coordinating team sections in mass disasters, in investigating bite and tooth marks, in gathering evidence and perhaps testifying as expert witnesses in courts of law, and, finally, in evaluating postmortem evidence in child abuse or battered adult cases that result in death.

▶ Dental assistants play an important role in the identification process by recording accurate data, making radiographs, and taking impressions. The accuracy of these records is critical to positive identification of individuals.

▶ Through a comparison of postmortem data and antemortem data, human remains may be identified. Other skeletal structures besides dentition may also be used to assist in the identification process.

▶ Mass disasters are responded to most efficiently by prepared teams, which include the forensic dental identification team. The team comprises four sections: postmortem exam, photography and radiography, antemortem data, and comparison.

▶ Identification kits contain supplies and equipment that are needed for mass identifications.

▶ When new removable dental prostheses and appliances are made, some form of identification (the individual's name or social security number) is marked on the prostheses. However, not all states require this invaluable identification tool.

▶ Tooth patterns are studied and evidence is carefully gathered and documented during bite injury investigation. This evidence is recognized by the courts as providing proof of the assailant's identity.

▶ Photographs, salivary samples taken from the wound, and impressions of the wound pattern are all part of bite mark protocol. These may later be compared to saliva and blood samples, dentition impressions, and photographs of a suspect.

▶ Evidence that is taken from samples is compared, using overlay methods, video superimposition, electron microscopy scans, transillumination, and alternative light photography.

▶ All health professionals are required by law to report any suspected cases of abuse. Many states give immunity or protect the person reporting an abuse case from any civil or criminal liability.

▶ Forensic dentists are involved in abuse cases when identification of bite and tooth marks is necessary.

▶ Dentists and dental auxiliaries may encounter child abuse victims among their patients.

▶ Signs of child abuse include overall poor care and neglect, unduly aggressive or withdrawn behavior, and physical signs of injury. These children should be interviewed by the dentist without the parents present.

BIBLIOGRAPHY

Averill DC, editor: *Manual of forensic odontology*, Colorado Springs, 1991, American Academy of Forensic Odontology.

Cottone JA, Standish SM, editors: *Outline of forensic dentistry*, Chicago, 1982, Yearbook Medical Publishers.

Warnick AJ: *Forensic dental identification team manual*, Lansing, 1989, Michigan Dental Association.

UNIT VIII LABORATORY PROCEDURES

39 Basic Dental Laboratory Procedures

LEARNING OBJECTIVES

You will have mastered the material in this chapter when you can:
▶ Define the key terms
▶ Identify rules for safety in the laboratory
▶ Explain techniques for infection control in the laboratory
▶ Explain the use of a dental laboratory prescription or work order
▶ Describe the function of MSDS in relation to the laboratory
▶ Identify basic equipment used in the laboratory within a dental practice

KEY TERMS

Alcohol lamp	Gypsum bins
Articulator	Investment oven
Bunsen burner	Laboratory prescription
Casting machine	Model trimmer
Casting oven	Sandblaster
Dental engine	Vacuum investing
Dental lathe	Vacuum machine
Gas torch	Vibrator

The laboratory in a dental office presents an opportunity for an assistant to become acquainted with equipment that is not found in the dental treatment room. Many laboratory procedures are performed in a commercial laboratory, but basic tasks may be performed by an assistant within the office. Perhaps the most common of these tasks are pouring impressions, trimming diagnostic models, and constructing custom-made trays. Baseplates, mouthguards, copings, and even waxed patterns for investment and casting procedures may be done in the office. The accessibility to a commercial laboratory, cost-effectiveness, skills of the staff, and the personal interests of the dentist will dictate the extent that various laboratory duties may be delegated to the assistant.

 The first successful commercial laboratory was organized in Boston by Dr. William H. Stowe, a dentist, and Frank F. Eddy, a toolmaker and machinist.

Rules for Safety in the Dental Laboratory

Since the laboratory is filled with the potential for accidents, a few basic rules should be followed to promote safety in this area.

1. No smoking should be a general rule. It is especially important not to smoke in the laboratory, since many flammable agents are used in this area.
2. Safety glasses must be worn when operating any rotary equipment, such as the dental lathe, model trimmer, or handpiece, when using the Bunsen burner, and when chipping away plaster or stone from models.
3. Hair should be pulled back and secured. Long hair can become entangled in rotary devices. Bending over a Bunsen burner can also create a potential hazard if hair is not secured.
4. Hanging jewelry or clothing, such as chains, ties, or scarves, should not be worn. Like long hair, any dangling clothing simply enhances the chance for an accident.
5. Do not lean over a Bunsen burner or a torch. Also, be certain to turn off these devices completely before leaving the area.
6. If a handpiece with an engine belt is used, change the belt frequently to avoid unexpected breaks in the belt. Maintain adequate tension on the belt to eliminate undue stress.

Complete information is needed, including the full name of the dentist to avoid confusion with dentists who have a similar name.

Details about the type of dental materials to be used in the case are recorded; including a shade button is helpful.

Specific instructions about the case must be detailed here. Drawings of prosthesis design may be placed here or on a special tooth chart on the back of the form.

Signature stamp may be used. Verification must be filed with the laboratory.

Include adequate time for return of lab case to be examined by the dentist before the patient's appointment.

LAB COPY

NAME _____ D.D.S.

ADDRESS _____ PHONE

CITY

SHARP LABORATORIES

3145 Professional Dr. —— Ann Arbor, Michigan 48104

971-5120

DATE: LAB CASE NO.

PATIENT'S NAME & NUMBER: AGE
SEX

TIME WANTED: FOR TRY IN METAL: BASE MAT.
☐ GOLD ☐
☐ CHROME ALLOY ☐

TIME WANTED: FOR FINISH MOULD
SHADE
MAKE

TYPE AND DESCRIPTION OF CASE
PLEASE GIVE COMPLETE INSTRUCTIONS

INSTRUCTIONS

℞

FURTHER INSTRUCTIONS AND DESIGN ON BACK OF FORM

DENTIST'S SIGNATURE _____ D.D.S.

LICENSE NO. _____

"This form designed and approved by the Michigan State Board of Dentistry in Compliance with Michigan Act No. 198, 1961."

FIG. 39-1 Laboratory requisition with major descriptions of information.

(Courtesy of Sharp Laboratory, Ann Arbor, Michigan.)

7. Keep electrical cords out of areas where water is used.
8. Turn off lathes, handpieces, model trimmers, and other rotary devices when they are not in use.
9. Use acceptable ventilation and exhaust systems when working with dental materials such as acrylic or when grinding on the lathe.
10. Follow OSHA guidelines for the handling of laboratory materials and substances.

Infection Control in the Dental Laboratory

Whether the setting is an office laboratory or a commercial laboratory, infection control guidelines must meet the requirements set by the Occupational Safety and Health Administration (OSHA). In addition, the National Association of Dental Laboratories has developed guidelines for its member laboratories based on these guidelines.

▶ Transferring a Patient Case to a Commercial Laboratory

Before dental materials are transferred to a commercial dental laboratory, the dental staff should rinse and disinfect (or sterilize, if appropriate) materials, including impressions, bite records, and preliminary denture set-ups. The prescription or work authorization form shown in Chapter 14 must accompany all laboratory cases and should be placed in a zip-lock bag to avoid contamination (Fig. 39-1). After disinfection or sterilization the materials should be placed in a plastic bag and heat sealed (Fig. 39-2).

Infection control protocol for exchanging a laboratory case between a dental practice and dental laboratories requires that the recommendations in Box 39-1 be followed.

▶ General Work and Production Areas

Special attention should be given to preventing the transmission of disease in the laboratory within the office. The following suggestions will aid in maintaining OSHA infection control standards as they apply to the dental laboratory.

1. Clean and disinfect work benches daily.
2. Disinfect work pans as soon as possible after removing an appliance to make certain that the pans have been decontaminated before being used again.
3. Do not eat or drink at laboratory work stations.
4. Do not use the same pumice for new work and repair work. For repair work, premeasure pumice in small amounts and discard it after each use.
5. Discard pumice that is used for new work at least once a week.
6. Wet pumice with a mixture of disinfectant and bacteriostatic soap. Do not use water alone.
7. Soak brush wheels and rag wheels in a disinfectant for 10 minutes, and allow to air dry overnight.
8. After pumice is used on a repair, disinfect the appliance for 10 minutes. These materials are surface disinfectants only, and when the material is cut or broken, the appliance must be disinfected again.

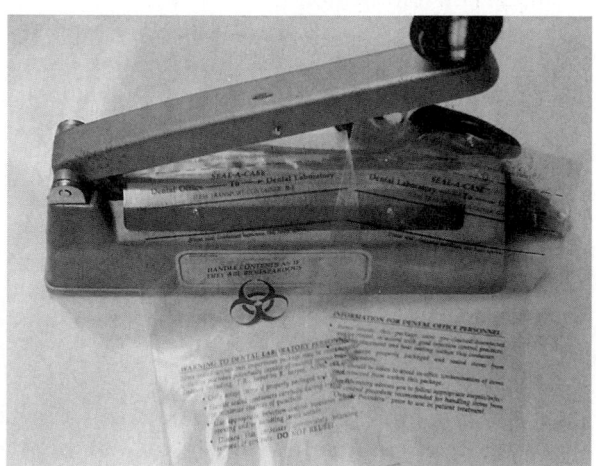

FIG. 39-2 Impressions are placed in a sealed plastic bag after disinfection and before they are transferred to the dental laboratory.

(Courtesy of Infection Control Service, Inc., Kent, Washington.)

BOX 39-1

INFECTION CONTROL PROTOCOL FOR TRANSFERRING LABORATORY CASES

▶ Do not give wet impressions to an ungloved delivery person or technician.
▶ Take care not to contaminate the delivery package. The laboratory may have to throw it away, and this will increase lab costs.
▶ Explain the infection control procedures that are followed in the office to the dental technicians. Identify the types of infection control materials that are used.
▶ Repeat infection control procedures each time the case is returned to the original laboratory or dental office for a try-in or adjustment to avoid cross-contamination.

9. Use universal precautions, masks, glasses or face shield, and gloves when operating mechanical devices. NOTE: Use dust-mist face masks in the laboratory. All face masks used in the dental laboratory should be approved by National Institute of Occupational Safety and Health (NIOSH).

10. Use an effective suction or vacuum system when an appliance is ground.

11. Keep disinfectant solutions readily available in the laboratory.

12. In states where denturism is legal, the denturist is responsible for following the same infection control procedures used in the dental treatment room regarding contact with patient's secretions.

Material Safety Data Sheets (MSDS)

The OSHA Hazard Communication Standard, Title 29 Code of Federal Regulations 1910.1200, requires that all dental professionals take certain steps to comply with the standard. Compliance instruction includes a training program that involves a review of a compiled list of hazardous chemicals, collection and maintenance of material safety data sheets (MSDS) (shown in Chapter 8), and proper labeling of all chemicals on site. It seems appropriate that this OSHA standard be reviewed in this chapter, since many of the hazardous materials used in the dental office are handled in the laboratory. Also, many dentists find it appropriate to have the data sheets displayed in this area of the office rather than the treatment or business areas.

▶ Hazardous Chemicals

The list of products that contain hazardous chemicals varies with the individual dental office and with the types of materials that are kept in each facility. Consequently, a standardized listing is not accurate for every office and must be customized to reflect products in each facility.

Certain products that are used daily include substances that are considered hazardous chemicals. A careful inspection of product labels provides information about the substances within the product that are considered to be hazardous. This form of labeling is a requirement of dental manufacturers when any product contains a hazardous chemical. The other source of information regarding hazardous chemicals is provided on the MSDS sheets. All manufacturers of products containing hazardous chemicals are legally obligated to provide the MSDS sheets for each product at the time of shipping to the purchaser.

A simple form that lists all hazardous chemicals in the dental office can be developed and made available to all dental personnel. This information could be set up as follows:

Chemical	Product	Manufacturing Company	Generic Area	MSDS on file
Mercury	Tytin	Kerr/Sybron Mfg.	Amalgam	Yes

PRECAUTIONS

Following certain specific precautions can minimize the risk from hazardous chemicals to dental personnel. The precautions regarding hazardous chemicals include handling the chemical properly in accordance with the manufacturer's or supplier's instructions. Always avoid skin contact, and minimize the chemical vapors in the air. Bottles of flammable chemicals should never be left open or used near open flames. The consumption of food or smoking in areas where chemicals are used is not allowed, and, when appropriate, protective eyewear and masks must be worn. All hazardous chemicals must be disposed of in accordance with MSDS instructions and applicable local, state, and federal regulations.

▶ Material Safety Data Sheets (MSDS)

As stated, MSDS are required to be provided by manufacturers/suppliers of hazardous chemicals to purchasers. It is also the responsibility of the manufacturer to provide accurate and proper information on the MSDS. The employer is also responsible for ensuring that the information on the sheet is complete. OSHA requires that MSDS include the following information:

- ▶ Product or chemical identity used on the label
- ▶ Manufacturer's or supplier's name and address
- ▶ Chemical and common names of each hazardous ingredient
- ▶ Name, address, and phone number for hazard and emergency information
- ▶ Preparation or revision date of MSDS
- ▶ The hazardous chemical's physical and chemical characteristics, such as vapor pressure and flashpoint
- ▶ Physical hazards, including the potential for fire, explosion, and reactivity
- ▶ Known health hazards
- ▶ OSHA-permissible exposure limit (PEL), American Conference of Government Industrial Hygienists (ACGIH) threshold limit value, threshold limit values (TLV), or other exposure limits
- ▶ Emergency and first-aid procedures
- ▶ Whether OSHA, National Toxicology Program (NTP), or International Agency for Research on Cancer (IARC) lists the ingredient as a carcinogen
- ▶ Precautions for safe handling and use
- ▶ Control measures, such as engineering controls, work practices, hygienic practices, and personal protective equipment that are required

‣ Primary routes of entry
‣ Procedure for spills, leaks, and cleanup

Dental professionals that maintain hazardous chemicals on the work premises are required to develop and maintain current files of MSDS on site and make them available to all personnel.

‣ Labeling

The Hazard Communication Standard requires labeling of all hazardous products. Certain products regulated by the Food and Drug Administration (FDA), such as impression materials, are exempt from the Hazard Communication Standard. Labels that are placed on the containers holding hazardous chemicals must not be removed for any reason. Chemicals that are transferred from the original container to a smaller container for use in the dental office should be labeled with the original label information. Many dental suppliers have labeling systems available for purchase. The information to include on the labels consists of the identity of the hazardous chemical, proper hazard warnings, and name and address of the manufacturer, importer, or other responsible party.

‣ Training Programs

Employers in a dental office are required by OSHA regulations to provide a written hazard communication program that includes specifics regarding meeting requirements for handling labeling and other forms of warning, MSDS, and employee information and training schedules. Employers are required to provide employees with information and training on all hazardous chemicals found in the dental office at any given time. If new products that are considered hazardous are purchased, training regarding these substances must be implemented.

The information employees are entitled to includes data that are reflected in the Hazard Communication Standard, work areas that contain hazardous chemicals, and the location of the written information regarding the program, lists of chemicals, and MSDS.

The training session for employees should include the means to determine the presence of a hazardous chemical in the work area, physical and health hazards of chemicals, how employees can protect themselves, and specific details of the hazard communication program of that office.

Dental Laboratory Equipment

In earlier chapters equipment that is common to the dental treatment rooms and the business office is discussed extensively. The dental assistant should have some awareness of the function of laboratory equipment.

A **dental lathe** is a common piece of equipment to any dental laboratory. In the office it is used to polish dentures, crowns, bridges, and inlays. Most lathes come supplied with a right and a left chuck onto which a variety of attachments can be placed, such as rag or chamois wheels, brushes, and burs. A splash hood must be included (with or without a light), a shield, and some form of exhaust to collect the debris that is created by the lathe. Fig. 39-3, *A*, illustrates a common set up found in many dental offices. Fig. 39-3, *B*, illustrates an assortment of polishing materials, brush wheels, and buffing wheels that are used with the dental lathe.

A 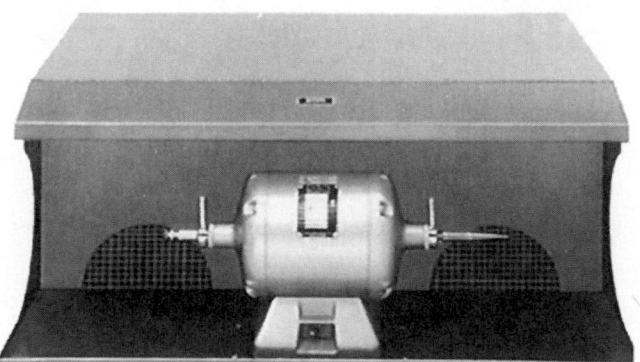 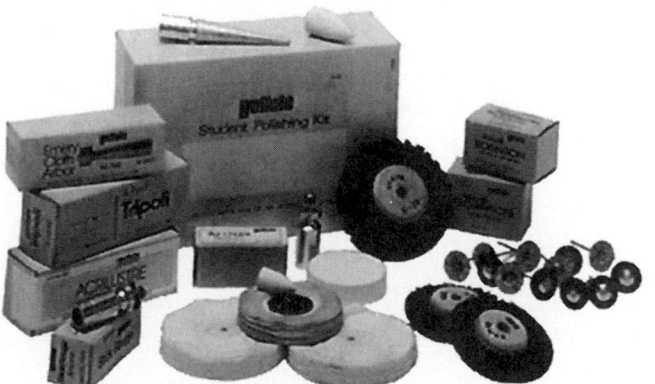 **B**

FIG. 39-3   *A,* Dental lathe with dust collector. *B,* Polishing wheels, and attachments for the lathe.

(Courtesy of Buffalo Dental Manufacturing Company, Inc., Syosset, New York.)

A **Bunsen burner** is frequently used in the dental office laboratory to warm waxes and to heat materials and solutions. The Bunsen burner that is illustrated in Fig. 39-4 provides an adjustable flame. A small tripod (Fig. 39-5) may be needed to hold a crucible when a solution is warmed; this may be placed over the Bunsen burner.

An **alcohol lamp** may be used to provide a small flame. The one shown in Fig. 39-6 is popular because it provides a flame at a right angle and it aids the operator in directing the flame to a specific area. As shown, the operator is able to melt wax on a baseplate in a specific region.

Air and **gas outlets** are needed in a laboratory. An air outlet is used frequently to dry impressions and other materials. A gas line is needed for the gas torch or Bunsen burner.

A **gas torch** may be used in some offices to provide a hot flame for casting or soldering procedures. Such a torch is frequently used in combination with oxygen to give a hot flame (Fig. 39-7).

A **vacuum machine** is used in the office to construct baseplates, custom trays, mouthguards, bruxism splints, temporary splints, and copings (Fig. 39-8, *A*). This device provides a heating element to warm the material to be used and a vacuum device that aids in the adaptation of the material to a model. Typically, the material to be used is placed into the holding frame, the heating element is placed into position and turned on, the material is softened to the desired level, and the vacuum is turned on, which allows the material to be adapted closely to a model. This procedure is described in detail in Chapter 40 for the construction of a mouthguard.

An automatic vacuum machine is available and becomes an effective piece of equipment for offices where a large number of acrylic trays, mouthguards, denture bases, relines, or copings are routinely constructed (Fig. 39-8, *B*).

A **vacuum mixing and investing machine** is a device that provides for the mixing of stone, plaster, and investment materials under a vacuum to give a smooth, dense finished product. The Vac-U-Spat is illustrated in Fig. 39-9 as it is used to prepare a mix of investment.

A **model trimmer** is a key piece of equipment in the dental laboratory. The primary use is for trimming casts both for diagnostic and working models. All trimmers come with the features identified in Fig. 39-10; more elaborate trimmers provide calibrated tables to enable trimming models at desired angles.

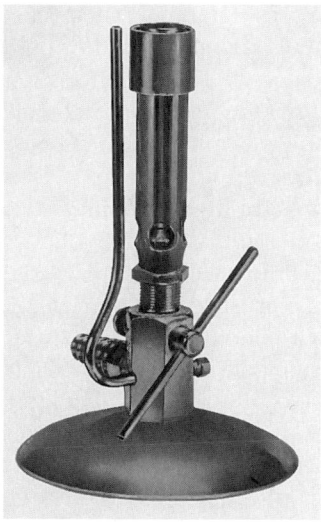

FIG. 39-4   Bunsen burner.

(Courtesy of Buffalo Dental Manufacturing Company, Inc., Syosset, New York.)

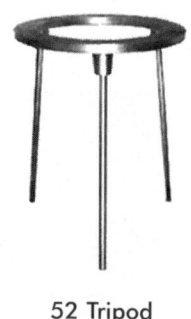

52 Tripod

FIG. 39-5   Small tripod.

(Courtesy of Buffalo Dental Manufacturing Company, Inc., Syosset, New York.)

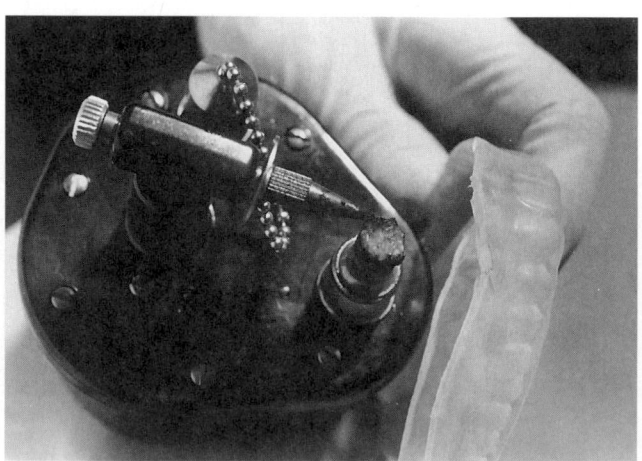

FIG. 39-6   Alcohol lamp.

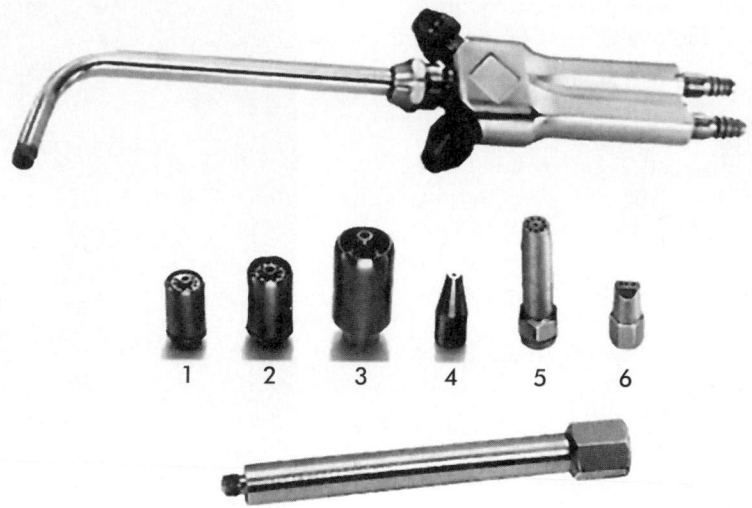

FIG. 39-7   Gas torch.

(Courtesy of Buffalo Dental Manufacturing Company, Inc., Syosset, New York.)

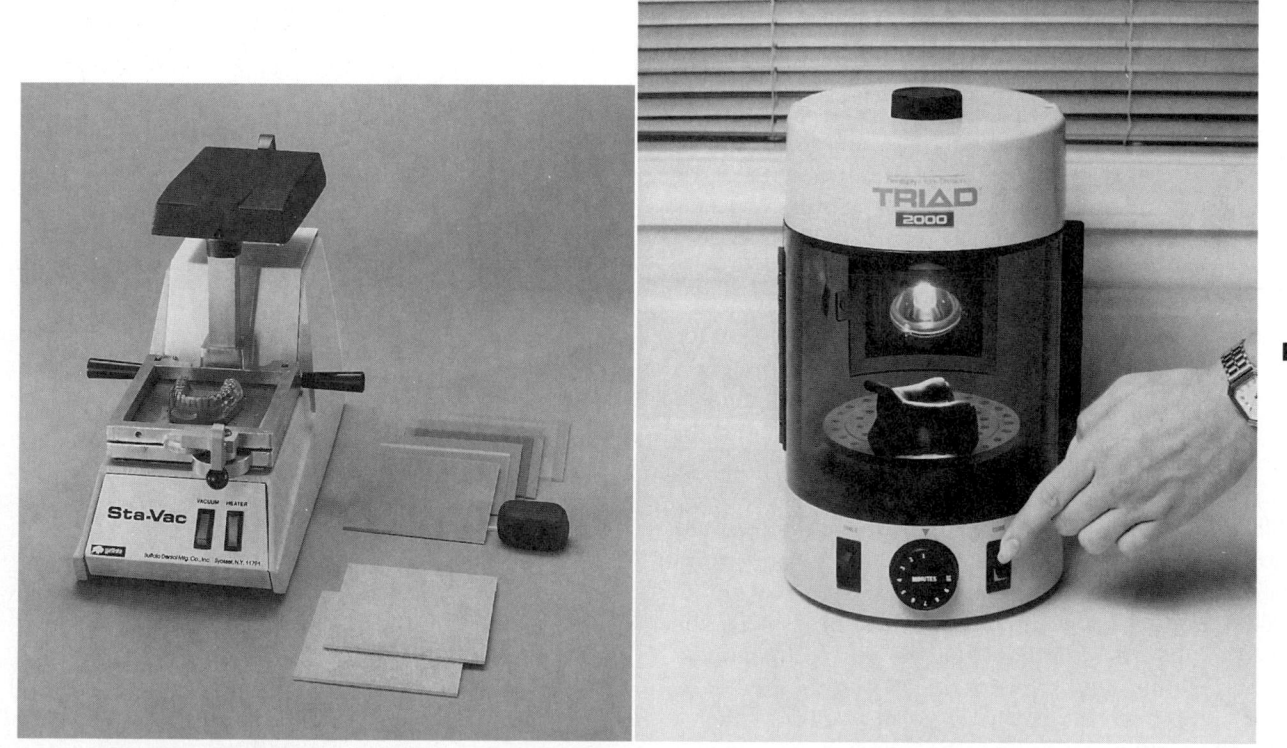

FIG. 39-8   *A,* Vacuum machine. *B,* Automatic vacuum machine.

(Courtesy of Dentsply International.)

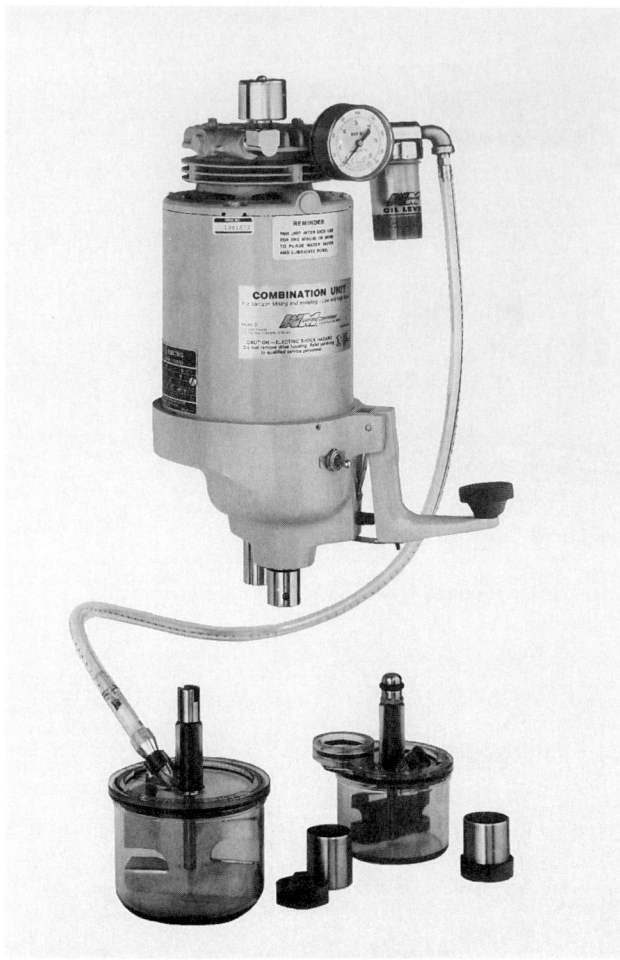

FIG. 39-9   Vac-u-Spat.

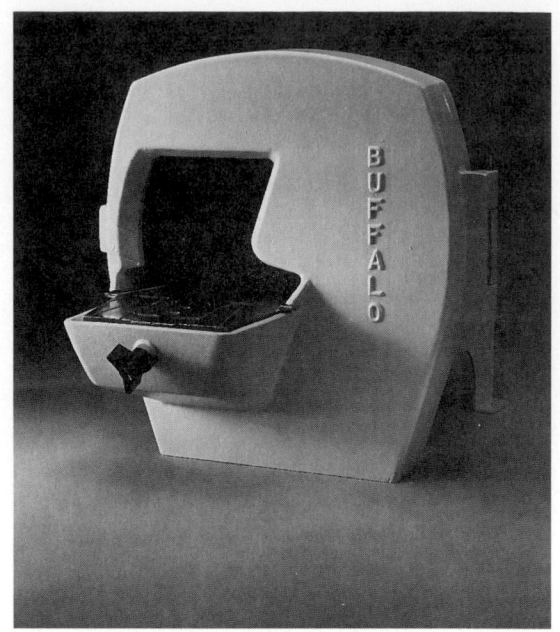

FIG. 39-10   Model trimmer.

(Courtesy of Buffalo Dental Manufacturing Company, Inc., Syosset, New York.)

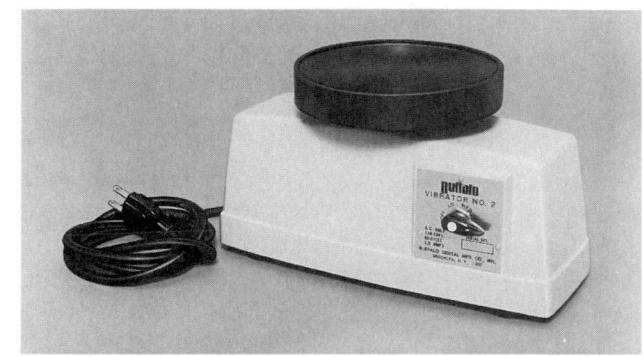

FIG. 39-11   Vibrator.

(Courtesy of Buffalo Dental Manufacturing Company, Inc., Syosset, New York.)

A small **vibrator** is an absolute necessity in any dental office. Fig. 39-11 illustrates a vibrator that is used for pouring impressions. Larger units can be purchased for heavier use. The vibrator should be covered with plastic wrap and carefully cleaned to avoid plaster buildup on the working surface.

Dental engines are a major category of equipment for the laboratory. A high-speed engine with a triple section arm is a standard version; a compact engine with a single arm is shown in Fig. 39-12. This handpiece is used for various extraoral duties, including cutting, trimming, and polishing.

Plaster/gypsum bins and laboratory benches are major pieces of equipment found in the laboratory. Plaster storage bins ensure a dry storage area for all gypsum products. The choice of lab benches is personal; they can be of different heights to accommodate standing, sitting, and wheelchairs. When the person is seated, the bench should be at or near elbow height. When the person is standing, the bench should be of a height that the operator will not need to bend over to work.

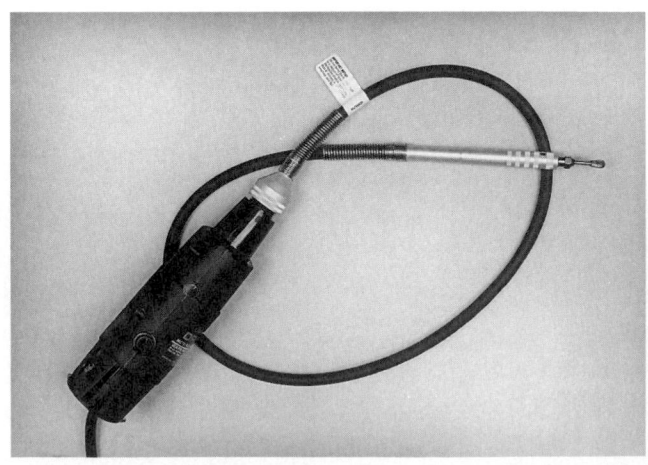

FIG. 39-12   Laboratory handpiece.

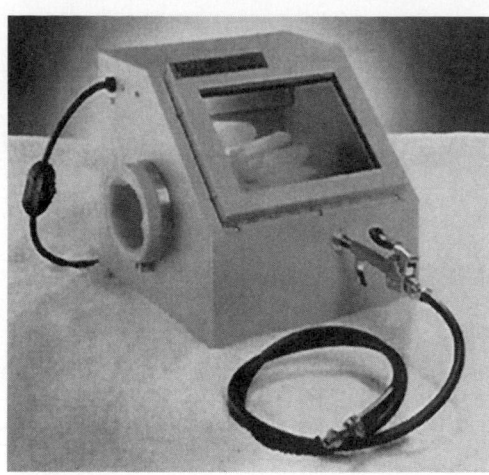

FIG. 39-13   Sandblaster.

(Courtesy of Buffalo Dental Manufacturing Company, Inc., Syosset, New York.)

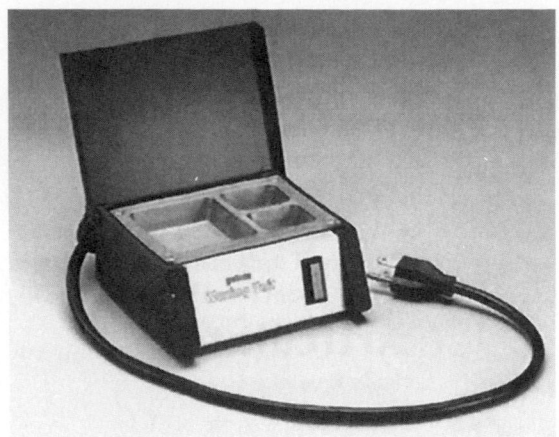

FIG. 39-14   Waxing unit.

(Courtesy of Buffalo Dental Manufacturing Company, Inc., Syosset, New York.)

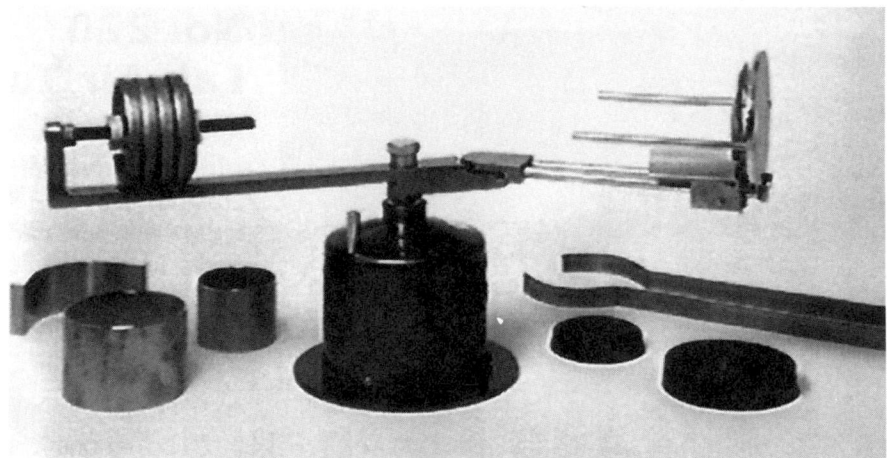

FIG. 39-15   Centrifugal casting machine.

(Courtesy of Buffalo Dental Manufacturing Company, Inc., Syosset, New York.)

On most laboratory benches some form of exhaust system will be installed. The office suite may have a central system or a countertop dust collector (see Fig. 39-3, *A*). This type of system produces a vacuum for suctioning porcelain, stone, metal, and other abrasives. The residue is collected in a water collection pan, which can be discarded.

Articulators may be used to articulate models for fixed prosthodontics, to analyze a case, or to mount denture setups for specialized relationships. The plain articulator allows for basic movements of opening and closing and for lateral movement. The more complex articulator allows the dentist to achieve special condylar movement and more precise alignment of the arches. This model

also may be used for face-bow relationships in prosthodontics with the addition of the face-bow mount (see Chapter 31).

A **sandblaster** (Fig. 39-13) provides a current of air to spray sand at a high velocity to etch or clean metal or hard surfaces. Commonly, these are used in a dental laboratory with a silica medium to clean castings or to etch the internal surface of a casting to aid in the identification of undercuts.

A **waxing unit** (Fig. 39-14) may be found in those offices where the dentist waxes patterns for investing. This heated unit melts the wax to a specific temperature and maintains the molten wax in this state.

In offices where the dentist or an in-house laboratory

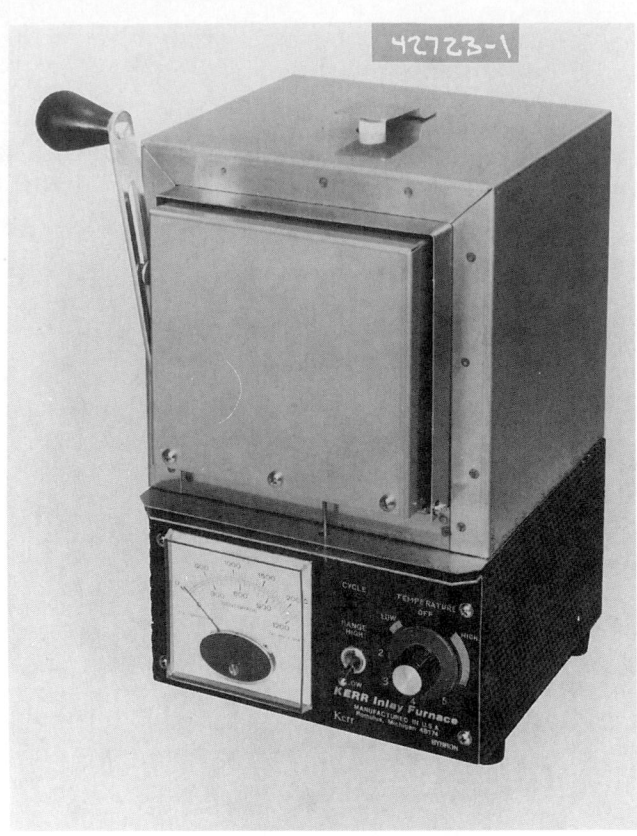

FIG. 39-16   Traditional casting oven.

(Courtesy of Kerr Manufacturing.)

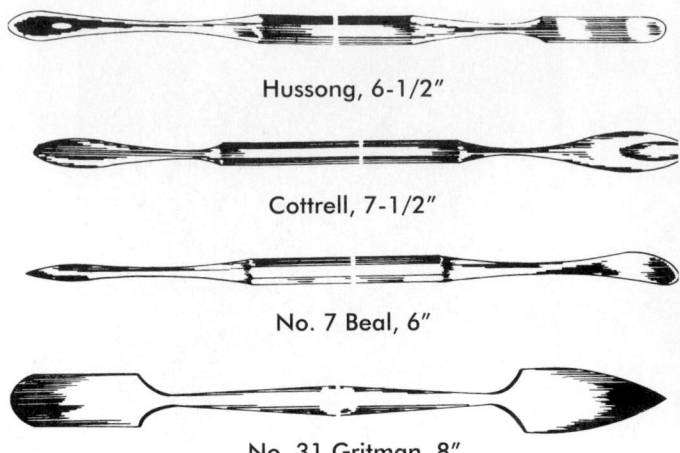

Hussong, 6-1/2"

Cottrell, 7-1/2"

No. 7 Beal, 6"

No. 31 Gritman, 8"

FIG. 39-17   Assorted laboratory instruments.

(Courtesy of Buffalo Dental Manufacturing Company, Inc., Syosset, New York.)

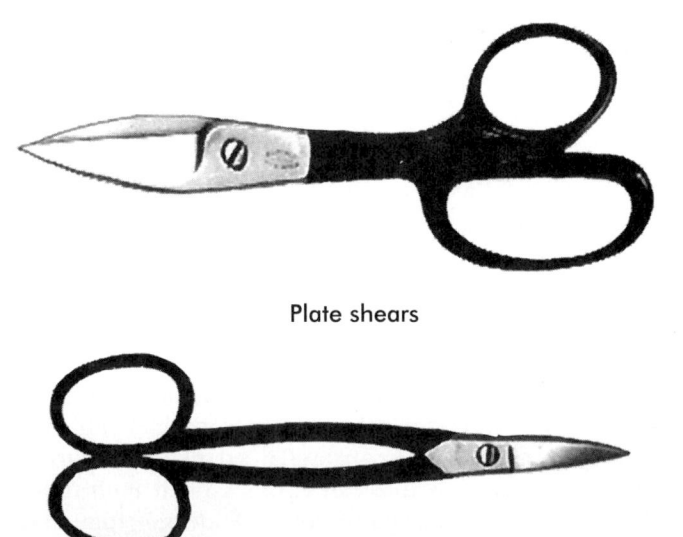

Plate shears

Plate shears

Diagonal cutting
nippers, wire, 5-1/2"

Plaster nippers, carbon steel
Plaster nippers, stainless steel

FIG. 39-18   Shears and nippers.

(Courtesy of Buffalo Dental Manufacturing Company, Inc., Syosset, New York.)

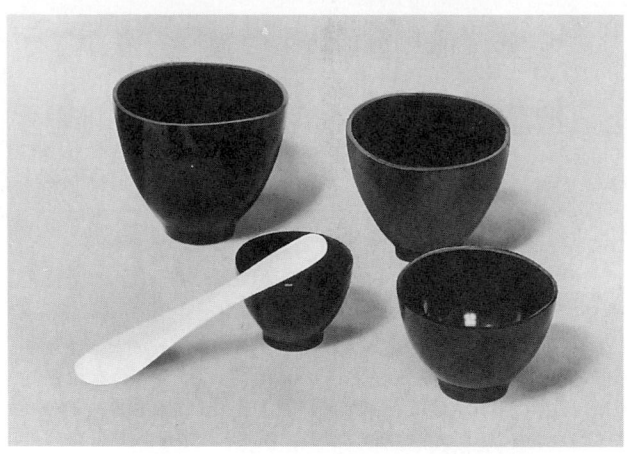

FIG. 39-19 Assorted rubber bowls.

technician is available, a **casting machine** will likely be found. Fig. 39-15 illustrates a typical centrifugal casting machine with an assortment of sprue bases and ring flasks. Tongs are used to transfer the flask from the **casting oven** in Fig. 39-16. Safety regulations require that this type of casting machine be embedded in a well so that it is not on the counter. An automatic casting machine and oven eliminate the manual steps required in the centrifugal-type casting machine.

Many small items are found in the dental laboratory. Perhaps the most widely used laboratory instruments are knives and spatulas. Laboratory spatulas may be flexible or rigid according to the materials to be mixed or to the operator's personal preference. In addition to these, an assortment of wax spatulas can be found. The most common, the #7 spatula, is used universally in waxing patterns or in many repairs. Carvers are also widely used in the laboratory to carve wax and prepare other devices. Fig. 39-17 illustrates an array of popular laboratory instruments.

It is frequently necessary to cut a variety of materials, such as copings, mouthguards, and plaster. To do this, heavy duty shears or nippers may be needed. Fig. 39-18 illustrates these shears and nippers.

Finally, the rubber bowl is used for many functions, to mix plaster, alginate, and a variety of other materials. It is a standard in any dental office (Fig. 39-19). These flexible bowls come in various sizes.

KEY POINTS

▶ The dental assistant may spend a minimal amount of time performing laboratory tasks or may find this is an activity that offers new variety to the daily tasks in the dental office. Regardless of the amount of time the dental assistant spends performing laboratory tasks, it is beneficial to become acquainted with the functions of common laboratory equipment.

▶ The dental assistant must understand the relationship between the dental practice and a commercial dental laboratory. The need for complete information on laboratory work orders, the routine to follow when transferring cases to and from the laboratory, and the role of the dental laboratory technician are all responsibilities the dental assistant must assume.

▶ Infection control is a major concern when dental materials are transferred to and from a commercial laboratory. OSHA guidelines must be followed before sending and upon receiving all materials.

▶ Record management, including laboratory prescription/requisition, MSDS, labeling, and employee training dates, is directly related to work in the dental office laboratory.

BIBLIOGRAPHY

Craig RG, O'Brien WJ, Powers JM: *Dental materials: properties and manipulation,* ed 5, St Louis, 1992, Mosby.

Department of Labor, Occupational Safety and Health Administration: *Occupational exposure to blood-borne pathogens,* Instruction CPL2-244B, December 6, 1991.

40 Advanced Dental Laboratory Procedures

LEARNING OBJECTIVES

You will have mastered the material in this chapter when you can:
▶ Define the key terms
▶ Define the purpose of diagnostic models
▶ Explain the procedure for pouring an alginate impression with a gypsum product for the purpose of creating a diagnostic model
▶ Identify the criteria for poured models
▶ Describe and demonstrate the procedure for trimming diagnostic models
▶ Explain the criteria for trimmed diagnostic models
▶ Explain the advantages for using a custom-made tray
▶ Describe and demonstrate the procedure for construction of custom-made trays
▶ Explain the criteria for clinically acceptable custom-made trays
▶ Explain the function of a mouthguard
▶ Describe the construction of a mouthguard
▶ Explain the criteria for a clinically acceptable mouthguard
▶ Describe the process of repairing a denture
▶ Describe the construction of a baseplate

Though the primary role of a dental assistant appears to be as a chairside assistant or a business office manager, he or she also routinely performs many laboratory duties. In the previous chapter the equipment common to most dental office laboratories was described; this chapter presents an opportunity to learn about the step-by-step procedure for constructing many of these laboratory devices, including diagnostic models that are made from alginate impressions, custom-made acrylic trays that are designed specifically to fit a patient's mouth, and mouthguards, as well as an overview of denture repairs and baseplate and bite rim construction.

Diagnostic Models

Probably few other laboratory projects are as frequently created as the construction of diagnostic models. **Diagnostic models** (described earlier in Chapter 24) are replicas of a patient's mouth that are studied to determine a diagnosis. In a specialty practice such as orthodontics this is a major responsibility for the dental assistant, but in a general dental practice it becomes a common routine for patients who are seeking major restorative treatment or an oral diagnosis.

The two basic parts to a set of diagnostic models are shown in Fig. 40-1. The **anatomic portion** includes all of the dental arch and alveolar processes, and the **art portion** provides a base for the models.

The steps in constructing a set of diagnostic models include the following:
  ▶ Assembling the armamentarium

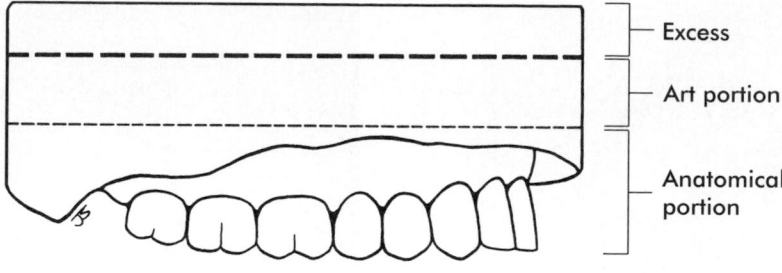

FIG. 40-1   Parts of a diagnostic model.

- Mixing the plaster and/or stone
- Pouring the impression
- Pouring the bases
- Removing the impression from the models
- Trimming the models
- Finishing the models
- Labeling the models

Purpose of Diagnostic Models

Properly trimmed diagnostic models that accurately represent the intraoral anatomy of a patient are invaluable in diagnosis and treatment of a patient. A well-trimmed set of models provides the purposes listed in Box 40-1.

Construction of Diagnostic Models

Before a set of diagnostic models can be produced, an alginate impression of the maxillary and mandibular arches must be obtained (see Chapter 24). The impressions are a negative reproduction of the intraoral anatomy, and the final result—the set of diagnostic models—is a positive reproduction.

POURING AN IMPRESSION

Diagnostic models are typically poured in plaster, but some dentists prefer that the anatomic portion be poured in stone and the base be poured in plaster. This ensures denser anatomic surfaces and a less dense base, which can be trimmed more easily.

Chapter 24 describes how the impressions are taken, rinsed, and sprayed with a disinfectant, wrapped in a paper towel, and placed in a plastic bag for 15 minutes. It is at this point that the laboratory activity begins for constructing a set of diagnostic models. All armamentarium for pouring an impression is assembled. The impressions are rinsed and air dried before pouring. The impressions may be dried with compressed air, but care should be taken not to use a high volume to avoid tearing the impression material.

Assembling the Armamentarium

Armamentarium for impression pouring includes the following materials (Fig. 40-2):

Model plaster or *snow white plaster*
White stone or *cast stone* (optional)
Scale to weigh powder
Graduated cylinder (100 ml)
Rubber bowls
Plaster spatula
Vibrator

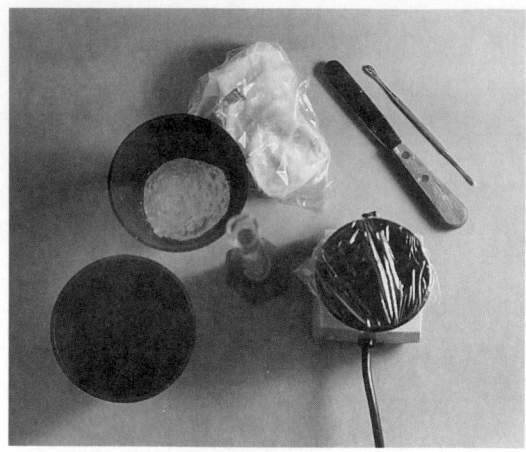

FIG. 40-2   Armamentarium for pouring an impression.

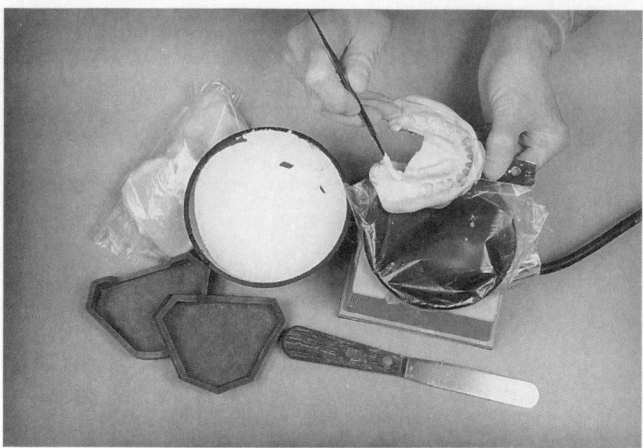

FIG. 40-3   Cover is placed on a vibrator before an impression is poured. Using a #7 spatula, the first increment of stone is poured into the impression at one heel and the impression is vibrated so that the material flows toward the anterior of the arch.

Base formers (optional)
#7 wax spatula
Maxillary and mandibular alginate impression
Waxed paper or glass slab

Mixing the Plaster or Stone

The anatomic parts of the models are poured in white rapid stone; the base portions are poured in white model plaster. The stone and plaster are mixed, using the following proportions:

Dental stone: 30 ml of water to 100 g powder
Model plaster: 50 ml of water to 100 g powder

1. Prepare a mix of white stone using the proper water to powder ratio. In most cases 200 g of dental stone powder and 60 ml of water are sufficient to pour the anatomic portion of both the maxillary and mandibular impressions. Refer to Chapter 11 for mixing gypsum materials.
2. The stone is mixed with a plaster spatula in a rubber bowl as described in Chapter 11.
3. When the mix is smooth and homogeneous, the bowl is held firmly on the vibrator until all the bubbles come to the surface.

Pouring the Impression

1. Place the mandibular impression on the vibrator. You may want to cover the vibrator with a piece of plastic or with a plastic bag to keep it clean (Fig. 40-3).
2. Using the #7 spatula, place a small amount of stone at one heel and allow the material to slowly flow toward the anterior of the arch (Fig. 40-3).
3. Vibrate the first portion of stone in the impression by tilting the tray until the stone flows to the heel

on the opposite side. As the material flows to the opposite side, allow it to flow into all of the embrasures.
4. Continue adding small increments until all occlusal surfaces are well covered. Adding small increments in this manner will help to eliminate voids and bubbles on the teeth of the model.
5. Once this is done, more stone can be added with the plaster spatula until the impression is filled to the top (Fig. 40-4).
6. At this point it is best to place the impression on the vibrator intermittently to prevent possible overflow onto the outside of the impression. The surface of the stone will be uneven. Do not try to smooth the surface. Leave it roughened for greater attachment to the base (Fig. 40-4).
7. Set the filled mandibular impression out of the way of the vibrator to prevent movement in the poured stone.
8. Pour the maxillary arch in the same manner by beginning in the tuberosity area.
9. Continue with steps 1 to 7, making certain the palate is thoroughly covered.

Pouring the Bases

Prepare a mix of model plaster using the proper water to powder proportions. Usually a separate mix of plaster is needed to fill each model base former. In most cases 250 g of model plaster powder and 125 ml of water will provide a large enough mix to fill a base former or provide an adequate mass to create a base. For a firmer mass, use less water.

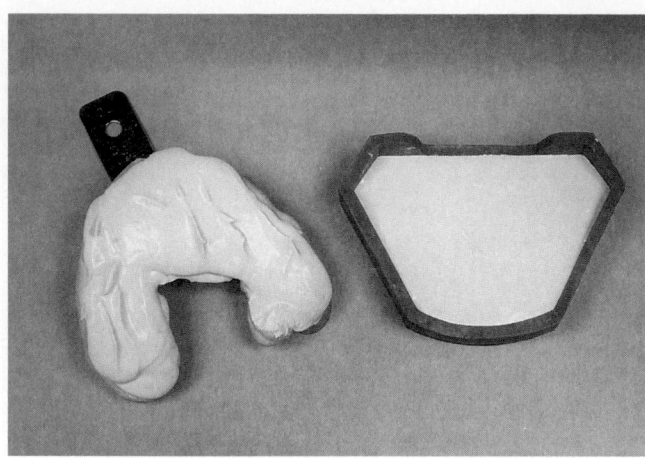

FIG. 40-4   Continue adding small increments, until all occlusal surfaces are well covered. Once this is done, more stone can be added with the plaster spatula until the impression is filled to the occlusal. The surface is left roughened and is set aside to prepare the base.

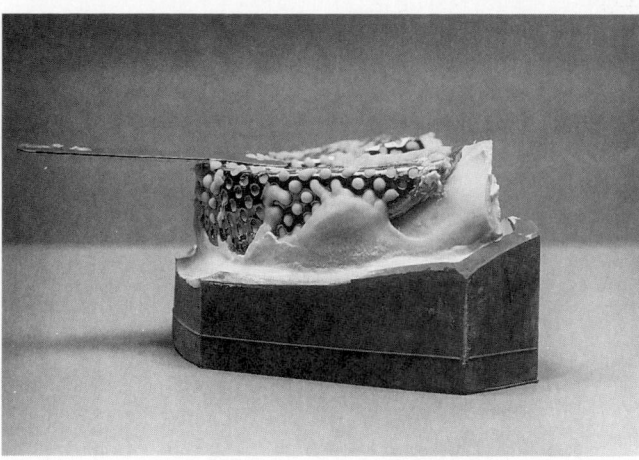

FIG. 40-5   The stone-filled impression is inverted onto the poured base. The impression is centered over the base former and is gently worked into the base material; the occlusal plane must be parallel with the base of the former.

1. Spatulate and vibrate the plaster mix until it is free of bubbles and lumps.
2. When the mix is smooth and homogeneous, the bowl is held firmly on the vibrator until all the bubbles come to the surface.
3. Place the base former on the vibrator and pour from the rubber bowl slowly and directly into the base former, so that bubbles rise to the surface.
4. Immediately after the model former is filled, invert the stone-filled impressions onto the freshly poured plaster surfaces (Fig. 40-5).
5. Gently work the stone-filled impressions slightly down into the plaster of the base former. A continuous union between the stone and the plaster must be formed. Avoid embedding (locking) the tray in the plaster mass by placing the impression into the plaster only until it reaches the edge of the tray.
6. Center the impression over the plaster base former, and position it on the plaster base so that the occlusal plane will be parallel to the bottom of the base in the final model (see Fig. 40-5).
7. Fill in voids at the posterior to ensure that the posterior areas, the heels of the mandibular, and the tuberosity areas of the maxillary model are well supported by plaster.
8. Smooth the open tongue space with the lab spatula and remove any excess plaster in this area. Some assistants like to place a piece of dampened paper towel in the tongue area to create a smooth surface, thus avoiding a large mass of plaster hardening in this area.

9. Complete this process for the opposing impression.
10. Allow the poured models to set undisturbed until the plaster and stone are hard.

An alternative method of pouring a base is described below. Some dentists prefer to create the base instead of using base formers. In some situations the base formers may be restrictive, and this method offers more freedom.

1. Prepare the mix. Spatulate and vibrate the plaster as described in the above procedure.
2. Insert the mass of plaster onto waxed paper or a large glass slab, and place it into a mound about 1 inch to 1½ inches high. The shape of the mass should resemble the shape of the impression tray, wider at the posterior and narrower in the anterior.
3. Gently place the stone-filled impression onto this mass. A continuous union between the stone and plaster must be formed. The same attention given to the posterior, the heels, the tuberosity, and the tongue areas when using the molds should be done in this method, too.
4. Center the impression in the mass, and position it so that the occlusal plane is parallel to the slab or countertop. As mentioned in the previous technique, do not embed the tray in the base plaster.
5. Smooth the outer edges of the plaster base, leaving not more than ¾ inch of plaster around the outer edge of the tray (Fig. 40-6, *A*).
6. Allow the model to remain undisturbed until the plaster or stone is hard. Complete this process for the opposing arch.

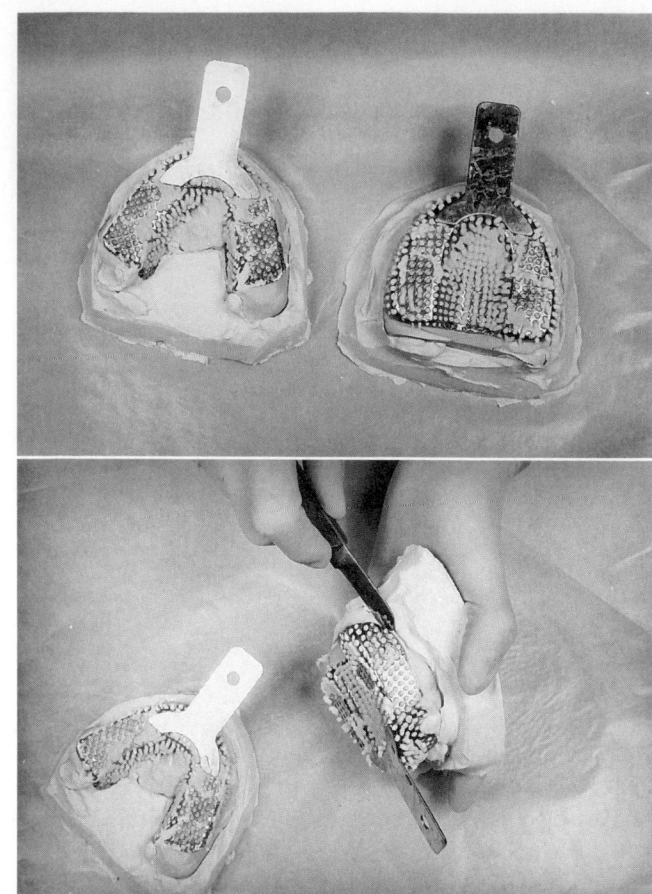

A

B

FIG. 40-6   *A,* Models poured and inverted onto a free form base. Note the ability to create a larger base for trimming. *B,* The impression is removed from the model by gently lifting the impression. A laboratory knife is used carefully, if it is needed, to break any undercut areas.

Removing Impressions from the Models

After the gypsum material has reached the final set, the impression can be removed from the model. This may be accomplished by gently lifting the impression from the model. If necessary a laboratory knife can be used to carefully break any undercuts and to push up on the impression, dislodging it from the stone model. Take care not to force the impression, since it is possible to fracture teeth during this process. If the impression is not removed in a timely manner, syneresis will occur in the alginate impression, making it more difficult to remove the dried impression from the model and thus creating a potential for fracture of the teeth as the impression is removed (Fig. 40-6, *B*).

Once the models have been separated, the alginate impression material can be discarded. The trays are cleaned, sterilized, and returned to the storage area for future use. A set of well-poured impressions is just one more step toward obtaining an accurate set of diagnostic models (Box 40-2).

BOX 40-2

CRITERIA FOR POURED MODELS

1. All plaster and stone surfaces must be free of voids and bubbles.
2. The union between the stone in the anatomic portion and the plaster base should be continuous and free of voids.
3. The anatomic portion of the cast (dental arch and alveolar process) must be centered on the plaster base to provide adequate plaster on all sides for proper trimming.
4. The occlusal plane of the dental arch should be parallel to the bottom of the rapid stone base.
5. The base must be thick enough to provide adequate plaster for trimming the casts to the proper height.
6. The anatomic portion of the cast must have sufficient vestibular and posterior extension to allow for proper depth of model trimming.
7. The tongue area on the mandibular model should be free of excess plaster or stone.

▶ Trimming Diagnostic Models

Several methods are used to trim models, and the following discussion describes one of these techniques. After a while the assistant becomes proficient at this procedure and may not need to use some of the suggested armamentarium. Many experienced professionals are capable of *eyeballing* many of the cuts. The procedure that is described is relatively simple to follow and produces excellent results. Regardless of the technique that is used, the maxillary model is trimmed first and the mandibular model is trimmed in occlusion with the maxillary model. Before beginning to trim the models, the assistant should have a thorough understanding of the terms *parallel* and *symmetrical.* **Parallel** means to be an equal distance apart at every point. **Symmetry** refers to having the same form, plane, or angle on opposite sides. To apply this to model trimming, the assistant must be able to visualize parallel relationships between two different points and to recognize symmetry in angles and cuts that are made on a model. The lines and angles in Fig. 40-7 illustrate the differences between parallel and nonparallel, and symmetry and asymmetry.

Assembling the Armamentarium

The following items comprise the armamentarium for trimming (Fig. 40-8):

Parallell lines

Nonparallell lines

Symmetrical lines   Nonsymmetrical outer lines

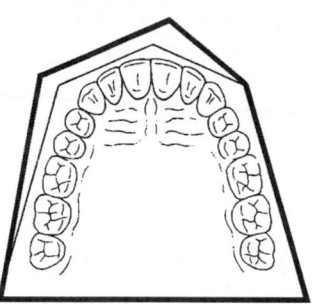

FIG. 40-7   Lines and angles illustrate parallelism and symmetry.

Model trimmer
Plastic protractor
Flexible millimeter ruler
Pencils, graphite and colored
Dividers
Miter square or *angle former*
Laboratory knife
#7 wax spatula
Wet-and-dry sandpaper

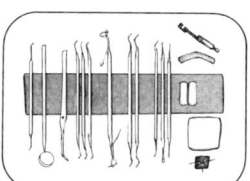

Preparing the Models

The following trimming procedure is done using models that have been placed in a plaster mass rather than in rubber molds. The preformed molds require less preparation, since they have some basic form and are relatively smooth on the sides. Regardless of the base form, the models must be soaked in water for 10 to 15 minutes to saturate them. A dry model will bind in the model trimmer and leave stone on the cutting wheel. Do not, however, leave the models standing in water for a long period or leave them under running water, since this causes surface roughness.

Be sure the table of the model trimmer is at 90 degrees to the wheel. Use a right angle to check accuracy (see Fig. 40-8). Most trimmers have an adjustment knob that

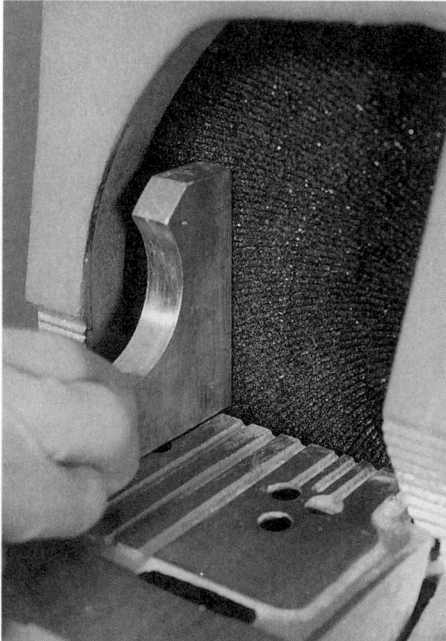

FIG. 40-8   The table of the model trimmer is examined to ensure that it is at a 90-degree angle in relation to the cutting wheel.

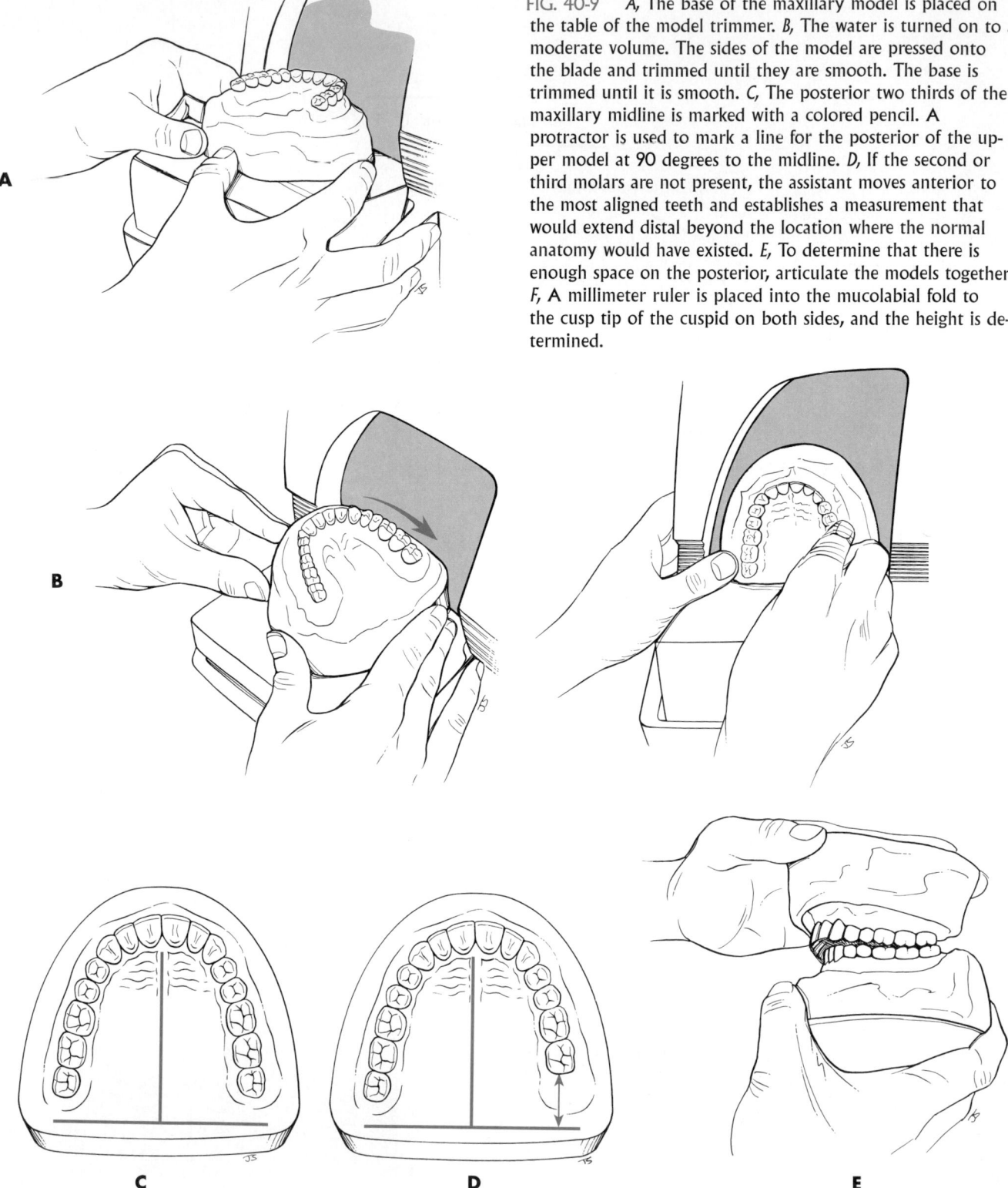

FIG. 40-9   *A,* The base of the maxillary model is placed on the table of the model trimmer. *B,* The water is turned on to a moderate volume. The sides of the model are pressed onto the blade and trimmed until they are smooth. The base is trimmed until it is smooth. *C,* The posterior two thirds of the maxillary midline is marked with a colored pencil. A protractor is used to mark a line for the posterior of the upper model at 90 degrees to the midline. *D,* If the second or third molars are not present, the assistant moves anterior to the most aligned teeth and establishes a measurement that would extend distal beyond the location where the normal anatomy would have existed. *E,* To determine that there is enough space on the posterior, articulate the models together. *F,* A millimeter ruler is placed into the mucolabial fold to the cusp tip of the cuspid on both sides, and the height is determined.

allows the table to be set at 90 degrees. Even a small variation of 3 to 4 degrees from 90 degrees will be noticeable in the trimmed models.

1. Begin with the maxillary model. Use a laboratory knife and #7 wax spatula to chip off plaster bubbles on the occlusal side of the teeth, and remove any excess on the heel of the model.
2. Place the base of the maxillary model on the table of the model trimmer (Fig. 40-9, *A*).
3. Turn on the water to a moderate volume. Too rapid a flow of water will cause spillover, and not enough flow will cause plaster or stone to remain on the wheel (Fig. 40-9, *B*).
4. Gently press the side of the model onto the blade and trim around the sides of the model until they are smooth. The width of the model must fit into the model trimmer window (Fig. 40-9, *B*). If it does not, remove more plaster from the sides of the model.

Determining the Midline of the Model

1. Mark the posterior two thirds of the maxillary midline with a colored pencil. This line is the midline of the maxillary model. Using the protractor, mark a line for the posterior of the upper model at 90 degrees to the midline. Mark this line 5 to 10 mm posterior to the distal end of the maxillary tuberosity (Fig. 40-9, *C*). NOTE: If the distal end of the maxillary tuberosity is not well defined or the second or third molars are not present, it may be

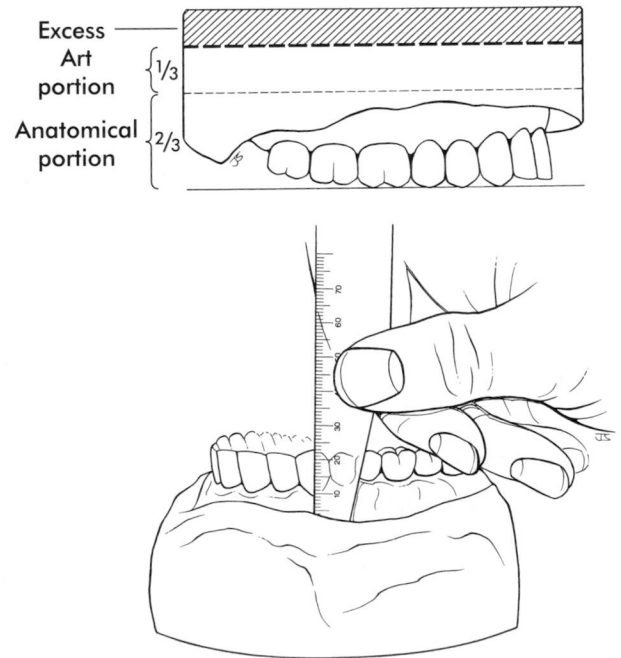

F

Continued.

FIG. 40-9, cont'd   For legend see opposite page.

necessary to move anterior to the most aligned teeth and to establish a measurement that would extend distal beyond the location where the normal anatomy would have existed (Fig. 40-9, *D*).

2. In a model with a Class II relationship, be sure there is sufficient stone posterior to the distal end of the maxillary tuberosity to allow trimming of the posterior end of the mandibular model parallel to the posterior end of the maxillary model without trimming into the nearest mandibular tooth.
3. To determine that there is enough space on the posterior end of the models, articulate the models together (Fig. 40-9, *E*). Don't guess; you'll regret it later.

Determining the Height of the Model

The model is divided into two parts, the anatomic and the art portions. In general, the anatomic portion equals two thirds of the total height of the model and one third of the art portion.

1. To determine the anatomic height, use a flexible millimeter ruler and measure the maxillary model from the base of the mucolabial fold to the cusp tip of the cuspid on both sides (Fig. 40-9, *F*).
2. If these measurements are not the same, average them. For example, if one side is 23 mm and the opposite side is 25 mm, the anatomic portion of the model is 24 mm. This represents two thirds of the total height of the maxillary model.

Therefore, if: $\quad \frac{2}{3} = 24$ mm (anatomic portion)
$\quad\quad\quad\quad\quad\quad \frac{1}{3} = 12$ mm (art portion)

Total height of
maxillary model $\quad = 36$ mm

3. Since the mandibular model will be the same height, the total height of the articulated models will be 72 mm.
4. If this is your first model trimming experience, you may wish to add 3 to 5 mm to this measurement on each arch to allow for potential error. This excess can always be removed after the maxillary base is trimmed.

Paralleling the Base with the Occlusal Plane

1. Set the dividers at the predetermined measurement using the millimeter ruler. In this case the measurement was 36 mm, so the opening of the dividers will be 36 mm.
2. Place the maxillary model on the flat surface of a lab bench with the occlusal plane contacting the surface of the bench.
3. Rock the model forward, so that the incisal edge of

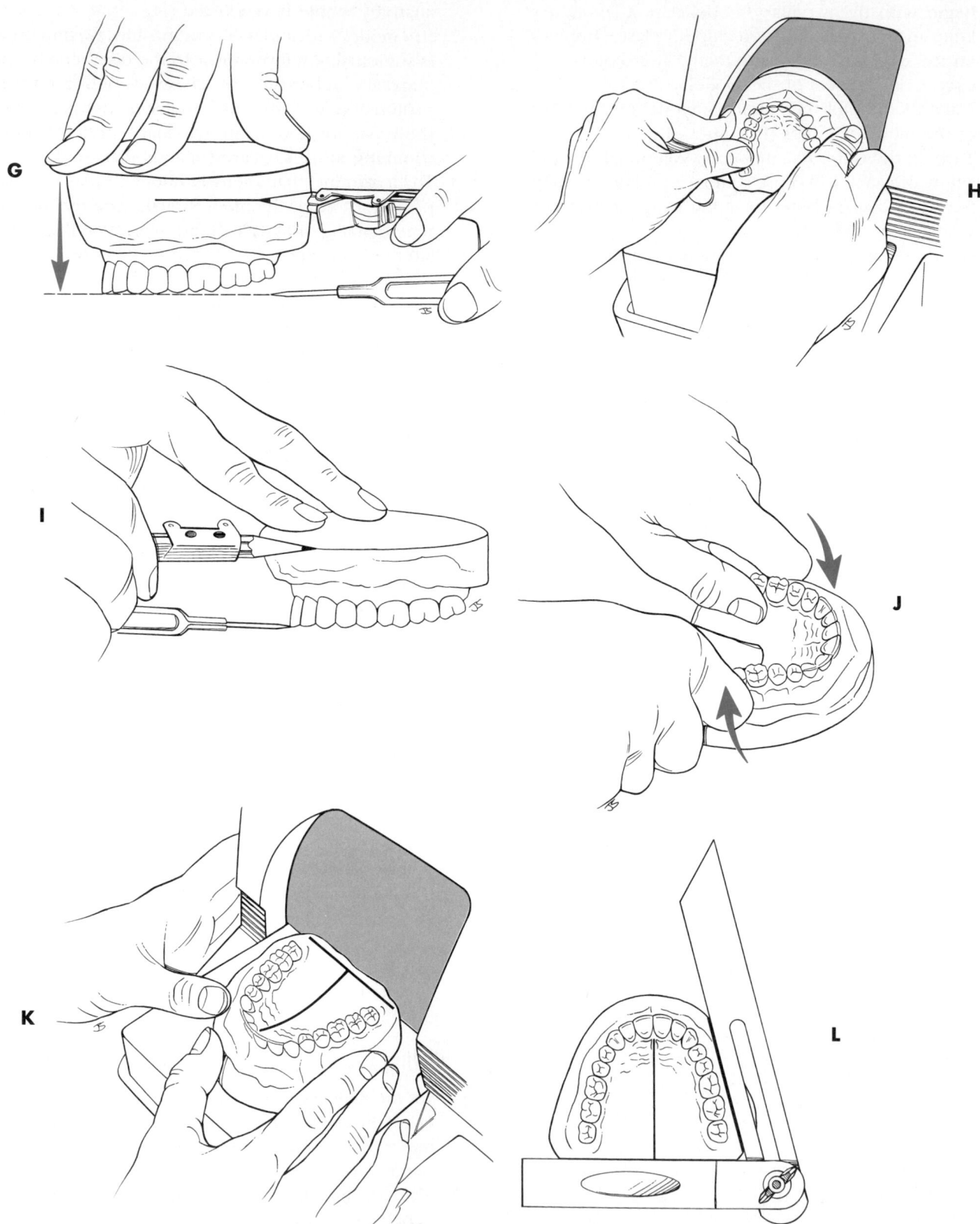

FIG. 40-9, cont'd   For legend see opposite page.

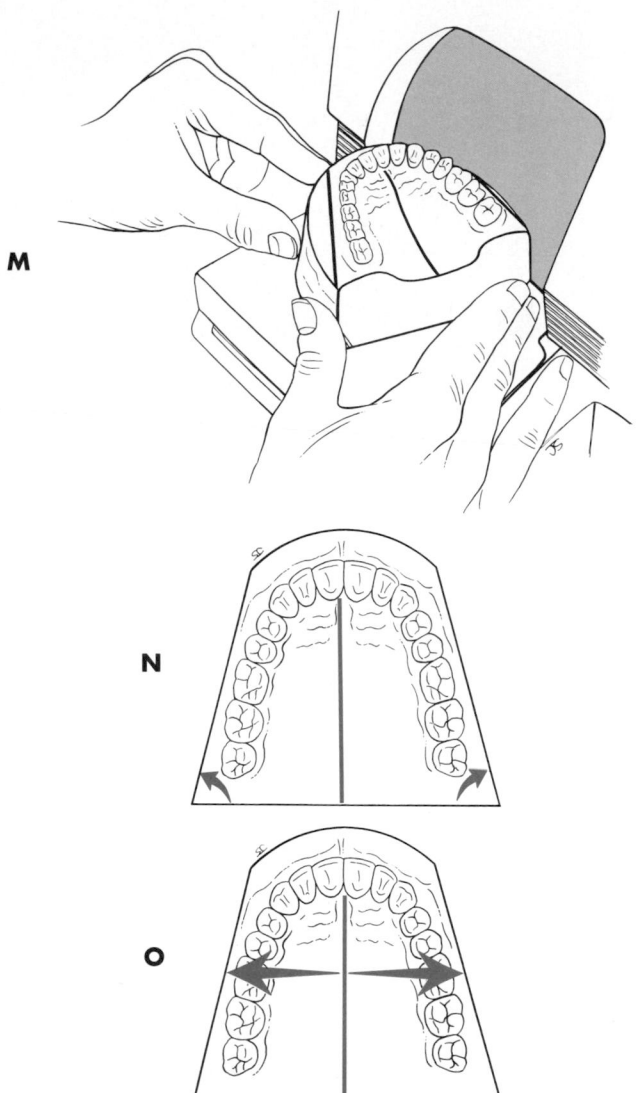

FIG. 40-9, cont'd   *G*, The model is placed on a flat surface and rocked forward toward the central incisors; a line is drawn with the dividers around the base of the model. *H*, The base of the model is trimmed down to the pencil line. *I*, The height of the model is assessed by placing it on the lab bench, rocking it forward, and measuring the height with the dividers. *J*, Bevels on the base are assessed by placing the base on the lab bench and rocking it laterally. *K*, The base surface of the maxillary model is placed on the model trimmer table and trimmed to the pencil line that was drawn perpendicular to the palatal midline. *L*, The angle former is laid parallel to the buccal plane of one side and marked with a line along the greatest depth of the buccal vestibule, which is approximately 5 mm from the buccal surface of the teeth. The angle former is turned over to the opposite side and the side of the model is marked in the same manner. *M*, The model base is placed on the table and trimmed to the pencil lines on both sides. *N*, Both trimmed sides should be at the same angle to the back of the model. *O*, The sides of the model should be an equal distance away from the palatal midline.

Continued.

the central incisors contacts the lab bench, and draw a line with the dividers around the base of the model (Fig. 40-9, *G*). The reason for rocking the model forward is to compensate for the **curve of Spee**, which causes the maxillary molars to dip downward to follow the curve in the mandibular molars. If this is not done, the base of the trimmed model will not be parallel to the occlusal plane.

4. Trim the top (base) of the model down to the pencil line drawn around the base (Fig. 40-9, *H*).
5. Recheck the height of the model by placing it on the lab bench, rocking it forward, and measuring the height with the dividers (Fig. 40-9, *I*). If it is not the correct height all around the base, return it to the trimmer and remove the excess.
6. To check for bevels on the base, place the base on the lab bench and rock laterally (Fig. 40-9, *J*). If there is movement, it indicates a bevel or unevenness in the base. Return the model to the trimmer and gently move the base laterally on the blade to remove the bevel.
7. Recheck the height before continuing.

Trimming the Back of the Model

1. Place the base surface (surface just trimmed) of the maxillary model on the model trimmer table.
2. Establish the back of the maxillary model by trimming in to the pencil line that was drawn perpendicular to the palatal midline (Fig. 40-9, *K*).

Trimming the Sides of the Model

1. Choose the side of the maxillary model with the best alignment of posterior teeth from cuspid through second molar.
2. Using the angle former laid parallel to the buccal surfaces, mark a line along the greatest depth of the buccal vestibule, which will be about 5 mm from the buccal surface of the teeth (Fig. 40-9, *L*).
3. In many cases this side cut line runs parallel to an imaginary line that connects the cusp tip of the cuspid to the mesial buccal cusp of the second permanent molar in the most well-aligned quadrant.
4. Turn the angle former over, so that it is parallel to the opposite side, and mark the opposite side of the model in the same manner and at the same angle to the back of the cast (Fig. 40-9, *L*).
5. Place the model base on the table, and trim the model in to the pencil lines on both sides (Fig. 40-9, *M*).
6. The trimmed sides are both at the same angle to the back of the model (Fig. 40-9, *N*).
7. The sides of the model should be an equal distance away from the palatal midline (Fig. 40-9, *O*).

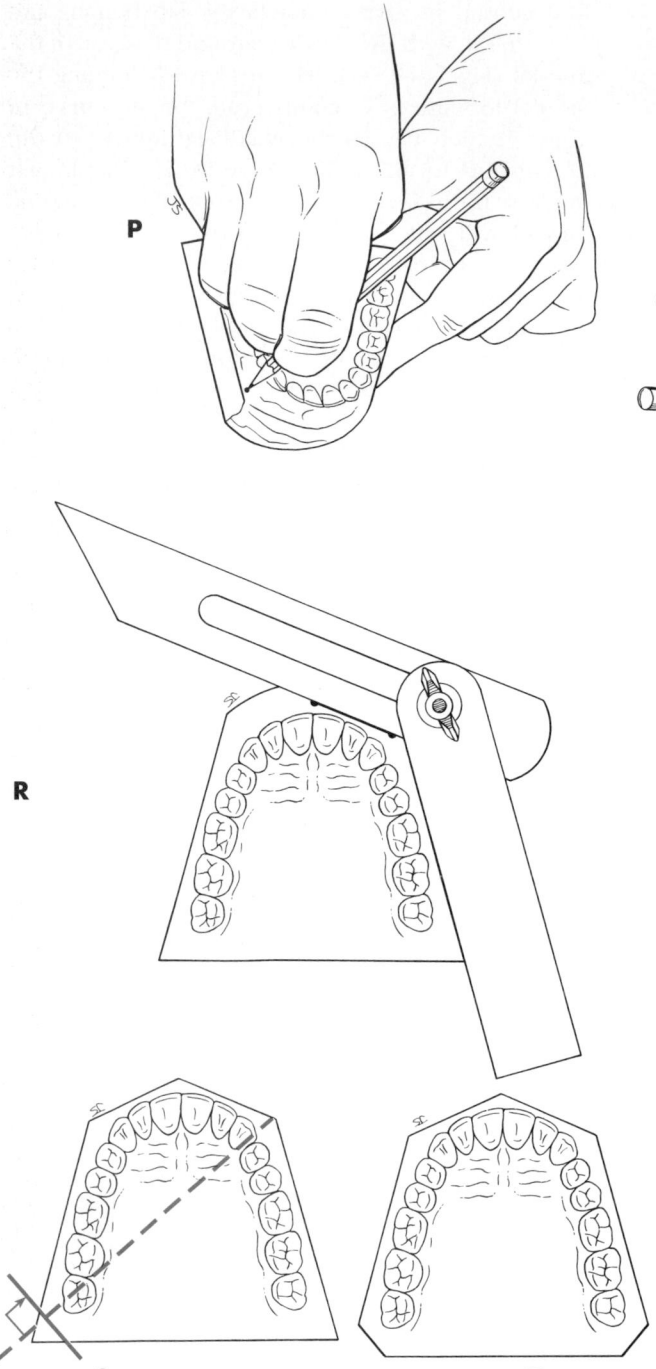

P   Q

R

S   T

FIG. 40-9, cont'd   *P,* The maxillary model is marked at the
deepest point of the buccal vestibule at the most normally positioned cuspid. *Q,* The midline of the maxillary cast is marked
on the anterior vestibule at about 5 mm from the labial of
the central incisors. *R,* Using the angle former a line is drawn
from the cuspid mark to the midline and then the same line is
drawn on the opposite side. *S,* A line at 90 degrees is drawn
to a bi-sector of the cuspid angle of the side and front cuts.
This is done on both sides and is trimmed to the pencil line. *T,*
The heel cuts should be symmetric in length from side to side
(⅜ inch to ⅝ inch wide) and at the same angle to the back.

Trimming the Anterior of the Model

1. Mark the maxillary model at the deepest point of the buccal vestibule at the most normally positioned cuspid (Fig. 40-9, *P*).
2. Mark the midline of the maxillary cast on the anterior vestibule. This point will be about 5 mm from the labial surface of the central incisors.
3. Using the angle former as a guide, draw a line from the cuspid mark to the midline (Fig. 40-9, *Q*).
4. With the angle former, draw the same line on the opposite side.
5. Trim the anterior to this line (Fig. 40-9, *R*). If there is an anterior protrusion of these teeth, it may be necessary to move the marked line out farther to avoid cutting into anatomy when the anterior cut is made.
6. The anterior cuts should follow the general contour of the anterior teeth, be of equal length, be at the same angle to the sides of the model, be cut to the greatest depth of the vestibule without cutting into the anterior teeth, and end anteriorly at the midline of the maxillary arch and posteriorly at a point directly buccal to the mesiodistal midline of the most normally positioned cuspid.

Trimming the Heels of the Model

1. Draw a line at 90 degrees to a bisector of the cuspid angle of the side and front cuts. Do this on both sides (Fig. 40-9, *S*).
2. Trim to the pencil line.
3. The heel cuts should be symmetric in length from side to side (⅜ to ⅝ inch wide) and at the same angle to the back and sides of the cast from side to side (Fig. 40-9, *T*).

Trimming the Mandibular Model

1. Occlude the maxillary and mandibular casts with the wax bite. Mark the back of the mandibular cast parallel to the back of the maxillary cast (Fig. 40-10, *A*).

2. With the casts occluded and the wax bite in place, place the models on table of the model trimmer with the maxillary model on the bottom (Fig. 40-10, *B*). Trim the back of the mandibular model just short of the line drawn on the mandibular model (Fig. 40-10, *C*). This cut will make the back of the mandibular model parallel to the back of the maxillary model. Since it is difficult to see the relationship of the backs of the models, do not bring the back of the mandibular model in all the way to the pencil line; this will be done later.

3. Place the articulated models on the bench top with the top of the maxillary model flat on the bench surface. Scribe a line that is twice the height of the maxillary model (measurement taken from step 1 of paralleling the base with the occlusal plane) up from the bench top, and mark the base of the mandibular model (Fig. 40-10, *D*).

4. Trim the base of the mandibular model to the pencil line. The base will be 90 degrees to the back of the mandibular model (Fig. 40-10, *E*). As with the maxillary model, examine the base of the model for bevels, and remove any unevenness if it exists.

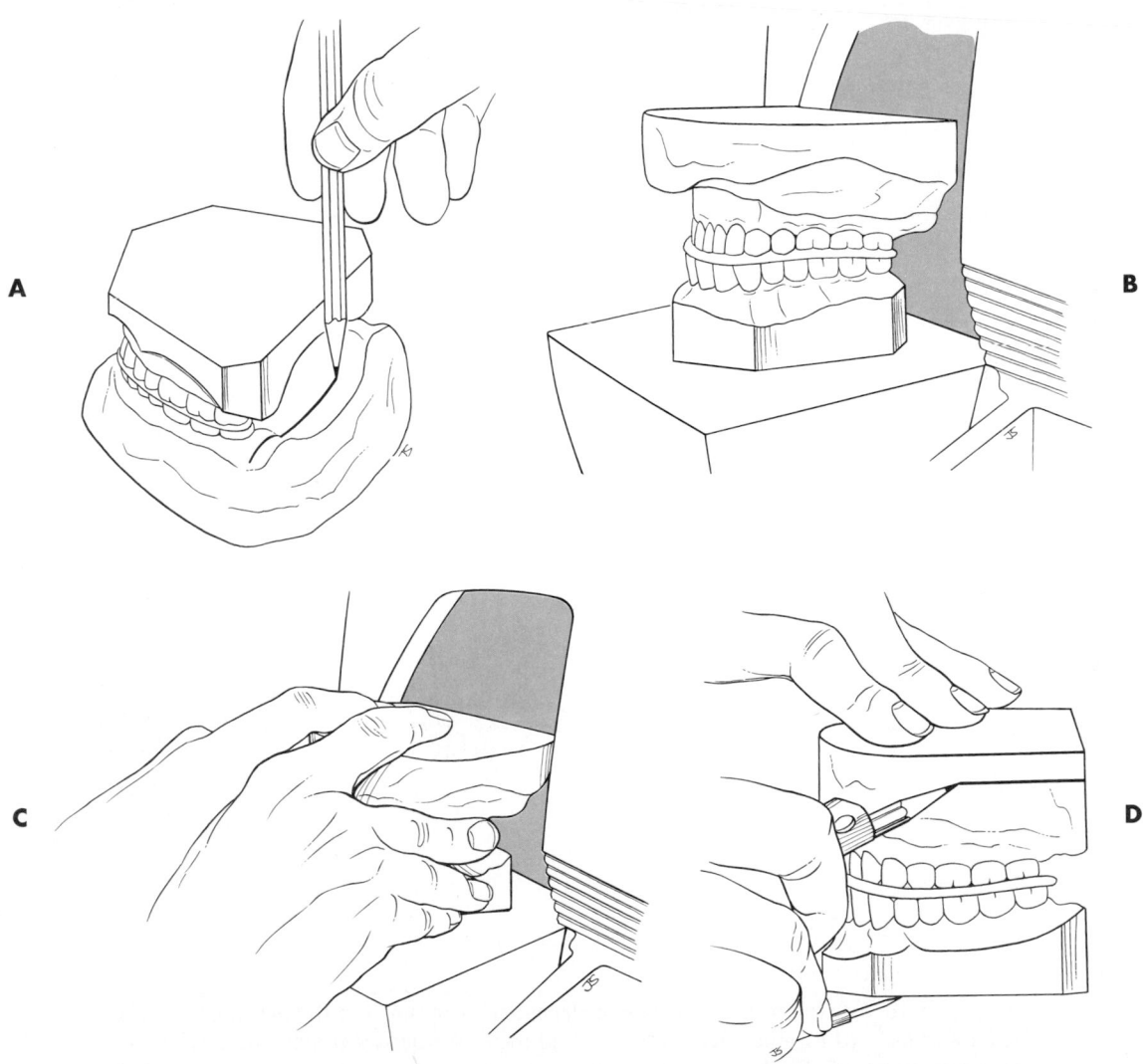

FIG. 40-10 *A,* The mandibular cast is marked parallel to the maxillary cast. *B,* The casts are occluded, with the wax bite in place. *C,* With the maxillary model on the bottom the back of the mandibular model is trimmed just short of the line drawn on the mandibular model. *D,* With the top of the maxillary model flat on the bench and the models articulated, a line is scribed that is twice the height of the maxillary model.

Continued.

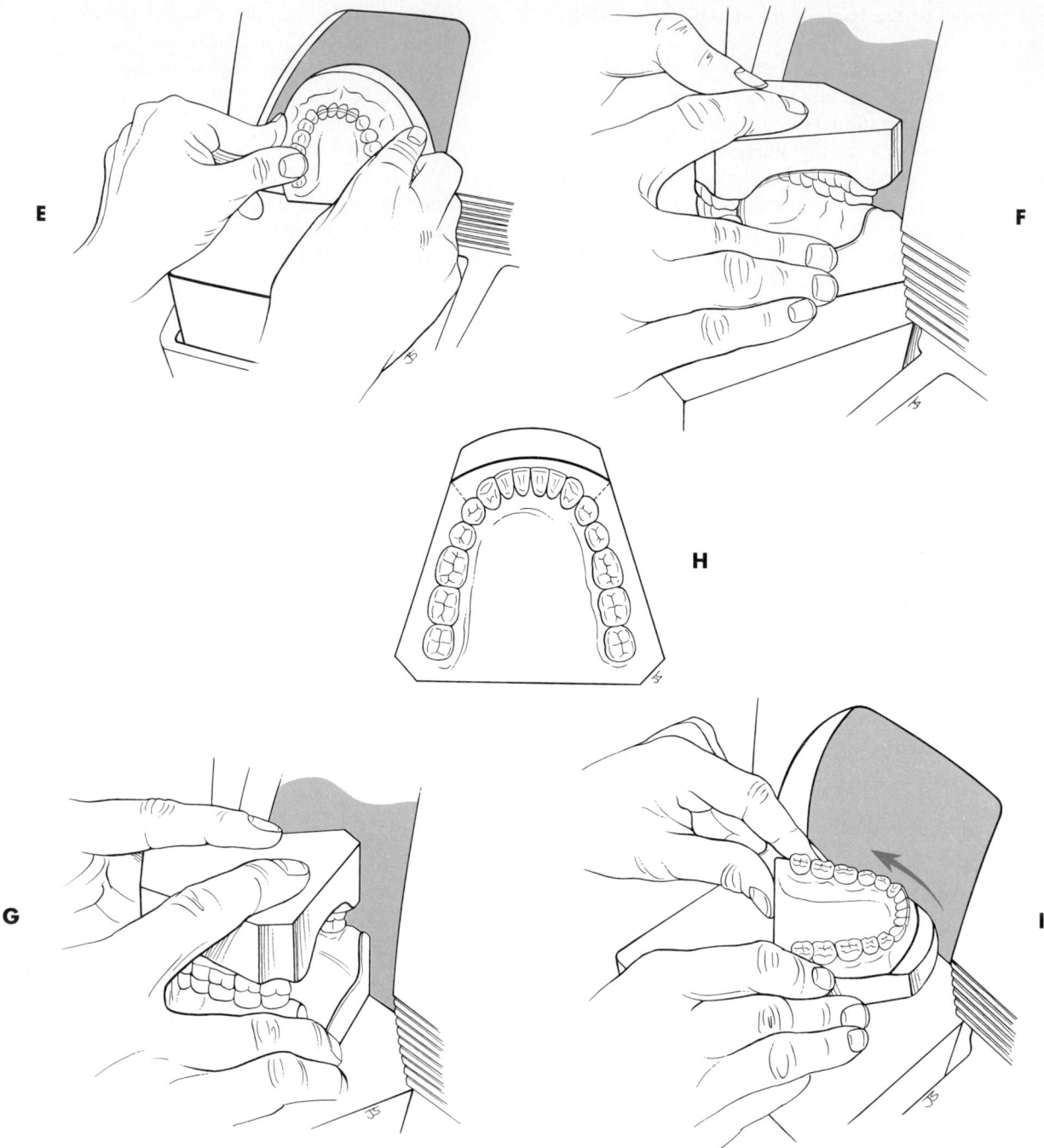

FIG. 40-10, cont'd   *E,* The base of the mandibular model is trimmed to the pencil line. *F,* The models are articulated together again; the back and then the sides are trimmed flush with the maxillary model. *G,* The heels of the mandibular cast are trimmed even with the maxillary cast. *H,* The models are separated, and an arc is marked on the mandibular model at the deepest point of the vestibule, from midline of the first premolar to the midline of the opposite premolar. *I,* The mandibular model is trimmed in an arc.

5. Then articulate the models together and place the flat base surface of the mandibular cast on the model trimmer table. Complete trimming the back of the model to the pencil line and flush with the back of the maxillary model.
6. With the models still articulated, trim the sides of the lower model flush with the sides of the maxillary model (Fig. 40-10, *F*).
7. Trim the heels of the lower cast to be (a) parallel to the opposite side of the model, (b) at the same angle to the back, and (c) equal in length (both being ⅜ inch to ⅝ inch long) (Fig. 40-10, *G*).
8. Before trimming the anterior of the mandibular model, separate the models and mark an arc on the mandibular model at the deepest point of the vestibule from midline of the first premolar to the midline of the opposite premolar (Fig. 40-10, *H*).
9. Trim the mandibular model in an arc that roughly follows the lower anterior teeth. Trim in close to the incisor teeth, but do not grind into the incisors (Fig. 40-10, *I*).

Finishing Procedures

1. Trim the capital (top of the maxillary model) and base (bottom of the mandibular model) as needed to establish the final height of the occluded models (with wax bite in place). The occlusal plane should be centered between the top and bottom of the occluded set of models (Fig. 40-11, *A*).
2. With a lab knife, trim the tongue space flat and smooth. Do not destroy the anatomy of the depth of the lingual tissue extension. Also, the extra plaster projections beyond the anatomic registration at the heel areas of the maxillary and mandibular models may be smoothed off with a lab knife.
3. Fill any voids or bubbles in the models with plaster or stone. The models should be saturated with water before the plaster is applied. A thick mix of plaster provides the best results. Allow the added plaster to dry before going on to the next step.
4. Smooth all flat surfaces under running water with a block wrapped in wet-and-dry sandpaper. Keep all

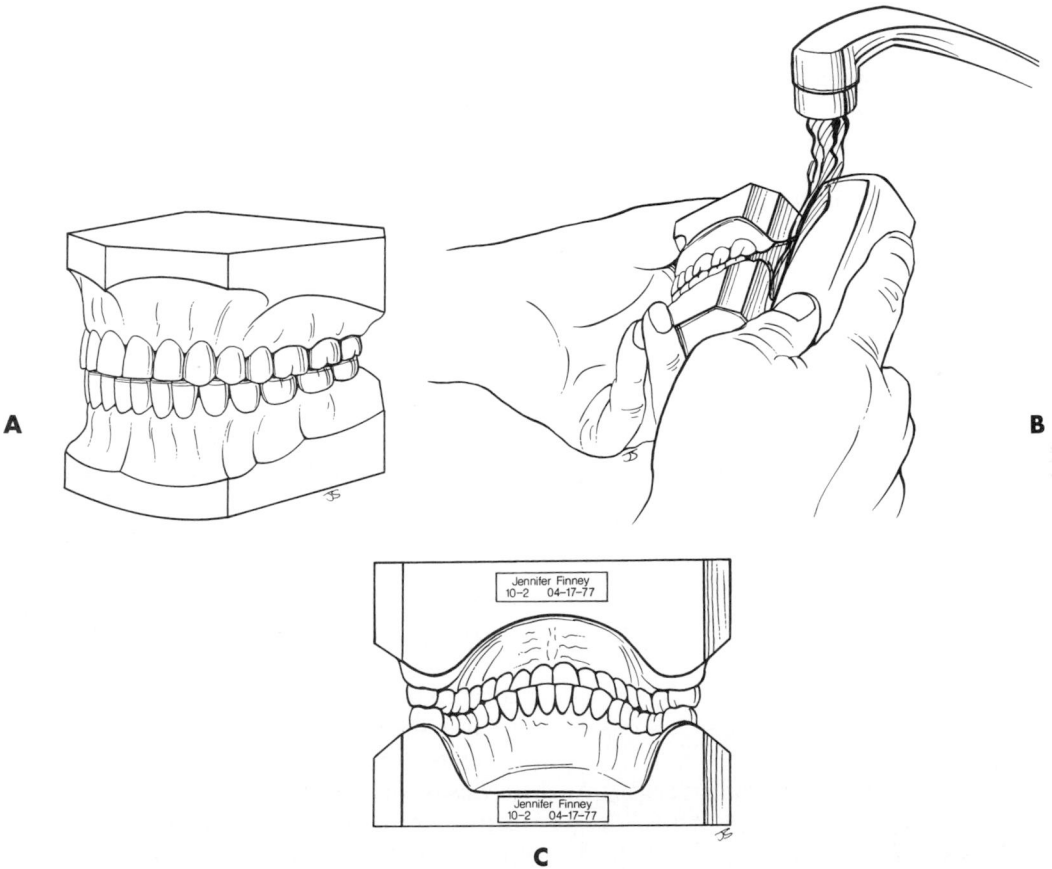

A   **B**

C

FIG. 40-11   *A,* The top of the maxillary model and base of the mandibular model are trimmed as needed to establish an accurate final height. The occlusal plane should be centered between both models. *B,* After a lab knife is used to trim the tongue space flat and smooth, all flat surfaces are smoothed under running water, using a block wrapped in wet-and-dry sandpaper. Keep all line angles sharp and parallel. *C,* Labels are typed for both models.

line angles sharp and parallel. Do not round the edges. Do not sand any anatomic portions of the models. An Arkansas stone or an arbor band on a handpiece or lathe can be used to remove excess plaster on flat surfaces (Fig. 40-11, *B*).

5. Remove any bubbles or imperfections with a #7 wax spatula.
6. Type labels for both models (Fig. 40-11, *C*). Include the patient's age at the time of the impression in years and months (10-2 indicates 10 years, 2 months). Print the date of the impression next to the patient's age. If possible, allow the models to

dry a day or two before labeling. The following is an example label:

Jennifer Finney
10-2   04-17-77

Criteria for Trimmed Diagnostic Models

The criteria for a well-trimmed set of models are practically universal and can be achieved with most techniques (Box 40-3).

Special Considerations

The procedure just described works well in most situations. There are times, however, when a set of models requires modifications in trimming, such as in missing teeth, severe malocclusion, or an asymmetric arch. To deal with these situations, keep in mind the criteria for acceptable models and attempt to meet as many of these criteria as possible. For instance, even though teeth may be missing, there should be some evidence of an alveolar ridge or perhaps teeth in the opposite arch for comparison. Therefore, as long as you treat the area as though it had all of the teeth present and do not destroy anatomic structure, you should be able to maintain symmetry.

In a situation where there is a crossbite or other types of malocclusion, always be certain to articulate the models together to anticipate the need to extend a buccal or anterior cut line. In such a situation you should be able to maintain the same angle, but you may find that the distance between the side cuts and the midline are about the same. However, you will have saved anatomy and attempted to preserve symmetry.

Construction of Custom-Made Acrylic Trays

Another common laboratory procedure for the dental assistant is the construction of a **custom-made tray** for a patient. The basic goal is to fabricate a tray that will accurately fit the patient's dental arches regardless of their configuration. This cannot always be accomplished with a standard stock tray. The custom-made tray has several advantages (Box 40-4).

Custom-made trays may be constructed for an arch, a segment, or an individual quadrant for a variety of purposes. Most commonly trays are constructed for the following types of treatment:

Quadrant trays are used for a final impression for a single crown, inlay, or small fixed bridge.

Full arch trays are used for a final impression for single or multiple crowns, inlays, bridges, or partial dentures.

BOX 40-3

CRITERIA FOR TRIMMED DIAGNOSTIC MODEL

1. Backs of the models must be located posterior to the maxillary tuberosity and posterior to the most posterior mandibular tooth.
2. Backs of the maxillary and mandibular models must be in the same plane.
3. When articulated in occlusion, backs of the models should set flush on a flat surface without any movement of the occlusion.
4. Base of the maxillary and mandibular models should be parallel to each other.
5. All of the angles should be symmetric from side to side.
6. All of the trimmed sides opposite each other should be the same height.
7. Art portion of the maxillary model should be one third of the total height of the model.
8. When articulated together, the models should be double the height of the maxillary model when the maxillary occlusal plane is parallel to a flat surface.
9. Occlusal plane should be between 0 and 5 degrees to the bases.
10. Occlusal plane should be centered in the total height of the model.
11. Midline of the maxillary model should be established at the posterior two thirds of maxillary palatal raphe.
12. Flat cuts and angles should be symmetric with the midline.
13. Vertical cut lines should be parallel to each other and at a 90-degree angle to the base.
14. Sides should be trimmed to the greatest depth of the vestibule without destroying anatomic structure.
15. Models should be finished with:
    Smooth sides and bases
    Bubbles and voids removed or filled
    Sharp line angles
    Smooth tongue space
16. Typed labels on both models that include the patient's name, age, and the date of the impression

ADVANTAGES OF CUSTOM-MADE TRAYS

Improved accuracy in the impression ensures a better fit of the tray.

A uniform thickness of the impression will be established between the tissues and tray walls to eliminate a potential for voids.

Use of stops eliminates the tray resting on occlusal or incisal surfaces and consequently prevents *burn–through* on dentulous trays.

Less impression material is required to fill the tray.

Tray design can be altered to compensate for missing teeth, unusual arch form, tori, or small mouth openings.

Full arch edentulous trays are used for final impressions for a complete denture.

Segment trays may be used for final impressions for anterior crowns, bridges, or laminates.

The steps in construction of a custom-made acrylic tray include the following:

▶ Preparing the model
▶ Adapting the spacer
▶ Mixing the material
▶ Adapting the material to the spacer
▶ Removing the tray from the model
▶ Finishing the tray

This section provides a general procedure for each of these steps. Basically, you will either construct a quadrant or segment tray with a handle, a full arch tray with a handle for an arch with teeth present, or a full

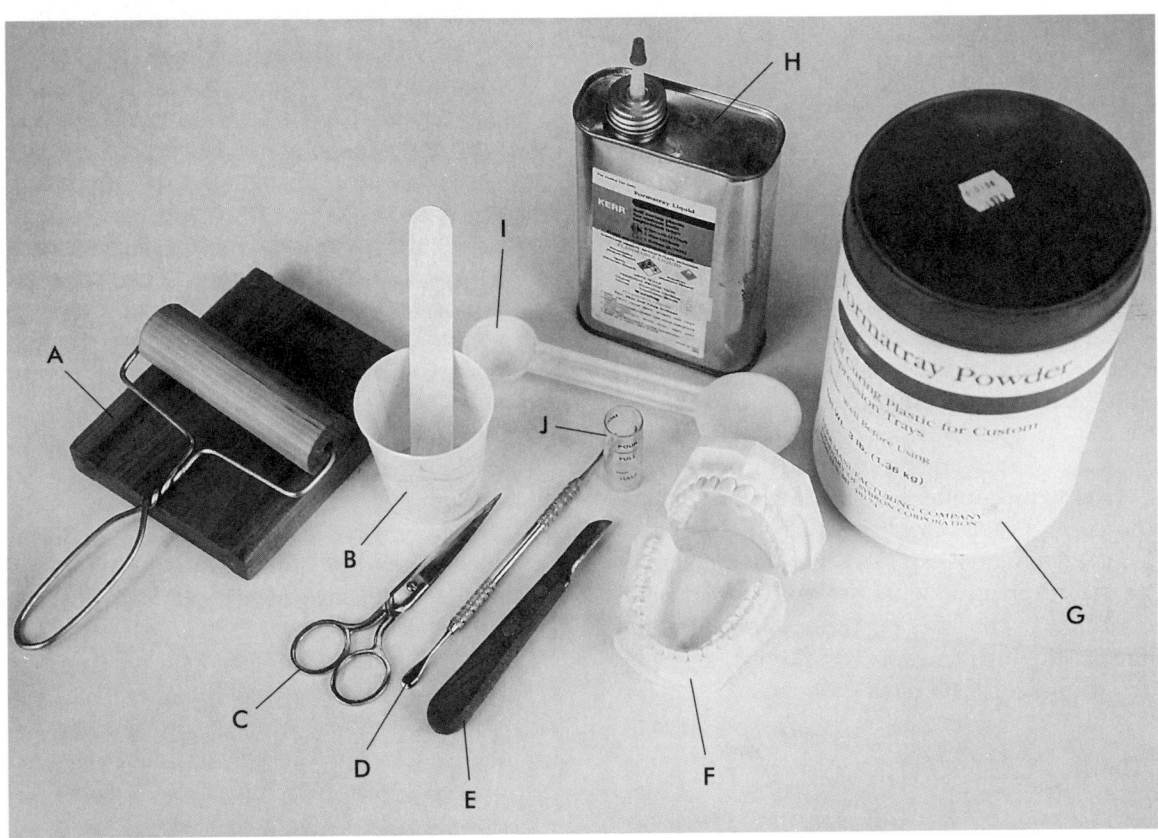

A. Roller and board (optional)
B. Paper cup and tongue blade
C. Scissors
D. #7 Spatula
E. Laboratory knife
F. Study models
G. Acrylic powder
H. Acrylic liquid
I. Powder measuring device
J. Liquid measuring device

Not shown: lining material; wax or nonasbestos liner; bunsen burner; or warm water as desired

FIG. 4-12 Armamentarium for acrylic tray construction.

arch tray with or without a handle for an edentulous arch.

Armamentarium

The armamentarium for constructing custom-made trays includes the following items (Fig. 40-12):

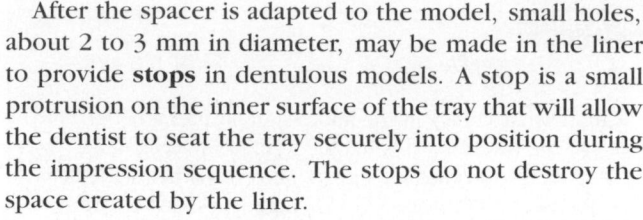

Study models
Acrylic powder and liquid
Powder and liquid measuring devices
Rubber bowl with water
Scissors
Colored pencil
Unwaxed cup
Nonasbestos casting liner or baseplate wax
Tongue blade
Bunsen burner
Wooden roller and board
Lubricant

▶ Preparing the Model

1. With a colored or indelible pencil mark the model for the location of the periphery of the tray.
   a. On models where teeth are present, the mark should be 2 to 3 mm below the cervical margin of the tooth on the buccal and lingual sides.
   b. On an edentulous mandibular model the line is drawn at the greatest depth of the vestibule on the buccal side, extending posterior to the retromolar area and then continuing on the lingual side at the same depth as the buccal.
   c. On an edentulous maxillary model the line is drawn at the greatest depth of the vestibule on the buccal side. On the posterior side the line connects the hamular notch to the fovea.
2. Soak the model for 5 minutes.

▶ Adapting the Spacer

The **spacer** is a method of controlling the amount of impression material that will ultimately occupy the space between the teeth and the tray walls and acts as a guide for adapting the acrylic to the model. The amount of space between the tray and teeth is determined by the thickness of the material used as a spacer. A well-adapted spacer should do the following:

▶ Provide uniform thickness of the spacer material
▶ Extend to the site of the tray periphery marked on the model
▶ Be contoured to compensate for malalignment of teeth or structures, such as a torus
▶ Be designed to eliminate the potential of undercuts

After the spacer is adapted to the model, small holes, about 2 to 3 mm in diameter, may be made in the liner to provide **stops** in dentulous models. A stop is a small protrusion on the inner surface of the tray that will allow the dentist to seat the tray securely into position during the impression sequence. The stops do not destroy the space created by the liner.

1. Cut a piece of baseplate wax that, when folded in half to provide two thicknesses, will cover the area previously outlined for which the tray is being constructed (Fig. 40-13, *A*).
   a. Quadrant tray — Cut a strip that will extend at least two teeth posterior and two teeth anterior to the tooth to be prepared for the restoration (Fig. 40-13, *B*).
   b. Full arch dentulous — fold a full sheet of baseplate wax in half and cut two thirds of the way through the wax at the midline, leaving the fold intact. When the wax is opened at the midline, the wax will resemble the shape of the arch (Fig. 40-13, *C*).
   c. Edentulous maxillary full arch — Cut enough material to cover the palatal area extending to the depth of the vestibule and posterior to cover the tuberosities (Fig. 40-13, *D*).
   d. Edentulous mandibular full arch — Cut strips to cover all of the ridge and flange areas and extend posterior to the retromolar area (Fig. 40-13, *E*).
2. Soften the wax in warm water or with a Bunsen burner. Do not overheat the wax, or it will begin to melt.
3. If a nonasbestos liner is used for a spacer, use two thicknesses of the liner. Dip the liner in water to soften it.
4. Adapt the spacer to the model with your fingers. NOTE: When constructing a full tray on a maxillary model, adapt the palatal area first to ensure adequate coverage.
5. Avoid the possibility of an undercut by filling in space in which the tray could become locked in place.
6. With a #7 spatula, scrape away some of the spacer on the tooth at the most distal and mesial ends of the quadrant covered by the liner (Fig. 40-13, *F*). These open spaces will create the *stops,* so that the acrylic will rest directly on the teeth.
   a. An extra stop is often placed in full arch dentulous trays in the lingual anterior area.
   b. Stops are not necessary on edentulous trays.

▶ Mixing the Acrylic

A self-curing acrylic is used to construct the tray. A nonwaxed cup should be used as a container for mixing. It can be discarded and will not distort during the exothermic reaction created by the material. Most materials come with powder and liquid measuring

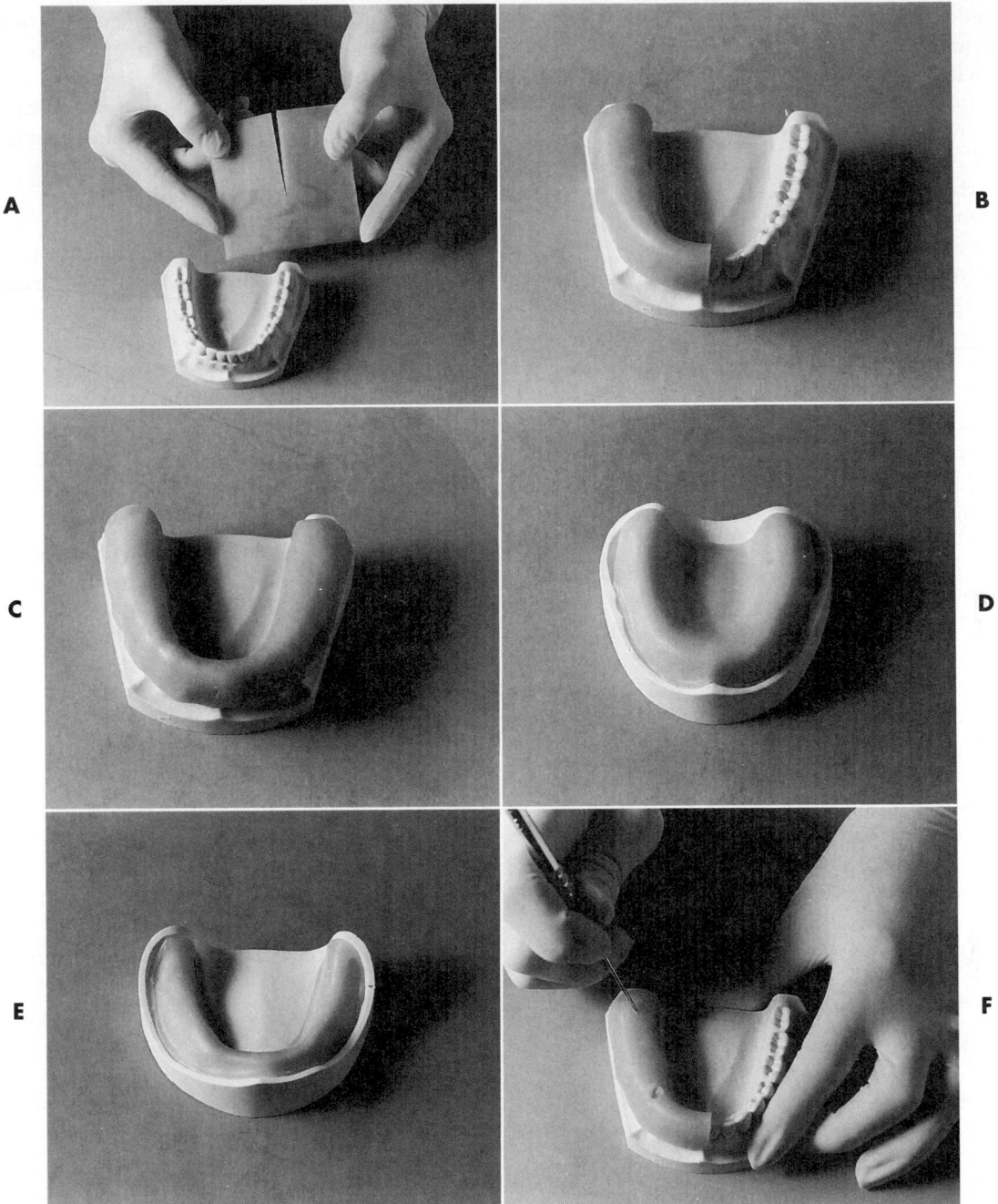

FIG. 40-13   *A,* A piece of baseplate wax is cut to cover the area previously outlined. *B,* Wax spacer in place for a quadrant tray. *C,* Wax spacer for a full arch dentulous tray. *D,* Wax spacer for an edentulous maxillary full arch tray. *E,* Wax spacer for an edentulous mandibular full arch tray. *F,* A #7 spatula is used to scrape away some of the spacer on the tooth at the most distal and mesial ends to create stops.

Continued.

devices and directions for the amounts to be used for a quadrant or full arch tray. Some materials indicate two consistencies of the material, one that is pourable and the other that is moldable. The mold consistency is the more popular technique and applies to the following:

1. If a roller and board are used, lightly coat the surface of each with petroleum jelly.
2. Measure powder and liquid.
   a. Quadrant tray:
      1 small scoop of powder
      Fill to the *½ mold* line to measure liquid for one small scoop of powder.
   b. All full arch trays:
      1 large scoop of powder
      Fill to the *full mold* line to measure liquid for one large scoop of powder.
3. Place measured liquid in a paper cup, and add powder.
4. Mix with a tongue depressor, until all of the powder particles are wetted.
5. Wait for the mix to lose its gloss (about 1 minute).
6. While waiting, lightly lubricate your fingers with petroleum jelly or cool water.
7. When the gloss is gone, test the mix by making an indentation in the center of the mass with the tongue depressor. If the indentation does not disappear, then the mix is ready to use. If the indentation flows back together, then wait a little while and retest (Fig. 40-13, *G*).
8. When the material is ready, remove it from the cup and roll it into a ball or a roll in your hand. Knead it to eliminate all folds in the roll or ball (Fig. 40-13, *H*).
9. If a roller and board are used, place the ball on the board, thick side up, and roll into a flat shape. This can be done in the palm of your hand. If done by hand, be certain it is uniform in thickness and does not show finger depressions. The shape of the rolled acrylic depends on the design of the tray.

▶ Adapting the Material to the Spacer

To adapt the material to a full arch dentulous model, the following procedure is suggested.

1. The material is shaped into a rope that is just slightly shorter than the length of the arch. Extra thickness is left in the middle of the rope, in the anterior region, to be used later to adapt a handle (Fig. 40-13, *I*).
2. Press the acrylic over the spacer.
3. Begin to adapt the material to the arch by working the material from the occlusal/incisal edge to the lingual edge and repeating the same procedure for the buccal side (Fig. 40-13, *J*).
4. Press firmly over the *stop* areas to be sure that the material contacts the model.

5. Pull out excess material from the anterior region to form a handle that extends about ½ inch to ¾ inch and is directed slightly toward the opposite arch (Fig. 40-13, *K*).
6. Either quickly remove the material from the model and trim with scissors to the proper length or leave the material on the model and cut off the excess with a lab knife (Fig. 40-13, *L*). Regardless of which instrument you use, make long cutting strokes to leave a smooth periphery.
7. Readapt the material to the model as quickly as possible to avoid distortion.
8. Keep pressing the material against the spacer until the material achieves its initial set. Be careful not to force acrylic into undercut areas on the model or it will be difficult to remove the tray from the model.

QUADRANT TRAY

1. The acrylic is shaped into a small rope that is approximately the length of the spacer (Fig. 40-13, *M*).
2. Press the acrylic over the spacer.
3. Begin to adapt the material to the quadrant by working the material from the occlusal/incisal edge to the lingual edge and then repeat the same procedure for the buccal side.
4. Press firmly over the *stop* areas to be sure that the material contacts the model.
5. Create a handle for a dentulous or quadrant tray by pulling some of the material perpendicular to the incisal edges and pinching it together. The handle should be about ¾ inch in length and nearly parallel with the occlusal plane (Fig. 40-13, *N*). Too long a handle will cause difficulty in positioning the tray and too short a handle will make it difficult for the operator to remove the tray.
6. As in the full arch tray, press the material against the spacer until the material achieves its initial set; be careful not to force acrylic into undercut areas.

MAXILLARY ARCH

For an edentulous model the following procedure is suggested.

1. Form the material into a *pancake* shape, with the posterior being wider than the anterior to conform to the shape of the arch. The material should be of an even thickness throughout (Fig. 40-13, *O*).
2. Place the acrylic on the model and adapt the acrylic with your fingers over the spacer, beginning in the palatal region and moving across to the alveolar ridge on both sides and down into the vestibule. By adapting the palate area first, any air trapped under the acrylic can be worked toward the periphery of the tray (Fig. 40-13, *P*).

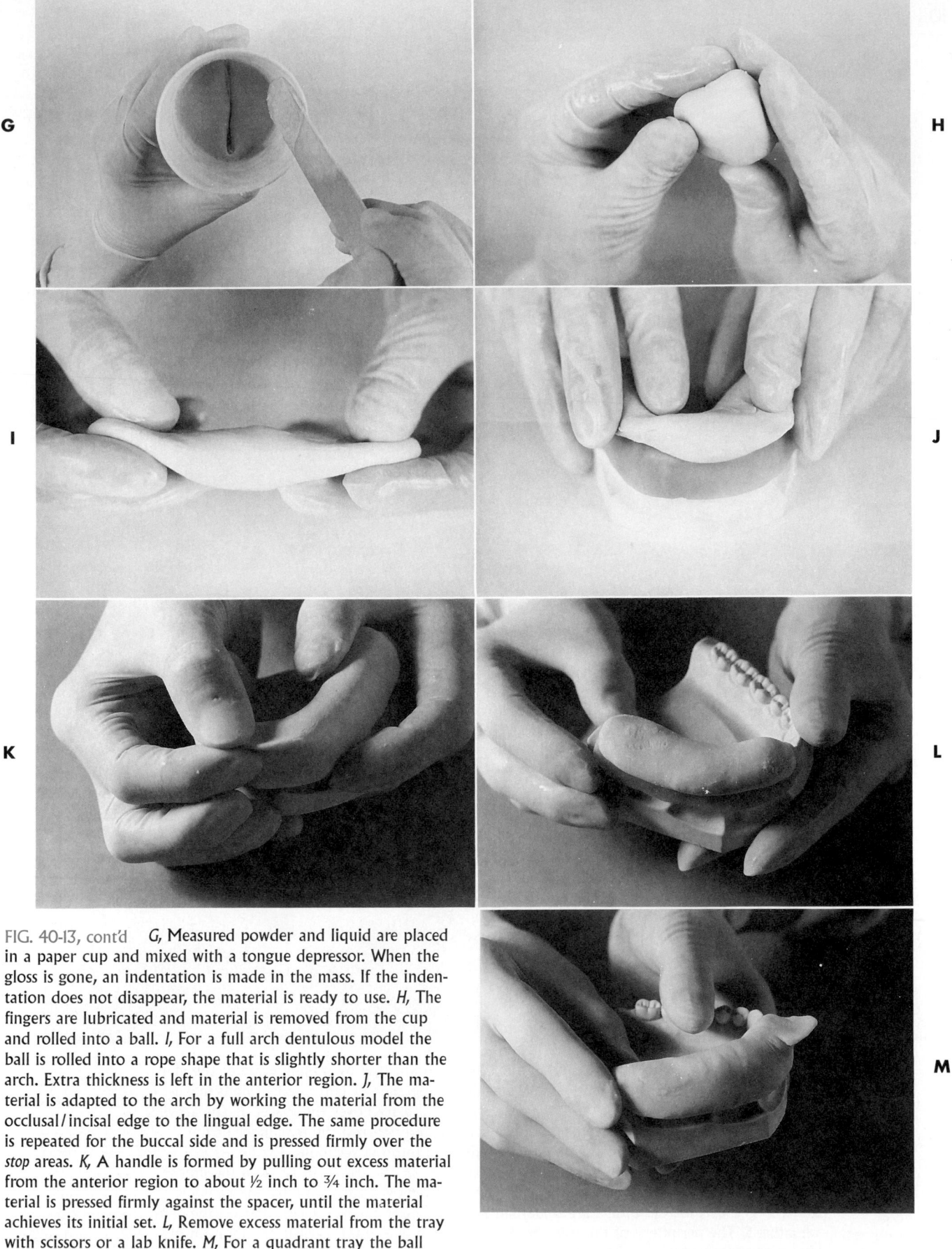

FIG. 40-13, cont'd   *G,* Measured powder and liquid are placed in a paper cup and mixed with a tongue depressor. When the gloss is gone, an indentation is made in the mass. If the indentation does not disappear, the material is ready to use. *H,* The fingers are lubricated and material is removed from the cup and rolled into a ball. *I,* For a full arch dentulous model the ball is rolled into a rope shape that is slightly shorter than the arch. Extra thickness is left in the anterior region. *J,* The material is adapted to the arch by working the material from the occlusal/incisal edge to the lingual edge. The same procedure is repeated for the buccal side and is pressed firmly over the *stop* areas. *K,* A handle is formed by pulling out excess material from the anterior region to about ½ inch to ¾ inch. The material is pressed firmly against the spacer, until the material achieves its initial set. *L,* Remove excess material from the tray with scissors or a lab knife. *M,* For a quadrant tray the ball is shaped into a small rope that is approximately the length of the spacer.   *Continued.*

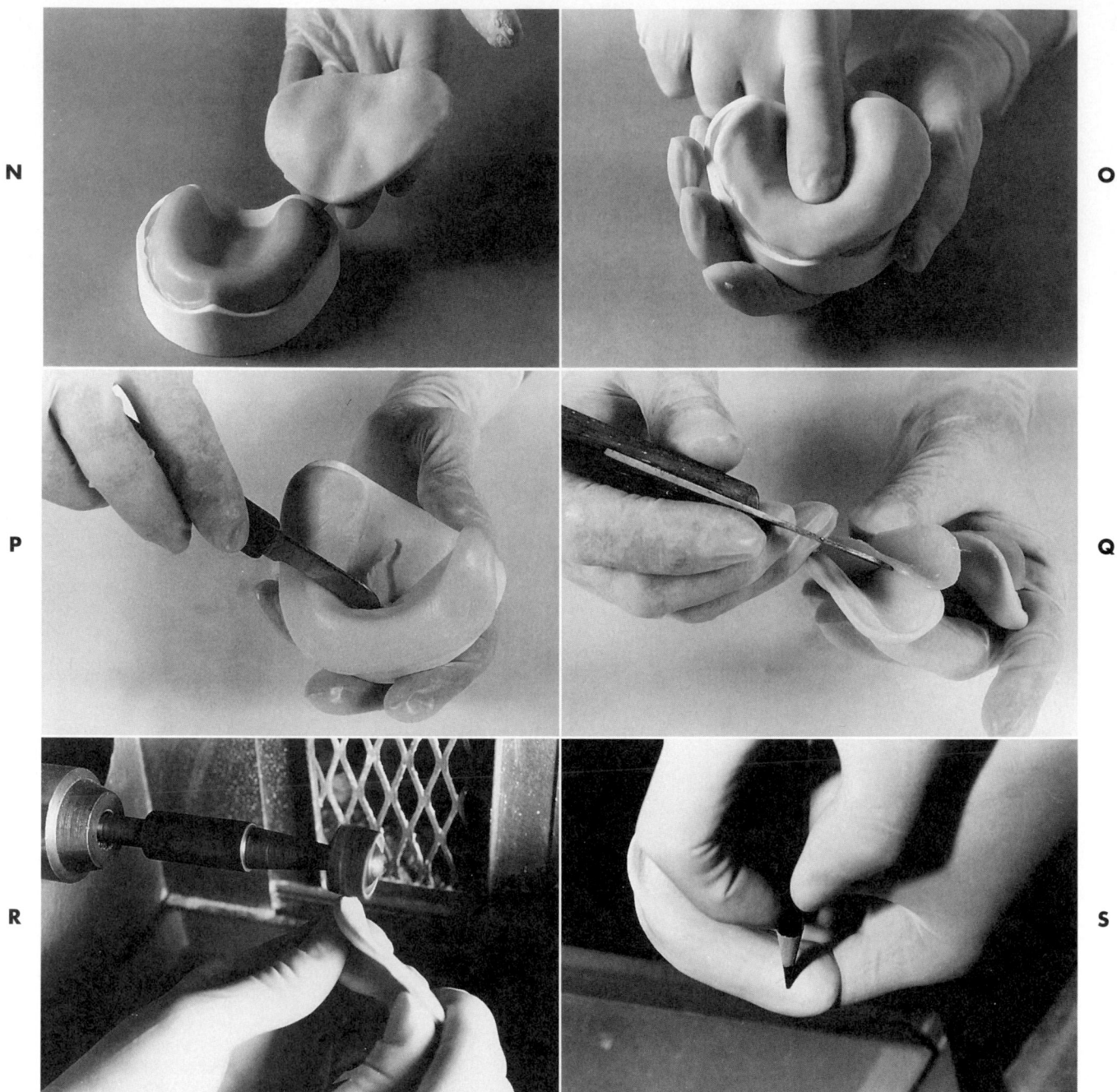

FIG. 40-13, cont'd   *N,* A handle is created for the quadrant tray by pulling some of the material perpendicular to the incisal edges and pinching it together. *O,* For an edentulous maxillary arch the material is formed into a *pancake* shape and placed over the spacer. *P,* The acrylic is placed on the model and adapted to the palatal region first; then the remainder of the material is placed over alveolar ridge on both sides and into the vestibule. The excess is trimmed from the lingual and buccal areas with a knife. *Q,* The tray is lifted from the model after 15 to 20 minutes, using a lab knife. The spacer is removed with a #7 spatula or lab knife. *R,* The peripheral borders are smoothed with an emery band or acrylic bur on the dental lathe. *S,* The periphery of the tray should abut to the line drawn earlier. The location of the stops is marked with a colored pencil.

MANDIBULAR ARCH

1. Form the material into a rope or *hot dog* shape that is long enough to extend the length of the arch, including the retromolar pad areas on both sides as shown in Fig. 40-13, *I* through *L*. Again, the material should be of even thickness.
2. Place the acrylic over the spacer and adapt the material with your fingers. By beginning at the crest of the alveolar ridge and pressing the material toward the vestibule on one side and then moving to the lingual side and adapting the material toward the floor of the mouth, you will be able to eliminate any that is trapped air on the crest of the tray.
3. Avoid pinching the sides of the acrylic, since this will distort the tray and may cause air to be trapped in the crest area.

With both edentulous acrylic trays the material is forced down into the vestibule and may extend beyond the spacer. If this occurs, trim off the excess before the material sets. Use a lab knife or scissors to trim to the proper length. To avoid distortion, readapt the material immediately. If the material is allowed to harden before it is trimmed, the excess can be removed later with a bur or arbor band on the lathe or handpiece.

▶ Removing the Tray from the Model

1. Remove the tray from the model after 15 to 20 minutes.
2. Remove the spacer material, and clean out the interior of the tray. Use warm water to remove excess wax or lift out the nonasbestos liner with a #7 spatula (Fig. 40-13, *Q*) if it adheres to the tray.
3. Clean the interior thoroughly with a toothbrush if necessary.
4. Smooth the peripheral borders with an emery band or acrylic bur on the dental lathe (Fig. 40-13, *R*). The periphery of the tray should abut the line drawn earlier. Avoid creating sharp edges on the tray that might cause discomfort to the patient.
5. Rinse and dry the interior of the tray to remove debris.
6. With a colored pencil, mark the location of the stops on the exterior of the tray (Fig. 40-13, *S*).

Box 40-5 lists criteria for clinically acceptable custom acrylic trays.

▶ Special Considerations

As in model trimming sometimes a model on which an acrylic tray is to be constructed presents special anomalies. Teeth may be missing or rotated or a torus may be present. Often, an area must be blocked out with wax or a nonasbestos type liner or the spacer must be adapted to the contours of the anatomy to design a tray that will compensate for these anomalies.

Mouthguard Construction

Today many patients actively participate in contact sports. A **mouthguard** is made of a resilient plastic material that is prepared directly from a cast of the patient's mouth. When the mouthguard is in place, the wearer is able to breathe and speak normally. One of the most common services a dentist can perform for this patient is the construction of a mouthguard. A mouthguard can prevent many injuries during contact sports (Box 40-6).

BOX 40-5

CRITERIA FOR CLINICALLY ACCEPTABLE CUSTOM ACRYLIC TRAYS

- ▶ It is free from voids or wrinkles.
- ▶ It has a uniform thickness.
- ▶ The peripheral borders are smooth and even.
- ▶ It is free from lateral rocking.
- ▶ Stops are well defined.
- ▶ Dentulous tray extends 2 to 3 mm below the cervical border.
- ▶ The border of the edentulous tray extends to the greatest depth of the vestibule.
- ▶ The full arch tray extends posterior to the maxillary tuberosity or the retromolar pad.
- ▶ A tray with full palatal coverage does not extend distal to the fovea area.
- ▶ Handles are at least ½ inch but no more than ¾ inch in length and are at an angle to provide easy removal from the mouth.
- ▶ Stops are marked on the exterior.
- ▶ Interior surface is free from debris.

BOX 40-6

FUNCTIONS OF A MOUTHGUARD

1. Prevent tooth injury by absorbing and deflecting blows to the teeth.
2. Prevent jaw fractures by creating a cushion between the teeth during the impact of a blow.
3. Shield the lips, tongue, and gingival tissues from laceration.
4. Reduce potential TMJ disorders by cushioning the lower jaw.
5. Prevent potential concussions by absorbing the shock of a blow to the mandible.

A variety of options are available to the patient. The first is to purchase a preformed mouthguard at the local pharmacy or sports store and follow the directions for adapting it to the mouth. Another option is to have the dentist adapt a preformed mouthguard to the patient's mouth (Fig. 40-14); this is done by heating the material in warm water, inserting the material into the mouth, and adapting it to the maxillary arch. These preformed mouthguards certainly provide some protection but are less accurate than a custom-made mouthguard, which is adapted to a model made from an impression of the patient's mouth. The procedure is relatively simple and is a common laboratory task for a dental assistant. The procedure described here uses a manual vacuum machine, but an automatic vacuum processor could be used if available.

Armamentarium

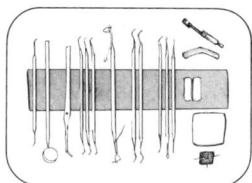

Maxillary model of patient's
  mouth
Laboratory engine
Large acrylic/cutting bur
Vacuum machine
Mouthguard material
Alcohol torch
Laboratory knife or scalpel
Laboratory shears
Bowl of water
Finishing bur
Chamois wheel

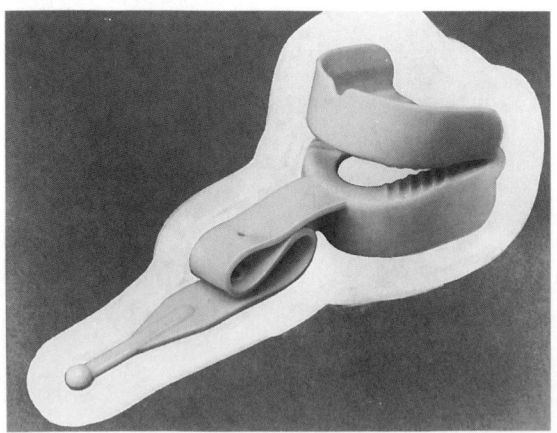

FIG. 40-14   Preformed mouthguard.

▶ Construction of the Mouthguard with a Vacuum Machine

1. Using the maxillary model of the patient, place a hole in the palatal region at the midline, distal to the rugae; this can be done with a large acrylic or cutting bur on a laboratory handpiece; it increases suction to the lingual area and provides better lingual adaptation. If a patient has a Class III malocclusion, the amount of space available for the mouthguard may be prohibitive and the dentist will then need to decide if it is feasible to construct such an appliance for the patient.
2. With a waxed or indelible pencil, mark a finish line for the mouthguard at the junction of the attached gingivae and oral mucosa (Fig. 40-15, *A*). NOTE: The mouthguard does not cover the palate.
3. Soak the cast in water for 3 to 4 minutes to eliminate the mouthguard material that adheres to the model.
4. Place the mouthguard material into the vacuum machine frame, secure the latch, and place the frame in position nearest the heater unit. The mouthguard material is supplied in various thicknesses from 0.08 inch for thin mouthguards to 0.15 inch for the thicker mouthguards are required by football regulations (Fig. 40-15, *B*).
5. Place the model on the base of the vacuum.
6. Turn on the heat and observe the material as it begins to warm and soften. It will begin to sag in the center as it warms. Do not allow it to warm too much, or it will become tacky and difficult to adapt. A sheet that is not warmed enough will not be able to adapt to the anatomic structure of the model (Fig. 40-15, *C*).
7. Once the sheet of material is adequately heated, pull the heated plastic sheet over the moist model and turn on the vacuum. This creates a suction that draws the material over the model.
8. Turn off the heat and push the heater unit to the side.
9. When the vacuum has drawn the material completely down over the model, about 2 to 3 minutes, turn off the vacuum.
10. With moist fingers adapt the material completely around the occlusal and palatal areas (Fig. 40-15, *D*).
11. Remove the material and model from the frame.
12. Allow the material to cool.
13. Remove the material from the model.
14. Using a sharp lab knife or scalpel, trim the material to the line marked on the model in step 2 (Fig. 40-15, *E*).
15. Using a finishing bur, as shown in Fig. 40-15, *F,* trim the peripheral borders of the mouthguard.

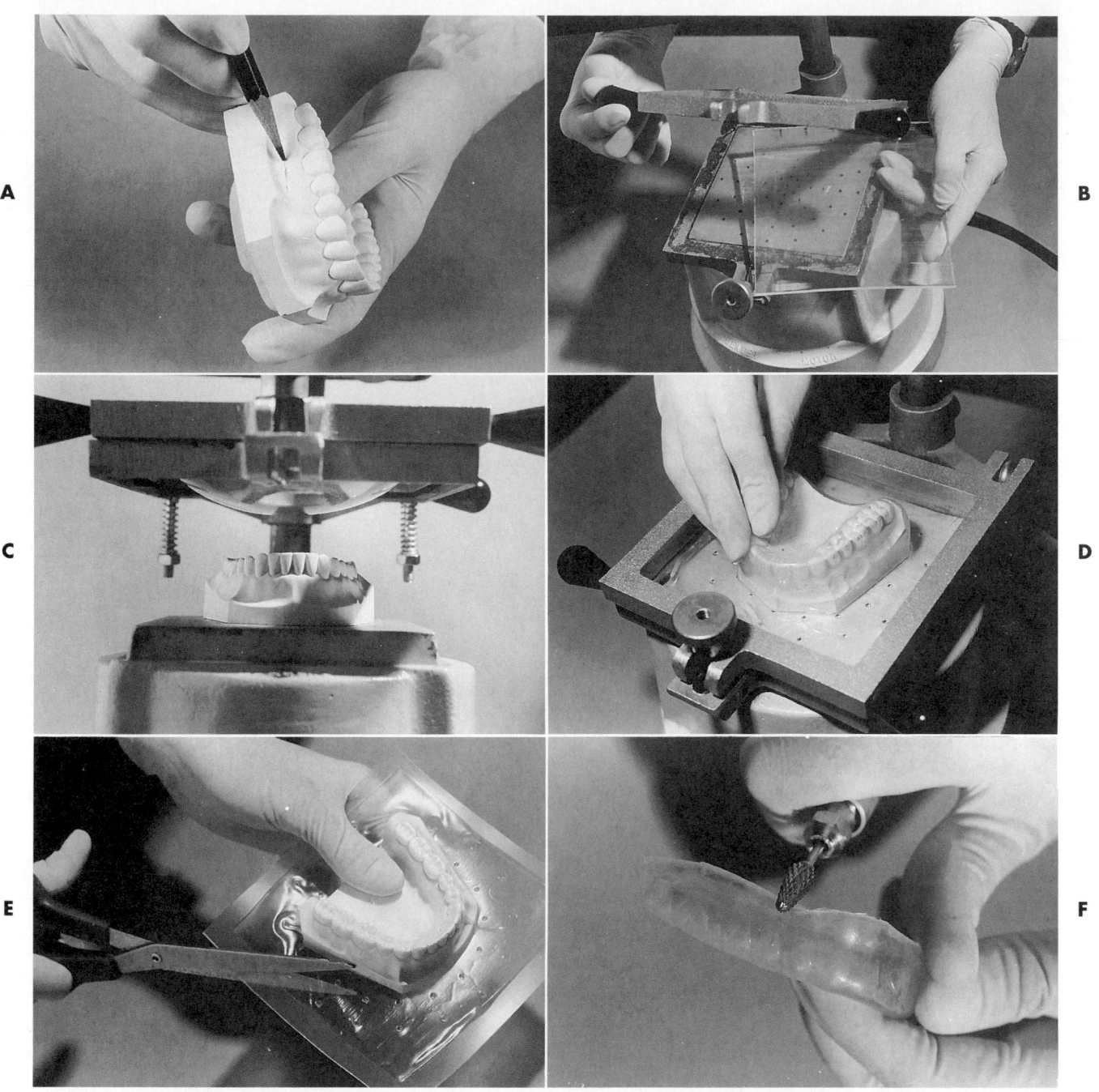

FIG. 40-15   *A,* A hole is made in the maxillary model with a large round acrylic bur. A line is scribed 3 to 4 mm below the cervical line to indicate periphery of the mouthguard. *B,* After the model has been soaked, the mouthguard material is placed into a vacuum machine. *C,* The material is heated until it begins to soften. *D,* After the suction has been used to adapt the mouthguard to the model, moistened fingers are used to adapt the material to the occlusal surfaces. *E,* The model is cut from the material. *F,* The periphery is trimmed with an acrylic bur.

Continued.

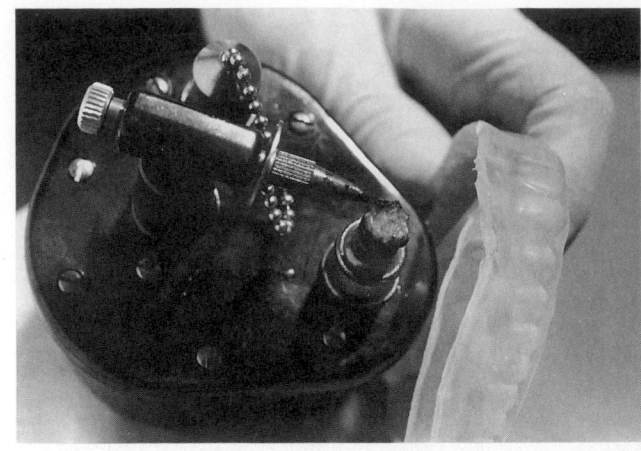
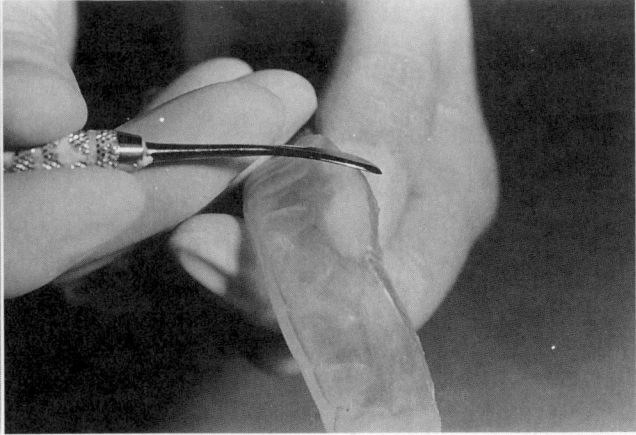

FIG. 40-15, cont'd   *G,* Using an alcohol lamp the peripheral edges are heated. *H, A* #7 spatula is used to smooth as necessary.

16. Use an alcohol torch to warm any rough edges (Fig. 40-15, *G* and *H*). A #7 wax spatula may be used to smooth the edges after heating, or the edges of the mouthguard may be placed over the flame, and with moistened fingers the edge can be contoured.

17. If neither of the procedures in the above step provides a smooth peripheral edge, then buff the edges of the mouthguard with a chamois wheel to ensure a smooth finish.

18. When the mouthguard is delivered to the patient, special home care instructions should be given; these include placing the mouthguard in a container of water when it is not being used or storing it on the model in a closed box.

The criteria for a clinically acceptable mouthguard are listed in Box 40-7.

Additional Laboratory Duties

Depending on the interest of a dentist, the skills of the staff, and the access to a commercial dental laboratory, other minor types of laboratory duties may be performed in a general dental office. Among these are denture repairs; bite rim construction; making wax patterns for crowns, bridges, or inlays; investing and casting; temporary restorations for fixed prosthetics; and temporary dentures. In specialty offices, such as orthodontics, small appliances might also be constructed. Since the construction of temporary restorations is an advanced function in many states and generally a chairside responsibility, this procedure is described in Chapter 32.

▶ Denture Repair

A common type of dental emergency is a fractured denture; this can result from accidental dropping or a change in the occlusal relationships. If the fracture is minor or a single acrylic tooth has been lost or broken, repair can be accomplished within the dental office. The use of cold curing resin simplifies the repair process. The steps for this type of repair are listed in Box 40-8 and illustrated in Fig. 40-16, *A* through *F*.

If the patient has a major repair that involves multiple fractures, the loss of teeth, or a new impression, repair might have to be done at a commercial dental laboratory. A minor repair can often be accomplished in a short time, sometimes while the patient waits. A more complicated procedure may require the doctor's evaluation and, with a new impression, specialized instructions to the laboratory. This, of course, would require a second appointment for the patient.

BOX 40-7

CRITERIA FOR A CLINICALLY ACCEPTABLE MOUTHGUARD

Close adaptation to anatomic structures
Uniform thickness throughout
Smooth peripheral borders
Extends to the maxillary tuberosity
Should not impinge on vestibular or gingival tissue
Should not impinge on frena

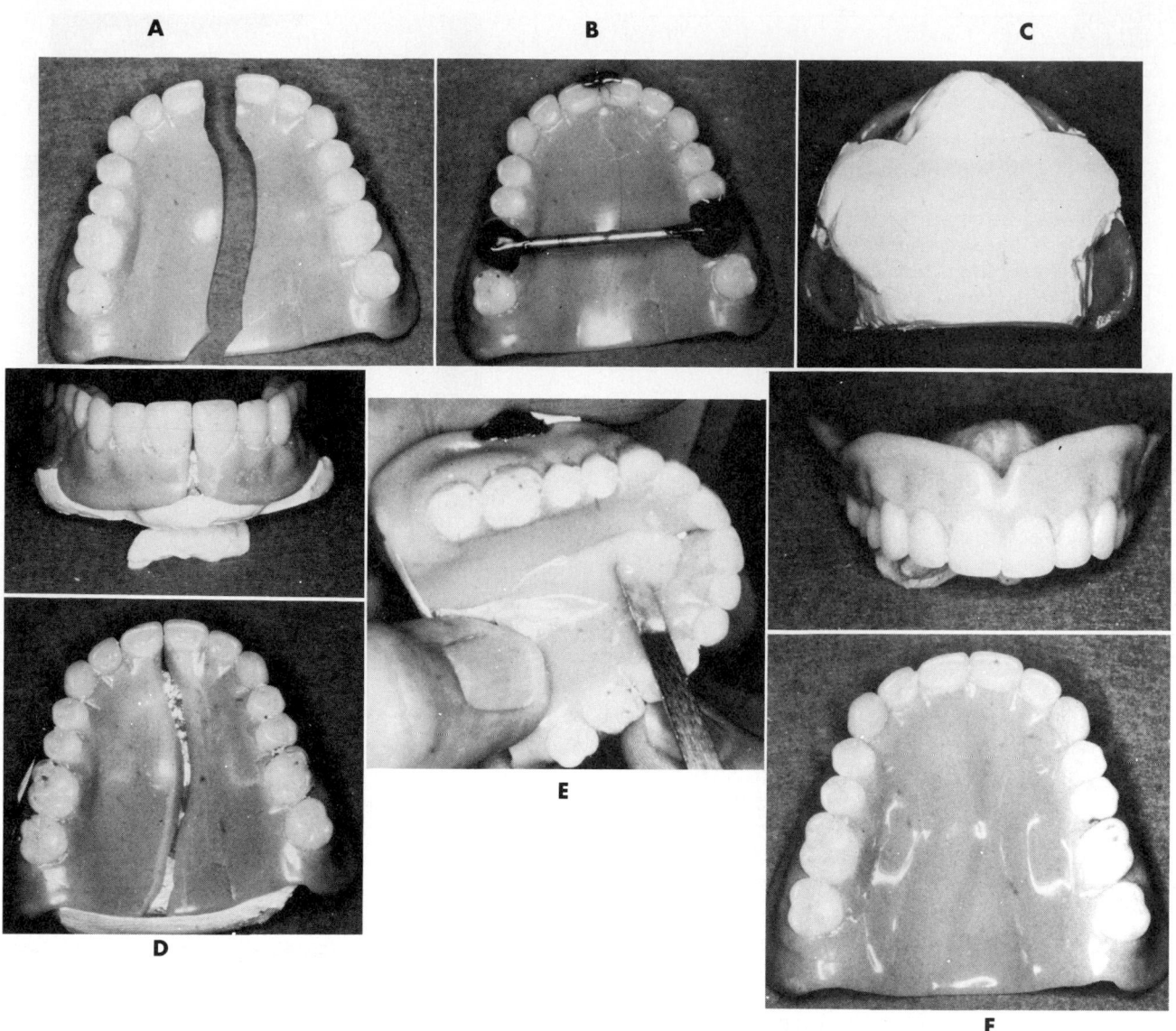

FIG. 40-16   *A,* The pieces are fit together and examined. *B,* The two parts are held together with sticky wax and a toothpick or an old bur. *C,* The inner surface of the denture is lightly lubricated and plaster is gently vibrated into this area. *D,* Acrylic resin is cut away from each side of the fracture, and the denture is replaced on the cast. *E,* The acrylic is flowed into the space that has been cut away, until the area is overfilled. *F,* After the acrylic resin has been polymerized, the denture is finished and polished.

(From Boucher: *Prosthodontic treatment for the edentulous patient*)

▶ Bite Rim Construction

A bite rim is an occluding surface built on a baseplate to establish a maxillomandibular relationship when arranging teeth in denture construction. This use of bite rims is discussed in greater detail in Chapter 31. Often bite rims are constructed in the dental office. Bite rims may be made by rolling a sheet of baseplate wax into a cylinder, which creates several layers of wax, or it may be made by using a preformed bite rim made of baseplate wax. The baseplate wax is shaped into a horseshoe form and adapted to the alveolar crest area of the baseplate.

The height of the wax for the bite rim must extend enough to simulate the height of the missing teeth. The width of the wax bite rim is determined by the contour of the patient's mouth. A final setup of the baseplates and

PROCEDURE FOR REPAIRING A FRACTURED DENTURE

1. Clean debris and food from the broken edges.
2. Hold the two parts together with the use of sticky wax and a toothpick or old bur.
3. Lightly lubricate the inner surface of the denture, and gently vibrate plaster into this area.
4. Remove the denture from the cast, and cut away acrylic resin from each side of the fracture.
5. Replace the denture onto the cast.
6. Paint the edges of the fracture with acrylic resin monomer, and mix the repair acrylic resin.
7. Flow the acrylic into the cutaway space, until the area is overfilled. The extra material will be needed to allow for finishing.
8. When the repair resin has been polymerized, excess material can be removed with large acrylic burs and finished as a denture base.
9. The plaster is removed, and the inner surface is finished.
10. The denture is polished and disinfected.

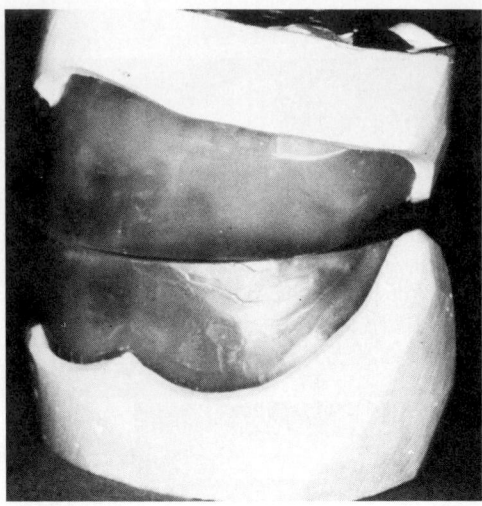

FIG. 40-17   Maxillary and mandibular bite rims have been contoured and adjusted for preliminary jaw relations.

bite rims is placed on an articulator (Fig. 40-17), and the dentist establishes the correct vertical and centric relationships from measurements taken of the patient at an earlier appointment. Once the set-up is completed, the patient is seen for an appointment to try in the set-up and determine if the centric and vertical relationships are correct.

KEY POINTS

▶ A dental assistant who has an interest and the skills to perform basic laboratory duties can be an asset to any office. The preparation of many laboratory devices can be done when the dentist is absent from the office or during procedures that do not require a chairside assistant, including pouring impressions, trimming models, preparing custom-made trays, mouthguards, baseplates, and bite rims, and repairing dentures.

▶ Pouring impressions and trimming a set of clinically accepted diagnostic models is common in many dental offices and in a specialty practice, such as orthodontics; it becomes a task that is performed many times each day. To trim a set of clinically acceptable models, specific guidelines are followed, resulting in an esthetic product that can be used for diagnosis, is symmetric, and provides definition between the art and anatomic portions of the models.

▶ Custom-made trays are used extensively in prosthodontics and are designed specifically to fit an individual patient. These trays may be made for a quadrant, full dentulous, or edentulous arch and can compensate for various anomalies in a patient's mouth. Specific criteria are followed to achieve a clinically acceptable custom-made acrylic tray.

▶ A mouthguard is a protective device used in contact sports. This device, designed on a cast of a patient's mouth, can prevent tooth fracture, damage to the dental arches, lacerations to soft oral tissues, TMJ dysfunction, and possible concussion.

▶ Other laboratory tasks that can be performed by qualified dental assistants include denture repair, baseplate and bite rim construction, and the various steps in creating a cast metal restoration.

BIBLIOGRAPHY

Barton RE, Matteson SR, Richardson RE: *The dental assistant,* ed 6 Philadelphia, 1988, Lea & Febiger.

Laboratory procedures manual, DEN 126, Washtenaw Community College, Ann Arbor, Michigan.

Zarb GA et al: *Boucher's prosthodontic treatment for edentulous patients,* St. Louis, 1990, Mosby.

EPILOGUE

41 The Beginning: Marketing Your Skills

LEARNING OBJECTIVES

You will have mastered the material in this chapter when you can:

▶ Determine your career goals

▶ Identify your personal assets and liabilities for a job

▶ Determine desirable characteristics for a job you might seek

▶ Identify personal priorities for a potential job

▶ Determine methods of marketing your skills

▶ Prepare data for job applications and interviews

▶ Explain how to advance on the job

Once a dental assistant has completed a program of study, thoughts turn to obtaining a certificate, a license, and ultimately a job. At times, a person may become apprehensive about the prospect of a national or state credentialing examination or about seeking a job. It is even possible to lose self-confidence. However, cultivating positive attitudes and taking time to reflect on career goals help in determining the kind of job to seek.

When you are ready to seek employment, it is assumed that you have completed your course of study, used the *Study Guide for Comprehensive Dental Assisting,* studied for a credentialing examination, and obtained or will shortly obtain the necessary credentials as an educated dental assistant and health care professional. Therefore,

this chapter discusses marketing the skills of a highly educated dental assistant.

Before the assistant ventures into the job market, your career goals must be determined. Obviously you are interested in dental assisting and have spent considerable time studying in this field. At this juncture you must explore ways that your career can develop in the future. A career path is based on careful planning and preparation but can be altered by unexpected opportunities and luck. To begin preparation, ask yourself a series of questions.

Where have I been? This question reviews your past, helps you to identify some of the reasons you arrived where you are, and can give you a sense of origin. For some individuals, looking at the past can be depressing, whereas others may yearn for the comfort of the past. Regardless of the impact of the past, reflection is worthwhile. Although some personal information is confidential and certain types of inquiries may not be made during a job interview, it is wise to be prepared for questions about your past employment. For instance, if you had worked at several jobs in the past, an inquiry may be made about the reason for having changed jobs frequently. You will want to explain your job history honestly.

Where am I now? This question seems obvious, yet you need to reassure yourself about where you are in your career path. You have just completed a course of study, you are secure or insecure in a personal/family relationship, and you are looking forward to work in the near or distant future. You need to know that where you are at present will enable you to continue on the career path.

Where am I going? This goal-oriented question helps you determine what you want to be doing in the near and distant future. For some individuals, getting a job and obtaining independence are all they desire. For others, the job may be the means to a future goal. To obtain a job now, to gain experience, to continue school, and ultimately to pursue teaching or dental school may represent several short-range goals that are needed to meet the final, long-range goal. Regardless of what your goals are, you need to realize they might change; being flexible in your goals will enable you to accept challenges along the way.

How am I going to get there? This question is used to

identify the route or steps that need to be identified to achieve your goals. For some, independence means a job or a job may mean security and self-worth. For others, additional education means a short-term job for support to return to school for another degree.

How will I know when I have arrived? Simply stated, this question seeks to have you define what success means to you. For some people this is ever changing. Success can be represented by money, tangible material items, or a feeling of security and satisfaction. No one answer is correct for this question. It is an individual response that only you can determine.

Before going on any job interview it is wise to spend some time by yourself or to share thoughts with peers about these questions. This introspection and sharing can help to build confidence in your plans and goals for a career.

Taking time to prepare yourself for your future career can influence a job interview. When a dentist or office manager asks you to describe yourself, your background, and your career goals, you will be prepared. To simply say, "Oh, there isn't much to tell," indicates you have not given your career much thought, and a potential employer might think you feel the same way about employment.

Self-Assessment

As you begin to seek employment, ask yourself, "What skills and characteristics can I bring to a job and to a prospective employer?" Take some time to write down your skills, strengths, and weaknesses with a prospective job in mind.

You may find as you begin this exercise that you seem to concentrate on your weaknesses. This is not uncommon. Parents, teachers, and associates share criticism willingly, thinking it will improve a person, but sincere praise might not be given as frequently. Criticism may be so common that, when praise *is* offered, it might be difficult to accept. Learn to accept praise, identify your positive characteristics, and develop your assets.

▶ Identifying Personal Assets and Liabilities

Where do you start? First, identify positive characteristics and skills. Then identify your liabilities, but be able to explain how these weaknesses can be overcome. For instance, if you are a person who is prompt, who is seldom absent, and who gives attention to detail, you possess characteristics that are sought in a new employee. If you find it difficult to trim a set of diagnostic models or if you have a problem with the paralleling technique when exposing maxillary molar radiographs,

---

BOX 41-1

DESIRABLE CHARACTERISTICS FOR NEW EMPLOYEES

Promptness	Good general health
Initiative	Creativity
Dependability	Willingness to accept change
Confidentiality	Willingness to work with a
Flexibility	team
Self-motivation	Effective organizational skills
Enthusiasm	Use of proper language skills
Honesty	in verbal and written commu-
Sense of humor	nication

---

these are skill deficiencies that can be improved with more experience. If a prospective employer were to ask about any weaknesses, you could explain that, although you did not do well trimming models in school, you are interested in improving this skill and are willing to expend some extra time on your own to do so. This positive attitude displays an interest in improving rather than an attitude of not caring. Characteristics commonly sought in new employees are identified in Box 41-1.

Marketing Your Skills

A well-educated, experienced dental assistant with the appropriate credentials has valuable bargaining power for obtaining a job that utilizes these skills and provides adequate compensation. Simply to state that you are a graduate of an accredited program is a credible assertion; however, to support this claim with valid data that demonstrate the positive effect you can have on the practice is likely to win you the job.

If a dentist were to state that he or she couldn't afford a well-educated dental assistant, your response might be "I don't believe you can afford *not* to have a well-educated assistant." Consider the following rebuttals to the dentist's reluctance.

1. As a credentialed assistant you have proven by some form of study and a valid test written by dental professionals that you have a basic understanding of dental knowledge and procedures.
2. Research has verified that a single qualified chairside assistant can increase productivity by 30% or more.
3. To delegate infection control to an inexperienced person with no formal knowledge of OSHA standards is opening the door to potential penalties and litigation.

4. Losses due to errors in infection control, claim form management, appointment scheduling, laboratory procedures, manipulation of dental materials, chairside techniques, and patient retention can be significantly reduced with a qualified educated assistant. Although an initial orientation period is necessary in any office, the educated assistant is already aware of procedures and materials that are used in dentistry.
5. Mature students who return to school from other careers, such as homemaking, teaching, and nursing, can bring with them maturity and many life experiences that are valuable assets to any dental assistant job.
6. An educated assistant will remain in the profession longer than an inexperienced person because they have a commitment to the profession through the educational process.
7. An educated assistant enters the interview process with at least 300 hours of clinical experience and many hours of practical laboratory experience.

You must develop a caring, positive, and firm attitude about your ability to become an asset to the office. If you feel uncomfortable about any of these statements, continue to research them and be prepared with some hard data that support your response. For instance, the statement in item no. 2 can be found in research from the 1940s and 1950s that was done by the University of Kentucky and University of Alabama. It is your responsibility, however, to live up to the claims you make.

Your skills, knowledge of dentistry, investment in your education, and credentials are all tools that can be used to achieve compensation commensurate with that of other allied health professionals who have similar backgrounds and responsibilities.

Job Priorities

Every one dreams of the ideal job. Yet many people are so excited to be given an interview that they take the first job offer without considering their needs and priorities.

Before applying for a job or preparing for the job interview decide what you need and want in a job. Several factors to consider are work environment, challenge of the job, responsibilities, location of the work place, salary, benefits, opportunities, and hours. The benefits package can be broken down into specific categories, and those that you consider high priority can be listed as separate items. Although a dentist is required to provide an employee with HBV vaccinations; clinic attire for patient exposure; and protective barriers, such as glasses, masks, and gloves, additional benefits that are often considered are identified in Box 41-2.

Once you have reviewed the various factors involved in job selection, decide on your own top five priorities for

BOX 41-2

POTENTIAL JOB BENEFITS

Uniform allowance (nonclinic)	Profit sharing
Retirement plan	Child care
Health insurance	Dues to professional organization
Vision insurance	Travel and expenses to professional meetings
Dental care/insurance (for self and family)	Special bonuses; holidays
	Production achievement

a job and then rate each of the job offers. A decision-making grid like the one that accompanies Box 41-3 might help.

The job offers are listed in the left vertical column and the priorities in the horizontal boxes at the top. Starting on the left the priorities are given a point value based on your personal needs. Each job is evaluated and the points totaled. If there is a tie, other characteristics can be added.

Data Preparation for Prospective Job

Job information may be obtained from many sources, including the dental assistant faculty, college placement department, private employment agencies, newspaper want ads, clinical rotations, and word of mouth. Regardless of the source of the prospective job, several documents are needed during the job search and interview. These include a letter of application, personal resume, job application, verification of credentials, and follow-up letters.

▶ Preparing a Resume

The resume, or personal vitae, is intended to relieve the letter of application of details regarding your background and qualifications for the job. A resume should include a career objective; education; credentials; work experience; extracurricular activities, memberships, and special service honors; as well as references. An example of a resume is shown in Fig. 41-1. Note the statement that references are available upon request. When you name anyone as a reference, you should contact that person in advance and confirm that he or she is willing to be a reference for you. These individuals should have dental experience and be able to verify your professional skills and personal characteristics.

A resume should be brief, complete, accurate, and attractively presented. The use of word processing

```
                                    RESUME

        PERSONAL DATA

        Name:          Deborah L. Benson

        Address:       5281 Kalamazoo Ave., S. E.
                       Grand Rapids, MI 49507

        Telephone No:   AC 616 - 111-2817        Soc. Sec. No:    369-38-5043

        Objective:  To obtain a job that will utilize my dental assisting skills to a maximum
                    in the practice of team dentistry.

        EDUCATION

        Kent Community College, Grand Rapids, Michigan
        Graduated, June 19--, Associate Degree in Dental Assisting, 3.42 Grade Point Average
        C.D.A.- May 28, 19--
        Related Courses:  Dental Science             Clinical Practice
                          Dental Laboratory Procedures    Dental Roentgenology
                          Dental Practice Management
        Member of:  Kent County Dental Ass't. Assoc., Michigan Dental Ass't. Assoc. and
                    American Dental Ass't. Assoc.


        South High School, Grand Rapids, Michigan
        Graduated, June 19--, College Preparatory

        EMPLOYMENT RECORD

        Clinical Practice:  January - June, 19--
        Xavier University, School of Dentistry
            DAU, Pedodontic, and Crown and Bridge Clinics
        Charles Allan, D.D.S. 123 Huron River Drive, S.E. Grand Rapids, Michigan
        James Richardson, D.D.S. 2608 Patricia, Wyoming, Michigan
        Charles Van Beek, D.D.S. 2426 Naubinway, Franklin, Michigan


        Summer Job:  June - September, 19--
        J. D. Jenks, D.D.S. 1334 Main S. E., Grand Rapids, Michigan

        REFERENCES
```

FIG. 41-1   Resume.

(From Finkbeiner BL, Patt JC: *Practice Management for the Dental Team,* ed 3, St Louis, 1991, Mosby.)

enables you to create original copies and use specialized features that will create a good initial image.

▶ Preparing a Letter of Application or Inquiry

A letter of application is the initial introduction of yourself; this may be one of the most important letters you will write. Basically, it is a sales letter that not only introduces you, but also verifies your skills, knowledge, and ability. Special attention should be given to the appearance, format, and content of the letter, since it might be a deciding factor in obtaining an interview with the prospective employer.

The goals of a letter of application should be to:
▶ Create interest
▶ Describe your abilities
▶ Request an interview

An example of a letter of application, which is sent as the cover letter to the resume, is shown in Fig. 41-2. Suggestions for writing a letter of application are shown in Box 41-3.

▶ Collecting Pertinent Data

Before the interview, collect all of the information you might need in a small notebook. This ensures that you will not forget anything during the interview. Such organization can eliminate the need to ask for a telephone directory or potential errors in data entry on the form. The information should include the following:
▶ Your name, address, phone numbers, and times you can be reached
▶ Complete names, addresses, and phone numbers of references
▶ Chronologic listing of former employment, addresses, and contact persons

5281 Kalamazoo Ave., S.E.
Grand Rapids, MI 49507
June 15, 19--

Joseph W. Lake, D.D.S.
611 Main Street S.E.
Grand Rapids, MI 49502

Dear Dr. Lake:

This letter is in response to your advertisement in the Grand Rapids News, June 12, 19--. You asked for a dental assistant who is skilled in four-handed dentistry, gets along with people, and possesses management capabilities. Consider me an applicant for this job.

You will see from the enclosed resume that I have taken courses at Kent Community College, Grand Rapids, Michigan to prepare me as a Registered Dental Assistant. I have successfully completed courses in dental assisting that will be valuable to your practice and have had considerable clinical and business office experience.

You may contact me at 111-2817 after 3:00 p.m. any day of the week. I am available for an interview at your convenience.

Sincerely,

Deborah L. Benson, R.D.A.

Enclosure

FIG. 41-2   **Letter of application.**

(From Finkbeiner BL, Patt JC: *Practice management for the dental team,* ed 3, St Louis, 1991, Mosby.)

(From Finkbeiner BL, Patt JC: *Practice management for the dental team,* ed 3, St Louis, 1991, Mosby.)

BOX 41-3

SUGGESTED CONTENT FOR LETTER OF APPLICATION

1. Create an impressive image. The letter must be keyed (typed), neat, free from smudges and wrinkles, and printed on bond paper. Review the letter and check for spelling, grammar, and other keyboarding errors.
2. Be brief. This letter is simply an introduction and an attention getter; it should stimulate interest in the reader to review the resume.
3. Be *you* oriented. The letter should emphasize what you can do for the practice from the dentist's point of view rather than from your point of view. Simply stated, do not begin each paragraph or sentence with "I."
4. Address the letter to a specific person, not "To Whom It May Concern." Take the time to find out the correct name of the prospective employer and, if you are answering a blind ad from the newspaper, use "Dear Doctor" as the salutation.
5. Be honest. Do not make any claims in the letter that you will not be able to substantiate.
6. Use an appropriate letter style. Styles such as block and modified block (left margins the same or indented) are more traditional and are well accepted.

Job Decision Making Grid

	Practice environment	Salary	Benefits	Location	Challenge	Hours	Total
Point value	6	5	4	3	2	1	
Job offer No. 1		✓	✓	✓		✓	13
Job offer No. 2	✓		✓	✓	✓		15
Job offer No. 3	✓	✓		✓			14

▶ List of your job priorities
▶ Questions you want to have answered during the interview

▶ Completing the Application

The type of dental assisting job for which you are applying will determine the detail and complexity of the application form. This form may be sent to you before an

EMPLOYMENT APPLICATION

All information listed on this application will be considered and handled as personal and confidential. Please write or print legibly.

Date _____

NAME _____ PHONE NO. _____

MAILING ADDRESS _____ SS# _____
No.   Street   City   State   Zip

How long have you lived in this area? _____ Are you over 18 yrs. of age and under 70? Yes _____ No _____

Are you known by Schools / References by another name? Yes _____ No _____ If yes by what name? _____

Position interested in: _____ If offered employment when can you start _____
(Date)

Will transportation to work be a problem for you? Yes _____ No _____

Can your vacation be arranged most any time? Yes _____ No _____ If no, when? _____

Is there any reason why you could not be bonded? Yes _____ No _____ Do you wish employment: Full time _____

Part time _____ Hours per week _____

Does the sight of blood bother you? Yes _____ No _____

Number of days missed from work/school in last year because of illness or injury: _____

List any physical defects or chronic diseases you think may interfere with your ability to perform the job you are presently applying for:

_____
_____
_____

EDUCATION

	Elementary	High	College/University	Professional
School Name				
Years Completed: (Circle)	4 5 6 7 8	9 10 11 12	1 2 3 4	1 2 3 4
Diploma/Degree				
Describe Course Of Study:				
Describe Specialized Training, Apprenticeship, Skills, Seminars, Courses, Extra-Curricular Activities				

SKILLS:

	(circle)			(circle)	
Typing (Speed _____)	Yes	No	Pour Models	Yes	No
Shorthand (Speed _____)	Yes	No	Cavitron	Yes	No
Bookkeeping - Pegboard	Yes	No	Cast Inlays	Yes	No
Dictation Equipment	Yes	No	Plaque Control Instruction	Yes	No
Handling Group Insurance	Yes	No	Oral Evacuator	Yes	No
Take X-Rays	Yes	No	Knowledge of Dental Instruments	Yes	No
Panoramic X-Rays	Yes	No	Knowledge of Dental Terms	Yes	No
Other: (Describe if yes)	Yes	No	Data Processing	Yes	No

_____
_____
_____
_____

This employer provides equal opportunity to all persons without regard to handicap, race, color, religion, sex, age or national origin.

Form 113 1980 SYCOM, Madison, WI Printed in U.S.A.   Over

FIG. 41-3   Application for employment.

(From Finkbeiner BL, Patt JC: *Practice management for the dental team,* ed 3, St Louis, 1991, Mosby.)

interview, or you may be asked to complete it the day of the interview.

Before the application form is completed, read through it thoroughly to avoid asking unnecessary ques-tions or duplicating your answers. The form may be typed (if presented in advance) or the directions may indicate that the form be written. The application can be a test of your ability to follow directions as well as a test of

EMPLOYMENT RECORD · List most recent employer first:

Name of Employer		
Address		
Supervisor & Telephone Number		
Title & Description of your job		
Dates of Employment	Start	Last
Earnings	Start	Last
Reason for leaving		

Name of Employer		
Address		
Supervisor & Telephone Number		
Title & Description of your job		
Dates of Employment	Start	Last
Earnings	Start	Last
Reason for leaving		

Name of Employer		
Address		
Supervisor & Telephone Number		
Title & Description of your job		
Dates of Employment	Start	Last
Earnings	Start	Last
Reason for leaving		

REFERENCES (not former employers or relatives):

NAME	ADDRESS	TYPE BUSINESS

In the course of making an employment decision, this employer makes it a practice to verify with previous employers information such as dates of employment, description of job duties, attendance records, reason for leaving, etc. If there are any employers you wish we not contact, please indicate their names below and reasons why:

_____

_____

_____

_____

I understand that if I am employed and any statement herein is not true, I may be released immediately, I will be paid only through the day of release and this employer may cancel any rights to accrued benefits.

_____   _____
Date   Signature

FIG. 41-3, cont'd   **Application for employment.**

neatness. Be prepared with a ballpoint pen to complete the form.

Be sure that you answer all of the questions. If a question does not relate to you, write N/A (not applicable) or draw a line through the question. This will indicate to the employer that you did read the question and did not overlook it.

Be truthful when answering each of the questions. Dates, names, and places need to be accurate. Your prepared notebook should aid you at this point. A commonly used application is shown in Fig. 41-3.

▶ Preparing for the Interview

A call from a potential employer for a personal interview is an exciting time, yet it is one that is filled with apprehension. You may not know anything about the prospective employer, but one thing is certain: you know about yourself, and now is the time to market your skills and abilities.

Dress appropriately, be well groomed, and be on time. Image is important, and rightfully so. Wear something that makes you feel good but is appropriate for the situation. Jeans may be natural for you, but they are not appropriate for a job interview.

During the interview you may be confronted with several questions, such as those that follow:

1. Tell me something about yourself. (If you did your homework earlier, this will be a breeze.)
2. Why do you think you would be a good employee?
3. What are your strengths? Your weaknesses?
4. How did you decide to enter dental assisting?
5. With what types of clinical procedures are you familiar?
6. In what type of work environment do you function well?
7. Are you certified? Licensed?
8. What types of clinical experience have you had?
9. Are you willing to work in various satellite offices?
10. Hypothetical questions that require you to respond to certain clinical and human relations situations.

In general, it is wise to pause after a question is asked to reflect on your answer. Take time and don't blurt out an answer—this is not a timed test. Write out your answers to the questions above and practice them verbally (in front of a mirror) to determine what your body language is telling the prospective interviewer.

Remember that the interview is a two-way street, and you should be given an opportunity to ask questions. Generally, as the interviewer comes to the conclusion of the questions, he or she will ask if you have questions. You may suggest that you had prepared some questions in advance and take a look at this list to ensure that all questions have been answered. Some of the following questions might be ones that you may want to cover:

1. What will be my responsibilities?
2. How does the staff work together as a team?
3. To whom do I report?
4. What types of evaluations will be used for my performance?
5. Could you explain the salary scale and advancement levels?
6. Would you describe the benefit package and when I would be eligible for these?
7. How do you practice four-handed dentistry?
8. What is your attitude toward continuing education for yourself and the staff?
9. How long has the position been available, and how many people have held the position in the last 3 or 4 years?
10. What is your practice philosophy?

When the interview is over, you may be given a tour of the facility. You may be asked to return to observe the office as the interview enters the final stages, or you may be asked to come for a working interview. Employers will generally interview several applicants before making a job offer to one of the candidates. If the interviewer does not offer, inquire when the interviews will be complete, when the decision will be made about the hiring, and whether you will receive a call or a letter regarding the final decision. You may be offered the job at the interview, and you can ask for a short time to think about the job offer if you wish. In either case, thank the interviewer for his or her time.

▶ Follow-up after the Interview

Once you have completed the interview, you will want to determine if the job is right for you. To evaluate the position and determine whether it is for you, return to the initial job evaluation grid that you completed earlier and perhaps review several questions that you have in mind about the job. These might include the following:

1. What will my responsibilities be? Do I have the skills for the job? Is it the area in which I am really interested?
2. What will my hours of work be? Do they provide regular lunch hours? Are these hours compatible with my family and personal responsibilities?
3. If I work overtime, will I be paid or receive compensatory time off?
4. What is in the benefit package? Medical insurance, vision, dental prescription plan?
5. Does the office appear to adhere to OSHA guidelines and acceptable infection control procedures?
6. Are there profit sharing, bonuses, retirement plans, or other remunerative packages?
7. What is the policy for sick days, personal leave days, and holidays?

8. When will I be eligible for vacation and how much time will I receive each year? Is there a specified time or is the time choice mine?

9. How am I evaluated, and is my performance evaluation correlated to a form of merit compensation?

10. Is there evidence that four-handed dentistry concepts are practiced in the office?

It is wise to write down the details of the interview that you want to remember, such as salary, hours, and duties.

Once you have reviewed your questions, evaluated the job, and determined how the offer fits into your priorities, you can decide if this job fits into your career path.

Within 1 or 2 days a follow-up letter should be sent to the interviewer. This is an indication to the interviewer that you are interested in the position, and this may place your application in priority. A sample letter is shown in Fig. 41-4. Avoid calling before the decision deadline to inquire about the job. After the decision deadline it is

---

5281 Kalamazoo Ave., S. E.
Grand Rapids, MI 49507
June 25, 19—

Joseph W. Lake, D.D.S.
611 Main Street S. E.
Grand Rapids, MI 49502

Dear Dr. Lake:

Thank you for the interview you gave me yesterday afternoon.

It was my privilege to see such a well-organized dental team. Because of my training, I am confident that I can become an efficient dental assistant and an asset to your dental team.

After you have had a chance to review my application, you will see that I have had considerable work experience.

I am available for work immediately. You may contact me any day of the week by calling 111-2817 after 3:00 p.m.

Sincerely,

Deborah L. Benson, R. D. A.

FIG. 41-4　Follow-up letter.

(From Finkbeiner BL, Patt JC: *Practice management for the dental team*, ed 3, St Louis, 1991, Mosby.)

Dear Dr. Martin:

Please accept my resignation as chairside assistant for your practice effective July 12, 19_ _.

Since I plan to return to school in August, I will need a few weeks to get things ready and to pre-pare for the fall term. I will be happy to orient my replacement if you wish.

Thank you for the opportunity to work with you these past 4 years. This job has provided me with a great deal of experience, and I have enjoyed working with you and the patients. My replacement has much to look forward to in this job.

Respectfully yours,

Jennifer McGinnis

FIG. 41-5   Letter of resignation.
(From Finkbeiner BL, Patt JC: *Practice management for the dental team,* ed 3, St Louis, 1991, Mosby.)

appropriate to call or write if you have received no response.

Advancing on the Job

Obtaining a job is one task, but getting ahead in the job and keeping the job is an even more important achievement. To perform well in a job, a person must have a complete job description and well-prepared directions for various tasks. This information can be provided in an employee procedure manual. In addition, a contract or written agreement between the employer and employee can serve to define the details of the employment and determine when the periodic evaluations will be performed.

To grow professionally, you must keep up with the changes in technology and be willing to participate in your professional organizations. Even if you have to pay for these activities yourself, you will find the benefits are worth the investment.

If you are unable to participate in courses or seminars offered by your professional organizations, you may want to enroll in classes in your local 4-year colleges, community colleges, or vocational schools. As you progress in your career, you may find that you will be assuming administrative or supervisory tasks. Consequently, you may want to take courses in management, small business administration, telecommunications, computer applications, or human relations. Once you are employed, you may find these courses enjoyable and be more relaxed than when you were in your earlier professional programs and were concerned about grades and completion.

Self-Evaluation

Periodically you will want to evaluate yourself and determine if you are maintaining your interest and skill level. This evaluation, done honestly, may point to areas in which you need improvement to progress to the professional level you initially expected to attain when you took the job. The evaluation forms in Tables 41-1 and 41-2 will help you in this self-evaluation of technical, as well as personal, development areas.

Changing Career Paths

It is possible that you may be employed in a job for 3 or 4 years, receive excellent evaluations from your employer, and yet one day think "I'm bored with this job. I'm leaving right now and not coming back." These thoughts are normal; however, do not act hastily. You have spent considerable time in the job, spent time and money on your education, and invested years with the practice. Before leaving a job, take the time to analyze the situation as you did when you applied for the job. If you continue to think that the job is not right for you, then take some action.

Analyze the reasons you are unhappy in the job. Sit down in a quiet place and decide whether it is the job itself, the co-workers, the employer, personality traits, value differences, money, or promotions or if are you simply bored and believe that you are not growing. Have you discussed these concerns with your employer? Are you ready for a change? Have you continued to learn on the job so that you are ready for the next step? Are you still enthusiastic about the profession? If the problem is one of boredom, what have you done to make the job challenging? Have you made an effort to look for opportunities to grow on the job?

Once you have determined your reasons for unhappiness in the job setting, spend some time looking at your goals. Remember, earlier it was stated that your goals change as you mature. Maybe you need to rethink your career goals. You might be ready to return to school to teach or even to go on to dental school. You may want a new environment in a large company or an institution in dental practice management or other areas.

Once you have reevaluated your career goals, consider your qualifications for attaining these goals. Will this new job opportunity be challenging and offer the priorities you have determined, or is the move simply lateral, doing different tasks in the same environment? Will the new job offer the challenges you are seeking?

Regardless of the reasons for leaving a job, you have the responsibility to your employer to submit a letter of termination and adequate notification for them to replace you. Fig. 41-5 is an example of a letter of resignation.

Attitudes for Continued Success

A highly qualified and educated dental assistant is the key to increased production, retention of patients, prevention of transmission of infectious diseases; the right individual can significantly decrease stress on the dental operating team. As you grow past your entry level position on the job, you will discover that your future success depends more and more on your attitude and human relations skills. To have completed a program of study in dental assisting, you have a good beginning.

Your willingness to be a team player and to cooperate with patients and staff and your good communication skills will be assets to the dental practice. Your initiative, self-motivation, creativity, and enthusiasm indicate an eagerness to accept leadership and challenges in the office. Your desire to learn, your curiosity, and your flexibility will enable you to attain new skills and to advance in your career.

Continue to market your skills, maintain an interest in new technologies, and accept changes no matter where you are on your career path. Good luck!

TABLE 41-1   SELF-EVALUATION OF PERSONAL CHARACTERISTICS

The following questions are designed for you to use in evaluation of your own personal characteristics. If you cannot honestly answer a question "yes," then you should spend time in self-improvement in these areas during the coming weeks. REMEMBER—be honest with yourself; you are the person who will benefit the most from such an evaluation.

	Yes	No	Sometimes
SELF-CONFIDENCE			
1. Do you communicate easily with people?			
2. Are you willing to continue with a job even though you are criticized?			
3. When you have made a decision, do you support your decision?			
4. Do you refrain from bragging?			
5. Do you accept new responsibilities easily?			
TACTFULNESS			
6. Do you think about what you say before saying it?			
7. Do you practice self-control?			
8. Do you avoid unnecessary interruptions of others' privacy?			
9. Do you make patients feel important?			
10. Are you patient with others?			
11. Do you have empathy for other people?			
DEPENDABILITY			
12. Are you always on time for work, school, and/or appointments?			
13. Do you pay attention to the details of your work?			
14. Do you avoid being absent except for serious illness?			
15. Do you follow through with your commitments?			
16. Do you stay with a job until it is finished?			
17. Do you always do the job assigned to you?			
INITIATIVE			
18. Do you look for work that needs to be done?			
19. Do you organize your time?			
20. Are you proud of your completed work?			
21. Are you eager to please other people?			
22. Do you accomplish more work than is assigned to you?			
JUDGMENT AND DECISION MAKING			
23. Are you eager to learn new things?			
24. Are you curious about the unknown?			
25. Do you examine all possibilities before making a decision?			
26. Do you evaluate the results of an action before taking it?			
27. Are you interested in continuing education?			
INTEGRITY			
28. Do you respect other people and their property?			
29. Do you avoid discussing confidential information?			
30. Do you refrain from gossip?			
31. Can you be trusted with money that belongs to the office?			
32. Do you tell the truth even though you may suffer the consequences?			
HUMAN RELATIONS			
33. Do you have a sense of humor?			
34. Are you a good listener?			
35. Do you maintain eye contact when talking to another person?			
36. Can you accept criticism?			
37. Do you avoid being overbearing?			
38. Do you speak first when meeting someone new?			
39. Do you think of others before yourself?			
40. Do you use a person's name when talking to him?			
41. Do you avoid frowning and smile naturally?			

TABLE 41-2   SELF EVALUATION: HYGIENE AND GROOMING CHARACTERISTICS

The following questions are designed for you to use in evaluation of your personal hygiene. If you cannot honestly answer a question "yes," then you should spend time in developing a daily routine that will improve your grooming and hygiene habits. REMEMBER—as a member of a health profession you must set a good example of optimum health.

	Yes	No	Sometimes
BODY HYGIENE			
1. Do you bathe daily?			
2. Do you use a deodorant daily?			
ORAL HYGIENE			
3. Do you brush your teeth at least twice daily?			
4. Do you have regular oral prophylaxis?			
5. Do you have your mouth restored to maximum dental health?			
6. Do you use floss to aid in destruction of plaque?			
HAIR			
7. Do you shampoo your hair regularly?			
8. Is your hair always neatly combed?			
9. Is your hair styled to keep it off your face and out of the field of operation?			
10. Is your scalp free of dandruff?			
HANDS			
11. Are your nails short, clean and well manicured?			
12. Do you avoid the use of nail polish?			
13. Are your hands smooth and always clean?			
EYES			
14. Do you have regular eye examinations?			
15. Your glasses or safety glasses are well fitted and clean?			
16. Do you avoid excessive eye makeup?			
FACE			
17. Do you avoid excessive use of makeup?			
18. Is your face clean and free of disease?			
19. Is your face free of dry, scaly areas?			
GENERAL HEALTH			
20. Do you get adequate sleep at night?			
21. Do you have an annual physical examination?			
22. Do you exercise daily?			
23. Do you participate in some form of recreation weekly?			
POSTURE			
24. Do you stand erect?			
25. Do you sit straight in a chair?			
26. Do you wear shoes that are comfortable and proper fitting?			
27. Are your feet free of disease?			
UNIFORM			
28. Do you wear clean, appropriate clothing daily?			
29. Are your shoes clean and highly polished?			
30. Is your uniform free of stains and repairs?			
31. Do you wear fresh underwear daily?			
32. Do you avoid excessive use of jewelry?			

Legal Provisions for Delegating Functions to Dental Assistants and Dental Hygienists*

This is a summary of the report of the Department of Educational Surveys of the American Dental Association. For the most recent legal provisions for delegating functions to dental assistants or hygienists, refer to the current dental law in your state.

American Dental Association Survey Center, 1993.

ABBREVIATIONS AND EXPLANATIONS USED IN THIS REPORT FOR

Dental Assisting and Dental Hygiene Education/Experience Requirements

NONE — may perform function without any specific education

ACCREDITED — graduate of a program accredited by the Commission on Dental Accreditation (CDA)

ACC/SPEC — graduate of a CDA accredited program that includes instruction in the specific function

APPROVED — graduate of a program approved by the state board but not accredited by the CDA

SPECIFIC — completion of a specific course approved by the state board in the function

EXPERIENCE — specified period of occupational experience may be required

ACC-NONE — graduate of a program accredited by the CDA OR the function may be performed without any specific education

ACC-AC/SPEC — graduate of a program accredited by the CDA OR of an accredited program that includes instruction in the specific function

ACC-EXP — graduate of a program accredited by the CDA OR a specific period of occupational experience may be required

ACC-APP — graduate of a program accredited by the CDA OR approved by the state board

ACC-SPEC — graduate of a program accredited by the CDA OR completion of specific course approved by the state board

AC/SPEC-SPEC — graduate of a CDA accredited program that includes instruction in the specific function OR completion of a specific course approved by the state board

APP-SPEC — graduate of a program approved by the state board OR completion of a specific course approved by the state board

ACC-AC/SPEC-SPEC — graduate of a program accredited by the CDA OR of an accredited program that includes instruction in the specific function OR completion of a specific course approved by the state board

ACC-AC/SPEC-APP — graduate of a program accredited by the CDA OR of an accredited program that includes instruction in the specific function OR approved by the state board

ACC-APP-SPEC — graduate of a program accredited by the CDA or approved by the state board OR completion of a specific course approved by the state board

APP-ACC-EXP — graduate of a program approved by the state board OR accredited by the CDA OR a specific period of occupational experience may be required

AC/SPEC-APP-SPEC — graduate of a CDA accredited program that includes instruction in the specific function OR approved by the state board OR completion of a specific course approved by the state board may be required

AC-AC/SPEC-AP-SP — graduate of a program accredited by the CDA OR of an accredited program that includes instruction in the specific function OR completion of a specific course approved by the state board may be required

AC-AC/SPEC-AP-EX — graduate of a program accredited by the CDA OR of an accredited program that includes instruction in the specific function OR approved by the state board OR a specific period of occupational experience may be required

N/AP — not applicable

N/R — non responsive

Dental Assisting Examination / Credential Requirements

NONE — an examination is not required for the performance of the specific function

WRITTEN — a written examination is required by the state board to perform the function

CLINICAL — a clinical examination is required by the state board to perform the function

WRIT/CLIN — written and clinical examinations are required by the state board to perform the function

CDA EXAM — Certified Dental Assistant Examination (CDAE) administered by the Dental Assisting National Board (DANB) is required by the state board to perform the function

WAIVED — examination can be waived based on credentials and/or experience

WRIT/CLIN-NONE — written and clinical exams are required OR exam may not be required to perform the function

WAIVED-NONE — examination can be waived based on credentials and/or experience OR exam may not be required to perform the function

WRIT-CDA EXAM — a written examination OR the CDAE administered by the DANB may be required to perform the function

WRIT-WAIVED — a written examination may be required OR the exam may be waived based on credentials and/or experience

WRIT/CLIN-CDA — written and clinical exams are required OR the CDAE administered by the DANB may be required by the state board to perform the function

WRIT-CDA-NONE — a written examination OR the CDAE administered by the DANB may be required to perform the function OR an exam may not be required to perform the function

WRIT-CLIN-CDA — a written or clinical exam OR the CDAE administered by the DANB may be required to perform the function

WRIT-CDA-WAIVED — a written exam OR the CDAE administered by the DANB OR the exam can be waived based on credentials and/or experience

N/AP — not applicable

N/R — non responsive

Dental Hygiene Examination/Credential Requirements

NONE — an examination is not required for the performance of the specific function

KNOWLEDGE — knowledge of the specific function is evaluated as part of the regular state/regional board written examination

PERFORMANCE — performance of the specific function is evaluated as part of the regular state/regional board clinical examination

KNOW/PER — knowledge and performance of the specific function are evaluated as part of the regular state/regional board written and clinical examinations

WRITTEN — in addition to the regular exam, a special written examination on the specific function is required

CLINICAL — in addition to the regular exam, a special clinical examination on the specific function is required

WRIT/CLIN — in addition to the regular exam, a special written and clinical examinations on the special function are required

WAIVED — examination can be waived based on credentials

PER-NONE — performance of the specific function is evaluated as part of the regular clinical exam OR an exam may not be required

PER-WAIVED — performance of the specific function is evaluated as part of the regular clinical exam OR the exam may be waived based on credentials

K/P-CLIN — knowledge and performance of the specific function are evaluated as part of the regular written and clinical examinations OR in addition to the regular exam, a clinical exam on the function is required

K/P-WAIVED — knowledge and performance of the specific function are evaluated as part of the regular written and clinical examinations OR the exam can be waived on credentials

WRIT-WAIVED — in addition to the regular exam, a special written and clinical examinations on the specific function are required OR the exam may be waived based on credentials

KNOW-WRIT-WAV — knowledge of the specific function is evaluated as part of the regular written exam OR in addition to the regular exam, a special written examination may be required OR an exam may be waived based on credentials

K/P-KNOW-PER — knowledge and performance of the specific function are evaluated as part of the regular written and clinical examinations OR knowledge of the function is evaluated as part of the written exam OR performance of the function is evaluated as part of the clinical exam

K/P-WRIT-WAV — knowledge and performance of the specific function are evaluated as part of the regular written and clinical examinations OR in addition to the regular exam, a special written exam may be required OR an exam may be waived based on credentials

N/AP — not applicable

N/R — non responsive

Dental Assisting and Dental Hygiene Supervision Requirements

DIRECT — dentist in office and evaluates patient during same visit

INDIRECT — dentist in office but may evaluate patient at a later time

GENERAL — dentist has authorized procedure but is not necessarily in office

NONE — no supervision is required

UNDEFINED — degree of supervision is not specified

N/AP — not applicable

N/R — non responsive

INSPECTING THE ORAL CAVITY: DENTAL ASSISTING

State	Permission	Required education	Required examination	Required supervision
Alabama	Yes	None	None	Direct
Alaska	Function not Listed	N/AP	N/AP	N/AP
Arizona	No	N/AP	N/AP	N/AP
Arkansas	No	N/AP	N/AP	N/AP
California	Yes	Acc-Ac/Spec-App	Writ/Clin	General
Colorado	Yes	None	None	Direct
Connecticut	No	N/AP	N/AP	N/AP
Delaware	Function not Listed	N/AP	N/AP	N/AP
District of Columbia	No	N/AP	N/AP	N/AP
Florida	Yes	Accredited	None	Direct
Georgia	Yes	None	None	Direct
Hawaii	Yes	None	None	Direct
Idaho	Yes	None	None	Direct
Illinois	No	N/AP	N/AP	N/AP
Indiana	DECLINES TO RESPOND			
Iowa	No	N/AP	N/AP	N/AP
Kansas	DECLINES TO RESPOND			
Kentucky	No	N/AP	N/AP	N/AP
Louisiana	Yes	None	None	Direct
Maine	No	N/AP	N/AP	N/AP
Maryland	No	N/AP	N/AP	N/AP
Massachusetts	Yes	None	None	General
Michigan	Yes	Accredited	Writ/Clin	Indirect
Minnesota	No	N/AP	N/AP	N/AP
Mississippi	Function not Listed	N/AP	N/AP	N/AP
Missouri	Yes	None	None	Direct
Montana	Function not Listed	N/AP	N/AP	N/AP
Nebraska	Function not Listed	N/AP	N/AP	N/AP
Nevada	No	N/AP	N/AP	N/AP
New Hampshire	No	N/AP	N/AP	N/AP
New Jersey	No	N/AP	N/AP	N/AP
New Mexico	No	N/AP	N/AP	N/AP
New York	No	N/AP	N/AP	N/AP
North Carolina	Yes	None	None	Direct
North Dakota	Function not Listed	N/AP	N/AP	N/AP
Ohio	Yes	None	None	Direct
Oklahoma	No	N/AP	N/AP	N/AP
Oregon*	Yes	None	None	Indirect
Pennsylvania*	No	N/AP	N/AP	N/AP
Rhode Island	No	N/AP	N/AP	N/AP
South Carolina	Yes	None	None	Direct
South Dakota	No	N/AP	N/AP	N/AP
Tennessee	DECLINES TO RESPOND			
Texas	Yes	None	None	Direct
Utah	No	N/AP	N/AP	N/AP
Vermont	Yes	Accredited	CDA Exam	Indirect
Virginia	No	N/AP	N/AP	N/AP
Washington	Yes	None	None	Direct
West Virginia	Yes	None	None	Direct
Wisconsin	Yes	None	None	Direct
Wyoming	Function not Listed	N/AP	N/AP	N/AP

*The rules for these states are either under review or the returned survey was incomplete. Therefore, the responses shown are from the responses that were reported in the 1990 report.

APPLYING TOPICAL ANESTHETIC AGENTS: DENTAL ASSISTING

State	Permission	Required education	Required examination	Required supervision
Alabama	Yes	None	None	Direct
Alaska	Function not Listed	N/AP	N/AP	N/AP
Arizona	Yes	N/R	N/R	Direct
Arkansas	No	N/AP	N/AP	N/AP
California	No	N/AP	N/AP	N/AP
Colorado	Yes	None	None	Direct
Connecticut	No	N/AP	N/AP	N/AP
Delaware	Function not Listed	N/AP	N/AP	N/AP
District of Columbia	No	N/AP	N/AP	N/AP
Florida	Yes	None	None	Direct
Georgia	Yes	None	None	Direct
Hawaii	Yes	None	None	Direct
Idaho	Yes	None	None	Direct
Illinois	Yes	Experience	None	Direct
Indiana	DECLINES TO RESPOND			
Iowa	Yes	None	None	Direct
Kansas	DECLINES TO RESPOND			
Kentucky	Yes	N/R	N/R	Direct
Louisiana	Yes	None	None	Direct
Maine	Yes	None	None	Direct
Maryland	No	N/AP	N/AP	N/AP
Massachusetts	Yes	None	None	Indirect
Michigan	Yes	None	None	Indirect
Minnesota	Yes	Acc-Spec	Written	Indirect
Mississippi	Function not Listed	N/AP	N/AP	N/AP
Missouri	Yes	None	None	Direct
Montana	Yes	None	None	Direct
Nebraska	No	N/AP	N/AP	N/AP
Nevada	Yes	None	None	Direct
New Hampshire	Yes	Acc-App	Writ/Clin-CDA	Direct
New Jersey	Yes	None	None	Direct
New Mexico	Yes	None	None	Direct
New York	No	N/AP	N/AP	N/AP
North Carolina	Yes	None	None	Direct
North Dakota	Yes	None	None	Direct
Ohio	Yes	None	None	Direct
Oklahoma	Yes	None	None	Direct
Oregon*	Yes	None	None	Indirect
Pennsylvania*	No	N/AP	N/AP	N/AP
Rhode Island	Yes	None	Waived	Direct
South Carolina	Yes	None	None	Direct
South Dakota	Yes	None	None	Direct
Tennessee	DECLINES TO RESPOND			
Texas	Yes	None	None	Undefined
Utah	Yes	None	None	Direct
Vermont	Yes	Acc/Spec	CDA Exam	Direct
Virginia	Yes	Acc-Spec	Written	Direct
Washington	Yes	None	None	Direct
West Virginia	No	N/AP	N/AP	N/AP
Wisconsin	Yes	None	None	Direct
Wyoming	Yes	None	None	Indirect

*The rules for these states are either under review or the returned survey was incomplete. Therefore, the responses shown are from the responses that were reported in the 1990 report.

REMOVING EXCESS CEMENT FROM CORONAL SURFACES OF TEETH: DENTAL ASSISTING

State	Permission	Required education	Required examination	Required supervision
Alabama	Yes	None	None	Direct
Alaska	Function not Listed	N/AP	N/AP	N/AP
Arizona	Yes	None	None	Direct
Arkansas	Yes	None	None	Direct
California	Yes	Ac-Ac/Spec-Ap-Sp	Writ/Clin	Direct
Colorado	Yes	None	None	Direct
Connecticut	No	N/AP	N/AP	N/AP
Delaware	Yes	N/R	N/R	Direct
District of Columbia	No	N/AP	N/AP	N/AP
Florida	Yes	Accredited	None	Direct
Georgia	Yes	None	None	Direct
Hawaii	Yes	None	None	Direct
Idaho	Yes	None	None	Direct
Illinois	Yes	Experience	None	Direct
Indiana	DECLINES TO RESPOND			
Iowa	No	N/AP	N/AP	N/AP
Kansas	DECLINES TO RESPOND			
Kentucky	Yes	N/R	N/R	Direct
Louisiana	Yes	None	None	Direct
Maine	Yes	None	None	Direct
Maryland	Yes	Ac-Ac/Spec-Ap-Sp	Writ-CDA-Waived	Direct
Massachusetts	Yes	None	None	Direct
Michigan	Yes	Accredited	Writ/Clin	Direct
Minnesota	No	N/AP	N/AP	N/AP
Mississippi	Function not Listed	N/AP	N/AP	N/AP
Missouri	Yes	None	None	Direct
Montana	Yes	None	None	Direct
Nebraska	Yes	None	None	Direct
Nevada	Yes	None	None	Direct
New Hampshire	Yes	Approved	Writ/Clin	Direct
New Jersey	Yes	App-Spec	Writ-CDA-None	Direct
New Mexico	Yes	None	None	Direct
New York	No	N/AP	N/AP	N/AP
North Carolina	Yes	Acc-Ac/Spec-App	None	Direct
North Dakota	Yes	Acc-Ac/Spec-App	CDA Exam	Direct
Ohio	No	N/AP	N/AP	N/AP
Oklahoma	Yes	None	None	Direct
Oregon*	Yes	Acc-App-Spec	Writ/Clin	Direct
Pennsylvania*	No	N/AP	N/AP	N/AP
Rhode Island	Yes	None	Waived	Direct
South Carolina	Yes	Acc-Exp	None	Direct
South Dakota	Yes	None	None	Direct
Tennessee	DECLINES TO RESPOND			
Texas	No	N/AP	N/AP	N/AP
Utah	Yes	None	None	Direct
Vermont	Yes	Acc/Spec	CDA Exam	Direct
Virginia	Yes	None	None	Direct
Washington	Yes	None	None	Direct
West Virginia	Yes	None	None	Direct
Wisconsin	Yes	None	None	Direct
Wyoming	Yes	None	None	Direct

*The rules for these states are either under review or the returned survey was incomplete. Therefore, the responses shown are from the responses that were reported in the 1990 report.

CEMENTING BANDS/BONDING BRACKETS: DENTAL ASSISTING

State	Permission	Required education	Required examination	Required supervision
Alabama	No	N/AP	N/AP	N/AP
Alaska	Function not Listed	N/AP	N/AP	N/AP
Arizona	No	N/AP	N/AP	N/AP
Arkansas	No	N/AP	N/AP	N/AP
California	No	N/AP	N/AP	N/AP
Colorado	Yes	None	None	Direct
Connecticut	No	N/AP	N/AP	N/AP
Delaware	No	N/AP	N/AP	N/AP
District of Columbia	No	N/AP	N/AP	N/AP
Florida	No	N/AP	N/AP	N/AP
Georgia	No	N/AP	N/AP	N/AP
Hawaii	No	N/AP	N/AP	N/AP
Idaho	Function not Listed	N/AP	N/AP	N/AP
Illinois	No	N/AP	N/AP	N/AP
Indiana	DECLINES TO RESPOND			
Iowa	No	N/AP	N/AP	N/AP
Kansas	DECLINES TO RESPOND			
Kentucky	No	N/AP	N/AP	N/AP
Louisiana	No	N/AP	N/AP	N/AP
Maine	No	N/AP	N/AP	N/AP
Maryland	No	N/AP	N/AP	N/AP
Massachusetts	No	N/AP	N/AP	N/AP
Michigan	No	N/AP	N/AP	N/AP
Minnesota	No	N/AP	N/AP	N/AP
Mississippi	No	N/AP	N/AP	N/AP
Missouri	No	N/AP	N/AP	N/AP
Montana	No	N/AP	N/AP	N/AP
Nebraska	No	N/AP	N/AP	N/AP
Nevada	Yes	None	None	Direct
New Hampshire	No	N/AP	N/AP	N/AP
New Jersey	No	N/AP	N/AP	N/AP
New Mexico	No	N/AP	N/AP	N/AP
New York	No	N/AP	N/AP	N/AP
North Carolina	No	N/AP	N/AP	N/AP
North Dakota	No	N/AP	N/AP	N/AP
Ohio	No	N/AP	N/AP	N/AP
Oklahoma	No	N/AP	N/AP	N/AP
Oregon*	No	N/AP	N/AP	N/AP
Pennsylvania*	No	N/AP	N/AP	N/AP
Rhode Island	No	N/AP	N/AP	N/AP
South Carolina	Function not Listed	N/AP	N/AP	N/AP
South Dakota	No	N/AP	N/AP	N/AP
Tennessee	DECLINES TO RESPOND			
Texas	No	N/AP	N/AP	N/AP
Utah	No	N/AP	N/AP	N/AP
Vermont	No	N/AP	N/AP	N/AP
Virginia	No	N/AP	N/AP	N/AP
Washington	Function not Listed	N/AP	N/AP	N/AP
West Virginia	Yes	None	None	Direct
Wisconsin	No	N/AP	N/AP	N/AP
Wyoming	Yes	None	None	Direct

*The rules for these states are either under review or the returned survey was incomplete. Therefore, the responses shown are from the responses that were reported in the 1990 report.

BENDING ARCHWIRES: DENTAL ASSISTING

State	Permission	Required education	Required examination	Required supervision
Alabama	Function not Listed	N/AP	N/AP	N/AP
Alaska	Function not Listed	N/AP	N/AP	N/AP
Arizona	No	N/AP	N/AP	N/AP
Arkansas	Yes	None	None	Direct
California	No	N/AP	N/AP	N/AP
Colorado	Yes	None	None	Direct
Connecticut	No	N/AP	N/AP	N/AP
Delaware	Function not Listed	N/AP	N/AP	N/AP
District of Columbia	No	N/AP	N/AP	N/AP
Florida	Yes	Accredited	None	Direct
Georgia	No	N/AP	N/AP	N/AP
Hawaii	No	N/AP	N/AP	N/AP
Idaho	Function not Listed	N/AP	N/AP	N/AP
Illinois	No	N/AP	N/AP	N/AP
Indiana	DECLINES TO RESPOND			
Iowa	Yes	N/R	N/R	N/R
Kansas	DECLINES TO RESPOND			
Kentucky	No	N/AP	N/AP	N/AP
Louisiana	No	N/AP	N/AP	N/AP
Maine	Yes	None	None	Direct
Maryland	Yes	Ac-Ac/Spec-Ap-Sp	Writ-CDA-Waived	Direct
Massachusetts	Yes	None	None	Direct
Michigan	No	N/AP	N/AP	N/AP
Minnesota	No	N/AP	N/AP	N/AP
Mississippi	No	N/AP	N/AP	N/AP
Missouri	No	N/AP	N/AP	N/AP
Montana	Function not Listed	N/AP	N/AP	N/AP
Nebraska	No	N/AP	N/AP	N/AP
Nevada	No	N/AP	N/AP	N/AP
New Hampshire	No	N/AP	N/AP	N/AP
New Jersey	No	N/AP	N/AP	N/AP
New Mexico	No	N/AP	N/AP	N/AP
New York	No	N/AP	N/AP	N/AP
North Carolina	No	N/AP	N/AP	N/AP
North Dakota	No	N/AP	N/AP	N/AP
Ohio	No	N/AP	N/AP	N/AP
Oklahoma	No	N/AP	N/AP	N/AP
Oregon*	No	N/AP	N/AP	N/AP
Pennsylvania*	No	N/AP	N/AP	N/AP
Rhode Island	No	N/AP	N/AP	N/AP
South Carolina	Yes	None	None	Direct
South Dakota	No	N/AP	N/AP	N/AP
Tennessee	DECLINES TO RESPOND			
Texas	No	N/AP	N/AP	N/AP
Utah	No	N/AP	N/AP	N/AP
Vermont	No	N/AP	N/AP	N/AP
Virginia	No	N/AP	N/AP	N/AP
Washington	Function not Listed	N/AP	N/AP	N/AP
West Virginia	Yes	None	None	Direct
Wisconsin	No	N/AP	N/AP	N/AP
Wyoming	No	N/AP	N/AP	N/AP

*The rules for these states are either under review or the returned survey was incomplete. Therefore, the responses shown are from the responses that were reported in the 1990 report.

EXPOSING RADIOGRAPHS: DENTAL ASSISTING

State	Permission	Required education	Required examination	Required supervision
Alabama	Yes	None	None	Direct
Alaska	Function not Listed	N/AP	N/AP	N/AP
Arizona	Yes	N/R	W/C-CDA-Waived	Direct
Arkansas	Yes	Acc-Spec	Written	Direct
California	Yes	Ac-Ac/Spec-Ap-Sp	Writ/Clin	Direct
Colorado	Yes	Specific	CDA Exam-None	General
Connecticut	Yes	None	None	Direct
Delaware	Yes	N/R	N/R	Direct
District of Columbia	No	N/AP	N/AP	N/AP
Florida	Yes	None	None	Direct
Georgia	Yes	None	None	Direct
Hawaii	Yes	None	None	Direct
Idaho	Yes	None	None	Direct
Illinois	Yes	Experience	None	Direct
Indiana	DECLINES TO RESPOND			
Iowa	Yes	Specific	Written	Direct
Kansas	Yes	None	None	Direct
Kentucky	Yes	Specific	N/R	Direct
Louisiana	Yes	Ac/Spec-App-Spec	None	Direct
Maine	Yes	None	Clinical	General
Maryland	Yes	Ac-Ac/Spec-Ap-Sp	Written	Direct
Massachusetts	Yes	Acc-Spec	Waived	General
Michigan	Yes	Specific	None	Indirect
Minnesota	Yes	Acc-Spec	Written	Indirect
Mississippi	Yes	Ac-Ac/Spec-Ap-Sp	Writ-CDA Exam	Direct
Missouri	Yes	None	None	Direct
Montana	Yes	None	Writ/Clin	Indirect
Nebraska	Yes	Ac/Spec-App-Spec	None	Direct
Nevada	Yes	None	None	Indirect
New Hampshire	Yes	Ac/Spec-Spec	Writ/Clin	Direct
New Jersey	Yes	Specific	Writ/Clin	Direct
New Mexico	Yes	Specific	Writ/Clin-CDA	Indirect
New York	Yes	None	None	Direct
North Carolina	Yes	Ac/Spec-App-Spec	Writ/Clin	Direct
North Dakota	Yes	Acc-Ac/Spec-App	CDA Exam	Direct
Ohio	Yes	None	None	Direct
Oklahoma	Yes	Specific	Writ/Clin	Direct
Oregon*	Yes	Specific	Writ/Clin	General
Pennsylvania*	Yes	None	Written	Direct
Rhode Island	Yes	Specific	Waived	Direct
South Carolina	Yes	Acc-Exp	CDA Exam	Direct
South Dakota	Yes	Specific	Written	Direct
Tennessee	DECLINES TO RESPOND			
Texas	Yes	None	Written	Direct
Utah	Yes	Specific	Written	Direct
Vermont	Yes	Ac-Ac/Spec-Sp-Ex	Writ/Clin-CDA	Indirect
Virginia	Yes	Specific	Written	Direct
Washington	Yes	None	None	Direct
West Virginia	Yes	None	None	Direct
Wisconsin	Yes	None	None	Direct
Wyoming	Yes	Ac-Ac/Spec-Ap-Ex	Waived-None	Indirect

*The rules for these states are either under review or the returned survey was incomplete. Therefore, the responses shown are from the responses that were reported in the 1990 report.

EXPOSING RADIOGRAPHS: DENTAL HYGIENE

State	Permission	Required education	Required examination	Required supervision
Alabama	Yes	Approved	None	Direct
Alaska	Yes	Accredited	Per-Waived	General
Arizona	Yes	Accredited	Performance	General
Arkansas	Yes	Accredited	Know/Per	Direct
California	Yes	Acc-Ac/Spec-App	Know/Per	Direct
Colorado	Yes	Accredited	Know/Per	General
Connecticut	Yes	Accredited	Knowledge	General
Delaware	Yes	Approved	Know/Per	General
District of Columbia	Yes	Accredited	Know/Per	General
Florida	Yes	Acc/Spec	None	General
Georgia	Yes	Accredited	Know/Per	Direct
Hawaii	Yes	Accredited	None	Direct
Idaho	Yes	Accredited	Know/Per	General
Illinois	Yes	Specific	K/P-Waived	Direct
Indiana	Yes	Accredited	Writ-Wavied	Direct
Iowa	Yes	Accredited	Know/Per	General
Kansas	Yes	Accredited	Know/Per	Direct
Kentucky	Yes	N/R	N/R	Direct
Louisiana	Yes	Accredited	Know/Per	Indirect
Maine	Yes	Accredited	Know/Per	General
Maryland	Yes	Acc-App	K/P-Writ-Wav	Indirect
Massachusetts	Yes	Accredited	Knowledge	General
Michigan	Yes	Accredited	Know/Per	General
Minnesota	Yes	Accredited	Know/Per	General
Mississippi	Yes	Accredited	Performance	N/R
Missouri	Yes	Accredited	Know/Per	Indirect
Montana	Yes	Accredited	Per-Wavied	General
Nebraska	Yes	Accredited	K/P-Waived	General
Nevada	Yes	Accredited	None	Direct
New Hampshire	Yes	Accredited	Knowledge	General
New Jersey	Yes	Accredited	Know/Per	Direct
New Mexico	Yes	Accredited	Know/Per	General
New York	Yes	Accredited	Know/Per	General
North Carolina	Yes	Approved	Knowledge	Indirect
North Dakota	Yes	Accredited	Know/Per	General
Ohio	Yes	Accredited	Know/Per	Direct
Oklahoma	Yes	Accredited	Knowledge	Direct
Oregon*	Yes	Accredited	Know/Per	General
Pennsylvania*	Yes	Accredited	Know/Per	Direct
Rhode Island	Yes	Accredited	Know/Per	Indirect
South Carolina	Yes	Accredited	None	Indirect
South Dakota	Yes	Accredited	Know/Per	Indirect
Tennessee	DECLINES TO RESPOND			
Texas	Yes	Accredited	Performance	General
Utah	Yes	Accredited	Know/Per	General
Vermont	Yes	Accredited	Knowledge	General
Virginia	Yes	Accredited	Know/Per	Direct
Washington	Yes	Accredited	None	General
West Virginia	Yes	Accredited	Know/Per	Direct
Wisconsin	Yes	Accredited	None	General
Wyoming	Yes	Accredited	Know/Per	General

*The rules for these states are either under review or the returned survey was incomplete. Therefore, the responses shown are from the responses that were reported in the 1990 report.

PERFORMING PULP VITALITY TESTING: DENTAL ASSISTING

State	Permission	Required education	Required examination	Required supervision
Alabama	Yes	None	None	Direct
Alaska	Function not Listed	N/AP	N/AP	N/AP
Arizona	Function not Listed	N/AP	N/AP	N/AP
Arkansas	Yes	None	None	Direct
California	Yes	Acc-Ac/Spec-App	Writ/Clin	Direct
Colorado	Function not Listed	N/AP	N/AP	N/AP
Connecticut	No	N/AP	N/AP	N/AP
Delaware	No	N/AP	N/AP	N/AP
District of Columbia	No	N/AP	N/AP	N/AP
Florida	Function not Listed	N/AP	N/AP	N/AP
Georgia	No	N/AP	N/AP	N/AP
Hawaii	No	N/AP	N/AP	N/AP
Idaho	Function not Listed	N/AP	N/AP	N/AP
Illinois	No	N/AP	N/AP	N/AP
Indiana	DECLINES TO RESPOND			
Iowa	No	N/AP	N/AP	N/AP
Kansas	DECLINES TO RESPOND			
Kentucky	Unanswered	N/R	N/R	N/R
Louisiana	No	N/AP	N/AP	N/AP
Maine	No	N/AP	N/AP	N/AP
Maryland	Yes	Ac-Ac/Spec-Ap-Sp	Written	Direct
Massachusetts	Yes	Accredited	CDA Exam	Direct
Michigan	No	N/AP	N/AP	N/AP
Minnesota	No	N/AP	N/AP	N/AP
Mississippi	No	N/AP	N/AP	N/AP
Missouri	No	N/AP	N/AP	N/AP
Montana	Function not Listed	N/AP	N/AP	N/AP
Nebraska	Function not Listed	N/AP	N/AP	N/AP
Nevada	No	N/AP	N/AP	N/AP
New Hampshire	Yes	Ac/Spec-Spec	Writ/Clin-CDA	Direct
New Jersey	No	N/AP	N/AP	N/AP
New Mexico	No	N/AP	N/AP	N/AP
New York	No	N/AP	N/AP	N/AP
North Carolina	No	N/AP	N/AP	N/AP
North Dakota	Yes	Acc-Ac/Spec-App	CDA Exam	Direct
Ohio	Yes	None	None	Direct
Oklahoma	No	N/AP	N/AP	N/AP
Oregon*	Function not Listed	N/AP	N/AP	N/AP
Pennsylvania*	No	N/AP	N/AP	N/AP
Rhode Island	No	N/AP	N/AP	N/AP
South Carolina	Function not Listed	N/AP	N/AP	N/AP
South Dakota	Yes	None	None	Direct
Tennessee	DECLINES TO RESPOND			
Texas	No	N/AP	N/AP	N/AP
Utah	No	N/AP	N/AP	N/AP
Vermont	Yes	Acc/Spec	CDA Exam	Indirect
Virginia	No	N/AP	N/AP	N/AP
Washington	Function not Listed	N/AP	N/AP	N/AP
West Virginia	No	N/AP	N/AP	N/AP
Wisconsin	Yes	None	None	Direct
Wyoming	Function not Listed	N/AP	N/AP	N/AP

*The rules for these states are either under review or the returned survey was incomplete. Therefore, the responses shown are from the responses that were reported in the 1990 report.

PERFORMING PULP VITALITY TESTING: DENTAL HYGIENE

State	Permission	Required education	Required examination	Required supervision
Alabama	Yes	N/R	None	Direct
Alaska	Yes	Accredited	None	General
Arizona	Function not Listed	N/AP	N/AP	N/AP
Arkansas	Yes	Accredited	Knowledge	Direct
California	Yes	Acc-Ac/Spec-App	Know/Per	General
Colorado	Yes	Accredited	None	General
Connecticut	No	N/AP	N/AP	N/AP
Delaware	Yes	Approved	Know/Per	General
District of Columbia	No	N/AP	N/AP	N/AP
Florida	No	N/AP	N/AP	N/AP
Georgia	No	N/AP	N/AP	N/AP
Hawaii	No	N/AP	N/AP	N/AP
Idaho	Function not Listed	N/AP	N/AP	N/AP
Illinois	Yes	Specific	K/P-Waived	Direct
Indiana	Function not Listed	N/AP	None	Direct
Iowa	No	N/AP	N/AP	N/AP
Kansas	Yes	Accredited	Know/Per	Direct
Kentucky	Unanswered	N/R	N/R	N/R
Louisiana	Function not Listed	N/AP	N/AP	N/AP
Maine	Yes	Accredited	Know/Per	General
Maryland	Yes	Acc-App	K/P-Writ-Wav	Indirect
Massachusetts	Yes	Accredited	Know/Per	Direct
Michigan	Yes	Accredited	Know/Per	General
Minnesota	No	N/AP	N/AP	N/AP
Mississippi	No	N/AP	N/AP	N/AP
Missouri	No	N/AP	N/AP	N/AP
Montana	Function not Listed	N/AP	N/AP	N/AP
Nebraska	No	N/AP	N/AP	N/AP
Nevada	No	N/AP	N/AP	N/AP
New Hampshire	Yes	Accredited	Know/Per	General
New Jersey	No	N/AP	N/AP	N/AP
New Mexico	No	N/AP	N/AP	N/AP
New York	Function not Listed	N/AP	N/AP	N/AP
North Carolina	No	N/AP	N/AP	N/AP
North Dakota	Yes	Accredited	Know/Per	General
Ohio	Yes	Accredited	Know/Per	Direct
Oklahoma	No	N/AP	N/AP	N/AP
Oregon*	Function not Listed	N/AP	N/AP	N/AP
Pennsylvania*	No	N/AP	N/AP	N/AP
Rhode Island	No	N/AP	N/AP	N/AP
South Carolina	Function not Listed	N/AP	N/AP	N/AP
South Dakota	Yes	Accredited	Know/Per	Direct
Tennessee	DECLINES TO RESPOND			
Texas	No	N/AP	N/AP	N/AP
Utah	Unanswered	N/R	N/R	N/R
Vermont	Yes	Accredited	None	General
Virginia	No	N/AP	N/AP	N/AP
Washington	Function not Listed	N/AP	N/AP	N/AP
West Virginia	Yes	Accredited	Knowledge	Direct
Wisconsin	Yes	Accredited	Know/Per	General
Wyoming	Function not Listed	N/AP	N/AP	N/AP

*The rules for these states are either under review or the returned survey was incomplete. Therefore, the responses shown are from the responses that were reported in the 1990 report.

MAKING ALGINATE IMPRESSIONS FOR STUDY CASTS: DENTAL ASSISTING

State	Permission	Required education	Required examination	Required supervision
Alabama	Yes	None	None	Direct
Alaska	Function not Listed	N/AP	N/AP	N/AP
Arizona	Yes	None	None	Direct
Arkansas	Yes	None	None	Direct
California	Yes	Acc-Ac/Spec-App	Writ/Clin	Direct
Colorado	Yes	None	None	General
Connecticut	Yes	None	None	Direct
Delaware	Yes	N/R	N/R	Direct
District of Columbia	No	N/AP	N/AP	N/AP
Florida	Yes	Accredited	None	Direct
Georgia	Yes	None	None	Direct
Hawaii	Yes	None	None	Direct
Idaho	Yes	None	None	Direct
Illinois	Yes	Experience	None	Direct
Indiana	DECLINES TO RESPOND			
Iowa	Yes	None	None	Direct
Kansas	DECLINES TO RESPOND			
Kentucky	Yes	N/R	N/R	Direct
Louisiana	Yes	None	None	Direct
Maine	Yes	None	None	General
Maryland	Yes	Ac-Ac/Spec-Ap-Sp	Writ-CDA-Waived	Direct
Massachusetts	Yes	None	None	Indirect
Michigan	Yes	None	None	Indirect
Minnesota	Yes	Acc-Spec	Written	Indirect
Mississippi	Yes	None	None	Direct
Missouri	Yes	None	None	Direct
Montana	Yes	None	None	Direct
Nebraska	No	N/AP	N/AP	N/AP
Nevada	Yes	None	None	Indirect
New Hampshire	Yes	Acc-App	Writ/Clin-CDA	Direct
New Jersey	Yes	App-Spec	Writ-CDA-None	Direct
New Mexico	Yes	None	None	Indirect
New York	No	N/AP	N/AP	N/AP
North Carolina	Yes	Acc-Ac/Spec-App	None	Direct
North Dakota	Yes	None	None	Direct
Ohio	Yes	None	None	Direct
Oklahoma	Yes	None	None	Direct
Oregon*	Yes	Acc-App-Spec	Writ/Clin-None	Indirect
Pennsylvania*	Yes	None	None	Direct
Rhode Island	No	N/AP	N/AP	N/AP
South Carolina	Yes	Acc-Exp	None	Direct
South Dakota	Yes	None	None	Direct
Tennessee	DECLINES TO RESPOND			
Texas	Yes	None	None	Undefined
Utah	Yes	None	None	Direct
Vermont	Yes	None	None	Indirect
Virginia	Yes	None	None	Direct
Washington	Yes	None	None	Direct
West Virginia	Yes	None	None	Direct
Wisconsin	Yes	None	None	Direct
Wyoming	Yes	None	None	Indirect

*The rules for these states are either under review or the returned survey was incomplete. Therefore, the responses shown are from the responses that were reported in the 1990 report.

MAKING ALGINATE IMPRESSIONS FOR STUDY CASTS: DENTAL HYGIENE

State	Permission	Required education	Required examination	Required supervision
Alabama	Yes	N/R	None	Direct
Alaska	Yes	Accredited	Per-Wavied	General
Arizona	Yes	Accredited	None	General
Arkansas	Yes	Accredited	Knowledge	Direct
California	Yes	Acc-Ac/Spec-App	Know/Per	Direct
Colorado	Yes	Accredited	None	General
Connecticut	Yes	Accredited	None	General
Delaware	Yes	Approved	Know/Per	General
District of Columbia	Yes	Accredited	Know/Per	General
Florida	Yes	Acc/Spec	None	General
Georgia	Yes	Accredited	None	Direct
Hawaii	Yes	Accredited	None	Direct
Idaho	Yes	Accredited	Know/Per	General
Illinois	Yes	Specific	K/P-Waived	Direct
Indiana	Function not Listed	N/AP	None	Direct
Iowa	Yes	Accredited	Knowledge	General
Kansas	Yes	Accredited	Know/Per	Direct
Kentucky	Yes	N/R	N/R	Direct
Louisiana	Yes	Accredited	Knowledge	Indirect
Maine	Yes	Accredited	Know/Per	General
Maryland	Yes	Acc-App	K/P-Writ-Wav	Indirect
Massachusetts	Yes	Accredited	Know/Per	General
Michigan	Yes	Accredited	None	General
Minnesota	Yes	Accredited	Know/Per	General
Mississippi	Yes	Accredited	None	Direct
Missouri	Yes	Accredited	Knowledge	Direct
Montana	Yes	Accredited	None	General
Nebraska	Yes	Accredited	K/P-Waived	General
Nevada	Yes	Accredited	None	Direct
New Hampshire	Yes	Accredited	Knowledge	General
New Jersey	Yes	Accredited	Knowledge	Direct
New Mexico	Yes	Accredited	None	General
New York	Yes	Accredited	Knowledge	Direct
North Carolina	Yes	Approved	None	Direct
North Dakota	Yes	Accredited	Know/Per	General
Ohio	Yes	Accredited	None	Direct
Oklahoma	Yes	Accredited	None	Direct
Oregon*	Yes	Accredited	Know/Per	General
Pennsylvania*	Yes	Accredited	None	Direct
Rhode Island	Yes	Accredited	Know/Per	Indirect
South Carolina	Yes	Accredited	None	Direct
South Dakota	Yes	Accredited	Know/Per	Indirect
Tennessee	DECLINES TO RESPOND			
Texas	Yes	Accredited	None	General
Utah	Yes	Accredited	None	General
Vermont	Yes	Accredited	None	General
Virginia	Yes	Accredited	None	Direct
Washington	Yes	Accredited	None	Direct
West Virginia	Yes	Accredited	None	Direct
Wisconsin	Yes	Accredited	Know/Per	General
Wyoming	Yes	Accredited	Know/Per	General

*The rules for these states are either under review or the returned survey was incomplete. Therefore, the responses shown are from the responses that were reported in the 1990 report.

CORONAL POLISHING: DENTAL ASSISTING

State	Permission	Required education	Required examination	Required supervision
Alabama	No	N/AP	N/AP	N/AP
Alaska	No	N/AP	N/AP	N/AP
Arizona	No	N/AP	N/AP	N/AP
Arkansas	Yes	Acc-Spec	Writ/Clin	Direct
California	Yes	Ac-Ac/Spec-Ap-Sp	Writ/Clin	Direct
Colorado	Yes	None	None	Direct
Connecticut	No	N/AP	N/AP	N/AP
Delaware	No	N/AP	N/AP	N/AP
District of Columbia	No	N/AP	N/AP	N/AP
Florida	No	N/AP	N/AP	N/AP
Georgia	Yes	None	None	Direct
Hawaii	No	N/AP	N/AP	N/AP
Idaho	Yes	Specific	Written	Direct
Illinois	No	N/AP	N/AP	N/AP
Indiana	DECLINES TO RESPOND			
Iowa	Yes	None	None	Direct
Kansas	DECLINES TO RESPOND			
Kentucky	No	N/AP	N/AP	N/AP
Louisiana	Yes	Ac/Spec-App-Spec	CDA Exam-Waived	Direct
Maine	No	N/AP	N/AP	N/AP
Maryland	No	N/AP	N/AP	N/AP
Massachusetts	Yes	Accredited	CDA Exam	General
Michigan	No	N/AP	N/AP	N/AP
Minnesota	Yes	Acc-Spec	Written	Indirect
Mississippi	Function not Listed	N/AP	N/AP	N/AP
Missouri	Yes	None	None	Direct
Montana	Yes	Specific	None	Direct
Nebraska	No	N/AP	N/AP	N/AP
Nevada	Yes	None	None	Direct
New Hampshire	No	N/AP	N/AP	N/AP
New Jersey	No	N/AP	N/AP	N/AP
New Mexico	Yes	Ac-Ac/Spec-Ap-Sp	None	Direct
New York	No	N/AP	N/AP	N/AP
North Carolina	No	N/AP	N/AP	N/AP
North Dakota	Yes	Acc-Ac/Spec-App	CDA Exam	Direct
Ohio	No	N/AP	N/AP	N/AP
Oklahoma	Yes	Specific	Writ/Clin	Direct
Oregon*	No	N/AP	N/AP	N/AP
Pennsylvania*	No	N/AP	N/AP	N/AP
Rhode Island	No	N/AP	N/AP	N/AP
South Carolina	Yes	Acc-Exp	None	Direct
South Dakota	Yes	N/R	N/R	Direct
Tennessee	DECLINES TO RESPOND			
Texas	No	N/AP	N/AP	N/AP
Utah	Yes	None	None	Direct
Vermont	Yes	Acc/Spec	CDA Exam	Direct
Virginia	Yes	None	None	Direct
Washington	Yes	None	None	Direct
West Virginia	No	N/AP	N/AP	N/AP
Wisconsin	Yes	None	None	Direct
Wyoming	Yes	None	None	Direct

*The rules for these states are either under review or the returned survey was incomplete. Therefore, the responses shown are from the responses that were reported in the 1990 report.

CORONAL POLISHING: DENTAL HYGIENE

State	Permission	Required education	Required examination	Required supervision
Alabama	Yes	Approved	Know/Per	Direct
Alaska	Yes	Accredited	Per-Waived	General
Arizona	Yes	Accredited	Performance	General
Arkansas	Yes	Accredited	Knowledge	Direct
California	Yes	Acc-Ac/Spec-App	Know/Per	General
Colorado	Yes	Accredited	Know/Per	None
Connecticut	Yes	Accredited	Performance	General
Delaware	Yes	Approved	Know/Per	General
District of Columbia	Yes	Accredited	Know/Per	General
Florida	Yes	Acc/Spec	Know/Per	Direct
Georgia	Yes	Accredited	Know/Per	Direct
Hawaii	Yes	Accredited	None	Direct
Idaho	Yes	Accredited	Know/Per	General
Illinois	Yes	Specific	K/P-Waived	Direct
Indiana	Yes	Accredited	Per-Waived	Direct
Iowa	Yes	Accredited	Know/Per	General
Kansas	Yes	Accredited	Know/Per	Direct
Kentucky	Yes	N/R	N/R	Indirect
Louisiana	Yes	Accredited	Know/Per	Direct
Maine	Yes	Accredited	Know/Per	General
Maryland	Yes	Acc-App	K/P-Writ-Wav	Indirect
Massachusetts	Yes	Accredited	Know/Per	General
Michigan	Yes	Accredited	Know/Per	General
Minnesota	Yes	Accredited	Know/Per	General
Mississippi	Yes	Accredited	Performance	N/R
Missouri	Yes	Accredited	Know/Per	Indirect
Montana	Yes	Accredited	Per-Waived	General
Nebraska	Yes	Accredited	K/P-Waived	General
Nevada	Yes	Accredited	Know/Per	Direct
New Hampshire	Yes	Accredited	Knowledge	General
New Jersey	Yes	Accredited	Know/Per	Direct
New Mexico	Yes	Accredited	None	General
New York	Yes	Accredited	Know/Per	General
North Carolina	Yes	Approved	Performance	Indirect
North Dakota	Yes	Accredited	Know/Per	General
Ohio	Yes	Accredited	Know/Per	Direct
Oklahoma	Yes	Accredited	Knowledge	Direct
Oregon*	Yes	Accredited	Know/Per	General
Pennsylvania*	Yes	Accredited	Know/Per	Direct
Rhode Island	Yes	Accredited	Know/Per	Indirect
South Carolina	Yes	Accredited	Performance	Indirect
South Dakota	Yes	Accredited	Know/Per	Indirect
Tennessee	DECLINES TO RESPOND			
Texas	Yes	Accredited	Performance	General
Utah	Yes	Accredited	Know/Per	General
Vermont	Yes	Accredited	Performance	General
Virginia	Yes	Accredited	Know/Per	Direct
Washington	Yes	Accredited	Know/Per	General
West Virginia	Yes	Accredited	Know/Per	Direct
Wisconsin	Yes	Accredited	Know/Per	General
Wyoming	Yes	Accredited	Know/Per	General

*The rules for these states are either under review or the returned survey was incomplete. Therefore, the responses shown are from the responses that were reported in the 1990 report.

APPLYING TOPICAL ANTICARIOGENIC AGENTS: DENTAL ASSISTING

State	Permission	Required education	Required examination	Required supervision
Alabama	Yes	None	None	Direct
Alaska	No	N/AP	N/AP	N/AP
Arizona	Yes	None	None	Direct
Arkansas	Yes	None	None	Direct
California	Yes	Acc-Ac/Spec-App	Writ/Clin	Direct
Colorado	Yes	None	None	Direct
Connecticut	No	N/AP	N/AP	N/AP
Delaware	Function not Listed	N/AP	N/AP	N/AP
District of Columbia	No	N/AP	N/AP	N/AP
Florida	Yes	None	None	Direct
Georgia	Yes	Specific	None	Direct
Hawaii	Function not Listed	N/AP	N/AP	N/AP
Idaho	Yes	None	None	Direct
Illinois	No	N/AP	N/AP	N/AP
Indiana	DECLINES TO RESPOND			
Iowa	Yes	None	None	Direct
Kansas	DECLINES TO RESPOND			
Kentucky	No	N/AP	N/AP	N/AP
Louisiana	Yes	None	None	Direct
Maine	No	N/AP	N/AP	N/AP
Maryland	Unanswered	N/R	N/R	N/R
Massachusetts	Yes	Accredited	CDA Exam	General
Michigan	Yes	Accredited	N/R	Indirect
Minnesota	Yes	Acc-Spec	Written	Indirect
Mississippi	Function not Listed	N/AP	N/AP	N/AP
Missouri	Yes	None	None	Direct
Montana	Yes	None	None	Direct
Nebraska	Yes	None	None	Direct
Nevada	Yes	None	None	Direct
New Hampshire	Yes	Acc-App	Writ/Clin-CDA	Direct
New Jersey	No	N/AP	N/AP	N/AP
New Mexico	Yes	None	None	Direct
New York	Function not Listed	N/AP	N/AP	N/AP
North Carolina	Yes	None	None	Direct
North Dakota	Yes	Acc-Ac/Spec-App	CDA Exam	Direct
Ohio	Yes	None	None	Direct
Oklahoma	Yes	Specific	Written	Direct
Oregon*	Yes	None	None	Indirect
Pennsylvania*	No	N/AP	N/AP	N/AP
Rhode Island	Yes	None	Waived	Direct
South Carolina	Yes	None	None	Direct
South Dakota	Yes	None	None	Direct
Tennessee	DECLINES TO RESPOND			
Texas	Yes	None	None	Undefined
Utah	Yes	None	None	Direct
Vermont	Yes	Acc/Spec	CDA Exam	Direct
Virginia	Yes	Acc-Spec	Written	Direct
Washington	Yes	None	None	Direct
West Virginia	No	N/AP	N/AP	N/AP
Wisconsin	Yes	None	None	Direct
Wyoming	No	N/AP	N/AP	N/AP

*The rules for these states are either under review or the returned survey was incomplete. Therefore, the responses shown are from the responses that were reported in the 1990 report.

APPLYING TOPICAL ANTICARIOGENIC AGENTS: DENTAL HYGIENE

State	Permission	Required education	Required examination	Required supervision
Alabama	Yes	N/R	None	Direct
Alaska	Yes	Accredited	Per-Waived	General
Arizona	Yes	Accredited	Performance	General
Arkansas	Yes	Accredited	Knowledge	Direct
California	Yes	Acc-Ac/Spec-App	Know/Per	Direct
Colorado	Yes	Accredited	None	None
Connecticut	Yes	Accredited	None	General
Delaware	Yes	Approved	Know/Per	General
District of Columbia	Yes	Accredited	Know/Per	General
Florida	Yes	Acc/Spec	None	General
Georgia	Yes	Accredited	None	Direct
Hawaii	Yes	Accredited	None	Direct
Idaho	Yes	Accredited	Know/Per	General
Illinois	Yes	Specific	K/P-Waived	Direct
Indiana	Yes	Accredited	None	Direct
Iowa	Yes	Accredited	Knowledge	General
Kansas	Yes	Accredited	Know/Per	Direct
Kentucky	Yes	N/R	N/R	Indirect
Louisiana	Yes	Accredited	Knowledge	Indirect
Maine	Yes	Accredited	Know/Per	General
Maryland	No	N/AP	N/AP	N/AP
Massachusetts	Yes	Accredited	Know/Per	General
Michigan	Yes	Accredited	Know/Per	General
Minnesota	Yes	Accredited	Know/Per	General
Mississippi	Yes	Accredited	None	Direct
Missouri	Yes	Accredited	None	Indirect
Montana	Yes	Accredited	None	General
Nebraska	Yes	Accredited	K/P-Waived	General
Nevada	Yes	Accredited	None	Indirect
New Hampshire	Yes	Accredited	Knowledge	General
New Jersey	Yes	Accredited	Knowledge	Direct
New Mexico	Yes	Accredited	Knowledge	General
New York	Yes	Accredited	Knowledge	General
North Carolina	Yes	Approved	None	Indirect
North Dakota	Yes	Accredited	Know/Per	General
Ohio	Yes	Accredited	None	Direct
Oklahoma	Yes	Accredited	None	Direct
Oregon*	Yes	Accredited	Know/Per	General
Pennsylvania*	Yes	Accredited	None	Direct
Rhode Island	Yes	Accredited	Know/Per	Indirect
South Carolina	Yes	Accredited	None	Indirect
South Dakota	Yes	Accredited	Know/Per	Indirect
Tennessee	DECLINES TO RESPOND			
Texas	Yes	Accredited	None	General
Utah	Yes	Accredited	Per-None	General
Vermont	Yes	Accredited	None	General
Virginia	Yes	Accredited	None	Direct
Washington	Yes	Accredited	Knowledge	General
West Virginia	Yes	Accredited	Knowledge	Direct
Wisconsin	Yes	Accredited	Know/Per	General
Wyoming	Yes	Accredited	Know/Per	General

*The rules for these states are either under review or the returned survey was incomplete. Therefore, the responses shown are from the responses that were reported in the 1990 report.

APPLYING PIT AND FISSURE SEALANTS: DENTAL ASSISTING

State	Permission	Required education	Required examination	Required supervision
Alabama	No	N/AP	N/AP	N/AP
Alaska	No	N/AP	N/AP	N/AP
Arizona	No	N/AP	N/AP	N/AP
Arkansas	No	N/AP	N/AP	N/AP
California	Yes	Ac-Ac/Spec-Ap-Sp	Writ/Clin	Direct
Colorado	Yes	None	None	Direct
Connecticut	No	N/AP	N/AP	N/AP
Delaware	Function not Listed	N/AP	N/AP	N/AP
District of Columbia	No	N/AP	N/AP	N/AP
Florida	No	N/AP	N/AP	N/AP
Georgia	Yes	Specific	None	Direct
Hawaii	No	N/AP	N/AP	N/AP
Idaho	Yes	Specific	Written	Direct
Illinois	No	N/AP	N/AP	N/AP
Indiana	DECLINES TO RESPOND			
Iowa	No	N/AP	N/AP	N/AP
Kansas	DECLINES TO RESPOND			
Kentucky	No	N/AP	N/AP	N/AP
Louisiana	No	N/AP	N/AP	N/AP
Maine	No	N/AP	N/AP	N/AP
Maryland	No	N/AP	N/AP	N/AP
Massachusetts	Yes	Accredited	CDA Exam	Direct
Michigan	Yes	Accredited	Writ/Clin	Direct
Minnesota	Yes	Acc-Spec	Written	Direct
Mississippi	Yes	None	N/R	N/R
Missouri	Yes	None	None	Direct
Montana	Function not Listed	N/AP	N/AP	N/AP
Nebraska	No	N/AP	N/AP	N/AP
Nevada	Yes	None	None	Direct
New Hampshire	Yes	Approved	Writ/Clin	Direct
New Jersey	No	N/AP	N/AP	N/AP
New Mexico	No	N/AP	N/AP	N/AP
New York	No	N/AP	N/AP	N/AP
North Carolina	Yes	Acc-Ac/Spec-App	None	Direct
North Dakota	No	N/AP	N/AP	N/AP
Ohio	Yes	Specific	Writ/Clin	Direct
Oklahoma	No	N/AP	N/AP	N/AP
Oregon*	No	N/AP	N/AP	N/AP
Pennsylvania*	No	N/AP	N/AP	N/AP
Rhode Island	Yes	Acc-Spec	None	Direct
South Carolina	Yes	Acc-Exp	None	Direct
South Dakota	No	N/AP	N/AP	N/AP
Tennessee	DECLINES TO RESPOND			
Texas	No	N/AP	N/AP	N/AP
Utah	Yes	None	None	Direct
Vermont	Yes	Acc/Spec	CDA Exam	Direct
Virginia	Yes	None	None	Direct
Washington	Yes	None	None	Direct
West Virginia	No	N/AP	N/AP	N/AP
Wisconsin	No	N/AP	N/AP	N/AP
Wyoming	No	N/AP	N/AP	N/AP

*The rules for these states are either under review or the returned survey was incomplete. Therefore, the responses shown are from the responses that were reported in the 1990 report.

APPLYING PIT AND FISSURE SEALANTS: DENTAL HYGIENE

State	Permission	Required education	Required examination	Required supervision
Alabama	Yes	Approved	Knowledge	Direct
Alaska	Yes	Accredited	Per-Waived	General
Arizona	Yes	Accredited	Performance	General
Arkansas	Yes	Accredited	Knowledge	Direct
California	Yes	Acc-Ac/Spec-App	Know/Per	General
Colorado	Yes	Accredited	None	None
Connecticut	Yes	Accredited	None	General
Delaware	Yes	Approved	Know/Per	General
District of Columbia	Yes	Accredited	Know/Per	Direct
Florida	Yes	Acc/Spec	None	Direct
Georgia	Yes	Accredited	None	Direct
Hawaii	Yes	Accredited	None	Direct
Idaho	Yes	Accredited	Know/Per	General
Illinois	Yes	Specific	K/P-Waived	Direct
Indiana	Function not Listed	N/AP	None	Direct
Iowa	Yes	Accredited	Knowledge	General
Kansas	Yes	Accredited	Know/Per	Direct
Kentucky	Yes	N/R	N/R	Indirect
Louisiana	Yes	Accredited	Knowledge	Indirect
Maine	Yes	Accredited	Know/Per	General
Maryland	Yes	Acc-App	K/P-Writ-Wav	N/R
Massachusetts	Yes	Accredited	Know/Per	General
Michigan	Yes	Accredited	Know/Per	General
Minnesota	Yes	Accredited	Know/Per	General
Mississippi	Yes	Accredited	None	Direct
Missouri	Yes	Accredited	None	Indirect
Montana	Yes	Accredited	None	General
Nebraska	Yes	Accredited	K/P-Waived	General
Nevada	Yes	Accredited	None	Direct
New Hampshire	Yes	Ac/Spec-Spec	Know/Per	Indirect
New Jersey	Yes	Acc-Spec	Know-Writ-Wav	Direct
New Mexico	Yes	Acc-Ac/Spec-App	None	General
New York	Yes	Accredited	Knowledge	General
North Carolina	Yes	Approved	None	Direct
North Dakota	Yes	Accredited	Know/Per	General
Ohio	Yes	Accredited	None	Direct
Oklahoma	Yes	Accredited	None	Direct
Oregon*	Yes	Ac/Spec-Spec	None	General
Pennsylvania*	Yes	Accredited	None	Direct
Rhode Island	Yes	Accredited	Know/Per	Indirect
South Carolina	Yes	Accredited	None	General
South Dakota	Yes	Accredited	Know/Per	Indirect
Tennessee	DECLINES TO RESPOND			
Texas	Yes	Acc-Spec	Written	General
Utah	Yes	N/R	N/R	General
Vermont	Yes	Accredited	None	General
Virginia	Yes	Accredited	None	Direct
Washington	Yes	Accredited	Knowledge	General
West Virginia	Yes	Accredited	Knowledge	Direct
Wisconsin	Yes	Accredited	Know/Per	General
Wyoming	Yes	Accredited	Know/Per	Direct

*The rules for these states are either under review or the returned survey was incomplete. Therefore, the responses shown are from the responses that were reported in the 1990 report.

PLACING PERIODONTAL DRESSINGS: DENTAL ASSISTING

State	Permission	Required education	Required examination	Required supervision
Alabama	Yes	None	None	Direct
Alaska	Function not Listed	N/AP	N/AP	N/AP
Arizona	No	N/AP	N/AP	N/AP
Arkansas	No	N/AP	N/AP	N/AP
California	Yes	Acc-Ac/Spec-App	Writ/Clin	Direct
Colorado	Yes	None	None	Direct
Connecticut	No	N/AP	N/AP	N/AP
Delaware	Function not Listed	N/AP	N/AP	N/AP
District of Columbia	No	N/AP	N/AP	N/AP
Florida	Yes	Accredited	None	Indirect
Georgia	Yes	Specific	None	Direct
Hawaii	Function not Listed	N/AP	N/AP	N/AP
Idaho	Yes	None	None	Direct
Illinois	No	N/AP	N/AP	N/AP
Indiana	DECLINES TO RESPOND			
Iowa	No	N/AP	N/AP	N/AP
Kansas	DECLINES TO RESPOND			
Kentucky	No	N/AP	N/AP	N/AP
Louisiana	Yes	Ac/Spec-App-Spec	CDA Exam-Waived	Direct
Maine	No	N/AP	N/AP	N/AP
Maryland	Yes	N/R	N/R	Direct
Massachusetts	Yes	None	None	Indirect
Michigan	Yes	Accredited	Writ/Clin	Direct
Minnesota	Yes	Acc-Spec	Written	Indirect
Mississippi	Function not Listed	N/AP	N/AP	N/AP
Missouri	No	N/AP	N/AP	N/AP
Montana	Function not Listed	N/AP	N/AP	N/AP
Nebraska	Yes	None	None	Direct
Nevada	Yes	None	None	Direct
New Hampshire	No	N/AP	N/AP	N/AP
New Jersey	Yes	App-Spec	Writ-CDA-None	Direct
New Mexico	No	N/AP	N/AP	N/AP
New York	No	N/AP	N/AP	N/AP
North Carolina	No	N/AP	N/AP	N/AP
North Dakota	Yes	Acc-Ac/Spec-App	CDA Exam	Direct
Ohio	Yes	None	None	Direct
Oklahoma	Yes	Specific	Written	Direct
Oregon*	Function not Listed	N/AP	N/AP	N/AP
Pennsylvania*	No	N/AP	N/AP	N/AP
Rhode Island	Yes	None	Waived	Direct
South Carolina	Yes	None	None	Direct
South Dakota	No	N/AP	N/AP	N/AP
Tennessee	DECLINES TO RESPOND			
Texas	Yes	None	None	Undefined
Utah	No	N/AP	N/AP	N/AP
Vermont	Yes	Acc/Spec	CDA Exam	Direct
Virginia	Yes	None	None	Direct
Washington	Yes	None	None	Direct
West Virginia	No	N/AP	N/AP	N/AP
Wisconsin	Yes	None	None	Direct
Wyoming	Yes	None	None	Direct

*The rules for these states are either under review or the returned survey was incomplete. Therefore, the responses shown are from the responses that were reported in the 1990 report.

PLACING PERIODONTAL DRESSINGS: DENTAL HYGIENE

State	Permission	Required education	Required examination	Required supervision
Alabama	Yes	N/R	None	Direct
Alaska	Yes	Accredited	None	Undefined
Arizona	Yes	Accredited	None	Direct
Arkansas	Yes	Accredited	Knowledge	Direct
California	Yes	Acc-Ac/Spec-App	Know/Per	General
Colorado	Yes	Accredited	None	General
Connecticut	No	N/AP	N/AP	N/AP
Delaware	Yes	Approved	Know/Per	General
District of Columbia	Yes	Accredited	Performance	Direct
Florida	Yes	Acc/Spec	None	General
Georgia	Yes	Specific	None	Direct
Hawaii	Yes	Accredited	None	Direct
Idaho	Yes	Accredited	Know/Per	General
Illinois	No	N/AP	N/AP	N/AP
Indiana	Function not Listed	N/AP	N/AP	Direct
Iowa	Yes	Accredited	Knowledge	General
Kansas	Yes	Accredited	Know/Per	Direct
Kentucky	Yes	N/R	N/R	Direct
Louisiana	Yes	Accredited	None	Direct
Maine	Yes	Accredited	Know/Per	Direct
Maryland	Yes	Acc-App	K/P-Writ-Wav	Indirect
Massachusetts	Yes	Accredited	Know/Per	General
Michigan	Yes	Accredited	Know/Per	General
Minnesota	Yes	Accredited	Know/Per	General
Mississippi	Function not Listed	N/AP	N/AP	N/AP
Missouri	Yes	Accredited	None	Direct
Montana	Yes	Accredited	None	General
Nebraska	Yes	Accredited	K/P-Waived	General
Nevada	Yes	Accredited	None	Direct
New Hampshire	No	N/AP	N/AP	N/AP
New Jersey	Yes	Accredited	Knowledge	Direct
New Mexico	No	N/AP	N/AP	N/AP
New York	Yes	Accredited	Knowledge	Direct
North Carolina	No	N/AP	N/AP	N/AP
North Dakota	Yes	Accredited	Know/Per	General
Ohio	Yes	Accredited	None	Direct
Oklahoma	Yes	Accredited	None	Direct
Oregon*	Yes	Accredited	None	General
Pennsylvania*	Yes	Accredited	None	Direct
Rhode Island	Yes	Accredited	Know/Per	Indirect
South Carolina	Yes	Accredited	None	Indirect
South Dakota	Yes	Accredited	Know/Per	Indirect
Tennessee	DECLINES TO RESPOND			
Texas	Yes	Accredited	None	General
Utah	Yes	Acc/Spec	N/R	General
Vermont	Yes	Accredited	None	General
Virginia	Yes	Accredited	None	Direct
Washington	Yes	Accredited	None	Direct
West Virginia	No	N/AP	N/AP	N/AP
Wisconsin	Yes	Accredited	Know/Per	Direct
Wyoming	Yes	Accredited	Know/Per	Direct

*The rules for these states are either under review or the returned survey was incomplete. Therefore, the responses shown are from the responses that were reported in the 1990 report.

REMOVING PERIODONTAL DRESSINGS: DENTAL ASSISTING

State	Permission	Required education	Required examination	Required supervision
Alabama	Yes	None	None	Direct
Alaska	Function not Listed	N/AP	N/AP	N/AP
Arizona	No	N/AP	N/AP	N/AP
Arkansas	Yes	None	None	Direct
California	Yes	Acc-Ac/Spec-App	Writ/Clin	Direct
Colorado	Yes	None	None	Direct
Connecticut	No	N/AP	N/AP	N/AP
Delaware	Yes	N/R	N/R	Direct
District of Columbia	No	N/AP	N/AP	N/AP
Florida	Yes	Accredited	None	Indirect
Georgia	Yes	None	None	Direct
Hawaii	Yes	None	None	Direct
Idaho	Yes	None	None	Direct
Illinois	Yes	Experience	None	Direct
Indiana	DECLINES TO RESPOND			
Iowa	No	N/AP	N/AP	N/AP
Kansas	DECLINES TO RESPOND			
Kentucky	No	N/AP	N/AP	N/AP
Louisiana	Yes	Ac/Spec-App-Spec	CDA Exam-Wavied	Direct
Maine	No	N/AP	N/AP	N/AP
Maryland	Yes	Ac-Ac/Spec-Ap-Sp	Writ-CDA-Waived	Direct
Massachusetts	Yes	None	None	Indirect
Michigan	Yes	Accredited	Writ/Clin	Direct
Minnesota	Yes	Acc-Spec	Written	Indirect
Mississippi	Function not Listed	N/AP	N/AP	N/AP
Missouri	Yes	None	None	Direct
Montana	Yes	None	None	Direct
Nebraska	Yes	None	None	Direct
Nevada	Yes	None	None	Direct
New Hampshire	Yes	Acc-App	Writ/Clin-CDA	Direct
New Jersey	Yes	App-Spec	Writ-CDA-None	Direct
New Mexico	Yes	None	None	Direct
New York	No	N/AP	N/AP	N/AP
North Carolina	Yes	Acc-Ac/Spec-App	None	Direct
North Dakota	Yes	Acc-Ac/Spec-App	CDA Exam	Direct
Ohio	Yes	None	None	Direct
Oklahoma	No	N/AP	N/AP	N/AP
Oregon*	Yes	None	None	Indirect
Pennsylvania*	No	N/AP	N/AP	N/AP
Rhode Island	Yes	None	Waived	Direct
South Carolina	Yes	None	None	Direct
South Dakota	Yes	None	None	Direct
Tennessee	DECLINES TO RESPOND			
Texas	Yes	None	None	Undefined
Utah	Yes	None	None	Direct
Vermont	Yes	Acc/Spec	CDA Exam	Direct
Virginia	Yes	None	None	Direct
Washington	Yes	None	None	Direct
West Virginia	Yes	None	None	Direct
Wisconsin	Yes	None	None	Direct
Wyoming	Yes	None	None	Direct

*The rules for these states are either under review or the returned survey was incomplete. Therefore, the responses shown are from the responses that were reported in the 1990 report.

REMOVING PERIODONTAL DRESSINGS: DENTAL HYGIENE

State	Permission	Required education	Required examination	Required supervision
Alabama	Yes	N/R	None	Direct
Alaska	Yes	Accredited	None	Undefined
Arizona	Yes	Accredited	None	Direct
Arkansas	Yes	Accredited	Knowledge	Direct
California	Yes	Acc-Ac/Spec-App	Know/Per	General
Colorado	Yes	Accredited	None	General
Connecticut	Yes	Accredited	None	General
Delaware	Yes	Approved	Know/Per	General
District of Columbia	Yes	Accredited	Performance	Direct
Florida	Yes	Acc/Spec	None	General
Georgia	Yes	Accredited	None	Direct
Hawaii	Yes	Accredited	None	Direct
Idaho	Yes	Accredited	Know/Per	General
Illinois	Yes	Specific	K/P-Waived	Direct
Indiana	Function not Listed	N/AP	N/AP	Direct
Iowa	Yes	Accredited	Knowledge	General
Kansas	Yes	Accredited	Know/Per	Direct
Kentucky	Yes	N/R	N/R	Direct
Louisiana	Yes	Accredited	None	Direct
Maine	Yes	Accredited	Know/Per	General
Maryland	Yes	Acc-App	K/P-Writ-Wav	Direct
Massachusetts	Yes	Accredited	Know/Per	General
Michigan	Yes	Accredited	Know/Per	General
Minnesota	Yes	Accredited	Know/Per	General
Mississippi	Function not Listed	N/AP	N/AP	N/AP
Missouri	Yes	Accredited	None	Direct
Montana	Yes	Accredited	None	Direct
Nebraska	Yes	Accredited	K/P-Waived	General
Nevada	Yes	Accredited	None	Direct
New Hampshire	Yes	Accredited	Knowledge	General
New Jersey	Yes	Accredited	Knowledge	Direct
New Mexico	Yes	N/R	None	Direct
New York	Yes	Accredited	Knowledge	Direct
North Carolina	Yes	Approved	None	Indirect
North Dakota	Yes	Accredited	Know/Per	General
Ohio	Yes	Accredited	None	Direct
Oklahoma	Yes	Accredited	None	Direct
Oregon*	Yes	Accredited	None	General
Pennsylvania*	Yes	Accredited	None	Direct
Rhode Island	Yes	Accredited	Know/Per	Indirect
South Carolina	Yes	Accredited	None	Indirect
South Dakota	Yes	Accredited	Know/Per	Indirect
Tennessee	DECLINES TO RESPOND			
Texas	Yes	Accredited	None	General
Utah	Yes	Acc/Spec	N/R	General
Vermont	Yes	Accredited	None	General
Virginia	Yes	Accredited	None	Direct
Washington	Yes	Accredited	None	Direct
West Virginia	Yes	Accredited	Knowledge	Direct
Wisconsin	Yes	Accredited	Know/Per	Direct
Wyoming	Yes	Accredited	Know/Per	Direct

*The rules for these states are either under review or the returned survey was incomplete. Therefore, the responses shown are from the responses that were reported in the 1990 report.

REMOVING SUTURES: DENTAL ASSISTING

State	Permission	Required education	Required examination	Required supervision
Alabama	Yes	None	None	Direct
Alaska	Function not Listed	N/AP	N/AP	N/AP
Arizona	No	N/AP	N/AP	N/AP
Arkansas	Yes	None	None	Direct
California	Yes	Acc-Ac/Spec-App	Writ/Clin	Direct
Colorado	Yes	None	None	Direct
Connecticut	No	N/AP	N/AP	N/AP
Delaware	Function not Listed	N/AP	N/AP	N/AP
District of Columbia	No	N/AP	N/AP	N/AP
Florida	Yes	Accredited	None	Direct
Georgia	Yes	None	None	Direct
Hawaii	Yes	None	None	Direct
Idaho	Yes	None	None	Direct
Illinois	Yes	Experience	None	Direct
Indiana	DECLINES TO RESPOND			
Iowa	No	N/AP	N/AP	N/AP
Kansas	DECLINES TO RESPOND			
Kentucky	Yes	N/R	N/R	Direct
Louisiana	Yes	None	None	Direct
Maine	Yes	None	None	Direct
Maryland	Yes	Ac-Ac/Spec-Ap-Sp	Writ-CDA-Waived	Direct
Massachusetts	Yes	None	None	Indirect
Michigan	Yes	Accredited	Writ/Clin	Direct
Minnesota	Yes	Acc-Spec	Written	Indirect
Mississippi	Function not Listed	N/AP	N/AP	N/AP
Missouri	Yes	None	None	Direct
Montana	Yes	None	None	Direct
Nebraska	Yes	None	None	Direct
Nevada	Yes	None	None	Direct
New Hampshire	Yes	Acc-App	Writ/Clin-CDA	Direct
New Jersey	Yes	App-Spec	Writ-CDA-None	Direct
New Mexico	Yes	None	None	Direct
New York	No	N/AP	N/AP	N/AP
North Carolina	Yes	Acc-Ac/Spec-App	None	Direct
North Dakota	Yes	Acc-Ac/Spec-App	CDA Exam	Direct
Ohio	Yes	None	None	Direct
Oklahoma	Yes	N/R	Writ/Clin	Direct
Oregon*	Yes	None	None	Indirect
Pennsylvania*	Yes	None	None	Direct
Rhode Island	Yes	None	Waived	Direct
South Carolina	Yes	None	None	Direct
South Dakota	Yes	None	None	Direct
Tennessee	DECLINES TO RESPOND			
Texas	Yes	None	None	Undefined
Utah	Yes	None	None	Direct
Vermont	Yes	Acc/Spec	CDA Exam	Direct
Virginia	Yes	None	None	Direct
Washington	Yes	None	None	Direct
West Virginia	Yes	None	None	Direct
Wisconsin	Yes	None	None	Direct
Wyoming	Yes	None	None	Direct

*The rules for these states are either under review or the returned survey was incomplete. Therefore, the responses shown are from the responses that were reported in the 1990 report.

REMOVING SUTURES: DENTAL HYGIENE

State	Permission	Required education	Required examination	Required supervision
Alabama	Yes	N/R	None	Direct
Alaska	Yes	Accredited	None	Undefined
Arizona	No	N/AP	N/AP	N/AP
Arkansas	Yes	Accredited	Knowledge	Direct
California	Yes	Acc-Ac/Spec-App	Know/Per	General
Colorado	Yes	Accredited	None	General
Connecticut	Yes	Accredited	None	General
Delaware	Yes	Approved	Know/Per	General
District of Columbia	Yes	Accredited	Performance	Direct
Florida	Yes	Acc/Spec	None	General
Georgia	Yes	Accredited	None	Direct
Hawaii	Yes	Accredited	None	Direct
Idaho	Yes	Accredited	Know/Per	General
Illinois	Yes	Specific	K/P-Waived	Direct
Indiana	Function not Listed	N/AP	N/AP	Direct
Iowa	No	N/AP	N/AP	N/AP
Kansas	Yes	Acc-Spec	None	
Kentucky	Yes	N/R	N/R	Direct
Louisiana	Yes	Accredited	None	Indirect
Maine	Yes	Accredited	Know/Per	General
Maryland	Yes	Acc-App	K/P-Writ-Wav	Direct
Massachusetts	Yes	Accredited	Know/Per	General
Michigan	Yes	Accredited	Know/Per	General
Minnesota	Yes	Accredited	Know/Per	General
Mississippi	Function not Listed	N/AP	N/AP	N/AP
Missouri	Yes	Accredited	None	Indirect
Montana	Yes	Accredited	None	General
Nebraska	Yes	Accredited	K/P-Waived	General
Nevada	Yes	Accredited	None	Indirect
New Hampshire	Yes	Accredited	Knowledge	General
New Jersey	Yes	Accredited	Knowledge	Direct
New Mexico	Yes	N/R	None	Direct
New York	Yes	Accredited	Knowledge	Direct
North Carolina	Yes	Approved	None	Indirect
North Dakota	Yes	Accredited	Know/Per	General
Ohio	Yes	Accredited	None	Direct
Oklahoma	Yes	Accredited	None	Direct
Oregon*	Yes	Accredited	None	General
Pennsylvania*	Yes	Accredited	None	Direct
Rhode Island	Yes	Accredited	Know/Per	Direct
South Carolina	Yes	Accredited	None	Direct
South Dakota	Yes	Accredited	Know/Per	Indirect
Tennessee	DECLINES TO RESPOND			
Texas	Yes	Accredited	None	General
Utah	Yes	N/R	N/R	General
Vermont	Yes	Accredited	None	General
Virginia	Yes	Accredited	None	Direct
Washington	Yes	Accredited	None	Direct
West Virginia	Yes	Accredited	None	Direct
Wisconsin	Yes	Accredited	Know/Per	General
Wyoming	Yes	Accredited	Know/Per	General

*The rules for these states are either under review or the returned survey was incomplete. Therefore, the responses shown are from the responses that were reported in the 1990 report.

MONITORING NITROUS OXIDE ANALGESIA: DENTAL ASSISTING

State	Permission	Required education	Required examination	Required supervision
Alabama	Yes	None	None	Direct
Alaska	Function not Listed	N/AP	N/AP	N/AP
Arizona	Yes	None	None	Direct
Arkansas	Yes	Specific	None	Direct
California	No	N/AP	N/AP	N/AP
Colorado	Yes	None	None	Direct
Connecticut	No	N/AP	N/AP	N/AP
Delaware	No	N/AP	N/AP	N/AP
District of Columbia	No	N/AP	N/AP	N/AP
Florida	Yes	Accredited	None	Direct
Georgia	Yes	Specific	None	Direct
Hawaii	Yes	N/R	N/R	N/R
Idaho	Yes	Specific	Written	Direct
Illinois	No	N/AP	N/AP	N/AP
Indiana	DECLINES TO RESPOND			
Iowa	No	N/AP	N/AP	N/AP
Kansas	Yes	Accredited	N/R	Direct
Kentucky	Yes	Acc/Spec	N/R	Direct
Louisiana	No	N/AP	N/AP	N/AP
Maine	Yes	None	None	Direct
Maryland	No	N/AP	N/AP	N/AP
Massachusetts	Yes	Accredited	CDA Exam	Direct
Michigan	No	N/AP	N/AP	N/AP
Minnesota	Yes	Acc-Spec	Written	Indirect
Mississippi	Function not Listed	N/AP	N/AP	N/AP
Missouri	Yes	Specific	Writ/Clin	Direct
Montana	Yes	None	None	Direct
Nebraska	No	N/AP	N/AP	N/AP
Nevada	No	N/AP	N/AP	N/AP
New Hampshire	No	N/AP	N/AP	N/AP
New Jersey	No	N/AP	N/AP	N/AP
New Mexico	No	N/AP	N/AP	N/AP
New York	No	N/AP	N/AP	N/AP
North Carolina	Yes	Specific	None	Direct
North Dakota	Yes	Acc-Ac/Spec-App	CDA Exam	Direct
Ohio	No	N/AP	N/AP	N/AP
Oklahoma	Yes	Specific	Writ/Clin	Direct
Oregon*	Yes	None	None	Direct
Pennsylvania*	No	N/AP	N/AP	N/AP
Rhode Island	No	N/AP	N/AP	N/AP
South Carolina	No	N/AP	N/AP	N/AP
South Dakota	No	N/AP	N/AP	N/AP
Tennessee	DECLINES TO RESPOND			
Texas	Yes	None	Written	Direct
Utah	Yes	None	None	Direct
Vermont	No	N/AP	N/AP	N/AP
Virginia	Yes	None	None	Direct
Washington	Yes	None	None	Direct
West Virginia	No	N/AP	N/AP	N/AP
Wisconsin	Yes	None	None	Direct
Wyoming	Function not Listed	N/AP	N/AP	N/AP

*The rules for these states are either under review or the returned survey was incomplete. Therefore, the responses shown are from the responses that were reported in the 1990 report.

MONITORING NITROUS OXIDE ANALGESIA: DENTAL HYGIENE

State	Permission	Required education	Required examination	Required supervision
Alabama	Yes	N/R	None	Direct
Alaska	No	N/AP	N/AP	N/AP
Arizona	Yes	Accredited	None	Direct
Arkansas	Yes	Acc-Spec	Writ-Waived	Direct
California	Yes	Acc-Ac/Spec-App	Know/Per	Direct
Colorado	Yes	Accredited	None	Direct
Connecticut	No	N/AP	N/AP	N/AP
Delaware	No	N/AP	N/AP	N/AP
District of Columbia	Yes	N/R	N/R	Direct
Florida	Yes	Acc/Spec	None	Direct
Georgia	Yes	Accredited	None	Direct
Hawaii	Yes	N/R	N/R	N/R
Idaho	Yes	Accredited	Know/Per	Indirect
Illinois	No	N/AP	N/AP	N/AP
Indiana	Yes	Accredited	None	Direct
Iowa	Yes	Accredited	Know/Per	General
Kansas	Yes	Acc/Spec	N/R	Direct
Kentucky	Yes	Acc/Spec	N/R	Direct
Louisiana	No	N/AP	N/AP	N/AP
Maine	Yes	Accredited	Know/Per	General
Maryland	No	N/AP	N/AP	N/AP
Massachusetts	Yes	Accredited	Know/Per	Direct
Michigan	No	N/AP	N/AP	N/AP
Minnesota	Yes	Accredited	Know/Per	General
Mississippi	Yes	Accredited	None	Direct
Missouri	Yes	Acc-Spec	Writ/Clin	Direct
Montana	Yes	Accredited	None	Direct
Nebraska	Yes	Acc-Spec	None	Direct
Nevada	Yes	Ac/Spec-App-Spec	None	Direct
New Hampshire	No	N/AP	N/AP	N/AP
New Jersey	No	N/AP	N/AP	N/AP
New Mexico	Yes	Accredited	None	Direct
New York	Function not Listed	N/AP	N/AP	N/AP
North Carolina	Yes	Approved	None	Indirect
North Dakota	Yes	Accredited	Know/Per	General
Ohio	Yes	Specific	None	Direct
Oklahoma	Yes	Accredited	None	Direct
Oregon*	Yes	Accredited	None	Direct
Pennsylvania*	No	N/AP	N/AP	N/AP
Rhode Island	No	N/AP	N/AP	N/AP
South Carolina	No	N/AP	N/AP	N/AP
South Dakota	Yes	Specific	None	Direct
Tennessee	DECLINES TO RESPOND			
Texas	Yes	Accredited	Written	Direct
Utah	Yes	N/R	None	Direct
Vermont	No	N/AP	N/AP	N/AP
Virginia	Yes	Accredited	None	Direct
Washington	Yes	Approved	Know/Per	Direct
West Virginia	No	N/AP	N/AP	N/AP
Wisconsin	Yes	Accredited	Know/Per	Direct
Wyoming	Function not Listed	N/AP	N/AP	N/AP

*The rules for these states are either under review or the returned survey was incomplete. Therefore, the responses shown are from the responses that were reported in the 1990 report.

PLACING MATRICES: DENTAL ASSISTING

State	Permission	Required education	Required examination	Required supervision
Alabama	Yes	None	None	Direct
Alaska	Function not Listed	N/AP	N/AP	N/AP
Arizona	Function not Listed	N/AP	N/AP	N/AP
Arkansas	Yes	None	None	Direct
California	Yes	Acc-Ac/Spec-App	Writ/Clin	Direct
Colorado	Yes	None	None	Direct
Connecticut	No	N/AP	N/AP	N/AP
Delaware	Function not Listed	N/AP	N/AP	N/AP
District of Columbia	No	N/AP	N/AP	N/AP
Florida	Yes	Accredited	None	Indirect
Georgia	Yes	None	None	Direct
Hawaii	Yes	None	None	Direct
Idaho	Yes	None	None	Direct
Illinois	Yes	Experience	None	Direct
Indiana	DECLINES TO RESPOND			
Iowa	No	N/AP	N/AP	N/AP
Kansas	DECLINES TO RESPOND			
Kentucky	Unanswered	N/R	N/R	N/R
Louisiana	Yes	Ac/Spec-App-Spec	CDA Exam-Waived	Direct
Maine	Yes	None	None	Direct
Maryland	Yes	Ac-Ac/Spec-Ap-Sp	Written	Direct
Massachusetts	Yes	Accredited	CDA Exam	Direct
Michigan	No	N/AP	N/AP	N/AP
Minnesota	No	N/AP	N/AP	N/AP
Mississippi	No	N/AP	N/AP	N/AP
Missouri	Yes	None	None	Direct
Montana	Yes	None	None	Direct
Nebraska	Yes	None	None	Direct
Nevada	No	N/AP	N/AP	N/AP
New Hampshire	Yes	Acc-App	Writ/Clin-CDA	Direct
New Jersey	Yes	App-Spec	W/C-CDA-None	Direct
New Mexico	Yes	None	None	Direct
New York	No	N/AP	N/AP	N/AP
North Carolina	Yes	Acc-Ac/Spec-App	None	Direct
North Dakota	Yes	Acc-Ac/Spec-App	CDA Exam	Direct
Ohio	No	N/AP	N/AP	N/AP
Oklahoma	No	N/AP	N/AP	N/AP
Oregon*	Yes	Acc-App-Spec	Writ/Clin-None	Direct
Pennsylvania*	No	N/AP	N/AP	N/AP
Rhode Island	Yes	None	Waived	Direct
South Carolina	Yes	None	None	Direct
South Dakota	Yes	None	None	Direct
Tennessee	DECLINES TO RESPOND			
Texas	Yes	N/R	N/R	N/R
Utah	No	N/AP	N/AP	N/AP
Vermont	Yes	Acc/Spec	CDA Exam	Direct
Virginia	Yes	None	None	Direct
Washington	Yes	None	None	Direct
West Virginia	No	N/AP	N/AP	N/AP
Wisconsin	Yes	None	None	Direct
Wyoming	Yes	None	None	Direct

*The rules for these states are either under review or the returned survey was incomplete. Therefore, the responses shown are from the responses that were reported in the 1990 report.

PLACING MATRICES: DENTAL HYGIENE

State	Permission	Required education	Required examination	Required supervision
Alabama	Yes	N/R	None	Direct
Alaska	Yes	Accredited	None	Undefined
Arizona	Function not Listed	N/AP	N/AP	N/AP
Arkansas	Yes	Accredited	Knowledge	Direct
California	Yes	Acc-Ac/Spec-App	Know/Per	Direct
Colorado	Yes	Accredited	None	General
Connecticut	No	N/AP	N/AP	N/AP
Delaware	Yes	Approved	Know/Per	General
District of Columbia	No	N/AP	N/AP	N/AP
Florida	Yes	Acc/Spec	None	Indirect
Georgia	Yes	Accredited	None	Direct
Hawaii	Yes	Accredited	None	Direct
Idaho	Yes	Accredited	Know/Per	General
Illinois	Yes	Specific	K/P-Waived	Direct
Indiana	Function not Listed	N/AP	N/AP	Direct
Iowa	No	N/AP	N/AP	N/AP
Kansas	Yes	Accredited	Know/Per	Direct
Kentucky	Yes	N/R	N/R	Direct
Louisiana	Yes	Accredited	None	Direct
Maine	Yes	Accredited	None	Direct
Maryland	Yes	Acc-App	K/P-Writ-Wav	Direct
Massachusetts	Yes	Accredited	Know/Per	Direct
Michigan	No	N/AP	N/AP	N/AP
Minnesota	No	N/AP	N/AP	N/AP
Mississippi	Function not Listed	N/AP	N/AP	N/AP
Missouri	Yes	Accredited	None	Indirect
Montana	Yes	Accredited	None	Direct
Nebraska	Yes	Accredited	K/P-Waived	General
Nevada	No	N/AP	N/AP	N/AP
New Hampshire	Yes	Accredited	Knowledge	General
New Jersey	Yes	Accredited	Knowledge	Direct
New Mexico	Yes	N/R	None	Direct
New York	Yes	Accredited	Knowledge	Direct
North Carolina	Yes	Approved	None	Indirect
North Dakota	Yes	Accredited	Know/Per	General
Ohio	No	N/AP	N/AP	N/AP
Oklahoma	No	N/AP	N/AP	N/AP
Oregon*	Yes	Accredited	None	General
Pennsylvania*	Yes	Accredited	None	Direct
Rhode Island	Yes	Accredited	Know/Per	Direct
South Carolina	Yes	Accredited	None	Direct
South Dakota	No	N/AP	N/AP	N/AP
Tennessee	DECLINES TO RESPOND			
Texas	Yes	Accredited	None	Direct
Utah	Yes	N/R	N/R	Undefined
Vermont	Yes	Acc-Ac/Spec-Spec	Writ/Clin-Wav	Direct
Virginia	Yes	Accredited	None	Direct
Washington	Yes	Approved	Know/Per	Direct
West Virginia	No	N/AP	N/AP	N/AP
Wisconsin	Yes	Accredited	Know/Per	Direct
Wyoming	Yes	Accredited	Know/Per	General

*The rules for these states are either under review or the returned survey was incomplete. Therefore, the responses shown are from the responses that were reported in the 1990 report.

REMOVING MATRICES: DENTAL ASSISTING

State	Permission	Required education	Required examination	Required supervision
Alabama	Yes	None	None	Direct
Alaska	Function not Listed	N/AP	N/AP	N/AP
Arizona	Function not Listed	N/AP	N/AP	N/AP
Arkansas	Yes	None	None	Direct
California	Yes	Acc-Ac/Spec-App	Writ/Clin	Direct
Colorado	Yes	None	None	Direct
Connecticut	No	N/AP	N/AP	N/AP
Delaware	Function not Listed	N/AP	N/AP	N/AP
District of Columbia	No	N/AP	N/AP	N/AP
Florida	Yes	Accredited	None	Indirect
Georgia	No	N/AP	N/AP	N/AP
Hawaii	Yes	None	None	Direct
Idaho	Function not Listed	N/AP	N/AP	N/AP
Illinois	Yes	Experience	None	Direct
Indiana	DECLINES TO RESPOND			
Iowa	No	N/AP	N/AP	N/AP
Kansas	DECLINES TO RESPOND			
Kentucky	Unanswered	N/R	N/R	N/R
Louisiana	Yes	Ac/Spec-App-Spec	CDA Exam-Waived	Direct
Maine	Yes	None	None	Direct
Maryland	Yes	Ac-Ac/Spec-Ap-Sp	Written	Direct
Massachusetts	Yes	Accredited	CDA Exam	Direct
Michigan	No	N/AP	N/AP	N/AP
Minnesota	No	N/AP	N/AP	N/AP
Mississippi	Function not Listed	N/AP	N/AP	N/AP
Missouri	Yes	None	None	Direct
Montana	Yes	None	None	Direct
Nebraska	Yes	None	None	Direct
Nevada	No	N/AP	N/AP	N/AP
New Hampshire	Yes	Acc-App	Writ/Clin-CDA	Direct
New Jersey	Yes	App-Spec	Writ-CDA-None	Direct
New Mexico	Yes	None	None	Direct
New York	No	N/AP	N/AP	N/AP
North Carolina	Yes	Acc-Ac/Spec-App	None	Direct
North Dakota	Yes	Acc-Ac/Spec-App	CDA Exam	Direct
Ohio	No	N/AP	N/AP	N/AP
Oklahoma	No	N/AP	N/AP	N/AP
Oregon*	Function not Listed	N/AP	N/AP	N/AP
Pennsylvania*	No	N/AP	N/AP	N/AP
Rhode Island	Yes	None	Waived	Direct
South Carolina	Yes	None	None	Direct
South Dakota	Yes	None	None	Direct
Tennessee	DECLINES TO RESPOND			
Texas	Yes	N/R	N/R	N/R
Utah	No	N/AP	N/AP	N/AP
Vermont	Yes	Acc/Spec	CDA Exam	Direct
Virginia	Yes	None	None	Direct
Washington	Function not Listed	N/AP	N/AP	N/AP
West Virginia	Yes	None	None	Direct
Wisconsin	Yes	None	None	Direct
Wyoming	Yes	None	None	Direct

*The rules for these states are either under review or the returned survey was incomplete. Therefore, the responses shown are from the responses that were reported in the 1990 report.

REMOVING MATRICES: DENTAL HYGIENE

State	Permission	Required education	Required examination	Required supervision
Alabama	Yes	N/R	None	Direct
Alaska	Yes	Accredited	None	Undefined
Arizona	Function not Listed	N/AP	N/AP	N/AP
Arkansas	Yes	Accredited	Knowledge	Direct
California	Yes	Acc-Ac/Spec-App	Know/Per	Direct
Colorado	Yes	Accredited	None	General
Connecticut	No	N/AP	N/AP	N/AP
Delaware	Yes	Approved	Know/Per	General
District of Columbia	No	N/AP	N/AP	N/AP
Florida	Yes	Acc/Spec	None	Indirect
Georgia	No	N/AP	N/AP	N/AP
Hawaii	Yes	Accredited	None	Direct
Idaho	Yes	Accredited	Know/Per	General
Illinois	Yes	Specific	K/P-Waived	Direct
Indiana	Function not Listed	N/AP	N/AP	Direct
Iowa	No	N/AP	N/AP	N/AP
Kansas	Yes	Accredited	Know/Per	Direct
Kentucky	Yes	N/R	N/R	Direct
Louisiana	Yes	Accredited	None	Direct
Maine	Yes	Accredited	None	Direct
Maryland	Yes	Acc-App	K/P-Writ-Wav	Direct
Massachusetts	Yes	Accredited	Know/Per	Direct
Michigan	No	N/AP	N/AP	N/AP
Minnesota	No	N/AP	N/AP	N/AP
Mississippi	Function not Listed	N/AP	N/AP	N/AP
Missouri	Yes	Accredited	None	Indirect
Montana	Yes	Accredited	None	Direct
Nebraska	Yes	Accredited	K/P-Waived	General
Nevada	No	N/AP	N/AP	N/AP
New Hampshire	Yes	Accredited	Knowledge	General
New Jersey	Yes	Accredited	Knowledge	Direct
New Mexico	Yes	N/R	None	Direct
New York	Yes	Accredited	Knowledge	Direct
North Carolina	Yes	Approved	None	Indirect
North Dakota	Yes	Accredited	Know/Per	General
Ohio	No	N/AP	N/AP	N/AP
Oklahoma	No	N/AP	N/AP	N/AP
Oregon*	Yes	Accredited	None	General
Pennsylvania*	Yes	Accredited	None	Direct
Rhode Island	Yes	Accredited	Know/Per	Direct
South Carolina	Yes	Accredited	None	Direct
South Dakota	No	N/AP	N/AP	N/AP
Tennessee	DECLINES TO RESPOND			
Texas	Yes	Accredited	None	Direct
Utah	Yes	Accredited	N/R	Undefined
Vermont	Yes	Acc-Ac/Spec-Spec	Writ/Clin-Wav	Direct
Virginia	Yes	Accredited	None	Direct
Washington	Function not Listed	N/AP	N/AP	N/AP
West Virginia	Yes	Accredited	Knowledge	Direct
Wisconsin	Yes	Accredited	Know/Per	Direct
Wyoming	Yes	Accredited	Know/Per	General

*The rules for these states are either under review or the returned survey was incomplete. Therefore, the responses shown are from the responses that were reported in the 1990 report.

PLACING RUBBER DAMS: DENTAL ASSISTING

State	Permission	Required education	Required examination	Required supervision
Alabama	Yes	None	None	Direct
Alaska	Function not Listed	N/AP	N/AP	N/AP
Arizona	No	N/AP	N/AP	N/AP
Arkansas	Yes	None	None	Direct
California	Yes	Acc-Ac/Spec-App	Writ/Clin	Direct
Colorado	Yes	None	None	Direct
Connecticut	No	N/AP	N/AP	N/AP
Delaware	Yes	N/R	N/R	Direct
District of Columbia	No	N/AP	N/AP	N/AP
Florida	Yes	Accredited	None	Indirect
Georgia	Yes	None	None	Direct
Hawaii	Yes	None	None	Direct
Idaho	Yes	None	None	Direct
Illinois	Yes	Experience	None	Direct
Indiana	DECLINES TO RESPOND			
Iowa	No	N/AP	N/AP	N/AP
Kansas	DECLINES TO RESPOND			
Kentucky	Yes	N/R	N/R	Direct
Louisiana	Yes	None	None	Direct
Maine	Yes	None	None	Direct
Maryland	Yes	Ac-Ac/Spec-Ap-Sp	Writ-CDA-Waived	Direct
Massachusetts	Yes	None	None	General
Michigan	Yes	Accredited	Writ/Clin	Indirect
Minnesota	Yes	Acc-Spec	Written	Indirect
Mississippi	Function not Listed	N/AP	N/AP	N/AP
Missouri	Yes	None	None	Direct
Montana	Yes	None	None	Direct
Nebraska	Yes	None	None	Direct
Nevada	Yes	None	None	Direct
New Hampshire	Yes	Acc-App	Writ/Clin-CDA	Direct
New Jersey	Yes	App-Spec	W/C-CDA-None	Direct
New Mexico	Yes	None	None	Direct
New York	No	N/AP	N/AP	N/AP
North Carolina	Yes	Acc-Ac/Spec-App	None	Direct
North Dakota	Yes	Acc-Ac/Spec-App	CDA Exam	Direct
Ohio	Yes	None	None	Direct
Oklahoma	Yes	Specific	Writ/Clin	Direct
Oregon*	Yes	Acc-App-Spec	Writ/Clin-None	Direct
Pennsylvania*	Yes	None	None	Direct
Rhode Island	Yes	None	Waived	Direct
South Carolina	Yes	None	None	Direct
South Dakota	Yes	None	None	Direct
Tennessee	DECLINES TO RESPOND			
Texas	Yes	None	None	Undefined
Utah	Yes	None	None	Direct
Vermont	Yes	Acc/Spec	CDA Exam	Direct
Virginia	Yes	None	None	Direct
Washington	Yes	None	None	Direct
West Virginia	Yes	None	None	Direct
Wisconsin	Yes	None	None	Direct
Wyoming	Yes	None	None	Direct

*The rules for these states are either under review or the returned survey was incomplete. Therefore, the responses shown are from the responses that were reported in the 1990 report.

PLACING RUBBER DAMS: DENTAL HYGIENE

State	Permission	Required education	Required examination	Required supervision
Alabama	Yes	N/R	None	Direct
Alaska	Yes	Accredited	None	Undefined
Arizona	No	N/AP	N/AP	N/AP
Arkansas	Yes	Accredited	Knowledge	Direct
California	Yes	Acc-Ac/Spec-App	Know/Per	Direct
Colorado	Yes	Accredited	None	General
Connecticut	Yes	Accredited	None	General
Delaware	Yes	Approved	Know/Per	General
District of Columbia	Yes	Accredited	Performance	Direct
Florida	Yes	Acc-Spec	None	Indirect
Georgia	Yes	Accredited	None	Direct
Hawaii	Yes	Accredited	None	Direct
Idaho	Yes	Accredited	Know/Per	General
Illinois	Yes	Specific	K/P-Waived	Direct
Indiana	Function not Listed	N/AP	N/AP	Direct
Iowa	No	N/AP	N/AP	N/AP
Kansas	Yes	Accredited	Know/Per	Direct
Kentucky	Yes	N/R	N/R	Direct
Louisiana	Yes	Accredited	None	Direct
Maine	Yes	Accredited	Know/Per	General
Maryland	Yes	Acc-App	K/P-Writ-Wav	Direct
Massachusetts	Yes	Accredited	Know/Per	General
Michigan	Yes	Accredited	Writ/Clin	Direct
Minnesota	Yes	Accredited	Know/Per	General
Mississippi	Function not Listed	N/AP	N/AP	N/AP
Missouri	Yes	Accredited	None	Indirect
Montana	Yes	Accredited	None	General
Nebraska	Yes	Accredited	K/P-Waived	General
Nevada	Yes	Accredited	None	Direct
New Hampshire	Yes	Accredited	Knowledge	General
New Jersey	Yes	Accredited	Knowledge	Direct
New Mexico	Yes	N/R	None	Direct
New York	Yes	Accredited	Knowledge	Direct
North Carolina	Yes	Approved	None	Indirect
North Dakota	Yes	Accredited	Know/Per	General
Ohio	Yes	Accredited	None	Direct
Oklahoma	Yes	Accredited	None	Direct
Oregon*	Yes	Accredited	None	General
Pennsylvania*	Yes	Accredited	None	Direct
Rhode Island	Yes	Accredited	Know/Per	Direct
South Carolina	Yes	Accredited	None	Direct
South Dakota	Yes	Accredited	Know/Per	Indirect
Tennessee	DECLINES TO RESPOND			
Texas	Yes	Accredited	None	General
Utah	Yes	Acc/Spec	None	Undefined
Vermont	Yes	Acc-Ac/Spec-Spec	Writ/Clin-Wav	Direct
Virginia	Yes	Accredited	None	Direct
Washington	Yes	Accredited	Knowledge	Direct
West Virginia	Yes	Accredited	Knowledge	Direct
Wisconsin	Yes	Accredited	Know/Per	Direct
Wyoming	Yes	Accredited	Know/Per	General

*The rules for these states are either under review or the returned survey was incomplete. Therefore, the responses shown are from the responses that were reported in the 1990 report.

REMOVING RUBBER DAMS: DENTAL ASSISTING

State	Permission	Required education	Required examination	Required supervision
Alabama	Yes	None	None	Direct
Alaska	Function not Listed	N/AP	N/AP	N/AP
Arizona	No	N/AP	N/AP	N/AP
Arkansas	Yes	None	None	Direct
California	Yes	Acc-Ac/Spec-App	Writ/Clin	Direct
Colorado	Yes	None	None	Direct
Connecticut	No	N/AP	N/AP	N/AP
Delaware	Function not Listed	N/AP	N/AP	N/AP
District of Columbia	No	N/AP	N/AP	N/AP
Florida	Yes	Accredited	None	Indirect
Georgia	Yes	None	None	Direct
Hawaii	Yes	None	None	Direct
Idaho	Yes	None	None	Direct
Illinois	Yes	Experience	None	Direct
Indiana	DECLINES TO RESPOND			
Iowa	Yes	None	None	Direct
Kansas	DECLINES TO RESPOND			
Kentucky	Yes	N/R	N/R	Direct
Louisiana	Yes	None	None	Direct
Maine	Yes	None	None	Direct
Maryland	Yes	Ac-Ac/Spec-Ap-Sp	Writ-CDA-Waived	Direct
Massachusetts	Yes	None	None	General
Michigan	Yes	Accredited	Writ/Clin	Indirect
Minnesota	Yes	Acc-Spec	Written	Indirect
Mississippi	Function not Listed	N/AP	N/AP	N/AP
Missouri	Yes	None	None	Direct
Montana	Yes	None	None	Direct
Nebraska	Yes	None	None	Direct
Nevada	Yes	None	None	Direct
New Hampshire	Yes	Acc-App	Writ/Clin-CDA	Direct
New Jersey	Yes	App-Spec	W/C-CDA-None	Direct
New Mexico	Yes	None	None	Direct
New York	No	N/AP	N/AP	N/AP
North Carolina	Yes	Acc-Ac/Spec-App	None	Direct
North Dakota	Yes	Acc-Ac/Spec-App	CDA Exam	Direct
Ohio	Yes	None	None	Direct
Oklahoma	Yes	Specific	Writ/Clin	Direct
Oregon*	Yes	Acc-App-Spec	Writ/Clin-None	Direct
Pennsylvania*	Yes	None	None	Direct
Rhode Island	Yes	None	Waived	Direct
South Carolina	Yes	None	None	Direct
South Dakota	Yes	None	None	Direct
Tennessee	DECLINES TO RESPOND			
Texas	Yes	None	None	Undefined
Utah	Yes	None	None	Direct
Vermont	Yes	Acc/Spec	CDA Exam	Direct
Virginia	Yes	None	None	Direct
Washington	Yes	None	None	Direct
West Virginia	Yes	None	None	Direct
Wisconsin	Yes	None	None	Direct
Wyoming	Yes	None	None	Direct

*The rules for these states are either under review or the returned survey was incomplete. Therefore, the responses shown are from the responses that were reported in the 1990 report.

REMOVING RUBBER DAMS: DENTAL HYGIENE

State	Permission	Required education	Required examination	Required supervision
Alabama	Yes	N/R	None	Direct
Alaska	Yes	Accredited	None	Undefined
Arizona	No	N/AP	N/AP	N/AP
Arkansas	Yes	Accredited	Knowledge	Direct
California	Yes	Acc-Ac/Spec-App	Know/Per	Direct
Colorado	Yes	Accredited	None	General
Connecticut	Yes	Accredited	None	General
Delaware	Yes	Approved	Know/Per	General
District of Columbia	Yes	Accredited	Performance	Direct
Florida	Yes	Acc-Spec	None	Indirect
Georgia	Yes	Accredited	None	Direct
Hawaii	Yes	Accredited	None	Direct
Idaho	Yes	Accredited	Know/Per	General
Illinois	Yes	Specific	K/P-Waived	Direct
Indiana	Function not Listed	N/AP	N/AP	Direct
Iowa	Yes	Accredited	None	General
Kansas	Yes	Accredited	Know/Per	Direct
Kentucky	Yes	N/R	N/R	Direct
Louisiana	Yes	Accredited	None	Indirect
Maine	Yes	Accredited	Know/Per	General
Maryland	Yes	Acc-App	K/P-Writ-Wav	Direct
Massachusetts	Yes	Accredited	Know/Per	General
Michigan	Yes	Accredited	Writ/Clin	Direct
Minnesota	Yes	Accredited	Know/Per	General
Mississippi	Function not Listed	N/AP	N/AP	N/AP
Missouri	Yes	Accredited	None	Direct
Montana	Yes	Accredited	None	General
Nebraska	Yes	Accredited	K/P-Waived	General
Nevada	Yes	Accredited	None	Direct
New Hampshire	Yes	Accredited	Knowledge	General
New Jersey	Yes	Accredited	Knowledge	Direct
New Mexico	Yes	N/R	None	Direct
New York	Yes	Accredited	Knowledge	Direct
North Carolina	Yes	Approved	None	Indirect
North Dakota	Yes	Accredited	Know/Per	General
Ohio	Yes	Accredited	None	Direct
Oklahoma	Yes	Accredited	None	Direct
Oregon*	Yes	Accredited	None	General
Pennsylvania*	Yes	Accredited	None	Direct
Rhode Island	Yes	Accredited	Know/Per	Direct
South Carolina	Yes	Accredited	None	Direct
South Dakota	Yes	Accredited	Know/Per	Direct
Tennessee	DECLINES TO RESPOND			
Texas	Yes	Accredited	None	General
Utah	Yes	Acc/Spec	None	Undefined
Vermont	Yes	Acc-Ac/Spec-Spec	Writ/Clin-Wav	Direct
Virginia	Yes	Accredited	None	Direct
Washington	Yes	Accredited	Knowledge	Direct
West Virginia	Yes	Accredited	Knowledge	Direct
Wisconsin	Yes	Accredited	Know/Per	Direct
Wyoming	Yes	Accredited	Know/Per	General

*The rules for these states are either under review or the returned survey was incomplete. Therefore, the responses shown are from the responses that were reported in the 1990 report.

FABRICATING TEMPORARY/INTERIM RESTORATIONS: DENTAL ASSISTING

State	Permission	Required education	Required examination	Required supervision
Alabama	Yes	None	None	Direct
Alaska	Function not Listed	N/AP	N/AP	N/AP
Arizona	Function not Listed	N/AP	N/AP	N/AP
Arkansas	No	N/AP	N/AP	N/AP
California	No	N/AP	N/AP	N/AP
Colorado	Yes	None	None	Direct
Connecticut	No	N/AP	N/AP	N/R
Delaware	Unanswered	N/R	N/R	N/AP
District of Columbia	No	N/AP	N/AP	N/AP
Florida	Function not Listed	N/AP	N/AP	N/AP
Georgia	Yes	None	None	Direct
Hawaii	Function not Listed	N/AP	N/AP	N/AP
Idaho	Function not Listed	N/AP	N/AP	N/AP
Illinois	Yes	Experience	None	Direct
Indiana	DECLINES TO RESPOND			
Iowa	Unanswered	N/R	N/R	N/R
Kansas	Unanswered	N/R	N/R	N/R
Kentucky	Yes	N/R	N/R	Direct
Louisiana	Yes	None	None	Direct
Maine	No	N/AP	N/AP	N/AP
Maryland	Unanswered	N/R	N/R	N/R
Massachusetts	Unanswered	N/R	N/R	N/R
Michigan	Yes	Accredited	Writ/Clin	Direct
Minnesota	No	N/AP	N/AP	N/AP
Mississippi	No	N/AP	N/AP	N/AP
Missouri	Yes	None	None	Direct
Montana	Function not Listed	N/AP	N/AP	N/AP
Nebraska	Yes	None	None	Direct
Nevada	Yes	None	None	Direct
New Hampshire	No	N/AP	N/AP	N/AP
New Jersey	Yes	App-Spec	Writ-CDA-None	Direct
New Mexico	Yes	None	None	Direct
New York	No	N/AP	N/AP	N/AP
North Carolina	Yes	None	None	Direct
North Dakota	Yes	Acc-Ac/Spec-App	CDA Exam	Direct
Ohio	Yes	None	None	Direct
Oklahoma	Unanswered	N/R	N/R	N/R
Oregon*	Unanswered	N/R	N/R	N/R
Pennsylvania*	Unanswered	N/R	N/R	N/R
Rhode Island	No	N/AP	N/AP	N/AP
South Carolina	Function not Listed	N/AP	N/AP	N/AP
South Dakota	Function not Listed	N/AP	N/AP	N/AP
Tennessee	DECLINES TO RESPOND			
Texas	Yes	None	None	Undefined
Utah	Unanswered	N/R	N/R	N/R
Vermont	Yes	Acc/Spec	CDA Exam	Direct
Virginia	No	N/AP	N/AP	N/AP
Washington	Function not Listed	N/AP	N/AP	N/AP
West Virginia	Function not Listed	N/AP	N/AP	N/AP
Wisconsin	No	N/AP	N/AP	N/AP
Wyoming	Function not Listed	N/AP	N/AP	N/AP

*The rules for these states are either under review or the returned survey was incomplete. Therefore, the responses shown are from the responses that were reported in the 1990 report.

FABRICATING TEMPORARY/INTERIM RESTORATIONS: DENTAL HYGIENE

State	Permission	Required education	Required examination	Required supervision
Alabama	Yes	N/R	None	Direct
Alaska	No	N/AP	N/AP	N/AP
Arizona	Function not Listed	N/AP	N/AP	N/AP
Arkansas	Function not Listed	N/AP	N/AP	N/AP
California	No	N/AP	N/AP	N/AP
Colorado	Yes	Accredited	None	General
Connecticut	No	N/AP	N/AP	N/AP
Delaware	Unanswered	N/R	N/R	N/R
District of Columbia	No	N/AP	N/AP	N/AP
Florida	No	N/AP	N/AP	N/AP
Georgia	Yes	Accredited	None	Direct
Hawaii	Unanswered	N/R	N/R	N/R
Idaho	Function not Listed	N/AP	N/AP	N/AP
Illinois	Yes	Specific	K/P-Waived	Direct
Indiana	Function not Listed	N/AP	N/AP	Direct
Iowa	Unanswered	N/R	N/R	N/R
Kansas	Unanswered	N/R	N/R	N/R
Kentucky	Yes	N/R	N/R	Direct
Louisiana	Yes	Accredited	None	Direct
Maine	No	N/AP	N/AP	N/AP
Maryland	No	N/AP	N/AP	N/AP
Massachusetts	Unanswered	N/R	N/R	N/R
Michigan	Yes	Accredited	Writ/Clin	Direct
Minnesota	No	N/AP	N/AP	N/AP
Mississippi	No	N/AP	N/AP	N/AP
Missouri	Yes	Accredited	None	Direct
Montana	Function not Listed	N/AP	N/AP	N/AP
Nebraska	Yes	Accredited	K/P-Waived	Direct
Nevada	Yes	Accredited	None	Direct
New Hampshire	No	N/AP	N/AP	N/AP
New Jersey	Yes	N/R	N/R	N/R
New Mexico	Yes	N/R	None	Direct
New York	Function not Listed	N/AP	N/AP	N/AP
North Carolina	Yes	Approved	None	Indirect
North Dakota	Yes	Accredited	Know/Per	General
Ohio	Yes	Accredited	None	Direct
Oklahoma	Unanswered	N/R	N/R	N/R
Oregon*	Unanswered	N/R	N/R	N/R
Pennsylvania*	Unanswered	N/R	N/R	N/R
Rhode Island	Yes	Accredited	Know/Per	Direct
South Carolina	Function not Listed	N/AP	N/AP	N/AP
South Dakota	Function not Listed	N/AP	N/AP	N/AP
Tennessee	DECLINES TO RESPOND			
Texas	Yes	Accredited	None	General
Utah	Unanswered	N/R	N/R	N/R
Vermont	Yes	Acc-Ac/Spec-Spec	Writ/Clin-Wav	Direct
Virginia	No	N/AP	N/AP	N/AP
Washington	Function not Listed	N/AP	N/AP	N/AP
West Virginia	No	N/AP	N/AP	N/AP
Wisconsin	No	N/AP	N/AP	N/AP
Wyoming	Function not Listed	N/AP	N/AP	N/AP

*The rules for these states are either under review or the returned survey was incomplete. Therefore, the responses shown are from the responses that were reported in the 1990 report.

PLACING TEMPORARY/INTERIM RESTORATIONS: DENTAL ASSISTING

State	Permission	Required education	Required examination	Required supervision
Alabama	Yes	None	None	Direct
Alaska	Function not Listed	N/AP	N/AP	N/AP
Arizona	Function not Listed	N/AP	N/AP	N/AP
Arkansas	Function not Listed	N/AP	N/AP	N/AP
California	Yes	Acc-Ac/Spec-App	Writ/Clin	Direct
Colorado	Yes	None	None	Direct
Connecticut	No	N/AP	N/AP	N/AP
Delaware	No	N/AP	N/AP	N/AP
District of Columbia	No	N/AP	N/AP	N/AP
Florida	Yes	Accredited	None	Direct
Georgia	Yes	None	None	Direct
Hawaii	Function not Listed	N/AP	N/AP	N/AP
Idaho	Yes	Specific	Written	Direct
Illinois	No	N/AP	N/AP	N/AP
Indiana	DECLINES TO RESPOND			
Iowa	No	N/AP	N/AP	N/AP
Kansas	DECLINES TO RESPOND			
Kentucky	No	N/AP	N/AP	N/AP
Louisiana	No	N/AP	N/AP	N/AP
Maine	No	N/AP	N/AP	N/AP
Maryland	No	Ac-Ac/Spec-Ap-Sp	Writ-CDA-Waived	Direct
Massachusetts	Yes	None	None	General
Michigan	Yes	Accredited	Writ/Clin	Direct
Minnesota	No	N/AP	N/AP	N/AP
Mississippi	No	N/AP	N/AP	N/AP
Missouri	Yes	None	None	Direct
Montana	Yes	None	None	Direct
Nebraska	Yes	None	None	Direct
Nevada	Yes	None	None	Direct
New Hampshire	No	N/AP	N/AP	N/AP
New Jersey	Yes	App-Spec	Writ-CDA-None	Direct
New Mexico	Yes	None	None	Direct
New York	No	N/AP	N/AP	N/AP
North Carolina	Yes	Acc-Ac/Spec-App	None	Direct
North Dakota	Yes	Acc-Ac/Spec-App	CDA Exam	Direct
Ohio	No	N/AP	N/AP	N/AP
Oklahoma	No	N/AP	N/AP	N/AP
Oregon*	No	N/AP	N/AP	N/AP
Pennsylvania*	Yes	None	None	Direct
Rhode Island	No	N/AP	N/AP	N/AP
South Carolina	Yes	Acc-Exp	None	Direct
South Dakota	No	N/AP	N/AP	N/AP
Tennessee	DECLINES TO RESPOND			
Texas	Yes	None	None	Undefined
Utah	No	N/AP	N/AP	N/AP
Vermont	Yes	Acc/Spec	CDA Exam	Direct
Virginia	No	N/AP	N/AP	N/AP
Washington	Yes	None	None	Direct
West Virginia	No	N/AP	N/AP	N/AP
Wisconsin	Yes	None	None	Direct
Wyoming	Function not Listed	N/AP	N/AP	N/AP

*The rules for these states are either under review or the returned survey was incomplete. Therefore, the responses shown are from the responses that were reported in the 1990 report.

PLACING TEMPORARY/INTERIM RESTORATIONS: DENTAL HYGIENE

State	Permission	Required education	Required examination	Required supervision
Alabama	Yes	N/R	None	Direct
Alaska	No	N/AP	N/AP	N/AP
Arizona	Function not Listed	N/AP	N/AP	N/AP
Arkansas	Function not Listed	N/AP	N/AP	N/AP
California	Yes	Acc-Ac/Spec-App	Know/Per	General
Colorado	Yes	Accredited	None	General
Connecticut	No	N/AP	N/AP	N/AP
Delaware	Yes	Approved	Know/Per	General
District of Columbia	No	N/AP	N/AP	N/AP
Florida	Yes	Acc/Spec	None	Direct
Georgia	Yes	Accredited	None	Direct
Hawaii	Yes	Accredited	None	Direct
Idaho	Yes	Accredited	Know/Per	Indirect
Illinois	Yes	Specific	K/P-Waived	Direct
Indiana	Function not Listed	N/AP	N/AP	Direct
Iowa	No	N/AP	N/AP	N/AP
Kansas	Yes	Accredited	Know/Per	Direct
Kentucky	Yes	N/R	N/R	Direct
Louisiana	Yes	Accredited	Knowledge	Indirect
Maine	Yes	Accredited	Know/Per	General
Maryland	No	N/AP	N/AP	N/AP
Massachusetts	Yes	Accredited	Know/Per	General
Michigan	Yes	Accredited	Writ/Clin	Direct
Minnesota	Yes	Accredited	Know/Per	General
Mississippi	No	N/AP	N/AP	N/AP
Missouri	Yes	Accredited	None	Direct
Montana	Yes	Accredited	None	General
Nebraska	Yes	Accredited	K/P-Waived	Direct
Nevada	Yes	Accredited	None	Direct
New Hampshire	No	N/AP	N/AP	N/AP
New Jersey	Yes	Accredited	Knowledge	Direct
New Mexico	Yes	N/R	None	Direct
New York	Yes	Accredited	Knowledge	Direct
North Carolina	Yes	Approved	None	Indirect
North Dakota	Yes	Accredited	Know/Per	General
Ohio	No	N/AP	N/AP	N/AP
Oklahoma	Yes	Accredited	None	Direct
Oregon*	Yes	Ac/Spec-Spec	None	General
Pennsylvania*	Yes	Accredited	None	Direct
Rhode Island	Yes	Accredited	Know/Per	Direct
South Carolina	Yes	Accredited	None	Direct
South Dakota	No	N/AP	N/AP	N/AP
Tennessee	DECLINES TO RESPOND			
Texas	Yes	Accredited	None	General
Utah	Yes	Acc/Spec	None	Undefined
Vermont	Yes	Acc-Ac/Spec-Spec	Writ/Clin-Wav	Direct
Virginia	No	N/AP	N/AP	N/AP
Washington	Yes	Accredited	None	Direct
West Virginia	No	N/AP	N/AP	N/AP
Wisconsin	Yes	Accredited	Know/Per	General
Wyoming	Yes	Accredited	Know/Per	General

*The rules for these states are either under review or the returned survey was incomplete. Therefore, the responses shown are from the responses that were reported in the 1990 report.

REMOVING TEMPORARY/INTERIM RESTORATIONS: DENTAL ASSISTING

State	Permission	Required education	Required examination	Required supervision
Alabama	Yes	None	None	Direct
Alaska	Function not Listed	N/AP	N/AP	N/AP
Arizona	Function not Listed	N/AP	N/AP	N/AP
Arkansas	No	N/AP	N/AP	N/AP
California	Yes	Acc-Ac/Spec-App	Writ/Clin	Direct
Colorado	Yes	None	None	Direct
Connecticut	No	N/AP	N/AP	N/AP
Delaware	Yes	N/R	N/R	N/R
District of Columbia	No	N/AP	N/AP	N/AP
Florida	Yes	Accredited	None	Indirect
Georgia	No	N/AP	N/AP	N/AP
Hawaii	Yes	None	None	Direct
Idaho	Yes	Specific	Written	Direct
Illinois	No	N/AP	N/AP	N/AP
Indiana	DECLINES TO RESPOND			
Iowa	No	N/AP	N/AP	N/AP
Kansas	DECLINES TO RESPOND			
Kentucky	No	N/AP	N/AP	N/AP
Louisiana	Yes	None	None	Direct
Maine	Yes	None	None	Direct
Maryland	No	N/AP	N/AP	N/AP
Massachusetts	Yes	None	CDA Exam	Direct
Michigan	Yes	Accredited	Writ/Clin	Direct
Minnesota	No	N/AP	N/AP	N/AP
Mississippi	No	N/AP	N/AP	N/AP
Missouri	Yes	None	None	Direct
Montana	Yes	None	None	Direct
Nebraska	Yes	None	None	Direct
Nevada	No	N/AP	N/AP	N/AP
New Hampshire	No	N/AP	N/AP	N/AP
New Jersey	No	N/AP	N/AP	N/AP
New Mexico	Yes	None	None	Direct
New York	No	N/AP	N/AP	N/AP
North Carolina	Yes	Acc-Ac/Spec-App	None	Direct
North Dakota	Yes	Acc-Ac/Spec-App	CDA Exam	Direct
Ohio	No	N/AP	N/AP	N/AP
Oklahoma	No	N/AP	N/AP	N/AP
Oregon*	No	N/AP	N/AP	N/AP
Pennsylvania*	No	N/AP	N/AP	N/AP
Rhode Island	No	N/AP	N/AP	N/AP
South Carolina	Function not Listed	N/AP	N/AP	N/AP
South Dakota	No	N/AP	N/AP	N/AP
Tennessee	DECLINES TO RESPOND			
Texas	Yes	None	None	Undefined
Utah	Yes	None	None	Direct
Vermont	Yes	Acc/Spec	CDA Exam	Direct
Virginia	No	N/AP	N/AP	N/AP
Washington	Yes	None	None	Direct
West Virginia	No	N/AP	N/AP	N/AP
Wisconsin	Yes	None	None	Direct
Wyoming	No	N/AP	N/AP	N/AP

*The rules for these states are either under review or the returned survey was incomplete. Therefore, the responses shown are from the responses that were reported in the 1990 report.

REMOVING TEMPORARY/INTERIM RESTORATIONS: DENTAL HYGIENE

State	Permission	Required education	Required examination	Required supervision
Alabama	Yes	N/R	None	Direct
Alaska	No	N/AP	N/AP	N/AP
Arizona	Function not Listed	N/AP	N/AP	N/AP
Arkansas	Yes	Accredited	Knowledge	Direct
California	Yes	Acc-Ac/Spec-App	Know/Per	General
Colorado	Yes	Accredited	None	General
Connecticut	No	N/AP	N/AP	N/AP
Delaware	Yes	Approved	Know/Per	General
District of Columbia	No	N/AP	N/AP	N/AP
Florida	Yes	Acc/Spec	None	Direct
Georgia	No	N/AP	N/AP	N/AP
Hawaii	Yes	Accredited	None	Direct
Idaho	Yes	Accredited	Know/Per	Indirect
Illinois	Yes	Specific	K/P-Waived	Direct
Indiana	Function not Listed	N/AP	N/AP	Direct
Iowa	No	N/AP	N/AP	N/AP
Kansas	Yes	Accredited	Know/Per	Direct
Kentucky	Yes	N/R	N/R	Direct
Louisiana	Yes	Accredited	Knowledge	Indirect
Maine	Yes	Accredited	Know/Per	General
Maryland	No	N/AP	N/AP	N/AP
Massachusetts	Yes	Accredited	Know/Per	Direct
Michigan	Yes	Accredited	Writ/Clin	Direct
Minnesota	No	N/AP	N/AP	N/AP
Mississippi	No	N/AP	N/AP	N/AP
Missouri	Yes	Accredited	None	Direct
Montana	Yes	Accredited	None	Direct
Nebraska	Yes	Accredited	K/P-Waived	Direct
Nevada	No	N/AP	N/AP	N/AP
New Hampshire	No	N/AP	N/AP	N/AP
New Jersey	No	N/AP	N/AP	N/AP
New Mexico	Yes	N/R	None	Direct
New York	Yes	Accredited	Knowledge	Direct
North Carolina	Yes	Approved	None	Indirect
North Dakota	Yes	Accredited	Know/Per	General
Ohio	No	N/AP	N/AP	N/AP
Oklahoma	No	N/AP	N/AP	N/AP
Oregon*	Function not Listed	N/AP	N/AP	N/AP
Pennsylvania*	Yes	Accredited	None	Direct
Rhode Island	Yes	Accredited	Know/Per	Direct
South Carolina	Yes	Accredited	None	Direct
South Dakota	No	N/AP	N/AP	N/AP
Tennessee	DECLINES TO RESPOND			
Texas	Yes	Accredited	None	General
Utah	Yes	Acc/Spec	None	Undefined
Vermont	Yes	Acc-Ac/Spec-Spec	Writ/Clin-Wav	Direct
Virginia	No	N/AP	N/AP	N/AP
Washington	Function not Listed	N/AP	N/AP	N/AP
West Virginia	No	N/AP	N/AP	N/AP
Wisconsin	Yes	Accredited	Knowledge	Direct
Wyoming	No	N/AP	N/AP	N/AP

*The rules for these states are either under review or the returned survey was incomplete. Therefore, the responses shown are from the responses that were reported in the 1990 report.

APPLYING CAVITY LINERS AND BASES: DENTAL ASSISTING

State	Permission	Required education	Required examination	Required supervision
Alabama	Yes	None	None	Direct
Alaska	Function not Listed	N/AP	N/AP	N/AP
Arizona	Function not Listed	N/AP	N/AP	N/AP
Arkansas	No	N/AP	N/AP	N/AP
California	Yes	Acc-Ac/Spec-App	Writ/Clin	Direct
Colorado	Yes	None	None	Direct
Connecticut	No	N/AP	N/AP	N/AP
Delaware	Function not Listed	N/AP	N/AP	N/AP
District of Columbia	No	N/AP	N/AP	N/AP
Florida	Yes	Accredited	None	Indirect
Georgia	Yes	Specific	None	Direct
Hawaii	No	N/AP	N/AP	N/AP
Idaho	No	N/AP	N/AP	N/AP
Illinois	No	N/AP	N/AP	N/AP
Indiana	DECLINES TO RESPOND			
Iowa	No	N/AP	N/AP	N/AP
Kansas	DECLINES TO RESPOND			
Kentucky	No	N/AP	N/AP	N/AP
Louisiana	Yes	Ac/Spec-App-Spec	CDA Exam-Waived	Direct
Maine	No	N/AP	N/AP	N/AP
Maryland	No	N/AP	N/AP	N/AP
Massachusetts	No	N/AP	N/AP	N/AP
Michigan	No	N/AP	N/AP	N/AP
Minnesota	Yes	Acc-Spec	Written	Indirect
Mississippi	No	N/AP	N/AP	N/AP
Missouri	No	N/AP	N/AP	N/AP
Montana	Function not Listed	N/AP	N/AP	N/AP
Nebraska	No	N/AP	N/AP	N/AP
Nevada	No	N/AP	N/AP	N/AP
New Hampshire	No	N/AP	N/AP	N/AP
New Jersey	No	N/AP	N/AP	N/AP
New Mexico	No	N/AP	N/AP	N/AP
New York	No	N/AP	N/AP	N/AP
North Carolina	Yes	Acc-Ac/Spec-App	None	Direct
North Dakota	No	N/AP	N/AP	N/AP
Ohio	Yes	None	None	Direct
Oklahoma	No	N/AP	N/AP	N/AP
Oregon*	No	N/AP	N/AP	N/AP
Pennsylvania*	No	N/AP	N/AP	N/AP
Rhode Island	Yes	None	Waived	Direct
South Carolina	No	N/AP	N/AP	N/AP
South Dakota	No	N/AP	N/AP	N/AP
Tennessee	DECLINES TO RESPOND			
Texas	No	N/AP	N/AP	N/AP
Utah	No	N/AP	N/AP	N/AP
Vermont	No	N/AP	N/AP	N/AP
Virginia	No	N/AP	N/AP	N/AP
Washington	No	N/AP	N/AP	N/AP
West Virginia	No	N/AP	N/AP	N/AP
Wisconsin	Yes	None	None	Direct
Wyoming	No	N/AP	N/AP	N/AP

*The rules for these states are either under review or the returned survey was incomplete. Therefore, the responses shown are from the responses that were reported in the 1990 report.

APPLYING CAVITY LINERS AND BASES: DENTAL HYGIENE

State	Permission	Required education	Required examination	Required supervision
Alabama	Yes	N/R	None	Direct
Alaska	No	N/AP	N/AP	N/AP
Arizona	Function not Listed	N/AP	N/AP	N/AP
Arkansas	No	N/AP	N/AP	N/AP
California	Yes	Acc-Ac/Spec-App	Know/Per	Direct
Colorado	Yes	Accredited	None	General
Connecticut	No	N/AP	N/AP	N/AP
Delaware	No	N/AP	N/AP	N/AP
District of Columbia	No	N/AP	N/AP	N/AP
Florida	Yes	Acc/Spec	None	Indirect
Georgia	Yes	Experience	None	Direct
Hawaii	No	N/AP	N/AP	N/AP
Idaho	Yes	Accredited	Know/Per	Indirect
Illinois	No	N/AP	N/AP	N/AP
Indiana	Function not Listed	N/AP	N/AP	Direct
Iowa	No	N/AP	N/AP	N/AP
Kansas	Function not Listed	N/AP	N/AP	N/AP
Kentucky	Yes	N/R	N/R	Direct
Louisiana	Yes	Accredited	None	Direct
Maine	No	N/AP	N/AP	N/AP
Maryland	No	N/AP	N/AP	N/AP
Massachusetts	No	N/AP	N/AP	N/AP
Michigan	No	N/AP	N/AP	N/AP
Minnesota	Yes	Accredited	Know/Per	General
Mississippi	No	N/AP	N/AP	N/AP
Missouri	No	N/AP	N/AP	N/AP
Montana	Function not Listed	N/AP	N/AP	N/AP
Nebraska	No	N/AP	N/AP	N/AP
Nevada	No	N/AP	N/AP	N/AP
New Hampshire	No	N/AP	N/AP	N/AP
New Jersey	No	N/AP	N/AP	N/AP
New Mexico	No	N/AP	N/AP	N/AP
New York	Function not Listed	N/AP	N/AP	N/AP
North Carolina	Yes	Approved	None	Indirect
North Dakota	No	N/AP	N/AP	N/AP
Ohio	Yes	Accredited	None	Direct
Oklahoma	No	N/AP	N/AP	N/AP
Oregon*	Function not Listed	N/AP	N/AP	N/AP
Pennsylvania*	Yes	Accredited	None	Direct
Rhode Island	Yes	Accredited	None	Direct
South Carolina	Yes	Accredited	None	Direct
South Dakota	No	N/AP	N/AP	N/AP
Tennessee	DECLINES TO RESPOND			
Texas	No	N/AP	N/AP	N/AP
Utah	No	N/AP	N/AP	N/AP
Vermont	No	N/AP	N/AP	N/AP
Virginia	No	N/AP	N/AP	N/AP
Washington	Function not Listed	N/AP	N/AP	N/AP
West Virginia	No	N/AP	N/AP	N/AP
Wisconsin	Yes	Accredited	Knowledge	Direct
Wyoming	Function not Listed	N/AP	N/AP	N/AP

*The rules for these states are either under review or the returned survey was incomplete. Therefore, the responses shown are from the responses that were reported in the 1990 report.

PLACING AMALGAM RESTORATIONS FOR CONDENSATION BY THE DENTIST: DENTAL ASSISTING

State	Permission	Required education	Required examination	Required supervision
Alabama	Yes	None	None	Direct
Alaska	Function not Listed	N/AP	N/AP	N/AP
Arizona	No	N/AP	N/AP	N/AP
Arkansas	No	N/AP	N/AP	N/AP
California	No	N/AP	N/AP	N/AP
Colorado	Yes	None	None	Direct
Connecticut	No	N/AP	N/AP	N/AP
Delaware	No	N/AP	N/AP	N/AP
District of Columbia	No	N/AP	N/AP	N/AP
Florida	No	N/AP	N/AP	N/AP
Georgia	No	N/AP	N/AP	N/AP
Hawaii	No	N/AP	N/AP	N/AP
Idaho	No	N/AP	N/AP	N/AP
Illinois	No	N/AP	N/AP	N/AP
Indiana	DECLINES TO RESPOND			
Iowa	No	N/AP	N/AP	N/AP
Kansas	DECLINES TO RESPOND			
Kentucky	Yes	N/R	N/R	Direct
Louisiana	No	N/AP	N/AP	N/AP
Maine	Yes	None	None	Direct
Maryland	No	N/AP	N/AP	N/AP
Massachusetts	Yes	None	None	Direct
Michigan	No	N/AP	N/AP	N/AP
Minnesota	No	N/AP	N/AP	N/AP
Mississippi	No	N/AP	N/AP	N/AP
Missouri	No	N/AP	N/AP	N/AP
Montana	Function not Listed	N/AP	N/AP	N/AP
Nebraska	No	N/AP	N/AP	N/AP
Nevada	No	N/AP	N/AP	N/AP
New Hampshire	No	N/AP	N/AP	N/AP
New Jersey	Yes	App-Spec	Writ-CDA-None	Direct
New Mexico	No	N/AP	N/AP	N/AP
New York	No	N/AP	N/AP	N/AP
North Carolina	No	N/AP	N/AP	N/AP
North Dakota	Function not Listed	N/AP	N/AP	N/AP
Ohio	Yes	Specific	Writ/Clin	Direct
Oklahoma	No	N/AP	N/AP	N/AP
Oregon*	No	N/AP	N/AP	N/AP
Pennsylvania*	Yes	None	None	Direct
Rhode Island	No	N/AP	N/AP	N/AP
South Carolina	No	N/AP	N/AP	N/AP
South Dakota	No	N/AP	N/AP	N/AP
Tennessee	DECLINES TO RESPOND			
Texas	No	N/AP	N/AP	N/AP
Utah	No	N/AP	N/AP	N/AP
Vermont	Yes	Acc/Spec	CDA Exam	Direct
Virginia	Yes	None	None	Direct
Washington	No	N/AP	N/AP	N/AP
West Virginia	No	N/AP	N/AP	N/AP
Wisconsin	No	N/AP	N/AP	N/AP
Wyoming	No	N/AP	N/AP	N/AP

*The rules for these states are either under review or the returned survey was incomplete. Therefore, the responses shown are from the responses that were reported in the 1990 report.

PLACING AMALGAM RESTORATIONS FOR CONDENSATION BY THE DENTIST: DENTAL HYGIENE

State	Permission	Required education	Required examination	Required supervision
Alabama	Yes	N/R	None	Direct
Alaska	No	N/AP	N/AP	N/AP
Arizona	No	N/AP	N/AP	N/AP
Arkansas	No	N/AP	N/AP	N/AP
California	No	N/AP	N/AP	N/AP
Colorado	Yes	Accredited	None	General
Connecticut	No	N/AP	N/AP	N/AP
Delaware	No	N/AP	N/AP	N/AP
District of Columbia	No	N/AP	N/AP	N/AP
Florida	No	N/AP	N/AP	N/AP
Georgia	No	N/AP	N/AP	N/AP
Hawaii	No	N/AP	N/AP	N/AP
Idaho	No	N/AP	N/AP	N/AP
Illinois	No	N/AP	N/AP	N/AP
Indiana	Function not Listed	N/AP	N/AP	Direct
Iowa	No	N/AP	N/AP	N/AP
Kansas	Function not Listed	N/AP	N/AP	N/AP
Kentucky	Yes	N/R	N/R	Direct
Louisiana	No	N/AP	N/AP	N/AP
Maine	Yes	Accredited	None	Direct
Maryland	No	N/AP	N/AP	N/AP
Massachusetts	Yes	Accredited	Know/Per	Direct
Michigan	No	N/AP	N/AP	N/AP
Minnesota	No	N/AP	N/AP	N/AP
Mississippi	No	N/AP	N/AP	N/AP
Missouri	No	N/AP	N/AP	N/AP
Montana	Function not Listed	N/AP	N/AP	N/AP
Nebraska	No	N/AP	N/AP	N/AP
Nevada	No	N/AP	N/AP	N/AP
New Hampshire	No	N/AP	N/AP	N/AP
New Jersey	Yes	Accredited	Knowledge	Direct
New Mexico	No	N/AP	N/AP	N/AP
New York	Function not Listed	N/AP	N/AP	N/AP
North Carolina	No	N/AP	N/AP	N/AP
North Dakota	Function not Listed	N/AP	N/AP	N/AP
Ohio	Yes	Specific	Writ/Clin	Direct
Oklahoma	No	N/AP	N/AP	N/AP
Oregon*	No	N/AP	N/AP	N/AP
Pennsylvania*	Yes	Accredited	None	Direct
Rhode Island	Yes	Accredited	Know/Per	Direct
South Carolina	No	N/AP	N/AP	N/AP
South Dakota	No	N/AP	N/AP	N/AP
Tennessee	DECLINES TO RESPOND			
Texas	No	N/AP	N/AP	N/AP
Utah	No	N/AP	N/AP	N/AP
Vermont	Yes	Acc-Ac/Spec-Spec	Writ/Clin-Wav	Direct
Virginia	Yes	Accredited	None	Direct
Washington	Yes	Approved	Know/Per	Direct
West Virginia	No	N/AP	N/AP	N/AP
Wisconsin	No	N/AP	N/AP	N/AP
Wyoming	Yes	Acc-Spec	K/P-Clin	Direct

*The rules for these states are either under review or the returned survey was incomplete. Therefore, the responses shown are from the responses that were reported in the 1990 report.

PLACING AND CONDENSING AMALGAM RESTORATIONS BY THE DENTAL ASSISTANT

State	Permission	Required education	Required examination	Required supervision
Alabama	No	N/AP	N/AP	N/AP
Alaska	Function not Listed	N/AP	N/AP	N/AP
Arizona	No	N/AP	N/AP	N/AP
Arkansas	No	N/AP	N/AP	N/AP
California	No	N/AP	N/AP	N/AP
Colorado	Yes	None	None	Direct
Connecticut	No	N/AP	N/AP	N/AP
Delaware	No	N/AP	N/AP	N/AP
District of Columbia	No	N/AP	N/AP	N/AP
Florida	No	N/AP	N/AP	N/AP
Georgia	No	N/AP	N/AP	N/AP
Hawaii	No	N/AP	N/AP	N/AP
Idaho	No	N/AP	N/AP	N/AP
Illinois	No	N/AP	N/AP	N/AP
Indiana	DECLINES TO RESPOND			
Iowa	No	N/AP	N/AP	N/AP
Kansas	DECLINES TO RESPOND			
Kentucky	Yes	N/R	N/R	Direct
Louisiana	No	N/AP	N/AP	N/AP
Maine	No	N/AP	N/AP	N/AP
Maryland	No	N/AP	N/AP	N/AP
Massachusetts	No	N/AP	N/AP	N/AP
Michigan	No	N/AP	N/AP	N/AP
Minnesota	No	N/AP	N/AP	N/AP
Mississippi	No	N/AP	N/AP	N/AP
Missouri	No	N/AP	N/AP	N/AP
Montana	Function not Listed	N/AP	N/AP	N/AP
Nebraska	No	N/AP	N/AP	N/AP
Nevada	No	N/AP	N/AP	N/AP
New Hampshire	No	N/AP	N/AP	N/AP
New Jersey	No	N/AP	N/AP	N/AP
New Mexico	No	N/AP	N/AP	N/AP
New York	No	N/AP	N/AP	N/AP
North Carolina	No	N/AP	N/AP	N/AP
North Dakota	No	N/AP	N/AP	N/AP
Ohio	Yes	Specific	Writ/Clin	Direct
Oklahoma	No	N/AP	N/AP	N/AP
Oregon*	No	N/AP	N/AP	N/AP
Pennsylvania*	Yes	None	None	Direct
Rhode Island	No	N/AP	N/AP	N/AP
South Carolina	No	N/AP	N/AP	N/AP
South Dakota	No	N/AP	N/AP	N/AP
Tennessee	DECLINES TO RESPOND			
Texas	No	N/AP	N/AP	N/AP
Utah	No	N/AP	N/AP	N/AP
Vermont	No	N/AP	N/AP	N/AP
Virginia	No	N/AP	N/AP	N/AP
Washington	No	N/AP	N/AP	N/AP
West Virginia	No	N/AP	N/AP	N/AP
Wisconsin	No	N/AP	N/AP	N/AP
Wyoming	No	N/AP	N/AP	N/AP

*The rules for these states are either under review or the returned survey was incomplete. Therefore, the responses shown are from the responses that were reported in the 1990 report.

PLACING AND CONDENSING AMALGAM RESTORATIONS BY THE DENTAL HYGIENIST

State	Permission	Required education	Required examination	Required supervision
Alabama	No	N/AP	N/AP	N/AP
Alaska	No	N/AP	N/AP	N/AP
Arizona	No	N/AP	N/AP	N/AP
Arkansas	No	N/AP	N/AP	N/AP
California	No	N/AP	N/AP	N/AP
Colorado	Yes	Accredited	None	General
Connecticut	No	N/AP	N/AP	N/AP
Delaware	No	N/AP	N/AP	N/AP
District of Columbia	No	N/AP	N/AP	N/AP
Florida	No	N/AP	N/AP	N/AP
Georgia	No	N/AP	N/AP	N/AP
Hawaii	No	N/AP	N/AP	N/AP
Idaho	No	N/AP	N/AP	N/AP
Illinois	No	N/AP	N/AP	N/AP
Indiana	Function not Listed	N/AP	N/AP	Direct
Iowa	No	N/AP	N/AP	N/AP
Kansas	DECLINES TO RESPOND			
Kentucky	Yes	N/R	N/R	Direct
Louisiana	No	N/AP	N/AP	N/AP
Maine	No	N/AP	N/AP	N/AP
Maryland	No	N/AP	N/AP	N/AP
Massachusetts	No	N/AP	N/AP	N/AP
Michigan	No	N/AP	N/AP	N/AP
Minnesota	No	N/AP	N/AP	N/AP
Mississippi	No	N/AP	N/AP	N/AP
Missouri	No	N/AP	N/AP	N/AP
Montana	No	N/AP	N/AP	N/AP
Nebraska	No	N/AP	N/AP	N/AP
Nevada	No	N/AP	N/AP	N/AP
New Hampshire	No	N/AP	N/AP	N/AP
New Jersey	No	N/AP	N/AP	N/AP
New Mexico	No	N/AP	N/AP	N/AP
New York	Function not Listed	N/AP	N/AP	N/AP
North Carolina	No	N/AP	N/AP	N/AP
North Dakota	No	N/AP	N/AP	N/AP
Ohio	Yes	Specific	Writ/Clin	Direct
Oklahoma	No	N/AP	N/AP	N/AP
Oregon*	No	N/AP	N/AP	N/AP
Pennsylvania*	Yes	Accredited	None	Direct
Rhode Island	Unanswered	N/R	N/R	N/R
South Carolina	No	N/AP	N/AP	N/AP
South Dakota	No	N/AP	N/AP	N/AP
Tennessee	DECLINES TO RESPOND			
Texas	No	N/AP	N/AP	N/AP
Utah	No	N/AP	N/AP	N/AP
Vermont	No	N/AP	N/AP	N/AP
Virginia	No	N/AP	N/AP	N/AP
Washington	Yes	Approved	Know/Per	Direct
West Virginia	No	N/AP	N/AP	N/AP
Wisconsin	No	N/AP	N/AP	N/AP
Wyoming	Yes	Acc-Spec	K/P-Clin	Direct

*The rules for these states are either under review or the returned survey was incomplete. Therefore, the responses shown are from the responses that were reported in the 1990 report.

CARVING AMALGAMS: DENTAL ASSISTING

State	Permission	Required education	Required examination	Required supervision
Alabama	No	N/AP	N/AP	N/AP
Alaska	Function not Listed	N/AP	N/AP	N/AP
Arizona	No	N/AP	N/AP	N/AP
Arkansas	No	N/AP	N/AP	N/AP
California	No	N/AP	N/AP	N/AP
Colorado	Yes	None	None	Direct
Connecticut	No	N/AP	N/AP	N/AP
Delaware	No	N/AP	N/AP	N/AP
District of Columbia	No	N/AP	N/AP	N/AP
Florida	No	N/AP	N/AP	N/AP
Georgia	No	N/AP	N/AP	N/AP
Hawaii	No	N/AP	N/AP	N/AP
Idaho	No	N/AP	N/AP	N/AP
Illinois	No	N/AP	N/AP	N/AP
Indiana	DECLINES TO RESPOND			
Iowa	No	N/AP	N/AP	N/AP
Kansas	DECLINES TO RESPOND			
Kentucky	Yes	N/R	N/R	Direct
Louisiana	No	N/AP	N/AP	N/AP
Maine	No	N/AP	N/AP	N/AP
Maryland	No	N/AP	N/AP	N/AP
Massachusetts	No	N/AP	N/AP	N/AP
Michigan	No	N/AP	N/AP	N/AP
Minnesota	No	N/AP	N/AP	N/AP
Mississippi	No	N/AP	N/AP	N/AP
Missouri	No	N/AP	N/AP	N/AP
Montana	Function not Listed	N/AP	N/AP	N/AP
Nebraska	No	N/AP	N/AP	N/AP
Nevada	No	N/AP	N/AP	N/AP
New Hampshire	No	N/AP	N/AP	N/AP
New Jersey	No	N/AP	N/AP	N/AP
New Mexico	No	N/AP	N/AP	N/AP
New York	No	N/AP	N/AP	N/AP
North Carolina	No	N/AP	N/AP	N/AP
North Dakota	No	N/AP	N/AP	N/AP
Ohio	Yes	Specific	Writ/Clin	Direct
Oklahoma	No	N/AP	N/AP	N/AP
Oregon*	No	N/AP	N/AP	N/AP
Pennsylvania*	Yes	None	None	Direct
Rhode Island	No	N/AP	N/AP	N/AP
South Carolina	No	N/AP	N/AP	N/AP
South Dakota	No	N/AP	N/AP	N/AP
Tennessee	DECLINES TO RESPOND			
Texas	No	N/AP	N/AP	N/AP
Utah	No	N/AP	N/AP	N/AP
Vermont	No	N/AP	N/AP	N/AP
Virginia	No	N/AP	N/AP	N/AP
Washington	No	N/AP	N/AP	N/AP
West Virginia	No	N/AP	N/AP	N/AP
Wisconsin	No	N/AP	N/AP	N/AP
Wyoming	No	N/AP	N/AP	N/AP

*The rules for these states are either under review or the returned survey was incomplete. Therefore, the responses shown are from the responses that were reported in the 1990 report.

CARVING AMALGAMS: DENTAL HYGIENE

State	Permission	Required education	Required examination	Required supervision
Alabama	No	N/AP	N/AP	N/AP
Alaska	No	N/AP	N/AP	N/AP
Arizona	No	N/AP	N/AP	N/AP
Arkansas	No	N/AP	N/AP	N/AP
California	No	N/AP	N/AP	N/AP
Colorado	Yes	Accredited	None	General
Connecticut	No	N/AP	N/AP	N/AP
Delaware	No	N/AP	N/AP	N/AP
District of Columbia	No	N/AP	N/AP	N/AP
Florida	No	N/AP	N/AP	N/AP
Georgia	No	N/AP	N/AP	N/AP
Hawaii	No	N/AP	N/AP	N/AP
Idaho	No	N/AP	N/AP	N/AP
Illinois	No	N/AP	N/AP	N/AP
Indiana	Function not Listed	N/AP	N/AP	Direct
Iowa	No	N/AP	N/AP	N/AP
Kansas	DECLINES TO RESPOND			
Kentucky	Yes	N/R	N/R	Direct
Louisiana	No	N/AP	N/AP	N/AP
Maine	No	N/AP	N/AP	N/AP
Maryland	No	N/AP	N/AP	N/AP
Massachusetts	No	N/AP	N/AP	N/AP
Michigan	No	N/AP	N/AP	N/AP
Minnesota	No	N/AP	N/AP	N/AP
Mississippi	No	N/AP	N/AP	N/AP
Missouri	No	N/AP	N/AP	N/AP
Montana	No	N/AP	N/AP	N/AP
Nebraska	No	N/AP	N/AP	N/AP
Nevada	No	N/AP	N/AP	N/AP
New Hampshire	No	N/AP	N/AP	N/AP
New Jersey	No	N/AP	N/AP	N/AP
New Mexico	No	N/AP	N/AP	N/AP
New York	Function not Listed	N/AP	N/AP	N/AP
North Carolina	No	N/AP	N/AP	N/AP
North Dakota	No	N/AP	N/AP	N/AP
Ohio	Yes	Specific	Writ/Clin	Direct
Oklahoma	No	N/AP	N/AP	N/AP
Oregon*	No	N/AP	N/AP	N/AP
Pennsylvania*	Yes	Accredited	None	Direct
Rhode Island	Unanswered	N/R	N/R	N/R
South Carolina	No	N/AP	N/AP	N/AP
South Dakota	No	N/AP	N/AP	N/AP
Tennessee	DECLINES TO RESPOND			
Texas	No	N/AP	N/AP	N/AP
Utah	No	N/AP	N/AP	N/AP
Vermont	No	N/AP	N/AP	N/AP
Virginia	No	N/AP	N/AP	N/AP
Washington	Yes	Approved	Know/Per	Direct
West Virginia	No	N/AP	N/AP	N/AP
Wisconsin	No	N/AP	N/AP	N/AP
Wyoming	Yes	Acc-Spec	K/P-Clin	Direct

*The rules for these states are either under review or the returned survey was incomplete. Therefore, the responses shown are from the responses that were reported in the 1990 report.

POLISHING AMALGAMS: DENTAL ASSISTING

State	Permission	Required education	Required examination	Required supervision
Alabama	No	N/AP	N/AP	N/AP
Alaska	Function not Listed	N/AP	N/AP	N/AP
Arizona	No	N/AP	N/AP	N/AP
Arkansas	No	N/AP	N/AP	N/AP
California	No	N/AP	N/AP	N/AP
Colorado	Yes	None	None	Direct
Connecticut	No	N/AP	N/AP	N/AP
Delaware	No	N/AP	N/AP	N/AP
District of Columbia	No	N/AP	N/AP	N/AP
Florida	Yes	Accredited	None	Direct
Georgia	No	N/AP	N/AP	N/AP
Hawaii	No	N/AP	N/AP	N/AP
Idaho	Yes	Specific	Written	Direct
Illinois	No	N/AP	N/AP	N/AP
Indiana	DECLINES TO RESPOND			
Iowa	No	N/AP	N/AP	N/AP
Kansas	DECLINES TO RESPOND			
Kentucky	Yes	N/R	N/R	Direct
Louisiana	No	N/AP	N/AP	N/AP
Maine	No	N/AP	N/AP	N/AP
Maryland	No	N/AP	N/AP	N/AP
Massachusetts	No	N/AP	N/AP	N/AP
Michigan	No	N/AP	N/AP	N/AP
Minnesota	Yes	Acc-Spec	Written	Indirect
Mississippi	No	N/AP	N/AP	N/AP
Missouri	Yes	None	None	Direct
Montana	Yes	None	None	Direct
Nebraska	No	N/AP	N/AP	N/AP
Nevada	No	N/AP	N/AP	N/AP
New Hampshire	No	N/AP	N/AP	N/AP
New Jersey	No	N/AP	N/AP	N/AP
New Mexico	Yes	Ac-Ac/Spec-Ap-Sp	Waived-None	Direct
New York	No	N/AP	N/AP	N/AP
North Carolina	No	N/AP	N/AP	N/AP
North Dakota	Yes	Acc-Ac/Spec-App	CDA Exam	Direct
Ohio	Yes	Specific	Writ/Clin	Direct
Oklahoma	No	N/AP	N/AP	N/AP
Oregon*	Yes	Acc-App-Spec	Writ/Clin-None	Direct
Pennsylvania*	Yes	None	None	Direct
Rhode Island	No	N/AP	N/AP	N/AP
South Carolina	Yes	Acc-Exp	None	Direct
South Dakota	No	N/AP	N/AP	N/AP
Tennessee	DECLINES TO RESPOND			
Texas	No	N/AP	N/AP	N/AP
Utah	No	N/AP	N/AP	N/AP
Vermont	Yes	Acc/Spec	CDA Exam	Direct
Virginia	No	N/AP	N/AP	N/AP
Washington	Yes	None	None	Direct
West Virginia	No	N/AP	N/AP	N/AP
Wisconsin	No	N/AP	N/AP	N/AP
Wyoming	No	N/AP	N/AP	N/AP

*The rules for these states are either under review or the returned survey was incomplete. Therefore, the responses shown are from the responses that were reported in the 1990 report.

POLISHING AMALGAMS: DENTAL HYGIENE

State	Permission	Required education	Required examination	Required supervision
Alabama	Yes	Approved	None	Direct
Alaska	Yes	Accredited	None	Undefined
Arizona	Yes	Accredited	None	General
Arkansas	Yes	Accredited	Knowledge	Direct
California	Yes	Acc-Ac/Spec-App	Know/Per	General
Colorado	Yes	Accredited	None	None
Connecticut	Yes	Accredited	None	General
Delaware	Yes	Approved	Know/Per	General
District of Columbia	No	N/AP	N/AP	N/AP
Florida	Yes	Acc/Spec	None	General
Georgia	Yes	Accredited	None	N/R
Hawaii	Yes	Accredited	None	Direct
Idaho	Yes	Accredited	Know/Per	General
Illinois	Yes	Specific	K/P-Waived	Direct
Indiana	Function not Listed	N/AP	N/AP	Direct
Iowa	Yes	Accredited	Know/Per	General
Kansas	Yes	Accredited	Know/Per	Direct
Kentucky	Yes	N/R	N/R	Direct
Louisiana	Yes	Accredited	None	Indirect
Maine	Yes	Accredited	Know/Per	General
Maryland	Yes	Acc-App	K/P-Writ-Wav	Direct
Massachusetts	Yes	Accredited	Know/Per	General
Michigan	Yes	Accredited	Know/Per	General
Minnesota	Yes	Accredited	Know/Per	General
Mississippi	Yes	Accredited	None	Direct
Missouri	Yes	Accredited	None	Indirect
Montana	Yes	N/R	N/R	N/R
Nebraska	Yes	Accredited	K/P-Waived	General
Nevada	Yes	Accredited	None	Direct
New Hampshire	Yes	Acc/Spec	Knowledge	General
New Jersey	Yes	Acc-Spec	Know-Writ-Wav	Direct
New Mexico	Yes	N/R	None	General
New York	Yes	Accredited	Knowledge	General
North Carolina	Yes	Approved	None	Indirect
North Dakota	Yes	Accredited	Know/Per	General
Ohio	Yes	Accredited	Know/Per	Direct
Oklahoma	Yes	Accredited	None	Direct
Oregon*	Yes	Accredited	None	General
Pennsylvania*	Yes	Accredited	None	Direct
Rhode Island	Yes	Accredited	Know/Per	Direct
South Carolina	Yes	Accredited	None	Direct
South Dakota	Yes	Accredited	Know/Per	Indirect
Tennessee	DECLINES TO RESPOND			
Texas	Yes	Accredited	None	General
Utah	Yes	Accredited	None	General
Vermont	Yes	Accredited	None	General
Virginia	No	N/AP	N/AP	N/AP
Washington	Yes	Accredited	Know/Per	General
West Virginia	Yes	Accredited	Knowledge	Direct
Wisconsin	Yes	Accredited	Know/Per	General
Wyoming	Yes	Acc-Spec	K/P-Clin	Direct

*The rules for these states are either under review or the returned survey was incomplete. Therefore, the responses shown are from the responses that were reported in the 1990 report.

PLACING AND FINISHING COMPOSITE RESIN RESTORATIONS: DENTAL ASSISTING

State	Permission	Required education	Required examination	Required supervision
Alabama	No	N/AP	N/AP	N/AP
Alaska	Function not Listed	N/AP	N/AP	N/AP
Arizona	No	N/AP	N/AP	N/AP
Arkansas	No	N/AP	N/AP	N/AP
California	No	N/AP	N/AP	N/AP
Colorado	Yes	None	None	Direct
Connecticut	No	N/AP	N/AP	N/AP
Delaware	No	N/AP	N/AP	N/AP
District of Columbia	No	N/AP	N/AP	N/AP
Florida	No	N/AP	N/AP	N/AP
Georgia	No	N/AP	N/AP	N/AP
Hawaii	No	N/AP	N/AP	N/AP
Idaho	No	N/AP	N/AP	N/AP
Illinois	No	N/AP	N/AP	N/AP
Indiana	DECLINES TO RESPOND			
Iowa	No	N/AP	N/AP	N/AP
Kansas	DECLINES TO RESPOND			
Kentucky	Yes	N/R	N/R	Direct
Louisiana	No	N/AP	N/AP	N/AP
Maine	No	N/AP	N/AP	N/AP
Maryland	No	N/AP	N/AP	N/AP
Massachusetts	No	N/AP	N/AP	N/AP
Michigan	No	N/AP	N/AP	N/AP
Minnesota	No	N/AP	N/AP	N/AP
Mississippi	No	N/AP	N/AP	N/AP
Missouri	No	N/AP	N/AP	N/AP
Montana	Function not Listed	N/AP	N/AP	N/AP
Nebraska	No	N/AP	N/AP	N/AP
Nevada	No	N/AP	N/AP	N/AP
New Hampshire	No	N/AP	N/AP	N/AP
New Jersey	No	N/AP	N/AP	N/AP
New Mexico	No	N/AP	N/AP	N/AP
New York	No	N/AP	N/AP	N/AP
North Carolina	No	N/AP	N/AP	N/AP
North Dakota	No	N/AP	N/AP	N/AP
Ohio	Yes	Specific	Writ/Clin	Direct
Oklahoma	No	N/AP	N/AP	N/AP
Oregon*	No	N/AP	N/AP	N/AP
Pennsylvania*	No	N/AP	N/AP	N/AP
Rhode Island	No	N/AP	N/AP	N/AP
South Carolina	No	N/AP	N/AP	N/AP
South Dakota	No	N/AP	N/AP	N/AP
Tennessee	DECLINES TO RESPOND			
Texas	No	N/AP	N/AP	N/AP
Utah	No	N/AP	N/AP	N/AP
Vermont	No	N/AP	N/AP	N/AP
Virginia	No	N/AP	N/AP	N/AP
Washington	No	N/AP	N/AP	N/AP
West Virginia	No	N/AP	N/AP	N/AP
Wisconsin	No	N/AP	N/AP	N/AP
Wyoming	No	N/AP	N/AP	N/AP

*The rules for these states are either under review or the returned survey was incomplete. Therefore, the responses shown are from the responses that were reported in the 1990 report.

PLACING AND FINISHING COMPOSITE RESIN RESTORATIONS: DENTAL HYGIENE

State	Permission	Required education	Required examination	Required supervision
Alabama	No	N/AP	N/AP	N/AP
Alaska	No	N/AP	N/AP	N/AP
Arizona	No	N/AP	N/AP	N/AP
Arkansas	No	N/AP	N/AP	N/AP
California	No	N/AP	N/AP	N/AP
Colorado	Yes	Accredited	None	General
Connecticut	No	N/AP	N/AP	N/AP
Delaware	No	N/AP	N/AP	N/AP
District of Columbia	No	N/AP	N/AP	N/AP
Florida	No	N/AP	N/AP	N/AP
Georgia	No	N/AP	N/AP	N/AP
Hawaii	No	N/AP	N/AP	N/AP
Idaho	No	N/AP	N/AP	N/AP
Illinois	No	N/AP	N/AP	N/AP
Indiana	Function not Listed	N/AP	N/AP	Direct
Iowa	No	N/AP	N/AP	N/AP
Kansas	DECLINES TO RESPOND			
Kentucky	Yes	N/R	N/R	Direct
Louisiana	No	N/AP	N/AP	N/AP
Maine	No	N/AP	N/AP	N/AP
Maryland	No	N/AP	N/AP	N/AP
Massachusetts	No	N/AP	N/AP	N/AP
Michigan	No	N/AP	N/AP	N/AP
Minnesota	No	N/AP	N/AP	N/AP
Mississippi	No	N/AP	N/AP	N/AP
Missouri	No	N/AP	N/AP	N/AP
Montana	Function not Listed	N/AP	N/AP	N/AP
Nebraska	No	N/AP	N/AP	N/AP
Nevada	No	N/AP	N/AP	N/AP
New Hampshire	No	N/AP	N/AP	N/AP
New Jersey	No	N/AP	N/AP	N/AP
New Mexico	No	N/AP	N/AP	N/AP
New York	Function not Listed	N/AP	N/AP	N/AP
North Carolina	No	N/AP	N/AP	N/AP
North Dakota	No	N/AP	N/AP	N/AP
Ohio	Yes	Specific	Writ/Clin	Direct
Oklahoma	No	N/AP	N/AP	N/AP
Oregon*	No	N/AP	N/AP	N/AP
Pennsylvania*	Yes	Accredited	None	Direct
Rhode Island	No	N/AP	N/AP	N/AP
South Carolina	No	N/AP	N/AP	N/AP
South Dakota	No	N/AP	N/AP	N/AP
Tennessee	DECLINES TO RESPOND			
Texas	No	N/AP	N/AP	N/AP
Utah	No	N/AP	N/AP	N/AP
Vermont	No	N/AP	N/AP	N/AP
Virginia	No	N/AP	N/AP	N/AP
Washington	Yes	Accredited	Knowledge	Direct
West Virginia	No	N/AP	N/AP	N/AP
Wisconsin	No	N/AP	N/AP	N/AP
Wyoming	Yes	Acc-Spec	K/P-Clin	Direct

*The rules for these states are either under review or the returned survey was incomplete. Therefore, the responses shown are from the responses that were reported in the 1990 report.

PLACING AND PACKING RETRACTION CORDS: DENTAL ASSISTING

State	Permission	Required education	Required examination	Required supervision
Alabama	Yes	None	None	Direct
Alaska	Function not Listed	N/AP	N/AP	N/AP
Arizona	Function not Listed	N/AP	N/AP	N/AP
Arkansas	Yes	None	None	Direct
California	No	N/AP	N/AP	N/AP
Colorado	Yes	None	None	Direct
Connecticut	No	N/AP	N/AP	N/AP
Delaware	Unanswered	N/R	N/R	N/R
District of Columbia	No	N/AP	N/AP	N/AP
Florida	Yes	Accredited	None	Direct
Georgia	No	N/AP	N/AP	N/AP
Hawaii	Function not Listed	N/AP	N/AP	N/AP
Idaho	Function not Listed	N/AP	N/AP	N/AP
Illinois	No	N/AP	N/AP	N/AP
Indiana	DECLINES TO RESPOND			
Iowa	No	N/AP	N/AP	N/AP
Kansas	Unanswered	N/R	N/R	N/R
Kentucky	Unanswered	N/R	N/R	N/R
Louisiana	Yes	Ac/Spec-App-Spec	CDA Exam-Waived	Direct
Maine	Yes	None	None	Direct
Maryland	No	N/AP	N/AP	N/AP
Massachusetts	Unanswered	N/R	N/R	N/R
Michigan	No	N/AP	N/AP	N/AP
Minnesota	No	N/AP	N/AP	N/AP
Mississippi	Unanswered	N/R	N/R	N/R
Missouri	No	N/AP	N/AP	N/AP
Montana	Function not Listed	N/AP	N/AP	N/AP
Nebraska	Yes	None	None	Direct
Nevada	Yes	None	None	Direct
New Hampshire	No	N/AP	N/AP	N/AP
New Jersey	Yes	App-Spec	Writ-CDA-None	Direct
New Mexico	No	N/AP	N/AP	N/AP
New York	No	N/AP	N/AP	N/AP
North Carolina	Yes	Acc-Ac/Spec-App	None	Direct
North Dakota	No	N/AP	N/AP	N/AP
Ohio	No	N/AP	N/AP	N/AP
Oklahoma	Unanswered	N/R	N/R	N/R
Oregon*	Unanswered	N/R	N/R	N/R
Pennsylvania*	Unanswered	N/R	N/R	N/R
Rhode Island	No	N/AP	N/AP	N/AP
South Carolina	Function not Listed	N/AP	N/AP	N/AP
South Dakota	Function not Listed	N/AP	N/AP	N/AP
Tennessee	DECLINES TO RESPOND			
Texas	Unanswered	N/R	N/R	N/R
Utah	Unanswered	N/R	N/R	N/R
Vermont	No	N/AP	N/AP	N/AP
Virginia	No	N/AP	N/AP	N/AP
Washington	Yes	None	None	Direct
West Virginia	No	N/AP	N/AP	N/AP
Wisconsin	No	N/AP	N/AP	N/AP
Wyoming	No	N/AP	N/AP	N/AP

*The rules for these states are either under review or the returned survey was incomplete. Therefore, the responses shown are from the responses that were reported in the 1990 report.

PLACING AND PACKING RETRACTION CORDS: DENTAL HYGIENE

State	Permission	Required education	Required examination	Required supervision
Alabama	Yes	Approved	None	Direct
Alaska	Function not Listed	Accredited	N/AP	N/AP
Arizona	Function not Listed	N/AP	N/AP	N/AP
Arkansas	Yes	Accredited	None	Direct
California	Yes	Acc-Ac/Spec-App	Know/Per	Direct
Colorado	Yes	Accredited	None	General
Connecticut	No	N/AP	N/AP	N/AP
Delaware	Unanswered	N/R	N/R	N/R
District of Columbia	No	N/AP	N/AP	N/AP
Florida	Yes	Acc/Spec	Knowledge	Direct
Georgia	No	N/AP	N/AP	N/AP
Hawaii	Unanswered	N/R	N/R	N/R
Idaho	Function not Listed	N/AP	N/AP	N/AP
Illinois	No	N/AP	N/AP	N/AP
Indiana	Function not Listed	N/AP	N/AP	Direct
Iowa	No	N/AP	N/AP	N/AP
Kansas	Unanswered	N/R	N/R	N/R
Kentucky	Unanswered	N/R	N/R	N/R
Louisiana	Yes	Accredited	None	Direct
Maine	Yes	Accredited	Know/Per	Direct
Maryland	No	N/AP	N/AP	N/AP
Massachusetts	Unanswered	N/R	N/R	N/R
Michigan	No	N/AP	N/AP	N/AP
Minnesota	No	N/AP	N/AP	N/AP
Mississippi	Unanswered	N/R	N/R	N/R
Missouri	No	N/AP	N/AP	N/AP
Montana	Function not Listed	N/AP	N/AP	N/AP
Nebraska	Yes	Accredited	K/P-Waived	Direct
Nevada	Yes	Accredited	None	Direct
New Hampshire	No	N/AP	N/AP	N/AP
New Jersey	Yes	Accredited	Knowledge	Direct
New Mexico	No	N/AP	N/AP	N/AP
New York	Function not Listed	N/AP	N/AP	N/AP
North Carolina	Yes	Approved	None	Indirect
North Dakota	No	N/AP	N/AP	N/AP
Ohio	No	N/AP	N/AP	N/AP
Oklahoma	Unanswered	N/R	N/R	N/R
Oregon*	Unanswered	N/R	N/R	N/R
Pennsylvania*	Unanswered	N/R	N/R	N/R
Rhode Island	No	N/AP	N/AP	N/AP
South Carolina	Function not Listed	N/AP	N/AP	N/AP
South Dakota	Function not Listed	N/AP	N/AP	N/AP
Tennessee	DECLINES TO RESPOND			
Texas	Unanswered	N/R	N/R	N/R
Utah	Unanswered	N/R	N/R	N/R
Vermont	No	N/AP	N/AP	N/AP
Virginia	No	N/AP	N/AP	N/AP
Washington	Yes	Accredited	Knowledge	Direct
West Virginia	Function not Listed	N/AP	N/AP	N/AP
Wisconsin	No	N/AP	N/AP	N/AP
Wyoming	Function not Listed	N/AP	N/AP	N/AP

*The rules for these states are either under review or the returned survey was incomplete. Therefore, the responses shown are from the responses that were reported in the 1990 report.

PERFORMING SUPRAGINGIVAL SCALING: DENTAL ASSISTING

State	Permission	Required education	Required examination	Required supervision
Alabama	No	N/AP	N/AP	N/AP
Alaska	No	N/AP	N/AP	N/AP
Arizona	No	N/AP	N/AP	N/AP
Arkansas	No	N/AP	N/AP	N/AP
California	No	N/AP	N/AP	N/AP
Colorado	No	N/AP	N/AP	N/AP
Connecticut	No	N/AP	N/AP	N/AP
Delaware	No	N/AP	N/AP	N/AP
District of Columbia	No	N/AP	N/AP	N/AP
Florida	No	N/AP	N/AP	N/AP
Georgia	No	N/AP	N/AP	N/AP
Hawaii	No	N/AP	N/AP	N/AP
Idaho	No	N/AP	N/AP	N/AP
Illinois	No	N/AP	N/AP	N/AP
Indiana	DECLINES TO RESPOND			
Iowa	No	N/AP	N/AP	N/AP
Kansas	DECLINES TO RESPOND			
Kentucky	No	N/AP	N/AP	N/AP
Louisiana	No	N/AP	N/AP	N/AP
Maine	No	N/AP	N/AP	N/AP
Maryland	No	N/AP	N/AP	N/AP
Massachusetts	No	N/AP	N/AP	N/AP
Michigan	No	N/AP	N/AP	N/AP
Minnesota	No	N/AP	N/AP	N/AP
Mississippi	No	N/AP	N/AP	N/AP
Missouri	No	N/AP	N/AP	N/AP
Montana	No	N/AP	N/AP	N/AP
Nebraska	No	N/AP	N/AP	N/AP
Nevada	No	N/AP	N/AP	N/AP
New Hampshire	No	N/AP	N/AP	N/AP
New Jersey	No	N/AP	N/AP	N/AP
New Mexico	No	N/AP	N/AP	N/AP
New York	No	N/AP	N/AP	N/AP
North Carolina	No	N/AP	N/AP	N/AP
North Dakota	No	N/AP	N/AP	N/AP
Ohio	No	N/AP	N/AP	N/AP
Oklahoma	No	N/AP	N/AP	N/AP
Oregon*	No	N/AP	N/AP	N/AP
Pennsylvania*	No	N/AP	N/AP	N/AP
Rhode Island	No	N/AP	N/AP	N/AP
South Carolina	No	N/AP	N/AP	N/AP
South Dakota	No	N/AP	N/AP	N/AP
Tennessee	DECLINES TO RESPOND			
Texas	No	N/AP	N/AP	N/AP
Utah	No	N/AP	N/AP	N/AP
Vermont	No	N/AP	N/AP	N/AP
Virginia	No	N/AP	N/AP	N/AP
Washington	No	N/AP	N/AP	N/AP
West Virginia	No	N/AP	N/AP	N/AP
Wisconsin	No	N/AP	N/AP	N/AP
Wyoming	No	N/AP	N/AP	N/AP

*The rules for these states are either under review or the returned survey was incomplete. Therefore, the responses shown are from the responses that were reported in the 1990 report.

PERFORMING SUPRAGINGIVAL SCALING: DENTAL HYGIENE

State	Permission	Required education	Required examination	Required supervision
Alabama	Yes	Approved	Know/Per	Direct
Alaska	Yes	Accredited	Per-Waived	General
Arizona	Yes	Accredited	Performance	General
Arkansas	Yes	Accredited	Know/Per	Direct
California	Yes	Acc-Ac/Spec-App	Know/Per	Direct
Colorado	Yes	Accredited	Know/Per	None
Connecticut	Yes	Accredited	Performance	General
Delaware	Yes	Approved	Know/Per	General
District of Columbia	Yes	Accredited	Know/Per	Direct
Florida	Yes	Acc/Spec	Know/Per	Direct
Georgia	Yes	Accredited	Know/Per	Direct
Hawaii	Yes	Accredited	None	Direct
Idaho	Yes	Accredited	Know/Per	General
Illinois	Yes	Specific	K/P-Waived	Direct
Indiana	Function not Listed	Accredited	Per-Waived	Direct
Iowa	Yes	Accredited	Know/Per	General
Kansas	Yes	Accredited	Know/Per	Direct
Kentucky	Yes	Accredited	N/R	Indirect
Louisiana	Yes	Accredited	Know/Per	Direct
Maine	Yes	Accredited	Know/Per	General
Maryland	Yes	Acc-App	K/P-Writ-Wav	Indirect
Massachusetts	Yes	Accredited	Know/Per	General
Michigan	Yes	Accredited	Know/Per	General
Minnesota	Yes	Accredited	Know/Per	General
Mississippi	Yes	Accredited	Performance	N/R
Missouri	Yes	Accredited	Know/Per	Indirect
Montana	Yes	Accredited	Per-Waived	General
Nebraska	Yes	Accredited	K/P-Waived	General
Nevada	Yes	Accredited	Know/Per	Direct
New Hampshire	Yes	Accredited	Knowledge	General
New Jersey	Yes	Accredited	Know/Per	Direct
New Mexico	Yes	Accredited	Know/Per	General
New York	Yes	Accredited	Know/Per	General
North Carolina	Yes	Approved	Performance	Indirect
North Dakota	Yes	Accredited	Know/Per	General
Ohio	Yes	Accredited	Know/Per	Direct
Oklahoma	Yes	Accredited	Knowledge	Direct
Oregon*	Yes	Accredited	Know/Per	General
Pennsylvania*	Yes	Accredited	Know/Per	Direct
Rhode Island	Yes	Accredited	Know/Per	Indirect
South Carolina	Yes	Accredited	Performance	Indirect
South Dakota	Yes	Accredited	Know/Per	Indirect
Tennessee	DECLINES TO RESPOND			
Texas	Yes	Accredited	Performance	General
Utah	Yes	Accredited	Know/Per	General
Vermont	Yes	Accredited	Performance	General
Virginia	Yes	Accredited	Know/Per	Direct
Washington	Yes	Accredited	Performance	General
West Virginia	Yes	Accredited	Know/Per	Direct
Wisconsin	Yes	Accredited	Know/Per	General
Wyoming	Yes	Accredited	Know/Per	General

*The rules for these states are either under review or the returned survey was incomplete. Therefore, the responses shown are from the responses that were reported in the 1990 report.

PERFORMING SUBGINGIVAL SCALING: DENTAL HYGIENE

State	Permission	Required education	Required examination	Required supervision
Alabama	Yes	Approved	Know/Per	Direct
Alaska	Yes	Approved	Per-Waived	General
Arizona	Yes	Accredited	Performance	General
Arkansas	Yes	Accredited	Know/Per	Direct
California	Yes	Acc-Ac/Spec-App	Know/Per	Direct
Colorado	Yes	Accredited	Know/Per	None
Connecticut	Yes	Accredited	Performance	General
Delaware	Yes	Approved	Know/Per	General
District of Columbia	Yes	Accredited	Know/Per	General
Florida	Yes	Acc/Spec	Know/Per	General
Georgia	Yes	Accredited	Know/Per	Direct
Hawaii	Yes	Accredited	None	Direct
Idaho	Yes	Accredited	Know/Per	General
Illinois	Yes	Specific	K/P-Waived	Direct
Indiana	Function not Listed	Accredited	Per-Waived	Direct
Iowa	Yes	Accredited	Know/Per	Indirect
Kansas	Yes	Accredited	Know/Per	Direct
Kentucky	Yes	N/R	N/R	Indirect
Louisiana	Yes	Accredited	Know/Per	Direct
Maine	Yes	Accredited	Know/Per	General
Maryland	Yes	Acc-App	K/P-Writ-Wav	Indirect
Massachusetts	Yes	Accredited	Know/Per	General
Michigan	Yes	Accredited	Know/Per	Indirect
Minnesota	Yes	Accredited	Know/Per	General
Mississippi	Yes	Accredited	Performance	N/R
Missouri	Yes	Accredited	Know/Per	Indirect
Montana	Yes	Accredited	Per-Waived	General
Nebraska	Yes	Accredited	K/P-Waived	General
Nevada	Yes	Accredited	Know/Per	Direct
New Hampshire	Yes	Accredited	Knowledge	General
New Jersey	Yes	Accredited	Know/Per	Direct
New Mexico	Yes	Accredited	Know/Per	General
New York	Yes	Accredited	Know/Per	General
North Carolina	Yes	Approved	Performance	Indirect
North Dakota	Yes	Accredited	Know/Per	General
Ohio	Yes	Accredited	Know/Per	Direct
Oklahoma	Yes	Accredited	Knowledge	Direct
Oregon*	Yes	Accredited	Know/Per	General
Pennsylvania*	Yes	Accredited	Know/Per	Direct
Rhode Island	Yes	Accredited	Know/Per	Indirect
South Carolina	Yes	Accredited	None	Indirect
South Dakota	Yes	Accredited	Know/Per	Indirect
Tennessee	DECLINES TO RESPOND			
Texas	Yes	Accredited	Performance	General
Utah	Yes	Accredited	Know/Per	General
Vermont	Yes	Accredited	Performance	General
Virginia	Yes	Accredited	Know/Per	Direct
Washington	Yes	Accredited	Performance	General
West Virginia	Yes	Accredited	Know/Per	Direct
Wisconsin	Yes	Accredited	Know/Per	General
Wyoming	Yes	Accredited	Know/Per	General

*The rules for these states are either under review or the returned survey was incomplete. Therefore, the responses shown are from the responses that were reported in the 1990 report.

ROOT PLANING: DENTAL HYGIENE

State	Permission	Required education	Required examination	Required supervision
Alabama	Yes	Approved	Know/Per	Direct
Alaska	Yes	Accredited	None	General
Arizona	Yes	Accredited	Performance	General
Arkansas	Yes	Accredited	Know/Per	Direct
California	Yes	Acc-Ac/Spec-App	Know/Per	General
Colorado	Yes	Accredited	Know/Per	None
Connecticut	Yes	Accredited	Performance	General
Delaware	Yes	Approved	Know/Per	General
District of Columbia	No	N/AP	N/AP	N/AP
Florida	Yes	Acc/Spec	Know/Per	Direct
Georgia	Yes	Accredited	Know/Per	Direct
Hawaii	Yes	Accredited	None	Direct
Idaho	Yes	Accredited	Know/Per	General
Illinois	Yes	Specific	K/P-Waived	Direct
Indiana	Function not Listed	Accredited	Per-Waived	Direct
Iowa	Yes	Accredited	Know/Per	General
Kansas	Yes	Accredited	Know/Per	Direct
Kentucky	Yes	N/R	N/R	Direct
Louisiana	Yes	Accredited	Know/Per	Direct
Maine	Yes	Accredited	Know/Per	General
Maryland	Yes	Acc-App	K/P-Writ-Wav	Indirect
Massachusetts	Yes	Accredited	Know/Per	General
Michigan	Yes	Accredited	Know/Per	General
Minnesota	Yes	Accredited	Know/Per	General
Mississippi	Yes	Accredited	Performance	N/R
Missouri	Yes	Accredited	Know/Per	Indirect
Montana	Yes	Accredited	Per-Waived	General
Nebraska	Yes	Accredited	K/P-Waived	General
Nevada	Yes	Accredited	Know/Per	Direct
New Hampshire	Yes	Accredited	Knowledge	General
New Jersey	Yes	Accredited	Know/Per	Direct
New Mexico	Yes	Accredited	Know/Per	General
New York	Yes	Accredited	Know/Per	General
North Carolina	Yes	Approved	Performance	Indirect
North Dakota	Yes	Accredited	Know/Per	General
Ohio	Yes	Accredited	Know/Per	Direct
Oklahoma	Yes	Accredited	Knowledge	Direct
Oregon*	Yes	Accredited	Know/Per	General
Pennsylvania*	Yes	Accredited	Know/Per	Direct
Rhode Island	Yes	Accredited	Know/Per	Indirect
South Carolina	Yes	Accredited	Performance	Indirect
South Dakota	Yes	Accredited	Know/Per	Indirect
Tennessee	DECLINES TO RESPOND			
Texas	Yes	Accredited	None	General
Utah	Yes	Accredited	Per-None	General
Vermont	Yes	Accredited	Performance	General
Virginia	Yes	Accredited	Know/Per	Direct
Washington	Yes	Accredited	Performance	General
West Virginia	Yes	Accredited	Know/Per	Direct
Wisconsin	Yes	Accredited	Know/Per	General
Wyoming	Yes	Accredited	Know/Per	General

*The rules for these states are either under review or the returned survey was incomplete. Therefore, the responses shown are from the responses that were reported in the 1990 report.

CLOSED GINGIVAL CURETTAGE: DENTAL HYGIENE

State	Permission	Required education	Required examination	Required supervision
Alabama	Yes	Approved	Know/Per	Direct
Alaska	Yes	Accredited	None	General
Arizona	Yes	Accredited	Performance	General
Arkansas	Yes	Accredited	Knowledge	Direct
California	Yes	Acc-Ac/Spec-App	Know/Per	Direct
Colorado	Yes	Accredited	Know/Per	None
Connecticut	No	N/AP	N/AP	N/AP
Delaware	No	N/AP	N/AP	N/AP
District of Columbia	No	N/AP	N/AP	N/AP
Florida	Yes	Acc/Spec	Know/Per	Direct
Georgia	Yes	Accredited	Know/Per	Direct
Hawaii	Yes	Accredited	None	Direct
Idaho	Yes	Accredited	Know/Per	General
Illinois	Yes	Specific	K/P-Waived	Direct
Indiana	Function not Listed	N/AP	N/AP	N/AP
Iowa	Yes	Accredited	Know/Per	General
Kansas	Yes	Accredited	Know/Per	Direct
Kentucky	Yes	N/R	N/R	Direct
Louisiana	Function not Listed	N/AP	N/AP	N/AP
Maine	Yes	Accredited	Know/Per	General
Maryland	No	N/AP	N/AP	N/AP
Massachusetts	Yes	Accredited	Know/Per	General
Michigan	Yes	Accredited	Know/Per	Direct
Minnesota	No	N/AP	N/AP	N/AP
Mississippi	Yes	Accredited	Performance	N/R
Missouri	Yes	Acc-Spec	Writ/Clin	Direct
Montana	Yes	Accredited	N/R	General
Nebraska	Yes	Accredited	K/P-Waived	General
Nevada	Yes	Accredited	Know/Per	Direct
New Hampshire	No	N/AP	N/AP	N/AP
New Jersey	Yes	Accredited	Knowledge	Direct
New Mexico	Yes	Accredited	Know/Per	General
New York	Function not Listed	N/AP	N/AP	N/AP
North Carolina	No	N/AP	N/AP	N/AP
North Dakota	Yes	Accredited	Know/Per	General
Ohio	Yes	Accredited	Know/Per	Direct
Oklahoma	Yes	Accredited	Writ/Clin	Direct
Oregon*	Yes	Accredited	Know/Per	General
Pennsylvania*	Yes	Accredited	Know/Per	Direct
Rhode Island	No	N/AP	N/AP	N/AP
South Carolina	No	N/AP	N/AP	N/AP
South Dakota	Yes	Accredited	Know/Per	Indirect
Tennessee	DECLINES TO RESPOND			
Texas	No	N/AP	N/AP	N/AP
Utah	Yes	Accredited	Per-None	General
Vermont	No	N/AP	N/AP	N/AP
Virginia	No	N/AP	N/AP	N/AP
Washington	Yes	Accredited	Knowledge	Direct
West Virginia	Yes	Accredited	Know/Per	Direct
Wisconsin	No	N/AP	N/AP	N/AP
Wyoming	Yes	Accredited	Know/Per	General

*The rules for these states are either under review or the returned survey was incomplete. Therefore, the responses shown are from the responses that were reported in the 1990 report.

ADMINISTRATION OF NITROUS OXIDE ANALGESIA: DENTAL HYGIENE

State	Permission	Required education	Required examination	Required supervision
Alabama	Yes	N/R	None	Direct
Alaska	No	N/AP	N/AP	N/AP
Arizona	Yes	Accredited	None	Direct
Arkansas	Yes	Acc-Spec	Writ-Waived	Direct
California	Yes	Acc-Ac/Spec-App	Know/Per	Direct
Colorado	No	N/AP	N/AP	N/AP
Connecticut	No	N/AP	N/AP	N/AP
Delaware	No	N/AP	N/AP	N/AP
District of Columbia	No	N/AP	N/AP	N/AP
Florida	No	N/AP	N/AP	N/AP
Georgia	No	N/AP	N/AP	N/AP
Hawaii	No	N/AP	N/AP	N/AP
Idaho	Yes	Accredited	Know/Per	Indirect
Illinois	No	N/AP	N/AP	N/AP
Indiana	No	N/AP	N/AP	N/AP
Iowa	No	N/AP	N/AP	N/AP
Kansas	Yes	Acc/Spec	N/R	Direct
Kentucky	No	N/AP	N/AP	N/AP
Louisiana	No	N/AP	N/AP	N/AP
Maine	No	N/AP	N/AP	N/AP
Maryland	No	N/AP	N/AP	N/AP
Massachusetts	No	N/AP	N/AP	N/AP
Michigan	No	N/AP	N/AP	N/AP
Minnesota	No	N/AP	N/AP	N/AP
Mississippi	No	N/AP	N/AP	N/AP
Missouri	Yes	Acc-Spec	Writ/Clin	Direct
Montana	No	N/AP	N/AP	N/AP
Nebraska	No	N/AP	N/AP	N/AP
Nevada	Yes	Ac/Spec-App-Spec	None	Direct
New Hampshire	No	N/AP	N/AP	N/AP
New Jersey	No	N/AP	N/AP	N/AP
New Mexico	No	N/AP	N/AP	N/AP
New York	Function not Listed	N/AP	N/AP	N/AP
North Carolina	No	N/AP	N/AP	N/AP
North Dakota	No	N/AP	N/AP	N/AP
Ohio	No	N/AP	N/AP	N/AP
Oklahoma	Yes	Specific	Writ/Clin	Direct
Oregon*	Yes	Ac/Spec-Spec	None	Indirect
Pennsylvania*	No	N/AP	N/AP	N/AP
Rhode Island	No	N/AP	N/AP	N/AP
South Carolina	No	N/AP	N/AP	N/AP
South Dakota	Yes	Specific	None	Direct
Tennessee	DECLINES TO RESPOND			
Texas	No	N/AP	N/AP	N/AP
Utah	Yes	N/R	None	Direct
Vermont	No	N/AP	N/AP	N/AP
Virginia	No	N/AP	N/AP	N/AP
Washington	Yes	Approved	Know/Per	Direct
West Virginia	No	N/AP	N/AP	N/AP
Wisconsin	No	N/AP	N/AP	N/AP
Wyoming	No	N/AP	N/AP	N/AP

*The rules for these states are either under review or the returned survey was incomplete. Therefore, the responses shown are from the responses that were reported in the 1990 report.

ADMINISTERING LOCAL ANESTHETIC AGENTS BY INFILTRATION: DENTAL HYGIENE

State	Permission	Required education	Required examination	Required supervision
Alabama	No	N/AP	N/AP	N/AP
Alaska	Yes	Specific	Writ/Clin	Direct
Arizona	Yes	Approved	Performance	Direct
Arkansas	No	N/AP	N/AP	N/AP
California	Yes	Acc-Ac/Spec-App	Know/Per	Direct
Colorado	Yes	Acc-Ac/Spec-Spec	None	Direct
Connecticut	No	N/AP	N/AP	N/AP
Delaware	No	N/AP	N/AP	N/AP
District of Columbia	No	N/AP	N/AP	N/AP
Florida	No	N/AP	N/AP	N/AP
Georgia	No	N/AP	N/AP	N/AP
Hawaii	Yes	Acc-Ac/Spec-Spec	None	Direct
Idaho	Yes	Acc/Spec	Writ/Clin	Indirect
Illinois	No	N/AP	N/AP	N/AP
Indiana	No	N/AP	N/AP	N/AP
Iowa	No	N/AP	N/AP	N/AP
Kansas	No	N/AP	N/AP	N/AP
Kentucky	No	N/AP	N/AP	N/AP
Louisiana	No	N/AP	N/AP	N/AP
Maine	No	N/AP	N/AP	N/AP
Maryland	No	N/AP	N/AP	N/AP
Massachusetts	No	N/AP	N/AP	N/AP
Michigan	No	N/AP	N/AP	N/AP
Minnesota	No	N/AP	N/AP	N/AP
Mississippi	No	N/AP	N/AP	N/AP
Missouri	Yes	Acc-Spec	Writ/Clin	Indirect
Montana	Yes	Acc-Ac/Spec	Writ/Clin	Direct
Nebraska	No	N/AP	N/AP	N/AP
Nevada	Yes	Ac/Spec-App-Spec	None	Direct
New Hampshire	No	N/AP	N/AP	N/AP
New Jersey	No	N/AP	N/AP	N/AP
New Mexico	Yes	Accredited	Writ/Clin	Direct
New York	Function not Listed	N/AP	N/AP	N/AP
North Carolina	No	N/AP	N/AP	N/AP
North Dakota	No	N/AP	N/AP	N/AP
Ohio	No	N/AP	N/AP	N/AP
Oklahoma	Yes	Specific	Writ/Clin	Direct
Oregon*	Yes	Ac/Spec-Spec	None	General
Pennsylvania*	No	N/AP	N/AP	N/AP
Rhode Island	No	N/AP	N/AP	N/AP
South Carolina	No	N/AP	N/AP	N/AP
South Dakota	Yes	Specific	None	Direct
Tennessee	DECLINES TO RESPOND			
Texas	No	N/AP	N/AP	N/AP
Utah	Yes	Acc-App-Spec	Writ/Clin	Undefined
Vermont	No	N/AP	N/AP	N/AP
Virginia	No	N/AP	N/AP	N/AP
Washington	Yes	Approved	Know/Per	Direct
West Virginia	No	N/AP	N/AP	N/AP
Wisconsin	No	N/AP	N/AP	N/AP
Wyoming	Yes	Acc-Ac/Spec	K/P-Waived	Indirect

*The rules for these states are either under review or the returned survey was incomplete. Therefore, the responses shown are from the responses that were reported in the 1990 report.

ADMINISTERING LOCAL ANESTHETIC AGENTS BY BLOCK: DENTAL HYGIENE

State	Permission	Required education	Required examination	Required supervision
Alabama	No	N/AP	N/AP	N/AP
Alaska	Yes	Specific	Writ/Clin	Direct
Arizona	Yes	Approved	Performance	Direct
Arkansas	No	N/AP	N/AP	N/AP
California	Yes	Acc-Ac/Spec-App	Know/Per	Direct
Colorado	Yes	Acc-Ac/Spec-Spec	None	Direct
Connecticut	No	N/AP	N/AP	N/AP
Delaware	No	N/AP	N/AP	N/AP
District of Columbia	No	N/AP	N/AP	N/AP
Florida	No	N/AP	N/AP	N/AP
Georgia	No	N/AP	N/AP	N/AP
Hawaii	No	N/AP	N/AP	N/AP
Idaho	Yes	Acc/Spec	Writ/Clin	Indirect
Illinois	No	N/AP	N/AP	N/AP
Indiana	No	N/AP	N/AP	N/AP
Iowa	No	N/AP	N/AP	N/AP
Kansas	Yes	Acc/Spec	N/R	Direct
Kentucky	No	N/AP	N/AP	N/AP
Louisiana	No	N/AP	N/AP	N/AP
Maine	No	N/AP	N/AP	N/AP
Maryland	No	N/AP	N/AP	N/AP
Massachusetts	No	N/AP	N/AP	N/AP
Michigan	No	N/AP	N/AP	N/AP
Minnesota	No	N/AP	N/AP	N/AP
Mississippi	No	N/AP	N/AP	N/AP
Missouri	No	N/AP	N/AP	N/AP
Montana	Yes	Acc-Ac/Spec	Writ/Clin	Direct
Nebraska	No	N/AP	N/AP	N/AP
Nevada	Yes	Ac/Spec-App-Spec	None	Direct
New Hampshire	No	N/AP	N/AP	N/AP
New Jersey	No	N/AP	N/AP	N/AP
New Mexico	Yes	Accredited	Writ/Clin	Direct
New York	Function not Listed	N/AP	N/AP	N/AP
North Carolina	No	N/AP	N/AP	N/AP
North Dakota	No	N/AP	N/AP	N/AP
Ohio	No	N/AP	N/AP	N/AP
Oklahoma	Yes	Specific	Writ/Clin	Direct
Oregon*	Yes	Ac/Spec-Spec	None	General
Pennsylvania*	No	N/AP	N/AP	N/AP
Rhode Island	No	N/AP	N/AP	N/AP
South Carolina	No	N/AP	N/AP	N/AP
South Dakota	Yes	Specific	None	Direct
Tennessee	DECLINES TO RESPOND			
Texas	No	N/AP	N/AP	N/AP
Utah	Yes	Acc-App-Spec	Writ/Clin	Undefined
Vermont	No	N/AP	N/AP	N/AP
Virginia	No	N/AP	N/AP	N/AP
Washington	Yes	Approved	Know/Per	Direct
West Virginia	No	N/AP	N/AP	N/AP
Wisconsin	No	N/AP	N/AP	N/AP
Wyoming	Yes	Acc-Ac/Spec	K/P-Waived	Indirect

*The rules for these states are either under review or the returned survey was incomplete. Therefore, the responses shown are from the responses that were reported in the 1990 report.

PLACING SUTURES: DENTAL HYGIENE

State	Permission	Required education	Required examination	Required supervision
Alabama	No	N/AP	N/AP	N/AP
Alaska	No	N/AP	N/AP	N/AP
Arizona	No	N/AP	N/AP	N/AP
Arkansas	No	N/AP	N/AP	N/AP
California	No	N/AP	N/AP	N/AP
Colorado	Yes	Accredited	None	General
Connecticut	No	N/AP	N/AP	N/AP
Delaware	No	N/AP	N/AP	N/AP
District of Columbia	No	N/AP	N/AP	N/AP
Florida	No	N/AP	N/AP	N/AP
Georgia	No	N/AP	N/AP	N/AP
Hawaii	No	N/AP	N/AP	N/AP
Idaho	No	N/AP	N/AP	N/AP
Illinois	No	N/AP	N/AP	N/AP
Indiana	Function not Listed	N/AP	N/AP	Direct
Iowa	No	N/AP	N/AP	N/AP
Kansas	No	N/AP	N/AP	N/AP
Kentucky	No	N/AP	N/AP	N/AP
Louisiana	No	N/AP	N/AP	N/AP
Maine	No	N/AP	N/AP	N/AP
Maryland	No	N/AP	N/AP	N/AP
Massachusetts	No	N/AP	N/AP	N/AP
Michigan	No	N/AP	N/AP	N/AP
Minnesota	No	N/AP	N/AP	N/AP
Mississippi	Function not Listed	N/AP	N/AP	N/AP
Missouri	No	N/AP	N/AP	N/AP
Montana	No	N/AP	N/AP	N/AP
Nebraska	Function not Listed	N/AP	N/AP	N/AP
Nevada	No	N/AP	N/AP	N/AP
New Hampshire	No	N/AP	N/AP	N/AP
New Jersey	No	N/AP	N/AP	N/AP
New Mexico	No	N/AP	N/AP	N/AP
New York	Function not Listed	N/AP	N/AP	N/AP
North Carolina	No	N/AP	N/AP	N/AP
North Dakota	No	N/AP	N/AP	N/AP
Ohio	No	N/AP	N/AP	N/AP
Oklahoma	No	N/AP	N/AP	N/AP
Oregon*	No	N/AP	N/AP	N/AP
Pennsylvania*	No	N/AP	N/AP	N/AP
Rhode Island	No	N/AP	N/AP	N/AP
South Carolina	No	N/AP	N/AP	N/AP
South Dakota	No	N/AP	N/AP	N/AP
Tennessee	DECLINES TO RESPOND			
Texas	No	N/AP	N/AP	N/AP
Utah	No	N/AP	N/AP	N/AP
Vermont	No	N/AP	N/AP	N/AP
Virginia	No	N/AP	N/AP	N/AP
Washington	No	N/AP	N/AP	N/AP
West Virginia	No	N/AP	N/AP	N/AP
Wisconsin	No	N/AP	N/AP	N/AP
Wyoming	No	N/AP	N/AP	N/AP

*The rules for these states are either under review or the returned survey was incomplete. Therefore, the responses shown are from the responses that were reported in the 1990 report.

LEVEL OF SUPERVISION REQUIRED IN THE FOLLOWING SETTINGS: DENTAL HYGIENE

State	Dental office	Long-term care facility	School systems	Home-bound care	State institutional facility
Alabama	Direct	Direct	Direct	Direct	Direct
Alaska	General	General	General	General	General
Arizona	Dir/Indir/Gen	General	Non Responsive	General	General
Arkansas	Direct/General	Indirect	Undefined	Undefined	Indirect
California	Direct	Direct	Direct	Direct	Direct
Colorado	None	None	None	None	None
Connecticut	General	General	General	General	General
Delaware	General	General	General	General	General
District of Columbia	General	General	General	General	General
Florida	General	General	General	General	General
Georgia	Direct	Direct	Non Responsive	Direct	Non Responsive
Hawaii	Direct	General	General	General	General
Idaho	General	General	General	General	General
Illinois	Direct	Direct/General	Direct	Direct/General	Direct/General
Indiana	Direct	Direct	None	Direct	Direct
Iowa	General	General	Undefined	General	General
Kansas	Direct	Direct	Direct	Direct	Direct
Kentucky	Indirect	Indirect	Indirect	Indirect	Indirect
Louisiana	Direct	Non Responsive	Non Responsive	Non Responsive	General
Maine	Direct	Undefined	None	Undefined	Undefined
Maryland	Indirect	Indirect	Indirect	Indirect	Indirect
Massachusetts	General	General	General	General	General
Michigan	General	General	General	General	General
Minnesota	Dir/Indir/Gen	Dir/Indir/Gen	Dir/Indir/Gen	Dir/Indir/Gen	Dir/Indir/Gen
Mississippi	Direct	Indirect	Indirect	Indirect	Indirect
Missouri	General	General	General	General	General
Montana	General	General	General	General	General
Nebraska	General	General	General	General	General
Nevada	Direct	General	General	General	Undefined
New Hampshire	General	General	General	General	General
New Jersey	Direct	General	General	Direct	General
New Mexico	General	General	General	General	General
New York	Direct/General	Direct/General	General	Non Responsive	Direct/General
North Carolina	Indirect	Indirect	Indirect	Indirect	Indirect
North Dakota	Direct/General	General	Direct/General	Direct/General	General
Ohio	Indirect	Undefined	General	Undefined	Undefined
Oklahoma	Direct	Direct	Direct	Direct	Direct
Oregon*	General	General	General	General	General
Pennsylvania*	Direct	General	General	General	General
Rhode Island	Indirect	Indirect	Indirect	Indirect	Indirect
South Carolina	Direct	Indirect/Gen	General	Indirect/Gen	Indirect/Gen
South Dakota	Dir/Indir/Gen	Dir/Indir/Gen	Non Responsive	Non Responsive	Dir/Indir/Gen
Tennessee	DECLINES TO RESPOND				
Texas	General	General	General	General	General
Utah	General	General	Undefined	General	General
Vermont	General	General	General	General	General
Virginia	Direct	Direct	Direct	Direct	Direct
Washington	Direct/General	None	Undefined	Undefined	None
West Virginia	Direct	Direct	Direct	Direct	Direct
Wisconsin	General	General	None	General	General
Wyoming	General	General	Undefined	Undefined	Undefined

*The rules for these states are either under review or the returned survey was incomplete. Therefore, the responses shown are from the responses that were reported in the 1990 report.

NUMBER OF STATES WITH PROVISIONS FOR DELEGATING SPECIFIC EXPANDED FUNCTIONS TO DENTAL ASSISTANTS AND/OR HYGIENISTS

	Assisting	Hygiene
Inspecting the oral cavity	20/48	N/A
Applying topical anesthetic agents	36/48	N/A
Removing excess cement from coronal surfaces of teeth	38/48	N/A
Cementing bands/bonding brackets	4/48	N/A
Bending archwires	9/48	N/A
Exposing radiographs	47/49	50/50
Performing pulp vitality testing	11/47	19/48
Making alginate impressions for study casts	43/48	49/50
Coronal polishing	23/48	50/50
Applying topical anticariogenic agents	33/47	49/50
Applying pit and fissure sealants	19/48	49/50
Placing periodontal dressings	25/48	42/50
Removing periodontal dressings	37/48	48/50
Removing sutures	40/48	46/50
Monitoring nitrous oxide analgesia	24/49	34/50
Placing matrices	31/47	37/50
Removing matrices	28/47	36/50
Placing rubber dams	41/48	46/50
Removing rubber dams	41/48	47/50
Fabricating temporary/interim restorations	17/40	18/41
Placing temporary/interim restorations	22/48	36/50
Removing temporary/interim restorations	22/48	29/50
Applying cavity liners and bases	11/48	15/50
Placing amalgam restorations for condensation by the dentist	10/48	13/50
Placing and condensing amalgam restorations	4/48	6/48
Carving amalgams	4/48	6/48
Polishing amalgams	15/48	47/50
Placing and finishing composite resin restorations	3/48	6/49
Placing and packing retraction cords	11/39	12/39
Performing supragingival scaling	—	49/50
Performing subgingival scaling	N/A	49/50
Root planing	N/A	48/50
Closed gingival curettage	N/A	34/50
Administration of nitrous oxide analgesia	N/A	13/50
Administering local anesthetic agents by infiltration	N/A	16/50
Administering local anesthetic agents by block	N/A	15/50
Placing sutures	N/A	1/50

NOTE: The number to the left of the (/) is the total number of jurisdictions which permit delegation of the function. The number to the right of the (/) is the total number of jurisdictions which provided information on the specific function.

N/A—Not applicable as an expanded function.

NUMBER OF STATES REQUIRING FORMAL TRAINING AND/OR EXAMINATION BEFORE DELEGATING SPECIFIC EXPANDED FUNCTIONS TO DENTAL ASSISTANTS AND/OR DENTAL HYGIENISTS

	Formal training in the expanded function		Examination required	
	Assisting	Hygiene	Assisting	Hygiene
Inspecting the oral cavity	4/20	N/A	3/20	N/A
Applying topical anesthetic agents	5/36	N/A	5/36	N/A
Removing excess cement from coronal surfaces of teeth	12/38	N/A	9/38	N/A
Cementing bands/bonding brackets	—	N/A	—	N/A
Bending archwires	2/9	N/A	1/9	N/A
Exposing radiographs	27/47	49/50	27/47	42/50
Performing pulp vitality testing	6/11	18/19	6/11	15/19
Making alginate impressions for study casts	10/43	47/49	6/43	25/49
Coronal polishing	12/23	49/50	9/23	47/50
Applying topical anticariogenic agents	10/33	47/49	9/33	29/49
Applying pit and fissure sealants	12/19	47/49	8/19	29/49
Placing periodontal dressings	10/25	40/42	9/25	20/42
Removing periodontal dressings	12/37	45/48	10/37	23/48
Removing sutures	11/40	42/46	10/40	20/46
Monitoring nitrous oxide analgesia	12/24	30/34	7/24	12/34
Placing matrices	12/31	33/37	10/31	18/37
Removing matrices	11/28	33/36	9/28	18/36
Placing rubber dams	13/41	43/46	11/41	24/46
Removing rubber dams	13/41	44/47	11/41	24/47
Fabricating temporary/interim restorations	5/17	15/41	4/17	6/41
Placing temporary/interim restorations	9/22	33/36	6/22	18/36
Removing temporary/interim restorations	7/22	26/29	6/22	16/29
Applying cavity liners and bases	6/11	13/15	4/11	4/15
Placing amalgams for condensation by the dentist	3/10	11/13	3/10	7/13
Placing and condensing amalgams	1/4	5/6	1/4	3/6
Carving amalgams	1/4	5/6	1/4	3/6
Polishing amalgams	9/15	44/47	7/15	24/47
Placing and finishing composite resin restorations	1/3	5/6	1/3	3/6
Placing and packing retraction cords	4/11	13/12	2/11	6/12
Performing supragingival scaling	—	50/49	—	48/49
Performing subgingival scaling	N/A	49/49	N/A	47/49
Root planing	N/A	48/48	N/A	45/48
Closed gingival curettage	N/A	33/34	N/A	30/34
Administration of nitrous oxide analgesia	N/A	11/13	N/A	6/13
Administering local anesthetic agents by infiltration	N/A	16/16	N/A	11/16
Administering local anesthetic agents by block	N/A	15/15	N/A	10/15
Placing sutures	N/A	1/1	N/A	—

NOTE: The number to the left of the (/) is the total number of jurisdictions which require formal training or examinations. The number to the right of the (/) is the total number of jurisdictions which permit delegation of the function.

N/A—Not applicable as an expanded function.

NUMBER OF STATES REQUIRING SPECIFIC SUPERVISION OF
DENTAL ASSISTANTS AND DENTAL HYGIENISTS WHEN PERFORMING FUNCTION

	Direct		Indirect	
	Assisting	Hygiene	Assisting	Hygiene
Inspecting the oral cavity	15/20	N/A	3/20	N/A
Applying topical anesthetic agents	30/36	N/A	5/36	N/A
Removing excess cement from coronal surfaces of teeth	38/38	N/A	—	N/A
Cementing bands/bonding brackets	4/4	N/A	—	N/A
Bending archwires	8/9	N/A	—	N/A
Exposing radiographs	36/47	16/50	7/47	7/50
Performing pulp vitality testing	10/11	9/19	1/11	1/19
Making alginate impressions for study casts	32/43	22/49	8/43	4/49
Coronal polishing	21/23	16/50	1/23	7/50
Applying topical anticariogenic agents	28/33	15/49	3/33	8/49
Applying pit and fissure sealants	18/19	19/49	—	6/49
Placing periodontal dressings	21/25	22/42	3/25	4/42
Removing periodontal dressings	32/37	26/48	4/37	4/48
Removing sutures	36/40	20/46	3/40	5/46
Monitoring nitrous oxide analgesia	22/24	27/34	1/24	2/34
Placing matrices	29/31	25/37	1/31	3/37
Removing matrices	26/28	24/36	1/28	3/36
Placing rubber dams	36/41	27/46	3/41	4/46
Removing rubber dams	36/41	28/47	3/41	3/47
Fabricating temporary/interim restorations	16/17	14/18	—	1/18
Placing temporary/interim restorations	20/22	21/36	—	3/36
Removing temporary/interim restorations	19/22	20/29	1/22	3/29
Applying cavity liners and bases	9/11	11/15	2/11	3/15
Placing amalgam restorations for condensation by the dentist	10/10	13/13	—	—
Placing and condensing amalgams	4/4	6/6	—	—
Carving amalgams	4/4	6/6	—	—
Polishing amalgams	14/15	18/47	1/15	4/47
Placing and finishing composite resin restorations	3/3	6/6	—	—
Placing and packing retraction cords	11/11	11/12	—	1/12
Performing supragingival scaling	—	17/49	—	7/49
Performing subgingival scaling	N/A	16/49	N/A	9/49
Root planing	N/A	17/48	N/A	6/48
Closed gingival curettage	N/A	18/34	N/A	1/34
Administration of nitrous oxide analgesia	N/A	11/13	N/A	2/13
Administering local anesthetic agents by infiltration	N/A	11/16	N/A	3/16
Administering local anesthetic agents by block	N/A	11/15	N/A	2/15
Placing sutures	N/A	1/1	N/A	—

NOTE: The number to the left of the (/) is the total number of jurisdictions that have required supervision. The number to the right of the (/) is the total number of jurisdictions which permit delegation of the function.

N/A—Not applicable as an expanded function.

NUMBER OF STATES REQUIRING SPECIFIC SUPERVISION OF DENTAL ASSISTANTS AND DENTAL HYGIENISTS WHEN PERFORMING FUNCTION—cont'd

	General		None	
	Assisting	Hygiene	Assisting	Hygiene
Inspecting the oral cavity	2/20	N/A	—	N/A
Applying topical anesthetic agents	—	N/A	—	N/A
Removing excess cement from coronal surfaces of teeth	—	N/A	—	N/A
Cementing bands/bonding brackets	—	N/A	—	N/A
Bending archwires	—	N/A	—	N/A
Exposing radiographs	4/47	26/50	—	—
Performing pulp vitality testing	—	10/19	—	—
Making alginate impressions for study casts	2/43	24/49	—	—
Coronal polishing	1/23	25/50	—	1/50
Applying topical anticariogenic agents	1/33	25/49	—	1/49
Applying pit and fissure sealants	—	23/49	—	1/49
Placing periodontal dressings	—	16/42	—	—
Removing periodontal dressings	—	18/48	—	—
Removing sutures	—	20/46	—	—
Monitoring nitrous oxide analgesia	—	4/34	—	—
Placing matrices	—	8/37	—	—
Removing matrices	—	8/36	—	—
Placing rubber dams	1/41	14/46	—	—
Removing rubber dams	1/41	15/47	—	—
Fabricating temporary/interim restorations	—	3/18	—	—
Placing temporary/interim restorations	1/22	12/36	—	—
Removing temporary/interim restorations	—	6/29	—	—
Applying cavity liners and bases	—	2/15	—	—
Placing amalgam restorations for condensation by the dentist	—	1/13	—	—
Placing and condensing amalgams	—	1/6	—	—
Carving amalgams	—	1/6	—	—
Polishing amalgams	—	22/47	—	1/47
Placing and finishing composite resin restorations	—	1/6	—	—
Placing and packing retraction cords	—	1/12	—	—
Performing supragingival scaling	—	24/49	N/A	1/49
Performing subgingival scaling	N/A	23/49	N/A	1/49
Root planing	N/A	24/48	N/A	1/48
Closed gingival curettage	N/A	13/34	N/A	1/34
Administration of nitrous oxide analgesia	N/A	—	N/A	—
Administering local anesthetic agents by infiltration	N/A	1/16	N/A	—
Administering local anesthetic agents by block	N/A	1/15	N/A	—
Placing sutures	N/A	1/1	N/A	—

NOTE: The number to the left of the (/) is the total number of jurisdictions that have required supervision. The number to the right of the (/) is the total number of jurisdictions which permit delegation of the function.

N/A—Not applicable as an expanded function.

NUMBER OF STATES REQUIRING SPECIFIC SUPERVISION OF DENTAL ASSISTANTS AND DENTAL HYGIENISTS WHEN PERFORMING FUNCTION—cont'd

	Undefined	
	Assisting	Hygiene
Inspecting the oral cavity	—	N/A
Applying topical anesthetic agents	1/36	N/A
Removing excess cement from coronal surfaces of teeth	—	N/A
Cementing bands/bonding brackets	—	N/A
Bending archwires	—	N/A
Exposing radiographs	—	—
Performing pulp vitality testing	—	—
Making alginate impressions for study casts	1/43	—
Coronal polishing	—	—
Applying topical anticariogenic agents	1/33	—
Applying pit and fissure sealants	1/19	—
Placing periodontal dressings	1/25	1/42
Removing periodontal dressings	1/37	1/48
Removing sutures	1/40	1/46
Monitoring nitrous oxide analgesia	—	—
Placing matrices	—	2/37
Removing matrices	—	2/36
Placing rubber dams	1/41	2/46
Removing rubber dams	1/41	2/47
Fabricating temporary/interim restorations	1/17	—
Placing temporary/interim restorations	1/22	1/36
Removing temporary/interim restorations	1/22	1/29
Applying cavity liners and bases	—	—
Placing amalgam restorations for condensation by the dentist	—	—
Placing and condensing amalgams	—	—
Carving amalgams	—	—
Polishing amalgams	—	1/47
Placing and finishing composite resin restorations	—	—
Placing and packing retraction cords	—	—
Performing supragingival scaling	—	—
Performing subgingival scaling	N/A	—
Root planing	N/A	—
Closed gingival curettage	N/A	—
Administration of nitrous oxide analgesia	N/A	—
Administering local anesthetic agents by infiltration	N/A	1/16
Administering local anesthetic agents by block	N/A	1/15
Placing sutures	N/A	—

NOTE: The number to the left of the (/) is the total number of jurisdictions that have required supervision. The number to the right of the (/) is the total number of jurisdictions which permit delegation of the function.

N/A—Not applicable as an expanded function.

STATES WHICH RECOGNIZE MORE THAN ONE CATEGORY OF DENTAL ASSISTANTS

Arizona	Expose radiographs
Arkansas	Registered dental assistant
California	Registered dental assistant Registered dental assistant—extended functions
Idaho	Take impressions for study casts Expose and develop radiographs Apply topical medicaments as prescribed by the dentist Assist by the placement of rubber dams Remove excess cement from coronal surfaces of teeth Pre-select orthodontic bands, wires and temporary crowns Place matrix bands Remove sutures Remove/replace ligature wires on orthodontic appliances
Iowa	Certified in dental radiology
Maryland	Certified dental radiation technologist
Michigan	Non-licensed dental assistant Registered dental assistant
Minnesota	Registered dental assistant
Mississippi	Radiology
New Mexico	Certified dental assistant Non-certified dental assistant Dental assistant certified in dental radiography
North Dakota	Certified dental assistant Registered dental assistant
Ohio	Advanced qualified personnel Basic qualified personnel
Oklahoma	Expose intra- and extra-oral radiographs Apply topical fluoride Polishing coronal surfaces of teeth Placing periodontal dressings Assisting in the administration of nitrous oxide Placing and removing rubber dams
Oregon	X-ray certification Expanded function dental assistant Expanded function orthodontic assistant
South Dakota	Radiograph only Monitoring of nitrous oxide Expanded functions
Vermont	Dental assistant trainee Certified dental assistant Traditional dental assistant Expanded functions dental assistant
Virginia	Radiology Application of fluoride topical anesthetic Desensitizing agents
Wyoming	Expose radiographs

STATES WHICH RECOGNIZE MORE THAN ONE CATEGORY OF DENTAL HYGIENISTS

Alaska	Administer local anesthetic agents
Arizona	Regular dental hygienist Hygienist certified in local anesthesia Hygienist certified in expanded function
California	Registered dental hygienists Registered dental hygienists in extended functions
New Mexico	Apply pit and fissure sealants Administer local anesthesia
Wyoming	Expanded functions

Glossary

Abandonment withdrawing a patient from treatment without giving reasonable notice or providing a competent replacement.

ABCs of emergency care levels of emergency care to determine airway, breathing, and circulation.

Abrade to wear away by friction.

Abrasion abnormal wearing away of a substance or tissue by a mechanical process. Grinding or wearing away of a tooth tissue by mastication, improper brushing methods, bruxism, or other causes.

Abscess localized accumulation of pus in a cavity formed by tissue disintegration.

Acid etching process by which the prism structure of the enamel surface is altered by applying acids such as phosphoric, lactic, or chelating agents (ethyldiaminetetraacetic acid [EDTA]; the effect is to leave a cleansed surface of enamel microporosities that provide a source of mechanical retention for a filling or orthodontic bonding material.

ACLS advanced cardiac life support; process that includes BLS, plus the use of adjunctive equipment to support ventilation, establishment of an IV fluid lifeline, drug administration, cardiac monitoring, defibrillation, control of cardiac arrhythmias, and postresuscitation care.

Acrylic crown temporary restoration constructed from acrylic that provides full coverage to restore function and esthetics to a prepared tooth, protect the tooth from thermal changes, and eliminate mesial drift and trauma.

Acute herpetic gingivostomatitis inflammation of the gingivae and oral mucosa caused by the invasion of the herpes virus. Distinguished by red and swollen gingivae, red mucosa, evidence of vesicles and ulcers, pain, and increased temperature. Common in childhood; duration about 14 days.

ADA American Dental Association; national professional organization for dentists.

ADAA American Dental Assistants' Association; national professional organization for dental assistants.

Adenopathy enlargement of the glandular organs and tissues generally attributed to a disease process.

ADHA American Dental Hygienists' Association; national professional organizations for dental hygienists.

Adjustment modification made upon a dental prosthesis in preparation for and/or following its use by the patient.

Advanced bell eruption enamel organ formation creating the crown of the tooth.

Advanced functions duties delegated by a dentist allowing a dental auxiliary to perform specific intraoral tasks. Special restrictions and educational requirements are identified by individual state dental practice acts to define the delegations of advanced functions.

Afferent message impulse message carried by afferent nerves toward the brain from peripheral areas.

Air/water syringe apparatus of metal, glass, or plastic material consisting of a nozzle, or needle, barrel, and plunger or rubber bulb, through which air, water, or a combination of the two may be delivered under pressure to the desired area.

Aluminum crown temporary metal crown designed to be placed on a tooth to provide function, protect the tooth from thermal changes, and eliminate mesial drift and trauma.

Alveolar crest most coronal portion of the alveolar bone.

Alveolar process portion of the maxillae or mandible that forms the dental arch and serves as the bony support for the teeth. Its cortical covering is continuous with the compact bone of the body of the maxillae or mandible, whereas the trabecular portion is continuous with the spongiosa of the body of the jaws.

Alveolar ridge bony ridge (alveolar process) of the maxillae or mandible, which contains the alveoli (sockets of the teeth).

Amalgam alloy, one of the constituents being mercury; dental amalgam is a combination of alloys commonly including silver, tin, and optionally copper or zinc mixed with mercury.

Amalgam tattoo localized area of blue-gray pigmentation caused by an accidental or unavoidable implantation of dental amalgam into the oral tissues.

Ameloblast cell from which tooth enamel is formed.

Anaphylactic shock severe allergic reaction resulting from an injection of a substance to which an individual has become sensitized.

Anatomic crown portion of dentin covered by enamel.

Anatomic position body position is vertical, facing forward with hands to the sides and the palms facing forward to assist in body part identification.

Anesthesiologist specialist in anesthesiology.

Angioedema spontaneous swelling of the lips, cheeks, eyelids, tongue, soft palate, pharynx, and glottis, frequently associated with allergy to foods or drugs and lasting from several hours to several days. Involvement of the glottis results in obstruction of the airway.

Angle's classification of malocclusion classification of the different forms of malocclusion set up by Edward Angle, an orthodontist (1855-1930). Class I: normal anteroposterior relationship of mandible to maxilla. The mesiobuccal cusp of the maxillary first permanent molar occludes with the buccal groove of the mandibular first permanent molar. Class II: the posterior relationship of the mandible to the maxilla. The mesiobuccal cusp of the maxillary first permanent molar occludes mesial to the buccal groove of the mandibular first permanent molar. Divisions of this classification may exist. Class III: the anterior relationship of the mandible to the maxilla. The mesiobuccal cusp of the maxillary first permanent molar occludes distal to the buccal groove of the mandibular first permanent molar; subdivisions may occur.

Anode positive terminal of an x-ray tube. The anode consists of a tungsten target embedded in a copper stem and set at an angle to the cathode. The anode is the location where x-rays originate in the tube, thus it is often called the target or focal spot.

Anterior situated in front of; the forward position.

Antisepsis prevention of infection of a body surface, usually skin or oral mucosa, through the application of an antimicrobial agent.

Antiseptic antimicrobial agent for application to a body surface, usually skin or oral mucosa, in an attempt to prevent or minimize infection at the area of application.

ANUG abbreviation for acute necrotizing ulcerative gingivitis, a recurrent periodontal disease primarily involving the interdental papillae, which undergo necrosis and ulceration.

Apex end of the root.

Apexification process of induced root development of apical closure of the root by hard tissue deposition.

Apexogenesis treatment of a vital pulp by a pulp capping or pulpotomy (removal of the coronal portion of the pulp) to permit continued closure of the open apex and growth of the root.

Apical foramen channel located at the conical tip of the root or roots of each tooth through which the pulp receives its vascular and neural supply.

Apicoectomy surgical procedure whereby the apical portion of the root is removed, usually after the root canal filling has been completed.

Appointment schedule list printed list denoting patient appointments in chronologic order for each day. This posting of activities is placed in treatment rooms and other frequently used areas.

Archwire wire applied to two or more teeth through fixed attachments to cause or guide tooth movement orthodontically. Full archwire extends from the molar region on one side of the arch to the opposite side; sectional archwire extends to include only a few teeth on one side or an anterior segment.

Arkansas stone natural abrasive stone used to sharpen instruments.

Armamentarium all materials and instruments needed for any given procedure.

Articular meniscus fibrous cartilage found in the articular capsule.

Articulation contact relationship of the maxillary and mandibular teeth when moving into and away from centric occlusion.

Articulator mechanical device that simulates the temporomandibular joints and jaw members to which maxillary and mandibular casts may be attached.

Asepsis without infection; free from viable pathogenic microorganisms.

Aseptic technique process of producing asepsis or destruction of pathogenic microorganisms, such as sterilization by dry heat or steam under pressure.

Assault intentional, unlawful act of bodily injury to another by force or unlawfully directing force toward another person so as to create a reasonable fear of imminent danger, coupled with the apparent present ability to do the harm threatened if not prevented. A completed assault is battery. In a dental setting, the unconsented touching of the body would be assault and battery.

Assignment specific procedure given to a dental auxiliary by the dentist which is to be performed on a designated patient of record. The dentist need not be physically present either in the office or in the treatment room at the time the procedure is performed.

Atrium (pl., atria); a chamber or cavity communicating with another structure.

Attachment width distance in millimeters from the base of the pocket to the mucogingival line. Indicates width of attached gingiva.

Attrition normal loss of tooth substance due to friction caused by physiologic forces.

Autogenous infection self-produced infection; originating within the body.

Avulsed tooth tooth that has been abnormally luxated from its alveolar support, commonly as a sequela to trauma; also "evulsed."

AW attachment width.

Axial line or plane running parallel to the long axis of an object.

Bar metal segment of greater length than width that serves to connect two or more parts of a removable partial denture.
Labial bar a major connector located labial to the dental arch joining two or more bilateral parts of a removable partial denture.
Lingual bar a major connector located lingual to the dental arch joining two or more bilateral parts of a mandibular removable partial denture.
Palatal bar a major connector that crosses the palate and unites two or more parts of a maxillary removable partial denture.

Base 1. foundation or support on which something rests; the point of attachment of a part; the principal ingredient of a material. 2. consistency of a dental cement which provides a thick plasticized material that is placed under restorations.

Baseplate temporary substance representing the base of a denture that is used for making maxillomandibular (jaw) relation records and for the arrangement of teeth.

Bass technique toothbrushing technique used in periodontal disease: the bristles are positioned in the sulcus, in contact with the gingiva and tooth simultaneously, and with gentle vibration the brush is moved in short back and forth strokes. The brush is advanced around the mouth, on the cheek and tongue surfaces, until all areas have been thoroughly brushed.

Battery completed assault.

Behavior management techniques various procedures used in the management of patients, most commonly children. Procedures include communication, psychology, and sometimes drug administration.

Bell stage third stage of formation of the enamel organ.

Bicuspidization surgical procedure used in endodontic treatment when severe bone loss is confined to the furcation area. The process creates two bicuspids (premolars) from a mandibular molar.

Bifurcation division into two parts or branches, as any two roots of a tooth.

Bilateral pertaining to both sides.

Binangle instrument having two offsetting angles in its shank. The angles keep the cutting edge or the face of the nib within 3 mm of the axis of the shaft.

Biomechanical cleansing process of flushing a root canal with sodium hypochlorite to clean and remove debris from the canal.

Biopsy removal of a tissue specimen or other material from the living body for microscopic examination to aid in establishing a diagnosis.

Bisecting technique intraoral radiographic technique in which the x-ray beam is directed perpendicular to a line bisecting the long axis of the tooth and the film plane.

Bitewing (interproximal projection) intraoral radiograph depicting the crowns of maxillary and mandibular teeth and interdental bone crests. A bitewing radiograph is made using a film positioned by special tabs on which the teeth are closed.

Black, G. V. noted scientist and dentist responsible for creation of Black classification of tooth nomenclature and cavity classification.

Blade part of an instrument bearing a cutting edge; it begins at the terminal angle of the shank and ends at the cutting edge.

Bleaching use of a chemical oxidizing agent (sometimes in combination with heat) to lighten tooth discolorations.

Blood pressure pressure exerted on arterial walls by the blood when the heart is in systole (systolic pressure), and the pressure maintained by the elasticity of the arteries when the heart is in diastole (diastolic pressure). A consistent arterial pressure greater than 140/90 is considered abnormally high and is suggestive of hypertensive vascular disease.

Bonding 1. adhesion of orthodontic attachments to the teeth without use of an interposed band or the adhesion of a restorative, such as composite material, to the tooth. 2. The bonding technique involves the placement of an acid etchant on the enamel surface of the tooth. The etched enamel provides a slightly porous surface for the bonding material to adhere. The composite resin material then adheres to the bonded resin.

Bone swaging lateral displacement of alveolar bone into an adjacent vertical bony defect.

Border molding shaping of an impression material by the manipulation or action of the tissues adjacent to the borders of an impression.

Boxing (an impression) enclosure of an impression by the building up of vertical walls to produce the desired size and form of the base of the cast, and to preserve certain details of the impression.

Bracket small metal attachment fixed to a band for the purpose of fastening the arch-wire to the orthodontic band.

Bridge colloquial description for a fixed or nonremovable partial denture. This type of prosthesis replaces one or more teeth and is intended to be permanently attached to the tooth or root abutments.

Broach instrument with numerous protruding barbs from a metal shaft. It is generally used to engage the dental pulp for extirpation.

Buccal pertaining to or adjacent to the cheek.

Bud stage first stage of formation of the enamel organ that has developed from the lamina dura.

Bunsen burner small laboratory burner consisting of a vertical metal tube connected to a gas source, which produces a very hot flame from a mixture of gas and air let in through adjustable holes at the base.

Bur rotary cutting instrument of steel or tungsten carbide; supplied with cutting heads of various shapes.

Burnish to condense and polish under the sliding pressure of a smooth hand instrument, as in finishing the surface of a gold restoration.

Calculus mineralized plaque; a hard, rough deposit on the tooth surface.

Calorie unit for measurement of heat created when the body burns or metabolizes food that has been eaten.

Canal portion of the root that contains the pulp tissue and is bounded by dentin.

Candidosis infection with *Candida albicans;* also known as candidiasis and thrush.

Cap stage second stage of formation of the enamel organ.

Capitation 1. practice of dentistry financed by a set fee per person per given period of time. A form of contracted dental care, usually by a corporation, institution, or other group. 2. System by which the contracting dentist, assuming the financial risk, is compensated at a fixed per capita rate, usually on a monthly basis, in return for agreeing to provide specific, predetermined dental services as appropriate and necessary to eligible subscribers.

Carbohydrate any group of organic nutrients including sugars, starches, and cellulose, containing carbon, hydrogen, and oxygen only, with the ratio of hydrogen to oxygen atoms usually 2:1 and releasing 4 kcalories per gram.

Caries decay or death of tissue; in dentistry it refers to the infectious disease that progressively destroys tooth substance, beginning on the enamel by demineralization or on the cementum.

Caries removal the process of arresting the decay through mechanical removal.

Carotid arteries either one of the two main right and left arteries of the neck.

Carpule cylindrical device that holds medication before and during administration.

Cartridge *see* Carpule.

Casting machine mechanical device used for throwing or forcing a molten metal into a refractory mold.

Cathode negative terminal of an x-ray tube. The cathode consists of a helical tungsten filament within a molybdenum reflector cup. The function of the cathode is to produce a cloud of electrons.

Cavity classification carious lesions are classified according to the surfaces of a tooth on which they occur (labial, buccal, occlusal, etc.), type of surface (pit and fissure or smooth surface), and numerical grouping.

Cavity wall one of the enclosing sides of a prepared cavity. Walls take the names of the surface of the tooth adjoining the involved surface toward which it is placed.

CDA Certified Dental Assistant; a person who has met specific criteria and who has successfully completed a credentialing examination.

CDC Centers for Disease Control and Prevention.

Cementoenamel junction junction of the enamel of the crown and the cementum of the root of a tooth (cervical line). The area above the junction corresponds to the anatomic crown of the tooth; the area apical to the junction constitutes the anatomic root of the tooth.

Cementoblasts cells that form the cementum.

Cementum specialized, calcified connective tissue that covers the anatomic root of a tooth, giving attachment to the periodontal ligament.

Central incisors cutting teeth; the first of the four anterior teeth of either jaw.

Central nervous system portion of the nervous system consisting of the brain and spinal cord.

Centric occlusion relationship of opposing occlusal surfaces that provides the maximum planned contact and/or intercuspation. It should exist when the mandible is in centric relation to the maxillae.

Centric relation most retruded physiologic relation of the mandible to the maxillae, a position that can exist at various degrees of jaw separation and that occurs on the terminal hinge axis.

Centrix syringe type of syringe designed to assist in the application of a resin filling material into a cavity preparation.

Cephalogram extraoral radiographic examination of the head. It is most frequently used in orthodontics to measure and study maxillofacial growth or relationships of maxilla and mandible. A cephalogram is made by placing the patient's head in a special positioner that maintains precise alignment of head to film.

Chairside assistant dental health care worker whose primary responsibility is to assist the dentist or independently perform clinical treatment for the patient.

Charters' technique method of toothbrushing in which the brush is held horizontally, with the bristles lying against the teeth and gingivae and pointed in a coronal direction at 45 degrees so that the bristles lie half on the teeth and half on the gingivae. A vibratory cycle of a very constricted diameter is negotiated so that the brush head moves circularly but the brush bristles remain fairly stationary while being agitated. The circular vibration loosens debris and pumps the bristles into interproximal areas to massage the tissues.

Chisel instrument designed after the carpenter's chisel. 1. As a hand cutting instrument the device is used for cutting or cleaving hard tissue; the instrument is beveled with a cutting edge on one side only; it can have a straight or angled shank. 2. As a scaler the instrument has a single blade perpendicular to the long axis of the instrument shank and handle and is used in a pulling action to remove calculus.

Chuck device, commonly made of metal, inside the head of high speed handpieces that is used as a retentive mechanism to hold a bur or stone in place.

Cingulum portion of incisor teeth and canines, occurring on the lingual or palatal aspects, that forms a convex protuberance at the cervical third of the anatomic crown. Represents the lingual or palatal developmental lobe of these teeth.

Circumvallate papillae large V-shaped projections on the dorsal surface of the tongue.

Civil law statutory law as opposed to common law or judge-made law (such as case law). The Dental Practice Act is a civil law.

Claim form statement listing services rendered, the date of the services, and itemization of fees. The completed and signed form serves the carrier as the basis for payment of benefits.

Clasp part of a removable partial denture that acts as a direct retainer and/or stabilizer for the denture by partially encircling or contracting an abutment tooth.

Classification of motions classification system that identifies the extent of involvement of the body in completing a dental motor task.

    class 1: motions of the fingers only;

    class 2: motions of the fingers and wrist;

    class 3: motions of the fingers, wrist, and elbow;

    class 4: motions of the fingers, wrist, elbow, and upper arm;

    class 5: motions of the fingers, wrist, elbow, upper arm, and body.

Clearance condition in which bodies may pass each other without hindrance; also, the distance between bodies.

Cleft vertical soft tissue defect in which the gingival margin dips sharply and abruptly in an apical direction, then moves back up again.

Client-centered therapy Rogerian concept of humanistic psychology that places the client at the center of all decision making.

Clinical chart legal record of all existing dental conditions and treatment performed for a specific patient.

Clinical crown that portion of enamel visibly present in the oral cavity; the portion of a tooth that is occlusal to the deepest part of the gingival crevice.

Clinical examination visual and tactile scrutiny of the tissues of and surrounding the oral cavity.

Closed panel in a prepayment plan, a group of dentists sharing office facilities who provide stipulated services to an eligible group for a set premium. For beneficiaries of plans using closed panels, choice of dentists is limited to panel members. Dentists must accept any beneficiary as a patient.

Cold sterilization means of killing some microorganisms by immersion in a cold chemical solution.

Collimation restricting the size of the x-ray beam by absorbing divergent x-rays with metal tubes or diaphragms interposed in the path of the beam. Rectangular collimators limit the primary beam to approximate the size of intraoral radiographic film.

Communication technique of conveying thoughts or ideas between two people or groups of people.

Composite resinous filling material formed by a reaction of an ether bisphenol A with acrylic resin monomers; initiated by a benzoyl peroxide amine system to which inorganic fillers (glass beads and rods of either aluminum, silicate, quartz, or tricalcium phosphate) are added.

Compressive strength amount of resistance of a material to fracture under compression or biting forces.

Compules premeasured units of dental materials such as a single paste resin filling material.

Concave curved like the inner surface of a sphere.

Condyle rounded process at the end of the ramus of the mandible that articulates in the glenoid fossa.

Conscious sedation sedative technique whereby the patient is awake and can respond to simple commands.

Consent concurrence of wills; permission.

Contact area point at which abutment teeth touch each other.

Contact point point at which teeth in the opposing arch touch each other.

Continuing care maintenance care; continued periodic re-examination and supervision of periodontal care after completion of treatment procedures.

Contra-angle instrument that has two or more offset angles of such a degree that the end of the instrument is kept within 3 mm of the long axis of the shaft; attachment for burs, stones, and disks to provide easy access to all posterior surfaces of the teeth.

Convenience form modifications necessary, beyond basic outline form, to facilitate proper instrumentation for the preparation of the cavity or insertion of the restorative material; also, the placing of starting points or slight undercuts to retain the first portions of restorative material while succeeding portions are placed.

Conventional radiography use of x-radiation and x-ray film to record an image.

Convex having a surface or boundary that curves or bulges outward, as the exterior of a sphere.

Copayment amount or percentage of the total approved amount that the subscriber is obligated to pay. This is not to be confused with deductible amount.

Coronal pulp portion of the pulp that resides in the crown of the tooth.

Coronal suture joins the frontal and parietal bones.

Coronaplasty occlusal equilibration.

Coronoid process thin triangular rounded eminence originating from the anterosuperior surface of the ramus of the mandible. Provides insertion for the various fiber bundles of the temporal muscle.

Corrosion electrolytic or chemical attack of a surface. Usually refers to the attack of a metal surface.

CPR cardiopulmonary resuscitation.

Credential letter or certificate given to a person to verify that the person has the right to assume a certain authority or perform an activity.

Crevicular fluid sulcular fluid; characteristic fluid in the gingival sulcus that is similar but not identical to tissue fluid.

Cribriform plate alveolar bone that forms the tooth socket and to which the periodontal ligament is attached (radiographically the lamina dura).

Crista galli projection of the ethmoid bone in the anterior cranial fossa that assists in attaching the dura mater of the brain.

Crossbite occlusion that exists when the line of occlusion of the mandibular teeth is anterior and/or buccal to the maxillary teeth.

Cross-contamination transfer of impurities, infection, or disease from one source to another.

Cross-infections transfer of infection from one source to another.

Curet spoon-shaped scaler used to debride and smooth tooth roots and cut away diseased soft tissue lining the gingival sulcus.

Curettage surgical removal of diseased soft tissue lining the gingival sulcus.

Curetting use of curet scalers to remove subgingival calculus from the root surface of the tooth.

Curing light visible light source used to activate the polymerization of resin restorative materials.

Curve of Spee 1. anatomic curvature of the occlusal alignment of teeth, beginning at the tip of the lower canine, following the buccal cusps of the natural premolars and molars, and continuing to the anterior border of the ramus, as described by von Spee. 2. The curve of the occlusal surfaces of the arches in vertical dimension, brought about by a dipping downward of the mandibular premolars, with a corresponding adjustment of the upper premolars.

Cusp notably pointed or rounded eminence on or near the masticating surface of a tooth.

Cuspidor small sinklike device located near the dental chair into which the patient expectorates.

Cuspids canines; the four pointed teeth in humans, situated one on each side of each jaw, distal to the lateral incisor; form the keystone of the arch.

Custom-made tray acrylic tray customized for an individual patient arch; used in taking final impressions.

Cyst pathologic space in bone or soft tissue containing fluid or semifluid material, generally lined by epithelium.

Daily journal sheet financial record used as a legal document to indicate the listing of activities for each patient seen in the office during the day.

Data information, especially that put into a computer.

DDS Doctor of Dental Science; Doctor of Dental Surgery.

DE double-ended, as in a double-ended hand-cutting instrument.

Debride to remove mechanically.

Deciduous dentition that which will be shed. Term pertains specifically to the first dentition of humans or animals. The teeth constituting the first dentition.

Deductible stipulated sum the covered person must pay toward the cost of dental treatment before the benefits of the program go into effect. The deductible may be annual or payable only once and may vary in amount from program to program.

Defamation of character false communication of information about a person that results in injury to a person's reputation by verbal (slander) or written (libel) word.

Defendant party against whom relief or recovery is sought in a lawsuit.

Deformation distortion; disfigurement.

Dental amalgam alloy, one of the constituents of which is mercury, used for dental restorations and dies.

Dental assistant auxiliary to the dentist.

Dental engine electric motor that, by means of a continuous-cord drive over pulleys, or other styles, actuates a handpiece that holds a rotary instrument.

Dental hygienist person educated in an accredited school and licensed by the state where residing to provide health services, such as scaling and polishing teeth, health education and training, and radiography, under the direction of a licensed dentist.

Dental laboratory technician one skilled in the art of executing the dentist's prescription for the mechanical fabrication of dental appliances.

Dental lathe machine for producing rotary motion that uses a grinding or polishing wheel. The object that is revolved by it may be fashioned to a circular pattern with the instrument, which is stationary.

Dental practice act legal standards for the practice of dentistry developed through legislative action within the state. Defines minimum educational standards, requirements for licensure/registration, and the criteria for license revocation or suspension for a dentist, hygienist, and in several states the dental assistant.

Dental public health specialty of dentistry concerned with preventing and controlling dental diseases and promoting dental health on a community-wide basis.

Dental stools seat with four or five casters and some form of back or abdominal support used by dental health care workers at chairside.

Dental unit piece of equipment in which are assembled various dynamic instruments used in dental treatment, such as dental handpieces, operatory light, bracket table, HVE hoses, saliva ejector, water supply, electric outlets, compressed air, and miscellaneous instruments.

Dentifrice pharmaceutical preparation provided as a paste, gel, or powder and used in conjunction with a toothbrush to clean and polish the teeth. Contains a mild abrasive, detergents, binders, flavoring agents, and sometimes a caries-preventive agent such as fluoride.

Dentin portion of the tooth that lies subjacent to the enamel and cementum. Consists of an organic matrix on which mineral (calcific) salts are deposited; pierced by tubules containing filamentous protoplasmic processes of the odontoblasts that line the pulpal chamber and canal. It is of mesodermal origin.

Dentinal tubules space in the dentin in which odontoblasts are found and are active.

Dentinocemental junction line of union of the cementum and dentin of the tooth.

Dentist one whose profession is to treat diseases and injuries of the teeth and oral cavity and to construct and insert restorations of and for the teeth, jaws, and mouth.

Dentition natural teeth in position in the dental arches.

Denture artificial substitute for missing natural teeth and adjacent tissues.

Developmental groove fine depressed line in the enamel of a tooth that marks the union of the lobes of the crown in its development.

Diagnosis translation of data gathered by clinical and radiographic examination into an organized, classified definition of the conditions present.

Diagnostic model reproduction of the dental arches and surrounding tissues; produced from impressions.

Diastema abnormal space between two adjacent teeth in the same dental arch.

Diet analysis documentation of food intake that is analyzed for quality and content to ensure a balanced diet and controlled oral health.

Digitized radiography use of a small camera and computer to record an image electronically.

Dimensional change percentage of shrinkage or expansion of a dental material or other substance.

Direct contact method of disease transmission caused by coming into contact with the infected person.

Direct supervision dentist has designated a patient of record upon whom services are to be performed and has described the procedure to be performed.

Direct vision ability to see an object with the naked eye without the use of a mirror to reflect the image.

Disaccharide any of a class of carbohydrates, including lactose and sucrose, that yields two monosaccharides on hydrolysis.

Discrimination showing of partiality or prejudice in treatment; specific action or policy directed against the welfare of a certain person or group of persons.

Disinfection act of destroying some pathogenic microorganisms.

Distal away from the median sagittal plane of the face and following the curvature of the dental arch.

Distal end most posterior part of a removable dental restoration or denture flange.

DMD Doctor of Dental Medicine.

Donor tissue tissue (gingiva, mucosa, or bone) moved to a new location in a grafting procedure.

Dorsal pertaining to the back or to the posterior part of an organ.

Ductile ability of a material to be stretched or elongated without fracture.

ECG/EKG electrocardiogram; electrocardiograph.

Ectoderm stage layer of cells that develops into the nervous system, specialty organs, epidermal tissue, and mucous membranes.

Edentulous without any natural teeth. The state of the oral cavity after all teeth have been lost.

Elastics rubber bands used to apply force to the tooth during orthodontic treatment.

Electrical properties two properties, corrosion and galvanism, are found in dental materials. When two metals come in contact with each other in the oral cavity an electrical reaction occurs.

Electrosurgery unit high-frequency electrical source used to cut or alter tissues in the oral cavity.

Embrasure opening, as in a wall. The space between the curve proximal surfaces of the teeth.

EMS Emergency Medical Service.

Enamel hard, glistening tissue covering the anatomic crown of the tooth composed primarily of hexagonal rods of hydroxyapatite, sheathed in an organic matrix and oriented with the long axis approximately at a right angle to the surface.

Endoderm innermost of the three primary germ layers of an embryo, developing into the intestinal tract and associated structures.

Endodontic file small metal hand instrument with tightly spiraled blades used to clean and shape a root canal.

Endodontics branch of dental practice that applies the knowledge of endodontology (root canal therapy).

Endotracheal tube tube inserted into the trachea, which delivers gases to the lungs.

EPA Environmental Protection Agency.

Epilepsy general term for a variety of disorders characterized by abnormalities of consciousness and convulsions due to brain damage. Drugs used in the treatment of symptoms (e.g., hydantoin sodium, diphenylhydantoin sodium) promote gingival hyperplasia.

Epinephrine hormone secreted by the adrenal medulla that stimulates hepatic glycogenolysis, causing an elevation in the blood sugar, vasodilation of blood vessels of the skeletal muscles, vasoconstriction of the arterioles of the skin and mucous membranes, relaxation of bronchiolar smooth muscles, and stimulation of heart action. Used in local anesthetics for its vasoconstrictive action.

Erosion chemical or mechanical destruction of tooth tissue; the action can create concavities of various shapes at the cementoenamel junction of teeth.

Erythema patchy, circumscribed, or marginated macular redness of the skin or mucous membranes due to hyperemia or inflammation.

Esthetics branch of philosophy dealing with beauty, especially with the components color and form.

Ethics 1. science of moral obligation; a system of moral principles, quality, plus practice. 2. The moral obligation to render to the patient the best possible quality of dental service and to maintain an honest relationship with other members of the profession and humankind in general.

Ethmoid bone spongy bone that forms the roof of the nasal fossae and a portion of anterior fossa of the skull that opens into the nasal cavity.

Etiology 1. causative factors. 2. The factors implicated in the causation of disease. 3. The study of the factors causing disease.

  Local factors environmental influences that may be implicated in the causation and/or perpetuation of a disease process.

  Systemic factors generalized biologic factors that are implicated in the causation, modification, and perpetuation of a disease entity. Within the oral cavity, the actions of the systemic factors are modified by interaction with local factors.

Excise cut away entirely.

Exodontia pertaining to the extraction of teeth.

Exothermic reaction chemical reaction that gives off heat as the chemicals react.

Expert witness witness called to explain to the judge and jury what happened based on the patient's record and to offer an opinion as to whether the dental care met acceptable standards.

Explorer instrument with fine, sharp tip used to feel the surface characteristics of a tooth.

Extension for prevention principle of cavity preparation stated by G. V. Black in 1891. To prevent the recurrence of decay, he advocated extension of the preparation subgingivally and axially and occlusally into an area that is readily polished and cleaned.

Extracoronal dressing temporary restoration that encircles all or part of the remaining tooth.

Extraction removal of a tooth from the oral cavity by means of elevators and/or forceps.

  Serial extraction of selected primary teeth over a period of years (often ending with removal of the first premolar teeth) to relieve crowding of the dental arches during eruption of the lateral incisors, canines, and premolars.

Extrinsic muscle muscles attached to the trunk and a limb.

Eyewash OSHA-required device used to flush the eyes with water when exposed to contaminants.

Face bow caliper-like device used to record the relationship of the maxillae and/or the mandible to the temporomandibular joints.

Face bow fork part of the face bow assemblage used to attach the occlusion rim to the face bow proper.

Facial term used to designate the surface of the tooth toward the face (synonyms: buccal, labial).

Fact witness witness who must provide only firsthand knowledge, not hearsay.

False pocket excessively deep sulcus caused by gingival swelling without apical migration of the epithelial attachment.

Fat adipose tissue of the body; fatty acids, or lipids, are the most concentrated form of the energy-releasing nutrients, providing 9 kcalories per gram.

Fat soluble soluble in fats or solvents for fats; in nutrition a group of vitamins classified according to their method of metabolism.

Federal Dentaire Internationale international organization that produced a tooth identification system (FDI Tooth Numbering System) based on a two-digit system; the first digit indicates the arch, dentition, and location and the second digit refers to the specific tooth.

Felony crime that is punishable by imprisonment for more than 1 year.

Festoon large roll of marginal gingiva, usually around the facial surface of a tooth.

Fiberoptics transmission of light along a course of flexible material (plastic or glass). The intense light may be used to transilluminate teeth in diagnosing caries, to augment visualization of the operative field when incorporated in a handpiece, and to accelerate the initiator incorporated in visible (white) light–polymerized composites.

Fibroblast cell found within fibrous connective tissue, varying in shape from stellate (young) to fusiform and spindle shaped. Associated with the formation of collagen fibers and ground substance of connective tissue.

Fibroma benign tumor composed primarily of fibrous connective tissue.

Filiform papillae projections of small pointed areas that are found on the dorsum of the anterior two thirds of the tongue.

Filtration use of absorbers for selectively screening out unwanted low-energy x-rays from the primary beam. Federal law requires at least 2.5 mm added aluminum filtration for x-ray machines operating at 70 to 90 kVp.

Finish degree of finish of a polished surface; the removal of excess restorative material from the margins and contours of a restoration; polishing the restoration.

First molars primary and permanent teeth with four or five cusps and multiple roots.

First premolars secondary teeth, also referred to as first bicuspids, located between the canines and first molars; usually have two cusps; replace the molars of the primary dentition.

Fixed appliance   orthodontic appliance that is cemented to the teeth or attached by means of an adhesive material.

Fixed cabinetry   nonmobile cabinetry found in the dental suite.

Fixed fee   type of third-party coverage that establish a specific fee for specific treatment; no charge-backs are acceptable for participants.

Fixed prosthodontics   phase of prosthodontics that deals with the replacement and/restoration of teeth by artificial substitutes that are not readily removable.

Flap surgery   incision and elevation of all or a portion of soft tissue in an area, completion of other procedures in conditions of good access and visibility, then repositioning and suturing of the soft tissue.

Flasking   process of investing the cast and a wax denture in a flask preparatory to molding the denture-base material into the form of the denture.

Flooding   technique used to control the uncooperative patient to reduce anxieties.

Flossing   mechanical cleansing of tooth surfaces with waxed or unwaxed tape or floss.

Flow   to move in a manner similar to a liquid stream.

Fluoride   salt of hydrofluoric acid topically applied or added to the drinking water and dentifrices. Fluoride helps in the reduction of dental caries by combining with the hydroxy-apatite of the hard tooth structure to form fluoroapatite, which is more resistant to carious breakdown.

Foliate papillae   small indistinct papillae found on the folds of the posterior area of the sides of the tongue.

Fones technique   toothbrushing technique in which the teeth are occluded, the brush is at a right angle to the teeth, and large, sweeping, scrubbing circles are described. With the jaws parted, the palatal and lingual surfaces of the teeth are scrubbed using smaller circles. Occlusal surfaces are brushed in an anteroposterior direction.

Foot control   device activated by the foot to operate dental handpieces.

Foramen   1. natural opening in a bone or other structure. 2. Natural opening in the root, usually at or near the apical end.

Foramen magnum   large opening in the base of the occipital bone.

Fossa   pit, hollow, or depression.

Four-handed dentistry   technique of chairside operation in which four hands are kept busy working in the oral cavity simultaneously.

Framework   skeletal portion of a prosthesis (usually metal) around which and to which are attached the remaining portions of the prosthesis to produce the finished restoration (partial denture).

Fraud   intentional perversion of truth for the purpose of inducing another, in reliance on it, to part with something valuable or to surrender a legal right; deliberate deception; deceit; trickery.

Free gingival junction   area where the free gingiva meets the sulcus area.

Free-way space   distance between the occluding surfaces of the maxillary and mandibular teeth when the mandible is in its physiologic rest position. This can be determined by calculating the difference between the rest vertical dimension and the occlusal vertical dimension.

Frenectomy   1. excision of a frenum. 2. Surgical detachment and/or excision of a frenum from its attachment into the mucoperiosteal covering of the alveolar processes.

Frenum   (pl., frena); fold of mucous membrane attaching the cheeks and lips to the mandibular and maxillary mucosa and limiting the motions of the lips and cheeks.

Frontal bone   bone that forms the forehead.

Frontal plane   vertical plane that passes through the body from the head to the feet and is perpendicular to the sagittal plane.

Fructose   very sweet sugar ($C_6H_{12}O_6$) occurring in many fruits and honey and used as a preservative for foodstuffs and as an intravenous nutrient. Also called fruit sugar and levulose.

Fulcrum   support upon which a lever rests when force is applied.

Full coverage crown   restoration that reproduces the entire surface anatomy of the clinical crown and fits over a prepared tooth.

Full-thickness flap   mucoperiosteal flap.

Functional occlusion   1. occlusion in which attention is directed specifically to performance and is differentiated from structure and appearance. 2. Any tooth contacts made within the functional range (according to the size) of the opposing tooth surfaces. An occlusion that occurs during function.

Fungiform papillae   small circular papillae that are found in the anterior two thirds of the dorsal area of the tongue.

Furcation   region of division of the root portion of a tooth. **Root**   the interradicular bone resorption in multirooted teeth due to periodontal disease.

Furcation involvement   extension of periodontal disease into the area where the tooth roots separate.

Galactose   simple sugar $CH_2OH (CHOH)_4 CHO$ commonly occurring in lactose.

Galvanism   direct current created by a battery. An electromotive force of 500 mV may exist in the mouth.

General anesthetic   irregular, reversible depression of the cells of the higher centers of the central nervous system that makes the patient unconscious and insensible to pain.

General practitioner   licensed dentist who performs all types of dental treatment.

Geographic tongue   presence of maplike areas on the tongue that are smooth and red with a whitish yellow perimeter.

Gingival graft   excision and moving of a piece of gingiva or thick mucosa from one area to another.

Gingival retracting clamp   rubber dam clamp that provides retraction of the gingival tissue.

Gingival sulcus   space between the free gingiva and the tooth.

Gingivectomy   surgical removal of gingival tissue.

Gingivectomy knife   instrument, with specially designed blades used to incise gingival tissue.

Gingivitis   inflammation of the gingiva; usually a result of poor oral hygiene and an accumulation of bacterial plaque on the teeth.

Gingivoplasty   plastic surgery of the gingiva to shape it to physiologic contour.

Glenoid fossa   fossae in the temporal bone in which condyles of the mandible articulate with the skull.

Glossitis inflammation of the tongue.

Glucose six-carbon (hexose) sugar; the principal sugar in blood, serving as a major source of metabolic energy.

Grand mal epileptic seizure that is seen as generalized involuntary muscular contraction and cessation of respiration with tonic and clonic spasms of the muscles.

Granulation tissue highly vascular connective tissue formed in response to inflammation.

Granuloma localized mass of granulation tissue.

Grit degree of roughness based on size and shape of abrasive particle. Larger sizes and irregular shapes are rougher.

Hand-over-mouth method of behavior management in pediatric dentistry.

Handpiece instrument used to hold rotary instruments in the dental engine or condensing points in mechanical condensing units. It is connected by an arm, cable, belt, or tube to the source of power (motor, air, water).

Harassment troubling, worrying, or tormenting another person with repeated questions, comments, or attacks.

HBV viral form of hepatitis B that is transmitted in contaminated serum in blood transfusions or by the use of contaminated needles and instruments.

Headgear orthodontic apparatus encircling the head or neck and providing attachment for an intraoral appliance in use of extraoral anchorage.

Heimlich maneuver emergency procedure to dislodge food or other obstruction from the trachea, thereby preventing asphyxiation.

Hemisection complete sectioning through the crown of a tooth into the furcation region.

Herpes simplex infection caused by the herpes simplex virus.

Hidden transfer technique commonly used to transfer the anesthetic syringe out of the view of the patient.

Hierarchy of needs pyramid of needs, described by Dr. Abraham H. Maslow, that motivate behavior: physiologic, safety, social, ego, and self-actualization.

Hoe scaler that resembles a garden hoe.

HVE system high-velocity evacuation system used to remove oral fluids and debris.

Hygoformic device used to isolate the mandibular teeth and remove fluids from the oral cavity.

Hyperemia congestion; increased and excessive amount of blood in a tissue. The hyperemia may be active or passive.

Hyperglycemia increase in the concentration of sugar in the blood. It is a feature of diabetes mellitus.

Hyperplasia thickening or enlargement of the tissue caused by an abnormal increase in the number of normal cells in tissue.

Hypertension abnormal elevation of systolic and/or diastolic arterial pressure. Systolic hypertension is generally related to emotional stress, sclerosis of the aorta and large arteries, or aortic insufficiency. Diastolic hypertension may be due to obscure causes (essential), renal disease, or endocrine disorders.

Hypoglycemia condition existing when the concentration of blood sugar (true blood sugar) is 40 mg/100 ml or less. Symptoms may not occur even when the concentration is considerably less. Symptoms include nervousness, hunger, weakness, vertigo, and faintness. Hypoglycemia may occur in the fasting state and following the injection of insulin.

Hypotension abnormally low tension, especially low blood pressure.

Imaging creating a picture.

Immediate denture complete or removable partial denture constructed for insertion immediately following the removal of natural teeth.

Implant denture that receives its stability and retention from a substructure that is partially or wholly implanted under the soft tissues of the denture basal seat.

Incisal relating to the cutting edge of the anterior teeth, incisors, or canines.

Incise cut into.

Incisive papilla The elevation of soft tissue covering the foramen of the incisive or nasopalatine canal.

Index (pl., indices) scoring system in which a number describes a designated oral condition; for example, oral hygiene, periodontal disease, caries.

Indirect contact method of transmitting infection or disease without coming into direct contact with the source of the contaminant.

Indirect vision use of a dental mouth mirror to provide vision of the treatment site.

Infection invasion of tissues of the body by disease-producing microorganisms and the resultant reaction of the tissues to the microorganisms and/or their toxins.

Infection control policies and procedures to minimize risk of transmitting infectious diseases.

Inferior situated below or lower than a point of reference.

Inflammation cellular and vascular response or reaction to injury, characterized by pain, redness, swelling, heat, and disturbance of the function; can be acute or chronic.

Informed consent form signed by a patient who has been provided sufficient information, in understandable language, to make an intelligent decision about whether to proceed with the treatment prescribed. The patient is given ample opportunity to ask questions.

Infrabony pocket pocket with base below the level of the alveolar crest.

Inhalation drawing of air or other vapor into the lungs.

Initial phase of treatment conservative, nonsurgical actions taken as a first step toward elimination of periodontal disease.

Insertion act of implanting, placing, or introducing a needle or other device into the tissues.

Instrument exchange method of transferring instruments between the dental assistant and operator; a method of reducing unnecessary movement at chairside to decrease fatigue and time and motion.

Instrument formula method of naming and describing hand instruments. A three- or four-digit number denoting the width and length of the blade, angle of the blade, and angle of cutting edge.

Instrument number number assigned by the dental manufacturer relating to the instrument formula.

Instrumentation 1. instruments and supplies for use in a treatment procedure. 2. The process of using dental instruments during dental treatment.

Interdental aids devices used to mechanically remove certain dental deposits from tooth surfaces.

Interdental knife *see* Periodontal knife.

Interdental papilla   part of the gingivae filling the interproximal spaces between adjacent teeth, consisting partly of free and partly of attached gingivae.

Interim denture   dental prosthesis to be used for a short interval for reasons of esthetics, mastication, occlusal support, convenience, or to condition the patient to the acceptance of an artificial substitute for missing natural teeth until more definitive prosthetic therapy can be provided.

Interim dressing   material placed in a tooth or on oral tissues to provide protection and function until healing takes place or a permanent restoration is placed.

Intracoronal dressing   temporary dressing placed within the coronal portion of the tooth until a permanent restoration can be placed.

Intravenous conscious sedation   anesthetic procedure in which anesthesia or analgesia is obtained without loss of consciousness.

Intrinsic muscle   muscles that have an origin and insertion within a structure.

Invasion of privacy   wrongful intrusion into one's private activities such as to cause humiliation or mental suffering.

Inventory   itemized compilation of materials on hand.

Investment oven   device used to heat an invested mold to eliminate a wax pattern and expand a mold during the burnout procedure.

Irrigation   use of a syringe or nozzle to flush a pocket, root canal, or other tissue site prior to placing medications or dressings.

Isolation   separation of one area from another to prevent transmission of fluids or disease.

Jacksonian epilepsy   form of epilepsy that includes spasms seen in one area of the body or group of muscles.

Keyes technique   use of salt, baking soda, and hydrogen peroxide to prevent or control periodontal disease.

Kilovolt peak (kVp)   crest value in kilovolts of the potential difference of a pulsing potential generator. A kilovolt is a unit of electromotive force, equal to 1000 volts, that drives electric current through a circuit. High kilovoltage is essential for the production of dental x-rays.

Labial   of or pertaining to a lip.

Laboratory requisition/prescription   directions given to a laboratory technician by a licensed dentist for the construction of a dental prosthesis.

Lacrimal bone   small fragile bone of the face found in the anterior portion of the medial wall of the orbit.

Lambdoid suture   area that denotes the union of the occipital and the parietal bones of the skull.

Lamina dura   dense cortical bone lining the alveolus as it appears on a radiograph; white line between the dark periodontal ligament space and light gray trabecular alveolar bone on a radiograph.

Laminate   restoration made by forming a thin sheet or layer of dental material, such as porcelain to form a restoration; commonly used in anterior teeth for esthetic purposes.

Lateral   position either to the right or the left of the midsagittal plane.

Lateral incisor   second incisor; tooth distal to the central incisor.

Law   standard, rule, or set of rules of conduct established and enforced by the government of a society.

LDH   Licensed Dental Hygienist.

Ledger card   accounting form for keeping track of debits, expenditures, credits, and charges.

Lesion   pathologic disturbance of a tissue resulting in the loss of continuity, enlargement, or function.

Leukoplakia   white lesion formed on the oral mucous membrane from surface epithelial cells.

Liability   state of being bound by law or justice to do something or to make something good; legal responsibility.

Licensure   credential granted to a candidate by the state after the candidate has met the necessary requirements to practice in the profession.

Lichen planus   disease of unknown etiology characterized by a lacy pattern on the buccal mucosa or a bilateral network of raised white or bluish white porcelain-like delicate lines or series of small dots.

Ligature tie   wire or threadlike substance used to tie a tooth to an orthodontic appliance.

Line angle   angle formed by the junction of two walls along a line; designated by combining the names of the walls forming the angle.

Lingual   pertaining to the tongue.

Lingual groove   vertical groove located on the middle of lingual surface of maxillary molar teeth.

Lobe   in dental anatomy a portion of a tooth formed from a distinct point for the initiation of calcification.

Local anesthesia   loss of pain sensation over a specific area of the anatomy without loss of consciousness.

Longitudinal plane   invisible vertical line that dissects the body, object, or organ.

Lubricant   oil or water used to protect a surface from heat during an abrasive cutting procedure.

Luting   attaching one object to another with wax or other dental material.

Maintenance   continuing care after completion of treatment procedures.

Malleable   capable of being extended or beaten into thin sheets by blows from a hammer or pressure from a roller.

Malocclusion   malposition or imperfect contact of the mandibular and maxillary teeth. Often associated with other dentofacial deformities.

Malpractice   in medicine and dentistry, a professional person's act or failure to act that was the proximate cause of an injury to a patient and that was below the standard of care required.

Mamelon   rounded end of one of the enamel-forming groups on the incisal edge of incisors. These are usually worn away with use.

Mandible   lower jaw; a horseshoe-shaped bone, bilaterally consisting of a vertical component (ramus), a horizontal component joined in the midline (body and symphysis), and a condyle that articulates to the temporal bone of the skull (TMJ).

Mandibular foramen   opening on the medial aspect of the vertical ramus of the mandible approximately midway between the mandibular and gonial notches; may be located posterior to the middle of the ramus. It contains interior alveolar vessels and the inferior alveolar nerve.

Mandrel   part of the handpiece that holds a disk, stone, or cup. It is usually a shaft with a screw at the end to change the disk.

Marginal ridge ridge or elevation of enamel that forms the boundary of the occlusal surface of a tooth.

Master cone solid substance, usually gutta-percha or silver, used to fill the space once occupied by the pulp in endodontic treatment.

Maxilla irregularly shaped bone forming half of the upper jaw (made up of the two maxillae).

Meatus opening through a body part.

Mechanical properties properties that relate to the amount of stress a dental material can withstand within the oral cavity.

Medial in a direction toward or forward of the midline or middle of an object or the body.

Mental protuberance extended growth area on the anterior inferior surface (chin) of the mandibular midline.

Mesial situated in the middle; median, toward the middle line of the body or toward the center line of the dental arch.

Mesoderm middle germ layer of the embryo that produces connective tissue, blood, bone, cartilage, and muscle.

Metabolism reactions within an organism that yield energy or synthesize necessary substances.

Metal base metallic portion of a denture base forming a part or all of the basal surface of the denture. It serves as a base for the attachment of the acrylic resin part of the denture base and the teeth.

Midsagittal plane invisible vertical line or plane that divides the body through the sagittal suture into equal right and left portions.

Milliampere (mA) unit of electric current; 1/1000 of an ampere. In radiography, milliamperage determines the number of electrons available at the filament.

Mineral organic substance that is important in regulating body functions.

Misdemeanor crime classified as less serious, commonly punishable by a fine but may include imprisonment for less than 1 year or both.

Mixed dentition complement of teeth in the jaws after the eruption of some of the permanent teeth but before all the deciduous teeth are absent.

Mobile cabinetry equipment that can be moved about the treatment area to provide close working surfaces and drawers for chairside assisting in four-handed dentistry.

Mobility how far beyond normal the tooth moves in its socket.

Model trimmer grinding device with an abrasive wheel used for trimming or shaping (grinding) plaster or stone casts or models.

Modeling behavior management technique that allows one person through observation to learn a desired response from another person.

Modified Stillman's technique toothbrushing technique developed to simply massage the gingiva; the modified Stillman's method now includes cleaning the entire tooth. It is recommended for those patients with gingival recession and/or puffy gingival tissue.

Monangle having only one angle, such as a chisel.

Monitor screen attached to a computer to show data output.

Monosaccharide simple sugar.

Motion economy elimination of unnecessary movement.

Mould 1. form in which an object is cast or shaped. 2. The term used to specify the shape of an artificial tooth or teeth.

Mouthguard resilient intraoral device worn during participation in contact sports to reduce the potential for injury to the teeth and associated tissue.

Mucobuccal fold mucobuccal reflection; line of flexure of the oral mucous membrane as it passes from the mandible or maxillae to the cheek.

Mucocele epithelium-lined sac containing mucus.

Mucogingival defect improper shape of the gingiva or alveolar mucosa.

Mucolabial fold line of flexure of the oral mucous membrane as it passes from the mandible or maxillae to the lip.

Mucoperiosteal full-thickness flap all soft tissue in an area is incised and elevated.

Mucosal split-thickness flap epithelium and part of the underlying connective tissue are incised and separated from the remaining connective tissue and periosteum.

Muscles of facial expression frequently called the mimetic muscles; variable in contour, widely distributed over the scalp and face, and especially concentrated about the orbits, outer ear, and lips. As a group they have only one bony origin in the facial skeleton. The muscles form a circular rim around the perimeter of the facial bones and extend anteriorly as a tube of tissue in which the lumen narrows and terminates in the orbicularis oris.

Muscles of mastication powerful muscles that elevate and rotate the mandible so that the opposing teeth may occlude for mastication.

Muscle trimming shaping of an impression material by the manipulation or action of the tissues adjacent to the borders of an impression.

Nasal aperture opening of the nasal cavity in the skull.

Nasal bones bones that form the bridge of the nose.

Nasal conchae three scroll-like bones—the superior and middles bones, which rise from the ethmoid bone, and the inferior bone, which emanates from the facial bone.

Necrosis death of a cell or group of cells in contact with living tissue.

Negligence performance of an act that a reasonably careful person under similar circumstances would not do or, conversely, the failure to perform an act that a reasonably careful person would do under similar circumstances.

Nitrous oxide N_2O; laughing gas; nitrogen monoxide; nitrogen monoxidum. A gas with a sweet odor and taste; used as an analgesic and sedative agent in combination with oxygen for the performance of minor operations. It is sometimes called laughing gas because it may excite a hilarious delirium preceding insensibility.

Nonsuccedaneous referring to permanent teeth that do not replace primary teeth.

Nonverbal communication gesture or movement that indicates a reaction from another person, such as frowning, striking back with a fist, or folded arms.

Nutrient substance that provides nourishments and affects the metabolic and nutritive activities of the body.

Oblique slanting or change from horizontal.

Obturation act of closing or occluding.

Obturator prosthesis used to close a congenital or acquired opening in the palate.

Occipital bone bone in the posterior area of the skull that lies between the parietal and temporal bones. Forms the posterior base of the skull.

Occlusal pertaining to the contacting surfaces of opposing units (teeth or occlusion rims). Pertaining to the masticating surfaces of the posterior teeth.

Occlusal clearance condition in which the opposing occlusal surfaces may glide over one another without any interfering projection.

Occlusal equilibration reshaping of the occlusal or incisal surfaces of selected teeth to improve the bite; coronaplasty.

Occlusal load bite force.

Occlusion 1. act of closure or state of being closed. 2. Any contact between the incising or masticating surfaces of the upper and lower teeth.

Odontoblasts cell that forms the surface layer of the dental papilla that forms dentin of the tooth. Odontoblasts continue production for years after eruption.

Office policy written statement of the dentist's philosophy and policies defining the responsibilities of the patient and office staff.

OH 1. oral hygiene; number describing the oral hygiene condition of a tooth 2. Abbreviation used in charting to indicate overhang in a restoration.

Onlay cast type restoration that is retained by frictional or mechanical factors in the prepared tooth; restores one or more cusps and adjoining occlusal surfaces of the tooth.

Oral histology microscopic study of oral tissues.

Oral hygiene aids assortment of materials, devices, and substances used intraorally to maintain good oral health.

Oral hygiene score rating given to indicate the amount of plaque present in a patient's mouth. The oral hygiene score can be figured using the following formula: total number of disclosed tooth surfaces divided by the total number of tooth surfaces times 100% equals the oral hygiene score. The lower the score, the more likely the oral hygiene habits are satisfactory.

Oral pathology branch of dentistry that deals with the study of oral diseases, especially the nature and function of the disease.

Orbit bony cavity containing the eye; eye socket.

Origin less movable of the two points of attachment of a muscle, usually the end attached to the more rigid part of the skeleton.

Orthodontic band thin metal ring, usually stainless steel, that secures orthodontic attachments to a tooth.

Orthodontics area of dentistry concerned with the supervision, guidance, and correction of the growing and mature dentofacial structures, including conditions that require movement of teeth and correction of malrelationships and malformations of related structures.

Orthognathic surgery surgery to alter relationships of dental arches and/or supporting bones, usually accomplished in conjunction with orthodontic therapy.

OSHA Occupational Safety and Health Administration.

Osseous surgery bone surgery. May be augmentive (bone added) or resective (bone taken away).

Osteitis inflammation of the bone.

Osteoblasts cuboidal cells associated with the growth and development of bone. In active growth osteoblasts form a continuous layer on old bone similar to a sheet of epithelial

cells; when the bone growth is arrested, the cells assume an elongated appearance like fibroblasts.

Osteoclasts large multinucleated cells associated with the resorption of bone. Seen in irregular concavities within marginal areas of bone undergoing resorption.

Outline form shape of the area of the tooth surface included within the cavosurface margins of a prepared cavity.

Output concerning computers, end result after manipulation of information.

Overbite vertical overlapping of maxillary over mandibular teeth, usually measured perpendicular to the occlusal plane.

Overdenture complete or partial removable denture supported by retained roots to provide improved support, stability, and tactile and sensation and to reduce ridge resorption.

Overjet horizontal projection of maxillary teeth beyond the mandibular teeth, usually measured parallel to the occlusal plane. When not otherwise specified, the term is generally assumed to refer to central incisors and is measured from the labial surface of the lower central incisors to the labial surface of the upper central incisors at the level of the upper incisor edge. Unique conditions may sometimes require other measuring techniques.

Oxygenating agent substance that liberates oxygen. Applied to tissues to kill anaerobic microorganisms.

Palatine bone pair of bones in the skull that form the posterior part of the palate, a portion of the nasal cavity, and the floor of the eye.

Palatine raphe line that delineates each half of the palate.

Palm grasp method of using the entire palm to hold a dental instrument; primarily used on bulky instruments such as a rubber dam clamp forceps.

Palm-and-thumb grasp grasp that is similar to the hold on a knife when one is whittling wood; the handle rests in the palm and is grasped by the four fingers while the thumb rests on an adjoining object.

Palmer Notation System tooth-numbering system that codes the teeth with numbers and letters using brackets to indicate the arch.

Panoramic radiographic method in which a continuous image of both maxillary and mandibular dental arches and associated structures are obtained.

Papilloma benign neoplasm of epithelium characterized by a warty appearance.

Papoose board means of restricting movements of an uncooperative child; consists of a flat board with soft fabric ties to deter the use of the limbs.

Parallel extending in the same direction and at the same distance apart at every point so as never to meet, as in lines or planes.

Paralleling technique intraoral radiographic technique in which the film is held parallel to the long axis of the tooth or teeth being radiographed while the x-ray beam is directed perpendicular (at a right angle) to the teeth and film.

Paranasal sinuses general term that encompasses the maxillary, ethmoidal, frontal, and sphenoidal sinuses found in the head and face region.

Parietal bone one of two bones that assist in forming the top and sides of the skull.

Partial denture dental prosthesis, replacing one or more teeth; can be removed from the mouth and replaced at will.

Patient education providing knowledge, i.e., dental information, to a patient to enhance dental health.

PD pocket depth; distance from the gingival margin to the base of a pocket.

Pediatric dentistry branch of dentistry that includes educating the child to accept dentistry; restoring and maintaining the primary, mixed, and permanent dentitions; applying preventive measures for dental caries and periodontal disease; and preventing, intercepting, and correcting various problems of occlusion.

Pen grasp grasp in which the instrument is held somewhat as a pen is held, with the handle in contact with the thumb and first two fingers.

Percolation process of filtration; seeping of a fluid through another substance.

Periapical around the apex; in radiography, the type of film used to record images of the teeth and surrounding structures.

Periapical abscess abscess involving the apical region of the root, alveolus, and surrounding bone as a sequela of pulpal disease.

Periapical radiograph radiograph illustrating the tooth apices and surrounding structure in a specific intraoral area.

Pericoronitis inflammation of the tissue flap over a partially erupted tooth, commonly a third molar.

Periodontal disease episodic, site-specific infection of the dental supporting structures.

Periodontal dressing periodontal pack; bandage for oral soft tissue.

Periodontal knife interdental knife; surgical instrument with two beveled blades for incising marginal and interdental gingiva.

Periodontal ligament space dark line between light gray dentin and cementum and alveolar bone on a radiograph. Indicates the space in which the soft ligament is located.

Periodontal pack *see* Periodontal dressing.

Periodontal probe hand instrument with millimeter calibrations used for measuring pocket depth, attachment width, and size of soft tissue lesions.

Periodontics art and science of examination, diagnosis, and treatment of diseases affecting the periodontium; a study of the supporting structures of the teeth, including not only the normal anatomy and physiology of these structures, but also the deviations from normal.

Periodontist dentist with additional specialized education and training in diagnosis and treatment of the supporting structures of the teeth.

Periodontitis inflammation of the periodontium that extends beyond the gingiva.

Periodontium tissues that invest (or help to invest) and support the teeth, i.e., the gingivae, cementum of the tooth, periodontal ligament, and alveolar and supporting bone.

Periphery limit, boundary, or circumferential margin of a denture base.

Permanent dentition thirty-two teeth of adulthood that either replace or are added to the complement of deciduous teeth.

Petit mal recurrent disorder of cerebral function resulting in some form of seizure. Petit mal seizure symptoms may range from no noticeable change in behavior to loss of consciousness and other functions.

Phase part of a procedure or series of procedures that extend over time.

Physiologic contour tissue shape that best promotes tissue health.

Pit and fissure sealants resinous material designed for application to the occlusal surfaces of posterior teeth to seal the surface irregularities and prevent ingress of oral fluids, food, and debris.

Pocket pathologically deepened sulcus.

Plaintiff person or party who institutes a suit in court.

Pocket depth (PD) distance in millimeters from the gingival margin to the base of a pocket.

Point angle angle formed by the junction of three walls at a common point; designated by combining the names of the walls forming the angle.

Polymerize to chain together similar molecules to form a compound of high molecular weight.

Polysaccharide group of nine or more monosaccharides joined by a glycosidic bonds, such as starch and cellulose.

Post and core metal casting usually with a post in the canal or root, designed to retain an artificial crown.

Posterior situated behind.

Posterior palatal seal soft tissues along the junction of the hard and soft palates on which pressure within the physiologic limits of the tissues can be applied by a denture to aid in the retention of the denture.

PPO preferred provider organization.

Predetermination administrative procedure whereby a dentist submits a treatment plan to the carrier before treatment is initiated. Then the carrier returns the treatment plan, indicating the patient's eligibility, covered service amounts payable, application of appropriate deductibles, copayment factors, and maximums. Under some programs, predetermination by the carrier is required when covered charges are expected to exceed a certain amount, commonly $100. Synonyms: preauthorization, precertification, preestimate of cost, pretreatment estimate, prior.

Preset trays armamentarium trays set up in sequence of use.

Press-roll technique toothbrushing technique that involves placement of the toothbrush at the gingival line and with pressure rolling the bristles toward the occlusal line.

Prevention action taken to deter or forego an occurrence or disease.

Primary carrier the plan covering the patient as the employee.

Primary consistency state to which a dental material is mixed to allow the material to achieve flow and act as a luting agent.

Primary dentition teeth that erupt first and are usually replaced by the permanent teeth.

Process in anatomy, a marked prominence or projection of a bone. In dentistry, a series of operations that convert a wax pattern, such as that of a denture base, into a solid denture base of another material.

Prognosis 1. foretelling of the probable course of a disease; a forecast of the outcome of a disease. 2. A forecast of the probable result of a regimen of treatment.

Prophylaxis   prevention of disease.

Prosthesis   artificial replacement of one or more teeth and/or associated structures.

Prosthodontics   prosthetic dentistry; the part of dentistry pertaining to the restoration and maintenance of oral function, comfort, appearance, and health of the patient by the replacement of missing teeth and contiguous tissues with artificial substitutes. Prosthodontics has three main branches: removable prosthodontics, fixed prosthodontics, and maxillofacial prosthetics.

Fixed   the branch of prosthodontics concerned with the replacement and/or restoration of teeth by artificial substitutes that are not readily removable.

Removable   branch of prosthodontics that is concerned with the replacement and restoration of teeth and tissues with a prosthesis that can be readily removed.

Protein   any one of a group of complex organic nitrogenous compounds; the principal constituent of cell protoplasm. Polymers of amino acids that are joined by peptide or amide bonds.

Proximal   surface of a tooth that is adjacent to another tooth.

Psychomotor seizure   epileptic seizure that affects the temporal lobe and results in reduced motor activity.

Pulp   organ made up of blood vessels, nerves, and cellular elements, including odontoblasts, that forms dentin. It normally occupies the central portion of teeth.

Pulp canal   space in the radicular portion of the tooth occupied by the pulp.

Pulp chamber   pulp cavity; space occupied by the pulp.

Pulpal floor   flat bottom or enclosing base of the prepared cavity nearest the pulp.

Pulpectomy   pulp extirpation. The complete removal of pulp from the pulp chamber and root canal.

Pulpitis   inflammation of the pulpal tissue of a tooth.

Pulpotomy   surgical amputation of the dental pulp coronal to the dentinocemental junction.

Pyrexia   fever; elevation of the body temperature.

Quadrant   one fourth of a circle. In dentistry, one fourth of the total dentition, consisting of all the teeth in half of one jaw, extending from the midline circumferentially around the arch and including the last molar. The four quadrants are the maxillary right, maxillary left, mandibular left, and mandibular right.

Quality assurance   maintaining optimal performance in a procedure. In radiology it describes certain tests to ensure that the radiographic system is functioning properly and that the radiographs produced are acceptable.

Radiation   emission and propagation of energy through space or a medium in the form of waves or particles.

Radiation safety   methods used to protect persons from accidental injury from exposure to radiation; also includes methods to reduce exposure in dental and medical settings.

Radiograph   visible image produced on a radiation-sensitive film emulsion by exposing the film to radiation and chemicals so that a negative is produced. Also called an x-ray film, radiogram, roentgenogram, and roentgenograph.

Radiology   branch of medical science that deals with the use of radiant energy in the diagnosis and treatment of disease.

Radiolucent   producing dark images on film because a large

amount of radiation interacts with the film. Also refers to structures that are easily penetrated by x-rays.

Radiopaque   producing light images on film because only a small amount of radiation interacts with the film. Also refers to structures that absorb or attenuate radiation.

Ramus   The portions of the mandible that extend upward and backward from the horseshoe-shaped body and terminate in two processes: the articular condyloid process and the coronoid process.

Rapport   feeling of reciprocal interest and concern.

RDA   1. Registered Dental Assistant. 2. Recommended Dietary Allowances of the Food and Nutrition Board of the National Research Council.

Reamer   instrument with a tapered metal shaft, more loosely spiraled than a file; used to enlarge and clean root canals.

Rebase   process of refitting a denture by replacing the denture base material without changing the occlusal relations of the teeth.

Recall   procedure of advising or informing a patient to have oral health reviewed or reexamined; an important phase of preventive dentistry.

Recession   loss by apical migration.

Recipient tissue   tissue bed; area to which tissue (gingiva, mucosa, or bone) is added in a grafting procedure.

Reconstructive phase   portion of periodontal treatment in which the teeth and arches are brought to physiologic form. As they are indicated, reconstruction includes procedures for removal of decay; restoration of teeth with fillings, inlays and onlays; endodontics; orthodontics; oral and maxillofacial surgery; implant therapy; and fixed and removable prosthodontics.

Reflect   to push back tissues from an area.

Reline   to resurface the tissue side of a denture with new base material to make it fit more accurately.

Removable appliance   orthodontic appliance designed to be removed and replaced by the patient.

Reparative dentin   dentin of an irregular nature formed below a carious lesion as a means of preserving pulpal integrity.

Replant   to replace a tooth or teeth that have been removed from the alveolus either intentionally or unintentionally, as in an accident.

Resistance form   shape given to a prepared cavity to enable the restoration and remaining tooth structure to withstand masticatory stress.

Resorption   loss by melting away, especially bone loss.

Respondeat superior   principle that holds an employer liable for the negligent acts of an employee when carrying out the employer's orders or serving the employer's interest.

Rest   rigid (stabilizing) extension of a fixed or removable partial denture that contacts a remaining tooth or teeth to dissipate vertical or horizontal forces.

Retention form   provision made in a cavity preparation to prevent displacement of the restoration.

Retentive properties   ability of a dental material to resist movement or displacement under axial stress.

Retromolar pad   mass of tissue located at the distal termination of the mandibular residual ridge.

Reverse transfer   act of transferring instruments or handpieces in an opposite direction; specifically transferring an earlier used handpiece with the pickup portion of the hand and receiving the used handpiece with the delivery portion of the hand.

Ridge remainder of the alveolar process and its soft tissue covering after the teeth are removed.

Root planing use of instruments, primarily curets, to smooth the root surface until it feels like glass.

Root resection removal of one root of a multirooted tooth.

Rubber dam thin sheet of latex rubber used to isolate a tooth or teeth and keep them dry during a dental procedure.

Saccharin white crystalline powder having a taste about 500 times sweeter than cane sugar, used as a calorie-free sweetener.

Saddle part of a complete or partial denture that rests on the oral mucosa and to which the teeth are attached.

Sagittal plane anteroposterior median plane of the body.

Salient important to the issue at hand.

Saliva ejector tubular plastic- or metal-tipped suction tube attached to either a water or air pressure vacuum system; evacuates fluids from the oral cavity during a dental procedure.

Salivary glands glands that secrete saliva. Three major groups of salivary glands contribute their secretions to form the whole saliva; accessory mucous glands found within oral mucosa contribute also in small part. The primary glands are the parotid, submaxillary, and sublingual.

Sandblaster device used in conjunction with air and small sand particles to reduce the smoothness on a surface.

Sanitization act of making something sanitary, or clean and free of dirt.

Scaler instrument used to remove calculus from teeth.

Scaling use of instruments with cutting blades to remove calculus from the tooth surface.

SE single ended, as a dental instrument with only one working end.

Second molars seventh tooth from the midline in each quadrant of the permanent dentition.

Second premolars fifth tooth from the midline in each quadrant of the permanent dentition.

Secondary carrier company insuring the dependent employee when the patient is the spouse or dependent child of the employee covered by the primary carrier.

Secondary consistency state to which a dental material is mixed that allows the material to be thick, rolled, or doughy before placement in increments into the prepared tooth.

Secondary dentition *see* Permanent dentition.

Sedation production of a sedative effect; the act or process of calming.

See-ability ergonomic positioning of the dental equipment, patient, and dental health team to enable the dental team to see the site of operation without undue stress on any of the parties involved.

Segments any of the parts into which a body naturally separates or is divided, either actually or by an imaginary line; the oral cavity is divided into six segments, two anterior and four posterior.

Selective absorption act of selectively absorbing, reflecting, or transmitting electromagnetic radiation depending on structure (atomic number, density, and thickness).

Sensory message impression conveyed by an afferent nerve to a sensory nerve center.

Separator instrument or device used to wedge teeth apart.

Septum Interdental (interdental alveolar septum) the portion of the alveolar process extending between the roots of adjacent teeth.

Nasal thin, vertical bony septum separating the right and left nasal cavities.

Shade selection tooth color selection. The determination of the color (hue, brilliance, saturation, translucency) of the artificial tooth or set of teeth for a given patient.

Shaft part of the instrument that is grasped by the hand.

Shank portion of the instrument that unites the shaft or handle with the working point or blade.

Shearing strength maximum stress an object can withstand before fracture when a shearing force is applied.

Sickle scaler with two curved or straight blades, triangular in cross section, and a pointed tip. Used to debride supragingival deposits.

Sinus cavity, recess, or hollow space.

Soft copy electronic record.

Solubility capability of being dissolved.

Sorption condition of being absorbed.

Spacer material used between two surfaces to allow for the placement of another material. Commonly used as a nonasbestos liner between a dentulous or edentulous model prior to fabricating a custom acrylic impression tray. The spacer allows room for placement of final impression material.

Specialty a branch of dentistry in which the professional is specially qualified after having completed an advanced program of study and having met specified criteria.

Sphenoid bone irregular, wedge-shaped bone located at the base of the skull in front of the temporal bone and the basilar portion of the occipital bone. Sphenoid body is more or less cuboidal and hollowed out interiorly to form the sphenoidal air sinuses. Extending from the body laterally are two great wings and two lesser wings. Projecting below the body are two pterygoid processes. The lateral surfaces of the pterygoid processes give origin to the external pterygoid muscles, whereas the medial surfaces give origin to the internal pterygoid muscles.

Splint device, usually plastic, that fits over or is attached to teeth to broaden the area over which occlusal/incisal forces are distributed.

Splinting ligating, tying, or joining of periodontally involved teeth to one another to stabilize and immobilize the teeth, thus preventing them from being adversely affected by occlusal forces. Splinting includes acrylic resin bite guards, orthodontic band splints, wire ligation, provisional splints, and fixed prostheses.

Stainless steel crown preformed steel crown used for the restoration of badly broken down primary teeth and first permanent molars.

Standard of care predetermined level of care that is acceptable to the community of professionals.

State board of dentistry group of individuals responsible for the implementation of dental laws and rules within a state.

Statutory law law enacted by a legislative body; such a law must conform to state and federal constitutions.

Stent 1. Device used to hold a skin graft placed to maintain a body orifice, cavity, or space. An acrylic resin appliance used as a positioning guide or support. 2. An appliance that maintains tissue, such as a skin transplant, in a predetermined position.

Sterilization act or process of rendering sterile; the process of freeing from germ life.

Stomatitis inflammation of the soft tissues of the oral cavity resulting from mechanical, chemical, thermal, viral, radiation, or allergic causes or as a secondary manifestation of a systemic disease; aphthous stomatitis refers to common canker sore or recurrent ulcers of the mouth that appear to be a manifestation of recurrent herpes simplex.

Stop 1. Passive support. 2. An extension from a prosthesis that affords vertical support for a restoration.

Strain 1. Deformation induced by an external force. 2. Deformation expressed as a pure number or ratio resulting from the application of a load. 3. A traumatic stretching or compression of tissues such as the ligaments, capsule, or musculature associated with a joint.

Stress 1. Force induced by or resisting an external force; measured in terms of force per unit area. 2. The force of energy directed against a tissue structure or against the function of tissue as the result of injury and trauma associated with fracture, burn, infection, surgical procedure, pharmacologic action, or anxiety states. 3. In prosthodontics, forcibly exerted pressure, such as the pressure of the maxillary teeth against the mandibular teeth, and the pressure contact of an ill-fitting removable partial denture on the supporting teeth or ridge structures.

Subgingival below the gingival margin.

Subscriber person, usually the employee, who represents the family unit in relation to the prepayment plan. Other family members are dependents. Synonym: certificate holder.

Subtraction radiography use of a computer to compare a series of radiographs or printed images of an area and indicate differences between them.

Succedaneous referring to teeth that replace the deciduous teeth after they have been shed (the permanent incisors, cuspids, and premolar teeth are referred to as succedaneous teeth).

Succinct brief but complete.

Sucrose crystalline disaccharide carbohydrate found in many plants, mainly sugar cane, sugar beet, and maple, and used widely as a sweetener, preservative, and in the manufacture of plastics and cellulose.

Sulcular fluid crevicular fluid; characteristic fluid in the gingival sulcus that is similar but not identical to tissue fluid.

Sulcus temperature gauge device that electronically measures and records the temperature of the sulcular fluid.

Superior in a direction above or higher than a specified point.

Supine position of the body lying on the back with the face up.

Suprabony pocket pocket with base above the level of the alveolar crest.

Supragingival above the gingival margin.

Surgery treatment of disease, injury, or deformity by the use of manual or automatic instruments; removing parts or tissue by cutting.

Surgical phase portion of periodontal treatment in which surgery of the periodontal soft tissue and alveolar bone is completed.

Surveying process of studying the parallelism or lack of parallelism of the teeth and associated structures to determine a path for the placement of a restoration with the least interference and most stability.

Suture 1. Union between two bones formed in a membrane, the uniting medium (which tends to disappear eventually) being a fibrous membrane continuous with the periosteum. 2. Surgical stitch or seam. 3. Materials with which body structures are sewn, as after an operation or injury. 4. To sew up a wound.

Svedopter retraction device provided with an assortment of tongue blades; capable of retraction and evacuation of fluids.

Swaging *see* Bone swaging.

Symmetric evenly balanced or uniformly developed.

Symphysis line of fusion of the lateral halves of the anterior portion of the mandible at the midline. Present only in fetal life. The mandibular symphysis is a large joint of the suture type, with intramembranous ossification.

Syncope swooning or fainting; temporary suspension of consciousness caused by cerebral anemia.

Synovial lubricating fluid of the joints.

Table of allowance list of specified amounts that will be paid toward the cost of dental services rendered; the patient pays the difference between the allowance and the actual cost of service.

Template pattern or mold; a curved or flat plate used as an aid in setting teeth.

Temporal bone lateral bone of the skull composed of squamous and mastoid portions.

Temporary restoration *see* Interim dressing.

Temporomandibular joint 1. joint formed by the two condyles of the mandible. 2. The bilateral articulation between the glenoid or mandibular fossae of the temporal bones and condyles (condyloid processes) of the mandible. The structures that make up the temporomandibular joint include the mandibular fossae of the temporal bones, articular disks, mandibular condyles, and articular tubercles of the zygomatic process of the temporal bone.

Tensile strength 1. resistance to a pulling force. 2. The amount of stress a material is able to withstand when being pulled lengthwise before permanent deformation results.

Third molars eighth tooth from the midline in each quadrant of the permanent dentition.

Three-quarter crown cast restoration that covers most of the clinical crown, commonly with the exception of the buccal surface, and fits over the prepared tooth.

Tissue bed *see* Recipient tissue.

Tissue conditioning preparation of soft oral tissues, by the use of soft liners, prior to construction or rebasing of a new complete or partial denture.

Toe tip end of instrument blade.

Tonic-clonic seizures epileptic spasms of tonic nature, muscular contractions, and clonic contraction and relaxation of muscles.

Topical anesthesia form of local anesthesia whereby free nerve endings in accessible structures are rendered incapable of stimulation by applying a suitable solution directly to the surface of the area.

Tort wrong committed against another person or another's property, generally resolved through a civil trial with a monetary settlement for damages being made rather than imprisonment.

Torus bulging projection of bone; mandibularis torus is a bony enlargement unilaterally or bilaterally on the lingual aspect of the mandible in the canine-premolar region of a small percentage of people; palatinus torus appears in the midline of the hard palate in about one fifth of the people.

TPR temperature, pulse, and respiration.

Transverse plane imaginary plane passing through the two condyles around which the mandible may rotate without translateral movement.

Transverse ridge 1. elevation or prominence formed by the union of two triangular ridges crossing transversely the occlusal surface of lower premolars (buccal and lingual ridge cusps). 2. Ridge found on maxillary molar running from buccal to lingual.

Traumatic occlusion bite with such poor distribution of forces in one or more areas that injury to the periodontium results.

Treatment plan sequence of procedures planned for the treatment of a patient.

Trendelenburg position position in which the patient is on the back with the head and chest lowered and the legs elevated.

Trial point radiograph intermediate radiograph for determining the placement of a master cone.

Triangular ridge elevation or prominence on the occlusal surface of posterior teeth that extends from the point of a cusp to the approximate center of the crown.

Trifurcation division into three parts or branches, as the three roots of a maxillary first molar.

Trigeminal nerve fifth cranial nerve; a mixed motor and sensory nerve connected with the pons through three roots (motor, proprioceptive, and large sensory), the latter root expanding into the trigeminal ganglion, from which arise the ophthalmic, masseteric, and mandibular divisions.

Triple angle refers to three angles of a shank of a dental instrument; commonly found in a hoe or scaler.

Try in preliminary insertion of a removable denture wax-up (trial denture), or of a partial denture casting or of a finished restoration to determine factors such as fit, esthetics, and maxillomandibular relation.

Tubercle a small rounded nodule or elevation on the surface of the skin, bone, or other tissue.

UCR usual, customary, and reasonable fee.

Unilateral one sided.

Universal Numbering System numbering system used to code or identify teeth by using numbers and letters.

Universal precautions combination of devices and techniques used to protect patients and dental health care workers from infectious diseases.

Vacuum investing investing of a pattern within a vacuum to form a mold.

Varix distended vein that has bulged enough to elevate the overlying mucosa.

Vasoconstrictor vasopressor; an agent that causes a rise in blood pressure by constricting the blood vessels. In local areas it causes constriction of the arterioles and capillaries.

Ventral pertains to the lower or underneath portion of the body; opposite of dorsal.

Ventricle one of two lower chambers of the heart that contract when filled with blood to force blood into the arteries.

Vertical dimension length of the face as determined by the amount of separation of the jaws.

Vestibule portion of the oral cavity that is bounded on one side by the teeth, gingivae, and alveolar ridge (in the edentulous mouth, the residual ridge) and on the other by the lips and cheeks.

Vincent's infection *see* ANUG.

Viscosity resistance of a liquid against forces acting to make it move.

Vitamin one of a number of unrelated organic substances that occur in small amounts in food and are required for normal metabolic activity. The vitamins may be water or fat soluble.

Vomer flat, trapezoidal bone that forms the posteroinferior part of the nasal septum.

Water soluble dissolves in water; in nutrition refers to a group of vitamins classified according to their method of metabolism.

Wettability measure of the affinity of a liquid for a solid as indicating by spreading of a drop.

Winged/wingless clamps metal clamps placed on a tooth to stabilize a rubber dam in the mouth. Wing clamps have lateral extensions capable of holding the dam; wingless clamps require the dam be placed on the tooth before attaching the clamp since there are no projections to attach the dam.

Wire edge fine light burr (roughness) left on a instrument blade as a result of sharpening.

Yield point 1. place on the stress-strain curve where marked permanent deformation occurs; it is just beyond the proportional limit. 2. The point where permanent deformation starts in a metal.

Zygomatic arch zygomatic process of the temporal bone. Bowlike prominence created at the side of the head by the temporal process of the zygoma uniting with the zygomatic process of the temporal bone.

Zygomatic bone malar; quadrangular bone on each side of the face that unites the frontal and superior maxillary bones with the zygomatic process of the temporal bone. It forms the cheek prominence, a portion of the lateral wall and floor of the orbit, and parts of the temporal fossa and infratemporal fossa.

Index

in oral and maxillofacial surgery, 859
supporting tissues in, 82
tooth development and eruption in, 83-85
tooth identification in, 79
tooth morphology in, 68
tooth numbering systems in, 69-71
tooth surfaces in, 72-73
Intravenous administration, 254
of anesthesia
in oral and maxillofacial surgery, 867
in oral surgery, 887-888, 889
of glucose, 271
in sedation, 1140
Intrinsic stains, 121
Intrinsic tongue muscles, 58, 1140
Intruded teeth, 819
Invasion of privacy, 352-353, 1140
Inventory, defined, 1140
Inventory control, 404
Inverted cone bur, 492, 494
Investment materials, 333
Investment mixing machine, 754, 755, 1008
Investment of wax pattern, 754-755
Investment oven, 1140
Iodine, 100
as germicide, 264
in obturation, 845
recommended dietary allowance of, 91
source, function and effect of, 94
Iodophors, 172, 175
Ionizing radiation, 178, 179, 180
Ionomer filling material, 313
Ionomer restorations, 408
IPA system; see Individual Practice Association system
Ipecac syrup, 250
Iridium, 336
Iron, 99, 250
full cast, 740
recommended dietary allowance of, 91
source, function and effect of, 93
surgery and, 108
in vegetarian diet, 107
Irreversible acute pulpitis, 814
Irreversible hydrocolloid, 319, 328
Irreversible pulpitis, 816
Irrigation, 1140
in endodontics, 836
for oral hygiene, 943
in periodontics, 970-974
water, 654, 655
Irritation fibroma, 140-141
Ischemia, transient, 748
Ismelin; see Guanethidine
Isoflurane, 866
Isolation, 546-566
in amalgam procedure, 694
cellulose wafer in, 564, 565
in cement temporary, 798, 799
cotton rolls in, 564-565
defined, 1140
in endodontics, 828
hygroformics in, 564, 565
mouth prop in, 566
purpose of, 546-547
rubber dam, 547-564; see also Rubber dam isolation
svedopters in, 564, 565
Isoniazid, 108
Isoproterenol, 249
Isordil; see Isosorbide
Isosorbide, 249
Isuprel; see Isoproterenol

IV administration; see Intravenous administration
Ivory band, 680, 681
Ivory matrix retainer, 680, 681

J

Jacket, porcelain, 725
Jacksonian epilepsy, 641, 1140
Jaw, 41-42
in removable prosthodontics, 782-785
stiffness of, 892
Jaw projection, 223
Jewelry, 1003
Job
advancement in, 1052
application for, 1048-1049
data preparation for, 1045-1052
priorities of, 1045
sources of, 20-22
Jo-Dandy, 493, 498
Joint prosthesis, 631
Journal sheet
daily, 1135
financial, 389, 390
Judging as barrier to communication, 362
Judgment and decision making, 1053
Judicial decisions, 341, 342-343
Jugular chain, 603, 605
Jugular vein, 52
Juvenile periodontal disease, 961
Juvenile periodontitis, 119

K

Kanamycin, 249
Kantrex; see Kanamycin
Kaon; see Potassium chloride
Kaposi's sarcoma, 144
Keflex; see Cephalexin
Kells CE, 12-13
Kells E, 178
Kennedy classification system for partially edentulous mouth, 765
Ketone, 166
Keyes technique, 1140
in periodontics, 974
Kidney disease, 863
Kidneys, 38
Kilocalories, 89
Kilovoltage, 182, 1140
Kilpatrick H, 19
Kinetic energy, 179, 182
Knife, 478
amalgam, 973, 984
gingivectomy, 1138
gold, 478
interdental, 1139
in periodontics, 973, 983
periodontal, 973, 983, 1143
Knoop hardness test, 279
Korotkoff sounds, 596, 598
K-style files, 831, 833
kVp; see Kilovoltage

L

Labeling
as barrier to communication, 362
food, 101-103
of hazardous chemicals, 155, 156, 1006, 1007

of prescription, 267
Labial, defined, 1140
Labial bar, 1132
for partial denture, 768, 769
Labial commissure, 55
Labial frenum, 55
torn, 998-999
Labial glands, 50
Labial mucosa, 607, 608
Labial surface, 72, 73
of denture, 770
Labial tubercle, 55
Labiomental groove, 55
Laboratory procedures, 1003-1013
advanced; see Advanced laboratory procedures
asepsis in, 174-175
in dental suite, 428
equipment in, 1007-1013
for fixed prosthodontics, 739, 751
infection control in, 1005-1006
material safety data sheets in, 1006-1007
prescriptions in, 1005
for removable prosthodontics
final, 785-786, 787
interim, 776, 780-782, 785
requisitions in, 1004, 1140
for clinical records, 386
safety in, 1003-1005
Laboratory technician, 8, 1136
Lacrimal bone, 39, 1140
Lacrimal fossa, 41
Lacrimal gland, 41
Lacrimal sac, 41
Lactase, 89
Lactose, 95
intolerance of, 107
Lambdoid suture, 41, 1140
Lamina, 83, 84
Lamina dura, 82, 111, 112
defined, 1140
in radiographic examination, 619, 620
Laminate, 723-725, 1140
Laminate veneer, 408
Lamp, alcohol
in laboratory, 1008
in mouthguard construction, 1038
Lamprene; see Clofazimine
Lanoxin; see Digoxin
Large intestine, 89
Larodopa; see Levodopa
Lasers, 488-489
Lasix; see Furosemide
Latch-type bur, 494
Latch-type contra-angle, 490, 491
Latch-type shank device, 699
Latent period of radiation, 185
Lateral, defined, 1140
Lateral burnisher, 681
Lateral excursion, 43
Lateral flap displacement, 978
Lateral incisor, 1140
Lateral jaw projection, 223
Lateral pterygoid muscle, 44-45, 46
Lathe, 1007, 1136
Laughing gas, 865
Law, 342-345
defined, 1140
statutory, 1146
Lawsuit, 344
Laxatives, 250
LDH; see Licensed Dental Hygienist
Lead apron
ALARA concept and, 188
disinfection of, 221